www.harcourt-international.com

Bringing you products from all Harcourt Health Sciences companies including Baillière Tindall, Churchill Livingstone, Mosby and W.B. Saunders

▶ **Browse** for latest information on new books, journals and electronic products

▶ **Search** for information on over 20 000 published titles with full product information including tables of contents and sample chapters

▶ **Keep up to date** with our extensive publishing programme in your field by registering with **eAlert** or requesting postal updates

▶ **Secure online ordering** with prompt delivery, as well as full contact details to order by phone, fax or post

▶ **News** of special features and promotions

If you are based in the following countries, please visit the country-specific site to receive full details of product availability and local ordering information

USA: **www.harcourthealth.com**

Canada: www.harcourtcanada.com

Australia: www.harcourt.com.au

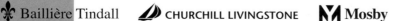 Baillière Tindall   CHURCHILL LIVINGSTONE   Mosby   W.B. SAUNDERS

Total burn care

Second edition

Commissioning Editor: Paul Fam
Project Development Manager: Tim Kimber
Project Manager: Scott Millar
Designer: Andy Chapman

Total burn care
Second edition

Edited by

David N Herndon, MD, FACS

Director of Burn Services
Professor of Surgery & Pediatrics
Jesse H Jones Distinguished Chair
    in Surgery
The University of Texas Medical Branch

Chief of Staff & Director of Research
Shriners Burns Hospital for Children
815 Market Street
Galveston, Texas
USA

W. B. SAUNDERS

London • Edinburgh • New York • Philadelphia • St Louis • Sydney • Toronto 2002

W.B. SAUNDERS
An imprint of Harcourt Publishers Limited

© Harcourt Publishers Limited 2002

[WB] is a registered trademark of Harcourt Publishers Limited

The right of David N Herndon to be identified as editor of this work has been asserted by him in accordance with the Copyright, Designs and Patents Act 1988

First published 1996
Reprinted 1996, 1997, 2000
Second edition 2002

ISBN 0-7020-2612-3

British Library Cataloguing in Publication Data
A catalogue record for this book is available from the British Library

Library of Congress Cataloging in Publication Data
A catalog record for this book is available from the Library of Congress

Note
Medical knowledge is constantly changing. As new information becomes available, changes in treatment, procedures, equipment and the use of drugs become necessary. The editors, contributors and the publishers have taken care to ensure that the information given in this text is accurate and up to date. However, readers are strongly advised to confirm that the information, especially with regard to drug usage, complies with the latest legislation and standards of practice.

Typeset by Phoenix Photosetting, Lordswood, Chatham, Kent
Printed in China

The
Publisher's
policy is to use
**paper manufactured
from sustainable forests**
I

Contents

Immediate care

The burn wound

Inhalation injury

Response to injury

Contributors

Naoki Aikawa, MD, DMSc, FACS
Professor and Chairman, Department of Emergency and
Critical Care Medicine
Keio University Hospital
Tokyo, Japan

Craig S Amin, PhD
Research Associate (Surgery)
Department of Surgery
Loyola University Medical Center
Maywood, Illinois
USA

Carlos Angel, MD
Assistant Professor of Surgery
Department of Surgery
The University of Texas Medical Branch
Galveston, Texas
USA

Juan P Barret, MD
Plastic and Reconstructive Surgeon
Department of Surgery
University Hospital Groningen
Groningen
The Netherlands

Robert E Barrow, PhD
Professor of Surgery, University of Texas Medical Branch
Co-ordinator of Research
Shriners Burns Hospital
Galveston, Texas
USA

Debra A Benjamin, RN, MSN
Assistant Director of Clinical Research and Medical Staff
Administration
Shriners Burns Hospital
Galveston, Texas
USA

Palmer Q Bessey, MD
Professor of Surgery
Weill Cornell Medical College
New York Presbyterian Hospital
Rochester, New York
USA

Patricia E Blakeney, Ph.D.
Clinical Psychologist, Clinical Professor
Department of Surgery
Shriners Burns Hospital
Galveston, Texas
USA

Stephen Boyce, MD
Shriners Hospitals for Children
Cincinnati, Ohio
USA

Michael C Buffalo, RN, ACPNP
Associate Nursing Director of Outpatient and Perioperative Care
Shriners Burns Hospital
Galveston, Texas
USA

Jason H Calhoun, MD
Professor and Chairman of Orthopedics and Rehabilitation
Department of Orthopedics and Rehabilitation
University of Texas Medical Branch
Galveston, Texas
USA

Dai H Chung, MD
Chief, Section of Pediatric Surgery
Assistant Professor of Surgery
The University of Texas Medical Branch
Galveston, Texas
USA

William G Cioffi, Jr, MD, FACS
Chief, Division of Trauma and Burns
Rhode Island Hospital
Providence, Rhode Island
USA

Kumudika Iyanthi de Silva, PhD
Research Associate (Surgery)
Burn and Shock Trauma Institute
Loyola University Medical Center
Maywood, Illinois
USA

Robert H Demling, MD
Professor of Surgery, Harvard
Brigham and Women's Hospital
Boston, Massachusetts
USA

Kumudika I de Silva, Phd
Research Associate
Burn and Shock Trauma Institute
Loyola University Medical Center
Maywood, Illinois
USA

Matthias B Donelan, MD, FACS
Assistant Professor of Surgery
Assistant Clinical Professor of Surgery
Newton-Wellesley Hospital
Newton, Massachusetts
USA

William R Dougherty, MD, FACS
Director
Lehigh Valley Hospital Regional Burn Center
Allentown, PA
USA

Patricia L Edgar, RN
Certified Infection Control Professional
Director, Infection Control
Shriners Burns Hospital
Galveston, Texas
USA

Loren H Engrav, MD
Professor and Chief of Plastic Surgery
University of Washington
Harborview Medical Center
Seattle, Washington
USA

E Burke Evans, MD
Professor Orthopedics
Department of Orthopedics and Rehabilitation
University of Texas Medical Branch
Galveston, Texas
USA

James A Fauerbach, PhD
Assistant Professor, John Hopkins University School of Medicine
Chief Psychologist
Baltimore Regional Burn Center
Baltimore, MD
USA

John C Fitzpatrick, MD
Staff Surgeon
US Army Institute of Surgical Research
Fort Sam, Houston, Texas
USA

Richard L Gameli, MD, FACS
The Robert J Freeark Professor of Surgery
Professor and Chairman, Department of Surgery
Director, Burn and Shock Trauma Institute
Chief, Burn Center
Loyola University Medical Center
Maywood, Illinois
USA

Aziz Ghahary, PhD
Associate Professor of Surgery
University of Alberta
Edmonton, Alberta
Canada

Warren Gold, MD
Clinical Fellow
Shriners Burns Hospital
Galveston, Texas
USA

Cleon W Goodwin, MD
Commander and Director
US Army Institute of Surgical Research
Fort Sam Houston, Texas
USA

Mary Gordon, RN, MS
Burn Clinical Nurse Specialist
Shriners Burns Hospital
Galveston, Texas
USA

David G Greenhalgh, MD, FACS
Chief of Burns, Professor of Surgery
Shriners Hospital for Children
Sacramento, California
USA

C Edward Hartford, MD
Professor, Department of Surgery
University of Colorado Health Sciences Center
Denver, Colorado
USA

Leslie C Hannon, Certified Orthotist-Prosthetist
Manager of Orthotics
Hanger Prosthetics-Orthotics
Galveston, Texas
USA

Hal K Hawkins, MD, PhD
Associate Professor, Pathology and Pediatrics
Shriners Burns Hospital
Galveston, Texas
USA

John P Heggers, PhD, BCLD, CWS(AAWM), FAAM
Director of Clinical Microbiology
Professor of Surgery (Plastic), Microbiology & Immunology
Shriners Burns Hospital
Galveston, Texas
USA

David M Heimbach, MD, FACS
Director, Burn Center
University of Washington
Harborview Medical Center
Seattle, Washington
USA

Ambrosio Hernandez, MD
Chief Resident
Department of Surgery
The University of Texas Medical Branch
Galveston, Texas
USA

David N Herndon, MD, FACS
Jesse H Jones Distinguished Chair in Burn Surgery
University of Texas Medical Branch
Chief of Staff and Director of Research
Shriners Burns Hospital
Galveston, Texas
USA

Marsha Hildreth
Director, Dietary/Support Services
Shriners Burns Hospital
Galveston, Texas
USA

Maureen A Hollyoak MBBS, M Med Sci, FRACS
Clinical Associate Professor
Royal Brisbane Hospital
Herston, Brisbane
Queensland
Australia

Ted T Huang, MD
Clinical Professor of Surgery
University of Texas Medical Branch
Shriners Burns Hospital
Galveston, Texas
USA

John L Hunt, MD
Co-Director, Burn Unit, Parkland Memorial Hospital
Professor
Department of Surgery
UT Southwestern Medical Center
Dallas, Texas
USA

Marc G Jeschke, MD, MMS
Surgical Resident
Klinik und Poliklinik für Chirurgie
Klinikum der Universität Regensburg
Regensburg
Germany

Stephen B Jones, PhD
Professor of Physiology (Surgery)
Department of Physiology and the Burn and
Shock Trauma Institute
Loyola University Medical Center
Maywood, Illinois
USA

Gordon L Klein, MD, MPH
Professor of Pediatrics and Preventive Medicine
Department of Pediatrics
University of Texas Medical Branch and
Shriners Burn Hospital
Galveston, Texas
USA

George C Kramer, PhD
Professor, Resuscitation Laboratories, Dept of Anesthesiology
University of Texas Medical Branch
Shriners Burns Hospital
Galveston, Texas
USA

Hugo A Linares, MD
Chief of Research Pathology (retired)
Shriners Burns Institute
Galveston, Texas
USA

Tjøstolv Lund, MD, PhD
Department of Anesthesia and Intensive Care
National Burn Center
Haukeland University Hospital
Bergen, Norway

Arnold Luterman, MD
University of South Alabama
Department of Surgery
Mobile, Alabama
USA

Robert L McCauley, MD
Chief, Plastic & Reconstructive Surgery
Shriners Burns Hospital
Galveston, Texas
USA

Roberta Mann, MD
Director of Burn Center
Torrance Memorial Burn Center
Torrance, California
USA

Janet A Marvin, RN, MN
Director of Nursing
Shriners Hospital for Children
Galveston, Texas
USA

Arthur D Mason Jr, MD
Consultant
US Army Institute of Surgical Research
Brooke Army Medical Center
Fort Sam Houston, Texas
USA

Walter J Meyer, III, MD
Professor in Child Psychiatry
Head, Department of Psychology and Psychiatry Services
Shriners Burns Hospital
Galveston, Texas
USA

Stephen M Milner, MD, BDS, FRCS, FACS
Associate Professor of Plastic Surgery and Director, Regional
Burn Center
The Plastic Surgery Institute
Southern Illinois University School of Medicine and
Memorial Medical Center
Springfield, Illinois
USA

Joseph M Mlakar, MD
Director
St Josephs Burn Center
Fort Wayne, Indiana
USA

Ron P Mlcak, RRT, MS
Director of Respiratory Care
Shriners Burns Hospital
Galveston, Texas
USA

William W Monafo, BA, MD
Professor of Surgery Emeritus
Washington University School of Medicine
St Louis, Missouri
USA

Dan Morgan, Certified Prosthetist, BS Physical Therapy
Certified Prosthetist-Orthotist, Manager
Hanger Prosthetics-Orthotics
Galveston, Texas
USA

Stephen E Morris, MD, FACS
Assistant Professor of Surgery
University of Utah School of Medicine
Department of Surgery
Salt Lake City, Utah
USA

Elise M Morvant, MD
Assistant Professor of Anesthesiology and Pediatrics
University of Texas Medical Branch
Galveston, Texas
USA

David W Mozingo, MD
Associate Professor of Surgery
University of Florida
Department of Surgery
Gainesville, Florida
USA

Michael J Muller, MBBS, M Med Sci, FRACS
Clinical Associate Professor
Royal Brisbane Hospital
Herston, Brisbane
Queensland
Australia

Thomas Muehlberger, MD, PhD, FRCS
Attending Plastic Surgeon
Department of Plastic and Reconstructive Surgery
Hannover Medical School
Hannover, Germany

Andrew M Munster, MD, FRCS, FACS (Eng & Ed)
Professor of Surgery & Plastic Surgery
Baltimore Regional Burn Center
Johns Hopkins Bayview Medical Center
Baltimore, Maryland
USA

Sheila Ott, OTR
Occupational Therapist
University of Texas Medical Branch
Galveston, Texas
USA

David R Patterson, PhD, ABPP, ABPH
Professor of Rehabilitation Medicine
Harborview Medical Center
Department of Rehabilitation Medicine
Seattle, Washington
USA

Lynn A Peterson, CRNA
Administrative Director of Anesthesia
Chief CRNA
Shriners Burns Hospital
Galveston, Texas
USA

Donald S Prough, MD
Professor and Chair
Department of Anesthesiology
University of Texas Medical Branch
Galveston, Texas
USA

Basil A Pruitt, Jr, MD
Clinical Professor of Surgery
The University of Texas Health Science Center
Department of Surgery
San Antonio, Texas
USA

Gary F Purdue, MD
Professor of Surgery
UT Southwestern Medical Center
Parkland Memorial Hospital
Dallas, Texas
USA

John P Remensynder, MD
Associate Professor of Surgery
Plastic and Reconstructive Surgery Visiting Surgeon
Harvard Medical School
Massachusetts General Hospital
Boston, Massachusetts
USA

Rhonda S Robert, PhD
Psychologist, Assistant Professor
Shriners Burns Hospital
Galveston, Texas
USA

Daniel K Robie, MD
Chief of Pediatric Surgery
Assistant Professor of Surgery
Tripler Army Medical Center
Honolulu, Hawaii
USA

Martin C Robson, MD
Professor Emeritus of Surgery
Department of Surgery
University of South Florida
Tampa, Florida
USA

Jeffrey R Saffle, MD, FACS
Professor of Surgery
University of Utah Health Center
Salt Lake City, Utah
USA

Roger E Salisbury, MD
Professor of Surgery, NY Medical College
Chief, Plastic and Reconstructive Surgery, Director
Westchester Burn Center
Valhalla, New York
USA

Arthur P Sanford, MD
Assistant Professor, Department of Surgery
The University of Texas Medical Branch
Shriners Burns Hospital
Galveston, Texas
USA

Paul G Scott PhD
Professor of Biochemistry
University of Alberta
Edmonton, Alberta
Canada

Michael Serghiou, OTR
Director, Rehabilitation Services
Shriners Burns Hospital
Galveston, Texas
USA

Ravi Shankar, PhD
Associate Professor of Surgery and Cell Biology
Department of Surgery
Loyola University Medical Center
Maywood, Illinois
USA

Robert L Sheridan, MD, FACS
Director of Trauma, Massachusetts General Hospital
Associate Professor of Surgery
Harvard Medical School
Assistant Chief of Staff
Shriners Burns Hospital
Boston, Massachusetts
USA

Edward R Sherwood, MD, PhD
Assistant Professor
University of Texas Medical Branch
Consultant Medical Staff
Shriners Burns Hospital
Galveston, Texas
USA

Yotaro Shinozawa, MD, PhD
Professor of Emergency Medicine
Department of Emergency and Critical Care Medicine
Tohoku University Graduate School of Medicine
Sendai, Japan

Kazutaka Soejima, MD
Department of Plastic & Reconstructive Surgery
Tokyo Women's Medical University
Tokyo
Japan

Marcus Spies, MD
Burn Fellow, Shriners Burns Hospital
Department of Surgery
University of Texas Medical Branch
Galveston, Texas
USA

Steven J Thomas, MD
Research Burn Fellow
Shriners Burns Institute
Galveston, Texas
USA

Chris R Thomas, MD
Professor of Psychiatry and Behavioral Sciences
University of Texas Medical Branch
Galveston, Texas
USA

Ronald G Tompkins, MD, ScD
Massachusetts General Hospital
Boston, Massachusetts
USA

Daniel L Traber, PhD
Professor of Anesthesiology
University of Texas
Medical Branch
Galveston, Texas
USA

Edward E Tredget, MD, MSC, FRCSC
Professor of Surgery
University of Alberta Hospital
Alberta, Canada

Cynthia Villarreal, BS Pharmacy
Director of Pharmacy
Shriners Burns Hospital
Galveston, Texas
USA

Peter M Vogt, MD, PhD
Professor of Plastic Surgery, Chief of Staff
Department of Plastic and Reconstructive Surgery
Hannover Medical School
Hannover, Germany

Thomas L Wachtel, MD, MMM, CPE, FACS, FCCM
Clinical Professor of Surgery
Medical Director, trauma
Paradise Valley, Arizona
USA

Glenn D Warden, MD
Professor of Surgery
University of Cincinnati College of Medicine
Chief of Staff, Shriners Burns Hospital
Shriners Burns Hospital
Cincinnati, Ohio
USA

Petra M Warner, MD
Assistant Professor
University of Cincinnati College of Medicine and
Shriners Burns Institute
Cincinnati, Ohio
USA

W Geoff Williams, MD
Assistant Professor
Division of Plastic and Reconstructive Surgery
Shriners Burns Hospital
Galveston, Texas
USA

Steven E Wolf, MD
Assistant Professor, Department of Surgery
Shriners Burns Hospital
Galveston, Texas
USA

Lee C Woodson, MD, PhD
Associate Professor LE Hughes University of
Texas Medical Branch
Chief, Anesthesiology
Shriners Burns Hospital
Galveston, Texas
USA

Bruce E Zawacki, MD, MA
Emeritus Associate Professor of Surgery and of
Religion/Social Ethics
University of Southern California School of Medicine and of
Religion/Social Ethics
Los Angeles, California
USA

Preface

In the last 15 years, burn care has improved to the extent that persons with burns covering 80% of their total body surface can frequently survive. In the 5 years since the publication of the first edition of this book, basic and clinical sciences have continued to provide information, further elucidating the complexities of burn injuries and opportunities for improvement in care. In this edition, as in the last, advances in the treatment of burn shock, inhalation injury, sepsis, hypermetabolism, the operative excision of burn wounds, scar reconstruction, and rehabilitation are reviewed. Burn care demands attention to every organ system as well as to the patient's psychological and social status. The scope of burn treatment extends beyond the preservation of life and function; and the ultimate goal is the return of burn survivors, as full participants, back into their communities.

The second edition has been extensively updated with massive additions of new data and references that have led to vast decreases in mortality and improvement in morbidity since the last edition.

This book was prepared to consider the complex management of burned patients from injury through rehabilitation; it incorporates treatments of injuries from diverse sources and addresses the concerns of a variety of burn care professionals who act in concert. A major theme throughout is that advances defined in basic science laboratories need to progress through prospective randomized studies to their clinical application. *Total Burn Care* is designed as a text on the management of burned patients, not only for surgeons, anesthesiologists, and residents but also nurses and allied health professionals. This book will hopefully serve as a sophisticated instruction manual to guide those with less experience through difficult experiences in burn care. It is anticipated that it will additionally stimulate knowledgeable scientists and experienced clinicians to pose new questions and to join together in pursuing randomized and prospective studies.

Contributors have been selected from a small number of institutions in order to provide a unified approach with a sharp focus and minimal duplication. Themes covered elsewhere in the literature have been condensed and the bibliographies selected to assure the reader ready access to the expanded literature on current burn care. The final organization of the book reflects neither the importance of the subject matter nor the order of application following injury.

The support of the staff of WB Saunders is gratefully acknowledged, as is the Shriners Burns Institute, contributors' universities, and the teaching hospitals which have provided clinical opportunities and the laboratories for research.

DAVID N HERNDON
October 2001

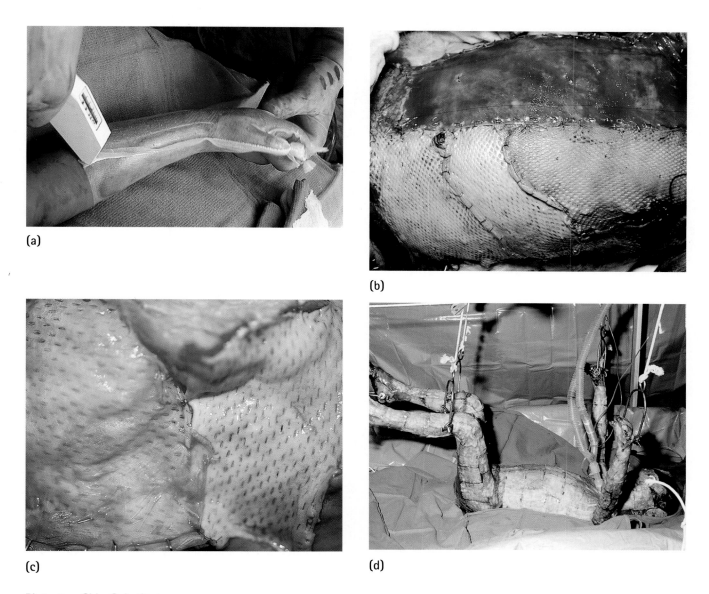

Plate 1 – Skin Substitutes

(a) **Biobrane.** The use of Biobrane has revolutionized care for 2nd degree burns. Advantages of Biobrane include decreased pain and elimination of dressing changes.

(b) **Integra.** Dermal and skin substitutes can be used as temporary cover for severe burns. Integra, a bilaminar skin substitute, can replace homografts as temporary cover. The silastic superficial layer can be removed after 3 weeks and a super-thin autograft then placed on top. The entire wound can be covered with Integra, which is subsequently autografted when donor sites are available.

(c) **AlloDerm.** Other dermal substitutes are also available for wound closure. The use of AlloDerm, a commercially available human homodermis, with a super-thin autograft overlay promotes rapid healing of the donor site and recropping quickly becomes possible.

(d) **CEA.** By means of cultured epidermal autograft techniques, the entire body can be covered and closed in one operative setting. Skeletal traction is used to manipulate patients after the application of cultured epidermal autograft.

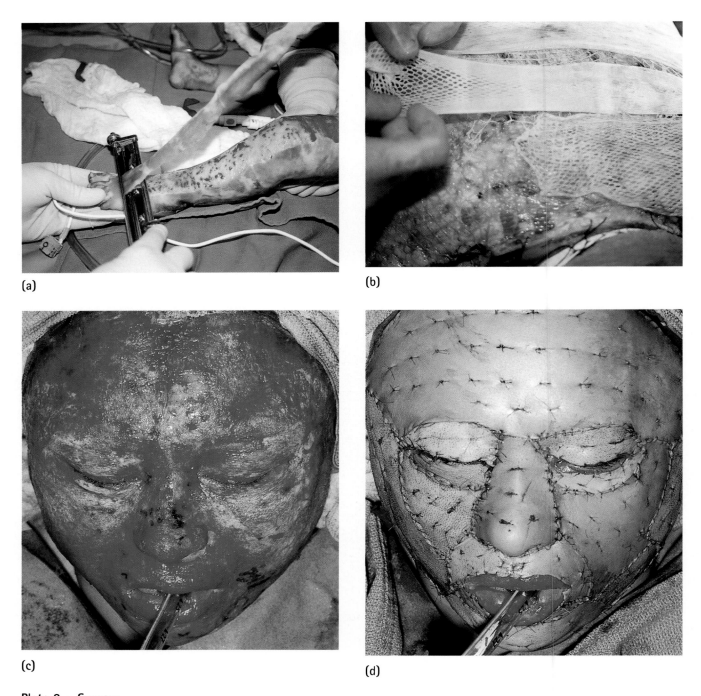

Plate 2 – Surgery

(a) **Excision.**

(b) **4:1 graft.** The "Sandwich" technique. 4:1 meshed autografts are covered with 2:1 or sheet homografts as a temporary cover. Homografts desiccate when the 4:1 autograft is completely healed.

(c) **Face excision.** Full thickness burns to the face. Appearance after early excision.

(d) **Face graft.** The same patient as shown in Plate 4c after sheet autografting to the face following esthetic units. It is very important to graft the face following these units to provide the best cosmetic outcome. Note the quilting stitches help to immobilize the grafts after surgery.

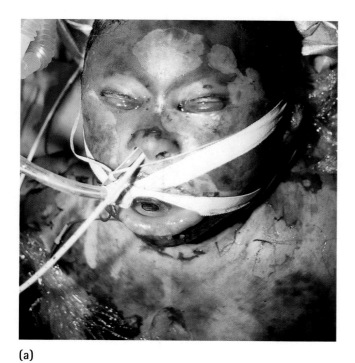

(a)

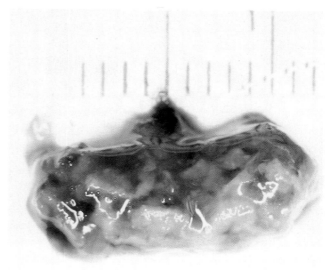

(b)

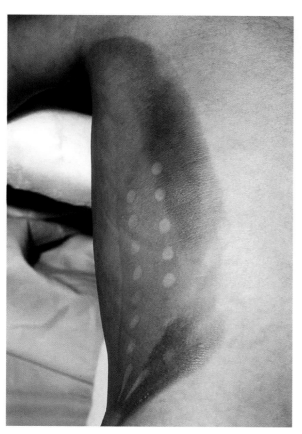

(c)

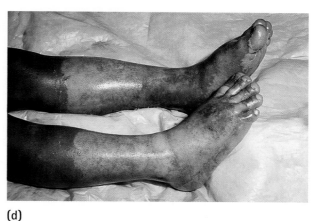

(d)

Plate 3 – Inhalation Injury & Abuse

(a) **Smoke inhalation injury.** Smoke inhalation injury with severe edema to the face following an 85% TBSA burn. Management of the airway with early prophylactic endotracheal intubation is paramount.

(b) **Tracheal cast.** Smoke inhalation induced tracheal cast. Vigorous treatment of aerosolized heparin/Mucomyst and pulmonary toilet is required.

(c) **Abuse.** Contact burn in which the markings of an iron are clearly visible.

(d) **Abuse.** Classic "stocking" pattern resulting from feet being immersed in very hot water. The initial history given by the mother of the 21 month old was that an older sibling had turned on hot water, and the patient herself dipped her feet into the tub.

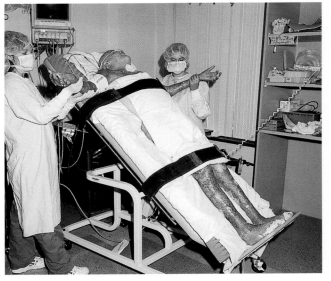

(a)

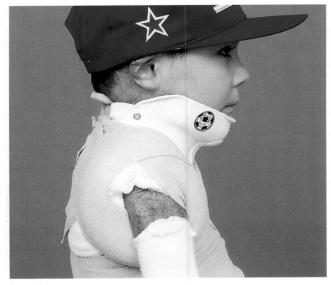

(b)

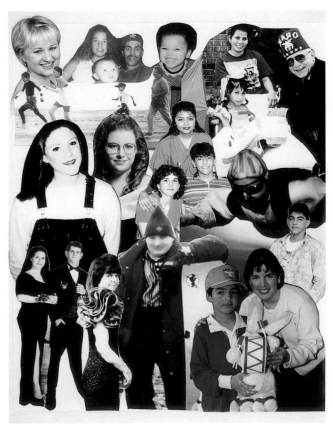

(c)

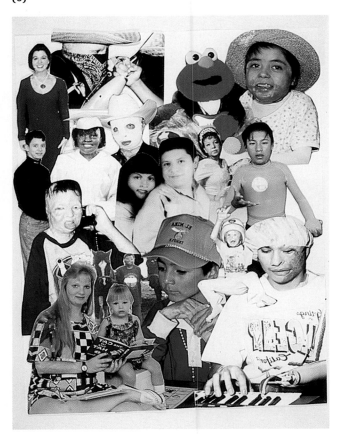

(d)

Plate 4 – Miscellaneous

(a) **Tilt table.** All patients, regardless of burn size, location, and severity, must be started on a program of early mobilization and ambulation.

(b) **Splinting.** Neck collars must be worn at all times when not exercising. If there are grafted areas on the chest, they must be protected. When scars on the neck exist, patients should sleep without a pillow in order to maximize neck extension.

(c), (d) **Collage.** Survivors of severe burn injuries can return to active, interesting, and productive lives in spite of scars and amputations. Recovery is a long and difficult process challenging the physical and psychological resilience of the individual. Burn care professionals must provide guidance and support to survivors and to their families during the years of recovery.

Introduction

History of the treatment of burns

Steven Thomas
Robert E Barrow
David N Herndon

The first direct evidence of treating burns was found depicted in the cave paintings of Neanderthal man; many historic references have occurred since. Documentation of burn care, found in the Egyptian Smith papyrus of 1500 BC advocated a salve of resin and honey.[1] In the sixth century BC, the Chinese used tinctures and extracts from tea leaves. Nearly 200 years later, Hippocrates described the use of rendered pig fat and resin which was impregnated in bulky dressings. This was alternated with warm vinegar soaks augmented with tanning solutions made from oak bark. Celsus, in the first century AD, mentioned the use of wine and myrrh, a lotion used probably for its bacteriostatic properties. Galen, who lived from AD 130–210, used vinegar and an open exposure technique.[1] The Arabian physician Rhases recommended the use of cold water for the alleviation of pain associated with burns. Ambroise Paré (AD 1510–1590), advocated a variety of ointments and poultices from medieval excremental alchemy, and effectively treated burns with onions and described a procedure for early burn wound excision. Guilhelmus Fabricius Hildanus, a German surgeon, who made unique contributions to the treatment of contractures, published *De Combustionibus* in 1607, which discussed the pathophysiology of burns. In 1797, Edward Kentish published an essay describing pressure dressings as a means to relieve pain and burn blisters. Around this period, Marjolin identified squamous cell carcinomas that developed in chronic open burn scars. In the early nineteenth century, Dupuytren[2] (**Figure 1**) reviewed the care of 50 burn patients treated with occlusive dressings and developed a classification of burn depth that remains in use today. He was perhaps the first to recognize gastric and duodenal ulceration as a complication of severe burns, a problem discussed in more detail in 1842 by Curling of London.[3]

Dr Truman G Blocker Jr (**Figure 2**) pointed out the value of a

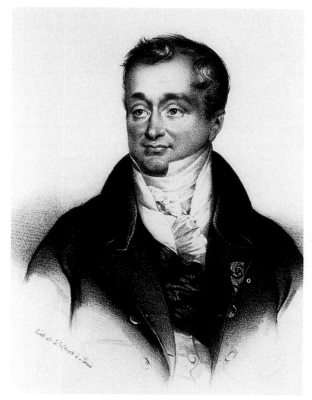

Fig. 1 Dupuytren.

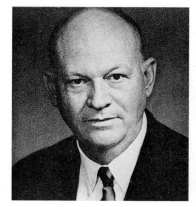

Fig. 2 Truman G Blocker Jr.

multidisciplinary team approach to burn care and used this team approach in treating the victims of the 1947 Texas City Disaster, still known as the deadliest industrial accident in American history. He was known for his pioneering research in treating burns and treated children 'by cleansing and exposing the burn wounds and feeding them as much as they could tolerate.' In 1962, his dedication to treating burned children convinced the Shriners of North America to build their first burn institute for children in Galveston, Texas.[4]

Most major advances in burn care have occurred within the last 5 decades. Between 1942 and 1952, shock, sepsis, and multiorgan failure caused a 50% mortality rate in children with burns covering 50% of their total body surface area (TBSA).[5] Recently, burn care survival in children has improved such that a greater than 95% TBSA burn can be survived 50% of the time.[6] Improvements have been made in resuscitation, control of infection, support of the hypermetabolic response, nutritional support, prevention of stress ulcers, treatment of major inhalation injuries, early closure and coverage of the burn wound, and the multidisciplinary team approach to burn care and rehabilitation.

Resuscitation

The foundation leading to our current fluid and electrolyte management began with studies of Frank P Underhill (**Figure 3**) who, as Professor of Pharmacology and Toxicology at Yale, studied 20 individuals burned in a 1921 fire at the Rialto Theater.[7] Underhill found that blister fluid had a composition similar to plasma which could be replicated by a salt solution containing protein. He suggested that burn patients died from loss of fluid and not, as previously thought, from toxins. Lund and Browder (**Figures 4** and **5**) in 1944, estimated burn surface areas and developed diagrams in which physicians could easily draw the burned areas and derive a

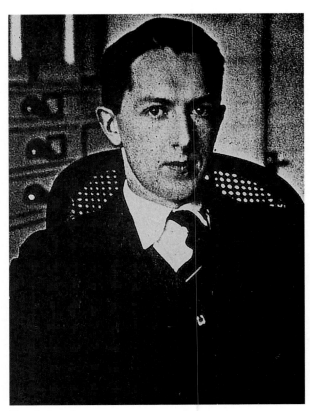

Fig. 4 Lund.

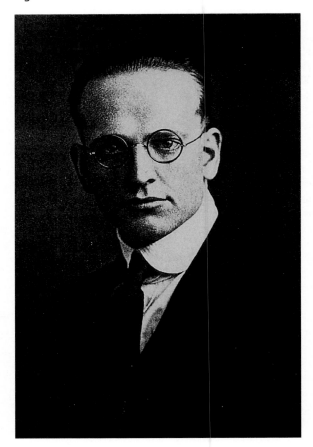

Fig. 5 Browder.

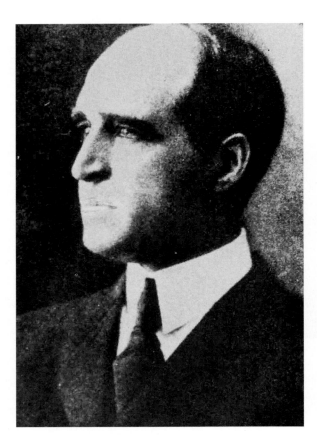

Fig. 3 Frank P Underhill.

quantifiable percent of total body surface area burned.[8] This led to the development of fluid replacement strategies based on surface area burned. Knaysi *et al.*[9] proposed a simple 'rule of nines' for evaluating the percentage of body surface area burned. In 1946, Drs Oliver Cope and Francis Moore (**Figures 6** and **7**) were able to quantify the amount of fluid required for adequate resuscitation by analyzing young adults who were trapped inside the burning Coconut Grove Nightclub in Boston. They postulated that the interstitial space was a major recipient of plasma loss, causing swelling in both injured and uninjured tissues in proportion to %TBSA burned.[10] Moore concluded that additional fluid, over that collected from the sheets and evaporative water loss, was needed in the first 8 hours after burn to replace 'third space' loss, and developed a formula for replacement of fluid based on percent body surface area burned[11] (**Table 1**). Kyle and Wallace[12] (**Figure 8**) modified fluid

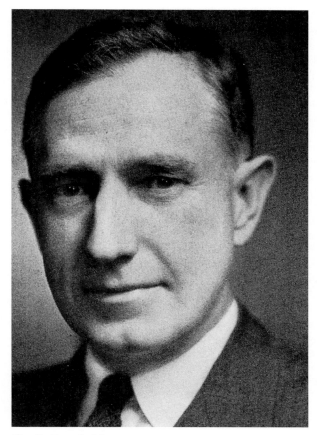

Fig. 7 Francis Moore.

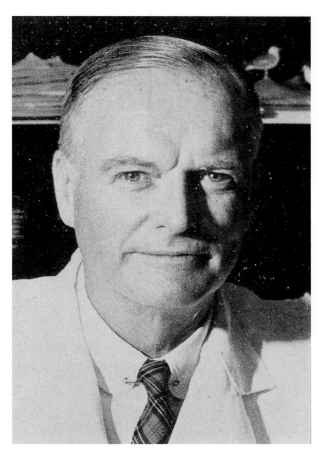

Fig. 6 Oliver Cope.

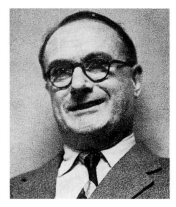

Fig. 8 Wallace.

Table 1			
Formula	Crystalloid volume	Colloid volume	Free water
Evans	1.0 ml/kg/% burn Normal Saline	1.0 ml/kg/% burn	2.0 liters
Brooke	1.5 ml/kg/% TBSA Lactated Ringers	0.5 ml/kg/% TBSA burn	2.0 liters
Parkland	4 ml/kg/% TBSA	None	None
Modified Brooke	2 ml/kg/% burn first 24 hours		
Hypertonic (Monafo)	250 mEq/LNa+ in volume to maintain urine output @ 30 ml/hr		
Warden	Lactated Ringers + 50 mEq NaHCO^3 (180 mEqNa +/L for 8h)		
	8 h post burn: LR to maintain U/O @30–50 ml/h		
SBH-Galveston	5000 ml/m^2 burned + 1500 ml/m^2 total	None	None

replacement formulas for use in children. They showed that the heads of children were relatively larger and the legs were relatively shorter than adults. Evans (**Figure 9**) and his colleagues[13] made recommendations relating fluid requirements to body weight and surface area burned. Normal saline (1.0 ml/kg/% burn) plus colloid (1.0 ml/kg/% burn) along with 2000 ml D5W to cover insensible water losses was infused over the first 24 hours after burn. One year later, Reiss *et al.*[14] presented the Brooke formula which modified the Evans formula by substitution of lactated Ringer's for normal saline and decreasing the amount of colloid given. Baxter and Shires[15] (**Figures 10** and **11**) developed a formula without colloid which is now referred to as the Parkland formula. This is perhaps the most widely used formula today and recommends 4 ml of Ringer's lactate/kg/% TBSA burned/24 h postburn. All of these formulas (**Table 1**) advocate giving half of the fluid in the first 8 hours and the other half in the subsequent 16 hours after burn. The greatest quantity of salt is given in the first 24 hours postburn. After that, more hypotonic solutions are given to replace evaporative water loss. Baxter and Shires discovered that after cutaneous burn, fluid is not only deposited in the interstitial space but also marked intracellular edema develops. There is a disruption of sodium–potassium pump activity, resulting in an inability to remove fluid from cells. They also showed that protein, given in the first 24 hours post-injury, was not necessary and postulated that, if used, it would leak out of the vessels and cause edema to exacerbate. This was later substantiated in studies of burn patients with smoke inhalation injuries.[16]

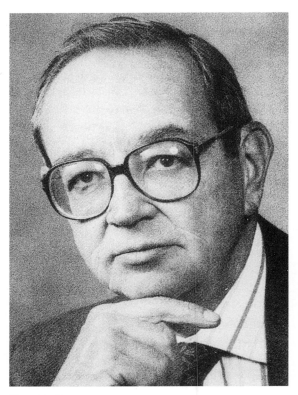

Fig. 10 Baxter.

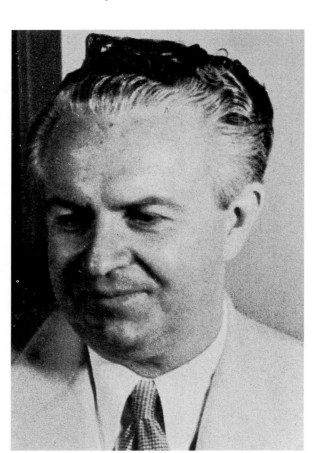

Fig. 9 Evans.

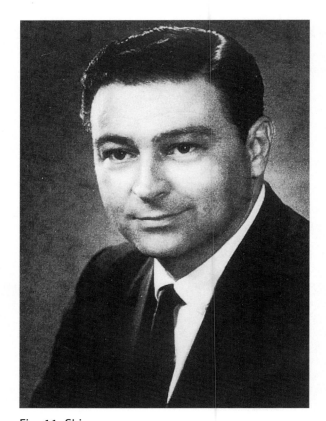

Fig. 11 Shires.

Control of infection

Another major advancement in burn care that decreased mortality was the control of infection. Between 1966 and 1975, 60–80% of patients with burns over 50% of their total body surface died of bacterial sepsis. With the introduction of efficacious topical antimicrobials, burn wound sepsis decreased. Early excision and coverage further decreased morbidity and mortality from burn wound sepsis. In 1965, Carl Moyer[17] (**Figure 12**) proposed using 0.5% silver nitrate soaks as a potent topical antibacterial agent. He also advocated the use of crystalloid resuscitations and was one of the first to test hypertonic salt solutions.

Mafenide acetate (Sulfamylon), a drug used by the Germans for treatment of open wounds in World War II, was adapted for treating burns at the Institute of Surgical Research in San Antonio by microbiologist Robert Lindberg in association with John Moncrief[18] (**Figure 13**). This antibiotic would penetrate third degree eschar and was extremely effective against a wide spectrum of wound pathogens, significantly reducing burn wound sepsis. Simultaneously, Charles Fox[19] (**Figure 14**) in New York, developed silver sulfadiazine (Silvadene), which was almost as efficacious and had fewer complications than Sulfamylon, with Sulfamylon being more efficacious in penetrating eschar than Silvadene. Sulfamylon, however, is a carbonic anhydrase inhibitor which causes systemic acidosis and compensatory hyperventilation and may lead to pulmonary edema. Because of its success in controlling infection in burns combined with minimal side effects, silver sulfadiazine has become the mainstay of topical antimicrobial therapy. We have used nystatin in combination with Silvadene to control *Candida*.[20]

Hypermetabolic response to trauma

Major decreases in mortality have been the result of a better understanding of how to support the hypermetabolic response to severe burns. This response is characterized by an increase in the metabolic rate and peripheral catabolism. The catabolic response was described by Sneve[21] as exhaustion and emaciation. He recommended a nourishing diet and exercise. Cuthbertson (**Figure 15**) described the negative nitrogen and phosphorus balance after long bone trauma. Cope *et al.*[22] quantified the metabolic rate in patients with moderate burns, and Francis Moore[23] advocated the maintenance of body cell mass by continuous feeding to prevent catabolism after trauma and injury. Over the last 20 years the

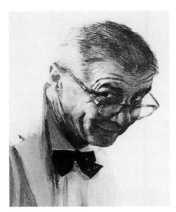

Fig. 12 Carl Moyer.

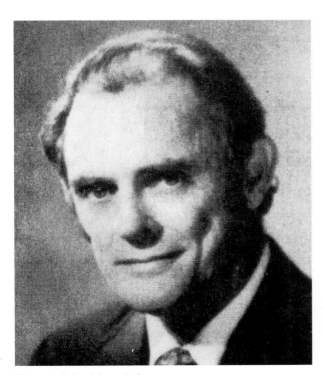

Fig. 13 John Moncrief.

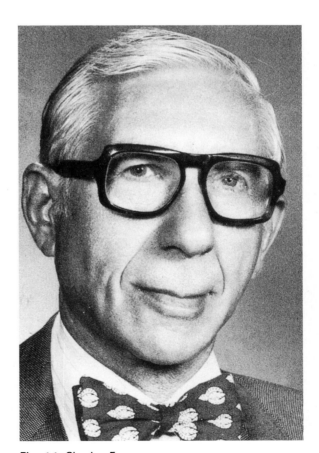

Fig. 14 Charles Fox.

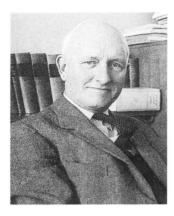

Fig. 15 Cuthbertson.

hypermetabolic response to burn has been shown to cause increased metabolism, negative nitrogen balance, glucose intolerance, and insulin resistance. In 1974, Douglas Wilmore (**Figure 16**) and colleagues[24] defined catecholamines as the primary mediator of this response. He showed that catecholamines were 5- to 6-fold elevated after major burns which caused an increase in peripheral lipolysis and catabolism of peripheral protein. Hart et al.[25] further showed that the metabolic response rose with increasing burn size reaching a plateau at a 40% TBSA burn. Bessey, in 1984, demonstrated that the stress response required not only catecholamines but cortisol and glucagon as well. Wilmore et al.[26] examined the effect of ambient temperature on the hypermetabolic response to burns and found that burn patients desired an environmental temperature of 33°C

and that they were striving for a core temperature of 38.5°C. Thus, warming the environment from 28° to 33°C decreased the hypermetabolic response substantially, but did not abolish it. Wilmore suggested that the wound itself served[27] as the afferent arm of the hypermetabolic response and that its avidity for glucose and other nutrients, at the expense of the rest of the body, stimulated the stress response. He felt that heat was produced by biochemical inefficiency, which was later defined by Robert Wolfe[28] as futile substrate cycling. Wolfe et al. also demonstrated that burned patients were glucose-intolerant and insulin-resistant[29] with an increase in glucose transport to the periphery, but a decrease in glucose uptake into the cells.[30]

Nutritional support

Shaffer and Coleman advocated high caloric feedings as early as 1909. Wilmore (1971) supported supranormal feedings with intake as high as 8000 kcal/day. P William Curreri[31] (**Figure 17**) retrospectively looked at a number of burned patients to quantify the amount of calories required to maintain body weight over a period of time. In a study of nine adults with 40% TBSA, he found that when they were given a maintenance feeding at -25 kcal/kg and added an additional 40 kcal/% TBSA burned per day, their body weight could be maintained during acute hospitalization. Sutherland[32] proposed that children should receive 60 kcal/kg body weight plus 35 kcal/% TBSA burn per day. Herndon et al.[33] subsequently showed that supplemental parenteral nutrition increases both immune deficiency and mortality, and recommended continuous enteral feeding as a standard treatment for burns.

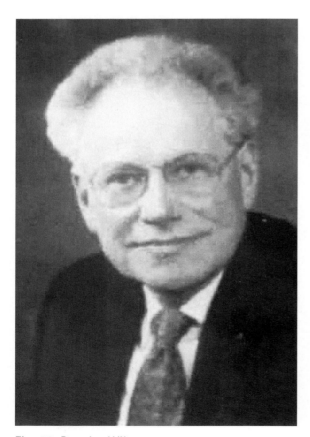

Fig. 16 Douglas Wilmore.

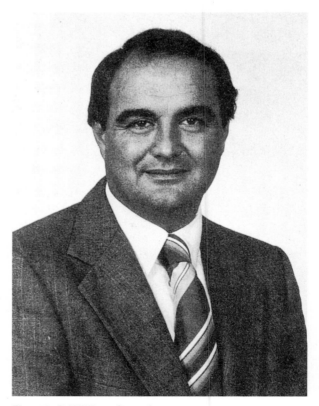

Fig. 17 P William Curreri.

Stress ulcers

Dupuytren and Curling defined acute gastrointestinal ulcers as major problems after burn. Czaja, McAlhany, and Pruitt[34] (shown in **Figure 18**) at the Institute of Surgical Research in San Antonio studied the stomachs of burn patients and found gastric erosions in 86% of all burns over 40% TBSA. The incidence of gastric erosion was reduced by scheduling antacids to treat the low pH. This led to the now traditional protocol of measuring gastric pH on an hourly basis and alternating Maalox and/or Amphogel to adjust the gastric pH. This has virtually eliminated gastric ulcers as a problem in patients with a major burn. Continuous enteral feeding also helps maintain the integrity of gut mucosae, decreases bacterial translocation, and minimizes the need for antacids.

Early excision

One of the most effective therapies in decreasing mortality from major thermal injuries has been the early excision of the burn wound and its coverage by various techniques.[35] Jackson (**Figure 19**) and colleagues[36] pioneered excision and grafting, beginning in 1954 with burns of 3% TBSA and gradually increasing up to burns covering 30% TBSA. Janzekovic[37] (**Figure 20**) working alone in Yugoslavia in the 1960s developed the concept of removing deep second degree burns by tangential excision with a simple uncalibrated knife. She treated 2615 patients with deep second degree burns by tangential excision of eschars between the third and fifth day postburn. She then covered the excised wound with autografts which allowed patients to return to work within a week or so from the time of injury. William Monafo[38] (**Figure 21**) was one of the first Americans to advocate the use of excision and grafting techniques for larger burns. Dr John Burke[39] (**Figure 22**), at

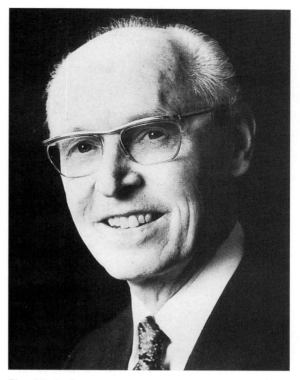

Fig. 19 Jackson.

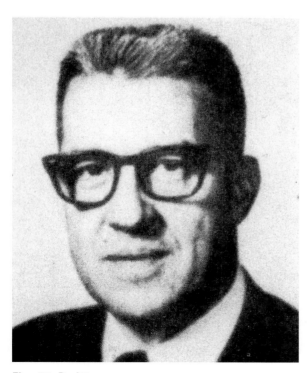

Fig. 18 Pruitt.

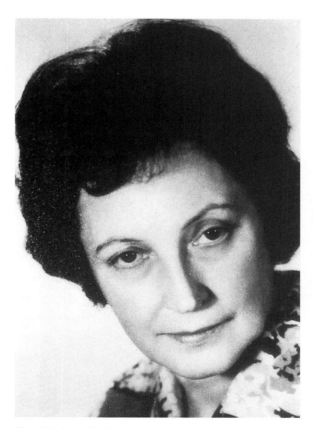

Fig. 20 Janzekovic.

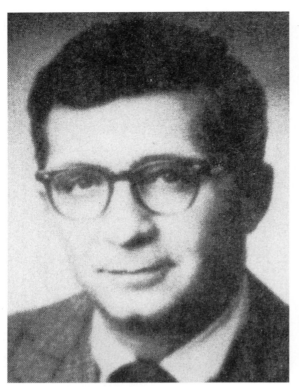

Fig. 21 William Monafo.

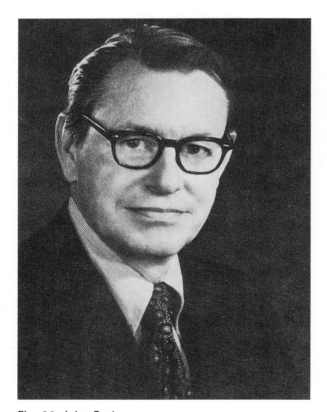

Fig. 22 John Burke.

Massachusetts General Hospital in Boston, reported an unprecedented survival after massive excision to the level of fascia in children with burns over 80% TBSA. He practiced early burn excision throughout the early 1970s and 1980s using a combination of tangential excision for the smaller burns (Janzekovic's technique) and excision to the level of fascia for the larger burns. He showed a decrease in length of hospital stay and mortality in massively burned patients. Lauren Engrav et al.[40] compared tangential excision versus nonoperative treatment in burns of indeterminate depth. Their randomized prospective study, conducted in 1983 showed that when deep second-degree burns of <20% TBSA were grafted early, patients could return to work quicker, had shorter hospitalization, and less hypertrophic scaring. Herndon et al.,[41] in a randomized prospective study, showed a decrease in mortality in massively burned adults with third-degree burns when they were treated with early excision of the total burn wound as opposed to conservative treatment. Herndon et al.[42] also reported that massively burned children with 95% TBSA burns may have a 50% survival rate after early burn wound excision.

Skin grafting

Progress in skin grafting techniques has paralleled the developments in wound excision. A Swiss medical student, JI Reverdin, performed reproducible skin grafts[43] in 1869. The method gained widespread attention throughout Europe for a brief period, but since the results were extremely variable the method fell into disrepute. JS Davis[44] resurrected this technique in the United States during the 1930s and reported the use of 'small deep grafts' later known as pinch grafts. Split-thickness skin grafts were accepted during the 1930s due in part to improved and reliable instruments. The 'Humby knife', developed in 1936, was the first reliable dermatome, but was cumbersome. Padgett and Hood developed an adjustable dermatome which had cosmetic advantages. Padgett[45] also developed a system for categorizing skin grafts into four types based upon thickness. Tanner and colleagues,[46] in 1964, revolutionized burn wound grafting with the development of the meshed skin graft. J Wesley Alexander[47] (**Figure 23**) gave us a simple method of widely expanding autograft skin and then covering it with cadaver skin. This has since been the mainstay in the treatment of massively burned individuals. Jack Burke[48] developed artificial skin in 1981, which is marketed today as Integra™. It consists of a bi-layer of artificial skin made of a collagen network and covered with a layer of plastic. He first used this on very large burns covering over 80% of the TBSA. David Heimbach (**Figure 24**) led one of the early Multicenter Randomized Clinical Trials using Integra™.[49] The development of tissue cultured grown skin by Bell et al.,[50] in combination with an artificial dermis, perhaps offers us the best opportunity for better future outcomes.

Pulmonary injury

The latest area to advance in the treatment of major burns has been an improvement in the treatment of the concomitant pulmonary injury. Shirani, Pruitt, and Mason[51] (**Figure 25**) reported that smoke inhalation injury and pneumonia, in addition to age and burn size, greatly increased burn mortality. The realization that the physician should not under-resuscitate burn patients with an

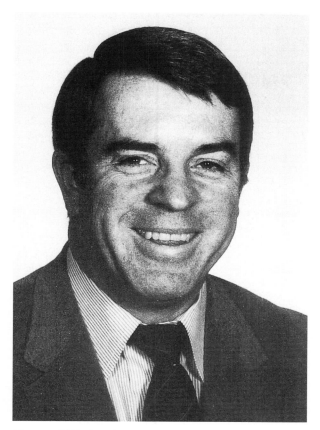

Fig. 23 J Wesley Alexander.

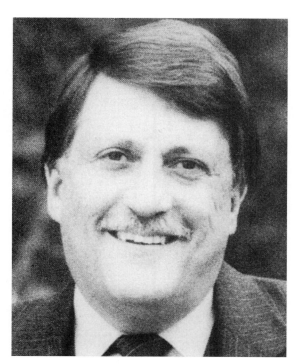

Fig. 24 David Heimbach.

inhalation injury has been emphasized by Navar *et al.*[52] and Herndon *et al.*[53] A patient with a major inhalation injury requires 2 ml/kg/% TBSA burn more fluid in the first 24 hours postburn to maintain adequate urine output and organ perfusion. Multicenter studies looking at patients with adult respiratory distress have advocated respiratory support at low peak pressures to reduce the incidence of barotrauma. It is now standard care for patients with smoke inhalation injury to receive tidal volumes of 6–8 ml/kg with a PEEP of 7.5 mmHg with peak pressures being kept at the minimum needed to maintain Pco_2 <60 and pH<7.25.

A high-frequency oscillating ventilator advocated by Cioffi[54] and Cortiella *et al.*[55] has added the benefit of pressure ventilation at low tidal volumes with a rapid inspiratory minute volume that provides a vibration that may encourage inspissated sputum to travel up the airway. The use of heparin, N-acetylcysteine, and bronchodilator aerosols have decreased mortality at least in pediatric populations.[56,57]

Conclusion

The evolution of burn treatments has been extremely exciting over the last 40 years. It is our hope that the next 10 years will witness the development of an artificial skin which combines the concepts of Burke *et al.*[58] with the tissue culture technology described by Bell.[50] We hope to see further improvements in the treatment of smoke inhalation injuries through the development of arterial venous CO_2 removal and extracorporeal membrane oxygenation devices.[59] Perhaps even lung transplants will fit into the treatment regimen for end-stage pulmonary failure. Further decreases in mortality can be expected, but further advances in understanding how to rehabilitate patients better and return them to a fruitful life are necessary. Our goals continue to strive for a better understanding of the pathophysiology of contractures and hypertrophic scar formation in order to best treat scar formation and how to modulate it in a positive fashion over the next decade.

References

1. Majo G. *The Healing Hand.* Harvard University Press, Harvard, 1973.
2. Dupuytren G. Lecons orales de clinque chirorjica faites a' l' Hotel–Dieu de Paris. Vol. I: pp 413–516. Vol. II: 1–80, Baillière, Paris, 1832.
3. Curling TB. On acute ulceration of the duodenum in cases of burn. *Med Chir Trans London* 1842; **25**: 260–281
4. Blocker TG Jr. Talk given to plastic surgery residents. Galveston, Texas, October 1, 1981, unpublished.

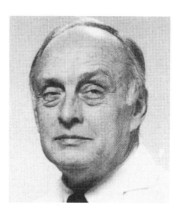

Fig. 25 Mason.

5. Bull JP, Fischer AJ. A study of mortality in a burns unit: a revised estimate. *Ann Surg* 1954; **139(95)**: 269–274.

6. Wolf SE *et al.* Mortality determinants in massive pediatric burns. *Ann Surg* 1997; **225(5)**: 554–569.

7. Underhill FP. The significance of anhydremia in extensive surface burns. *JAMA* 1930; **95**: 852.

8. Lund CC, Browder NC. The estimation of areas of burns. *Surgical Gyn Obstet* 1944; **79**: 352–358.

9. Knaysi GA, Crikelair GF, Cosman B. The rule of nines: it's history and accuracy. Presented to the *Am. Soc. Plast. & Reconstruct. Surg.*, New York City, November 6, 1967.

10. Cope O, Moore FD. The redistribution of body water. *Ann Surg* 1947; **126**: 1016.

11. Moore FD. The body-weight burn budget. Basic fluid therapy for the early burn. *Surg Clin North Am* 1970; **50(6)**: 1249–1265.

12. Kyle MJ, Wallace AB. Fluid replacement in burnt children. *Br J Plast Surg* 1951; 194–204.

13. Evans EI *et al.* Fluid and electrolyte requirements in severe burns. *Ann Surg* 1952; **135**: 804.

14. Reiss *et al.* Fluid and electrolyte balance in burns. *JAMA* 1953; **152**: 1309.

15. Baxter CC, Shires GT. *Ann NY Acad Sci* 1968; **150**: 874.

16. Tasaki O, Goodwin C, Saitoh D, *et al.* Effects of burns on inhalation injury. *J Trauma* 1997; **43(4)**: 603–607.

17. Moyer CA *et al.* Treatment of large human burns with 0.5 per cent silver nitrate solution. *Arch Surg* 1965; **90**: 812.

18. Lindberg RB, Moncreif JA, Switzer WE, Order SE, Mills W Jr. The successful control of burn wound sepsis. *J Trauma* 1965; **5(5)**: 601–616.

19. Fox CL Jr, Ruppole B, Stanford W. The control of *Pseudomonas* infection in burns with silver sulfadiazine. *Surg Gynecol Obstet* 1969; **128**: 1021.

20. Heggers JP, Robson MC, Herndon DN, Desai MH. The efficacy of nystatin combined with topical microbial agents. *J Burn Care Rehabil* 1989; **10(6)**: 508–511.

21. Sneve H. The treatment of burns and skin grafting. *JAMA* 1905; **45**: 1–8.

22. Cope O, Nardi GL, Quijano M, Rovit RL, Stanbury JB, Wright A. Metabolic rate and thyroid function following acute thermal trauma in man. *Ann Surg* 1953; **137**: 165–174.

23. Moore FD. *Burns in Metabolic Care of the Surgical Patient.* WB Saunders, Philadelphia, 1959.

24. Wilmore DW, Long JM, Mason AD, Skreen RW, Pruitt BA Jr. Catecholamines: mediators of hypermetabolic response to thermal injury. *Ann Surg* 1974; **180**: 653–669.

25. Hart DW *et al.* Determinants of skeletal muscle catabolism after severe burn. *Ann Surg* 2000; **232(4)**: 455–465.

26. Wilmore DW, Mason AD, Johnson DW, Pruitt BA. Effect of ambient temperature on heat production and heat loss in burn. *J Appl Physiol* 1975; **38**: 593–597.

27. Wilmore DW, Aulick LH, Mason AD, Pruitt BA. Influence of the burn wound on local and systemic responses to injury. *Ann Surg* 1977; **186**: 444–445.

28. Wolfe RR, Durkot MJ, Wolfe MH. Effect of thermal injury on energy metabolism, substrate kinetics and hormonal concentration. *Cric Shock* 1982; **9**: 383–394.

29. Wolfe RR *et al.* Glucose metabolism in severely burned patients. *Metabolism* 1979; **28(10)**: 1031–1039.

30. Wilmore DW, Smith RJ, O'Dwyer ST. The gut: a central organ after surgical stress. *Surgery* 1988; **104**: 917–923.

31. Curreri PW *et al.* Dietary requirements of patients with major burns. *J Am Diet Assn* 1974; **65**: 415.

32. Sutherland AB. Nitrogen requirements in the burn patient: a reappraisal. *Burns* 1977; **2**: 238–244.

33. Herndon DN *et al.* Increased mortality with intravenous supplemental feeding in severely burned patients. *J Burn Care Rehabil* 1989; **10(4)**: 309–313.

34. Czaja AJ, McAlhany JC, Pruitt BA. Acute gastroduodenal disease after thermal injury. An endoscopic evaluation of incidence and natural history. *N Engl J Med* 1974; **291(18)**: 925–929.

35. Tompkins RG *et al.* Significant reductions in mortality for children with burn injuries through the use of prompt eschar excision. *Ann Surg* 1988; **208(5)**: 577–585.

36. Jackson D, Topley E, Cason JS, Lowbury EJC. Primary excision and grafting of large burns. *Ann Surg* 1960; **152**: 167–189.

37. Janzekovic Z. A new concept in the early excision and immediate grafting of burns. *J Trauma* 1970; **10**: 1103–1108.

38. Monafo WW. Tangential excision. *Clin Plast Surg* 1974; **1**: 591–601.

39. Burke JF *et al.* Primary burn excision and immediate grafting: a method of shortening illness. *J Trauma* 1974; **14**: 389–395.

40. Engrav LH, Heimbach DM, Reus JL, Harner TJ, Marfin JA. Early excision and grafting versus nonoperative treatment of burns of indeterminate depth. A randomized prospective study. *J Trauma* 1983; **23**: 1001–1004.

41. Herndon DN, Barrow RE, Rutan RL, Rutan TC, Desai MH. A comparison of conservative versus early excision. *Ann Surg* 1989; **209**: 547–553.

42. Herndon DN, Gore DC, Cole M, *et al.* Determinants of mortality on pediatric patients with greater than 70% full-thickness total body surface area thermal injury treated by early total excision and grafting. *J Trauma* 1987; **27**: 208–212.

43. Reverdin JL. Greffe epidermique. *Bulletin de la Societe' Imperiale de Chirurgie de Paris* 1869; **101**: 511–515.

44. Davis JS. The use of small deep skin grafts. *JAMA* 1914; **63**: 985–989.

45. Padgett FC. Indications for determination of the thickness for split skin grafts. *Am J Surg* 1946; **72**: 683–693.

46. Tanner JC, Vandeput J, Olley JF. The mesh skin graft. *Plast Reconst Surg* 1965; **34**: 287–292.

47. Alexander JW, MacMillan BG, Law E, Kittur DS. Treatment of severe burns with widely meshed skin autograft and meshed skin allograft overlay. *J Trauma* 1981; **21(6)**: 433–438.

48. Burke JF, Yannas IV, Quimby WC, Bondoc CC, Jung WK. Successful use of a physiologically acceptable artificial skin in the treatment of extensive burn injury. *Ann Surg* 1981; **194**: 413–428.

49. Heimbach D *et al.* Artificial dermis for major burns: a multi-center randomized clinical trial. *Ann Surg* 1988; **208(3)**: 313–320.

50. Bell E, Ehrlich HP, Buttle DJ, *et al.* Living tissue formed *in vitro* and accepted as skin-equivalent tissue of full-thickness. *Science* 1981; **211**: 1052.

51. Shirani KZ, Pruitt BA, Mason AD. The influence of inhalation injury and pneumonia on burn mortality. *Ann Surg* 1987; **205**: 82.

52. Navar PD, Saffle JR, Warden GD. Effect of inhalation injury on fluid resuscitation requirements after thermal injury. *Am J Surg* 1985; **150(6)**: 716–720.

53. Herndon DN, Barrow RE, Traber DL, Rutan RL, Abston S. Extravascular lung water changes following smoke inhalation and massive burn injury. *Surgery* 1987; **102(2)**: 324–349.

54. Cioffy WG *et al.* Ventilatory support following burns and smoke-inhalation injury. *Resp Care Clin N Am* 1997; **3(1)**: 21–49.

55. Cortiela J, Mlcak R, Herndon DN. High frequency percussive ventilation in pediatric patients with inhalation injury. *J Burn Care Rehabil* 1999; **20(3)**: 232–235.

56. Herndon DN, Traber DL, Pollard P. Pathophysiology of inhalation injury. In: Herndon DN (ed) *Total Burn Care.* WB Saunders Co., London, 1996, pp. 175–183.

57. Desai MH, Mlcak R, Richardson J, Nichols R, Herndon DN. Reduction in mortality in pediatric patients with inhalation injuries with aerosolized Heparin/N-acetylcysteine. *J Burn Care Rehabil* 1998; **19(3)**: 210–212.

58. Burke JF, Yannas IV, Quimby WC, Bondoc CC, Jung WK. Successful use of a physiologically viable artificial skin in the treatment of extensive burn injury. *Ann Surg* 1981; **194**: 413–428.

59. Zwischenberger JB, Cardenas VJ, Tao W, Niranjan SC, Clark JW, Bidani A. Intravascular membrane oxygenation and carbon dioxide removal with IVOX: can improved design and permissive hypercapnia achieve adequate respiratory support during severe respiratory failure: *Artificial Organs* 1994; **18**: 833–839.

Chapter 1

Teamwork for total burn care: achievements, directions, and hopes

David N Herndon, Patricia E Blakeney

Introduction

Major burn injury evokes strong emotional responses in most lay persons and health professionals who are confronted by the spectre of pain, deformity, and potential death associated with significant burns. Severe pain and repeated episodes of sepsis followed by predictable outcomes of either death or a survival encumbered by pronounced disfigurement and disability has been the expected pattern of sequelae to serious burn injury for most of mankind's history.[1] However, these dire consequences have, over time, been ameliorated so that, while burn injury is still intensely painful and sad, the probability of resultant death has been significantly diminished. As illustrated in **Table 1.1**, during the decade prior to 1952, a 50% mortality rate occurred in young adults (15–44 years of age) with total body surface area (TBSA) burns of 46% or greater.[2] Forty years later, statistics from the pediatric and adult burn units in Galveston, Texas indicated that the 50% mortality rate accom-

Table 1.1 Percent of total body surface area (TBSA) burn for an expected 50% mortality in 1952 and 1993		
Age (years)	1952 (% TBSA)	1993* (% TBSA)
0–14	49	98
15–44	46	72
45–64	27	51
>65	10	25

* Galveston Burn Unit.

panied a 70% or greater TBSA for the same age group. Improved survival has been the primary focus of burn treatment advancement in the past few decades.

Such improvement in forestalling death is a direct result of the maturation of the science of burn care. Scientifically sound analyses of patient data have led to the development of formulas for fluid resuscitation[3–6] and nutritional support.[7,8] Clinical research has demonstrated the utility of topical antimicrobials in delaying onset of sepsis, thereby contributing to decreased mortality of burn patients.[9] Prospective randomized clinical trials have determined the efficacy of early surgical therapy in improving survival for many burned patients by decreasing blood loss and by diminishing the occurrence of sepsis.[10–15] Basic science and clinical research have contributed to decreased mortality by describing pathophysiology related to inhalation injury and suggesting treatment methods which have decreased the incidence of pulmonary edema and pneumonia.[16–19] Scientific investigations of the hypermetabolic response to major burn injury have led to improved management of this life-threatening phenomenon, resulting not only in diminished loss of life but also promising improved quality of life.[20–35]

Melding scientific research with clinical care has been promoted throughout the recent history of burn care, in large part because of the aggregation of burned patients into single purpose units staffed by dedicated health care personnel. Dedicated burn units were first established in Great Britain in order to facilitate nursing care.[36] The first US burn center was established at the Medical College of Virginia in 1947 followed that same year by the US Army Surgical Research Unit, later renamed the US Army Institute of Surgical Research.[36] Directors of both of these centers and later the founders of the Burn Hospitals of Shriners Hospitals for Children emphasized the importance of collaboration between clinical care and basic scientific disciplines.[1] The organizational design of these centers stimulated the formation of a self-perpetuating feedback loop of clinical and basic scientific inquiry.[36] Scientists in such a system receive first-hand information about clinical problems while clinicians receive provocative ideas about patient responses to injury from experts of other disciplines.[1] Advances in burn care over the last 50 years attest to the value of a dedicated burn unit organized around the concept of a collegial group of basic scientists, clinical researchers, and clinical care givers, all asking questions of each other, sharing observations and information, and together seeking solutions to improve the welfare of their patients.

Findings of the group at the Army Surgical Research Institute pointed out the necessity of involving many disciplines in the treatment of patients with major burn injuries and stressed the utility of a team concept.[1] The International Society of Burn Injuries and its journal, *Burns*, and the American Burn Association with its publication, *Journal of Burn Care and Rehabilitation*, have publicized to widespread audiences the notion of successful multidisciplinary work by burn teams.

Members of a burn team

As illustrated by a perusal of the contents of either of the afore-mentioned journals and by the contents of this volume, the burn team can include epidemiologists, molecular biologists, microbiologists, physiologists, biochemists, pharmacists, pathologists, endocrinologists, nutritionists, and numerous other scientific and medical specialists. Burn injury is a complex systemic injury, and the search for improved methods of treatment leads to inquiry from many approaches. Each scientific finding stimulates new questions and potential involvement of additional specialists.

At times, the burn team can be thought of as including the environmental service workers responsible for cleaning the unit, the volunteers who may assist in a variety of ways to provide comfort for patients and families, the hospital administrator, and many others who support the day-to-day operations of a burn center and impact significantly on the well-being of patients and staff. The traditional concept of the burn team, however, connotes the multidisciplinary group of direct-care providers. Burn surgeons, nurses, dietitians, and physical and occupational therapists are the skeletal core; most burn units include anesthesiologists, respiratory therapists, pharmacists, and social workers. In recent years, as mortality rates have decreased, interest has intensified in the quality of life for burn survivors, both acutely in the hospital and for the long term. Consequently, more burn units have added psychologists, psychiatrists, and, more recently, exercise physiologists to their burn team membership. In pediatric units, child life specialists and school teachers are significant members of the team of care takers as well.

Infrequently mentioned as members of the team, but obviously important in influencing the outcome of treatment, are the patient and the family of the patient. Persons with major burn injuries contribute actively to their own recovery, and each brings individual needs and agendas into the hospital setting which influence the ways in which treatment is provided by the professional care team.[37] The patient's family members often become active participants: obviously so in the case of children, but also in the case of adult patients. Family members become conduits of information from the professional staff to the patient; they act, at times, as spokespersons for the patient, and at other times, they become advocates for the staff in encouraging the patient to cooperate with dreaded procedures.

With so many diverse personalities and specialists potentially involved, it may appear absurd to purport to know what or who constitutes a burn team. Yet references to the 'burn team' are plentiful, and there is common agreement on some specialists whose expertise is required for excellent care of significant burn injury.

Surgeons

A burn surgeon is the key figure of the burn team. Either a general surgeon or a plastic surgeon or, perhaps, both with expertise in providing emergency and critical care, as well as the techniques of skin grafting and amputations, provides leadership and guidance for the rest of the team which may include several surgeons. The surgeon's leadership is particularly important during the early phase of patient care when moment-to-moment decisions must be made based on the surgeon's knowledge of the physiological responses to the injury, the current scientific evidence, and the appropriate medical/surgical treatment. The surgeon must not only possess knowledge and skill in medicine but also must be able to communicate clearly, both receiving and giving information, with a diverse staff of experts in other disciplines. The surgeon alone cannot provide comprehensive care but must be wise enough to know when and how to seek counsel as well as how to give directions clearly and firmly to direct activities surrounding patient care. The senior surgeon of the team is accorded the most authority and control of any member of the team and, thus, bears the responsibility and receives the accolades for the success of the team as a whole.[37]

Nurses

The nurses of the burn team represent the largest single disciplinary segment of the burn team, providing continuous coordinated care to a patient.[36] The nursing staff is responsible for technical management of the 24-hour physical treatment of the patient. As well, they provide emotional support to the patient and patient's family and control the therapeutic milieu that allows the patient to recover. The nursing staff is often the first to identify changes in the patient's condition and initiate therapeutic interventions.[36] Because recovery from a major burn is a rather slow process, burn nurses combine the qualities of sophisticated intensive care nursing with the challenging aspects of psychiatric nursing. Nursing case management can play an important role in burn treatment, extending the coordination of care beyond the hospitalization through the lengthy period of out-patient rehabilitation.

Anesthesiologists

An anesthesiologist who is an expert in the altered physiological parameters of the burned patient is critical to the survival of the patient, who usually undergoes multiple surgical procedures acutely. Anesthesiologists on the burn team must be familiar with the phases of burn recovery and the physiological changes to be anticipated as the burn wounds heal.[1] Anesthesiologists play significant roles in facilitating comfort for burned patients, not only in the operating room but also in the painful ordeals of dressing changes, removal of staples, and physical exercise.

Respiratory Therapists

Inhalation injury, prolonged bed rest, fluid shifts, and the threat of pneumonia concomitant with burn injury render respiratory therapists essential to the patient's welfare.[36] They evaluate pulmonary mechanics, perform therapy to facilitate breathing, and closely monitor the status of the patient's respiratory functioning.

Rehabilitation Therapists

Occupational and physical therapists begin to plan therapeutic interventions at the patient's admission to maximize functional recovery. Burned patients require special positioning and splinting, early mobilization, strengthening exercises, endurance activities, and pressure garments to promote healing while controlling scar formation. These therapists must be very creative in designing and applying the appropriate appliances. Knowledge of the timing of application is necessary. In addition, rehabilitation therapists must become expert behavioral managers for their necessary treatments are usually painful to the recovering patient who will resist in a variety of ways. While the patient is angry, protesting loudly, or pleading for mercy, the rehabilitation therapist must persist with aggressive treatment in order to combat quickly forming and very strong scar contractures. The same therapist, however, typically is rewarded with adoration and gratitude from an enabled burn survivor.

Nutritionists

A nutritionist or dietitian monitors daily caloric intake and weight maintenance and recommends dietary interventions to provide optimal nutritional support to combat the hypermetabolic response of burn injury. Caloric intake as well as intake of appropriate vitamins, minerals, and trace elements must be managed to promote wound healing and facilitate recovery.

Psychosocial Experts

Psychiatrists, psychologists, and social workers with expertise in human behavior and psychotherapeutic interventions provide continuous sensitivity in caring for the emotional and mental well-being of patients and their families. These professionals must be knowledgeable about the process of burn recovery as well as human behavior in order to make optimal interventions. They serve as confidants and supports for the patients, families of patients, and on occasion, for other burn team members.[38] They often assist colleagues from other disciplines in developing behavioral interventions with problematic patients which allow the colleague and the patient to achieve therapeutic success.[42] During initial hospitalization, these experts attend to managing the patient's mental status, pain tolerance, and anxiety level to provide comfort to the patient and also to facilitate physical recovery. As the patient progresses toward rehabilitation, the role of the mental health team becomes more prominent in supporting optimal psychological, social, and physical rehabilitation.

Functioning of a burn team

Gathering together a group of experts from diverse disciplines will not constitute a team.[43] In fact, the diversity of the disciplines, in addition to individual differences of gender, ethnicity, values, professional experience, and professional status render such teamwork a process fraught with opportunities for disagreements, jealousies, and confusion.[44] The process of working together to accomplish the primary goal, i.e. a burn survivor who returns to a normally functional life, is further complicated by the requirement that the patient and family of the patient collaborate with the professionals. It is not unusual for the patient to attempt to diminish his immediate discomfort by pitting one team member against another or 'splitting' the team. Much as young children will try to manipulate parents by going first to one and then to the other, patients, too, will complain about one staff member to another or assert to one staff member that another staff member allows less demanding rehabilitation exercises or some special privilege.[45] Time must be devoted to a process of trust-building among the team members. It is imperative that the team communicate – openly and frequently – or the group will lose effectiveness.

The group becomes a team when they have common goals and tasks to be accomplished and when they share, as individual members, overlapping values that will be served by accomplishing their goals.[39,40] The team becomes an efficient work group through a process of establishing mechanisms of collaboration and cooperation which facilitate focusing on explicit tasks rather than on covert distractions of personal need and interpersonal conflict.[40,41]

Work groups develop best in conditions that allow each individual to feel acknowledged as valuable to the team.[46,47]

A burn team has defined and shared goals with clear tasks. For the group of burn experts to become an efficient team, skillful leadership that facilitates the development of shared values among team members and ensures the validation of the members of the team as they accomplish tasks is necessary. The burn team consists of many experts, each with specialized knowledge; for that expertise to be fully beneficial, every expert voice must be heard and acknowledged. There will be disagreement, but the disagreement should be offered in a respectful manner, ideally resulting in increased understanding and new perspectives which can lead to improved care for the patient.[48]

The acknowledged formal leader of the team is the senior surgeon who may find the arduous job of medical and social leadership difficult and perplexing. Empirical studies, with remarkable consistency, indicate that the required functions for successful leadership can be grouped into two somewhat incompatible clusters:

- to direct the group toward tasks and goal attainment; and
- to facilitate the interaction of the group members, enhancing their feelings of worth.[40,47–51]

Task-oriented behavior by the leader may at times clash with the needs of the group for emotional support. During those times, the team may inadvertently impede the successful performance of both the leader and the team as the group seeks alternate means of establishing feelings of self-worth. When the social/emotional needs of the group are not met, the group begins to spend more time attempting to satisfy individual needs and less time pursuing task-related activity.

Studies of group behavior demonstrate that high-performance teams are characterized by synergy between task accomplishment and individual need fulfillment.[40,49] Since one formal leader cannot always attend to task and interpersonal nuances, groups allocate, informally or formally, leadership activities to multiple persons.[40,41,47,50] The literature in organizational behavior indicates that the most effective leader is one who engages the talents of others and empowers them to utilize their abilities to further the work of the group.[40,41,50] Failure to empower the informal leaders limits their abilities to contribute fully.

For the identified leader of the burn team, i.e. the senior surgeon, to achieve a successful, efficient burn team, it is important that the leader be prepared to share leadership with one or more 'informal' leaders in such a way that all leadership functions are fulfilled.[40,41,47,50,52] The prominence and the identity of any one of the informal leaders will change according to situational alteration. The successful formal leader will encourage and support the leadership roles of other members of the team, developing a climate in which the team members are more likely to cooperate and collaborate toward achievement beyond individual capacity.

For many physicians, the concept of sharing leadership and power appears at first to be threatening, for it is the physician, after all, who must ultimately write the orders and be responsible for the patient's medical needs.[53] However, sharing power does not mean giving up control.[50] The physician shares leadership by seeking information and advice from other team members and empowers them by validating the importance of their expertise in the decision-making process. The physician, however, maintains control of the patient's care and medical treatment.

Summary and hopes for the future

Centralized care provided in designated burn units has promoted a team approach to both scientific investigation and clinical care which has demonstrably improved the welfare of burn patients. Multidisciplinary efforts are imperative for the continued increase in understanding of and therapeutic responses to the emotional, psychological, and physiological recovery and rehabilitation of the burned person. Tremendous scientific and technological advances have led to dramatically increased survivability for burn victims.

Our hopes for the future are that by following the same model of collaboration, scientists and clinicians will pursue solutions to the perplexing problems the burn survivor must encounter. Physical discomforts such as itching still interfere with rehabilitation of the patient. New techniques for controlling hypertrophic scar and for reconstructive surgeries could do much to diminish the resultant disfigurement.[54] The combined use of anabolic agents[35] and supervised strength and endurance training[29] are currently being investigated as future means of enhancing the well-being of survivors of massive burn injury. Further development of psychological expertise within burn care, and increased public awareness of the competence of burn survivors, may ease the survivor's transition from incapacitated patient to functional member of society. We hope that burn care in the future will continue to devote the same energy and resources which have resulted in such tremendous advances in saving lives to improving the capacity for preserving optimal quality of life for survivors.

References

1. Artz CP, Moncrief JA. The burn problem. In: Artz CP, Moncrief JA eds. *The Treatment of Burns*, 2nd edn. Philadelphia, PA: WB Saunders Co., 1969: 1–21.
2. Bull JP, Fisher AJ. A study of mortality in a burns unit: a revised estimate. *Ann Surg* 1954; **139**: 269–74.
3. Evans EI, Purnell OJ, Robinett PW, Batchelor A, Martin M. Fluid and electrolyte requirements in severe burns. *Ann Surg* 1952; **135**: 804–17.
4. Baxter CR, Marvin JA, Curreri PW. Fluid and electrolyte therapy of burn shock. *Heart Lung* 1973; **2**: 707–13.
5. Artz CR. Burns updated. *J Trauma* 1976; **16**: 2–15.
6. Carvajal HE. Fluid therapy for acutely burned child. *Compr Ther* 1977; **3**: 17–24.
7. Curreri PW, Richmond D, Marvin JA, Baxter CR. Dietary requirements of patients with major burns. *J Am Diet Assoc* 1974; **65**: 415–17.
8. Hildreth MA, Herndon DN, Desai MH, Duke MA. Reassessing caloric requirements in pediatric burn patients. *J Burn Care Rehab* 1988; **9**: 616–18.
9. Lindbergh RB, Pruitt BA Jr, Mason AD Jr. Topical chemotherapy and prophylaxis in thermal injury. *Chemotherapy* 1976; **3**: 351–9.
10. Janzekovic Z. A new concept in the early excision and immediate grafting of burns. *J Trauma* 1975; **15**: 42–62.
11. Burke JF, Bandoc GC, Quinby WC. Primary burn excision and immediate grafting: a method for shortening illness. *J Trauma* 1974; **14**: 389–95.
12. Engrav LH, Heimbach DM, Reus JL, Harnar TJ, Marvin JA. Early excision and grafting vs. nonoperative treatment of burns of indeterminant depth: A randomized prospective study. *J Trauma* 1983; **23**: 1001–4.
13. Herndon DN, Barrow RE, Rutan RL, *et al.* A comparison of conservative versus early excision therapies in severely burned patients. *Ann Surg* 1989; **209**: 547–53.
14. Desai MH, Herndon DN, Broemeling L, Barrow RE, Nichols RJ Jr, Rutan RL. Early burn wound excision significantly reduces blood loss. *Ann Surg* 1990; **211**: 753–62.
15. Desai MH, Rutan RL, Herndon DN. Conservative treatment of scald burns is superior to early excision. *J Burn Care Rehab* 1991; **12**: 482–4.
16. Shirani KZ, Pruitt BA Jr, Mason AD Jr. The influence of inhalation injury and pneumonia on burn mortality. *Ann Surg* 1987; **205**: 82–7.
17. Herndon DN, Barrow RE, Traber DL, *et al.* Extravascular lung water changes following smoke inhalation and massive burn injury. *Surgery* 1987; **102**: 341–9.
18. Herndon DN, Barrow RE, Linares HA, *et al.* Inhalation injury in burned patients: effects and treatment. *Burns* 1988; **14**: 349–56.
19. Cioffi WG Jr, Rue LW III, Graves TA, *et al.* Prophylactic use of high-frequency percussive ventilation in patients with inhalation injury. *Ann Surg* 1991; **213**: 575–82.
20. Wilmore DW, Long JM, Mason AD Jr, *et al.* Catecholamines: mediator of the hypermetabolic response to thermal injury. *Ann Surg* 1974; **180**: 653–69.
21. Herndon DN, Stein MD, Rutan TC, Abston S, Linares H. Failure of TPN supplementation to improve liver function, immunity, and mortality in thermally injured patients. *J Trauma* 1987; **27**: 195–204.
22. Herndon DN, Barrow RE, Stein M, *et al.* Increased mortality with intravenous supplemental feeding in severely burned patients. *J Burn Care Rehab* 1989; **10**: 309–13.
23. Low A, Jeschke M, Barrow R, Herndon D. Attenuating growth delay with growth hormone in severely burned children. *Seventh Vienna Shock Forum*. Vienna, Austria, November 1999.
24. Low JA. Growth hormone prevents delay in height development in burned children. *59th Annual Meeting of the American Association for the Surgery of Trauma*. Boston, MA, September 1999.
25. Low JFA, Barrow RE, Mittendorfer B, Jeschke MG, Chinkes DL, Herndon DN. The effect of short-term growth hormone treatment on growth and energy expenditure in burned children. *Pediatrics* 2000 (in press).
26. Low JFA, Herndon DN, Barrow RE. Effect of growth hormone on growth delay in burned children: a 3-year follow-up study. *Lancet* 1999; **354**: 1789.
27. Cucuzzo N, Herndon DN. The effects of aerobic exercise in the rehabilitation or severely burned children. *Proceedings of the American Burn Association* 21: 203. Las Vegas, NV, March 2000.
28. Cucuzzo N, Farmer S, Sesostris I, Herndon DN. Three repetition maximum strength testing in burned children. *Proceedings of the American Burn Assoc* 21: 205. Las Vegas, NV, March 2000.
29. Cucuzzo NA, Ferrando AA, Herndon DN. A comparison of a progressive resistance exercise program and traditional outpatient therapy for severely burned children. *Med Sci Sports Exerc* 2000 (in press).
30. Hart DW, Wolf SE, Chinkes DL, *et al.* Determinants of catabolism after severe burn. Presented at the Amer Surg Assoc, Philadelphia, PA, April 2000.
31. Hart DW, Wolf SE, Chinkes DL, *et al.* Determinants of catabolism after severe burn. *Ann Surg* 2000 (in press).
32. Hart DW, Wolf SE, Mlcak R, *et al.* Persistence of muscle catabolism after severe burn. Presented at the Society of University Surgeons, Toronto, Canada, 2 November 2000.
33. Hart DW, Wolf SE, Mlcak R, *et al.* Persistence of muscle catabolism after severe burn. *Surgery* 2000 (in press).
34. Hart DW, Wolf SE, Ramzy PI, *et al.* Anabolic effects of oxandrolone following severe burn. Presented at the Society of Critical Care Medicine, Orlando, FL, February 2000.
35. Hart DW, Wolf SE, Ramzy PI, *et al.* Anabolic effects of oxandrolone following severe burn. *Lancet* 2000 (in press).
36. Rutan RL. On the shoulders of giants. Galveston, TX: Shriners Burns Institute, 1994, unpublished manuscript.
37. Shakespeare PG. Who should lead the burn care team? *Burns* 1994; **19(6)**: 490–4.
38. Morris J, McFadd A. The mental health team on a burn unit: a multidisciplinary approach. *J Trauma* 1978; **18(9)**: 658–63.
39. Miller EJ, Rice AK. Selections from: Systems of organization. In: Coleman AD, Bexton WH, eds. *Group Relations Reader*. Sausalito, CA: Grex, 1975; 43–68.
40. Harris PR, Harris DL. High performance team management. *Leadership and Organization – Development Journal* 1989; **10(4)**: 28–32.
41. Yank GR, Barber JW, Hargrove DS, Whitt PD. The mental health treatment team as a work group: team dynamics and the role of the leader. *Psychiatry* 1992; **55**: 250–64.
42. Hughes TL, Medina-Walpole AM. Implementation of an interdisciplinary behavior management program. *J Am Geriatr Soc* 2000; **48(5)**: 581–7.
43. Schofield RF, Amodeo M. Interdisciplinary teams in health care and human services settings: are they effective. *Health and Social Work* 1999; **24(3)**: 210.
44. Fallowfield L, Jenkins V. Effective communication skills are the key to good cancer care. *Eur J Cancer* 1999; **35(11)**: 1592–7.
45. Perl E. Treatment team in conflict: the wishes for and risks of consensus. *Psychiatry* 1997; **60(2)**: 182.
46. Pawlicki RE, Bertera JF, Nicholson M. Practice management: what constitutes an excellent team member. *Am J Pain M* 1994; **4(4)**: 175–7.
47. Litterer JA. *The Analysis of Organizations*, 2nd edn. New York: John Wiley & Sons, 1973.
48. Van Norman G. Interdisciplinary team issues. Internet Publication, Univ of Washington, 1999.
49. Fleishman EA, Mumford MD. Zaccaro SJ, Levin KY, Korotkin AL, Hein MB. Taxonomic efforts in the description of leader behavior: a synthesis and

functional interpretation. Special Issue: Individual Differences and Leadership: *Leadership Quarterly* 1991; **2(4)**: 245–87.

50. Hollander EP, Offermann LR. Power and leadership in organizations: relationships in transition. *Am Psychol* 1990; **45(2)**: 179–89.

51. Krantz J. Lessons from the field: an essay on the crisis of leadership in contemporary organizations. *J Appl Behav Sci* 1990; **26(1)**: 4944.

52. Glaser EM, Van Eynde DE. Human resource development, team building, and a little bit of 'Kiem Tau': Part 1. *Organization Development Journal* 1989; 20–4.

53. Fiorelli JS. Power in work groups: team members' perspectives. *Hum Relat* 1988; **41(1)**: 1–12.

54. Constable JD. The state of burn care: past, present, and future. *Burns* 1994; **20(4)**: 316–24.

Chapter 2

Epidemiological, demographic, and outcome characteristics of burn injury

Basil A Pruitt Jr, Cleon W Goodwin, Arthur D Mason Jr

Introduction

In 1998, there were 146 941 deaths from all injuries in the United States which in a total population of 270 248 524 represents a crude, all-injury death rate of 54.36 and an age-adjusted death rate of 48.26 per 100 000 population respectively. Within that all-injury total, the magnitude of the public health problem represented by burns is indicated by the fire and burn deaths reported for the United States as a whole, and each state individually, by the National Center for Injury Prevention and Control. In 1998, there were 3813 fire and burn deaths recorded in the United States, which represents a fire/burn crude death rate of 1.41 and an age-adjusted death rate of 1.19 per 100 000 population respectively. Fire/burn deaths in individual states in 1998 ranged from 290 and 289 in Texas and California, respectively, to a low of 3 and 2 in Wyoming and Rhode Island, respectively. The age-adjusted fire and burn death rates in 1998 ranged from 3.69 to 3.58 per 100 000 in Mississippi and Alaska, respectively, to a low of 0.3 and 0.12 per 100 000 in Utah and Rhode Island, respectively.[1]

Fire and burn deaths occur with greatest frequency in residential fires, especially in multifamily dwellings and in low income census tracts.[2] Eighty-one percent of fire-related deaths occur in the home.[3] In 1995, 3600 deaths and approximately 18 600 injuries were attributed to residential fires.[3] It has been reported that approximately 12 individuals die in a residential fire each day, with young children and the elderly being the most likely victims.[4,5] In the 5-year period, 1991 to 1995, children of less than 5 years, and adults of 65 or more years, had averaged annualized death rates five to six times higher than the national average for all ages.[3] Young children have difficulty escaping from a fire because of dependency, and the elderly because of preexisting diseases and decreased agility.

Epidemiology and demography

Geographic location, presumably because of regional differences in construction and heating devices as well as economic status, influences death rates from house fires. House fire death rates are higher in the eastern part of the United States, particularly the Southeast, as compared to the West.[6] There are marked seasonal differences in house fire deaths. From 1991 to 1995, residential fire-related deaths were highest during the cold winter months (December–February) when greatest use is made of heating and lighting devices, and lowest in the warm summer months (June–August).[3] Unattended and/or improperly positioned cooking and heating devices are the leading causes of residential fires.[7] House fires cause only approximately 4% of burn admissions, but the 12% fatality rate of patients hospitalized for burns sustained in house fires is higher than the 3% fatality rate for patients with burns from other causes. This difference is presumably the effect of associated inhalation injury.[8,9]

Playing with matches, cigarette lighters, and other ignition devices has been incriminated as the cause of 1 in 10 residential fire deaths.[6] House fire death rates show little gender prominence except for an increased incidence in males aged 2 to 5, a group that has the highest rate of non-fatal burns due to unsupervised play with matches.[10] In fact, among children of 9 years or less, child-play fires are the leading cause of residential fire-related death and injury. Careless smoking, which accounts for 1 in 4 residential fire deaths, is the most common cause of such fatalities.[11] Alcohol and drug intoxication, which contribute to careless smoking behavior by impairing mentation, have been reported to be a factor in 40% of residential fire deaths, which appears to contribute to the high weekend frequency of house fires.[12] Arson is the second most common cause of residential fire deaths.[11] Defective or inappropriately used heating devices, which are the third most common cause, account for 1 in 6 residential fire deaths overall, and an even greater proportion in low income areas.[11] The effect of low income on fire and burn deaths is also related to residence in older buildings, crowded living conditions, and absence of smoke detectors. Nearly 800 children, aged 14 and less, died as a consequence of fire and burn related injury in 1996.[13] Flames and burns were considered to be responsible for one-fourth of all fire-related deaths in children. As a reflection of the effect of economic status, minority children aged 0 to 19 are more than three times as likely to die in a residential fire than white children.[5] As income increases, racial differences in house fire death rates decrease.[14]

During the 5-year period, 1991 to 1995, the residential fire-related death rate in the United States decreased from 1.3 to 1.1 per 100 000 population.[3] This change has been attributed to the combined effects of improved building design, the use of safer appliances and heating devices, and the increased use of smoke and fire detectors. Data from the Centers for Disease Control Behavioral Risk Factor Surveillance System (BRFSS) indicate that the presence of smoke alarms in households in the United States is high, i.e. more than 78% of households in all 50 states. In 1995, 93.6% of all US households claimed to have at least one smoke alarm.[3] There are almost half as many fire-related deaths in homes with smoke alarms as compared to homes without those devices.[15,16]

The economic consequences of residential fires are also great. In 1995, property damage and other direct costs attributable to such fires were estimated to exceed four billion dollars.[17] The health care costs of burn injuries are also prodigious. Each year in the United States 60 000 to 80 000 people require in-hospital care for burns. The average cost of hospital care of a patient injured by flame and/or smoke inhalation ranges from $29 560 to $117 506 with much higher costs incurred by patients with extensive burns. The length of hospital stay ranges from one day to hundreds of days (mean 8.7) and for patients 80 years and above is more than twice as long as that for children under 5.[17] The estimated cost of a fire-related death, which includes the loss of future productivity ranges from $250 000 to 1.5 million dollars.[18,20,21]

Unlike fire deaths, the precise number of burn injuries that occur in the United States is unknown. Twenty-one states require that burn injuries be reported, but two require that only burns associated with assaults or arson be reported, and seven require that only larger burns (usually those involving more than 15% of the total body surface area) be reported.[22] Consequently, the total number of burns must be estimated by extrapolation of data collected in less than one-half of the states to the entire population. Such estimates have ranged from 1.4 million to 2 million injuries due to burns and fires each year.[6,23] Because of the general improvement in living conditions in the United States, an annual incidence of approximately 1.25 million is considered to be a realistic estimate at the present time.[24] The majority of those burns are of limited extent (more than 80% of burns involve less than 20% of the total body surface area).[23] However, as recently as the 1980s, it was estimated that in the United States, 270–300 patients per million population (67 500–75 000) per year sustained burns which – because of extent, associated injury or comorbid conditions – required admission to a hospital.[2] In light of the overall decrease in the incidence of burns, it is currently estimated that only 190–263 patients per million population (51 300–71 100) will require admission to a hospital annually.[19,24]

A review of 1994 Pennsylvania statewide hospital discharge data identified 3173 cases with a fire or burn diagnosis for a rate of 263 per million population.[19] Sixty-eight percent of the patients were males and 70% of the patients were white. Hospital discharge rates showed three distinct peaks, i.e. patients of less than 5 years, patients between 25 and 39 years, and patients 65 years and older. The discharge rate for males was slightly more than twice that of females and the rate for blacks was more than twice that for whites. Scalds and hot substances were the cause of the burn in 58% of the patients. Fire and flame sources accounted for 34% of the burns (clothing ignition 15%, conflagration 12%, and controlled fire

7%). Two percent of the burns were self-inflicted and 2% were the consequence of an assault.

A smaller subset of approximately 20 000 burn patients with even more severe injuries, as defined by the American Burn Association (**Table 2.1**), are best cared for in a burn center.[25] Those patients consist of 42 per million population with major burns and 40 per million population having lesser burns but a complicating co-factor.[2] There are 139 self-designated burn care facilities in the United States, and 17 in Canada which are distributed in close relationship to population density and contain a total of 2120 beds (**Figure 2.1**).[26] As described below, the geographic distribution of burn centers necessitates the use of aeromedical transfer by both rotary and fixed wing aircraft to transport patients requiring burn center care to those facilities from distant and remote areas.

In addition to economic status[27] and geographic location[27,28] the risk of being burned and the predominant cause of burn injury are related to age[29], occupation, and participation in recreational activities.[30] Scald burns are the most frequent form of burn injury overall and cause over 100 000 patients to seek treatment in hospital emergency rooms.[31,32]

High risk populations

Children

It has been estimated that 83 000 children, aged 14 and under, were treated in hospital emergency rooms for burn-related injuries in 1997. Of those injuries, 59 000 were thermal burns and 24 000 scald burns.[13] An average of 16 children with scald burns die each year, and those aged 4 and less account for nearly all of those deaths.[13] Of the children aged 4 and under who are hospitalized for burn-related injuries, 65% have scald burns, 20% contact burns, and the remainder flame burns. The majority of scald burns in children, especially those aged 6 months to 2 years, are from hot foods and liquids, particularly coffee which may be dispensed at temperatures of up to 180°F (82.2°C) and spilled in the kitchen or other places where food is prepared and served.[13] Hot tap-water burns,

---

Table 2.1 American Burn Association major burn injury criteria

1. Second and third degree burns greater than 10% of the total body surface area in patients under 10 or over 50 years of age.
2. Second and third degree burns greater than 20% of the total body surface area in other age groups.
3. Significant burns of face, hands, feet, genitalia, or perineum and those that involve skin overlying major joints.
4. Third degree burns greater than 5% of the total body surface area in any age group.
5. Inhalation injury.
6. Significant electric injury including lightning injury.
7. Significant chemical injury.
8. Burns with significant preexisting medical disorders that could complicate management, prolong recovery, or affect mortality (e.g. diabetes mellitus, cardiopulmonary disease).
9. Burns with significant concomitant trauma (may require initial treatment in a trauma center).
10. Burn injury in patients who will require special social and emotional or long-term rehabilitative support, including cases of suspected child abuse and neglect.

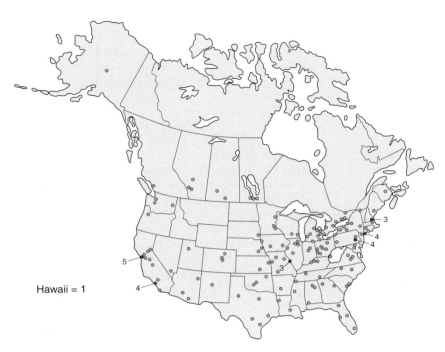

Hawaii = 1

Fig. 2.1 Burn care facilities in North America 1999–2000. The numbers indicate facilities in areas where these are concentrated.

which typically occur in the bathroom, tend to be more severe and cover a larger portion of the body surface than other scald burns. Consequently, such burns, which account for nearly one-fourth of all childhood scald burns, are associated with higher hospitalization and death rates than other hot liquid burns.[13] Ninety-five percent of burns among children due to the operation of microwave devices are scald burns resulting from the spillage of hot liquids or food.[13]

Among children (14 years and less), hair curlers and curling irons, room heaters, ovens and ranges, irons, gasoline, and fireworks are the most common causes of product-related burn injuries.[13] Nearly two-thirds of electric injuries in children aged 12 and under are caused by household electric cords and extension cords.[13] Contact with the current in wall outlets causes an additional 14% of such injuries.[13] Male children are at higher risk of burn-related death and injury than female children, and children aged 4 and under or with a disability are at the greatest risk of burn-related death and injury, especially from scald and contact burns.[13] Boys that are heavier than normal for their age are more burn-prone than their normal-sized counterparts. A recent retrospective study of 372 children admitted to a single burn center from January 1991 through July 1997 confirmed that males who were large for age on the basis of weight or height were over-represented in the burn population.[33] Interestingly, that same study indicated that male children at or under the fifth percentile for weight, and male and female children at or under the fifth percentile for height were also over-represented among pediatric burn patients. The authors considered the latter finding to reflect, at least in part, the effect of concomitant malnutrition or neglect.

The occurrence of tap-water scalds can be prevented by adjusting the temperature settings on hot water heaters or by installing special faucet valves so that water does not leave the tap at temperatures above 120°F (48.8°C).[13,34] Thermostatic valves, which shut the hot water off if the cold water fails, are the most dependable.[35] The results of a survey in Denmark indicated that the kitchen, not the bathroom, is the most common site of burn injury (39% of burns).[36] Those burns were most commonly due to contact with hot liquids.

The Elderly

The elderly represent an increasing sector of the population, the members of which have an increased risk of being burned and higher morbidity and mortality rates than younger patients. A recent review of medical records of patients admitted to a burn center during a 7-year period revealed that 221 (11%) of 1557 admissions were 59 years or older.[37] Ninety-seven (44%) of that group were women, a reflection of the higher percentage of women in the elderly population. Two-thirds of the injuries were caused by flames or explosions, 20% by scalds, 6% by electricity, 2% by chemicals, and 6% by 'other causes'. Forty-one percent of the injuries occurred in the bedroom and/or living room, 28% out of doors or in the work place, 18% in the kitchen, 8% in the bathroom, and 5% in the garage or basement. Seventy-seven percent of the patients had one or more preexisting medical conditions. Sixty-four patients (29%) had smoke inhalation. In 57% of patients judgment and/or mobility were impaired. Ten percent of patients tested positive for ethanol and 29% for other drugs by toxicology screening. Survival advantage was conferred by younger age, absence of inhalation injury, absence of preexisting medical conditions, and lesser extent of burn. A review of 111 octogenarians admitted to a burn center between 1983 and 1993 revealed that scalds caused 32% of injuries, flames 30%, contact 29%, bath immersion 7%, electricity 2%, and hot oil 1%.[38] In 18% a disease such as a stroke was considered to be directly responsible for the burn injury and in an additional 50% of the patients, a preexisting disease was considered to be contributory to the injury event. The average length of stay was almost twice that of younger adults and rehabilitation of survivors was markedly prolonged.

The Disabled

The disabled are a group of patients considered to be 'burn-prone'. The majority of burns in the disabled occur at home and are most often scalds. The effects of disability and preexisting disease in those patients are evident in the duration of hospital stay (27.6 days on average) and the death rate (22.2%) associated with the modest average extent of burn (10% of the total body surface area).[39]

Military Personnel

In wartime, military personnel are at high risk for burn injury, both combat related and accidental. The incidence of burn injury, which is related to both the type of weapons employed and the type of combat units engaged, has ranged from 2.3% to as high as 85% of casualties incurred in various periods of conflict over the past six decades (**Table 2.2**). The detonation of a nuclear weapon at Hiroshima in 1945 instantaneously generated an estimated maximum of 57 700 burn patients and destroyed many treatment facilities which thereby compromised the care of those burn patients.[40] In the Vietnam conflict, as a consequence of the total air superiority achieved by the US Air Force and the lack of armored fighting vehicle activity, patients with burn injury represented only 4.6% of all patients admitted to Army medical treatment facilities or quarters in Vietnam from 1963 to 1975.[41] The majority (58%) of the 13 047 burn patients treated in those years were non-battle injuries, with only 5536 (42%) being battle injuries. The overall incidence of burns as the cause of injury in all United States military forces in Vietnam during those years may well have been higher. Allen *et al.* reported that during calendar years 1967 and 1968 a total of 1963 military burn patients from Vietnam were admitted and treated at a burn unit established in a United States Army General Hospital in Japan.[42] In consonance with the data from US Army hospitals in Vietnam, the burns in 847 (43.2%) of those patients were the result of hostile action. In the Panama police action in late 1989, the low incidence of burn injury (only 6 or 2.3% of the total 259 casualties had burns) has been attributed to the fact that the action involved only infantry and airborne infantry forces using small arms weaponry.

As exemplified by the Israeli conflicts of 1973 and 1982, and the British Army of the Rhine experience in World War II between March 1945 and the end of hostilities in Northwest Europe, the personnel in armored fighting vehicles have been at relatively high risk for burn injury.[43,44] Burns have also been common injuries in war at sea. In the Falkland Islands campaign of 1982, 34% of all casualties from the British Navy ships were burns.[45] The increased incidence of burn injuries, 10.5% and 8.6% in the Israeli conflicts of 1973 and 1982 respectively as compared to the 4.6% incidence in the 1967 Israeli conflict, is considered to reflect what has been termed 'battlefield saturation with tanks and anti-tank weaponry'.[43,46] The decreased incidence of burn injuries, 8.6% in the 1982 Israeli conflict as compared to the 10.5% in the 1973 Israeli conflict, has been attributed to enforced use of flame retardant garments and the effectiveness of an automatic fire extinguishing system within the Israeli tanks.[46] Those factors have also been credited with reducing the extent of the burns that did occur. In the 1973 Israeli conflict, 29% of the patients with burns had injuries that involved 40% or more of the total body surface, and only 21% had burns of less than 10% of the body surface. In the 1982 Israeli conflict those same categories of burns represented 18% and 51%, respectively, of all burn injuries. Modern weaponry may have eliminated the differential incidence of burn injury between armored fighting vehicle personnel and the personnel of other combat elements. One of almost every five casualties had burns in both the British and Argentinian forces in the 1982 Falkland Islands conflict in which there was little if any involvement of armored fighting vehicles.[45,47] Conversely, there were only 36 (7.8%) burn casualties in the total 458 casualties sustained by US Forces in 1990 and 1991 during Operation Desert Shield/Storm in which there was extensive involvement of armored fighting vehicles.

Even though the risk of burn injury in the combat population is relatively high, the distribution of burn size in other than armored fighting vehicle personnel is comparable to that in the civilian population, i.e. more than 80% of the patients have burns of less than 20% of the body surface. Even so, the number of burns that can be rapidly generated necessitates that planning for combat casualty care include augmentation of in-theater medical treatment facilities with personnel having burn-specific expertise as was done in Operation Desert Shield/Storm. Even in peacetime noncombat munitions incidents are common in the US Army. In a recent 7-year period there were 742 noncombat munitions incidents reported in which 894 soldiers were injured.[48] The most common types of injuries were burns which occurred in 261 or 26.7% of all the patients injured. The high incidence of burn injury in military personnel in both war and peace will generate a subset of extensively burned patients who will require tertiary burn center care to ensure optimum functional outcome and maximum survival.

Table 2.2 Incidence of burn injury in armed conflict	Casualties	
Conflict	Percentage	Number
World War II Hiroshima 1945[40]	65–85	45 500–59 500
Vietnam Conflict 1965–1973[41]	4.6	13 047
Israeli Six Day War 1967[45]	4.6	
Yom Kippur War 1973[43]	10.5	
Falkland Islands War 1982		
British Casualties[46]	18.0	140
Argentinian Casualties[47]	17.5	34 of 194
Lebanon War 1982[43]	8.6	
Panama Police Action 1989	2.3	6 of 259
Operation Desert Shield/Storm 1990–1991	7.9	36 of 458

Burn etiologies

Burns from scalds and contacts with hot materials cause approximately 100 deaths per year.[6] The case fatality rate of scald injury is low (presumably due to the usually modest extent and limited depth of the burn), but scalds are major causes of morbidity and associated health care costs, particularly in children less than 5 years of age and in the elderly. Although deaths from scalds are relatively rare in patients between the ages of 5 and 64, both rates of hospitalization for burn injury and death rates are three times higher for blacks than for caucasians.[49]

Even though the burns of 30% of all patients requiring admission to a hospital are caused by scalding due to hot liquids,[50,51] flame is the predominant cause of burns in patients admitted to burn centers, particularly in the adult age group (**Table 2.3**). The misuse of fuels and flammable liquids is a common cause of burn injury. A recent retrospective review of admissions to one burn center for the multiyear period 1978 to 1996 identified 1011 (23.3% of 4339 acute admissions) as being gasoline related.[52] The average total extent of burn was 30% of the total body surface area with an average 14% full thickness burn component. One hundred and forty-four of those patients expired. The unsafe use of gasoline was implicated in 87% of patients in whom the cause of the burn could be identified, and in 90 or 63% of the 144 fatalities. The use of gasoline for purposes other than as a motor fuel, and any indoor use of a volatile petroleum product should be discouraged as part of any prevention program. In one epidemiologic study in New York state, the largest number of admissions in the teenage/early adult age group (15–24 years) was related to automobiles. Ignition of fuel following a crash, steam from radiators, and contact with hot engine and exhaust parts were the most frequent causes.[51] In a review of 178 patients who had been burned in an automobile crash, it was noted that slightly more than one-third had other injuries, most commonly involving the musculoskeletal system, and that approximately 1 in 6 had inhalation injury (1 in 3 of those

who died.).[53] A review of patients admitted to a referral burn center revealed that burns sustained while operating a vehicle involved an average of more than 30% of the total body surface and were associated with mechanical injuries (predominantly fractures) much more frequently than those burns incurred in the course of vehicle maintenance activities, which involved an average of less than 30% of the total body surface.[54]

Automotive-related flame burns can also be caused by fires and explosions resulting from 'carburetor-priming' with liquid gasoline; and such burns have been reported to account for 2% to 5% of burn unit admissions.[55] The burns sustained in boating accidents are also most often flash burns due to an explosion of gasoline or butane and typically affect the face and hands.[30] Bonfire and barbeque burns caused by flash ignition of a flammable liquid, which is used to start or accelerate a fire, affect those same areas as well as the anterior trunk.[56]

The ignition of clothing is the second leading cause of burn admissions for most ages.[51] The burn injury rate due to the ignition of clothing is influenced by poverty and is inversely related to income. The fatality rate of patients with burns due to the ignition of clothing is second only to that of patients with burns incurred in house fires.[51] Burns caused by ignition of synthetic fabrics which melt and adhere to the skin are commonly deeper than burns caused by other fabrics and typically exhibit a gravity-dependent 'runoff' pattern. More than three-quarters of deaths due to the ignition of clothing occur in patients above the age of 64.[6] Clothing ignition deaths, which were a frequent cause of death in young girls, have decreased as clothing styles have changed and are now rare among children with little overall gender difference. From 1975, when it was mandated that sleep-wear sizes 0 to 6X successfully pass a standard flame test, until 1999 when that law was repealed, the percentage of clothing burns caused by sleep-wear in children aged 0–12 decreased from 55% to 27%.[51,57] Sleep-wear related burns are being closely monitored to assess the affect of deregulation of sleep-wear garments on related burns.

Table 2.3 Admissions to US Army Institute of Surgical Research Burn Center, 1994–2000				
	Age groups (years)			
Cause of burn	0–15	16–40	Over 40	Total
Hot liquids	225	151	111	487
Gasoline, diesel, and kerosene	75	215	129	419
Open flame	72	118	109	299
Structural fires	15	40	60	115
Butane, propane, or natural/sewer gas explosions	10	54	42	106
Motor vehicles crashes	3	30	8	41
Smoking, clothing ignition	2	11	27	40
Bomb, shell, grenade simulator, and gunpowder explosions	9	49	6	64
Contact	53	26	25	104
Electrical*	9	46	12	67
Chemical	3	19	16	38
Welding	0	8	3	11
Intentional				
Self-inflicted	0	21	15	36
Suspected assault/abuse	3	13	8	24
Aircraft crashes	1	58	3	62
Train crashes	1	1	0	2
Sunburn	0	0	2	2
Total	481	860	576	1917
*One lightning injury				

Work related burns account for 20–25% of all serious burns. A Bureau of Labor Statistics survey in 1985 indicated that 6% of all work related thermal burns occurred in adolescent workers (16–19 years).[58] In a 1986 study in Ohio, it was noted that the majority of hospital-treated burns in the teenage/young adult group occurred on the job.[59] A study in that same year revealed that 6 out of 10 hospitalized burn injuries in employed men in Massachusetts were work related.[60] Restaurant related burns, particularly those due to deep fryers, represent a major and preventable source of occupational burn morbidity, and in restaurants account for 12% of work related injuries.[61] Almost 700 deaths annually are caused by occupation related burns.[61,62]

As would be anticipated, the risk of burn injury due to hot tar is greatest for roofers and paving workers. Of all accidents involving roofers and sheet metal workers, 16% are burns caused by hot bitumen, and 17% of those injuries are of sufficient severity to prevent work for a variable period of time. In the state of California, in 1979, 366 roofers and slaters sustained burn injuries.[63] The majority of hot tar burns involved the hand and upper limb.[64] Another occupation associated with an increased risk of burn injury is welding in which flash burns and explosions are the most common injury-producing events.

In the United States in 1988, there were 236 200 patients with chemical injuries of all types treated in emergency rooms. Of those patients, 35 000 or 15% were patients of all ages with chemical burns, and 6500 or 5% were children younger than 5 years with chemical burns. The limited extent of burns due to chemical contact is indexed by the fact that only 800, or 2%, of the chemical burns required admission to a hospital. The effect of age (in the very young, removal of the offending agent may be delayed) on the severity of chemical injury is evident in the fact that 400 of the patients requiring admission to a hospital for the care of chemical burn injuries were children younger than 5 years.[65] The greatest risk of injury due to strong acids occurs in patients who are involved in plating processes and fertilizer manufacture. The greatest risk of injury due to strong alkalis in the work place is associated with soap manufacturing and in the home with the use of oven cleaners. The greatest risk of phenol injuries is associated with the manufacture of dyes, fertilizers, plastics, and explosives. The greatest risk of hydrofluoric acid injury is associated with etching processes, petroleum refining, and air conditioner cleaning. Anhydrous ammonia injury is most common in agricultural workers, and cement injury is most common in construction workers. Injury due to petroleum distillates, which cause delipidation, is greatest in refinery and tank farm workers, while white phosphorus and mustard gas injuries are most frequent in military personnel.[66]

Nearly 1000 deaths are caused annually by electric current. One-third of electric injuries occur in the home and one-quarter occur on farms or industrial sites.[51] The greatest incidence of electrical injury caused by household current occurs in young children who insert uninsulated objects into electrical receptacles or bite or suck on electric cords in sockets.[2] Low-voltage direct current injury can be caused by contact with automobile battery terminals or by defective or inappropriately used medical equipment such as electrosurgical devices,[67] external pacing devices,[68] or defibrillators.[69] Although such injuries may involve the full-thickness of the skin, they are characteristically of limited extent. Caucasians, apparently because of employment patterns, are almost twice as likely to be injured by high-voltage electric current than are blacks.[62] Employees of utility companies, electricians, construction workers (particularly those working with cranes), farm workers moving irrigation pipes, oil field workers, truck drivers, and individuals installing antennae are at greatest risk of high-voltage electric injury.[2] The greatest incidence of electric injury occurs during the summer as a reflection of farm irrigation activity, construction work, and work on outdoor electrical systems and equipment.[10]

A total of 1318 deaths were caused by lightning in the United States from 1980 through 1995.[70] Of those who died, 1125 (85%) were male and 896 (68%) were 15 to 44 years of age. The annual death rate from lightning was greatest among patients aged 15 to 19 years (6 deaths per 10 million population; crude rate: 3 per 10 million) and is 7 times greater in males than females. The greatest number of deaths caused by lightning, 145 and 91, occurred in Florida and Texas, respectively. However, New Mexico, Arizona, Arkansas, and Mississippi had the highest crude death rates of 10, 9, 9, and 9 per 10 million population, respectively. Lopez and Holle note that National Oceanic and Atmospheric Administration data identified an average of 93 deaths and 257 injuries caused by lightning occurred each year during the period 1959–1990.[71] Those authors also cited a study based on national death certificate data for 1968–1985 which reported an average of 107 lightning deaths each year and an annual death rate of 6.1 per 10 million population.

Approximately 30% of persons struck by lightning die, with the greatest risk of death being in those patients with cranial burns or leg burns. Ninety-two percent of lightning associated deaths occur during the summer months (May–September) when thunderstorms are most common. Seventy-three percent of deaths occur during the afternoon and early evening when thunderstorms are most apt to occur. Fifty-two percent of patients who died from lightning injury were engaged in outdoor recreational activity such as golfing and fishing and 25% were engaged in work activities when struck. Sixty-three percent of lightning associated deaths occur within one hour of injury. Virtually all lightning injuries and deaths can be prevented by taking appropriate precautions. The recent decrease in lightning related deaths appears to be related to a decrease in the farm population, better understanding of the pathophysiology of lightning injury, and improved resuscitation techniques.

Fireworks are another seasonal cause of burn injury. Approximately 10% of patients with fireworks injuries require in-hospital care and approximately 60% of those injuries are burns.[72] These data can be used to estimate that 1.86 to 5.82 fireworks related burns per 100 000 persons occurred in the United States during the 4th of July holiday.[73] Extrapolation of the National Electronic Injury Surveillance System (NEISS) data indicates that 13 263 patients sustained burns in 1992 from fireworks and flares.[74] Sparklers, firecrackers, and bottle rockets caused the greatest number of burn injuries requiring hospital care.[75] Nearly 3000 children, aged 14 or less, sustained fireworks related injuries that required treatment in hospital emergency rooms in 1996.[13] Burns accounted for approximately 60% of those injuries, and principally involved the hands, head, and eyes. As expected, 75% of such injuries occur in the month surrounding 4th of July.[13] Males, especially those aged 10 to 14, are at the highest risk for fireworks related injuries. Children, aged 4 and under, are at highest risk for sparkler related injuries.[13] At the US Army Institute of Surgical Research Burn Center, only 4, or 0.1%, of 3628 burn patients admitted during a 15-year period had been burned by fireworks.

Burn injury can also be intentional, either self-inflicted or caused by assault. A retrospective review of 5758 burn patients treated at a regional burn center during a 12-year period identified 51 patients (26 males and 25 females) with a diagnosis of self-inflicted burns.[76] In 42 patients, in whom the injury was an attempt at suicide, the burn involved from 1% to 84% of the total body surface with an average extent of 22%. Twelve, or 28%, of those patients expired. There were nine patients in whom the injury was considered a form of self-mutilation. Those injuries involved 1–5% of the total body surface with an average extent of 1.4%. Forty-three percent of all the injuries occurred at home, and 14 occurred while the patient was in a psychiatric institution. Seventy-three percent of the patients had a history of psychiatric disease; and these were predominantly affective disorders or schizophrenia in the suicides, and personality disorders in the self-mutilators. Fifty-five percent of the suicides had previously attempted suicide; 66% of the self-mutilators had made at least one previous attempt at self-mutilation. The authors concluded that the very fact of self-burning warranted psychiatric assessment. Buddhist ritual burning caused by contact with smoldering incense is a traditional religious form of self-mutilation.[77] Squyres et al. reported their experience in treating 17 people over a 3-year period for self-inflicted burns.[78] The average extent of burn in those patients was 29.5% of the total body surface; and 59% of them had concomitant inhalation injury. All of those patients had a psychiatric disorder which, in 47% of the group, was related to substance abuse. The most frequently employed means of injury was ignition of a flammable liquid.

Assault by burning is most often caused by throwing liquid chemicals at the face of the intended victim or by the ignition of a flammable liquid with which the victim has been doused. Relatively uncommon is the infliction of burn injury by dousing the victim with hot water. Duminy and Hudson have reported their experience with 127 patients who had been intentionally injured with hot water.[79] The burns in those patients involved from 1% to 45% of the total body surface area with an average extent of 13.7%. The trunk and arms were burned in 116 of the patients, the head and neck in 84, and the legs in 27. The vast majority, 84, had only partial thickness injuries. Fifty-one of the 94 male patients and 12 of the 33 females had been assaulted by their spouses. In cases of spouse abuse, the face or genitalia are characteristically splashed with chemicals or hot liquids while cases due to abuse or neglect in elderly, disabled, and handicapped adults resemble those in child abuse cases.[80,81] In India, a common form of spouse abuse is burning by intentional ignition of clothing. When such burns are fatal they have been called 'dowry deaths' since they have been used to establish the widower's eligibility for a new bride and dowry.

Child abuse represents a special form of burn injury most commonly inflicted by parents but also perpetrated by siblings and child-care personnel. Child abuse has been associated with teenage parents, mental deficits in either the child or the abuser, illegitimacy, a single parent household, and low socioeconomic status (although child abuse can occur in all economic groups). Abuse is usually inflicted upon children younger than 2 years of age who, in addition to burns, may exhibit signs of poor hygiene, psychological deprivation, and nutritional impairment.[82] The most common form (approximately one-third of cases) of child abuse thermal injury is caused by cigarettes; such injuries, because of their limited extent, frequently do not require admission to a hospital.[83] Child abuse by burning has also been inflicted by placing a small child in a microwave oven. The burn injuries produced in that manner are typically present on the body parts nearest the microwave generating element, full-thickness in depth and sharply demarcated.[84] Child neglect, if not child abuse, is considered to be a factor in burns of the hand, particularly those on the dorsum of the hand, due to contact with a hot clothing iron.[85] Most often scalding causes the burns in abused children who require in-hospital care.[86] Such injuries are often associated with soft tissue trauma, fractures, and head injury. A distribution typical of child abuse immersion scald burns, i.e. feet, posterior legs, buttocks, and the hands, should heighten one's suspicion of child abuse. The presence of such burns mandates a complete evaluation of the circumstances surrounding the injury and the home situation. The importance of identifying child abuse in the case of a burn injury resides in the fact that if such abuse goes undetected and the child is returned to the abusive environment, there is a high risk of fatality due to repeated abuse.

Elder abuse can also take the form of burn injury. A congressional report published in 1991 indicated that 2 million older Americans are abused each year, and some estimates claim a 4% to 10% incidence of neglect or abuse of the elderly.[87] A recent retrospective review of 28 patients, 60 years and above, admitted to a single burn center during a calendar year, identified self-neglect in seven, neglect by others in three, and abuse by others in one.[88] Adult protective services were required in two cases. The authors of that study concluded that abuse was likely to be under-reported because of poor understanding of risk factors and a low index of suspicion on the part of the entire spectrum of healthcare personnel.

Patients may also sustain burns while in the hospital for diagnosis and treatment of other disease.[89] In addition to the electric injuries noted above, chemical burns have been produced by inadvertent application of glacial acetic acid, concentrated silver nitrate, iodine, or phenol solutions, and potassium permanganate crystals. Application of excessively hot soaks or towels or inappropriate use of heat lamps or a heating blanket are other causes of burn injury to patients.[90] Much more serious are the burns and inhalation injuries caused by electrocautery or laser devices, explosions of gases (including oxygen), or ignition of the instruments used for endotracheal and endobronchial procedures or anesthetic management.[91] A common cause of burn injury, particularly in disoriented hospital or nursing home patients, is the ignition of bed clothes and clothing by a burning cigarette. Smoking should be banned in health care facilities, or at least restricted to adequately monitored situations. A recent retrospective review of 4510 consecutive patients admitted to a burn center between January 1978 and July 1997 identified 54 patients who sustained burns while undergoing medical treatment.[92] Twenty-two patients sustained their injuries in a hospital or nursing home, most commonly (12 patients) as a consequence of a fire started by smoking activities. Fifty-eight percent of those patients expired. Another two patients were scalded while being bathed in nursing homes and one of those patients expired. Thirty-two patients were burned as a consequence of home medical therapy, including nine vaporizer scald burns, eight burns caused by ignition of therapeutic oxygen, and 11 caused by inappropriate application of heat. In contrast to other studies, no patients in this series sustained burns from medical lasers.

Burn patient transport and transfer

As noted above, the concordance of burn treatment facility location and population density necessitates that many patients requiring burn center care be transferred from other locations to such institutions. For transfer across short distances and in congested urban areas, ground transportation is frequently more expeditious than aeromedical transfer. Aeromedical transfer is indicated when the patient requires movement from a remote area or when such transfer will shorten the time during which the patient is in transit as compared to ground transportation. Helicopters are frequently employed for the aeromedical transfer of patients over distances of less than 200 miles (320 km). Vibration, poor lightning, restricted space, and noise make in-flight monitoring and therapeutic interventions difficult, a fact that emphasizes the importance of carefully evaluating the patient and modifying treatment as needed to establish hemodynamic and pulmonary stability prior to undertaking the transfer. When transfer requires movement over greater distances, fixed wing aircraft are utilized, ideally those in which an oxygen supply is available to support mechanical ventilation. The patient compartment of such an aircraft should be well lit, permit movement of attending personnel, and have some measure of temperature control.

In general, burned patients travel best in the immediate postburn period as soon as hemodynamic and pulmonary stability have been attained by resuscitation. This avoids the instability caused by infection, secondary hemorrhage, sepsis, or cardiac insufficiency, all of which may occur later in the severely burned patient's hospital course.[93] The importance of having an experienced burn physician accompany a patient during aeromedical transfer is indicated by the findings of a study in which the management problems encountered during 124 flights to transfer 148 burn patients were reviewed.[94] More than half the patients required therapeutic interventions by the surgeon of the burn team prior to undertaking aeromedical transfer. Such interventions most commonly involved placement or adjustment of a cannula or catheter, modification of fluid therapy, or endotracheal intubation and modification of ventilatory management. In slightly more than one-third of the patients, such interventions were considered necessary to correct physiologic instabilities which would have compromised patient safety during the transfer procedure. Six of the 124 patients required an escharotomy to relieve compression of the chest or a limb caused by a constricting eschar. The therapeutic alterations most commonly needed during the aeromedical transfer procedure itself were changes in fluid therapy, adjustment of a ventilator, and administration of parenteral medications exclusive of analgesics. The medical personnel effecting the burn patient transfer must bring with them all the equipment and supplies needed for pre-flight preparation and in-flight management of the patient.

Continuity and quality of care during the transport procedure are ensured by:

- physician-to-physician case review to assess the patient's need for and ability to tolerate aeromedical transfer,
- prompt initiation of the aeromedical transfer mission,
- examination of the patient in the hospital of origin by a burn surgeon from the receiving hospital and correction of organ dysfunction prior to undertaking aeromedical transfer,
- in-flight monitoring by burn experienced personnel.

During the 10-year period 1991–2000, US Army Institute of Surgical Research Burn Care Flight Teams using such a regimen completed 266 helicopter and fixed wing aeromedical transfer missions to transport 310 burn patients within the continental United States without any in-flight deaths. During the same period, the Institute carried out 12 intercontinental aeromedical transfer missions in which 17 burn patients were transported with only one in-flight death.

Outcome Analysis in Burn Injury

The importance of extent of injury in determining burn outcome was recognized by Holmes in 1860, and discussions expressing that extent as either a measured area or as a fraction of body surface appeared early in this century.[95–97] Formal expression of burn size as a percentage of total body surface area, however, awaited the work of Berkow in 1924.[98] Though accorded little recognition as such, this single advance in the understanding of thermal injury, along with the corollary understanding that burn size is a crucial determinant of pathophysiological response, made burns the first form of trauma whose impact could be measured and easily communicated. Techniques based on this understanding produced what were in effect the first trauma indices. Appreciation of the effect of burn size on outcome made assessment of the relationship between burn size and mortality, direct comparison of populations of burned patients, and rational assessment of therapy possible long before rigorous outcome analysis became feasible for any other form of injury.

The earliest comprehensive statistical technique used for such assessment was univariate probit analysis.[99,100] This approach, laborious in the days of paper files and rotary calculators, required that the population studied be arbitrarily partitioned into groups that were relatively similar in burn size and age. Such analyses yield equations describing the effect of burn size on mortality which are valid for only the particular age group studied. An early attempt to develop a multivariate evaluation was made by Schwartz, who used probit plane analysis to estimate the relative contributions of partial and full thickness burns to mortality. This approach also required arbitrary partitioning of the population.[101]

The advent of computers of suitable power and further development of statistical techniques have reduced the difficulty of analyzing burn mortality, removed the necessity for arbitrary partitioning, and made these techniques much more accessible.[102] Their use to assess outcome requires an understanding of the techniques themselves and of the population being analyzed. The analysis of a population of 8448 patients admitted for burn care to the United States Army Institute of Surgical Research or to its predecessor, the US Army Surgical Research Unit, between January 1, 1950 and December 31, 1991 illustrates the concepts underlying modern outcome analysis and depicts the trends in mortality that have been characteristic of most major burn centers in this country.

For validity, an important first step in such studies is to achieve as much uniformity as possible in the population to be analyzed. These patients reached the Institute between the day of injury and postburn day 531 (mean 5.86 days, median 1 day), with burns averaging 31% (range 1–100%, median 26%) of the total body surface. Their age distribution was biphasic, with one peak at 1 year of age and another aged 20; the mean age of the entire population was 26.5 years (range 0–97 years, median 23 years). From this group, 7893 (93.4%) who had flame or scald burns were selected, excluding patients with electric or chemical injuries.

This group included patients who sustained thermal injuries in Vietnam and were first transferred to Japan and then selectively transferred to the Institute. Arriving at the Institute relatively late in their courses, these survivors of temporal cohorts in which some deaths had already occurred exhibited inordinately low mortality. Outcome is inevitably biased toward survival as the postburn time of admission lengthens. To avoid this bias, the analysis focused on the 4870 patients with flame or scald injuries who reached the Institute on or before the second postburn day, excluding later arrivals. Burn size in these patients averaged 34% (range 1–100%, median 29%), and age was again biphasic, with peaks at 1 and 21 years and a mean of 27.1 years (range 0–93 years, median 24 years).

One object of the analysis was to evaluate changes in burn mortality during the four decades of experience included in the study. For reliable results, the techniques used required more patients than were available in some single years; a moving 5-year interval, advancing 1 year at a time, was used to group the data. The number of patients in each of the overlapping 5-year intervals is shown in **Figure 2.2**. In this and subsequent plots, the data for a 5-year interval are plotted at the first year of the interval, reflecting that year and the succeeding four. The number of admissions meeting the selection criteria was small in the early years of the Institute's experience and rose in somewhat linear fashion during the second and third decades to a sustained plateau of approximately 800 (160/year).

Mean patient age is shown in **Figure 2.3**. Between 1950 and 1965, most of the admissions were young soldiers; mean age approxi-

mated 22.5 years and was relatively stable. During the succeeding decade, this value rose to an irregular plateau centering on 30 years of age, a change reflecting a greater number of civilian emergency admissions and increasing age in the military population.

Figure 2.4 shows the variation in mean burn size during the study interval, and **Figure 2.5** shows the roughly parallel mortality. Mean burn size peaked in the two intervals spanning 1969 to 1974 and decreased steadily after that time. Mortality, principally due to burn wound sepsis, peaked at 46% during those years. The two data sets are shown together in **Figure 2.6** and suggest a crude index of the results of burn care in this population. There were two intervals in which percent mortality exceeded mean percent burn. The first occurred in the late 1950s and early 1960s, a time when burn wound sepsis due to *Pseudomonas aeruginosa* was uncontrolled. This was succeeded by a 6-year interval of good control of wound infection following the introduction of topical wound treatment with mafenide. In turn, this was followed by a second interval of poor control in the late 1960s and early 1970s, during which both *Pseudomonas* and a mafenide-resistant *Providencia stuartii* were major causes of sepsis; this endemic was controlled by the mid-1970s following changes in topical treatment and wound management.

Raw percent mortality, even in conjunction with burn size, is never an adequate index of the effectiveness of treatment, since the frequency of death after burn injury is also determined by prior

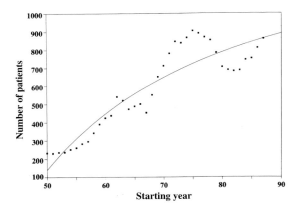

Fig. 2.2 Number of patients meeting study criteria. Values are plotted at the first year of each moving 5-year interval.

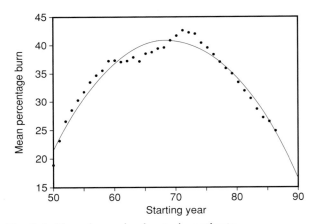

Fig. 2.4 Mean burn size in study patients.

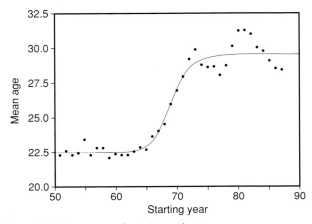

Fig. 2.3 Mean age of study patients.

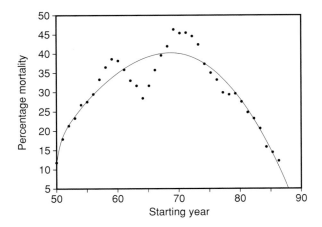

Fig. 2.5 Percentage mortality in study patients in each moving 5-year interval.

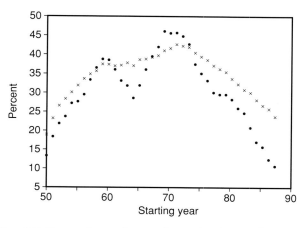

Fig. 2.6 Comparison of mean burn size (crosses) and percent mortality (circles).

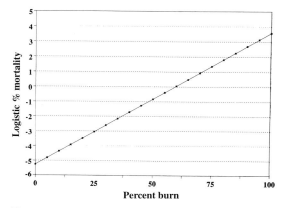

Fig. 2.8 Logistic transformation of the ordinate in Figure 2.6.

patient condition, age, inhalation injury, and the occurrence of pneumonia and burn wound sepsis. Each of these elements, except for prior condition, can be addressed in analysis, but only burn size, age, and the presence or absence of inhalation injury are known at the time of admission. In the present group, burn size and age were available for every patient, but data on inhalation injury were missing for patients admitted in the earlier years; we elected to use burn size and age for analysis. This choice does not exclude the impact of the complications, but does confound that impact with those of burn size and age.

For a uniform population of specific age, a plot of the relationship between burn size and percent mortality is S-shaped, or sigmoid – small burns produce relatively few deaths, but as burn size increases mortality rises steeply and then plateaus as it approaches its maximum of 100%. **Figure 2.7** illustrates this dose–response relationship for 50-year-old patients admitted to the Institute between 1987 and 1991. Such curves are mathematically intractable and are usually transformed to more easily managed straight lines for analysis. Several mathematical transformations have been used to accomplish this. As previously noted, the one used in early analyses was probit transformation; in the present study, a logistic transformation, illustrated in **Figure 2.8**, was used. The choice between these is one of convenience, as either one yields essentially the same information.[103,104]

The locations of a sequence of such curves for groups of patients of increasing age move first to the right (toward larger burn size) as age increases from infancy to young adulthood, and then to the left, passing through the infant location at around age 45 and continuing inexorably leftward with increasing age. These differing locations reflect the greater risk of burn mortality at the extremes of age. The cubic curve in **Figure 2.9** describes this curvilinear effect of age on mortality; the effect was least at age 21. For this population, the age function was relatively stable over the entire interval of study.

As we have noted, earlier analyses began by dividing the studied population into arbitrary age and burn size groups; probit analysis of the relationship between burn size and percent mortality in each age group then permitted estimation of the LD_{50}, the burn size lethal to half the selected age group. To accommodate both age and burn size simultaneously, without arbitrary partitioning of the population, multiple logistic regression was used for this study, with each member of the population entering the analysis as an individual data point.

The result of this three-dimensional form of analysis is most readily visualized as a plane lying within a cube. **Figure 2.10** shows the sigmoid response of mortality to burn size for three discrete ages, and **Figure 2.11** shows the curvilinear variation of mortality with age in patients entering this study between 1987 and

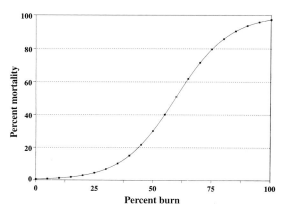

Fig. 2.7 Effect of burn size on percent mortality.

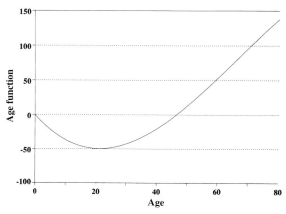

Fig. 2.9 Effect of age on mortality. Effect is minimal at age 21. Note that horizontal intersects share a common effect.

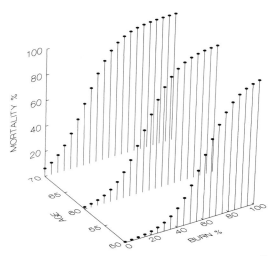

Fig. 2.10 Effect of burn size on percent mortality at three discrete ages (1987–1991).

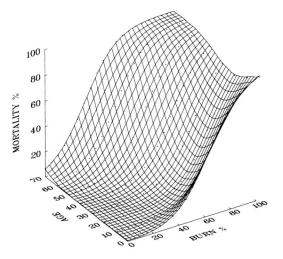

Fig. 2.12 Plane of percent mortality with age and burn size coodinates (1987–1991).

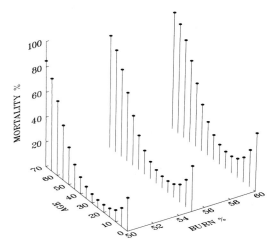

Fig. 2.11 Effect of age on percent mortality at three discrete burn sizes.

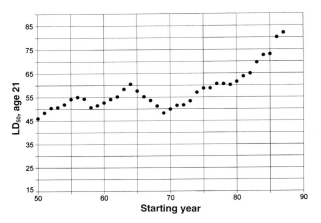

Fig. 2.13 LD_{50} in moving 5-year intervals in patients 21 years of age. Increasing values indicate improving prognosis.

1991. A best fitting plane which covers the tips of spikes representing all of the burn sizes and ages of interest is generated by the multiple logistic technique, and it is illustrated for these particular patients in **Figure 2.12**. The equation representing this plane is of the form shown below, in which L is the logistic of percent mortality and P the expected fractional mortality rate.

$$L = a_1 + a_2 \, (\% \text{ burn}) - a_3 \, (\text{age}) + a_4 \left(\frac{\text{age}^2}{100} \right) - a_5 \left(\frac{\text{age}^3}{10\,000} \right)$$

$$P = \frac{\exp^L}{1 + \exp^L}$$

The advantage of this approach, as opposed to previously used age and burn size partitioned analyses, is that it permits analysis of an entire population without artificial segmentation, and allows an explicit estimation of expected mortality for each member of the population. Serial applications of the technique were used to assess mortality in each of the moving 5-year intervals of the study.

Figure 2.13 reflects the changes in LD_{50} which were experienced by young adult patients during the four decades of the study. This value, indexing the mean likelihood of survival after burn injury, has increased steadily in all age groups since the mid-1970s. Many aspects of care have changed and improved during this time:

- early resuscitation became more widely understood and better practiced;
- topical chemotherapy with alternating applications of mafenide acetate and silver sulfadiazine, coupled with the use of a chlorhexidine-based wash solution (Hibiclens), permitted better control of wound infection;
- early wound excision came to be more generally practiced;
- the clinical facility was remodeled to permit single bed isolation;
- better infection control techniques limited cross contamination of wounds;
- new antibiotics, more effective against Gram-negative organisms, became available;
- inhalation injury and other pulmonary problems became

better understood and are now managed with better equipment;

■ improved grafting techniques and the use of biological dressings facilitated earlier coverage of large wounds.

In essence, we have learned, through integrated clinical and laboratory research, how to apply ordinary principles of trauma and wound care to this extraordinary injury. No single innovation has produced a 'step' improvement in mortality, but the aggregate effect has been steadily improving survival.

This improvement in survival is reflected in **Figures 2.14** and **2.15**, which depict early (1950–1963) and recent (1987–1991) mortality planes, respectively. The improvement is not uniform for all burn sizes or ages, nor would one expect this to be so. Small burns have never been lethal, except at the extremes of age; little improvement in survival could occur with such injuries. At the other extreme, very large burns in older patients have always been lethal and remain so. To define the age and burn size coordinates of the improvement in survival, one subtracts one mortality plane

from another; the result is itself a plane depicting the difference in mortality in age and burn size coordinates (**Figure 2.16**). The greatest differences occurred in the area of the LD$_{80}$ of the 1950–1963 mortality plane.

In the interval between 1992 and 1999, a total of 1951 patients were admitted for burn care. Among these, 1800 (92%) had sustained thermal injuries, and 1453 were admitted on or before the second postburn day. Mortality in these patients did not differ significantly from that observed between 1987 and 1991. Pooling these groups yielded an estimating equation based on 2194 patients and spanning 13 years. The relationship between predicted and observed mortality in this population is consistent over the probability spectrum (**Figure 2.17**).

Though this experience conforms with that of most burn centers in the United States, it should be noted that there are still many areas of the world where the survival of patients with burns of more than 40% of the total body surface is rare. During the half century covered by this study, 1555 (24%) of the studied patients died. Had the mortality experienced since 1987 prevailed through the whole interval, little more than half this number would have succumbed to their injuries. Mortality now is less than half that characterizing the first decade of the Institute's experience.

As previously noted, estimates of the annual total number of burns in the United States, for which there is little reliable information, range as high as 2 000 000. A more reliable, but still imperfect, previously cited estimate is that between 51 000 and 71 000 acutely burned patients are admitted to hospitals in the United States each year. **Figure 2.18** is based on composite data from several sources and depicts an estimate of the age and burn size distribution of these patients. Using the Institute's mortality experience between 1987 and 1999 as a basis for projecting expected mortality yields the data shown in **Figure 2.19**, which depicts the age and burn size distribution of the expected deaths.

According to this model, patients over 50 years of age with burns of 50% or less of the total body surface account for 19% of admissions and 50% of deaths; at the other age extreme, children under 5 years of age account for 19% of admissions and only 12.5% of deaths.

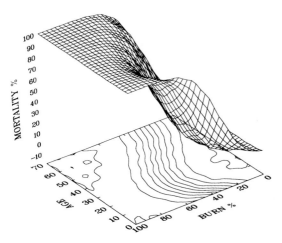

Fig. 2.14 Mortality plane for patients admitted between 1950 and 1963. Note location of contour lines in base of cube.

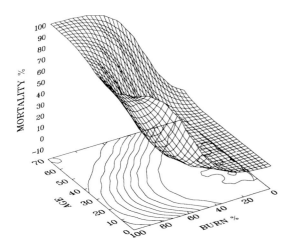

Fig 2.15 Mortality plane for patients admitted between 1987 and 1991. Note contour locations.

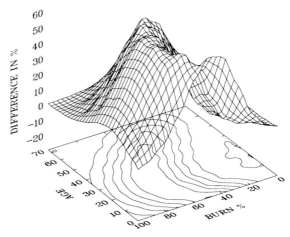

Fig. 2.16 Plane of differences in percent mortality between 1950 and 1963 and 1987 and 1991. Note location of peak.

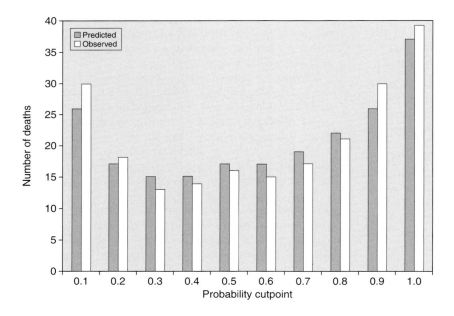

Fig. 2.17 Expected and observed deaths, 1987–1999.

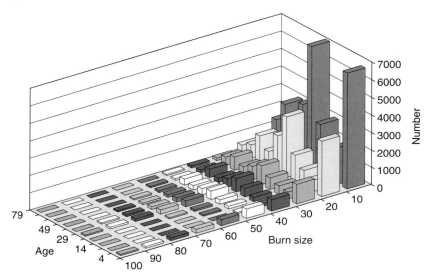

Fig. 2.18 Estimated age/burn size distribution of 71 000 annual hospital admissions.

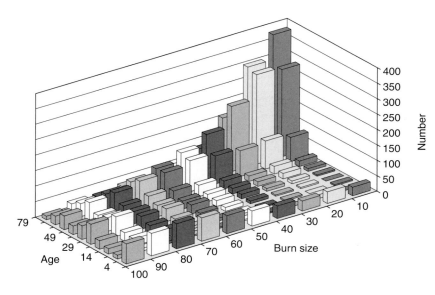

Fig. 2.19 Estimated age and burn size distribution of expected deaths among patients depicted in **Figure 2.16**.

Much has been accomplished in acute burn care during the last half-century, and further improvement in outcome will probably occur as inhalation injury and pneumonia come under control and new wound coverage techniques are developed, but such improvement will be harder won and smaller in magnitude. Preservation of function, reconstruction, and rehabilitation, areas which have received less attention in the past, appear the more likely primary targets of future burn research and may be expected to materially enhance the quality of life for burn survivors.

References

1. United States Fire/Burn Deaths and Rates per 100 000, E890–E899, E924, E958.1, 2, 7, E961, E968.0, E988.1, 2, 7. Office of Statistics and Programming, National Center for Injury Prevention and Control, Centers for Disease Control and Prevention, Atlanta, GA, 1998.
2. Pruitt BA Jr, Mason AD Jr, Goodwin CW. Epidemiology of burn injury and demography of burn care facilities. In: Gann DS. ed. *Problems in General Surgery*, Vol. 7, No. 2. Philadelphia: JB Lippincott, 1990: 235–251.
3. Deaths resulting from residential fires and the prevalence of smoke alarms – United States, 1991–1995. *Morbid Mortal Wkly Rep* 47(38): 803–806.
4. Karter MJ. 1991 US fire loss. *NFPA Journal* 1992; Sep–Oct: 30–43.
5. US DoH. *Injury Mortality: National Summary of Injury Mortality Data, 1984–1990*. US Department of Health and Human Services, Washington, DC, June 1993.
6. Baker SP, O'Neill B, Ginsberg NJ, Li G. Fire, burns and lightning. Chapter 12. *The Injury Fact Book*. 2nd ed. New York: Oxford University Press, 1992: 161–173.
7. Hall JR. The US fire problem and overview report. Leading causes and other patterns and trends. Quincy, Massachusetts, National Fire Protection Association, Fire Analysis and Research Division, 1998.
8. Feck GA, Baptiste MS, Tate CL Jr. Burn injuries: epidemiology and prevention. *Accid Anal Prev* 1979; **11**: 129–136.
9. Feck GA, Baptiste MS, Tate CL Jr. *An Epidemiologic Study of Burn Injuries and Strategies for Prevention*, Atlanta, GA. Department of Health and Human Services, Public Health Services, Centers for Disease Control, 1978.
10. Baker SP, O'Neill B, Ginsberg NJ, Li G. Unintentional injury. *The Injury Fact Book*; 2nd ed. Chapter 4. New York: Oxford University Press, 1992: 39–64.
11. *Fire in the United States, 1983 to 1990*. 8th ed. National Fire Data Center, Emmitsburg, MD, October 1993.
12. Runyan CW, Bangdiwala SI, Linzer MA, *et al*. Risk factors for fatal residential fires. *N Engl J Med* 1992; **327**: 859–863.
13. Burn Injury Fact Sheet, National Safe Kids Campaign, 1301 Pennsylvania Avenue NW, Suite 1000, Washington, DC, 20004–1707.
14. Mierley MC, Baker SP. Fatal house fires in an urban population. *JAMA* 1983; **249**: 1466–1468.
15. Ahrens M US experience with smoke detectors and other fire detectors. Quincy Massachusetts. National Fire Protection Association, Fire Analysis and Research Division, 1997.
16. Marshall S, Runyan CW, Bangdiwala SI, Linzer MA, Sacks JJ, Butts JD. Fatal residential fires: who dies and who survives. *JAMA* 1998; **279**: 1633–1637.
17. Karter MJ Jr. Fire loss in the United States during 1995. Quincy Massachusetts: National Fire Protection Association, Fire Analysis and Research Division, 1996.
18. Anonymous. *Burns Causes and Costs: A Burn Foundation Report*. Burn Foundation, Philadelphia, PA, 1989.
19. Forjuoh SN. The mechanisms, intensity of treatment, and outcomes of hospitalized burns: issues for prevention. *J Burn Care Rehabil* 1988; **19**: 456–460.
20. Rice DP, MacKenzie EJ, *et al*. Cost of Injury in the United States: a Report to Congress. Institute for Health and Aging. University of California, San Francisco, CA, An Injury Prevention Center, The Johns Hopkins University, 1989.
21. Hall JR. *The Total Cost of Fire in the United States through 1991*. Quincy, MA: National Fire Protection Association 1993: 1–20.
22. Hammond J. The status of statewide burn prevention legislation. *J Burn Care Rehabil* 1993; **14**: 473–475.
23. Pruitt BA Jr, Goodwin CW. Thermal Injuries. In: Davis JH, Sheldon GF, eds. *Surgery; A Problem-Solving Approach*, 2nd edn. Chapter 17. St Louis: Mosby, 1995: 644.
24. Brigham PA, McLoughlin E. Burn incidence and medical care use in the United States: estimate, trends, and data sources. *J Burn Care Rehabil* 1996; **17**: 95–107.
25. Resources for optimal care of patients with burn injury. In: *Resources for Optimal Care of the Injured Patient*, Chapter 14. Chicago, IL: The American College of Surgeons, 1990: 58.
26. Burn Care Resources in North American, 1999–2000 Ed. Chicago, IL: American Burn Association, 625 N Michigan Ave, Ste 1530, Chicago, IL 60611.
27. Henson DA, Rode H, Bloch CE. Primus stove burns in Cape Town: a costly but preventable injury. *Burns* 1988; **20**: 251–252.
28. Rioja LF, Alonso PE, Soria MD, *et al*. Incidence of ember burns in Andalusia (Spain). *Burns* 1988; **20**: 251–252.
29. Iregbulem LM, Nnabuko BE. Epidemiology of childhood thermal burns in Enugu, Nigeria. *Burns* 1993; **19**: 223–226.
30. Shergill G, Scerri GV, Regan PJ, Roberts AHN. Burn injuries in boating accidents. *Burns* 1993; **19**: 229–231.
31. Graitcer PL, Sniezek JE. Hospitalizations due to tap water scalds, 1978–1985. *Morbid Mortal Wkly Rep* 1988; **37**: 35–38.
32. Milo Y, Robinpour M, Glicksman A, *et al*. Epidemiology of burns in the Tel Aviv area. *Burns* 1993; **19**: 352–357.
33. Barillo DJ, Burge TS, Harrington DT, *et al*. Body habitus as a predictor of burn risk in children: do fat boys still get burned? *Burns* 1998; **24**: 725–727.
34. Baptiste MS, Feck G. Preventing tap water burns. *Am J Public Health* 1980; **70**: 727–729.
35. Stephen FR, Murray JP. Prevention of hot tap water burns – a comparative study of three types of automatic mixing valve. *Burns* 1993; **19**: 56–62.
36. Lindblad BE, Mikkelsen SS, Larsen TK, Steinke MS. A comparative analysis of burn injuries at two burns centers in Denmark. *Burns* 1994; **20**: 173–175.
37. McGill V, Kowal-Vern A, Gamelli RH. Outcome for older burn patients. *Arch Surg* 2000; **135**: 320–325.
38. Cadier MA, Shakespeare PG. Burns in octogenarians. *Burns* 1995; **21**: 200–204.
39. Backstein R, Peters W, Neligan P. Burns in the disabled. *Burns* 1993; **19**: 192–197.
40. Effects on Personnel Chapter XI. In: Glasstone S, ed. *The Effects of Nuclear Weapons*, Department of the Army Pamphlet. No. 39–3 United States Atomic Energy Commission, June 1957: 455–464.
41. Burns Sustained in Vietnam, 1965–1973. Data Tables Supplied by Department of the Army, The Chief of Military History and the Center of Military History; Washington, DC, 20314, 1980.
42. Allen BD, Whitson TC, Henjyoji EY. Treatment of 1963 Burned Patients at 106th General Hospital, Yokohama, Japan. *J Trauma* 1970; **10**: 386–392.
43. Shafir R. Burn Injury and Care in the Recent Lebanese Conflict. Presentation on behalf of The Surgeon General, Israeli Defense Forces and Staff. The Israeli Society of Plastic and Reconstructive Surgery, 1984.
44. Owen-Smith MS. Armoured fighting vehicle casualties. *J Royal Army Med. Corps* 1977; **123**: 65–76.
45. Chapman CW. Burns and plastic surgery in the South Atlantic campaign 1982. *J Royal Navy Med Serv* 1983; **69**(2): 71–79.
46. Eldad A, Torem M. Burns in the Lebanon War 1982: 'the Blow and the Cure'. *Military Medicine* 1990; **155**: 130–132.
47. Carlos Sereday, MD, Major, Argentine Navy Medical Corps. Personal communication, 1990.
48. Kopchinski B. US Army Noncombat Munitions Injuries. *Military Medicine* 2001; **166**: 135–138.
49. Rossignol AM, Boyle CM, Locke JA, Burke JF. Hospitalized burn injuries in Massachusetts: an assessment of incidence and product involvement. *Am J Public Health* 1986; **76**: 1341–1343.
50. Clark WR, Fromm BS. Burn mortality experienced at a regional unit. Literature review, *Acta Chir Scand* 1987; Suppl 357.
51. Baker SP, O'Neill B, Karpf RS. *The Injury Fact Book*. Lexington, MA: Lexington Books, 1984: 139–154.
52. Barillo DJ, Stetz CK, Zak AL, *et al*. Preventable burns associated with a misuse of gasoline. *Burns* 1998; **24**: 439–443.
53. Purdue GF, Hunt JL, Layton TR, *et al*. Burns in motor vehicle accidents. *J Trauma* 1985; **25**: 216–219.
54. Barillo DJ, Cioffi WG, McManus WF, *et al*. Vehicle-related burn injuries. *Proceedings of Association for the Advancement of Automotive Medicine*, 2340 Des Plaines Avenue, Suite 106, Des Plaines 1993; **11**: 209–218.
55. Renz BM, Sherman R. Automobile carburetors and radiator-related burns. *J Burn Care Rehabil* 1992; **1**: 414–421.
56. Regan PJ, Budny PG, Lavelle JR, *et al*. Bonfire and barbecue burns. *Burns* 1991; **17**: 306–308.
57. *Eighth Annual Flammable Fabrics Report*. Consumer Product Safety Commission, Washington, DC, 1980.
58. Occupational burns among restaurant workers – Colorado and Minnesota. *Morb Mortal Wkly Rep* 1993; **42**: 713–716.
59. Chatterjee BF, Barancik JI, Fratianne RB, *et al*. Northeastern Ohio Trauma Study V: Burn injury. *J Trauma* 1986; **26**: 844–847.
60. Rossignol AM, Locke JA, Boyle CM, Burke JF. Epidemiology of work-related burn injuries in Massachusetts requiring hospitalization. *J Trauma* 1986; **26**: 1097–1101.

61. Personck ME. Profiles in safety and health: eating and drinking places. *Monthly Labor Review* 1991; **114**: 19–26.

62. Baker SP, O'Neill B, Ginsberg NJ, *et al.* Occupational injury. *The Injury Fact Book*, 2nd ed. Chapter 9. New York: Oxford University Press, 1992: 114–133.

63. Pruitt BA Jr, Edlich RF. Treatment of bitumen burns (Letter) *JAMA* 1982; **247**: 1565.

64. Renz BM, Sherman R. Hot tar burns: 27 hospitalized cases. *J Burn Care Rehabil* 1994; **15**: 341–345.

65. Acute chemical hazards to children and adults. *NEISS Data Highlights*. Vol. 12, January–December 1988. Washington, DC. Directorate for Epidemiology, US Consumer Product Safety Commission.

66. Mozingo DW, Smith AA, McManus WF, *et al.* Chemical burns. *J Trauma* 1988; **28**: 642–647.

67. Leeming MN, Ray C Jr, Howland WS. Low-voltage direct current burns. *JAMA* 1970; **214**: 1681–1684.

68. Pride HB, McKinley DF. Third-degree burns from the use of an external cardiac pacing device. *Crit Care Med* 1990; **18**: 572–573.

69. Reisin L, Baruchin AM. Iatrogenic defibrillator burns. *Burns* 1990; **16**: 128.

70. Lightning-associated deaths – United States 1980–1995. *Morb Mortal Wkly Rep* May 22 1998; **47**: 391–394.

71. Lopez RE, Holle RL. Demographics of lightning casualties. *Semin Neurol* 1995; **15**: 286–295.

72. Kale D, Harwood B. Fireworks injuries, 1981. *NEISS Data Highlights*. January–December 1981. Washington, DC: Directorate for Epidemiology, US Consumer Products Safety Commission.

73. McFarland LV, Harris JR, Kobayashi JM, *et al.* Risk factors for fireworks-related injury in Washington state. *JAMA* 1984; **251**: 3251–3254.

74. Injuries associated with selected consumer products treated in hospital emergency departments calendar 1992. *NEISS Data Highlights*, Vol. 16, 1992. Washington, DC: Directorate for Epidemiology, US Consumer Products Safety Commission.

75. Berger LR, Kalishman S, Rivara FP. Injuries from fireworks. *Pediatrics* 1985; **75**: 877–882.

76. Sonneborn CK, Vanstraelen TM. A retrospective study of self-inflicted burns. *Gen Hosp Psychiatry* 1992; **14**: 404–407.

77. Budny PG, Regan PJ, Riley P, *et al.* Ritual burns – the Buddhist tradition. *Burns* 1991; **17**: 335–337.

78. Squyres V, Law EJ, Still JM Jr. Self-inflicted burns. *J Burn Care Rehabil* 1993; **14**: 476–479.

79. Duminy FJ, Hudson DA. Assault inflicted by water. *Burns* 1993; **19**: 426–428.

80. Krob MJ, Johnson A, Jordan MH. Burned-and-battered adults. *J Burn Care Rehabil* 1986; **7**: 529–531.

81. Bowden ML, Grant ST, Vogel B, *et al.* The elderly, disabled and handicapped adult burned through abuse and neglect. *Burns* 1988; **14**: 447–450.

82. O'Neill JA Jr, Meacham WF, Griffin PP, *et al.* Patterns of injury in the battered child syndrome. *J Trauma* 1973; **13**: 332–339.

83. Showers J, Garrison KM. Burn abuse: a four-year study. *J Trauma* 1988; **28**: 1581–1583.

84. Surrell JA, Alexander RM, Kohle SD, *et al.* Effects of microwave radiation on living tissues. *J Trauma* 1987; **27**: 935–939.

85. Batchelor JS, Vanjari S, Budny P, Roberts AHN. Domestic iron burns in children: a cause for concern? *Burns* 1994; **20**: 74–75.

86. Purdue GF, Hunt JL, Prescott PR. Child abuse by burning – an index of suspicion. *J Trauma* 1988; **28**: 221–224.

87. Elder abuse: what can be done? Select Committee on Aging, US House of Representatives, Washington DC, Government Printing Office, 1991.

88. Bird PE, Harrington DT, Barillo DJ, *et al.* Elder abuse: a call to action. *J Burn Care Rehabil* 1998; **19**: 522–527.

89. Pegg SP. Can burns injuries occur in hospital? Presented at 9th Congress of the International Society for Burn Injuries, 30 June 1994, Paris, France. Abstract 87 in 9th *Congress of International Society for Burns Injuries*, Abstracts Volume.

90. Sadove RC, Furgasen TG. Major thermal burn as a result of intraoperative heating blanket use. *J Burn Care Rehabil* 1992; **13**: 443–445.

91. Chang BW, Petty P, Manson PN. Patient fire safety in the operating room. *Plast Reconstr Surg* 1994; **93**: 519–521.

92. Barillo DJ, Coffey EC, Shirani KZ, Goodwin CW. Burns caused by medical therapy. *J Burn Care Rehabil* 2000; **21**: 269–273.

93. Pruitt BA Jr, FitzGerald BE. A military perspective. In: Bowers JZ, Purcell EF, eds. *Emergency Medical Services: Measures to Improve Care.* Port Washington, NY: Independent Publishers Group, 1980: 223–244.

94. Treat RC, Sirinek KR, Levine BE, Pruitt BA Jr. Air evacuation of thermally injured patients: principles of treatment and results. *J Trauma* 1980; **20**: 275–279.

95. Holmes T, ed. *A System of Surgery, Theoretical and Practical*, Vol. I. London: JW Parker & Son, 1860: 723.

96. Suzuki S. The injuries in modern naval warfare. *Boston Med Surg J* CXXXVII(24): 610, December 9, 1897.

97. Weidenfeld LB. *Medizinisches Vademecus*. 1912: 206–224.

98. Berkow SG. Method of estimating extensiveness of lesions (burns and scalds) based on surface area proportions. *Arch Surg*, January 1924; 8(pt 1): 138–148.

99. Bull JP, Squire JR. A study of mortality in a burns unit: standards for the evaluation of alternative methods of treatment. *Ann Surg*, August 1949; **130**(2): 160–173.

100. Bull JP, Fisher AJ. A study of mortality in a burns unit: a revised estimate. *Ann Surg* 1954; **139**(3): 269–274.

101. Schwartz MS, Soroff HS, Reiss E, Artz CP. An evaluation of the mortality and the relative severity of second and third-degree injuries in burns. Research Report Nr. 12–56. In: Research Reports. US Army Surgical Research Unit, Form Sam Houston, TX, December 1956.

102. SPSS for Windows, ver.9.0, SPSS Inc., Chicago, IL.

103. Finney DJ. *Probit Analysis*. 3rd ed. Cambridge: Cambridge University Press, 1971.

104. Hosmer DW, Lemeshow S. *Applied Logistic Regression*. New York: John Wiley & Sons, 1989.

Immediate care

Chapter 3

Prevention of burn injuries
John L Hunt
Gary F Purdue

Introduction

The word 'prevent' comes from the Latin word 'praevenire', which means to anticipate. The prefix 'pre' means before and 'venire' means to come. During the last century in the United States, burn treatment had always come before burn prevention. Since burns, then as now, represent such a small percent of all traumatic injuries, burn prevention has not been viewed as a high priority heath issue by a large portion of society.

Burns are still referred to as accidents by many in the medical community and society in general.[1] Believing that burns and other traumatic injuries are 'accidents' ('accident-prone' individual) implies the individual has little or no fault in the injury cause. The word accident means an event that takes place without one's foresight or proceeds from an unknown cause, an unfortunate occurrence, or mishap, especially one resulting in an injury. Synonyms include misadventure, mischance, misfortune, mishap, and disaster. The word injury is a more appropriate term. It is derived from the Latin word 'juris', which means not right. An injury represents damage that occurs as a result of an exposure to a physical or chemical agent at a rate greater than what the body can tolerate. Unfortunately the designation of traumatic injuries as accidents is still perpetrated in the E codes which are the supplementary classification of external causes of injury. An example is E893, Accident caused by ignition of clothing; or E898.1, Accident caused by other, burning by: candle, cigar, pipe or cigarette.

Historical perspective

The medical community in Great Britain in the first decade of the 20th century was well aware that burn injuries and deaths represented a serious public health issue.[2] Scalds and burns were noted to occur predominately in children. Unguarded fires and the flammability of flannelette, a cotton garment, were recognized as common causes of burns in children and old women. Legislation was enacted making parents liable to a fine if a child younger than 8 years was injured or died as a result of an unguarded open fire. In a review of over 3600 patients with flame burns and scalds, two-thirds occurred in and around the home, one-third were at work, 50% were children, 82% were the result of clothing fires; cottons were the common fabrics and the number of scalds about equaled that from burns, but the former were more likely to survive.[3] Approximately 50% of home accidents were judged to be preventable.

Research was conducted on the design and flammability of clothing. Fabrics were treated with tin, antimony, and titanium to make them relatively flame-retardant. Statistics on common locations and causes for home 'accidents' identified the kitchen and cooking, scald burns from children pulling over containers with hot liquids, and the use of flammable liquids. Burns as a result of a seizure were recognized. Prevention efforts included education and 'propaganda' (film, radio, newspapers, exhibits, posters), better design of housing and improving living conditions (decreasing overcrowding), safer methods of heating houses (central heating and electric fires), use of nonflammable materials in girls and women clothing, and better design of fireguards for coal fires. Better design of teapots, cups, and cooking utensils rendering them more difficult to tilt over. One author, in 1946, expressed quite clearly that carelessness, neglect of normal precautions, and stupidity were human factors associated with burns.[4] It was recognized that accurate and comprehensive burn data were lacking, but necessary if long-term prevention policies were to be enacted.

Injury control

The five key areas in injury control are:

1. epidemiology,
2. prevention,
3. injury biomechanics (physical and functional responses of the victim to the injury),

4. treatment,
5. rehabilitation.[5]

The major components of epidemiology include measurement of both the frequency and distribution of the injury. This in turn is analyzed and interpreted. Next, risk factors are identified, an intervention strategy is developed and tested and, lastly, the results analyzed.

Burn injury magnitude

In the US in 1995 the leading causes of injury deaths in their order of magnitude were motor vehicle, firearm, poisoning, fall, suffocation, drowning, and finally fire/burn.[6] Under the age of 15 years, burns ranked third. Approximately 90% of all burns and fire deaths are unintentional. An intentional burn would be a forced immersion in hot water or self-immolation. Since 1985 the age-adjusted death rate for burns/fires in the US has decreased by 33%.[6] Even so the US continues to have the highest per capita burn death rate of any industrialized nation in the world, two to three times that of many European countries. Between 1993 and 1995 in the US there were 18.7 burn deaths per million population compared with 15 and 5.5 in Canada and Switzerland, respectively. In 1993 one fire death occurred approximately every 113 minutes. The highest fatality rates are seen in children 4 years or younger and adults over the age of 55. Together these account for one-third of all fire deaths. Males suffer nearly twice as many fire deaths and injuries in almost all age groups. In 1996 there were 1 975 000 fires reported in the US, resulting in 25 550 injuries and 4990 deaths, and with an approximate cost estimate of $9.4 billion. Residential fire statistics for 1996 revealed that 69.8% of all fires, 70.4% of deaths, and 61.4% of fire injuries occurred in family dwellings. Apartments accounted for 23%, 15.8%, and 31% of the total fires, deaths, and injuries, respectively. The two leading causes of one- and two-family dwellings fires were cooking (15.9%) and heating (15.2%). Apartments had fewer fires as a result of heating-related problems (4.8%), but cooking was the leading cause (33.1%). Apartments were felt to have fewer heating fires because central heating was more common and more often better maintained than in family dwellings. Burn and fire prevention has been steadily improving in hotels and motels. Only 16 hotel/motel fire deaths were reported in 1996 and over 60% were related to smoking. Data from 1996 revealed that 94 fireman died and 87 150 injuries occurred while on duty. This represents a 34.8% decline in mortality and an 11.8% decrease in fatal fire injuries over the last 10 years.[6] Most industrialized nations throughout the world surpass the US in practicing fire prevention. In the United States more emphasis has been placed on improving technology, fire suppression, and fire service delivery mechanisms.

Risk factors

The host is the principal focus of injury prevention. Common burn risk factors include age – spill scalds and immersions in the very young, and flame in the elderly – and gender, with males sustaining more burns.[8] Medical conditions associated with physical or mental illness include arthritis and stroke, where the victim is slow or unable to escape the burn event; diabetes, peripheral neuropathy with decreased or no lower extremity pain perception; dementia, confusion, forgetfulness; and psychiatric, depression

(suicide). Other risk factors include alcohol, drugs (narcotic dependency affecting coordination and perception), and medications such as tranquilizers, barbiturates, lack of or inadequate seizure medication.

Injury Prevention Comes of Age

The science of injury prevention took form in the middle of the last century. In 1961, Gibson was the first to classify the energy sources involved in any injury event into five physical agents: kinetic or mechanical, chemical, thermal, electrical, and radiation.[7] A common form of mechanical energy associated with a burn is a motor vehicle collision. Three risk factors associated with any injury are

1. the vector or energy source and the way it is delivered,
2. the host or injured person, and
3. the environment, both physical and social.

A seminal article in modern injury science was published by Haddon in 1968.[8] He identified three phases of an injury event:

1. Pre-event: preventing the causative agent from reaching the susceptible host.
2. Event: includes transfer of the energy to the victim. Prevention efforts in this phase operate to reduce or completely prevent the injury.
3. Post-event: determines the outcome once the injury has occurred. This includes anything that limits ongoing damage or repairs the damage. This phase determines the ultimate outcome.

Haddon then created a matrix of nine cells which enabled the three events of the injury to be analyzed against the factors related to the host, agent or vector, and environment[9] (**Figure 3.1**). This matrix is a very useful tool for analyzing an injury-producing event and recognizing the factor(s) important in its prevention. Risk factors and potential intervention strategies can be identified. Haddon also proposed 10 general strategies for injury control (**Table 3.1**).

Burn Intervention Strategy

The emergence of the science of prevention has turned attention away from individual 'blame' and the attitude that society has no part in the promotion of prevention to the concept that sociopolitical involvement is necessary.[10]

All burn injuries should be viewed as preventable. Public health is defined as the effort organized by society to protect, promote, and restore the people's health.[11] The public health model of injury prevention and control is divided into

- surveillance,
- interdisciplinary education and prevention programs,
- environmental modifications,
- regulatory action,
- support of clinical interventions.

Primary prevention is preventing the event from ever occurring. Secondary prevention includes the acute care, rehabilitation, and reducing the degree of disability or impairment as much as possible. Tertiary prevention concentrates on preventing or decreasing disability. Disability prevalence and productive activity loss are important outcome measures. There are both active and passive prevention strategies. Passive or environmental intervention is

	AGENT or VECTOR	HOST	ENVIRONMENT	
			Physical	**Social**
PRE-EVENT	Fire safe cigarette	Control seizure	Non-slip tub surface	Legislation-Factory preset water heater thermostats
EVENT	Sprinklers, smoke detectors	Flame retardant cloths	Fire escapes	Fire drill education
POST-EVENT	Water	First aid antibiotics	EMS	Emergency & Rehabilitation services

Figure 3.1 The Haddon matrix for burn control

Table 3.1 General strategies for burn control

1. Prevent creation of the hazard (stop producing firecrackers)
2. Reduce amount of hazard (decrease chemical concentration in commercial products)
3. Prevent release of the hazard (child-resistant butane lighters)
4. Modify rate or spatial distribution of the hazard (vapor-ignition-resistant water heaters)
5. Separate release of the hazard in time or space (small spouts for hot water faucet)
6. Place barrier between the hazard and the host (install fence around electrical transformers, fire screen)
7. Modify nature of the hazard (use low conductors of heat)
8. Increase resistance of host to hazard (treat seizure disorder)
9. Begin to counter damage already done by hazard (first aid, rapid transport, and resuscitation)
10. Stabilization, repair, rehabilitation of host: example (provide acute care – burn center and rehabilitation)

automatic; little to no cooperation or action is required by the host. This is the most effective prevention strategy. Examples include building codes requiring smoke alarms, sprinkler installation, and factory-adjusted water heater temperature. Active prevention measures are voluntary, emphasize education to encourage people to change their unsafe behavior, and require repetitive educational measures to maintain individual action. Herein lies its weakness. Project Burn Prevention was a program funded by the Consumer Product Safety Commission (CPSC) in 1975.[12] It was undertaken to determine if a burn prevention program would decrease burn deaths by utilizing an educational program and media messages involving a large population base. The authors concluded that there was no reduction of burn incidence or severity in their study with either the school education program or media campaign. Education to bring about and maintain personal responsibility was not sufficient. Active prevention is the least effective and most difficult strategy to maintain, especially over a long period. Examples

are a home fire drill plan, and wearing goggles and gloves when handling toxic chemicals. Passive strategies are not always successful: a water heater thermostat may be raised by a homeowner and a sprinkler system or smoke alarm must be maintained. Once surveillance data have been established and collected, then prioritizing high-risk burn groups is necessary in order to identify intervention strategies.

The four E's of Intervention are Engineering, Economic, Enforcement, and Education.[13] Engineering – focuses on the physical environment (product safety design) and the vector. Examples include fire-resistant upholstery and bedding, child-resistant multi-purpose lighters (including cigarette), and insulated electric wire. Economic – influences behavior, i.e. monetary incentives such as insurance rate reduction if a home has smoke alarms or sprinklers. Enforcement – influences behavior with laws, building codes, and regulations, i.e. requiring fire escapes, sprinklers/smoke alarms in motels, hotels, and homes (**Table 3.2**). Education – influences

Table 3.2 Components of a hotel/motel safety program

1. Fire sprinklers
2. Smoke/fire detectors
3. Automatic alarm system
4. Manual alarm system (pull-boxes in stairwells and near elevators)
5. Fire department standpipes (a vertical pipe usually noted in stairwells and acts as a reserve in order to secure a uniform pressure in a water supply system)
6. Emergency lights
7. Emergency exit system
8. Exit signs
9. Pressurized stairways (a fan blows air in from the exterior thus creating a positive pressure in the stairway to keep smoke from entering into the stairway and blocking the exit path. This is unnecessary if the stairway is open to the exterior of the building)
10. Smoke control systems
11. Portable fire extinguishers
12. Staff fire emergency response plan
13. Staff training

behavior through knowledge and reasoning. Examples include pamphlets, public television programs, CPSC News Alerts. These active measures are the least effective.

In any prevention program the results must be evaluated.[14] If a prevention program does not achieve the stated goal(s), possible reasons include (1) the technique or measurement used may be inappropriate to identify the reduction caused by the prevention strategy; (2) faulty program design; and (3) study design may have been good, but the program was carried out inappropriately.

With this background in the epidemiology and prevention of injuries, important areas of challenge and opportunity in burn prevention both past, present, and future will be discussed.

Flammable clothing

In the decade of the 1940s, publicity surrounding children sustaining burns to their legs as a result of the ignition of Gene Autry cowboy suits or 'chaps' (made of highly flammable-brushed rayon), awoke both the medical and lay community in the US to the dangers of flammable clothing.[15] This was soon reinforced when burns resulting from 'torch sweaters' worn by girls began to suddenly appear. Extensive research was conducted to determine fabric flammability.[16,17] Wool burns very slowly and does not ignite. It melts with a red glow, retracts from the heat source, and finally extinguishes itself. On the other hand, cotton burns like a torch and is completely destroyed in a matter of seconds. Raised cut materials were known to be very flammable. While rayon ignites easily, it does not burn as intensely as cotton. A combination of cotton and wool burns less than either by itself. Silk produces a red glow but usually goes out quite quickly. Nylon simply melts but will cling to the underlying surface. Loose-fitting clothing, particularly if the individual is in an upright position and air currents are created by moving, tends to make the burn worse. A close nap or closely woven material is more flame-retardant than loose weave textiles.

In 1953 legislation regulating the manufacture and sale of wearing apparel of highly flammable clothing (the Flammability Fabrics Act) was passed in the US. As a result of the Act, contracts were awarded to Burn Units to collect epidemiologic data regarding flammable fabric burns, flammability testing methods were improved and standardized, and flame-retardant fabrics were developed. The initial Act covered only fabrics that came in contact with the body and therefore excluded industrial fabrics. The Act was amended in 1967 to include articles of wearing apparel and interior furnishings such as paper, plastic, rubber, synthetic film, and synthetic foam. In the US the chemical agent TRIS was the common additive used to make flame-retardant clothing. TRIS was banned in 1977 by the CPSC, not because of the lack of scientific proof of its effectiveness but because a 'two-year feeding study' in rodents conducted by the National Cancer Institute revealed that the agent caused cancer.[18,19] Did TRIS and flame-retardant sleepwear result in a decline of clothing flame burns?[20] Analysis of 6000 burns admitted to 15 burn centers in the United States between 1965 and 1969 revealed that 86% of all flame burns involved fabrics.[21] In 1977, McLoughlin et al. reported a decrease in sleepwear burns at the Shrines Burn Institute in Boston, MA.[22] It was recognized, however, that accurate national statistics to support their experience were lacking. Other explanations were proposed – the change in referral patterns of patients, improved public education on the hazards of sleepwear, behavior changes not

directly related to the flammability of sleepwear, changes in clothing design, and finally that burn injuries were still occurring but were less severe. Clothing burns involve three factors: flammability, the behavior of the wearer, and the heat source.[23] During this same period, make-up of clothing changed. By 1985, 87% of children's sleepwear was made of synthetics and only about 13% of sleepwear was made of cotton. In 1996, sleepwear standards for children were amended by the CPSC. Sleepwear for children 9 months or younger and tight-fitting garments (up to size 14 and not exceeding specified measurements for specific areas of the body) can now be sold even though they do not meet the flammability standards ordinarily applied to such sleepwear. In 1999 the CPSC stated that it had not identified sufficient data to support claims of additional injuries as a result of relaxed standards in children's sleepwear. The commission emphasized that sleepwear standards were designed to protect children from burn injuries if they came in contact with an open flame such as match or stove. Flame-resistant or snug-fit clothing does not apply for sleepwear in sizes of 9 months and under because infants wearing these sizes are 'insufficiently mobile to expose themselves to sources of fire'.[24] What about the children that do not voluntarily expose themselves to an open flame? The safest sleepwear is a snug-fitting, flame-resistant garment. Hang tags must be attached to clothing stating that the garment should fit snugly, is not flame-resistant, and a loose-fitting garment is more likely to catch fire. In 1999 a rash of clothing burns occurred in girls, ages 2.5–11, wearing large loose-fitting cotton T-shirts as nightdresses. The victims had been playing with either matches or a lighter.[25]

Hot water burns

All tap water scald burns are preventable. In 1983 the Washington state legislature required all new home water heaters be preset to 49°C (120°F).[26] The time of exposure to this temperature is sufficiently long that the victim, usually a child or elderly disabled person, is able to be removed or can climb out of the water before a severe burn can occur. An educational program was instituted to inform people to voluntarily decrease the water temperature. Follow-up in 1988 revealed there had indeed been a reduction in pediatric burns caused by hot water. Voluntary reduction of thermostat temperatures to a safe level by manufacturers has not been uniformly successful. Mandatory regulations to lower water heater temperature would be the most effective strategy, but until society is educated and convinced of its benefit, change will be slow. Other prevention methods to reduce tap water scald burns include inserting shut-off valves in the water circuit to detect temperatures over a certain level, and the use of liquid-crystal thermometers in bathtubs to alert the care giver of the water temperature.[27,28] Unfortunately prevention of spill burns from various hot liquids, which represent the largest percentage of pediatric burns, is more problematic. Most spill scald burns will not be prevented by adjusting hot water thermostats. Negligence on the part of the care giver(s) is the key issue. Preventive measures must depend on education, but how successful will behavior modification be when care givers or family members forget to keep hot liquids such as coffee, soup, or tea, grease or electric cords attached to pots, or deep fryers out of the reach of children? Success can be achieved through a combination of education, legislation, and/or litigation regarding product safety.[29,30] Examples include ovens with a door that can be opened and climbed on by a child and an oven that is not secured to the wall. The child's weight on an open door can tip the oven forward, spilling hot liquids.[31] The first example might appear obvious and involves common sense, but common sense is not always so common. The second involves product design and installation.

Fire-safe cigarettes

A cigarette when left unattended and not even puffed can burn as long as 20–40 minutes. In 1993, 30–45% of residential fire deaths were caused by the careless use of cigarettes. In 1996, smoking was the cause in 4.8% of 191 729 residential fires, 10.6% of all fire injuries, 17% of deaths, and 4.1% of the $2.6 billion lost.[6] Smoking was the cause of 30% of single and 15% of multiple fire fatalities. The combination of apartments and smoking represents an even more deadly fire environment: cigarettes accounted for 7.2% of all fires, 26% of the injuries, and 27% of the deaths in this scenario. Fires that began in bedding or upholstered furniture were attributed to cigarettes in 44% and 63% of cases, respectively. When smoking is combined with alcohol use there is an even greater risk of burn/fire injuries and fatalities.[32] Statistics collected between 1986 and 1987 revealed that positive blood alcohol levels were 7.8 times more common in fire injuries than noninjuries. Consumption of five or more drinks per occasion was associated with an increased risk of a fire fatality. The odds ratio of a fire injury in a house where members collectively smoked from 1 to 9 cigarettes per day was 1.5 relative to households with no smokers, from 10 to 19 cigarettes per day the odds ratio was 6.6, and if greater than 20 cigarettes per day the odds ratio was 3.6. The data revealed that smoking appeared to be the more important risk factor. Smoking continues to be pervasive in society, especially in both teenagers and older age groups. Although cigarette smoking is slowly on the decrease in some industrialized societies, it is increasing in developing countries. It is likely that smoking will remain a leading cause of fire injuries and fatalities for years to come.

The concept of a fire-safe cigarette was explored in the early part of the 1920s. For the most part the concept remained dormant until 1984 when the Cigarette Safety Act created a technical study group on cigarette and little cigar fire safety.[33] This group was to determine if a fire-safe cigarette could be made and would it be commercially feasible. A report in 1987 confirmed that this could indeed be done by reducing the cigarette circumference, lowering the tobacco density, making the paper less porous, and reducing the citrate in the paper.[34] Two important facts emerge regarding cigarette-related burns:

1. Burn data on nonfatal cigarette fire injuries are lacking on the national level.
2. Legal liability may very well turn out to be the most effective means of decreasing both nonfatal and fatal burns associated with cigarettes.

Litigation against tobacco manufacturers for production of cigarettes, a known cause of fire injuries and deaths, when the technology for a safer cigarette has been available for years, is a distinct possibility.[35] Possible collusion to discourage the development of a fire-safe cigarette has been reported. On 11 January 2000, Philip Morris companies announced the development of a new type of cigarette paper that contains bands of paper that slow the rate of combustion. This technology was first reported to be available more than a decade ago. The production of a safe cigarette should

not be voluntary, but be required by law. Everyone is encouraged to read the article titled 'How the tobacco industry continues to keep the home fires burning' by Andrew McGuire.[36]

Carbon monoxide (CO) inhalation is the leading cause of fatal poisoning in the industrialized world.[37] Burn injuries and fatalities are often associated with CO intoxication. Heating systems are the most common cause of a fatal CO poisoning followed by charcoal grills, gas water heaters, stoves, lanterns, and gas ranges. A CO alarm near all sleeping areas represents an effective event-prevention strategy.

Smoke detectors/alarms

Without question the use of smoke alarms has had the greatest impact in decreasing fire deaths in the US.[38] Unfortunately the statistics are not all encouraging. In 1966, the percent of residential fire deaths in homes with an operating smoke alarm was 13%, 11.5% of deaths occurred in homes with a nonoperating alarm, and 38.5% in houses without an alarm.[6] Smoke alarm performance was not much better in one- and two-family dwelling fire fatalities: 10% had operating alarms, 10% had alarms present but not operating, and no alarm was present in 42%. Socioeconomic factors associated with lack of functioning smoke detectors include living in a non-apartment dwelling, an annual income of less than $20 000, being unmarried, and living in a non-metropolitan county, and homes with children younger than age 5. Smoke detector ownership was most often associated with not living in public housing, higher education (completing high school), maternal age (not a teenager), practice fire drills, and larger homes.[39–41]

In 1985, McLoughlin published *Smoke Detector Legislation*.[42] Her conclusions were that smoke detector installation in new houses *appears* to be effective when mandated by a building code. Mallonee *et al.* in 1996 collected data on a smoke detector giveaway program in Oklahoma City, OK.[43] The target area for intervention had the highest rate of injuries related to residential fires in the city. The number of injuries per 100 000 population was 4.2 times higher than the rest of the city. A total of 10 100 smoke alarms were distributed to 9291 homes. Over the next 4 years the annualized injury rate per 100 000 population decreased by 80% in the target area, as compared to only 8% in the rest of the city. The authors concluded that target intervention with a smoke-alarm-give away program reduced residential fire injuries. Smoke alarms represent intervention before the burn event occurs. Sprinklers are an intervention strategy that works during the event. Smoke detector legislation has been proven to be an effective prevention strategy. Building codes mandating installation in new homes has been proven to be a practical solution. While 'retrofit' laws would appear to be unenforceable, the practical solution is to require installation when a house is sold or an apartment rented. Installation in existing homes represents the ultimate goal, but this will not be accomplished by legislation. Maintenance of alarms is just as difficult.

Fire sprinklers

Sprinklers complement smoke detectors.[44] Automatic fire sprinklers have been in use in the US since the later part of the 19th century. They are the most effective way of limiting the spread of fire in the early stages. In 1996 residential sprinklers were found in less than 2% of residential fires.[6] The National Fire Prevention Association estimates that occupants with a smoke alarm in the home have a 50% better change of surviving a fire than those without a smoke detector. Adding sprinklers increases the chances of surviving a fire to nearly 97%. One sprinkler is adequate to control fire in over 90% of the documented sprinkler activations in all residential fires. In 1978, San Clemente, California was the first jurisdiction in the United States to require residential sprinklers in all new structures. In 1985, Scottsdale, Arizona required a sprinkler system in every room of all new industrial, commercial, and residential building. The cost in a new 2000 square foot home in 1986 was $1.14/foot^2 and in 1996 it was $0.59–0.70/foot^2.[45] Installation in an 1800 foot^2 home would be about 1.7% of the total cost. In 1988 only about half of all hotels and motels had sprinkler systems. **Table 3.2** lists components of a hotel/motel fire safety program if the structure is over 75 feet.[46] It is estimated that 75% of high-rise and 50% of low-rise hotels have sprinkler systems. In hotels less than three stories, sprinkler requirements may not apply. Over 200 communities in the US have residential sprinkler laws.

Evaluating the Effect of Burn Prevention

Successful burn prevention includes collecting, analyzing, and then interpreting burn statistics including mortality and even more importantly burn morbidity. Heretofore, much of this has been done on a local level and without a national perspective in mind. The ongoing collection of data will allow:

1. identification of the magnitude of the type of burn injury,
2. monitor the trend of specific areas of burn injuries that need attention and are prevalent,
3. identify if new injury problems arise,
4. develop the methodology to evaluate burn prevention or intervention efforts.

Many successful burn prevention programs have been developed on the local level using locally generated data. Behavior modification on a local level can be instituted more quickly than waiting for national societal initiatives and legislation. Unfortunately, local efforts affect only a few. Prevention research should generate information, which can be useful on a national level. There must be rigorous methods of evaluating research so the conclusions may be shared. Many burn prevention programs have had an insufficient number of subjects, no controls, inadequate or short follow-up periods, no control for confounders and, of utmost importance, few use mortality and morbidity as outcome measures. While it might be difficult to conduct prospective, randomized, and double-blinded studies (Class I research), nevertheless rules of good scientific research should be followed.[47] Studies with a single hypothesis should be conducted over an adequate length of time. The prevention goal should be realistic and achievable and the results must be carefully analyzed. Since the incidence of both burn injuries and deaths is decreasing throughout the United States, no single burn unit or community will have a large enough patient population to conduct meaningful prospective studies. Peck and Maley determined the population requirements necessary to conduct adequate statistical studies.[48] To conduct a study necessary to show a decrease in injuries by 50% and 10% (alpha level of 0.05 and power of 0.08) requires a population of 9330 and 295 082, respectively. To realize a 50% and 10% reduction in burn deaths would require a population of 4 672 000 and 148 175 000, respectively. Wanda *et al.* published a review article on the effectiveness of prevention interventions in house fire injuries.[49] Various types of intervention programs were reviewed, including school, preschool, community, education programs, fire response-training programs for children, office-based counseling, home inspection programs, smoke detector giveaway campaigns, and smoke detector legislation. The important conclusion was that fire-related injuries must use morbidity and mortality as outcome measures. There was wide variability regarding study design, data sources, and outcome measures.

Prevention strategies must be coordinated on a national level. While passive prevention programs are the most effective, they are often slow to implement. Active prevention is not always easy, and requires time, significant organization support, and money. Unfortunately in the US it is unusual for a fire department to spend more than 5% of its budget on fire prevention.[50] Active and passive measures are not mutually exclusive though and both must be utilized. While all burns *should* be preventable, unfortunately the aphorism 'it is easier said than done' is true.

References

1. Doege TC. Sounding board: an injury is no accident. *N Engl J Med* 1978; **9**: 509–10.
2. Colebrook L, Colebrook V. The prevention of burns and scalds. *Lancet* 1949; **11**: 181–8.
3. Colebrook L, Colebrook V, Bull JP, Jackson DM. The prevention of burning accidents. *Br Med J* 1956; **1**: 1379–86.
4. Editorial. Death in the fire place. *Lancet* 1946; **Dec 7**: 833–4.
5. Hennekens CH, Buring JE *Epidemiology in Medicine*. Boston: Little Brown, 1987: 3–13, 178–94.
6. *Fire in the United States 1987–1996*, 17th ed. National Fire Data Center.
7. Bonnie RJ, Fulco CE, Liverman CT. *Reducing the Burden of Injury. Advancing Prevention and Treatment*. National Academy Press, 1999.
8. Haddon W. The changing approach to the epidemiology, prevention, and amelioration of trauma: the transition to approaches etiologically rather than descriptively based. *Am J Public Health* 1968; **58**: 1431–8.
9. Haddon W. Advances in the epidemiology of injuries as a basis for public policy. *Public Health Rep* 1980; **95**: 411–21.
10. McKinlay JB. The promotion of health through planned sociopolitical change: challenges for research and policy. *Soc Sci Med* 1993; **36**: 109–17.
11. Barss P, Smith GS, Barker S, Mohan D. *Injury Prevention. Epidemiology, Surveillance, and Policy*. New York: Oxford University Press, 1998.
12. McLoughlin E, Vince CJ, Lee AM, Crawford JD: Project burn prevention: outcome and implications. *Am J Public Health* 1982; **72**: 241–7.
13. Budnick LD. Injuries. In: Cassens BJ, ed. *Preventive Medicine and Public Health*. Media, PA: Harwal, 1992: 165–73.
14. McLoughlin E. Issues in evaluation of fire and burn prevention programs. *J Burn Care Rehabil* 1982; **3**: 281–4.
15. Burnett WE, Caswell HT. Severe burns from inflammable cowboy pants. *JAMA* 1946; **130**: 935–6.
16. Crikelair GF. Flame-retardant clothing. *J Trauma* 1966; **6**: 422–7.
17. Crikelair GF, Agate F, Bowe A. Gasoline and flammable and nonflammable clothing studies. *Pediatrics* 1976; **58**: 585–94.
18. United States Consumer Product Safety Commission. *CPSC Bans TRIS-Treated Children's Garments*. News Release, 7 April 1977.
19. Blum A, Ames BN. Flame-retardant additives as possible cancer hazards. *Science* 1977; **95**: 7–23.
20. Knudson MS, Bolieu SL, Larson DL, Brown RD. Children's sleepwear flammability standards: have they worked? *Burns* 1979; **6**: 255–60.
21. Feller I, Tholen D, Cornell RG. Improvements in burn care, 1965 to 1979. *JAMA* 1980; **244**: 2074–8.
22. McLoughlin E, Clarke N, Stahl K, Crawford JD. One pediatric burn unit's experience with sleepwear-related injuries. *Pediatrics* 1977; **60**: 405–9.
23. Oglesbay FB. The flammable fabrics problem. *Pediatrics* 1969; **44**: 827–95.
24. Cusick JM, Grant EJ, Kucan JO. Children's sleepwear: relaxation of the Consumer Product Safety Commission's flammability standards. *J Burn Care Rehabil* 1997; **18**: 469–76.
25. Wilson DI, Bailie FB. Night attire burns in young girls – the return of an old adversary. *Burns* 1999; **25**: 269–71.

26. Erdmann TC, Feldman KW, Rivara FP, Heimbach DM, Wall HA. Tap water burn prevention. The effect of legislation. *Pediatrics* 1991; **88**: 572–7.

27. Maley M. Scald burns associated with tap water. *J Burn Care Rehabil* 1989; **10**: 172–3.

28. Katcher ML, Landry GL, Shapiro MM. Liquid-crystal thermometer use in pediatric office counseling about tap water burn prevention. *Pediatrics* 1980; **83**: 766–71.

29. Feldman KW, Schaller RT, Feldman JA, McMillon M. Tap water scald burns in children. *Pediatrics* 1978; **62**: 1–7.

30. Webne S, Kaplan FJ, Shaw M. Pediatric burn prevention: an evaluation of the efficacy of a strategy to reduce tap water temperature in a population at risk for scalds. *Dev Behavior Pediatr* 1989; **10**: 187–91.

31. Still JS, Craft-Coffman B, Law E, Colon-Santini J, Grant J. Burns of children caused by electric stoves. *J Burn Care & Rehabil* 1998; **19**: 364–5.

32. Ballard JE, Koepsell TD, Rivara F. Association of smoking and alcohol drinking with residential fire injuries. *Am J Epidemiol* 1990; **135**: 26–34.

33. Botkin JR. The fire-safe cigarette. *JAMA* 1988; **260**: 226–9.

34. Brigham PA, McGuire A. Progress towards a fire-safe cigarette. *J Public Health Policy* 1996; **16**: 433–9.

35. Barillo DJ, Brigham PA, Kayden DA, Heck RT, McManus AT. The fire-safe cigarette: a burn prevention tool. *J Burn Care Rehabil* 2000; **21**: 164–70.

36. McGuire A. How the tobacco industry continues to keep the home fires burning. *Tobacco Control* 1999; **8**: 67–9.

37. Varon J, Marik PE, Fromm RE, Gueler A. Carbon monoxide poisoning: a review for clinicians. *J Emergency Med* 1999; **17**: 87–93.

38. DiGuiseppi C, Roberts I, Spears N. Smoke alarm installation and function in inner London council housing. *Arch Dis Child* 1999; **81**: 400–3.

39. Gorman RL, Charney E, Holtzman NA, Roberts KB. A successful city-wide smoke detector give-away program. *Pediatrics* 1985; **75**: 14–18.

40. Shaw KN, McCormick MC, Kustra SL, Ruddy RM, Casey RD. Correlates of reported smoke detector usage in an inner-city population: participants in a smoke detector give-away program. *Am J Public Health* 1988; **78**: 650–3.

41. Miller RE, Reisinger KS, Blatter MM, Wucher F. Pediatric counseling and subsequent use of smoke detectors. *Am J Public Health* 1982; **72**: 392–3.

42. McLoughlin E, Marchone M, Hanger L, German PS, Baker SP. Smoke detector legislation: its effect on owner-occupied homes. *Am J Public Health* 1985; **75**: 858–62.

43. Mallonee S, Istre GR, Rosenberg M, Reddish-Douglas M, Jordan F, Silverstein P, Tunell W. Surveillance and prevention of residential-fire injuries. *N Engl J Med* 1996; **335**: 27–31.

44. Council on Scientific Affairs. Preventing death and injury from fires with automatic sprinklers and smoke detectors. *JAMA* 1987; **2577**: 1618–20.

45. McLoughlin E, McGuire A. The causes, cost, and prevention of childhood burn injuries. *AJDC* 1990; **144**: 677–83.

46. The American Fire Sprinkler Association, Dallas, Texas, July 2000.

47. Wards L, Tenebein M, Moffatt MEK. House fire injury prevention update. Part II. A review of the effectiveness of preventive interventions. *Injury Prevention* 1999; **5**: 217–25.

48. Peck MD, Maley MP. Population requirements for statistical analysis of efficacy of burn prevention programs. *J Burn Care Rehabil* 1991; **12**: 282–4.

49. Wanda L, Tenenbein M, Moffatt MEK. House fire injury prevention update. Part II. A review of the effectiveness of preventive interventions. *Injury Prevention* 1999; **5**: 217–25.

50. Stambaugh H, Schaenman P. International concepts of fire protection: ideas that could help US prevention. *J Burn Care Rehabil* 1988; **9**: 312–13.

Chapter 4

Care of outpatient burns
C Edward Hartford

Introduction

Although there has been a remarkable decline in the incidence of burn injuries in the United States during the past several decades, approximately 1.25 million individuals still sustain a burn injury each year.[1] Currently, fewer than 45 000 of these victims require hospitalization and there are about 4500 burn-related deaths annually.[1] Therefore, thermal trauma typically results in an injury of low mortality in which the majority of care can be safely rendered in an ambulatory setting.

The outcome of burns treated in the outpatient setting is usually good. If, however, care is suboptimal, protracted morbidity or compromised function can result. The goals of therapy are to minimize pain and the risk of infection, achieve wound healing in a timely fashion, preserve physical function, minimize cosmetic deformity, and affect physical and psychosocial rehabilitation in the most expeditious manner.

Who can be managed as an outpatient?

When the patient is first evaluated, information is immediately available from which an accurate prognosis can be derived. These prognostic factors – and a huge dose of common sense – determine the initial treatment venue. The prognostic factors include: age of patient; extent of the burn; depth of the burn; premorbid diseases; and co-morbid disorders which include respiratory complications, associated trauma, distribution of the burn, and the injuring agent. Additionally, when outpatient care is an option the patient's social situation needs to be assessed. In some instances, it may be prudent to initiate care in the hospital so that potential, complicating medical problems can be sorted out.

Age

Patients between 5 and 20 years of age have the most favorable outcome from burns. The LA_{50} for this age cohort is 94.5% total body surface area (TBSA) of burn.[2] Younger individuals, especially infants, have an increase in morbidity as well as mortality from burn injury. In this group, child abuse or neglect must be included in the psychosocial analysis.[3,4] The peak incidence of nonaccidental burn injury is 13–24 months of age.[5] Burns that are particularly suspicious are those whose appearance suggests an injury from a cigarette, hot iron, or immersion in hot water. The latter injury is identified by sharp demarcation between the burned and unburned skin. The absence of splash marks and scalding which has occurred in an institution should also heighten one's suspicion. Even with trivial injury, if the burn was sustained under suspicious circumstances or the history does not correspond with the nature or distribution of the burn, the patient should be hospitalized for their protection. Cases of suspected abuse or neglect must be referred to the appropriate social services agency.

Any patient over the age of 70 years with burns is in danger of dying regardless of the extent of the burn.[2] The LA_{50} for this age group is 29.5% TBSA of burn. Therefore, admitting the older patient to a hospital to assess their response to the injury can prove invaluable before treatment is continued as an outpatient.

Extent of the Burn

The larger the percent of body surface area involved by the burn, the worse the prognosis. The percent of the body surface area can be roughly estimated by the 'rule of nines',[6] or more accurately by the technique of Lund and Browder[7] (**Figure 4.1**). A helpful adjunct in estimating the area of the burn is that the patient's palm approximates 1% of their body surface area.

Any burned patient who requires intravenous fluid resuscitation should be admitted to a hospital. This includes adults and older children with burns in excess of 15% of the body surface area, as well as younger children (under 5 years of age) and infants with burns in excess of 10% of the body surface area.[8] In some instances, due to premorbid dehydration caused by physical activity, an arid or semi-arid climate, alcohol, or diuretics, some patients with smaller burns may need supplemental intravenous fluids for optimal care.

Depth of the Burn

The deeper the burn, the worse the prognosis. However, depth of small area burns is less important in determining the need to initiate care in a hospital than the extent of the burn.

When a burn is first evaluated it is often difficult to determine its depth. The superficial injury of sunburn or its equivalent is easy to identify. Likewise, it is easy to discern a waxen, dry, inelastic, insensate, cadaveric-appearing wound as a full-thickness burn. However, it is extremely difficult to distinguish the subtle differences between a superficial partial-thickness burn, which will heal spontaneously within 3 weeks, and a deep partial-thickness burn which takes longer to heal. This is especially true for weeping wounds in which the blisters have ruptured. Initially, these wounds appear superficial and are perfused. However, with time, as the injured small blood vessels in the wound thrombose, the wound takes on the ischemic, cadaveric appearance of a deeper injury.[9,10] This change does not reflect invasive infection but merely the natural evolution of the wound.

Premorbid Diseases

Preexisting medical conditions often have a profound influence upon the clinical course and outcome of a burn injury. While any medical disorder may have an adverse effect, there are a number of conditions that occur frequently among the burned and which may play a significant role in causation or outcome. For instance, any condition or habit that alters an individual's mental state may lead to a burn injury. These include seizure disorders, senility and psychiatric illnesses as well as the use of sedatives, controlled substances, and alcohol. These usually obligate hospital admission. Medical conditions that are known to enhance morbidity of patients with burns include renal failure, congestive heart failure, cardiac dysrhythmias, hypertension, chronic obstructive pulmonary disease, diabetes mellitus, sequelae of alcoholism, conditions which require the use of steroids, morbid obesity, and immune system compromise.[11] The clinical status of any of these disorders must be determined and their potential influence on the outcome assessed before determining whether the patient can be safely managed as an outpatient.

Co-morbid Disorders

Respiratory complications

Synchronous lung injury substantially magnifies the burned patient's risk and may occur even with no or trivial cutaneous burn injury.[12,13] Since adverse respiratory sequelae from inhalation injury, upper respiratory obstruction, and carbon monoxide poisoning may not be immediately apparent,[14] a period of monitored observation is warranted. Overnight observation is usually sufficient.

Associated trauma

Burns frequently occur with other forms of trauma. If the burn involves only a small area of the body, the associated trauma will dictate whether a patient needs to be hospitalized.

Distribution of the burn

The location of the burn may have a profound effect on the patient's activities of daily living, and dictate the setting in which the patient receives care. For instance, the edema from a small-area superficial burn of the face may result in swelling of the eyelids, hampering the patient's vision (**Figure 4.2**). Likewise, burns of the hands, feet, or those involving the perineum or adjacent areas may severely limit an individual's autonomy. While burns in these areas may not necessarily demand care in a hospital, there must be consideration of the assistance available to the patient when contemplating outpatient ambulatory care.

Because of fluid flux into the tissues beneath a burn, patients with circumferential burns of an extremity are in danger of ischemia of underlying and distal tissues from increased tissue pressure.[15] Except for those with very superficial burns, all patients with circumferential burns of an extremity should be admitted to the hospital and monitored for evidence of elevated tissue pressure. Since the clinical signs of compartment syndrome and ischemia in a burned extremity are unreliable,[16] the author advocates measuring the tissue pressure by direct methods. Alternatively, a Doppler ultrasonic flowmeter can be used to assess the circulatory status of the extremity.[16]

Burns across joints do not, for that reason alone, require admission to a hospital.

Injuring agent

Patients exposed to low-voltage electricity, arbitrarily defined as less than 1000 volts (the most frequent source being household currents of 110 or 220 volts), are in great danger of dying at the accident scene from a cardiac dysrhythmia, usually ventricular fibrillation.[17] Following low-voltage electrical exposure, the most frequent residual electrocardiographic abnormality is a nonspecific

BURN DIAGRAM　Shriners Burns Institute – Galveston Unit

Age: _____ Sex: _____ Date of admission _____

Type of burn:　Flame ☐　Electrical ☐　　Scald ☐　Chemical ☐　Inhalation injury ☐

Date of burn: _____

Date completed: _____

Completed by: _____

Date revised: _____

Revised by: _____

Approved by: _____

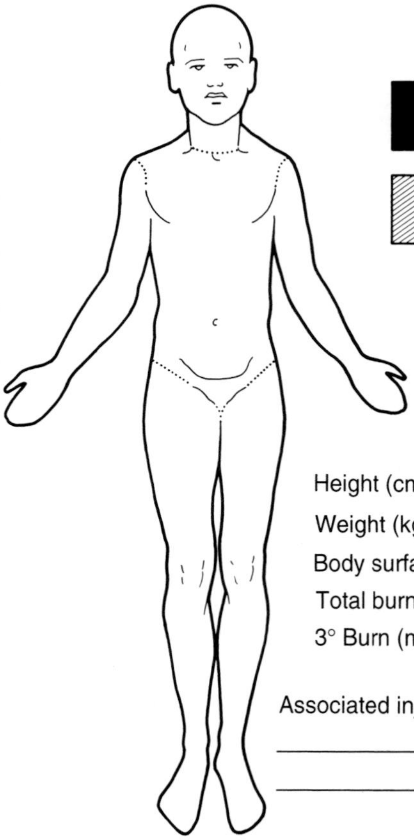

■ 3rd°

▨ 2nd°

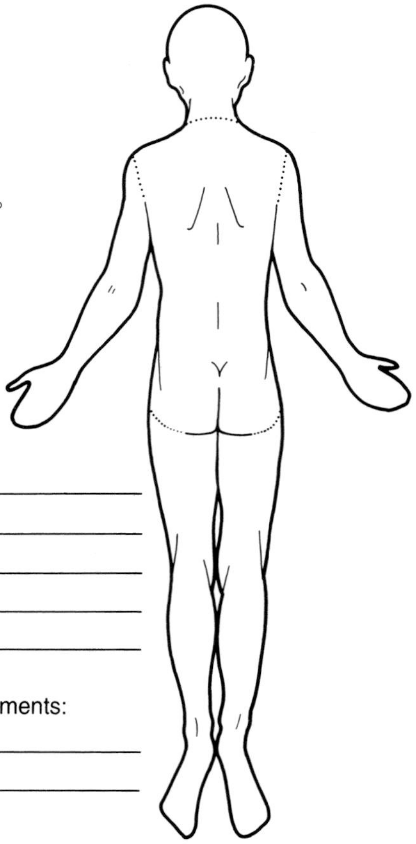

Height (cm) _____

Weight (kg) _____

Body surface (m²) _____

Total burn (m²) _____

3° Burn (m²) _____

Associated injuries/comments:

_____

_____

BURN ESTIMATE – AGE VS. AREA

Area	Birth–1 year	1–4 years	5–9 years	10–14 years	15 years	Adult	2°	3°	TBSA %
Head	19	17	13	11	9	7			
Neck	2	2	2	2	2	2			
Ant. trunk	13	13	13	13	13	13			
Post. trunk	13	13	13	13	13	13			
R. buttock	2.5	2.5	2.5	2.5	2.5	2.5			
L. buttock	2.5	2.5	2.5	2.5	2.5	2.5			
Genitalia	1	1	1	1	1	1			
R.U. arm	4	4	4	4	4	4			
L.U. arm	4	4	4	4	4	4			
R.L. arm	3	3	3	3	3	3			
L.L. arm	3	3	3	3	3	3			
R. hand	2.5	2.5	2.5	2.5	2.5	2.5			
L. hand	2.5	2.5	2.5	2.5	2.5	2.5			
R. thigh	5.5	6.5	8	8.5	9	9.5			
L. thigh	5.5	6.5	8	8.5	9	9.5			
R. leg	5	5	5.5	6	6.5	7			
L. leg	5	5	5.5	6	6.5	7			
R. foot	3.5	3.5	3.5	3.5	3.5	3.5			
L. foot	3.5	3.5	3.5	3.5	3.5	3.5			
						TOTAL			

Fig. 4.1 Chart used to calculate the surface area involved by burn. It takes into account that, as one grows from infancy to adulthood, the relative surface area of the head decreases while the relative surface area of the lower extremities increases. Modified from Lund and Browder.[7]

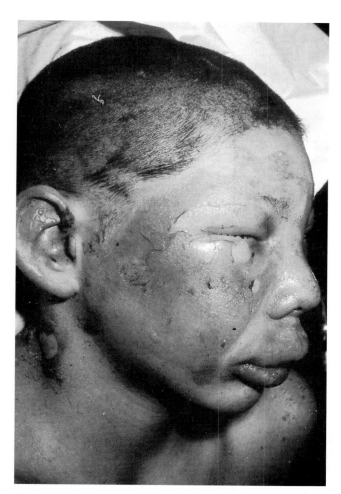

Fig. 4.2 Swelling caused by a burn that healed spontaneously without scar. For several days the edema of the eyelids prevented the patient from seeing.

change in the ST-T wave segment[18] and the most troublesome dysrhythmias are among the atrial fibrillation-flutter group.[19] If the electrocardiogram is normal or becomes normal during observation, the chances of a subsequent dysrhythmia or cardiac arrest are virtually nil.

The tissue damage from low levels of electrical energy is usually small and most patients do not need to be hospitalized. Occasionally, however, the damage to a child's lip, tongue, gums and dentition from sucking on a defective energized electrical cord may preclude efficient oral alimentation. In this cirumstance, hospitalization to establish satisfactory oral intake is probably wise.

Patients who sustain tissue damage from contact with high-voltage electricity generally require admission.

Brushing off dry chemicals or copious lavage with water of wet chemicals are the appropriate emergency treatment.[20,21] No one knows how long lavage should be continued, but up to 1 hour has been recommended.[22] One guide is the presence of pain, the supposition being that, as long as there is pain, the chemical is still active and continuing to cause damage.

In some instances, there are specific antidotes for the pain caused by a chemical. For example, with hydrofluoric acid, the injured tissues should be injected with calcium gluconate.[23] Hydrofluoric acid also serves as a good example of the many chemicals that are absorbed into the body with the potential to cause organ injury. Exposure of concentrated hydrofluoric acid to as little as 3% of the body surface area can result in a fatal dysrhythmia from hypocalcemia due to calcium binding to absorbed fluoride ion.[24] Since it is impossible to remember the systemic sequelae of all the chemicals to which an individual might be exposed, the physician should identify the chemical and seek information from the local poison control center.

After emergency local wound care, the treatment of the residual wound from a chemical is the same as the treatment for any wound.

Social circumstances

Patients whose injuries may be nonaccidental need to be admitted to a hospital for their protection.

Before a patient is discharged from emergency care, the physician should ascertain that there are satisfactory resources available for supervision and care, and a way in which the patient can readily reaccess medical care. Therefore, the distance the patient lives from care needs to be taken into consideration. For outpatients a visiting nurse can be invaluable in providing wound care and monitoring for wound complications, as well as assessing the patient's physical progress and social situation.

Treatment

Cooling the Burn

The first objective in burn wound care is to dissipate the heat. As long as the temperature in the tissues is above 45°C injury continues to occur.[25] The first step is to remove the source of heat. Both clinical and experimental evidence indicate a beneficial effect from immediate active cooling of the wound to dissipate heat.[26] Cool tap water or saline at about 8°C (46.4°F) applied in any practical manner (e.g. compress, lavage, or immersion) is as effective as any other product or method.[27-29] Colder substances, such as ice, may be detrimental.[30] The period of time that is required for active cooling is brief.[31] Typically, by the time most patients present for care, the tissues have already cooled spontaneously.

Active cooling also has several potential advantages beyond dissipation of heat. First, cooling stabilizes skin mast cells, decreasing histamine release and, thereby, decreasing edema of the wound. Secondly, in the first several hours after the injury, cooling is an effective way of controlling the pain of partial-thickness burns.[32,33] In cooling for pain control, cool, but not ice-cold,[34,35] moist compresses are applied to the painful wound. This method is applicable in the management of virtually all patients whose wounds can be safely cared for in an ambulatory setting. Because of the limited surface area of burn among these patients, the detrimental systemic effects of active cooling, e.g. hypothermia from accelerated heat loss, should not occur. However, since water conducts heat 23 times faster than air, it makes good sense to monitor the patient's core temperature during active cooling of the wound.

Pain Control

Burn wounds are painful. The most severe pain occurs with partial-thickness wounds devoid of the superficial layers of epithelium. Initially it is intense and can prove to be unbearable. The pain spontaneously moderates after several hours but intensifies when wounds are manipulated during dressing changes, wound care, and physical activity. While eschar-covered burns may be insensate, when the eschar separates spontaneously or is removed or cut into, the exposed viable tissues are painful.[36]

Narcotics are typically required as first-line treatment. In the emergency setting, small incremental doses of morphine can be given intravenously and titrated to effect. Subsequently, acetaminophen with codeine or similar analgesics, alone or in combination, is usually effective. Provided alteration of platelet function is not a concern, nonsteroidal anti-inflammatory drugs (NSAIDs) may be effective. Analgesics can be supplemented with short-acting benzodiazepines, such as midazolam, to enhance sedation and prevent loss of memory and anxiolysis. Most patients will require supplemental analgesics for sleep, wound dressing changes, and physical therapy.

Clearance of these classes of drugs is accelerated among those who regularly abuse alcohol or controlled substances.[37,38] Therefore, remarkable amounts of analgesics and sedatives may be required.

If a patient's pain cannot be controlled by oral medication, the patient may need to be admitted to a hospital. In the hospital setting, effective pain control can usually be obtained by the patient-controlled analgesia method. Even with patient-controlled analgesia, supplemental analgesia and sedation will often be required when wound dressings are changed.

Topically applied or injected local anesthetics are not recommended in the management of burns.

Local Burn Wound Care

Loose, devitalized tissue is gently trimmed away, a practice known as epluchage. This process should not cause pain or bleeding.

Blisters

Recommendations for the management of blisters are varied and range from leaving blisters intact,[39] to removing the blistered skin immediately,[40] or delaying removal.[41]

Those who advocate removal of blistered skin cite laboratory studies that show that the blister fluid exhibits several potentially detrimental effects.[40] Immune function is depressed by impaired function of polymorphonuclear leukocytes and lymphocytes. Blister fluid adversely affects neutrophil chemotaxis, opsonization, and intracellular killing. Inflammation is enhanced by the presence of metabolites of arachidonic acid in the blister fluid. A plasmin inhibitor in the blister fluid decreases vascular patency. Finally, blister fluid may provide a medium for the growth of bacteria. Based on these considerations, the case can be made that blistered skin should be removed to facilitate healing.

Conversely, this author recommends leaving burn blisters intact. Blisters form in the stratum spinosum layer of the epidermis. An intact blister usually indicates a superficial partial thickness wound, which will heal spontaneously within 3 weeks. If, under these circumstances, the blistered skin is removed, the wound is converted from an absolutely painless one to a painful, open wound exposed to colonization by bacteria and potential infection.[39] An infection in a burn wound covered by an intact blister rarely occurs. Therefore, this author prefers to leave blisters intact, and recommends that they be dressed for protection and not covered with medication.

Blistered skin violated by needle aspiration or by spontaneous rupture also has the potential for bacterial contamination and infection. Attempts to use the loose skin of a ruptured blister as a protective dressing are often ineffective.

If the blister remains intact, and the wound is a superficial partial-thickness burn, spontaneous resorption of the fluid will begin in about 1 week. The blistered skin will gradually wrinkle and collapse onto the healing wound surface and become firm and inelastic. One should not be in a hurry to remove this protective layer.

Persistence of the blister, with no signs of spontaneous resorption of the fluid after several weeks, usually signifies that the underlying wound is either deep partial-thickness or full-thickness.

There is often concern about large blisters in locations that limit range of motion, such as in the palm of the hand. Many advocate needle aspiration of the fluid. The author does not. Experience has shown that full range of motion of the hand is virtually always restored.

Cleansing the wound

For cleansing and to remove residual dirt, the wound is gently washed with room temperature or tepid (100°F) water and a mild, bland soap. Chlorhexidine gluconate soap is desirable because of its antimicrobial activity against common skin flora.[42]

In the treatment of burns from tar and asphalt, after cooling to dissipate heat, the solidified tar and asphalt can be removed by solvents that have a close structural affinity to these substances. Therefore, substances related to petrolatum (an oleaginous colloid suspension of solid microcrystalline waxes in petroleum oil) are effective. Medi-Sol™ Adhesive Remover is a citrus-based nontoxic, nonirritating Category I Medical Device solvent authorized by the FDA for use on the skin. It is an effective product for the removal of tar and asphalt.[43] It can be obtained from Orange-Sol Medical Products Division (1400 N Fiesta Blvd, Bldg. 100, Gilbert, AZ 85233–1000, phone 602–497–8822).

Medi-Sol™ Adhesive Remover is liberally applied and then removed by gentle wiping. Polysorbates alone or in combination with topical antibiotics[44] and topical antibiotics in petrolatum base[45] can be used but are less effective, and repetitive applications are usually required.

Topical Agents

There is a long tradition of applying substances to burn wounds in an attempt to prevent infection.[46] A large variety of antiseptics, antibiotics, and topical antibacterial (antimicrobial) agents have been advocated. Most of these agents have adverse local or systemic effects, or impede wound healing, or both. Additionally, there is no published evidence that the use of any topical agent designed to prevent or control infection will favorably influence the outcome of small burns.[47–49] In spite of this, many physicians feel obligated to apply one of these agents to the wound. All published comparative studies show no advantage of these agents over petrolatum-impregnated gauze.[50] However, if the treating physician believes that the use of a topical antimicrobial agent is desirable, and most do, there are several choices. Antiseptics, detrimental to wound healing, should be avoided. Among the topical agents introduced for the treatment of burns during the past 4 decades, 1% silver sulfadiazine ointment has the fewest side-effects and is probably the current best recommendation. However, if the patient is allergic to sulfa products, silver sulfadiazine should not be used. Because sulfonamides are known to increase the possibility of kernicterus, silver sulfadiazine is not used on pregnant women, nursing mothers, and infants less than 2 months of age. Because silver sulfadiazine impedes epithelization, it should be discontinued when healing partial-thickness wounds are devoid of necrotic tissue and evidence of reepithelization is seen (**Figure 4.3**).

Alternatively, there has been increasing interest in the use of combinations of antibiotics in ointment for the treatment of small-area burns. These drugs have no clinically discernible detrimental effect on wound healing. These antimicrobial combinations include triple antibiotic ointment (neomycin, 3.5 mg/g; bacitracin zinc, 400 units/g; and polymyxin B sulfate, 5000 units/g) and polysporin (polymyxin B sulfate, 10 000 units/g; and bacitracin zinc, 500 units/g). These antibiotic combinations have efficacy against the Gram-positive cocci and some of the aerobic Gram-negative bacilli that most frequently colonize small burn wounds. Occasionally, small superficial pustules caused by a yeast develop on the surrounding uninjured skin. Stopping the antimicrobial agent results in clearing of these lesions. This author now uses these agents almost exclusively in the management of small area burns when a topical antimicrobial is used.

Dressing the wound

Because there are virtually no objective studies on the subject, dogmatic recommendations for dressing small burn wounds cannot be made. Dressings serve three purposes: (1) to absorb drainage; (2) to provide protection and a measure of isolation of the wound from the environment; and (3) to decrease wound pain. In most instances this author prefers to dress wounds and makes the following suggestions.

Superficial partial-thickness burns, the equivalent of sunburn, with intact epidermis, require neither topical medication nor a dressing.

For relatively small superficial partial-thickness burns devoid of epithelium, it is generally conceded that topical antibacterial agents are not necessary.[47–49] Nonmedicinal white petrolatum-impregnated fine mesh or porous mesh gauze (Adaptic®), or fine mesh absorbent gauze impregnated with 3% bismuth tribromophenate in nonmedicinal petrolatum blend (Xeroform®) are satisfactory wound covers. If the burn is deeper and contains adherent necrotic tissue, a topical antimicrobial agent may be used.

For practical reasons, most burns of the face are treated without dressing. These wounds may also be treated without topical medication, allowing the wounds to dry and form a crust. Because the dry wound is often uncomfortable and heals more slowly than moist wounds, many physicians prefer to use a thin layer of bland ointment combined with a topical antibiotic, e.g. Baciquent® (bacitracin in anhydrous lanolin, mineral oil, and white petrolatum). The ointment is applied to the wound after gentle cleansing with water twice daily, or more frequently as needed, particularly in a dry climate. Bacitracin has activity against Gram-positive bacteria. Occasionally it causes a contact dermatitis that impedes wound healing.

Since one purpose of dressings is to absorb drainage, the thickness of the dressing is determined by the amount of drainage generated between dressing changes. In weeping superficial partial-thickness wounds, the amount of drainage is greatest soon after the injury. As the character of the wound changes and healing begins, drainage decreases. Lint-free, coarse mesh gauze, usually starting with about 20 thicknesses, is preferred by the author.

The dressing is held in place with an elastic gauze bandage (e.g. Kling® or Kerlix®) wrapped with sufficient tightness to hold the gauze in place but not so tightly as to impede circulation. Many use Flexinette® to secure the dressing. Stockinette, semi-impervious to liquid, can be used as an outer layer to help prevent the drainage from soaking through the dressing. As an alternative, a cohesive flexible bandage (Coflex®, Coban®, Co-wrap®) can be used as an outer layer to hold a dressing securely in place and prevent drainage from seeping through. Joints are dressed to facilitate range of motion and fingers are dressed separately (**Figure 4.4**). However, among infants and young children, an effective way to hold the hand and fingers in extension is with a multilayer covering of one of the cohesive flexible bandages. This kind of a dressing functions as a 'soft' splint.

The frequency with which dressings are changed is arbitrary and dictated by the volume of drainage. Recommendations range from twice daily, to as infrequently as once a week. Those who advocate twice-daily dressing changes do so based on the use of topical antimicrobials whose half-life is about 8 hours. Those who use petrolatum, antibiotic combinations in ointment, or bismuth-impregnated petrolatum gauze recommend less frequent dressing changes, some extending the period to as long as 5 or 7 days.[50,51]

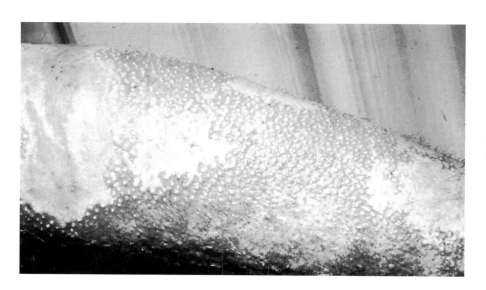

Fig. 4.3 Healing partial-thickness burn showing prominent islands of squamous epithelium that have emerged from epidermal appendages. Epithelium will expand to resurface the wound. When islands of squamous epithelium appear in a wound, spontaneous reepithelization is imminent.

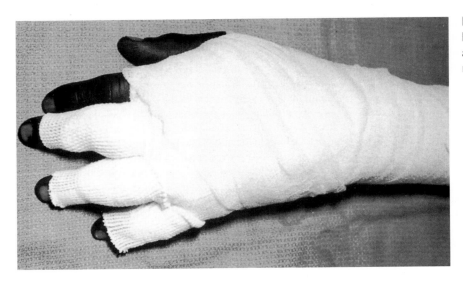

Fig. 4.4 Completed dressing of the hand. All joints should be dressed to allow as much functional range of motion as possible.

For in-patients, the author prefers once daily dressing changes to permit daily inspection and cleansing of the wound. Moreover, after about 24 hours, wound dressings are often saturated or disheveled. Daily dressing changes may be used in the care of outpatients even if the patient or another lay person is responsible for the inspection, cleansing, and redressing of the wound. Cleansing of the wound can often be incorporated into general body cleansing each day. The person responsible for wound care should be instructed in the clinical manifestations of wound infections.

In the management of burns among pediatric outpatients, the author now has an extensive and satisfying experience with the use of triple antibiotic ointment and dressing changes done at 3- to 4-day intervals. In many instances these dressings are changed and the progress of healing checked at clinic visits. Therefore, parents do not need to deal with the disquieting chore of changing their child's dressings and inflicting pain on them.

Synthetic Wound Dressings

The use of synthetic wound coverings is becoming more popular in the treatment of superficial partial-thickness burn wounds. The purported advantages are less pain, use of less pain medication, shorter wound healing time, improved compliance with scheduled outpatient visits and lower costs.

Biobrane®

There are two prospective randomized clinical trials of small numbers of patients that show that in the treatment of superfical partial-thickness burns the use of Biobrane® results in less pain, a lower pain medication requirement, and shorter healing time when compared to those patients treated with 1% silver sulfadiazine.[52,53]

Biobrane® is a bilayer fabric composed of an inner layer of knitted nylon threads coated with porcine collagen and an outer layer of rubberized silicone, pervious to gases but not to liquids and bacteria.[54] Wounds on which Biobrane® is to be applied must be carefully selected. They must be fresh, not infected, free of eschar and debris, moist, have a sensate surface, and demonstrate capillary blanching and refill. It is applied snugly to the cleansed wound overlapping itself or unburned skin and held in place with sterile strips of adhesive tape. The key to the successful use of Biobrane® is adherence to the wound. Therefore, the burned area must be dressed or splinted, especially across a joint, to prevent shearing of the Biobrane® from the wound surface. Satisfactory adherence usually occurs in about 2–4 days. If, at follow-up, the Biobrane® is found to be loose, the nonadherent area can be trimmed away and new Biobrane® applied. If sterile fluid accumulates beneath the synthetic dressing, it can be aspirated; however, if the fluid is purulent, the Biobrane® must be opened to permit complete drainage. Biobrane® is left intact until the wound has reepithelized. Then it can be gently teased away. If the wound surface has residual necrotic tissue, Biobrane® will not adhere.

Hydrocolloid dressings

Hydrocolloid dressings are described as wafers, powders, or pastes composed of materials such as gelatin, pectin, and carboxymethyl-cellulose. They provide a moist environment favorable for wound healing and a barrier against exogenous bacteria and fluids. They have been effective in the treatment of small-area partial-thickness burns.[55,56] In comparison to wounds treated with 1% silver sulfadiazine, those treated with hydrocolloid occlusive dressings had more rapid wound healing, less pain, and needed fewer dressing changes. As a result, the cost of care was lower. There are a number of products made by different manufactures that are probably suitable, e.g. Cutinova® Thin (Beiersdorf-Jobst), DuoDerm® CGF Border Sterile Dressing (ConvaTec), RepliCare® Hydrocolloid Dressing (Smith-Nephew), Restore® Wound Care Dressing (Hollister). Hydrocolloid dressings may be left in place for several days at a time.

Other wound dressing materials

Numerous wound dressing products have been introduced and advocated for the treatment of burns, especially small burns. Most of the clinical information about the efficacy of these products is anecdotal. However, information in medical publications can be accessed through the cost-free National Library of Medicine's Internet Grateful Med service. (The internet address is *http://igm.nlm.nih.gov/* Click on MEDLINE. On the search screen use the name of the product and burns as the subjects.)

Elevation of the Burned Area

One of the most effective ways to reduce the incidence of infection in burns is to eliminate edema from the burned part. Burn injury elicits edema in the tissues immediately subjacent to the wound. Additionally, there is a great tendency for the patient to hold the injured part immobile in a dependent position. To eliminate edema, the injured part should be exercised regularly and, when not in use, maintained slightly above the level of the heart. Merely elevating a leg off the floor to the level of the hip when in the sitting position is not sufficient. Holding the burned forearm flexed and dependent in a sling will enhance edema. Specific instructions and a demonstration of the proper position should be explicit.

The most efficient position for the injured part is just slightly above the level of the heart. To elevate the burned part higher above the heart does not further enhance removal of excess tissue fluid.[57]

Patients with small burns who experience persistent edema beyond 3 days are spending too much time with the part dependent.

When burns involve the lower extremity, walking and holding the leg in the dependent position often elicit severe pain. To diminish this effect, support, such as with a rubberized elastic bandage (Ace Bandage®), applied from the level of the toes to above the burn should be used. This will also aid in reducing the accumulation of edema during walking.

Instructions and Follow-up Care

Before patients are released from emergency care, they are instructed in wound care, positioning, physical therapy, the clinical manifestations of infection, a convenient way to reaccess medical care (usually by telephone), and given pain medication.

We examine most patients within the next several days. This allows reinspection of the wound, assessment of the patient's compliance with instructions and reinforcement of the principles of wound care. Often, because of pain during emergency care, the patient is distracted from fully understanding instructions. If concern remains, more frequent visits are scheduled until the physician is certain that care is being followed appropriately. After that, the patient can be seen at weekly intervals.

Definitive Wound Closure

A primary objective in burn care is to have all wounds healed within 1 month. Usually, this goal is easily achieved in an ambulatory setting. Burn wounds that heal spontaneously from the depth of the wound within 3 weeks have an excellent result. When this occurs, the skin functions normally with good elasticity, a nil incidence of hypertrophic scarring (scars that are red, raised, and indurated), and little, if any, alteration in pigmentation. The longer spontaneous healing takes the worse the result. With longer healing periods, there is an increasing likelihood of developing hypertrophic scarring[58] and unsightly alterations in pigmentation. In addition, wounds that take a very long time to heal may have unstable epithelium.

It is the surgeon's responsibility to make certain that burn wounds either heal spontaneously or are closed surgically in a timely fashion. If it is apparent that a wound will not heal spontaneously within 3 or 4 weeks: a better outcome[59,60] can usually be anticipated by surgically removing the residual necrotic tissue and any granulation tissue by tangential excision[61] and applying a skin graft. In many instances it is obvious immediately or within several days as to whether spontaneous healing will occur within 3 or

4 weeks. Among wounds in which the subtle differences between superficial and deep partial-thickness burns are not initially discernable, by 2 weeks after injury it is usually apparent whether or not the wound will heal spontaneously within the next 7–10 days. At 2 weeks after injury, those wounds which are devoid of necrotic tissue and have evidence of squamous reepithelization will usually heal spontaneously within the desirable time frame. The beginning of reepithelization can be detected by seeing tiny opalescent islands of epithelium throughout the wound (see **Figure 4.3**).

Infection and Use of Systemic Antibiotics

There is no evidence that systemic antibiotic prophylaxis will decrease the incidence of infection in small burn wounds.[62] Antibiotics should be used when there is evidence of infection.

The burn itself elicits inflammation. Therefore, the early manifestation of infection in the wound may be quite subtle. Mild erythema, edema, pain, and tenderness, all classic signs of infection, may be present without infection. However, when these manifestations increase over baseline, especially in the presence of lymphangitis and fever, treatment for infection should be instituted. Mainstays of treatment for infection include elevation and rest of the infected wound to control swelling and systemic antibiotic therapy. If the infection progresses the patient should be hospitalized and antibiotics given intravenously.

Infections in the outpatient setting are usually caused by common skin flora. Those most frequently implicated are staphylococci. If there is evidence of infection a culture of the surface of the wound should be obtained to identify the offending organism and narrow the spectrum of antibiotic therapy. While some burn care physicians advocate the use of burn wound biopsy quantitative culture rather than a wound surface culture,[63] this author has not found biopsy cultures to be necessary in the treatment of outpatient burns.

Among patients with burns treated in an ambulatory setting, it is quite unusual to develop systemic sepsis. However, patients should be instructed to take their temperature twice daily, once in the morning shortly after they get up from sleep, and again late in the afternoon before they eat supper. Localized infection will be reflected in fever in the afternoon. Sustained fever is suggestive of systemic sepsis. Temperatures above 38°C, especially if accompanied by symptoms of malaise and anorexia, should be reported to the physician and the patient called in for examination.

A change in the appearance of the wound during the first several days is more likely to indicate a decrease in perfusion of the wound than wound infection. This is frequently observed with scald burns. Any further burn wound discoloration, such as the appearance of gray or black spots, especially if there are other manifestations of infection, should raise concern for invasive infection. This rarely occurs among those treated as outpatients. However, if it does occur, the patient should be hospitalized, the wound biopsied for histologic and microbiological studies,[64] and treatment for infection instituted.

Burns, even minor ones, are tetanus-prone wounds.[65] Tetanus prophylaxis should be provided unless the patient has received tetanus immunization within 5 years.[66]

Pruritus

Itching is an annoying, often unrelenting manifestation of healing and healed burn wounds.

Most burn patients develop pruritus. The incidence is higher among children. The lower extremities are most frequently affected and more frequently than the upper. The face is seldom involved.[67]

Postburn itching interferes with everything. Scratching often results in repetitive superficial wounding of both skin-grafted and spontaneously healed wounds. Triggered and enhanced by environmental extremes, especially heat, physical activity, and stress, pruritus is most intense in the period immediately after wounds are healed. In most instances, it gradually diminishes and eventually stops. There are a few patients in whom it persists beyond 18 months. Patients with prolonged and chronic itching may harbor a psychogenic component.

The sensation of itch is most likely a primary sensory modality rather than, as widely held in the past, a *forme fruste* of pain.[68] Histamine, whose synthesis is known to be increased in healing and inflamed wounds,[69] as well as bradykinin and a series of endopeptides, have all been implicated in the genesis of itching.[70,71] Because the precise mechanism of pruritus is not known, the likelihood is that there are multiple causative factors.

Since there are no controlled trials defining the best treatment, management is by trial and error. However, antihistamines, cool compress, and lotions are the corner stones of most attempts to relieve burn-related itching. The antihistaminic diphenhydramine hydrochloride is the most frequently prescribed first treatment.[72] This drug has an added benefit of providing mild sedation. Other antihistamines, such as cyproheptadine hydrochloride, may also be tried. Analgesics of any kind may be helpful by altering perception of itching in the central nervous system. Combinations of antihistamines and analgesics may be tried. Many patients find comfort in an air-conditioned environment. Cool compresses also may temporarily interrupt the itching cycle. A variety of topical agents, including aloe vera,[73] which has antiinflammatory and antimicrobial properties and skin moisturizing creams, such as Vaseline Intensive Care®, Eucerin®, Nivea®, mineral oil, cocoa butter, and even lard, have been effective. Any lotion free of alcohol is probably helpful. Hydroxyzine hydrochloride, a drug used to provide relief from anxiety and emotional tension, is used by many to help ameliorate itching. In addition, many patients prefer loose, soft clothing made from cotton.

The staff at the Shriners Burns Hospital, Galvaston, Texas, uses the following protocol for the treatment of itching.

Step 1: Use moisturizing body shampoo and lotions.
Step 2: Diphenhydramine 1.25 mg/kg/dose PO q 4 h scheduled.
Step 3: Hydroxyzine 0.5 mg/kg/dose PO q 6 h *and* diphenyhydramine 1.25 mg/kg/dose PO q 6 h. Alternate medication so that patient is receiving one itch medicine every 3 hours while awake.
Step 4: Hydroxyzine 0.5 mg/kg/dose PO q 6 h *and* cyproheptadine 0.1 mg/kg/dose PO q 6 h *and* diphenhydramine 1.25 mg/kg/dose PO q 6 h. Alternate medication so that patient is receiving one itch medicine every 2 hours while awake.

Phillips and Robson[74] advocate using penicillin in pruritus management. They observed that postburn hypertrophic scars were much more frequently colonized with beta-hemolytic streptococcus, *Staphylococcus aureus*, and *Staph. epidermidis* compared to matched healed wounds without hypertrophic scarring. Therefore, to decrease the inflammation caused by these microorganisms, a root cause of itching, they used the following regimen: low-dose oral penicillin, 250 mg twice daily, to control the beta-hemolytic streptococcus, and applied an aloe vera cream. As noted above, aloe vera has both anti-inflammatory and antimicrobial properties.

Traumatic Blisters in Reepitheliazed Wounds

As the wounds reepitheliazed, the delicate thin layer of epithelium is fragile and easily damaged. Itching and other mild forms of trauma may cause small blisters. Patients need to be cautioned about this potential and assured that the epithelium will gain strength and that this will not be a long-term problem. If these blisters rupture, leaving small superficial wounds, the wounds may be left exposed to form a crust. Alternatively, Adaptic® or Xeroform® and a light dressing or one of the hydrocolloid wafer products may be used.

Rehabilitative Physical Care

Measures to preserve strength and restore function should be incorporated into the initial treatment plan when the patient is first seen.[75] Before leaving emergency care, the patient's physical activity should be discussed and a program for range of motion exercises and muscle strengthening outlined – both verbally and in writing.

At each subsequent follow-up visit, function and strength should be assessed. If there is lack of compliance or if the patient's function begins to deteriorate, the patient should be referred for supervised physical or occupational therapy, or both. If the injury extends across a joint, or involves the hand or distal portion of the lower extremity, it is advisable to have therapists involved from the outset. When there are burns of the face that have the potential for facial dysfunction, it may be prudent to have the patient evaluated and treated by a speech pathologist.

The potential for development of contractures and hypertrophic scars among the burned treated as outpatients is the same as for those treated as in-patients.[75] The principles of prevention and treatment of these complications apply in both settings.

Outpatient treatment of moderate and major burns

Some patients classified as having moderate or even major burn injuries (**Table 4.1**)[76] are suitable for treatment in the ambulatory setting.[77] The purported advantages include less cost, less chance of exposure to antibiotic-resistant microorganisms, and a more psychologically comfortable environment for the patient. In spite of these benefits, caution should be exercised in selecting patients with moderate and major thermal injury for early discharge from the hospital. On the other hand, as convalescence progresses, many of these patients can have the terminal phase of their acute burn care completed safely as outpatients.

The conditions that need to be met in order to consider ambulatory care for any patient include: intravenous fluid resuscitation must be completed; there must be no ongoing complication; there must be no wound or systemic manifestation of sepsis; adequate enteral nutrition must be established; and pain control must be satisfactory with medication taken by mouth. Additionally, arrangements need to be made for wound care and physical and/or occupational therapy.

Table 4.1 Classification of burn severity

Minor burn

15% TBSA or less in adults

10% TBSA or less in children and the elderly

2% TBSA or less full-thickness burn in children or adults without cosmetic or functional risk to eyes, ears, face, hands, feet, or perineum

Moderate burn

15–25% TBSA in adults with less than 10% full-thickness burn

10–20% TBSA partial-thickness burn in children under 10 and adults over 40 years of age with less than 10% full-thickness burn.

10% TBSA or less full-thickness burn in children or adults without cosmetic or functional risk to eyes, ears, face, hands, feet, or perineum

Major burn

25% TBSA or greater

20% TBSA or greater in children under 10 and adults over 40 years of age

10% TBSA or greater full-thickness burn

All burns involving eyes, ears, face, hands, feet, or perineum that are likely to result in cosmetic or cosmetic impairment

All high-voltage electrical burns

All burn injury complicated by major trauma or inhalation injury

All poor risk patients with burn injury

TBSA, total body surface area.

Acknowledgments

Martha George, BA, Alden H Harken, MD, and Maureen L Smith, RN, MSN provided valuable assistance in the preparation of this manuscript.

References

1. Brigham PA. *Burn Incidence and Treatment in the United States: 2000 Fact Sheet.* Chicago, IL: American Burn Association, 2000.
2. Saffle JR, Davis B, Williams P. Recent outcomes in the treatment of burn injury in the United States: report from the American Burn Association Patient Registry. *J Burn Care Rehabil* 1995; 16: 219–32.
3. Rosenberg NM, Marino D. Frequency of suspected abuse/neglect in burn patients. *Pediatr Emerg Care* 1989; 5: 219–21.
4. Guzzetta PC, Randolph J. Burns in children: 1982 *Ped Rev* 1983; 4: 271–8.
5. Uchiyama N, German J. Pediatric considerations. In: Achauer BM, ed. *Management of the Burned Patient.* Norwalk, CT: Appleton & Lange, 1987: 203–9.
6. Evans EI, Purnell OJ, Robinett PW, Batchelor A, Martin, M. Fluid and electrolyte requirements in severe burns. *Ann Surg* 1952; 135: 804–15.
7. Lund CC, Browder NC. The estimate of areas of burns. *Surg Gynecol Obstet* 1944; 79: 352–8.
8. Herndon DN, Rutan RL, Rutan TC. Management of the pediatric patient with burns. *J Burn Care Rehabil* 1993; 14: 3–8.
9. deCamara DL, Raine TJ, London MD, Robson MC, Heggers JP. Progression of thermal injury: a morphologic study. *Plast Reconstr Surg* 1982; 69: 491–9.
10. Gatti JE, LaRossa D, Silverman DG, Hartford CE. Evaluation of the burn wound with perfusion fluorometry. *J Trauma* 1983; 23: 202–6.
11. Krob MJ, D'Amico FJ, Ross DL. Do trauma scores accurately predict outcomes for patients with burns? *J Burn Care Rehabil* 1991; 12: 560–3.
12. Heimbach DM, Waeckerle JF. Inhalation injuries. *Ann Emerg Med* 1988; 17: 1316–20.
13. Thompson PB, Herndon DN, Traber DL, Abston S. Effect of mortality of inhalation injury. *J Trauma* 1986; 26: 163–5.
14. McManus WF, Pruitt BA Jr. Thermal injuries. In: Mattox KL, Moore EE, Feliciano DV, eds. *Trauma.* Norwalk, CT: Appleton & Lange, 1988: 675–89.
15. Waymack JP, Pruitt BA Jr. Burn wound care. *Adv Surg* 1990; 23: 261–89.
16. Moylan JA Jr, Inge WW Jr, Pruitt BA Jr. Circulatory changes following circumferential extremity burns evaluated by the ultrasonic flowmeter: an analysis of 60 thermally injured limbs. *J Trauma* 1971; 11: 763–70.
17. Hooker DR, Kouvenhoven WB, Langworthy OR. The effect of alternating electrical currents on the heart. *Am J Physiol* 1933; 103: 444–54.
18. Solem L, Fischer RP, Strate RG. The natural history of electrical injury. *J Trauma* 1977; 17: 487–92.
19. Baxter CR. Present concepts in the management of major electrical injury. *Surg Clin N Am* 1970; 50: 1401–18.
20. Curreri PW, Asch MJ, Pruitt BA Jr. The treatment of chemical burns: specialized diagnostic, therapeutic, and prognostic considerations. *J Trauma* 1970; 10: 634–42.
21. van Rensburg LC. An experimental study of chemical burns. *S Afr Med J* 1962; 36: 754–9.
22. Gruber RP, Laub DR, Vistnes LM. The effect of hydrotherapy on the clinical course and pH of experimental cutaneous chemical burns. *Plast Reconstr Surg* 1975; 55: 200–4.
23. Dibbell DG, Iverson RE, Jones W, Laub DR, Madison MS. Hydrofluoric acid burns of the hand. *J Bone Joint Surg* 1970; 52-A: 931–6.
24. Greco RJ, Hartford CE, Haith LR Jr, Patton ML. Hydrofluoric acid-induced hypocalcemia. *J Trauma* 1988; 28: 1593–6.
25. Moritz AR, Henriques FC Jr. Studies of thermal injury II. The relative importance of time and surface temperature in the causation of cutaneous burns. *Am J Pathol* 1947; 23: 695–720.
26. Davies JW. Prompt cooling of burned area: a review of benefits and the effector mechanisms. *Burns Incl Therm Inj* 1982; 9: 1–6.
27. Blomgren I, Eriksson E, Bagge U. The effect of different colling temperatures and immersion fluids on post-burn oedema and survival of the partially scalded hairy mouse ear. *Burns Incl Therm Inj* 1985; 11: 161–5.
28. Saranto JR, Rubayi S, Zawacki BE. Blisters, cooling, antithromboxanes, and healing in experimental zone-of-stasis burns. *J Trauma* 1983; 23: 927–33.
29. Jandera V, Hudson DA, deWet PM, Innes PM, Rode H. Cooling the burn wound: evaluation of different modalities. *Burns* 2000; 26: 256–70.
30. Swada Y, Urushidate D, Yotsuyangl T, Ishita K. Is prolonged and excessive cooling of a scalded wound effective? *Burns* 1997; 23: 55–8.
31. Demling RH, Mazess RB, Wolberg W. The effect of immediate and delayed cool immersion on burn edema formation and resorption. *J Trauma* 1979; 19: 56–60.
32. King TC, Zimmerman JM. First-aid cooling of the fresh burn. *Surg Gynecol Obstet* 1965; 120: 1271–3.
33. Ofeigsson OJ. Water cooling: first-aid treatment for scalds and burns. *Surgery* 1965; 57: 391–400.
34. Pushkar NS, Sandorminsky BP. Cold treatment of burns. *Burns Incl Thermal Inj* 1982; 9: 101–10.
35. Purdue GF, Layton TR, Copeland CE. Cold injury complicating burn therapy. *J Trauma* 1985; 25: 167–8.
36. Osgood PF, Szyfelbein SK. Management of burn pain in children. *Pediatrc Clin N Am* 1989; 36: 1001–13.
37. Goldstein JA. Mechanism of induction of hepatic drug metabolizing enzymes: recent advances. *Trends Pharmacol Sci* 1984; 5: 290.
38. Jaffe JH. Drug addiction and drug abuse. In: Gilman AG, Rall TW, Nies AS, Taylor P, eds. *Goodman and Gilman's The Pharmacological Basis of Therapeutics*, 8th edn. New York: Pergamon Press, 1990: 522–73.
39. Swain AH, Azadian BS, Wakeley CJ, Shakespeare PG. Management of blisters in minor burns. *Br Med J (Clin Res)* 1987; 295: 181.
40. Rockwell WB, Ehrlich HP. Should burn blister fluid be evacuated? *J Burn Care Rehabil* 1990; 11: 93–5.
41. Demling RH, LaLonde C. Burn trauma. In: Blaisdell FW, Trunkey DD, eds. *Trauma Management*, Vol. IV. New York: Thieme Medical, 1989: 55–6.
42. Demling RH. Burns. *N Engl J Med* 1985; 313: 1389–98.
43. Stratta RJ, Saffle JR, Kravitz M, Warden GD. Management of tar and asphalt injuries. *Am J Surg* 1983; 146: 766–9.
44. Demling RH, Buerstatte WR, Perea A. Management of hot tar burns. *J Trauma* 1980; 20: 242.
45. Ashbell TS, Crawford HH, Adamson JE, Horton CE. Tar and grease removal from injured parts. *Plast Reconstr Surg* 1967; 40: 330–1.
46. Hartford CE. The bequests of Moncrief and Moyer: an appraisal of topical therapy of burns – 1981 American Burn Association presidential address. *J Trauma* 1981; 21: 827–34.
47. Hunter GR, Chang FC. Outpatient burns: prospective study. *J Trauma* 1976; 16: 191–5.
48. Miller SF. Outpatient management of minor burns. *Am Fam Physician* 1977; 16: 167–72.
49. Nance FC, Lewis VL Jr, Hines JL, Barnett DP, O'Neill JA. Aggressive outpatient care of burns. *J Trauma* 1972; 12: 144–6.

50. Heinrich JJ, Brand DA, Cuono CB. The role of topical treatment as a determinant of infection in outpatient burns. *J Burn Care Rehabil* 1988; **9**: 253–7.

51. Haynes BW Jr. Outpatient burns. *Clinics Plastic Surg* 1974; **1**: 645–51.

52. Gerding RL, Emerman CL, Effron D, Lukens T, Imbembo AL, Fratianne, RB. Outpatient management of partial-thickness burns: Biobrane® versus 1% silver sulfadiazine. *Ann Emerg Med* 1990; **19**: 121–4.

53. Barret JP, Dziewulski P, Ramy PI, Wolf SE, Desi MH, Herndon DN. Biobrane versus 1% silver sulfadiazine in second-degree pediatric burns. *Plast Reconstr Surg* 2000; **105**: 62–5.

54. Tavis MJ, Thornton JW, Bartlett RH, Roth JC, Woodroof EA. A new composite skin prosthesis. *Burns Incl Thermal Inj* 1980; **7**: 123–30.

55. Wyatt D, McGowan DN, Najarian MP. Comparison of a hydrocolloid dressing and silver sulfadiazine cream in the outpatient management of second-degree burns. *J Trauma* 1990; **30**: 857–65.

56. Hermans MH. Hydrocolloid dressing (Duoderm) for the treatment of superficial and deep partial thickness burns. *Scand J Plast Reconstr Surg Hand Surg* 1987; **21**: 283–5.

57. Matsen FA III. *Compartmental Syndromes.* New York: Grune & Stratton, 1980: 57–8.

58. Deitch EA, Wheelahan TM, Rose MP, Clothier J, Cotter J. Hypertrophic burn scars: analysis of variables. *J Trauma* 1983; **23**: 895–8.

59. Engrav LH, Heimbach DM, Reus JL, Harnar TJ, Marvin JA. Early excision and grafting vs. nonoperative treatment of burns of indeterminant depth: a randomized prospective study. *J Trauma* 1983; **23**: 1001–4.

60. Burke JF, Bondoc CC, Quinby WC Jr, Remensnyder JP. Primary surgical management of the deeply burned hand. *J Trauma* 1976; **16**: 593–8.

61. Janvekovic Z. A new concept in the early and immediate grafting of burns. *J Trauma* 1970; **10**: 1103–8.

62. Durtschi MB, Orgain C, Counts GW, Heimbach DM. A prospective study of prophylactic penicillin in acutely burned hospitalized patients. *J Trauma* 1982; **22**: 11–14.

63. Loebl EC, Marvin JA, Heck EL, Curreri PW, Baxter CR. The method of quantitative burn-wound biopsy cultures and its routine use in the care of the burned patient. *Am J Clin Pathol* 1974; **61**: 20–4.

64. Pruitt BA Jr. The diagnosis and treatment of infection in the burn patient. *Burns Incl Thermal Inj* 1984; **11**: 79–91.

65. Larkin JM, Moylan JA. Tetanus following a minor burn. *J Trauma* 1975; **15**: 546–8.

66. Committee on Trauma, American College of Surgeons. *A Guide to Prophylaxis Against Tetanus in Wound Management*, 1984 revision. The American College of Surgeons, 1984.

67. Bell L, McAdams T, Morgan R, *et al.* Pruritus in burns: a descriptive study. *J Burn Care Rehabil* 1988; **9**: 305–8.

68. Herndon JH Jr. Itching: the pathophysiology of pruritus. *Int J Dermatol* 1975; **14**: 465–84.

69. Kahlsen G, Rosengren E. New approaches to the physiology of medicine. *Physical Rev* 1968; **48**: 155–96.

70. Keele CA, Armstrong D. *Substances Producing Pain and Itch.* London: Edward Arnold, 1964: 297–8.

71. Robson MC, Jellema A, Heggers JP, Hagstrom WJ. Care of the healed burn wound: a prospective randomized study. San Antonio, TX: American Burn Association, 1980; 94 (Abstract).

72. Gordon MD. Pruritus in burns. *J Burn Care Rehabil* 1988; **9**: 305–11.

73. Heimbach DM, Engrav LH, Marvin J. Minor burns: guidelines for successful outpatient management. *Postgrad Med* 1981; **69**: 22–32.

74. Phillips LG, Robson MC. Comments from Detroit Receiving Hospital, Detroit, Michigan. *J Burn Care Rehabil* 1988; **9**: 308–9.

75. Helm PA, Kevorkian G, Lushbaugh M, Pullium G, Head MD, Cromes GF. Burn injury: rehabilitation management in 1982. *Arch Phys Med Rehabil* 1982; **63**: 6–16.

76. Guidelines for service standards and severity classification in the treatment of burn injury. Appendix B to Hospital Resources Document. *ACS Bulletin* 1984; **69**: 25–8.

77. Warden GD, Kravitz M, Schnebly A. The outpatient management of moderate and major thermal injury. *J Burn Care Rehabil* 1981; **2**: 159–61.

Chapter 5

Burn disaster management

Thomas L Wachtel

Introduction

Burns are among the worst trauma problems that can befall man. When fire encounters objects and materials that burn, they are destroyed in a relatively short time. The action of fire on living organisms may be lethal within a few seconds. If a fire is not immediately lethal, it initiates a pathological condition called a burn that is considered the most complex trauma that can assail a human organism.[1] The larger a burn injury, the more severe the consequences and the higher the chance of an adverse outcome or even death. The utilization of resources for burned patients is extraordinarily high as well, when compared to other trauma victims.[2] In addition, advances in science and technology have increased the risk of accidents that result in a transfer of thermal energy to people located nearby. The number of casualties from such accidents increases as more powerful sources of energy are harnessed.[3] Because of growth in the fields of transportation and technology, we are now confronted with a potentially rapid growth in the absolute number of burns a mass disaster as well as an increase in the possible dangers surrounding the use of thermic energy of unprecedented power such that the magnitude and consequences could be appalling.[4–7] The potential for modern-day fire catastrophes involving urban areas, high-rise buildings, large crowds collected at community events, and worldwide terrorism poses a serious challenge to fire technology and to society.[8] Such disasters normally exceed the resources of local health care providers and facilities.[3]

A disaster is a situation where there are unforeseen serious and immediate threats to public health.[9] Masellis has divided the management of rescue operations into two separate entities – thermal agent (fire) disaster and burn disaster. They are linked by the common denominator of fire as well as causal force (**Figure 5.1**). A fire disaster is a serious and sudden vast ecological breakdown in the relationship between man and his environment on such a scale that the stricken community needs extraordinary efforts to cope with the disaster, and often requires outside help or international aid.[10] There have been 25 such fires in the United States in the 20th century that have caused tremendous destruction of life and property. These sentinel fires have led to changes in public opinion and important advances in fire prevention.[8] Fire disasters include losses of material goods and losses of human life resulting from massive heat production. These losses can be quantified by the extent of damage to material property and the number of people who are injured and dead.[1] One specific aspect of a fire disaster is that the number of people involved is always high. A fire causing 25 or more deaths is termed a fire catastrophe.[8] Fire disasters with large numbers of burned victims will escalate clinical care and logistical problems several fold and require application of the principles of disaster management.[11] The consequences of a major fire disaster can be broadly predicted, even though specific measures for dealing with injured victims will vary from region to region.[12] For example, of all disasters with more than 20 dead at the scene, 70% are classified as explosions and fires due to train crashes, air crashes, and underground disasters.[9] The most severe

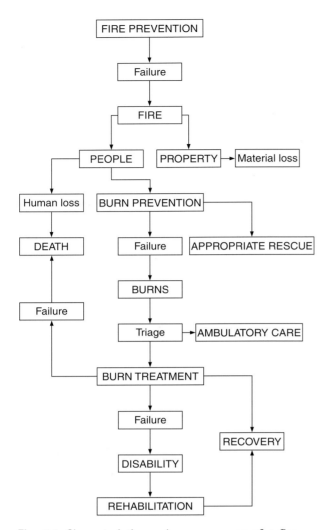

Fig. 5.1 Characteristics and consequences of a fire. Disasters increase the magnitude of the human and material losses and damages.

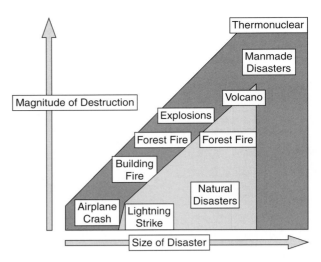

Fig. 5.2 Burn disaster sources and magnitude of destruction.

A major disaster plan is intended to provide optimal treatment of victims of a major accident when there are too many patients to be treated by routine emergency services.[15] The number of people injured in a burn disaster is defined as the sum of the number admitted to hospitals with burns and the number killed outright.[9,12] For rural and wilderness areas, that number may be as few as one or two. For an urban burn center, in a large tertiary hospital, the ability to care for a larger number of burned victims may be enhanced. Eventually, however, even the resources of a sophisticated burns center in a multispecialty hospital within a mature trauma system will become exhausted, and the previous planning, preparedness, training, response, relief, rehabilitation, and reconstruction for a major burn emergency or burn disaster situation will be overwhelmed.[16] The solution will require either secondary triage of burned victims to other more distant burn and tertiary facilities (**Figure 5.3**) or transportation of staff, supplies, and equipment to the site of the disaster.[2] The management of mass burns remains a highly complex problem of organization.[6] The characteristics and principles of a burn disaster are shown in **Table 5.1**.

Very large disasters remain uncommon.[12] Despite the potential for mass disasters, conflagrations have become less frequent in the US since the 1940s.[8] The incidence of major fires in Europe, however, has increased in recent years.[12] The severity of injuries among those admitted to hospitals suggests that either victims were able to escape rapidly and, thus, sustained relatively small burns (<30% total body surface area [TBSA]) to exposed areas of skin, or that timely escape was impossible and victims were engulfed and sustained lethal injuries (>70% TBSA).[12] One explanation is that a great number of victims are trapped in indoor fires and failed to escape. The morbidity and elevated immediate death rate in indoor disasters was mainly due to hypoxia, inhalation injuries, intoxication, and inhalation of poisonous compounds.[9,17] The effect of hydrogen cyanide and carbon monoxide has been postulated as a cause of incapacity and inability to react, and accounts for high indoor death rates.[9] No rescue people reached the severely injured in time.[9]

of such fires are liquefied petroleum gas disasters.[9] Local factors will influence exactly how the victims are managed in a burn disaster. Burn disaster management is necessary when the number of burn casualties exceeds local resources.

A burn disaster can be defined as the overall effect of massive action from a known thermal agent on living people. It is characterized by an excessive number of seriously burned patients with a high rate of disability and death[1] (**Figure 5.1**). Burn disasters are most frequently man-made as opposed to natural disasters (e.g. a volcanic eruption, lightning strike) and, in general, are comparatively confined to a limited geographical area (**Figure 5.2**). Earthquake-related flame burns and scalds are infrequent, but when they occur they are usually combined with mechanical trauma.[13] The initial information needed in order to respond to a disaster revolves around a definition of the event and the geography in question. This includes information about the location as well as means of access to the location, such as points of egress from a room, a building, a field, a town or a country.[14]

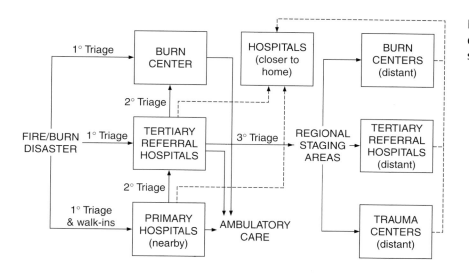

Fig. 5.3 Triage scheme for a fire/burn disaster: 1° = primary; 2° = secondary; 3° = tertiary.

Table 5.1 Characteristics and principles of a burns disaster[1]

The place the disaster occurs is not always accessible and care and assistance may not be adequate

The time interval between the accident and initiation of care must be less than 2 hours

The burns are mainly very extensive and the general condition of the victims is precarious

Triage of victims must be effected only by specialists, as only specialists are able to evaluate the immediate gravity of the burn

Inhalation of combustion gases, fumes, and hot air causes damage to the airways; and this alone can jeopardize survival

Hypovolemic shock induces a state of tissue hypoxia with irreversible damage to various organs and systems

The burn is often associated with other serious problems such as vast wounds, fractures, electrical injuries, or blast injury lesions

The overall assessment of the damage to people must be made not only on the basis of the number of dead but also on the number of people burned and suffering risk of disability

---

The diversity of fire disasters serves to illustrate the scale and nature of problems faced by medical services in dealing with mass burn casualties.[12,18–20] For truly effective disaster management, the key is prevention and preparedness rather than a *post hoc* fire fighting type of emergency response.[10,21] Disaster medicine is the study of collaborative applications of various health disciplines to the prevention, immediate response to, and rehabilitation of health problems that arise from a disaster.[10] For this kind of scientific approach and technical underpinning, special studies, surveys and applied research, social and natural science investigations, and managerial applications are necessary[10] (**Table 5.2**). Training people for disaster management requires courses on disaster health, in addition to innate humanitarian compassion.[10] Furthermore, epidemiology has proved most promising in disaster management.[10] Disaster epidemiology links data collection, analysis of the disaster, analysis of risk factors for adverse social and health effects, clinical investigation of the impact of diagnostic and therapeutic methods, the effectiveness of various types of the assistance, and the long-term influence of relief operations on restoration of pre-disaster conditions.[10] Practical application of disaster medicine is a continuous cycle of planning for disasters, exercising the plan, utilizing the practiced plan should a disaster arise, and examining the response to either an exercise or a real disaster in detail in an after-action assessment (**Figure 5.4**).

The disaster plan

Fortunately, few people will have a chance to exercise their disaster plan in a real burn disaster, but everyone must plan for such a contingency. The burn component must be integrated into overall local, regional, national, and international disaster plans. Effective disaster planning will not only lessen property loss and social disruption caused by disaster impacts, but will also reduce suffering and the distress of casualities.[22] Despite evidence available from past disasters, adequate provision for the management of burned casualties is still lacking in most disaster plans.[12] Disaster planning should emphasize that most burns are either minor or very extensive.[22] New developments in the organization of emergency

Table 5.2 The 10 principles for the scientific basis of disaster management[10]

Prevention
Preparedness
Disaster profiles
Disease patterns
Planning and preparation for effective multidisciplinary response
Mobilization of multisectorial manpower resources
Risk assessment
Post-emergency phase
Reconstructive phase
Community and local/national institution involvement

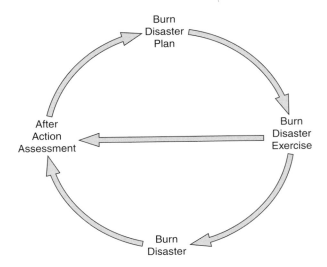

Fig. 5.4 The cycle of burn disaster management.

medical service systems dictate that new approaches to disaster planning preparedness are essential in order to implement current concepts of emergency medical care delivery.[11,14] The important aspects of modern disaster management from the medical perspective include:

- the utilization of medical triage and treatment protocols in order to effect control and transportation of patients;
- early notification of all hospitals that could potentially receive patients;
- transportation of patients to appropriate hospitals utilizing an existing point-of-entry plan.

This enables burn victims to be transported to facilities with burn treatment capability and available beds.[14] Three distinct phases of relief operations are necessary: immediate assistance, first aid, and organized relief. Immediate assistance is provided in the first 2–3 hours by people on the spot (trained volunteers, physicians, and nurses) and is fundamental to the prognosis of fire disaster victims. A timely, rational, safe, and effective intervention is the main guarantee *quo ad vitam* for the victims of a fire disaster.[10] A more complex body of organized relief may not be able to reach a disaster scene for at least 6 or 7 hours. Entire systems must be tested in training programs so that they are made intelligible to the public, supported by management resources, implemented properly, and promulgated to all potential first rescue workers.[23] When burn casualties exceed the local ability to provide adequate care, a major disaster should be declared so that facilities can prepare for upcoming casualties.[2]

Not all fire disasters result in mass burn casualties.[12] However, when a burn disaster involves many hundreds of patients, it will usually be necessary to have burn teams from many countries participate in order to achieve optimal care for burned victims.[3,24] Collaboration is possible, especially when such teams have made advance plans for transporting their team and equipment to a site many thousands of kilometers from their home bases.[3] The joint work of the Soviet and US physicians during the Ufa train explosion demonstrates the efficacy of international cooperation. In planning for the care of victims of future disasters, such international cooperation should be illustrious.[25]

Planning aimed at mitigating the effects on people (in terms of suffering, disability, and risk to life) must be related to a more complete evaluation of involved damage.[1] The operational rescue plan must be developed along three lines: immediate care, medical rescue within 3 hours, and use of specific equipment and means for the rescue of burned patients. Factors that influence the evolution of a disaster include:[1]

- the unpredictability of when disasters occur;
- the moment of a disaster (day/night, festivity, etc.);
- the characteristics of a disaster (explosion, collapse of building, production of toxic gases and fumes, forest fire, etc.);
- the area where a disaster occurs (city, non-urban area, accessibility, presence of material suitable for relief operations, etc.);
- the type of building involved (civil dwelling, hotel, office, hospital, etc.);
- the number of people injured and the type of trauma;
- the population's degree of preparedness to manage a disaster situation.

Communication

Online voice communication with a trauma center, trauma surgeon, burn center, burn coordinator, and burn surgeon is important. Disaster plans should utilize existing communication venues and have the ability to expand (i.e. bring in additional equipment and staff). Communications must be fast, practiced, and limited in scope. A point-of-entry plan must communicate the type of disaster: burns, burns and other trauma, trauma, spinal cord injuries, acute medical complications, poisoning, behavioral crisis, neonatal patients, or pediatric victims. A consideration that impacts on incident management is the existence and utilization of a centralized reporting and notification mechanism,[14] such as the enhanced 911 centralized communication system for fire, police, and emergency medical services in the United States. The system should have the capability to contact metropolitan area ambulance services and hospitals individually or collectively through the centralized communication system. This feature allows for central collection of hospital bed availability data, relay of relevant information on the status of the disaster to hospitals, centralized coordination of the disaster response, and direction of ambulances carrying triaged patients to appropriate facilities.[14] The benefits of a comprehensive system with a centralized communications component are shown in **Table 5.3**.

A central data bank that stores up-to-date information on the capacity of each burn center to accept patients is imperative for disaster management. Valuable information is also provided concerning hospital capability, intensive care/burn intensive care availability, equipment availability (fluidized beds, etc.), and technical procedures. The information should be utilized on a daily basis for the distribution of burns within the geographical area under nondisaster circumstances. Such a system can then be extremely useful in the event of a disaster when the distribution of patients is urgent. The French telematic data bank for burns also includes an epidemiologic file that forms the basis for prevention campaigns. It is compatible with the International Society for Burn

Table 5.3 Benefits of a comprehensive system with a centralized communications component[14]

Improved notification of the incident

Consistent initial and follow-up information

Timeliness of response

Better management of the incident

Accuracy in the collection of pertinent information concerning the incident

Analysis of the information to determine the correct level of response, triage to hospitals and specialty centers

Utilization of transport vehicles

Ultimate outcome of burned victims

Injuries and the European organization.[26] A German system that is used on a daily basis responds extremely well. It was not used primarily in the Ramstein air disaster, and that was a reason for criticism of their disaster management. It *was* used for secondary triage and for consultation on burned patients. The United States' system, National Disaster Management System (NDMS), was activated during Operation Desert Storm and is used by some regions for the distribution of burn patients. The Italian ARGO satellite system combines a coordination center, data collection center, transportation center, and burn center into a meshed sub-network. It is expandable and allows the organization to care for severely burned patients. The telecommunication system has high standards of reliability and survival to guarantee continuity of communications from and to a disaster area. It is divided into telephone, fax, video telecommunications networks, and a territorial data collection network. The information is continually updated and links with a national organization capable of rapid mobilization of carriers for the transport of patients. The ARGO satellite system allows immediate contact between specialized burn centers and the physicians treating patients in the disaster area so that support is available for staff in the field. It functions as a radio telephone in an ambulance and as an ordinary portable telephone carried by a physician.[27]

The Plan for a Disaster Scene

There is a practical need for a disaster plan.[28] Of the 14 disasters studied by Arturson, only in the San Juanico tragedy was a disaster plan in place.[9] Preventive measures were usually lacking in all disasters investigated, and mistakes were observed frequently.[9] Advance planning includes availability of well-trained leadership for disaster situations.[9] Sorting or triage is performed most effectively by a clinician experienced in the care of burns, as doctors without such experience frequently overestimate the proportion of the body surface burned.[2] Expert triage may minimize the requirement for specialized burn beds since moderate to severe burns, which are best cared for in specialized burn centers, seem to be fewer in numbers following severe fire disaster.[9] The French burn system, for example, incorporates this philosophy into a uniform triage system.[26] Where current disaster plans had been well rehearsed, effective dispersal, immediate care, and secondary transfer of severely burned patients was efficient and resulted in good outcomes.[29] When the plans are not rehearsed and expert triage is not present at the disaster site, the burden of triage falls on the nearest hospital.[30]

The initial task for a disaster plan is to forecast methods to iden-

tify all burned victims. A search and rescue effort involved in a disaster primarily revolves around finding, extricating, and/or transporting victims, including the injured and the dead as well as the noninjured.[22] Fire services are well positioned and structured to undertake this search and rescue role. They may need to be augmented with heavy rescue units and additional personnel. There should be significant pre-disaster planning and training for organized search and rescue, involving the fire service and a variety of local groups. Seldom does one specific community group assume complete responsibility. Timeliness is essential and stress inherent. Widespread damage to structures will result in large numbers of casualities and trapped people within an immediate disaster zone. It can be anticipated that people who are trapped will attempt to free themselves, and untrapped survivors will go to their aid. A concentrated effort to rescue trapped persons during the first few hours after a disaster will yield greater dividends in lives saved than any larger or more highly developed effort made later.[22] A larger burn disaster may require that trained rescuers operate solely in a supervisory role while large numbers of untrained workers are added to a trained nucleus in order to rapidly expand rescue capability.

Most disaster plans emphasize a restriction of treatment, at the site or in the emergency department/accident ward, to lifesaving measures and initial prioritization with early transfer to more sophisticated resources where reassessment can take place.[31] Prior disasters and international responses to them underscore the need for a coordinated response to major burn disasters and the positive results of international cooperation.[3,25] Delays in the dispersal of casualties may be avoided by prior planning, especially if international transfer of patients is envisioned.[12] Recent incidents involving mass burn casualties have demonstrated that the specific needs of severely burned victims demand a comprehensive plan that follows the guidelines of the Advanced Burn Life Support (ABLS) course for initial care, assessment of burn size and depth, resuscitation, evaluation for other injuries, care of the burn wound, etc.[32]

The positive effect of a previous disaster on the preparedness of the people involved is substantial.[33] A disaster plan must incorporate details of disasters occurring in several scenarios. These may be unique to an individual area, but all should include preparations for explosions.[9,19,28,31,34–38] Particular procedures regarding both medical assistance and general behavior, and those that rescue workers have to perform, must include educational campaigns, refresher courses, and training sessions aimed at citizens of every social extraction starting at school age.[1] As an example, burn disaster from a forest fire would depend on the fire typology; and the variability depends on meteorological conditions. Specific details for an incident command system that were developed for fighting forest fires in California, USA, are generally useful for organizing and implementing action for all fire and burn disasters, irregardless of size or complexity.[11] The essential figure is usually a firefighter, but other people may be involved.[39] The number of victims may range from only a dozen (France, 1986) to very many (71 dead, 2000 injured – Australia, 1983; 50 000 homeless – China, 1987).

A disaster response system can be activated for industrial accidents, such as those that occur at petrochemical industries, foundries, and the like.[40] The preparation phase is characterized by mapping the industries at risk of potential flammable or toxic substances most frequently used in an area and which transit avenues are used. This requires the collaboration of other experts such as engineers, chemists, physicists, toxicologists, etc., in order to coordinate all necessary data for potential fire disasters and effective disaster planning. A training phase should be carried out in close collaboration with agencies and people likely to be involved in self-protection, extinguishing of a fire, and rescue of burned victims. A didactic phase through organized meetings of volunteer personnel is required.[40] Burn centers and hospitals whose catchment area includes oil rigs or hazardous materials should plan for appropriate contingencies.[41]

A disaster plan may have to be tailored to meet the specific needs of an area or a site. In a fire disaster, the number of people involved may be so high that it is impossible to consider all victims for immediate transfer to existing specialized burn centers. Because of the limited number of beds available and because a disaster may occur some distance away,[3,42–44] the organization and establishment of a field hospital may be required. To be effective, a field hospital must have easy transport, rapid assembly, and the possibility of administering complete and effective treatment to patients. Multi-unit nomadic tents may offer the best facilities.[43,44] The reduced weights of these tents, their ease of packing, and their limited bulk represent considerable advantages, especially with regard to transportation and rapidity and simplicity of assembly. The modular composition means that their size can be adapted according to the effective needs of a disaster situation.[44] The organization and establishment of a field hospital must be based on a very precise predetermined plan that defines all the logistic and sanitary activities of a field hospital that are required to manage a disaster immediately and long term.[44]

It is important to exercise a disaster plan through coordination of simulated disasters (**Figure 5.4**) involving all of the relevant public safety agencies, prehospital ambulance providers, hospital-based personnel, and proceed-out teams.[14,21] As one team reported: 'The whole operation went very smoothly. This was partly because the staff had been through several "dummy runs" of a detailed civil accident procedure and partly because they had several hours to prepare for the first casualties to arrive.'[44]

Effective disaster management can only be accomplished when a thorough disaster planning process has been conducted.[45] Such a process must include all elements and all recognized emergency response and relief agencies that could play a role in responding to a disaster.[11,14,46,47] The most important outcome of a planning exercise is that each of the agencies be educated as to the roles and responsibilities of the others so that essential links between agencies can be established.[14]

Transportation: How Will They Arrive?

Transportation considerations depend on the number of victims and their conditions, identification of toxic substances, and other factors. Emergency transport of burned victims may be sporadic and *de novo* in a fire disaster, but more often it will involve medical rescue services such as fully equipped ambulances, helicopters, fixed wing aircraft, and water rescue craft. Most victims are transported by ground vehicles (ambulances, private vehicles, commandeered buses, trucks, etc.). For fire disasters that are up to 100 miles from medical facilities, the use of helicopter services that are fully equipped flying ambulances, often permanently based at hospitals and used exclusively for emergency purposes, are an invaluable mechanism for transport. Numerous factors have led to the creation and development worldwide of medical air

rescue services and, in particular, to the widespread use of helicopter services.[48] Over 300 hospitals in the world have their own helicopter ambulances and fixed wing aircraft used exclusively for emergency transport.[48] The Italian model of helicopter rescue service is acquiring growing recognition.[48] The Italian medical evacuation is made through a single nationwide telephone number in Italy that connects qualified multilingual personnel, including physicians and other specialists, to local rescue services, hospitals, civil and military authorities, and other organizations involved in disaster relief. A sophisticated software program provides, in real time, all necessary information for rescue operations within a specific region, and if the need arises, for inter-regional coordination and transport.[48,49]

The main aim of a helicopter rescue service is to guarantee prompt arrival (maximum time 20 minutes) of a medical team specialized in resuscitation and provided with all the equipment normally available in a hospital intensive care unit. The necessary emergency therapy can be carried out on the spot or continued during transport of a patient. The transport is not necessarily to the nearest hospital, but to the hospital best equipped to receive a patient.[48,50] The communication coordination system, activated by the regional operative headquarters, coordinates transportation by ground, helicopter, or a fixed wing aircraft for long-distance transport.

Under most circumstances, transportation must be carried out in coordination with other rescue organizations. The transport of a victim to the nearest hospital for more thorough assessment and life-saving treatment (e.g. airway management) may occur pending possible placement in a specialized burn center. This phase is often difficult because of lack of beds for burned patients in a region, especially in the case of those requiring extensive care, and must be planned in the transportation phase of a disaster plan.

Timing and coordination of transport of burned patients is critical;[51] and delays may occur, especially if national or international transportation by air is envisioned, unless communication and cooperation are assured by prior agreements.[12] The personnel and material conditions, as well as the mode of transport, should be an integral part of an emergency disaster plan. A burn team must consider the consequences of aeromedical transport in order to determine whether it is safe for a burned patient or what measures should be used in order to effect a safe transfer.[52] Burn casualties can best tolerate transfer on the day of the accident, so long as it does not take more than 60 minutes; and later transfers should take place by the end of the third or fourth post-accident day before sepsis can fully develop.[6] The result of an extensive traffic jam must be anticipated in a disaster plan since it may hinder the arrival of patients as well as physicians and staff who are not on duty, but who are inbound to staff or relieve current staff.[28] Long delays in transportation of patients have been the rule in most disasters.[9]

Facilities

The relative scarcity of specialized facilities and expertise for the treatment of extensive burns is of particular concern, such that involvement of distant centers may be anticipated following large disasters.[12] Even a moderate disaster might fill all available burn beds and saturate the total burn capacity of a wide area. It is vital to plan for supporting hospitals in a primary inner circle and for the designated burn centers and tertiary hospitals in an outer circle to be included[9,53] (see **Figure 5.3**). Following very large disasters, optimal care of severely burned victims will be achieved only if distant burn centers are also involved.[54] Prior awareness of the location and capacity of specialized facilities will enhance the successful dispersal of casualties.[55]

The role played by specialized burn treatment units is significant.[6] Burn centers seldom plan to have low levels of occupancy that would enable them to accommodate mass burn casualties, so the emergency plan for a burn center must include emergency evacuation of existing burn, trauma, surgical, and other patients to have available beds for mass burn casualties. The hospital must establish a control center, discharge or move patients to alternate care, organize beds for the incoming mass casualties, and pull in extra staff, often without the knowledge of how many casualties to expect. Multiple injuries, including burns and inhalation injuries, may occur in mass casualties from explosions. A burn center should receive logistical support from the sponsoring hospital in order to provide the best treatment for a large number of burned casualties. Logistical support requires work from the hospital staff who are concerned with sterilization, pharmacy, medical and nursing care, radiological diagnosis, and intensive care.[28] Little things, such as availability of urine dosimeters, are important!

Traditionally, hospitals have seen their role, during a burn disaster, as related to the medical management of patients admitted to them because of an incident. An expanded role has included sending teams of physicians and nurses to disaster scenes in order to aid in triage and medical management.[56,57] The role of a hospital in disaster management can be expanded further to include a strong focus on leadership within the medical component of a disaster. On-site medical management can be organized in one of two ways:

- via 'proceed-out teams' of physicians who go directly to the scene; or
- through medical direction given by radio to trained prehospital life support teams at the scene.[14]

Another responsibility that may be given to a hospital is the coordination with and medical guidance of the fire, rescue, police, and public safety components of a disaster response.[14] Few major hospitals have full comprehensive specialty services, including burn units; and major disaster plans should recognize such limitations and obtain prior consent for referral.[15] Within a hospital, the disaster plan must bring additional operating rooms online as needed for semi-urgent care of burned victims, while reserving one or two for lifesaving procedures that may be required. The goal is to match hospital resources with the needs of burned victims. In some cases, this will be driven by priorities; in others, a first-come-first-served basis will be installed.

As an alternative to designated burn centers, patients with burns may be managed in a general hospital without any particular facility for the management of burns.[58] In this case, a hospital disaster plan must be activated. The reception area and initial treatment area ought to be available for the majority of burned victims. Additional personnel should be summoned. A hospital is obliged to clear hospital beds, particularly on surgical wards and intensive care units, by transfer or discharge. If the expertise, supplies, and equipment are not adequate, secondary triage to adequate facilities is necessary.

Personnel

As part of an overall disaster plan, it must be ensured that a sufficient number of people have adequate training for initial resuscitation of burned victims. Often the medical and hospital staff that are willing to help have little experience in burn care. It has been found that training of personnel is rare, especially concerning communication links.[9] Training in preventive measures typically is absent, and disasters display the lack of training of personnel to cope with a tragedy.[9,35] Education concerning simple management of minor and moderate burns should be given on a broad basis to doctors and nurses outside of burn care facilities.[9] The Advanced Burn Life Support Course is an excellent tool for training such individuals.[32] Burn center staff must be available for advisory and consultation services by telephone or telex.[6] Expert triage is important, but health care professionals must be able to work effectively in primitive conditions together with other emergency helpers.[9] When admitting patients and rendering qualified specialized medical aid at a hospital, the participation of mixed physicians teams (surgeon, burn specialist, resuscitation, therapist, etc.) is advisable.

A plan that places a single care giver, usually a nurse, with each patient is optimal. That nurse, then, stays with a burned patient through all of the initial steps of care and insures intravenous (IV) fluid administration, pain control, tetanus toxoid administration, airway maintenance, ventilation, and documentation.

Often the first thing that is asked by a burn patient is to contact relatives.[59] That task should be delegated to someone other than hands-on care givers for the burn casualty, capable of understanding the burn injury and empathetic with relatives and friends. The handling of families, as well as mass media,[60,61] must be an integral part of every disaster plan. Major mass burn disasters, such as the Piper Alpha and Ramstein tragedies, involve the wounded and relatives from many countries.[41,59,63,64] Multilingual support personnel are essential under these circumstances.

Research on human behavior in critical situations has identified three different kinds of reaction: rational action, panic, and resignation. The two normal reactions when a way of escape can be seen are rational action and panic.[65] When positive action will lead to safety, resignation is a pathologic form of behavior. It is difficult to plan for the psychological reactions to a fire/burn disaster. The two main elements of this drama that have to be understood are the actual fire and the mass of people.[65] Nevertheless, experts with psychological training should be utilized for the development of psychological support for burn victims, their families and friends, rescue workers, and health care workers. Immediate sessions for debriefing of the rescue workers should be put in place. Psychological support for health care workers will be necessary because of their high levels of stress and extended hours of work. The psychological support teams in the fire and burn disaster simulations can help a team rehearse the decisions that must be made in the care of large numbers of burn casualties so that the team is less likely to suffer emotional stress at the precise moment when technical skill and emotional equilibrium are most needed.[65]

The effect of a previous disaster can have a profound effect on responsible staff.[33] The disasters in Armenia and Chernobyl emphasized to the Soviet Health Ministry officials the importance of having contingency plans made in advance of any accident. That experience led to the rapid triage and transport of victims from the accident site to medical centers in surrounding towns following the Ufa train disaster. The Soviet experience during the Ufa incident demonstrated that such an organization of public health services permitted the rendering of aid to the majority of victims in a rapid and appropriate time frame.[3] The Italian military have become interested in their role in disaster relief.[46,47] Physicians and other staff members who are not familiar with burn care must have some means to assess the extent of burns and initiate therapy. Vitale *et al.* have prepared a clinical file and protocol for general doctors and for nonspecialized hospital physicians to assist burn patients.[66] Such a file should be incorporated into a disaster plan.

Supplies/Equipment

A disaster plan must be tailored to the supplies and equipment that are available. For example, fiberoptic bronchoscopy may be useful in the early diagnosis of inhalation injury, but may not be available for use during a disaster.[28] An alternate plan for an individual hospital may be the need to transport some burn victims to facilities that have the capability of proper care due to the availability of appropriate equipment. Problems in rendering aid in such extreme situations exemplify the necessity of having an organization with a separate department of catastrophe medicine.[3] A plan must assure that the management of individual patients will be optimal under a variety of organizational structures. Compromises may be necessary in extreme circumstances, but the ideal is to develop a plan to avoid them whenever possible (i.e. patients with eyelid/facial burns are seen within 4 hours by an ophthalmic surgeon who has proper supplies and equipment or sufficient supplies and equipment are available to start physiotherapy within 48 hours).[58] Even when personnel are available, there may be a lack of specific materials. A practical kit for various procedures in the first few hours after severe burns is helpful.[67] It must incorporate the following basic features:[68]

- easy to transport to the scene of a disaster;
- easy to keep in good condition at a medical/surgical post;
- long-lasting;
- simple to use;
- robust and lightweight enough for air transport.

The contents of an emergency kit should be an integral part of a disaster preparation and be approved by burn experts on a planning committee. Preparing a kit that includes all the necessary supplies for initial care of burned patients is a significant investment of time and money to initiate and maintain. Air dropping a kit was lifesaving for immediate surgical treatment and resuscitation of burned victims in remote areas without direct access to rescue teams or made up for deficiencies in medicines and medical supplies in hospitals that have admitted people with severe burns who were not immediately transferable to other hospitals.[69] Pre-positioned supplies were of significant benefit at Landstuhl Army Hospital during the Ramstein air disaster.

Education

An educational program must be based on a precise method that starts with analysis of a problem of health and safety and then encompasses epidemiological, behavioral, and educational diagnoses.[70] Health education and training programs assume particular importance in burn disaster planning. They must include the clinical, technical, and operational aspects of a disaster. Implementation of these plans must follow well-defined programs of teaching at schools, starting with primary school level, through education at civil defense courses, periodic refresher courses for physicians, nurses, volunteers, Red Cross personnel, fire brigades, police, etc., in addition to periodic exercises with simulated fire

disasters that involve the general population and local rescue forces.[23,49] Training methods may use brochures, stickers, coloring albums, posters, notices, and a variety of audiovisual means, particularly videotapes. Videotapes can recreate and simulate situations and propose actions for assistance to victims.[23] An interactive video using ordinary documentary film with educational elements can train a student in prevention as well as every element of burn care. Multimedia presentations improve a user's attention and achieve greater educational effectiveness than a usual mono-medium message; and they should be used in initial as well as refresher courses.[23]

The level of prevention achieved depends on the number and effectiveness of public education and information programs that have been pursued.[70] The role of health education is to facilitate the learning of behavior patterns that will reduce risk factors and increase protection factors by means of identification of motivational elements related to behavior.[70]

Prevention

The most notable immediate reward for good burn disaster planning is the template that is established for burn prevention programs. Inspection of public buildings at the time of their initial construction and after any remodeling is necessary in order to ensure proper fire prevention methods. Failure to observe this axiom was crucial in the Stardust disaster.[71] Attention should be paid to methods of egress, as well as fire-fighting capability such as water hose reels and fire-resistant materials.[71] Posting fire escape plans within rooms of public buildings, providing adequate fire egress instructions and facilities, having fire drills in public facilities (schools, office building, hospitals,[19] operating rooms,[21] ships, airplanes,[18] etc.) are important aspects of training as well as prevention. There must be proper liaison between disaster planning departments and fire services. A fire department has to ensure that they have proper equipment to fight fires and rescue victims from all facilities in their catchment area, including high-rise buildings, hospitals, and schools. They should be aware of buildings with hazardous materials, fuel, and explosives in their area. Inspections must include adherence to statutory building regulations and the laws that make these regulations effective. Fire services and local authorities are required to be adequately staffed, properly equipped, and appropriately trained.

Trauma Systems

Burn centers should be integrated into large hospitals that are able to obtain assistance from several other specialty units from within the hospital.[28] Trauma centers must begin to fill the gap that exists between resources for emergency medical systems and a disaster response.[14] With leadership from trauma systems, meaningful planning can be accomplished among pre-hospital emergency medical systems, hospitals, and the public safety community.[14] This shift in disaster management responsibility from the public safety sector to the medical community incorporates advances made in the organization of emergency medical services.[14]

The disaster

A disaster plan is especially important for burned patients; and thus, it may be helpful to illustrate the operation of such plans through examples from actual major burn disasters. Most burn disasters and burn casualties occur in more urban and populated areas.[9,28,35,43,63,65,72] The Ural train–gas pipeline catastrophe was an exception.[3,36,37,73–75] Thus, the arrival of the first casualty will usually occur shortly after an incident; and the flow thereafter will be proportional to the number of casualties, the distance of the incident from the receiving facilities, the ease of triage, and the transportation available. The aim of all health workers concerned with mass burns is to give each burned patient the same care they would receive if they were the only patient burned and to save and cure as many of those afflicted as possible.[6] There may be overriding conditions that may make this impossible. It is imperative when this situation occurs that a reassessment of secondary triage to other burn care facilities be entertained. The operation of a rescue plan must take into account the types, kinds, and numbers of burn victims and the type of intervention required.[1]

Putting the Disaster Plan into Action

Immediate care is usually delivered by people on the scene of a disaster – relatives, friends, and passersby – people who may have witnessed the disaster or people who have arrived immediately at the scene. Their help is an automatic reaction derived from affection, friendship, or a spirit of human solidarity.[1] In the case of burn disasters, the first responders must know how to approach a fire, how to enter a burning building that may be full of smoke or toxic fumes, how to rescue a person whose clothes are on fire, how to treat burn wounds and associated trauma immediately, and how to provide medical relief.[1] One of the most troublesome confounding problems is establishing the number of casualties and the size of their burns.

Often the major management problem is a lack of information from the site of the accident.[31] The focus of patient assessment and care responsibilities shifts from hospitals to the scene of a disaster where triage, evaluations, and medical management of multiple casualties occur.[14,76] Burn disaster activities should all be coordinated centrally through one resource center utilizing a centralized communication hub with central medical emergency direction capabilities (**Table 5.3**). On-scene patient management is generally organized in two distinct phases: patient triage and ambulance staging.[14] On-scene management, when organized and conducted properly, allows for controlled treatment of patients, optimal allocation of resources, and maximization of the utility of these resources for patients.[77] Guidelines for immediate care of burn victims include:

- self-control;
- self-protection;
- qualitative assessment of burns;
- quantitative assessment of a patient's burns;
- intravenous fluid therapy;
- analgesic therapy;
- bladder catheterization;
- pressure relieving incisions (escharotomy);
- reexamination of patient;
- hospital transfer.[23]

Organized relief refers to the mobilization of all civil defense and military forces that are ready to intervene in the event of a burn disaster.[46,47] These forces arrive at the scene of an accident as rapidly as possible, but usually not within the first 3 hours. They are equipped with the necessary means and structures to enable them to perform their rescue action during the first 48–72 hours after a disaster until all the people have been evacuated.[1] These forces are trained to manage the general details of fire disasters. Special units are composed of personnel trained in the emergency care of severely burned patients and equipped with specific means and materials. These units should be in charge of preliminary triage, preparing a preliminary evacuation plan, contacting dispatching stations, selecting means of transport, organizing first aid posts, and clearing the area of the dead.[1]

All assistance to patients who have been exposed to fire and have extensive burns must be specific, precise, considerate, and timely.[23] Using an established Burns Mass Disaster plan enabled improved mortality for 10 badly burned victims that were airlifted to a burns center, 1000 kilometers away.[78] Communication, triage, treatment, transport, staffing, and supply are the basic problems that confront health care workers caring for mass burns.

Control/Communications Center

A region-wide disaster network should be developed, linking the communications of multiple hospitals so that each could receive all communications relevant to a disaster from the central communications center, and air and ground transportation units would be included in the link. This requires rigid communications discipline in order to ensure that only pertinent voice communication is transmitted. Priority triage of victims can be accomplished by radio contact between central communication physicians and referring physicians in local hospitals. Through this system, secondary patient triage, hospital notification, and medical control of patients coming from a disaster, as well as mobilization of ground and aeromedical transportation, can be affected. Burned patients can be secondarily transferred to burn centers with available beds, equipment, and personnel so that optimal care can be delivered to each patient.

Accounting for patients is the main function of the control/communication center after initial communications between a disaster scene and facilities have diminished. Transmittal of pertinent information regarding the condition of those patients being transferred from one facility to another tertiary care facility is important. Equally important is to accurately account for the dead. This information is crucial for handling families and friends. Appropriate communication to the media is an issue of public trust, but must follow approved public relations protocols.[60]

Triage

The primary inflow

Triage ought to be conducted in a simple, straightforward, and experienced manner. Triage should be prognostic with a view to singling out those among the burned who are likely to survive.[6] The two most important aspects of triage have to do with who will perform triage and where. The initial triage will most likely be at the site of a burn disaster by bystanders followed shortly by other first responders. The triage area is an important consideration. A safe triage area must be secured so that additional burn victims are not created because of lack of scene safety. The lobby of a hotel might serve as a good triage area, since it has good access and egress, appropriate space to work, and serves as a known location to all rescue workers and medical personnel. With lack of sophistication at the scene, burn victims may be taken to the nearest hospital emergency department or accident ward for triage[14] before they are transported to tertiary burn centers.[14,31,36,64,65,75] Sorting should, ideally, be performed at the site by an expert in burns.[2,65,79] Expert triage may minimize the requirement for specialized burn beds.[12] Few casualties with burn wounds of 30–70% TBSA (14% of those admitted) were encountered following fire disaster.[12] Since bed availability in specialized centers is limited, it is clear that accurate triage is essential.[12] The rapid evacuation of casualties to nearby hospitals is a realistic aim for all but the most isolated locations, aided by the fact that most burn victims are themselves initially mobile and cooperative[46] (see **Figure 5.3**).

The organization of salvage work is affected by the number of casualties, the seriousness of their injuries, and the general conditions of a disaster.[6] The actual triage of patients will be influenced not only by the total number of casualties and bed availability but also by such factors as depth and locations of wounds, complications such as inhalation injury, and extremes of age.[12,26] With effective triage, the demand for specialized burn care can be minimized. In the case of the Ramstein disaster, the triage sites formed *de novo* where large numbers of patients were encountered, medical personnel congregated naturally, and supplies could be obtained for initial resuscitation. The patients were then carried a short distance to staging areas for helicopter pick up or for ambulance or bus loading. In the Ramstein disaster, complete triage on the scene was not possible. Most of the victims were transported by a 'load and go' system to nearby hospitals. The triage response of emergency services at the air base was criticized.[9,63,64]

Because of the nature of some burn disasters, it is important to establish triage stations somewhat removed from an immediate scene.[14] This would be in response to hazards to the rescue and triage personnel such as bomb threats and potential explosions, interference by a crowd, or simply the fact that better facilities for triage are nearby and available.

Patients must be triaged into categories for systematic referral to appropriate facilities. The triage category is based on the severity of injury and the potential for salvage. The overall goal is to do the most good for the most people. In general, when resources are unlimited and a disaster plan incorporates additional resources, even the most severely injured burn victim will receive optimal care if the triage is accomplished in the most favorable manner. Where resources are limited, triage may require a method for selecting casualties on a true priority basis. It may mean developing an expectant category for those so severely injured that they are not likely to survive.

The problem of triage can be simplified and facilitated by a flexible adaptation of certain formulas. The gravity of burns can be expressed in terms of the extent of TBSA burned and age of the patient. In Czechoslovakia, the sum of age and extent of burn that is greater than 90 has established an empirical 50% chance of survival. By flexibly bringing this number up or down, depending on the overall situation, one can extend or narrow the number of burn casualties who ought to be transported first.[6] Immediate triage is essential in the presence of large numbers of burned patients. It has been observed that if a long period elapses before rescue teams could start triage and resuscitation, most of the severely injured die and many of the initially moderately injured develop serious complications.[9] Triage may identify five important groups for victims of burn disasters[2] (**Table 5.4**).

Secondary triage

The Ural mountain train–gas pipeline explosion (Ufa train disaster) was a classic example of the need for secondary triage. During the initial stages following the Ufa train accident, victims were evacuated to nearby settlements where first aid was rendered, aseptic bandages placed, and fluid resuscitation started. During the second stage, victims were evacuated by medical vehicles and helicopters to Ufa and Techelyabinsk. Total evacuation took 16 hours and 45 minutes, and 806 people were admitted to hospitals and burn centers.[3] Helicopters from a nearby military training base airlifted survivors to hospitals in the regional cities of Ufa, Asha, Gorky, and Chelyabinsk. Aeroflot organized a series of special flights, evacuating 160 of the most badly burned, including 37 children, to hospitals in Moscow.[75] In the Ramstein disaster, rapid initial transport to supporting hospitals was instituted, but further transport to designated hospitals was not thought to have been carried out properly. The result was that some hospitals and burn centers were overloaded with patients while nearby hospitals and burn centers did not get any patients at all.[9,63,64] Secondary or tertiary transfers could have relieved the problem. The result of good secondary triage is that none of the institutions will be overly taxed in providing disaster response; this will allow uninterrupted care of all patients, including the patients who are already in a facility.

Once patients are re-triaged to a specialty center, a surgeon directing a major disaster plan may not be able to personally see and assign priorities to a large number of patients because the true priority cannot be assigned until the last patient has arrived. Therefore, a first-come-first-served policy may be effective, reserving some resources for severe emergency problems. To reexamine each of the patients thoroughly by removing all dressings is dis-

Table 5.4 Triage criteria and care plans[2]	
Triage criteria	**Care plan**
Minor burns/non-critical sites: <10% TBSA for children; <20% TBSA for adults	Dress wounds; tetanus prophylaxis; out-patient care
Minor burns/critical sites (hands, face, perineum)	Admit, early operations, special wound care, short hospital stay
20–60% TBSA burned	Requires intravenous fluids/careful monitoring. Burn units, trained personnel
Extensive burns (>60% TBSA burned); inhalation injury/associated trauma; associated medical illnesses	Mortality high; may be placed in expectant category; pain medication; psychological support
Minor burns/inhalation injury/associated injuries	Administer oxygen, measure carboxyhemoglobin, + or – intubate, ventilate, care of associated injuries

tressing for the patients and time-consuming for surgeons. Surgeons, therefore, may make hurried and incomplete examinations from which some minor mistakes may result. Further, the senior surgeon directing the surgical management of a major accident should stay out of the operating theater, freeing himself of all routine commitments for the day until the last patient has left the operating theater.[15] The senior surgeon must, however, keep control of the surgical needs of the patients, interface with relatives, and arrange for transfers of patients to other hospitals if an overload occurs in the receiving hospital and also to eventually transfer patients closer to their homes when their care can be directed safely and appropriately from a hospital closer to home (see **Figure 5.3**).

Forty-seven patients from the Ramstein disaster were re-triaged at the Homburg-Saar trauma center using Plan A (natural disasters, fires and explosions/departments of surgery, anesthesia, and radiology), Level II (20–50 victims, activates additional staff and an executive team of department chairs) of their hospital disaster plan. Forty-two patients arrived together on a bus less than 1 hour after the crash and activated the main secondary triage. Secondary triage took place in the triage zone of the trauma center by six emergency room shock teams. Twenty-four victims had deep dermal or full-thickness burns up to 90%. Eleven had additional trauma. Twenty-two were classified second priority and eight with minor injuries went home after first aid treatment in the out-patient department. Patients were prepared for transfer to nearby hospitals; but this proved to be unnecessary. Four intensive care units were reinforced with additional staff. Six burn victims were transferred by helicopter to German and American burn centers during the following 48 hours. After discussion with burn center physicians, five patients with severe injuries (burns in combination with other injuries) were not transferred and expired of multiple organ failure.[64] A thorough burn disaster plan addresses the contingency of disproportions between capacities and facilities as well as the ethical problems in mass burn disasters.[5,80] Secondary triage or tertiary triage may occur when burn victims can be repatriated to their domestic hospitals. Eleven of the 22 hospitalized patients at the Homburg trauma center following the Ramstein disaster were transferred to their domestic hospitals.

Treatment

Initial care: the ABCs

The first order of treatment is to ensure an adequate airway and ventilation for each burned victim. This is most often a problem in patients with inhalation injury or mechanical trauma to the face, neck, or chest. Patients with respiratory problems must be identified immediately and those with inhalation injuries must be noted very early in order to reduce mortality and morbidity.[58] Intubation and ventilation may be required at the scene and at any time thereafter for inadequate airway or breathing. Firemen are usually the best-trained rescue personnel and are capable of initiating care of burned victims. The kind of assistance provided by the first rescuers is of primary importance for the prognosis of casualties. First responders must carry out the first triage of urgent cases, taking into consideration a high number of poly-traumatized patients. They must also initiate all medical and surgical procedures necessary for preliminary resuscitative therapy and initial local treatment of burns.[1]

Patients with all but minor burns should receive prompt fluid replacement in order to counteract the loss of protein-rich fluid into interstitial tissues.[2] In the Ufa train disaster, first aid was rendered to victims at the site of the accident by local inhabitants and the medical staff of hospitals located in nearby settlements. Within 12 hours, 25 teams of emergency first aid personnel from the city of Ufa and Civil Defense Medical Brigades provided additional care. Effective early management extends the time available for dispersal of casualties.[12] The two fundamental conditions for prognosis are the time interval between the accident and commencement of infusion therapy and the quality of therapy administered.[66] Effective fluid therapy during the first 24 hours provides an interval in which transfer of patients may be organized.[12] Fluid therapy should be based on the simplest, most expedient effective way of treating a problem. The extent of a burn should be assessed in terms of the percentage of the TBSA using a patient's hand (fingers together) as representing 1%.[2] The sum of the partial-thickness and full-thickness burns is used when calculating fluid requirements. The Baxter-Shires formula of 4 ml Ringer's lactate/kg body weight 1% TBSA second and third degree burn/24 hours is effective and should be started within half an hour for adults with burns greater than 20% TBSA, for children with burns greater than 10% TBSA, and patients up to the age of 4 years with burns greater than 5% TBSA. Diuresis at 0.5–0.7 ml/kg/h should be maintained.[6] The substitution of IV resuscitation by enteral therapy is possible for small burns.[6] No colloids should be administered for the first 24 hours.

Junior staff can set up IV infusion, administer analgesics, obtain baseline blood samples and radiographs, arrange photographic documentation, begin monitoring fluid balance, and prepare chronological documentation.[2] Adequate resuscitation was the key to a better survival rate among similar groups of patients whose medical treatment was otherwise the same in two burn units in Spain.[9,34] The Ufa train disaster provided an example of the consequences of a long delay in fluid resuscitation.[9]

Initially, burned areas should be simply covered with a clean sheet. If a patient must remain for a period before triage, the initial facility may wish to cover a wound with dressings impregnated with silver sulfadiazine or some other effective topical agent and gauze to hold the dressings in place for the transfer. The efficient work of a nursing staff in treating patients with topical antimicrobials before an exact diagnosis of depth and extent of burns is known wastes time, because the wounds will need to be uncovered in order to allow the receiving medical staff to confirm the diagnosis of size and depth of burn.[28] One must exercise judgment as to how long to leave a burn wound unprotected from topical antimicrobials so that a physician can evaluate the burn wound. Physicians may well be consumed in life-saving measures for other burned victims for some extended period. The same could be said for the need for escharotomies. Detailed assessment of casualties will obviously take some time. Such assessment is, therefore, only practical in a clinical environment where facilities and personnel are available for management of fluid therapy and for treatment of urgent complications.[12] Early debridement of burn tissue is not necessary initially, but can be carried out within the first 5 days postburn once a patient has reached an appropriate facility. The management of burns should involve debridement and wound coverage as soon as possible.[28] However, this is a function of the tertiary receiving hospital/burn center and should only be considered as part of the eventual care of the patient, not the initial resuscitation.

Methods of treatment must be modified, and medications must

be standardized and reduced to basics.[9] Initially, no prophylactic antibiotics are administered, but prophylaxis against stress ulcers should be given. Although antibiotics are not used in many burn centers for prophylaxis because of the development of resistant organisms,[81] in a situation where a large number of patients with burns arrive at a general hospital, which would be unlikely to have an endogenous supply of resistant organisms (or the capability of early detection of burn wound sepsis), it would seem advisable to use prophylaxis.[58]

Psychological Considerations

Psychological training must be given by expert psychoanalysts using group work techniques.[65] An effort should be made to reduce psychological interference that might hinder the organization of rescue work and burn care. Initially, people must trust their rescue workers and be guided by them. This assists in the escape from disaster and lessens the psychological impact. The best psychological first aid is to assist and organize escape from a disaster. During and immediately after a fire/burn disaster, civic education in schools by mass media and through other means of communication may help lessen the psychological impact of a disaster on a community. Psychological support must be tailored to the situation of a fire/burn disaster. As in the case of the Ramstein disaster, the audience at the air show was family-oriented with many school children witnessing the holocaust and experiencing the panic of the event. Therefore, great energy was spent in psychological debriefs in the schools where the children attended and in other public forums.

Patients admitted to a hospital should have supportive psychological counseling given early, throughout their hospital stay, and for follow-up after discharge in order to minimize the late emotional disturbances.[58] Professionally trained teams of experienced rescue workers help to control emotional problems such as panic caused by a fire disaster.[58] Most of these patients will have major emotional problems.[41,59] 'They are agitated, anxious, very dependent, and out of action. Their faces are not looking good. They have seen their friends go up in flames. Some survivors had heard hundreds of men screaming that they were going to die. Psychologists and social workers were drafted to offer emotional and practical help to survivors and brief families, as well as support the nurses looking after them.'[59] It is only later, as the drama of the first days dies down, that nurses start to feel the strain. Talking among the health care givers about an incident helps.[59] Psychological support for victims, relatives, rescuers, and health workers must not be forgotten.[82] Advisors from Bradford and Kent, who had developed special services to help the bereaved in response to the Bradford fire and the Zeebrugge ferry disasters were available to help.[59] Apart from the casualties themselves, the greatest concern was for the bereaved relatives, most of them with no body to grieve over and no ritual funeral rites to help them mourn. Many bereaved families were desperate to speak to people in the hospitals in order to find out all they could about missing relatives, now presumed dead.[59] Professionals must be available to help these people during and after a disaster.

Staffing

Initial staffing

Medical staff on duty must be able to undertake emergency care of initial victims prior to arrival of additional staff, as was the case

with the Hipercor victims when traffic conditions delayed the arrival of off-duty burns and surgical staff as well as additional hospital staff to care for burned patients.[28] This can create an overwhelming task for health care providers. In the Ufa train disaster the average number of patients per health care team was 12–15.[3] Within a very short period, initial medical people (physicians, nurses, and members of voluntary organizations) must respond to victims of a burn disaster site. These medical personnel are supported by public and private organizations in the area, hospitals, casualty departments, clinics, fire brigades, and police; and they are coordinated by local authorities.[1]

When admitting patients and rendering qualified, specialized medical aid at a hospital, the participation of mixed physician teams is advisable.[3] A senior surgeon should calculate the number of hours of operating room time required for proper care of all patients. A priority must be established for initial care and for any dressing changes and re-operations that are required. From that calculation, staffing requirements for the operating rooms, as well as for postoperative anesthetic care, intensive care, and ward care, can be established. A senior surgeon should act as coordinator and get surgeons working as soon as patients arrive, keeping two operating theaters reserved for lifesaving operations.[15] Such calculations will drive the requirements for equipment and supplies and, with some foresight, drive the re-supply rate.

In the San Juanico tragedy, in which about 7000 people were injured, 2000 were hospitalized, 625 had severe burns, 300 died immediately, 250 died in hospitals later, and 60 000 were evacuated, 7000 people were involved in the rescue work during the first 48 hours. Of these, 200 were firefighters, 1000 were physicians, 1300 were paramedics, 1800 were nurses, 2000 were military personnel, and 750 were drivers and helicopter pilots.[9,35]

Volunteers will come! Assistance from volunteers may occur spontaneously from a crowd or community as it did at Ramstein and Piper Alpha or respond to a formal request as in the Ufa train disaster. 'You'll see the basic goodness in people when this sort of thing happens. Everyone rallies around. They don't think of payment. We had no problem with staffing, people just appeared. Although only a skeleton staff was on duty, the switchboard was flooded with nurses offering their services.'[59] Volunteers may need supervision and oversight to assure that they do not become overwhelmed or psychologically dysfunctional.

At Ramstein, the townspeople in Landstuhl heard the jet airplanes stop flying and many helicopters start flying and sensed a disaster. They responded to the Landstuhl Army Hospital and served as clean-up crews, traffic control, stretcher-bearers, and many other functions without being asked and often without any supervision. They just did the right things to help the effort. After needs were assessed in the Bashkir train–gas pipeline disaster, two pediatric burn teams were sent to assist in the care of burned children. These teams integrated with the host nation's medical personnel to care for the burn victims.[36,75] The US team arrived 2 weeks after the disaster.[75] The cooperative effort allowed an increased frequency of dressings and more aggressive, rapid, and complete debridement of wounds. New techniques were introduced such as the use of a free hand skin graft knife, an air-driven dermatome, a skin graft mesher, and the use of dilute epinephrine solution for topical control of bleeding. Additional splints were made. One aspect of the burn care at Children's Hospital Nine was the role of parents providing much of the care of their children.

They were present virtually all of the time on the wards. For those children whose parents were missing or children orphaned because of the disaster, others acted as surrogates. They fed the children, changed the beds and clothing, transported them around the hospitals, and received them directly from the dressing and operating rooms still partially anesthetized.[75] Soviet medical and paramedical staff slowly realized the large number of patients involved, the extent of their injuries, and the logistics of their care. The result was acceptance of medical help offered by burn care teams from the US, UK, France, Israel, and Cuba, which illustrated the importance of having access to international medical support following disasters of such magnitude that local (regional and national) medical resources were exhausted.[9] Full and immediate use should be made of colleagues called out under a major disaster plan or they will disappear.

Relief staffing

Relief personnel must replace or be assigned to the effort when the initial staff become exhausted. With so many serious cases, often the usual number of staff must be doubled. Usually there is no difficulty in finding them. Nurses often volunteer their services and the response is great.[59] A plastic surgeon who had been attending a burn conference heard news of the Piper Alpha disaster and along with six other burn specialists from all over the country came to help treat burns. At Ramstein, off-duty hospital personnel augmented the initial staff and provided the relief staff needed to care for burned and mechanically traumatized victims.

Supply

Replenishing supplies used up in the care of many burned patients initially comes from warehousing facilities at or near the burn unit or hospital. Transport of additional supplies becomes crucial since the care of burned patients has high resources requirements for IV fluids, pain medications, topical antibiotics, and the like. If re-supply cannot be effected, then there will be a decline in the care of burn victims or a need for secondary triage to a facility equipped and supplied to provide optimal care.

As the US team joined the burn surgeons at Children's Hospital Nine in caring for children from the Ufa train disaster, certain ideas and materials also necessarily came along. Project Hope provided over 7000 kg of badly needed medical supplies, drugs, and equipment, all of which arrived during the 2 weeks while the US team was in the then Soviet Union. Such material aid permitted the Soviet surgeons to carry out usual therapy more effectively and the US team to introduce some new ideas and techniques.[75] The Brooke Army team brought tons of much needed supplies with them as well.[25] Authorities need to act on guidelines that provide for the stockpiling of specific mobilization materials in the most convenient location, the management of ambulance services, traffic control, the use of local and regional mass media, and the general means of transportation.[1] At Ramstein, contingency supplies specifically for a mass disaster were brought in and used for the care of burned patients.

Transportation

Coordination and mobilization of necessary transportation mechanisms (i.e. ground ambulance and/or aeromedical helicopter) and avoidance of calling in unneeded ambulances to a scene, which tends to confuse scene management, are essential.[14] The same control may be necessary for leapfrogging facilities to not overload one hospital at any given time.[83] Most patients will be transported by ground vehicles, particularly if a disaster is in an urban area. Remoteness of areas, traffic congestion, and the need for secondary triage may provide good reasons for aeromedical transfer. For a helicopter service in Italy, 2.5% of approximately 2500 flights concerned the secondary transport of burn victims while 0.5% provided direct medical assistance to burned patients at the scene of accidents.[84] Careful preparations by a hospital requesting transfers can be performed prior to air medical evacuation (**Table 5.5**). The size of a helicopter (or airplane) affects the optimal therapeutic access to various anatomical parts, monitoring of a patient, ventilatory assistance, and the number of patients that can be transported at one time. Larger helicopters with advanced instrumentation and excellent air speed effect the transportation during adverse meteorological conditions.[84]

Table 5.5 Specific protocol for preparing burned patients for medical evacuation[84]
Cannulation of several venous routes of which one should be central if possible (followed by chest radiograph)
Monitoring of diuresis
Insertion of nasogastric tube
Sedation and/or analgesia
Cleansing of wounds
Tracheal intubation (if necessary)
Application of sanitary devices to prevent excessive heat loss

After-action assessment

Disaster management must include the overall assessment of the consequences of a disaster. This assessment must be as accurate as possible whether it refers to a presumed or actual event.[1] Awareness of the scale and nature of past disasters may aid in the formulation of new plans for dealing with mass burn causalities in the future.[12] Uniform language and a framework to report and analyze disaster incidents is important and will contribute to evaluations that are more accurate.[14] The study of 10 major fire-related public transport aircraft accidents led to changes in cabin interior materials and potential filters that could provide satisfactory respiratory protection.[85] Modifications and revisions to disaster plans and disaster management can be effectively accomplished by initiating a mechanism of post-incident evaluation of disaster exercises and actual disaster responses. The central coordination of the response can be the focal point for this evaluation, which must include all of the emergency medical services and the resources involved in a disaster response.[56]

All of the agencies and individuals involved in a burn disaster should be assembled routinely, immediately following incidents in order to critique the events while the facts are clear in the minds of the providers.[14] Information included in these sessions, although sometimes subjective, is usually quite candid and complete; and when combined with taped and written recordings of the incidents, it provides important lessons about the strengths and weaknesses of the management of the response.[14] Relevant lessons learned include the knowledge that all public service agencies are integrally involved in successful management of a burn disaster and must be kept informed of current burn disaster plans. A multi-agency mass disaster plan that had been formulated and rehearsed in preparation for the Pan American Games was used when a pilotless aircraft struck a hotel.[86] Such a critique depends on reliable information for successful management of the next disaster. From an in-depth review, individual facilities are able to effect changes such as directing online communications to an admitting office, preparing intensive care units and operating rooms, as well as establishing a person with authority to make decisions for the hospitals' ability to accept patients without questioning their fiscal resources. Major internal changes can be effected, based on data and corrections made to allow a hospital to accept burn disaster victims at any hour that a disaster may occur. The practical benefit of these evaluation sessions is the fact that changes in disaster plans and operational management are made based on information learned during a disaster response critique.[14] Critiques often identify problems on notification of hospitals and burn centers concerning the nature and extent of injuries, as well as the number of patients they should expect. Organized relay of pertinent patient information to hospital staff or mobilization of appropriate physicians, specialists, and staff is key. Matching patients with specific injuries, such as burns, to facilities capable of treating these specific problems, such as burn centers, is the mark of a well-designed and effectively managed disaster plan. In addition, forensic information is obtained that may be useful for disaster planning as well as for industrial change.[86,87]

Some important, but previously unknown, statistics have been generated from after-action reports. The total number of injured patients was more than six times higher and the number of casualties admitted to hospitals was nearly 20 times greater following outdoor disasters than indoor disasters.[9] The immediate death rate at the site was very high (74%) in indoor fires compared to outdoor disasters (35%), but the hospital death rate was lower following indoor disasters.[9,12] Sixty percent of burn victims of indoor disasters sustained burns covering less than 30% of their TBSA.[9] In a significant number of patients with very extensive burns (greater than 70% TBSA), they occurred after outdoor fires, while very few were admitted with extensive burns after indoor fires.[2] Those who failed to escape from indoor fires died rapidly from a combination of hypoxia and inhalation of poisonous compounds.[88,89] The poor prognosis of burn victims with large burns sustained in mass disasters has been emphasized and is reflected in the high mortality following outdoor disasters.[12,34,90] The number of burn victims admitted with burns in the 30–70% TBSA range was consistently low, which is more important since patients with this burn size potentially obtain the greatest benefit from referral to a burn center.[12] In an indoor disaster of another kind, the MGM Grand Hotel fire in Las Vegas resulted in 300 hospital admissions for smoke inhalation, but no burn injuries.[91] After-action reports will allow analysis of the environmental impact of the disaster, the vulnerability of the territory, and the information, education, and participation of the population.[71] In emergencies, human behavior is a decisive factor in the creation of dangerous or harmful situations and it plays a basic role in the evolution of the effects of a disaster.[71] Retrospective studies of are less helpful, but can direct future planning of burns mass disasters.[92]

A bonus lesson learned from after-action reporting was that burn teams working together could exchange new ideas and techniques with colleagues from other parts of the world who are not familiar with such techniques.[3,93] The effect of the combined efforts of the Soviet and US Army medical teams who worked together at the largest hospital in the city of Ufa was that the team was able to effectively care for a large number of patients. Prior to this event, neither the hospital nor the Soviet physicians working at the hospital had had significant burn care experience.[3] Other follow-on studies directed comparative studies of the microbial spectrum of burn wounds and medicinal sensitivities of the microorganisms.[94] The lessons learned provide a framework for burn disaster management should a group be asked to provide assistance in the future.[25] All of these data are important in planning for the next burn disaster.

References

1. Masellis M. Thermal agent disaster and fire disaster; definition, damage, assessment and relief operations, chapter 1. In: Masellis M, Gunn SWA, eds. *The Management of Mass Burn Casualties and Fire Disasters: Proceedings of the First International Conference on Burns and Fire Disasters*. Dordrecht: Kluwer Academic, 1992: 7–12.
2. Griffiths RW. Management of multiple casualties with burns. *Br Med J* 1985; **291**: 917–18.
3. Kulyapin AV, Sakhautdinov VG, Temerbulatov VM, Becker WK, Waymack JP. Bashkiria train-gas pipeline disaster; a history of the joint USSR/USA collaboration. *Burns* 1990; **16(5)**: 339–42.
4. Abend M, Bubke O, Hotop S, Krawehl-Nakath C, Willy C, Sohns T, van Beuningen D. Estimating medical resources required following a nuclear event. *Comput Biol Med* 1999; **29(6)**: 407–21.
5. Kumar P, Jagetia GC. A review of triage and management of burns victims following a nuclear disaster. *Burns* 1994; **20(5)**: 397–402.
6. Simko S. Reflections on the organization of mass burns treatment. *Acta Chir Plast* 1981; **23(3)**: 197–200.
7. Sorensen B. Management of burns occurring as mass casualties after nuclear explosion. *Burns* 1979; **6**: 33–6.
8. Layton TR, Elhauge ER. US fire catastrophes of the 20th century. *J Burn Care Rehabil* 1982; **3(1)**: 21–8.
9. Arturson G. Analysis of severe fire disasters, chapter 4. In: Masellis M, Gunn SWA, eds. *The Management of Mass Burn Casualties and Fire Disasters: Proceedings of the First International Conference on Burns and Fire Disasters*. Dordrecht: Kluwer Academic, 1992: 24–33.
10. Gunn SWA. The scientific basis of disaster medicine, chapter 2. In: Masellis M, Gunn SWA, eds. *The Management of Mass Burn Casualties and Fire Disasters: Proceedings of the First International Conference on Burns and Fire Disasters*. Dordrecht: Kluwer Academic, 1992: 13–18.
11. Firescope California. *Fire Service Field Operations Guide*, ICS 420–1. Incident Command System Publication, April 1999.
12. Mackie DP, Koning HM. Fate of mass burn casualties; implications for disaster planning. *Burns* 1990; **16(3)**: 203–6.
13. Nakamori Y, Tanaka H, Oda J, Kuwagata Y, Matsuoka T, Yoshioka T. Burn injuries in the 1995 Hanshin-Awaji earthquake. *Burns* 1997; **23(4)**: 319–22.
14. Jacobs LM, Goody MM, Sinclair A. The role of a trauma center in disaster management. *J Trauma* 1983; **23**: 697–701.
15. Bliss AR. Major disaster planning. *Br Med J* 1984; **288**: 1433–4.
16. Gunn SWA. *Multilingual Dictionary of Disaster Medicine and International Relief*. Dordrecht: Kluwer Academic, 1990.
17. Woolley WD, Smith PC, Fardell PJ, Murrell JM, Rogers SP. The Stardust Disco Fire, Dublin 1981: studies of combustion products during simulation experiments. *Fire Safety Journal* 1984; **7**: 267.
18. Hill IR. An analysis of factors impeding passenger escape from aircraft fires. *Avia Space Environ Med* 1990; **61(3)**: 261–5.
19. Servais J. Fire emergency in a hospital, chapter 17. In: Masellis M, Gunn SWA, eds. *The Management of Mass Burn Casualties and Fire Disasters: Proceedings of the First International Conference on Burns and Fire Disasters*. Dordrecht: Kluwer Academic, 1992: 113–15.
20. Trovato B. Fire services at a motor racing track, chapter 16. In: Masellis M, Gunn SWA, eds. *The Management of Mass Burn Casualties and Fire Disasters: Proceedings of the First International Conference on Burns and Fire Disasters*. Dordrecht: Kluwer Academic, 1992: 110–12.
21. Halstead MA. Fire drill in the operating room. Role playing as a learning tool. *AORN J* 1993; **58(4)**: 697–706.
22. Alley EE. Problems of search and rescue in disasters, chapter 26. In: Masellis M, Gunn SWA, eds. *The Management of Mass Burn Casualties and Fire Disasters:*

Proceedings of the First International Conference on Burns and Fire Disasters. Dordrecht: Kluwer Academic, 1992: 175–6.

23. Masellis ML. Management of mass burn casualties in disasters. *Ann Medit Burns Club* 1988; **1**: 155–9.

24. Remensnyder JP, Ackroyd FP, Astrozjinikova S, *et al.* Burned children from the Bashkir train–gas pipeline disaster I. Acute management at Children's Hospital 9, Moscow. *Burns* 1990; **16(5)**: 329–32.

25. Becker WK, Waymack JP, McManus AT, Shaikhutdinov M, Pruitt BA Jr. Bashkirian train–gas pipeline disaster: the American military response. *Burns* 1990; **16(5)**: 325–8.

26. Costagliola M, Laguerre J, Rouge D. Infobrul – the value of a telematic databank for burns and burns centers in the event of a disaster, chapter 32. In: Masellis M, Gunn SWA, eds. *The Management of Mass Burn Casualties and Fire Disasters: Proceedings of the First International Conference on Burns and Fire Disasters.* Dordrecht: Kluwer Academic, 1992: 190–4.

27. Martinelli G. The ARGO satellite system: a network for severe burns and disasters, chapter 44. In: Masellis M, Gunn SWA, eds. *The Management of Mass Burn Casualties and Fire Disasters: Proceedings of the First International Conference on Burns and Fire Disasters.* Dordrecht: Kluwer Academic, 1992: 7–12.

28. Morrell PAG, Nasif FE, Domenech RP, Carol ES, Roda JAB. Burns caused by the terrorist bombing of the department store hipercor in Barcelona: Part 1. *Burns* 1990; **16(6)**: 423–5.

29. Mackie DP, Hoekstra MJ, Baruchin AM. The Amsterdam air disaster – management and fate of casualties. *Harefuah* 1994; **126(8)**: 484–5.

30. Ortenwall P, Sager-Lund C, Nystrom J, Martinell S. Disaster management lessons can be learned from the Gothenburg fire. *Lakartidningen* 2000; **97(13)**: 1532–9.

31. Allister L, Hamilton GM. Cardowan coal mine explosion: experience of a mass burns event. *Br Med J* 1983; **287**: 403–5.

32. Demuth MW, Dimick AR, Gillespie RW, *et al. Advanced Burn Life Support Course.* Chicago, IL: American Burn Association, 2000.

33. Sharpe DT, Foo IT. Management of burns in major disasters. *Injury* 1990; **21(1)**: 41–4; discussion 55–7.

34. Arturson G. The Los Alfaques disaster: a boiling-liquid, expanding-vapour explosion. *Burns* 1981; **7**: 233–51.

35. Arturson G. The tragedy of San Juanico – the most severe LPG disaster in history. *Burns* 1987; **13(2)**: 87–102.

36. Herndon DN. A survey of the primary aid response to the Bashkir train-gas pipeline disaster. *Burns* 1990; **16**: 323–4.

37. Benmeir P, Levine I, Shostak A, Oz V, Shemer J, Sokolova T. The ural train-gas pipeline catastrophe: the report of the IDF medical corps assistance. *Burns* 1991; **17(4)**: 320–2.

38. Brusco M. Fire in port, chapter 13. In: Masellis M, Gunn SWA, eds. *The Management of Mass Burn Casualties and Fire Disasters: Proceedings of the First International Conference on Burns and Fire Disasters.* Dordrecht: Kluwer Academic, 1992: 89–92.

39. Bovio G. Forest fires and the danger to firefighters, chapter 7. In: Masellis M, Gunn SWA, eds. *The Management of Mass Burn Casualties and Fire Disasters: Proceedings of the First International Conference on Burns and Fire Disasters.* Dordrecht: Kluwer Academic, 1992: 51–9.

40. Colombo D, Foti F, Volonte M, Micucci G. Rescue of the burn patients and on-site medical assistance by a helicopter rescue service, chapter 42. In: Masellis M, Gunn SWA, eds. *The Management of Mass Burn Casualties and Fire Disasters: Proceedings of the First International Conference on Burns and Fire Disasters.* Dordrecht: Kluwer Academic, 1992: 249–50.

41. Rayner C. Offshore disaster on a fixed installation – the Piper Alpha disaster of 6 July 1988. In: Zellner PR, ed. *Die Versorgung des Brandverletzten in Katastrophenfall.* Darmstadt: Steinkopff Verlag, 1990: 33–7.

42. Dioguardi D, Brienza E, Altacera M. The role of information sciences in the management of disasters. *Ann Medit Burns Club* 1988; **1**: 165–7.

43. Dioguardi D, Brienza E, Portincasa A, Di Lonardo A, Matarrese V. A proposal for the strategic planning of medical services in the case of major fire disasters in the city of Bari. *Ann Medit Burns Club* 1989; **2(3)**: 147–50.

44. Brienza E, Madami LM, Catalano F, Del Zotti M. Organizational criteria for setting up a field hospital after a fire disaster, chapter 33. In: Masellis M, Gunn SWA, eds. *The Management of Mass Burn Casualties and Fire Disasters: Proceedings of the First International Conference on Burns and Fire Disasters.* Dordrecht: Kluwer Academic, 1992: 195–7.

45. Jenkins AL. Disaster planning, chapter 15. In: *Emergency Department Organization and Management.* St Louis: Mosby, 1978: 243–61.

46. Cuccinello G. The commitment of the Italian Army Medical Corps to relief of the civilian population in the event of public disasters, chapter 29. In: Masellis M, Gunn SWA, eds. *The Management of Mass Burn Casualties and Fire Disasters: Proceedings of the First International Conference on Burns and Fire Disasters.* Dordrecht: Kluwer Academic, 1992: 133–9.

47. Di Martino M. The organization of the Italian Army Medical Corps in relation to contributions to civil defense in the event of disasters, chapter 30. In: Masellis M, Gunn SWA, eds. *The Management of Mass Burn Casualties and Fire Disasters: Proceedings of the First International Conference on Burns and Fire Disasters.* Dordrech: Kluwer Academic, 1992: 185–6.

48. Bianchi M, Minniti U. The use of helicopters in integrated rescue work and medical transport, chapter 41. In: Masellis M, Gunn SWA, eds. *The Management of Mass Burn Casualties and Fire Disasters: Proceedings of the First International Conference on Burns and Fire Disasters.* Dordrecht: Kluwer Academic, 1992: 246–8.

49. Meurant J. Communications in the prevention of natural and man-made disasters: the role of the national and international Red Cross and Red Crescent organizations, chapter 60. In: Masellis M, Gunn SWA, eds. *The Management of Mass Burn Casualties and Fire Disasters: Proceedings of the First International Conference on Burns and Fire Disasters.* Dordrecht: Kluwer Academic, 1992: 317–27.

50. Treat RC, Sirinek KR, Levine BA, Pruitt BA Jr. Air evacuation of thermally injured patients: principles of treatment and results. *J Trauma* 1980; **20(4)**: 270–5.

51. Judkins KC. Aeromedical transfer of burned patients: a review with special reference to European civilian practice. *Burns* 1988; **14(3)**: 171–9.

52. Heredero FXS. Physiopathology of burn disease during air evacuation, chapter 40. In: Masellis M, Gunn SWA, eds. *The Management of Mass Burn Casualties and Fire Disasters: Proceedings of the First International Conference on Burns and Fire Disasters.* Dordrecht: Kluwer Academic, 1992: 243–5.

53. Wachtel TL, Cowan ML, Reardon JD. Developing a regional and national burn disaster response. *J Burn Care Rehabil* 1989; **10(6)**: 561–7.

54. Bayer M. Rampenbestrijiding verliep uitzonderlijk snel. *Alert* 1988; **10**: 2.

55. Editorial. Burn care facilities in the UK. *Burns* 1989; **15(2)**: 183–6.

56. Baker F. The management of mass casualty disasters. *Top Emerg Med* 1979; **1**: 149–57.

57. Orr S, Robinson W. The Hyatt disaster: two physicians' perspectives. *J Emerg Nursing* 1982; **8**: 6–11.

58. Duignan JP, McEntee GP, Scully B, Corrigan TP. Report of a fire disaster – management of burns and complications. *Irish Med J* 1984; **77**: 8–10.

59. Hicks H. No stranger to disaster. *Nurs Times* 1988; **84(29)**: 16–17.

60. Melorio E. Mass media and serious emergencies, chapter 56. In: Masellis M, Gunn SWA, eds. *The Management of Mass Burn Casualties and Fire Disasters: Proceedings of the First International Conference on Burns and Fire Disasters.* Dordrecht: Kluwer Academic, 1992: 301–4.

61. Mosca A, Amico M, Geraci V, Masellis M. The role of the mass media burn prevention campaigns – psychological considerations, chapter 58. In: Masellis M, Gunn SWA, eds. *The Management of Mass Burn Casualties and Fire Disasters: Proceedings of the First International Conference on Burns and Fire Disasters.* Dordrecht: Kluwer Academic, 1992: 311–13.

62. Ellinger K, Quintel M, Das Ramstein Ungluck. *Notarzt* 1989; **5**: 68.

63. Kossman T, Trentz O. Das Flugschau-Ungluck in Ramstein: Erfahrungbericht uber die Akutversorgung des Verletztenkontingents des Universitatsklinikums Homburg/Saar. In: Zellern PR, ed. *Die Versorgung des Brandveniertzten in Katastrophenfall.* Darmstadt: Steinkopff Verlag, 1990: 79–83.

64. Kossmann T, Wittling I, Buhren V, Sutter G, Trantz O. Transferred triage to a level 1 trauma center in a mass catastrophe of patients; many of them burns. *Acta Chir Plast* 1991; **33(3)**: 145–50.

65. Amico M, Geraci V, Mosca A, Masellis M. Psychological reactions in the disaster emergencies: hypotheses and operative guidelines, chapter 50. In: Masellis M, Gunn SWA, eds. *The Management of Mass Burn Casualties and Fire Disasters: Proceedings of the First International Conference on Burns and Fire Disasters.* Dordrecht: Kluwer Academic, 1992: 278–81.

66. Vitale R, D'Arpa N, Conte F, Cucchiara P, Guzzetta C, Masellis M. Clinical file and protocol for general doctors and for non-specialized hospital doctors to assist burn patients, chapter 34. In: Masellis M, Gunn SWA, eds. *The Management of Mass Burn Casualties and Fire Disasters: Proceedings of the First International Conference on Burns and Fire Disasters.* Dordrecht: Kluwer Academic, 1992: 198–221.

67. Di Salvo L, Vitale R, Masellis M. Therapeutic kit and procedures for fluid resuscitation in disasters, chapter 38. In: Masellis M, Gunn SWA, eds. *The Management of Mass Burn Casualties and Fire Disasters: Proceedings of the First International Conference on Burns and Fire Disasters.* Dordrecht: Kluwer Academic, 1992: 231–8.

68. Caruso E, Crabai P, Donati L, Klinger M, Garbin S, Zaza R. Ready-to-use emergency kit for treatment of severe burns: definition and specifications, chapter 39. In: Masellis M, Gunn SWA, eds. *The Management of Mass Burn Casualties and Fire Disasters: Proceedings of the First International Conference on Burns and Fire Disasters.* Dordrecht: Kluwer Academic, 1992: 239–42.

69. Donati L. Campiglio GL, Garbin S, Zara R, La Rosa F, Crabai P, Caruso E. Burn patients in major emergencies. The preparation of air-drop kits for emergency surgical-resuscitation use. *Minerva Chir* 1993; **48(9)**: 479–83.

70. Costanzo S. Health education in disaster medicine, chapter 20. In: Masellis M,

Gunn SWA, eds. *The Management of Mass Burn Casualties and Fire Disasters: Proceedings of the First International Conference on Burns and Fire Disasters*. Dordrecht: Kluwer Academic, 1992: 133–9.

71. McCollum ST. Lessons from the Dublin 1981 fire catastrophe, chapter 6. In: Masellis M, Gunn SWA, eds. *The Management of Mass Burn Casualties and Fire Disasters: Proceedings of the First International Conference on Burns and Fire Disasters*. Dordrecht: Kluwer Academic, 1992: 45–50.

72. Pietersen CM, Huerta SC. *Analysis of the LPG Incident at San Juan Ixhuatepec, Mexico City*. The Hague: TNO, 1984.

73. Pietersen CM. De ramp met de pepleiding in de Sovjet Unie. *Alert* 1989; **9**: 3.

74. Fedorov VD, Alekseev AA. Medical care of mass burn victims: the Vishnevsky principles and organization in the Ufa disaster, chapter 35. In: Masellis M, Gunn SWA, eds. *The Management of Mass Burn Casualties and Fire Disasters: Proceedings of the First International Conference on Burns and Fire Disasters*. Dordrecht: Kluwer Academic, 1992: 222–3.

75. Remensnyder JP, Ackroyd FP, Astrozjnikova S, *et al.* Burned children from the Bashkir train-gas pipeline disaster II. Follow-up experience at Children's Hospital 9, Moscow. *Burns* 1990; **16(5)**: 333–6.

76. Mazzarella B, Scanni E, Carideo P, Maresca A, Vivona G, Sorrentino A. On-site treatment of severely burned patients, chapter 36. In: Masellis M, Gunn SWA, eds. *The Management of Mass Burn Casualties and Fire Disasters: Proceedings of the First International Conference on Burns and Fire Disasters*. Dordrecht: Kluwer Academic, 1992: 224–6.

77. Cohen E. Triage 1982. *J Emerg Med Ser* 1982; **7**: 24–8.

78. Wu WT, Ngim RC. Anatomy of a burns disaster: the Miri Bank explosion. *Ann Acad Med Singapore* 1992; **21(5)**: 640–8.

79. Barclay TL. Planning for mass burn casualties. In: Wood C, ed. *Accident and Emergency Burns: Lessons from the Bradford Disaster*. London: Royal Society of Medicine Services Roundtable III, 1986.

80. Roding H. Ethical problems in mass burn disasters. *Zentralbl Chir* 1981; **106(18)**: 1204–9.

81. Alexander JW. Control of infection following burn injury. *Arch Surg* 1971; **103**: 435–43.

82. Anantharaman V. Burns mass disasters: aetiology, predisposing situations and initial management. *Ann Acad Med Singapore* 1992; **21(5)**: 635–9.

83. Jacobs LM, Ramp JM, Breay JM. An emergency medical system approach to disaster planning. *J Trauma* 1979; **19(3)**: 157–62.

84. Landiscina M, Bile L, Bollini C, Magatti MF. The burn patients and medically assisted helicopter transport, chapter 43. In: Masellis M, Gunn SWA, eds. *The Management of Mass Burn Casualties and Fire Disasters: Proceedings of the First International Conference on Burns and Fire Disasters*. Dordrecht: Kluwer Academic, 1992: 251–2.

85. Trimble EJ. The management of aircraft passenger survival in fire. *Toxicology* 1996; **115(1–3)**: 41–61.

86. Clark MA, Hawley DA, McClain DL, Pless JE, Marlin DC, Standish SM. Investigation of the 1987 Indianapolis Airport Ramada Inn incident. *J Forensic Sci* 1994; **39(3)**: 644–9.

87. Salomone J III, Sohn AP, Ritzlin R, Gauthier JH, McCarty. Correlations of injury, toxicology, and cause of death to Galaxy Flight 203 crash site. *J Forensic Sci* 1987; **32(5)**: 1403–15.

88. Davis JWL. Toxic chemical versus lung tissue – an aspect of inhalation injury revisited. *J Burn Care Rehabil* 1986; **7(3)**: 213–22.

89. Clark WR Jr, Nieman GF. Smoke inhalation. *Burns* 1988; **14(4)**: 473–94.

90. Sharpe DT, Roberts AH, Barclay TL, *et al.* Treatment of burns casualties after fire at Bradford City football ground. *Br Med J* 1985; **291**: 945–8.

91. Buerk CA, Batdorf JW. Cammack V, *et al.* The MGM Grand Hotel fire. *Arch Surg* 1982; **117**: 641–5.

92. Ngim RC. Burns mass disasters in Singapore – a three decade review with implications for future planning. *Singapore Med J* 1994; **35(1)**: 47–9.

93. Remensynder JP, Astrozjnikova S. Bell L, *et al.* Progress in a Moscow children's burn unit: a joint Russian–American collaboration. *Burns* 1995; **21(5)**: 323–35.

94. Men'shikov DD, Zalogueva GV, Gerasimova LI, Orlova Nia, Ianisker Gia, Sidorova IV. The microfloral wound dynamics of the victims in the railroad disaster in Bashkiria. *Zh Mikrobiol Epidemiol Immunobiol* 1991; **7**: 32–5.

Chapter 6

Pre-hospital management, transportation, and emergency care

Ronald P Mlcak

Michael C Buffalo

Introduction

Advances in trauma and burn management over the past three decades have resulted in improved survival and reduced morbidity from major burns. The cost of such care, however, is high; it requires conservation of resources such that only a limited number of burn intensive care units with the capabilities of caring for such labor-intensive patients can be found – hence regional burn care has evolved. This regionalization has led to the need for effective prehospital management, transportation, and emergency care. Progress in the development of rapid, effective transport systems has resulted in marked improvement in the clinical course and survival for victims of thermal trauma.

For burn victims, there are usually two phases of transport. The first is the entry of the burn patient into the emergency medical system with treatment at the scene and transport to the initial care facility. The second phase is the assessment and stabilization of the patient at the initial care facility and transportation to the burn intensive care unit.[1] With this perspective in mind, this chapter reviews current principles of optimal pre-hospital management, transportation, and emergency care.

Pre-hospital care

Prior to any specific treatment, a patient must be removed from the source of injury and the burning process stopped. As the patient is removed from the injuring source, care must be taken so that a rescuer does not become another victim.[2] All care givers should be aware of the possibility that they may be injured by contact with the patient or the patient's clothing. Universal precautions, including wearing gloves, gowns, masks, and protective eye wear, should be used whenever there is likely contact with blood or body fluids. Burning clothing should be removed as soon as possible to prevent further injury.[3] All rings, watches, jewelry, and belts should be removed as they can retain heat and produce a tourniquet-like effect with digital vascular ischemia.[4] If water is readily available, it should be poured directly on the burned area. Early cooling can reduce the depth of the burn and reduce pain, but cooling measures must be used with caution, since a significant drop in body temperature may result in hypothermia with ventricular fibrillation or asystole. Ice or ice packs should never be used, since they may cause further injury to the skin or produce hypothermia.

Initial management of chemical burns involves removing saturated clothing, brushing the skin if the agent is a powder, and irrigation with copious amounts of water, taking care not to spread chemical on burns to adjacent unburned areas. Irrigation with water should continue from the scene of the accident through emergency evaluation in the hospital. Efforts to neutralize chemicals are contraindicated due to the additional generation of heat, which would further contribute to tissue damage. A rescuer must be careful not to come in contact with the chemical, i.e. gloves, eye protectors, etc., should be worn.

Removal of a victim from an electrical current is best accomplished by turning off the current and by using a nonconductor to separate the victim from the source.[5]

On-site assessment of a burned patient

Assessment of a burned patient is divided into primary and secondary surveys. In the primary survey, immediate life-threatening conditions are quickly identified and treated. The primary survey is a rapid, systematic approach to identify life-threatening conditions. The secondary survey is a more thorough head-to-toe evaluation of the patient. Initial management of a burned patient should be the same as for any other trauma patient, with attention directed at airway, breathing, circulation, and cervical spine immobilization.

Primary Assessment

Exposure to heated gases and smoke from the combustion of a variety of materials results in damage to the respiratory tract. Direct heat to the upper airways results in edema formation, which may obstruct the airway. Initially, 100%-humidified oxygen should be given to all patients when no obvious signs of respiratory distress are present. Upper airway obstruction may develop rapidly following injury, and the respiratory status must be continually monitored in order to assess the need for airway control and ventilator support. Progressive hoarseness is a sign of impending airway obstruction. Endotracheal intubation should be done early before edema obliterates the anatomy of the area.[3]

The patient's chest should be exposed in order to adequately assess ventilatory exchange. Circumferential burns may restrict breathing and chest movement. Airway patency alone does not assure adequate ventilation. After an airway is established, breathing must be assessed in order to insure adequate chest expansion. Impaired ventilation and poor oxygenation may be due to smoke inhalation or carbon monoxide intoxication. Endotracheal intubation is necessary for unconscious patients, for those in acute respiratory distress, or for patients with burns of the face or neck which may result in edema which causes obstruction of the airway.[3] The nasal route is the recommended site of intubation. Assisted ventilation with 100%-humidified oxygen is required for all intubated patients.

Blood pressure is not the most accurate method of monitoring a patient with a large burn because of the pathophysiologic changes which accompany such an injury. Blood pressure may be difficult to ascertain because of edema in the extremities. A pulse rate may be somewhat more helpful in monitoring the appropriateness of fluid resuscitation.[6]

If a burn victim was in an explosion or deceleration accident, there is the possibility of a spinal cord injury. Appropriate cervical spine stabilization must be accomplished by whatever means necessary, including a cervical collar to keep the head immobilized until the condition can be evaluated.

Secondary Assessment

After completing a primary assessment, a thorough head-to-toe evaluation of a patient is imperative.[7] A careful determination of trauma other than obvious burn wounds should be made. As long as no immediate life-threatening injury or hazard is present, a secondary examination can be performed before moving a patient; precautions such as cervical collars, backboards, and splints should be used.[8] Secondary assessment should examine a patient's past medical history, medications, allergies, and the mechanisms of injury.

There should never be a delay in transporting burn victims to an emergency facility due to an inability to establish intravenous (IV) access. If the local/regional emergency medical system (EMS) protocol prescribes that an IV line is started, then that protocol should be followed. The pre-hospital burn life support course recommends that if a patient is less than 60 minutes from a hospital, an IV is not essential and can be deferred until a patient is at a hospital. If an IV line is established, Ringer's lactate solution should be infused at 500 ml/h in an adult and 250 ml/h in a child 5 years of age or over. In children younger than 5 years of age no IV lines are recommended.[4]

Pre-hospital care of wounds is basic and simple, because it requires only protection from the environment with an application of a clean dressing or sheet to cover the involved part. Covering wounds is the first step in diminishing pain. If it is approved for use by local/regional EMS, narcotics may be given for pain, but only intravenously in small doses and only enough to control pain. Intramuscular or subcutaneous routes should never be used, since fluid resuscitation could result in unpredictable patterns of uptake.[4] No topical antimicrobial agents should be applied in the field.[4,9] The patient should then be wrapped in a clean sheet and blanket to minimize heat loss and to control temperature during transport.

Transport to Hospital Emergency Department

Rapid, uncontrolled transport of a burn victim is not the highest priority, except in cases where other life-threatening conditions coexist. In the majority of accidents involving major burns, ground transportation of victims to a hospital is available and appropriate. Helicopter transport is of greatest use when the distance between an accident and a hospital is 30–150 miles or when a patient's condition warrants.[10] Whatever the mode of transport, it should be of appropriate size, and have emergency equipment available as well as trained personnel, such as a nurse, physician, paramedic, or respiratory therapist.

Assessment and emergency treatment at initial care facility

The assessment of a patient with burn injuries in a hospital emergency department is essentially the same as outlined for a pre-hospital phase of care. The only real difference is the availability of more resources for diagnosis and treatment in an emergency department. As with other forms of trauma, the primary survey begins with the ABCs, and the establishment of an adequate airway is vital. Endotracheal intubation should be accomplished early if impending respiratory obstruction or ventilatory failure is anticipated, because it may be impossible after the onset of edema following the initiation of fluid therapy. Securing an endotracheal tube may be difficult because traditional methods often do not adhere to burned skin, and tubes are easily dislodged. One method of choice includes securing an endotracheal tube with woven tape under the ears as well as over the ears.[11] While doing assessments and making interventions for life-threatening problems in the primary survey, precautions should be taken to maintain cervical spine immobilization until injuries to the spine can be ruled out.

Following a primary survey, a thorough head-to-toe evaluation of a patient should be done. This includes obtaining a history as thorough as circumstances permit. The history should include the mechanism and time of the injury and a description of the surrounding environment, such as whether injuries were incurred in an enclosed space, the presence of noxious chemicals, the possibility of smoke inhalation, and any related trauma. A complete physical examination should include a careful neurological examination, as evidence of cerebral anoxic injury can be subtle. Patients with facial burns should have their corneas examined with fluorescent staining. Routine admission laboratories should include a complete blood count, serum electrolytes, glucose, blood urea nitrogen (BUN), and creatine. Pulmonary assessment should include arterial blood gases, chest X-rays, and carboxyhemoglobin.[12]

All extremities should be examined for pulses, especially with circumferential burns. Evaluation of pulses can be assisted by use of a Doppler ultrasound flowmeter. If pulses are absent, the involved limb may need urgent escharotomy for release of the constrictive, unyielding eschar (**Figure 6.1**). In circumferential chest burns, escharotomy may also be necessary to relive chest wall restriction and improve ventilation. Escharotomies may be performed at the bedside under IV sedation using electrocautery. Mid-axial incisions are made through the eschar but not into subcutaneous tissue of the eschar in order to assure adequate release. Limbs should be elevated above the heart level. Pulses should be monitored for 48 hours.[12]

If pulses are still present, but appear endangered, chemical escharotomy with enzymatic ointments (Accuzyme, collagenase, Elase) can be effective. Enzymatic escharotomy in hand burns may be preferred since surgical incisions risk exposure of superficial nerves, vessels, and tendons. Enzymatic escharotomy is indicated only during the first 24–48 hours postburn, and it should be used only in combination with a topical antimicrobial agent or sepsis can occur. With enzymatic escharotomy, there is usually a spike in temperature, which subsides after the enzyme is removed.

Evaluation of Wounds

After the primary and secondary surveys are completed and resuscitation is underway, a more careful evaluation of burn wounds is performed. The wounds are gently cleaned, and loose skin and in large wounds blisters are debrided (see care of outpatient burns, chapter 4). Blister fluid contains high levels of inflammatory mediators, which increase burn wound ischemia. The blister fluid is also a rich media for subsequent bacterial growth. Deep blisters on the palms and soles may be aspirated instead of debrided in order to improve patient comfort. After burn wound assessment is complete, the wounds are covered with a topical antimicrobial agent and appropriate burn dressings or a biological dressing is applied.

An estimate of burn size and depth assists in making a determination of severity, prognosis, and disposition of a patient. Burn size directly affects fluid resuscitation, nutritional support, and surgical interventions. The size of a burn wound is most frequently estimated by using the rule-of-nines method (**Figure 6.2**). A more accurate assessment can be made of a burn injury, especially in children, by using the Lund and Browder chart, which takes into account changes brought about by growth (**Figure 6.3**).[4,9] The American Burn Association identifies certain injuries as usually

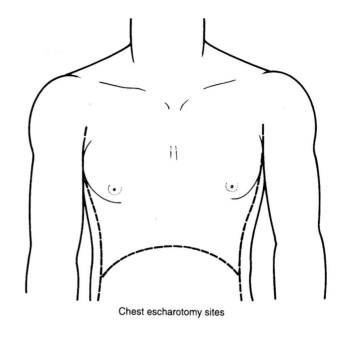

Chest escharotomy sites

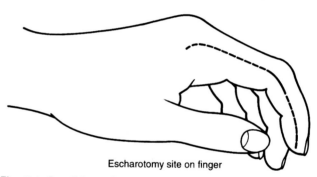

Escharotomy site on finger

Fig. 6.1 Possible escharotomy sites.

requiring a referral to a burn center. Patients with these burns should be treated in a specialized burn facility after initial assessment and treatment at an emergency department. Questions about specific patients should be resolved by consultation with a burn center physician (**Table 6.1**).[4,13]

Fluid Resuscitation

Establishment of IV lines for fluid resuscitation is necessary for all patients with major burns including those with inhalation injury or other associated injuries. These lines are best started in the upper extremity peripherally. A minimum of two large caliber IV catheters should be established through nonburned tissue if possible, or through burns if no unburned areas are available. Ringer's lactate solution should be infused at 2–4 ml/kg/% total body surface area (TBSA) which is burned.[1,4,9] Children must have additional fluid for maintenance.[14]

Taking into account the increased evaporative water loss in the formula for fluid resuscitation for pediatric patients, the initial resuscitation should begin with 5000 ml/m^2/% TBSA burned/day + 2000 ml/m^2/BSA total/day 5% dextrose in Ringer's lactate. This formula calls for one-half of the total amount to be given in the first

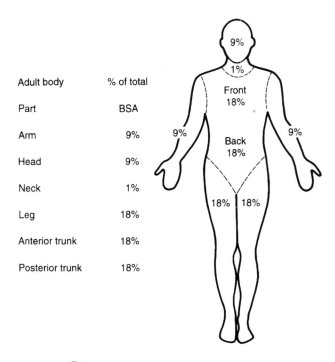

Adult body	% of total
Part	BSA
Arm	9%
Head	9%
Neck	1%
Leg	18%
Anterior trunk	18%
Posterior trunk	18%

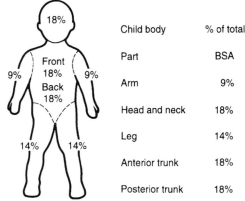

Child body	% of total
Part	BSA
Arm	9%
Head and neck	18%
Leg	14%
Anterior trunk	18%
Posterior trunk	18%

Fig. 6.2 Estimation of burn size using the Rule of Nines.

Table 6.1 Criteria for transfer of a burn patient to a burn center
Second degree burns greater than 10% total body surface area (TBSA)
Third degree burns
Burns that involve the face, hands, feet, genitalia, perineum, and major joints
Chemical burns
Electrical burns including lightning injuries
Any burn with concomitant trauma in which the burn injuries pose the greatest risk to the patient
Inhalation injury
Patients with preexisting medical disorders that could complicate management, prolong recovery, or affect mortality
Hospitals without qualified personnel or equipment for the care of critically burned children

8 hours post-injury with the remainder given over the following 16 hours (**Table 6.2**).[14]

All resuscitation formulas are designed to serve as a guide only. The response to fluid administration and physiologic tolerance of a patient is the most important determinant. Additional fluids are commonly needed with inhalation injury, electrical burns, associated trauma, and delayed resuscitation. The appropriate resuscitation regimen administers the minimal amount of fluid necessary for maintenance of vital organ perfusion; the subsequent response of the patient over time will dictate if more or less fluid is needed so that the rate of fluid administration can be adjusted accordingly. Inadequate resuscitation can cause diminished perfusion of renal and mesenteric vascular beds. Fluid overload can produce undesired pulmonary or cerebral edema.

Urine Output Requirements

The single best monitor of fluid replacement is urine output. Acceptable hydration is indicated by a urine output of more than 30 ml/h in an adult (0.5 ml/kg/h) and 1 ml/kg/h in a child. Diuretics are generally not indicated during an acute resuscitation period. Patients with high-voltage electrical burns and crush injuries with myoglobin and/or hemoglobin in the urine have an increased risk of renal tubular obstruction. Sodium bicarbonate should be added to IV fluids in order to alkalinize the urine, and urine output should be maintained at 1–2 ml/kg/h as long as these pigments are in the urine.[14] The addition of an osmotic diuretic such as mannitol may also be needed to assist in clearing the urine of these pigments.

Additional Assessments and Treatments

Decompression of stomach

To combat the problem of gastric ileus, a nasogastric tube should be inserted in all patients with major burns in order to decompress the stomach. This is especially important for patients being transported at high altitudes.[13] Additionally, all patients should be restricted from taking anything by mouth until after the transfer has been completed. Decompression of the stomach is usually necessary because an anxious, apprehensive patient will swallow considerable amounts of air and distend the stomach. Narcotics also diminish peristalsis of the gastrointestinal tract and result in distension.

A patient must be kept warm and dry. Hypothermia is detrimental to traumatized patients and can be avoided or at least minimized by the use of sheet and blankets. Wet dressings should be avoided.

The degree of pain experienced initially by the burn victim is inversely proportional to the severity of the injury.[8] No medication

Table 6.2 Burn fluid resuscitation formula
Fluid administration – Ringer's lactate
First 24 hours: 5000 ml/m^2 burn + 2000 ml/body area m^2, administer half in 8 hours and the remaining half in 16 hours
Second 24 hours: 3750 ml/m^2 + 1500 ml/body area m^2 administer half in 8 hours and the remaining half in 16 hours
Adjust the above rates to maintain a urine output of 1 ml/kg/h

Age	0–1	1–4	5–9	10–14	15
A – $\frac{1}{2}$ of head	$9\frac{1}{2}$%	$8\frac{1}{2}$%	$6\frac{1}{2}$%	$5\frac{1}{2}$%	$4\frac{1}{2}$%
B – $\frac{1}{2}$ of one thigh	$2\frac{3}{4}$%	$3\frac{1}{4}$%	4%	$4\frac{1}{4}$%	$4\frac{1}{2}$%
C – $\frac{1}{2}$ of one leg	$2\frac{1}{2}$%	$2\frac{1}{2}$%	$2\frac{3}{4}$%	3%	$3\frac{1}{4}$%

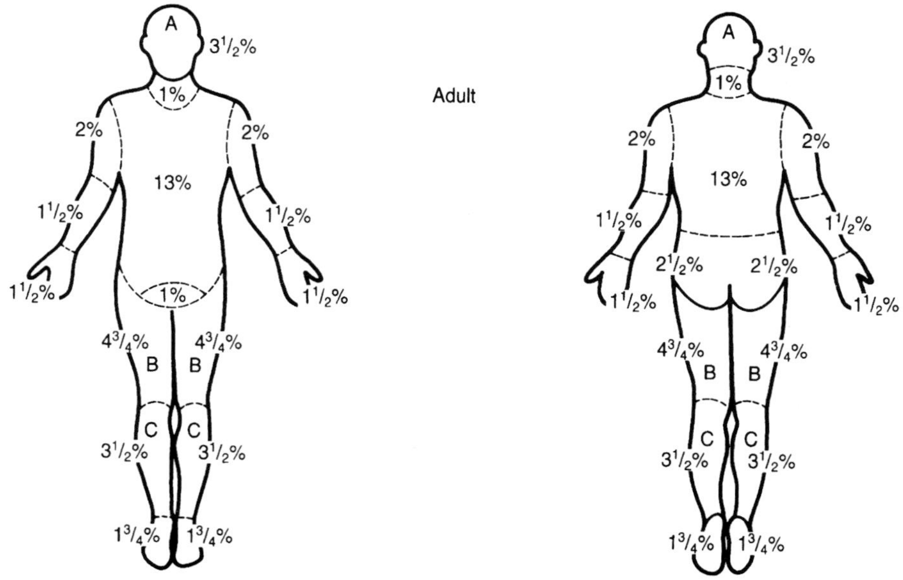

Fig. 6.3 Estimation of burn size using the Lund and Browder method.

for pain relief should be given intramuscularly or subcutaneously. For mild pain, aspirin 650 mg orally every 4–6 hours may be given. For severe pain, morphine, 1–4 mg intravenously every 2–4 hours, is the drug choice, although meperidine (Demerol) 10–40 mg by IV push every 2–4 hours may be used.[10] Recommendations for tetanus prophylaxis are based on the patient's immunization history. All patients with burns should receive 0.5 ml of tetanus toxoid. If prior immunization is absent or unclear, or if the last booster was more than 10 years ago, 250 units of tetanus immunoglobulin is also given.[4]

Transportation guidelines

The primary purpose of any transport teams is not to bring a patient to an intensive care unit but to bring that level of care to the patient as soon as possible. Therefore, the critical time involved in a transport scenario is the time it takes to get the team to the patient. The time involved in transporting a patient back to a burn center becomes secondary. Communication and teamwork are the keynotes to an effective transport system.

When transportation is required from a referring facility to a specialized burn center, a patient can be fairly well stabilized before being moved. Initially, the referring facility should be informed that all patient referrals require physician-to-physician discussion. Pertinent information needed will include patient demographic data; time, date, cause and extent of burn injury; weight and height; baseline vital signs; neurological status; laboratory data; respiratory status; previous medical and surgical history; and allergies.

A referring hospital is informed of specific treatment protocols regarding patient management prior to transfer. To ensure patient stability the following guidelines are offered:

- Establish two IV sites, preferably in an unburned upper extremity, and secure IV tubes with sutures.
- Insert a Foley catheter and monitor for acceptable urine output (30 ml/h adult, 1 ml/kg/h child).
- Insert a nasogastric tube and ensure that the patient remains NPO.
- Maintain body temperature between 38 and 39.0°C rectally.
- Stop all narcotics.
- For burns less than 24 hours old, only use lactated Ringer's solution. The staff physician will advise on the infusion rate, which is calculated based on the percentage of total body surface area burned.

Following physician-to-physician contact and collection of all pertinent information, the physicians will make recommendations regarding an appropriate mode of transportation. The options are based on distance to a referring unit, patient complexity, and comprehensiveness of medical care required. Options include:

- Full medical intensive care unit transport with a complete team, consisting of a physician, a nurse, and a respiratory therapist from the burn facility;
- Medical intensive care transport via fixed wing or helicopter with a team from a referring facility;
- Private plane with medical personnel to attend patient;
- Commercial airline;
- Private ground ambulance;
- Transport van with appropriate personnel.

Transport Team Composition

Because stabilization and care for a burned patient is so specialized, team selection is of the utmost importance. Traditionally, these patients were placed in an ambulance with an emergency medical technician and transported with few efforts made to stabilize the patient prior to transfer. As levels of care and technology have evolved, the need for specialized transport personnel has been increasingly observed. Today most transport teams are made up of one or more of the following health care members: a registered nurse, a respiratory therapist, and/or a staff physician or house resident. Because a large number of burned patients require some type of respiratory support due to inhalation injury or carbon monoxide intoxication, the respiratory therapist and nurse team has proven to be an effective combination. The background and training of nurses and therapists differ in many ways, so such a team provides a larger scope of knowledge and experience when both are utilized. Team members ideally should be cross-trained so that each member can function at the other's level of expertise.

Training and Selection

Since the transport team will work in a high stress environment, often with life or death consequences, these individuals must be carefully selected. The selection process should involve interviews with a nursing administrator, a director of respiratory therapy, and a medical director of a transport program.

Minimum requirements for transport team members should include:

1. Transport nurse qualifications:
   - a registered nurse;
   - minimum of 6 months burn care experience;
   - current cardiopulmonary resuscitation (CPR) certification;
   - advanced cardiac life support (ACLS) or pediatric advanced life support (PALS) certification;
   - able to demonstrate clinical competency;
   - observe two transports;
   - a valid passport for international response.
2. Transport respiratory therapist qualifications:
   - registered/certified respiratory therapist with 6 months burn care experience;
   - licensed by appropriate regulatory agency as a respiratory care practitioner;
   - have current CPR certification;
   - have ACLS or PALS certification;
   - able to demonstrate clinical competency;
   - observe two transports;
   - demonstrate a working knowledge of transport equipment;
   - a valid passport for international response.

Because all of the care rendered by a transport team outside a hospital is given as an extension of care from a transporting/receiving facility, specific steps must be taken to protect staff and physicians from medical liability and to provide consistent care for all patients. Strict protocols are used to guide all patient care; team members should be in constant communications with an attending physician regarding a patient's condition and the interventions to be considered. Team members must be proficient at a number of procedures, which may be needed during transport or while stabilizing a patient prior to transport. To keep up with current technology and changes, team members should be included in discussions of recent transports and current management techniques, so that they can discuss patient care issues, receive ongoing in-service education, and participate in a review of the quality of transports.

Modes of Transportation

Once the need for transport of a burned patient is established, the decision must be rendered concerning what type of transportation vehicle is to be used (**Table 6.3**). There are two models of transport commonly used: ground (ambulance/transport vehicle), air (helicopter, fixed wing), or a combination of both. Factors to be considered when selecting a mode of transportation are the condition of the patient and the distance involved. The level of the severity of the burn mandates the speed with which the team must arrive in order the stabilize and transport a patient.[15]

Ground transport

Ground transport should be considered to cover distances of 70 miles or less; however, sometimes a patient's condition may require air transport, particularly helicopter transport, even though the distance is within the 70-mile range. The ground transport vehicle should be modified with special equipment needed for intensive care transport, and there must be enough room to comfortably seat team members and equipment.

Table 6.3 Transport criteria: mode and team composition, burns ≤ 6 days postburn				
Weight	% Burn	Distance (miles)	Team*	Transport mode
≤3	Any	75	C	Van, helicopter
		76-250	C	Turboprop airplane
		≥251	C	Learjet
3.1-20	≥10	75	N-RT	Van, helicopter
		76-500	N-RT	Commercial flight or turboprop airplane
		≥501	N-RT	Commercial airplane or Learjet
	≥10	75	C	Van, helicopter
		76-250	C	Turboprop airplane
		≥251	C	Learjet
20≥20	≤20	75	N	Commercial flight or turboprop airplane
		76-500	N-RT	
		≥501	N-RT	Commercial airplane or Learjet
	≥20	75	N	Van, helicopter
		76-500	C	Turboprop plane
		≥501	C	Jet

*C, Complete team (doctor, nurse, respiratory therapist); N, nurse; RT, respiratory therapist.

If any of the following criteria exist, the transport shall be changed to the fastest mode with a complete team:
- depressed mental status,
- drug depression,
- respiratory support,
- unstable cardiovascular system,
- presence of associated diseases,
- decreased urine output unresponsiveness to appropriate fluid administration,
- absent or marginal venous access,
- hypothermia unresponsive to corrective measures.

Table 6.4 Altitude's effects on blood gas values				
Altitude	Pressure	Tracheal Po$_2$	Alveolar Po$_2$	Alveolar Pco$_2$
Sea level	760	149	103	40
5000 feet	632	122	79	38
10 000 feet	523	100	61	36
15 000 feet	429	80	46	33
20 000 feet	349	63	33	30

Air transport

Air transport is used primarily when long distances or the critical nature of an injury separate a team from a patient. Air transport, however, does present its own unique set of problems. Aviation physiology is a specialty unto itself, and the gas laws play an important role in air transport and must be taken into consideration.

Dalton's law states that in a mixture of gases, the total pressure exerted by the mixture is equal to the sum of the pressures each would exert alone.[16] This is important when changing a patient's altitude because as altitude increases, barometric pressure decreases. The percentage of nitrogen, oxygen, and carbon dioxide remain the same, but the partial pressures they exert change (**Table 6.4**).[17]

Altitude is an important factor in the oxygenation of a transported patient and constant monitoring by a team is required under such circumstances. Boyle's law states that the volume of gas is inversely proportional to the pressure to which it is subject at a constant temperature. This gas law significantly affects patients with air leaks and free air in the abdomen, because as altitude increases, the volume of air in closed cavities also increases.[18] For this reason, all air that can be reached should be evacuated prior to an increase in altitude. Intrathoracic air and gastric air must be removed via functional chest tubes or nasogastric tubes and periodically checked during transport. Other factors that should be considered during air transport are reduced cabin pressure, turbulence, noise and vibration, changes in barometric pressure, and acceleration/deceleration forces. Physiologic changes which affect a patient and team members include middle ear dysfunction, pressure-related problems with sinuses, air expansion in a gastrointestinal tract, and motion sickness. Utilizing transport vehicles that have pressurized cabins can reduce or eliminate most of these problems.[19]

Helicopters and fixed wing aircraft

Helicopters and fixed wing aircraft both have advantages and disadvantages related to patient care. Helicopters are widely used for short-distance medical air transport. Medical helicopters, because they are usually based on hospital premises, have no need to use airport facilities or ambulance services and, thereby, reduce team response time. Helicopters are able to land close to a referring hospital. Additionally, helicopters provide ease in loading and unloading patients and equipment.[15] The disadvantages of helicopter transport include its limited range, usually less than 150 miles[20] and its non-pressurized cabin which limits the altitude at which patients can be safely carried. The low-altitude capabilities also subject the aircraft to variability in weather (i.e. fog, rain, and reduced visibility); therefore, helicopter flights experience much more interference due to the weather. Other disadvantages include

noise, vibrations, reduced air speed, small working space, lower weight accommodation, and high maintenance requirements.[15]

When long distances must be traveled (greater than 150 miles) or when increased altitude is necessary, fixed wing aircraft are considered as a viable mode of transport for patients. The advantages of using fixed wing aircraft include: long range capabilities, increased speed, ability to fly in most weather conditions, control of cabin pressure and temperature, larger cabin space, and more liberal weight restrictions. Disadvantages of fixed wing aircraft include the need for an airport with adequate runway length, difficulty in loading and unloading patients and equipment, and the pressure of air turbulence and noise.

Equipment

Because medical equipment used in intensive care units has evolved tremendously in the last 10 years, there is no reason that these advances should not be extended to the equipment, which is used in a transport program. **Tables 6.5** and **6.6** outline the drugs and equipment used in our successful transport system. The transport team must be able to provide ICU level care whenever needed. Most hospitals are well stocked and able to provide necessary supplies for initial patient stabilization and resuscitation; however, specialty items relating to the care of burn patients may not be present or adequate to meet the needs of burn victims. It is imperative that adequate equipment be available to handle any situation, which may arise during a transport process (**Figure 6.4**). Extra battery packs and electrical converters on fixed wing aircraft are recommended due to long transport times and delays caused by unforeseeable circumstances of weather or logistics.

Portable Monitor

A portable ECG monitor capable of monitoring two pressure channels should accompany all patients in transport. This allows for continuous monitoring of heart rate, rhythm, and arterial blood pressure. The second pressure channel may be used for patients with a pulmonary artery catheter or those who need intracranial pressure monitoring. This monitor should be small and lightweight but able to provide a display bright enough to be seen from several feet away. The monitor should have its own rechargeable power supply which continuously charges while connected to an alternat-

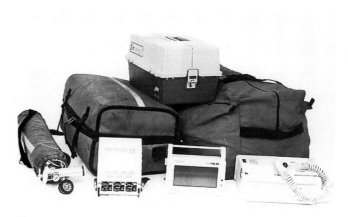

Fig. 6.4 Typical equipment used in transport of a patient.

Table 6.5 Medical equipment used in a transport system

Monitor bag	Quantity
Pressure bag	1
EKG cable	1
Pressure cable	2
Oxygen saturation cables	2
Oxygen saturation probes	2
Stapler	1
Staple remover	1
Stethoscope	1
EKG pads (adult/pedi)	9 each
Blood pressure tubing (NIBP)	1
Safe-cuff (NIBP – various sizes)	1 each
Automatic blood pressure cuffs	1 each
Temperature probe – rectal	1
Thermometer	1
Thermometer covers	1 box
Defibrillator jell tube	1
Sphygmomanometer	1
GI/GU bag	
Salem sumps (10,12,14,16fr)	1 each
Feeding tube 8fr	1
Surgilube	5
Clean gloves	20
Umbilical tape	1 jar
60 ml catheter tip syringe	2
Guaiac cards	10
Guaiac reagent	1 bottle
Diastix	1 bottle
Benzoin swabs	5
Cal stat	1 bottle
Tongue blades	10
Cotton swabs	10
Foley's temp. (8,10,12,16fr)	1 each
Sterile gloves	10
pH paper	1
Respiratory equipment	
Resuscitation bag adult/pedi	1 each
Oxygen mask adult/pedi	1 each
Venturi mask adult/pedi	1 each
T-Tube adapters	2
CPR microshield	1
Cricothyrotomy catheter sets	1
Tracheostomy tubes (00-8.0)	1 each
Endotracheal tubes (3.0-8.0)	2 each
Laryngoscope handles (1g.sm.)	2 each
Laryngoscope blades (Miller – Sizes 0-4)	1 each
Laryngoscope blades (MacIntosh – Sizes 0-4)	2
Magill forceps adult/pedi	1
Stylets adult/pedi	1
Airways (sm, med, lg)	1
PEEP valves	2
Wright respirometer	1
Pleural drainage set	1
Heimlick valves	2
Siemens Minimed III	1
Defibrillator	1
Batteries (C & D)	4 each
Prepodyne swabs	4
Skin degreaser	1 bottle
Nebulizer kit	2
1″ tape roll	1
Nipple adapters	2
E cylinder regulator	2
E cylinder wrench	2
Suction catheters (8-14fr)	5 each
Suction pump	1
Hard tip suction device	1
Adapters (15 & 22mm)	2 each
Normal saline vials	10
Vaponephrine solution	1 bottle
Goggles	1
Clean gloves	10
Humid vent adapters	2
Oxygen tanks aluminum	6
Oxygen tubing	2
TXP transport ventilator	1
Protocol Propag 106	1
Defibrillator battery support system	1

ing current (AC) power supply. One suitable unit is the Protocol Systems Propaq 106 portable monitor (**Figure 6.5**). This monitor has two pressure channels; it provides a continuous display of ECG, heart rate, systolic, diastolic, and mean blood pressure; it can display temperature and oxygen saturation; and it is also capable of operating a noninvasive blood pressure cuff. High and low alarms for each monitored parameter can be set, silenced, or disabled by a trained operator.

Infusion Pump

Continuous delivery of fluids and pharmacological agents must not be interrupted during transport. Infusion pumps can be easily attached to stretchers and are usually capable of operating for several hours on internal batteries. These devices should have alarms to warn of infusion problems and should be as small and lightweight as possible (**Figure 6.6**).

Ventilator

Size, weight, and oxygen consumption are the primary concerns in selecting transport ventilators. A weight under 5 pounds (2.2 kg) is desirable, and a ventilator's dimensions should make it easy to mount or to place on a bed. Orientation of controls should be along a single plane, and inadvertent movement of dials should be difficult.[21] The ventilator breathing circuit and exhalation valve should be kept simple, and incorrect assembly should be impossible. The TXP transport ventilator (Percussionaire Corporation, Sand Point, ID) is a portable pressure-limited time-cycled ventilator and is approved for in-flight use by the US Air Force (**Figure 6.7**). The transport ventilator weighs 1.5 pounds (0.68 kg), can be set to provide respiratory rates of between 6 and 250 breaths per minute, and provides tidal volumes of between 5 and 1500 cc. This ventilator is powered entirely by oxygen and requires no electrical power. All timing circuit gases are delivered to the patient so that operation of the ventilator does not consume additional oxygen. The I : E ratios are preset at the factory from 1 : 1 at frequencies of 250 cycles per minute to 1 : 5 at a rate of 6 cycles per minute. As a result, breath stacking and undesired overinflation due to air trapping may be avoided.[22]

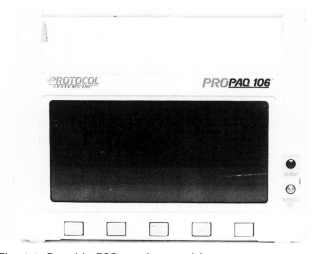

Fig. 6.5 Portable ECG monitor used in transport.

Table 6.6 Burn transport supply list

Medications	Quantity	Medications	Quantity
Epinephrine	2	Compazine	2
Atropine sulfate	2	Hep-Lock flush	5
Sodium bicarbonate	2	Heparin	1
Calcium chloride	2	Lidocaine	
D50	2	(injectable/cardiac strip)	1
Lidocaine	2	Narcan	4
Bretylol	2	Albumin	2
Isoproterenol	2	Regular insulin	1
Dopamine	4	Benadryl	4
Dobutrex	2	Chloral hydrate suppository	2
Calcium gluconate	2	Chloral hydrate 500 mg/10 ml	2
Lasix	10	Tylenol 650 mg/25ml	2
Potassium chloride	4	Tylenol suppository	2
Ranitidine	2	Lacri-Lube tube	2
Benadryl (injectable)	4	Maalox	1
Polysporin ointment	2	Phenergan	2
Elase ointment	2	Thorazine	2
Medical equipment	**Quantity**	**Medical Equipment**	**Quantity**
IV bag 1			
D5.3NS 1000ml	2	Needle holder	1
D10W 500 ml	1	Hemostat	1
Lactated Ringer's solution	2	0-silk suture	3
48" Pressure tubing	2	Staples (10, 11, 15)	1
IV start pack	2	Solution sets (10gtts,ml)	2
T-piece	4	Solution sets (60gtts/ml)	2
Stopcocks	4	Minimed full set	2
Y-ports	2	Minimed half set	2
Scissors	1	Betadine (bottle)	1
IV bag 2			
D5W 250 ml	2	Syringes (1, 3, 5, 10, 35 ml)	10 each
Normal saline 250 ml	2	Needles (22g, 20g, 19g, 16g)	10 each
Pressure transducers	2	IV catheters (16g, 18g, 20g, 22g)	6 each
60 ml Luer-lock syringe	2	Medicuts (18g, 20g, 22g)	1 each
Side pouch			
Kerlix 6"	10	Burn dressing (1g)	2
Ace wraps (6", 4", 3")	6 each	1" tape roll	1
Space blanket	1	2" tape roll	1
Urometer	1	4 x 4's (box)	2

Stabilization

One of the primary reasons for a specialized transport team is to be able to transport a patient in as stable condition as possible. Current practice has evolved to embrace the concept that events during the first few hours following burn injury may affect the eventual outcome of the patient; this is especially true with regard to fluid management and inhalation injury. Stabilization techniques performed by the transport team have been expanded to include procedures that are usually not performed by nursing or respiratory personnel. Such techniques include interpreting radiographs and laboratory results and then conferring with fellow team members, referring physicians, and the team's own medical staff in order to arrive at a diagnosis and plan for stabilization. The transport team may perform such procedures as venous cannulation, endotracheal intubation, arterial blood gas interpretation, and management of mechanical ventilators. Team members may request new radiographs, in order to assess catheter or endotracheal tube placement or to assess the pulmonary system's condition. Team members may

aid in the diagnosis of air leaks (pneumothorax) and evacuate the pleural space of the lung by needle aspiration as indicated. All of these procedures may be immediately necessary and life-saving. Cross-training of all team members to be able to perform the others' jobs is recommended in order to safeguard patients in the event that any team member becomes incapacitated during transport. All these skills can be learned via experience in a burn intensive care unit, through formal training seminars, and via a thorough orientation program. Mature judgment, excellent clinical skills, and the ability to function under stress are characteristics needed when selecting candidates for a transport program.

Patient assessment prior to transport to a specialized burn care unit from a referring hospital

Initial assessment upon arrival of a flight team should include a list of standard procedures for determining a burned patient's current condition. First, a thorough review of the patient's history con-

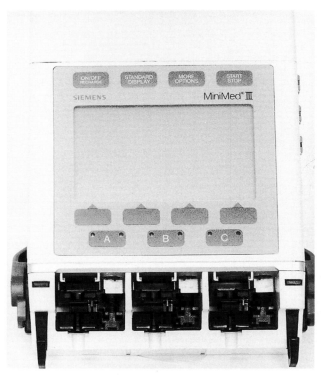

Fig. 6.6 Portable IV pump used in transport.

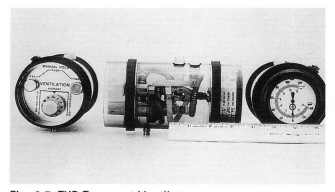

Fig. 6.7 TXP Transport Ventilator.

cerning the accident and past medical history must be done. This process provides the transport team with an excellent base from which to begin to formulate a plan of action. The patient will certainly have been diagnosed by a referring physician; however, a transport team often finds problems overlooked in initial evaluations. Since burn care is a specialized field, modes of treatment may very greatly outside the burn treatment community. Frequently, a referring hospital is not well versed in the treatment of burn victims and should not be expected to display the expertise found among clinicians who work with such patients everyday. Thus, the next step in stabilizing a burn patient is a physical assessment done by a transport team. These procedures should always be performed in the same order and in a structured fashion. Assessment of a burn patient begins with the ABCs of a primary survey, including airway, breathing, circulation, cervical spine

immobilization, and a brief baseline neurological examination. All patients should be place on supplemental oxygen prior to transport in order to minimize the effects of altitude changes on oxygenation. Two IV lines should be started peripherally with a 16-gauge catheter or larger. Ideally, IV lines should be placed in nonburn areas but may be placed through a burn if they are the only sites available for cannulation. Intravenous lines should be sutured in place because venous access may not be available after the onset of generalized edema. The fluid of choice for initial resuscitation is lactated Ringer's solution.

In addition to initial stabilization procedures, blood should be obtained for initial laboratory studies if not already done. Initial diagnostic studies include hematocrit, electrolytes, urinalysis, chest X-ray, arterial blood gas, and carboxyhemoglobin levels. Any correction of laboratory values must be done prior to transfer and verified with repeat studies. Electrocardiographic monitoring should be instituted on any patient prior to transfer. Electrode patches may be a problem to place because the adhesive will not stick to burned skin. If alternative sites for placement cannot be found, an option for monitoring is to insert skin staples and attach the monitor leads to them with alligator clips. This provides a stable monitoring system, particularly for the agitated or restless patient who may displace needle electrodes. A Foley catheter with a urimeter should be placed to accurately monitor urine output. Acceptable hydration is indicated by a urine output of more than 30 ml/h in an adult (5 ml/kg/h) and at least 1 ml/kg/h in a child.

With the exception of escharotomies, open chest wounds, and actively bleeding wounds, management during transport consists of simply covering wounds with a topical antimicrobial agent or a biological dressing. Wet dressings are contraindicated because of the decreased thermoregulatory capacity of patients sustaining large burns and the possibility of hypothermia. To combat the problem of a gastric ileus, a nasogastric tube should be inserted in all burn patients in order to decompress the stomach. This is especially important for patients being transferred at high altitudes. Hypothermia can be avoided or minimized by the use of heated blankets and/or aluminized Mylar space blankets. The patient's rectal temperature must be kept between 37.5 and 39.0°C.

A clear, concise, chronological record of the mechanism of injury and assessment of airway, breathing, and circulation should be kept in the field and en route to the hospital. This information is vital for a referring facility to better understand and anticipate the condition of the patient. Additionally, all treatments, including invasive procedures, must be recorded, along with a patient's response to these interventions.

Summary

Burn injuries present a major challenge to a health care team, but an orderly, systematic approach can simplify stabilization and management. A clear understanding of the pathophysiology of burn injuries is essential for providing quality burn care in the pre-hospital setting, at the receiving health care facility, and at the referring hospital prior to transport. After a patient has been rescued from an injury-causing agent, assessment of the burn victim begins with a primary survey. Life-threatening injuries must be treated first, followed by a secondary survey, which documents and treats other injuries or problems. Intravenous access may be established in concert with logical/regional medical control and appropriate fluid resuscitation begun. Burn wounds should be covered with clean, dry sheets; and the patient should be kept warm with blankets to prevent hypothermia. The patient should be transported to an emergency room in the most appropriate mode available.

At the local hospital, it should be determined if a burn patient needs burn center care according to the American Burn Association Guidelines. In preparing for organizing a transfer of a burn victim, consideration must be given to the continued monitoring and management of the patient during transport. In transferring burn patients, the same priorities developed for pre-hospital management remain valid. During initial assessment and treatment and throughout transport, the transport team must ensure that the patient has an adequate airway, breathing, circulation, fluid resuscitation, urine output, and pain control. Ideally, transport of burn victims will occur through an organized, protocol-driven plan, which includes specialized transport mechanisms and personnel. Successful transport of burn victims, whether in the pre-hospital phase or during interhospital transfer, requires careful attention to treatment priorities, protocols, and details.

References

1. Boswick JA, ed. *The Art and Science of Burn Care*. Rockville, MD: Aspen Publishers, 1987.
2. Dimick AR. Triage of burn patients. In: Wachtel TL, Kahn V, Franks HA, eds. *Current Topics in Burn Care*. Rockville, MD: Aspen Systems, 1983: 15–18.
3. Wachtel TL. Initial care of major burns. *Postgrad Med* 1989; **85(1)**: 178–96.
4. American Burn Association. *Advanced Burn Life Support Providers Manual*. Chicago, IL: American Burn Association, 1994.
5. American Burn Association. Radiation injury. *Advanced Burn Life Support Manual*. Appendix 1 Chicago, IL: American Burn Association, 1994.
6. Bartholomew CW, Jacoby WD. Cutaneous manifestations of lightning injury. *Arch Dermatol* 1975; **26**: 1466–8.
7. Committee on Trauma, American College of Surgeons. Burns. In: *Advanced Trauma Life Support Course Book*. Chicago: American College of Surgeons, 1984: 155–63.
8. Rauscher LA, Ochs GM. Pre-hospital care of the seriously burned patient. In: Wachtel TL, Kahn V, Franks HA, eds. *Current Topics in Burn Care*. Rockville, MD: Aspen Systems, 1983: 1–9.
9. Goldfarb JW. The burn patient, Air Medical Crew National Standards Curriculum, Phoenix, 1988, ASHBEAMS.
10. Marvin JA, Heinback DM. Pain control during the intensive care phase of burn care. *Crit Care Clin* 1985; **1**: 147–57.
11. Mlcak RP, Helvick B. Protocol for securing endotracheal tubes in a pediatric burn unit. *J Burn Care Rehabil* 1987; **8**: 233–7.
12. Herndon DN, Desai MH, Abston S. *et al. Residents Manual*. Galveston: Shriners Burns Hospital, and the University of Texas Medical Branch, 1992: 1–17.
13. Collini FJ, Kealy GP. Burns: a review and update. *Contemp Surg* 1989; **34**: 75–7.
14. Herndon DN, Rutan R, Rutan T. The management of burned children. *J Burn Care Rehabil* 1993; **14**: 3–8.
15. Roy LR, Cunningham W. Transport. *Neonatal and Pediatric Respiratory Care*. St Louis: CV Mosby, 1988: 321.
16. McPhearson SP. *Respiratory Therapy Equipment*, 3rd edn. St Louis: CV Mosby, 1986.
17. *US Navy Flight Surgeons' Manual*. Government publication, 1968.
18. Jacobs B. *Emergency Patient Care, Pre-Hospital Ground and Air Procedures*. New York: Macmillan, 1983.
19. McNeil EL. *Airborne Care of the Ill and Injured*. New York: Springer-Verlag, 1983.
20. *Federal Regulations for Pilots*. Government publication, 1987.
21. Branson RD. Intrahospital transport of critically ill; mechanical ventilation of patients. *Resp Care* 1992; **37**: 775–93.
22. Johanningman JA, Branson RD, Cambell RS, Hurst JM. Laboratory and clinical evaluation of the Max transport ventilator. *Resp Care* 1990; **35**: 952–9.

Chapter 7

Pathophysiology of burn shock and burn edema

George C Kramer, Tjøstolv Lund
David N Herndon

Introduction and historical notes

If left untreated cutaneous thermal injury greater than one-third of the total body surface area (TBSA) invariably results in the severe and unique derangement of cardiovascular function called burn shock. Shock is defined as an abnormal physiologic state in which the flow of blood is insufficient to maintain adequate nutritive perfusion to meet cellular needs. Before the 19th century, it was demonstrated that after a burn, fluid is lost from the blood so that the blood becomes thicker; and in 1897, saline infusions for severe burns were first advocated.[1,2] However, a real understanding of burn pathophysiology was not reached until the work of Frank Underhill.[3] He demonstrated that unresuscitated burn shock correlates with greatly increased hematocrit values in burned patients, which are secondary to fluid and electrolyte loss after burn injury. The increased hematocrit values occurring shortly after severe burn were interpreted as a plasma volume deficit. Cope and Moore showed that the hypovolemia of burn injury resulted from fluid and protein translation into burned and nonburned tissues.[4]

Throughout the 20th century, both animal and clinical studies have established the importance of fluid resuscitation for burn shock. Investigations have focused on the rapid and massive fluid sequestration in the burn wound and the resultant hypovolemia. We now have an extensive experimental database on the circulatory and microcirculatory alterations associated with burn shock

and edema generation in both the burn wound and nonburned tissues. During the last decade, research has focused on identifying and defining the release mechanisms and effects of the many inflammatory mediators produced and released after burn injury.[5]

It is now recognized that burn shock is a complex process of circulatory and microcirculatory dysfunction, not easily or fully repaired by fluid resuscitation. Severe burn injury results in significant hypovolemic shock and substantial tissue trauma, both of which cause the formation and release of many local and systemic mediators.[6–8] Burn shock results from the interplay of hypovolemia and mediator action and continues as a significant pathophysiologic state, even if hypovolemia is corrected. Increases in pulmonary and systemic vascular resistance (SVR) and myocardial depression occur despite adequate preload and volume support.[8–12] These physiologic changes can further exacerbate the whole body inflammatory response into a vicious cycle of accelerating organ dysfunction.[7,8,13]

This chapter examines our present understanding of the pathophysiology of the early events in burn shock, focusing on the many facets of organ and systemic effects directly resulting from the hypovolemia and circulating mediators. Inflammatory shock mediators, both local and systemic, that are implicated in the pathogenesis of burn shock include histamine, serotonin, kinins, oxygen free radicals, and products of the eicosanoid acid cascade – prostaglandins, thromboxanes, and interleukins. Additionally, certain hormones and mediators of cardiovascular function are elevated several-fold after burn injury; these include epinephrine, norepinephrine, vasopressin, angiotensin II, and neuropeptide-Y. Most certainly other mediators and factors are also involved. Understanding the complex mechanism of the pathophysiologic actions of these mediators may be of great relevance when optimally effective therapies are designed. The hope is that an improved early treatment of burn shock, perhaps through individualized fluid resuscitation protocols and methods of mediator blockade, can be developed to ameliorate or eliminate the incidence of organ dysfunction. Effective burn resuscitation and treatment of burn shock remain major challenges in modern medicine.

Hypovolemia and rapid edema formation

Initially, burn shock is hypovolemic in nature and characterized by the hemodynamic changes similar to those that occur after hemorrhage, including decreased plasma volume, cardiac output, urine output, and an increased systemic vascular resistance with resultant reduced peripheral blood flow.[6,8,14–16] Following the development of hypovolemia, hemoconcentration occurs. In severe cases a transient increase in hematocrit and hemoglobin concentration will appear, even though adequate fluid resuscitation is provided. As in the treatment of other forms of hypovolemic shock, the primary initial therapeutic goal is to promptly restore vascular volume and to preserve tissue perfusion in order to minimize tissue ischemia. However, burn resuscitation is complicated not only by the severe burn wound edema but also by severe and sustained edema in nonburned soft tissue that is unique to thermal trauma. Large volumes of resuscitation solutions are required to maintain vascular volume during the first few hours after an extensive burn. The rapid edema formation and weight gain slows during the first few hours, but can continue through the first 24 hours[16,17] or longer within the thermally injured tissue.

By definition, edema develops when the rate by which fluid is filtered out of the microvessels exceeds the flow in the lymph vessels draining the same tissue mass. The edema formation appears to follow a biphasic pattern. An immediate and rapid increase in the water content of burn tissue is seen in the first hour after burn injury.[15,17] A second and more gradual increase in fluid extravasation occurs during the first 12–24 hours after burn injury in both the burned skin and nonburned soft tissue.[7,17] The amount of edema formation in burned skin depends on the type and extent of injury,[15,18] whether fluid resuscitation is given, and also on the type and amount of fluid administered.[19] Without sustained fluid infusion the edema fluid is somewhat self-limited as plasma volume and capillary pressure decrease. However, during resuscitation, maintenance of blood volume, blood flow, and capillary pressure can cause continuous fluid extravasation. The edema development in thermally injured skin is characterized by the extremely rapid increase of tissue water content, which can double within the first hour after burn.[15,20] Leape found a 70–80% water content increase in a full-thickness burn wound 30 minutes after burn injury, with 90% of this change occurring in the first 5 minutes.[16,21,22] There was little increase in burn wound water content after the first hour in the nonresuscitated animals. In resuscitated animals or animals with small wounds, adequate tissue perfusion continues to 'feed' the edema for several hours. Demling *et al.* used dichromatic absorptiometry to measure edema development during the first week after

an experimental partial-thickness burn injury on one hind limb in sheep.[17] Although edema was rapid with over 50% occurring in the first hour, maximum water content did not occur until 12–24 hours after burn injury.

Normal microcirculatory fluid exchange

An understanding of the physiologic mechanisms of the rapid formation of burn edema requires a basic knowledge of normal microvascular physiology. Under normal physiologic conditions, the pressure in arterioles, capillaries, and venules causes a filtration of fluid into the interstitial space of all tissues. This fluid is then partially reabsorbed into the circulation at the venous end of capillaries and venules, while the remaining net filtration is removed from the interstitial space by lymphatic drainage.[23,24] Fluid transport across the microcirculatory wall in normal and pathological states is quantitatively described by the Landis–Starling equation (**Figure 7.1**):

$$J_v = K_f\,[(P_c - P_{if}) - \sigma(\pi_p - \pi_{if})]$$

This equation describes the physical forces and physiologic mechanisms that govern fluid transfer between vascular and extravascular compartments. J_v is the volume of fluid that crosses the microvasculature barrier; K_f is the capillary filtration coefficient, which is the product of the capillary surface area and hydraulic conductivity of the capillary wall; P_c is the capillary hydrostatic pressure; P_{if} is the interstitial fluid hydrostatic pressure; π_p is the colloid osmotic pressure of plasma; π_{if} is the colloid osmotic pressure of interstitial fluid; σ is the osmotic reflection coefficient. Edema occurs when the lymphatic drainage (J_L) does not keep pace with the increased J_v.

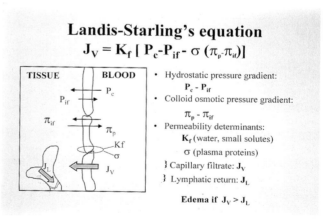

Landis-Starling's equation
$$J_V = K_f\,[\,P_c\text{-}P_{if}\text{-}\sigma\,(\pi_p\text{-}\pi_{if})]$$

Fig. 7.1 Microvascular 'Starling pressures' in thermally injured cutaneous tissue. During normal conditions the Starling forces result in a slight pressure imbalance favoring filtration with lymph flow (J_L) exactly equal to fluid filtration (J_v). In burned skin, all Starling forces are altered, creating a large increase in J_v, which exceeds J_L and causes rapid edema. Data shown represent Starling forces in burned skin before injury and at 5 minutes postburn just prior to starting resuscitation.

Mechanisms of burn edema

By analyzing the factors interrelating the physiological determinants of transmicrovascular fluid flux (i.e. Landis–Starling equation), edema may theoretically be formed by:

- increased K_f;
- increased P_c;
- decreased P_{if};
- decreased σ;
- decreased π_p; and
- increased π_{if}.

Burn edema may be unique among other types of edema, because in burn edema all of these variables seem to change significantly in the direction required to increase fluid filtration. Each variable is discussed individually.

Capillary Filtration Coefficient (K_f)

Burn injury causes direct and indirect mediator-modulated changes of the barrier properties of the capillary wall, which are reflected as large increases in both protein and water permeability. Arturson and Mellander showed that K_f in the scalded hind limb immediately increases two to three times, suggesting that the hydraulic conductivity (water permeability) of the capillary wall increases.[25] However, K_f is a function of both hydraulic conductivity and the capillary surface area. Thus, local vasodilation and microvascular recruitment would also likely contribute to the increased K_f in addition to an increased hydraulic conductivity. Measuring K_f and the rate of edema formation (J_v) allowed Arturson and Mellander to determine the changes in transcapillary pressures necessary to account for the increased capillary filtration. Their calculations indicated that a transcapillary pressure gradient of 100–250 mmHg was required to explain the extremely rapid edema formation that occurred in the first 10 minutes after a scald injury. They concluded that only a small fraction of the early formation of burn edema could be attributed to the changes in K_f and permeability. Arturson and Mellander suggested that osmotically active molecules generating sufficiently large osmotic reabsorption pressures are released from burn-damaged cells. On the other hand, subsequent studies described below show that very large increases in filtration force could be directly attributed to changes in P_c and particularly P_{if} in burned injury skin.

Capillary Pressure (P_c)

In most forms of shock, capillary pressure decreases as a result of arteriolar vasoconstriction. However, studies in which P_c was estimated by vascular occlusion methods, in the scalded hind limb of dogs, showed that P_c doubled to 45–50 mmHg during the first 30 minutes after burn injury and slowly returned to baseline over 3 hours.[26] We are unaware of studies that have measured P_c in nonburned skin, but it is likely that P_c decreases in nonburned tissue as a result of the documented increase in peripheral resistance.

Interstitial Hydrostatic Pressure (P_{if})

An initial surprising, but now well-verified, finding established that P_{if} in dermis becomes highly negative after thermal injury. Using a micropipette and tissue oncometer, dermal P_{if} was found to rapidly reduce from its normal value of −1 mmHg to less than −100 mmHg in isolated skin preparations.[18] This generation of a strongly

negative interstitial fluid hydrostatic pressure constitutes a 'suction force' or imbibition pressure adding to the capillary pressure in promoting fluid filtration from the intravascular to the interstitial space. *In vivo* measurements show a temporary reduction of −20 to −30 mmHg; presumably, this number is less negative because fluid extravasation relieves the imbibition pressure. After resuscitation, P_{if} can increase to a positive value of 1–2 mmHg or remain negative.[27–29] The interstitial compliance, i.e. the relation between P_{if} and tissue volume, is markedly altered after burn injury and fluid resuscitation. This may account for the sustained edema of burn injury that can last for days. The mechanism behind the negative-pressure generation may be related to the denaturation of collagen[28,29] and to changes in the compliance of thermally injured tissue. Recently, the release of adhesional forces (β_1-integrins) between the interstitial matrix fibers and cells were found to cause an imbibition pressure to develop following different inflammatory reactions.[30]

These data suggest that the highly negative P_{if} is the predominant mechanism responsible for both the initial rapid development of edema and the sustained edema in burn injured skin. The changes in interstitial space compliance (pressure–volume-relationship) induced by the thermal insult may also be responsible for the sustained edema in burn injured skin.

Osmotic Reflection Coefficient (σ)

The osmotic reflection coefficient is an index of the proportion of the full osmotic pressure generated by plasma proteins that is effectively exerted across the capillary wall. A σ of 1.0 represents a membrane impermeable to protein; a σ of 0 represents a membrane that is completely permeable to protein. In skin, the normal σ of albumin is reported to be 0.85–0.95.[31,32] Increased capillary permeability to protein causes a reduced σ, an effective reduction in the reabsorptive oncotic gradient across the capillary wall, and a resulting increase in net fluid filtration. Studies of lymph sampled from burned skin are consistent with the large and sustained increases in capillary permeability,[15,31,32] while a transient and smaller increase in capillary permeability occurs over 8–12 hours post-injury in other soft tissue not directly burned.[32] Pitt *et al.* estimated the σ for skin from dog hind paw using the lymph washdown technique and reported a normal σ of 0.87 for albumin and a reduction to 0.45 after scald injury.[26]

Plasma Colloid Osmotic Pressure (π_p)

The normal plasma protein concentration of 6–8 g/dl and its associated π_p of 25–30 mmHg produce a significant transcapillary reabsorptive force partially outweighing the fluid filtration out of the microvasculature.[14,24] Plasma colloid osmotic pressure decreases in nonresuscitated burn injured animals as protein-rich fluid extravasates into burn wounds, while protein-poor transcapillary reabsorption takes place in nonburned tissue.[14,33–35] Plasma is further diluted, and π_p is further reduced after crystalloid resuscitation. Zetterstrom and Arturson found that plasma oncotic pressure was reduced to half of the normal values in burn patients. π_p can decrease so rapidly with resuscitation that the transcapillary colloid osmotic pressure gradient ($\pi_p-\pi_{if}$) will approach zero or even reverse to favor filtration and edema.[33,35] Although it is likely that some hypoproteinemia after major burn injury is inevitable, animal and clinical studies that used early colloid resuscitation maintained π_p at higher levels than crystalloid resuscitation alone.[7,34,36] Also, it is clear that the degree of hypoproteinemia and reduced π_p correlates with the total volume of fluid resuscitation.[34] Initial therapy with colloid solution is advocated by some clinicians,[7] while the majority wait 8–24 hours post-injury, reasoning that normalization of microvascular permeability in injured tissue must occur before colloid therapy is cost-effective.[8]

Interstitial Colloid Osmotic Pressure (π_{if})

The π_{if} in skin is normally 10–15 mmHg or about one-half that of plasma in humans.[24,37] It is commonly claimed that prenodal lymph fluid has a composition similar to interstitial fluid.[24] Experimental studies in animals using lymph as representative of interstitial fluid show that the colloid osmotic pressure in lymph from burned skin initially increases 4–8 mmHg indicating increased permeability.[32] However, more direct measurements of π_{if} using wick sampling[19,35,37] or tissue sampling technique[24] show only modest initial increases in π_{if} of 1–4 mmHg in the early nonresuscitated phase of burn injury. With resuscitation, π_p falls and then π_{if} decreases as the protein concentration of capillary filtrate remains less than plasma despite an increased permeability and a reduced σ. Compared with nonburned skin, the π_{if} remains significantly higher in the burn wound, supporting the view that sustained increases in protein permeability contribute to the persistence of burn edema.[24,27,37] However, compared with the large changes in P_c and particularly P_{if}, the increased capillary protein permeability is not the predominant mechanism for the early rapid rate of edema formation in burned injury skin.[28]

Nonburned tissue

Generalized edema in soft tissue not directly injured is characteristic after a major burn. Brouhard *et al.* reported increased water content in nonburned skin even after a 10% burn, with the maximum increase occurring at 12 hours postburn.[38] Arturson reported an increased transcapillary fluid flux (lymph flow) from nonburned tissue and a transient increase in permeability, as measured by an increase in the lymph concentration of plasma protein and macromolecular dextran infused as a tracer.[15,20,31] Harms extended these findings by measuring changes in lymph flow and protein transport of noninjured soft tissue for 3 days after injury.[32] He found that skin and muscle permeability were elevated for up to 12 hours postburn for molecules the size of albumin and immunoglobulin G, while capillary permeability of the lung's microvascular showed no increase. Maximum increased lymph flow and tissue water content were observed to correlate with the severe hypoproteinemia occurring during the early resuscitation period.[8,36] The sustained increase in water content and the elevated lymph flow of the nonburned tissue are likely the results of the sustained hypoproteinemia.[31–34]

Demling and colleagues postulated that the edema could be partially attributed to an alteration in the interstitium.[39] They suggested that interstitial protein washout increases the compliance of the interstitial space and that water transport and hydraulic conductivity across the entire blood–tissue–lymph barrier increased with hypoproteinemia. Several clinical and animal studies have established that maintaining more normal protein levels can ameliorate the overall edema formation.[7,40] Nonburn edema can also be limited by using nonprotein colloids such as dextran, if the colloid osmotic gradient is increased above normal.[8,36] However, it is not known if either the correction of hypoproteinemia or the use of albumin or dextran can lead to improved clinical outcome. It has been shown that the use of colloids has no beneficial effect on edema in the burn wound.[27,36]

Altered cellular membranes and cellular edema

In addition to a loss of capillary endothelial integrity, thermal injury also causes change at the membrane level of other cells. Baxter demonstrated that in burns of >30% total body surface area (TBSA) there is a systemic decrease in cellular transmembrane potentials as measured in skeletal muscle away from the site of injury.[10] It would be expected that the directly injured cell would have a damaged cell membrane, increasing sodium and potassium fluxes, resulting in cell swelling. However, this process also appears in cells that are not directly heat-injured. Micropuncture techniques have demonstrated partial depolarization in the normal skeletal muscle membrane potential of –90 mV to levels of –70 to –80 mV; cell death occurs at –60 mV. The decrease in membrane potentials is associated with an increase in intracellular water and sodium.[41–43] Similar alterations in membrane functions and cellular edema have been reported in hemorrhagic shock,[41,43] and also in the liver and endothelial cells.[44,45] A circulating shock factor(s) is likely to be responsible for the membrane depolarization,[46] but surprisingly, the molecular characterization of such a circulating factor has not been reported. Early investigators of this phenomenon postulated that a decrease in ATP levels or ATPase activity was the mechanism for membrane depolarization; however, other research suggests that it may result from an increased sodium conductance in membranes or an increase in sodium–hydrogen antiport activity.[42,45] Resuscitation of hemorrhage rapidly restores depolarized membrane potentials to normal, but resuscitation of burn injury only partially restores the membrane potential and intracellular sodium concentrations to normal levels, demonstrating that hypovolemia alone is not totally responsible for the cellular swelling seen in burn shock.[47] Membrane depolarization may be caused by different factors in different states of shock. Very little is known about the time course of the changes in membrane potential in clinical burns. More importantly, we do not know the extent to which altered membrane potentials affect total volume requirements and organ function in burn injury or even shock in general.

Mediators of burn injury

Several local and circulating mediators are produced or released after thermal injury. These mediators play important roles in the pathogenesis of edema and the cardiovascular abnormalities of burn injury. Many mediators alter vascular permeability directly or indirectly by increasing the microvascular hydrostatic pressure and surface area via the arteriolar vasodilation superimposed on an already altered membrane. The exact mechanism(s) of mediator-induced injury are of considerable clinical importance, as this understanding would allow for the development of pharmacologic modulation of burn edema and shock by mediator inhibition.

Histamine

Histamine is most likely to be the mediator responsible for the early phase of increased capillary permeability seen immediately after burn. Histamine causes large endothelial gaps to transiently form as a result of the contraction of venular endothelial cells.[48]

Histamine is released from mast cells in thermally injured skin; however, the increase in histamine levels and its actions are only transient. Histamine can also cause a rise in capillary pressure (P_c) by arteriolar dilation and venular contraction. Statistically significant reductions in burn edema have been achieved with histamine blockers and mast cell stabilizers when tested in acute animal models.[48] Friedl et al. have demonstrated that the pathogenesis of burn edema in the skin of rats appears to be related to the interaction of histamine with xanthine oxidase and oxygen radicals.[49] Histamine and its metabolic derivatives increased the catalytic activity of xanthine oxidase (but not xanthine dehydrogenase) in rat plasma and in rat pulmonary artery endothelial cells. In thermally injured rats, levels of plasma histamine and xanthine oxidase rose in parallel, in association with the uric acid increase. Burn edema was greatly attenuated by treating rats with the mast cell stabilizer cromolyn, complement depletion, or the H_2 receptor antagonist cimetidine, but was unaffected by neutrophil depletion.[50–52] Despite encouraging results in animals, beneficial antihistamine treatment of human burn injury has not been demonstrated.

Prostaglandins

Prostaglandins are potent vasoactive autocoids synthesized from the arachidonic acid released from burned tissue and inflammatory cells. They contribute to the inflammatory response of burn injury.[53,54] Macrophages and neutrophils infiltrate the wound and release prostaglandin as well as thromboxanes, leukotrienes, and interleukin-1. These wound mediators have both local and systemic effects. Prostaglandin E_2 (PGE_2) and leukotrienes LB_4 and LD_4 directly and indirectly increase microvascular permeability.[55] Prostacyclin (PGI_2) is produced in burn injury and is also a vasodilator, but may cause direct increases in capillary permeability as well. PGE_2 appears to be one of the more potent inflammatory prostaglandins, causing the postburn vasodilation in wounds, which, when coupled with the increased microvascular permeability, contributes to edema.[56,57]

Thromboxane

Thromboxane A_2 (TXA_2) and its metabolite thromboxane B_2 (TXB_2) are produced locally in the burn wound by platelets.[48] Vasoconstrictor thromboxanes may inhibit edema formation; however, by decreasing blood flow they can contribute to a growing zone of ischemia under the burn wound, and can cause the conversion of a partial-thickness wound to a deeper full-thickness wound. The serum level of TXA_2 and TXA_2/PGI_2 ratios are increased significantly in burn patients.[58,59] Heggers showed the release of TXB_2 at the burn wound was associated with local tissue ischemia, and that thromboxane inhibitors prevented the progressive dermal ischemia associated with thermal injury and thromboxane release.[60,61] The TXA_2 synthesis inhibitor anisodamine also showed beneficial macrocirculatory effects by restoring the hemodynamic and rheological disturbances towards normal. Demling showed that topically applied ibuprofen (which inhibits the synthesis of prostaglandins and thromboxanes) decreases both local edema and prostanoid production in burned tissue without altering systemic production.[62] On the other hand, systemic administration of ibuprofen did not modify early edema, but did attenuate the postburn vasoconstriction that impaired oxygen delivery to tissue in burned sheep.[63]

Kinins

Kinins, specifically bradykinin, are local mediators of inflammation that increase venular permeability. It is likely that bradykinin production is increased after burn injury, but its detection in blood or lymph can be difficult owing to the simultaneous increase in kininase activity and the rapid inactivation of free kinins. The generalized inflammatory response after burn injury favors the release of bradykinin.[64] Pretreatment of burn-injured animals with aprotinin, a general protease inhibitor, should have decreased the release of free kinin, but no effect on edema was noted.[65] On the other hand, pretreatment with a specific bradykinin receptor antagonist reduced edema in full-thickness burn wound in rabbits.[66]

Serotonin

Serotonin is released early after burn injury.[67] This agent is a smooth-muscle constrictor of large blood vessels. Antiserotonin agents such as ketanserin have been found to decrease peripheral vascular resistance after burn injury, but have not been reported to decrease edema.[67] On the other hand, the pretreatment effect of methysergide, a serotonin antagonist, reduces the hyperemic or increased blood flow response in the burn wounds of rabbits, along with reducing the burn edema.[66] However, methysergide did not prevent increases in the capillary reflection coefficient or permeability.[68] Ferrara et al. found a dose-dependent reduction of burn edema when methysergide was given preburn to dogs, but claimed that this was not attributable to blunting of the regional vasodilator response.[68] Zhang et al. reported a reduction in nonnutritive skin blood flow after methysergide administration to burned rabbits.[69]

Catecholamines

Catecholamines are released in massive amounts after burn injury.[7,70,71] On the arteriolar side of the microvessels these agents cause vasoconstriction, which tends to reduce capillary pressure, particularly when combined with the hypovolemia and the reduced venous pressure of burn shock.[48] Reduced capillary pressure may limit edema and induce interstitial fluid to reabsorb from nonburned skin, skeletal muscle, and visceral organs in nonresuscitated burn shock. Further, catecholamines, via β-agonist activity, may also partially inhibit increased capillary permeability induced by histamine and bradykinin.[48] These potentially beneficial effects of catecholamines may not be operative in directly injured tissue and may also be offset in nonburned tissue by the deleterious vasoconstrictor and ischemic effects. The hemodynamic effects of catecholamines will be discussed later in the chapter.

Oxygen Radicals

Oxygen radicals play an important inflammatory role in all types of shock, including burn shock. These short-lived elements are highly unstable reactive metabolies of oxygen; each one has an unpaired electron, making them strong oxidizing agents.[72] Superoxide anion (O_2^-), hydrogen peroxide (H_2O_2), and hydroxyl ion (OH^-) are produced and released after any inflammatory reaction or reperfusion of ischemic tissue. The hydroxyl ion is believed to be the most potent and damaging of the three. The formation of the hydroxyl radical requires free ferrous iron (Fe_2) and H_2O_2. Evidence that these agents are released after burn injury is the increased lipid peroxidation found in circulating red blood cells and biopsied tissue.[51,72,73] Nitric oxide (NO) simultaneously generated with the superoxide anion can lead to the formation of peroxynitrite

(ONOO⁻). The presence of nitrotyrosine in burn skin, found in the first few hours after injury, suggests that peroxynitrite may play a deleterious role in burn edema.[74] On the other hand, the blockade of NO synthase did not reduced burn edema, while treatment with the NO precursor arginine reduces burn edema.[75] NO may be important for maintaining perfusion and limiting the zone of stasis in burn skin.[76] Although the pro- and anti-inflammatory roles of NO remain controversial, it would appear that the acute beneficial effects of NO generation outweigh any deleterious effect in burn shock.

Antioxidants, namely agents that either directly bind to the oxygen radicals (scavengers) or cause their further metabolism, have been evaluated in several experimental studies.[77,78] Catalase, which removes H_2O_2, and superoxide dismutase (SOD), which removes radical O_2^-, have been reported to decrease the vascular loss of plasma after burn injury in dogs and rats.[51,77] Demling showed that large doses of deferoxamine (DFO), an iron chelator, when used for resuscitation of 40% TBSA in sheep, prevented systemic lipid peroxidation and decreased the vascular leak in non-burned tissue while also increasing oxygen utilization.[79] However, DFO may have accentuated burned tissue edema, possibly by increasing the perfusion of burned tissue.

The plasma of thermally injured rats showed dramatic increases in levels of xanthine oxidase activity, with peak values appearing as early as 15 minutes after thermal injury. Excision of the burned skin immediately after the thermal injury significantly diminished the increase in plasma xanthine oxidase activity.[49,51] The skin permeability changes were attenuated by treating the animals with antioxidants (catalase, SOD, dimethyl sulfoxide, dimethylthiourea) or an iron chelator (DFO), thus supporting the role of oxygen radicals in the development of vascular injury as defined by increased vascular permeability.[51] Allopurinol, a xanthine oxidase inhibitor, markedly reduced both burn lymph flow and levels of circulating lipid peroxides, and further prevented all pulmonary lipid peroxidation and inflammation.[73] This suggests that the release of oxidants from burned tissue was in part responsible for local burn edema, as well as distant inflammation and oxidant release.[73] The failure of neutrophil depletion to protect against the vascular permeability changes and the protective effects of the xanthine oxidase inhibitors (allopurinol and lodoxamide tromethamine) suggest that xanthine oxidase is the more likely source of the oxygen radicals involved in the formation of burn edema. These data suggest that the vascular injury, defined by an increased vascular permeability of burn injury, is in part related to the activation of xanthine oxidase and the generation of toxic oxygen metabolites that damage microvascular endothelial cells.[49,51]

Platelet Aggregation Factor

Platelet aggregation (or activating) factor (PAF) can increase capillary permeability and is released after burn injury.[65,80] Ono et al. showed in scald-injured rabbits that TCV-309 (Takeda Pharmaceutical Co. Ltd, Japan), a PAF antagonist, infused soon after burn injury blocked edema formation in the wound and significantly inhibited PAF increase in the damaged tissue in a dose-dependent manner. In contrast, the SOD content in the group treated with TCV-309 was significantly higher than that of the control group.[80] These findings suggest that the administration of large doses of a PAF antagonist immediately after injury may reduce burn wound edema and the subsequent degree of burn shock by suppressing PAF and superoxide radical formation.

Angiotensin II and Vasopressin

Angiotensin II and vasopressin, or antidiuretic hormone (ADH), are two hormones that participate in the normal regulation of extracellular fluid volume by controlling sodium balance and osmolality through renal function and thirst.[48] However, during burn shock where sympathetic tone is high and volume receptors are stimulated, both hormones can be found in supranormal levels in the blood. Both are potent vasoconstrictors of the terminal arterioles, but have little effect on the venules. Angiotensin II may be responsible for the selective gut ischemia; and gut mucosal ischemia may play a pivotal role in bacterial translocation and the development of sepsis and even multi-organ failure.[81-83] In severely burn-injured patients, angiotensin II levels were elevated two to eight times normal in the first 1–5 days after burn injury with peak levels occurring on day 3.[84] Vasopressin had peak levels of 50 times normal upon admission and declined towards normal over the first 5 days after burn injury. Along with catecholamines, vasopressin may be largely responsible for increased system vascular resistance and left heart afterload, which can occur in resuscitated burn shock. Sun et al. used vasopressin-receptor antagonist in rats with burn shock to improve hemodynamics and survival time, while vasopressin infusion exacerbated burn shock.[85]

Corticotropin–releasing Factor

Corticotropin-releasing factor (CRF) has proven to be efficacious in reducing protein extravasation and edema in burned rat paw. CRF may be a powerful natural inhibitory mediator of the acute inflammatory response of the skin to thermal injury.[86]

Other approaches to pharmacological attenuation of burn edema

Many reports on edema-reducing attempts using known burn mediator-blocking agents are presented above. However, there are other investigations attempting to ameliorate or inhibit the fluid extravasation induced by thermal injury. Among these are high-dose ascorbic acid (vitamin C) found to be efficient in reducing fluid needs both in burn-injured patients and experimental animals when administered postburn.[87,88] Topically applied local anesthetic lidocaine/prilocaine cream has been reported to be effective in reducing albumin extravasation in small burns in experimental animals.[89] The inositol triphosphate analog α-trinositol has also been found effective in reducing postburn edema when administered after injury.[90-92] Even though α-trinositol showed promising effects in animal experiments and also seemed to reduce pain in pilot clinical projects, its routine clinical application is not established. So far only the high-dose vitamin C regimen has found a place in clinical practice, but its use is not yet widespread.

Hemodynamic consequences of acute burns

The cause of reduced cardiac output (CO) during the resuscitative phase of burn injury has been the subject of considerable debate. There is an immediate depression of cardiac output before any detectable reduction in plasma volume. The rapidity of this response suggests a neurogenic response to receptors in the thermally injured skin or increased circulating vasoconstrictor mediators. Soon after injury a developing hypovolemia and reduced venous return undeniably contributes to the reduced cardiac output. But the subsequent persistence of reduced CO after apparently adequate fluid therapy, as evidenced by a reduction in heart rate and restoration of both arterial blood pressure and urinary output, has been attributed to circulating myocardial depressant factor(s), which possibly originate from the burn wound.[11,12] Demling et al. showed a 15% reduction in CO despite an aggressive volume replacement protocol after a 40% scald burn in sheep.[17] However, there are also sustained increases in catecholamine secretion and elevated systemic vascular resistance for up to 5 days after burn injury.[70,84] Michie et al. measured CO and SVR in anesthetized dogs resuscitated after burn injury.[93] They found that CO fell shortly after injury and then returned toward normal; however, reduced CO did not parallel the blood volume deficit. They concluded that the depression of CO resulted not only from blood volume decreases but also from an increased SVR and from the presence of a circulating myocardial depressant substance. Thus, there may be two factors other than reduced volume and venous return that significantly affect CO after burn injury: increased SVR and depressed myocardial contractility. On the other hand, patients suffering major burn injury tend to have supranormal CO (sometimes more than double) 3–6 days post-injury. This is secondary to the establishment of a hypermetabolic state.

Increased Systemic Vascular Resistance and Organ Ischemia

Cardiac output may remain below normal after adequate volume replacement in burn patients and experimental animals. Sympathetic stimulation and hypovolemia result in the release of catecholamines, vasopressin, angiotensin II, and neuropeptide-Y after burn injury.[84,85] These agents act primarily on the arteriolar smooth muscle, causing vasoconstriction, which is systemically manifested by increased afterload and SVR. The increased SVR after burn injury is also partly the result of increased blood viscosity secondary to the hemoconcentration.

Hilton and others performed a series of experiments in anesthetized dogs in which infusion of various peripheral vasodilators improved CO after burn injury.[93,94] They demonstrated a reduction in the peripheral vascular resistance and an augmented CO after verapamil, but the myocardial force of contraction remained depressed. Pruitt et al. examined the hypothesis that increased sympathetic activity is responsible partly for reduced CO in a group of burned patients.[95] They showed an improvement of CO with the vasodilator hydralazine. CO increased from 77% of baseline after-burn to 110% with treatment, and SVR decreased by 50% from elevated burn levels.[96]

There are several organs particularly susceptible to ischemia, organ dysfunction, and organ failure when burn resuscitation is delayed or inadequate. These include the kidney and the gastrointestinal tract. Renal ischemia can result directly from hypovolemia and increased sympathetic tone, but elevations in serum-free hemoglobin and particularly myoglobin correlate with increased renal failure.[97,98] Renal failure rates are on the decline due to standardized regimens of aggressive fluid therapy, but when therapy is delayed or associated with hypotension, acute renal failure is not uncommon.[97,98]

Sustained vasoconstriction of the gastrointestinal tract can occur even with adequate resuscitation.[82,99] Bacterial and endotoxin translocation may reduce mucosal pH and can contribute to the development of sepsis and is a consequence of visceral ischemia.

Cerebralopathies are not uncommon after large cutaneous burns, particularly in children, but the exact cause remains unclear. Studies in anesthetized sheep subjected to a 70% TBSA scald show that cerebral autoregulation is well maintained in the immediate postburn period, but 6 hours after resuscitation cerebral vascular resistance was inappropriately increased in proportion to perfusion pressure, resulting in reductions of cerebral blood flow of 50%.[100]

Pulmonary Edema

In large burns, there is also a pronounced increase in pulmonary vascular resistance (PVR) that corresponds with the increased SVR.[8,36] Also, pulmonary edema is not an uncommon finding, but it occurs more often after, than during, the fluid-resuscitation phase of burn injury. It results mainly from increased capillary pressure secondary to the increased PVR, which has components of both pre- and postcapillary vasoconstriction. Pulmonary wedge pressure is increased more than left atrial pressure after experimental burn injury due to postcapillary venular constriction.[36,101] It is likely that some left heart failure also contributes to the increased capillary pressure. However, the developing hypoproteinemia may be the greatest contributing factor to postburn pulmonary edema.[102] There is no evidence of increased capillary permeability from analysis of lung lymph sampled in large animal models after 40% TBSA injury, although rat studies suggest that albumin sequestration increases in the lungs after a 30% cutaneous scald.[51] Clinical studies suggest that in the absence of inhalation injury, the lungs do not necessarily develop edema.[103–105] This is consistent with the finding of little or no change in the microvascular permeability of the lung, and the fact that lung lymph rate may increase considerably to prevent interstitial fluid accumulation. Pulmonary dysfunction associated with inhalation injury is discussed in a separate chapter.

Myocardial Dysfunction

Myocardial function can be compromised after burn injury due to the right heart overload and direct depression of contractility shown in isolated heart studies.[106,107] Increases in the afterload of both the left and right heart result from SVR and PVR elevations. The left ventricle compensates and CO can be maintained with increased afterload by augmented adrenergic stimulation and increased myocardial oxygen extraction. However, the right ventricle has a minimal capacity to compensate for increased afterload. In severe cases, desynchronization of the right and left ventricles is deleteriously superimposed on a depressed myocardium.[108] Burn injury greater than 45% TBSA can produce intrinsic contractile defects. Several investigators reported that aggressive early and sustained fluid resuscitation failed to correct left ventricular contractile and compliance defects.[107–109] These data suggest that hypovolemia is not the sole mechanism underlying the myocardial defects observed with burn shock. Serum from patients failing to sustain a normal CO after thermal injury have exhibited a markedly negative inotropic effect on in vitro heart preparations.[110] In other patients with large burn injuries and normal cardiac indices, little or no depressant activity was detected.

Sugi et al. studied intact, chronically instrumented sheep after a 40% TBSA flame burn injury and associated smoke-inhalation injury, and after smoke-inhalation injury alone. They found that maximal elastance (E_{max}) was reduced after either burn injury or inhalation injury, showing decreased contractility in an intact animal.[111,112] Horton *et al.* demonstrated decreased left ventricular contractility in isolated, coronary perfused, guinea pig hearts harvested 24 hours after burn injury.[113] This dysfunction was more pronounced in hearts from aged animals and was not reversed by resuscitation with isotonic fluid. It was largely reversed by treatment with 4 ml/kg of hypertonic saline dextran (HSD), if administered during the initial 4–6 hours of resuscitation.[114,115] These authors also effectively ameliorated the cardiac dysfunction of thermal injury with infusions of antioxidants, arginine, and calcium channel blockers.[116-118] Cioffi and colleagues observed persistent myocardial depression after burn in a similar model when the animals received no resuscitation after burn injury.[119] In these studies, immediate and full resuscitation totally reversed abnormalities of contraction and relaxation after burn injury. However, resuscitation is often delayed in burn-injured patients due to a variety of circumstances. Murphy *et al.* showed elevations of troponin-1, a serum marker for cardiac injury, in patients with a TBSA > 18%, despite good cardiac indices.[120] Resuscitation and cardiac function studies emphasize the importance of early and adequate fluid therapy and suggest that functional myocardial depression after burn injury may not occur in patients receiving prompt and adequate volume therapy.

The primary mechanisms by which burn shock alters myocardial cell membrane integrity and impairs mechanical function remains unclear. Oxygen-derived free radicals may play a key causative role in the cell membrane dysfunction that is characteristic of several low-flow states. Horton *et al.* showed that a combination therapy of the free radical scavengers SOD and catalase significantly improved burn-mediated defects in left ventricular contractility and relaxation when administered along with adequate fluid resuscitation (4 ml/kg/% of burn). Antioxidant therapy did not alter the volume of fluid resuscitation required after burn injury.[116]

Summary and conclusion

Thermal injury results in massive fluid shifts from the circulating plasma into the interstitial fluid space, causing hypovolemia and swelling of the burned skin. When burn injury exceeds 25% TBSA there is also edema generation of noninjured tissues and organs. Fluid extravasation is caused by changes in all of the Starling forces. The rapid swelling immediately following injury is secondary to the development of strongly negative interstitial fluid pressure (imbibition pressure) and to a lesser degree by an increase in microvascular pressure and permeability. The type of fluid resuscitation, timing, and total volume infused influence these fluid shifts. Due to the complexity and interrelation of many variables, mathematical modeling with computer simulation of fluid and solute shifts and mass balances might be of help both to evaluate the relative importance of the known alterations and to help designing future studies.[121]

Secondary to the thermal insult there is release of inflammatory mediators and stress hormones. Circulating mediators deleteriously increase microvascular permeability and alter cellular membrane function by which water and sodium enter cells. Circulating mediators may also impair cardiac contractility, whereas increased vasoconstrictors further aggravate ischemia from the hypovolemia and cardiac dysfunction. The end result of a complex chain of events is decreased intravascular volume, increased systemic vascular resistance, decreased cardiac output, end-organ ischemia, and metabolic acidosis. Early excision of the devitalized tissue may reduce the local and systemic effects of mediators released from burned tissue, thus potentially preventing a progressive derangement. Without early and full resuscitation therapy these derangements result in acute renal failure, vascular ischemia, cardiovascular collapse, and death.

Resuscitation itself has complications: edema in both the burn wound and particularly in the noninjured soft tissue is increased by resuscitation. Burn edema is a serious complication, and might contribute to decreased tissue oxygen diffusion and further ischemic insult to already damaged cells. The increased tissue pressure caused by the established edema may further compromise blood flow, again potentiating the tissue damage and increasing the risk of infection. Research should continue to focus on methods to ameliorate the severe edema and vasoconstriction that exacerbate tissue ischemia. The success of this research will require identification of key (circulatory) factors that alter physical properties of the interstitium, capillary permeability, cause vasoconstriction, depolarize cellular membranes, and depress myocardial function. Hopefully, methods to prevent the release and to block the activity of specific mediators can be further developed in order to reduce the morbidity and mortality rates of burn shock.

References

1. Cockshott WP. The history of the treatment of burns. *Surg Gynecol Obstet* 1956; 102: 116–24.
2. Haynes BW. The history of burn care. In: Boswick JAJ, ed. *The Art and Science of Burn Care*, 1987; 3–9.
3. Underhill FP, Carrington GL, Kapsinov R, Pack GT. Blood concentration changes in extensive superficial burns, and their significance for systemic treatment. *Arch Intern Med* 1923; 32: 31–9.
4. Cope O, Moore FD. The redistribution of body water and fluid therapy of the burned patient. *Ann Surg* 1947; 126: 1010–45.
5. Youn YK, LaLonde C, Demling R. The role of mediators in the response to thermal injury. *World J Surg* 1992; 16(1): 30–6.
6. Aulick LH, Wilmore DW, Mason AD, Pruin BA. Influence of the burn wound on peripheral circulation in thermally injured patients. *Am J Physiol* 1977; 233: H520–6.
7. Settle JAD. Fluid therapy in burns. *J Roy Soc Med* 1982; 1(75): 7–11.
8. Demling RH. Fluid replacement in burned patients. *Surg Clin North Am* 1987; 67: 15–30.
9. Demling RH, Will JA, Belzer FO. Effect of major thermal injury on the pulmonary microcirculation. *Surgery* 1978; 83(6): 746–51.
10. Baxter CR. Fluid volume and electrolyte changes of the early postburn period. *Clin Plast Surg* 1974; 1(4): 693–709.
11. Baxter CR, Cook WA, Shires GT. Serum myocardial depressant factor of burn shock. *Surg Forum* 1966; 17: 1–3.
12. Hilton JG, Marullo DS. Effects of thermal trauma on cardiac force of contraction. *Burns Incl Therm Inj* 1986; 12: 167–71.
13. Clark WR. Death due to thermal trauma. In: Dolecek R. Brizio-Molteni L, Molteni A, Traber D, eds. *Endocrinology of Thermal Trauma*. Philadelphia. PA: Lea & Febiger, 1990: 6–27.
14. Lund T, Reed RK. Acute hemodynamic effects of thermal skin injury in the rat. *Circ Shock* 1986; 20: 105–14.
15. Arturson G. Pathophysiological aspects of the burn syndrome. *Acta Chir Scand* 1961; 274(Supp 1): 1–135.
16. Leape LL. Kinetics of burn edema formation in primates. *Ann Surg* 1972; 176: 223–6.
17. Demling RH, Mazess RB, Witt RM, Wolberg WH. The study of burn wound edema using dichromatic absorptiometry. *J Trauma* 1978; 18: 124–8.
18. Lund T, Wiig H, Reed RK. Acute postburn edema: role of strongly negative interstitial fluid pressure. *Am J Physiol* 1988; 255: H1069.
19. Onarheim H, Lund T, Reed R. Thermal skin injury: II. Effects on edema formation and albumin extravasation of fluid resuscitation with lactated Ringer's, plasma, and hypertonic saline (2400 mosmol/l) in the rat. *Circ Shock* 1989; 27(1): 25–37.

20. Arturson G, Jakobsson OR. Oedema measurements in a standard burn model. *Burns* 1985; 1: 1–7.
21. Leape LL. Early burn wound changes. *J Pediatr Surg* 1968; 3: 292–9.
22. Leape LL. Initial changes in burns: tissue changes in burned and unburned skin of rhesus monkeys. *J Trauma* 1970; 10: 488–92.
23. Landis EM, Pappenheimer JR. Exchange of substances through the capillary walls. In: Hamilton WF, Dow P, eds. *Handbook of Physiology*, Vol 2 Sect. 2. Baltimore: Williams and Wilkins, 1963: 961–1034.
24. Aukland K, Reed RK. Interstitial-lymphatic mechanisms in the control of extracellular fluid volume. *Physiol Rev* 1993; 73(1): 1–78.
25. Arturson G, Mellander S. Acute changes in capillary filtration and diffusion in experimental burn injury. *Acta Physiol Scand* 1964; 62: 457–3.
26. Pitt RM, Parker JC, Jurkovich GJ, Taylor AE. Analysis of altered capillary pressure and permeability after thermal injury. *J Surg Res* 1987; 42(6): 693–702.
27. Kinsky MP, Milner SM, Button B, Dubick MA, Kramer GC. Resuscitation of severe thermal injury with hypertonic saline dextran: effects on peripheral and visceral edema in sheep. *J Trauma* 2000 (in press).
28. Lund T, Onarheim H, Reed RK. Pathogenesis of edema formation in burn injuries. *World J Surg* 1992; 16: 2–9.
29. Lund T, Onarheim H, Wiig H, Reed RK. Mechanisms behind increased dermal imbibition pressure in acute burn edema. *Am J Physiol* 1989; 256(4 Pt 2): H940–8.
30. Reed RK, Woie K. Integrins and control of interstitial fluid pressure. *News Physiol Sci* 1997; 12: 42–8.
31. Arturson G. Microvascular permeability to macromolecules in thermal injury. *Acta Physiol Scand* 1979; 463(Suppl): 111–222.
32. Harms B, Kramer G, Bodai B, Demling R. Microvascular fluid and protein flux in pulmonary and systemic circulations after thermal injury. *Microvasc Res* 1982; 23: 77–86.
33. Zetterstrom H, Arturson G, Plasma oncotic pressure and plasma protein concentration in patients following thermal injury. *Acta Anaesth Scand* 1980; 24: 288–94.
34. Demling RH, Kramer GC, Harms B. Role of thermal injury-induced hypoproteinemia on edema formation in burned and nonburned tissue. *Surgery* 1984; 95: 136–44.
35. Pitkanen J, Lund T, Aanderud L, Reed RK. Transcapillary colloid osmotic pressures in injured and non-injured skin of seriously burned patients. *Burns* 1987; 13(3): 198–203.
36. Kramer GC, Gunther RA, Nerlich ML, Zweifach SS, Demling RH. Effect of dextran 70 on increased microvascular fluid and protein flux after thermal injury. *Circ Shock* 1982; 9: 529–43.
37. Lund T, Reed RK. Microvascular fluid exchange following thermal skin injury in the rat: changes in estravascular colloid osmotic pressure, albumin mass, and water content. *Circ Shock* 1986; 20: 91–104.
38. Brouhard BH, Carvajal HF, Linares HA. Burn edema and protein leakage in the rat. I. Relationship to time of injury. *Microvasc Res* 1978; 15: 221–8.
39. Neumann M, Demling RH. Colloid vs crystalloid: a current perspective. *Intens Crit Care Digest* 1990; 9(1): 3–6.
40. Kramer G, Harms B, Bodai B, Demling R, Renkin E. Mechanisms for redistribution of plasma protein following acute protein depletion. *Am J Physiol* 1982; 243: H803–9.
41. Shires GT, Cunningham JN Jr, Baker CRF, Reeder SF, Illner H, Wagner IY, Maher J. Alterations in cellular membrane dysfunction during hemorrhagic shock in primates. *Ann Surg* 1972; 176(3): 288–95.
42. Nakayama S, Kramer GC, Carlsen RC, Holcroft JW, Cala PM. Amiloride blocks membrane potential depolarization in rat skeletal muscle during hemorrhagic shock (abstract). *Circ Shock* 1984; 13: 106–7.
43. Arango A, Illner H, Shires GT. Roles of ischemia in the induction of changes in cell membrane during hemorrhagic shock. *J Surg Res* 1976; 20(5): 473–6.
44. Holliday RL, Illner HP, Shires GT. Liver cell membrane alterations during hemorrhagic shock in the rat. *J Surg Res* 1981; 31: 506–15.
45. Mazzoni MC, Borgstrom P, Intaglietta M, Arfors KE. Lumenal narrowing and endothelial cell swelling in skeletal muscle capillaries during hemorrhagic shock. *Circ Shock* 1989; 29(1): 27–39.
46. Evans JA, Darlington DN, Gann DS. A circulating factor(s) mediates cell depolarization in hemorrhagic shock. *Ann Surg* 1991; 213(6): 549–57.
47. Button B, Baker RD, Vertrees RA, Allen SE, Bodwick MS, Kramer GC. Quantitative assessment of a circulating depolarizing factor in shock. *Shock* 2000; 15: 239–244.
48. Goodman-Gilman A, Rall TW, Nies AS, Taylor R. *The Pharmacological Basis of Therapeutics*. New York: Pergamon Press, 1990.
49. Friedl HS, Till GO, Tentz O, Ward PA. Roles of histamine, complement and xanthine oxidase in thermal injury of skin. *Am J Pathol* 1989; 135(1): 203–17.
50. Boykin Jr JV, Manson NH. Mechanisms of cimetidine protection following thermal injury. *Am J Med* 1987; 83(6A): 76–81.
51. Till GO, Guilds LS, Mahrougui M, Friedl HP, Trentz O, Ward PA. Role of xanthine oxidase in thermal injury of skin. *Am J Pathol* 1989; 135(1): 195–202.
52. Tanaka H, Wada T, Simazaki S, Hanumadass M, Reyes HM, Matsuda T. Effects of cimetidine on fluid requirement during resuscitation of third-degree burns. *J Burn Care Rehabil* 1991; 12(5): 425–9.
53. Harms B, Bodai B, Demling R. Prostaglandin release and altered microvascular integrity after burn injury. *J Surg Res* 1981; 31: 27–8.
54. Anggard E, Jonsson CE. Efflux of prostaglandins in lymph from scalded tissue. *Acta Physiol Scand* 1971; 81: 440–3.
55. Arturson G. Anti-inflammatory drugs and burn edema formation. In: May R, Dogo G, eds. *Care of the Burn Wound*. Basel: Karger, 1981: 21–4.
56. Arturson G, Hamberg M, Jonsson CE. Prostaglandins in human burn blister fluid. *Acta Physiol Scand* 1973; 87: 27–36.
57. LaLonde C, Knox J, Daryani R. Topical flurbiprofen decreases burn wound-induced hypermetabolism and systemic lipid peroxidation. *Surgery* 1991; 109: 645–51.
58. Huang YS, Li A, Yang ZC. Roles of thromboxane and its inhibitor anisodamine in burn shock. *Burns* 1990; 4: 249–53.
59. Herndon DN, Abston S, Stein MD. Increased thromboxane B2 levels in the plasma of burned and septic burned patients. *Surg Gynecol Obstet* 1984; 159(3): 210–13.
60. Heggers JP, Loy GL, Robson MC, Del Beccaro EJ. Histological demonstration of prostaglandins and thromboxanes in burned tissue. *J Surg Res* 1980; 28: 11–15.
61. Heggers JP, Robson MC, Zachary LS. Thromboxane inhibitors for the prevention of progressive dermal ischemia due to thermal injury. *J Burn Care Rehabil* 1985; 6: 46–8.
62. Demling RH, LaLonde C. Topical ibuprofen decreases early postburn edema. *Surgery* 1987; 5: 857–61.
63. LaLonde C, Demling RH. Inhibition of thromboxane synthetase accentuates hemodynamic instability and burn edema in the anesthetized sheep model. *Surgery* 1989; 5: 638–44.
64. Jacobsen S, Waaler BG. The effect of scalding on the content of kininogen and kininase in limb lymph. *Br J Pharmacol* 1966; 27: 222.
65. Hafner JA, Fritz H. Balance antiinflammation: the combined application of a PAF inhibitor and a cyclooxygenase inhibitor blocks the inflammatory take-off after burns. *Int J Tissue React* 1990; 12: 203.
66. Nwariaku FE, Sikes PJ, Lightfoot E, Mileski WJ, Baxter C. Effect of a bradykinin antagonist on the local inflammatory response following thermal injury. *Burns* 1996; 22(4): 324–7.
67. Carvajal H, Linares H, Brouhard B. Effect of antihistamine, antiserotonin, and ganglionic blocking agents upon increased capillary permeability following burn edema. *J Trauma* 1975; 15: 969–75.
68. Ferrara JJ, Westervelt CL, Kukuy EL, Franklin EW, Choe EU, Mercurio KK, Lippton HL, Flint LM. Burn edema reduction by methysergide is not due to control of regional vasodilation. *J Surg Res* 1996; 61(1): 11–16.
69. Zhang XJ, Irtun O, Zheng Y, Wolfe RR. Methysergide reduces nonnutritive blood flow in normal and scalded skin. *Am J Physiol* 2000; 278(3): E452–61.
70. Wilmore DW, Long JM, Mason AD, Skreen RW, Pruitt BA. Catecholamines: mediator of the hypermetabolic response to thermal injury. *Ann Surg* 1974; 80: 653–9.
71. Hilton JG. Effects of sodium nitroprusside on thermal trauma depressed cardiac output in the anesthesized dog. *Burns Incl Therm Inj* 1984; 10: 318–22.
72. McCord J, Fridovieh I. The biology and pathology of oxygen radicals. *Ann Intern Med* 1978; 89: 122–7.
73. Demling RH, LaLonde C. Early postburn lipid peroxidation: effect of ibuprofen and allopurinol. *Surgery* 1990; 107: 85–93.
74. Rawlingson A, Greenacre SA, Brain SD. Generation of peroxynitrite in localized, moderate temperature burns. *Burns* 2000; 26(3): 223–7.
75. Lindblom L, Cassuto J, Yregard L, Mattsson U, Tarnow P, Sinclair R. Importance of nitric oxide in the regulation of burn oedema, proteinuria and urine output. *Burns* 2000; 26(1): 13–17.
76. Lindblom L, Cassuto J, Yregard L, Mattsson U, Tarnow P, Sinclair R. Role of nitric oxide in the control of burn perfusion. *Burns* 2000; 26(1): 19–23.
77. Slater TF, Benedetto C. Free radical reactions in relation to lipid peroxidation, inflammation and prostaglandin metabolism. In: Berti F, Veto G, eds. *The Prostaglandin System*. New York: Plenum Press, 1979: 109–26.
78. McCord JM. Oxygen-derived free radicals in post ischemic tissue injury. *N Engl J Med* 1978; 312: 159–63.
79. Demling R, Lalonde C, Knox J, Youn YK, Zhu D. Fluid resuscitation with deferoxamine prevents systemic burn-induced oxidant injury. *J Trauma* 1991; 31(4): 538–43.
80. Ono I, Gunji H, Hasegawa T, Harada H, Kaneko F, Matsuzaki M. Effects of a platelet activating factor antagonist on edema formation following burns. *Burns* 1993; 3: 202–7.
81. Fink MP. Gastrointestinal mucosal injury in experimental models of shock, trauma, and sepsis. *Crit Care Med* 1991; 19(5): 627–41.

82. Cui X, Sheng Z, Guo Z. Mechanisms of early gastro-intestinal ischemia after burn: hemodynamic and hemorrheologic features [Chinese]. *Chin J Plast Surg Burns* 1998; **14**(4): 262–5.

83. Tadros T, Traber DL, Heggers JP, Herndon DN. Angiotension II inhibitor DuP753 attenuates burn and endotoxin-induced gut ischemia, lipid perioxidation, mucosal permability, and bacterial translocation. *Ann Surg* 2000; **231**(4): 566–76.

84. Crum RL, Dominie W, Hansbrough JF. Cardiovascular and neuroburnoral responses following burn injury. *Arch Surg* 1990; **125**: 1065–70.

85. Sun K, Gong A, Wang CH, Lin BC, Zhu HN. Effect of peripheral injection of arginine vasopressin and its receptor antagonist on burn shock in the rat. *Neuropeptides* 1990; **1**: 17–20.

86. Kiang JG, Wei-E T. Corticotropin-releasing factor inhibits thermal injury. *J Pharmacol Exp Ther* 1987; **2**: 517–20.

87. Tanaka H, Matsuda H, Shimazaki S, Hanumadass M, Matsuda T. Reduced resuscitation fluid volume for second-degree burns with delayed initiation of ascorbic acid therapy. *Arch Surg* 1997; **132**(2): 158–61.

88. Tanaka H, Lund T, Wiig H, Reed RK, Yukioka T, Matsuda H, Shimazaki S. High dose vitamin C counteracts the negative interstitial fluid hydrostatic pressure and early edema generation in thermally injured rats. *Burns* 1999; **25**(7): 569–74.

89. Jonsson A, Mattsson U, Tarnow P, Nellgard P, Cassuto J. Topical local anesthetics (EMLA) inhibit burn-induced plasma extravasation as measured by digital image colour analysis. *Burns* 1998; **24**(4): 313–18.

90. Lund T, Reed RK. Alpha-Trinositol vitamin inhibits edema generation and albumin extravasation in thermally injured skin. *J Trauma* 1994; **36**(6): 761–5.

91. Ferrara JJ, Kukuy EL, Gilman DA, Choe EU, Franklin EW, Flint LM. Alpha-trinositol reduces edema formation at the site of scald injury. *Surgery* 1998; **123**(1): 36–45.

92. Tarnow P, Jonsson A, Mattsson U, Rimback G, Cassuto J. Inhibition of plasma extravasation after burns by D-myo-inositol-1,2,6-triphosphate using digital image colour analysis. *Scand J Plast Reconstr Surg Hand Surg* 1998; **32**(2): 141–6.

93. Michie DD, Goldsmith RS, Mason AD Jr. Effects of hydralazine and high molecular weight dextran upon the circulatory responses to severe thermal burns. *Circ Res* 1963; **13**: 46–8.

94. Hilton JG. Effects of verapamil on thermal trauma depressed cardiac output in the anesthetized dog. *Burns Incl Therm Inj* 1984; **10**: 313–17.

95. Pruitt PAJ, Mason ADJ, Moncrief JA. Hemodynamic changes in the early post burn patients: The influence of fluid administration and of a vasodilator (hydralazine). *J Trauma* 1971; **11**: 36.

96. Minifee PK, Barrow RE, Abston S, Desai MH, Herndon DN. Improved myocardial oxygen utilization following propranolol infusion in adolescents with post-burn hypermetabolism. *J Pediatr Surg* 1989; **24**(8): 806–11.

97. Holm C, Horbrand F, von Donnersmarck GH, Muhlbauer W. Acute renal failure in severely burned patients. *Burns* 1999; **25**(2): 171–8.

98. Chrysopoulo MT, Jeschke MG, Dziewulski P, Barrow RE, Herndon DN. Acute renal dysfunction in severely burned adults. *J Trauma* 1999; **46**(1): 141–4.

99. Tokyay R, Zeigler ST, Traber DL, Stothert JC, Loick HM, Heggers JP, Herndon DN. Postburn gastrointestinal vasoconstriction increases bacterial and endotoxin translocation. *J Am Physiol* 1993: 1521–7.

100. Shin C, Kinsky MP, Thomas JA, Traber DL, Kramer GC. Effect of cutaneous burn injury and resuscitation on the cerebral circulation. *Burns* 1998; **24**: 39–45.

101. Demling RH, Wong C, Jin LJ, Hechtman H, Lalonde CKW. Early lung dysfunction after major burns: role of edema and vasoactive mediators. *J Trauma* 1985; **25**(10): 959–66.

102. Demling RH, Niehaus G, Perea A, Will JA. Effect of burn-induced hypoproteinemia on pulmonary transvascular fluid filtration rate. *Surgery* 1979; **85**: 339–43.

103. Tranbaugh RF, Lewis FR, Christensen IM, Elings VB. Lung water changes after thermal injury: the effects of crystalloid resuscitation and sepsis. *Ann Surg* 1980; **192**: 47–9.

104. Tranbaugh RF, Elings VB, Christensen JM, Lewis FR. Effect of inhalation injury on lung water accumulation. *J Trauma* 1983; **23**: 597.

105. Herndon DN, Barrow RE, Traber DL, Rutan TC, Rutan RL, Abston S. Extravascular lung water changes following smoke inhalation and massive burn injury. *Surgery* 1987; **102**(2): 341–9.

106. Martyn JAJ, Wilson RS, Burke JF. Right ventricular function and pulmonary hemodynamics during dopamine infusion in burned patients. *Chest* 1986; **89**: 357–60.

107. Adams HR, Baxter CR, Izenberg SD. Decreased contractility and compliance of the left ventricle as complications of thermal trauma. *Am Heart J* 1984; **108**(6): 1477–87.

108. Merriman TW Jr, Jackson R. Myocardial function following thermal injury. *Circ Res* 1962; **11**: 66–9.

109. Horton JW, White J, Baxter CR. Aging alters myocardial response during resuscitation in burn shock. *Surg Forum* 1987; **38**: 249–51.

110. Baxter CR, Shires GT. Physiological response to crystalloid resuscitation of severe burns. *Ann NY Acad Sci* 1968; **150**: 874–94.

111. Sugi K, Newald J, Traber LD. Smoke inhalation injury causes myocardial depression in sheep. *Anesthesiology* 1988; **69**: A111.

112. Sugi K, Theissen JL, Traber LD, Herndon DN, Traber DL. Impact of carbon monoxide on cardiopulmonary dysfunction after smoke inhalation injury. *Circ Res* 1990; **66**: 69–75.

113. Horton JW, Baxter CR, White J. Differences in cardiac responses to resuscitation from burn shock. *Surg Gynecol Obstet* 1989; **168**(3): 201–13.

114. Horton JW, White DJ, Baxter CR. Hypertonic saline dextran resuscitation of thermal injury. *Ann Surg* 1990; **211**(3): 301–11.

115. Horton JW, Shite J, Hunt JL. Delayed hypertonic saline dextran administration after burn injury. *J Trauma Injury: Injury, Infect Crit Care* 1995; **38**(2): 281–6.

116. Horton JW, White J, Baxter CR. The role of oxygen derived free radicles in burn-induced myocardial contractile depression. *J Burn Care Rehab* 1988; **9**(6): 589–98.

117. Horton JW, Garcia NM, White J, Keffer J. Postburn cardiac contractile function and biochemical markers of postburn cardiac injury. *J Am Coll Surg* 1995; **181**: 289–98.

118. Horton JW, White J, Maass D, Sanders B. Arginine in burn injury improves cardiac performance and prevents bacterial translocation. *J Appl Physiol* 1998; **84**(2): 695–702.

119. Cioffi WG, DeMeules JE, Gameili RL. The effects of burn injury and fluid resuscitation on cardiac function *in vitro*. *J Trauma* 1986; **26**: 638–43.

120. Murphy JT, Horton JW, Purdue GF, Hunt JL. Evaluation of troponin-1 as an indicator of cardiac dysfunction following thermal injury. *Burn Care Rehabil* 1997; **45**(4): 700–4.

121. Bert J, Gyenge C, Bowen B, Reed R, Lund T. Fluid resuscitation following a burn injury: implications of a mathematical model of microvascular exchange. *Burns* 1997; **23**: 93–105.

Chapter 8

Fluid resuscitation and early management
Glenn D Warden

Introduction

Proper fluid management is critical to the survival of the victim of a major thermal injury. In the 1940s, hypovolemic shock or shock-induced renal failure was the leading cause of death after burn injury. Today, with our current knowledge of the massive fluid shifts and vascular changes that occur during burn shock, mortality related to burn-induced volume loss has decreased considerably. Although a vigorous approach to fluid therapy has ensued in the last 20 years and fewer deaths are occurring in the first 24–48 hours postburn, the fact remains that approximately 50% of the deaths occur within the first 10 days following burn injury from a multitude of causes, one of the most significant being inadequate fluid resuscitation therapy.[1] Knowledge of fluid management following burn shock resuscitation is also important and is often overlooked in burn education.

Burn shock resuscitation

The history of burn resuscitation began over a century ago; however, complete appreciation of the severity of fluid loss in burns was not apparent until the enlightening studies of Frank P Underhill,[2] who studied the victims of the Rialto Theater fire in 1921. His concept that burn shock was due to intravascular fluid loss was further elucidated by Cope and Moore,[3] who conducted studies on patients from the Coconut Grove disaster in 1942. They developed the concept of burn edema and introduced the body-weight burn budget formula for fluid resuscitation of burn patients. In 1952, Evans[1] developed a burn surface area–weight formula for computing fluid replacement in burns which became the first simplified formula for fluid resuscitation for burn patients. Surgeons at the Brooke Army Medical Center modified the original Evans formula and this became the standard for the next 15 years.

A number of methods for accomplishing adequate volume replacement therapy have been advocated in the more than 40 years since the introduction of the Evans' formula in 1952. This chapter will review the various methods advocated and present the rationale of each. Importantly, properly utilized, each resuscitation formula can be effective in the resuscitation of the burn patient in the immediate postburn period, provided that close attention is paid to the individual's clinical response to therapy and that fluid replacement therapy is modified according to this response. The fact that patients respond to a wide variety of resuscitative efforts is testimony to the fact that burn patients are very resilient and can be overwhelmed only under the most unfavorable circumstances.[4]

Pathophysiology of Burn Injury

Modern fluid resuscitation formulas originate from experimental studies in the pathophysiology of burn shock. Burn shock is both hypovolemic shock and cellular shock, and is characterized by specific hemodynamic changes including decreased cardiac output, extracellular fluid, plasma volume, and oliguria. As in the treatment of other forms of shock, the primary goal is to restore and preserve tissue perfusion in order to avoid ischemia. However, in burn shock, resuscitation is complicated by obligatory burn edema, and the voluminous transvascular fluid shifts which result from a major burn are unique to thermal trauma.

Although the exact pathophysiology of the postburn vascular changes and fluid shifts is unknown, one major component of burn shock is the increase in total body capillary permeability. Direct thermal injury results in marked changes in the microcirculation. Most of the changes occur locally at the burn site, when maximal edema formation occurs at about 8–12 hours post-injury in smaller burns and 12–24 hours post-injury in major thermal injuries. The rate of progression of tissue edema is dependent upon the adequacy of resuscitation.

Multiple mediators have been proposed to explain the changes in vascular permeability seen postburn. The mediators can produce either an increase in vascular permeability or an increase in microvascular hydrostatic pressure.[5,6] Most mediators act to increase permeability by altering membrane integrity in the venules. The early phase of burn edema formation, lasting for minutes to an hour, has been thought by some investigators to be the result of mediators, particularly histamine and bradykinin. Other mediators implicated in the changes in vascular permeability seen postburn include vasoactive amines, products of platelet activation and the complement cascade, hormones, prostaglandins, and leukotrienes. Vasoactive substances are also released which may act primarily by increasing microvascular blood flow or vascular pressures, further accentuating the burn edema.[7,8] Histamine is released in large quantities from mast cells in burned skin immediately after injury.[9] Histamine has been clearly demonstrated to increase the leakage of fluid and protein from systemic micro vessels, its major effect being on venules in which an increase in the intracellular junction space is characteristically seen.[10] However, the increase in serum histamine levels after burn is transient, peaking in the first several hours post-injury, indicating that histamine is only involved in the very early increase in permeability. The use of H_1 receptor inhibitors, e.g. diphenhydramine, has only limited success in decreasing edema. Recently, the use of an H_2 receptor antagonist has been reported to decrease burn edema in an animal model.[11]

Serotonin is released immediately postburn as a result of platelet aggregation and acts directly to increase the pulmonary vascular resistance and indirectly to amplify the vasoconstrictive effect of norepinephrine, histamine, angiotensin-2, and prostaglandin.[12] The use of ketanserin, a specific serotonin antagonist in a porcine burn shock model, improved cardiac index, decreased pulmonary pressure, and reduced arteriovenous oxygen content differences compared to a control group in the early postburn period. Serotonin antagonists should be investigated further as possible adjuvant therapeutic agents during burn shock resuscitation.[13] Prostaglandins, vasoactive products of arachidonic acid metabolism, have been reported to be released in burn tissue and to be at least in part responsible for burn edema. Although these substances do not directly alter vasopermeability, increased levels of vasodilator prostaglandins such as prostaglandin E_2 (PGE_2) and prostacyclin (PGI_2) result in arterial dilatation in burned tissue, increased blood flow and intravascular hydrostatic pressure in the injured microcirculation, and thus accentuate the edema process. Concentrations of PGI_2 and the vasoconstrictor thromboxane A_2 (TXA_2) have been demonstrated in burned tissue, burn blister fluid, lymph, and wound secretion.[14,15] However, the use of prostaglandin inhibitors has produced variable results in animal studies. Arturson[16] reported a decrease in burn lymph and protein flow with the use of a prostaglandin inhibitor, indomethacin. Those results have not been corroborated by other investigators and the role of thromboxane and the prostaglandins still needs to be elucidated.

The activation of the proteolytic cascades, including those of coagulation, fibrinolysis, the kinins, and the complement system, has been demonstrated to occur immediately following thermal injury. Kinins, specifically bradykinins, are known to increase vascular permeability, primarily in the venule. Rocha and co-workers[17] report increased kinin levels in burn edema fluid in the rat. The release of other mediators and the generalized inflammatory response after burns favors the activation of the kallikrein–kinin system, with the release of bradykinin into the circulation.[18]

Elevation of proteolytic activity has been demonstrated in both animals and in burn patients.[19] Pretreatment with protease inhibitors significantly decreases free kinin levels but appears to have little effect on the edema process.

The end result of the changes in the microvasculature due to thermal injury is disruption of normal capillary barriers separating intravascular and interstitial compartments, and rapid equilibrium of these compartments. This results in severe depletion of plasma volume with a marked increase in extracellular fluid clinically manifested as hypovolemia.

In addition to a loss of capillary integrity, thermal injury also causes changes at the cellular level. Baxter[20] has demonstrated that in burns of >30% total body surface area (TBSA), there is a systemic decrease in cell transmembrane potential, involving nonthermally injured cells as well. This decrease in cell transmitting potential, as defined by the Nernste equation, results from an increase in intracellular sodium concentration. The cause of this is thought to be a decrease in sodium ATPase activity responsible for maintaining the intracellular–extracellular ionic gradient. Baxter further demonstrated that resuscitation only partially restores the membrane potential and intracellular sodium concentrations to normal levels, demonstrating that hypovolemia with its attendant ischemia is not totally responsible for the cellular swelling seen in burn shock. In fact, the membrane potential may not return to normal for many days postburn despite adequate resuscitation. If resuscitation is inadequate, cell membrane potential progressively decreases, resulting ultimately in cellular death. This may be the final common denominator in burn shock during the resuscitation period.

Although the etiology of burn shock is not totally understood, many authors have studied the fluid volume shifts and hemodynamic changes that accompany burn shock. Early work by Moyer,[21] and Baxter and Shires,[22] established the definitive role of crystalloid solutions in burn resuscitation and delineated the fluid volume changes in the early postburn period. Moyer's original studies in 1965,[21] demonstrated that burn edema sequestered enormous amounts of fluid, resulting in the hypovolemia of burn shock. In addition, he described the first crystalloid-only resuscitation formula used to treat burn shock. He noted that burn shock recovery occurred in the majority of patients studied, although hemoconcentration remained unchanged and the hematocrit was unresponsive to fluid administration despite adequate resuscitation. This became the first objective evidence that burn shock is not simply due to hypovolemia but is also influenced by extracellular sodium depletion. Baxter and Shires[22] in 1968, using radioisotope dilution techniques, defined the fluid volume changes of the postburn period in relation to cardiac output. They first demonstrated that edema fluid in the burn wound is isotonic with respect to plasma fluid and contains protein in the same proportions as that found in blood. This confirmed Arturson's earlier findings that in major burns there is complete disruption of the normal capillary barrier, with free exchange between plasma and extravascular extracellular compartments. They measured changes in fluid compartment volumes in burned primates and dogs and demonstrated that in untreated (unresuscitated) animals, a 30–50% extracellular fluid (ECF) defect persisted at 18 hours postburn. Plasma volume decreased 23% to 27% below controls, although red cell mass changed only about 10% over the same 18-hour period. Thus, the greatest volume loss was functional intravascular extracellular fluid. Cardiac output was initially depressed very soon after injury to a level of about 25% of controls at 4 hours after a 30% TBSA burn. By 18 hours, however, the cardiac output had stabilized at around 40% of control, despite persistent defects in plasma and ECF volumes. On the basis of studies using different volumes of resuscitation fluids, they arrived at an optimal response in terms of cardiac output and restoration of ECF at the end of 24 hours in a canine model. Clinical studies using similar sodium and fluid loads immediately followed, confirming efficacy in restoring ECF to within 10% of controls within 24 hours. This became the basis for the Baxter or Parkland formula.[20] Mortality was comparable to that obtained with a colloid-containing resuscitation formula.

Baxter went on to demonstrate that during the first 24 hours postburn, plasma volume changes were independent of the type of infused fluid, whether crystalloid or colloid, but at approximately 24 hours post-injury, an infused amount of colloid would increase the plasma volume by the same amount. His findings prove that colloid-containing solutions are an unnecessary component of fluid resuscitation in the first 24 hours. He recommended their use only after capillary integrity was restored, to correct the persistent plasma volume deficit of about 20% as measured externally. While the fluid shifts were being defined by Baxter in terms of crystalloid resuscitation, Moncrief and Pruitt[4] worked to characterize the hemodynamic alterations that occur in burn shock with and without fluid resuscitation. Their efforts culminated in the Brooke formula modification which utilized 2 cc/kg/% burn during the first 24 hours. Fluid needs were initially estimated according to the modified Brooke formula, but the actual volume for resuscitation was based on clinical response. In their study, resuscitation permitted an average decrease of about 20% in both extracellular fluid and plasma volume, but no further loss accrued in the first 24 hours. In the second 24 hours postburn, plasma volume restoration occurred with the administration of colloid. Blood volume, however, was only partially restored and an ongoing loss of 9% of the red cell mass per day was found. Cardiac output, initially quite low, rose over the first 18 hours postburn, despite plasma volume and blood volume defects. These results were quite consistent with those demonstrated by Baxter in his animal studies. Peripheral vascular resistance during the initial 24 hours was initially very high but decreased as cardiac output improved, and in fact the changes were reciprocal. Once plasma volume and blood volume loss ceased, cardiac output rose to supranormal levels where it remained until healing or grafting occurred.

Moylan and associates[23] in 1973, using a canine model, defined the relationships between fluid volumes, sodium concentration, and colloid in restoring cardiac output during the first 12 hours post-injury. No significant colloid effect on cardiac output was noted in the first 12 hours post-injury. In addition, 1 mEq of sodium was found to exert an effect on cardiac output equal to 13 times that of 1 ml of salt-free volume. This experiment established the fact that any combination of sodium and volume within the broad limits of the study would effectively resuscitate a thermally injured patient.

Arturson's landmark studies in 1979[16] on vascular permeability characterized the nature of the 'leaky capillary' in the postburn period. He demonstrated in a canine model that increased capillary permeability is found both locally and in nonburned tissue at distant sites when the TBSA burn exceeded 25%. He proposed that the burn wound is characterized by rapid edema formation due to dilatation of the resistance vessels (precapillary arterioles); increased extravascular osmotic activity, due to the products of thermal injury; and increased microvascular permeability to macromolecules. The increased permeability permits molecules of up to 350 000 molecular weight to escape from the microvasculature, a size which allows essentially all elements of the vascular space except red blood cells to escape from it. Further studies by Demling and co-workers[24] have demonstrated that in 50% TBSA burns, one-half of the initial fluid resuscitation requirement may end up in nonthermally injured tissues.

Resuscitation from Burn Shock

Fluid resuscitation is aimed at supporting the patient throughout the initial 24-hour to 48-hour period of hypovolemia. The primary goal of therapy is to replace the fluid sequestered as a result of thermal injury. The critical concept in burn shock is that massive fluid shifts can occur even though total body water remains unchanged. What actually changes is the volume of each fluid compartment, intracellular and interstitial volumes increasing at the expense of plasma volume and blood volume. In light of all the studies on different fluid regimens, the question still remains: 'What is the best formula for resuscitation of the burn patient?'

It is quite clear that the edema process is accentuated by the resuscitation fluid. The magnitude of edema will be affected by the amount and type of fluid administered.[25] The National Institutes of Health consensus summary on fluid resuscitation in 1978 was not in agreement in regard to a specific formula; however, there was consensus in regard to two major issues – the guidelines used during the resuscitation process and the type of fluid used. In regard to the guidelines, the consensus was to give the least amount of fluid necessary to maintain adequate organ perfusion. The volume infused should be continually titrated so as to avoid both under-resuscitation and over-resuscitation.[26,27] As for the optimum type of fluid, there is no question that replacement of the extracellular salt lost into the burned tissue and into the cell is essential for successful resuscitation.[19,21]

Crystalloid resuscitation

Crystalloid, in particular lactated Ringer's solution with a sodium concentration of 130 Meq/L, is the most popular resuscitation fluid currently utilized. Proponents of the use of crystalloid solution alone for resuscitation report that other solutions, specifically colloids, are no better and are certainly more expensive than crystalloid for maintaining intravascular volume following thermal injury.[4] The most common reason given for not using colloids is that even large proteins leak from the capillary following thermal injury. However, capillaries in nonburned tissues do continue to sieve proteins, maintaining relatively normal protein permeability characteristics.

The quantity of crystalloid needed is in part dependent upon the parameters used to monitor resuscitation. If a urinary output of 0.5 cc/kg of body weight/hour is considered to indicate adequate perfusion, approximately 3 cc/kg/% burn will be needed in the first 24 hours. If 1 cc/kg of body weight/hour of urine is deemed necessary, then of course considerably more fluid will be needed and in turn more edema will result. The Parkland formula recommends 4 cc/kg/% burn in the first 24 hours, with one-half of that amount administered in the first 8 hours[9] (**Table 8.1**). The modified Brooke formula recommends beginning burn shock resuscitation at

2 cc/kg/% burn in the first 24 hours (**Table 8.1**). In major burns, severe hypoproteinemia usually develops with these resuscitation regimens. The hypoproteinemia and interstitial protein depletion may result in more edema formation.

Hypertonic saline

Hypertonic salt solutions have been known for many years to be effective in treating burn shock.[28,29] Rapid infusion produces serum hyperosmolarity and hypernatremia with two potentially positive effects.[28,32] The hypertonic serum reduces the shift into the extracellular space of intravascular water. Proposed benefits include decreased tissue edema and fewer attendant complications, including escharotomies for vascular compromise or endotracheal intubation to protect the airway. Monafo[28] reported that the resuscitation of burn patients with salt solution of 240–300 mEq/L resulted in less edema because of the smaller total fluid requirements than with lactated Ringer's solution. Urine output was the indicator used during resuscitation. Demling and colleagues[30] in an animal model demonstrated that the net fluid intake was less if burned animals were resuscitated with hypertonic saline to the same cardiac output compared with lactated Ringer's. Urine output was much higher with hypertonic solution. Interestingly, soft-tissue interstitial edema in burned and nonburned tissue, as reflected by lymph flow, was increased with hypertonic saline similar to that of lactated Ringer's (LR). This can be explained by a shift of intracellular water into extracellular space as the result of the hyperosmolar solution. Extracellular edema can therefore occur at the same time as intracellular fluid defect. This may give the external appearance of less edema. Although several studies to date have reported that this intracellular water depletion does not appear to be deleterious, the issue remains controversial. Shimazaki et al.[31] resuscitated 46 patients with either LR or hypertonic saline. The sodium infusions were equivalent, but the free water load was greater with LR; 50% of the latter required endotracheal intubation. The hypertonic serum also delivers a more concentrated ultrafiltrate within the kidney. This increases urine volume and salt clearance without marked increases in the required volume of free water.

There is no consensus regarding the type of osmolarity of hypertonic resuscitation fluid. Caldwell et al.[32] in 1979 reported a series of 37 patients with greater than 30% burns treated with either LR or hypertonic lactated saline (HLS), but no colloid. Total sodium balance was the same but the HLS group received 30% less free water and the reduced weight gain was maintained for 7 days. Subsequent reports from this institution reported successful HLS resuscitation in the elderly and children but no improvement in late mortality.[39,36,40]

Bartolani et al.[41] randomized 40 patients to receive LR or HLS. HLS patients received more sodium, but less total fluid than the LR group. The observed higher mortality with HLS was attributed to larger burns in this group.

The role of colloid in association with hypertonic saline (HSS) resuscitation is also unclear. Most physicians reserve colloid for the second 24 hours, if at all, unless the patient remains poorly perfused after large infusions of crystalloid. Griswold et al.[42] reported resuscitation of 47 patients with HSS resuscitation. Of these, 29 were also given colloid as albumin or fresh frozen plasma based on burn severity, premorbid state, or poor response to HSS resuscitation. This group had larger burns, greater mean age, and higher incidence of inhalation injury, but required only 57% of the fluid volume predicted by the Parkland formula, compared to 75% of predicted volume in the HSS alone group. Both groups maintained urine volumes of 1 ml/kg/h with no significant difference in hematocrit or serum sodium levels. Jelenko et al.[43] also reported in a small series that patients given HSS and albumin required fewer escharotomies, fewer days of mechanical ventilation, and less total fluid than patients resuscitated with LR or HSS alone. Gunn et al.[33] in a series of 51 randomized patients found no difference in fluid requirements or weight gain if they were given LR or hypertonic saline, if fresh frozen plasma was administered to maintain serum albumin levels above 2 g/dl, but all patients received hypotonic enteral feedings during resuscitation.

Yoshioka et al.[34] reviewed 53 patients treated with greater than 30% burns resuscitated with LR, LR and colloid, or HLS. Fluid requirements were 4.8 ml/kg/% TBSA with LR, 3.3 ml/kg/% TBSA with LR and colloid, and 2.2 ml/kg/% TBSA with HLS. The total sodium requirements were increased 30% with LR compared to the other groups. Oxygen extraction, measured as A-VO$_2$ difference, was improved with HLS, but reduced with LR-colloid, perhaps because of protein leak across the alveoli.

Table 8.1 Formulas for estimating adult burn patient resuscitation fluid needs (Warden GD. World J Surg 1992; 16: 16–23.[51])			
Colloid formulas	**Electrolyte**	**Colloid**	**D5W**
Evans	Normal saline 1.0 cc/kg/% burn	1.0 cc/kg/% burn	2000 cc
Brooke	Lactated Ringer's 1.5 cc/kg/% burn	0.5 cc/kg	2000 cc
Slater	Lactated Ringer's 2 L/24 hours	Fresh frozen plasma 75 cc/kg/24 hours	
Crystalloid formulas			
Parkland	Lactated Ringer's	4 cc/kg/% burn	
Modified Brooke	Lactated Ringer's	2 cc/kg/% burn	
Hypertonic saline formulas			
Hypertonic saline solution (Monafo)	Volume to maintain urine output at 30 cc/h Fluid contains 250 mEq Na/L		
Modified hypertonic (Warden)	Lactated Ringer's + 50 mEq NaHCO$_3$ (180 mEq Na/L) for 8 hours to maintain urine output at 30–50 cc/h		
	Lactated Ringer's to maintain urine output at 30–50 cc/h beginning 8 hours postburn		
Dextran formula (Demling)	Dextran 40 in saline – 2 cc/kg/h for 8 hours		
	Lactated Ringer's – volume to maintain urine output at 30 cc/h		
	Fresh frozen plasma – 0.5 cc/kg/h for 18 hours beginning 8 hours postburn		

Vigorous administration of hypertonic saline solutions can produce a serum sodium above 160 mEq/dl or serum osmolarity greater than 340 mOs/dl, followed by a rapid fall in urine output.[35] Bowser-Wallace et al.[36] and Crum et al.[37] have reported 40–50% of patients treated with HLS developed hypernatremia with serum sodium greater than 160 mEq/L requiring switch to hypotonic fluids. Huang et al.[38] reported a series of deaths associated with hypernatremia and hyperosmolarity following hypertonic saline resuscitation. Serial determinations of serum sodium and serum osmolarity are required to prevent complications including sudden anuria, brain shrinkage with tearing of intracranial vessels, or excessive brain swelling following rapid correction of serum hyperosmolarity. Current recommendations are that the serum sodium levels should not be allowed to exceed 160 mEq/dl during its use. Of interest, Gunn and associates,[33] in a prospective randomized study of patients with 20% TBSA burns evaluating HSL versus LR solution, were not able to demonstrate decreased fluid requirements, improved nutritional tolerance, or decreased percent weight gain.

Warden et al., at the Shriners Hospital for Children, have utilized a modified hypertonic solution in major thermal injuries >40% TBSA burn. The resuscitation fluid contains 180 mEq Na$^+$ (lactated Ringer's + 50 mEq NaHCO$_3$). The solution is utilized until the reversal of metabolic acidosis has occurred, usually by 8 hours postburn. The volume administered is begun at a rate calculated by the Parkland formula (4 cc/kg/% burn); however, volume is titrated to maintain urine output at 30–50 cc/h. After 8 hours the resuscitation is completed utilizing LR to maintain urine output at 30–50 cc/h. This hypertonic formula can be used in infants and in the elderly without the accompanying risk of hypernatremia.[44,45]

Colloid resuscitation

Plasma proteins are extremely important in the circulation since they generate the inward oncotic force that counteracts the outward capillary hydrostatic force. Without protein, plasma volume could not be maintained and massive edema would result. Protein replacement was an important component of early formulas for burn management. The Evans formula, advocated in 1952, used 1 cc/kg of body weight/% burn each for colloid and LR over the first 24 hours. The Brooke formula was clearly based on estimate rather than determined scientifically, but the formula used 0.5 cc/kg/% burn as colloid and 1.5 cc/kg/% burn as LR. The burn budget of Moore similarly used a substantial amount of colloids.[3] Considerable confusion exists concerning the role of protein in a resuscitation formula. There are three schools of thought:

1. Protein solutions should not be given in the first 24 hours because during this period they are no more effective than salt water in maintaining intravascular volume and they promote accumulation of lung water when edema fluid is being absorbed from the burn wound.[46]
2. Proteins, specifically albumin, should be given from the beginning of resuscitation along with crystalloid; it should usually be added to salt water.
3. Protein should be given between 8 and 12 hours postburn using strictly crystalloid in the first 8–12 hours because of the massive fluid shifts during this period. Demling demonstrated experimentally that restoration and maintenance of plasma protein contents were not effective

until 8 hours postburn, after which adequate levels can be maintained with infusion.[47] Because nonburned tissues appear to regain normal permeability very shortly after injury and because hypoproteinemia may accentuate the edema, the action advocated by the first school appears to be least appropriate.

The choice of the type of protein solution can be confusing. Heat-fixed protein solutions, e.g. Plasmanate, are known to contain some denatured and aggregated protein, which decreases the oncotic effect. Albumin solutions would clearly be the most oncotically active solutions. Fresh frozen plasma, however, contains all the protein fractions that exert both the oncotic and the nononcotic actions. The optimal amount of protein to infuse remains undefined. Demling[47] uses between 0.5 and 1 cc/kg/% burn of fresh frozen plasma during the first 24 hours, beginning at 8–10 hours postburn.[48,49] He emphasizes that all major burns require large amounts of fluid, but notes that older patients with burns, patients with burns and concomitant inhalation injury, and patients with burns in excess of 50% TBSA not only develop less edema but also better maintain hemodynamic stability with the addition of protein.

Slater and co-workers[44] have recently utilized fresh frozen plasma during burn shock. They use lactated Ringer's, 2 liters for 24 hours, and fresh frozen plasma, 75 ml/kg/24 h (**Table 8.1**). Although the volume of fresh frozen plasma is calculated, the volume infused is titrated to maintain an adequate urine output. Although the authors are utilizing colloid early in the burn shock period, they emphasize that most burn patients have received LR in significant volumes during field management.

Dextran resuscitation solutions

Dextran is a colloid consisting of glucose molecules which have been polymerized into chains to form high molecular weight polysaccharides.[49] This compound is commercially available in a number of molecular sizes. Dextran, which has an average molecular weight of 40 000 daltons, is referred to as low molecular weight dextran. British dextran has a mean molecular weight of 150 000, whereas the dextran used predominantly in Sweden has a molecular weight of 70 000. Dextran is excreted at the kidneys, with 40% removed within 24 hours. The remainder is slowly metabolized. Demling and associates have utilized dextran 70 in a 6% solution to prevent edema in nonburned tissues. Dextran 70 carries some risk of allergic reaction and can interfere with blood typing. Dextran 40 actually improves the microcirculatory flow by decreasing red cell aggregation.[50] Demling and colleagues[49] demonstrated that the net requirements to maintain vascular pressure at the baseline levels with dextran 40 were about half those seen with LR alone during the first 24 hours postburn. These authors have used an infusion rate of dextran 40 and saline of 2 cc/kg/h along with sufficient LR to maintain adequate perfusion. At 8 hours an infusion of fresh frozen plasma at 0.5–1.0 cc/kg/% TBSA burn over 18 hours is instituted along with necessary additional crystalloid (**Table 8.1**).

In the young pediatric burn patient with major burn injury, colloid replacement is frequently required as serum protein concentration rapidly decreases during burn shock. The Shriners Hospitals for Children in Cincinnati and Galveston both routinely utilize colloid during resuscitation of children with major thermal injuries.[51,52]

Special Considerations in Burn Shock Resuscitation

Fluid resuscitation in the thermally injured pediatric patient

The burned child continues to represent a special challenge, since resuscitation therapy must be more precise than that for an adult with a similar burn. In addition, children have a limited physiological reserve. We have demonstrated that children require more fluid for burn shock resuscitation than adults with similar thermal injury; fluid requirements for children averaged 5.8 cc/kg/% burn.[53] In addition, children commonly require intravenous resuscitation for relatively small burns of 10–20% TBSA. Baxter[45] found similar resuscitation requirements in the pediatric age group. Graves and associates[54] substantiated that children received 6.3 ± 2 cc/kg/% TBSA burn. At the Shriners Burns Hospital, Cincinnati, we have utilized the Parkland formula with the addition of maintenance fluid, to the resuscitation fluid volume, 4 ml/kg × % TBSA burn per 24 hours + 1500 cc/m² BSA per 24 hours. This is the formula used to begin burn shock resuscitation and to compare the amount of fluid needed by a particular pediatric burn patient with that needed by an unburned pediatric patient (**Table 8.2**). This is similar to the results reported by Graves and co-workers[54] who found that if maintenance fluids were subtracted from the resuscitation fluid requirements, the resulting resuscitation volumes would approach 4 cc/kg/% burn. At the Shriners Burns Hospital in Galveston, fluid requirements are estimated according to a formula based on total BSA and BSA burned in square meters.[52] Total fluid requirements for the first day are estimated as follows: 5000 ml/m² BSA burned per 24 hours + 2000 ml/m² BSA per 24 hours.

Inhalation injury

The presence of inhalation injury increases the fluid requirements for resuscitation from burn shock after thermal injury.[55] We have demonstrated that patients with documented inhalation injury require 5.7 cc/kg/% burn, as compared to 3.98 cc/kg/% burn in patients without inhalation injury. These data confirm and quantitate that inhalation injury accompanying thermal trauma increases the magnitude of total body injury and requires increased volumes of fluid and sodium to achieve resuscitation from early burn shock.

Choice of Fluids and Rate of Administration

It is clear that all the solutions reviewed are effective in restoring tissue perfusion. However, it makes no more sense to use one particular fluid for all patients than it does to use one antibiotic for all infections. Most patients with burns of <40% TBSA and patients with no pulmonary injury can be resuscitated with isotonic crystalloid fluid. In patients with burns of >40% TBSA and in patients with pulmonary injury, hypertonic saline can be utilized in the first 8 hours postburn, following which lactated Ringer's is infused to complete burn shock resuscitation. In the pediatric and elderly burn patient population, utilizing a lower but still hypertonic concentration of sodium, i.e. 180 mEq/L, still gives the benefits of hypertonic resuscitation without the potential complications of excessive sodium retention and hypernatremia.

In patients with massive burns, young pediatric patients, and burns complicated by severe inhalation injury, a combination of fluids may be utilized to achieve the desired goal of tissue perfusion while minimizing edema. In treating such patients, we have utilized the regimen of modified hypertonic (lactated Ringer's + 50 mEq NaHCO₃) saline fluid containing 180 mEq Na/L for the first 8 hours. After correction of the metabolic acidosis, which generally requires 8 hours, the patients are given LR only for the second 8 hours. In the last 8 hours, a 5% albumin in LR is utilized to complete resuscitation. The resuscitation solution used in Galveston for pediatric patients is an isotonic glucose-containing solution to which a moderate amount of colloid (human serum albumin) is added. The solution is prepared by mixing 50 ml of 25% human serum albumin (12.5 g) with 950 ml in a LR solution.

The monitoring of burn shock resuscitation is initiated by first responders and is generally concluded once the patient's fluid needs have decreased to a maintenance rate, based upon body size and evaporative water loss. Factors influencing monitoring needs include the extent and depth of burn, the presence of inhalation injury, associated injuries, preexisting medical illnesses, and patient age. The monitoring process can be classified based upon the intensity and frequency of observations, as well as the methods employed. While the level of monitoring must be individualized for each patient, one must weigh the risks and benefits of each modality. Young, healthy patients with minor burns may only require the occasional periodic assessment of vital signs, whereas those with more extensive burns and/or other risk factors may require more invasive techniques. A recent survey of 251 burn centers throughout the United States, Canada, United Kingdom, Australia, and New Zealand revealed that only 12% frequently used pulmonary artery catheter (PAC) monitoring during fluid resuscitation in patients with >30% TBSA burns.[56] Moreover, only 60% of the respondents who addressed treatment goals following PAC insertion indicated that they utilized predetermined physiologic parameters to direct fluid therapy.

Clinical monitoring of burn shock resuscitation has traditionally relied on clinical assessment of cardiovascular, renal, and biochemical parameters as indicators of vital organ perfusion. Heart rate, blood pressure, and electrocardiographic recordings are the primary modalities for monitoring cardiovascular status in any patient. Fluid balance during burn shock resuscitation is typically monitored by measuring hourly urine output via an indwelling urethral catheter. It has been recommended that urine output be maintained between 30 and 50 ml/h in adults,[22] and between 0.5 and 1.0

Table 8.2 Formulas for estimating pediatric resuscitation needs			
Cincinnati	4 ml × kg × % TBSA burn	1st 8 hours	Lactated Ringer's + 50 mg NaHCO₃
Shriners Burns Hospital	+		
	1500 cc × m² BSA	2nd 8 hours	Lactated Ringer's
		3rd 8 hours	Lactated Ringer's + 12.5 g albumin
Galveston	5000 ml/m² BSA burn	Ringer's lactate	
Shriners Burns Hospital	+	+	
	2000 ml/m² BSA	12.5 g albumin	

ml/kg/h in patients weighing less than 30 kg;[26] however, there have been no clinical studies identifying the optimal hourly urine output to maintain vital organ perfusion during burn shock resuscitation.

Because large volumes of fluid and electrolytes are administered both initially and throughout the course of resuscitation, it is important to obtain baseline laboratory measurements of complete blood count, electrolytes, glucose, albumin, and acid–base balance.[57] Laboratory values should be repeated as clinically indicated throughout the resuscitation period. These parameters are generally sufficient to assess the physiologic response of most burn patients during burn shock resuscitation. While clinical interpretation of the data should rely on the evaluation of trends rather than on isolated measurements, there have been no studies demonstrating which tests should be performed, how often they should be repeated, or the effect of frequent laboratory testing on the success of resuscitation.

Invasive hemodynamic monitoring permits the direct, and sometimes continuous, measurement of central venous pressure (CVP), pulmonary capillary wedge pressure (PCWP), and pulmonary vascular hemodynamics as well as the calculation of cardiac output (CO), systemic vascular resistance (SVR), oxygen delivery (DO_2), and oxygen consumption (VO_2). The decision to perform such monitoring requires consideration of risks, cost-effectiveness, and impact on clinical outcome. The Swan–Ganz catheter is most commonly utilized in patients in whom routine monitoring is felt to be ineffective, when there is a history of preexisting cardiac disease, or when there are other complicating factors.

PAC-guided therapy has been studied most extensively in trauma and critically ill surgical patients. Kirton and Civetta[58] performed a critical literature review to determine if the use of the PAC in trauma patients altered outcome. They concluded that hemodynamic data derived from the PAC appeared to be beneficial to ascertain cardiovascular performance, to direct therapy when noninvasive monitoring was felt to be inadequate, or when the endpoints of resuscitation were difficult to define. These findings were echoed at the 1997 Pulmonary Artery Catheter Consensus Conference; however, there was no unanimity that PAC-guided therapy altered mortality in trauma patients.[59]

Studies of PAC use for monitoring burn shock resuscitation are limited. Retrospective analyses of adult patients with extensive burn injuries have concluded that PCWP is a more reliable indicator of circulatory volume than CVP,[60] and that CO is more accurate in assessing the efficacy of resuscitation than hourly urine output.[61] These findings were supported by Dries and Waxman[62] who noted that urine output and vital signs monitoring did not correlate with PCWP, cardiac index (CI), SVR, DO_2, or VO_2. They concluded that PAC monitoring may be beneficial in patients at high risk for adverse outcomes due to suboptimal resuscitation. Most recently, Schiller and Bay have reported their retrospective experience in 95 patients treated over a 4-year period during which an attempt was made to maximize circulatory endpoints.[63] They concluded that early invasive monitoring facilitated more aggressive resuscitation and resulted in increased survival, and that the inability to achieve hyperdynamic endpoints predicted resuscitation failure.

PAC-guided monitoring has also been used to aid in achieving predetermined therapeutic endpoints during the resuscitation and management of trauma and critically ill patients. In a series of prospective randomized class II trials, Shoemaker et al.[64,65] demonstrated that patients resuscitated to hyperdynamic endpoints (i.e.

increased CI, DO_2I, VO_2I) had decreased mortality, ICU stay, and ventilator days compared to patients who were resuscitated to normal hemodynamic values. Recent studies by Fleming[64] and Bishop[65] have not only supported these conclusions but also demonstrated a decreased incidence of organ failures.

While the data supporting hyperdynamic resuscitation are impressive, there is also strong evidence that such therapeutic goals are not associated with improved outcome. Two trials in critically ill patients[66,67] were unable to demonstrate any benefit of PAC monitoring on patient outcome. These studies were supported by prospective randomized trials[68,69] which demonstrated no statistical differences in survival, organ failure, or ICU days between the control and hyperdynamic groups.

In an evidence-based review of these and other citations, Cooper et al.[70] concluded that the existing literature had inconsistent results regarding the efficacy of goal-oriented hemodynamic therapy. This conclusion was underscored by Elliott[71] who cited a meta-analysis of seven studies in which no significant differences in mortality were noted between control and hyperdynamic resuscitation groups.

The most appropriate endpoints in burn shock resuscitation are also unresolved. As such, the goal of achieving hyperdynamic resuscitation remains controversial. While Aikawa[72] was able to resuscitate 19/21 patients (90.5%) using the PAC to reach normal hemodynamic endpoints, Bernard[73] demonstrated that the ability to sustain a supranormal CI was associated with enhanced tissue perfusion and survival. This was supported by Schiller et al.[74] who demonstrated that an inadequate or unsustained response to hyperdynamic resuscitation was associated with nonsurvival. A follow-up study by these authors[75] also demonstrated significantly reduced mortality in those patients where PAC-guided resuscitation assisted in achieving hyperdynamic endpoints. The ability to achieve adequate oxygen delivery with hyperdynamic burn shock resuscitation has also been recently evaluated by Barton et al.[76] While patients achieved significant increases in VO_2I and DO_2I, they required 63% more fluid than predicted by the Parkland formula, a mean resuscitation volume of 9.07 ml/kg/% TBSA burn, and a mean of 50.4 hours to complete resuscitation.

More than 20 human studies in critically ill patients have demonstrated that blood lactate (BL) levels are highly accurate as a guide to the efficacy of resuscitation.[71,77] Blood lactate levels directly reflect anaerobic metabolisms as a consequence of hypoperfusion, and normalizing levels have long been associated with improved survival from nonburn shock.[78] In other studies, BL has been demonstrated to distinguish survivors from nonsurvivors.[79,80] In two prospective, goal-directed studies in critically ill patients, BL proved superior to not only MAP and urine output but also to DO_2, VO_2, and CI.[81,82]

It is important to emphasize that all of the resuscitation formulas are only guidelines for burn shock resuscitation. The Parkland formula, for instance, decreases the volume administered by 50% at 8 hours postburn. The relationship between the fluid volume required and time postburn depicted by the smooth curve in **Figure 8.1** represents the influence of temporal changes in microvascular permeability and edema volume on fluid needs. That curve is contrasted with the abrupt changes in fluid infusion rate as prescribed by the formula. The formulas are utilized as starting points for volume replacement and to compare the individual patient with the 'average' burn patient.

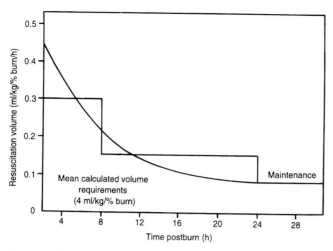

Fig. 8.1 Physiological curve of fluid requirements compared to Parkland formula, emphasizing that formulas are only guidelines for fluid therapy during burn shock (from Warden GD. *World J Surg* 1992; **16**: 21–23[51]).

An interesting question is, 'When has burn shock resuscitation been completed successfully?' It is obvious that resuscitation is completed when there is no further accumulation of edema fluid, which generally occurs between 18 and 30 hours postburn. The resuscitation fluids are utilized until the volume of infused fluid needed to maintain adequate urine volume of 30–50 cc/h in adults and 1 cc/kg/h in children equals the maintenance fluid volume. The maintenance fluid requirements following burn shock resuscitation include the patient's normal maintenance volume plus evaporative water loss.

Failure of Burn Shock Resuscitation

In certain patients, failure of burn shock resuscitation still occurs despite administration of massive volumes of fluid. Such patients are characterized by either extreme age and exceptionally extensive tissue trauma or by major electrical injury, major inhalation injury, delay in initiating adequate fluid resuscitation, or underlying disease that limits metabolic and cardiovascular reserve.[83] In these patients, refractory burn shock and resuscitation failure remain major causes of early mortality despite advances in emergency care and transport, resuscitation regimens, and physiologic stabilization.

We have used plasma exchange in patients with major thermal injuries who failed to respond to conventional fluid volumes during resuscitation from burn shock.[84] The indications for plasma exchange are ongoing fluid requirements exceeding twice those predicted by the Parkland formula despite conversion to hypertonic lactated saline resuscitation fluid. During a 3-year period, 22 patients underwent plasma exchange during burn shock resuscitation. A therapeutic response was documented in 21 of the 22 patients, characterized by a sharp decrease in fluid requirements from a mean of 260% above the predicted hourly volume by the resuscitation formula to within calculated requirements at a mean time of 2.3 hours following plasma exchange. Only one patient, who had a 100% TBSA burn (88% full-thick-

ness), failed to respond to plasma exchange and expired at 18 hours postburn. Slater and Goldfarb[85] have substantiated the beneficial effect of plasma exchange in sustaining patients during the immediate postburn period when patients fail to respond appropriately to conventional fluid resuscitation. This modality offers an alternative management technique for the treatment of refractory burn shock.

Fluid replacement following burn shock resuscitation

Although the heat-injured microvessels may continue to manifest increased vascular permeability for several days, the rate of loss is considerably less than that seen in the first 24 hours. Burn edema by this time is near maximal and the interstitial space may well be saturated with sodium. Additional fluid requirements will depend on the type of fluid used during the initial resuscitation. If hypertonic salt resuscitation has been utilized during the entire burn shock period, a hyperosmolar state is produced and the addition of free water will be required to restore the extracellular space to an isoosmolar state.

If colloid has not been utilized during burn shock and the serum oncotic pressure is low due to intravascular protein depletion, protein repletion is frequently needed. The amount of protein varies with the resuscitation utilized. Requirements of 0.3–0.5 cc/kg/TBSA burn of 5% albumin during the second 24 hours are utilized with the modified Brooke formula. The Parkland formula replaces the plasma volume deficit with colloid. This deficit varies from 20 to 60% of the circulating plasma volume. We have utilized colloid replacement based on a 20% plasma volume deficit during the second 24 hours (circulating plasma volume × 20%).

In addition to colloid, the patients should receive maintenance fluids. In burn patients the maintenance fluids include an additional amount for evaporative water loss. The total daily maintenance fluid requirements in the adult patient following burn shock can be calculated by the following formula: basal (1500 cc/m^2) + evaporative water loss [(25 + % burn) × m^2 × 24] = total maintenance fluid (m^2 = total body surface area in square meters). This fluid may be given via the intravenous route or with enteral feeding. The solution infused intravenously should be 50% normal saline with potassium supplements. With the loss of intracellular potassium during burn shock, the potassium requirements in adults are about 120 mEq/day. In the pediatric patient, increased fluids are required due to the differences in BSA to weight ratios compared to adults. In addition, children also require relatively larger volumes of urine for excretion of waste products. At the Cincinnati Shrine Unit, the maintenance fluid requirements are calculated by the following formula: (35 + % burn) × BSA × 24 (evaporative water loss) + 1500 ml × BSA per day (maintenance fluids). In Galveston, the recommended fluids needs are estimated as follows: 3750 ml/m^2 BSA per day (burn-related losses) + 1500 ml/m^2 BSA per day (maintenance fluids).

Following the initial 24–48 hours postburn period of resuscitation, urinary output is an unreliable guide to adequacy of hydration.[86] Respiratory water losses, osmotic diuresis secondary to accentuated glucose intolerance, osmotic diuresis secondary to high protein, high caloric feedings, and derangements in the ADH mechanisms all contribute to increased fluid losses despite an adequate urine output. In general, patients with major thermal injuries will require a urine output of 1500–2000 cc/24 hours in adults, and 3–4 ml/kg/h in children.

The measurement of serum sodium concentration is not only a means of diagnosing dehydration but also the best guide for planning and following successful fluid replacement. Other useful laboratory indices of the state of hydration and guides of therapy include body weight change, serum and urine nitrogen concentrations, serum and urine glucose concentrations, the intake and output record, and clinical examination.

Continuous colloid replacement may be required to maintain colloid oncotic pressure in very large burns and in the pediatric burn patient. Maintaining serum albumin levels above 2.0 g/dl is desirable.

The electrolyte calcium, magnesium, and phosphate must also be monitored. Although the replacement of these electrolytes has been studied in detail in burn patients, maintaining the values within normal limits is desirable and varies in each patient.

Summary

The volume necessary to resuscitate burn patients is dependent upon injury severity, age, physiological status, and associated injury. Consequently, the volume predicted by a resuscitation formula must commonly be modified according to the individual's response to therapy. In optimizing fluid resuscitation in severely burned patients, the amount of fluid should be just enough to maintain vital organ function without producing iatrogenic pathological changes. The composition of the resuscitation fluid, within limitations, in the first 24 hours postburn probably makes very little difference; however, it should be individualized to the particular patient. The utilization of the beneficial properties of hypertonic, crystalloid, and colloid solutions at various times postburn will minimize the amount of edema formation. The rate of administration of resuscitation fluids should maintain urine outputs of 30–50 cc in adults and 1–2 cc/kg in children. When a child weighs 30–50 kg, the urine output should be maintained at the adult level. Fluid resuscitation based on our current knowledge of the massive fluid shifts and vascular changes that occur following burn injury has markedly decreased mortality related to burn-induced volume loss. The failure rate for adequate resuscitation is <5% even for patients with burns >85% TBSA. These improved statistics, however, are derived from experience in burn centers where there is substantial knowledge of the pathophysiology of burn injury. Inadequate volume replacement in major burns is, unfortunately, common when clinicians lack sufficient knowledge and experience in this area.

Areas of burn shock research that need further attention include:

1. the definition of the postburn course of capillary permeability changes, and identification of humoral or cellular factors influencing these changes;
2. the identification and evaluation of pharmacological agents that can significantly alter capillary leakage;
3. elucidation of the relationships between resuscitation fluid composition and pulmonary function changes; and
4. the effect of resuscitation on late organ dysfunction, such as post-resuscitation wound, renal, and pulmonary complications.[87]

References

1. Artz CP, Moncrief JA. The burn problem. In: Artz CP, Moncrief JA, eds. *The Treatment of Burns.* Philadelphia: WB Saunders, 1969: 1–22.
2. Underhill FP. The significance of anhydremia in extensive surface burn. *JAMA* 1930; **95**: 852–7.
3. Moore FD. The body-weight budget: basic fluid therapy for the early burn. *Surg Clin North Am* 1970; **50**: 1249–65.
4. Pruitt BA Jr, Mason AD Jr, Moncrief JA. Hemodynamic changes in the early post burn patients: the influence of fluid administration and of a vasodilator (hydralazine). *J Trauma* 1971; **11**: 36–46.
5. Majno G, Palide GE. Studies on inflammation. I. The effect of histamine and serotonin on vascular permeability. *J Cell Biol* 1961; **11**: 571–8.
6. Majno G, Shea SM, Leventhal M. Endothelial contractures induced by histamine type mediators. *J Cell Biol* 1969; **42**: 647–72.
7. Anggard E, Jonsson CE. Efflux of prostaglandins in lymph from scalded tissue. *Acta Physiol Scand* 1971; **81**: 440–47.
8. Sevitt S. Local blood flow in experimental burns. *J Pathol Bact* 1949; **61**: 427–34.
9. Leape L. Initial changes in burns: tissue changes in burned and unburned skins of Rhesus monkeys. *J Trauma* 1970; **10**: 488–92.
10. Carvajal HF, Brouhard BH, Linares HA. Effect of antihistamine-antiserotonin and ganglionic blocking agents upon increased capillary permeability following burn trauma. *J Trauma* 1975; **15**: 969–75.
11. Boykin JV Jr, Crute SL, Haynes BW Jr. Cimetidine therapy for burn shock: a quantitative assessment. *J Trauma* 1985; **25**: 864–70.
12. VanNeuten JM, Janssen PAJ, VanBeck J. Vascular effects of ketanserin (R 41 468), a novel antagonist of 5-HT$_2$ serotonergic receptors. *J Pharmacol Exp Ther* 1981; **218**: 217–80.
13. Holliman CJ, Meuleman TR, Larsen KR, Port JD, Stanley TH, Pace AL, Warden GD. The effect of ketanserin, a specific serotonin antagonist, on burn shock hemodynamic parameters in a porcine burn model. *J Trauma* 1983; **23**: 867–74.
14. Heggers JP, Loy GL, Robson MC, DelBaccaro EJ. Histological demonstration of prostaglandins and thromboxanes in burned tissue. *J Surg Res* 1980; **28**: 110–17.
15. Herndon DN, Abston S, Stein MD. Increased thromboxane B$_2$ levels in the plasma of burned and septic burned patients. *Surg Gynecol Obstet* 1984; **159**: 210–13.
16. Arturson G. Microvascular permeability to macromolecules in thermal injury. *Acta Physiol Scand Suppl* 1979; **463**: 111–22.
17. Rocha E, Silva M, Antonio A. Release of bradykinin and the mechanisms of production of thermic edema (45°C) in the rat's paw. *Med Exp* 1960; **3**: 371–8.
18. Holder IA, Neely AN. Hageman factor-dependent kinin activation in burns and its theoretical relationship to postburn immunosuppression syndrome and infection. *J Burn Care Rehabil* 1990; **11(6)**: 496–503.
19. Neely AN, Nathan P, Highsmith RF. Plasma proteolytic activity following burns. *J Trauma* 1988; **28**: 362–7.
20. Baxter CR. Fluid volume and electrolyte changes in the early post-burn period. *Clin Plast Surg* 1974; **1**: 693–703.
21. Moyer CA, Margraf HW, Monafo WW. Burn shock and extravascular sodium deficiency: treatment with Ringer's solution with lactate. *Arch Surg* 1965; **90**: 799–811.
22. Baxter CR, Shires GT. Physiological response to crystalloid resuscitation of severe burns. *Ann NY Acad Sci* 1968; **150**: 874–94.
23. Moylan JA, Mason AB, Rogers PW, Walker HL. Postburn shock: a critical evaluation of resuscitation. *J Trauma* 1973; **13**: 354–8.
24. Demling RH, Mazess RB, Witt RM, Wolbert WH. The study of burn wound edema using dichosmatic absorptionmetry. *J Trauma* 1978; **18**: 124–8.
25. Hilton JG. Effects of fluid resuscitation on total fluid loss following thermal injury. *Surg Gynecol Obstet* 1981; **152**: 441–7.
26. Schwartz SL. Consensus summary on fluid resuscitation. *J Trauma* 1979; **19(11 Suppl)**: 876–7.
27. Shires GT. Proceedings of the Second NIH Workshop on Burn Management. *J Trauma* 1979; **19(11 Suppl)**: 862–3.
28. Monafo WW. The treatment of burn shock by the intravenous and oral administration of hypertonic lactated saline solution. *J Trauma* 1970; **10**: 575–86.
29. Monafo WW, Halverson JD, Schechtman K. The role of concentrated sodium solutions in the resuscitation of patients with severe burns. *Surgery* 1984; **95**: 129–35.
30. Demling RH, Gunther RA, Haines B, Kramer G. Burn edema Part II: Complications, prevention, and treatment. *J Burn Care Rehabil* 1982; **3**: 199–206.
31. Shimazaki S, Yukioka T, Matsuda H. Fluid distribution and pulmonary dysfunction following burn shock. *J Trauma* 1991; **31**: 623–6.
32. Caldwell FT, Bowser BH. Critical evaluation of hypertonic and hypotonic solutions to resuscitate severely burned children: a prospective study. *Ann Surg* 1979; **189**: 546–52.
33. Gunn ML, Hansbrough JF, Davis JW, Furst SR, Field TO. Prospective randomized

trial of hypertonic sodium lactate vs. lactated Ringer's solution for burn shock resuscitation. *J Trauma* 1989; **29**: 1261–7.

34. Yoshioka T, Maemura K, Ohhashi Y, Sugimoto H, Takahashi M, Sugimoto T. Effect of intravenously administered fluid on hemodynamic change and respiratory function in extensive thermal injury. *Surg Gynecol Obstet* 1980; **151**: 503–7.

35. Shimazaki S, Yoshioka T, Tanaka N, Sugimoto T, Onji. Body fluid changes during hypertonic lactated saline solution therapy for burn shock. *J Trauma* 1977; **17**: 38–43.

36. Bowser-Wallace BH, Cone JB, Caldwell FT Jr. A prospective analysis of hypertonic lactated saline vs. Ringer's lactate-colloid for the resuscitation of severely burned children. *Burns Incl Therm Inj* 1986; **12**: 402–9.

37. Crum R, Bobrow B, Shackford S, Hansbrough J, Brown MR. The neurohumoral response to burn injury in patients resuscitated with hypertonic saline. *J Trauma* 1988; **28**: 1181–7.

38. Huang PP, Stucky FS, Dimick AR, Treat RC, Bessey PQ, Rue LW. Hypertonic sodium resuscitation is associated with renal failure and death. *Ann Surg* 1995; **221**: 543–54.

39. Bowser-Wallace BH, Cone JB, Caldwell FT Jr. Hypertonic lactated saline resuscitation of severely burned patients over 60 years of age. *J Trauma* 1985; **25**: 22–6.

40. Bowser-Wallace BH, Caldwell FT Jr. Fluid requirements of severely burned children up to 3 years old: hypertonic lactated saline vs. Ringer's lactate-colloid. *Burns Incl Therm Inj* 1986; **12**: 549–55.

41. Bartolani A, Governa M, Barisoni D. Fluid replacement in burned patients. *Acta Chir Plast* 1996; **38**: 132–6.

42. Griswold JA, Anglin BL, Love RT Jr, Scott-Conner C. Hypertonic saline resuscitation: efficacy in a community-based burn unit. *South Med J* 1991; **84**: 692–6.

43. Jelenko C III, Williams JB, Wheeler ML, Callaway BD, Fackler VK, Albers CA, Barger AA. Studies in shock and resuscitation. I: use of a hypertonic, albumin-containing, fluid demand regimen (HALFD) in resuscitation. *Crit Care Med* 1979; **7**: 157–67.

44. Du G, Slater H, Goldfarb IW. Influence of different resuscitation regimens on acute weight gain in extensively burned patients. *Burns* 1991; **17**: 147–50.

45. Baxter CR. Problems and complications of burn shock resuscitation. *Surg Clin North Am* 1978; **58**: 1313–22.

46. Goodwin CW, Dorethy J, Lam V, Pruitt BA Jr. Randomized trial of efficacy of crystalloid and colloid resuscitation on hemodynamic response and lung water following thermal injury. *Ann Surg* 1983; **197**: 520–31.

47. Demling RH. Fluid resuscitation. In: Boswick JA Jr, ed. *The Art and Science of Burn Care*. Rockville, MD: Aspen, 1987: 189–202.

48. Demling RH, Kramer GD, Harms B Role of thermal injury-induced hypoproteinemia on edema formation in burned and non-burned tissue. *Surgery* 1984; **95**: 136–44.

49. Demling RH, Kramer GC, Gunther R, Nerlich M. Effect of non-protein colloid on post-burn edema formation in soft tissues and lung. *Surgery* 1985; **95**: 593–602.

50. Gelin LE, Solvell L, Zederfeldt B. The plasma volume expanding effect of low viscous dextran and Macrodex. *Acta Chir Scand* 1961; **122**: 309–23.

51. Warden GD. Burn shock resuscitation. *World J Surg* 1992; **16**: 16–23.

52. Carvajal HF. Fluid therapy for the acutely burned child. *Compr Ther* 1977; **3**: 17–24.

53. Merrell SW, Saffle JR, Sullivan JJ, Navar PD, Kravitz M, Warden GD. Fluid resuscitation in thermally injured children. *Am J Surg* 1986; **152**: 664–9.

54. Graves TA, Cioffi WG, McManus WF, Mason AD Jr, Pruitt BA Jr. Fluid resuscitation of infants and children with massive thermal injury. *J Trauma* 1988; **28**: 1656–9.

55. Navar PD, Saffle JR, Warden GD. Effect of inhalation injury on fluid resuscitation requirements after thermal injury. *Am J Surg* 1985; **150**: 716–20.

56. Mansfield MD, Kinsell J. Use of invasive cardiovascular monitoring in patients with burns greater than 30 percent body surface area: a survey of 251 centres. *Burns* 1996; **22**: 549–51.

57. Fabri PJ. Monitoring of the burn patient. *Clin Plast Surg* 1986; **13**: 21–7.

58. Kirton OC, Civetta JM. Do pulmonary artery catheters alter outcome in trauma patients? *New Horizons* 1997; **5**: 222–7.

59. Pulmonary artery catheter consensus conference: Consensus statement. *Crit Care Med* 1997; **25**: 910–25.

60. Aikawa N, Martyn JA, Burke JR. Pulmonary artery catheterization and thermodilution cardiac output determination in the management of critically burned patients. *Am J Surg* 1978; **135**: 811–17.

61. Agarwal N, Petro J, Salisbury RE. Physiologic profile monitoring in burned patients. *J Trauma* 1982; **23**: 577–83.

62. Dries DJ, Waxman K. Adequate resuscitation of burn patients may not be measured by urine output and vital signs. *Crit Care Med* 1991; **19**: 327–9.

63. Schiller WR, Bay RC. Hemodynamic and oxygen transport monitoring in management of burns. *New Horizons* 1996; **4**: 475–82.

64. Fleming AW, Bishop M, Shoemaker W, et al. Prospective trial of supranormal values as goals of resuscitation in severe trauma. *Arch Surg* 1992; **127**: 1175–81.

65. Bishop MH, Shoemaker WC, Appel PL, et al. Prospective, randomized trial of survivor values of cardiac index, oxygen delivery, and oxygen consumption as resuscitation endpoints in severe trauma. *J Trauma* 1995; **38**: 780–7.

66. Pearson KS, Gomez MN, Moyers JR, Carter JG, Tinkler JW. A cost/benefit analysis of randomized invasive monitoring of patients undergoing cardiac surgery. *Anesth Analg* 1989; **69**: 336–41.

67. Ontario Intensive Care Study Group. Evaluation of right heart catheterization in critically ill patients. *Crit Care Med* 1992; **20**: 928–33.

68. Yu M, Levy MM, Smith P, Takiguchi SA, Miyasaki A, Myers SA. Effect of maximizing oxygen delivery on morbidity and mortality rates in critically ill patients: A prospective, randomized, controlled study. *Crit Care Med* 1993; **21**: 830–8.

69. Gattinoni L, Brazzi L, Pelosi P, et al. A trial of goal-oriented hemodynamic therapy in critically ill patients. *N Engl J Med* 1995; **333**: 1025–32.

70. Cooper AB, Goig GS, Sibbald WJ. Pulmonary artery catheters in the critically ill. An overview using the methodology of evidence-based medicine. *Crit Care Clin* 1996; **12**: 777–94.

71. Elliott DC. An evaluation of the end points of resuscitation. *J Am Coll Surg* 1998; **187**: 536–47.

72. Aikawa N, Ishbiki K, Naito C, et al. Individualized fluid resuscitation based on haemodynamic monitoring in the management of extensive burns. *Burns* 1982; **8**: 249–55.

73. Bernard F, Gueugniaud P-Y, Bertin-Maghit M, Bouchard C, Vilasco B, Petit P. Prognostic significance of early cardiac index measurements in severely burned patients. *Burns* 1994; **20**: 529–31.

74. Schiller WR, Bay RC, McLachlan JG, Sagraves SG. Survival in major burn injuries is predicted by early response to Swan–Ganz-guided resuscitation. *Am J Surg* 1995; **170**: 696–700.

75. Schiller WR, Bay RC, Garren RL, Parker I, Sagraves SG. Hyperdynamic resuscitation improves survival in patients with life-threatening burns. *J Burn Care Rehabil* 1997; **18**: 10–16.

76. Barton RG, Saffle JR, Morris SE, Mone M, Davis B, Shelby J. Resuscitation of thermally injured patients with oxygen transport criteria as goals of therapy. *J Burn Care Rehabil* 1997; **18**: 1–9.

77. Mizock BL, Falk JL. Lactic acidosis in critical illness. *Crit Care Med* 1992; **20**: 80–93.

78. Bakker J, Coffemils M, Leon M, et al. Blood lactate levels are superior to oxygen derived variables in predicting outcome in human septic shock. *Chest* 1991; **99**: 956–62.

79. Weil MH, Afifi AA. Experimental and clinical studies on lactate and pyruvate as indicators of the severity of acute circulatory failure (shock). *Circulation* 1970; **41**: 989–1001.

80. Henning RJ, Weil MH, Weiner F. Blood lactate as a prognostic indicator of survival in patients with acute myocardial infarction. *Circ Shock* 1982; **9**: 307–15.

81. Boyd I, Grounds RM, Bennett ED. A randomized clinical trial of the effect of deliberate perioperative increase of oxygen delivery on mortality in high-risk surgical patients. *JAMA* 1993; **270**: 2699–707.

82. Abramson D, Scalea TM, Hitchcock R, et al. Lactate clearance and survival following injury. *J Trauma* 1993; **35**: 584–8.

83. Pruitt B Jr. Fluid and electrolyte replacement in the burned patient. *Surg Clin NA* 1978; **58**: 1291–312.

84. Warden GD, Stratta R, Saffle JR Jr, Kravitz M, Ninnemann JL. Plasma exchange therapy in patients failing to resuscitate from burn shock. *J Trauma* 1983; **23**: 945–51.

85. Schnarrs R, Cline C, Goldfarb I, Hanrahan J, Jacob H, Slater H, Gaisford J. Plasma exchange for failure of early resuscitation in thermal injuries. *J Burn Care Rehabil* 1986; **7**: 230–3.

86. Warden GD, Wilmore D, Rogers P, Mason D, Pruitt B. Hypernatremic state in hypermetabolic burn patients. *Arch Surg* 1973; **106**: 420–3.

87. Pruitt BA Jr. Fluid resuscitation of extensively burned patients. *J Trauma* 1981; **21**(Suppl): 690–2.

The burn wound

Chapter 9

Evaluation of the burn wound management decisions

David Heimbach, Roberta Mann, Loren Engrav

Introduction

In addition to the extent of burn and the age of the patient, the depth of burn is a primary determinant of mortality following thermal injury. Burn depth is also the primary determinant of the patient's long-term appearance and function. For many years burns were treated by daily washing, removal of loose dead tissue, and some sort of topical nostrum until they healed by themselves or, eventually, granulation tissue appeared in the base of the wound. Superficial dermal burns healed within 2 weeks and deep dermal burns healed over many weeks if infection was prevented. Full-thickness burns lost their eschar in 2–6 weeks by collagenase production from bacteria and mechanically by daily debridement. When the granulating bed became free of debris and relatively uninfected, split-thickness skin grafts were applied, usually some

3–8 weeks after injury, and a 50% graft take was considered to be acceptable. Repeated graftings eventually closed the wound. The prolonged and intense inflammatory response made hypertrophic scar and contractures part of normal burn treatment. Vigorous physical therapy, nutritional support, psychosocial support, and pain management were required on a daily basis for many weeks in order to yield a satisfactory result.

Modern treatment involves early surgical removal of the burn. Rather than waiting for spontaneous separation, the eschar is now surgically removed early in the burn course and the wound closed with grafting techniques and acute flaps individualized to each patient.

When nonoperative treatment is the routine, the accurate assessment of burn depth is of little importance save for predicting mortality. On the other hand, with aggressive surgical treatment, an accurate estimation of burn depth becomes crucial. Burns which heal within 3 weeks generally do so without hypertrophic scarring or functional impairment, although long-term pigment changes are common. Burns which take longer than 3 weeks to heal often produce unsightly hypertrophic scars and frequently lead to functional impairment, as well as providing only a thin, fragile epithelial cover for many weeks or months. State of the art care now, at least in patients with small and moderate burns, involves early excision and grafting of all burns which will not heal within 3 weeks.[1-5] The challenge is to determine which burns will heal within 3 weeks.

An understanding of burn depth requires an understanding of skin thickness. The anatomy and pathophysiology of the skin is well covered in another chapter. The standard technique for determining burn depth has long been clinical observation of the wound. Unfortunately, the difference in burn depth between a burn which heals in 3 weeks and a deep dermal burn which will heal only after many weeks, or a full-thickness burn which will not heal at all, may be only a matter of only a few tenths of a millimeter. Further, a burn is a dynamic process for the first few days, and a burn which appears shallow on day 1 may appear deep by day 3. Finally, the kind of topical wound care used can dramatically change the appearance of the burn. Because of these limitations, and because of its increased importance in planning definitive burn wound care, interest has been stirred and technology has brought numerous devices and techniques to determine burn depth more precisely than clinical observation.

Estimation of burn depth

Clinical Observation

Despite modern technology, clinical observation still remains the standard for diagnosis. Very shallow (heal in less than 2 weeks) and very deep (full-thickness charred burns) present little difficulty even to inexperienced observers. Superficial dermal burns involve only the papillary dermis and characteristically form blisters with fluid collection at the interface of the epidermis and dermis. Blistering may not occur for some hours following injury and burns thought to be first degree may subsequently be diagnosed as superficial dermal burns by day 2. Once blisters are removed, the wound is pink and wet and is quite painful as currents of air pass over it. The wound is hypersensitive to touch and the patient will rarely permit more than one diagnostic adventure with a pin to test sensation. These wounds blanch with pressure, and the blood flow to the dermis is increased over that of normal skin. Obvious charred full-thickness burns are leathery, firm, depressed when compared to adjoining normal skin, and are insensitive to light touch and pinprick. Unfortunately for the clinician, there are many burns whose depth is intermediate between these obvious ones.

Deep dermal burns extend into the reticular dermis and generally will take 3 or more weeks to heal. They also blister, but the wound surface is usually a mottled pink and white color immediately following the injury. The patient complains of discomfort rather than pain. When pressure is applied to the burn, capillaries refill slowly or not at all. The wound is often less sensitive to pinprick than the surrounding normal skin.[6,7] By the second day the wound may be white and is usually fairly dry.

Noncharred full-thickness burns can masquerade with many of the clinical findings of a deep dermal burn. Like deep dermal burns, they may be mottled in appearance. They rarely blanch on pressure, and may have a dry, white appearance. In some cases the burn may be translucent with clotted vessels visible in the depths. Some full-thickness burns, particularly immersion scalds, may have a red appearance, and can be confused by the uninitiated as a superficial dermal burn. They can be distinguished, however, because these red, full-thickness burns do not blanch with pressure.

Evaluation by an experienced surgeon as to whether an apparent deep dermal burn will heal in 3 weeks is about 50% accurate[8] – tossing a coin is about as useful a technique. In experienced hands, however, early excision and grafting provides better results than nonoperative care for such 'indeterminate' burns.[2]

An intense search for a more precise diagnosis of burn depth has been mounted ever since it became important to determine whether the patient would benefit from early operation. A number of techniques have been used based on the physiology of the skin and alterations produced by burning. These techniques take advantage of:

- the ability to detect dead cells or denatured collagen (biopsy, ultrasound, vital dyes);
- altered blood flow (fluorescein, laser Doppler, and thermography);
- the color of the wound (light reflectance); and
- physical changes, such as edema (magnetic resonance imaging). A brief review of each follows.

Burn Wound Biopsy

Histologic wound biopsy would seem to be the most precise diagnostic tool.[9] However, biopsies leave permanent scars in partial-thickness wounds, they are expensive, and they require an experienced pathologist to tell live from denatured collagen and cells. Further, the burn wound is dynamic during the first several days, and even in the 1950s Douglas Jackson reported that 7 days were necessary to obtain reproducible results.[10] Another day or two is required to obtain permanent sections, and there is no guarantee that areas adjacent to the biopsy are the same depth. For these reasons, biopsies are rarely used in clinical practice; to the author's knowledge, no studies have determined correlation with biopsy and time to healing. Using of an *in vitro* model, Ho-Asjoe *et al.*[11] found the use of cryosections and an immunofluorescent staining method to be quicker and more clear-cut than standard light microscopic techniques. This preliminary report will require further investigation to transform the method from an experimental model to standard practice in the clinical setting.[11]

Ultrasound

Moserová, using an industrial ultrasound device in 1982, was able to detect differences between normal pig skin and that scalded for 5 and 15 seconds.[12] His initial work was expanded as technology improved. Cantrell[13] was able to detect denatured from normal collagen in pigskin. One problem with this technique is that collagen denatures at 65°C while the epidermal cells, from which the burn must heal, are killed at about 47°C. As a result, apparent depth is likely to be underestimated by ultrasound. Further refinements in instrumentation have enabled Brink[14] to reach a significant correlation between ultrasound burn depth and histology in pigs ($r = 0.90$). Unfortunately, in the clinical arena Wachtel,[15] in five burned patients, reported that ultrasound comparisons with clinical evaluation and histopathological studies of burn wound biopsies of the same burned areas failed to show any substantive improvement in predicting the depth of burn by ultrasonic scanning techniques. Perhaps more precise instruments will continue to improve resolution.

Vital Dyes

In experimental small mammal models, India ink can provide a one-time demonstration of blood flow to the skin.[16–18] India ink, however, kills the animal on injection; so, while a useful experimental technique, it has no role in patient wound assessment.

A vital dye directly applied to the burn wound would be useful in detecting dead tissue and also in determining the depth of excision. Davies[19] described important characteristics of such a dye. It should stain only dead tissue, not be removable with wound treatment, be nontoxic, provide a sharp demarcation between living and dead tissue, penetrate all dead tissue, and be compatible with topical treatments usually used in burn care. Zawacki[20] in 1970 studied patent blue V and tetracycline for the diagnosis of burn depth but the results were subjective. In a rat model, Davies and his co-workers evaluated methylene blue, toluidine blue, trypan blue, Evans blue and Disulfine Blue sulfan blue marker dyes. Methylene blue, which is metabolized to a colorless compound by living cells, was selected for preliminary testing in patients. When mixed with silver sulfadiazine and applied topically, a significant blue discoloration appeared within 48 hours which remained after vigorous washing. Excision was carried down to dermis, which was unstained. They reported 'encouraging' results in this preliminary study, but the authors have no more recent reports listed in the *Index Medicus*. Immediately following this report with methylene blue, brief clinical use of this technique in our burn center did not produce a satisfactorily sharp demarcation to guide excision.

Fluorescein Fluorometry

Fluorescein, injected systemically, is delivered through a patent's circulation and fluoresces under ultraviolet light. It has been widely used to determine viability of flaps,[21,22] intestine, and even whole extremities.[23] The use of fluorescein fluorescence to determine burn depth was first reported in 1943.[24] Because treatment plans were not altered based on burn depth, the technique lay fallow until more precise instruments could measure the magnitude of fluorescence – a fiberoptic perfusion fluorometer. Gatti[25] studied 63 burns with the fluorometer after intravenous (IV) administration of sodium fluorescein. The fluorescein kinetics were monitored for 1 hour within the first 48 hours and again between the third and sixth days postburn, and compared to the kinetics in adjacent normal skin. Depth of burn was confirmed by biopsy and healing characteristics. Fluorometric analysis during both study periods consistently distinguished between partial-thickness and full-thickness burns. Partial-thickness burns uniformly exhibited fluorescence within 10 minutes; full-thickness burns showed nil. Enthusiasm for this technique must be tempered by the knowledge that when this technique was reported in 1982, most burn surgeons excised only full-thickness burns, leaving partial-thickness burns to heal on their own. Therefore, there was an advantage to distinguishing between partial- and full-thickness burns. Gatti's report was confirmed with high-speed Polaroid photography in 1984, but again the fluorescein technique was best at distinguishing full-thickness (no fluorescence) from nonfull-thickness burns.[26,27]

A report by Black[28] in 1986 could not confirm significant differences between partial- and full-thickness burns using a similar technique. In both rat and human models, 59 burn sites (eight rats) and 37 burn sites (seven patients) were assessed. Readings were taken for 3 hours on the rats and 1 hour on the patients during the first 48 hours, and the procedure was repeated for 5 days postburn. Maximum values during these periods were determined for burn and nonburn sites, and background levels were subtracted from these values. The rate of fluorescein uptake and the peak times for burn and nonburn sites were then compared. Actual depth of burn was determined by whether or not healing had occurred. The results showed no significant difference between partial-thickness and full-thickness burns using fluorometry, as standard deviations in both models for both depths of burn were too large to distinguish between groups, let alone be predictive in any given burn. In porcine burns the intensity of ICG fluorescence measured at the surface of the wound for burns of similar age was shown to decrease exponentially with the depth of the burn. The enhanced fluorescence of partial-thickness burns is attributable to increased permeability, and the decreased signal associated with deeper injuries is attributable to vascular occlusion.[29,30]

The studies remain inconclusive. Our own experience with fluorescein indicates that it confirms the clinical diagnosis in very deep and very shallow burns, areas where there is little confusion, but that it cannot distinguish between intermediate and deep dermal burns, where the distinction is crucial in operative planning.

Laser Doppler Flowmetry

The laser Doppler has been used since 1975 for monitoring the cutaneous circulation. Light from a helium–neon laser is carried by fiberoptics to the skin where it interacts with both stationary structures and moving blood cells within a sample volume of approximately 1 mm.[3] Back-scattered light from the moving cells is shifted in velocity using the Doppler principle, while back-scattered light from stationary objects remains at its original frequency. The mixing of these light waves is translated to an

electrical signal, and mathematical estimation of blood flow can be made in normal versus study areas of skin. The laser Doppler has the advantage of being easy to use, noninvasive (although the probe must be held against the skin), and provides immediate results. In some studies, the skin was heated to 40°C (to ensure maximal vasodilatation).

Sorensen's group in Denmark first reported the use of a laser Doppler on a burn unit. In a first study, the investigators measured skin blood flow in burned patients at rest and after applying a topical heat load at 44°C and found a close relationship between burn depth and the combination of flow level and ability to vasodilate.[31] They also measured skin blood flow in 15 burned patients on the third day postburn and compared results to a punch biopsy taken from the same point. They found an excellent correlation between biopsy and laser, but only good correlation between laser and clinical assessment for full-thickness burns. Nonetheless, the authors felt that their results were encouraging.

Initial studies in our burn center showed excellent correlation with full-thickness burns (no flow) and shallow burns (normal or increased flow) but considerable variation from patient to patient with comparable burns as well as at different times in the same area in the same patient with moderate and deep dermal burns. Readings varied particularly with temperature (immediately after bathing, in a warm room, etc.); the state of anxiety (catecholamine response); and elevation of an extremity (cutaneous blood flow essentially disappeared as the hands were elevated).

In further studies, we followed the cutaneous circulation over time in burned patients and rats.[32] We asked whether measuring changes in cutaneous blood flow might help predict the ultimate fate of burns which were not obviously shallow or deep. A laser Doppler flowmeter was used to study cutaneous perfusion for at least 72 hours in partial-thickness wounds on patients with burns of less than 15% total body surface area (TBSA) and in experimental wounds of similar size on rats. Clinical wounds which healed without grafting consistently showed elevated perfusion levels which increased further within 72 hours. Wounds that eventually required grafting had lower perfusion levels with no obvious pattern of increase. Differences between average flow levels for healing and nonhealing burns were statistically significant throughout the study period. Perfusion levels in experimental wounds were stratified according to burn severity (scalds for 1, 3, 5, 10 seconds), with shallower wounds showing a pattern of increase similar to the clinical wounds. While the means were significantly different in these studies ($p = 0.05$), individual burns showed enough overlap that absolute levels of flow were not predictive for any given patient; however, the trend toward increased flow for healing burns and flat flow for nonhealing burns was quite constant, and if the patient can be followed for several days, the method has merit in deciding who would benefit from excision and grafting after day 3. Similar findings (significant group differences but considerable individual overlap) were reported recently by O'Reilly and colleagues.[33] Clinical studies using the laser Doppler to determine burn depth are ongoing, and refinements of the technology continue; however, its use has not become standard in everyday clinical decision making (to graft or not to graft).

Park *et al.* also used a laser Doppler flowmeter, concluding that there was also a significant correlation between initial flow measurements and the depth of burn wounds. They concluded that laser Doppler flow measurements performed early after burn injury are useful in predicting the depth of burn wounds.[34] Extending previous laser studies, Yeong studied flux of flow, representing maximal dilitation in response to heat in burned human skin and using discriminate analysis to conclude that that there could be a 94% accuracy in predicting whether burns would heal within 3 weeks compared to an experienced physician's decision making of 70%.[35]

Thermography

Diminished blood flow to deep dermal and full-thickness burns makes them cooler to touch,[36] a finding confirmed by thermography in 1974 by Hackett.[37] Initial studies of thermography as a tool for predicting the need for excision and grafting of deep dermal wounds in 30 patients were presented with guarded optimism by Mason in 1981, suggesting that thermography might be more accurate than clinical judgment.[38] Thermography, like the laser Doppler, is highly dependent on room and patient temperature, the patient's anxiety and stress level, and area of the body considered.[39] Despite these drawbacks, Cole[40,41] compared thermography to clinical assessment of 32 burned hands. Superficial and deep partial-thickness burns were treated conservatively, with excision and grafting of those which had not healed only after 2–3 weeks after injury. This delayed surgery group and the healed group were retrospectively analyzed to determine the predictive value of the initial clinical and thermographic assessments of the depth of the burns. Full-thickness burns were excised and grafted within 5 days and were not included in the study. Initial thermographic assessment correctly predicted the outcome (whether healed or excised and grafted) in 33 of 36 burns. This relationship was highly significant. Initial clinical assessment of depth had no significant relationship with the time taken to heal. In agreement with other methods, Liddington reported that thermography was most accurate after 3 days following burning.[42]

Light Reflectance

The skin is relatively transparent to short wavelength infrared light, and reduced hemoglobin absorbs more of the light than oxygenated hemoglobin. Anselmo and Zawacki in 1973[43] reasoned that thrombosed vessels in full-thickness burns would become visible in infrared light and could be distinguished from the open vessels of partial-thickness burns. Computer analysis of infrared photographs was encouraging, and they extended their work, publishing results in 1977[44] of computer analyses of photographs taken with red, green, and infrared filtered light. A mainframe computer generated ratios of the green/infrared, red/infrared, and red/green images point by point over the entire surface. The authors felt that these images could accurately distinguish shallow, deep dermal, and full-thickness burns. Unfortunately, wound analysis was very expensive and time-consuming, so it was too slow for clinical decision making.

Based on their work, we devised a portable, noninvasive (the wound is not touched) electronic device which could instantaneously measure the spectral characteristics of red, green, and infrared light reflected from the burn.[45] The burn depth indicator (BDI) was essentially 100% accurate for shallow and full-thickness wounds. For intermediate wounds, using the endpoint of wound healing as less than or more than 3 weeks, clinical assessments by two experienced surgeons were compared to readings from the device. In about one-third of cases the surgeons were unwilling to commit themselves to a prediction. In the cases where the surgeons were willing to make a prediction, they were incor-

rect about 25% of the time. The BDI was significantly more accurate than the clinical assessment in those predicted not to heal by the surgeons and maintained an accuracy of 79% in the wounds where the surgeons would not make a prediction. Of importance, and not usually addressed in many other studies, are the dynamic qualities of the burn wound. The light reflectance device clearly showed changes each day for the first 3–4 days, and its accuracy, like that of the surgeons, was best on day 3.

We have extended our studies with light reflectance[46,47] and now can produce real-time false-colored television and Polaroid pictures of the wound, providing green-colored wounds which will certainly heal, yellow-colored wounds if unlikely to heal in 3 weeks, and red-colored wounds which will definitely not heal in 3 weeks. Recently Eisenbeiss *et al.* presented a similar noninvasive imaging method for objective determination of the depth of burn wounds. The authors' method is easy to use and enables even the nonspecialized physician to determine the burn depth at a very early time and to make available an objective documentation for quality management. Practicality remains to be seen.[48]

Magnetic Resonance Imaging

Full-thickness burns result in slower resorption of wound edema than partial-thickness burns. Since proton magnetic resonance imaging (MRI) parameters correlate with tissue water content, Koruda[49] determined whether proton MRI could distinguish them. Early after burning the MRI could distinguish higher water content in partial- and full-thickness rat burns than in adjacent normal skin. By 48 hours the partial-thickness burn had returned to control values, while the full-thickness burn remained edematous. Unfortunately the rat skin had to be excised in order to use the MRI, so useful clinical application is still some time away.

Summary

Based on this review of widely differing techniques, it becomes apparent that precise determination of burn depth awaits further refinement of instrumentation, and clinical assessment remains the not-so-golden standard. In addition to the appearance of the wound, other factors can help determine the need for operation. These factors are discussed below and include the type of burn, the age of the patient, and the circumstances surrounding the injury.

Scalds

In civilian practice, scalds, usually due to hot water, are the most common cause of burns. Despite educational programs, the epidemiology and incidence of scalds worldwide changes very little.[50-57] Water at 140°F (60°C) will create a deep dermal or full-thickness burn in 3 seconds, and at 156°F (68.8°C) the same burn will occur in 1 second.[58] Freshly brewed coffee from an automatic percolator is generally about 180°F (82.2°C). Boiling water always causes deep burns; soups and sauces, which are thicker in consistency and remain in contact longer with the skin, invariably cause deep burns. In general, exposed areas tend to be burned less deeply than areas covered with clothing. Clothing retains the heat and keeps the liquid in contact with the skin for a longer period of time. As a result scalds are generally a mosaic of superficial and indeterminate dermal burns.[59] Therefore, unless the burns are obviously deep, we treat them nonoperatively for 10–14 days and then excise areas which will be unlikely to heal within the 3-week window.

The wisdom of this plan was confirmed by Desai[60] who randomized children with scald burns to early (within 72 hours) versus late excision (waiting 2 weeks), showing that early operation required considerably more blood replacement without any clinical benefit.

Immersion scalds are deep and serious burns.[61–64] Although the water may not be as hot as with a spill scald, the duration of contact is usually longer and these burns frequently occur in small children or in elderly or infirm patients with thin skin. For this reason, many States have initiated legislation to set home and public hot water heaters to maximum temperatures below 130°F (54.4°C).[65]

Intentional scalds and head injuries are the most common forms of reported child abuse,[66–70] and in our burn center, deliberate scalds occur in about 2% of all the children admitted. Detailed descriptions of this tragic consequence are available elsewhere in this book, but the physician must be alert that the history provided matches the distribution and probable cause of the burn. Such burns are usually deep, and many will require excision and grafting. Although water temperature may not be as high as a spill scald, the duration of the burn is considerably longer. Deliberate scalds have also been reported as a form of female-to-male assault.[71,72]

Scald burns from grease or hot oil are generally deep dermal or full-thickness. Cooking oil and grease, when hot enough to use for cooking, may be in the range of 350°F (176.7°C). Often the victim tries to carry a burning pot of grease out of doors and douses himself. In this circumstance, the grease is at about 400°F (204.4°C), and the burns are invariably suitable for early excision and grafting.[73,74]

Tar and asphalt burns are a special kind of scald. The 'mother pot' at the back of the roofing truck maintains tar at a temperature of 400–500°F (204–260°C). Burns caused by tar directly from the 'mother pot' are invariably full-thickness. By the time the tar is spread on the roof, its temperature has diminished to the point where most of the burns are deep dermal in nature.[75–77] Unfortunately, initial evaluation is difficult because of the adherent tar.[78] Tar can be removed by application of a petroleum-base ointment under a dressing. The dressing is changed and the ointment reapplied every 2–4 hours until the tar has dissolved. Only then can the extent of the injury and the depth of the burn be accurately estimated. Most tar burns are suitable for early excision and grafting.

Flame burns

Flame burns are the next most common injuries seen. Although the incidence of injuries from house fires has decreased with the advent of smoke detectors, careless smoking, improper use of flammable liquids, automobile accidents, and clothing ignited from stoves or space heaters still exact their toll. In one study of several burn centers, 28% of flame burns occurred in patients with high blood ethanol levels, and 51% of victims in fires behaved inappropriately when trying to escape.[79] Patients whose bedding or clothes have been on fire rarely escape without some full-thickness burns.

Flash burns

Flash burns are next in frequency. Explosions of natural gas, propane, gasoline, and other flammable liquids cause intense heat for a very brief time. For the most part, clothing, unless it ignites, is protective in flash burns, and flash burns generally have a distribution involving all exposed skin, with the deepest areas facing the source of ignition. For the most part, flash burns are dermal in depth, being superficial or deep in proportion to the amount and kind of fuel that explodes. While such burns will generally heal without extensive skin grafting, they may be very large in extent and may be associated with significant thermal damage to the upper airway.

Contact burns

Contact burns result from hot metals, plastic, glass, or hot coals. Such burns are usually limited in extent but are invariably very deep. Contact burns, especially in patients who were unconscious at the time of injury, or in patients dealing with molten materials, are frequently fourth degree. It is common for patients involved in industrial accidents to have both severe contact burns and crush injuries since these accidents commonly occur from presses or from hot, heavy objects. The increased use of wood-burning stoves with surface temperatures hot enough to ignite paper or wood brings an increasing number of toddlers with deep palm burns, as the toddler trips and falls with hands outstretched against the stove.[80] Left alone, such burns heal from the edges with contracture of the palm leading to permanent disability. An aggressive approach with excision and grafting using thick split-thickness grafts[80] or full-thickness grafts[81] is warranted. Particularly vexing are contact burns following motor vehicle accidents where the patient is trapped against a muffler or engine block. Such burns are often fourth degree, and may well require acute flap coverage.[82]

Electrical burns

Electrical burns are in reality thermal burns from very high intensity heat and from explosion of cell membranes.[83] Electricity as it meets the resistance of body tissues is converted to heat in direct proportion to the amperage of the current and the electrical resistance of the body parts through which it passes.[84] The smaller the size of the body parts through which the electricity passes, the more intense the heat and the less the heat is dissipated. Therefore, fingers, hands, forearms, feet, and lower legs are frequently totally destroyed, whereas larger volume areas, like the trunk, usually dissipate enough current to prevent extensive damage to viscera unless the entrance or exit wound is on the abdomen or chest.[85–87] Arc electrical burns are common in addition to the usual entrance and exit wounds. These occur when current takes the most direct path, rather than a longer path of seeming less resistance. These deep and destructive wounds occur at joints which are in close apposition at the time of injury. Most common are burns of the volar aspect of the wrist, the antecubital fossa when the elbow is flexed, and the axilla if the shoulder is adducted as current passes from upper extremity to trunk. While cutaneous manifestations of electrical burns may appear limited, the skin injury is only the tip of the iceberg; massive underlying tissue destruction may take place.

There are two reasons for early operation in the patient with electrical burns. Massive deep tissue necrosis may lead to acidosis or myoglobinuria which will not clear with standard resuscitation techniques. In this unusual circumstance, major debridement and amputations may be needed urgently. Far more commonly, the deep tissues undergo swelling and the risk of compartment syndrome further compromising damaged tissue is real. Careful monitoring is mandatory, and escharotomies and fasciotomies should be performed at the slightest suggestion of progression.[88] Any progression of median or ulnar nerve deficit in the electrically injured hand is an indication for immediate median and ulnar nerve release at the wrist. The use of a technetium scan to help identify damaged and necrotic muscle has been advocated,[89,90] but has not achieved widespread use. In our experience, they have been overly sensitive in detecting damage to deep, unexposed muscle groups which, left alone, will fibrose and not require excision.

If immediate decompression or debridement is not required, we feel that definitive operations can be done between days 3 and 5, before bacterial contamination occurs and after the tissue necrosis is delineated. Extraordinary measures, such as vascular grafts[91,92] to replace clotted arteries, and emergent free flaps[93,94] may sometimes be indicated, but the surgeon is cautioned that they may actually increase morbidity and prolong the patient's recovery when one of the newer prostheses might give better function than a hand or foot with poor sensation and motor function.

Chemical burns

Chemical burns, usually caused by strong acids or alkali, are most often the result of industrial accidents, drain cleaners, assaults, and the improper use of harsh solvents. In contrast to thermal burns, chemical burns cause progressive damage until the chemicals are inactivated by reaction with the tissue or dilution by flushing with water. Although individual circumstances vary, acid burns may be more self-limiting than alkali burns. Acid tends to 'tan' the skin, creating an impermeable barrier which limits further penetration of the acid. Alkalis, on the other hand, combine with cutaneous lipids to create soap and thereby continue 'dissolving' the skin until they are neutralized. A full-thickness chemical burn may appear deceptively superficial, clinically causing only a mild brownish discoloration of the skin. The skin may appear to remain intact during the first few days postburn, and only then begin to slough spontaneously. Unless the observer can be absolutely sure, chemical burns should be considered deep dermal or full-thickness until proven otherwise.

Burns caused by wet cement can be vexing.[95–97] Workers often kneel in wet cement or spill cement inside boots or gloves and do not become symptomatic for some hours. By the time they seek medical help, the wounds are often deep and, in our experience, most often need grafting.

Hydrofluoric acid (HF) burns are potentially very destructive. HF penetrates through the skin and causes deep tissue destruction by combining with cellular calcium.[98,99] HF is widely used in the computer chip industry, in cleaning solvents, and in paint removers. As with cement, the worker may not become symptomatic for several hours after exposure, when severe pain develops, usually of involved fingers. Delayed or inadequate treatment can lead to amputation. Older recommendations of calcium-containing topical gels[100,101] and direct injection of calcium gluconate into the involved tissue have now largely been replaced by intra-arterial perfusion of calcium ions into vessels serving the injured area.[102–105] Such treatment is almost magical, with immediate cessation of pain and minimal tissue destruction.

Burns in the elderly

As people age, their skin atrophies with thinning of the dermis and disappearance of skin appendages.[106] These are some of the many factors which make burn mortality in the geriatric patient disproportionate to the rest of the population with similar burns.[107–110] The thin skin also makes the diagnosis of burn depth difficult, although the best rule of thumb is to assume that there are no shallow burns in the elderly. Survivors with burns larger than 40% TBSA are rare, and modern surgical and intensive care techniques have only marginally influenced mortality in smaller burns.[109–112] The dilemma of nonoperative versus aggressive early operation is not resolved for the elderly population. An aggressive surgical approach[1,113–115] appears to cut down on hospital time, as it does in all patients, but does not appear to have any better survival or function than a conservative approach[116] which emphasizes early discharge and home care for smaller burns.

In the elderly, grafts on fat often do not survive; all donors, even when taken at 0.008 inch are very slow to heal. Our current plan is to excise to fascia full-thickness burns which will not heal from the periphery or by contraction, and to graft them with 2:1 meshed grafts taken at 0.008 inch from the back. Indeterminate burns are generally left to heal or granulate, as outpatients if possible. Occasionally narrow burns can be excised and the skin surgically closed,[117] but closure with any tension invites dehiscence and infection.

Conclusion

Although there are many different types of burn wounds, the extent of tissue destruction is always a function of the temperature of the heat source, the duration of contact, and the thickness of the involved skin. Burns which are unlikely to heal in less than 3 weeks should be treated by early excision and grafting (within 7 days of injury). Benefits of this approach include reduction in length of hospital stay, earlier return to work or school, and optimal functional and cosmetic results. Research is ongoing to determine reliable methods of defining burn depth, so that those patients who need grafting may be treated expeditiously and so that the risks of operation can be avoided in those who do not.

References

1. Deitch E. A policy of early excision and grafting in elderly burn patients shortens the hospital stay and improves survival. *Burns Incl Therml Inj* 1985; **12**: 109–14.
2. Engrav L, Heimbach D, Reus J, Harner T, Marvin JA. Early excision and grafting vs. nonoperative treatment of burns of indeterminant depth: a randomized prospective study. *J Trauma* 1983; **23**: 1001.
3. Frist W, Ackroyd F, Burke J, Bondoc C. Long-term functional results of selective treatment of hand burns. *Am J Surg* 1985; **149**: 516–21.
4. Gray D, Pine R, Harner T. Early excision versus conventional therapy in patients with 20 to 40% burns. *Am J Surg* 1982; **149**: 76.
5. Thompson P, Herndon DN, Abston S, Rutan T. Effect of early excision on patients with major thermal injury. *J Trauma* 1987; **27**: 205–7.
6. Jackson D. Second thoughts on the burn wound. *J Trauma* 1969; **9**: 839.
7. Bajaj SP, Nield DV, Rayment R, Khoo CT. A simple modification of the pinprick test for the assessment of burn depth in children. *Burns Incl Therml Inj* 1988; **14**: 468–72.
8. Hlava P, Moserov AJ, Konigov AR. Validity of clinical assessment of the depth of a thermal injury. *Acta Chir Plast* 1983; **25**: 202–8.
9. Sevitt S. *Burns Pathology and Therapeutic Applications.* London: Butterworth, 1910: 57.
10. Jackson D. The diagnosis of the depth of burning. *Br J Surg* 1953; **40**: 588–96.
11. Ho-Asjoe M, *et al.* Immunohistochemical analysis of burn depth. *J Burn Care Rehabil* 1999; **20(3)**: 207–11.

12. Moserová J, Hlava P, Malinsky J. Scope for ultrasound diagnosis of the depth of thermal damage. Preliminary report. *Acta Chir Plast* 1982; 24: 235–42.

13. Cantrell JH. Can ultrasound assist an experienced surgeon in estimating burn depth? *J Trauma* 1984; 24: S64–70.

14. Brink JA, Sheets PW, Dines KA. Quantitative assessment of burn injury in porcine skin with high-frequency ultrasonic imaging. *Invest Radiol* 1986; 21: 645–51.

15. Wachtel TL, Leopold GR, Frank HA, Frank DH. B-mode ultrasonic echo determination of depth of thermal injury. *Burns Incl Therml Inj* 1986; 12: 432–7.

16. Zawacki B. Reversal of capillary stasis and prevention of necrosis in burns. *Ann Surg* 1974; 180: 98.

17. Robson MC, Heggers JP. The effect of prostaglandins on the dermal microcirculation after burning, and the inhibition of the effect by specific pharmacological agents. *Plast Reconstr Surg* 1979; 63: 781.

18. Kaufman T, Hurwitz D, Heggers JP. The india ink injection technique to assess the depth of experimental burn wounds. *Burns* 1984; 10: 405.

19. Davies M, Adendorff D, Rode H, van de Reit IS. Colouring the damaged tissues on the burn wound surface. *Burns* 1980; 6: 156.

20. Zawacki BE, Walker HL. An evaluation of patent blue V, brophenol blue and tetracycline for the diagnosis of burn depth. *Plast Reconstr Surg* 1970; 54: 459–65.

21. Silverman D, LaRossa D, Barlow C. Quantification of tissue fluorescein delivery and prediction of flap viability with the fiberoptic dermofluorometer. *Plast Reconstr Surg* 1980; 66: 545.

22. Silverman D, Norton K, Brousseau D. Serial fluorometric documentation of fluorescein dye delivery. *Surgery* 1985; 97: 185.

23. Hurford WE, Silverman DG. Evaluation of ischemic extremities by quantitative fluorescence assessment. *Surg Forum* 1982; 323: 442–3.

24. Dingwall JA. A clinical test for differentiating second from third degree burns. *Ann Surg* 1943; 118: 427–9.

25. Gatti J, LaRossa D, Silverman D, Hartford C. Evaluation of the burn wound with perfusion fluorometry. *J Trauma* 1983; 23: 202–6.

26. Grossman A, Zuckerman A. Intravenous fluorescein photography in burns. *J Burn Care Rehabil* 1984; 5: 65.

27. Zuckerman A. Fluorescein fluorescence photography for the evaluation of burns. *J Biol Photogr* 1983; 51: 33–5.

28. Black KS, Hewitt CW, Miller DM. Burn depth evaluation with fluorometry: is it really definitive? *J Burn Care Rehabil* 1986; 7: 313–17.

29. Schomacker KT, *et al.* Biodistribution of indocyanine green in a porcine burn model: light and fluorescence microscopy. *J Trauma* 1997; 43(5): 813–19.

30. Jerath MR, *et al.* Burn wound assessment in porcine skin using indocyanine green fluorescence. *J Trauma* 1999; 46(6): 1085–8.

31. Alsbjørn B, Micheels J, Sørensen B. Laser Doppler flowmetry measurements of superficial dermal, deep dermal and subdermal burns. *Scand J Plast Recon Surg* 1984; 18: 75–9.

32. Green M, Holloway GA, Heimbach DM. Laser Doppler monitoring of microcirculatory changes in acute burn wounds. *J Burn Care Rehabil* 1988; 9: 57–62.

33. O'Reilly TJ, Spence RJ, Taylor RM, Scheulen JJ. Laser Doppler flowmetry evaluation of burn wound depth. *J Burn Care Rehabil* 1989; 50: 1–60.

34. Park DH, *et al.* Use of laser Doppler flowmetry for estimation of the depth of burns. *Plast Reconstr Surg* 1998; 101(6): 1516–23.

35. Yeong EK, *et al.* Improved accuracy of burn wound assessment using laser Doppler. *J Trauma* 1996; 40(6): 956–61.

36. Watson AC, Vasilescu CT. Thermography in plastic surgery. *J R Coll Surg Edinb* 1972; 17: 247.

37. Hackett MEJ. The use of thermography in the assessment of depth of burn and blood supply of flaps, with preliminary reports on its use in Dupuytren's contracture and treatment of varicose ulcer. *Br J Plas Surg* 1974; 27: 311.

38. Mason B, Graff A, Pegg S. Colour thermography in the diagnosis of the depth of burn injury. *Burns* 1981; 7: 197.

39. Henane R, Bittel J, Banssilon V. Partitional calorimetry measurements of energy exchanges in severely burned patients. *Burns* 1981; 7: 180.

40. Cole R, Jones S, Shakespeare P. Thermographic assessment of hand burns. *Burns* 1990; 16: 60–3.

41. Cole R, Shakespeare P, Chissell H, Jones S. Thermographic assessment of burns using a nonpermeable membrane as wound covering. *Burns* 1991; 17: 117–22.

42. Liddington MI, Shakespeare PG. Timing of the thermographic assessment of burns. *Burns* 1996; 22(1): 26–8.

43. Anselmo VJ, Zawacki BE. Infrared photography as a diagnostic tool for the burn ward. *Proc Soc Photo-optical Instr Engrs* 1973; 8: 181.

44. Anselmo VJ, Zawacki BE. Multispectral photographic analysis – a new quantitative tool to assist in the early diagnosis of thermal burn injury. *Ann Biomed Eng* 1977: 179–83.

45. Heimbach D, Afromowitz M, Engrav L. Burn depth estimation – man or machine. *J Trauma* 1984; 24: 373.

46. Afromowitz MA, Van LGS, Heimbach DM. Clinical evaluation of burn injuries using an optical reflectance technique. *IEEE Trans Biomed Eng* 1987; 34: 114–27.

47. Afromowitz MA, Callis JB, Heimbach DM, DeSoto LA, Norton MK. Multispectral imaging of burn wounds: a new clinical instrument for evaluating burn depth. *IEEE Trans Biomed Eng* 1988; 35: 842–50.

48. Eisenbeiss W, Marotz J, Schrade JP. Reflection-optical multispectral imaging method for objective determination of burn depth. *Burns* 1999; 25(8): 697–704.

49. Koruda MJ, Zimbler A, Settle RG. Assessing burn wound depth using in vitro nuclear magnetic resonance (NMR). *J Surg Res* 1986; 40: 475–81.

50. Cason C. A study of scalds in Birmingham. *J R Soc Med* 1990; 83: 690–2.

51. Fallat ME, Rengers SJ. The effect of education and safety devices on scald burn prevention. *J Trauma* 1993; 34: 560–3.

52. Chen T, Yang J, Tsai Y, Noordhoff M. Pediatric burns – 2 year survey of cases admitted to the Chang Gung Memorial Hospital. *Chang Keng I Hsueh* 1989; 12: 45–50.

53. Langley J, Dodge J, Silva P. Scalds to preschool children. *NZ Med J* 1981; 93: 84–7.

54. Lindblad B, Terkelsen C. Scalding accidents among children – an epidemiologic study. *Ugeskr Laeger* 1990; 152: 1590–1.

55. Langley J, Tobin P. Childhood burns. *NZ Med J* 1983; 96: 681–4.

56. Raine P, Azmy A. A review of thermal injuries in young children. *J Pediatr Surg* 1983; 18: 21–6.

57. Tejerina C, Reig A, Codina A. An epidemiological study of burn patients hospitalized in Valencia, Spain during 1989. *Burns* 18: 15–18.

58. Moritz A, Henriques F. Studies of thermal injury II. The relative importance of time and surface temperature in the causation of cutaneous burns. *Am J Pathol* 1947; 23: 695.

59. Irei M, Baston S, Bonds E. The optimal time for excision of scald burns in toddlers. *J Burn Care Rehab* 1986; 7: 508–10.

60. Desai MH, Rutan RL, Herndon DN. Conservative treatment of scald burns is superior to early excision. *J Burn Care Rehabil* 1991; 12: 482.

61. Ding YI, Pu SS, Pan ZL. Extensive scalds following accidental immersion in hot water pools. *Burns Incl Therm Inj* 1987; 13: 305–3.

62. Graitcer PL, Sniezek JE. Hospitalizations due to tap water scalds. *MMWR CDC Surveill Summ* 1987; 37: 35–8.

63. Tennant WG, Davison PM. Bath scalds in children in the south-east of Scotland. *J R Coll Surg Edinb* 1991; 36: 319–22.

64. Walker A. Fatal tapwater scald burn in the USA 1979–1986. *Burns* 1990; 16: 49–52.

65. Erdmann T, Feldman K, Rivara F, Heimbach D, Wall H. Tap water burn prevention: the effect of legislation. *Pediatrics* 1991; 88: 572–7.

66. Caniano D, Beaver B, Boles E. Child abuse: an update on surgical management in 256 cases. *Ann Surg* 1986; 203: 219–24.

67. Kumar P. Child abuse by thermal injury – a retrospective study. *Burns* 1984; 10: 344.

68. Ledbetter D, Tapper D. Injuries caused by child abuse. *Compr Ther* 1989; 15: 9–13.

69. Renz BM, Sherman R. Child abuse by scalding. *J Med Assoc Ga* 1992; 81: 574–8.

70. Renz BM, Sherman R. Abusive scald burns in infants and children: a prospective study. *Am Surg* 1993; 59: 329–34.

71. Purdue G, Hunt J. Adult assault as a mechanism of burn injury. *Arch Surg* 1990; 125: 268–9.

72. Krob MJ, Johnson A, Jordan MH. Burned-and-battered adults. *J Burn Care Rehabil* 1986; 7: 529–31.

73. Pegg S, Seawright A. Burns due to cooking oils – an increasing hazard. *Burns Incl Therm Inj* 1983; 9: 362–9.

74. Hayes LC, Ward RS, Suffle JR, *et al.* Grease burns at fast-food restaurants. Adolescents at risk. *J Burn Care Rehabil* 1991; 12: 203–8.

75. Wachtel TL, Frank HA, Shabbazz A. Scalds from molten tar: an industrial hazard. *J Burn Care Rehabil* 1988; 9: 218–19.

76. Hill M, Achauer B, Martinez S. Tar and asphalt burns. *J Burn Care Rehabil* 1984; 5: 271.

77. Demling R, Buerstatte W, Perea A. Management of hot tar burns. *J Trauma* 1980; 20: 242.

78. James N, Moss A. Review of burns caused by bitumen and the problems of its removal. *Burns* 1990; 16: 214–16.

79. Byrom R, Word E, Tewksbury C, Edlich R. Epidemiology of flame burn injuries. *Burns Incl Therm Inj* 1984; 11: 1–10.

80. Yanofsky N. Upper extremity burns from wood stoves. *Pediatrics* 1984; 73: 722–6.

81. Merrell S, Saffle J, Schnebly A. Full-thickness skin grafting for contact burns of the palm in children. *J Burn Care Rehabil* 1986; 7: 501–7.

82. Gibran NS, Engrav LH, Heimbach DM, Swiontkowski MF, Foy HM. Engine block burns: Dupuytren's 4th, 5th and 6th burns. *J Trauma* 1994; 37(2): 176–81.

83. Lee RC, Kolodney MS. Electrical injury mechanisms: electrical breakdown of cell membranes. *Plast Reconstr Surg* 1987; **80**: 672–9.

84. Sances A, Myklebust J, Larson S. Experimental electrical injury studies. *J Trauma* 1981; **21**: 589.

85. Xue-Wei W. Successful treatment of a case of electrical burn of the abdomen complicated with intestinal perforation. *Burns* 1981; **8**: 28.

86. Yang J, Tasi YC, Noordhoff MS. Electrical burn with visceral injury. *Burns* 1985; **11**: 207.

87. Zhu ZX, Yu DC, Wang Y, Zhao L. Successful treatment of a severe electrical injury involving the stomach. *Burns* 1993; **19**: 80–2.

88. Edlich R, Rodeheaver G, Halfacre S. Technical consideration for fasciotomies in high voltage electrical injuries. *J Burn Care Rehabil* 1980; **1**: 22.

89. Holliman C, Saffle J, Kravitz M, Warden G. Early surgical decompression in the management of electrical injuries. *Am J Surg* 1982; **144**: 733.

90. Hunt J, Lewis S, Parkey R, Baxter C. The use of technetium-99m stannous pyrophosphate scintigraphy to identify muscle damage in acute electric burns. *J Trauma* 1979; **19**: 409.

91. Bartle EJ, Wang XW, Miller GJ. Early vascular grafting to prevent upper extremity necrosis after electrical burns: anastomotic false aneurysm, a severe complication. *Burns Incl Therm Inj* 1987; **13**: 313–17.

92. Wang XW, Bartle EJ, Roberts BB. Early vascular grafting to prevent upper extremity necroses after electric burns: additional commentary on indications for surgery. *J Burn Care Rehabil* 1987; **8**: 391–4.

93. Wang XW, Barle EJ, Roberts BB, *et al.* Free skin flap transfer in repairing deep electrical burns. *J Burn Care Rehabil* 1987; **8**: 111–14.

94. Yang JY, Noordhoff MS. Early adipofascial flap coverage of deep electrical burn wounds of upper extremities. *Plast Reconstr Surg* 1993; **91**: 819–25.

95. Early S, Simpson R. Caustic burns from contact with wet cement. *JAMA* 1985; **254**: 528–9.

96. Feldberg L, Regan PJ, Roberts AH. Cement burns and their treatment. *Burns* 1992; **18**: 51–3.

97. Peters W. Alkali burns from wet cement. *Can Med Assoc J* 1984; **130**: 902–4.

98. Bertolini JC. Hydrofluoric acid: a review of toxicity. *J Emerg Med* 1992; **10**: 163–8.

99. Anderson WJ, Anderson JR. Hydrofluoric acid burns of the hand: mechanism of injury and treatment. *J Hand Surg* 1988; **13**: 52–7.

100. Bracken W, Cuppage F, McLaury R, Kirwin C, Klaassen C. Comparative effectiveness of topical treatments for hydrofluoric acid burns. *J Occup Med* 1985; **27**: 733–9.

101. Chick L, Borah G. Calcium carbonate gel therapy for hydrofluoric acid burns of the hand. *Plast Reconstr Surg* 1990; **86**: 935–40.

102. Siegel DC, Heard JM. Intra-arterial calcium infusion for hydrofluoric acid burns. *Aviat Space Environ Med* 1992; **63**: 206–22.

103. Vance MV, Curry SC, Kunkel DB, Ryan PJ, Ruggeri SR. Digital hydrofluoric acid burns: treatment with intraarterial calcium infusion. *Ann Emerg Med* 1986; **15**: 890–6.

104. Velvart J. Arterial perfusion for hydrofluoric acid burns. *Hum Toxicol* 1983; **2**: 233–8.

105. Pegg S, Siu S, Gillett G. Intra-arterial infusions in the treatment of hydrofluoric acid burns. *Burns Incl Therm Inj* 1985; **11**: 440–3.

106. Gilchrest BA. Age-associated changes in the skin. *J Am Geriat Soc* 1982; **20**: 139–42.

107. Ostrow LB, Bongard FS, Sacks ST, McGuire A, Trunkey DD. Burns in the elderly. *Am Fam Physician* 1987; **35**: 149–54.

108. Saffle J, Larson C, Sullivan J, Shelby J. The continuing challenge of burn care in the elderly. *Surgery* 1990; **108**: 534–43.

109. Tejerina C, Reig A, Codina J, Safont J, Mirabet V. Burns in patients over 60 years old: epidemiology and mortality. *Burns* 1992; **18**: 149–52.

110. Zoch G, Meissl G, Bayer S, Kyral E. Reduction of the mortality rate in aged burn patients. *Burns* 1992; **18**: 153–6.

111. Anous MM, Heimbach DM. Causes of death and predictors in burned patients more than 60 years of age. *J Trauma* 1986; **26**: 135–9.

112. Li B, Hsu W, Shih T. Causes of death in aged burn patients: analysis of 36 cases. *Burns* 1990; **16**: 207–10.

113. Tompkins R, Burke J, Schoenfeld D. Prompt eschar excision: a treatment system contributing to reduced burn mortality. *Ann Surg* 1986; **204**: 272–81.

114. Deitch E, Clothier J. Burns in the elderly: an early surgical approach. *J Trauma* 1983; **23**: 891–4.

115. Kara M, Peters WJ, Douglas L, Morris S. An early surgical approach to burns in the elderly. *J Trauma* 1990; **30**: 430–2.

116. Housinger T, Saffle J, Ward S, Warden G. Conservative approach to the elderly patient with burns. *Am J Surg* 1984; **148**: 817–20.

117. Ikeda J, Sugamata A, Jimbo, Yukioka T, Makino K. A new surgical procedure for aged burn victims: applications of dermolipectomy for burn wounds and donor sites. *J Burn Care Rehabil* 1990; **11**: 27–31.

Chapter 10

Wound care
William W Monafo
Palmer Q Bessey

After a burne the scarre which remaineth is uncommonly rough, unequall and ill-favored.

(Ambrose Paré, 1510–1590)

Introduction

Wound care comprises but one of the many burn care components, as the size of this volume attests but it is arguably the most pivotal one. The management of extensive burn wounds is one of the last areas in modem surgical practice that still relies heavily on uncontrolled clinical observations or anecdotal personal experience. There are innumerable procedural details which, alone or in specific combination or order, may be important or not and may either help or hinder, but which must – and sooner rather than later – result in permanent wound closure. It is of course impossible to communicate these details fully or in precise chronological sequence even were space unlimited. What follows is thus necessarily incomplete; it is meant, however, to communicate the essentials of burn wound care, at least from a single viewpoint. Major reasonable alternatives are noted as the treatment algorithm unfolds during the days or weeks (not months, any longer!) of acute phase convalescence that ends with wound closure. Subsequently, rehabilitation and recovery or maintenance of function become the focus of care.

When possible, the biological basis or the perceived, evidence-based rationale of a particular method or procedure is given in the hope it will accomplish more than did the unhelpful response of a prominent burn surgeon who, when asked why he was proceeding so would reply 'because its the best way we have'.

Cutaneous wound healing

It is axiomatic that intelligent wound management is not possible unless it is guided by the relevant biology of wound healing, a subject presently in a phenomenal growth phase at the molecular and biochemical level. A brief commentary on cutaneous wound healing is therefore in order.

Dermal (Partial-Thickness or Second Degree) Burns

The epidermis provides an important physical barrier to environmental microorganisms; its lipid components constitute another, if imperfect barrier – this to the loss of water vapor. Epidermal cells lining the skin appendages and at the perimeter of a wound provide the reservoir from which reepithelization occurs. The skin appendages are sparser in the deeper, reticular dermal zone than in the superficial papillary zone. So-called deep dermal burns or scalds that extend down into the reticular dermis therefore require longer to reepitheliaze – 21 days or more by clinical convention.

Hypertrophic scar and contractures that limit function are common sequelae of deep dermal burns. A useful clinical rule of thumb is that the longer the reepithelization time of dermal burns the worse the functional and/or cosmetic result. **Table 10.1** lists some of the characteristics of superficial versus deep dermal burns.

As healing occurs, complex interactions, mediated in part by various cytokines, peptide growth factors, and proteases, take place between activated epidermal cells and the subjacent dermal matrix and its population of fibroblasts, inflammatory, and endothelial cells.[1] As these interactions become more fully understood, pharmacological, or even gene therapy, which accelerates epithelialization will likely become widely available. In a clinical trial, a 10% reduction in 'healing time' (i.e. reepithelialization) resulted after topical application of epidermal growth factor (EGF) to split-skin graft donor sites.[2] Experimentally, gene transfer of EGF accelerates wound repair.[3] Therapy with human growth hormone in severely burned children has been shown to speed donor site closure, probably by its effect on increasing levels of insulin-like growth factor-1 (IGF-1).[4] The modulation of wound repair by nutritional, metabolic, or pharmacological therapy is discussed in detail elsewhere in this volume (Chapter 21).

Full-Thickness Burns (Subdermal or Third Degree Burns)

Full-thickness burns require a surgical procedure for closure unless they are of limited area and can reasonably be allowed to close by a combination of wound contraction and reepithelialization. The necrotic soft tissue layer ('eschar') which forms varies in thickness depending on the burn depth but may extend into the subcutaneous fat or beyond. Wound closure cannot occur while eschar remains *in situ*. Spontaneous eschar separation is due primarily to the action of bacterial proteases and therefore does not occur in sterile full-thickness burns; full-thickness burn eschars in gnotobiotic rodents remained in place for 8 months or more![5] Clinically, eschar separation is delayed in proportion to the efficacy of the wound antiseptic measures employed.[6] The thinner eschar that forms over deep dermal burns will, however, separate spontaneously even in the absence of microorganisms as reepithelialization proceeds beneath it.

Wound Contraction

Deep wounds that remain open for several weeks are seen to progressively decrease in surface area, provided infection is absent and nutrition is reasonably maintained. This phenomenon is termed 'wound contraction' and appears to be due to contractile forces generated in the wound bed – possibly by differentiated fibroblasts containing contractile protein, the so-called 'myofibroblasts', a phenotype that can be induced by transforming growth factor-β-1.[7] Epithelial ingrowth from the wound perimeter in full-thickness burns typically contributes minimally (10% or less) to the area decrease.

Contraction is of course desirable in one sense because as it proceeds both the risk of infection and the metabolic drain which results from the wound losses of water vapor and body fluids decrease.[8] From a functional or cosmetic standpoint, however, wound contraction near important joints, the eyelids, or mouth is clearly highly undesirable and to be avoided. Some factors that can alter the rate of wound contraction are schematically depicted in **Figure 10.1**. As shown, successful split-thickness skin grafts will slow contraction, while full-thickness ones essentially abolish it. The clinical reality is, however, that split-thickness grafts are necessary to attain coverage in extensive burns because their donor sites reepithelialize in 10–14 days, can be re-cropped, and do not require surgical closure. Small full-thickness grafts may be necessary during acute phase care on the eyelids and periorbitally to prevent or correct severe ectropion or on deep palmar burns in infants.[9]

Hypertrophic scar burns are the prototypical cause of hypertrophic scar, a phenomenon unique to man; this lack of a simple animal experimental model explains the slowness of progress in the understanding of its biological basis. Hypertrophic scar occurs regularly after injury to the reticular dermis, but with a severity that is highly variable and unpredictable. The most widely used therapy for these scars is the near-continuous wearing of elastic compression garments, as discussed elsewhere in this volume; a comparatively rapid therapeutic response in some patients to topical silicone gel sheeting has also been observed.[10]

From the point of view of acute wound care, however, it is important to note that hypertrophic scar infrequently forms beneath split-thickness skin grafts applied in sheets; although it regularly forms in deep dermal burns that are allowed to close

Table 10.1 Clinical characteristics of superficial dermal and deep dermal burns		
	Superficial	Deep
Blisters	Yes	Yes
Anatomical depth	Papillary dermis	Reticular dermis
Early analgesia	No	Yes
Color	Pink	Ivory, white, mottled
Capillary refill	Yes	No
Reepithelialization time	<21 days	>21 days
Hypertrophic scar	Rare	Frequent
Wound contraction	Minimal	Potentially significant

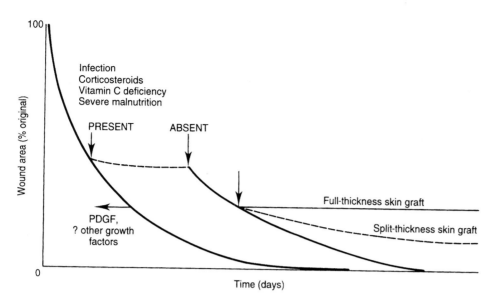

Fig. 10.1 A schematic representation of wound contraction showing the effects of infection, severe malnutrition, and other factors which impede spontaneous decrease in wound surface area. As shown, split-thickness grafts impede but do not prevent subsequent wound contraction, while full-thickness grafts essentially abolish it.

spontaneously, at the perimeter of sheet grafts and in the interstices of the widely used expanded meshed grafts (**Plate 1a, b**). The mesh graft technique, although it speeds wound coverage, yields even more unsatisfactory cosmetic results than sheet grafts – which themselves are less than ideal because of their poor color match and the halo of hypertrophic scar that may frame them.

Wound care

Initial Assessment: an Individualized Care Plan is Essential

The clinical assessment of burn depth frequently changes during the first post-injury week. This has particular significance if near-immediate surgical wound closure is planned. Whether an apparent increase in depth is due to an inevitable, progressive occlusion of the circulation in the 'zone of stasis' at the wound periphery where endothelial injury has occurred, or to the compression of the dermal vessels by the edema attending injury and/or resuscitation, or whether it simply represents the ±30% inaccuracy of most clinical observations cannot be determined in an individual instance. Conversely, superficial dermal burns, especially those on the dorsum of the hands, are frequently misdiagnosed initially as deep dermal, which can lead to unnecessary surgery.

The clinician should formulate an appropriate, individualized care plan within the first hours or days postburn that includes an achievable timetable for wound closure. The plan must include which if any burns are to be treated surgically, if so in what sequence and using which donor sites. In the interim preceding wound closure, a protocol of daily wound care – based to the extent possible on physiologic principles – is also necessary, as is a team of nurses and other personnel to carry it out. A single set of standard procedures for basic bedside wound care is highly desirable, as multiple methods typically lead to confusion and anxiety among nursing personnel and can be important factors in staff turnover. Attending surgeons should agree upon the essentials of their protocol and ensure that the rationale of its components is clearly understood by all team members. When variance becomes necessary, team members need to be informed of the reasons for change.

The Bandage

A burn dressing has three principal functions:

- *Protective.* When skin is thermally injured the physical barrier of the epidermis to microorganisms is lost, as well as its mild antiseptic property. The result is that the environmental flora proliferates readily on the wound surface. In small burns, an effective dressing can isolate the wound so that few if any organisms are ever recoverable. As the wound area increases, however, the efficacy of a dressing's barrier function decreases.
- *Metabolic.* An occlusive dressing reduces evaporative heat loss and minimizes cold stress and shivering. Because the principal cutaneous water vapor barrier resides in the epidermis, even superficial burns result in water vapor loss (with its attendant caloric requirement of 0.58 Cal./Kg water lost).[8] Intact eschar provides only a partial impediment, while excised or granulating wounds lose water vapor maximally.[11] Evaporative loss from exposed burns may be several-fold higher than the 'normal' 150 ml/24 hours; and the air currents generated by air-fluidized beds may increase the evaporative loss by much as 10-fold and thus impose a large caloric demand and fluid replacement requirement. An occlusive dressing (usually of cotton gauze) of reasonable thickness will impede water vapor loss appreciably, particularly if it is in turn kept covered with a dry blanket. Biological dressings such as cadaver allograft and an ever-increasing number of commercially available (and expensive) synthetic dressings and bioengineered skin substitutes can also minimize the loss; but their cost-effectiveness and efficacy are debatable, especially in major burns. Minimizing the nutritional demand is vital in the supportive care of patients with major burns, as discussed in detail elsewhere in this volume.
- *Comfort.* Superficial burns are initially extraordinarily sensitive to air currents; and deeper burns become progressively more tender with time as nerves reinnervate

them. Open wounds drain. A bandage eliminates air currents from the wound surface, absorbs and contains wound secretions that would otherwise soil bed linen, etc., and if properly constructed may also provide splinting action to help maintain a desirable position of function.

Dressing Materials

A convenient, satisfactory dressing which can be rapidly applied consists of rolls of 36-layer, loose-weave cotton gauze 9 inches in width, pre-cut into 5-foot lengths (Hermitage Hospital Products, Niantic, CT). For small limbs, rolls of the same material 4.5 inches in width are convenient. These dressings are in turn held in place with a spiral bandage of bias-cut stockinette, usually 6 inches in width, which is also pre-cut and rolled. The dressings and stockinette are sterilized in packages of 10. For the face, an inner layer of 1-inch vaginal packing is useful for accurately covering the bridge of the nose, the chin, and for padding the ears to prevent pressure necrosis.

Over fresh skin grafts, nonadherent synthetic plastic gauze (Exudry™, Frastec Corp., New York, NY) can be used. This material is available either in rolls over which the aforementioned dressings can be applied, or as a self-contained, prefabricated absorbent pad bonded to an inner, Exudry™ layer. This material adheres minimally to a wound or graft and is available in other configurations as well.

Despite their cost, the physiological (and psychological) benefits of occlusive burn dressings speak persuasively for their routine use. Alternatives such as allograft, xenograft, and biological or other synthetic materials are discussed in detail in Chapters 18 and 20.

Wound Hygiene

The French word *débridement* ('unbridling', i.e. as in escharotomy or fasciotomy) has, in North America at least, come to signify both the formal surgical excision of devitalized tissue (including, but not limited to burns) as well as the simple piecemeal removal of bits and fragments of separating eschar, ruptured bleb fragments, foreign material, etc., during the routine dressing change at the bedside. Burn dressings are typically replaced daily or more frequently, especially if drainage is profuse. The thin eschar that forms over deep dermal burns also tends to separate piecemeal as epithelialization occurs beneath it. Systematic, gentle wound cleansing with removals of bits of slough, exudate, etc., would seem eminently reasonable, although evidence of benefit does not exist to our knowledge. Hopefully this practice is worth the not inconsiderable pain, apprehension, and expense with which it is associated.

Topical antimicrobial agents

General Background

Burn injury not only damages the normal skin barrier but also impairs host immunological defenses. Because the eschar is frequently several centimeters or more distant from patent microvasculature, systemically administered antimicrobial agents may not achieve therapeutic levels by diffusion to the wound surface, where microbial numbers are usually greatest. Topically applied antimicrobials provide high concentrations of drug at the wound surface; they penetrate eschar variably, a property that should be considered in their selection. Normal skin harbors a sparse bacterial flora, consisting mainly of diphtheroids and *Staphylococcus epidermidis* and, occasionally, *S. aureus*.

Gram-negative bacteria are not usually present in normal skin. The burn wound flora changes in the post-injury interval, depending in part on the topical and/or systemic antimicrobial therapy being used and on the efficacy with which cross-contamination is prevented. After a variable initial period (days) when the wound is apparently sterile or contains only normal flora, Gram-positive organisms, mainly *S. aureus*, typically predominate. Subsequently, Gram-negative species appear. In most centers isolates of *Proteus*, *Klebsiella*, *Escherichia coli* and other enteric flora predominate, with *Pseudomonas* species being less frequent.[12,13] Anaerobes are infrequent, but can be encountered when large volumes of necrotic muscle are present, as in high-voltage electrical injury.

The goal of *prophylactic* topical therapy is initially to delay and later to minimize wound colonization.[13] If successful, this will reduce or eliminate the development of invasive wound infections. Prophylactic usage should be differentiated from that aimed at treating established or imminent invasive infection. Prophylactic agents do not need to penetrate the eschar deeply, as environmental fallout is the source of contamination. They should have activity against common wound pathogens as listed above, should not retard wound healing (although some of them do so, to some extent,[14]) and they should have low toxicity, which implies that systemic absorption is low. None of the topical antimicrobials, either alone or in combination, will *eliminate* colonization of major burn wounds. Frequent clinical observation is necessary in order to ensure that basic wound hygienic measures are being satisfactorily carried out, that the frequency of dressing changes is appropriate, and that the clinical appearance of the wounds is satisfactory.

When an established burn wound infection is present, the spectrum of activity of a proposed agent must include the organisms responsible. Concerns about toxicity, patient comfort, cost, and other factors require careful assessment. In most instances, eradication of an invasive infection will require the use of one or more topical agents, which penetrate eschar readily, as by definition microbial invasion of previously normal, unburned tissue exists. Systemic antibiotics of appropriate spectrum are also necessary; in relatively localized infections, sub-eschar antibiotic infusions and/or surgical excision are sometimes efficacious. Invasive burn wound infections with *Staphylococcus* or *Pseudomonas* species have been frequently treated with topical mafenide acetate, which penetrates eschar readily.[15] Other agents may also be of benefit in these potentially lethal infections.[16]

Specific Agents

As already noted, topical therapy in most instances is prophylactic. Frequent clinical inspection is the best method of noting the clinical response. Wound surveillance bacterial culture results require clinical correlation because the distinction between colonization, which is frequent, and invasive infection, which is now uncommon, is partly a clinical one. In general, quantitative wound biopsy cultures, which exceed 100 000 organisms per gram, are consistent with, although not diagnostic of, invasive infection. The microscopic visualization of organisms invading normal tissue in a wound biopsy specimen is diagnostic, but gives no information as to the extent of the infection.[15]

Silver sulfadiazine

Silver sulfadiazine is easily the most frequently used prophylactic agent in burn patients. It is a white, highly insoluble compound that is synthesized from silver nitrate and sodium sulfadiazine.[13,17] It is available in 1% concentration in a water-soluble cream base. The cream is relatively painless to apply and does not stain bed linens or other objects, which it contacts. Silver sulfadiazine has *in vitro* activity against a wide range of organisms including *S. aureus*, *E. coli*, *Klebsiella* species, *Pseudomonas aeruginosa*, *Proteus* species and *Candida albicans*. The drug penetrates eschar poorly. Its precise mechanism of action is unclear.

The toxicity commonly associated with sulfonamides, such as crystalluria and methemoglobinemia, is rare after silver sulfadiazine treatment. The most common toxicity is a transient leukopenia occurring within several days of the initiation of therapy and is associated with a disproportionate decrease in circulating neutrophils; the incidence is from 5 to 15% of patients treated.[18] The leukopenia can reach alarmingly low levels – less than 1000 mm². Despite these observations, no increase in the incidence of infectious complications has been identified. The leukopenia typically recovers spontaneously, whether or not the agent has been discontinued. Although it has been suggested that leukocyte margination in the wound independent of any drug effect might alone explain the leukopenia, more recent data suggest that there is a direct toxic effect on bone marrow.[19] Cutaneous sensitivity reactions, typically in the form of a maculopapular rash, occur in less than 5% of patients and rarely require discontinuing the drug. Acute hemolytic anemia has been reported in a burn patient treated with silver sulfadiazine who lacked the enzyme glucose-6 phosphatase.[20]

Clinical trials have suggested that silver sulfadizine reduces wound bacterial density and delays colonization with Gram-negative bacteria, but treatment failures occur with some frequency in large burns (>40–50% body surface area). The agent is usually applied on a daily or twice-daily basis. When it is used on superficial dermal burns, a yellow-gray 'pseudo eschar' typically forms after several days, which can be confusing to inexperienced personnel. This film, several millimeters thick, results from interaction between the cream and the wound exudate and is harmless; it is easily lifted away, revealing a healthy, superficial wound bed beneath it.

Mafenide acetate

Mafenide was introduced as a topical burn treatment in the mid-1960s. It is available in a water-soluble cream base at 11.1% concentration, and also, more recently, as a 5% solution. It has excellent antibacterial activity against most Gram-positive species, including *Clostridia*, but limited activity against some staphylococci, particularly methicillin-resistant strains. It has a broad activity against most Gram-negative pathogens commonly isolated from burn wounds, but, importantly, has minimal antifungal activity.[21] Early enthusiasm for its prophylactic use was soon tempered because of its systemic toxicity and by the considerable pain that occurs on application. The drug is so rapidly absorbed through open wounds that local concentrations are sharply reduced, requiring usually twice-daily applications.

Mafenide is a potent carbonic anhydrase inhibitor; hyperchloremic metabolic acidosis is frequent when it is used continuously on extensive burns.[22] Moderate to severe hyperventilation as respiratory compensation for the acidosis is characteristic and the

$Paco_2$ is persistently subnormal. Minute ventilation may approach or exceed 50 L/min. Pulmonary complications are a hazard with its continuous use and toxicity increases in frequency to the wound area and treatment duration. A maculopapular rash occurs in about 5% of patients but can usually be controlled with antihistamines and may not require discontinuing the drug. Although the use of mafenide as a prophylactic agent has decreased for the reasons cited, its excellent eschar penetration makes it useful for the short-term control of invasive burn wound infections. In some centers, the drug is still used prophylactically but toxicity is minimized or avoided by alternating it with silver sulfadizine, usually at 12-hour intervals.

0.5% Silver nitrate solution

One-half percent silver nitrate solution was introduced as an effective topical agent in the mid-1960s.[23] Together with the near-simultaneous introduction of topical mafenide, the modern era of topical burn wound therapy had begun. Shortly thereafter, silver sulfadizine was synthesized and would become available; most recently, still another silver preparation, Acticoat™ has appeared. Silver nitrate is effective against most strains of *Staphylococcus* and *Pseudomonas*, and also has activity against many of the Gram-negative aerobes that commonly colonize burn wounds. Concentrations much above 5% are histotoxic. Most biologically important silver salts, especially the chloride and proteinate, are highly insoluble. The agent, or at least the silver moiety, does not therefore penetrate eschar significantly and silver absorption is minimal; although trace amounts have been detected in blood and tissue following protracted application, there is no significant direct toxicity. But the hypotonic solution (29.4 mmol Ag/L) leaches electrolyte, especially sodium from the wound surface. As much as 350 mmol of sodium/day/m² of body surface area treated may be lost. Continuous oral and/or intravenous (IV) electrolyte supplementation is therefore essential. Hyponatremia or hypokalemia may occur rapidly, especially in infants or children with large burns.

The other important, but fortunately infrequent, complication of this agent is methemoglobinemia, which occurs as a result of nitrate reduction by wound bacteria (usually Gram-negative species) with subsequent systemic absorption of the toxic nitrite. The diagnosis should be suspected if the skin or blood appears cyanotic or 'gray' but the arterial oxygen content is normal. Confirmation of the diagnosis by blood methemoglobin measurement should lead to prompt withdrawal of the agent. Additional specific treatment with reducing agents may also be required.

Silver nitrate is relatively painless on application. It is typically used to saturate gauze dressings similar to those described above. The dressings should be rewet with the silver nitrate at 2-hourly intervals to prevent silver concentrations reaching histotoxic levels. The agent stains everything it touches brown or black, including bed linens, floors, etc. Although silver nitrate is an effective prophylactic agent, it is presently not widely used routinely, principally because of its staining property. Its therapeutic effect is approximated by silver sulfadiazine, which is easier to use.

Cerium nitrate–silver sulfadiazine

This agent was introduced in the mid 1970s but is not now commercially available in the US, although it is available in several western European and South American countries.[24,25] It is easily prepared by combining commercially available silver sulfadiazine with a solution of cerium nitrate. Cerium, one of the lanthanide 'rare earth' series of elements has antimicrobial activity *in vitro* and is relatively non-toxic. Wound bacteriostasis may be more efficient with its use in major burns compared to silver sulfadiazine alone.[24] The *in vitro* antimicrobial spectrum of this agent is qualitatively similar to that of silver nitrate or silver sulfadiazine. It has been suggested that the efficacy of the cerium nitrate–silver sulfadiazine combination might be due in part to an effect on immune function. Cell-mediated immunity appears to be relatively preserved in burned rodents treated with topical cerium nitrate alone or in combination with silver sulfadiazine.[26] Others have reported highly favorable mortality data in burn patients who have been briefly immersed in a bath of cerium nitrate shortly after admittance to the hospital; they suggest that improved immune function is responsible for their results.[27] Methemoglobinemia due to nitrate reduction and absorption, as with silver nitrate, is also rarely observed with this agent, the cerium moiety of which is absorbed to a limited extent. Electrolyte disturbances are not associated with the use of cerium nitrate–silver sulfadiazine.

Wasserman *et al.* reported excellent results in patients with massive burns treated with cerium nitrate–silver sulfadiazine cream.[28] That report parallels our own prior experience using the cream in patients with very large, ostensible 'lethal' injuries.[29] Boecks *et al.* also report favorable clinical results, although others are less enthusiastic.[30,31] A randomized, prospective clinical trial in high-risk burn patients comparing the cerium nitrate–silver sulfadiazine combination to silver sulfadiazine alone is currently being organized.[32]

Acticoat

This material, which has recently become available commercially, consists of a sheet of thin, flexible rayon/polyester to which is bonded polyethylene mesh that has been coated with a nanocrystalline film of pure silver.[33] When exposed to body fluids or wound exudate, silver ions are released in an even, sustained manner over at least 24 hours and possibly 48 hours. The antimicrobial spectrum of Acticoat is broad, similar to that of silver nitrate. The silver that ionizes from the plastic sheet may have an atomic structure that differs from conventional silver ions as the result of the 'sputtering' process used to coat the film and may be more bactericidal as a result. Preliminary clinical trials have been promising.[34] The material is relatively painless to apply and can be left in place for 48 hours, or possibly longer; to date, no significant toxicity has been reported.

Nitrofurazone

A water-soluble cream base containing 0.2% nitrofurazone is available. The agent has *in vitro* activity against a number of burn wound pathogens including *Staphylococcus*, but does not have significant activity against *Pseudomonas*. Severe cutaneous allergic reactions may occur. The agent may be useful in the treatment of invasive wound infection caused by *Enterobacter cloacae*.[35]

Chlorhexidine

Chlorhexidine gluconate combined with 0.5% silver nitrate appears to be comparably effective to silver sulfadiazine.[36] A diphosphanilate chlorhexidine conjugate, although having an even broader antimicrobial spectrum, causes troublesome pain on application. Plasmid-mediated resistance does not appear to occur with chlorhexidine, in contrast to the sulfonamides.

Povidone–iodine

This compound is inappropriate for use on major burn wounds, both because of its relative inactivation by wound exudate and because renal dysfunction due to systemic absorption of the iodine moiety is a significant hazard.[37] Rarely, iodine-induced thyroid dysfunction can also occur after topical therapy with this agent.[38]

Nystatin

The topical antifungal nystatin can be used to control candidal growth on burn wounds.[39] Yeast and/or other fungal wound colonization may be related to selection pressures exerted by antibiotic use and/or the use of topical agents ineffective against these organisms such as Sulfamylon. Colonization by *C. albicans* does not appear to increase mortality. Fortunately, invasive fungal infection is uncommon.

Other agents

The topical antibiotic mupirocin may be useful to treat methicillin-resistant staphylococci.[40] Polymyxin B and bacitracin ointments are used occasionally by some on small areas but nephrotoxicity and/or ototoxicity are a hazard with their prolonged use over wide areas.

Combination therapy

The simultaneous use of combinations of topical agents is not unreasonable in selected patients, although in instances, the efficacy of such combinations (mafenide and nystatin, for example) may paradoxically be decreased.[39] The results of *in vitro* sensitivity testing methods such as the agar well procedure in an attempt to determine the optimal topical agent or combination of agents should be cautiously interpreted.[41] The results depend importantly on the solubility in agar of the agents tested rather than, as desired, the true sensitivity of the organism. Silver or cerium compounds, for example, tend to fare poorly in this system due to their poor solubility/diffusivity.

Surgical wound closure

Perspective

During the past 30 years, the treatment of deep burns by experienced burn surgeons has changed dramatically.[42] Previously, nearly all large, deep burns were treated expectantly: eschar was permitted to slough spontaneously and the wounds were left to ultimately granulate before they were skin-grafted. Split-thickness skin grafts were procured and applied in many instances, not in sheets, but using a variety of free-hand techniques and/or the unreliable dermatomes then available. Small patches or 'stamps' of graft, or even smaller 'pinch' grafts were used to maximize epithelial perimeter and, hopefully, minimize graft loss from the heavily contaminated wounds. Weeks or, frequently, months passed before wound closure could be achieved with these methods, even in burns that today would be considered minor or trivial. Survival was all but unprecedented if the burn surface area exceeded more than 40% of the body surface area.

Perceptive surgeons were of course fully cognizant of the many disadvantages associated with such passive, expectant therapy. It was clearly contrary to the fundamental principle in the treatment of other types of wounds which had been learned, nearly forgotten, then relearned during two World Wars: the prompt excision of all devitalized tissue. This axiom clearly seemed applicable to burn treatment, but numerous practical clinical constraints prevented its general application.

In the early post World War II years, surgical therapy was in practice being used only for burns that by modern standards would be considered trivial.[43] In more extensive burns, effective measures for controlling wound microbial growth were lacking and dense wound colonization almost invariably occurred within the first few days and commonly then was the source of invasive infection of normal tissue at the burn margins, systemic sepsis, and death. Physiological monitoring was near nonexistent, whether in the operating room or on the ward; ventilatory support postoperatively consisted primarily of oxygen administration and tracheostomy if necessary. There were few safe, effective antibiotics and the importance of nutritional support was ill-appreciated.

The terrible odors which emanated from the wounds disappeared virtually overnight when effective topical therapy was introduced in the mid-1960s.[6,23] This one advance, more than any other, re-awakened widespread interest by the surgical community in burn care with its many previously unaddressed problems: *pari passu*, many other important advances were occurring, particularly in the area of critical care medicine, which was in the process of becoming its own specialty; an ever-growing menu of potent and relatively safe antibiotics was appearing; precision power dermatomes that made procuring skin grafts of precise thickness and in long sheets an easy matter were available; mesh-expansion techniques of the grafts, which improved take and minimized the requisite donor area were developed;[44] sophisticated continuous physiological monitoring was introduced for use both within and without the operating room and effective mechanical ventilation came into common use; and perhaps most importantly, the incalculable benefit of concentrating severely burned patients in dedicated treatment centers where experienced and interested personnel could interact was generally recognized and widely implemented. These and other factors contributed to the dramatic overall improvement in burn care that has occurred. It is not possible to calculate the individual contribution of those nonsurgical advances to the reduction in burn mortality and morbidity, but we suspect they may be generally underestimated, particularly, perhaps, by enthusiastic surgeons.[45,46]

The Modern Era

An aggressive, earlier and more frequent use of definitive surgical therapy for deep burns has become the norm in the Western world.[47-50] The vastly improved early physiological status of the modern-day patient and the ready availability of in-depth logistic support from many areas of the hospital now permits the excision and skin-grafting by an experienced team of even near-total deep burns in one or more stages without incurring perioperative mortality. What previously had been a frustrating, necessarily hypothetical debate about the virtue of prompt surgical wound treatment has become standard practice. When the deep burns are not life-threatening, early, aggressive surgical wound closure clearly has benefit. *The question remains open, however, as to the timing and extent to which surgical wound closure should be utilized in patients with burns so extensive that survival is problem-atic.* Before discussing the various surgical options, it is useful to briefly outline the most commonly used operative techniques.

Methods of Surgical Wound Closure

General anesthesia is usually required; IV ketamine or inhalational techniques are both useful. Regional anesthesia may occasionally also be suitable, as for limb burns with adjacent available donor skin for graft harvest. We prefer to utilize the main hospital-operating suite because of the rapid availability of personnel and expertise should complications occur intraoperatively. Depending on the magnitude of the wound to be treated, an adequate supply of cross-matched blood must be available. Estimates ranging widely from 172 to 616 ml of blood loss per 1% total body surface area excised have been reported.[51,52] If appreciable blood loss is anticipated, preoperative transfusion with packed red blood cells in order to minimize or avoid intraoperative transfusion should be considered. Succinyl choline administration is contraindicated because it can trigger potentially rapidly lethal hypokalemia. Anesthesia in burn patients is discussed in detail elsewhere in this book.

The operating room ambient temperature should be maintained in the low 90s°F in patients with large burns in order to avoid severe hypothermia, which is a particular hazard in children because of their relatively larger surface area for heat loss. In order to reduce the severity of the intraoperative temperature drift which often occurs despite the high ambient temperature, our practice is to change the dressings shortly preoperatively on those wounds not to be excised or grafted; only the planned donor site and wounds to be treated are exposed intraoperatively. The rate of body temperature recovery to normal postoperatively may correlate with survival, a slow return boding ill.[53]

Primary closure of excised burns or donor sites

Small deep burns on lax skin areas such as the buttock, female breast, or the limbs or torso in the elderly can on occasion be excised and closed primarily, particularly if cosmesis is not an issue. In the elderly also, donor sites harvested from lax skin areas can at times be closed primarily, thus avoiding donor site conversion to full-thickness injury or its delayed epithelialization, two not uncommon complications in the elderly.

Amputation

When a major portion of a limb, hand, or digit has been destroyed, or its potential for functional recovery is judged to be nil, amputation may be appropriate or even life-saving, especially when doing so eliminates the deep burn and the stump can be closed primarily.

Tangential excision

The 'tangential' or so-called 'laminar' method of sequentially shaving the eschar from the wound surface until a viable-tissue plane is reached was popularized in the 1970s.[54,55] It is particularly suitable for the excision of deep dermal or shallow, superficial full-thickness burns. The procedure is usually performed using a hand-held blade equipped with a calibrated depth guard, such as the small Goulian knife or the larger, more cumbersome Humby knife (**Plate 2**). In experienced hands, tangential excision is rapid and permits salvage of viable reticular dermis, although hemorrhage may be considerable. On limbs, a tourniquet probably helps to reduce blood loss, although it makes the differentiation of viable from non-viable tissue more difficult.[56]

Dermatome excision

For broad, relatively flat burn deep burns, a power dermatome such as the Brown, with its depth gauge set appropriately, is convenient for rapidly performing tangential excision on extensive, confluent areas above the wrist or ankle, or on the torso, usually at the level of the subcutaneous fat. The method is also useful in deep dermal injuries, but is not suitable for use on the hand, foot, or face.

Degloving (avulsion)

For deep burns that extend well into the subcutaneous fat and are circumferential, a degloving technique is rapid and highly effective, if aesthetically disturbing. Linear escharotomies placed 180° apart on a limb, and/or at the wound margins otherwise, facilitate the maneuver, which is performed using toothed surgical clamps such as the Kocher to obtain purchase sufficient to permit degloving, which is best terminated at the level of wrist or ankle.

Cold scalpel, electrocautery

Formal excision to any depth with the scalpel and/or the Bovie electrocautery unit, using the latter at either cutting or coagulation settings as necessary, is of course commonly used. Laser methods for wound excision have offered no clear advantages of either speed or hemostasis and necessary safety precautions further complicate their use.

Enzymatic debridement

Proteases (sutilains) elaborated by *Bacillus subtilis* (Travase™) have been championed periodically as an effective, nonsurgical, and relatively bloodless means of eschar removal. This approach has not gained wide acceptance, particularly in the treatment of extensive burns, in part because bacteremia may occur with its use in the presence of wound colonization. There is also the hypothetical disadvantage that proteolysis occurring in marginally viable tissue could increase burn depth unnecessarily. Enzymatic debridement has also been used to substitute for surgical escharotomy in acute burns with edema-induced vascular compromise, particularly in hand burns. We lack personal experience with this application of enzymatic debridement, which is clearly less rapid and definitive than is surgical escharotomy, which provides immediate tissue decompression and restoration of blood flow.

Hemostasis

As noted already, the blood loss associated with burn wound excision and skin grafting is commonly brisk. Limb tourniquets and topically applied or subcutaneously injected dilute epinephrine solution on donor sites and/or the wound bed are both used to minimize blood loss and are safe and probably effective.[57] Manual compression and elevation, the electrocautery, and topical thrombin spray are also useful adjuncts. Large vessels are ligated as necessary using absorbable material. Probably the most important determinant of the magnitude of blood loss, however, is the duration of the operation. We arbitrarily limit total operative time to 2 hours, as blood loss correlates strongly with operative time. The early surgical excision of burn wounds, i.e. within the first few days post-injury, appears to minimize attendant blood loss, presumably because the inflammatory response at the wound margins

has incompletely developed.[51] Clearly, as excision incurs hemorrhage and may increase the overall transfusion requirement as well, the risk of viral disease transmission, although small, is increased concomitantly. Although blood transfusion also has an immunosuppressive effect, its impact in this setting appears to be small, at least in the US, as the declining mortality and morbidity of burns in the present era of aggressive surgical wound excision attests.[58]

Skin graft procurement

A variety of precision dermatomes, most gas-powered, are presently available for both graft procurement and wound debridement in burn patients; the Padgett and Brown instruments are among the most widely used. It is worth noting that the Goulian, hand-held instrument, equipped with a shim of appropriate depth can be extremely useful in procuring skin grafts from the scalp and other relatively inaccessible areas (**Plate 3**). Since the introduction of the Tanner-Vandeput instrument for the mesh-expansion of skin grafts, other, similar devices have become available that provide a variety of expansion ratios and permit the meshing of long sheets of graft without the use of plastic carriers. For most purposes, a 1.5:1 or 2:1 expansion ratio provides a reasonable compromise between the reduction of the donor site area that must be cropped and the time required for epithelial outgrowth to completely close the grafted wound (< about 7 days). Greater expansion ratios – up to 6:1 – can be useful in patients with extensive burns but complete wound epithelialization by them when fully expanded may require several weeks; widely meshed grafts, which are fragile, can be protected with overlay biological dressings of cadaver allograft.[59]

Surgical Wound Closure in Patients with Non-Life Threatening Burns

Most burn patients do not have injuries that carry a significant mortality risk. The average burn size in a typical US burn center is about 20% total body surface area (TBSA) or somewhat less.[60] About two-thirds of the patients admitted to burn centers have burns of 30% TBSA or less.[45] In such patients, if they are less then 50 years of age, the survival rate exceeds 97%. Deaths from such injuries occur almost exclusively in the elderly or there is coexistent inhalation injury. Further, the deep component of such burns is often appreciably smaller than the TBSA. But even when all of the injury is full-thickness or deep dermal and would benefit from prompt surgical closure, there will be ample skin graft donor sites available for wound closure; few patients will have a physiological status that contraindicates operation, even if attended by brisk hemorrhage. In short, delaying the surgical therapy that will in any case be necessary eventually in such patients offers no advantage and many disadvantages. With delay, the wound microbial density will be higher, the pain and apprehension associated with dressing changes and physical therapy more prolonged, and length of stay and cost increased. The only prerequisites to prompt surgical therapy are an adequate bank blood supply and an experienced surgical and anesthetic team.

The excision and grafting of such injuries within a few days postburn is routine in many, if not most burn centers, including our own, where it has been standard for more than 20 years. The take of skin grafts in these patients should be uniformly good – i.e. approaching 100% – so that prompt and permanent wound closure is regularly achieved with one or, occasionally two operative procedures. But it should be emphasized that, theoretical considerations aside, the impediments to successful wound closure increase in parallel with the increasing extent of the burn. In trials comparing early with delayed surgical therapy in the same institution, hospital stay was reduced with early surgery only when the burn area was small – averaging 6% TBSA.[61]

Management of the Deep Dermal Component of 'Small' Burns

Although successful wound closure within a few days shortens hospital stay and reduces early pain, one can question whether it: (1) provides better long-term function, or (2) lessens the incidence and severity of hypertrophic scar compared to an approach that treats the deep dermal burn component expectantly and allows those wounds to heal spontaneously? These, after all, are the two most important goals of therapy in this patient population, since mortality is not the overriding issue. A straightforward answer to this question is not possible. Enthusiastic advocates of early surgical therapy have tended to disregard the evidence that intensive physical therapy that is begun initially and continued well beyond the acute phase may well be the most important determinant of the end functional result. There is no question that function is recovered sooner in wounds that have been promptly closed surgically because relatively painless joint movement is facilitated; but this difference narrows toward imperceptibility with time, provided that appropriate physical therapy is continued in those whose deep dermal burns are permitted to close spontaneously, as has been found in prospective studies of hand burns.[62,63] Unfortunately, in dorsal hand burns at least, the severity of the residual hypertrophic scar does not seem to be influenced by the rapidity (i.e. from a few days to a few weeks) with which wound closure has occurred. Nevertheless, on balance we still prefer to treat most deep dermal burns, including those of the hands by early tangential excision and skin grafting, although enthusiasm has waned somewhat as controlled follow-up data such as those just cited have appeared. It needs to be stressed again that an experienced surgical-physical therapy team is mandatory if the operative approach is used for the results to be acceptable.

Burns >30% TBSA: Staged versus Early Total Wound Closure

Although only about one-third of the hospitalized burn population have injuries exceeding 30% TBSA, one-half or more of all burn deaths occur in this cohort.[60] As burn size increases within the cohort, and/or if inhalation injury coexists, the mortality probability also increases.

Early total excision

Would mortality from extensive injuries be reduced if all the deep burns (i.e. full-thickness plus deep dermal) were surgically closed within a few days post-injury, before wound bacterial colonization has become well established? This concept has a not inconsiderable number of credible advocates, including the Editor of this volume. But given the tendency during the first few days to over-diagnose deep dermal burns that are more superficial and would otherwise heal rapidly, this approach inevitably further increases an already wide donor–recipient site skin disparity. Several operative sessions are usually necessary within the first few days to complete the excision and cover the wounds. A combination of

autologous skin grafts harvested from what little unburned areas remain and a variety of temporary wound covers, most frequently cadaver allograft, must then be employed to achieve the stated goal of wound closure. There is a clear consensus that extensive excised wounds should not be left open in these immunocompromised patients. With modern supportive care and an experienced operative team, even near total burns can be so treated surgically without early postoperative mortality. But does this logistically complex approach reduce mortality?

Only two prospective, randomized trials of early total excision have been reported; to our knowledge in one, there was no survival advantage with excision performed within 24 hours of injury.[64] In the controls, surgical therapy was not begun until the 10–14th day postburn. Although there was a small reduction in hospital stay (of 3.3 days in excised patients), the reduction in stay was observed only in a cohort with burns <15% TBSA. Based on these disappointing results, the authors abandoned early excision. As noted elsewhere in this chapter, others have also observed a significant reduction in hospital stay (usually a close correlate of near complete wound closure) only in small burns.[61]

In the second, more recent trial, 85 adults with burns ranging from 30 to 98% TBSA were treated either by excision of all deep burns within 72 hours or by a method described as 'conservative operative debridement with gradual wound closure', a method that would appear to be considerably different and far less aggressive than the staged excisional approach described below;[65] the wounds in the control group were not treated surgically until at least 3 weeks post-injury. There was no survival difference in the two groups considered as a whole, whether or not inhalation injury coexisted. (Advocates of early massive excision had hoped it would blunt the excessive mortality in that highly lethal combination of injuries.) In a subgroup of young patients, aged 17–30 years, who did not have inhalation injury, mortality in the 22 who were treated with excision was 9%, versus 45% in the conservatively treated cohort of 11 patients, a statistically significant difference. Although this data subset might appear to support early massive excision, the passive and essentially outmoded surgical approach used in the controls, together with the pooled, wide range of burn size necessary for the demonstration of a significant mortality difference, the skewed distribution of injury severity in favor of the excised group, and the small numbers, particularly of controls in this subset, suggests that the putative benefit of early total excision on mortality was not clearly established in this study.

The alternative: staged surgical wound closure

An alternative, qualitatively and temporally less aggressive approach than that just described is presently used in many if not most burn centers for patients with massive burns in whom unburned donor skin is in short supply. In this approach, staged excisions of unequivocally full-thickness burn areas are carried out at approximately 7-day intervals beginning within 10 days postburn, depending on physiological status and on clinically certain estimates of burn depth. The excised wounds are closed with autologous skin grafts. Progressive, permanent wound closure is thus achieved by a series of operative procedures in which unequivocally full-thickness burns are treated first and in which some or all burns of indeterminate depth may be permitted to epithelialize. Careful planning of the sequence in which available donor sites are utilized is essential, as is ingenuity in harvesting donor skin from relatively inaccessible anatomical areas. An interval of 7–10 days between operative procedures is usual. We and others have found that topical wound therapy using silver sulfadiazine cream that is modified by the addition of 2.2% cerium nitrate is particularly useful because the adherent eschar that usually forms is relatively resistant to bacterial colonization and can safely be left in place until it can be excised and closed with autologous skin as it becomes available.[28–30] Although temporary wound covers are at times used, the necessity for their routine use is much reduced with this approach.

It needs emphasis that, whatever their bias or belief, few if any contemporary burn surgeons delay for long the excision and grafting of large areas of unequivocally full-thickness burns, irrespective of total burn extent. One review of a large series of 200 patients with burns of 30% TBSA or more is reasonably representative of the experience in most hands with staged excision.[48] Eighty-eight percent of those who survived had initial excision of full-thickness burns between the 4th and 31st status postburn days (mean 13.5 days). Survivors in whom excision was performed relatively late had a predominance of deep dermal injury which was permitted to epithelialize spontaneously and smaller full-thickness burns that were grafted later. The nonsurvivors had bigger burns and a higher incidence of inhalation injury; excision could be performed in only 43%, as the remainder were judged too unstable to tolerate operation. Thus, outcome appeared to be determined principally by factors other than the surgical approach to wound therapy.

Envoi

Notwithstanding the numerous advances in supportive care that have made reasonably prompt surgical burn wound closure at a time of election a realistic option, the 'rough, unequal and ill-favored' scars that Paré lamented centuries ago unfortunately still remain largely as unsightly as they then were. A significant mortality probability should exist only in those relatively few patients with extensive burns and/or who have inhalation injury as well. Hypertrophic scar is the single most important unresolved problem in burn care today.

References

1. Clark RAF, Ed. *The Molecular and Cellular Biology of Wound Repair*, 2nd edn. New York; Plenum Press, 1996.
2. Brown GI, Nanney LB, Griffen J, *et al.* Enhancement of wound healing by topical treatment with epidermal growth factor. *N Engl J Med* 1989; **321**: 76–9.
3. Andree C, Swain WF, Page CP, *et al. In vivo* transfer and expression of a human epidermal growth factor gene accelerates wound repair. *Proc Natl Acad Sci USA* 1994; **91**: 12188–92.
4. Ramirez RJ, Wolf SE, Barrow RE, Herndon DN. Growth hormone treatment in pediatric burns. *Ann Surg* 1998; **228**: 439–48.
5. Dugan RC, Nance FC. Enzymatic burn wound debridement in conventional and germ-free rats. *Surg Forum* 1977; **2X**: 33–4.
6. Moyer CA, Brentano L, Gravens DL, Margraf HW, Monafo WW. Treatment of large human burns with 0.5% silver nitrate solution. *Arch Surg* 1965; **90**: 812–67.
7. Serini G, Bochaton-Paillat M-C, Ropray P, *et al.* The fibronectin domain ED-A is crucial for myofibroblastic phenotype induction by transforming growth factor-beta I. *J Cell Biol* 1998; **142**: 873–81.
8. Cone JB, Wallace BH, Caldwell FT. The effect of staged wound closure on the rates of heat production and heat loss of burned children and young adults. *J Trauma* 1988; **28**: 968–72.
9. Schwanholt C, Greenhalgh DG, Warden GD. A comparison of full-thickness versus split-thickness autografts for the coverage of deep palm burns in the very young pediatric burn patient. *J Burn Care Rehabil* 1993; **14**: 29–33.
10. Ahn ST, Monafo WW, Mustoe TA. Topical silicone gel: for the prevention and treatment of hypertrophic scars. *Arch Surg* 1991; **126**: 499–504.
11. Caldwell FT. Etiology and control of postburn hypermetabolism: the 1991 Presidential address to the American Burn Association. *J Burn Care Rehabil* 1991; **12**: 385–401.
12. Smith DJ, Thomson PD. Changing flora in burn and trauma units: historical perspective. *J Burn Care Rehabil* 1992; **13**: 276–80.
13. Monafo WW, West MA. Current treatment recommendations for topical burn therapy. *Drugs* 1990; **40**: 364–73.
14. White MG, Asch MJ. Acid base effects of topical mafenide acetate in the burned patient. *Arch Surg* 1984; **119**: 183–8.
15. Pruitt BA, McManus AT, Kim SH, *et al.* Burn wound infections: current status. *World J Surg* 1998; **22**: 135–45.
16. Wassennan D, Ioannovich JD, Hinzmann RD, *et al.* Interferon gamma in the prevention of severe, burn-related infections: a European phase 3 multicenter trial. *Crit Care Med* 1998; **26**: 434–39.
17. Fox CL. Silver sulfadiazine: a new topical therapy for *Pseudomonas* in burns. *Arch Surg* 1968; **96**: 184–8.
18. Smith-Choban P, Marshall WJ. Leukopenia secondary to silver sulfadiazine: frequency, characteristics and clinical consequences. *Am Surg.* 1987; **53**: 515–17.
19. Gamelli RI, Paxton TP, O'Reilly M. Bone marrow toxicity by silver sulfadiazine. *Surg Gyn Obstet* 1993; **177**: 115–20.
20. Eldad A, Neuman A, Weinberg A, *et al.* Silver sulfadiazine-induced hemolytic anemia in a glucose-6-phosphatase-deficient burn patient. *Burns* 1991; **17**: 430–2.
21. Lindbergh RB, Moncrief JA, Mason AD. Control of experimental and clinical burn wound sepsis by topical application of Sulfamylon compounds. *Ann NY Acad Sci* 1968; **150**: 950–72.
22. White MG, Asch MJ. Acid-base effects of topical mafenide acetate in the burned patient. *Arch Surg* 1984; **119**: 183–8.
23. Monafo WW. *The Treatment of Burns: Principles and Practice.* St Louis: Warren H. Green. 1971; 267.
24. Fox CL, Monafo WW, Ayvazian VH, *et al.* Topical chemotherapy for burns using cerium salts and silver sulfadiazine. *Surg Gyn Obstet* 1977; **144**: 668–72.
25. Hermans RP. Topical treatment of serious infections with special reference to the use of a mixture of silver sulfadiazine and cerium nitrate. *Burns* 1984; **11**: 59–62.
26. Peterson VM, Hansbrough JF, Wang XW, *et al.* Topical cerium nitrate cream prevents postburn immunosuppression. *J Trauma* 1985; **25**: 1039–44.
27. Scheidegger D, Sparkes BG, Luschern, *et al.* Survival in major burn injuries treated by one bathing in cerium nitrate. *Burns* 1992; **18**: 296–300.
28. Wassermann D, Schlotterer M, Lebreton F, *et al.* Use of topically applied silver sulfadiazine plus cerium nitrate in major burns. *Burns* 1989; **15**: 257–60.
29. Monafo WW, Robinson HN, Toshioka T, Ayvazian VH. Lethal burns: a progress report. *Arch Surg* 1978; **113**: 397–401.
30. Boecks W, Blondeel PN, Vandersteen K, *et al.* Effect of cerium nitrate-silver sulfadiazine on deep dermal burns: a histological hypothesis. *Burns* 1992; **18**: 456–62.
31. Munster Am, Helvig E, Rowland S. Cerium nitrate-silver sulfadiazine cream in the treatment of burns: a prospective evaluation. *Surgery* 1980; **88**: 658–60.
32. Allgower M. Personal communication, 1999.
33. Yin HQ, Langford R, Burrell RE. Comparative evaluation of the antimicrobial activity of Acticoat antimicrobial barrier dressing. *J Burn Care Rehabil* 1999; **20**: 195–200.
34. Tredgett EE, Shankowsky HA, Pannu R, *et al.* A matched-pair, randomized study evaluating the efficacy and safety of Acticoat silver coated dressing in the treatment of burn wounds. *J Burn Care Rehabil* 1998; **19**: 531–37.
35. Munster AM. Treatment of invasive *Enterobacter cloacae* burn wound sepsis with topical nitrofurazone. *J Trauma* 1998; **24**: 524–5.
36. Lawrence JC, Cason JS, Kidson A. Evaluation of phenoxetol-chlorhexidine cream as a prophylactic agent in burns. *Lancet* 1982; **1**: 1037–49.
37. Hunt JL, Sato R, Heck EL, Baxter CR. A critical evaluation of povidone-iodine absorption in thermally injured patients. *J Trauma* 1980; **20**: 127–31.
38. Rath T, Meissi G. Induction of hyperthyroidism in burn patients treated topically with povidone-iodine. *Burns* 1988; **14**: 320–2.
39. Heggers JP, Robson MC, Herndon DM, Desai MH. The efficacy of nystatin combined with topical microbial agents in the treatment of burn wound sepsis. *J Burn Care Rehabil* 1989; **10**: 508–11.
40. Strock LL, Lee EJ, Rutan RL, *et al.* Topical Bactroban (mupirocin) efficacy in treating burn wounds infected with methicillin-resistant *Staphylococci. J Burn Care Rehabil* 1990; **11**: 454–60.
41. Nathan P, Law EJ, Murphy DF, MacMillan BG. A laboratory method for selection of topical antimicrobial agents to treat infected burn wounds. *Burns* 1977; **4**: 177–87.

42. Monafo WW. Then and now: 50 years of burn treatment. *Burns* 1992; **18**: S7–10.

43. Cope O, Langohr JL, Moore FD, Webster RC. Expeditious care of full-thickness burn wounds by surgical excision and grafting. *Ann Surg* 1947; **125**: 1–21.

44. Klassen H. *History of Free Skin Grafting*. Berlin: Springer-Verlag, 1981: 190.

45. Monafo WW. Initial management of burns. *N Engl J Med* 1996; **335**: 1581–6.

46. Ryan CM, Schoenfeld DA, Thorpe WP, *et al.* Objective estimates of the probability of death from burn injuries. *N Engl J Med* 1998; **338**: 362–6.

47. Demling RH. Improved survival after massive burns. *J Trauma* 1983; **23**: 179–84.

48. McManus WF, Mason AD, Pruitt BA. Excision of the burn wound in patients with large burns. *Arch Surg* 1989; **124**: 718–20.

49. Monafo WW, Bessey PQ. Benefits and limitations of burn wound excision. *World J Surg* 1992; **16**: 37–42.

50. Tompkins RG, Remensnyder JP, Burke JF, *et al.* Significant reductions in mortality for children with burn injuries through the use of prompt eschar excision. *Ann Surg* 1988; **208**: 577–85.

51. Desai, MH, Herndon, DM, Broemeling L, *et al.* Early burn wound excision significantly reduces blood loss. *Ann Surg* 1990; **211**: 753–62.

52. Housinger TA, Lang D, Warden GD. A prospective study of blood loss with excisional therapy in pediatric burn patients. *J Trauma* 1993; **34**: 262–3.

53. Shiozaki T, Kishikawa M, Hiraide A, *et al.* Recovery from postoperative hypothermia predicts survival in extensively burned patients. *Am J Surg* 1993; **165**: 326–31.

54. Monafo WW, Aulenbacher CE, Pappalardo C. Early tangential excision of the eschars of major burns. *Arch Surg* 1972; **104**: 503–8.

55. Monafo WW. Tangential excision. *Clin Plast Surg* 1974; **1**: 591–601.

56. Marano M, O Sullivan G, Madden M, *et al.* Tourniquet technique for reduced blood loss and wound assessment during excision of burn wounds of the extremity. *Surg Gynecol Obstet* 1990; **171**: 249–50.

57. Musgrave M, Beveridge M, Fish J, Cartotto R. Minimizing blood loss in surgery. *J Burn Care Rehabil* 2000; **21 (No I, Part 2)**: S135.

58. Wolfe SE, Rose JK, Desai M, *et al.* Mortality determinants in massive pediatric burns: an analysis of 103 children with > 80% TBSA burns (>70% full-thickness). *Ann Surg* 1997; **225**: 554–69.

59. Alexander JW, McMillan BG, Law E, Kittur DS Treatment of severe burns with widely meshed autograft and meshed skin allograft overlay. *J Trauma* 1981; **21**: 433–8.

60. Saffle JR, Davis B, Williams P. American Burn Association Registry Participant Group. Recent outcomes in the treatment of burn injury in the United States: a report from the American Burn Association Patient Registry. *J Burn Care Rehabil* 1995; **16**: 219–32.

61. Engrav LH, Heimbach DM, Reuss JL, *et al.* Excision and grafting vs. nonoperative treatment of burns of indeterminate depth: a prospective, randomized study. *J Trauma* 1983; **23**: 1001–4.

62. Salisbury RE, Wright P. Evaluation of early excision of dorsal burns of the hand. *Plast Reconstr Surg* 1982; **69**: 670–5.

63. Goodwin CW, Maguire MS, McManus WF, Pruitt BA. Prospective study of burn wound excision of the hands. *J Trauma* 1983; **23**: 510–17.

64. Sorensen B, Fisker NP, Steensen JP, Kalaja E. Acute excision or exposure treatment. Final results of a three-year-old randomized controlled clinical trial. *Scand J Plast Reconstr Surg* 1984; **18**: 87–93.

65. Herndon DN, Barrow RE, Rutan RL, *et al.* A comparison of conservative versus early excision therapies in severely burned patients. *Ann Surg* 1989; **209**: 547–53.

Chapter 11

Treatment of infection in burns

John P Heggers, Hal Hawkins, Patricia Edgar
Cynthia Villarreal, David N Herndon

Microbial identification of the burn wound pathogen

Infection is a most undesirable partner in any operative procedure, and more particularly in the thermal injury. Therefore, the purpose of this chapter is to attempt to provide the new burn surgeon, and possibly re-familiarize the practicing burn surgeon, with the techniques, methodology, and terminology as it applies to the microbiology of the burn wound. There are several major benchmarks that must be adhered to in order to achieve reliable clinical microbiology results in its association with the thermal injury. The first and most important canon to remember is the selection of a proper specimen for culture. This entails obtaining a culture, which is free from contamination from the normal flora that may be present on the surface of the injured skin after the injury. This should include any leukocyte-laden exudate.[1]

Secondly, the size or amount of the specimen plays a very significant role in the appropriate identification of the etiologic agent. The use of prophylactic antimicrobials, both topical and systemic, should be noted so appropriate inhibitors or sufficient dilutions can be prepared or reagents added to void the drug interactions. The specimen should be collected and placed in a sterile container with appropriate media for transport to the laboratory.[2]

Presumptive examination of burn wound specimens

Most if not all specimens should be examined immediately. Tissue specimens should be homogenized or impression smears should be prepared: other body fluids transudates and exudates should be examined immediately after collection.

One of the most important techniques available to the burn surgeon is the Gram stain. This procedure is the primary road sign providing presumptive evidence as to the potential etiologic agent responsible for infection as well as providing a possible empirical use of both topical and systemic antibacterial therapy to control or eliminate the microbe, and most importantly what approach the laboratory should employ for successful isolation and identification of the etiologic agent of infection.

The preparation of the specimen for staining is made by aseptically transferring the suspect material to an aseptically clean clear glass slide. If the specimen is dry, a drop of water is placed on the slide first in order to emulsify the specimen for proper staining. *Caution*: Make sure there is sufficient specimen for both the Gram stain and the culture as well. **If the quantity of the specimen is insufficient, culture first, then Gram stain if possible**. A thin film is made, fixed by air-drying and then heat fixation, by passing the slide a few times through a flame or placing the slide on the rack above the incinerator (Oxford Labware, St Louis, MO).

The Gram-stain procedure is simple, consisting of four basic steps:

- Flood the slide with crystal violet for 10 seconds to 1 minute. (Times vary dependent for each stain employed, age of stain, authors' procedure, and outline). Rinse with tap water.
- Flood then with Gram's iodine for 10 seconds to 1 minute. Rinse with tap water.
- Carefully decolorize with 95% ethanol or acetone alcohol combination 10–20 seconds. (Acetone–alcohol may be used for a more rapid decolorization.)
- Counterstain with safranin 10–30 seconds. Air dry or blot with bibulous paper.

Two basic reactions will be noted. Organisms that stain blue or purple are classified gram-positive (i.e. staphylococci) and those that stain red are classified gram-negative (i.e. *Escherichia coli*).[2] (For an explanation concerning the mechanisms of the Gram reaction, it is suggested the reader review *Medical Microbiology* by Baron and Jennings, pages 28–34.[3]) Specimens collected should be placed in an appropriate sterile container, transport, or holding medium. There are several available for the more fastidious and anaerobic pathogens. Further discussion concerning the proper media will be addressed during the description of the frequently encountered pathogens.

All specimens taken at the time of surgical intervention should be inoculated to a variety of solid and liquid media. However, the only reliable method is a tissue biopsy, which is the true indicator of the potential pathogen in surgical sepsis. Quantitative counts should be performed using a modified Robson–Heggers technique.[4] The liquid medium employed is generally an enriched thioglycolate medium (THIO) or brain heart infusion broth (BHIB), supplemented to facilitate the recovery of anaerobes as well as the aerobic pathogens.[2,3,5] Aliquots of the serial-diluted specimens are subsequently inoculated to sheep blood agar (SBAP) with phenethyl alcohol (PEA), and MacConkey's agar (MACA). SBAP is an enriched medium that contains nutrient supplements, allowing a wide variety of organisms to reproduce. The SBAP with PEA is a selective medium, in that it will permit the growth of *Bacteroides fragilis*, *B. melaninogenicus*, *Clostridium perfringens* (*welchi*) and *Peptostreptococcus anaerobius* and should inhibit the growth of the facultative enterics, such as *Proteus mirabilis* and *E. coli*. MACA is a differential medium, distinguishing between lactose- and nonlactose-fermenting enteric organisms.

Each inoculated plate should be incubated in the suspected organism's appropriate atmospheric conditions.

A review of the resident and transient microbial flora that live as parasites and/or symbionts in and on man, will help to evaluate their significance as potential pathogens when encountered in surgical specimen (**Tables 11.1** and **11.2**).

Microbial identification

It is the design of the remaining portion of this chapter to reacquaint the burn surgeon with some of the major distinguishing characteristics of those pathogens encountered in burn wound sepsis.

The nomenclature and listing of the following microorganisms is a composite of *Bergey's Manual*[6] and NCDC's proposed changes.

A. Gram-positive cocci = facultative aerobic to anaerobic
1. Spherical cells in pairs and clusters, no chains
   a. *Micrococcus* spp. – differentiation from *Staphylococcus aureus*
   b. *Staphylococcus* spp.
   c. *Peptococcus* spp. (anaerobe)
2. Spherical cells in pairs, clumps, and chains
   a. *Streptococcus* spp.

Table 11.1 Frequently encountered gram–positive organisms according to organ association and probability of pathogenesis found in burn wounds*

Organism	Soft tissue skin	Upper respiratory tissue	Lower respiratory tissue	Endocardial	Gastro-intestinal tissue	Urogenital tract	Bone and joint
S. aureus	NF, P	P, NF	P	P	P	NF, P	P
S. epidermidis	NF, P	NF, P	P	P	P	NF, P	P
S. spp.	NF	NF, P	P	P	NF, P	NF, P	P
Str. pyogenes	P, NF	P, NF	P	P	P	P	P
Other strep	NF	NF	P	P	NF	NF, P	P
Enterococcus	P	P	P	P	NF, P	NF, P	P
Corynebacterium	NF	P	P	P	–	P	–
Diphtheroids	NF	NF	–	P	NF	NF	–
Micrococci	NF	NF	–	–	–	–	–
Candida albicans	NF	NF	P	P	NF	P, NF	P

NF, Normal flora; P, pathogens; – normally not found; however, these organisms should not be ignored when encountered.
* Modified from Heggers J. Microbiology for surgeons. In: Kerstein MD, ed. *Management of Surgical Infections*. Mt Kisco, NY: Futura Publishing Co., 1980: 27–55.

Table 11.2 Frequently encountered gram-negative organisms according to tissue association and potential of pathogenesis found in burn wounds*

Organism	Soft tissue skin	Upper respiratory tissue	Lower respiratory tissue	Endocardial	Gastro-intestinal tissue	Urogenital tract	Bone and joint
Fermentors (enterics)							
Escherichia coli	NF, P	NF, P	P	P	NF, P	NF, P	P
Klebsiella pneumoniae; Enterobacter cloacae, aerogenes	NF, P	NF, P	P	P	NF, P	NF, P	P
Proteus spp.	NF, P	P	P	P	NF, P	NF, P	P
Morganella morganii	P	–	P	–	P	P	P
Serratia marcescens	NF, P	–	P	P	P	P	P
Providencia spp.	P	–	P	–	P	P	P
Other enterics	NF, P	NF, P	P	P	NF, P	P	P
Nonfermentors							
Aeromonas hydrophilia	P	P	P	P	NF, P	P	P
Pseudomonas aeruginosa	P	NF, P	P	P	NF, P	P	P
Acinetobacter spp.	NF	NF	P	–	NF	NF	P
Achromobacter xylosoxidans	P	P	P	P	NF, P	P	P

* NF, normal flora; P, pathogens; –, normally not found; however, these organisms should not be ignored when encountered. Modified from Heggers J. Microbiology for surgeons. In: Kerstein MD, ed. *Management of Surgical Infections*. Mt Kisco, NY: Futura Publishing Co., 1980: 27–55.

  b.   *Enterococcus* spp.
  c.   *Peptostreptococcus* spp. (anaerobe)
B. Gram-positive bacilli
  1.   Aerobic (asporogenous) bacilli
    a.   *Corynebacterium*
    b.   *Listeria*
  2.   Spore-forming bacilli
    a.   *Bacillus* (aerobe)
    b.   *Clostridium* (anaerobe)
C. Gram-negative aerobic rods
  1.   Nonfermentors
    a.   *Pseudomonas aeruginosa*
    b.   *Burkholderia* spp.
    c.   *Acinetobacter* spp.
    d.   *Stenotrophomonas maltophilia*
D. Gram-negative facultatively anaerobic rods (glucose fermentors)
  1.   Enterobacteriaceae
    a.   *Escherichia coli*
    b.   *Enterobacter cloacae*
    c.   *Klebsiella pneumoniae*
    d.   *Serratia marcescens*
    e.   Other enteric organisms
  2.   Vibrionaceae
    a.   *Aeromonas hydrophilia*
  3.   Other miscellaneous Gram-negative rods.

Gram-Positive Cocci – Pairs, Clusters

The *Micrococcus* spp. as a rule are considered amphibionts or non-pathogenic; however, with the increasing frequency of prosthetic valve transplants these organisms are becoming more important. Another major reason for differentiating this genus is because of its similarity to the staphylococci.

Micrococci, a gram-positive cocci which generally forms tetrads, as opposed to the formation of grape-like clusters, is often seen mixed with staphylococci. Nonhemolytic colonies are prevalent and produce a wide variety of color (i.e. *M. luteus*).

Colonies vary from yellow and orange to red and even violet in color. There are three distinct species to be considered and they are *M. luteus*, *M. roseus*, and *M. varians*. Cultural differences are presented in **Table 11.3**.[7]

Table 11.3 Characteristics differentiating *Micrococcus* species from *Staphylococcus aureus**

Test	*M. varians*	*M. roseus*	*M. luteus*	*S. aureus*
Catalase	+	+	+	+
Coagulase	–	–	–	+
Acid from glucose aerobically	+	–	–	+
Acid from glucose anaerobically	–	–	–	+
15% NaC1	–	–	–	+
5% NaC1	+	+	+	+

+, positive; –, negative.
* Modified from Heggers J. Microbiology for surgeons. In: Kerstein MD, ed. *Management of Surgical Infections*. Mt Kisco, NY: Futura Publishing Co., 1980: 27–55.

The micrococci are normal inhabitants of the skin and the frequency of isolation in a burn wound is between 5 and 10%. They are considered nonpathogenic in a burn wound and are more frequently considered wound contaminants. While all are catalase positive, their distinct growth requirements are essential components of delineating the specific organisms.

The genus *Staphylococcus* is composed of several important pathogens, which include *Staph. aureus, Staph. epidermidis, Staph. saprophyticus, Staph. haemolyticus, Staph. hyicus hyicus, Staph. simulans,* and *Staph. cohnii.* All have a variable hemolytic activity. Although *Staph. aureus* usually produces golden or cream-colored colonies and *Staph. epidermidis* produces white to dull gray colonies, as do the other staphylococci, the color is not trustworthy for identification. The coagulase test is usually the differential test for separating these two species. It can be implemented best by either slide or tube method. However, should this slide method prove negative, true coagulase negativity then must be confirmed by the tube test. **Tables 11.4a** and **11.4b** compare some of the major key reactions for proper identification among the staphylococci. The slide screening test using human plasma is a presumptive determination which examines for 'bound' coagulase, while the confirmatory tube test employs rabbit plasma, which tests for 'free' coagulase. However, one must be sure the microbe being tested is a gram-positive cocci, since citrate-positive organisms such as *Pseudomonas, Serratia* and *Enterococcus* species utilize citrate and release calcium, which can cause a clot to form.[2,3]

Strains of *Staph. aureus* as well as other *Staphylococcus* species produce a wide variety of metabolites. Some are pathognomonic and also toxigenic, while those with minimal toxicity or no toxic effects at all, are of some diagnostic significance. Most of the human pathogens produce α- and β-lysins. Some exotoxins, which are produced by the pathogenic strains of staphylococci, include a pyrogenic toxin, a dermonecrotizing toxin, a lethal toxin, and leukocidin, which is presumably similar to the δ-lysin. Only *Staph. aureus* produces an enterotoxin, which is the cause of staphylococcal food poisoning while α-hemolysin does not lyse human red cells; it will lyse sheep red blood cells and rabbit red cells, while horse red cells are lysed only by δ-lysin. Other antigenic nontoxic metabolites produced by the staphylococci are coagulase, protease, lipase, deoxyribonuclease, fibrinolysin, gelatinase, in addition to hyaluronidase, phosphate, and staphylokinase.

Staph. aureus and the other members of the *Staphylococcus* species usually will develop resistance to antibiotics rather rapidly. The majority of the staphylococci strains isolated from hospital patients are resistant to penicillin, methicillin, cephalosporins, and the aminoglycosides. The former resistance is mediated by a β-lactamase or penicillinase, whereas methicillin is considered resistant to β-lactamase.[8]

Staph. epidermidis is a resident of human skin and mucous membranes and resembles *Staph. aureus* microscopically. *Staph. epidermidis* is tolerant of high NaCl concentrations as is *Staph. aureus.* However, it differs from *Staph. aureus* in that it is mannitol-, coagulase- and thermonuclease-negative. It is equally as pathogenic as *Staph. aureus,* and has been the principal etiologic agent in disease entities such as subacute bacterial endocarditis, infected surgical prosthesis, infections following bone marrow transplantation, or other states of immunosuppression such as in the thermal injury. Typically, *Staph. epidermidis* is resistant to penicillinase-resistant penicillins such as methicillin and cephalosporins, a similar case to *Staph. aureus.* Methicillin resistance is genetically mediated through a transposon.[8,9] Methicillin-resistant *Staph. epidermidis* (MRSE) delivers its genetically resistant code to a previously liable *Staph. aureus,* which subsequently becomes methicillin-resistant (MRSA).[9] *Staph. saprophyticus* resembles the other staphylococci but it is distinguished from them because of its resistance to nonobiocin; *Staph. saprophyticus* is also resistant to nalidixic acid (**Table 11.4a** and **11.4b**).

In burn wound infections the predominate gram-positive agent responsible during 1988–1989 was *Staph. aureus* (53.8%) followed by *Staph. hyicus hyicus* (24.0%); the other staphylococci accounted for the remaining 22.2% (**Table 11.5**). The staphylococci accounted for over 82% of the gram-positive isolates. Ten years later (Jan to Dec 1999) the predominant gram-positive agent was *Staph. epidermidis* (46.8%) followed by *Staph. aureus* (23.7%), and *Staph. haemolyticus* (23.5%). As usual the staphylococci accounted for 81.9% of the gram-positive isolates, the same percentage as 10 years ago (**Table 11.5**). The gram-positive isolates accounted for 58.2% of the total isolates. The staphylococci, more especially the MRSE and MRSA, are responsible for graft loss when the colony count of the graft bed is >10⁵ CFUs per gram of tissue.[10]

Staphylococcal diseases

All *Micrococcus* and *Staphylococcus* grow especially well on SBAP. Suspect colonies should be tested for catalase from a nutrient agar culture because blood agar can give a positive catalase reaction leading to an incorrect presumptive identification. Mannitol salt sugar (7.5% NaCl) with a nutrient agar overlay may be employed to confirm anaerobic fermentation of mannitol and NaCl tolerance, previously discussed above, as represented in **Table 11.3**.[6,7,11] Most common infections where the etiologic agent *Staphylococcus* spp. are encountered and are considered pathognomonic are septicemia; cellulitis; impetigo; scalded skin syndrome; and postoperative wound infections. However, the most serious staphylococcal infections are puerperal sepsis, pneumonia, osteomyelitis, endocarditis, and burn wound infections. Staphylococcal pseudomembranous enterocolitis will occur most frequently as a complication of antibiotic therapy.

Toxic shock syndrome

The toxic shock syndrome (TSS) was first described as such in 1978.[12] The disease is characterized by sudden onset of fever, vomiting, diarrhea, shock, and a diffuse macular erythematous rash, followed by desquamation of the skin on the hand and feet as well as hyperemia of various mucous membranes. However, the role of TSS has not been completely elucidated in the burn patient. It has been our experience that while burn patients may be infected with a TSS potential *Staph. aureus,* no other serious or untoward complications have been observed. In fact treatment of their burn wounds was not any different than those patients infected with a nontoxic TSS *S. aureus.*[13–15]

Streptococcaceae

The *Streptococcus* spp., however, appear as short and long chains of cocci and sometimes as diplococci as in the case of *Strep. (Diplococcus) pneumoniae,* which often appear as tear-drop or lancet diplococci. The streptococci are catalase-negative and pro-

Table 11.4 Differentiation of clinically important *Staphylococcus* species[+]

(a) Clinically important species

Character	S. aureus	S. epidemidis	S. saprophyticus
Coagulase*	+	−	−
Hemolysis	+	V	−
Novoabiocin resistance**	−	−	+
Phosphatase*	+	+	V
Acid, aerobically, from D-(+)-trehalose*	+	−	+
D-Mannitol	+	−	V
Maltose	+	−	V
Sucrose*	+	+	+
D-(+)-xylose* or L-(+)-arabinose	−	−	+
Xylitol	−	−	−
Anaerobic growth in thioglycollate	+	−	V
Nitrate/DNase	+/+	+	+>−
Identification accuracy based on the above characters	>95%	+w/−w	−/−
		>95%	>90%

(b) Other clinically important *Staphylococcus* species[+]

Character	S. simulans	S. haemolyticus	S. hyicus hyicus	S. hominis
Coagulase*	−	−	V	−
Hemolysis	V	+>+	V	−>+
Novoabiocin resistance**	−	−	−	−
Phosphatase*	V	−>+	V	−>+
Acid, aerobically, from D-(+) trehalose*	+>−	+	+	+>−
D-Mannitol*	+>−	+,−	+	−
Maltose	−>+	+	+	+
Sucrose*	+	+	V	+
D-(+)-xylose* or L-(+)-arabinose	−	−	V	−
Xylitol	−	−	V	−
Anaerobic growth in thioglycollate	+	+>+,+	+	−>+
Nitrate/DNase	+/w	d/ds	+/+	d/−w
Identification accuracy based on the above characters	>90%	>85%	>85%	>80%

[+] Modified from Holt J, Krieg NR, Sneath PHA, Staley JT, Williams ST, eds. *Bergey's Manual of Determinative Bacteriology*. 9th ed. Baltimore, MD: Williams & Wilkins, 1994.

* Characters recommended by the ICSB Subcommittee on the Taxonomy of Staphylococci and Micrococci.

** Minimal inhibitory concentration > 1.6 μg/ml.

V, Variable; w, weak reaction; +w, positive to weak reaction; −w, negative to weak reaction; d, delayed reaction; ds, tests differentiates subspecies; +, positive reaction; −, negative reaction.

Table 11.5 10-year comparison of gram-positive organisms isolated from pediatric burns

Organism	Jan–Dec 1999		Overall % of the group	1988–1989*		Overall % of the group
	No	%		No	%	
S. aureus	257	19.4	23.7	4402	44.2	53.8
S. epidermidis	508	38.4	46.8	1305	13.1	
S. hyicus hyicus	–	–		1961	19.7	24.0
S. haemolyticus	255	19.3	23.5	–	–	
Total staph	1085	81.9		8185	82.2	
Ec. faecalis	156	11.8	95.8	925	9.3	67.1
Ec. faecium	73	5.5		269	2.6	
Other GPO	–	–		584	5.9	32.9
Total strep	239	18.1		1778	17.8	
Total GPO	1324	100.0		9963	100.0	
Total isolates	2273	58.2		12.696	67.8	

*From Heggers JP, McCauley RL, Herndon DN. *Antimicrobial Therapy in Burn Patients. Part 1, Surgical Rounds*, 1992; July: 613–17.

duce a variety of hemolytic activity in the presence of blood. The types of hemolysis produced on SBAP are frequently used as an initial means of identification for the streptococci: α-hemolytic streptococci manifest a green discoloration of blood agar surrounding a small grayish colony which is resistant to dissolution by bile. *Strep. pneumoniae*, now classified as a member of the *Streptococcus* family, produces an α-hemolysis, characteristic of the viridans group. It is bile-soluble (autolysis by bile) and has Optochin sensitivity (TAXO P disk, BBL). The Optochin disk is impregnated with ethyl-dryocupreine HCl and then placed on an

SBAP inoculated with *Strep. pneumoniae*; inhibition of growth is observed after overnight incubation of 37°C in a 5–10% CO_2 atmosphere. Other α-hemolytic streptococci are not inhibited.[2,3,6] Both the enterococci and viridans streptococci fall into this particular multifarious streptococci. The viridans group is obviously more susceptible to penicillin than those of the enterococci group. Another dominant characteristic is the hemolysis they produce, which is considered a virulence factor, and quantitatively this group of organisms do not lend themselves to the standard rule of less than 10^5 for any tissue closure. The mere presence of a few β-hemolytic streptococci can cause a wound infection, failure of a primary closure, and loss of a skin graft. The major species that can be diagnosed with this particular type of hemolysis are *Strep. pyogenes*, 'β'-hemolytic streptococci group A and *Strep. agalactiae* 'β'-hemolytic streptococci group B, just to mention a few. There are those that subsist in the remaining Lancefield's groups that demonstrate the same type of hemolytic action.[2,5] Presumptive identification of *Strep. pyogenes* can be made by sensitivity to bacitracin, since 90% of all *Strep. pyogenes* are sensitive to bacitracin. However, *Strep. agalactiae* is CAMP-positive and hippurate-positive (**Table 11.6**). The remaining streptococci are variable in their ability to tolerate salt and temperature requirements. They all proliferate well in a reduced O_2 environment, with a CO_2 tension of 3–5%, on SBAP. As recounted earlier, hemolysis is the passport for identifying these microbes. For proper discriminating characteristics and sensitivity to SXT, see **Table 11.6**.[13–15]

The genus *Enterococcus (Ec.)* was established in 1984.[3,6] However, *Ec. faecalis* and *Ec. faecium* were the only two recognized species. Since that time, 12 additional species have been classified within the enterococci group; however, only *Ec. durans* and *Ec. avium* have been isolated from human infections.[2,6,12]

The majority of the enterococci are frequently nonhemolytic, termed γ-hemolysis. However, there are some strains that produce a β- or α-hemolysis on blood agar. These microorganisms are distinguished by their capability to grow in high salt concentrations and hydrolyze esculin, resulting in black discoloration of the medium.[2,3,6]

All members of the enterococci group besides tolerating 6.5% NaCl and being bile esculin (BE)-positive are also pyrolidonylarylamidase (PYR)- and leucine aminopeptidase (LAP)-positive. The species are separated into three groups based on specific biochemical reactions. Group I does not hydrolyze arginine but forms acid in a manitol, sorbitol, and sorbose broth. The important species here is *Ec. avium*. Group II on the other hand hydrolyzes arginine and forms acid in manitol and sorbitol broth only. The significant species in this group are *Ec. faecalis* and *Ec. faecium*. Group III, which includes *Ec. durans*, is negative for all tests described above.[2,6]

While it is important to recognize the pathogenicity of the streptococci, it must be recognized that the enterococci are predominant etiologic agents of the burn wound infections, accounting for 67.1% of burn wound infections among the streptococci and only 12% among the total Gram-positives during 1988–1989. Among the other streptococci, *Strep. mitis*, *Strep. anguis*, and others are responsible for the remaining 32.9% of burn wound infections caused by the streptococci. However, there was a shift in the isolates for the enterococci in 1999 favoring *Ec. faecalis* at 9.3%, followed by *Ec. faecium* at 2.6%. The enterococci accounted for 11.8% of the total Gram-positive agents, which is similar to that in 1988 and 1989 combined. Both enterococci accounted for 95.8% of those streptococci isolated during this time frame (Jan to Dec 1999) (**Table 11.5**).

While this portion of the chapter deals with the identification and isolation of Gram-positive organisms, it has been our experience over the years that the predominate organisms isolated from the burn wound are the Gram-positive cocci (**Table 11.5**).

Peptococcaceae

The anaerobic gram-positive cocci are a part of the indigenous microflora of the skin gastrointestinal, genitourinary, and oral

---

Table 11.6 Biological characteristics of the *Streptococcus* spp.*

Lancefield group	Representative species	Hemolytic reaction	Bacitracin sensitivity	CAMP reaction	Na hippurate	Bile esculin	6.5% NaCl	SXT sensitivity	Optochin bile solubility
A	*Str. pyogenes*	b[a](rarely[b])	S	−	−	−	−	V	−
B	*Str. agalactiae*	b>a[c]>g[b]	R	+	+	−	V	R	−
C	*Str. equi*	b>a>g	R	−	−	−	−	S	−
D	Enterococci								
	Ec. faecalis	g>b>a	R	−	V	+	+	S	
	Ec. faecium								
	Other								
	Ec. bovis	g>b>a	R	−	−	+	−	S	
	Ec. equinus								
G	*Str. canis*	b>g>a	R	−				S	
H	*Str. sanguis*	a>b>g	R	−				S	
K	*Str. salivarius*	a>b>g	R	−				S	
Nongroupable	Viridans	a>b>g	V	−	−	−	−	S	−
E	*Str. uberis*	g>a	R	V	+	+	−	S	−
None	*Str. pneumoniae*	a	V	−	−	−	−	−	+

* Modified from Heggers J. Microbiology for surgeons. In: Kerstein MD, ed. *Management of Surgical Infections*. 1980, Mt Kisco, NY: Futura Publishing Co., 1980: 27–55.
[a] Beta hemolysis (b);
[b] gamma hemolysis (g);
[c] alpha hemolysis (a).
V, Variable; R, resistant; S, sensitive; −, negative; +, positive.

cavity systems. They have been reported as pathogens in almost every type of human infection.[3,12] The anaerobic gram-positive cocci are divided into two respective genera which include the *Peptococcus* spp. (*Staphylococcus*-like) and the *Peptostreptococcus* spp. (*Streptococcus*-like). As the names indicate, their morphological features are similar to their aerobic counterparts of infection.[16]

The *Peptococcus* genus contains six diverse species and the *Peptostreptococcus* genus contains five different species. The distinguishing reactions are presented in **Table 11.7**. On anaerobic blood agar plates, both genera (genesus) appear as small gray to white colonies after 48–72 hours incubation. Occasional strains of both may be β-hemolytic or α-hemolytic. *Peptococcus* unlike *Peptostreptococcus* does not produce a sharp pungent odor which is believed to be a identifying characteristic. In THIO broth, colonies appear as small discrete compact bodies uniformly growing throughout the medium, sometimes producing gas[16] (**Table 11.7**). However, with early excision and grafting these agents are rarely encountered in today's burn wound infections. Yet in developing countries, where early excision and grafting is not a reality, such organisms could be potentially dangerous.

Nonsporogenous Gram-Positive Rods

The major asporogenous bacilli most frequently encountered is the *Corynebacterium* sp., which is felt to be a normal inhabitant of the skin, respiratory tract, and/or vaginal tract (**Table 11.1**). They are small, gram-positive rods which form Chinese-like characters or palisades. Methylene blue stains often are helpful in identifying the metachromatic granules of these microbes. The colonies on blood agar are usually very small, dry and nonhemolytic, often referred to as diphtheroids. The only *Corynebacterium* sp. considered to be of the pathogenic type is *Corn. diphtheriae*. When this organism is suspected as the etiologic agent, specimens should be inoculated to Loeffler's medium and blood tellurite agar. Colonies emerge as black or gray in color. Though fluorescent antibodies can identify the organism as *Corn. diphtheriae*, only the Elek plate will identify the toxigenic groups responsible for the infection[3,6,7] (**Table 11.8**). A strip filter paper is impregnated with diphtheria antitoxin (100 U/ml) and is placed on a plate of enrichment medium with tellurite. Then the suspect microbe is inoculated to the plate perpendicular to the strip. The toxin from the organism diffuses through the medium as does the antitoxin. At the point of contact a thin precipitate forms at a 45° angle to the inoculation.

Table 11.7 Biological reactions of the anaerobic gram-positive cocci*

	Hemolysis	Catalase	Esculin hydrolysis	Gas	Indole	Nitrate	Tween 80 growth stimulant	Gelatin liquid
Peptococcus species								
P. asacccharolyticus	−	−	−	+	+	−	+	−
P. constellatus	−	−	+	−	−	V	−	−
P. magnus	−	−	−	−	−	−	+	−
P. morbillorum	b[a]	−	−	−/+	−	−	+	+
P. prevotii	b	V	−/+	−/+	−	−	+	−
P. variables	−	−	−	−/+	−	−	+	+
Peptostreptococcus species								
P. anaerobius	b	−	−	+	−	−	+	−
P. intermedius	a[b]	−	+	+	−	−	+	−
P. micros	b	−	−	−/+	−	−	+	−
P. parvulus	−	−	−	+	−	−	+	+
P. productus	a or b	−	+	+	−	−	−	−

* Modified from Heggers J. Microbiology for surgeons. In: Kerstein MD, ed. *Management of Surgical Infections*. Mt Kisco, NY: Futura Publishing Co., 1980: 27–55.

[a] Beta hemolysis (b); [b] alpha hemolysis (a).

V, variable; −, negative; +, positive; −/+, reaction more negative than positive.

Table 11.8 Some characteristics of the gram-positive nonsporogenous bacilli*

Genus	Hemolysis	Aerobic 5–10% CO₂	Anaerobic	Facultative	Esculin	Catalase	Indole	Acid fast	Motility
Corynebacterium	V	+	+	+		+	V	−	−
Listeria	b[a]	+	−	+	+	+	−	−	+[b]
Nocardia	−	+	−	−	+			−	−
Erysipelothrix	a	+	−	−	−	−	−	+	−
Lactobacillus	−	−	+	+		−	−	−	−
Actinomyces	+[c]	−	+	+	+	−	−	−	−
Propionibacterium	−	−	+	−	+		V	−	
Bifidobacterium	−	−	−		+	−	−	−	−

* Modified from Heggers J. Microbiology for surgeons. In: Kerstein MD, ed. *Management of Surgical Infections*. Mt Kisco, NY: Futura Publishing Co., 1980: 27–55.

[a] *L. monocytogenes* only; [b] at 20–25°C; [c] Rabbit blood alpha>beta.

V, variable; −, negative; +, positive.

Diphtheria antitoxin (DAT) is a necessary essential in the treatment of these infections.

An organism which provokes a monocytic response in rabbits, but usually not in humans, can cause a severe meningitis in humans. This organism is called *Listeria monocytogenes*, which stains equally as a Gram-positive rod or coccobacillus, often forming palisades, as observed with the diphtheroids. *L. myocytogenes* is β-hemolytic on blood agar, and the specimen may require a few days at 4°C before primary isolation. *Listeria* is motile at room temperature, a feature the *Corynebacterium* does not possess[3,6,7] (**Table 11.8**).

Nocadia is a gram-variable or gram-positive branching filamentous rod. This organism, like its anaerobic partner (*Actinomyces*) produces sulfur granules that appear as tiny pale yellowish flecks composed of dainty branching hyphae. The media of choice for this microbe are Sarbound's dextrose agar and SBAP. Species belonging to the *Nocardia* genus are acid-fast or partially acid fast. **Table 11.8** presents some of the predominant characteristics of *Nocardia*.[3,6]

Erysipelothrix rhusiopathiae (*insidiosa*), the etiologic agent of erysipeloid in man, is adumbrated as a slender Gram-positive rod with a tendency to form filaments. On SBAP it produces an α-hemolysis and the colonies are translucent with a bluish sheen, as seen by reflected light. However, it grows better on horse blood agar combined with a trypticase soy agar overlay. Indole is negative and its catalase is not produced (**Table 11.8**).[3,6,16]

One of the anaerobic partners of the asporogenous Gram-positive rods is the *Actinomyces* genus. This group of microbes resembles the *Corynebacterium* in that they produce diphtheroid-like characters. But, filamentous compositions are usually present after 18–48 hours after anaerobic incubation. Like *Nocardia*, *Actinomyces* requires several days to a few weeks to make its demeanor obvious. Therefore, any specimen processed without an initial Gram stain will most decidedly disclose a negative response after 48 hours incubation.[3,6,16]

Propionibacterium (*Corynebacterium*) *acnes* and species of *Bifidobacterium* (*Endobacterium* and *Arachinia*) are generally categorized as anaerobic diphtheroids. This class of microbes are often encountered with other facultative or anaerobic organisms, thus questioning their pathogenic potential. However, if an active disease process is either in an acute or chronic state, and if any of these microbes are isolated with relative frequency, the clinician must consider them as the etiologic agent until further evidence to the contrary is obtained.[3,6,16] The etiologic agents described above are notorious infectious agents which have a worldwide distribution, and could possibly be encountered in a burn injury. Although, the frequency of occurrence has been negligible, this might be explained by the fact that most of these agents are sensitive to penicillin G, except in the case of *Erysipelothrix*, which is sensitive to erythromycin.

Spore-forming bacilli

The endospore-forming rods exist in two separate genera: those that are aerobic and those that are anaerobic. The aerobic variety is the *Bacillus* sp. and has been given the nom de plume of contaminant because of its ubiquitousness with one exception, *B. anthracis*, the cause of anthrax. It grows readily on solid media with a ground glass look and 'Medusahead' colony formation is characteristic. *B. anthracis* is not often found in burn wound infec-

tions, unless contact with contaminated soil has occurred. This organism is now becoming a bioterroristic agent.

The Gram stain often unveils a bacillus with square ends. Kingsley[17] employed PEA and chloral hydrate (CH) as a selective media to identify *B. anthracis* from other *Bacillus* sp. (**Table 11.9**). *Bacillus* sp. other than *B. anthracis* have recently been implicated as etiologic agents that are involved in bacteremia, septicemia, meningitis, and bronchopneumonia.[17–20] Turnball *et al.* provided evidence of a severe necrotic enterotoxin being produced by *B. cereus*.[20] As with the diphtheroids, the isolation of a *Bacillus* sp. in any specimen must not be taken lightly.

Table 11.9 Biological characteristics of the genus *Bacillus**

	SBAP hemolysis	Nitrate reduction	Motility	CH	PEA
B. anthracis	−	+	−	−	−
B. cereus	+	+	V	+	+
B. subtilis	+	+	+	V	+
B. megaterium	+	−	+	+	−

*Modified from Heggers J. Microbiology for surgeons. In: Kerstein MD, ed. *Management of Surgical Infections*. Mt Kisco, NY: Futura Publishing Co., 1980: 27–55. SBAP, Sheep blood agar; CH, chloral hydrate; PEA, phenylethyl alcohol; V, variable; −, negative; +, positive.

The anaerobic correlate is the genus *Clostridium*. Clostridia, like the aerobic gram-positive *Bacillus*, are also ubiquitous in nature. All species can produce *spores*. However, they are rarely seen in clinical specimens unless the tissue samples are necrotic. Those infections considered as exogenous are caused by this group: tetanus, gas gangrene (myonecrosis), botulism, food-borne gastrointestinal symptoms, and cellulitis. Predisposing constituents giving rise to endogenous infections include surgery, and any underlying disease entities such as leukemia, carcinoma, diabetes, as well as the use of immunosuppressive drugs. The necrotizing and hemolytic exotoxin of *Cl. perfringens* can be seen by the presence of an opalescence with the use of egg yolk agar. *Cl. perfringens* is commonly associated with myonecrosis and can probably be differentiated from *Cl. bifermentans*, *Cl. novyi*, and *Cl. septicum*, because of its distinctive 'double zone' hemolysis.[16]

Anaerobic infections in burned patients are usually associated with avascular muscle found in electrical injuries, frost bite, or cutaneous flame burns with concomitant crush-type injuries.[21–25] The high risk of developing tetanus (*C. tetani*), even with small burns, has led to the accepted practice of tetanus prophylaxis (tetanus toxoid 0.5 ml) as a routine part of the admission protocol for most burn centers.[26,27] In addition, if prior immunization is absent or unclear, or their last booster was more than 10 years ago, 250 units of tetanus antitoxin is also given. This is not unlike the administration of DAT (see page 127, Nonsporogenous).

Gram-negative aerobic rods

This family of gram-negative rods contains a distinctive group of etiologic agents of burn wound infections. Of this group aggregation, the *Pseudomonas* species are most repeatedly encountered and are chronic or acute. Earlier confrontations with this group of microbes were ignored as they were categorized as 'saprophytes'. This group of organisms are gram-negative and motile. They utilize carbohydrates oxidatively rather than through fermentation.

Since 1960, *Pseudomonas aeruginosa* has been recognized as a major burn pathogen.[28,29] Since that time it has increased its presence not only in burns but in other forms of trauma.[30] However *Ps. aeruginosa* is not the only documented pathogen among this group; other *Pseudomonas* species have been involved in nosocomial infection. After employing solutions of aqueous chlorohexidine, many infections due to *Burkholderia cepacia* occurred in a London hospital.[31] The microorganism had somehow contaminated the chlorhexidine solution. The contamination of a water supply in a hospital by *Stenotrophomonas multivorans* (formerly *Pseudomonas*) gave rise to a sequence of infections within that environment.[32] Twenty-two multiformities of surgical wounds and urinary tract conditions yielded *Ps. maltophilia* as reported by Gilardi,[33] with all species of *Pseudomonas* showing alterations in their susceptibility patterns with a prominent tendency toward resistance to newly developed antibiotics. This organism, however, is no longer called either a pseudomonad or *Xanthomonas* but has been placed in the genus *Stenotrophomonas*.[2,3,6,33] While similar to *Ps. aeruginosa* it is oxidase-negative, whereas *Ps. aeruginosa* is positive. *Sten. maltophilia* was the second most commonly isolated organism in burn wounds compared with *Ps. aeruginosa*. However, it has been our experience that *Acinetobacter* has replaced it. It is very adapt at rapidly developing a broad-spectrum antibiotic resistance. This resistance can emerge by changes to the expression of the chromosomal β-lactamase inducible populations and can be selected during therapy with broad-spectrum cephalosporins, sometimes causing clinical failure. Those organisms that fall into this select group include *Ps. aeruginosa*, *Stenotrophomonas*, *Enterobacter*, *Serratia*, *Citrobacter*, and *Morganella*, to mention a few.[2,3,6,31–33]

Alcaligenes faecalis, another gram-negative motile rod, is often considered *persona non grata* among the pathogenic organisms. However, it must be considered as an opportunistic pathogen[3,6] (**Table 11.10**). Its natural habitat is similar to *Ps. aeruginosa* in that it maintains a very close relationship with soil and water. Additionally in hospital settings it has been isolated from respirators, nebulizers, IV solutions, and hemodialysis systems.

Acinetobacter sp. are part of the indigenous flora of the respiratory, skin, as well as the gastrointestinal and genitourinary tracts of man and animals. They have been isolated from a diversity of clinical sources, including upper and lower respiratory tracts, urinary tract, surgical and burn wounds, and in bacteremias secondary to IV catheterization. Also occasional cases of septicemia or pneumonia have occurred in attenuated patients. Many of these patients who develop infections with this microorganism have had various manipulations including the use of respiratory therapy equipment, tracheal intubation, or bladder or central venous line catheterization (**Table 11.10**). While an agent of low virulence it has a predilection for infecting patients with dysfunctional host defense mechanisms. It develops a high degree of antimicrobial resistance. This resistance may be a direct result of previous antimicrobial therapy. While current taxonomy for *Acinetobacter* accepts only one species, *Acin. calcoaceticus*, it should be recognized that two biochemically distinct varieties exist within the species. Those species that form acid from dextrose are called *Acin. calcoaceticus* var. *anitratus*, while those that do not are called var. *Iwoffi*. It has been our experience that the *anitratus* variety is the one most resistant to antibiotics in the 1990s; however, to date (1999–2000) the majority of our *Acinetobacter* isolates have been a multiresistant *Acin. baumanni/hemolyticus*[34] sensitive only to imipenem/ampicillin-sulbactam. However, to date we have not experienced any major problems with this agent. In fact its incidence has been negligible.

Achromobacter sp. are frequently isolated from blood, the ear, urine, the respiratory tract, surgical and burn wounds, as well as feces. Some of the *Achromobacter* features necessary for identification can be found in **Table 11.10**. *Achromobacter* sp. are opportunistic pathogens, frequently found in the hospital water supply. As with all of the above it has a predilection for water.

Aeromonas (*Aer. hydrophila*) has been implicated as an etiological agent of human gastroenteritis. It produces several types of enterotoxins. Based on the results of laboratory studies, *Aer. hydrophila* has been shown to produce additional factors such as hemolysins (cytotoxins), endotoxin,[35] leukocidin,[36] and phospholipases.[37] Each of these factors, as well as any combination, may contribute to the pathogenesis of disease mediated by *Aer. hydrophila*. Fatal and nonfatal water-borne *Aeromonas* infections are associated with various clinical manifestations including septicemia,[38–46] meningitis,[42] endocarditis,[42] corneal ulcers,[43] peritonitis,[44] and wound infections.[45,46] Most strains of *Aer. hydrophila* are hemolytic on blood agar, and their culture filtrates lyse 1% suspensions of rabbit blood cells. These observations indicate that hemolysin produced by *Aer. hydrophila* may play an important role in the pathogenesis of disease. The significance of this microorganism as a human pathogen is better recognized now as more clinical laboratories are using proper diagnostic tests such as the indophenol oxidase test. In addition, *Aer. hydrophila* has been shown to be invasive in HEp-2 cell monolayers[47] and adherent to

Table 11.10 Biological responses of *Pseudomonas* and other gram-negative rods*									
Genus	Hemolysis	Motile	Oxidase	Citrate	Urea	Nitrate	Oxidase glucose	Arginine dehydrolase	Growth on SS
Pseudomonas	b	+	+	+	V	+	+	V	+
Alcaligenes	a	+	+	–/+	–	–	–	–	–
Acinetobacter	–	–	–	–	–	+	–	+
Achromobacter	+	+		+			+		+
Aeromonas	+	+		–	+	– (acid/gas) fermented	–	+

* Modified from Heggers J. Microbiology for surgeons. In: Kerstein MD, ed. *Management of Surgical Infections*. Mt Kisco, NY: Futura Publishing Co., 1980: 27–55.
SS, Shigella Salmonella Agar; a, alpha hemolysis; b, beta hemolysis; V, variable; +, positive; –, negative; –/+, more negative than positive.

human blood cells.[48] These also may be important virulence properties of the organism. Three cases of *Aer. hydrophila* burn wound infection have been reported by Purdue and Hunt.[49] Because of the aquatic nature of these organisms, infections may be related to trauma and concomitant exposure to water and soil. All three of the cases included a history of extinguishing the fire with dirty water or by rolling in dirt. These actions should alert the physician to consider *Aer. hydrophila* as a possible etiologic agent of infection.

Gram-negative facultatively anaerobic rods (Enteric Bacteria)

The largest and most repeatedly encountered group of microorganisms populating any burn wound environment along with the *Staphylococcus* sp. are the enterics, and they are found in the family of Enterobacteriaceae. This family contains 12 individual genera. Many of these organisms were previously categorized as nonpathogens and among these were the *Klebsiella–Enterobacter* group, *Serratia marcescens*, *Providencia* species and *Erwinia* species.[3,6,50]

Esch. coli, probably the most well known enteric, has been responsible for a wide diversity of infectious processes. Among these are: (1) frequently severe and sometimes fatal infections such as appendicitis, cystitis, pyelitis, peritonitis, septicemia, and gall bladder infections; (2) surgical and burn wound sepsis, and epidemic diarrhea of children and adults; and (3) 'travelers' diarrhea'. *Esch. coli* can be identified from other members of Enterobacteriaceae by its response to the classical IMVIC (indole, methyl red, Voges–Proskauer and citrate) reaction (++−) (**Table 11.11**).

The *Klebsiella–Enterobacter* group (K–E) are also gram-negative rods that are either motile or nonmotile. Fifty-one percent of moderately ill hospitalized patients had either *Kl. pneumoniae*, *Ent. aerogenes*, or *Ent. cloacae* isolated from their oropharyngeal space.[51] *Kl. pneumoniae* and its family are fast becoming a regular pathogen in nosocomial infections.[52] It is interesting that earlier isolation of the K–E group flora was thought to be part of the normal flora of the bronchial tree. The tribe Klebsiella is currently comprised of the genera *Klebsiella*, *Enterobacter*, and *Serratia*. Since the initial identification in 1823 of *Ser. marcescens*, it has maintained a valueless position as a 'saprophyte'.[53] It was primarily considered so harmless it was used to examine bacterial drift and settling rates in New York subways in 1964.[54] The idea seemed so very logical since *Ser. marcescens* produces a predominant chromogenic red pigment. However, 3 years later, Davis *et al.* reported that 94% of all the isolates from urinary tract infections were due

to *Ser. marcescens*.[54] He also discovered that the mortality rate in these patients was 33%. Thirty-five occurrences of *Ser. marcescens* bacteremia were reported in military personnel returning from Vietnam with accompanying burn wound infections.[55] The ubiquitousness of this microorganism has made it a serious pathogenic agent. It has been isolated on heart values after cardiac surgery,[56,57] in surgical and burn wound infections, in sepsis after splenectomy, and repeatedly in nosocomial outbreaks and disseminated by poor hygienic practices.[58,59] **Table 11.11** examines of its some predominant biochemical responses.

The remaining enterics consist of three additional genera: *Proteus*, *Providencia*, and *Morganella*. The genus *Proteus* is composed of two species: *Prot. mirabilis* and *Prot. vulgaris*. Both species can be found in massive concentrations in the feces of individuals undergoing oral antibiotic therapy. This group of organisms are often accountable for surgical and burn wound infections, intra-abdominal infections, as well as bacteremias and urinary tract infections. Some key biological features can be found in **Table 11.11**. The genus *Providencia* is composed of three species: *Prv. alcalifaciens*, *Prv. stuartii* and *Prv. rettgeri* which were formerly in the genus *Proteus*. *Providencia* species, like *Ser. marcescens*, have a broad range of pathologic involvement, from nosocomial infections[60,61] to septicemias, postoperative incisional wounds, burn wounds, pneumonias, and urinary tract infections.[60] These gram-negative bacilli fall into the general category of the paracolon bacteria and are categorized as a member of the genus *Proteus*, which is classified in Bergey's manual as *Prot. inconstans*.[6,50] The biological responses of this group of organisms are listed in **Table 11.11**. *Prv. stuartii* has been incriminated in numerous infections of patients in a burn unit, to include urinary tract infections as well.

Morganella morganii is the only species in the genus *Morganella* and was considered earlier a member of the genus *Proteus*. *M. morganii* has been co-joined with wound infections as well as urinary tract infections.

The *Erwinia* genus consists of 13 distinct species, all of which have been identified as plant pathogens, albeit *Erw. herbicola* which has managed to become pathogenic for man. The principal controversy ruminating around this organism lies in its ability to mimic *Esch. coli*. *Erwinia* are identical to all other gram-negative motile bacteria belonging to the Enterobacteriaceae.[6,50] Graevenitz and Strouse have reported *Erwinia* in human wound infections.[62,63] The enterics are not fastidious and require minimal medium for growth, and will grow on SBAP, MACA, gram-negative enrichment broth (GN broth), eosin methylene blue agar (EMB), as well

Table 11.11 Biological responses of some of the major Enterobacteriaceae*

Organism	Indole	MR	VP	Citrate	Urease	Motility	Arginine dihydrolase	KCN	H$_2$S
E. coli	+	+	−	−	−	V	V	−	−
Citrobacter	V	+	−	+	V	+	+	V	V
Klebsiella spp.	−	−	+	+	V	−	−	+	−
Enterobacter spp.	−	V	V	+	V	+	V	V	−
Ser. marcescens	−	V	+	+	−	+	−	+	−
Proteus spp.	+	+	−	V	+	+	?	V	V
Providencia	+	+	−	+	−	+	?	+	−
Morganella	+	+	−	−	+	+	−	+	−

* Modified from Heggers J. Microbiology for surgeons. In: Kerstein MD, ed. *Management of Surgical Infections*. Mt Kisco, NY: Futura Publishing Co., 1980: 27–55.
MR, Methyl red test; VP, Voges–Proskauer test; V, variable; −, negative; +, positive; ?, uncertain.

as nutrient agar. On MACA and EMB, lactose fermenters incorporate the dye contained in the media, while the nonlactose fermenters do not and therefore appear colorless. Triple sugar iron agar (TSI) slants are used to further identify the enterics based on biochemical changes in the medium[6,50] (**Table 11.12**).

Table 11.12 TSI reaction for some Enterobacteriaceae				
Organism	Slant	Butt	H$_2$S	Gas
Escherichia	A[b](K)[c]	A	–	+(–)
Citrobacter	A or K	A	V	+
K/E[a] group	A or K	A	–	+
Serratia spp.	K or A	A	–	–
Proteus vulgaris	A(K)	A	+	+
P. mirabilis	K(A)	A	+	+
M. morganii	K	A	–	–
Providencia	K	A	–	+/–
Prv. rettgeri	K	A	–	–

Butt, bottom of the test tube;
[a] *Klebsiella/Enterobacter* group; [b] acid reaction; [c] alkaline reaction; (), occasional; V, variable; –, negative; +, positive; +/–, more positive than negative.

Like the gram-positive clinical isolates, the gram-negative isolates from the burn wound are equally selective. While man's environment is overwhelmed with microbes, only a select smattering of gram-negative rods predominate, which specifically includes the pseudomonads and enterics, with *Ps. aeruginosa* being the predominant isolate, followed by *Esch. coli* and the other enterics. In comparing the gram-negative isolates for 1999 with those identified in a 1988–1989 study, we observed an increase in the number of *Ps. aeruginosa* isolates (53.4%) over 1988–1989 (33.6%), almost a 20% increase (**Table 11.13**). Another interesting observation was the appearance of *Acinetobacter baum/haem*, accounting for 46.8% of the nonfermentors and combined with *Ps. aeruginosa*, accounting for 53.4% of the total gram-negative isolates (**Table 11.13**). This appearance of *Acinetobacter* spp, in the ICU setting was experienced worldwide.

Miscellaneous gram-negative rods

Two species of some consequence in burn wound infections of man are *Flavobacterium meningosepticum* and *Chromobacterium violaceum*. Other members of this genera are natural inhabitants of soil, water, and vegetable, and are classified as contaminants.[6,50] *Fl. meningosepticum* is a gram-negative bacillus that is nonmotile and aerobic with a strictly respiratory type of metabolism. It grows at 37°C and produces a yellow to orange pigment on solid media. It is catalase-, oxidase-, and phosphatase-positive. Acid is produced from carbohydrates but no gas is produced. *Fl. meningosepticum* is widely distributed in soil and water, and is found in raw meats, milk, and other foods, in the hospital environment, and in human clinical material. Biochemical identification is presented in **Table 11.14**. It is consistently resistant to many antibiotics and has been isolated from burn wound with relative inconsistency, but when isolated it should be regarded as a pathogen.

Chrom. violaceum is a gram-negative bacillus that is motile and produces a violet ring in nutrient broth, with ideal growth at 30–35°C usually requiring 7 days for its total growth at 37°C, whereas *Fl. meningosepticum* is Gram-negative, 7 days nonmotile, and produces a yellow pigment on solid media also requiring 7 days for full development (although at room temperature). No pigment is produced at 37°C nor is there hemolysis, though the agar may exhibit a lavender/green discoloration as a result of proteolytic enzymatic activity. One major problem with this group of organisms is their natural habitat. Their close living arrangements with their human hosts give them a tactical advantage not only for the development of tolerance but resistance. Misuse or abuse of parenteral or enteral antibiotics can provide an environment for the formation of resistance. Consumers of food products generated through antibiotic feeding as well as unlicensed antibiotic usage are prime targets for the development of resistant organisms.

Table 11.13 10-Year comparison of gram-negative organisms isolated from pediatric burns						
Organism	Jan–Dec 1999		Overall %	1988–1989*		Overall % of
	No	%	of the group	No	%	the group
Ps. aeruginosa	334	35.2	53.4	1591	33.6	33.6
Ac. baum/haem	173	18.2	46.8	–	–	
E. coli	130	13.7		990	21.0	
K. pneumoniae	83	8.8	35.9	714	15.1	50.6
Ent. cloacae	105	11.1		384	8.1	
Ser. marcescens	22	2.3		304	6.4	
Other GNR	102	10.7		723	15.8	
Total GNR	949	100.0		4.733	100.0	
Total isolates	2273	41.8		14,696	32.2	

*From Heggers JP, McCauley R, Herndon DN. *Antimicrobial Therapy in Burn Patients. Part 1, Surgical Rounds*, 1992; July: 613–617.

Table 11.14 Key biochemical responses for the pathogenic genera *Chromobacterium* and *Flavobacterium*									
Species	Oxidase	Motility	Growth at 37°C	Indole	NO$_2$ to NO$_3$	Casein	Arginine dihydrolase	H$_2$S lead acetate strip	O-F media glucose maltose
Chr. violaceum	V	+	+	–	+	+	+	–/W[a]	–
Fl. meningosepticum	+	–	+	+	–	+	–	+	+

[a] = Weak reaction.
O-F, oxidation fermentation; V, Variable; +, positive; –, negative.

Gram-negative anaerobic bacilli

The most repeatedly confronted organisms in this group which may play a fearful role in surgical and burn wound infections are *Bacteroides* sp. and *Fusobacterium* sp. They are considered normal flora of the human body, beginning at the oropharyngeal cavity and ending at the gastrointestinal (GI) and urogenital tracts. Numerically they account for the major population in the oropharyngeal region in a 5:1 ratio over the aerobes and facultative anaerobes, while in the urogenital and GI tract the ratio is more dynamic at a 1000:1.[2,6,16,50] Yet when one scrutinizes the current statistics of anaerobic infections related to locality, all but 2–5% of surgical wound infections occurring in the oropharyngeal area are caused by the anaerobic[64] flora. Those occurring in the GI and urogenital tract are only responsible for about 10–15% of the wound infections.[65,66] Prior surgery, malignant neoplasms, arteriosclerosis, diabetes mellitus, prior antibiotic therapy, alcoholism, improper debridement, and steroid and immunosuppressive therapy are commonly major contributors associated in these types of wound infections.[65,66] Specimens collected for anaerobic organisms should be placed in appropriate transport tubes void of atmospheric O_2 or remain in syringes with attached needles containing suspect aspirates sealed off with a rubber stopper. **Table 11.15** examines some of the biochemical responses of this group of organisms. However, with the advent of the early excision and grafting, the incidence of anaerobic infections in the thermal injury has been reduced to a nonentity; therefore anaerobic cultures are uneconomical. Culturing for these anaerobes would be futile, as they require vascular tissue for survival. Their presence would only be observed if such tissue were to remain.

Fungi (Myceteae)

Until the advent of topical antimicrobial agents, fungal infections were not common in burned patients. However, the incidence of mycotic invasion has doubled since the implementation of topical antimicrobial agents to control bacterial colonization.[67,68] The burn wound is the most commonly infected site, although local or disseminated fungal infections of the respiratory tract, urinary tract, GI tract, and vagina are increasingly common.[67,69,70] *Candida* sp. are the most common nonbacterial colonizers of the burn wound, although true fungi such as *Aspergillus*, *Penicillium*, *Rhizopus*, *Mucor*, *Rhizomucor*, *Fusarium*, and *Curvularia* are not uncommon and have a much greater invasive potential than the yeasts.[71–74] (**Table 11.16**).

Early diagnosis of fungal infection is difficult as clinical symptoms frequently mimic low-grade bacterial infections. Routine culture techniques may require from 7 to 14 days to identify fungal contaminants, delaying the initiation of treatment as these pathogens are frequently not recovered in culture.[68] In contrast to bacterial sepsis, venous blood cultures may not reflect the causative organism.[74,75] Arterial blood cultures and retinal examination for characteristic candidal lesions can be useful. The isolation of *Candida* from three organs is usually required for the diagnosis of candidal sepsis.[69] Serum antibody titers to *Candida* have recently been advocated to assist in the early diagnosis.[76] Premortem diagnosis, confirmed with sufficient time to implement appropriate treatment, occurs in less than 40% of infected patients.[77] Because of their relatively large size, *Candida* are usually filtered out of blood at the capillary level. Organisms are usually seen in the urine when sepsis from a distant site occurs. Candidal sepsis is considered when *Can. albicans* can be isolated from three different tissue sites, i.e. blood, wound, urine, bronchial washings, or by a positive retinal examination. Candidal spores are omnipresent in the burned patient, appearing in stools, nasopharynx swabs, urine samples, and cultures of intact integument; however, fewer than 20% of patients with candidal wound colonization develop widespread candidiasis.[73,78] Only when the controlling bacterial populations are eradicated by systemic antibiotics or the host becomes immunosuppressed does candidal infection occur,[79] frequently following a bacterial sepsis. There is a 3–5% incidence of candidemia in the burned population[69,71,78,80] and a comparable rate of burn wound invasion.[71] Candidal infections occur most commonly in patients with large burn injuries who are hospitalized for long periods of time and have received multiple courses of antibiotics. Prophylactic treatment with oropharyngeal and topical nystatin have therefore become recommended.[69] However, fluconazole may be more effective in some cases.[78,79]

Unlike candidal infections, true fungal infections occur early in

Table 11.16 Colonization, infection, and invasive potential of the fungi

	Filamentous fungi	*Candida*
Incidence		
Colonization	2–4.4%	30–40%
Infection	1–2%	5–7%
Dissemination	1–2%	2–4%
Time of occurrence	Early	Late
Mortality		
With invasive infection	90–100%	80–100%

Table 11.15 Biochemical responses of the Bacteroidaceae

Organism	Hemolysis	Fermenter glucose	Indole	Catalase	20% Bile agar	Esculin hydrolysis	Black pigment	Kanamycin (1 MG disk)	H₂S
Bacteroides									
distasonis	–	+	–	+	+	+	–	R	–
fragilis	–	+	–	+	+	+	–	R	–
vulgatus	–	+	–	V	+	V	–	R	–
melaninogenicus									
Fusobacterium									
mortiferum	V	+	–	–	+	+	–	S	–
necrophorum	–	–	+	–	–	–	–	S	+
nucleatum	Green	–	+	–	–	–	–	S	+

V, variable; R, resistant; S, sensitive; +, positive; –, negative.

the hospital course of patients with specific predisposing characteristics. Most frequently, burned patients infected with fungi are exposed to spores in the environment by either rolling on the ground or jumping into surface water at the time of injury. Other environmental foci have been cited as the source of nosocomial fungal infection, including bandaging supplies left open to air, heating, and air conditioning ducts and floor drains.[81–83] Once colonized, broad nonbranching hyphae extend into subcutaneous tissue, stimulating an inflammatory response. This phenomena is diagnostic of fungal wound infection. Vascular invasion is common and often accompanied by thrombosis and avascular necrosis, clinically observed as rapidly advancing dark discolorations of the wound margins or well-described lesions.[68,72] Systemic dissemination of the infection occurs with invasion of the vasculature. **Table 11.17** provides information regarding this distribution of *Can. albicans* and other yeast isolates along with other pathogenic and saprophytic fungi which caused fungemia during the 1999 era. *Candida* accounted for 58% of fungemias encountered, followed by the true fungi which accounted for the remaining 42% of the fungemias (**Table 11.17**).

Table 11.17 Yeasts and fungi isolated from pediatric burn wounds from January 1, 1999 to December 31, 1999

Organisms	Jan–Dec 1999 No	%	Overall % of the group
C. albicans	64	97	
G. candidum	2	3.0	58%
Total yeast	66	100.0	
Total isolates	114		
Aspergillus sp.	13	27.1	
Fusarium sp.	10	20.8	
Penicillin sp.	9	18.7	
Curvularia sp.	6	12.5	42%
Bioplaris sp.	5	10.4	
Scedosporium sp.	3	6.3	
Rhizomucor sp.	2	4.2	
Total fungi	48	100.0	
Total isolates	114		

Viruses

Viral infections are being clinically recognized more frequently in burned patients. Prospective and retrospective assays of sera have documented a large incidence of subclinical viral infection. Retrospectively, Linneman[84] assayed stored sera of burned children and found a fourfold increase in antibodies to cytomegalovirus (CMV) in 22% of patients, 8% had increased herpes simplex titers, and 5% demonstrated a rise in varicella zoster titers. The study continued in a prospective manner, with 33% of the children developing CMV infection, 25% developing herpetic infections, and 17% developing adenovirus infection. CMV infection typically occurs approximately 1 month postburn and clinically presents as a fever of unknown origin and lymphocytosis.[85] Rarely are patients with less than 50% total body surface area (TBSA) burn infected. CMV infection frequently occurs concurrently with bacterial and fungal infections, but rarely alters the patient's clinical course. CMV inclusions may be identified in the cells of multiple organs, but have not been reported in the burn

wound.[86] The burned patients who most commonly contract the infection are known to have received multiple blood transfusions, which represent a major source of contamination.

Most commonly, herpetic lesions appear in healing partial-thickness burns or split-thickness donor sites, although other epithelial surfaces such as the oral or intestinal mucosa can be involved. In the latter case, herpetic lesions may lead to erosion and perforation. The clinical manifestations of lesions may be preceded by unexplained fever unresponsive to routine antibiotic coverage.[87] Partial-thickness burns and donor sites infected with herpes may 'convert' to full-thickness injuries requiring skin grafting for ultimate closure. Necrotizing hepatic and adrenal lesions may lead to multisystem organ failure. Mortality in patients with disseminated infection is about twice that expected for patients of similar age and burn size. Split-thickness grafts provide adequate coverage of previously infected herpetic wounds.[88]

Chickenpox (varicella zoster) infection is a frequent occurrence in school-aged children and is rapidly spread through inhalation of the virus. Varicella infections can be life-threatening in an immunocompromised host and mini-epidemics have occurred within pediatric burn units.[88] The characteristic fluid-filled lesions appear in healed or healing partial-thickness burn, as well as uninjured epithelium and mucous membranes. Due to the fragility of the newly healed or healing skin, the vesicles are much more destructive in the injured than in the uninjured skin, and may present as hemorrhagic, oozing pockmarks which are prone to secondary infection and subsequent scarring. New, neovascularized skin grafts may be lost and further grafting procedures should be delayed until the lesions are quiescent. Herpes simplex and zoster are consistently treated with systemic acyclovir or SV$_\Lambda$Galtrex.

Parasitic infections

In this age of the New Millennium when our world has been capsulized and world travel is now commonplace, we therefore must include a discussion of those organisms endemic to the patients origin which could complicate the burn injury. In our repertoire of lab examinations we did include a stool sample for ova and parasites. However, based on a study conducted by Barret *et al.* in 1999,[89] the authors concluded that patients being admitted from developing countries where parasitism is endemic should be treated empirically with antiparasite drug, preferably metronidazole or mebendazole (**Table 11.18**). They should be subsequently tested 2 weeks post-therapy. **Table 11.18** provides a list of those important parasites and recommended therapies frequently encountered from patients admitted from endemic developing countries and their recommended therapy. **Figures 11.1a,b–11.7a,b** are schematic representations of the most common endemic parasites. Recently it was noted that burn patients with smoke inhalation are at serious risk of mortality due to an *Ascaris* infection.[90]

Histopathologic approach based on clinical findings

An open wound is a favorable target for bacterial colonization. The term colonization indicates only the presence of viable bacteria on the surface of the wound or in the burn eschar. Although potentially dangerous, wound colonization does not imply that locally destructive or systemic infection is present. If the microorganisms successfully invade into viable tissue, they will produce a locally

Table 11.18 Drugs and dosages for treating parasitic infections

Organism or infection	Drug	Dosage	Follow-up
Ancylostoma duodenale	Mebendazole or Pyrantel pamoate or Albendazole	100 mg BID × 3 days 11 mg/kg (max 1 g) × 3 days 400 mg once	Fecal examination 2–4 wk post therapy If eggs are rare in fecal concentrations. There is no need to repeat therapy
Ascaris lumbricoides	Mebendazole or Pyrantel pamoate or Albendazole	100 mg BID × 3 days 11 mg/kg once (max 1 g) 400 mg once	Fecal examination 2–4 wk post therapy
Balantidium coli	Tetracycline or	500 mg QID × 10 days Children (8 years): 10 mg/kg/day OID × 10 days (max 2 g/day)	At least three negative fecal examinations 1 month after therapy
	Iodoquinol or	650 mg TID × 20 days Children: 40 mg/kg/day in three doses × 20 days	
	Metronidazole	750 mg TID × 5 days Children: 35–50 mg/kg/day in three doses × 5 days	
Blastocystis	Clinical significance is controversial: Metronidazole	750 mg TID × 10 days Children: 30–40 mg/kg/day in three doses × 10 days	Fecal examinations 2 wk to 1 month after therapy (must include permanent stain)
	or Iodoquinol	650 mg TID × 20 days Children: 30–40 mg/kg/day in three doses × 20 days	
Diphyllobothrium latum	Praziquantel or Niclosamide	10–20 mg/kg once 2 g once Children 11–34 kg: 1 g once >34 kg: 1.5 g once	Fecal examinations for eggs and proglottids 1 and 3 months after therapy
Entamoeba histolytica Asymptomatic cyst Passer	Iodoquinol or	650 mg/kg TID × 20 days Children: 30–40 mg/kg/day in three doses × 20 days	Fecal examinations 2 wk to 1 month after therapy (must include permanent stained smear)
	Paromomycin or Diloxanide	25–35 mg/kg TID × 7 days 500 mg TID × 10 days Children: 20 mg/kg/day in three doses × 10 days	
Invasive amebiasis	Metronidazole or	750 mg TID × 10 days Children: 35–50 mg/kg TID × 10 days	Monitor clinical response to therapy; follow-up with CT, ultrasonography,
	Tinidazole	600 mg BID or 800 mg TID × 5 days Children: 50 mg/kg or 60 mg/kg (max 2 g) every day × 3 days	and radionuclide scans
Enterobius vermicularis	Pyrantel pamoate or	11 mg/kg once (max 1 g); repeat after 2 wk Children: 1 mg/kg once (max 1 g); repeat after 2 wk	Monitor clinical response; follow-up with Scotch tape check of perianal area if symptoms persist (may take four to six consecutive negative tapes to rule out infection)
	Mebendazole or	100 mg once, repeat after 2 wk Children: 100 mg once; repeat after 2 wk	
	Albendazole	400 mg once; repeat after 2 wk	
Giardia lamblia	Metronidazole or	250 mg TID × 5 days Children: 15 mg/kg/day in three doses × 5 days	Fecal examinations 2 wk to 1 month after therapy (must include permanent stained smear or ELISA or DFA exam);
	Tinidazole or	2 g once Children: 50 mg/kg once (max 2 g)	Entero-Test if stools are negative and patient is symptomatic
	Furazolidone or	100 mg QID × 7–10 days Children: 6 mg/kg/day in for doses × 7–10 days	
	Paromomycin	25–35 mg/kg/day in three doses × 7 days	

Table 11.18 Drugs and dosages for treating parasitic infections –, *continued*

Organism or infection	Drug	Dosage	Follow–up
Necator americanus	Mebendazole or Pyrantel pamoate or Albendazole	100 mg BID × 3 days 11 mg/kg once (max 1 g) 400 mg once	Fecal examinations 2–4 wk post therapy; if eggs are in fecal concentrations, there is no need to repeat therapy
Pediculus humanus	1% Permethrin or 0.5% Malathion or Pyrethrins with piperonyl butoxide	Apply lotion to body, allow to remain for 10 mm, then bathe Topically Topically with second application 1 wk later	Examine clothing and bedding for nits and lice
Sarcoptes scabiei	5% Permethrin Ivermectin or 10% Crotamiton	Massage from head to soles of feet; wash off after 8 to 14 h 200 µg/kg p.o. once Topically	Monitor clinical course. May need mild steroid cream in sensitive individuals
Strongyloides stercoralis	Ivermectin or Thiabendazole or Albendazole	200 µg/kg/day × 1–2 days 25 mg/kg BID × 2 days (max 3 g/day) 400 mg p.o. every day × 3 days	Fecal examinations and/or culture 1 month after therapy
Taenia saginata	Praziquantel or Niclosamide	5–10 mg/kg p.o. once 2 g (1.0 g p.o. and then 1 h later 1.0 g) Children: 11–34 kg: 1 g >34 kg: 1.5 g	Fecal examinations for eggs or proglottids 1 month after therapy
T. solium	Praziquantel or Niclosamide	5–10 mg/kg p.o. once Same as for *T. saginata*	Fecal examinations for eggs or proglottids 1 mo after therapy
Trichinella spiralis	Mebendazole Plus Corticosteroids	200–400 mg TID × 3 days, 400–500 mg TID × 10 days 20–60 mg/days p.o.	Monitor clinical course; muscle biopsy in severe cases
Trichomonas vaginalis	Metronidazole or Tinidazole	2 g once or 250 mg TID or 375 mg BID p.o. × 7 days Children: 5 mg/kg TID × 7 days 2 g once Children: 50 mg/kg once (max 2 g)	Pelvic examination 1 month after therapy
Trichuris trichiura	Mebendazole or Albendazole	100 mg BID × 3 days 400 mg once	Fecal examinations 2–4 wk after therapy

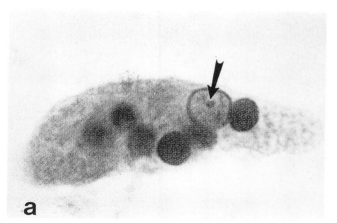

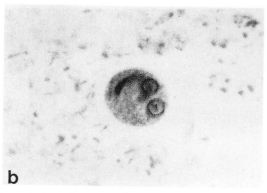

Fig. 11 .1 (a) *Entamoeba histolytica*, trophozoite with several ingested erythrocytes. The nuclear karyosome is slightly eccentric (arrow) (× 970 trichrome stain). (b) *Entamoeba histolytica* cyst with two nuclei present with several chromatoidal bars (× 970 iron hematoxylin stain).

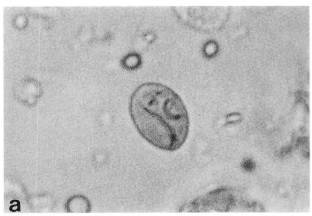
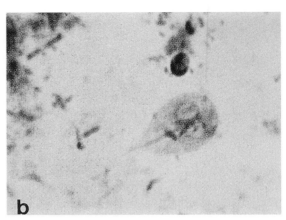

Fig. 11 .2 (a) *Giardia lamblia* cysts (× 970 iodine-stain) Note Voodoo mask appearance. (b) *Giardia lamblia* trophozoite, two karyosomes with candal flagella dividing the body in half (× 970 iron hematoxylin).

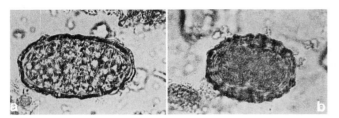

Fig. 11.3 (a) *Ascaris lumbricoides* infertilized egg (× 430) unstained; (b) fertilized egg of *A. lumbricoides* (× 430).

destructive infection (a septic burn wound) and may disseminate either viable bacteria or their toxic products systemically via blood or lymphatic vessels (burn wound sepsis). Evidently, the progression from simple colonization of the wound eschar to invasion of viable tissue is favored by a series of factors, which may be related to the patient (extension and depth of the burn, age, presence of prior disease, local condition of the wound), the microorganism

(density, motility, toxins, antimicrobial resistance), or the caregiver (iatrogenic causes). Systemic signs of infection may be obscured by metabolic or physiologic dysfunction in patients with severe burns. Therefore, it is essential to recognize the early signs of local burn wound infection. The burn wound should be examined at least once daily for signs of local wound infection[15,18,19] (**Table 11.19**).

Burn wound sepsis is suspected when a burn wound is the site of proliferating microorganisms exceeding 10^5/g tissue, and when there is invasion of subjacent unburned tissue.[29,91] The presence of microorganisms within the eschar or in necrotic tissue cannot be considered diagnostic of burn wound sepsis, but such colonization has the potential to invade viable tissue. Although a quantitative culture result of 10^5 viable microorganisms per gram of tissue correlates with a high probability of invasion of viable tissue, this is not necessarily the case. Therefore, burn wound culture should be accompanied by histologic study of a tissue sample from the same area when invasion of viable tissue is suspected.[92,93] It is strongly advised that continuous monitoring of the burn wound be con-

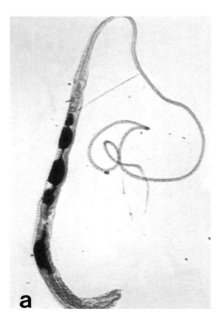
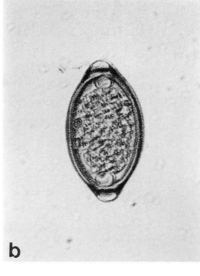

Fig. 11.4 (a) *Trichuris trichiuria* (*Trichocephalus*) adult female worm (×430 iron hematoxylin stain); (b) Fertilized *T. trichiuria* egg with usual polar plugs (×430 iodine stain).

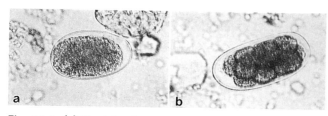

Fig. 11.5 (a) Unstained unsegmented *Necator americanus* egg (×430). (b) Segmented *N. americanus* with developing embryo (×430 iodine stain).

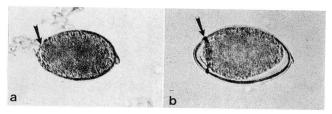

Fig. 11.6 (a) Iodine–stained *Diphyllobothrium latum* with operculum (arrow, ×430); (b) Immature unstained egg of *D. latum* with operculum (arrow, ×430).

Table 11.19 Burn wound infection: local signs*
Black or dark brown focal areas of discoloration
Enhanced sloughing of burned tissue or eschar
Partial-thickness injury converted to full-thickness necrosis
Purplish discoloration or edema of skin around the margins of the wound
Presence of ecthyma gangrenosa
Pyocyanotic appearance of subeschar tissue
Subcutaneous tissue with hemorrhagic discoloration
Variable-sized abscess formation and focal subeschar inconsistency

* Reproduced with permission from Heggars JP, Robson MC. Infection control in burn patients. *Clin Plas Surg* 1986; **13**: 39–47.

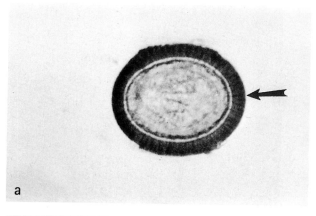

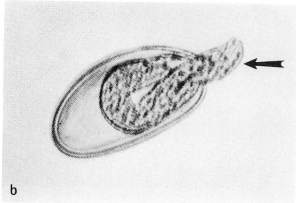

Fig. 11.7 (a) Unstained egg of *Taenia saginata* surrounded by mucous sheath (arrow, ×430); (b) Lava of a fully embrynoted egg (×430 iodine stain).

ducted to evaluate the possibility of bacterial invasion. The burned and unburned areas should be inspected daily for the presence of hemorrhagic, vesicular, or necrotic areas, and for gray, dark brown, or black spots as well as other unusual changes (**Table 11.19**). The suspected areas should be biopsied and the sample subjected to microbiological cultures and histopathologic studies. The specimens for both laboratories should be taken from adjacent areas. One biopsy sample divided in half usually suffices. The only requisite is that the specimen for histology must include surrounding viable tissue (**Figure 11.8a,b**).

Biopsies for histologic study are fixed in buffered formaldehyde, embedded in paraffin, and sections are collected on poly-lysine-coated or other adhesive slides. Sections are stained with hematoxylin and eosin, with the Brown and Hopps tissue Gram stain, and with methenamine silver, along with appropriate positive controls consisting of burn tissue that contains bacteria and fungi. When clinical suspicion of invasive wound infection is high and rapid surgical intervention is contemplated, frozen sections are prepared to allow rapid diagnosis. Necrotic subcutaneous tissue is difficult to study by frozen section, but the use of a commercial frozen sectioning aid (Instrumedics) has allowed us to provide frozen sections of consistently high quality from burned tissue. The frozen sections, like the routinely processed ones, are stained with hematoxylin and eosin, with the Brown and Hopps Gram stain, and with the methenamine silver stain for fungus. The controls should be frozen sections of infected tissue. This technique allows the samples to be evaluated for infection within approximately 2 hours of the time the biopsy is taken, depending on the number of samples. Findings on frozen sections are routinely confirmed by subsequent study of routinely processed tissue (**Figure 11.8c,d**).

Histologic diagnosis of invasive infection requires precise differentiation between tissue necrosis due to thermal injury and that due to invading microorganisms. The presence of microorganisms within the necrotic portion of a burn wound represents a hazard, but can represent saprophytic growth of organisms with

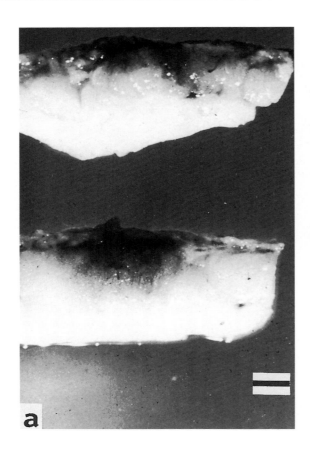

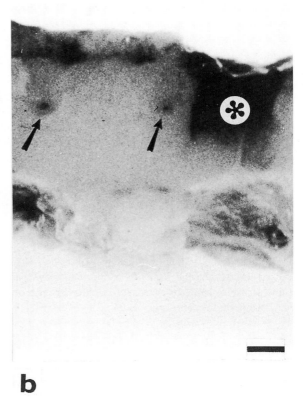

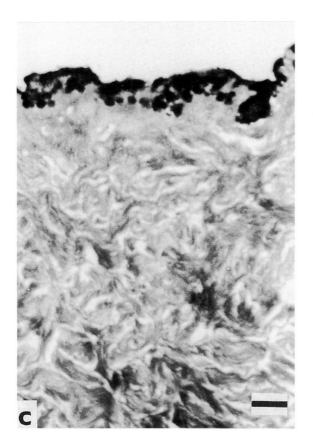

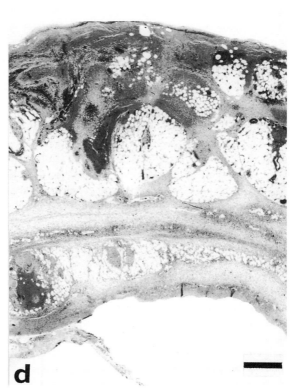

low pathogenic potential, and does not correlate well with clinical signs of sepsis. Necrosis is identified primarily on the basis of loss of nuclear staining (karyolysis) or prominent condensation of nuclear chromatin (pyknosis), or nuclear fragmentation (karyorrhexis). The presence of bacteria within intact, viable tissue, or surrounded by intact tissue is the basis for a diagnosis of invasion of viable tissue. The presence of polymorphonuclear neutrophils alone is not indicative of infection, since they often accumulate in sterile burn wounds. In fact, a band of neutrophils often is seen between the necrotic and viable tissue in a burn wound, or as a distinct necrotic remnant within the necrotic zone. In wounds infected by *Pseudomonas* species, bacteria may be seen in large numbers within the muscular walls of necrotic arteries. When fungi invade viable tissue, they often produce a wavefront of necrosis. This pattern is usually recognizable by the presence of fungal hyphae extending like fingers to the border between necrotic and intact tissue, and does represent dangerous invasion of viable tissue (see Chapter 36). The likelihood of bacterial invasion of viable tissue increases with burn depth. The morphologic sequence of increasingly dangerous infection includes the presence of clusters of bacteria on the specimen surface, clusters within the exudate and coagulum covering the wound, the presence of colonies of bacteria within necrotic hair follicles (connected to the surface), the presence of bacteria in clusters within the upper, middle, or deep portions of necrotic dermal tissue, colonization of necrotic subcutaneous tissue, and bacterial invasion into viable dermal or subcutaneous tissue (**Figure 11.8a,b**).

The evaluation of sepsis should include microbiological and histopathologic evaluation, along with clinical assessment of the patient. Blood cultures may be negative, or the selection of organisms isolated in culture may be altered by antibiotic therapy. The burn wound biopsy allows the location of bacterial growth to be determined, and the risk to the patient to be assessed more accurately. The biopsy also can detect abnormalities other than wound infection, and can uncover the presence of fungal or viral infections. These infections have a lower yield of culture isolation, may require special techniques for detection, and can occur as contaminants. Without biopsy, fungal and viral infections are difficult to recognize early. As antibacterial therapy becomes more effective, fungal wound infection is emerging as a cause of serious disease in a larger proportion of patients. If a viral infection is suspected, a Tzanck smear is very valuable. This procedure is very simple to perform. The suspected lesion, ideally the base of a freshly uncovered vesicle, is scraped firmly with the edge of a glass slide, and the resulting material is smeared on another slide and stained with a rapid Giemsa stain, or with Wright's stain or with methylene blue. The smear is examined under high magnification for the presence of multinucleated giant cells. This simple procedure allows rapid diagnosis of herpes virus infection (**Figure 11.9a,b,c,d**).

Clinical findings

Understanding Sepsis: New Findings, New Theories

Epidemiology of sepsis

Sepsis engendered by severe microbial infections continues to be a dominant and ravaging problem for patients around the world. Significant advancement has been achieved in the past 10 years in the evolution of consensus definitions for terms that had formerly been applied differently by divergent investigators: systemic inflammatory response syndrome (SIRS), sepsis (basically SIRS with infection), severe sepsis (basically sepsis with hypotension), and septic shock (severe sepsis with evidence of decreased perfusion and hypotension despite a fluid bolus). The terms are now considered to reflect a logical progression observed in a patient who, over time, is getting worse, commencing with SIRS and advancing toward septic shock. Roughly 400 000 cases of sepsis occur in the United States each year, with about 30–35% mortality. Sepsis is the 13th leading cause of morbidity and mortality in the US and it is the 11th leading cause of mortality for patients who are over 65.[94]

Another View of Sepsis: Changes for the Millennium

This hypothesis is constant with the concept that the pathophysiology of sepsis consists of a systemic response somewhat out of control. In this analysis, there is a local infection with a secondary systemic inflammatory involvement, which is the prime motivator of multiple organ failure. In fact, most evidence clearly shows that traumatized or septic patients have highly elevated levels of anti-eicosanoid mediators which classifies them immunocompromised. In other words the macrophages from these patients are tolerant to the lipopolysaccharide (LPS) of the microbial invaders and become anergic. The severity of trauma correlates with the degree of immunosuppression.

The key postulate is that evolution would have favored local inflammation and did a reversal on the systemic response (i.e. anti-inflammation). Based on this concept, local inflammation is necessary to control microbial invasion at the site of injury or infection, while an anti-inflammatory systemic response is required to eliminate damaging eicosanoid mediators in uninjured tissue. It should be realized that the neutralization of a single mediator could salvage patients with severe sepsis. The clinical diagnosis of sepsis can be made when clinical symptoms appear and a septic source can be identified. There are several cardinal signs of sepsis which embody both gram-negative as well as gram-positive involvement (**Table 11.20**). Constant surveillance of these signs can provide adjunctive information concerning the etiologic agent of sepsis. A septic source can be documented as: (1) burn wound biopsy with >10^5 organisms/g tissue and/or histologic evidence of viable tissue invasion; (2) positive blood culture; (3) urinary tract

Fig. 11.8 (opposite) *Burn wound infection.* (a) Discoloration of the subcutaneous tissue associated with *Pseudomonas* sp. invasion of viable tissue in a full-thickness burn. Gross anatomy. Bar = 3 mm. (b) Burn wound infection with bacterial vasculitis (arrows). The asterisk indicates the site of the punch biopsy. Note that the lower level of the punch biopsy reaches the viable tissue beyond the vasculitis level. Gross anatomy. Bar = 2 mm. (c) Superficial bacterial colonization (black discoloration). Gram stain. Bar = 50 μm. (d) Sections of skin showing necrosis and bacterial invasion reaching subcutaneous adipose tissue. Gram stain. Bar = 500 μm.

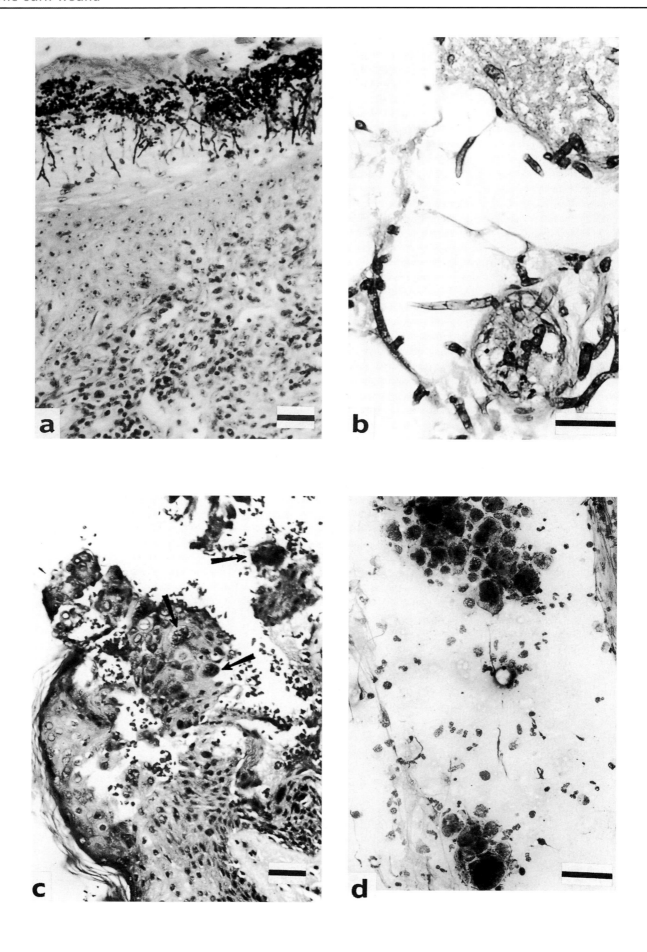

Table 11.20 Additional cardinal signs of burn wound sepsis*
Gram-negative sepsis
Burn wound biopsy >10⁵ organisms/g tissue and/or histologic evidence of viable tissue invasion
Rapid onset – well to ill in 8–12 hours
Increased temperature to 100–103°F (38°–39°C) or may remain within normal limits (37°C)
WBC may be increased
Followed by hypothermia – 94°F (34°–35°C) plus a decrease in WBC
Decreased bowel sounds (ileus)
Decreased BP and urinary output
Wounds develop focal gangrene
Satellite lesions away from burn wound
Mental obtundation
Gram-positive sepsis
Burn wound biopsy >10⁵ organisms/g tissue and/or histologic evidence of viable tissue invasion
Symptoms develop gradually
Increased temperature to 105°F or higher (>40°C)
WBC 20 000–50 000
Decreased hematocrit
Wound macerated in appearance, ropy and tenacious exudate
Anorexic and irrational
Decreased bowel sounds (ileus)
Decreased BP and urinary output
* Five or more signs or symptoms are definitive diagnostic parameters.

infection with $>10^5$ organisms/ml urine; (4) pulmonary infection with positive bacteria and white cells on a Class III or better sputum specimen. In addition to the identification of a septic source, at least five or more of the following criteria should be met: tachypnea (>40 breaths/min in adults), prolonged paralytic ileus, hyper or hypothermia (<36.5°C or >38.5°C), altered mental status, thrombocytopenia (<50 000 platelets/mm³), leukocytosis or penia (<3.5 or >15.0 cells/mm³), unexplained acidosis or hyperglycemia. Local evidence of invasive wound infection includes black or brown patches of wound discoloration, rapid eschar separation, conversion of wounds to full-thickness, spreading periwound erythema, punctate hemorrhagic subeschar lesions, and violaceous or black lesions in unburned tissue (ecthyma gangrenosum) (**Table 11.19**). When a patient exhibits signs and symptoms of sepsis, immediate institution of antibiotics is obligatory irrespective of the absence of confirmatory cultures. A delay of 3–4 days in a patient with a major burn wound result in an inordinately high morbidity. Specific antibiotic treatment should be administered if routine surveillance has identified the predominant organism (**Figures 11.10a,b,c,d and 11.11a,b**).

If we compare **Figure 11.10b** (reproduced from the 1st edition of this book) with **Figure 11.10a** for the year 1999 we see a drastic downward shift in susceptibility for *Esch. coli* for amikacin, aztreonam, and imipenem. This represents an overall 10–20% decrease in susceptibility. **Figure 11.10c** showing *Kl. pneumoniae* susceptibility patterns for 1988–1989 demonstrates a similar fluctuation when compared to **Figure 11.10a**. *Enterobacter cloacae*, on the other hand, has shown an increased resistance to amikacin and aztreonam when compared to the 1988–1989 results, while imipenem still remains effective for gram-negative coverage of the enterics (**Figure 11.10d**).

Of interest is the rapid development of resistance to the quinolone levofloxacin for *Ent. cloacae*, and more specifically *Esch. coli*, which demonstrates a >60% resistance. It is also interesting to note that in our earlier report *Ps. aeruginosa* had a reputable susceptibility to imipenem (**Figure 11.16b**, 1988–1989). As of 1999, it is 60% resistant (**Figure 11.11a**). The only agent consistently effective for these multiresistant organisms is colistin, followed by piperacillin/tazobactam. Two other major pathogens which over the past 10 years have gained notoriety are *Acinetobacter baum/haem*, *Stenotrophomonas* (*Xanthomonas*) *maltophila*. While ampicillin, sublactam, and imipenem are fairly effective against *Ac. baum/haem*, ceftazadine and trimethoprim/sulfamethoxazole appear to be the drugs of choice for *Sten. maltophila*. One major word of caution, however, empirical susceptibilities are temporary directives and should be an initial guide and should be altered for each agent's specific susceptibility response as soon as susceptibilities are available to prevent untoward complications.

Subacute Bacterial Endocarditis

Bacteremia associated with burn wound manipulations as well as such procedures as tooth extraction, endotracheal intubation, and sigmoidoscopy can be transient.[95,96] In healthy patients, transient bacterial showers are of little consequence. However, patients with a prior history of valvular heart disease are prone to the development of valvular vegetations. Burned patients, although usually young healthy adults prior to injury, develop a generalized immunosuppression and experience a significant number of invasive procedures which may increase the risk for endocarditis. The incidence of bacterial endocarditis appears to be increasing as we become more adapt at treating major burn injuries. However, its development is usually occult and like suppurative thrombophlebitis, and frequently not noted until there are persistent positive blood cultures.[97] Patients whose risk factor is high for the development of bacterial endocarditis are those with repetitive bacteremias, which may occur after continual instrumentation or surgical intervention. These patients should be closely monitored for the development of heart murmurs, and if found, should undergo echocardiography to determine the presence of vegetations. Blood cultures should be randomly taken for 72 hours, then

Fig. 11.9 (opposite) *Burn wound infection.* (a) Superficial fungal colonization involving superficial areas of epidermis. PAS stain. Bar = 50 μm. (b) Fungal invasion of subcutaneous adipose tissue. PAS stain. Bar = 50 μm. (c) Herpes virus infection. The arrows indicate some inclusion bodies. HE stain. Bar = 50 μm. (d) Herpes virus infection. Tzanck smear. Bar = 50 μm.

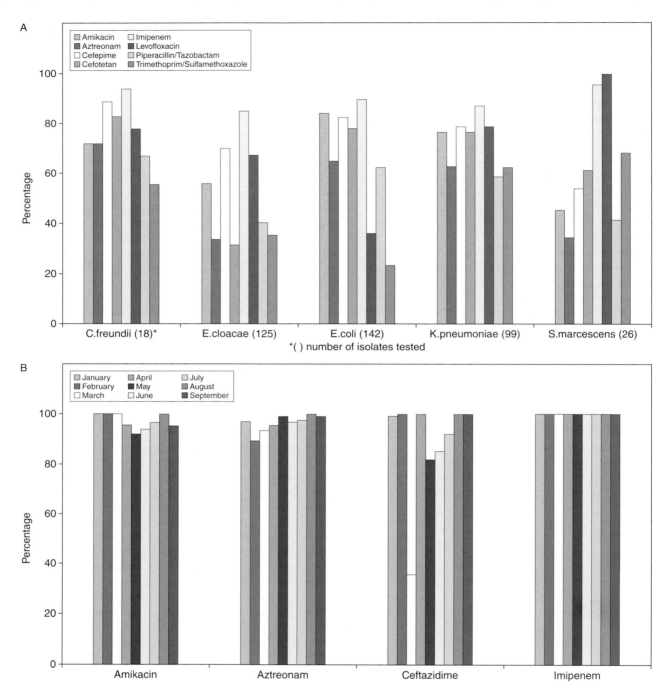

Fig. 11.10 (a) Antimicrobial susceptibility for the enterics January 1,1999 through December 31, 1999.
(b) Susceptibility patterns for *Esch. coli* against amikacin and miscellaneous β-lactam antibiotics (1996).

appropriate broad-spectrum antibiotics initiated and continued for the next 6 weeks.

Cannula Infections and Suppurative Thrombophlebitis

Infectious complications associated with IV and intra-arterial catheters represent a major problem irrespective of the constant attention to aseptic technique for insertion and appropriate mainte-nance.[97] The burned patient appears to be especially susceptible to this complication; catheter infection rates have been reported rang-

ing from 8 to 57%.[98,99] Suppurative thrombophlebitis may be con-firmed in up to 5% of patients hospitalized for burns over 20% TBSA.[100] A recent prospective study documented a 50% correla-tion between organism cultured from the catheter tips and hubs within 48 hours of insertion, and the incidence of catheter infection was inversely proportional to the distance of the insertion site from the burn wound.[101] It is interesting to note that the bacteria cultured from infected catheters could be traced to the skin in 96% of the cases. There data tend to support the hypothesis that catheter infec-tions primarily arise from burn wound contaminants migrating

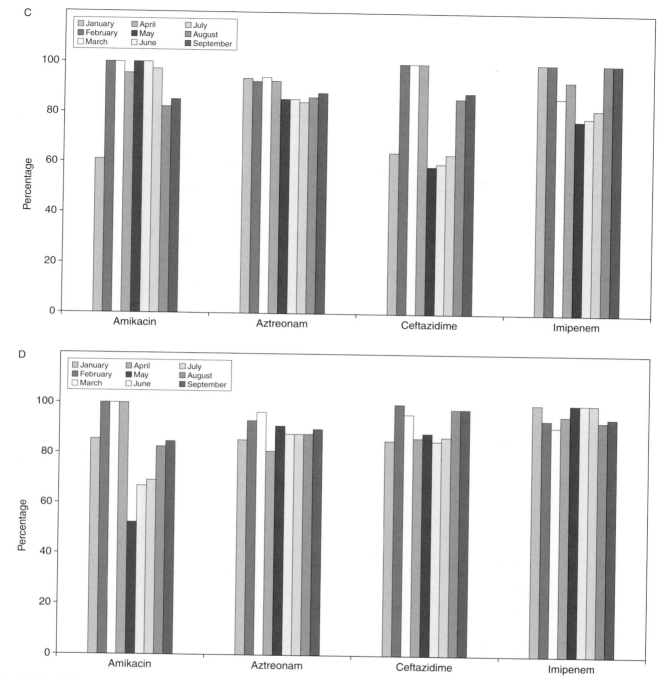

Fig. 11.10 (c) Susceptibility patterns for *Kl. pneumoniae* against amikacin and miscellaneous β-lactam antibiotics. (d) Susceptibility patterns for *Ent. cloacae* against amikacin and miscellaneous β-lactam antibiotics.

down the catheter to the tip. Strict aseptic technique for insertion of intravascular catheters, the use of Teflon catheters, and rotation of the catheter site, tubing, and apparatus every 72 hours have been related with a decrease in catheter injections rates.[102–104]

Suppurative thrombophlebitis should be suspected in those patients who have persistent positive blood cultures without signs of local infection. Often suppuration can occur after the time of catheter removal so cultures at the time of removal may be an unreliable predictor of infection. Gross clinical signs of suppurative thrombophlebitis are frequently not present.[105] Careful records of

previously cannulated sites can allow for sequential venotomy and examination for ultraluminal pus and histologic examination for intimal colonization. Upon confirmation of the diagnosis, immediate operative excision is essential to prevent progressive sepsis. Entire excision of a vein to the port of entry into the central circulation may be required because of the tendency of phlebitis to spring to vein valves, leaving an apparently normal vein in between the infected foci. The subcutaneous tissue and skin should be packed open where grossly purulent vein is removed and allowed to granulate and close by secondary intention.

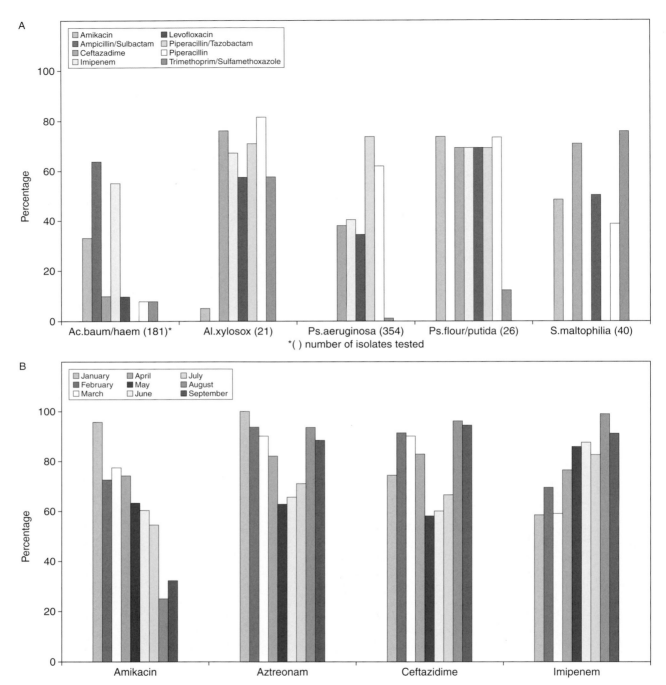

Fig. 11.11 (a) Antimicrobial susceptibilities for nonfermentors January 1, 1999 through December 31, 1999. (b) Susceptibility patterns for *Ps. aeruginosa* against amikacin and miscellaneous β-lactam antibiotics.

Suppurative Chondritis

Burns to the ear represent a clinical management challenge. Full-thickness injuries can injure the cartilage of the ear, resulting in autoamputation of a part or the entire external auricle. Because of the auricles comparatively low blood supply, chondritis frequently follows the progression of tissue ischemia. Chondritis is usually seen 3–5 weeks following the injury but may be seen earlier and may occur following partial- and full-thickness injuries. Since the introduction of mafenide acetate, which has become the topical agent of choice for burned cartilaginous surfaces, the incidence of

suppurative chondritis has significantly decreased. Characteristically, the patient will complain of dull pain. The ear will become warm, red, tender, and edematous. Appropriate antibiotics should be initiated immediately and if there is an identifiable site, immediate incision and drainage of the abscess should be undertaken and culture and sensitivity obtained. Should induration and tenderness continue, a more extensive debridement is imperative. Generally the helix is bivalved at the posterior helical margin and all necrotic cartilage debrided. Difficulty may arise in distinguishing between viable and necrotic tissue and frequently normal cartilage is sacrificed in order to ensure debridement. However, infected cartilage is usually soft, while normal cartilage will feel granular on curettage. If appropriate adequate excision of the necrotic tissue is not performed, suppurative chondritis can proceed to invade the mastoid bone, creating a potential for intracranial abscess formation.

Suppurative Sinusitis

An infection of this type has become more obvious recently because of constant long-term transnasal intubation and the use of nasogastric or nasoduodenum tubes for enteral feeding. The diagnosis is usually delayed due to clinically inapparent symptoms and only after more frequent causes of fever are ruled out does it become evident. Diagnosis is confirmed based on X-rays or CT scans. Therapy with broad-spectrum antibiotics is initiated; however, surgical drainage of the involved sinuses may be necessary if the infection is unresponsive to the antibiotics. Oral intubation and orogastric feeding may be utilized as a temporary measure; but, if sinusitis becomes complicated and if prolonged treatment is necessary, then a tracheostomy and/or gastrostomy is indicated.

Pneumonia

Pneumonia is the septic complication most frequently encountered in all critically ill patients. Airborne pneumonia, or bronchopneumonia, is the most common type of pulmonary sepsis. This form of pneumonia occurs relatively early (usually in the second postburn week) and begins as a bronchiolitis secondary to bacterial entry into the tracheobronchial tree with spread of infection to adjacent alveoli in a nonrandom manner most frequently involving the dependent portions of the lung. The causative organisms reflect the flora of the burn wound. Predisposing factors appear to be burn size; the occurrence of aspiration; the presence of a tracheostomy or nasotracheal tube; inhalation injury; or other complications such as septicemia and ileus from disturbances of fluid and electrolyte balance.[106] The performance of a tracheostomy or the placement of a nasotracheal tube in a burn patient is associated with a high incidence of necrotizing ulcerative tracheobronchitis, the occurrence rate being greater in the case of tracheostomy. The tracheobronchial infection is a result of both mechanical trauma to the tracheal wall by either the tip of the endotracheal tube or the tube cuff, if such is needed to assist ventilation, and the flora of the burn wound, which readily gain access to the tracheobronchial tree.

The mucosal and mural infection may spread distally to involve alveoli and cause bronchopneumonia. Bronchopneumonia is associated with a lower mortality than is hematogenous pneumonia. This septic complication can be minimized by meticulous aseptic tracheobronchial toilet by use of effective gastric decompression to prevent emesis and aspiration during periods of ileus, and by limiting endotracheal intubation and the duration of intubation to those patients with specific indications. Lung function should be monitored on a scheduled basis in all patients with extensive burns, particularly those with inhalation injury, and daily roentgenograms of the chest obtained. When a pulmonary infiltrate characteristic of bronchopneumonia is identified on a chest roentgenogram, an endobronchial culture should be obtained by the Leuken's tube technique, inhalation therapy should be intensified, and antibiotic therapy begun with the agent showing greatest effectiveness against the predominant organism, as determined by the bacterial surveillance program.

A solitary infiltrate occurring relatively late in the postburn course is the usual presenting sign of hematogenous infection versus pneumonia, but if the primary infection remains unidentified and untreated, multiple infiltrates may appear in a random distribution related to the pulmonary vasculature. Late-appearing pulmonary infiltrates, particularly a solitary infiltrate, and simultaneous recovery of a positive blood culture necessitate a search for an extrapulmonary site of infection. Sources of hematogenous pneumonia include a burn wound that has developed invasive infection, previously cannulated veins in which suppurative thrombophlebitis has developed, inapparent perforation of a viscus, such as a posteriorly penetrating Curling's ulcer, and occult soft-tissue infections, such as an injection site abscess. The primary source of infection must be treated, the patient given systemic antibiotics to which the causative organism is sensitive, and respiratory function supported if necessary.[12]

Sputum examination

Microscopic examination and culture of expectorated sputum remain the mainstays of the laboratory evaluation of pneumonia. Procurement of expectorated sputum is a noninvasive technique that can be carried out at no risk to the patient, provides samples of lower respiratory tract secretions for immediate evaluation, and in the majority of cases allows the clinician to make a presumptive diagnosis. Examination of the sputum should include observation of the color, amount, consistency, and odor of the specimen. Mucopurulent sputum is most commonly found with bacterial pneumonia or bronchitis. Scant or watery sputum is more often noted in viral and other atypical pneumonias. 'Rusty' sputum suggests alveolar involvement and has been most commonly associated with pneumococcal pneumonia. Dark red, mucoid sputum suggests Friedlander's pneumonia caused by encapsulated *Kl. pneumoniae*. Foul-smelling sputum is associated with mixed anaerobic infections most commonly seen with aspiration.[12]

In all cases of acute pneumonia, a Gram stain of the sputum should be prepared. In order to maximize the diagnostic yield of the sputum examination, only samples free of oropharyngeal contamination should be reviewed. As a guide, the number of neutrophils and epithelial cells should be quantitated under low power (100×), with further examination reserved for samples containing >25 neutrophils and <10 epithelial cells. Such samples contain minimal oropharyngeal contamination. Samples with more epithelial cells and fewer neutrophils are nondiagnostic and should be discarded. The morphologic and staining characteristics of any bacteria seen should be recorded and an estimate made of the predominant organisms. Where no bacterial predominance exists, this should be noted as well. The sputum Gram stain is helpful to identify organisms other than the pneumococci. Small gram-negative coccobacillary organisms are characteristic of *Haemophilus influenzae*. Staphylococci appear as gram-positive cocci in tetrads and grape-like clusters. Organisms of mixed morphology are characteristic of anaerobic infection. Few bacteria are seen with legionnaires' disease, mycoplasma, pneumonia, and viral pneumonia.

In a recent study, Ramzy et al, attempted to establish the relationship of the burn wound flora to microbial pathogens in the tracheobronchial tree.[107] It has important implications for antimicrobial therapy in the severely burned patient. Management of septic complications is bolstered by surveillance quantitative wound cultures (QWC) and bronchial lavage fluid (BLF) cultures. In 30 (48%) of the 62 BLF cultures, there was a match between the organism identified in the BLF and the QWC. When strict quantitative criteria were applied, the match rate was only 9 (14%) of 62. Burn size and inhalation injury had no significant effect on match rate. Whereas the microbial pathogens were similar in the QWC and BLF, linear regression showed no value of QWC in predicting BLF culture results. The difference between qualitative and quantitative match rates suggests cross-colonization between the burn wound and tracheobronchial tree, but little to no cross-infection. The QWC and BLF cultures must be performed independently in determining antimicrobial specificity in the burned patient.

Nosocomial pneumonia is the leading cause of death from hospital-acquired infections. The estimated prevalence of nosocomial pneumonia within the intensive care setting ranges from 10 to 65%, with fatality rates greater that 25% reported in most studies. Ventilator-associated pneumonia (VAP) specifically refers to pneumonia that develops more than 48 hours after intubation (that is, late-onset VAP) in mechanically ventilated patients who had no clinical evidence suggesting the presence or likely development of pneumonia at the time of intubation. VAP that occurs within 48 hours of intubation is frequently the result of aspiration and usually yields a better prognosis than late-onset VAP, which is more often caused by antibiotic-resistant bacteria. The clinical importance of VAP is demonstrated by several investigations suggesting that it is an independent determinant of death for critically ill patients who require mechanical ventilation.

A consensus appears to be emerging that specific bacterial pathogens associated with high levels of antibiotic resistance (for example *Ps. aeruginosa*, *Acinetobacter* species, and methicillin-resistant *Staph. aureus* [MRSA]) are associated with greater mortality than are the more antibiotic-sensitive pathogens (for example, *H. influenzae* and methicillin-sensitive *Staph. aureus*). Even within the same species, those bacteria that are antibiotic-resistant are frequently associated with greater mortality in patients with VAP than are antibiotic-sensitive strains.

Recently, several groups of investigators have demonstrated that mortality was greater among patients with VAP who were judged to be receiving inadequate antibiotic therapy (based on the findings of cultures of lower airway specimens obtained by either bronchoalveolar lavage (BAL), a protected specimen brush (PSB), or tracheal aspiration) than among patients receiving antibiotics to which the isolated bacteria were sensitive. More important, these studies also suggested that the increased risk or mortality persisted despite changes made to the initial antibiotic therapy after reviewing the findings from lower airway cultures. The various authors of these studies independently concluded that the microbiologic cause of VAP and the antimicrobial resistance patterns of the isolated pathogens represented important determinants of patient outcomes.[108,109] These studies demonstrated that the hospital mortality rate was greater for patients who received an inadequate antibiotic regimen, initiated before obtaining the results of cultures from respiratory secretions, blood, or pleural fluid, than for patients who received an antibiotic regimen that provided adequate antimicrobial protection against all pathogens identified from cultures. More important, the study by Luna *et al.* found that subsequent changes in antibiotic therapy, based on the results of BAL fluid cultures, did not reduce the risk of hospital mortality in patients for whom inadequate antibiotic therapy was initially prescribed.[108,109]

Our present understanding of the treatment of VAP suggests an association between inadequate initial empiric antibiotic therapy and an increased risk of hospital mortality. The initial selection of empiric antibiotics appears to be one of the most important determinants of clinical outcome for patients with VAP. Microbiologic surveillance, through the use of cultures of lower respiratory tract secretions obtained bronchoscopically or otherwise, may help identify the early development of resistance to empirically prescribed antibiotics.[108]

Urinary Tract Infections

Urinary tract infections are usually associated with prolonged and often unnecessary catheterization. It is seldom essential to leave a catheter in place for more than a few days, and this device is often misused in the burn patient. Routine monitoring of urine from indwelling catheters should be done by needle aspirates through the rubber catheter with a 25-gauge needle on a regular basis two to three times a week (**Figures 11.12** and **11.13**). It is our practice not to use antimicrobial irrigations to prevent urinary tract infections, feeling that they are not particularly effective and may lead to infection by antibiotic-resistant organisms. When infection occurs patients should be treated with appropriate systemic antibiotics. Candiduria is often insignificant but may reflect active infection or septicemia, especially when mycelia can be demonstrated. When present, an active infection with *Candida* species usually responds to low doses of amphotericin B, fluconazole, or itraconazole.

Sources of Intra-abdominal Infections

Regional enteritis

The onset of regional enteritis may be acute, especially in the young, and can mimic acute appendicitis. The correct diagnosis of early regional enteritis can only be made at the time of operation, which reveals a thickened bowel wall and mesenteric lymph node involvement. However, the diagnosis is usually established by contrast radiography. Perforation as the result of an ulcer burrowing through the entire thickness of the bowel wall may occur. Usually the perforation is confined and may result in abscesses or internal fistulas. Rarely does the ulcer perforate freely into the peritoneal cavity. Perianal or perirectal abscesses and fistulas are also common manifestations of regional enteritis. Systemic antibiotics are often of value in the management of suppurative complications. Surgery is indicated to drain abdominal abscesses, to correct fistulas, and for free perforation. The principal complications of surgery are enterocutaneous fistula, intraperitoneal or wound sepsis, and prolonged postoperative ileus.

Necrotizing enterocolitis in neutropenic patients

Necrotizing enterocolitis occurs in patients who are severely granulocytopenic from any cause. Left upper quadrant abdominal pain is usual. Irritation of the adjacent diaphragm may result in pain referred to the left shoulder. Splenic enlargement and tenderness are often present, with high, spiking temperatures. Radiographic examination may reveal an elevated left hemidiaphragm, basilar pulmonary infiltrates, atelectasis, or a left pleural effusion. Shift of the colon and stomach down and to the right, and extraintestinal gas, either diffusely mottled or producing an air–fluid level in the left upper quadrant, may also be seen. Ultrasonography, CT, and

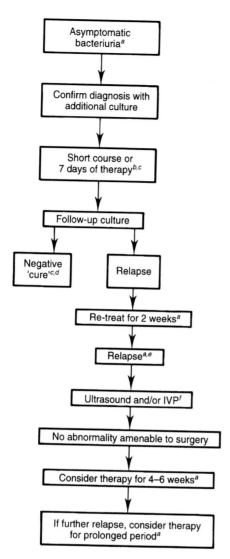

Fig. 11.12 Management of asymptomatic bacteria. [a]Consider no therapy in nonpregnant adults without obstructive uropathy or symptoms of urinary tract infection. [b]Consider ultrasound and/or intravenous pyelogram (IVP) in all children and men with correction of significant lesions. [c]Follow-up culture required only in pregnancy, in children, and in adults with obstructive uropathy. [d]Follow-up cultures monthly in pregnant women and at 6 weeks and 6 months in children. [e]Evaluate men for chronic bacterial prostatitis. [f]Delay 2 months postpartum in pregnant women. [g]Consider ultrasound and/or IVP after three to four reinjections.

MRI are the preferred diagnostic techniques for the evaluation of suspected splenic abscess. Initial antibiotic therapy should have a broad spectrum of activity. A combination of antibiotics that has activity against streptococci and both aerobic and anaerobic gram-negative bacilli would be appropriate initial antimicrobial therapy.

Acute cholecystitis

Acute cholecystitis is usually superimposed on a histologic picture of chronic cholecystitis. Ninety-five percent of all the gallbladders removed for acute cholecystitis exhibit fibrosis, flattening of the mucosa, and clusters of chronic inflammatory cells as sequelae of previous disease. Rokitansky–Aschoff sinuses are present in over 112 of the cases. These sinuses represent mucosal herniations presumably related to increased hydrostatic pressure during previous episodes of cystic duct obstruction. The early acute changes may be only edema and venous congestion. This is followed by focal necrosis and an influx of neutrophils as secondary bacterial proliferation occurs. This may then be followed by actual gangrene or perforation (**Figure 11.14**).

Initial obstruction of the cystic duct may be accompanied by a mild epigastric pain followed by reflex nausea and vomiting. If the obstruction is transient, these symptoms subside within 1–2 hours. With persistent obstruction the findings of acute cholecystitis evolve. Pain shifts to the right upper quadrant and becomes increasingly severe. Signs of peritoneal irritation may be present, and in a small number of patients the pain may radiate to the right shoulder or scapula. The gallbladder is palpable in 30–40% of the cases. Moderate temperature elevations and minimal icterus occur in two-thirds of patients. However, repeated chills and fever, jaundice, or hypotension would suggest suppurative cholangitis as a consequence of common duct obstruction. Most patients with acute cholecystitis have a complete remission within 1–4 days. However, approximately 25–30% of patients require surgery or develop some complication.

In the presence of cholecystitis and cholelithiasis, appreciable numbers of various bacteria may be found in the bile and walls of the gallbladder, even in the absence of symptoms. The organisms found in the biliary tract are commonly the same as the normal intestinal flora, namely, the enteric gram-negative bacilli, including *Esch. coli*, *Klebsiella*, *Enterobacter*, and *Proteus* spp., as well as the enterococci. In addition, recent studies have demonstrated the frequent recovery of anaerobic organisms including *Bacteroides*, *Clostridia*, and *Fusobacterium* spp. When present these anaerobes are frequently involved in polymicrobic infections, mixed with other anaerobes and aerobic gram-negative bacilli.

An appropriate initial antibiotic regimen includes an aminoglycoside (amikacin) or a cephalosporin in addition to an agent such as clindamycin or metronidazole, to treat for *Bact. fragilis*. Available evidence suggests that perioperative antibiotics are a helpful adjunct to surgery to prevent postoperative infectious complications. Because wound infection is thought to be due to contamination of the incision with infected bile at the time of operation, prophylactic antibiotics should be given in a manner that will achieve high blood and tissue concentrations at the time of surgery. Immediate surgery is indicated for gangrenous cholecystitis, perforation with peritonitis, and suspected pericholecystis abscess. In these patients, cholecystectomy with intraoperative cholangiography is the procedure of choice.

Cholangitis

Cholangitis can be defined as varying degrees of inflammation and/or infection involving hepatic and common bile ducts. Since the mucosa of the gallbladder is contiguous with the common bile duct via the cystic duct, it is not surprising that varying degrees of choledochitis occur as a limited cholangitis with cholecystitis. In

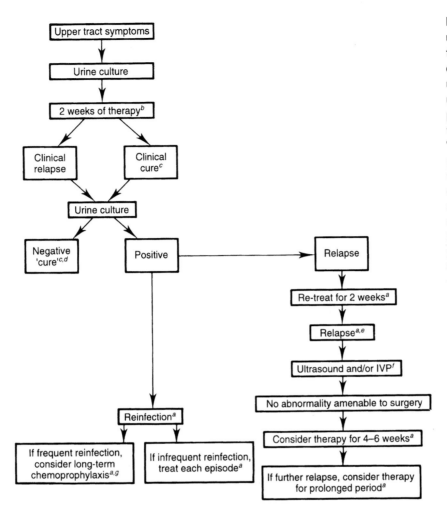

Fig. 11.13 Management of upper urinary tract infections. [a]Consider no therapy in nonpregnant adults without obstructive uropathy or symptoms of urinary tract infection. [b]Consider ultrasound and/or intravenous pyelogram (IVP) in all children and men with correction of significant lesions. [c]Follow-up culture required only in pregnancy, in children, and in adults with obstructive uropathy. [d]Follow-up cultures monthly in pregnant women and at 6 weeks and 6 months in children. [e]Evaluate men for chronic bacterial prostatitis. [f]Delay 2 months postpartum in pregnant women. [g]Consider ultrasound and/or IVP after three to four reinfections.

fact, specimens of the common duct taken at the time of cholecystectomy for acute cholecystitis usually show localized edema and inflammation. However, this disease is indistinguishable from uncomplicated acute cholecystitis.

In a manner similar to that described for cholecystitis, obstruction of the common duct results in increased pressure, edema, congestion, and necrosis of the walls of the biliary tree followed by rapid proliferation of bacteria within the biliary tree. In most instances, obstruction is due to gallstones. However, obstruction may be due to prior biliary tract surgery, tumor, chronic calcific pancreatitis, and parasitic infections. The onset is usually acute, with high fever, chills, diffuse pain, and tenderness over the liver. Jaundice is usually prominent. In some cases, shock and other findings of gram-negative bacteremia may be present; collectively, 85% of the patients fulfill Charcot's triad of fever, chills, and jaundice. There is usually marked leukocytosis with an increase in immature forms. The serum bilirubin level is often higher than 4 mg/dl and the serum alkaline phosphatase level is significantly higher than that encountered in acute cholecystitis. Biochemical and even clinical evidence of disseminated intravascular coagulation may be present.

Recent studies using detailed aerobic and anaerobic culture techniques suggest that the bacteriologic findings in cholangitis are similar to those in acute obstructive cholecystitis. gram-negative

enteric bacilli and anaerobic bacteria are the most common isolates. Unlike uncomplicated cholecystitis, bacteremia occurs in approximately 50% of cases. Bacteremia and shock occur commonly and perhaps are best included as part of the clinical picture of obstructive cholangitis. Prompt institution of appropriate antibiotic therapy is mandatory, since these severe infections are frequently complicated by bacteremia and shock. Based on the bacteriologic findings described above and on the known *in vitro* susceptibilities of these organisms, an appropriate regimen would be clindamycin or metronidazole plus an aminoglycoside or cephalosporin antibiotic. Prompt operative intervention with decompression of the common duct is mandatory in all but those few patients who respond promptly to antibiotics.

Infection control programs

The major role of local burn wound infection in sepsis suggests that the diagnosis and treatment of infections should focus primarily on the burn wound. Wound colonization will progress to infection only when the surface bacterial counts exceed some critical number. Accurate quantification of the burned patient's bacterial load is therefore the foundation of infection surveillance. This is achieved through routine cultures of sputum, urine, and wound. Quantitative cultures obtained on a routine basis will provide the

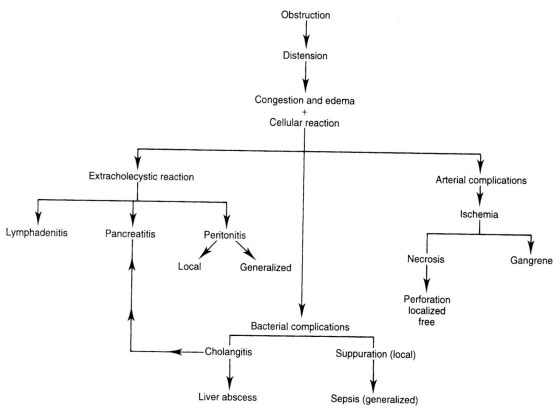

Fig. 11.14 Pathogenesis of acute cholecystitis.

monitoring of the progress of bacterial colonization, provide guidance in the event empiric antibiotic therapy becomes necessary, and will also provide for prompt intervention against bacterial invasion. Cultures of sputum, urine, and the wound should be obtained three times weekly. We routinely biopsy any adherent eschar and use swab cultures for other open wounds.

It is impractical to define all of the major advances that have been made in controlling the complication of burn wound infection. Evidence of such progress includes a general acceptance that the burn wound serves as the site of primary invasion for the majority of instances of local or generalized infection.[29,91] This is primarily because the burned skin has lost its defensive properties. Infection control of the burned patient is an enormous task that must be considered as a individual entity and not looked upon simply as the control of burn infections. Major burn wounds usually become infected within 3–5 days after admission; it is obvious that the infection arises from the patient's own bacterial flora and is not an exogenous occurrence. This is a controversial concept and repeatedly causes conflicts among hospital practitioners of infection control and members of the burn care team.

To conceive infection control in this select patient population, the burn wound must be recognized as the site of microbial colonization which may progress to invasion with systemic dissemination if not restrained. Further recognition that this colonization initially arises from the patient's own resident and transient bacteria is sovereign.[4,29,91,110–112] Although bacteria may not normally be recovered from the skin surface or from the sweat glands, they can be identified in the hair follicles, and particularly near the orifices

of the sebaceous glands. Bacteria of this normal endogenous skin flora are resistant to heat injury in practically the same degrees as are the skin cells. The bacteria on the surface are heat killed, as are the tissue cells of the surface, and initial swab cultures are usually sterile. Moreover, the bacteria in the hair follicles and sebaceous glands may survive (dependent on the extent of the burn injury), and the quantitative counts of biopsied specimens may show the same numbers of bacteria per gram of tissue (10^3) as found in the tissue prior to burning.[91,106,112] As these bacteria increase in number following the thermal injury and reach levels of greater than 10^5 bacteria per gram of tissue, they will erupt from the hair follicles and sebaceous glands and begin transmigrating through the tissue invading the dermal–subcutaneous boundary. Perivascular growth is accompanied by thrombosis of vessels and necrosis of any remaining dermal elements, transforming partial-thickness burns to full-thickness burn injuries. Levels of bacterial growth which exceed 10^5 bacteria per gram of tissue constitute localized burn wound infection, and levels greater than 10^8–10^9 bacteria per gram of tissue may be associated with lethal burns.[4,29,91,112,113] As the levels of bacterial growth increase so does the incidence of septicemia.[4,114]

Maintaining wounds at low contamination levels diminishes the frequency and duration of septic episodes caused by wound flora. This is accomplished by cleansing a wound two to three times per day by either showering or tubbing the patient. Some burn facilities still emerse patients in a tub to remove the debris and exudate that has accumulated between dressing changes; however, most burn facilities no longer advocate this cleaning technique because of the potential seeding of surface bacteria to the open burn wound. We, along with other burn facilities, have exclusively used the shower technique to wash down the debris from the patients. It is important to note that wound cleansing can be quite painful and the associated hematogenous seeding can cause a bacteremia. Therefore the technique of early excision may prevent these disadvantages. An alternative treatment for small second degree burns is to use a biological dressing. Biological dressings contain no toxins or bacterial properties. However, they provide a wound environment that prevents desiccation, reduces bacterial proliferation, diminishes or prevents loss of heat, water, protein, and red blood cells, and encourages the process of rapid wound healing. Biological dressings also diminish pain. Some examples of synthetic skin substitutes include Biobrane™, Opsite, and Omiderm.

Daily inspection of the wound is essential. Burn wound biopsies should be taken from any area of the wound which has changed in appearance, as described in **Table 11.19**. Bacterial sepsis is often preluded by changes in the color, odor, or amount of exudate from the wound, while fungal invasion is clinically conspicuous by a rapidly emerging and spreading dark discoloration. Consequently, the burn wound must be closely assessed for these manifestations. Few histologically demonstrated fungal infections are initially determined by culture; therefore treatment should be predicated on the identification of invasive hyphae by histological examination and may subsequently be confirmed by culture.

There is a controversy over the best method to determine infections, with some burn centers using surface cultures and others using contact plates. The area of greatest concern is the identification of the organism. We have found quantitative biopsies to be quite useful. Robson found that when colony counts were less than 10^2 graft survival was greater than 90%, but when colony counts were greater than 10^5 only 60% graft survival was observed.[115] We have routinely modified our topical antimicrobial therapy, alternating between silver sulfadiazine and mafenide acetate when colony counts are greater than 10^5. Mafenide acetate is more successful at penetrating the necrotic dermis than is silver sulfadiazine. This technique has been demonstrated to be successful in decreasing wound colony counts. However, early excision and grafting has been more rewarding. Quantitative swabs, smear cultures, and or contact plates (Rodak®) provide information regarding the potential infectious agent, while quantitative wound biopsies are a better determinant of bacterial loads. Quantitative cultures showing high bacterial counts correlate with histological evidence of burn wound infection in approximately 80% of cases.[4,91,116] If quantitative biopsies reveal greater than 10^3 organisms/g of tissue, a change in topical therapy is indicated. If bacterial counts exceed 10^5 organisms/g of tissue, localized burn wound infection should be considered and a histological examination performed. If histological evidence of invasion is present, systemic antibiotics should be consistent with the etiological agent of injection and the wound should be excised.[91–93]

Additional measures can be taken to diminish the incidence of burn wound colonization. The microorganisms initially populating the burned wound represent a mixture of endogenous resident flora and exogenous contaminants seeded by contact with the environment and attending personnel. Immunosuppressed burned patients should be protected from exposure to these environmental contaminants. However, the most elaborate methods of isolation have failed effectively to minimize the incidence of infection, although they have significantly reduced the incidence of cross-contamina-tion.[117–120] The most effective means of decreasing exposure of burned patients to exogenous bacteria is strict observation of appropriate hand washing among the health care providers. Waterproof gowns and gloves should be worn whenever direct contact with body fluids and wound exudates are unavoidable, thus protecting both the patient and the health care provider from inadvertent contamination. All dressing materials should be maintained as patient-specific. Intravenous pumps and poles, blood pressure devices, monitoring equipment, bedside tables and beds should be cleaned on a daily basis with antibacterial solutions. Terminal cleaning, following the discharge of the patient, should include the walls, ceiling, baseboards, and floors. Mattresses should be covered with vinyl and frequently inspected for cracks in their surfaces. Air filters should be repeatedly monitored for bacterial and fungal growth. Most units now house severely burned patients within individual, self-contained isolation rooms. However, common areas exist even within these units, predominantly the bathing or showering facilities. These areas should be conscientiously cleansed between patients with an effective bactericidal agent that is more specifically directed at those bacteria which predominate in each individual unit. Disposable or single-use sterilizable instruments should be used for blunt debridements and the use of any other type of instruments should be discouraged.

Pediatric Nosocomial Infection

The current epidemiology of pediatric nosocomial infections and the challenges practitioners face in the next millennium as they deal with this complication require further study. Bloodstream infection continues to be the most common nosocomial infection in most pediatric intensive care units (PICUs) and surveillance studies; other common nosocomial infections include ventilator-associated pneumonia, urinary tract infection, and surgical site infection. The most common organism isolated from bloodstream infection is coagulase-negative staphylococci. In the PICU, urinary tract infections are caused mainly by *Candida*, followed by *Esch. coli*. Other pathogens, such as respiratory syncytial virus, are also a concern as a cause of nosocomial infection in PICUs. It must be emphasized that viral pathogens need more attention as a cause of nosocomial infection due to their high incidence in the pediatric population.[121] Risk factors such as immunocompromise and increased number of portals of entry while in the PICU must be addressed. Proposed intervention measures to reduce fungal infections in the PICU include the use of HEPA filters and positive pressure ventilation. At the Boston Children's Hospital, the use of HEPA filters has been very successful in reducing the incidence of fungal infections. The challenge for the future in the management of pediatric nosocomial infection includes improving ways to measure nosocomial infection rates in infants and children, investigating new and multiresistant pathogens, controlling antibiotic use, and developing strategies effective for different providers of pediatric care.

A team from the Centers for Disease Control (CDC) measured background rates of infection in a high-risk nursery and performed a cohort study from 6 February through 8 March 1999. The investigators identified 24 of 105 patients (23%) who met the CDC's National Nosocomial Infections Surveillance System (NNISS) definition of nosocomial infection. Statistical analyses showed that patients with sepsis were more likely to have younger gestational age, low median birthweight, lower Apgar scores, a central venous catheter (CVC), total parenteral nutrition, and blood transfusion. Patients receiving IV injections were also at significant risk for sepsis. The high-risk nursery utilization rate of CVCs was greater than the NNIS 90th percentile. Twenty-three percent of patients with nosocomial sepsis died.[122]

Antimicrobial therapy

It is evident that the human population is not germ-free; ergo, health is not the absence of bacteria but more like a delicate balance between man and his microbes, including those of the environment. The intact skin and the mucous membrane are man's most significant defense; any alterations of the integument disturbs this defense as well as the balance with the microbial flora. Infection occurs when the microbes gain access to the underlying tissue and achieve a critical number. The major objective of the burn surgeon is to prevent this microbial invasion when and wherever possible, and when contamination occurs, to reduce the microbial levels so that wound healing can proceed unretarded.[113]

Resident and transient microbes of the skin are the etiological agents of infection, and antimicrobials are designed to eliminate the offenders. With the discovery of antimicrobials, the solution to the abrogation of wound infections seemed to be resolved. However, it soon became evident that even though the antimicrobials may provide a balance between man and his microbes through their ability to render the microbe ineffective and prevent burn wound infections, the microbes soon overcame this obstacle.

The use of therapeutic antimicrobials can provide precise delivery of a specific agent to eliminate the offending microbe since its sensitivity has already been determined, whereas prophylactic or perioperative antimicrobials cannot easily be selected. Usually the decision is based on the common occurrence of those predominating pathogens found among the burn patient population. While the quality of the surgical outcome can be severely compromised by infection, the actual numbers of these infections have been relatively small.[34,116,123]

Preventing infection in burn patients requires two defensive maneuvers. The first echelon of protection or prophylaxis is the establishment of techniques that will effectively obstruct burn wound contamination.[34,124–126]

1. Total area disinfection with appropriate cleansers should include the wound and encompassing areas.
2. Exclusion of the potential source of infection by debridement with grafting, provided the graft bed contains <10^5 bacteria per gram of tissue.[34,116,125]
3. Topical antimicrobial therapy: the appropriate selection of an agent for the specific microbial flora can be attained through agar well susceptibility assays and the utilization of the appropriate antimicrobial necessary for restraining local wound contamination and potential sepsis.[127–129]

The second echelon of this antimicrobial approach is:

1. Preliminary topical and systemic antimicrobial therapy should be introduced when sepsis is suspected and should be directed against those organisms common to burn populations. This approach is based on the microbiology data accumulated regarding the studies on the whole burn population.[119]

2. Enhance the burn patient's local and general ability to resist microbial burn invasion and resistance through appropriate resuscitative therapies and, in particular, nutritional therapies.[130]
3. Immunological procedures augmenting host resistance should be utilized such as administration of cryoprecipitates if appropriate.

The Use of Topical Antimicrobial Compounds and Agents

One of the most effective means to achieve a microbial balance in a colonized or infected wound is the proper use of prophylactic topical agents. Maintaining wounds at low colonization levels diminishes the frequency and duration of septic episodes caused by wound flora,[89] which subsequently reduces the caloric and fluid demands required by the patient during each septic episode. The introduction of topical antimicrobial agents resulted in a significant reduction in burn mortality to date.[128,131] However, no single agent is thoroughly effective against all organisms and each possesses its own advantages and disadvantages. Almost all currently used topical agents retard wound heating, and the application of some increases the patient's metabolic rate. Their effectiveness is measured by their ability to inhibit bacterial growth *in vitro* and reduce wound colony counts *in vivo*. Recent studies have demonstrated that some agents used in the past are no longer effective in inhibiting bacterial growth *in vitro*.[132] Wounds in which the quantitative culture counts remain less than 10^2 organisms/g tissue may remain dressed in the topical agent of choice. However, should the colony count show an increase beyond that point, a change in the topical agent is strongly recommended.

Sodium hypochlorite (NaOCl)

Currently the most effective topical antibacterial for cleansing a wound is sodium hypochlorite (NaOCl).[133] It transcends the topical antimicrobial effects and tissue toxicity of such products of povidone–iodine, acetic acid, and hydrogen peroxide.[67] While povidone–iodine is bactericidal at 1 and 0.5% concentration, it is toxic to fibroblasts; acetic acid at 0.25% is toxic to fibroblasts and not bactericidal; while hydrogen peroxide at 3% and 0.3% is toxic to fibroblasts only – the 3% is bactericidal.[28,133]

Studies by Heggers and his co-workers[134] clearly defined the efficacy of NaOCl at a concentration of 0.025% which was found to be bactericidal and nontoxic to fibroblasts and did not inhibit wound healing, provided appropriate buffers are used. However, the NaOCl is only effective over a 24-hour time frame after the buffer (0.3 N NaH_2HPO_4) is added to the NaOCl.[135] NaOCl soaks are most beneficial in reducing the bacterial numbers in a wound. NaOCl is a broad-spectrum antiseptic and is bactericidal for *Ps. aeruginosa*, *Staph. aureus*, as well as other gram-negative and gram-positive organisms.[68,134] It is effective against MRSA, MRSE, and the enterococci. NaOCl can be used separately or in concert with other antibacterials to control colonization or infection. NaOCl also enhances wound healing and increases wound breaking strength when compared to mafenide acetate.[134]

Silver nitrate (AgNO₃)

Formerly used as a 10% solution, silver nitrate ($AgNO_3$) was found to be toxic at this concentration. It has now been reinstated as a

0.5% solution which is nontoxic. In its current form it apparently does not injure regenerating epithelium in the wound, and is bacteriostatic against *Staph. aureus*, *Esch. coli*, and *Ps. aeruginosa*. $AgNO_3$ is most effective when the wound is carefully cleansed of all emollients and other debris, and debrided of all dead tissue. Multilayered coarse-mesh dressings should be placed over the wound and saturated with the $AgNO_3$ solution. Like silver sulfadiazine, $AgNO_3$ has limited penetration since the element silver is rapidly bound to the body's natural chemical substances, such as Cl^-.[127,128,131,136] Since it is hypotonic in nature, it can cause osmolar dilution, resulting in hyponatremia and hypochloremia. Serum electrolytes must be monitored very carefully.

Notable detriments to the use of $AgNO_3$ include that it is expensive, light-sensitive, and turns black upon contact with tissues and other Cl^- containing compounds, particularly if allowed to dry. $AgNO_3$ also requires special handling; if allowed to dry or covered with an impervious dressing, hyperpyrexia could occur.

Klebsiella species, the *Providencia* species, and other Enterobacteriaceae are not as susceptible as other bacteria. *Ent. cloacae* can cause methemoglobinemia by converting nitrate to nitrite as well as other nitrate-positive organisms.[127,128,131,136]

Silver sulfadiazine

Silver sulfadiazine (Silvadene®, Thermazine®, Flamazine®, SSD, and Burnazine®) is a 1% water-soluble cream combining sulfadiazine with silver. The silver ion binds with the DNA of the organism, consequently releasing the sulfonamide which interferes with the intermediary metabolic pathway of the microbe.[106,114,119,120] It is most effective against *Ps. aeruginosa*, the enterics, and equally effective as any antifungal drug against *Can. albicans*. *Staph. aureus* and some strains of the *Klebsiella* species have been less effectively controlled. Recently there have been reports of *Ps. aeruginosa* resistance.[137] Silver sulfadiazine can be applied with equal effectiveness using either the closed or open methods. Antimicrobial effectiveness has been observed to last for up to 24 hours. More frequent changes are required if a creamy exudate forms on the wound. Some of the benefits of this topical agent are its ease of use and its ability to reduce pain. It has some tissue-penetrating ability, but is limited to the surface epidermal layer.[127,136] However, it is not associated with acid–base disturbances or pulmonary fluid overload, as is mafenide acetate.[128,131] Silver sulfadiazine can be used separately or in combination with other antibacterials as well as enzymatic escharotomy compounds. It can be combined with nystatin, which enhances the antifungal capability of this agent.

By itself, silver sulfadiazine has been shown to retard wound healing; however, in conjunction with nystatin or *Aloe vera*, the wound retardant effect is reversed. The breaking strength is not affected; in fact it may be enhanced when combinations are employed (unpublished data, 1994). One detriment may be a reported granulocyte reduction. However, this appears to be reversible.[127,128,131,136]

Mafenide acetate

Mafenide acetate (Sulfamylon®) is available both in a 10% water-soluble cream or a 5% solution and has more substantial bacteriological data to support its efficacy than any of the other topical antimicrobial. Mafenide acetate has been shown to be effective against a broad range of microorganisms, especially against all strains of *Ps. aeruginosa* and *Clostridium*.[128,131,138]

After the wound has been cleansed of debris, mafenide acetate is applied to the wound like 'butter' (Lindberg's Butter). The treated burn surface is left exposed for maximal antimicrobial potency.[128,131,138] The cream is applied a minimum of two times a day and is reapplied if it is rubbed off between each application. Advantages of the cream is its ability to control *Ps. aeruginosa* wound infections, ease of application, and the absence of the need for dressings. Additionally, it has an ability to permeate the burn eschar to circumvent the colonization of the burn. The 5% solution is applied to an eight-ply gauze dressing, to the point of saturation, then changed every 8 hours. It has been proclaimed to have effective tissue-penetrating ability and appears to be especially effective after the dead tissue is removed from the granulating bed.[128,136,138,139] However, there are several detrimental aspects to the use of mafenide acetate. Protracted use, with the low environmental pH, favors the growth of *Can. albicans*. Mafenide acetate is converted to *p*-sulfamyl-vanzoic acid by monoamide oxidase, which is a carbonic anhydrase inhibitor, subsequently causing metabolic acidosis in the patient. In the unburned patient, respiratory alkalosis is present; therefore an imbalance is not present. On the other hand, if an inhalation injury exists with its concomitant respiratory acidosis and is associated with metabolic acidosis initiated by this drug, the end result can be fatal. This complication can also be seen when treatment with mafenide acetate occurs during septic episodes with metabolic acidosis, or if it is applied over a large area of the body surface.[128,131,138,140] Another detrimental problem encountered with mafenide acetate is that it is painful when applied to superficial partial-thickness burns with intact free nerve endings. This disadvantage is not particularly relevant since mafenide acetate was not designed for minor burns and is not painful on large full-thickness injuries. Its requirement to remain uncovered for antimicrobial activity may also be considered a disadvantage if a dressing is required. The 5% aqueous solution of mafenide acetate can be used in a wet dressing covered by the splint.[128,131,138,140]

It has been shown by others that fatality in major burns can be reduced by 33%.[73,74] As with silver sulfadiazine, mafenide acetate can be used individually or in conjunction with other antimicrobials. However, mafenide acetate retards wound healing and reduces the breaking strength of healed wounds.[127]

Povidone–iodine

A 10% ointment of povidone–iodine was designed after the demonstration of its broad spectrum of antimicrobial attributes in liquid form. Although its active antimicrobial component is iodine, there has been no documentation associated with skin hypersensitivity or toxic effects. It has a broad spectrum of antibacterial and antifungal activities.[127,128,131,133,141,142] Povidone–iodine ointment can be employed effectively in both the closed and open techniques. Quantitative bacteriological assessments imply that iodine is most efficacious when it is administered every 6 hours. Used in this approach, it is effective in controlling and/or preventing colonization.

Some problems have been encountered when using this drug. It can cause pain when applied. Recent studies intimate that it may be absorbed more extensively than was previously thought and could cause toxicity and renal failure, as well as acidosis. Concomitantly, it has been shown to be cytotoxic to fibroblasts as previously described.[127,128,131,133,141,142] However, it is a highly effective disinfectant when used on intact skin.

Gentamicin sulfate

Garamycin, or gentamicin sulfate, is available as a 0.1% water-soluble cream and is chemically similar to other aminoglycosides, such as kanamycin and neomycin. It has a broad spectrum of antimicrobial activity. Its use in wounds was based on its microbiocidal capabilities against *Ps. aeruginosa*. However, its topical application and abuse rapidly initiated gentamicin resistance.[127,128,131,133,141,142]

Bacitracin/polymyxin

Topical *antibiotics*, such as bacitracin/polymyxin, have been unproductive in controlling infection, specifically in grafting procedures. Lowbury made a very astute statement when he said, 'It was gratifying to have a topical chemoprophylactic agent which was not an antibiotic, the use of which would cause the emergence of antibiotic resistance.'[126,143] Many surgeons rely on this topical

agent for skin graft coverage because it is nontoxic and is similar to petrolatum gauze dressings, which were previously considered as a dressing for grafts. These two combined antibiotics have little or no effect on localized burn wound infections[144] (**Table 11.21**).

Nitrofurantoin

The topical antimicrobial Furacin was previously used and had questionable value therapeutically. However, in the past decade, researchers have shown that Furacin, or nitrofurantoin, was effective in the treatment of MRSA and other methicillin-resistant staphylococci. While Furacin was effective 75% of the time for most gram-negatives other than *Ps. aeruginosa*, bacitracin/polymyxin was only 21% effective[144,145] (**Table 11.22**).

Mupirocin (Bactroban®, Beecham Laboratories)

Mupirocin is one of several antibiotics derived from the fermentation of *Ps. fluorescens* and is also known as pseudomonic acid A. While the antimicrobial activity derived from cultures of *Ps. fluorescens* was first reported over a century and a half ago, this activity could not be adapted as an antimicrobial agent until Fuller *et*

Table 11 .21 Mean sensitivity zones of topical antibacterials against 126 biotypes of gram-positive isolates in the NAWD procedure

Organism	Number tested	Silvadene®	Sulfamylon®	Nitrofurazone	Bactroban	Polymyxin	Silva–Nystatin	Modified Dakin's	Silver nitrate
S. aureus	18	16±2.72*	27±4.79	32±4.24	25±16.32	4±7.42	14±5.34	3±4.12	16±2.94
S. auricularis	2	18	23±3.53	27±9.89	18±10.60	0	15±1.41	4±5.65	18±2.82
S. epidermidis	50	20±3.10	27±7.62	36±7.26	30±14.86	0	18±3.87	3±5.3	19±2.92
S. haemolyticus	35	19±0.98	31±5.26	35±6.10	20±16.54	0	18±3.46	3±4.86	18±1.84
S. sciuri	1	30	30	31	40	0	27	8	17
S. simulans	3	18±1.52	23±6.11	36±5.50	23±25.16	0	18±1.00	0	19±1.52
S. warneri	1	19	28	40	12	0	18	0	13
E. faecalis	9	17±4.69	25±3.67	22±2.40	28±6.00	0	17±4.64	1±3.00	12±1.99
E. faecium	7	11±2.73	28±4.04	23±3.73	29±9.81	0	11±5.68	0	11±2.82
Total	126	100%S	97.6%	98.4%	88.9S	3%	94.4%S	12.7%S	96.8%S
					6.3%R	97%R	2.4%l	12%l	2.4%l
					4.8%l		3.2%R	3.26R	0.8%R

*Mean value ± standard deviation

Table 11.22 Mean sensitivity zones of topical antibacterials against 79 biotypes of gram-negative Isolate in the NAWD Procedure

Organism	Number tested	Silvadene®	Sulfamylon®	Nitrofurazone	Bactroban	Polymyxin	Silva–Nystatin	Modified Dakins	Silver nitrate
A. baumanii	8	17±3.00*	23±2.55	21±3.02	16±3.07	8±0.64	17±3.02	12±3.02	15±2.21
A. lowffii	1	16	33	30	37	8	16	12	14
C. freundii	3	16±2.08	21±3.46	25±3.79	24±7.57	3±4.62	13±3.79	6±11.00	12±3.79
E. cloacae	7	13±2.7	19±3.73	23±0.79	26±1.57	8±3.78	11±5.86	6±4.38	10±2.21
E. coli	9	14±4.35	14±7.30	27±4.16	24±4.05	2±3.53	12±6.51	4±6.56	10±6.91
P. aeruginosa	25	16±5.03	29±6.13	6±8.15	11±6.79	1±2.23	14±4.75	9±7.55	17±4.73
P. fluorescens	8	14±1.67	23±4.70	9±7.07	12±1.82	2±3.7	16±0.52	7±5.78	16±2.00
P. maltophilia	1	18	20	16	18	9	13	10	15
Other	7	11±5.76	21±4.05	23±2.62	21±6.18	4±4.59	9±6.41	8±8.44	7±7.01
Total	79	92.4%S	97.5%S	75%S	91.1%S	3.8%S			
		3.8%l	2.5%l	3.8%l	3.8%l				
		3.8%R		21.2%R	5.1%R				

*Mean value ± standard deviation
Summary of results

al.[146] executed a more complete isolation and purification of pseudomonic acid A. It is this exploration, along with research associating the antimicrobial activity of mupirocin to an inhibition of microbial isoleucyl t-RNA synthetase, that causes inhibition of protein synthesis, which has made the clinical application of mupirocin possible.[146,147]

In vitro studies have subsequently established that mupirocin has omnipotent inhibitory activity against the gram-positive microbes, specifically *Staph. aureus* and *Staph. epidermidis*. Mupirocin's efficiency in the treatment of infection or colonization due to *Staph. aureus*, whether methicillin-sensitive or not, has been shown in various clinical settings.[146–148] Rode and co-workers[149] have provided additional data regarding the efficacy of mupirocin in the treatment of established wound infections, with *Staph. aureus* resistant to systemic methicillin, topical mafenide acetate, and povidone–iodine.

Recent *in vitro* and *in vivo* endeavors have shown mupirocin to be as efficacious in methicillin-resistant burn wound infections.[144] Mupirocin, while not sanctioned for gram-negative organisms, has been shown to be 75% effective against most enteric organisms and is significantly better than bacitracin/polymyxin[144] (**Table 11.21**).

Table 11.22 presents data on a study which confirmed that the antimicrobial effectiveness of several topicals and silver sulfadiazine had a comparable antimicrobial activity to that of mupirocin for the gram-negative organisms *Ps. aeruginosa*, *Esch. coli*, and *Kl. pneumoniae*, along with *Staph. aureus* (**Table 11.21**). Mupirocin inhibits wound healing when compared to controls by a half-life of 2 days, while the breaking strength is significantly enhanced over the control ($p<0.05$) (unpublished data 1994).

Nystatin (Mycostatin®, Squibb; Nilstat®, Lederle)

Nystatin is an antifungal antibiotic produced by *Streptomyces noursei*. Nystatin exerts its antifungal activity by binding to sterols in the fungal cell membrane. The drug is not active against organisms (e.g. bacteria) that do not contain sterols in their cell membrane. As a result of this binding, the membrane is no longer able to function as a selective barrier, and potassium and other cellular constituents are lost. Nystatin has fungistatic or fungicidal activity against a variety of pathogenic and nonpathogenic yeasts and fungi. *In vitro*, nystatin concentrations of approximately 3 μg/ml inhibit *Can. albicans* and *Can. guilliertnondi*. Concentrations of 6.25 μg/ml are required to inhibit *Can. krusei* and *Geotrichum lactis*. In general, there is little difference between minimum inhibitory and fungicidal concentrations for a particular organism. Nystatin is not active against bacteria, protozoa, or viruses.

Oral administration

Nystatin is used orally for the treatment of intestinal candidiasis. In patients with coexisting intestinal candidiasis and vulvovaginal candidiasis, nystatin may be administered orally, in conjunction with intravaginal application of an antifungal agent. While there is limited evidence that by reducing intestinal candidal colonization, combined oral and intravaginal antifungal therapy may provide some improvement in mycologic response and reduction in recurrence rate of vulvovaginal candidiasis, most evidence suggests that combined therapy does not substantially reduce the risk of recurrence compared with intravaginal therapy alone.

Cutaneous and mucocutaneous infections

For the treatment of cutaneous or mucocutaneous candidal infections, nystatin may be applied topically as cream, lotion, or ointment to affected areas 2–4 times daily. The cream or lotion formulations are preferred to the ointment for use in moist, intertriginous areas. In the treatment of candidiasis, conditions that favor growth of yeast and release of its irritating endotoxin, such as use of occlusive dressings and ointment formulations, should be avoided. Concomitant therapy should include attention to proper hygiene and skin care to prevent spread of infection and reinfection. In addition, the affected areas should be kept dry and exposed to air, if possible. Nystatin may be combined with SSD to increase the antimicrobial spectrum.

Discussion

The therapeutic effectiveness of topical antimicrobials can best be monitored by quantitative bacteriological analysis of the burn wound.[4,111,150] Previously, there were no *in vitro* tests available to support the selection of the most effective topical antimicrobial agent for any given organisms causing burn wound infection. Studies by Nathan and colleagues,[129] as well as by others,[145,151] recently provided evidence of a reproducible susceptibility method for testing pathogenic bacteria against the various topical antimicrobial agents. The bacterial isolates are spread over an agar surface with 6-mm wells cut into the agar; and then the topical antimicrobials are introduced into wells. Subsequently, the zones of inhibition can predict the agent's capability to provide the equilibrium between patient and bacteria. While current data are generated and new agents discovered, the microbes continue to alter their susceptibility. Therefore, at no time will the legendary 'topical antimicrobial agent of choice' be available therapeutically.[145,151]

Though topical antimicrobial therapy has significantly diminished the occurrence of invasive burn wound sepsis, we must search for other prophylactic and preventative methods to prevent burn wound infection. Bacterial control is imperfect at best and all wounds, as well as the patient as a whole, must be scrupulously monitored with adjunctive burn wound biopsies when indicated, with blood and other body fluid cultures, coupled with early excision and grafting to prevent, diagnose, and treat the infection in a timely manner.[4,29,34,114,116,124,128]

Significant advances have been made in recent years in the treatment of neoplastic diseases, prevention of graft rejection in transplant patients, and trauma and burn treatment. This has resulted in an increased number of patients affected by an immunocompromised system, which are much more susceptible to opportunistic infections. Depletion of the number of neutrophils, defects in neutrophil function, and T-cell defects all predispose the host to fungal infections. Aspergillosis and hyalohyphomycosis (specifically *Fusarium*) are the most common angioinvasive fungal infections in burn patients. Barret *et al.* examined the curative effects of direct application of nystatin powder on severely burned children affected by angioinvasive fungal infection.[152] The topical treatment of the wounds with nystatin powder at a concentration of 6 000 000 units/g proved to be effective in eradicating the invasive fungal infections. This new regimen of topical treatment not only is effective superficially but also eradicates invasive clusters of fungi in deep wound tissues, as documented by pathological examination. The application of the powder is easy and did not produce pain or discomfort. It did not impair wound healing and all previously autografted areas healed uneventfully.[152]

In a recent *in vitro* study conducted at the Shriner's Childrens Hospital to assess the efficacy of eight of the topical agents (as described above) against multiresistant gram-positive and gram-negative isolates, Silvadene® and mafenide acetate still remained extremely effective against both groups of organisms as determined by a modified NAWD. Among 126 gram-positive isolates, Silvadene® was effective 100% of the time, followed by nitrofurazone (98.4%), then Sulfamylon® (97.6%). Silver nitrate was 96.8% effective, while Silva-Nystatin was effective 94.4% of the time. Bactroban® susceptibility has been markedly reduced (88.9%) since Strocks et al's, study in 1990[144] (**Table 11.21**). Of the 79 gram-negative isolates tested, which included 25 clinical isolates of *Ps. aeruginosa*, susceptibility to Sulfamylon® was 97.5%, followed by Silvadene® at 92.4%, Bactroban® at 91.1% (an increase of 16% over the Strock et al. study).[144] The only other two topicals showing an antimicrobial effect were Silva-Nystatin (84.8%) and silver nitrate (83.5%) (**Table 11.22**).

Gold et al. (unpublished data) examined the role of topical antimicrobials in decreasing morbidity and mortality in major burn injuries (>50% TBSA). Of 39 patients studied who were treated with topical antimicrobials, which included Silvadene®, Sulfamylon®, nitrofurazone, and Bactroban®, 38 survived for a mortality rate of 2.5% (**Table 11.23**).

New topicals on the horizon

Grapefruit seed extract

What is grapefruit seed extract (GSE)? It is an acidic liquid that contains polyphenolic compounds which include quercetin, cam-pherol glycoside, and neohesperidin extract from grapefruit seeds to mention a few. The polyphenols are unstable but are converted into more stable substances that belong to a class of chemicals known as quaternary ammonium compounds. GSE features the best of both worlds: the quaternary compounds derived from the seed exhibit a broad-spectrum antimicrobial activity while void of any toxic side-effects of the chemically derived quaternaries.

Reagor et al. examined the antimicrobial effects of GSE using the NAWD technique.[153] These investigators tested 67 multiresistant clinical isolates and found that all organisms tested were equally susceptible (**Table 11.24a,b**). Heggers et al. tested the safety and efficacy of GSE in tissue culture and determined that concentrations up to 1:256 were toxic to keratinocytes and epidermal cells the agent was still bactericidal. Its bactericidal properties effectively destroy the bacterial membrane, causing the cytoplasmic constituents to leak out of the cell. What is unique is that at concentrations of 1:512 GSE was nontoxic and still bactericidal. It has potential as a future topical agent.[154]

Tea tree oil

Tea tree oil is termed 'the aboriginal antimicrobial'. Recently, Australian investigators demonstrated a broad-spectrum antimicrobial effect on both Gram-positive and Gram-negative organisms.

Acticoat®

Acticoat® A.B. Dressing consists of two sheets of high-density polyethylene mesh coated with ionic silver with a rayon/polyester core. Acticoat® A.B. Dressing provides broad-spectrum antimicrobial, bactericidal coverage against VRE, MRSA, *Ps. aeruginosa*, *Candida*, and approximately 150 other organisms. It can remain

Table 11.23 *In vitro* antimicrobial susceptibilities of topical agents as determined by the NAWD technique

Culture	No of samples	SSD Mean	SD	MA Mean	SD	FD Mean	SD	MU Mean	SD
All gram-positive	39	19.7[b,c,d]	3.3	25.3[a,c,d]	6.8	33.6[a,b]	6.2	30.6[a,b]	14.9
All gram-positive	37	15.4[b]	5.8	24.2[a,c]	7.2	18.2[b]	8.5	19.7	7.7
Esc. coli	6	16.3[c]	3.1	17.2[c]	6.1	27.0[a,b]	4.8	23.8	4.9
Ps. aeruginosa	12	16.1[b]	6.4	31.4[a,c,d]	4.6	9.5[b]	8.2	13.1[b]	5.8
S. epi	11	21.9[b]	3.0	24.5[a,c]	9.3	35.5[b]	2.6	30.7	14.2

*39 patients entered into the study.
38 patients survived for a 2.5% mortality rate.
Abbreviations: a: *p*<0.05 vs SSD, b: *p*<0.05 vs MA, c: *p*<0.05 vs FD, d: *p*<0.05 vs MU.

Table 11.24a Mean sensitivity zones of topical anti-bacterials against 27 biotypes of gram-positive isolates

Organism	Number tested	Zone sizes (in mm) Silvadene®	Sulfamylon®	Bactroban®	Nitrofurazone	Silva-Nystatin	GSE® Conc.
S. aureus	11	20±0.59*	33±1.1	37±6.3	33±1.0	16±0.62	24±0.35
S. epidermidis	7	22±0.46	33±0.69	30±4.5	34±5.0	19±0.61	26±1.1
S. haemolyticus	16	20±0.24	31±1.7	30±4.4	37±0.51	16±0.44	22±0.21
S. capitis	2	24±0.50	30±2.0	52±3.0	41±4.0	27±1.5	27±4.0
S. sciuri	1	20	33	14	38	15	22
S. salvarius	1	21	43	45	30	15	29
E. casseliflavus	1	14	28	40	25	11	26
E. faecalis	6	15±0.43	29±1.2	27±0.99	15±2.4	10±0.8	24±0.42
E. faecium	1	17	13	43	15	11	31

*Mean value ± standard error of the mean

Table 11.24b Mean sensitivity zones of topical anti-bacterials against 40 biotypes of gram-negative Isolates

Organism	Number tested	Zone sizes (in mm)					
		Silvadene®	Sulfamylon®	Bactroban®	Nitrofurazone	Silva-Nystatin	GSE® Conc.
Ps. aeruginosa	15	18±0.69*	34±1.0	12±0.62	9±0.55	17±0.75	16±0.24
P. fluor/putida	1	17	32	14	7	17	16
P. rettgeri	4	15±0.29	27±0.65	22±0.48	17±0.82	12±0.29	16±0.29
P. stuartii	1	15	23	25	18	12	15
M. morganii	2	14±0.50	23±2.5	16±1.5	25±0.50	10±0.0	18±1.0
Esch. coli	3	16±0.0	18±0.67	24±0.33	29±1.2	15±0.88	16±0.0
K. pneumoniae	1	19	24	23	24	15	16
Ac. baum/haem	14	16±0.40	26±0.72	15±0.36	18±0.78	13±0.32	17±0.0
E. taylorae	2	13±4.0	23±4.0	23±7.5	23±1.5	11±3.5	18±1.5
Ent. cloacae	17	12±0.56	23±0.91	25±1.2	22±1.4	10±0.48	16±0.11

*Mean value ± standard error of the mean

intact for several days on the wound, if there is minimal exudation.[172]

Mode of Action of Antimicrobials

Prior to the initiation of any antimicrobial therapy, each burn surgeon must consider four major essentials:

- each antimicrobial must be selected based on its effect and its specificity for the microbe present;
- this decision should be made on the basis of culture and susceptibility data;
- the time, dosage, route of administration, and duration of treatment should be in accordance with what is required to make the organism powerless; and
- local and systemic host-resistant factors should be taken into consideration.

Other factors to be considered are patient age, type of operation, length of operation, and underlying disease factors, to mention just a few.[127] **Table 11.25** summarizes the mode of action of the classes of antimicrobials.

It is essential to define the terms 'antibiotic', 'antimicrobial', and 'chemotherapeutic' agents, which have become interchangeable in medicine today.

- *Antibiotic*: life destructive; a biological substance produced by a living microbe with the capacity to inhibit or kill bacteria in dilute concentrations.
- *Antimicrobial*: suppression of growth or killing of bacteria; compounds possessing this antibacterial activity are usually synthesized in a laboratory, e.g. sulfonamides.
- *Chemotherapeutic*: life destructive; a chemical substance or combination of the above, e.g. carbolic acid, phenol, sodium hypochlorite, or acyclovir.[127] The mechanisms of action are mobile. Intermediary inhibition is accomplished by chemical substances that inhibit metabolism, e.g. sulfonamides, which act as analogs of p-aminobenzoic acid, thereby averting the synthesis of folic acid; silver sulfadiazine action is primarily due to silver toxicity to the microbe coupled with the action of sulfa. However, some antimicrobials such as penicillins require the bacteria to be in an actively metabolizing state and interact between the cell wall and cell membrane in order to be effective;

otherwise, they have little or no effect on a microbe whose cell wall is completely developed. Other antimicrobials, such as colistin or the polymyxins, affect the bacterial membrane. These antibiotics contain both lipophilic and lipophobic chemical molecules, giving them the ability to disrupt the lipid–protein interface which is the foundation of the microbial membrane. This disruption prevents the membrane from freely diffusing nutrients necessary for cell survival. Consequently, permanent binding of the cytoplasmic membrane by this type of antimicrobial is biocidal.

Antibiotic interference, which inhibits protein synthesis, occurs via two major biosynthetic pathways of microbial inhibition. One interferes with transcription, the process by which an encoded message is transferred to a messenger RNA (mRNA). The other occurs when RNA is in the process of protein synthesis. Consequently, protein synthesis may be inhibited by one or both of the above mechanisms. All aminoglycosides bind to the 30S ribosomal subunit, therefore inhibiting peptide bond composition, which eventually forms an inactive 70S ribosome. Chloramphenicol binds to the microbe's 50S ribosome, thus preventing the attachment of the active aminoacyl end of the aminoacyl-tRNA. Those antibacterials responsible for DNAse inhibition include nalidixic acid, novobiocin, and the quinolones (i.e. ciprofloxacin), which are variable in their interaction, and may interfere with transcription, DNA polymerase, and interaction with purine analogues, respectively[123,127] (**Table 11.24**).

The activities described above against the invading bacteria are not selective for just the bacteria. Those antibiotics which affect membrane, RNA, DNA, and intermediary metabolism of the bacteria also attack a host's metabolic process, thus interfering with a host's healing process.

Systemic antimicrobial therapy: the rationale

The employment of systemic antibiotics can be separated into three major approaches: perioperative, prophylactic, and therapeutic. While the use of systemic antibiotics is extremely essential in burn surgery when compared to other surgical services, it is important that we define a few terms.

- *Perioperative*: may be also considered prophylaxis; however, it involves the administration of systemic

Table 11.25 The metabolic effects of antimicrobials

Interrupts cell wall synthesis
  Aztreonam
  Bacitracin
  Cephalosporins
  Imipenem
  Penicillins
  Vancomycin
Interrupts cell membrane permeability
  Amphotericin B
  Grapefruit seed extract
  Nystatin
  Polymyxin B
  Polymyxin E (colistin)
Interrupts protein synthesis
  Amikacin
  Azithromycin
  Chloramphenicol
  Erythromycin
  Gentamicin
  Kanamycin
  Lincomycin
  Linezolid
  Neomycin
  Rifampin
  Streptomycin
  Telithromycin
  Tobramycin
Interrupts DNA synthesis
  Ciprofloxacin
  Griseofulvin
  Levofloxacin
  Nalidixic acid
  Norfloxacin
  Novobiocin
Interrupts intermediary metabolism
  Mafenide acetate
  Nitrofurans
  Silver sulfadiazine
  Sulfonamides
  Trimethoprim
  Acticoat

antibiotics as a protective measure for any type of surgical intervention. The time frame for administration should be short-lived and dosing is usually limited to one to time doses, depending on the operative procedure.

■ *Prophylactic*: a precautionary or preventative measure designed to preserve health and prevent the possible spread of disease (i.e. penicillin prophylaxis for 72 hours to prevent streptococcal infections in burns, tetanus toxoid for tetanus).

■ *Therapeutic*: the administration of antibiotics for the treatment of infection. Depending on the infection, therapy may continue for several days.[127]

As discussed above, prophylactic penicillin is usually administered to circumvent the emergence of *Strep. pyogenes* or Group A streptococci, and other β-hemolytic streptococci which are frequently responsible for graft loss, surgical and burn wound sepsis,

and other sequelae related to these infections. Cellulitis resulting from a streptococcal infection usually resolves under penicillin therapy. One can easily confirm this sequelae by a skin scraping of cellulitis lesion and a Gram stain. The presence of gram-positive cocci in chains is confirmation that the existing cellulitis is caused by streptococci.[4,13,34,127]

Any article dealing with the prevention or treatment of surgical and burn wound infections will inescapably encounter some controversy. Independent of the most conspicuous questions regarding indications, choice of antibiotic, route of administration, timing and duration, and the prophylactic or perioperative administration of antibiotics are the foundational concerns which impinge on such vehemently argued issues as excessive use of the medication, real risks versus potential benefits, and, last but not least, the ascending costs of hospital care.

Krizek and his colleagues published papers in 1975 and in 1985 where they described the fluctuation in use of antimicrobials.[155,156]

While major changes were observed for other areas of surgery, there has been little change in the use of antibiotics for burns when considering all burns; but there appears to be a significant demarcation when one reviews their use for in-patient burns. The responders in the 1985 survey showed a 16% decrease in their use of prophylactic antimicrobial therapy, which appears somewhat incongruent with current methodologies in burn care (i.e. early excision and grafting). However, it might also be reflective of the burn size treated by the surgeon.[95]

The general consensus regarding burn injuries is dependent on the size and the environment in which the incident occurred. A little burn (<10%) caused by scalding water might be considered a clean wound, which would require no antimicrobial coverage. However, a large flame burn due to a gas heater explosion in a garage should be considered a dirty wound, possibly contaminated or colonized with exogenous microbes present in the garage environment. This can be compounded by contaminated devices or substances in the environment used to extinguish the flames (old blankets, etc).

Burn size and the circumstances surrounding the event must influence the burn surgeon's decision to use or not use antibiotics.[155,156] Sasaki *et al.*[95] showed that several of the burn wound manipulations were responsible for bacteremias; not only do the trauma and tangential excision induce a bacteremia in approximately 50% of the cases when compared to other methods of manipulation, but routine instrumentation can also cause bacteremia.[95,157,158] The bigger the size of the initial burn, the greater the increase in the incidence of bacteremia. Those patients with a positive blood culture had an average TBSA injury of 46.6%, while those with a 25.5% TBSA injury had negative blood cultures.[95] A better understanding in determining when and when not to use antimicrobial agents may be provided by the definition of several terms:

■ *Bacteremia*: the transient presence of microorganisms in blood (i.e. bacteria in blood after brushing one's teeth or after sigmoidoscopy).[157–159]

■ *Septicemia*: the invasion of the bloodstream by pathogenic bacteria from a local foci of infection which provides an active multiplication of these bacteria and which is frequently accompanied by hyperthermia, hypothermia, and prostration.[159] This is a clinical diagnosis predicated on any three of the cardinal clinical and laboratory criteria for sepsis.

- *Colonization*: the presence of bacteria demonstrated by bacterial counts less than 10^5 bacteria per gram of tissue with no evidence of invasion, based on histopathologic data.[29,91] This can be monitored by quantitative biopsies and kept in control by the use of topical antibacterials.
- *Burn wound sepsis*: the presence of bacteria: where bacterial biopsy counts exceed 10^5 bacteria per gram of tissue[29,91,92] (**Table 11.20**).

Determination of the use of antimicrobial agents must be based on the knowledge of existing microorganisms which are present not only on the injured skin, but in the wound ready for closure. All wounds containing β-hemolytic streptococci or with a bacterial count >10^5 should be treated with an appropriate systemic or topical antimicrobial, or both, prior to closure.[123–125]

Administration of systemic antimicrobials

The plethora of experimental and clinical data compiled over the past 25 years clearly indicates that *in vivo* use of systemic antibiotics, when delivered more than 3–4 hours post-surgery, is totally ineffective.[116,123,127] Selecting a suitable antibiotic must be predicated on several factors:

- the possible pathogenic organism that could or can establish a burn wound infection;
- susceptibility patterns of etiologic agents characteristic of each hospital environment; and
- the kind of wound, i.e. incisional, traumatic, or burn wound.[116,123]

The risk of burn wound infection directly corresponds to the quantitative number of pathogenic organisms surviving in a wound. Determining the number of viable microbes present in burn tissue, or other biological body fluid, via quantitative analysis, furnishes confirmatory data which determines the extent of contamination or infection.[34,124]

Pharmacokinetics

The precise description of the pharmacokinetics of any drug can be extremely complex; the clinician can benefit considerably from the estimates that are fairly accurate and yet comprehensible. It is the aim of this chapter to be useful in the construction of therapeutic regimens and in the modification of these regimens for individualization of antimicrobial therapy.[160] More extensive discussions of pharmacokinetics can be found in several excellent books.[161,162]

It is important to note here, that in attempting to provide an adequate dosing regimen for a burn patient, the surgeon should take into consideration the hypermetabolic state of the patient. Such hypermetabolism necessitates higher dosages than normal since excretion rates are enhanced.[105,106,117,127]

The time-dependent interactions of antibacterial agents are important to both effectiveness and toxicity. The interactions of drugs and microorganisms depend on achieving antibiotic concentrations immediately adjacent to the bacteria, and consequently these levels depend on human drug interactions which include absorption, distribution, metabolism, excretion, and clinical status. Additionally, the serum and tissue concentrations of drugs may correlate with dose-related toxicities. Consequently, time-dependent interactions with humans can also be used to construct dosing regimens.

Volume of distribution

The volume of distribution (V_D) of a drug is interpreted as that volume in which the total amount of drug in the body (A) would have to be uniformly divided in order to give an observed plasma concentration (C_p).

$$V_D = \frac{A}{C_P}$$

Consequently, if 140 mg of gentamicin were given to a 70 kg patient and the serum concentration was found to be 8 µg/ml (= 8 mg/l), then the volume of distribution would be (140 mg) ± (8 mg/liter) = 17.5 liters.

The V_D is often represented in terms of body weight (l/kg). If expressed as l/kg, then the actual V_D is obtained simply by multiplying V_D per kg by the body weight.

If we modify the equation above, the dose (or amount) necessary to produce any desired serum concentration can be calculated with a drug whose V_D is known or the serum concentration that can be expected with any chosen dose. Thus, if the goal is to produce a serum concentration of gentamicin at 10 µg/ml (= 10 mg/l) in a 70 kg man, and the V_b is known to be 0.25 l/kg, then the dose must = (V_D) (C_P) = (0.25 l/kg) (70 kg) (10 mg/l) = 175 mg.

The volume of distribution need not and usually does not correspond to any actual anatomic or physiologic space. It is simply a mathematical tool.

Most antimicrobial agents have a V_D of between 0.15 l/kg and 0.40 l/kg. However, a few have larger V_D. The important clinical use of the V_D is that it provides an initial or loading dose that promptly delivers a therapeutic serum concentration. The V_D is also useful, as addressed below, in calculating subsequent or maintenance doses to attain therapeutic and yet safe serum concentrations.

Half-life

The half-life of a drug is interpreted as the time required for the serum concentration to fall to one-half its original concentration as it is being eliminated from the body.

Usually the half-life associated with a drug is the half-life of the predominant phase of drug elimination that absorption of the drug has been completed. It is also given that the fall in the serum concentration is parallel to the fall in the total concentration of drug in the body. The half-life of a drug remains constant over time if there has been no change in the processes of drug elimination, which the surgeon must anticipate when administering antibacterial therapy to a burn patient. During each half-life, 50% of the total amount of drug in the body is eliminated, and the serum concentration falls by 50%.

The half-lives of antimicrobial agents are variable. All of the current β-lactam antibiotics except ceftriaxone have very short half-lives (usually <1.5 hours). The aminoglycosides half-lives are somewhat longer (2–3 hours). Ceftriaxone, flucytosine, sulfisoxazole, and vancomycin have half-lives of 3–6 hours. Sulfamethoxazole, tetracycline, and trimethoprim have half-lives of 6–12 hours. Doxycycline has a relatively long half-life of 20 hours.

Clinically, a drug's half-life is prolonged in renal and hepatic dysfunction. The half-life may also be influenced by age, with extensions of the half-life in the newborn and the elderly, and with shortened half-lives in young children when compared with young adult values. Other drugs administered concomitantly can also alter a drug's half-life. However, it must be kept in mind that one is treating a thermally injured individual who is infected.

Repetitive dosing

With repetitive dosing of a drug at regular intervals, the peak serum concentrations and the trough concentrations rise to a steady state, and after this steady state is reached, the peak and trough serum concentrations remain constant if the dose remains constant and of course if there is no change in the rate of drug elimination. The attainment of a plateau or steady state is also applicable to continuous dosing at a constant rate where the serum concentrations climb until a steady state is reached and remain constant.

The rate at which the steady state is achieved is exclusively a function of the half-life of drug elimination and is dependent on the rate of drug delivery. Consequently, giving more per dose or per unit of time ultimately provides a higher concentration at the steady state but the steady state is still reached at the same time. A useful interpretation is that the steady state is achieved after four half-lives. In actuality, after one half-life the peak and trough of the mean serum concentration is about 50%, after three half-lives 88%, and after four half-lives 94% of the ultimate plateau levels. Therefore, when a dosage change is made or when a drug is discontinued, the new steady state is achieved after about four half-lives.

Clearly, the principle of a steady state has greater significance clinically with a half-life of several hours or longer than with a half-life of 1 hour or less. Generally, in antimicrobial chemotherapy, a loading dose must be considered whenever the half-life of the chosen drug is estimated to be 3 hours or longer. A loading dose should also be considered whenever the half-life of the chosen drug is estimated to be extended beyond 3 hours by hepatic or renal dysfunction.

Treatment of infections in burns

The major role of the antibiotic is to eliminate the potential agent of infection in the burn patient. The systemic treatment of an infection is often begun based on the empiric knowledge of the most common types of microbial infections seen in the burn population and the antibiotics that are most efficacious in their treatment. These infections will be divided into gram-negative and gram-positive bacterial infections in order to discuss the best antimicrobial therapy in their treatment.

Gram-positive bacterial infections

The three most common gram-positive organisms causing burn wound infections are the streptococci, staphylococci, and enterococci (**Table 11.5**).

Streptococcal infections

Immediately post-admission for a burn wound, patients are prophylaxed with the natural penicillins for 72 hours to prevent the emergence of the β-hemolytic streptococci of group A or B (*Strep. pyogenes* or *Strep. agalactiae*). Cellulitis may develop due to

streptococcal infection but can be treated with the natural penicillins. The natural penicillins, which consist of penicillin G and penicillin V, are usually bactericidal in action. Like most other β-lactam antibiotics, the antibacterial activity of the drugs results from inhibition of mucopeptide synthesis in the bacterial cell wall. Resistance to these antibiotics is due to the production of β-lactamases and/or intrinsic resistance. β-lactamases can inactivate the drugs by hydrolyzing the β-lactam ring of the penicillin antibiotic. Intrinsic resistance can result from the presence of a permeability barrier in the outer membrane of the organism or alteration in the properties of the target enzymes (penicillin-binding proteins). Should resistance or tolerance to the penicillins develop, then culture and sensitivity data would be utilized to select a therapeutic antibiotic to treat the streptococcal infection appropriately.[8,160]

Staphylococcal infections

Staphylococcus aureus and *Staph. epidermidis* are natural pathogens found on the skin and therefore are the most common cause of infections in the burn population (**Table 11.1**). These microbes generally produce penicillinases that break the penicillin ring and make the natural penicillins ineffective against these bacteria. These types of infections are generally treated by penicillinase-resistant penicillins that are termed 'methicillin-sensitive', and by vancomycin for those staphylococcal infections that are termed 'methicillin-resistant'.[4,123]

Penicillinase-resistant penicillins are active against many strains of *Staph. aureus* and *Staph. epidermidis* that are resistant to other commercially available penicillins because 60–95% of clinical isolates of *Staph. aureus* and 10–70% of clinical isolates of *Staph. epidermidis* produce penicillinases and are resistant to natural penicillins. These antibiotics include the parenteral antibiotics methicillin, nafcillin, and oxacillin, and the oral antibiotics cloxacillin, dicloxacillin, nafcillin, and oxacillin.[4,123,160]

Nafcillin is the most frequently used IV penicillinase-resistant penicillin since adverse renal effects have been reported most frequently with patients receiving IV methicillin, and hepatotoxicity has been reported most frequently in patients receiving IV oxacillin. As with other penicillins, hypersensitivity reactions are among the most frequent adverse reactions to penicillinase-resistant penicillins.[4,123,160]

Dicloxacillin is the most completely absorbed penicillinase-resistant penicillin from the GI tract and is therefore the most frequently used oral form of these antibiotics. Dosage adjustments are generally unnecessary when nafcillin or dicloxacillin are used in patients with renal impairment. *In vitro* studies indicate that a synergistic bactericidal effect can occur against penicillinase-producing and nonpenicillinase-producing *Staph. aureus* susceptible to penicillinase-resistant penicillins when nafcillin is used in conjunction with gentamicin or tobramycin.[160]

Vancomycin, alone or in conjunction with other anti-infectives, is generally considered the treatment of choice for infections caused by methicillin-resistant staphylococci. In the burn population, wherein methicillin-resistant staphylococci are reported with increasing frequency, initial therapy for suspected staphylococci infections should include vancomycin. Vancomycin is bactericidal and appears to bind to the bacterial cell wall, causing blockage of glycopeptide polymerization. This effect, which occurs at a site different from that affected by the penicillins, produces immediate inhibition of cell wall synthesis and secondary damage to the cytoplasmic membrane. Vancomycin is administered only by slow IV infusion. It is very irritating to tissue and therefore cannot be given intramuscularly. It is also not appreciably absorbed from the GI tract and cannot be given orally for the treatment of systemic infections. It must be given slowly over at least 1 hour since rapid IV administration has resulted in a hypotensive reaction referred to as the 'red man's syndrome' or 'red neck syndrome'. The reaction is characterized by a sudden decrease in blood pressure which can be severe and may be accompanied by flushing and/or a maculopapular or erythematous rash on the face, neck, chest, and upper extremities; the latter manifestation may also occur in the absence of hypotension.[123,160] Vancomycin must be carefully dosed and serum levels of the drug monitored since there is a narrow therapeutic versus toxic serum concentration range for this drug.

The burn patient also exhibits an increased creatinine clearance of this drug because of the hypermetabolic state after the burn trauma. Because of the wide interpatient variability of vancomycin elimination in the burn patient, the dosage must be individualized to provide optimal serum concentrations. The appropriate peak therapeutic blood level is 20–40 µg/ml in the treatment of staphylococci sepsis, with a trough of between 5 and 10 µg/ml. Toxic trough levels higher than 10 µg/ml are thought to be the cause of the nephrotoxicity, which may be manifested by transient elevations in the BUN or serum creatinine clearance, and the presence of hyaline and granular casts and albumin in the urine. Toxic peak levels of greater than 50 µg/ml are thought to cause ototoxicity. Vancomycin may cause damage to the auditory branch of the eighth cranial nerve. Permanent deafness has occurred. Tinnitus may precede the onset of deafness and necessitates discontinuance of the drug. Deafness may progress despite cessation of vancomycin therapy.[123,160]

Infections caused by MRSA (methicillin-resistant *Staph. aureus*) or methicillin-resistant *Staph. epidermidis* (MRSE) can be treated with vancomycin in conjunction with rifampin and/or an aminoglycoside. However, because of the additive toxicities with the concurrent systemic use of ototoxic or nephrotoxic drugs such as the aminoglycosides, their use should be carefully monitored.[160]

Staphylococcus aureus isolates with intermediate resistance to vancomycin glycopeptide-intermediate *Staph. aureus* (GISA) were first identified in 1996. Several more cases have been reported to date. Transfer of vancomycin resistance from *Enterococcus* to *Staphylococcus* species has not occurred *in vivo* as expected from *in vitro* experimentation. One proposed mechanism of glycopeptide resistance in *Staph. aureus* is cell wall thickening, causing vancomycin to bind less avidly. Despite the small number of reported GISA cases, it is imperative to assess the utility of currently marketed and investigational agents active against *Staph. aureus* in the event that glycopeptide antimicrobial agents are not a viable treatment option. Acronyms such as 'GISA', 'VISA', and 'VRSA' have been used to identify isolates of MRSA with reduced susceptibility to vancomycin. The difference in terminology reflects the differences in the definitions and the current state of confusion about the significance of such strains among infection control practitioners, infectious disease specialists, and microbiologists.

VRSA, or vancomycin-resistant *Staph. aureus*, has been used in the literature by European and Japanese investigators to identify isolates that have vancomycin minimum inhibitory concentrations (MICs) of 4–8 µg/ml frequently associated with treatment failures.

The interpretive criteria published by the National Committee for Clinical Laboratory Standards (NCCLS) employs the acronyms GISA and VISA (vancomycin-intermediate *Staph. aureus*). NCCLS defines organisms that require inhibitory concentrations of vancomycin ≤4 µg/ml as '*susceptible*'; those requiring from 8 to 16 µg/ml for inhibition are called 'intermediate susceptible'; while those requiring higher concentrations (≥32 µg/ml) are defined as '*resistant*'. Consequently, in the continental United States, VRSA earmarks only those strains of *Staph. aureus* with vancomycin MICs of ≥32 µg/ml, unlike our European and Japanese colleagues.

The term 'GISA' is technically a more precise description of the isolates we encountered today, because most are considered intermediate to both vancomycin and teicoplanin, which are glycopeptides and may be confusing to many clinicians. **Table 11.26** provides a few key techniques for recognizing GISA strains of *Staph. aureus*. Uniquely, antibiograms may provide an insight into identifying a GISA isolate. The majority of GISA strains of *Staph. aureus* are consistently resistant to penicillin, oxacillin, clindamycin, erythromycin, ciprofloxacin, and rifampin, while most are susceptible to trimethoprim/sulfamethoxazole, chloramphenicol, and tetracycline.[163]

Chloramphenicol

Reports of success and failure exist on the use of chloramphenicol in the treatment of *Staph. aureus* infections. In the United States, chloramphenicol is available in parenteral formulation only; it distributes widely into human tissues with measurable amounts detectable in most body fluids, including cerebrospinal fluid. Adverse effects of chloramphenicol include aplastic anemia, bone marrow suppression, and gray baby syndrome, thus limiting its potential use in oncology patients and infants.

Table 11.26 Key techniques for identifying GISA strains of *Staph. aureus*

Technique	Results	Comment
E-test	Vancomycin MIC≥6 µg/ml on Mueller-Hinton agar	Hold test for 24 h
Broth microdilution[a]	Vancomycin MIC = 8–16 µg/ml in Mueller-Hinton broth	Final reading should be done at 24 h
Brain heart infusion agar containing 6 µg/ml of vancomycin	Growth in 24 h	A positive results is presence of one or more colonies[c]

a. Any commercial microdilution panels (i.e. MicroScan®, Vitek®).
b. Any commercial source (i.e. BBL).
c. Use ATCC 25923, *Staph. aureus* as a negative control, and ATCC 51299, *Ec. faecalis* as a positive control.

Rifampin

This drug is highly active against staphylococci, but resistance develops rapidly when it is used as a single agent. In combination, rifampin is useful with minocycline, TMP-SMX, quinupristin/dalfopristin (Synercid®), and other agents. Cytochrome P-450 metabolized drugs can have their concentrations significantly affected by this P-450 inducer, with many drug interactions thus possible.

Quinupristin/dalfopristin (Synercid®)

One agent recently approved by the FDA for vancomycin-resistant *Ec. faecium* is quinupristin/dalfopristin, a streptogramin antibacterial with good *in vitro* activity against MRSA strains. This combination product is a 30:70 mixture of quinupristin and dalfopristin. Quinupristin is a pristinamycin la (group B streptogramin). Dalfopristin acts synergistically with quinupristin. Nichols reported the use of quinupristin/dalfopristin in skin and soft-tissue MRSA infection. Clinical success in response to *Staph. aureus* was achieved in nearly 71% of patients treated with vancomycin/oxacillin (*n* = 221), compared with almost 60% of patients treated with quinupristin/dalfopristin (*n* = 229). Bacteriological success in the treatment of MRSA infection occurred in 33% of vancomycin/oxacillin-treated and in 49% of quinupristin/dalfopristin-treated patients.[164] The number of patients with bacterial success is small and does not yield a conclusion. Unfortunately, the use of everninomycin in animals has led to the emergence of enterococci resistant to quinupristin/dalfopristin. Adverse effects of quinupristin/dalfopristin include injection-site reactions, GI intolerance, arthralgias/myalgias, and elevated liver function test results.

Enterococcal bacterial infections

The enterococcal microbial isolates most frequently isolated from burn wounds at Shriners Burns Hospital were *Ec. faecalis* and *Ec. faecium*. Enterococcal bacteria, unlike other gram-positive microorganisms, are not very susceptible to any of the penicillin antibiotics. Presently the only antibiotic that appears to be 98–100% effective against the gram-positive organisms that are methicillin-resistant, such as the enterococci, is vancomycin. The carbapenem antibiotic, imipenem, and the aminoglycoside, gentamicin, are synergistic against the enterococci but vancomycin is still the superior agent. Recently, Heggers *et al.* conducted a study to find alternative antibiotics that would be equally effective against VRE to include both species of *Enterococcus* (*faecalis* and *faecium*) of the 30 different isolates. Both chloramphenicol and tetracycline proved to be extremely effective against both VREs, whereas Synercid® is only effective against the VRE *Ec. faecium*. The above two antibiotics are equally effective against MRSA, VISA, and GISA isolates of staphylococci.

Gram-negative bacterial infections

The four most common gram-negative microbial isolates in the burn population at Shriners Burns Hospital were *Ps. aeruginosa*, *Esch. coli*, *Kl. pneumoniae*, and *Ent. cloacae*, in that order. The antibiotic arsenal used and its efficacy is quite varied based on the individual susceptibility of the microbial isolate to each antibiotic agent singly and in combination with other antibiotics.

Aminoglycosides

The aminoglycosides, and in particular gentamicin, were historically the antibiotics of choice in the treatment of gram-negative infections. The synergistic activity with the penicillinase-resistant penicillins and vancomycin in the treatment of staphylococci infections further standardized its premier status before the advent of the newer extended-spectrum penicillins, the third-generation cephalosporins, the monobactams, the carbapenems, and the quinolones[123,160] (**Figures 11.10a,b,c,d** and **11.11a,b**).

Aminoglycosides are usually bactericidal in action. Although the exact mechanism has not been fully elucidated, the drugs appear to inhibit protein synthesis in susceptible bacteria by irreversibly binding to 30S ribosomal units. The aminoglycosides consist of amikacin, gentamicin, kanamycin, neomycin, netilmicin, paromomycin, and tobramycin. The aminoglycosides, narrow therapeutic blood serum range is a critical factor in dosing the burn population since their hypermetabolic state makes dosing an individual function based on the patient's blood levels and their creatinine clearance. As with vancomycin, ototoxicity and nephrotoxicity occur most frequently with toxic serum levels and the additive toxicities of their concurrent use should be carefully monitored.[123,160]

The recommended therapeutic trough levels for gentamicin and tobramycin are between 1 and 2 µg/ml and 5–10 µg/ml for amikacin, and the acceptable peak levels are 4–10 µg/ml for gentamicin and tobramycin and 20–30 µg/ml for amikacin. An increased risk of toxicity occurs in gentamicin and tobramycin with prolonged peak serum concentrations of > 10–12 µg/ml and 30–35 µg/ml with amikacin and/or trough concentrations in gentamicin and tobramycin > 2 µg/ml and > 10 µg/ml with amikacin. Although gentamicin was used IV or IM extensively in the burn population, resistance due to increased permeability of the bacterial cell wall, alterations in the ribosomal binding site, or the presence of a plasmid-mediated resistance factor which is acquired by conjugation, led to the increased usage of tobramycin and finally amikacin, since amikacin is not a suitable substrate for most of the aminoglycoside-modifying enzymes produced by plasmid-mediated resistance.

Routine surveillance of *Ps. aeruginosa* and *Acinetobacter baum/haem* susceptibilities have shown that piperacillin tazobactam (Zosyn®) and ampicillin-sublactam are consistently effective against the above two organisms, respectively.

Extended-spectrum penicillins

The advent of the extended-spectrum penicillins and their reputed synergistic effect with aminoglycosides brought a new era of antibiotic therapy in burn infections. The extended-spectrum penicillins which consist of carbenicillin, mezlocillin, piperacillin, and ticarcillin are more active than the other penicillins against gram-negative bacilli because they are more resistant to inactivation by β-lactamases produced by gram-negative bacteria and/or because they more readily penetrate the outer membranes of these organisms. Extended-spectrum penicillins reportedly vary in their rate of bactericidal action and in their completeness of this effect. This appears to result partly from differences in drug-induced morphologic effects on susceptible bacteria and subsequent formation of bacterial variants with varying degrees of osmotic stability. The extended-spectrum penicillins should therefore never be used alone in the treatment of gram-negative infections. A synergistic effect between extended-spectrum antibiotics and aminoglycosides is generally unpredictable and should be confirmed with appropriate *in vitro* studies (**Figures 11.10a,b,c,d** and **11.11a,b**).

The combination of ticarcillin with clavulanic acid, a β-lactamase inhibitor, results in a synergistic bactericidal effect against many strains of β-lactamases producing bacteria. Clavulanic acid has a high affinity for, and irreversibly binds to, certain lactamases that can inactivate the extended-spectrum penicillins.

The usage of extended-spectrum penicillins in the treatment of gram-negative bacterial infections provided the burn population with a much less toxic antibiotic as compared to the aminoglycosides, since the most frequent adverse reactions to extended-spectrum penicillins were hypersensitivity reactions, GI effects, and local reactions.

Third-generation cephalosporins

The third-generation cephalosporins were the first antibiotics since the introduction of aminoglycosides that could be used alone in the treatment of gram-negative infections. The third-generation cephalosporins are β-lactam antibiotics that are usually bactericidal and like the penicillins their activity results from inhibition of mucopeptide synthesis in the cell wall. β-Lactam antibiotics bind to several enzymes in the bacterial cytoplasmic membrane that are involved in cell wall synthesis and cell division, which results in the formation of defective cell walls and osmotically unstable spheroplasts. The target enzymes have been classified as penicillin-binding proteins (PBPs) and appear to vary substantially among bacterial species. The β-lactam antibiotics spectra of activity is based on the affinity of these antibiotics for different PBPs in susceptible organisms. The third-generation cephalosporins, which consist of cefixime, cefoperazone, cefpodoxime, ceftazidime, ceftizoxime, ceftriaxone, and moxalactam, have an expanded spectrum of activity against gram-negative bacteria compared with the first- and second-generation cephalosporins.

The most frequent adverse reaction to cephalosporins reported are hypersensitivity reactions (approximately 5%). Other less frequent adverse reactions reported are hematologic effects, renal and genitourinary effects, hepetic effects, GI effects, and local effects (**Figures 11.10a,b,c,d** and **11.11a,b**).

With the emergence of more resistant organisms in both gram-positive and gram-negative bacteria, the demand for newer antibiotics becomes paramount. A newer cephalosporin under development, cefepime, has a broad spectrum of activity against gram-positive and gram-negative bacteria. In this study we compared the activity of cefepime (Cpe) to that of ceftriaxone (Cax), ceftazadine (Caz), and cefotaxime (Cft) on organisms isolated in a pediatric burn hospital. A total of 95 isolates were tested: 54 gram-negative rods and 41 methicillin-resistant staphylococci. Cpe susceptibility was determined using the E-test and compared with the Baxter Microscan breakpoint panels for gram-negatives and gram-positives (Caz is not included on the gram-positive panel). Of the gram-negative rods, 94% were sensitive to cefepime, 44% were sensitive to Cax, 85% were sensitive to Caz, and 41% were sensitive to Cft. The staphylococci showed sensitivities of 78% to cefepime, 54% to Cax, and 73% to Cft. These results show that Cpe is a better choice against gram-negative organisms than the other cephalosporins, a slightly better choice against staphylococci than Cft, and a better choice against staphylococci than Cax.

Miscellaneous β-lactam antibiotics

Aztreonam (AZT) is termed a synthetic monobactam antibiotic because, unlike the other β-lactam antibiotics which are bicyclic, it is a monocyclic β-lactam antibiotic. The antibacterial activity of aztreonam also results from inhibition of mucopeptide synthesis in the bacterial cell wall, but in addition aztreonam has a high affinity for PBP-3.[160] Although AZT has a narrow spectrum of activity, it is active *in vivo* against many of the gram-negative bacteria most frequently found in burn units, including most Enterobacteriaceae and *Ps. aeruginosa*. At Shriners Burns Hospital, *Ps. aeruginosa* exhibited a 90–100% susceptibility to aztreonam in 1999 (see **Figure 11.11b**).[165] Aztreonam has a high degree of stability against hydrolysis by bacterial β-lactamases including both plasmid-mediated and chromosomally mediated enzymes (**Figure 11.11b**). Adverse effects reported with AZT are similar to those reported with other β-lactam antibiotics and the drug is generally well tolerated.

Imipenem/cilastatin sodium is a combination of imipenem, a carbapenem antibiotic, with cilastatin sodium, a specific and reversible inhibitor of dehydropeptidase I which inactivates imipenem by hydrolyzing the β-lactam ring. Imipenem is usually bactericidal in action. Like other β-lactam antibiotics the antibacterial activity of imipenem results from inhibition of mucopeptide synthesis in the bacterial cell wall. Imipenem has an affinity for and binds to most PBPs of susceptible organisms. Imipenem is able to penetrate the outer membrane of most gram-negative bacteria and gain access to the PBPs more readily than many other currently available β-lactam antibiotics. *In vitro* studies also indicate that imipenem may have a postantibiotic inhibitory effect against some susceptible organisms such as *Staph. aureus*, *Esch. coli*, and *Ps. aeruginosa*. At Shriners Burns Hospital, *Esch. coli*, *Kl. pneumoniae*, and *Ent. cloacae* all showed susceptibility of 90–100% to imipenem/cilastatin sodium. *Ps. aeruginosa* showed a susceptibility of 80–100% to imipenem/cilastatin sodium. *In vitro* studies indicate that imipenem is a potent inducer of β-lactamases and can reversibly derepress inducible, chromosomal, mediated β-lactamases in *Ps. aeruginosa*, and Enterobacteriaceae. Although these enzymes inactivate AZT and most cephalosporins, adverse effects reported with imipenem and cilastatin are similar to those reported with other β-lactam antibiotics; and the drug is generally well tolerated although adverse central nervous system (CNS) effects, including seizures and myocloma, have been reported with IV imipenem and cilastatin sodium (**Figures 11.10a,b,c,d** and **11.11a,b**).

Quinolones

The quinolones class of antibiotics includes the parenteral antibiotics (ciprofloxacin and ofloxacin) and the oral antibiotics (ciprofloxacin, levofloxacin, enoxacin, lomefloxacin, nalidixic acid, norfloxacin, and ofloxacin). Ciprofloxacin IV is one of the most effective quinolones in the treatment of serious Gram-negative and Gram-positive infections. It is usually bactericidal in action and works by inhibiting DNA synthesis. Susceptibility of *Ent. cloacae* at Shriners Burns Hospital to ciprofloxacin can be produced *in vitro* in some organisms including some strains of the Enterobacteriaceae, *Ps. aeruginosa*, *Staph. aureus*, and *Ec. faecalis* by serial passage in the presence of increasing concentrations of the drug. Strains of MRSA, which are resistant to ciprofloxacin, have been reported with increasing frequency, and such strains can emerge at relatively rapid rates. The most frequent adverse effects of the drug involve the GI tract or the CNS problems.

Background

Several studies in children with cystic fibrosis have found that the use of ciprofloxacin was efficacious. From 1 January 1993 to 31 December 1997 56 pediatric burn patients at Shriners Hospital for Children were treated with ciprofloxacin when cultures proved resistant to other antibiotics. The hypothesis was that ciprofloxacin treatment is justified in the case of multiresistant organisms in burn populations. The burn area was 65% of the TBSA. The average patient age was 8.4 years. Of the 56 patients who received ciprofloxacin, 50 received the recommended dose. Biopsy specimens were assessed for quantitative bacteriology and antibiotic sensitivity. Radiologic review was conducted to examine for arthropathy. All patients showed unequivocal reduction in quantitative bacterial counts, and susceptibility to ciprofloxacin remained stable without the development of resistance. Of the 56 patients treated, 42 had a major reduction in their quantitative wound biopsies from 10^6 to fewer than 100 colonies per gram of tissue, while the remaining 14 were observed to have a 2- to 3-log decrease. No arthropathy was detected in any of the 56 patients receiving ciprofloxacin. Review of the patients' charts showed no documented adverse events associated with the use of ciprofloxacin. All patients survived their thermal injury and the complications associated with it without any untoward problems or complications of arthropathy.

On the basis of these data, ciprofloxacin therapy in the treatment of immunosuppressed pediatric burn patients is efficacious and does not cause arthropathy.[166]

Polymyxins

Colistimethate sodium is not routinely used as a systemic antimicrobial due to the dose-related nephrotoxicity, pseudomembranous colitis, and transient neurological disturbances associated with its use. The development of multiply-resistant *Ps. aeruginosa* sensitive only to colistimethate sodium led to its incorporation into the antimicrobial armamentarium at Shriners Hospital for Children. A bioassay for monitoring therapeutic serum levels through the use of *Bordetella bronchiseptica* in which the antimicrobial disk zone diameters were associated with known colistimethate sodium concentrations. The individual serum colistimethate sodium concentrations were then plotted at steady state. Thus, efficacious as well as safe serum concentrations of 100 µg/ml or less were determined. Patient creatinine clearance was monitored, as was intake and output, and sensorium to monitor for kidney function, diarrhea, and sensorium. Patient demographics are listed in **Table 11.27**. It was found that the antibiotic was efficacious in reducing *Ps. aeruginosa* colony counts in the doses administered with no toxicities.

Rotating antibiotic classes

One study examined the importance of whether scheduled changes of antibiotic classes targeted at the empiric treatment of gram-negative bacterial infections can reduce the occurrence of inadequate antimicrobial treatment and influence antibiotic resistance in ICUs. It was observed that in ICU patients who are treated for infectious diseases empirically, treatment is inadequate in roughly 25% of those cases which result in increased risk or mortality. Inadequate treatment is often due to undertreatment of antibiotic-resistant gram-negative bacilli. In an 18-month study in an adult ICU, empiric antibiotic treatment of bacterial infections were targeted with the recommendation for a 6-month interval for rotating antibiotics. In the first 6-month interval, ceftazidime was the recommended empiric agent; in the second period, ciprofloxacin; and in the third interval, cefepime. This rotational schedule led to a decrease in administration of inadequate antibiotic treatment for nosocomial gram-negative bacterial infections, with the rate of inadequate treatment falling to 1.6% by the end of the 18-month study. One rotational approach is to change the classes of antibiotics every 3 months, with monthly surveillance of organisms' susceptibility patterns.

Antifungals

Amphotericin B

Chemistry. Amphotericin B is an antifungal antibiotic produced by *Streptomyces nodosus*. The drug is an amphoteric polyene macrolide which occurs as a yellow to orange, odorless or practically odorless powder and is insoluble in water and in anhydrous alcohol. Each mg of amphotericin B contains no less than 750 µg of anhydrous drug. Amphotericin B for injection is commercially available as a sterile, buffered, lyophilized yellowish powder which contains sodium desoxycholate as a solubilizing agent.

Fungi. *In vitro*, amphotericin B concentrations of 0.03–1.0 µg/ml usually inhibit *Aspergillus fumigatus*, *Paracoccidioides brasiliensis*, *Coccidioides immitis*, *Cryptococcus neoformans*, *Histoplasma capsulatum*, *Mucor mucedo*, *Rhodotorula* spp., and *Sporothrix schenckii*. *Blastomyces dermatitidis* may require slightly higher drug concentrations for inhibition. The MIC of amphotericin B for *Candida* varies with species and strains; the MIC for *Can. albicans* and *Can. guilliermondil* is 0.2–1.9 µg/ml, and for strains of *Can. tropicalis* the MIC ranges from 0.2 to 25 µg/ml. It has been suggested that to successfully treat a systemic fungal infection, serum amphotericin B concentrations should be maintained at twice the *in vitro* MIC for the infecting fungus.

Protozoa. Amphotericin B is active *in vitro* and *in vivo* against *Leishmania braziliensis*. The drug is also active *in vitro* and *in vivo* against *L. mexicana* and *L. donovani*, including antimony-resistant strains of the organisms. *In vitro*, amphotericin B concentrations of

Table 11.27 Dosing, efficacy, and toxicity of colistimethate sodium in the treatment of multiresistant *P. aeruginosa* in pediatric burns

Gender	Age (Yr)	Wt. (kgs)	TBSA (%)	Dose (mg/kg/day)	Freq.	Duration (days)	Steady-State serum conc.	Efficacy	Toxicity
Female	16	47.5	95	5.2	Q12h	10	1 µg/ml	+	−
Male	7	17.3	85	5.2	Q8h	15	100 µg/ml	+	−
Female	16	51	MVA	4.7	Q12h	9		+	−
Male	16	43	88	5.2	Q8h	7		+	−
Female	4	26	65	5.2	Q8h	28	200 µg/ml	+	−

1 μg/ml result in complete elimination of *L. donovani* promastogites in human monocyte-derived macrophages and *L. donovani* promastogites in cell-free media. The drug is also active *in vitro* against *L. tropica*.

Absorption. Amphotericin B is poorly absorbed from the GI tract and must be given parenterally to treat systemic fungal infections. Immediately after completion of IV infusion of 30 mg of amphotericin B, average peak serum concentrations of 1 μg/ml can be achieved; with a dose of 50 mg, average peak serum concentrations will approximately be 2 μg/ml. Immediately after infusion, no more than 10% of the amphotericin B dose can be accounted for in serum. Average minimum serum concentrations of approximately 0.4 μg/ml have been reported when doses of 30 mg were given daily or when doses of 60 mg were given every other day.

Elimination. The elimination half-life of amphotericin B in patients whose renal function is normal prior to therapy is approximately 24 hours. Then after the first 24 hours, the rate at which amphotericin B is eliminated decreases. Over a 7-day period, the cumulative urinary excretion of a single dose of amphotericin B is about 40% of the administered drug. Following long-term administration of the drug, the elimination half-life of amphotericin B was 15 days, which suggests that slow release of the drug from the peripheral compartment may have accounted for the long half-life. It has been estimated that only about 3% of a total dose of amphotericin B is excreted in urine unchanged. The drug can be detected in blood up to 4 weeks and in urine up to 4–8 weeks after discontinuance of therapy. Amphotericin B is not hemodialyzable.

Adverse effects. Most patients who receive IV amphotericin B experience several of the following reactions: headache, chills, fever, hypotension, tachypnea, malaise, muscle and joint pain, anorexia, weight loss, dyspepsia, cramping, epigastric pain, and nausea and vomiting. Most of these reactions are considered to be dose-related, and they are usually less severe when the drug is administered slowly or on alternate days. Antipyretics, antihistamines, and antiemetics provide some symptomatic relief from many of the adverse effects of amphotericin B. The febrile reaction, which is sometimes accompanied by shaking chills, usually appears 1–3 hours after the start of IV infusion of amphotericin B and thus can be differentiated from chills due to bacterial infection; the febrile reaction usually subsides within 4 hours after discontinuance of the IV infusion.

Other acute reactions (e.g. hypotension, nausea, vomiting, tachypnea) appear 1–3 hours after initiating IV infusion of amphotericin B; the severity of these reactions may decrease with subsequent doses of the drug. Intravenous administration of corticosteroids prior to or during amphotericin B therapy reportedly decreases the severity of febrile reactions. Nephrotoxicity occurs in about 80% or more of the patients receiving the drug IV. Although nephrotoxicity of amphotericin B involves several mechanisms, including direct vasoconstriction, the drug appears to have a lytic action on cholesterol-rich lysosomal membranes of renal tubular cells.[160,162]

Fluconazole

Chemistry. Fluconazole is a synthetic triazole-derivative antifungal agent. The drug is structurally related to imidazole-derivative antifungal agents (e.g. butoconazole, clotrimazole, ketoconazole, micronazole), since it contains a five-membered azole ring attached by a carbon–nitrogen bond to other aromatic rings. However, imidazoles have two nitrogens in the azole ring and fluconazole and other triazoles (e.g. itraconazole, terconazole) have three nitrogens in the ring.

Spectrum. Fluconazole is active against fungi, including yeasts and dermatophytes. Fluconazole does not appear to have antibacterial activity.

Absorption. The pharmacokinetics of fluconazole are similar following IV or oral administration. The drug is rapidly and almost completely absorbed from the GI tract, and there is no evidence of first-pass metabolism. Oral bioavailability of fluconazole exceeds 90% in healthy, fasting adults; peak serum concentrations of the drug generally are attained within 1–2 hours after oral administration. The rate and extent of GI absorption of fluconazole are not affected by food.

Unlike some imidazole-derivative antifungal agents (e.g. ketoconazole), GI absorption of fluconazole does not appear to be affected by gastric pH. Studies in healthy, fasting adults indicate that peak serum concentrations, areas under the concentration–time curves (AUCs), time to peak serum concentrations, and elimination half-life of fluconazole are not affected substantially by concurrent administration of drugs that increase gastric pH.

In healthy, fasting adults who received a single 1 mg/kg oral dose of fluconazole, peak serum concentrations of the drug averaged 1.4 μg/ml. Following oral administration of a single 400-mg dose of fluconazole in healthy, fasting adults, peak serum concentrations average 6.72 μg/ml (range: 4.12–8.1 μg/ml). In healthy adults receiving 50 or 100 mg doses of fluconazole given once daily by IV infusion over 30 minutes, serum concentrations of the drug 1 hour after dosing on the sixth or seventh day of therapy range from 2.14 to 2.81 or 3.86–4.96 μg/ml, respectively.

Elimination. The serum elimination half-life of fluconazole in adults with normal renal function is approximately 30 hours (range 20–50 hours). Serum elimination or half-life of the drug is 22 hours after the first day of therapy and 23.8 and 28.6 hours after 7 and 26 days of therapy, respectively.

In patients with impaired renal function, plasma concentrations of fluconazole are higher and the half-life prolonged; elimination half-life of the drug is inversely proportional to the patient's creatinine clearance. In addition, there is limited evidence that elimination of the drug may be impaired in geriatric patients. The elimination half-life of fluconazole reportedly is not affected by impaired hepatic function.

Renal clearance of the drug averages 0.27 ml/min/kg in adults with normal renal function. Approximately 60–80% of a single oral or IV dose of fluconazole is excreted in urine unchanged, and about 11% is excreted in urine as metabolites. Small amounts of the drug are excreted in feces.

Fluconazole is removed by hemodialysis and peritoneal dialysis. The amount of the drug removed during hemodialysis depends on several factors (e.g. type of coil used, dialysis flow rate).

Adverse effects. Fluconazole generally is well tolerated. Adverse effects have been reported in about 5–30% of patients receiving fluconazole for 7 days or longer and have been severe enough to require discontinuance of the drug in about 1–2.8% of patients. Fever, edema, pleural effusion, oliguria, hypotension, arthralgia/myalgia, anaphylaxis, and finger stiffness have been reported rarely in patients receiving fluconazole. Hypokalemia, which required potassium replacement therapy and/or discontinuance of fluconazole, has occurred occasionally, including in several neutropenic patients with acute myeloid leukemia. Increased serum creatinine and BUN concentrations also have been reported.[160,162]

Itraconazole

Sporanox® is the brand name for itraconazole, a synthetic triazole antifungal agent. Itraconazole is a 1:1:1:1 racemic mixture of four diastereomers (two enantiomeric pairs), each possessing three chiral centers. Itraconazole's molecular formula is $C_{35}H_{38}Cl_2N_8O_4$; and it has a molecular weight of 705.64. It is a white to slightly yellowish powder. It is insoluble in water, very slightly soluble in alcohols, and freely soluble in dichloromethane. It has a pKa of 3.70 and a log partition coefficient of 5.66 at pH 8.1.

Mechanism of action. *In vitro* studies have demonstrated that itraconazole inhibits the cytochrome P-450-dependent synthesis of ergostol, which is a vital component of fungal cell membranes.

Pharmacokinetics and metabolism. The oral bioavailability of itraconazole is maximal when Sporanox® (itraconazole) capsules are taken with a full meal. The pharmacokinetics of itraconazole were studied using six healthy male volunteers who received, in a crossover design, a single 100 mg dose of itraconazole as a polyethylene glycol capsule, with or without a full meal. The same six volunteers also received 50 mg or 200 mg with a full meal in a crossover design. In this study, only itraconazole plasma concentrations were measured. Steady-state concentrations were reached within 15 days following oral doses of 50–400 mg daily.

Precautions. Hepatic enzyme test values should be monitored in patients with pre-existing hepatic function abnormalities. Hepatic enzyme test values should be monitored periodically in all patients receiving continuous treatment for more then 1 month or at any time a patient develops signs or symptoms suggestive of liver dysfunction. Patients should be instructed to report any signs and symptoms that may suggest liver dysfunction so that the appropriate laboratory testing can be done. Such signs and symptoms may include unusual fatigue, anorexia, nausea and/or vomiting, jaundice, dark urine, or pale stool.

Drug interactions. Both itraconazole and its major metabolite, hydroxyitraconazole, are inhibitors of the cytochrome P-450 3A enzyme system. Coadminstration of Sporanox® and drugs primarily metabolized by the cytochrome P-450 3A enzyme system may result in increased plasma concentrations of the other drug that could increase or prolong both its therapeutic and adverse effects.

Adverse reactions. There have been rare cases of reversible idiosyncratic hepatitis reported among patients taking Sporanox® (itraconazole) capsules. Sporanox® has been associated with rare cases of serious hepatotoxicity, including fatalities, primarily in patients with serious underlying medical conditions taking multiple medications. If clinical signs and symptoms develop that are consistent with liver disease and may be attributed to itraconazole, Sporanox® should be discontinued.[167]

Terbinafine

Lamisil® (terbinafine hydrochloride) tablets contain the synthetic allylamine antifungal compound terbinafine hydrochloride. Chemically, terbinafine hydrochloride is (E)-N-(6,6-dimethyl-2-hepten-4ynyl)-N-methyl-1-naphthalenemethanamine hydrochloride. It has the empirical formula $C_{21}H_{26}ClN$, and a molecular weight of 327.90.

Pharmacokinetics. Following oral administration, terbinafine is well absorbed (>70%) and the bioavailability of Lamisil® (terbinafine hydrochloride) tablets as a result of first-pass metabolism is approximately 40%. Peak plasma concentrations of 1 µg/ml appear within 2 hours after a single mg dose; the AUC is approximately 4.56 µg/ml. An increase in the AUC of terbinafine of less than 20% is observed when Lamisil® is administered with food. No clinically relevant age-independent changes in steady-state plasma concentrations of terbinafine have been reported.

Microbiology. Terbinafine hydrochloride is a synthetic allylamine derivative. Terbinafine hydrochloride is hypothesized to act by inhibiting squalene epoxidase, thus blocking the biosynthesis of ergosterol, an essential component of fungal cell membranes. *In vitro*, mammalian squalene epoxidase is only inhibited at higher (4000-fold) concentrations than is needed for inhibition of the dermatophyte enzyme.

Warnings. Rare cases of symptomatic hepatobiliary dysfunction, including cholestatic hepatitis, have been reported. Treatment with Lamisil® (terbinafine hydrochloride) tablets should be discontinued if hepatobiliary dysfunction develops (see Precautions). There have been isolated reports of serious skin reactions (e.g. Stevens–Johnson syndrome and toxic epidermal necrolysis). If progressive skin rash occurs, treatment with Lamisil® should be discontinued.

Drug interactions. *In vitro* studies with human liver microsomes showed that terbinafine does not inhibit the metabolism of tolbutamide, ethinylestradiol, ethoxycoumarin, and cyclosporine. *In vivo* drug–drug interaction studies conducted in normal volunteer subjects showed that terbinafine does not affect the clearance of antipyrine, digoxin, and the antihistamine terfenadine. Terbinafine does not affect the clearance of warfarin or warfarin's effect on prothrombin time. Terbinafine decreases the clearance of IV-administered caffeine by 19%. Terbinafine increases the clearance of cyclosporine by 15%.

Adverse reactions. Reported adverse events observed in three US/Canadian placebo-controlled trials. The adverse events reported encompass GI symptoms including diarrhea, dyspepsia, and abdominal pain, liver test abnormalities, rashes, urticaria, pruritus, and taste disturbances. In general, the adverse events were mild, transient, and did not lead to discontinuation from study participation. Rare adverse events based on worldwide experience with Lamisil® (terbinafine hydrochloride) tablet use include: symptomatic idiosyncratic hepatobiliary dysfunction (including cholestatic hepatitis), serious skin reactions (see Warnings), severe neutropenia, thrombocytopenia, and allergic reactions (including anaphylaxis). Rarely, Lamisil® may cause taste disturbance (including taste loss) which usually recovers within several weeks after discontinuation of the drug. Other adverse reactions which have been reported include malaise, fatigue, vomiting, arthralgia, myalgia, and hair loss.

Dosage and administration. Lamisil® (terbinafine hydrochloride), one 250 mg tablet, should be taken once daily for 6 weeks by patients with fingernail onychomycosis. Lamisil®, one 250 mg tablet, should be taken once daily for 12 weeks by patients with toenail onychomycosis. The optimal clinical effect is seen some months after mycological cure and cessation of treatment. This is related to the period required for outgrowth of healthy nail.[167]

Factors rendering antimicrobials neutralized

The bindings of antimicrobials to the proteins of tissue has been a subject of major concern for microbiologists and surgeons alike. This binding accounts for the reduced tissue levels which are occasionally noted when therapeutic doses of the aminoglycosides and cephalosporins are administered. Insoluble acid proteins, along with intracellular proteins, such as nucleic acids, are the components responsible for such an event.[15,127,160] Polymyxins bind to the phospholipids of the tissue membrane, while soluble intracellular protein binding occurs with such drugs as penicillin, and calcium and magnesium concentrations.[127] Among other factors that diminish the activity of antimicrobials are blood flow, intracellular location of bacteria, and pH. Anaerobic and hypercapneic conditions have been shown to render antibacterials such as the aminoglycosides inactive or less responsive against facultative organisms. Albeit, non-protein-bound drugs diffuse exceedingly well into locations containing blood clots, but such a condition can significantly reduce the antibacterial effect upon staphylococcal organisms present at the time of surgery.[20,160] Moreover, inert substances, such as fecal material, can render aminoglycosides inactive or alter the antimicrobial potential.[20,160]

The appearance of antimicrobial-resistant bacteria has been considered to be the result primarily of a predictable process, i.e. the development of a spontaneous mutation of the microbe with an occurrence rate of one organism in 10 million to 1 billion cell divisions, and with discriminative proliferation of the resistant organism in the presence of the antibiotic. Even more devastating is the phenomenon called 'infectious drug resistance'. This is a process where a genetic marker called a plasmid or transporon carrying an antibiotic-resistant factor is transferred from a resistant organism to a nonresistant one of the same species or of a different species.[123,160]

Lacey[8] has reported on the ecological relationship between the staphylococci and man, which presents some threatening concerns. Both *Staph. aureus* and *Staph. epidermidis* reside in cohabitation on the body surface and in the nasopharyngeal cavities of man; it is in the realm of possibility that the reservoir for these resistant plasmids could have originated in *Staph. epidermidis*, which subsequently is then transferred to *Staph. aureus*. The encoding of the plasmid tetracycline resistance in *Staph. epidermidis* is similar to

that of *Staph. aureus*. The most probable site for transfer is on the surface of skin of the host.[9,168]

In a study by Siegel *et al.*[169] on the continuous nontherapeutic use of antimicrobials in food-producing animals, the incidence of drug resistance was monumental. Organisms isolated from the feces of both bovine and swine demonstrated a minimum of 50% resistance to dihydrostreptomycin and oxytetracycline, which was elevated to 90% in most cases.

The delivery of tetracycline was found by Burton and colleagues[170] to magnify the colonization of the intestinal tract of humans by a resistant *Esch. coli* of bovine origin. The use of this antibacterial subsequently provided the mechanism of these drug-resistant factors to *Esch. coli* which were resident flora in man, as it usually does in food-producing animals.[169] WHO has recently established a ruling on how antibiotics are to be used in the food-processing industry (*Reuters Medical News*, 14 June 2000). **Table 11.28** outlines the rules WHO has established.

Table 11.28 WHO recommendation for antimicrobial use in food animals

1. Creation of national systems to monitor antimicrobial usage in food animals.
2. Obligatory prescriptions for all antimicrobials used for disease control in food animals.
3. Termination or rapid phasing-out of the use of antimicrobials for growth promotion if they are also used for treatment of humans in the absence of a public health safety evaluation.
4. Pre-licensing safety evaluation of antimicrobials with consideration of potential resistance to human drugs.
5. Monitoring of resistance to identify emerging health problems and timely corrective actions to protect human health.
6. Guidelines for veterinarians to reduce overuse and misuse of antimicrobials in food animals.

Summary

Topical and systemic antibacterials are powerful chemotherapeutic agents. However, they cannot, and will never, render man germ-free. The incidence of infection in operative procedures has changed little in the decades since the discovery of antimicrobials, and is most obviously not the result of visitation from without.[34,116,124,171] Antimicrobials should be used with therapeutic accuracy, observing there are many pitfalls.[123,127,171] As previously stated 'SHOOT WITH A RIFLE NOT A SCATTER GUN'.

Acknowledgments

The authors wishes to acknowledge Ms Cassie Maness for her devoted and conscientious efforts in the preparation of this manuscript. We would also like to acknowledge our Graphic Arts Department: Ms Sandra Baxter, our medical illustrator, who provided timely and precise illustrations of the data, and Mr Lewis Milutin Jr and Ms Tina Garcia for their photographic expertise. We also wish to acknowledge our fellow co-workers in Clinical Microbiology – Ms Edith Carino, Joyce Washington, Lana McCoy and Mr Thanh Dang for their devoted efforts in making this chapter come to fruition. Also included are the members of the Pharmacy team who maintained constant vigilance over the therapeutic administration of antibiotics.

References

1. Robson MC, Heggers JP. Surgical infection. 1. Single bacterial species or polymicrobic in origin. *Surgery* 1969; **65**: 608.
2. Balows A, Hausler WJ Jr, Herrmann KL, Isenberg HD, Shadomy HJ, eds. *Manual of Clinical Microbiology*, 5th edn. Washington, DC: American Society for Microbiology, 1991.
3. Baron S, Jennings PM. *Medical Microbiology*, 3rd edn. New York: Churchill Livingstone, 1991.
4. Heggers JP, Robson MC, eds. *Quantitative Bacteriology: Its Role in the Armamentarium of the Surgeon*, 1st edn. Boca Raton, FL: CRC Press, 1991.
5. Dowell VR Jr, Lombard GL, Thompson FSM, Armfield AY. Media for isolation; characterization and identification of obligately anaerobic bacteria. Washington DC: U.S. Department of Health, Education & Welfare, NCDC, 1977; 1–46.
6. Holt JG, Krieg NR, Smeath PHA, Staley JT, Williams ST, eds. *Bergey's Manual of Determinative Bacteriology*, 9th edn. Baltimore: Williams & Wilkins, 1994.
7. Gibbs BM, Skinner FA, eds. *Identification Methods for Microbiologists, Part A*. New York: Academic Press, 1966.
8. Lacey RW. Antibiotic resistance plasmids of *Staphylococcus aureus* and their clinical importance. *Bacteriol Rev* 1975; **39**: 1–32.
9. Heggers JP, Phillips LG, Boertman JA, *et al.* The epidemiology of methicillin-resistant *Staphylococcus aureus* in a burn center. *J Burn Care Rehab* 1988; **9**: 610–12.
10. Mowlavi A, Andrews K, Herndon DN, Heggers JP, Milner S. The effects of hyperglycemia on skin graft survival in the burn patient. *Ann Plast Surg* (in press).
11. Ellner PD. *Current Procedures in Clinical Bacteriology*, 2nd edn. Springfield, IL: Charles C. Thomas, 1978.
12. Mandell GL, Douglas RG Jr, Bennett JE, eds. *Principles and Practice of Infectious Diseases*, 3rd edn. *Vol 2*. New York: Churchill Livingstone, 1990.
13. Robson MC, Heggers JP. Surgical infection. 11. B-hemolytic streptococcus. *J Surg Res* 1969; **9**: 289.
14. Christie R, Atkins NE, Munch-Peterson E. A note on a lytic phenomenon shown by Group B streptococci. *Austr J Exp Biol* 1944; **22**: 197.
15. Gunn BA. SXT and Taxo A disks for presumptive identification of Group A and B streptococci in throat cultures. *J Clin Microbiol* 1976; **4**: 192.
16. Smith LDS, Holderman LV. *The Pathogenic Anaerobic Bacteria*, 2nd edn. Springfield, IL: Charles C. Thomas, 1968.
17. Kingsley RF. Selective medium for *Bacillus anthracis. J Bacteriol* 1966; **92**: 784.
18. Pennington JE, Gibbons ND, Strobeek JE, *et al. Bacillus* species infection in patients with hemotolic neoplasia. *JAMA* 1976; **235**: 1473.
19. Turnbull PCB, French TA, Dowsett EG. Severe systemic and pyogenic infections with *Bacillus cereus. Br Med J* 1977; **1**: 1628.
20. Turnball PCB, Nottingham JF, Ghosh AC. A severe necrotic enterotoxin produced by certain food, food poisoning and other clinical isolates of *Bacillus cereus. Br J Exp Pathol* 1977; **58**: 273.
21. McManus WF, Goodwin CW, Mason AD Jr, Pruitt BA Jr. Burn wound infection. *J Trauma* 1981; **21**: 3133–8.
22. Brook I, Randolph JG. Aerobic and anaerobic bacterial flora of burns in children. *J Trauma* 1981; **21**: 558–63.
23. Hartford CE, Ziffren SE. Electrical injury. *J Trauma* 1971; **11**: 331–6.
24. Gorbach SL, Thadepalli H. Isolation of *Clostridium* in human infections: evaluation of 114 cases. *J Infect Dis* 1975; **131 (Suppl)**: S81–5.
25. Davies DM. Gas gangrene as a complication of burns. *Scand J Plast Reconstr Surg* 1979; **12**: 73–5.
26. Sherman RT. The prevention and treatment of tetanus in the burn patient. *Surg Clin N Am* 1970; **50**: 1277–81.
27. Larkin JM, Moylan JA. Tetanus following a minor burn. *J Trauma* 1975; **15**: 546–8.
28. Artz CP, Moncrief JA. *The Treatment of Burns*. Philadelphia: WB Saunders, 1969.
29. Teplitz C. The pathology of burn and fundamentals of burn wound sepsis. In: Artz CP, Moncrief JA, Pruitt BA Jr, eds. *Burns: A Team Approach*. Philadelphia: WB Saunders Co, 1979; 45–94.
30. Heggers JP, Bames ST, Robson MC, *et al.* Microbial flora of orthopaedic war wounds. *Milit Med* 1969; **134**: 602.
31. Speller DCE, Stephens ME, Viant AC. Hospital infection by *Pseudomonas cepaci. Lancet* 1971; **1**: 1798.
32. Bassett DCJ, Stokes KJ, Thomas WRO. Wound infection with *Pseudomonas multivarons. Lancet* 1970; **1**: 1188.
33. Gilardi GL. *Pseudomonas maltophilia* infections in man. *Am J Clin Pathol* 1969; **51**: 58.
34. Robson MC. Quantitative bacteriology and the burned patient. In: Heggers JP, Robson MC, eds. *Quantitative Bacteriology: Its Role in the Armamentarium of the Surgeon*. Boca Raton, FL: CRC Press, 1991: 97–108.
35. Rigney MM, Zilinsky JW, Rouf MA. Pathogenicity of *Aeromonas hydrophila* in red leg disease in frogs. *Curr Microbiol* 1978; **1**: 175–9.
36. Scholz D, Scharmann W, Blobet H. Leucocidic substances from *Aeromonas hydrophila. Zbl Bakt Hyg 1 Abt Orig A* 1974; **228**: 312–16.
37. Bemheimer AW, Avigad LS, Avigad G. Interactions between aerolysin, erythrocyte membranes. *Infect Immun* 1975; **11**: 1312–19.
38. von Graevenitz A, Mensch AH. The genus *Aeromonas* in human bacteriology: report of 30 cases and review of the literature. *N Engl J Med* 1968; **278**: 245.
39. D'Alauro F, Ansinelli R. *Aeromonas hydrophila* septicemia in a previously healthy man. *JAMA* 1978; **240**: 1139.
40. Harris RL, Fainstein V, Elting L, Hopfer RL, Bodey GP. Bacteremia caused by *Aeromonas* species in hospitalized cancer patients. *Rev Infect Dis* 1985; **7**: 314–20.
41. Qadri SMH, Gordon LP, Wende RD, Williams RP. Meningitis due to *Aeromonas hydrophila. J Clin Microbiol* 1976; **3**: 102–4.
42. Davis WA, Kane JG, Garagusi VF. Human *Aeromonas* infections. *Medicine* 1987; **57(3)**: 267–77.
43. Feaster FT, Nisbet RM, Barber JC. *Aeromonas hydrophila* corneal ulcer. *Am J Ophthal* 1978; **85**: 114–17.
44. Salton R, Schick S. *Aeromonas hydrophila* peritonitis. *Cancer Chemother Rep* 1973; **57**: 489–91.
45. Hanson PG, Standridge J, Jarett F, Maki DG. Fresh-water wound infection due to *Aeromonas hydrophila. J Am Med Assoc* 1977; **238**: 1053–4.
46. Fulghum DD, Linton WR Jr, Taplin D. Fatal *Aeromonas hydrophila* infection of the skin. *Southern Med J* 1978; **71(6)**: 739–74.
47. Lawson MA, Burke V, Chang BJ. Invasion of KEp-2 cells by fecal isolates of *Aeromonas hydrophila. Infect Immun* 1985; **47**: 680–3.
48. Atkinson HM, Trust TJ. Hemagglutination properties and adherence ability of *Aeromonas hydrophila. Infect Immun* 1980; **27**: 938–46.
49. Purdue GF, Hunt JL. *Aeromonas hydrophila* infection in burn patients. *Burns* 1988; **14(3)**: 220–1.
50. Edwards PR, Ewing WH. *Identification of Enterobacteriaceae*, 3rd edn. Minneapolis: Burgess Publishing, 1972.
51. Johnson WG, Pierce AK, Sanford JP. Changing pharyngeal bacterial flora of hospitalized patients. *N Engl J Med* 1969; **281**: 1137.
52. Selden R, Lee S, Wang WLL, *et al.* Nosocomial *Klebsiella* infections: intestinal colonization as a reservoir. *Ann Int Med* 1971; **74**: 657.
53. Bizo A. *Serratia marcescens* vescicula tenuissima lactic primo roses: dehine rubro repleta. *Bil ital gl legg sc* 1823; **30**: 288.
54. Davis JT, Foltz E, Blakemore WS. *Serratia marcescens*: a pathogen of increasing clinical importance. *JAMA* 1970; **214**: 2190.
55. Heniyoji EY, Whitson TC, Obashi DK, Allen BC. Bacteremia due to *Serratia marcescens. J Trauma* 1971; **11**: 417.
56. Alexander RH, Reichenbach DD, Merindino KA. *Serratia marcescens* endocarditis. *Arch Surg* 1969; **98**: 287.
57. Quintilani R, Gifford RH. Endocarditis from *Serratia marcescens. JAMA* 1969; **208**: 2055.
58. Hall A, Inguagiato GJ, Park C. *Serratia marcescens* septicemia complicating splenectomy in a child. *Virginia Med Month* 1971; **98**: 605.
59. Dutton AAC, Ralston M. Urinary tract infection in a male urological ward with special reference to the mode of infection. *Lancet* 1957; **1**: 115.
60. Middleton JE. The sensitivity *in vitro* of the *Providencia* group of enteric bacteria to 14 antibiotics and nitrofurantoin. *J Clin Pathol* 1958; **1**: 270.
61. Solberg CO, Matsen JM. Infection with providence bacilli. A clinical and bacteriologic study. *Am J Med* 1971; **50**: 241.
62. Von Graebenitz A, Strouse A. Isolation of *Erwinia* species from human sources. *Antonie van Leeuwenhoek* 1966; **32**: 429.
63. Von Graevenitz A. *Erwinia* species isolates. *Ann NY Acad Sci* 1970; **174**: 436.
64. Nichols RE, Smith J. Clinical aspects of anaerobic infections in the surgical patient. *Am J Med Technol* 1975; **41**: 87.
65. Feiner JM, Dowell VR Jr. Bacteroides bacteremia. *Am J Med* 1971; **50**: 878.
66. Dowell IR, Jr, Lombard GL. *Presumptive Identification of Anaerobic Nonspore Forming Gram-negative Bacilli*. Washington, DC: US Department of Health, Education and Welfare, NCDC, 1980: 1–13.
67. Becker WK, Cioffi WG Jr, McManus AT, *et al.* Fungal burn wound infection. A 10-year experience. *Arch Surg* 1991; **126(1)**: 44–8.
68. Bruck HM, Nash G, Foley FD, *et al.* Opportunistic fungal infection of the burn wound with phycomycetes and *Aspergillus. Arch Surg* 1971; **102**: 476–82.
69. Desai MH, Herndon DN, Abston S. *Candida* infection in massively burned patients. *J Trauma* 1981; **21(3)**: 237–9.
70. Nash G, Foley FD, Goodwin MN Jr, *et al.* Fungal burn wound infection. *JAMA* 1971; **215**: 1664–6.

71. Spebar MJ, Lindberg RB. Fungal infection of the burn wound. *Am J Surg* 1981; **21(3)**: 237–9.

72. Spebar MJ, Lindberg RB. Fungal infection of the burn wound. *Am J Surg* 1979; **138**: 879–82.

73. Burdge JJ, Rea F, Ayers L. Noncandidal, fungal infections of the burn wound. *J Burn Care Rehabil* 1988; **9(6)**: 599–601.

74. Pruitt BA Jr. Phycomycotic infections. *Probl Gen Surg* 1984; 664–78.

75. Neame P, Rayner D. Mucormycosis: a report of 22 cases. *Arch Pathol* 1960; **70**: 261–8.

76. Kobayashi K, Mukae N, Matsunaga Y, Motchi M. Diagnostic value of serum antibody to *Candida* in an extensively burned patient. *Burns* 1990; **16(6)**: 414–17.

77. Goldstein E, Hoeprich PD. Problems in the diagnosis and treatment of systemic conditions. *J Infect Dis* 1980; **125**: 190–3.

78. Kidson A, Lowbury EJL. *Candida* infection of burns. *Burns* 1980; **6**: 228–30.

79. Solomhin JS, Simmons RL. *Candida* infection in surgical patients. *World J Surg* 1980; **4**: 381–94.

80. Prasad JK, Feller IF, Thomson PD. A ten year review of *Candida* sepsis and mortality in burn patients. *Surgery* 1987; **101**: 213–16.

81. Mead JH, Lupton GP, Dillavou CL, *et al.* Cutaneous rhizopus infection. *JAMA* 1979; **242**: 272–4.

82. Del Pelacio Hemandez A. Nosocomial infection by *Rhizomucor pusillus* in a clinical haematology unit. *J Hosp Infect* 1983; **4(1)**: 45–9.

83. Gartenberg G, Bottone EJ, Keusch FT, *et al.* Hospital acquired mucormycosis (*Rhizopus rhizopodiformis*) of skin and subcutaneous tissue: epidemiology, mycology and treatment. *N Engl J Med* 1978; **299**: 1115–18.

84. Linneman CC Jr, MacMillan BC. Viral infections in pediatric burn patients. *Am J Dis* 1983; **135**: 750–3.

85. Deepe GS Jr, MacMillan BC, Linnemann CC Jr. Unexplained fever in burned patients due to cytomegalovirus infection. *JAMA* 1982; **248**: 2299–301.

86. Goodwin CW, McManus WF. Viral infections in burned patients. *Immunology* 1985; **12**: 3–4, 8–9.

87. Edgar P, Kravitz M, Heggers JP, *et al.* Herpes simplex in pediatric burn patients. *Proc Am Burn Assoc* 1990; **22**: 56.

88. Weintraub WH, Lilly AB, Randolph JG. A chickenpox epidemic in a pediatric burn unit. *Surgery* 1974; **76**: 490–4.

89. Barret JP, Dardano AN, Heggers JP, McCauley RL. Infestations and chronic infections in foreign pediatric patients with burns: is there a role for specific protocols? *J Burn Care Rehabil* 1999; **20**: 482–6.

90. Heggers JP, Muller MJ, Elwood E, Herndon DN. *Ascariasis pneumonitisi*: a potentially fatal complication in smoke inhalation injury. *Burns* 1995; **21**: 149–51.

91. Teplitz C, Davis D, Mason AD, Moncrief JA. Pseudomonas burn wound sepsis. 1. Pathogenesis of experimental pseudomonas burn wound sepsis. *J Surg Res* 1964; **4**: 200–16.

92. Pruitt BA, Foley FD. The use of biopsies in burn patient care. *Surgery* 1973; **73**: 887–97.

93. Parks DH, Linares HA, Thompson PD. Surgical management of burn wound sepsis. *Surg Gynec Obstet* 1981; **153**: 374–6.

94. Wendt C, Messer SA, Hollis RJ, Pfaller MA, Wenzel RP, Herwaldt LA. Molecular epidemiology of Gram-negative bacteremia. *Clin Infect Dis* 1999; **28(3)**: 605–10.

95. Sasaki TM, Welch GW, Herndon DN, *et al.* Burn wound manipulation induced bacteremia. *J Trauma* 1979; **19(1)**: 46–8.

96. Beard CH, Ribeiro CD, Jones DM. The bacteremia associated with burns surgery. *Br J Surg* 1975; **62**: 638–41.

97. Hamory BH. Nosocomial sepsis related to intravascular access. *Crit Care Nurs Q* 1989; **11(4)**: 58–65.

98. Samsoondar W, Freeman JB, Coultish I, *et al.* Colonization of intravascular catheters in the intensive care unit. *Am J Surg* 1985; **149**: 730–2.

99. Maki DG, Jarrett F, Sarafin HW. A semiquantitative culture method for identification of catheter related infection in the burn patient. *J Surg Res* 1977; **22**: 513–20.

100. Stein JM, Pruitt BA Jr. Suppurative thrombophlebitis: a lethal iatrogenic disease. *N Engl J Med* 1970; **282**: 1452–5.

101. Franceschi D, Gerding RL, Phillips G, Fratianne RB. Risk factors associated with intravascular catheter infection in burned patients; a prospective randomized study. *J Trauma* 1989; **29(6)**: 811–16.

102. Smallman L, Burdon DW, Alexander-Williams J. The effect of skin preparation and care on the incidence of superficial thrombophlebitis. *Br J Surg* 1980; **67**: 861–2.

103. Sheth NK, Franson TR, Rose HD, *et al.* Colonization of bacteria on polyvinyl chloride and Teflon intravascular catheters in hospitalized patients. *J Clin Microbiol* 1983; **18**: 1061–3.

104. Maki DG, Botticelli JT, LeRoy ML, *et al.* Prospective study of replacing administration sets for intravenous therapy at 48 to 72 hour intervals. *JAMA* 1987; **258**: 1777–81.

105. Pruitt BA Jr, Stein JM, Foley FD, *et al.* Intravenous therapy in burn patients: suppurative thrombophebitis and other life threatening complications. *Arch Surg* 1970; **100**: 399–404.

106. Artz CP, Moncrief JA. *The Treatment of Burns*. Philadelphia: WB Saunders, 1969.

107. Ramzy PI, Herndon DN, Wolf SE, Heggers JP. Comparison of organisms found by bronchoalveolar lavage and quantitative wound culture in severely burned children. *Arch Surg* 1998; **133**: 1275–80.

108. Luna CM, Vukacich P, Niederman MS, *et al.* Impact of BAL data on the therapy and outcome of ventilator-associated pneumonia. *Chest* 1997; **111**: 676–85.

109. Kollef MH. Ventilator-associated pneumonia: the importance of initial empiric antibiotic selection. *Infect Med* 2000; **17(4)**: 265–8, 278–83.

110. Heggers JP, Robson MC, Ko F, *et al.* Transient and resident microflora of burn unit personnel and its influence on burn wound sepsis. *Infect Control* 1982; **3**: 471–4.

111. Pruitt BA Jr, McManus AT. Opportunistic infections in severely burned patients. *Am J Med* 1984; **76**: 146–53.

112. Robson MC. Bacterial control in the burn wound. *Clin Plast Surg* 1979; **6(4)**: 515–22.

113. Burke JR, Quinby WC, Bondoc CC, *et al.* The contribution of a bacterial isolated environment to the prevention of infection in seriously burned patients. *Ann Surg* 1977; **186**: 377–87.

114. Perez-Cappelano R, Manelli JC, Dalayret D, *et al.* Evaluation of the septicaemic risk by quantitative study of the cutaneous flora in patients with burns. *Burns* 1976; **3**: 42–5.

115. Robson MC, Krizek TS. Predicting skin graft survival. *J Trauma* 1973; **13(3)**: 213–17.

116. Robson MC, Krizek TJ, Heggers JP. Biology of surgical infection. In: Ravitch MM ed. *Current Problems in Surgery*. Chicago: Yearbook Medical Publishers, 1973: 1–62.

117. Robson MC. Burn sepsis. *Crit Care Clin* 1988; **4(2)**: 281–98.

118. Levenson SM, Alpert S, DelGuerico L, *et al.* The use of whole and partial body isolators for the care of severely burned patients. *Ann NY Acad Sci* 1968; **150(3)**: 1009–11.

119. Lowbury ESL, Babb SR, Ford PM. Protective isolation in a burn unit: the use of plastic isolators and air curtains. *J Hyg* 1971; **69**: 529–46.

120. Nance FC, Lewis V, Bomside GH. Absolute barrier isolation and antibiotics in the treatment of experimental burn wound sepsis. *J Surg Res* 1970; **10**: 33.

121. O'Rourke E. Pediatric nosocomial infections. Program and abstracts from the 39th ICAAC, 26–29 September 1999, San Francisco, CA.

122. Alonso-Echanove J. Increasing rates of nosocomial sepsis in a high-risk nursery (HRN) in Calif., Colombia 1999. Program and abstracts from the 39th ICAAC, 26–29 September 1999; San Francisco, CA.

123. Heggers JP. The use of antimicrobials agents. In: Krizek TJ, Robson MC, eds. *Clinics in Plastic Surgery*, Vol. 6. Philadelphia, PA: WB Saunders, 1979; 545–51.

124. Robson MC, Duke WF, Krizek TJ. Rapid bacterial screening in the treatment of civilian wounds. *J Surg Res* 1973; **14**: 426.

125. Robson MC. Wound healing and wound closure. In: Heggers JP, Robson MC, eds. *Quantitative Bacteriology: Its Role in the Armamentarium of the Surgeon*. Boca Raton, FL: CRC Press, 1991: 43–53.

126. Lowbury EJL. Wits versus genes: the continuing battle against infection. *J Trauma* 1979; **19**: 33–45.

127. Heggers JP. Antimicrobial agents. In: Heggers JP, Robson MC, eds. *Quantitative Bacteriology: Its Role in the Armamentarium of the Surgeon*, Boca Raton, FL: CRC Press, 1991: 115–25.

128. Moncrief JA. Topical antibacterial treatment of the burn wound. In: Artz CP, Moncrief JA, Pruitt, BA Jr, eds. *Burns, A Team Approach*. Philadelphia, PA: WB Saunders, 1979: 250–69.

129. Nathan P, Law EJ, Murphy DF, McMillan BG. A laboratory method for selection of topical antimicrobial agents to treat infected burn wounds. *Burns* 1979; **4**: 177–87.

130. Piotech JB, Meakins JL. Predicting infection in surgical patients. In: Simmon RL, ed. *Surgical Clinics in North America*, Vol. 59. Philadelphia, PA: WB Saunders, 1979: 185–97.

131. Moncrief JA, Lindberg RB, Switzer WE, Pruitt BA. The use of a topical sulfonamide in the control of burn wound sepsis. *J Trauma* 1966; **6(3)**: 407–19.

132. Holder IA, Schwab M, Jackson L. Eighteen months of routine topical antimicrobial susceptibility testing of isolates from burn patients: results and conclusions. *J Antimicrob Chemother* 1979; **5**: 455–63.

133. Lineweaver W, McMorris S, Soucy D, Howard R. Cellular and bacterial toxicities of topical antimicrobials. *Plast Reconstr Surg* 1985; **75**: 394–6.

134. Heggers JP, Sazy JA, Stenberg BD, McCauley RL, Strock LL, Robson MC, Herndon DN. Bactericidal and wound healing properties of sodium hypochlorite. *J Burn Care Rehabil* 1991; **12**: 420–4.

135. Fader RC, Maurer A, Stein MD, Abston S, Herndon DN. Sodium hypochlorite decontamination of split-thickness cadaveric skin infected with bacteria and yeast with subsequent isolation and growth of basal cells to confluency in tissue culture. *Antimicrob Agents Chemother* 1983; **24**: 181–5.

136. Robson MC. The use of topical agents to control bacteria. In: Dimick AR, ed. *The Burn Wound in Practical Approaches to Burn Management*. Deerfield, IL: Flint Laboratories, Travenol, Inc., 1977: 17–19.

137. Heggers JP, Robson MC. The emergence of silver sulfadiazine resistant *Pseudomonas aeruginosa*. *Burns* 1978; **5**: 184–87.

138. Moncrief JA. The status of topical antibacterial therapy in the treatment of burns. *Surgery* 1968; **63**: 862.

139. Kucan IO, Smoot EC. Five percent mafenide acetate solution in the treatment of thermal injuries. *J Burn Care Rehabil* 1993; **14**: 158–63.

140. Lindberg RB, Moncrief JA, Mason AD Jr. Control of experimental and clinical burn wound sepsis by topical application of sulfamylon compounds. *Ann NY Acad Sci* 1968; **150**: 950.

141. Georgiade NG, Harris WA. Open and closed treatment of burns with Povidone-iodine. In Polk HC Jr, Ebrenkranz NJ, eds. *Therapeutic Advances and New Clinical Impressions: Medical and Surgical Antisepsis with Betadine Microbicides*. Yonkers, NY: Purdue Frederick, 1972.

142. Krizek TJ, Davis JH, DesPrez JD, et al. Topical therapy of burns – experimental evaluation. *Plast Reconstr Surg* 1967; **39**: 248.

143. Livingston DH, Cryer HG, Miller FB, Malangoni MA, Polk HC, Weiner LJ. A randomized prospective study of topical antimicrobial agents on skin grafts after thermal injury. *J Plast Reconstr Surg* (in press).

144. Strock LL, Lee M, Rutan RL, Desai MH, Robson MC, Herndon DN, Heggers JP. Topical Bactroban® (Mupirocin): efficacy in treating NIRSA wounds infected with methicillin-resistant Staphylococci. *J Burn Care Rehabil* 1990; **11**: 454–9.

145. Heggers JP, Carino ES, Sazy JA, et al. A topical antimicrobial test system (TOPITEST®): Nathan's agar well revisited. *Surg Res Comm* 1990; **8**: 109–16.

146. Fuller AT, Mellows G, Woodford M, et al. Pseudomonic acid, an antibiotic produced by *Pseudomonas fluorescens*. *Nature (Lond.)* 1971; **234**: 416–17.

147. Buchvald J. An evaluation of topical mupirocin in moderately severe primary and secondary skin infections. *J Int Med Res* 1988; **16**: 66–70.

148. Denning DW, Driffith DH. Eradication of low-level resistant *Staphylococcus aureus* skin colonization with topical mupirocin. *Infect Control Hosp Epider* 1988; **9(6)**: 261–3.

149. Rode H, DeWet PM, Shepard GH, et al. Bacterial efficacy of mupirocin in multi-antibiotic resistant *Staphylococcus aureus* burn wound infection. *J Antimicrob Chemother* 1988; **21**: 589–95.

150. Pruitt BA Jr, Foley F. The use of biopsies in burn patient care. *Surgery* 1973; **73**: 8878–97.

151. Heggers JP, Robson MC, Herndon DN, Desai MH. The efficacy of nystatin combined with topical microbial agents in the treatment of burn wound sepsis. *J Burn Care Rehabil* 1989; **10**: 508–11.

152. Barret JP, Ramzy PI, Heggers JP, Villarreal C, Herndon DN, Desai MH. Topical nystatin powder in severe burns: a new treatment for angioinvasive fungal infections refractory to other topical and systemic agents. *Burns* 1999; **25(6)**: 505–8.

153. Reagor L, Gusman J, McCoy L, Carino E, Heggers JP. The effectiveness of grapefruit seed extract (GSE®) as an antibacterial agent. I. An *in vitro* agar assay. *J Alternative Complem Med* (submitted).

154. Heggers JP, Cottingham J, Gusman J, et al. The effectiveness of grapefruit seed extract (GSE®) as an antibacterial agent. II. Safety and efficacy. *J Alternative Complem Med* (submitted).

155. Krizek TJ, Koss N, Robson MC. The current use of prophylactic antibiotics in plastic and reconstructive surgery. *Plast Reconstr Surg* 1975; **55**: 21–33.

156. Krizek TJ, Gottlieb LJ, Koss H, Robson MC. The use of prophylactic antibacterials in plastic surgery: a 1980's update. *Plast Reconstr Surg* 1985; **76**: 953–63.

157. Richards JH. Bacteremia following irritation of foci of infection. *J Am Med Assoc* 1932; **99**: 1496–7.

158. LeFrock JL, Ellis CA, Turchik JB, Weinstein L. Transient bacteremia associated with sigmodoscopy. *N Engl J Med* 1973; **289**: 467–9.

159. Bennington, JL ed. *Saunders Dictionary and Encyclopedia of Laboratory Medicine and Technology*. Philadelphia, PA: WB Saunders, 1984; **167**: 1375.

160. Kucers A, Bennett McK N. *The Use of Antibiotics*, 4th Ed. Philadelphia, PA: JB Lippincott, 1987: 1–1678.

161. Rowland M, Tozer TN. *Clinical Pharmacokinetics: Concepts and Applications*. Philadelphia: Lea & Febiger, 1980.

162. *Physicians Desk Reference* 48th edn. Montvale NJ: Medical Economics Comp Inc., 1994: 517–19, 1095–6.

163. Tenover FC. VRSA, VISA and GISA: the dilemma behind the name game. *Clin Micro Newsletter* 2000; **22**: 49–53.

164. Nadler H, Dowzicky MJ, Feger C, Pease MR, Prokocime P. Quinupristin/dalfopristin: a novel selective-spectrum antibiotic for the treatment of multi-resistant and other Gram-positive pathogens. *Clin Micro Newsletter* 1999; **21**: 103–12.

165. Heggers JP, Linares H, Edgar P, Villarreal C, Herndon DN. Treatment of infections in burns in total burn care. In: Herndon DN, ed. *Total Burn Care 1st edn* London: Bailliere Tindall, 1996: 98–135.

166. Heggers JP, Villarreal C, Edgar P, et al. Ciprofloxacin the quinolone as a therapeutic modality in pediatric burn wound infections: efficacious or contraindicated. *Arch Surg* 1998; **133**: 1247–50.

167. *Physician's Desk Reference*, 54th edn. Montvale, NJ: Medical Economics Co., 2000: 1460, 2020.

168. Shanson DC, Kensit JG, Duke R. Outbreak of hospital infection with a strain of *Staphylococcus aureus* resistant to gentamicin and methicillin. *Lancet* 1976; **2**: 1347.

169. Siegel D, Huber WB, Enloe F. Continuous non-therapeutic use of antibacterial drugs in feed and drug resistance of gram-negative enteric flora of food producing animals. *Antimicrob Agents Chemother* 1974; **6**: 697–706.

170. Burton GC, Hirsh DC, Blendin DC, et al. The effects of tetracycline on the establishment of *Escherichia coli* of animal origin and the *in vivo* transfer of antibiotic resistance in the intestinal tract of man. In: Skinner FA, Carr JE, eds. *Normal Microbial Flora on Man*. New York: Academic Press, 1973: 507–21.

171. Barret J, Dardano AN, Heggers JP. Infections. In Herndon DN, Barret JP, ed. *A Color Atlas of Burn Care*, 1st edn. London: Bailliere Tindall, 2000: 110–21.

172. Burrell RE, Heggers JP, Davis GJ, Wright JB. Efficacy of silver-coated dressings as bacterial barriers in a rodent burn sepsis model. *Wounds* 1999; **11**: 64–71.

Chapter 12

Operative wound management
Michael J Muller, David Ralston, David N Herndon

Interventional wound management is the cornerstone of modern burn care. Much has changed in this area with many advantages for the patient being realized as a consequence. Skin grafting of granulation tissue, following eschar separation, has been replaced with operative intervention within hours of injury. Skin substitutes, dermal replacement, and cultured skin technology allow individualization of patient management for optimum results.

The burn wound

The natural history of a full-thickness burn wound is to promote an inflammatory response at the junction of the eschar and the underlying viable tissue. At this interface, bacterial proliferation in the eschar attracts polymorphonuclear leukocytes (neutrophils) that release large quantities of proteolytic enzymes and inflammatory mediators. Subsequent enzymatic action results in separation of the eschar from the now granulating interface. If the burn is large, the inflammatory response at the burned site becomes generalized. This effect is described fully elsewhere. Briefly, mediators such as prostanoids, thromboxane, histamine, cytokines, and tumour necrosis factor are all produced and released from the burned site. The serum levels of these mediators become measurable and increase in proportion to the area of the burn. The hypermetabolic response with protein catabolism, increased metabolic rate, increased susceptibility to infection, marked weight loss, and poor wound healing continue until the outpouring of mediators abates. While topical antimicrobial agents such as mafenide acetate and silver sulfadiazine have decreased the frequency and severity of systemic sepsis, these agents prolong eschar separation and therefore the hypermetabolic response.

Treatment of full-thickness burns by awaiting spontaneous eschar separation and subsequent skin grafting is a prolonged process associated with much pain and suffering, severe metabolic derangements, multiple septic episodes, and lengthy hospitalization. In the modern era, this technique should be limited to those who are so infirm that any other method cannot be contemplated.

Beneficial effects of operative wound management

Prompt wound closure has been shown repeatedly to improve survival, decrease length of hospital stay, and curb expenditure in burned patients of all ages. Children particularly have benefited from more timely and extensive surgical intervention.[1,2] There has been a remarkable increase in the burn size associated with a 50% mortality risk over recent decades such that it is now unusual for a child to succumb to burn injury of any size, even if it is associated with a smoke inhalation injury (**Table 12.1a,b**). Improving nutritional support and control of sepsis have also played a part in this achievement. Early surgery, however, has contributed most toward this major advance. Burke[3] reported on results of total excision of full-thickness burns in 1974. He applied homografts (cadaver skin) to seal the wound, controlled rejection by adding immunosuppressives, and cared for his patients in laminar flow chambers. Children with massive burns began surviving their injuries where they had never previously done so. Improved mortality, shorter hospital stay, and fewer metabolic complications were noted by others when early excision was retrospectively compared with late excision.[4] When 32 children, average age 7 years and mean burn size 65% total body surface area (TBSA) who underwent either total excision to fascia or serial debridement were studied: mortality, overall blood loss, and cumulative operating time were equivalent.[5] The early excision group, however, had their length of hospital stay almost halved (97 ± 8 days vs. 57 ± 5 days). Since that time, hundreds of children with burns >30% TBSA treated with early excision have exhibited a length of hospital stay less than 1 day/% TBSA burned.[6]

Mortality of adult burn patients at Massachusetts General Hospital declined from 24% in 1974 to 7% for 1979–1984 after prompt eschar excision and immediate wound closure was instituted as standard therapy in 1976.[7] Logistical regression analysis showed that this treatment significantly improved survival ($p<0.001$). Thirty adult patients admitted to the Galveston Burn Unit with very large burns were randomized to receive either early total or staged excision. In patients with no inhalation injury, mortality was decreased with early excision. Total blood requirements were similar between groups, negating an often used argument against excisional therapy. This study was expanded to include 85 patients, aged 17–55 years.[8] Those patients aged 17–30 years without inhalation injury showed significantly reduced mortality if treated by early excision (9%), than if treated conservatively (45%). Patients with a concomitant inhalation injury or age greater than 30 years, however, derived no survival benefit from early excision.

Munster and colleagues[9] demonstrated a statistically significant decrease in length of hospital stay that significantly correlated with a decrease in the interval between surgical interventions over a 14-year period at his institution. Other variables such as burn size, inhalation injury, and age remained static during this time (**Table 12.2**); they found that mortality rate decreased significantly while burn indices remained constant. The average annual increase of hospital charges for burn care grew at 9.6%, which was substantially lower than the hospital as a whole (10.8%). Active surgical intervention in burn care can be associated with cost containment and fewer lives lost.

Table 12.1a Mortality and pediatric burn patients

Burn size	<20%	20–40%	41–60%	61–100%
1980–1986	<0.1	1%	8%	32%
	n=1003	n=283	n=124	n=114
1987–2001	<0.1	1%	4%	18%
	n=1812	n=699	n=373	n=304

Table 12.1b Mortality and burn size: survival with larger burns is now far more likely

Age (years)	Burn size of 50% 1942–1952* (% TBSA)	Mortality 1980–1991† (%TBSA)
0–14	49	98
15–44	46	70
45–64	27	46
>65	10	19

% TBSA, percentage of total body surface area burned.
*Bull & Fisher.[1]
†Muller and Herndon.[2]

Table 12.2 Hospital stay and interval between surgeries: length of stay can be greatly reduced by timely return to the operating room (from Munster et al.[9])

	LOS (days)	Surgical interval (days)
1979	23	14
1990	14*	6

LOS = Length of hospital stay.
*LOS significantly decreased as the interval between surgical interventions decreased

Older burn patients have been shown to benefit from an early surgical approach. Deitch[10,11] operated upon 114 consecutive patients with an average age of 68 years, and showed a reduction of 40% in mean length of hospital stay when compared to national averages, and mortality was less than predicted. Many studies[12–16] show that early excision can be safely performed in the elderly, with clear benefit of reductions in duration of hospitalization and the number of septic episodes. Saffle[14] showed that the number of preexisting medical conditions in the elderly had no effect on survival, a salient point when planning treatment. The elderly also benefit from aggressive surgical treatment of their donor site wounds. They very commonly have loose and mobile skin. If donor sites or burns are situated on the lower abdomen, the flank, or thigh, they are amenable to excision and repair in the same manner as a reduction abdominoplasty.[17] This has the effect of reducing the area of open wound and decreasing the metabolic demand placed on their physiology.

Hypertrophic scar formation is common, with dark-skinned people and children being more prone to its development. However, the most important determinant of hypertrophic scarring is delayed wound healing. Deitch[18] has clearly shown that if wounds take more than 10 days to heal then the risk is significant and it rises to 80% if healing is delayed beyond 21 days. Surgery is therefore indicated for those whose wounds fail to heal promptly. Operative treatment is also an effective means of limiting the duration of pain that burn patients must endure. The ghastly experience of wound debridement in the tub by picking at the eschar, sometimes for many weeks, has been recounted by many as the worst part of their burn experience. Excisional therapy of the burn wound is humane, lifesaving, offers improved cosmetic and functional results, is cost-effective, and more swiftly returns the patient to their normal environment.

Techniques of burn wound excision

Excising a Small, Deep Burn

Once a burn wound is determined to be 'deep', operative intervention is indicated without further delay. 'Deep' burns are those which are clearly full-thickness or are deep dermal burns unlikely to heal within 14–21 days. They are typically flame and contact burns and are commonly situated on the extremities. Heimbach[19] observed that deep partial-thickness burns did not convert to full-thickness when topical antimicrobials were used to control infection. Although these wounds did eventually heal after many weeks, they showed persistent blistering, pruritus, hypertrophic scar formation, and poor functional results. These observations prompted a prospective trial of early excision and grafting versus nonoperative treatment of burns of indeterminate depth of less than 20% TBSA.[20] Shorter hospitalization, lower cost, less time away from work, but greater use of blood products were seen in those treated operatively. Those patients treated nonoperatively required more late grafts for closure and developed more hypertrophic scarring. There was no difference in need for reconstructive procedures, range of motion, or contour irregularities.

Tangential Excision

Tangential excision removes necrotic tissue while preserving as much of the underlying viable tissue as possible. Body contours are better preserved than with fascial level excision and therefore this is the usual method for small burns. The technique of tangential excision was originally described by Janzekovic[21] who observed that deep donor sites could be overgrafted with thinner split-thickness skin harvested from another area. She then extended this concept to dermal burns by excising thin layers of burn until living tissue was reached (**Figure 12.1a,b,c**). Split skin grafts were immediately applied. This technique of tangential excision and autografting of dermal burns was a major advance. Prior

to this time only full-thickness burns were excised and usually as a formal integumentectomy, taking subcutaneous fat and accompanying lymphatics down to the underlying layer of investing fascia (fascial excision). Janzekovic analyzed the results of the use of tangential technique of excision in over 2000 patients. She found that hospital stay, pain, and reconstructive procedures were all decreased compared to fascial excision.[22]

A number of different instruments can be used to perform tangential excision. The Rosenberg knife, Goulian knife, Watson knife, and powered dermatome all have their place depending on the anatomical arrangements; the powered dermatome is particularly useful for larger areas on flat surfaces such as the back. The Watson knife is probably the most popular instrument for tangential excision (**Figure 12.2**). The technique is aided by traction and counter-traction to place the area under tension. To ensure adequate depth is obtained, the excised tissue can be grasped as it appears from the top of the instrument and traction applied. Partial-thickness injuries are debrided to a white, shiny dermal surface with punctate bleeding that is fine and copious if the burn depth is superficial and less frequent from larger vessels for deep partial-thickness burns. Healthy fat has a yellow glistening appearance and it is imperative excision continues, layer by layer, until this appearance is obtained. Dullness, punctate hemorrhages, purple discoloration, or thrombosed vessels indicate nonviable tissue upon which grafts will fail and deeper excision is mandatory. When excision is performed on limbs following exsanguination with a rubber bandage and control of arterial inflow with a pneumatic tourniquet, these features are especially important. In particular, staining of the dermis with hemoglobin from lysed red cells indicates a need for deeper excision.

Controlling blood loss

Tangential excision can lead to copious blood loss unless measures are taken to limit potential hemorrhage. The simplest measure is to operate within 24 hours of injury. Vasoactive metabolites, particularly the potent vasoconstrictor thromboxane, are in abundance during this time and do much to limit blood loss.[23] This proposition is supported by a prospective trial of 318 children and adolescents with burns >30% TBSA. The average blood loss per surface area excised (ml/cm²) was compared at various postburn periods of

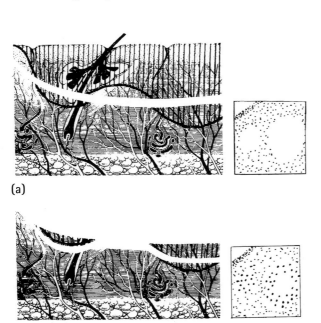

(a)

(b)

(c)

Fig. 12.1 (a,b,c) Schematic representation of tangential excision; sequential slices are taken until punctate haemorrhage is evident. (Adapted from Janzekovic[21] with permission.)

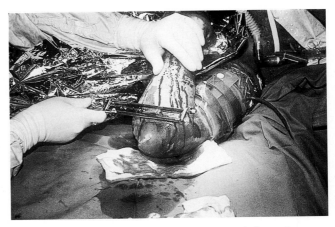

Fig. 12.2 Tangential excision using a hand dermatome; the sterilizable silicone tourniquet has been deflated.

excision. The entire full-thickness burn, with the exception of the face and perineum, was tangentially excised with a hand knife with contiguous partial-thickness burn removed to punctate bleeding with serial passes of an electric dermatome. Patients whose blood pressure was greater or less than 40% of baseline, urine output less 0.75 ml/kg/h, or developed pulmonary edema intraoperatively, or whose hematocrit was >48 or <24% were not included in the analysis. Overall mortality was 5% for an average size burn of 60% TBSA. Notably, early excision had no adverse effect on mortality and no intraoperative deaths were recorded. Very early excision led to a halving of blood loss for both large and small burns[24] (**Figure 12.3**). Further adjunctive measures to limit blood loss include tourniquets for the extremities, pre-debridement tumescence with weak (1 : 5 000 000) epinephrine (adrenaline) solution (**Figure 12.4**), topical application of epinephrine 1 : 10 000–1 : 20 000 via either spray or cannula, topical application of thrombin, fibrin sealant, autologous platelet gel, calcium-enriched alginate sheets, epinephrine-soaked (~1 : 400 000) lap-pads (sponges), and immediate bandaging with delayed grafting.

Exsanguination by firm application of a rubber bandage and use of a sterilizable, silicone tourniquet protected by a plastic sleeve allows for bloodless, unhurried debridement. This is a boon for the hand and fingers. The technique requires close attention to detail and some practice to recognize adequacy of debridement using the appearance of the wound bed as described above. The tourniquet can be released briefly to check adequacy of debridement and then quickly reinflated. The larger vessels are controlled by electrocautery or ligation and the wound is then flooded with a strong epinephrine solution, covered with sheets of calcium alginate. The tourniquet is released after 5–8 minutes. The limb should then be held elevated for about 10 minutes. Pre-excisional tumescence with epinephrine saline can be used almost everywhere except the digits. This technique is particularly useful for the trunk, scalp, and face. An infuser device speeds the process and certainly saves operator thumb strain. Pressure-bags, 'pitkin' syringes, and liposuction infusers can all be used. Delayed grafting is used in some centers to limit blood loss. If delayed grafting is undertaken, the wound bed needs to be kept moist and clean. A number of means are available: the wounds can be covered with bulky cotton dressings with tubing through the dressing to the wound surface used for continuous or intermittent irrigation with saline and added antibiotics. The patient returns to the operating room within 72 hours and undergoes a second procedure of harvest and application of skin grafts.

Techniques of wound closure

If the burn is small and donor sites are plentiful, skin grafts can be applied as 'sheet' or unmeshed skin. This technique requires experienced personnel to attend to the graft every few hours for a number of days to ensure that seromas and hematomas are controlled and expressed. Another less labor-intensive technique is to mesh the graft at a ratio of 1 : 1 or 1.5 : 1, but not to expand or stretch the mesh. If performed carefully, blood and seroma will drain away from the wound and a good cosmetic appearance is left. These grafts are best laid perpendicular to the long axis of limbs, particularly across joint flexural creases, which is in line with the general rule of placing potential scars perpendicular to the dominant muscle contraction in the area. This will decrease the degree of contracture if it occurs. Possible exceptions are the dorsum of the hand and forearm where some clinicians argue that longitudinally placed grafts are cosmetically superior.

If burns are huge and donor sites scarce, then areas such as the scalp, scrotum, and axillae may need to be harvested. These are meshed at a ratio of 4 : 1 or 6 : 1 and widely expanded. The wound is then sealed by an overlay of unexpanded, 1.5 : 1 meshed, fresh or frozen partial-thickness allografts. These are applied at 90° to the autograft in a sandwich pattern as described by Alexander *et al.*[25] (**Figure 12.5**). The cellular immune depression associated with massive burns makes rejection phenomena to the allograft uncommon. Fresh allografts, stored at 2–4°C in nutrient media, achieve an adherence rate of 95%. Even in large burns the face, neck, and hands are sheet grafted with thick split-skin if at all possible.

Advances in Wound Closure

Cultured skin has a definite place in modern burn care. Munster has shown that use of cultured epithelial autografts (CEA) in the

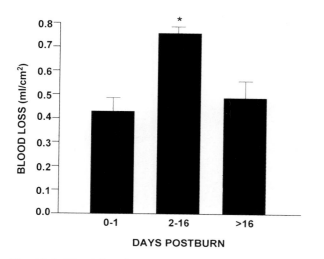

Fig. 12.3 Blood loss is almost halved by operating within 24 hours of injury. (Adapted from Desai MH *et al.*[24] with permission.)

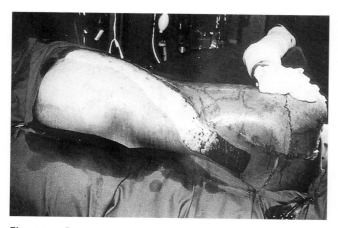

Fig. 12.4 Pre-excisional instillation of a weak epinephrine solution decreases blood loss. Epinephrine was injected under all the donor site except the superior end, which is the only area bleeding.

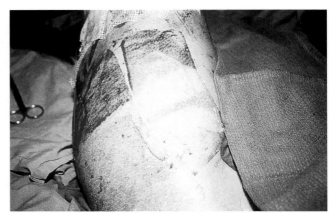

ALLOGRAFT

AUTOGRAFT

EXCISED WOUND

Fig. 12.5 Schematic representation of 'sandwich' technique of allograft overlay. (Adapted from Alexander JW *et al.*[25] with permission.)

massively burned decreased mortality.[26] Herndon[27] compared the use of CEA with wide mesh autograft and allograft overlay in a group of children with enormous burns, >90% TBSA. Use of CEA was associated with a much better cosmetic result at the expense of a longer length of hospital stay and more reconstructive procedures. Successful use of CEA in the massively burned, critically ill, (usually) ventilated patient is difficult. CEA is most often supplied as sheets measuring 10 cm × 15 cm. Unfortunately, it is very thin with 10–15 cell layers being the norm. This has all the strength of wet tissue paper and is very prone to shearing (**Figure 12.6**). As CEA in this patient group is most usually applied to a wound bed devoid of dermis, anchoring of the epithelial layer is delayed and consequently shearing and blistering is common for many months. Long-term survival of CEA is therefore particularly problematic on the posterior surfaces of these massively burned patients and goes some way towards explaining the 5–50% long-term engraftment CEA rates reported in the literature. CEA does have a definite place in wound management of the massively burned and biopsies should be procured on admission and sent immediately to commence the process of culture. Areas that are less prone to shearing such as the anterior surfaces of the torso and thighs are particularly appropriate for its use (**Figure 12.7a,b**). Wound excision should not be delayed whilst waiting delivery of the CEA. The wound

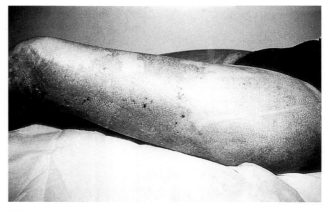

(a)

(b)

Fig. 12.7 (a) Cultured epithelial autograft (CEA) being applied to the anterior thigh. (b) Well-healed wounds following engraftment of CEA.

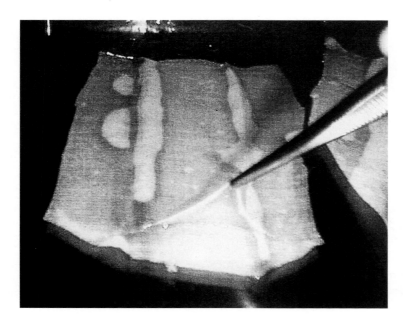

Fig. 12.6 Cultured epithelial autograft is very thin and delicate.

should be temporarily closed with fresh allograft until the CEA arrives.

In patients with smaller burns, and especially if dermal elements can be left, CEA as sheets and, more recently, delivered as a cell suspension as early as day 4 seems to have a role. Certainly, the donor site morbidity is minimal and the early results quite promising.

Donor site

Selecting the best donor site region and depth is a matter of careful judgment and much controversy; even more so is the method of donor-site management. There is general agreement that, if at all possible, the face and neck should be resurfaced by grafts harvested from the 'blush' area above the line of the nipple for the best color match. Small burns in other areas allow the donor site to be hidden on the upper thigh or buttock. In children, some favor the scalp for all applications as regrowth of hair hides the area. Unfortunately, for some, this does not come with a lifelong guarantee. The upper lateral thigh over the area of the greater trochanter is a good compromise. The area is usually hidden from view and effective pressure garment therapy can be applied against the underlying bony structure if hypertrophic scar eventuates. The buttock donor site is easier to hide but effective pressure therapy is less assured. Good quality grafts of consistent depth are obtained by use of a powered dermatome and certainly avoids the saw-tooth pattern often seen following use of a hand knife to harvest split-skin grafts. When the burn size is huge, some unusual donor sites need to be used. The axillae and the scrotum in males provide useful amounts of skin graft after tumescence to produce a tight surface for harvest. The soles of the feet can also be used. It is best to shave and discard a first layer of keratin and then harvest the grafts for definitive use.

Selection of depth of split-skin grafts is influenced by a number of factors. The overall burn size may predicate a need for recropping and wide expansion of meshed grafts. Thinner grafts of 6/1000th inch in adults should then be harvested. Massively burned patients can sometimes have such limited available donor-site area that recropping may have to be performed repeatedly to achieve wound closure. Even if harvesting is performed at as shallow a depth as possible, there is a point at which any subsequent recropping is of largely nonviable skin.[28] This loss of the donor sites' regenerative capabilities has drastic implications, not only for the closure of the original burn but also for the ability to perform reconstructive procedures at some later time.

Donor-Site Management

Donor sites are covered by scarlet red gauze, followed by dry gauze and compression bandages if anatomically possible. Bandages are removed 6 hours later and donor sites exposed. If donor sites fail to dry or develop excess moisture, a 40 watt heat lamp is positioned 18 inches away. Heat is applied for 20 minutes each hour until dry. Smaller donor sites can be treated with occlusive or adherent dressings such as Opsite™ or Biobrane™. These dressings can be applied to larger areas with innovation and effort but they carry the risk of promoting infection if fluid accumulates beneath the occlusive layer. This can lead to conversion to full-thickness wounds. Another technique is to use alginate sheets or hydrocolloid fiber dressings. They have the advantage of promoting moist wound healing and may diminish donor-site wound pain.

The trapped moisture does lend itself to gram-negative infection, however, and this should be carefully monitored. The slightest hint of green exudate mandates immediate removal and treatment with topical antimicrobials. Split-thickness skin graft donor sites heal primarily by epithelialization from the remaining epithelial elements. Healing is rapid with thin split-skin grafts as the residual hair follicles, sweat glands, and sebaceous glands are close together but with thicker skin grafts healing is delayed. The time to healing depends on depth of harvest, vascularity of the donor site, wound management, and general patient factors such as age, sepsis and vasopressors. The dermis heals with scar formation and there is no regeneration of harvested dermis. This has implications particularly for patients who require harvesting of healed donor sites. There is also a greater risk of hypertrophic scarring after harvesting of deeper grafts.

Management of specific burns

Scald Burns

Hot water scald burns of small or moderate size have been shown to be the exception to the general rule of early excision. Young children who had scald burns up to 20% TBSA required less area to be excised and had smaller blood transfusion requirements if operated upon in the second and third week postburn.[29] Earlier operation resulted in greater blood transfused and later operation led to much increased hospital stay (**Table 12.3**). A subsequent prospective trial randomized 24 children to early or late excision if their hot water scald injury had caused burns of clinically indeterminate depth.[30] No patient experienced a significant wound infection or systemic sepsis. Only half of the delayed excision group ultimately required surgical intervention and a significantly smaller area of excision was necessary for the remainder (**Table 12.4**).

In light of the foregoing evidence, children with hot water scald burns <20% TBSA can be appropriately treated with a topical antimicrobial such as silver sulfadiazine for about 2 weeks in the reasonable expectation of healing of most of the wound in the majority. This approach needs to be balanced by the knowledge that the longer a wound remains exposed to the environment, the greater the inflammatory response and subsequent scarring. Trauma, desiccation, and invasion by microorganisms almost certainly play a part in this process. A number of techniques are now available to cover the partial-thickness wound. When successful,

Table 12.3 Scald burn excision. Retrospective analysis of children with scald burns <30% TBSA. Nonoperative treatment for 14 days did not prolong length of stay. Operative blood loss was reduced (from Irei *et al.*[29])				
Day 1st surgery	0–5	6–10	11–20	>20
n	37	14	19	15
Weight (kg)	12.2±0.4	11.9±0.4	11.1±0.5	11.1±0.8
TBSA (%)	27±3	20±2	24±3	26±4
Blood loss (ml)	890±150*	400±70	430±140	240±160
Length of stay (days)	24±2	26±2	31±3	51±7*

Data presented as mean±SEM.
*Significantly different to all other groups.

Table 12.4 Early versus late excision of scald burns. Prospective, randomization to early or delayed wound excision led to half the patients healing spontaneously if surgery was delayed (from Desai et al.[30])

	n	Age	Burn size (% TBSA)	Postburn day excised	% Excised	Blood loss (TBBT)
Early excision	12	1.8±0.4	28±3	3±1	21±4	1.2±0.3
Late excision	6/12[†]	1.9±0.5	24±3	16±1	8±2*	0.3±0.1*

Data expressed as means ± SEM; TBBT, total body blood turnover.
*Significantly different compared with early excision.
[†]Only 6 of 12 underwent excision.

they have the added advantage of eliminating a great deal of the pain associated with dressing changes. These techniques are based on adherent wound dressings in the form of skin substitutes such as Biobrane™ and Transcyte™. Glycerol or cryopreserved allograft can also be used. More superficial wounds can be covered by a polyurethane membrane such as Omiderm™. These techniques can be used on patients with burns up to about 30% TBSA. The authors favor Biobrane™ for smaller and more superficial wounds that are pink, moist, and blanch readily.[31] Biobrane™ is a nylon/silicone bilaminated composite skin substitute. At the time of the first wound dressing, all loose skin and creams are removed to leave a clean, moist surface. The skin substitute is applied under some tension (like cling wrap on a bowl) and either stapled to itself on the extremities or taped to nonburned skin. A dry, nonadherent dressing should be applied and, where possible, firmly bandaged. The material works by becoming densely adherent to the exposed dermis, thus acting like a neoepidermis. Accumulation of fluid and nonadherence needs to be dealt with promptly or an abscess-like state can develop with pus trapped between the skin and the material. A few days of inactivity by the patient helps the development of adherence. The material needs to be applied in the first day or two postburn and the normal amount of vigilance is required to watch for invasive gram-positive infection. A toxic patient with increasing, throbbing wound pain and surrounding cellulitis are signs of this serious condition. Removal of the material, application of topical antimicrobial and appropriate systemic therapies are immediately indicated. Slightly deeper partial-thickness scald burns up to 40% TBSA can be treated by tangential excision and application of Transcyte™. Transcyte is basically Biobrane™ that has been placed in a culture medium of fibroblasts derived from fetal foreskin for a week. They adhere to the material and produce ground substances, collagen and growth factors. These substances, it is said, have a modulating effect on the inflammatory response in the wound bed. It is then frozen and so has to be defrosted prior to use. Transcyte™ is at least five times more expensive than Biobrane™ and while no hard evidence exists as yet that it yields any significant added benefit, the clinical impression is that it delivers a better cosmetic result. Transcyte™ probably also achieves better adherence rates than Biobrane™. The postoperative care of either material needs to be attentive with regular examination and preemptive trimming as required. It is important that creams, gels, and ointments are not allowed in contact with the material as this prevents or loosens adherence and leads to failure. This is particularly important if the standard wound dressing is tullegras or similar. Transcyte™ and Biobrane™ can also be used as temporary wound cover for excised full-thickness wounds and in place of allograft as the overlay for widely meshed autograft.

Adherence is more likely to occur and continue if the level of excision is fascia rather than subcutaneous fat – especially in very large burns.

Patients with very large scald burns, >40% TBSA, require total excision and immediate wound coverage. This may be with a combination of autograft, skin substitute, allograft, and dermal replacement (see later). Those with massive scald injury, >60% TBSA, require the same approach as the massive flame burn with selective fascial excision, widely meshed autograft and allograft overlay, dermal replacement material, and perhaps CEA.

The Very Large Burn

Patients with deep (flame) burns between 50 and 70% TBSA pose unique challenges with many conflicting demands for available donor sites. This is even more so when the patient has suffered a concomitant smoke inhalation and is likely to require ventilation for some weeks. In general, a fascial excision is indicated unless *very* healthy deep dermis can be left. This may be possible in areas of thick dermis such as the back. Near total excision should be completed in the first few days after injury and certainly by the fifth day postburn. The back, buttocks, and posterior thighs are covered with autograft taken at 6/1000th in adults, thinner in children, which is meshed at an expansion ration of 4 or 6 : 1. This is left on the carrier, if a Zimmer™ system is used, and applied to the wound bed and then painstakingly spread. A bulb syringe is a useful tool to 'float' the spaghetti-like graft into appropriate position. 'Fresh' allograft is the best option as an overlay. The central intravenous sites – subclavian and femoral – are covered with at least a 10 cm diameter patch of narrowly meshed, 1.5 : 1 autograft as is the tracheostomy site.

Consideration needs to be given to the use and extent of dermal replacement such as Integra™. Dermal replacement is an expensive option, but one that leaves an excellent result – when it works. Integra™ is, to date, the material with which most units have experience. It is a bilaminar composite that has a neodermis of bovine collagen held in a matrix pattern with shark cartilage chondroitin-6-sulphate. A layer of rubberized silicone is press sealed onto this and acts as a neoepidermis. The silicone layer does not drape and bend very well and is prone to delamination by movement over joints or by external shearing forces such as rough hands. For these reasons, Integra™ lends itself to application on flat, anterior surfaces away from joints. The abdomen, anterior thigh, forearm, leg, and male chest are such sites. Meticulous operative technique is essential with every point of excessive electrocautery that results in tissue necrosis leading to an area that fails. Topical epinephrine, and pinpoint accuracy with monopolar and selective use of bipolar electrocautery are the hemostatic methods of choice. Integra™ is best held in place by attaching an elastic netting material (Surginet™) over it. Further protection is then afforded by Exudry™ dressings. The neodermis is then revascularized from the underlying wound. This process takes 2–3 weeks to complete but is usually underway by 3–5 days. The neodermis usually becomes a plum color due to suffusion through the matrix of red cells from minor hemorrhage. This is normal and should be left alone. Actual hematomas are recognized by lifting of the material associated with a very dark red color. The area overlying the hematoma is best excised and the edges stapled down. The Integra™ can be replaced or the area treated with silver nitrate 0.5% soaked gauze. It must be remembered that the neodermis is inert and nonviable with no resistance to infection until neovascularization has occurred. This window of extreme vulnerability lasts about 5 days but the risk of delamination and shearing continues until the silicone neoepidermis has been replaced by epidermis. The neodermis is vascularized when it becomes a 'straw' color. Close inspection with magnification will reveal telangiectatic vessels dotted about. The second stage operation involves gentle removal of the silicone layer and application of 4–6/1000th inch autograft which can be meshed up to an expansion of 3:1. If shortage of donor sites necessitates expansion then the harvest needs to include as little dermis as possible otherwise a mesh pattern will permanently remain. It is said that CEA can be used for epidermal cover of Integra™ neodermis.[31] It is probably best to delay this procedure to ensure adequate vascularization and enhance CEA engraftment. The author's experience with this technique in very large and massive burns with multiresistant organisms resident upon them has not been gratifying. There is benefit in performing staged, sequential replacement of the silicone layer with ultra-thin, unmeshed autograft in sick patients with very large burns. Engraftment and graft survival seems to be more reliable in the long term and the cosmetic result enhanced – less haste but more progress. Debate continues regarding the role of Integra™ in wound coverage of patients with burns >70% TBSA. The incidence of failure due to infection rises dramatically as the burn size tops 75% TBSA. Decisions regarding its use will be influenced by the availability, or otherwise, of 'fresh' allograft. Integra™ does have a role in the management of medium to very large burns. It cannot be stated too strongly that Integra™ cannot be left abutting unexcised wound. It all has to be removed or infection will spread relentlessly from the edge and lead to failure.

Areas such as the knee and axilla do not suit the application of Integra™ due to movement causing delamination. Widely meshed autograft with allograft overlay can be interposed between sheets of Integra™ over these areas with good effect. Selective use of dermal replacement in areas of increased likelihood of success leaves autograft available for use on important structures such as the hand. The hands are then managed at a separate operating session on day 4 or 5 when burn edema has detumesced and the operator is fresh. While unmeshed grafts are preferable, especially for the fingers, an expansion ratio of 1.5:1 leaves an acceptable result and allows blood and serous exudate egress through the interstices without hindrance.

Massive Burns

The operating room

The safe management of a patient undergoing a massive burn debridement requires commitment and cooperation from a large

group of individuals. The procedures are long, intense, and performed under conditions that are physically and emotionally stressful. The room becomes crowded as the surgical team alone can number 6–8.

A very important perioperative issue for safe management of a patient undergoing a massive burn excision is the maintenance of body temperature. The patient is usually completely exposed and has little intact skin, especially after donor skin harvest. These areas are moist and evaporation leads to rapid heat loss. Convective heat loss also occurs at a great rate. To combat these sources of heat loss, a number of strategies can be used. The operating room should be warmed to 32°C. The latent heat of evaporation of water is 31.5°C. Above this temperature, the energy source for evaporation will come from the environment rather than the patient. This temperature, or higher, is definitely required during the process of patient preparation when the patient is being washed. Radiant heaters are also very helpful for perioperative thermoregulation. An indwelling bladder catheter temperature probe is essential to accurately monitor the patient's core temperature. Other adjunctive measures include the use of 'space blankets' – aluminum foil coverings on areas not being accessed – plastic sheeting over the head and face, and all intravenous fluids being given at 38°C through a warming coil. Repeated applications of warm blankets are also useful as are warm air blowers. Once these adjunctive measures have been put in place, the ambient temperature can often be decreased to a more comfortable (sic) 28–32°C! The operating room staff should be reminded to take fluids themselves each 30 minutes. Failure to do so leads to severe dehydration and a sickening headache.

The patient

Good vascular access is required and subclavian central and femoral arterial lines are favored. These lines need to be sutured securely to prevent dislodgment during positioning of the patient. Special attention to prevention of pressure areas is needed. The patients are often operated upon for many hours and so are at great risk of pressure necrosis. Gel pads under the heels, elbows, and occiput and an 'egg-crate' dimpled foam mattress or a dacron-filled mattress are essential. A customized, stainless steel surgical table with a channel at the periphery, which drains fluids towards an outlet, is very useful. The ability to obtain Trendelenburg and reverse Trendelenburg positions, along with the ability to raise and lower the whole table is essential. Scales for weighing the patient incorporated into the table are very helpful. Clipping and shaving of body hair in and around the wound and in donor sites is followed in many units with a total body wash with povidone–iodine detergent solution. The patient is then laid upon sterile drapes. This is more easily accomplished with children than with enormous adults.

The operation

During this process, loose skin and blisters are removed and cloudy burn blister fluid sent for microbiological examination. Two electrocautery dispersive plates are placed, usually under the buttocks or thighs. Donor skin harvest is performed early in the procedure and is often proceeded by instillation of 0.9% or 0.45% saline solution, preferably with added epinephrine, to assist in the process.

Excision commences with the patient in the prone position. Tangential or fascial excision, as appropriate, of the shoulders, back, buttocks, and upper thighs is performed. Wide meshed autograft with allograft or Biobrane™ overlay is applied. If insufficient autograft its available, the excised wound is covered with unexpanded, 1 : 1.5 meshed fresh allograft. Other alternatives include skin substitutes, such as Biobrane™ or Transcyte™, or cryopreserved allograft. Dermal replacement material is prone to failure due to infection in massive burns particularly on posterior surfaces, but can be used selectively on anterior flat surfaces. Multiple layers of bulky gauze dressings are applied over the antibiotic-impregnated gauze, in the case of allografts, or Exudry™ dressings if Biobrane™ was used. Thick silk sutures are inserted in a row along the flanks and tied in a loop. Tapes are then tied to the loops and tied over the bulky gauze dressing as a bolster. Another alternative is to apply multiple layers of chlorhexidine-impregnated, Vaseline gauze (Bactigras™), held with multiple staples. The patient is then placed in the supine position. Sterilizable, silicone tourniquets are often used on the limbs to decrease blood loss. Weak epinephrine clysis, topical 1 : 10 000 epinephrine irrigation, topical 5–20% thrombin solution spray, epinephrine-soaked lappads/sponges, and compression bandaging are all techniques used to limit blood loss during debridement. Electrocautery is used after a period of compression bandaging to control the residual, larger bleeding points.

Fascial-level excision is required for those areas where fat has been burned and in those with massive burns. This involves surgical removal of the full-thickness of integument, including all the subcutaneous fat, down to the layer of investing fascia. The advantages of this technique are that grafts take very well on fascia and blood loss is reduced. Episodes of sepsis lead to ischemic necrosis of subcutaneous fat subsequent to poor peripheral perfusion and microvascular stasis. This becomes problematic in patients with very large burns and leads to late graft loss and these ischemic areas become portals for invasive wound sepsis. The disadvantages of fascial excision are lymphedema and contour deformities. All lymphatics are excised, so lymphedema of dependent parts is often troublesome. The excised fat never regenerates and can give a spindly appearance to the areas excised while any increase in body fat is deposited in the remaining beds of adipose tissue. Moon faces and thick necks can result. Fascial excision is also indicated for life-threatening invasive wound sepsis particularly with fungi and yeast such as aspergillus and candida and also for large areas with failed graft take in a critically ill patient with massive burns.

Patients return to the operating room as soon as donor sites are healed for further autografting and replacement of nonadherent allograft or infected skin substitute. Massively burned children when treated with recombinant human growth hormone (GH), showed donor-site wound healing accelerated by 25% even if the patients presented infected and malnourished. There is a transient hyperglycemia in a third of patients that require insulin. The GH-treated patients require less infused albumin to maintain normal serum levels and this is an indication of the net positive protein balance induced.[33] The usual hospital stay for a 30 kg patient with a 60% TBSA burn of 42 days was reduced to 32 days. This tremendous decrease in length of hospital stay realizes a net saving of 15% in total costs. Salutary effects have also been documented in a group of patients treated nonoperatively. Mortality dropped from 45 to 8%.[34] Whilst it must be acknowledged that two European studies in critically ill adults of mixed etiology showed increased mortality among the GH-treated groups, this experience has not been repeated in the massively burned, pediatric population in North America.[35]

Other anabolic agents have shown promise as a means of speeding wound healing in severely injured, catabolic burn patients. Oxandrolone in a dose of 20 mg/day has demonstrated a positive effect on protein kinetics and wound healing in both animal models and clinical trials. Emaciated, massively burned children whose presentation was delayed by, on average, 30 days were also greatly aided by oxandrolone 0.2 mg/kg/day. Protein kinetics were normalized, further weight loss prevented, and wound healing was enhanced. No virilism, hirsutism, or hepatic dysfunction was noted (unpublished data). Donor-site wound healing was accelerated by 20% in oxandrolone-treated severely burned adults[36] compared to nontreated. While these pharmacological agents provide great support to the massively burned, they are only an adjunct to early, near-total excision and prompt wound coverage.

Operative management of burns in special areas

The Hand
Full-thickness burns should be excised and grafted as soon as practicable after diagnosis. However, the role of early operation for partial-thickness hand burns is contentious.[37–40] If donor skin is available, and the depth of the burn indicates that wound healing will not be complete in 10 days, then excision and grafting is reasonable and advantageous. Thick split-thickness skin grafts have been widely used to resurface hands. However, a prospective trial by Heimbach et al. demonstrated no difference between 15/1000th inch and 25/1000th inch skin graft, on assessment by blinded observers (unpublished data). The thinner graft will obviously induce less donor-site morbidity and obviate the need for overgrafting. If wide area coverage in huge burns is paramount or wounds will quickly heal, other techniques can be used. These include topical antimicrobials covered with dressings or a plastic glove, enclosing the hand in a plastic bag filled with topical antimicrobials, or application of a Biobrane™ glove.[41]

The Face
Facial burns that are obviously full-thickness and obviously require operative management are less problematic than those that are deep dermal with small patches of full-thickness injury. The face that needs grafting can be scheduled for operation as soon as swelling has subsided, but usually no earlier than day 5 postburn. Some centers use facemasks to exert pressure so that the grafts can be applied to a surface that more closely resembles the norm. This is a very labor-intensive exercise as the mask needs to be remolded each day to keep up with detumescence.

Selection of site and depth of donor skin harvest needs careful consideration. If at all possible, the donor skin should come from the 'blush' area above the line of the nipples for the best color match. While most favor the scalp, the potential problems of alopecia and hair growth from transplanted hair follicles are real concerns.[42] If the scalp is not available the other alternative is to harvest across the upper part of the back with subsequent overgrafting with a thin graft. Epinephrine clysis is a sensible preemptive measure to decrease blood loss especially if delivered in a large volume of saline.[43] This will make the harvesting process easier. If the skin over the upper back and shoulders is sun-damaged or freckled in fair-skinned individuals then other alternatives may need to be sought. It is best to remember also that the skin of the scalp of a bald man is usually quite thin and therefore not suitable as a donor site. If the upper back/shoulder region is selected, the donor site is best overgrafted with thin split-skin graft of, say, 6/1000th inch to prevent hypertrophic scar formation. Grafts should be taken as widely as possible so as to decrease the number of seams required.

Excising the face can be very bloody and loss of more than a total blood volume is not unknown – be prepared! Epinephrine clysis is essential to limit the exsanguinating hemorrhage. If the burn is obviously full-thickness, excision with needle-point electrocautery works well. If there is any doubt as to the depth, tangential excision with a Goulian knife is more appropriate as preservation of any viable dermal elements is essential for optimum results. Some centers delay the reconstructive phase of the procedure to decrease graft loss from hematoma formation. Temporary wound closure with cryopreserved allograft is a good option if this course is chosen.

Grafts should be placed in such a fashion as to mimic the esthetic units as much as possible. Glue is useful to 'spot-weld' around the edge of the grafts and is certainly faster than suturing. A narrow gauge (21) hypodermic needle inserted into the end of the glue nozzle limits 'runs' and increases accuracy (**Figure 12.8**). Magnification with loupes aids accurate excision and graft placement.

Deep dermal facial burns were shown by Tredgett[45] to be more prone to hypertrophic scarring if they took longer than 18 days to heal. This being the case, surgery can be planned for the third post-burn week. At operation, the first question to be answered is what to do with unhealed/unburned areas that do not completely cover a cosmetic unit. Folklore has it that excision of a whole cosmetic unit is essential for optimum results. It is difficult to find anyone who actually uses this approach, and it is one that has no appeal. The second question is what to do with the hair-bearing beard area in the adult male. If healing of this area is prolonged, folliculitis, which incites development of hypertrophic scar, is a common sequelae. Excision requires removing all hair follicles as grafting a partial-thickness excision results in hair erupting through the graft, with much infection and inflammation leading to hypertrophic scarring. The answer to this conundrum remains elusive. Skin substitutes can be used for the burned face in the same fashion as described for scald burns. Transcyte™, in particular, seems to offer benefit in this situation.[46] Exposure, desiccation, trauma to fragile tissues, and presence of microorganisms are all decreased. Wounds seem to be a little slower to heal but are much less erythematous (**Figure 12.9**).

Eyelids

Deep burns to the eyelids should be excised and grafted early. Delay inevitably leads to cicatricial ectropion, corneal exposure, and a threat to sight.[47] Postburn cicatricial ectropion is a dangerous condition, with unconscious, ventilated patients at particular risk. Release and full-thickness grafts to the lower lid and thick, split-thickness grafts to the upper lids should be undertaken as soon as the condition is diagnosed.[48] Unconscious patients can have their corneas protected by a combination of ophthalmic lubricants and cling-film stretched over the eye socket. This creates a moisture trap and prevents exposure keratitis (unpublished data).

Genital Burns

Hot water scald burns to the genitalia of both sexes, such as those in children, are best treated expectantly with spontaneous healing the usual result. Small, patchy full-thickness burns to the scrotum can be excised and closed to good effect. Most partial-thickness burns will heal spontaneously as scrotal skin is quite thick and contains multiple hair follicles. The very deep burn from flammable liquid or high-voltage electricity is often associated with full-thickness loss. Excision with electrocautery is recommended. If the tunica requires excision, temporary allografting of the testes, followed by delayed autografting is recommended. Circumcision of full-thickness burns to the foreskin works well and is appropriate as phimosis is a common sequelae. A deep burn to the glans may be best allowed to proceed to eschar separation, and grafting of resultant granulation tissue as severe hemorrhage accompanies surgical debridement. Full-thickness burns to the labia majora should be excised and grafted as a delayed procedure. This will decrease the degree of contracture that would certainly develop.

Perianal burns are seen in association with extensive burns in adults and in scalded children. Early excision is required for obvious full-thickness burns. Some centers recommend diversion of the fecal stream, preferably achieved laparoscopically, to aid

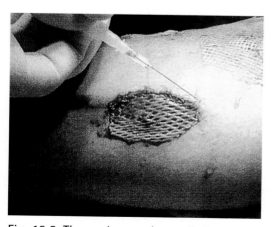

Fig. 12.8 Tissue glue can be applied accurately to the edge of the skin graft using a hypodermic needle.

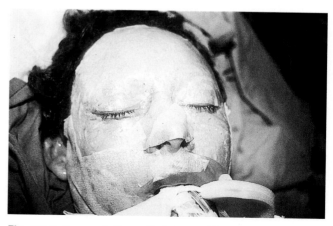

Fig. 12.9 Transcyte™ applied to a mid-dermal facial burn. Although not shown, the final result was excellent.

healing and graft take.[49] An alternative is to keep the stool liquid and maintain a rectal tube *in situ*. Another technique is to administer a bowel prep and follow surgery with an elemental diet and stool thickeners such as codeine. Bowel actions can thus be delayed for 5–7 days. If graft failure occurs, it is important to keep trying to achieve engraftment as the perianal, circular contracture that results from healing by secondary intention is difficult to fix.

The Breast

The nipple–areola complex, especially in females, is another area that requires extra attention. In general, it is best left unexcised as healing can occur from the deep glandular structures that are usually preserved. Sensation is also usually preserved and this is much appreciated by patients. Absence of a nipple is very noticeable and is often the one thing remarked upon by patients even though they have other areas of more extensive scarring. It needs to be made clear that excision of the breast mound in postpubertal, or the breast bud in prepubertal, females should be avoided if possible. Dermal replacement, such as Integra™, when applied on the female chest in juxtaposition to the unexcised areola, requires close attention. Acticoat™, Iodoflex granules™, or silver nitrate 0.5% soaked gauze can be used to attempt to control infection in this situation. The relatively avascular nature of the fat and connective tissue matrix that constitutes the majority of the nonlactating breast makes careful excision of all nonviable tissue even more important than usual. Retention dressings are useful for the isolated burn to decrease movement.

High–voltage electrical injury

High-voltage electrical injuries are devastating, particularly when the upper limb is affected.[50] The nature of the injuries also means that the effect on the resources of the treating hospital may also be significant. High voltage (>1000 volts) causes three patterns of injury that pose specific challenges. The patient who has had the current 'flash' over their skin will also be injured in other areas by flame burns from clothing that has been ignited. Contact points are likely to have had a concentration of energy and give a 'blown-out' appearance (**Figure 12.10**). When the high-voltage electrical injury has passed deeply along periosteum, nerves, and blood vessels, deep muscle necrosis is the rule. This tissue should be sought and excised. Radio-isotope scanning or positron emission tomograms are useful for identification of deep, devitalized tissue and so focus surgical attention.

Whilst controversy remains about the best time to reconstruct following electrical injury, the resulting defects often require complex reconstruction with either local, regional, or free flaps. The tendency for electrical injuries to be either underestimated or for the damage to progress, particularly if of a high voltage, means that the safe option is for reconstruction to be delayed for 3–5 days following single or multiple debridements.[50] Early debridement and reconstruction may be carried out but the muscle debridement needs to be aggressive to ensure no doubtful tissue is left and thus potentially viable tissue may be excised.[51] For this reason we favor an early sequential debridement technique.

Flap reconstruction is frequently required in electrical injuries due to the depth of the injury exposing structures not suitable for skin grafting (for example, exposed joints, tendons, and nerves). The judicious use of flap reconstruction may be preferable as a flap will import vascularity and allow vital structures such as nerves that are apparently nonviable to recover.[51] Flap selection depends on the condition of the patient and the extent of the injury. Local transposition (**Figure 12.11a,b**), advancement, adipofascial, and cross finger flaps may offer simple local reconstructive options assuming the local skin is uninjured.[52,53] For more extensive defects reverse pedicled flaps and free flaps may be required, assuming the inflowing vessels are not involved in the zone of injury. If local and regional vessels are damaged or unsuitable, a distant pedicled flap may be the only option and the groin flap is an excellent option for coverage of upper limb defects under these circumstances.[54] The disadvantage of the groin flap is that the hand is in a dependent position for a period of 10–14 days and this results in edema and joint stiffness. In electrical injuries affecting multiple sites, a combination of flaps may need to be used. Electrical injuries are always worse than they initially appear and usually require advanced tissue coverage techniques. Planning for these eventualities will enable a timely and appropriate operative approach.

Conclusion

Modern burn care is based on operative wound management. The evidence is clear that prompt excision and closure is lifesaving for patients with large burns. Skin substitutes and dermal replacement have made operative wound care even more appealing and offer an attractive alternative to topical antimicrobial therapy for partial-thickness wounds. Bioengineered composite skin replacement will soon make surgical management of burn wounds the norm.

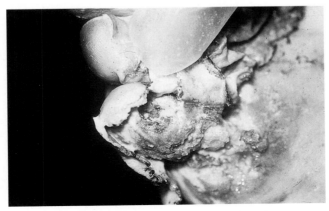

Fig. 12.10 'Blown-out' appearance of high-voltage electrical injury contact point.

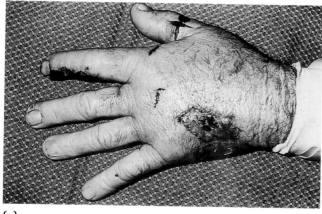

(a)

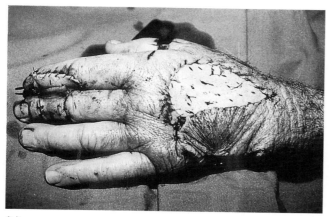

(b)

Fig. 12.11 (a) Low-voltage electrical burn to the dorsum of the left hand. Debridement of necrotic tissue left tendons without paratenon exposed. The wound was therefore not suitable for skin grafting. (b) Closure of the wound with a transposition flap and skin graft to secondary defect.

References

1. Bull JP, Fisher AJ. A study of mortality in a burns unit: a revised estimate. *Ann Surg* 1954; **139**: 269–74.
2. Muller MJ, Herndon DN. The challenge of burns. *Lancet* 1994; **343**: 216–20.
3. Burke JF, Bandoc CC, Quinby WC. Primary burn excision and immediate grafting: a method for shortening illness. *J Trauma* 1974; **14**: 389–95.
4. Pietsch JB, Netscher DT, Nagaraj HS, Groff DB. Early excision of major burns in children: effect on morbidity and mortality. *J Pediatr Surg* 1985; **20(4)**: 754–7.
5. Herndon DN, Parks DH. Comparison of serial debridement and autografting and early massive excision with cadaver skin overlay in the treatment of large burns in children. *J Trauma* 1986; **26(2)**: 149–52.
6. Herndon DN, Barrow RE, Rutan RL, Rutan TC, Desai MH, Abston S. A comparison of conservative versus early excision therapies in severely burned patients. *Ann Surg* 1989; **209**: 547–53.
7. Tompkins RG, Burke JF, Schoenfeld DA, Dondoc CC, Quinby WC, Behringen GC, Ackyroyd FW. Prompt eschar excision: a treatment system contributing to reduced burn mortality. *Ann Surg* 1986; **204(3)**: 272–81.
8. Thompson P, Herndon DN, Abston S, Rutan T. Effect of early excision on patients with major thermal injury. *J Trauma* 1987; **27(2)**: 205–7.
9. Munster AM, Smith-Meek M, Sharkey P. The effect of early surgical intervention on mortality and cost-effectiveness in burn care, 1978–91. *Burns* 1994; **20(1)**: 61–4.
10. Deitch EA, Clothier J. Burns in the elderly: an early surgical approach. *J Trauma* 1983; **23(10)**: 891–4.
11. Deitch EA. A policy of early excision and grafting in elderly burn patients shortens the hospital stay and improves survival. *Burns* 1985; **12**: 109–14.
12. Hara M, Peters WJ, Douglas LG, Morris SF. An early surgical approach to burns in the elderly. *J Trauma* 1990; **30(4)**: 430–2.
13. Scott-Conner CEH, Love R, Wheeler W. Does rapid wound closure improve survival in older patients with burns? *Ann Surg* 1990; **56**: 57–60.
14. Saffle JR, Larson CM, Sullivan J, Shelby J. The continuing challenge of burn care in the elderly. *Surgery* 1990; **108(3)**: 534–43.
15. Hunt JL, Purdue CF. The elderly burn patient. *Am J Surg* 1992; **164**: 472–6.
16. Lewandowski R, Pegg SP, Fortier K, Skimmings A. Burn injuries in the elderly. *Burns* 1993; **19(6)**: 513–15.
17. Ikeda J, Sugamata A, Jumbo Y, Yukioka T, Makino K. A new surgical procedure for aged burn victims: applications of dermolipectomy for burn wounds and donor sites. *J Burn Care Rehabil* 1990; **11(1)**: 27–31.
18. Deitch EA, Wheelahan TM, Rose MP, Clothier J, Cotter J. Hypertrophic burn scars: analysis of variables. *J Trauma* 1983; **23(10)**: 895–8.
19. Heimbach DM. Early burn excision and grafting. *Surg Clin N Am* 1987; **67(1)**: 93–107.
20. Engrav LH, Heimbach DM, Reus JL, Harnar TJ, Marvin JA. Early excision and grafting vs. nonoperative treatment of burns of indeterminant depth: a randomized prospective study. *Trauma* 1983; **23(11)**: 1001–4.
21. Janzekovic Z. A new concept in the early excision and immediate grafting of burns. *J Trauma* 1970; **10**: 1103–8.
22. Janzekovic Z. The burn wound from the surgical point of view. *J Trauma* 1975; **15**: 42–61.
23. Herndon DN, Abston S, Stein MD. Increased thromboxane B_2 levels in the plasma of burned and septic burned patients. *Surg Gynecol Obst* 1984; **159**: 210–13.
24. Desai MH, Herndon DN, Broemeling, Barrow RE, Nichols RJ Jr, Rutan RL. Early burn wound excision significantly reduces blood loss. *Ann Surg* 1990; **221**: 753–62.
25. Alexander JW, MacMillan BG, Law E, Kittur DS. Treatment of severe burns with widely meshed skin autograft and meshed skin allograft overlay. *J Trauma* 1981; **21(6)**: 433–8.
26. Munster MA. Cultured skin for massive burns. A prospective, controlled trial. *Ann Surg* 1996; **224(3)**: 372–5.
27. Barret JP, Wolf SE, Desai MH, Herndon DN. Cost-efficacy of cultured epidermal autografts in massive pediatric burns. *Ann Surg* 2000; **231(6)**: 869–76.
28. Huang KF, Linares HA, Evans MJ, *et al.* Can donor sites be harvested indefinitely? *Proc Am Burns Assoc* 1992;
29. Irei M, Abston S, Bonds E, Rutan T, Desai M, Herndon DN. The optimal time for excision of cald burns in toddlers. *J Burn Care Rehabil* 1986; **7(6)**: 508–10.
30. Desai MH, Rutan RL, Herndon DN. Conservative treatment of scald burns is superior to early excision. *J Burn Care Rehabil* 1991; **12**: 482–4.
31. Bannet JP, Dziewulski P, Ramzy PI, Wolf SE, Desai MH, Herndon DN. Biobrane versus 1% silver sulfadiazine in second-degree pediatric burns. *Plast Reconstr Surg* 2000; **105**: 62–5.
32. Boyce ST, Kagan RJ, Meyer NA, Yakuboff KP, Warden BD. Cultured skin substitutes combined with Integra artificial skin to replace skin autograft and allograft for the closure of excised full-thickness burns. *J Burn Care Rehabil* 1999; **20(6)**: 453–61.
33. Gilpin DA, Barrow RE, Rutan RL, Broemeling B, Herndon DN. Recombinant human growth hormone accelerates wound healing in children with large cutaneous burns. *Ann Surg* 1994; **220(1)**: 19–24.
34. Singh KP, Prasad R, Chari PS, Dash RJ. Effect of growth hormone therapy in burn patients on conservative treatment. *Burns* 1998; **24(8)**: 733–8.
35. Ramirez RJ, Wolf SE, Barrow RE, Herndon DN. Growth hormone treatment in pediatric burns: a safe therapeutic approach. *Ann Surg* 1998; **228(4)**: 439–48.
36. Demling RH, Orgill DP. The anticatabolic effects of the testosterone analog oxandrolone after severe burn injury. *J Crit Care* 2000; **15(1)**: 12–17.
37. Levine BA, Sirinek KR, Peterson HD, Pruitt BA. Efficacy of tangential excision and immediate autografting of deep second degree burns of the hand. *J Trauma* 1979; **19(9)**: 670–3.
38. Edstrom LE, Robson MC, Macchiaverna JR, Scala AD. Prospective randomized treatments for burned hands: non operative vs operative. *Scand J Plast Reconstr Surg* 1979; **13**: 131–5.
39. Salisbury RE, Wright P. Evaluation of early excision of dorsal burns of the hand. *Plast Reconstr Surg* 1982; **69(4)**: 670–5.
40. Frist W, Ackroyd F, Burke J, Bondoc C. Long term functional results of selective treatment of hand burns. *Am J Surg* 1985; **149**: 516–21.
41. McHugh TP, Robson MC, Heggers JP, Phillips LG, Smith DJ, McCallum MC.

Therapeutic efficacy of Biobrane in partial and full thickness thermal injury. *Surgery* 1986; **100(4)**: 661–4.

42. Barret JP, Dziewulski P, Wolf SE, Desai MH, Herndon DN. Outcome of scalp donor sites in 450 consecutive pediatric burn patients. *Plast Reconstr Surg* 1999; **103(4)**: 1139–42.

43. Huges WB, DeClement FA, Hensell DO. Intradermal injection of epinephrine to decrease blood loss during split thickness skin grafting. *J Burn Care Rehibil* 1996; **171(3)**: 243–5.

44. Sheridan RL, Szyfelbein SK. Staged high dose epinephrine clysis is safe and effective in extensive tangential burn excisions in children. *Burns* 1999; **25(8)**: 745–8.

45. Fraulin FO, Illmayer SJ, Tredget EE. Assessment of cosmetic and functional results of conservative versus surgical management of facial burns. *J Burn Care Rehabil* 1996; **17(1)**: 19–29.

46. Demling RH, DeSanti L. Management of partial thickness facial burns (comparison of topical antibiotics and bio-engineered skin substitutes). *Burns* 1999; **25(3)**: 256–61.

47. Barrow RE, Jeschke MG, Herndon DN. Early release of third-degree eyelid burns prevents eye injury. *Plast Reconstr Surg* 2000; **105(3)**: 860–3.

48. Astori IP, Muller MJ, Pegg SP. Cicatricial postburn ectropion and exposure keratitis. *Burns* 1998; **24(1)**: 64–7.

49. Quarmley CJ, Millar AJW, Rode H. The use of diverting colostomies in paediatric peri-anal burns. *Burns* 1999; **25(7)**: 645–50.

50. Hussmann J, Kucan JO, Russell RC, Bradley T, Zamboni WA. Electrical injuries – morbidity, outcome and treatment rationale. *Burns* 1995; **21(7)**: 530–5.

51. Chick LR, Lister GD, Sowder L. Early free flap coverage of electrical and thermal burns. *Plast Reconst Surg* 1992; **89(6)**: 1013–19.

52. Ramakrishnan KM, Jayaram V, Ramachandran K, Mathivanan T. Deepithelialized turnover flaps in burns. *Plastic Reconst Surg* 1988; **84(1)**: 172–3.

53. Jenkins AM, Pegg SP. Island flaps in the primary reconstruction of electrical burns. *Burns* 1987; **13(3)**: 236–40.

54. Lister GD, McGregor IA, Jackson IT. The groin flap in hand injuries. *Injury* 1973; **4(3)**: 229–39.

Chapter 13

Anesthesia for burned patients

Lee C Woodson, Edward R Sherwood
Elise M Morvant, Lynn A Peterson

Introduction

Continuous improvement in burn care since World War II has resulted in a steady increase in the rate of survival after large burn injury.[1] These improvements have been attributed to aggressive fluid resuscitation, early excision and grafting of burn wounds, more effective antimicrobials, advances in nutritional support, and development of burn centers. Now most patients with more than 80% total body surface area (TBSA) burned will survive if promptly treated. A recent study of risk factors for death following burn injuries identified three variables that can be used to estimate the probability of death: age greater than 60 years, burns over more than 40% of the total body surface area, and the presence of inhalation injury.[2] Mortality increased in proportion to the number of risk factors present: 0.3%, 3%, 33%, or approximately 90% mortality depending on whether zero, one, two, or three risk factors were present, respectively. The incidence of mortality is also influenced by significant coexisting disease or delays in resuscitation. Additionally, some burn patients develop refractory burn shock soon after injury and cannot be resuscitated.

Major burn injury results in pathophysiological changes in virtually all organ systems. **Table 13.1** lists some of the challenges presented by the acutely burned patient during the perioperative period. Several highly informative reviews of anesthetic management for burn surgery have been written during the past decade, each with its own special areas of concentration.[3–5]

Patients suffering burn injuries often require surgical treatment for years after the initial injury in order to correct functional and cosmetic sequelae. Anesthetic management for reconstructive burn surgery presents many special problems but this chapter will concentrate on the care of acute burn patients. The acute phase of burn injury is defined as the period from injury until the wounds have been excised, grafted, and healed.

Modern burn care depends on coordination of a multidisciplinary team including surgeons, intensivists, nurse clinicians, nutritionists, rehabilitation therapists, pulmonary care therapists, and anesthesia providers. Rational and effective anesthetic management of acute burn patients requires an understanding of this multidisciplinary approach so that perioperative care is compatible with the overall treatment goals for the patient. The current standard of

Table 13.1 Perioperative challenges in the acute burn patient

- Compromised airway
- Pulmonary insufficiency
- Altered mental status
- Associated injuries
- Limited vascular access
- Rapid blood loss
- Impaired tissue perfusion due to:
    - Hypovolemia
    - Decreased myocardial contractility
    - Anemia
- Decreased colloid osmotic pressure
- Edema
- Dysrhythmia
- Impaired temperature regulation
- Altered drug response
- Renal insufficiency
- Immunosuppression
- Infection/sepsis

Table 13.2 Major preoperative concerns in acutely burned patients

Age of patient
Extent of burn injuries (total body surface area)
Burn depth and distribution (superficial or full thickness)
Mechanism of injury (flame, electrical, scald, or chemical)
Airway patency
Presence or absence of inhalation injury
Elapsed time from injury
Adequacy of resuscitation
Associated injuries
Coexisting diseases
Surgical plan

surgical treatment calls for early excision and grafting of nonviable burn wounds, which may harbor pathogens and produce inflammatory mediators with systemic effects resulting in cardiopulmonary compromise. After an extensive burn injury, the systemic effects of inflammatory mediators on metabolism and cardiopulmonary function reduce physiological reserve and the patient's tolerance to the stress of surgery deteriorates with time. Assuming adequate resuscitation, extensive surgery is best tolerated soon after injury when the patient is most fit. However, it must be recognized that the initial resuscitation of patients with large burns results in large fluid shifts and may result in hemodynamic instability and respiratory insufficiency. Reynolds *et al.* reported that more than half of deaths after burn injuries occur due to failed resuscitation.[6] Effective anesthetic management of patients with extensive burn injuries requires an understanding of the pathophysiological changes associated with large burns and careful preoperative evaluation to assure that resuscitation has been optimized and an appropriate anesthetic plan has been formulated.

Preoperative evaluation of burn injury

The preoperative evaluation of burn patients requires knowledge of the continuum of pathophysiological changes that occur in these patients from the initial period after injury through the time that all wounds have healed. The dramatic changes that occur in all organ systems following burn injury directly affect anesthetic management. The following discussion will describe the pathophysiological changes that occur in the acutely burned patient as they relate to the preoperative evaluation. In addition to the routine features of the preoperative evaluation, evaluation of acute burn patients requires special attention to airway management and pulmonary support, vascular access, adequacy of resuscitation, and associated injuries. The severely burned patient presents with numerous preoperative concerns (**Table 13.2**).

The preoperative evaluation must be performed within the context of the planned operative procedure, which will depend on the location, extent, and depth of burn wounds, time after injury, presence of infection, and existence of suitable donor sites for autografting.

Initial Evaluation

Destruction of skin by thermal injury disrupts the vital functions of the largest organ in the body. The skin provides several essential protective and homeostatic functions (**Table 13.3**). Treatment of patients with burn injuries must compensate for loss of these functions, until the wounds are covered and healed. As a barrier to evaporation of water, the skin helps maintain fluid and electrolyte balance. Heat loss through evaporation and impairment of vasomotor regulation in burned skin diminishes effective temperature regulation. The skin's barrier function also protects against infection by invading organisms. Wound exudate rich in protein depletes plasma proteins when large body surface areas are injured.

In addition to loss of important functions of the skin, extensive burns result in an inflammatory response with systemic effects that alter function in virtually all organ systems. Preoperative evaluation of the burn patient is guided largely by a knowledge of these pathophysiological changes. Much of the morbidity and mortality associated with burn injuries are related to the size of the injury. The extent of the burn injury is expressed as the TBSA burned. Estimates of TBSA burned are used to guide fluid and electrolyte therapy and to estimate surgical blood loss. Percentage of the skin's surface that has been burned is estimated by the so-called rule of nines (see **Figure 4.1**). Estimates are modified for pediatric

Table 13.3 Functions of skin

1. Protection from environmental elements (e.g. radiation, mechanical irritation or trauma)
2. Immunological – antigen presentation, antibacterial products (sebum), barrier to entry of pathological organisms
3. Fluid and electrolyte homeostasis – helps maintain protein and electrolyte concentrations by limiting evaporation
4. Thermoregulation – helps control heat loss through sweating and vasomotor regulation of superficial blood flow
5. Sensory – extensive and varied sensory organs in skin provide information about environment
6. Metabolic – vitamin D synthesis and excretion of certain substances
7. Social – appearance of skin has strong influence on image and social interactions

Adapted from Williams WG, Phillips LG. Pathophysiology of the burn wound. In: Herndon DN, ed. *Total Burn Care*, 1st edn. London: WB Saunders, 1996: 64.

patients because of age-related differences in body proportions. A knowledge of the burn depth is also critical to anticipating physiological insult, as well as, planned surgical treatment. First degree or superficial second degree burns may heal without scarring or deformity and do not require surgical excision. Deeper second degree and third degree burns require surgical debridement and grafting with associated surgical blood loss.

Accurate estimates of blood loss are crucial in planning preoperative management of burn patients. With extensive wound excision or debridement, large amounts of blood can be lost rapidly. Adequate preparation in terms of monitors, vascular access, and availability of blood products is essential. Surgical blood loss depends on area to be excised (cm²), time since injury, surgical plan (tangential vs. fascial excision), and presence of infection.[7] Blood loss from skin graft donor sites will also vary depending on whether it is an initial or repeat harvest. These variables are valuable predictors of surgical blood loss, which is a critical factor in planning anesthetic management (**Table 13.4**).

Table 13.4 Calculation of Expected Blood Loss

Surgical procedure	Predicted blood loss
<24 h since burn injury	0.45 ml/cm² burn area
1–3 days since burn injury	0.65 ml/cm² burn area
2–16 days since burn injury	0.75 ml/cm² burn area
>16 days since burn injury	0.5–0.75 ml/cm² burn area
Infected wounds	1–1.25 ml/cm² burn area

Adapted from Desai et al., Ann Surg 1990.[7]

Airway and Pulmonary Function

Special attention must be paid to the airway and pulmonary function during preoperative evaluation. Burn injuries to the face and neck can distort anatomy and reduce range of mobility in ways that make direct laryngoscopy difficult or impossible. Specific alterations include impaired mouth opening, edema of the tongue, oropharynx, and larynx, as well as decreased range of motion of the neck. The tissue injury and sloughing present after severe facial burns may make mask ventilation difficult. Inhalation injury may impair pulmonary gas exchange and lead to respiratory insufficiency or failure.

The level of respiratory support must also be assessed. The level of required support may range from supplemental blow-by or mask oxygen to intubation and ventilation with high positive end-expiratory pressure (PEEP), and increased FIO_2 requirements. Lung injury can occur from smoke inhalation, systemic inflammation, and aggressive fluid resuscitation. Common pathologies include upper airway injury with stridor, bronchospasm, lower airway obstruction from mucus plugs and epithelial casts, as well as pulmonary edema due to acute lung injury or volume overload. With very high levels of PEEP or peak inspiratory pressure it must be determined if the anesthesia ventilator is adequate or if an ICU ventilator will need to be brought to the operating room. If the patient is intubated at the time of the preoperative evaluation it is essential to know what the indications for intubation were so that an appropriate plan for postoperative support can be made.

There is general recognition that smoke inhalation injury increases morbidity and mortality for burn patients.[8] The presence of an inhalation injury in combination with a cutaneous burn increases the volume of fluid required for resuscitation as much as 44%.[9] Numerous studies have also shown an increased incidence of pulmonary complications (pneumonia, respiratory failure, or ARDS) in patients with burns and inhalation injury when compared with burns alone.[10] Sequelae of inhalation injury include upper airway distortion and obstruction from direct thermal injury as well as impaired pulmonary gas exchange due to effects of toxic gases on lower airways and pulmonary parenchyma. These two components of the inhalation injury have separate time courses and pathophysiological consequences.

Foley described findings of 335 autopsies performed on patients who died from extensive burns.[11] Intraoral, palatal, and laryngeal burns were not uncommon among patients with inhalation injuries. The most common sites of laryngeal injury were the epiglottis and vocal folds where their edges were exposed. In contrast, thermal necrosis below the glottis and upper trachea was not observed in any of these patients. The lower airways are nearly always protected from direct thermal injury by the efficiency of heat exchange in the oro- and nasopharynx unless the injury involves steam or an explosive blast. This has been demonstrated in an experimental model.[12] Inhalation injury to the lower airways and pulmonary parenchyma is due to the effect of toxic or irritant gases.

Clinical suspicion of inhalation injury is aroused by the presence of certain risk factors such as history of exposure to fire and smoke in an enclosed space or a period of unconsciousness at the accident scene, burns including the face and neck, singed facial or nasal hair, altered voice, dysphagia, oral and/or nasal soot deposits, or carbonaceous sputum. The most immediate threat from inhalation injury is upper airway obstruction due to edema. Early or prophylactic intubation is recommended when this complication threatens. However, exposure to smoke does not always lead to severe injury and in the absence of overt evidence of respiratory distress or failure it may be difficult to identify patients who will experience progressive inflammation and ultimately require intubation of the trachea. In a retrospective study, Clark et al. reported that 51% of their patients exposed to smoke inhalation did not require intubation.[13] Unnecessary intubation in the presence of an inflamed laryngeal mucosa risks further damage to the larynx and subglottic area.[14,15]

Traditional clinical predictors of airway obstruction have been found to be relatively insensitive and inadequate for identifying early severe airway inflammation and often underestimate the severity of the injury.[16,17] More objective criteria for evaluation of the risk of airway obstruction are often needed. Hunt et al. found fiberoptic bronchoscopy to be a safe and accurate method for diagnosis of acute inhalation injury.[18] They described observations of severe supraglottic injuries associated with mucosal edema obliterating the piriform sinuses and causing massive enlargement of the epiglottis and arytenoid eminence. Haponic et al. made serial observations by nasopharyngoscopy in patients at risk for inhalation injury and found distortions of the upper airway described as compliant, edematous mucosa of the aryepiglottic folds, and arytenoid eminences that prolapsed to occlude the airway on inspiration.[19] Progressive upper airway edema in these patients was correlated with body surface area burned, resuscitative volume administered, and rate of infusion of resuscitative fluids. For patients who are at risk for inhalation injury but lack definitive indications for intubation, fiberoptic nasopharyngoscopy is effective in identifying laryngeal edema. Serial exams may help avoid unnecessary intubations and at the same time identify progressive inflammatory changes and allow intubation before severe airway obstruction and emergent conditions develop.

Lower airway and parenchymal injuries develop more slowly than upper airway obstruction. Prior to resuscitation, clinical signs and symptoms, chest X-ray, and blood gas analysis may be within normal limits despite significant injury that eventually progresses to respiratory failure requiring intubation and mechanical ventilation.[12,20]

Linares *et al.* studied the sequence of morphological changes following smoke inhalation in an experimental sheep model.[21] They observed four discrete but overlapping phases of injury described as exudative, degenerative, proliferative, and reparative. During the first 48 hours the *exudative phase* was characterized by PMN infiltration, interstitial edema, loss of Type I pneumocytes, and damage to the tracheobronchial epithelium in the form of focal necrosis, hemorrhage, and submucosal edema. The *degenerative phase* occurred between 12 and 72 hours and was characterized by progressive epithelial damage with shedding of necrotic tissue and formation of pseudomembranes and casts. Hyaline membranes developed over alveolar surfaces. Macrophages began to accumulate to begin absorption of necrotic debris. A *proliferative phase* was described between days 2 and 7 during which Type II pneumocytes and macrophages proliferated. After the fourth day *reparative* changes were observed with regeneration of epithelium from spared epithelium from the orifices of glands.

Demling and Chen have provided a lucid description of the pathophysiological changes following inhalation injury.[22] Decreased dynamic compliance increases the work of breathing. Increased closing volume and decreased functional residual capacity lead to atelectasis and shunt resulting in hypoxia. Airways become plugged by sloughed epithelium, casts, and mucus. Impaired ciliary action exacerbates the airway obstruction by decreasing the clearance of airway debris. These changes lead to further shunt and allow colonization and pneumonia. Treatment for inhalation injury is empiric and supportive with tracheal intubation and mechanical ventilation. The application of aggressive pulmonary toilet, high-frequency percussive ventilation, and respiratory therapy protocols designed to mobilize obstructing debris are also highly beneficial. The importance of strategies to limit ventilator-induced lung injury has been recognized.[23–27]

Carbon monoxide (CO) and cyanide are two major toxic components of smoke. The burn patient with evidence of inhalation injury should be evaluated for the presence of toxicity resulting from these compounds. CO binds hemoglobin 200 times more avidly than oxygen.[28] Therefore, CO markedly impairs the association of oxygen with hemoglobin and decreases oxygen-carrying capacity. CO also shifts the oxyhemoglobin dissociation curve to the left, thus decreasing the release of oxygen into tissues. These factors result in decreased oxygen delivery to tissues and, at critical levels, lead to anaerobic metabolism and metabolic acidosis. Signs and symptoms of CO poisoning include headache, mental status changes, dyspnea, nausea, weakness, and tachycardia. Patients suffering CO poisoning have a normal Pao_2 and oxygen saturation by routine pulse oximetry. They are not cyanotic. Carboxyhemoglobin must be detected by co-oximetry. Carboxyhemoglobin levels above 15% are toxic and those above 50% are often lethal. The major treatment approach is administration of 100% oxygen and, in severe cases, hyperbaric treatment to increase the partial pressure of oxygen in blood.[29]

Cyanide is also a component of smoke, resulting from the burning of certain plastic products.[30] Cyanide directly impairs the oxidative apparatus in mitochondria and decreases the ability of cells to utilize oxygen in metabolism. These alterations result in conversion to anaerobic metabolism and the development of metabolic acidosis. Signs and symptoms include headache, mental status changes, nausea, lethargy, and weakness. Hydrogen cyanide levels above 100 ppm are generally fatal. Treatment includes nitrates to increase methemoglobin levels. Methemoglobin competes with cytochrome oxidase for cyanide. However, excessive levels of methemoglobin lead to decreased oxygen-carrying capacity and may be toxic. Administration of sodium thiosulfate will cause production of thiosulfate, which decreases the toxicity of cyanide and increases its elimination.

Effect of burn injury on circulation

Thermal injury has profound effects on the systemic circulation, and hemodynamic management is a major component of perioperative care. It is critical for the anesthesiologist to assess the adequacy of postburn fluid resuscitation and the hemodynamic status of the patient. Important variables include blood pressure, heart rate, urine output, central venous pressure, base deficit, and blood lactate levels. In patients with pulmonary artery catheters, cardiac output, mixed venous oxygen saturation, cardiac and pulmonary filling pressures, and oxygen delivery parameters provide important information regarding the hemodynamic status of the burn patient. In addition, determination of blood hemoglobin level, fluid requirements, and the need for pressors or inotropes are important for developing an effective anesthetic plan.

After massive thermal injury, a state of burn shock develops due to intravascular hypovolemia and, in most cases, myocardial depression. This state of burn shock is characterized by decreased cardiac output, increased systemic vascular resistance, and tissue hypoperfusion.[31,32] Intravascular hypovolemia results from alterations in microvascular permeability in both burned and unburned tissues, leading to the development of massive interstitial fluid accumulation. Cutaneous lymph flow increases dramatically in the immediate postburn period and remains elevated for approximately 48 hours.[33] The forces responsible for this massive fluid shift involve all components of the Starling equilibrium:[34]

$$Q = kA \left[(P_c - P_i) + \sigma(\pi_i - \pi_c) \right]$$

The specific alterations include:

- an increased microvascular permeability coefficient (k) due primarily to the release of local and systemic inflammatory mediators;
- an increase in intravascular hydrostatic pressure (P_c) due to microvascular dilatation;
- decreased interstitial hydrostatic pressure (P_i);
- decreased intravascular oncotic pressure (π_c) due to leakage of protein from the intravascular space; and
- a relative increase in interstitial oncotic pressure due to a smaller decrease in interstitial oncotic pressure (π_i) compared to intravascular oncotic pressure (π_c).

The leakage of protein and fluid into the interstitial space often results in a washout of the interstitium and markedly increased lymph flow. The net effect of these changes is the development of massive edema during the first 24–48 hours after thermal injury with a concomitant loss of intravascular volume. The hypotension associated with burn injury is also due, in part, to myocardial depression. The inflammatory response to thermal injury results in the release of large amounts of inflammatory mediators such as tumor necrosis factor α (TNFα), interleukin-1 (IL-1), and prostaglandins. TNFα and IL-1 are known to have myocardial suppressant effects.[35,36] These factors, and other possibly unrecognized factors, are responsible for the depression in myocardial function that often results from burn injury.

If the patient survives the initial burn shock and is adequately resuscitated, a state of hyperdynamic circulation develops that is mediated by a variety of inflammatory mediators. This state of massive inflammation has been termed the systemic inflammatory response syndrome (SIRS) and is characterized by hypotension, tachycardia, a marked decrease in systemic vascular resistance, and increased cardiac output. SIRS has a continuum of severity ranging from the presence of tachycardia, tachypnea, fever, and leukocytosis to refractory hypotension and, in its most severe form, shock and multiple organ system dysfunction. In thermally injured patients, the most common cause of SIRS is the burn itself; however, sepsis, SIRS with the presence of infection or bacteremia, is also a common occurrence.

Burn patients require large volume fluid resuscitation in the immediate postburn period. This is due to a state of burn shock that develops in the immediate postburn period as described earlier. Several resuscitation protocols that utilize various combinations of crystalloids, colloids, and hypertonic fluids have been developed (**Table 13.5**). Isotonic crystalloid resuscitation is employed in most burn centers and generally provides adequate volume resuscitation. However, compared to colloids and hypertonic solutions, crystalloid resuscitation may require larger volumes and cause more tissue edema and hypoproteinemia. Therefore, interest has developed in analyzing colloid and hypertonic resuscitation regimens. Overall, colloid resuscitation within the first 24 hours of burn injury has not improved outcome compared to crystalloid resuscitation.[37,38] Furthermore, a recent meta-analysis indicated that mortality is higher in burned patients receiving albumin as part of the initial resuscitation protocol with a 2.4 relative risk of mortality compared to patients receiving crystalloid alone.[39] Because of the added cost with little benefit, colloid solutions have not been used routinely in the United States for initial volume resuscitation in burned patients.

The use of hypertonic saline, either alone or in conjunction with colloids, has also been advocated by some in the initial resuscitation of burned patients. Among the potential benefits are reduced volume requirements to attain similar levels of intravascular resuscitation and tissue perfusion compared to isotonic fluids.[40] Theoretically, the reduced volume requirements would decrease the incidence of pulmonary and tissue edema, thus reducing the incidence of pulmonary complications and the need for escharotomy. Hypertonic saline dextran solutions have been shown to expand intravascular volume by mobilizing fluids from intracellular and interstitial fluid compartments. Although hypertonic saline dextran solutions will transiently decrease fluid requirements, neither clinical nor experimental studies have shown an overall decrease in total resuscitation fluid needs.[41,42] Therefore, most burn centers continue to employ isotonic crystalloid fluids for initial resuscitation of patients in burn shock.

Several parameters have been used to assess the adequacy of volume resuscitation in burned patients (**Table 13.6**). Regardless of the parameter used, a critical factor is early volume resuscitation and establishment of tissue perfusion. Traditionally, urine output (0.5–1 ml/kg/h) and normalization of blood pressure (mean arterial blood pressure of greater than 70 mmHg) have been used as endpoints to indicate adequate volume replacement. However, recent studies indicate that these parameters may be poor predictors of adequate tissue perfusion. Jeng and colleagues showed that attaining urine outputs of greater than 30 ml/h and mean blood

---

Table 13.6 Criteria for adequate fluid resuscitation

- Normalization of blood pressure
- Urine output (1–2 ml/kg/h)
- Blood lactate (<2 mmol/liter)
- Base deficit (<−5)
- Gastric intramucosal pH (>7.32)
- Central venous pressure
- Cardiac index (CI) (4.5 liter/min/m²)
- Oxygen delivery index (DO$_2$I) (600 ml/min/m²)

Table 13.5 Formulas for estimating adult burn patient resuscitation fluid needs

Colloid formulas	Electrolyte	Colloid	D5W
Evans	Normal saline 1.0 ml/kg/% burn	1.0 ml/kg/% burn	2000 ml/24 h
Brooke	Lactated Ringer's 1.5 ml/kg/% burn	0.5 ml/kg	2000 ml/24 h
Slater	Lactated Ringer's 2 liter/24 h	Fresh frozen plasma	75 ml/kg/24 h
Crystalloid formulas			
Parkland	Lactated Ringer's	4 ml/kg/% burn	
Modified Brooke	Lactated Ringer's	2 ml/kg/% burn	
Hypertonic saline formulas			
Hypertonic saline solution (Monafo)	Volume to maintain urine output at 30 ml/h Fluid contains 250 mEq Na/liter		
Modified hypertonic (Warden)	Lactated Ringer's + 50 mEq NaHCO3 (180 mEq Na/liter) for 8 hours to maintain urine output At 30–50 ml/h		
Dextran formula (Demling)	Lactated Ringer's to maintain urine output at 30–50 ml/h beginning 8 hours postburn Dextran 40 in saline – 2 ml/kg/h for 8 hours		
	Lactated Ringer's – volume to maintain urine output at 30 ml/h		
	Fresh frozen plasma – 0.5 ml/kg/h for 18 hours beginning 8 hours postburn		

pressures of greater than 70 mmHg correlated poorly with global indicators of tissue perfusion such as base deficit and blood lactate levels.[43] In order to maintain perfusion of vital organs such as heart and brain, blood flow is often redistributed away from splanchnic organs. Persistent hypoperfusion of these organs ultimately results in tissue injury and may be a contributing factor to multisystem organ dysfunction. Recent studies have shown that normalization of blood pressure, heart rate, and urine output do not correlate with improved outcome.[44,45] Therefore, in the preoperative assessment of the burn patient, the anesthesiologist should not base the cardiovascular assessment strictly on these parameters.

Invasive cardiovascular monitors are not used routinely in burned patients to guide volume resuscitation. Most patients can be adequately resuscitated without their use. However, a small subset of patients, such as those with underlying cardiovascular disease or those that do not respond normally to volume resuscitation, may benefit from invasive monitoring. Some recent investigations have focused on the use of cardiac index and oxygen delivery as useful endpoints to guide volume resuscitation.[46,47] One way in which shock can be defined is oxygen debt. Therefore, maintaining an adequate cardiac index and oxygen delivery capacity such that oxygen delivery meets oxygen consumption provide useful criteria in guiding volume resuscitation. Bernard and colleagues have shown that patients surviving large burn injuries had higher cardiac indices and more effective oxygen delivery than nonsurvivors.[48] Some investigators have proposed the use of supranormal oxygen delivery as a means of assuring adequate tissue perfusion.[49,50] The preselected goals were a cardiac index of 4.5 l/m^2 and an oxygen delivery index of 600 ml/min/m^2. These values represent approximately 150% of normal cardiac index and oxygen delivery values. Attaining supraphysiological cardiac output and oxygen delivery has been shown to improve outcome in some studies. Schiller and colleagues demonstrated that maintaining a hyperdynamic hemodynamic state using fluids and inotropes improved survival in burn patients.[51] However, other investigations, including a meta-analysis, have shown that achieving supraphysiological levels of cardiac output and oxygen delivery did not improve mortality or decrease the incidence of organ failure in trauma and burn patients.[52-54] The use of inotropes to attain supraphysiological oxygen transport could be detrimental in some cases. One study that employed dobutamine to increase cardiac output and increase oxygen delivery demonstrated increased mortality.[55]

Blood lactate and base deficit provide indirect indices of global tissue perfusion. Lactic acid is a byproduct of anaerobic metabolism and is an indicator of either inadequate oxygen delivery or impaired oxygen utilization. In the absence of conditions such as cyanide poisoning or sepsis that alter oxygen utilization at the cellular level, lactate production serves as a useful marker of oxygen balance. Serum lactate levels have served as a useful marker of fluid resuscitation and tissue perfusion in burn patients.[56] A recent study showed serum lactate to be the most predictive index of adequate tissue perfusion and a lactate level of less than 2 mmol/l in the first 24–72 hours after burn injury correlated with increased survival.[57] Base deficit is another indirect indicator of global tissue perfusion. The base deficit is calculated from the arterial blood gas using the Astrup and Siggard-Anderson nomograms. Although it is not directly measured, base deficit provides a readily obtained and widely available indicator of tissue acidosis and shock. Base deficit has been shown to correlate closely with blood lactate and

provides a useful indicator of inadequate oxygen delivery. A retrospective study by Kaups et al. showed that base deficit was an accurate predictor of fluid requirements, burn size, and mortality rate.[58]

Lactate and base deficit serve as global markers of tissue perfusion and oxygen delivery. However, in burn patients, tissue perfusion is not uniform. Perfusion of the splanchnic beds is often sacrificed in order to maintain the perfusion of heart, brain, and kidneys. The use of gastric intramucosal pH (pH$_i$) has been advocated as a measure of splanchnic perfusion. Several studies have shown that measurement of pH$_i$ is useful in guiding resuscitation and that low pH$_i$ is a predictor of organ failure and death.[59] pH$_i$ is measured by gastric tonometry and can provide useful information regarding tissue perfusion.

Effect of burn injury on renal function

Acute renal failure (ARF) is a relatively common complication following burn injuries. The incidence of ARF following burn injury has been reported to range from 0.5 to 30% and is most dependent on the severity of the burn and the presence of inhalation injury.[60-62] The development of ARF is a poor prognostic indicator with mortality rates as high as 85% reported by some investigators.[63] However, Jeschke and colleagues have shown a decrease in mortality in pediatric burn patients with ARF to 56% since 1984.[64] Holm and colleagues observed that ARF could be divided into early and late categories. Early ARF was defined as occurring within 5 days of burn injury.[63] The most common apparent causes were hypotension and myoglobinuria. ARF occurring after 5 days of injury was defined as late. Here, sepsis was the most common cause with a small number of cases resulting from the administration of nephrotoxic drugs. Factors that will decrease the incidence of ARF and, if it occurs, associated mortality include adequate fluid resuscitation, early wound excision, and prevention of infection.[65] Regardless of the cause, it is critical to assess renal function in burn patients in order to develop a comprehensive anesthetic plan. Important areas of analysis include urine output, dialysis dependence, volume status, and electrolytes; also diuretic therapy should be noted. Scheduled doses of diuretics may need to be continued during the perioperative period to maintain urine output.

Thermoregulation in burn patients

Maintenance of proper body temperature is critical for optimizing wound healing and recovery in severely burned patients. The thermoregulatory system is controlled by three major components: afferent, central regulatory, and efferent limbs (**Figure 13.1**). Temperature is sensed by Aδ and C fibers present in skin and most other tissues in the body including central core tissues such as brain, deep abdominal, and thoracic viscera. Because the skin is in direct contact with the environment, its input plays an important role in thermal regulation. Of course, patients with large body surface area burns have had much of their skin removed. This removes some or all of the insulating properties of skin. However, Wallace and colleagues have shown that burn patients perceive changes in ambient temperature as effectively as normal controls.[66] An increase in the gradient of ambient temperature to skin temperature results in radiant heat loss that ultimately results in a sensation of cold. Changes in metabolic rate correlate most with the

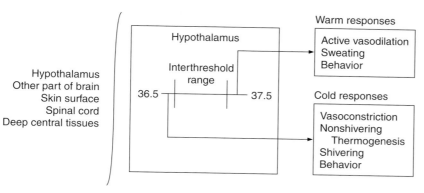

Fig. 13.1 Schematic demonstrating thermoregulatory control mechanisms. Afferent input from a variety of sites, most notably skin, central tissues, and brain, are processed in the central nervous system. Based on input, a variety of efferent thermoregulatory responses are initiated. (From Sessler DI. Temperature monitoring. In: Miller R, ed. *Anesthesia*, 3rd Edn. New York: Churchill Livingstone, 1990.)

patient's sensation of cold discomfort rather than ambient temperature. Burn patients respond with a brisk increase in heat generation and metabolic rate during periods of perceived cold discomfort.[66]

Central control of temperature is a complicated system that is not well understood. The hypothalamus plays an important role in temperature regulation, but the complete mechanism of temperature control is likely to be multifaceted and is an area of intense research. Regardless of the ultimate control mechanisms, temperature control can be divided into three main functions: *threshold*, *gain*, and *maximum response intensity*.

Threshold encompasses a set point at which responses to temperature change are initiated. In normal individuals the threshold range is generally near 36.5–37.5°C. In burn patients, the threshold set point is higher and the increase is proportional to the size of the burn. The work of Caldwell and colleagues predicts that the temperature set point will increase by 0.03°C per % TBSA burn.[67] This increase in temperature threshold appears to be due to the hypermetabolic state and the presence of pyrogenic inflammatory mediators such as TNF, IL-1, and IL-6 that are present after thermal injury. The elevated temperature set point can be decreased by administration of indomethacin, which suggests prostaglandins as a final common mediator of this response.[68,69]

Gain describes the intensity of response to alterations in temperature. In most cases the gain of thermoregulatory responses is very high with response intensity increasing from 10 to 90% with only a few tenths of a degree change in core temperature. This response is maintained in most burn patients, resulting in a further increase in metabolic rate.[66] However, work by Shiozaki and colleagues has shown that burn patients who are slow to respond to postoperative hypothermia are at increased risk of mortality.[70] The decreased responsiveness may be due, in part, to tissue catabolism, poor nutrition, or sepsis. In addition, the response to relative hypothermia is characterized by increased catecholamine release, tissue catabolism, and hypermetabolism. These responses further stress burn patients, and decrease their ability to respond to their primary injury.

The most important efferent responses to hypothermia are behavioral responses such as gaining shelter, covering up, and seeking a more desirable ambient temperature. In the acute postburn setting, most of these behaviors are impeded by positioning, sedation, and inability to seek a more favorable environment. Therefore, caregivers must be attentive to the patient's temperature and perception of cold so that measures can be undertaken to optimize the patient's temperature. Mechanisms of vasoconstriction, nonshivering heat production, and shivering remain intact in burn patients. However, these mechanisms are far less important than behavioral responses.

The induction of anesthesia results in relative ablation of thermoregulatory mechanisms and puts the patient at risk for developing hypothermia. Patients under general anesthesia exhibit a markedly decreased threshold for response to hypothermia (**Figure 13.2**). This is particularly important in burn patients given their high temperature set point and the deleterious effects of further stress responses and hypermetabolism in this patient population. Most anesthetics decrease nonbehavioral responses to hypothermia such as vasoconstriction, nonshivering thermogenesis, and shivering. Of course, behavioral responses are ablated during general anesthesia. Therefore, it is the responsibility of the intraoperative caregivers to monitor and maintain patient temperature. Actions such as maintaining higher ambient air temperature, covering extremities and head, applying warm blankets, utilizing radiant heaters, warming fluids and blood, and warming gases are usually effective in maintaining core temperature if applied aggressively. Ideally, hypothermia should be corrected prior to transport to the operating room. Hypothermia revealed in the preoperative evaluation may be due to inadequate resuscitation or metabolic instability. Either situation implies intolerance to anesthetic drugs or the stress of surgery.

Pharmacological considerations

General Considerations

Burn injury and its treatment result in physiological changes that may profoundly alter response to drugs. These changes alter both pharmacological and pharmacodynamic determinants of drug response. Altered drug response in burned patients may require

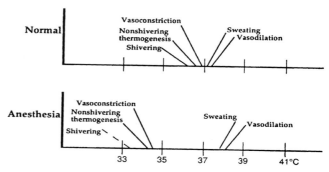

Fig. 13.2 Effects of anesthesia on thermoregulatory mechanisms. (From Sessler DI. Temperature monitoring. In: Miller R, ed. *Anesthesia*, 3rd edn. New York: Churchill Livingstone, 1990.)

deviation from usual dosages to avoid toxicity or decreased effi-cacy.[71] The complex nature of the pathophysiological changes, interpatient variation in the nature and extent of burn injuries, as well as the dynamic nature of these changes during healing and recovery make it difficult to formulate precise dosage guidelines for burn patients. However, an understanding of the systemic response to large burn injuries can help predict when altered drug response can be expected and how to compensate.

The two distinct phases of cardiovascular response to thermal injury can affect pharmacokinetic parameters in different ways. During the acute or resuscitation phase the rapid loss of fluid from the vascular space due to edema formation results in decreased car-diac output and tissue perfusion. Volume resuscitation during this phase dilutes plasma proteins and expands the extracellular fluid space especially, but not exclusively, around the burn injury itself. Decreased renal and hepatic blood flow during the resuscitation phase reduces drug elimination by these organs. Also, decreased cardiac output will accelerate the rate of alveolar accumulation of inhalation agents, which may result in an exaggerated hypotensive response during induction of general anesthesia.

After approximately 48 hours, the hypermetabolic and hyperdy-namic circulatory phase is established with increased cardiac output, oxygen consumption, and core temperature. During this phase, increased blood flow to the kidneys and liver may increase clear-ance of some drugs to the point where increased doses are required.[72]

Many drugs are highly protein bound. Drug effects and elimina-tion are often related to the unbound fraction of the drug which is available for receptor interaction, glomerular filtration, or enzy-matic metabolism. The two major drug-binding proteins have dis-parate response to burn injury. Albumin binds mostly acidic and neutral drugs (diazepam or thiopental) and is decreased in burn patients. Basic drugs (pKa>8, propranolol, lidocaine, or imipramine) bind to α-acid glycoprotein (AAG). AAG is consid-ered an acute phase protein and its concentration may double after burns. Since these drug-binding proteins respond in opposite ways to thermal injury it can be expected that changes in drug binding and function will depend on which of these proteins has the high-est affinity for the drug in question. Martyn et al. observed decreased plasma albumin concentration and increased plasma AAG concen-tration in burn patients.[73] These observations were associated with an increased unbound fraction for diazepam (bound by albumin) and a decreased unbound fraction for imipramine (bound by AAG).

Volume of distribution (V_d) can be changed by alterations of either extracellular fluid volume or protein binding. Large changes in both of these variables occur with thermal injuries. Drugs with high protein binding and/or a V_d in the range of the extracellular fluid volume may be associated with clinically significant alter-ations of V_d in burned patients. V_d is the most important determi-nant of drug response following a rapid loading dose. However, adjustments in dose to compensate for altered V_d are indicated only when V_d for the drug is small (<30 l) because with larger V_d only a small fraction of the drug is present in the plasma.[71]

Clearance is the most important factor determining the mainte-nance dose of drugs and can influence the response to drugs given by infusion or repeated bolus during anesthesia. Drug clearance is influenced by four factors:

- metabolism;
- protein binding;

- renal excretion; and
- novel excretion pathways.

The characteristic hepatic extraction of a particular drug influences changes in its clearance that occur after thermal injury. Drugs vary greatly in their extraction by the liver. Hepatic clearance of drugs highly extracted by the liver depends primarily on hepatic blood flow and is insensitive to alterations in protein binding. Clearance of these drugs may increase during the hyperdynamic phase when hepatic blood flow is increased. In contrast, clearance of drugs that have a low hepatic extraction coefficient is not affected by changes in hepatic blood flow but is sensitive to alterations in plasma pro-tein levels.[71] For these drugs it is the unbound fraction of the drug that is metabolized. As above, changes in unbound fraction depend on whether the drug is bound by albumin or AAG. Changes in pro-tein levels produce clinically significant pharmacokinetic changes only for drugs that are highly bound (80%).[74]

During resuscitation, renal blood flow may be reduced and renal excretion of drugs may be impaired. Later, during the hypermeta-bolic phase, renal blood flow is increased as a result of the elevated cardiac output. During this period excretion of certain drugs can be increased to the point that the dose may need to be increased. Loirat et al. reported increased glomerular filtration rates and reduced half-life of tobramycin in burn patients.[75] However, this was age-dependent and patients over 30 years of age did not have increased glomerular filtration or reduced half-life.

Burn patients may also experience altered drug clearance due to novel excretion pathways. Glew et al. found that 20% of a daily gentamicin dose was eliminated in the exudates lost to wound dressings.[76] In addition, rapid blood loss during surgery may speed elimination of drugs when blood loss and transfusion amount, essentially, to an exchange transfusion.

Hepatic clearance of drugs with low extraction coefficients is also sensitive to alterations of hepatic capacity (enzyme activity). There is evidence of impairment of hepatic enzyme activity in burn patients.[71] Phase I reactions (oxidation, reduction, or hydroxylation by the cytochrome P-450 system) are impaired in burn patients while Phase II reactions (conjugation) seem to be relatively preserved.[72] However, these generalizations do not always produce predictable alterations in pharmacokinetic parameters. For example, contradic-tory observations of morphine clearance in burn patients have been reported. Morphine metabolism is by glucuronidation. This is a Phase II reaction which is normally retained in thermally injured patients. Consequently, morphine clearance has been reported unchanged as predicted or decreased.[77,78] With so many variables involved, such as hepatic blood flow, V_d, plasma proteins, multiple drug exposure, and variation in burn injury, this inconsistency is not surprising. The key to effective drug therapy in burn patients is to monitor drug effects and carefully titrate the dose to the desired effect.

Muscle Relaxants

In terms of anesthetic management, the most profound and clini-cally significant effect of burn injuries on drug response relates to muscle relaxants. Burn injuries influence responses to both suc-cinylcholine and the nondepolarizing muscle relaxants. In burned patients, sensitization to the muscle relaxant effects of succinyl-choline can produce exaggerated hyperkalemic responses severe enough to induce cardiac arrest.[79] In contrast, burned patients are resistant to the effects of nondepolarizing muscle relaxants.

Cardiac arrest in burned patients after succinylcholine administration was first reported in 1958.[80] It was not until 1967, however, that an exaggerated hyperkalemic effect was identified as the cause of this phenomenon.[79,81] Several clinical studies have documented exaggerated increases in potassium concentrations after succinylcholine administration in burned patients. However, considerable individual variability exists; only a few patients in these series developed dangerously high potassium levels. The size of the increase was greater about 3–4 weeks after injury. The earliest exaggerated hyperkalemic response described occurred 9 days after injury and normal responses were observed in the remaining patients in this series for up to 14–20 days.[82] The shortest postburn interval associated with succinylcholine-induced cardiac arrest was 21 days.[83] Controversy surrounds recommendations regarding the safe use of succinylcholine after burn injury. Various authors recommend avoidance of succinylcholine at intervals ranging from 24 hours to 21 days after burn injury.[3,84] A recent series of letters to the editor of *Anesthesiology* illustrates the controversy surrounding this question.[85-87] In the absence of solid evidence one way or the other, most clinicians try to avoid the use of succinylcholine in the acute burn patient despite the acknowledgment that it is safe in terms of an exaggerated hyperkalemic response in the period immediately after injury.

An increase in the numbers of acetylcholine receptors and proliferation of these receptors away from the neuromuscular junction have been suggested as common mechanisms explaining both reduced sensitivity to nondepolarizing relaxants and exaggerated hyperkalemia after succinylcholine administration in burned patients. Under normal conditions, nicotinic acetylcholine receptors are concentrated at the neuromuscular junction; thus, the membrane-depolarizing effects of nicotinic cholinergic agonists are restricted to a small fraction of the muscle membrane. Denervation and immobilization increase the number of extrajunctional acetylcholine receptors and enlarge the area sensitive to acetylcholine.[84,88] As a result of receptor proliferation, a large portion of the membrane becomes sensitive to cholinergic agonists, and depolarization can cause release of potassium from a large area of the muscle cell surface rather than just the motor endplate. The resulting large-scale shift to intracellular potassium can generate life-threatening hyperkalemia. Similar changes have been suggested to occur after burn injuries.

Responses to nondepolarizing relaxants are also altered by burn injury. Three-to-fivefold greater doses are required to achieve adequate relaxation.[89] Resistance is apparent by 7 days after injury and peaks by approximately 40 days. Sensitivity returns to normal after approximately 70 days. Two reports described slight but measurable resistance to nondepolarizing relaxants persisting for more than a year after complete healing of the wounds. The mechanism of the altered response appears to involve pharmacodynamic rather than pharmacokinetic changes. Burns greater than 25% total body surface area require higher total dose and greater plasma concentrations of nondepolarizing blockers to achieve a given level of twitch depression.[90]

Resistance to nondepolarizing muscle relaxants may not be caused by changes in the numbers of acetylcholine receptors. Although Kim *et al.*[91] reported an increase in numbers of acetylcholine receptors in rat diaphragm after scald injuries, Marathe *et al.*[92] were unable to demonstrate increases in either receptor density or the ratio of extrajunctional to junctional receptors at a time when resistance to atracurium was maximal. Therefore, the mechanism of the altered response of burn patients to muscle relaxants has not been established. More recently, electrophysiological studies in a rat model of thermal injury revealed an increase in miniature end plate potential frequently, amplitude, and quantal content.[93] Enhanced neuromuscular transmission could antagonize nondepolarizing neuromuscular blockers and explain higher dosage requirements for these drugs.

Proliferation of acetylcholine receptors across the muscle membrane has been used to explain both resistance to nondepolarizing muscle relaxants and the exaggerated hyperkalemic response to succinylcholine. The observation of resistance of a patient to metocurine for up to 463 days after burn has been used to suggest that hyperkalemic responses to succinylcholine also could persist for more than a year.[94] However, the theoretical mechanism of the altered drug responses in burned patients is speculative; no pathologic hyperkalemic responses to succinylcholine in burned patients have been reported more than 66 days after burns.[84]

In contrast to other nondepolarizing neuromuscular blockers, mivacurium dosage requirements in pediatric patients appear to be unchanged by burn injury. The time to onset of drug action, degree of paralysis achieved by a specific dose, and rate of infusion required to maintain a given level of relaxation were all the same in burn patients as values reported for nonburned control patients.[95] Plasma cholinesterase activity is reduced in burn patients.[96] In a study by Martyn, the observation of an inverse relationship between plasma cholinesterase activity and recovery time from 25 to 75% twitch tension suggests that depression of metabolic degradation of mivacurium may compensate for other factors that induce resistance to relaxants.[95] This observation suggests that mivacurium can be administered to burn patients in normal doses that would avoid cardiovascular perturbations associated with required larger doses of other relaxants in burn patients.

Anesthetic management

Airway Management

If injuries do not preclude conventional airway management (i.e. mask fit, jaw lift, and mouth opening) standard induction and intubation procedures are appropriate. Hu *et al.* reported that gastric emptying was not delayed in patients with severe burns so that a rapid sequence induction is not necessary.[97] However, attention should be given to gastric residuals during enteric feeding. Development of sepsis can slow gastric emptying which can result in retained fluids in the stomach and risk of aspiration.

When burns include face and neck, swelling and distortion may make direct laryngoscopy difficult or impossible. In addition, loss of mandibular mobility may impair airway manipulation and make mask ventilation difficult. Fiberoptic intubation while maintaining spontaneous ventilation is a safe and reliable technique under these conditions. Fiberoptic intubation can be performed in awake adults but pediatric patients are unable to cooperate and must be sedated. Since most anesthetics cause collapse of pharyngeal tissues and airway obstruction they are unsuitable for fiberoptic intubation in patients whose airway would be difficult to manage with a mask.[98] Ketamine, however, is unique among anesthetic drugs because it maintains spontaneous ventilation and airway patency (**Figure 13.3**).[99,100]

Ketamine anesthesia has been found safe and effective for airway management in infants with difficult airways caused by

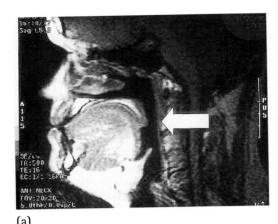

(a)

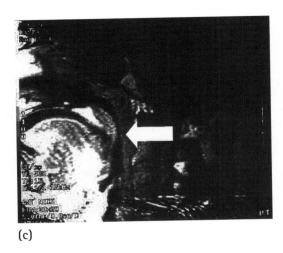

(c)

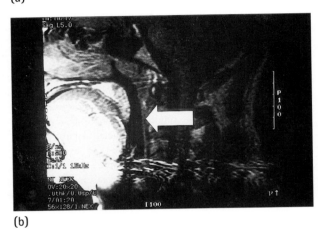

(b)

Fig. 13.3 Magnetic resonance images of a healthy volunteer during inspiration while conscious (a), or anesthetized with propofol (b) or ketamine (c). Anterior–posterior diameter of the pharynx at the level of the soft palate is marked by decreased during propofol anesthesia (b) but maintained during ketamine anesthesia (c).

congenital airway anomalies. Reports of successful nasotracheal intubation in infants with congenital airway malformations have been made both by manipulations guided by fiberoptic nasopharyngoscopy and the conventional technique of fiberoptic intubation with the endotracheal tube mounted on the fiberscope.[101,102] In the latter case an ultra-thin bronchoscope (2.7 mm) was required because a larger fiberscope would not fit through the appropriate-sized endotracheal tube. To facilitate intubation under ketamine anesthesia, topical anesthesia of the larynx with lidocaine prior to instrumentation of the larynx is advised. Since the ultra-thin bronchoscope lacks a working channel for administration of topical lidocaine, fiberoptic intubation with the 2.7 mm bronchoscope was preceded by nasopharyngoscopy with a 3.5 mm fiberscope for administration of topical lidocaine. At SBH Galveston we have also found this technique, utilizing two fiberscopes, effective in infants with burn injuries. Wrigley *et al.* evaluated the use of a 2.2 mm intubating fiberscope during halothane anesthesia in ASA 1 or 2 children aged 6 months to 7 years.[103] In this series of 40 patients a number of complications were experienced including laryngospasm and failure to achieve intubation with the fiberscope. This experience is in contrast to numerous reports of safe and effective airway management with ketamine.

Securing an endotracheal tube in a patient with facial burns presents a variety of problems and numerous techniques have been described.[104] Tape or ties crossing over burned areas will irritate the wound or dislodge grafts. A useful technique to avoid these problems involves the use of a nasal septal tie with one-eighth inch umbilical tape (**Figure 13.4**). The umbilical tape is placed around the nasal septum using an 8 or 10 French red rubber catheter that is passed through each naris and retrieved from the pharynx by direct laryngoscopy and McGill forceps. A length of umbilical tape is tied to each of the catheters and when the catheters are pulled back through the nose, each end of the umbilical tape is pulled out its respective naris producing a loop around the nasal septum. Before securing with a knot, care should be taken to assure that the uvula is not captured in the loop. A knot in the nasal septal tie should be snug enough to prevent excessive movement of the endotracheal tube but loose enough to prevent ischemic necrosis of the underlying tissues.

Airway management using a laryngeal mask airway (LMA) has also been used successfully during burn surgery for children. McCall *et al.* reported their experience with 141 general anesthetics administered to 88 pediatric burn patients.[105] Nineteen (13.5%) of the procedures were complicated by respiratory events such as unseating, desaturation, and partial laryngospasm that required intervention. Two of these events required intraoperative intubation without sequelae, while all other events resolved with therapy. Interestingly, the presence of preoperative respiratory problems or face/neck burns did not predict intraoperative respiratory problems. These authors suggest that, in patients with upper airway mucosal injury, LMA airway management may help avoid further laryngeal injury that might occur with intubation of the trachea.

Monitors

As with any critically ill patient suffering from multiorgan system involvement, the choice of monitors in a burned patient will

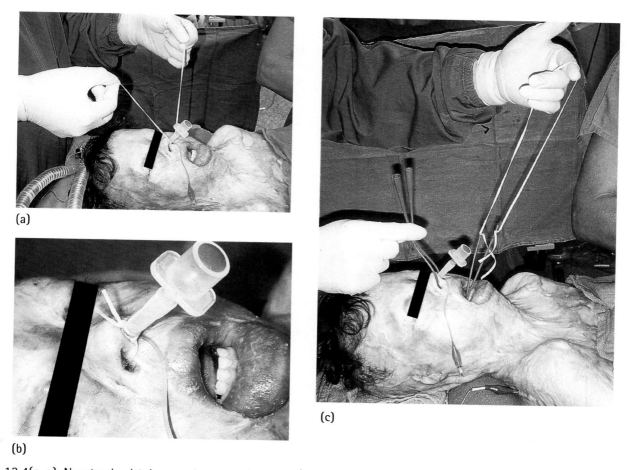

(a)

(b)

(c)

Fig. 13.4(a–c) Nasotracheal tubes can be secured with confidence by tying to umbilical tape tied in a loop around the nasal septum. This technique avoids irritating facial burn wounds or grafts and leaves the surgical field free of tape or ties.

depend on the extent of the patient's injuries, physiological state, and planned surgery. In addition to the preoperative pathophysiology associated with thermal injuries, perioperative monitoring must be adequate to assess rapid changes in blood pressure and tissue perfusion associated with the massive blood loss that can accompany excision of burn wounds. The minimum standards of the American Society of Anesthesiologists require monitoring of circulation, ventilation, and oxygenation. Standard monitors include electrocardiography (EKG), measurement of systemic blood pressure, pulse oximetry, capnography, and inspired oxygen concentration. The ability to measure body temperature should be readily available and is highly recommended for the burn patient.

Standard EKG gel electrodes usually will not adhere to burn patients because the skin is injured or covered with antibiotic ointment. For acute burn surgery, surgical staples and alligator clips are useful. Respiratory rate can be quantitated using bioimpedance from the EKG signal or from the capnogram. Pulse oximetry in burn patients can be difficult when transmission pulse oximetry sites are either burned or within the operative field. Reflectance pulse oximetry has been suggested as an alternative in these circumstances.[106]

If direct arterial pressure monitoring is not necessary, a blood pressure cuff can provide accurate measurements even if placed over bulky dressings applied to an extremity.[107] Systolic blood pressures obtained from the pressure at which the pulse oximetry signal returns during cuff deflation has also been found accurate.[108]

When blood loss is expected to be rapid and extensive, blood pressure may change more rapidly than the interval between cycles of noninvasive blood pressure measurement. In this case an arterial catheter can provide continuous and direct measurement of blood pressure. This monitor can provide much more information regarding the patient's circulatory status than just systolic and diastolic blood pressure. The arterial pressure wave form is influenced by preload, contactility, and vascular tone. Perioperative variation in the rate of rise of arterial pressure, the area under the pressure wave, position of the dicrotic notch, and beat to beat alterations in systolic pressure related to respiration all reflect clinically significant hemodynamic changes.[109] With experience, trends in these variables can help guide volume and vasoactive therapy. Display of the beat to beat arterial pressure allows measurement of systolic pressure variation (SPV). SPV is the difference between maximum and minimum systolic blood pressure during a single cycle of positive pressure mechanical ventilation. Several studies have correlated SPV with cardiac output response to volume infusion. Tavernier *et al.* recently reported that in septic patients on mechanical ventilation, SPV is a better predictor of left ventricular ejection volume response to volume loading than either pulmonary artery occlusion pressure or echocardiographic measurement of left ventricular end diastolic area.[110] Measurements are not as simple as merely 'eye-balling' the blood pressure trace because several variables influence SPV, including arrhythmias, tidal volume, and mechanical versus spontaneous ventilation. SPV provides a dynamic assessment of the interaction of preload and cardiac output.[111]

Arterial blood sampling for blood gas analysis also provides valuable information regarding pulmonary function and acid–base balance. Inadequate tissue perfusion may manifest as metabolic acidosis despite apparently adequate blood pressure.

In patients with large burns a central venous catheter serves several functions. Central venous pressure can be useful for titrating blood and fluid administration. Blood samples from a central vein are not truly mixed venous but trends in central venous oxygen tension can help identify inadequate tissue perfusion. A central venous catheter sutured into place also provides very secure intra-venous access and is an ideal route for administration of vasoactive infusions. A pulmonary artery catheter is usually not required for burn surgery. In some cases, however, the ability to more closely monitor ventricular function and oxygen supply/demand relation-ships may be helpful as when large doses of inotropes or high PEEP is required.

Urine output is the most useful perioperative monitor of renal function. Urine output of 0.5–1.0 ml/kg/h is often recommended as an end point for fluid management in acute burn patients. Adequate urine output is one measure of both renal and global per-fusion. When intraoperative transfusion is planned, examination of the urine may be the only reliable indicator of a transfusion reac-tion since signs and symptoms other than hematuria are masked by general anesthesia or hemodynamic changes associated with burn surgery. Myoglobinuria may also occur after burn injury and in this case a Foley catheter is necessary to monitor response to ther-apy. Diuretic therapy for myoglobinuria or any other indication will negate the usefulness of urine output as an index of perfusion.

Vascular Access

Securing adequate vascular access in the acutely burned patient is one of the more technically challenging procedures facing the anesthesia care team. In the pediatric age group the task can be even more difficult. Skin sites for insertion of vascular access catheters may be involved in the burn, and regional anatomy is often distorted by burn, edema, or scarring. Early in the course of an acute burn, shock leads to vasoconstriction, making cannulation of peripheral vessels nearly impossible. Later, once the patient has had several operative procedures, scarring in the area of access sites makes their placement difficult as well. Since burn patients undergo multiple debridement procedures it is necessary to attain vascular access many times in each patient. The need for frequent catheter changes between procedures to minimize catheter-related sepsis compounds the problem. The anesthesia care team is fre-quently involved in the maintenance of adequate access during the period of acute care and therefore must be facile in their place-ment. When a large portion of the surface area is burned, it becomes necessary to insert catheters through burned skin. Sutures are typically necessary to secure these catheters. If the burn is deep, it may have to debrided prior to line placement so that the catheter can be sutured to viable tissue.

For the operative excision of a large burn wound, an arterial catheter allows continuous blood pressure monitoring in the face of sudden and sometimes massive blood loss as well as during the titration of vasoactive drugs. It also allows easy intermittent access to blood samples for arterial blood gases, chemistries, and serial hematocrit determinations. For pediatric patients with large burns, arterial monitoring is essential. Additionally, if the use of topical or subcutaneous epinephrine is planned to help minimize blood loss, direct arterial pressure monitoring arterial aids in guiding therapy. Achieving arterial access is often complicated by overly-ing burn, skin graft, or scarring. In the latter case palpation of pulses can be difficult and the use of a Doppler probe is often very helpful.

The radial artery is the most frequently used site for monitoring, with large numbers of patients cannulated without complica-tions.[112] There is a relatively high rate of arterial occlusion: 8% with 20-gauge catheters and 34% with 18-gauge, but almost all completely recanalize.[113] Clearly, however, the catheter must be removed if distal hand or digit ischemia develops. In patients with severe hypotension the radial artery is not always easy to cannulate and blood pressure readings from the vessel can be inaccurate. Additionally, it is often difficult to maintain a radial arterial catheter for more than 48–72 hours, particularly in pediatric patients, and, unfortunately, the hands and forearms are typically involved in a large burn wound.

Accessing the femoral artery is easier in most patients, particu-larly those in low perfusion states because it is a larger and more central vessel.[114,115] The groin is often spared from injury, even in a large burn, and placement of a catheter in the femoral artery is not affected greatly by the presence of edema.[116] The duration of patency is twice that of a radial artery catheter, and the incidence of infection in a femoral artery catheter is similar to that of any other location, about 1%.[114] The risk of mechanical complications is smaller than that of more peripheral arteries because the arter-ial/catheter diameter ratio is larger. Still some recommend avoid-ing the femoral site unless no other site is available since loss of limb, or limb length discrepancy in children, is a devastating, if rare, complication.[117]

Other sites for arterial access include the dorsalis pedis, poste-rior tibial, and temporal arteries, none used with great frequency, and all distal enough to give inaccurate blood pressure readings, particularly in hypotensive patients. Use of the axillary artery has the disadvantages of a relatively higher rate of infection and diffi-culty in maintaining correct arm positioning for proper catheter function.[118]

The incidence of complications from arterial catheters has been cited as anywhere from 0.4 to 11%, with the higher rate seen most often in pediatric patients, particularly those under 1 year of age.[119–121] Early complications include bleeding, which is usually easily controlled, and hematoma formation, which is more common if the artery is transfixed during cannulation and is avoided by an adequate period of pressure applied to the site if bleeding occurs. Damping of the arterial waveform or clotting of the catheter is more common with small catheters or small arteries; this can be lessened somewhat by continuous heparin flushing systems.[122]

The incidence of catheter-related infections with arterial catheters is generally low, quoted at anywhere from 0.4 to 2.5% until 4 days duration. The incidence of infection gradually increases to 10% by 7 days, but stays constant thereafter. This relatively low rate of infection in comparison to central venous catheters confirms the clinical impression that catheter-related infections are less com-monly seen in the high-flow arterial system.[117,123]

Vascular insufficiency of the distal extremity occurs in 3–4% of patients in whom arterial catheters are placed.[118] Fortunately, most cases of ischemia resulting from vascular obstruction are evident immediately and resolve when the catheter is removed. The risk of ischemia can be minimized by selecting the smallest possible catheter that will give an accurate arterial waveform.[116] There is a marked increase in the incidence of arterial vasospasm when over 50% of the vessel lumen is occluded by the catheter.[124] This is certainly more of a problem in pediatric patients than adults. Predisposing factors to ischemia from arterial obstruction include hypotension, the use of vasoconstrictors, prolonged catheterization, age under 5 years, and insertion by cutdown.[125] Indeed, most reports of chronic sequelae have come in patients less than 1 year of age who were hypotensive at the time of catheter insertion. Other less commonly reported complications from arterial catheters include cutaneous damage, pseudoaneurysm formation, and septic arthritis of the hip.[126–128]

Central venous catheters are very useful for large volume resuscitation in patients with burns over 30% or more of their TBSA. As with arterial catheters, burn wound, edema, and scarring all hamper the placement of central venous catheters. Normal anatomic landmarks can be totally obliterated. The problem is compounded by the need for long-term access in patients with large burns who are also at high risk for central venous catheter infections and so will require frequent line changes. Ultrasound guidance has been used successfully to guide correct placement of appropriate-size catheters into central veins.

Catheters placed in the subclavian vein have a lower risk of infection than those placed in the internal jugular or femoral vein, but carry a higher risk of mechanical complications during their placement.[129] The internal jugular vein is typically more difficult to access in burn patients with facial and neck burns or edema and is associated with a higher infection risk. Additionally it is a difficult position in terms of patient comfort, particularly for pediatric patients. The femoral vein is a large central vein that is usually easy to cannulate. It has several advantages including no risk of pneumothorax, easier control of bleeding, less dependence on the supine position for placement, less anatomic distortion due to edema, and the inguinal region is often spared even in a large burn.[98] The risk of catheter-related infection is higher in the femoral vein than at other vascular access sites in some studies, and the risk of venous thrombosis is also quoted by some authors as being greater.[130–132]

Early complications with the placement of venous catheters include trauma, hematoma, bleeding, air embolus, pleural effusion, pneumothorax, or pericardial tamponade. Delayed complications include infection and thrombosis, which have been studied by many authors with often conflicting results. In one trial, 45 patients were randomized to either an upper extremity catheter group in which catheters were placed in the internal jugular or subclavian vein, or to a lower extremity catheter group in which catheters were placed in the femoral vein. No patients in the upper extremity group developed thrombosis, while six patients (25%) in the lower extremity group developed deep vein thrombosis. Additionally, another seven patients (29%) in the lower extremity group had nondiagnostic ultrasound findings.[132] In another trial involving pediatric patients, mechanical complications occurred in 9.5% of femoral venous catheters but only 1.8% of nonfemoral catheters.[133] A third study involved 162 femoral venous catheters

and 233 nonfemoral venous catheters; mechanical complications were equal in the two groups, 2.5% versus 2.1%. However, three of four patients who developed thrombosis were in the femoral group, as was the one patient who developed an embolus.[131] Conversely, 1449 femoral venous catheters were maintained in 313 burn patients with no pulmonary emboli. These catheters were changed every 3 days and the authors maintain that the femoral site can successfully be used as part of a site rotation for central venous access in burn patients.[134] Another 224 pediatric burn patients with femoral venous catheters had only a 3.5% incidence of mechanical complications including only one thrombus.[135] Finally, there has been a 20–46% incidence of femoral venous thrombosis found at autopsy in patients with femoral venous catheters left in place for a week or longer. A 67% incidence of thrombotic complications has been reported with internal jugular catheters and 61% with umbilical venous catheters when studied at autopsy.[136] It would seem safe to say that the femoral vein can be used for catheterization for short intervals with frequent line changes and diligent monitoring for thrombotic complications.[137]

When looking at the incidence of catheter-related infection from central venous catheters in burn patients, the answer is even less clear. There is an inherent difficulty when talking about the incidence of catheter-related infection in burn patients for several reasons. First, the patients with central venous catheters are the sickest patients. Secondly, the burn wound is a constant source of infection and pneumonia, and urinary tract infections are also fairly common in critically ill burn patients; in many patients catheter-related infection is a diagnosis of exclusion but burn patients always have at least one other obvious source of infection. Finally, since most catheter-related infections develop when bacteria migrate down the catheter tract from the skin, there is a higher risk of catheter infection when the insertion site is through or very near a burn wound.[138,139] To further cloud the picture, differing definitions of catheter-related infection make comparing different studies of the problem more difficult. Catheter-related infection in burn patients has been reported to have an incidence as low as 2.5% and as high as 22.4%.[138] One large study of 1183 burn patients and 1346 central venous catheters showed that the incidence of catheter-related infection was 19.5% with a mortality of 14.1%. These authors cite catheter-related infection as the second most common cause of sepsis in the burn patient after the burn wound.[140]

Many older studies recommend frequent catheter changes to decrease the incidence of infection, but several newer studies show no increase in infection out to as many as 7–10 days. Three large randomized trials demonstrated no difference in the incidence of catheter-related infections among groups who had lines placed at a new site every 7 days and groups who had their lines changed over a guidewire every 7 days.[130,143,144] The incidence of mechanical complications is clearly lower with guidewire exchange rather than changing to a new site. Several other trials have also indicated no advantage to routine changing of catheters before 7–10 days.[135,145,146] There are conflicting data in relation to incidence of infection and the site of the central venous catheter, although almost all studies agree that the incidence of infection is lowest if the subclavian approach is used.[130,133,146,147] Also, all studies that compared single lumen and multilumen catheters found a lower rate of infection with single lumen catheters.[129,146,147] Those that compared percutaneous catheter placement with placement via cutdown technique found a higher incidence of infection with cutdowns.[146–148]

Antibiotic-coated catheters have been studied clinically and show a lower rate of bacterial infection. Bacteria normally adhere to the surface of a catheter and secrete a polysaccharide film that resists both systemic antibiotics and attacks by polymorphonuclear cells, but bacteria cannot adhere to the surface of antibiotic-coated catheters. One big drawback is that current catheters must be bonded to antibiotic in solution prior to insertion, a time-consuming process that makes urgent placement of an antibiotic-coated catheter unlikely. Another problem is that their routine use may result in a higher incidence of fungal infection at catheter sites.[147]

Enough clinical evidence has accumulated that both the American Society of Anesthesiologists and the Centers for Disease Control (CDC) have developed guidelines for the prevention of catheter-related infections.[147,149,150] Both recommend single lumen catheters, use of the subclavian insertion site, barrier protection with strict sterile technique during placement, percutaneous placement with cutaneous asepsis, and catheter site dressing regimens with either sterile gauze or transparent dressings, changing dressings when clinically indicated. Both recommend against routine changing of the central venous catheter as a method to control catheter-related infection. Rather, they advise that a guidewire exchange can be used to replace a malfunctioning catheter if there is no infection at the insertion site. If a catheter-related infection is suspected, they recommend changing the catheter over a guidewire and culturing the tip; if the culture is positive, the catheter should be removed and a new catheter placed at a new site. If a catheter-related infection is documented, the use a guidewire exchange is not recommended; the infected catheter should be removed and a new catheter placed at a new site. The CDC also recommends the consideration of antibiotic-coated catheters for patients at high risk for infection, the avoidance of antibiotic ointment over the insertion site, and the strict avoidance of using total parenteral nutrition (TPN) catheters for any purpose other than TPN.

The operative debridement of a large burn wound is accompanied by rapid and sometimes considerable blood loss. Critical hypoperfusion of vital organs begins to occur when 20–30% of the blood volume is lost.[151] Irreversible shock and cellular damage can begin to occur within minutes depending on the continuing rate of loss. The achievement of a very rapid fluid infusion rate is critical in the resuscitation of the patient undergoing operative excision of the burn wound. Clearly, adequate venous access to achieve rapid infusion rates is imperative.

The flow of fluid through a tube was described by Poiseuille and is expressed by the formula:

$$Q = [\Delta P \times \pi r^4]/8nL$$

where Q is flow, ΔP is the pressure differential in the tube, r is the radius of the tube, n is viscosity of the fluid, and L is the length of the tube. From this formula, several relationships are established (**Table 13.7**). Flow through a tube can be increased by high pressure gradients, tubes of large diameter and short length, and the use of low-viscosity fluids. The most significant variable is the radius of the tube where changes result in exponential changes in flow: doubling the diameter of the tube increases flow 16 times. There have been a number of studies comparing flow rates of various catheters under different conditions. It is difficult to compare these studies directly since methods are not standardized. However, it is possible to gain from them valuable insight about the factors affecting flow. Large diameter, short catheters maximize flow, as

does a central venous location: flow is 20–40% less in a peripheral vein than in a central vein for the equivalent diameter and length catheter. Peripheral veins add resistance to flow before fluid is delivered to the central compartment.[152] Flow rates, however, are equal in hypovolemia and normovolemia for the same catheter size and length.

The high viscosity of blood diminishes flow rates considerably. Diluting one unit of packed red blood cells with 250 ml of normal saline can increase the flow of the blood by tenfold.[153] The application of a 300 mmHg pressure device to the blood unit can increase the flow rate another seven times. The diameter and length of the intravenous tubing system delivering fluid from the bag to the patient has profound effects on the rate of fluid delivery. Large-bore trauma tubing with an internal diameter of 5.0 mm allows fluid to flow three times as fast as standard blood infusion set tubing with an internal diameter of 4.4 mm, which is twice as fast as standard intravenous tubing with an internal diameter of 3.2 mm. The large-bore trauma tubing allows fluid flow rates of 1200–1400 ml/min.[154] Also, infusing blood or fluid through a 'piggyback' system into another access line can decrease flow by up to 90%.

Several large studies have shown introducer catheters to be superior to all other devices for the rapid infusion of blood and intravenous (IV) fluid (**Tables 13.8** and **13.9**). These catheters are typically of large diameter, with thin walls and no tapering so that for any given catheter size the inner diameter is largest.[151,155,156] This finding holds especially true for pediatric patients where vessel size is limited. The flow rate of a 4-French introducer catheter is greater than a 16-gauge IV catheter. However, the 4-French introducer, placed by the Seldinger technique, requires only a 21-gauge needle to be inserted into the vein for its placement.

Table 13.7 Factors that increase intravenous fluid flow

- Large catheter diameter
- Short catheter length
- Decrease fluid viscosity
- Add pressure device
- Large diameter of intravenous tubing
- Large vein size
- Central rather than peripheral vein
- Remove filters and stopcocks from tubing

Table 13.8 Introducer catheter sizes and flow rates (flow rates for normal saline under gravity)

Catheter size	Patient size	Flow rate
4 French	5–10 kg	285 ml/min
5 French	10–15 kg	380 ml/min
6 French	15–20 kg	480 ml/min
7 French	>20 kg	585 ml/min
8.5 French	>40 kg	805 ml/min

Table 13.9 Intravenous catheter sizes and flow rates (flow rates for normal saline under gravity)

Intravenous catheter	Flow rate
24 gauge	14 ml/min
22 gauge	24 ml/min
20 gauge	38 ml/min
18 gauge	55 ml/min
16 gauge	75 ml/min
14 gauge	93 ml/min

Patient Transport

The safe transport of a critically ill burn patient to and from the operating room can be a formidable task. A methodical approach will help to insure patient safety and the seamless maintenance of respiratory, hemodynamic, and general support. Hemodynamic status should be optimized prior to patient transport; pharmacological support may be required. The American Society of Anesthesiologists standards mandate evaluation, treatment, monitoring, and equipment appropriate to the patient's medical condition for any transport. Depending on the patient's condition, simple observation may be appropriate. Patients requiring supplemental oxygen should be monitored by pulse oximetry. Hemodynamic monitoring is guided by the patient's hemodynamic status. Sufficient battery power must be available for uninterrupted monitor and infusion pump function during transport.

Airway supplies should be readily available including a full oxygen cylinder, a self-inflating Ambu bag with mask, and intubation equipment. The patient's airway and ventilation as well as overall condition must be continually observed by the anesthesia care team. Drugs for resuscitation should accompany the patient on any transport. As discussed below, hypothermia is poorly tolerated by patients with an acute burn injury. It is imperative that patients be kept warm during transport in order to avoid increasing oxygen consumption and taxing limited metabolic reserve.

Selection of Anesthetic Agents

Many anesthetic agents have been used effectively for the induction and maintenance of anesthesia in burn patients. Intravenous agents (**Table 13.10**) can be used for both induction and maintenance and the specific agent used will depend primarily on the patient's hemodynamic and pulmonary status as well as the potential difficulty in securing the patient's airway. Ketamine has many advantages for use in the burn patient for induction and maintenance of anesthesia. As an induction agent, ketamine can be administered at a dose of 0.5–2.0 mg/kg. Except in patients that are catecholamine-depleted, ketamine generally preserves hemodynamic stability (**Figure 13.5**). In addition, ketamine preserves hypoxic and hypercapnic ventilatory responses and reduces airway

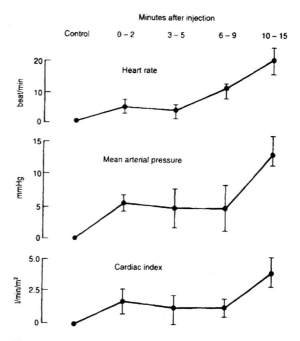

Fig. 13.5 Heart rate, mean arterial pressure, and cardiac index changes during a 15–minute period of ketamine administration to critically ill patients. (From Nolan JP. Intravenous agents. In: Grande CM *et al.*, eds. *Textbook of Trauma Anesthesia and Critical Care*. St Louis: Mosby Year Book, Inc., 1993.)

resistance.[157] Compared to other IV anesthetics, airway reflexes remain more intact after ketamine administration. However, some risk of aspiration remains. Patients who do not require ventilatory support can be allowed to breathe spontaneously, which provides an additional margin of safety should inadvertent extubation occur. In fact, some clinicians have reported the use of ketamine anesthesia without instrumentation of the airway.[158,159] Patients were allowed to breath spontaneously and the airway complication rate was comparable to that of intubated patients. The use of intramuscular ketamine can be beneficial in securing the airway in pediatric burn patients or uncooperative adults who do not have vascular access. Because ketamine preserves spontaneous ventilation and induces dissociative anesthesia, it provides good conditions for securing the airway by fiberoptic bronchoscopy. Addition of other anesthetic agents, particularly potent volatile agents or opioids, should be avoided until the airway is secured because these anesthetics depress respiratory drive and relax pharyngeal muscles thus increasing the risk of apnea, upper airway obstruction, or laryngospasm. Ketamine can also be utilized, either alone or in combination with other anesthetics, for maintenance of anesthesia either by infusion or intermittent bolus. Ketamine has potent analgesic properties and is used extensively in the operating room as well as for painful dressing changes and patient manipulations. A drying agent such as glycopyrrolate (2–5 µg/kg) is commonly given in combination with ketamine to reduce ketamine-induced secretions. In addition, benzodiazepines are often recommended in older children and adults to reduce the incidence of dysphoria sometimes associated with ketamine administration. Induction

Table 13.10 Dosage guidelines for the most commonly used intravenous anesthetic infusions

Anesthetic	Loading dose (mg/kg)	Infusion rate	
		Maintenance of anesthesia* (mg/min)	Sedation (mg/min)
Thiopental	2.0–4.0	10–20	1.0–5.0
Methohexital	1.5–3.0	5.0–8.0	0.5–2.5
Midazolam	0.2–0.4	0.1–1.0	0.035–0.7
Etomidate	0.2–0.4	1.0–2.0	0.5–1.0
Propofol	1.5–2.0	4.0–12.0	2.0–5.0
Ketamine	0.5–1.0	0.7–5.4	1.0–2.0

*Adjuvant to other agents (i.e. nitrous oxide, opioids).

†Infusion rate for midazolam is highly variable. Values in the table represent most commonly used doses.

‡Ketamine is contraindicated in head-injured patients. Its inclusion in this table pertains to use in other injuries.

From Nolan JP. Intravenous agents. In: Grande CM *et al.*, eds. *Textbook of Trauma Anesthesia and Critical Care*. St Louis: Mosby Year Book, Inc., 1993.

agents such as thiopental or propofol are more commonly used in patients returning for reconstructive procedures rather than in the acute phase of injury but are also sometimes chosen in patients with small burns and no evidence of airway or facial involvement when direct laryngoscopy is planned.

Volatile anesthetics may be used for both induction and maintenance of anesthesia in burn patients. In pediatric patients, mask induction with either halothane or sevoflurane is commonly used if the patient does not have injuries that may make airway manipulation difficult. In the acute setting, an anesthetic technique involving nasotracheal intubation after mask induction with halothane, nitrous oxide, and oxygen has been described.[160] The proponents particularly emphasize avoiding the potential problems associated with the ketamine-based technique. However, volatile agents produce dose-dependent cardiac depression and vasodilation (**Table 13.11**). In addition, hypoxic ventilatory drive is ablated by volatile anesthetics at low concentrations and a dose-dependent depression of hypercapnic drive also occurs. However, as maintenance agents volatile anesthetics have predictable wash-in and wash-out kinetics (**Figure 13.6**) and provide a useful adjunct to other agents when titrated to hemodynamic and ventilatory parameters. Of the volatile agents, nitrous oxide has the least impact on cardiovascular and respiratory function and can serve as a useful component of a balanced anesthetic if the patient's oxygen requirements permit (**Table 13.11**).

Opioids are important agents for providing analgesia for burn patients throughout the acute phase of injury and for providing postoperative analgesia in patients undergoing reconstructive procedures. The spectrum of opioids currently available provides a wide range of potencies, durations of action, and effects on the car-

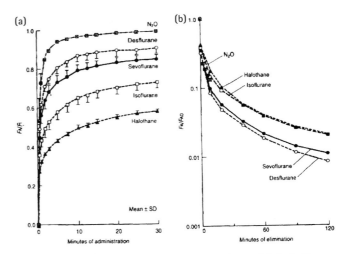

Fig. 13.6 (a) Wash-in curves of a variety of inhalation anesthetics. (b) Wash-out curve for volatile anesthetics. (From Yasuda N, *et al.* Comparison of kinetics of sevoflurane and isoflurane in humans. *Anesth Analg* 1991; 72: 316–24.)

diopulmonary system (**Table 13.12**). Burn patients experience intense pain even in the absence of movement or procedures, and opioids are the mainstay for providing analgesia in the acute phase of burn management. However, acute burn patients usually become tolerant to opioids because they receive continuous and prolonged administration of these drugs. Therefore, opioids should be titrated to effect in the acute burn patient. Most opioids have

Table 13.11 Cardiovascular effects of inhalation agents

Effect	Halothane	Enflurane	Isoflurane	Sevoflurane	Nitrous oxide
Contractility	↓↓	↓↓	↓	↓	±
Cardiac output	↓↓	↓	±	±	±
Systemic vascular resistance	±	↓↓	↓↓	↓↓	±
Mean arterial pressure	↓↓	↓↓	↓↓	↓↓	±
Heart rate	↓	±	↑↑	↑↑	±
Sensitization to catecholamines	↑↑↑	±	±	±	±
Baroreceptor reflexes	↓↓↓	↓↓↓	↓	↓	±

Table 13.12 Clinically relevant characteristics of the five most commonly used opioids

	Morphine	Meperidine	Fentanyl	Sufentanil	Alfentanil
Relative potency	1.0	0.1	100–200	700–1200	30–60
LD_{50} in dogs (mg/kg)	200	700	10	4.0	59.5–87.5
Analgesic dose	70–210 μg/kg	0.7–2.1 mg/kg	1.0–2.0 μg/kg	0.25 μg/kg	4.8 μg/kg
Anesthetic dose*	0.5–3.0 mg/kg	3.0–10 mg/kg	50–100 μg/kg	5.12 μg/kg	100–300 μg/kg loading dose + 25.50 μg/kg/h
MIC_{50}			15 ng/ml		270–400
MIC_{90}			25 ng/ml		
MIC_{95}			30 ng/ml		
Cardiovascular stability	±	– –	++++	++++	+++
Histamine release	++	+++	–	–	–
Respiratory depression	++	++	+++	+++	+++
Elimination half-life (h)	3.0	2.5	3.5	2.5	1.5

LD_{50} the dose that is lethal in 50% of subjects; $MIC_{50,90,95}$ minimum intra-arterial concentration that prevents response to sternotomy incision in 50%, 90%, and 95% of patients; –, no; +, yes.
*Doses used for cardiac surgery. Smaller doses combined with other drugs are sufficient for most trauma patients.
From Capan LM, *et al.* Principles of anesthesia for major trauma victim. In: Capan LM, *et al.*, eds. *Trauma Anesthesia*

little effect on cardiovascular function but they are potent respiratory depressants. Therefore, the ventilatory status of patients receiving opioids, particularly those with challenging airways, should be monitored closely.

Regional anesthesia can be used effectively in patients with small burns or those having reconstructive procedures. In pediatric or adult patients having procedures confined to the lower extremities, lumbar epidural or caudal anesthesia can provide a useful adjunct for control of postoperative pain. In cooperative adult patients with injuries confined to lower extremities, epidural or intrathecal anesthesia may be used if no contraindications exist. For upper extremity procedures, brachial plexus block may be considered as the primary anesthetic or as an adjunct for postoperative pain control.

Fluid Management

Overall, use of the traditional end points of blood pressure, heart rate, and urine output in conjunction with indicators of global perfusion such as base deficit or serum lactate will allow for the adequate management of fluid requirements both in the acute setting and in the operating room during burn wound excision as discussed extensively earlier in this chapter. The occasional patient may benefit from invasive monitoring with a pulmonary artery catheter to measure oxygen supply and consumption variables. Intraoperative fluid management incorporates the use of crystalloids, colloids, and blood products to maintain cardiac output, tissue perfusion, and oxygen delivery. Care must be taken not to overhydrate burn patients because of the increased risk of pulmonary and tissue edema. Tissue edema can increase the risk of skin graft failure.

Blood Transfusion

Hemorrhage is usually not a major concern during the immediate resuscitation phase in acutely burned patients unless other co-existing trauma exists. However, significant blood loss will occur when patients are taken to the operating room for excision and grafting of burn wounds. The amount of blood loss is determined by the age of the burn, the body surface area involved, and whether infection is present (see **Table 13.4**). In general, more blood loss will result as the time from initial injury increases and if wounds are infected. Controversy exists regarding transfusion triggers and targets. Some authors advocate allowing hematocrits to drop to 15–20% prior to transfusion in otherwise healthy patients undergoing limited excision and transfusing at a hematocrit of 25% in patients with preexisting cardiovascular disease.[161] The same group proposed maintaining hematocrits near 25% in patients with more extensive burns, and near 30% if the patients have preexisting cardiovascular disease. A small study by Sittig and Deitch showed fewer transfused units and no increase in adverse hemodynamic or metabolic effects in patients transfused at a hemoglobin of 6–6.5 g/dl compared to patients maintained at a hemoglobin near 10 g/dl.[162] However, in general, little data exist regarding the optimum management strategy for blood transfusion during burn wound excision.

Assessment of blood transfusion needs is best determined by evaluating the clinical status of the patient. Specifically, assessment of ongoing blood losses, preoperative hemoglobin levels, vital signs, and evidence of inadequate oxygen delivery such as hypotension, tachycardia, acidosis, and decreasing mixed venous oxygen tension provide important information regarding the oxygen balance in the patient. In addition, determination of the patient's oxygen content needs are important in determining the transfusion trigger for the patient. Patients with coexisting cardiac and pulmonary disease generally require higher oxygen-carrying capacity. Oxygen requirements will be determined by the type and severity of coexisting conditions. Overall, American Society of Anesthesiologists guidelines indicate that blood transfusion is rarely required at a hemoglobin of 10 g/dl or above and is almost always indicated at a hemoglobin of less than 6 g/dl.[163] For each patient, therefore, acceptable blood loss can be determined based on preexisting diseases, preoperative hematocrit (Hct), and the patients estimated blood volume (EBV) as follows:

$$\text{Acceptable blood loss} = \frac{\text{Hct now} - \text{Hct allowed}}{\text{Mean Hct}} \times \text{EBV}$$

Estimated blood volumes for different patient populations are indicated in **Table 13.13**.

Table 13.13 Average blood volumes	
Age	Blood volume (ml/kg)
Neonate	
Premature	95
Full-term	85
Infants	80
Adults	
Men	75
Women	65

During excision of large burn wounds, patients will often require one or more blood volumes of transfused blood to replace intraoperative blood losses. Massive blood transfusion can be associated with a variety of complications that will be discussed in the following sections.

Several means of decreasing surgical blood loss during burn wound excision may be employed such as the use of tourniquets on limbs and compression dressings at sites of burn wound excision or skin graft harvesting.[164] Some centers use epinephrine-soaked dressings or topical epinephrine spray to induce local vasoconstriction. Alternatively, subcutaneous tissues may be infiltrated with epinephrine-containing fluids. Overall, the use of topical or subcutaneous epinephrine in burn patients has not been associated with an increased incidence of side-effects or complications.[165] However, the effectiveness of this approach is unclear. A recent study showed that the use of topical epinephrine spray or subcutaneous epinephrine infiltration did not result in decreased blood loss during burn wound excision.[166] The data were quite variable, though, and the patients also received topical thrombin. A larger study examining the effects of subcutaneous epinephrine and topical thrombin might clarify this issue.

Blood Components

Several blood components are available for replacement of losses incurred during burn wound excision. These components include:

Whole blood

Whole blood consists of unfractionated blood and contains all of the components of blood including red blood cells, plasma, platelets, and white blood cells. However, whole blood stored for more than 24 hours does not contain functional white blood cells or platelets (**Table 13.14**). One unit of whole blood contains approximately 200 ml of red blood cells and 250 ml of plasma. Whole blood is available in some hospitals for large volume blood transfusions (trauma, liver transplantation, burns) and treatment of hypovolemic shock. However, because of the scarcity of blood products in most communities, whole blood is not readily available. Fractionation of whole blood into its individual components is a much more efficient and cost-effective means of maximizing blood usage. When available, however, whole blood provides an excellent means of volume expansion and providing oxygen carrying capacity in patients requiring large volume blood transfusion.

Table 13.14 Changes that occur during storage of whole blood in citrate–phosphate–dextrose

	Days of storage at 4°C			
	1	7	14	21
pH	7.1	7.0	7.0	6.9
PCO_2 (mmHg)	48	80	110	140
Potassium (mEq/l)	3.9	12	17	21
2,3-Diphosphoglycerate (μmol/ml)	4.8	1.2	1	1
Viable platelets (%)	10	0	0	0
Factors V and VII (%)	70	50	40	20

Packed red blood cells

Packed red blood cells (PRBCs) are the most common means of replacing RBC loss during surgical procedures. Most of the plasma and platelets are removed during processing so that PRBCs provide few plasma components, clotting factors, or platelets. A unit of PRBCs contains approximately 200 ml of red cells and 50 ml of residual plasma. A comparison of PRBC composition with whole blood is shown in **Table 13.15**. PRBCs provide oxygen-carrying capacity and, when reconstituted with crystalloid or plasma, volume resuscitation.

Table 13.15 Comparison of whole blood and packed red blood cells

Value	Whole blood	Packed red blood cells
Volume (ml)	517	300
Erythrocyte mass (ml)	200	200
Hematocrit (%)	40	70
Albumin (g)	12.5	4
Globulin (g)	6.25	2
Total protein (g)	48.8	36
Plasma sodium (mEq)	45	15
Plasma potassium (mEq)	15	4
Plasma acid (citric/lactic) (mEq)	80	25
Donor/recipient ratio	1 unit per patient	1 unit every 4–6 patients

Fresh frozen plasma

In the setting of burn injury, fresh frozen plasma (FFP) is most commonly used to replace clotting factors during massive blood transfusion. FFP will replace clotting factors as well as protein S and protein C by a factor of 2–3% per unit. The initial recommended volume is 10–15 ml/kg. The use of FFP varies among different burn centers. Plasma is frozen within 6 hours of collection and each unit provides approximately 250 ml of plasma containing normal levels of all coagulation factors. A National Institutes of Health consensus conference has recommended usage guidelines for FFP (**Table 13.16**).

Table 13.16 Indications for FFP according to National Institutes of Health guidelines

A. Replacement of isolated factor deficiencies (as documented by laboratory evidence)
B. Reversal of warfarin effect
C. In antithrombin III deficiency
D. Treatment of immunodeficiencies
E. Treatment of thrombotic thrombocytopenia purpura
F. Massive blood transfusion (only when factors V and VIII are 25% of normal)
G. Requirements for indications A and F would be a prothrombin and partial thromboplastin time of 1.5 times normal

In the setting of massive blood transfusion, FFP administration is indicated if active bleeding exists and laboratory evidence of coagulation factor depletion is shown. A volume of 2–6 units is generally used depending on the severity of the coagulopathy. In some burn centers, PRBCs are reconstituted with FFP on a one-to-one basis. Although this practice has not been shown to be deleterious compared to use of PRBCs reconstituted with crystalloid, there is no evidence that it decreases bleeding complications.[167] However, some practitioners argue that the use of FFP rather than crystalloid to reconstitute PRBCs results in less interstitial edema during the postoperative period and may enhance skin graft survival.

Platelets

Platelets are stored at room temperature to maximize viability. The incidence of bacterial contamination increases exponentially after 4 days. However, refrigerated platelets remain viable for only 24–48 hours. Platelets are obtained from either units of whole blood or by apheresis from a single donor. ABO-compatible platelets, particularly if from a single donor, should be used when possible because post-transfusion viability is improved. One unit of whole blood platelets contains approximately 5×10^{10} platelets in 50 ml of plasma. Most commonly, 6 units of platelets are combined into a single bag and transfused. A unit of single-donor platelets contains about 30×10^{10} platelets suspended in 200–400 ml of plasma. Therefore, 1 unit of single-donor platelets is equal to about 6 units of whole blood platelets. One unit of whole blood platelets will increase the platelet count by 5000–10 000/μl.

Cryoprecipitate

Cryoprecipitate is prepared by thawing FFP at 4°C and collecting the precipitate. Cryoprecipitate is rich in factors VIII and XIII, fibrinogen and von Willebrand's factor. In the setting of massive blood transfusion, it is used primarily to treat hypofibrinogenemia. Generally, cryoprecipitate is administered when plasma fibrinogen levels fall below 100 mg/dl. One unit of cryoprecipitate will increase plasma fibrinogen levels by 5–7 mg/dl.

Complications of Massive Blood Transfusion

Coagulopathy

Coagulopathy associated with massive blood transfusion is due to thrombocytopenia or depletion of coagulation factors. PRBCs are essentially devoid of platelets, and whole blood stored for more than 24 hours does not possess significant numbers of viable platelets. Whole blood contains essentially normal levels of coagulation factors with the exception of the volatile factors V and VIII. Because most plasma is removed from PRBCs, they provide a poor source of coagulation factors. Massive blood loss and transfusion with PRBCs or whole blood results in dilutional losses of both platelets and factors V and VIII.

Thrombocytopenia is the most common cause of nonsurgical bleeding after massive blood transfusion. In general, 15–20 units, or 2–4 blood volumes of blood or PRBCs, must be transfused before bleeding due to thrombocytopenia will develop (**Figure 13.7**). Observed platelet counts usually remain higher than calculated values due to release of platelets from sites of sequestration. Bleeding due to thrombocytopenia usually develops when the platelet count drops below 50–100 000 platelets/μl. Replacement of platelets usually requires transfusion of 6 units of whole blood platelets or 1 unit of single-donor platelets as described earlier in this chapter.

Development of coagulopathy due to depletion of coagulation factors is also possible during massive blood transfusion. Significant prolongation of the prothrombin (PT) and partial thromboplastin time (PTT) can result after transfusion of 10–12 units of PRBCs. Generally, FFP should be given to correct dilutional coagulopathy if the PT and PTT exceed 1.5 times normal

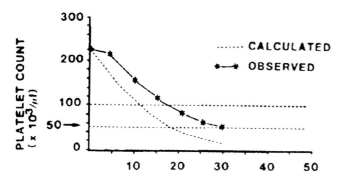

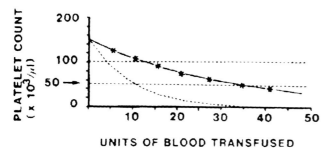

UNITS OF BLOOD TRANSFUSED

Fig. 13.7 Calculated versus observed mean platelet counts in two studies of platelet count after massive blood transfusion. (From Reed RL, *et al.* Prophylactic platelet administration during massive transfusion. *Ann Surg* 1986; 203: 46.)

levels. It is also important to know the fibrinogen level in massively transfused patients since hypofibrinogenemia can also result in prolongation of the PT and PTT. Fibrinogen may be replaced using cryoprecipitate.

Citrate toxicity

Citrate is universally used as an anticoagulant in the storage of blood because of its ability to bind calcium that is required for activation of the coagulation cascade. Citrate is metabolized by the liver and excreted by the kidneys. Patients with normal liver and kidney function are able to respond to a large citrate load much better than patients with hepatic or renal insufficiency. During massive blood transfusion, citrate can accumulate in the circulation, resulting in a fall in ionized calcium. Hypocalcemia can result in hypotension, reduced cardiac function, and cardiac arrhythmias. Severe hypocalcemia can also result in clotting abnormalities. However, the level of calcium required for adequate coagulation is much lower than that necessary to maintain cardiovascular stability. Therefore, hypotension and decreased cardiac contractility occur long before coagulation abnormalities are seen. During massive blood transfusion it is generally prudent to monitor ionized calcium, especially if hemodynamic instability is present in the hypocalcemic patient.

Potassium abnormalities

During the storage of whole blood or packed red cells, potassium leaks from erythrocytes into the extracellular fluid and can accumulate at concentrations of 40–80 mEq/l. Once the RBCs are returned to the *in vivo* environment, the potassium quickly reenters RBCs. However, during rapid blood transfusion, transient hyperkalemia may result, particularly in patients with renal insufficiency. The transient hyperkalemia, particularly in the presence of hypocalcemia, can lead to cardiac dysfunction and arrhythmias. In patients with renal insufficiency, potassium load can be minimized by the use of either freshly obtained blood or washed packed RBCs. Hypokalemia can also result from massive blood transfusion due to reentry of potassium into RBCs and other cells during stress, alkalosis, or massive catecholamine release associated with large volume blood loss. Therefore, potassium levels should be monitored routinely during large volume blood transfusions.

Acid–base abnormalities

During the storage of whole blood, an acidic environment develops due to the accumulation of lactate and citrate with a pH in the range of 6.5–6.7. Rapid transfusion of this acidic fluid can contribute to the metabolic acidosis observed during massive blood transfusion. However, metabolic acidosis in this setting is more commonly due to relative tissue hypoxia and anaerobic metabolism due to an imbalance of oxygen consumption and delivery. The anaerobic metabolism that occurs during states of hypovolemia and poor tissue perfusion results in lactic acidosis. Generally, administration of sodium bicarbonate is not indicated. The re-establishment of tissue perfusion and homeostasis is a much more important factor in re-establishing acid–base balance. In contrast, many patients receiving massive blood transfusion will develop a metabolic alkalosis during the post-transfusion phase. This is due to the conversion of citrate to sodium bicarbonate by the liver and is an additional reason to avoid sodium bicarbonate administration during massive blood transfusion except in cases of severe metabolic acidosis (base deficit >12).

Altered oxygen transport

During the storage of blood, red blood cell 2,3-diphosphoglycerate (DPG) levels decline. This results in a shift in the oxyhemoglobin dissociation curve to the left. Under these conditions, oxygen has a higher affinity for hemoglobin, and oxygen release at the tissue level is theoretically diminished. In clinical practice, this alteration in oxygen affinity has not been shown to be functionally significant.

Hypothermia

Rapid infusion of large volumes of cold (4°C) blood can result in significant hypothermia. When added to the already impaired thermoregulatory mechanisms in burn patients this can result in significant hypothermia. Potential complications of hypothermia include altered citrate metabolism, coagulopathy, and cardiac dysfunction. During large volume blood transfusion in burn patients, fluids should be actively warmed with systems designed to effectively warm large volumes of rapidly transfused blood. In addition, the room temperature should be elevated and the patient's extremities and head covered to minimize heat loss. Body temperature should be maintained at or above 37°C in burn patients.

Pulmonary complications

Pulmonary edema is a potential complication of massive blood transfusion. This may result from volume overload and/or pulmonary capillary leak due to inflammation and microaggregates present in transfused blood. Some studies have indicated that the incidence of pulmonary edema is more related to the patient's underlying injury than to blood transfusion per se. However, volume status should be monitored closely during large volume blood transfusion so that volume overload may be avoided.

Transfusion reactions

Hemolytic transfusion reactions are a relatively rare but devastating complication of blood transfusion. The incidence of transfusion reactions is approximately 1:5000 units transfused and fatal transfusion reactions occur at a rate of 1:100 000 units transfused. Most severe reactions result from ABO incompatibility. The most common cause of transfusing ABO-incompatible blood is clerical error. Therefore, most hospitals have developed policies that require multiple checks of the blood prior to transfusion. A list of blood types and associated circulating antibodies is shown in **Table 13.17**. Massive hemolytic transfusion reactions result from destruction of transfused erythrocytes by circulating antibodies and complement. Many of the common signs and symptoms of transfusion reactions (**Table 13.18**), such as chills, chest pain, and nausea, cannot be detected in the patient under anesthesia. The most commonly recognized signs of transfusion reaction in the anesthetized patient are fever, hypotension, hemoglobinuria, and coagulopathy. The steps involved in the treatment of hemolytic transfusion reaction are outlined in **Table 13.19**. The cornerstones of treatment are to stop the transfusion, protect the kidneys with aggressive hydration and alkalinization of urine, and treat existing coagulopathy.

Delayed hemolytic transfusion reactions can occur in patients that have received prior blood transfusions and result from a secondary immune response with production of antibodies to blood antigens. This reaction can occur from 2 to 21 days after transfusion and should be suspected in patients with unexplained

Table 13.17 Blood groups and cross-match

Blood group	Antigen on erythrocyte	Plasma antibodies	Incidence (%) Whites	Incidence (%) African-Americans
A	A	Anti-B	40	27
B	B	Anti-A	11	20
AB	AB	None	4	4
O	None	Anti-A Anti-B	45	49
Rh	Rh		42	17

Table 13.18 Frequency and signs and symptoms from hemolytic transfusion reactions in 40 patients

Sign or symptom	No. of patients
Fever	19
Fever and chills	16
Chest pain	6
Hypotension	6
Nausea	2
Flushing	2
Dyspnea	2
Hemogloburia	1

Table 13.19 Steps for the treatment of a hemolytic transfusion reaction

1. STOP THE TRANSFUSION
2. Maintain the urine output at a minimum of 75–100 ml/h by the following methods:
   a. Generously administer fluids intravenously and possibly mannitol, 12.5–50 g, given over a 5 to 15-minute period
   b. If intravenously administered fluids and mannitol are ineffective, then administer furosemide, 20–40 mg, IV
3. Alkalinize the urine; since bicarbonate is preferentially excreted in the urine, only 40–70 mEq/70 kg of sodium bicarbonate is usually required to raise the urine pH to 8, whereupon repeat urine pH determinations indicate the need for additional bicarbonate
4. Assay urine and plasma hemoglobin concentrations
5. Determine platelet count, partial thromboplastin time, and serum fibrinogen level
6. Return unused blood to blood bank for re-cross-match
7. Send patient blood sample to blood bank for antibody screen and direct antiglobulin test.
8. Prevent hypotension to ensure adequate renal blood flow

decreases in hematocrit during the postoperative period. Renal injury is less common than in acute hemolytic reactions but adequate hydration and alkalinization of urine are usually indicated. Febrile reactions are common following blood transfusion and are generally due to contaminating leukocytes and leukocyte antigens present in transfused blood. Pure febrile reactions usually do not require termination of the transfusion but the patient should be monitored closely to assure that a more severe transfusion reaction is not developing.

Infection

Infection is a major problem in burn patients due to disruption of the cutaneous barrier and immunosuppression. Blood transfusion adds to the infection risk. Graves and colleagues showed a significant correlation between the number of blood transfusions and infectious complications in burn patients.[169] The most common source of major infection from blood products is hepatitis. Hepatitis C is the most common offender, followed by hepatitis B. The incidence of hepatitis C is approximately 3 in 10 000 units transfused. The development of rigorous screening mechanisms has markedly decreased the incidence of HIV infection to 1 in 200 000–500 000 units transfused. CMV infection of blood products is very common and can be a problem in immunocompromised burn patients.

Postoperative care

After transfer of monitors and ventilatory support in the intensive care unit, a full report of the intraoperative anesthetic course is given, along with information about the patient's current condition and therapy. A chest radiograph is ordered to confirm endotracheal tube and central line position. Laboratory studies including arterial blood gas, blood chemistries, renal function tests, hematocrit, platelet count, and coagulation studies are sent soon after patient arrival to the intensive care unit. These studies are particularly important if massive transfusion was required in the operating room.

One of the most important issues in the immediate postoperative period for burn patients is adequate analgesia and sedation, particularly for the intubated and mechanically ventilated patient. Debridement of burned tissue and the harvesting of skin grafts are painful procedures that merit ample analgesic doses in order to insure patient comfort. It is not uncommon for burn patients to be quite tolerant to narcotic analgesics, especially after they have had several operative procedures, and in this case larger doses than normal are required.

Ongoing blood loss is unfortunately a common problem after the excision and grafting of a large burn wound, even when strict attention is placed on intraoperative hemostasis by surgical personnel. The burn wounds are necessarily excised down to bleeding tissue before skin grafts are applied. Massive intraoperative transfusion adds to the problem with dilutional thrombocytopenia and coagulopathy. Diligent postoperative care is needed to continually assess ongoing blood loss and transfuse additional blood products as they are indicated by clinical course and laboratory studies. Monitoring of central venous pressure and urine output also help in guiding postoperative blood and fluid therapy.

Adequate ventilation is essential in the postoperative period in order to minimize hypoxemia and hypercarbia. Blood gases and oxygen saturation can be used as guides to ventilator management. Patients with inhalation injury benefit not only from rational ventilator management but also from a program of inhaled bronchodilators and mucolytics combined with judicious airway suctioning. Extubated patients require supplemental oxygen for at least the first few hours postoperatively in order to maintain adequate oxygen saturation. Airway support may also be necessary initially in these patients until they are more alert and responsive.

Finally, burn patients must be recovered in a warm environment. Postoperative hypothermia can result in vasoconstriction, hypoperfusion, and metabolic acidosis. Radiant heaters, blood and fluid warmers, warm blankets, heated humidifiers for gas delivery, and high room temperature are all useful in the postoperative period to provide warmth to the recovering patient.

Summary

Anesthetic management of the burn patient presents numerous challenges. Anatomical distortions make airway management and vascular access difficult. Pathophysiological changes in cardiovascular function range from initial hypovolemia and impaired perfusion to a hyperdynamic and hypermetabolic state that develops after the resuscitative stage. These and other changes profoundly alter response to anesthetic drugs. Effective anesthetic management will depend on knowledge of the continuum of pathophysiological changes, technical skills, proper planning, and availability of proper resources. A team approach is necessary, keeping in mind that perioperative management should be consistent with ICU management and goals. This requires close communication with other members of the burn care team.

References

1. Saffle VR. Predicting outcomes of burns. *N Engl J Med* 1998; **338**: 387–8.
2. Ryan CM, Schoenfeld DA, Thorpe WP, Sheridan RL, Cassem EH, Tompkins RG. Objective estimates of the probability of death from burn injuries. *N Engl J Med* 1998; **338**: 362–6.
3. MacLennan N, Heimbach DM, Cullen BF. Anesthesia for major thermal injury. *Anesthesiology* 1998; **89**: 749–70.
4. Beushausen T, Mucke. Anesthesia and pain management in pediatric burn patients. *Pediatric Surg Int* 1997; **12**: 327–33.
5. Martyn JAJ ed. *Acute Management of the Burned Patient.* London: WB Saunders, 1990.
6. Reynolds EM, Ryan DP, Sheridan RL, Doody DP. Left ventricular failure complicating severe pediatric burn injuries. *J Pediatric Surg* 1995; **30**: 264–9.
7. Desai MH, Herndon DN, Broemeling L, Barrow RE, Nichols RJ, Rutan RL. Early burn wound excision significantly reduces blood loss. *Ann Surg* 1990; **211**: 753–9.
8. Thompson PB, Herndon DN, Traber DL, Abston S. Effect on mortality of inhalation injury. *J Trauma* 1986; **26**: 163–5.
9. Navar PD, Saffle JR, Warden GD. Effect of inhalation injury on fluid resuscitation requirements after thermal injury. *Am J Surg* 1985; **150**: 716–20.
10. Hollingsed TC, Saffle JR, Barton RG, Craft WB, Morris SE. Etiology and consequences of respiratory failure in thermally injured patients. *Am J Surg* 1993; **166**: 592–7.
11. Foley FD. The burn autopsy. *Am J Clin Pathol* 1969; **52**: 1–13.
12. Moritz AR, Henriques FC, McLean R. The effects of inhaled heat on the air passages and lungs: an experimental investigation. *Am J Pathol* 1945; **21**: 311–31.
13. Clark WR, Bonaventura M, Myers W. Smoke inhalation and airway management at a regional burn unit: 1974–1983. Diagnosis and consequences of smoke inhalation. *J Burn Care Rehabil* 1989; **10**: 52–62.
14. Muehlberger, T, Kunar D, Munster A, Couch M. Efficacy of fiberoptic laryngoscopy in the diagnosis of inhalation injuries. *Arch Otolaryngol Head Neck Surg* 1998; **124**: 1003–7.
15. Colice GL, Munster AM, Haponik EF. Tracheal stenosis complicating cutaneous burns: an underestimated problem. *Am Rev Respir Dis* 1986; **134**: 1315–18.
16. Clark CJ, Reid WH, Telfer ABM, Campbell D. Respiratory injury in the burned patient; the role of flexible bronchoscopy. *Anaesthesia* 1983; **38**: 35–9.
17. Haponic EF, Lykens MG. Acute upper airway obstruction in patients with burns. *Crit Care Rep* 1990; **2**: 28–49.
18. Hunt JL, Agee RN, Pruitt BA. Fiberoptic bronchoscopy in acute inhalation injury. *J Trauma* 1975; **15**: 641–9.
19. Haponic EF, Myers DA, Munster AM, Smith PL, Brih EJ, Wise RA, Bleecker ER. Acute upper airway injury in burn patients: serial changes of flow-volume curves and nasopharyngoscopy. *Am Rev Respir Dis* 1987; **135**: 360–6.
20. Lee JM, O'Connell DJ. The plain chest radiograph after acute smoke inhalation. *Clin Radiol* 1988; **39**: 33.
21. Linares HA, Herndon DN, Traber DL. Sequence of morphologic events in experimental smoke inhalation. *J Burn Care Rehabil* 1989; **10**: 27–37.
22. Demling RH, Chen C. Pulmonary function in the burn patient. *Semin Nephrol* 1993; **13**: 371–81.
23. Sheridan RL, Kacmarek RM, McEttrick MM, Weber JM, Ryan CM, Doody DP, Ryan DP, Schnitzer JJ, Topkins RG. Permissive hypercapnia as a ventilatory strategy in burned children: effect on barotrauma, pneumonia and mortality. *J Trauma* 1995; **39**(5): 854–9.

24. Cioffi WG Jr, Rue LW III, Graves TA, McManus WF, Mason AD Jr, Pruitt BA Jr. Prophylactic use of high-frequency percussive ventilation in patients with inhalation injury. *Ann Surg* 1991; **213**(6): 575–80; discussion 580–2.

25. Fitzpatrick JC, Cioffi WG Jr. Ventilatory support following burns and smoke-inhalation injury. *Respir Care Clin N Am* 1997; **3**(1): 21–49.

26. Reper P, Dankaert R, van Hille F, Van Laeke P, Duinslaeger L, Vanderkelen A. The usefulness of combined high-frequency percussive ventilation during acute respiratory failure after smoke inhalation. *Burns* 1998; **24**(1): 34–8.

27. Cortiella J, Mlcak R, Herndon DN. High frequency percussive ventilation in pediatric patients with inhalation injury. *J Burn Care Rehabil* 1999; **20**(3): 232–5.

28. Ernst A, Zibrak JD. Carbon monoxide poisoning. *N Engl J Med* 1998; **339**: 1603–8.

29. Tibbles P, Perrotta P. Treatment of carbon monoxide poisoning: a critical review of human outcome studies comparing normobaric oxygen with hyperbaric oxygen. *Ann Emerg Med* 1994; **24**: 269–76.

30. Clark CJ. Measurement of toxic combustion products in fire survivors. *J Roy Soc Med* 1982; **153**: 41–4.

31. Deitch EA. The management of burns. *N Engl J Med* 1990; **323**: 1249–53.

32. Horton JW, Baxter CR, White DJ. Differences in cardiac responses to resuscitation from burn shock. *Surg Gynecol Obstet.* 1989; **168**: 201–13.

33. Zetterstrom H, Arturson G. Plasma oncotic pressure and plasma protein concentration in patients following thermal injury. *Acta Anaesthesiol Scand* 1980; **24**: 288–94.

34. Kinsky MP, Guha SC, Button BM, Kramer GC. The role of interstitial Starling forces in the pathogenesis of burn edema. *J Burn Care Rehabil* 1998; **19**(1 Pt 1): 1–9.

35. Muller-Werdan U, Engelmann H, Werdan K. Cardiodepression by tumor necrosis factor-alpha. *Eur Cytokine Netw* 1998; **9**: 689–91.

36. Roberts AB, Vodovotz Y, Roche NS, Sporn MB, Nathan CF. Role of nitric oxide in antagonistic effects of transforming growth factor-beta and interleukin-1 beta on the beating rate of cultured cardiac myocytes. *Mol Endocrinol* 1992; **6**: 1921–30.

37. Alderson P, Schierhout G, Roberts I, Bunn F. Colloids versus crystalloids for fluid resuscitation in critically ill patients. *Cochrane Database Syst Rev* 2000; **2**: CD000567.

38. Nguyen TT, Gilpin DA, Meyer NA, Herndon DN. Current treatment of severely burned patients. *Ann Surg* 1996; **223**: 14–25.

39. The Albumin Reviewers (Alderson P, Bunn F, Lefebvre C, Li Wan Po A, Li L, Roberts I, Schierhout G). Human albumin solution for resuscitation and volume expansion in critically ill patients. *Cochrane Database Syst Rev* 2000; **2**: CD001208.

40. Guha SC, Kinsky MP, Button B, Herndon DN, Traber LD, Traber DL, Kramer GC. Burn resuscitation: crystalloid versus colloid versus hypertonic saline hyperoncotic colloid in sheep. *Crit Care Med* 1996; **24**: 1849–57.

41. Elgjo GI, Poli de Figueiredo LF, Schenarts PJ, Traber DL, Traber LD, Kramer GC. Hypertonic saline dextran produces early (8–12 hours) fluid sparing in burn resuscitation: a 24-hour prospective, double-blind study in sheep. *Crit Care Med* 2000; **28**: 163–71.

42. Suzuki K, Ogino R, Nishina M, Kohama A. Effects of hypertonic saline and dextran cardiac functions after burns. *Am J Physiol* 1995; **268**(2 Pt 2): H856–64.

43. Jeng JC, Lee K, Jablonski K, Jordan MH. Serum lactate and base deficit suggest inadequate resuscitation of patients with burn injuries: application of a point-of-care laboratory instrument. *J Burn Care Rehabil* 1997; **18**: 402–5.

44. Dries DJ, Waxman K. Adequate resuscitation of burn patients may not be measured by urine output and vital signs. *Crit Care Med* 1991; **19**: 327–9.

45. Wo CC, Shoemaker WC, Appel PL, Bishop MH, Kram HB, Hardin E. Unreliability of blood pressure and heart rate to evaluate cardiac output in emergency resuscitation and critical illness. *Crit Care Med* 1993; **21**: 218–23.

46. Schiller WR, Bay RC, Garren RL, Parker I, Sagraves SG. Hyperdynamic resuscitation improves survival in patients with life-threatening burns. *J Burn Care Rehabil* 1997; **18**: 10–16.

47. Holm C, Melcer B, Horbrand F, von Donnersmarck GH, Muhlbauer W. The relationship between oxygen delivery and oxygen consumption during fluid resuscitation of burn-related shock. *J Burn Care Rehabil* 2000; **21**: 147–54.

48. Bernard F, Gueugniaud PY, Bertin-Maghit M, Bouchard C, Vilasco B, Petit P. Prognostic significance of early cardiac index measurements in severely burned patients. *Burns* 1994; **20**: 529–31.

49. Bishop MH, Shoemaker WC, Appel PL, *et al.* Prospective, randomized trial of survivor values of cardiac index, oxygen delivery, and oxygen consumption as resuscitation endpoints in severe trauma. *J Trauma* 1995; **38**: 780–7.

50. Fleming A, Bishop M, Shoemaker W, *et al.* Prospective trial of supranormal values as goals of resuscitation in severe trauma. *Arch Surg* 1992; **127**: 1175–9.

51. Schiller WR, Bay RC, Garren RL, Parker I, Sagraves SG. Hyperdynamic resuscitation improves survival in patients with life-threatening burns. *J Burn Care Rehabil* 1997; **18**: 10–16.

52. Heyland DK, Cook DJ, King D, Kernerman P, Brun-Buisson C. Maximizing oxygen delivery in critically ill patients: a methodologic appraisal of the evidence. *Crit Care Med* 1996; **24**: 517–24.

53. Gattinoni L, Brazzi L, Pelosi P, Latini R, Tognoni G, Pesenti A, Fumagalli R. A trial of goal-oriented hemodynamic therapy in critically ill patients. SvO2 Collaborative Group. *N Engl J Med* 1995; **333**: 1025–32.

54. Durham RM, Neunaber K, Mazuski JE, Shapiro MJ, Baue AE. The use of oxygen consumption and delivery as endpoints for resuscitation in critically ill patients. *J Trauma* 1996; **41**: 32–9.

55. Hayes MA, Timmins AC, Yau EH, Palazzo M, Hinds CJ, Watson D. Elevation of systemic oxygen delivery in the treatment of critically ill patients. *N Engl J Med* 1994; **330**: 1717–22.

56. Porter JM, Ivatury RR. In search of the optimal end points of resuscitation in trauma patients: a review. *J Trauma* 1998; **44**: 908–14.

57. Holm C, Melcer B, Horbrand F, Worl HH, von Donnersmarck GH, Muhlbauer W. Haemodynamic and oxygen transport responses in survivors and non-survivors following thermal injury. *Burns* 2000; **26**: 25–33.

58. Kaups KL, Davis JW, Dominic WJ. Base deficit as an indicator or resuscitation needs in patients with burn injuries. *J Burn Care Rehabil* 1998; **19**: 346–8.

59. Robbins MR, Smith RS, Helmer SD. Serial pHi measurement as a predictor of mortality, organ failure, and hospital stay in surgical patients. *Am Surg* 1999; **65**: 715–19.

60. Davies MP, Evans J, McGonigle RJ. The dialysis debate: acute renal failure in burns patients. *Burns* 1994; **20**: 71–3.

61. Davies DM, Pusey CD, Rainford DJ, Brown JM, Bennett JP. Acute renal failure in burns. *Scand J Plast Reconstr Surg* 1979; **13**: 189–92.

62. Cameron JS. Disturbances of renal function in burnt patients. *Proc R Soc Med* 1969; **62**: 49–50.

63. Holm C, Horbrand F, von Donnersmarck GH, Muhlbauer W. Acute renal failure in severely burned patients. *Burns* 1999; **25**: 171–8.

64. Jeschke MG, Barrow RE, Wolf SE, Herndon DN. Mortality in burned children with acute renal failure. *Arch Surg* 1998; **133**: 752–6.

65. Chrysopoulo MT, Jeschke MG, Dziewulski P, Barrow RE, Herndon DN. Acute renal dysfunction in severely burned adults. *J Trauma* 1999; **46**: 141–4.

66. Wallace BH, Caldwell FT Jr, Cone JB. The interrelationships between wound management, thermal stress, energy metabolism, and temperature profiles of patients with burns. *J Burn Care Rehabil* 1994; **15**: 499–508.

67. Caldwell FT Jr, Wallace BH, Cone JB. The effect of wound management on the interaction of burn size, heat production, and rectal temperature. *J Burn Care Rehabil* 1994; **15**: 121–9.

68. Caldwell FT Jr, Graves DB, Wallace BH. Pathogenesis of fever in a rat burn model: the role of cytokines and lipopolysaccharide. *J Burn Care Rehabil* 1997; **18**: 525–30.

69. Caldwell FT Jr, Graves DB, Wallace BH. Chronic indomethacin administration blocks increased body temperature after burn injury in rats. *J Burn Care Rehabil* 1998; **19**: 501–11.

70. Shiozaki T, Kishikawa M, Hiraide A, Shimazu T, Sugimoto H, Yoshioka T, Sugimoto T. Recovery from postoperative hypothermia predicts survival in extensively burned patients. *Am J Surg* 1993; **165**: 326–30.

71. Jaehde U, Sorgel F. Clinical pharmacokinetics in patients with burns. *Clin Pharmacokinet* 1995; **29**: 15–28.

72. Bonate PL. Pathophysiology and pharmacokinetics following burn injury. *Clin Pharmacokinet* 1990; **18**: 118–30.

73. Martyn JA, Abernethy DR, Greenblatt DJ. Plasma protein binding of drugs after severe burn injury. *Clin Pharmacol Ther* 1984; **35**: 535–9.

74. Blaschke TF. Protein binding and kinetics of drugs in liver disease. *Clin Pharmacokinet* 1977; **2**: 32–44.

75. Loirat P, Rohan J, Baillet A, Beaufils F, David R, Chapman A. Increased glomerulofiltration rate in patients with major burns and its effect on the pharmacokinetics of tobramycin. *N Engl J Med* 1978; **299**: 915–19.

76. Glew RH, Moellering RC, Burke JF. Fentamicin dosage in children with extensive burns. *J Trauma* 1976; **16**: 819–23.

77. Perry S, Inturrisi CE. Analgesia and morphine disposition in burn patients. *J Burn Care Rehabil* 1983; **4**: 276–9.

78. Furman WR, Munster AM, Cane EJ. Morphine pharmacokinetics during anesthesia and surgery in patients with burns. *J Burn Care Rehabil* 1990; **11**: 391–4.

79. Tolmie JD, Joyce TH, Mitchell GD. Succinylcholine danger in the burned patient. *Anesthesiology* 1967; **18**: 467–70.

80. Moncrief JA. Complications of burns. *Ann Surg* 1958; **147**: 443–75.

81. Schaner PJ, Brown RL, Kirksey TD, Gunther RC, Ritchey CR, Gronert GA. Succinylcholine-induced hyperkalemia in burned patients. *Anesth Analg* 1969; **48**: 764–70.

82. Viby-Mogensen J, Hanel HK, Hansen E, Graae J. Serum cholinesterase activity in burned patients. II: Anaesthesia, suxamethonium and hyperkalaemia. *Acta Anaesthesiol Scand* 1975; **19**: 169–79.

83. McCaughey TJ. Hazards of anesthesia for the burned child. *Can Anaesth Soc J* 1962; **9**: 220–33.

84. Yentis SM. Suxamethonium and hyperkalemia. *Anaesth Intensive Care* 1990; **18**: 92–101.

85. Gronert GA. Letter to the editor: Succinylcholine hyperkalemia after burns. *Anesthesiology* 1999; **91**: 320.

86. MacLenna N, Heimbach DM, Cullen BF. Letter to the editor: Succinylcholine hyperkalemia after burns. *Anesthesiology* 1999; **91**: 320.

87. Martyn JA. Letter to editor in reply to: Succinylcholine hyperkalemia after burns. *Anesthesiology* 1999; **91**: 321–2.

88. Fambrough DM. Control of acetylcholine receptors in skeletal muscle. *Physiol Rev* 1979; **59**: 165–227.

89. Martyn JAJ, Szyfelbein SK, Ali HA, Matteo RS, Savares JJ. Increased d-tubocurarine requirement following major thermal injury. *Anesthesiology* 1980; **52**: 352–5.

90. Martyn JAJ, Liu LMO, Szyfelbein SK, Ambalavanar ES, Goudsouzian NG. The neuromuscular effects of pancuronium in burned children. *Anesthesiology* 1983; **59**: 561–4.

91. Kim C, Fuke N, Martyn JA. Burn injury to rat increases nicotinic acetylcholine receptors in the diaphragm. *Anesthesiology* 1988; **68**: 401–6.

92. Marathe PH, Haschke RH, Slattery JT, Zucker JR, Pavlin EG. Acetylcholine receptor density and acetylcholinesterase activity in skeletal muscle of rats following thermal injury. *Anesthesiology* 1989; **70**: 654–9.

93. Edwards JP, Hatton PA, Little RA, Pennington RA, Wareham AC. Increased quantol release of acetylcholine at the neuromuscular junction following scald injury in the rat. *Muscle Nerve* 1999; **22**: 1660–6.

94. Martyn JA, Matteo RS, Szyfelbein SK, Kaplan RF. Unprecedented resistance to neuromuscular blocking effects of metocurine with persistence after complete recovery in a burned patient. *Anesth Analg* 1982; **61**: 614–17.

95. Martyn JA, Goudsouzian NG, Chang Y, Szyfelbein SK, Schwartz AE, Patel SS. Neuromuscular effects of Mivacurium in 2- to 12-year-old children with burn injury. *Anesthesiology* 2000; **92**: 31–7.

96. Viby-Mogensen J, Hanel HK, Hansen E, Sorensen B, Graae J. Serum cholinesterase activity in burned patients I: biochemical findings. *Acta Anaesth Scand* 1975; **19**: 159–63.

97. Hu OY, Ho ST, Wang JJ, Lin CY. Evaluation of gastric emptying in severe, burn-injured patients. *Crit Care Med* 1993; **21**: 527–31.

98. Mathru M, Esch O, Lang J, Herbert ME, Chaljub G, Goodacre B, van Sonnenberg E. Magnetic resonance imaging of the upper airway: Effects of propofol anesthesia and nasal continuous positive airway pressure in humans. *Anesthesiology* 1996; **84**: 275–8.

99. Lang J, Herbert M, Esch, Chaljuh G, Mathru M. Magnetic resonance of the upper airway: Ketamine preserves airway potency compared to propofol anesthesia in human volunteers. *Anesth Anal* 1997; **84**: 542.

100. Wilson RD, Nichols RJ, McCoy NR. Dissociative anesthesia with CI-581 in burned children. *Anesth Analg* 1967; **46**: 719–24.

101. Alfery DD, Ward CF, Harwood IR, Mannino FL. Airway management for a neonate with congenital fusion of the jaws. *Anesthesia* 1979; **51**: 340–2.

102. Kleeman PP, Jantzen JP, Bonfils P. Clinical Reports: The ultra-thin bronchoscope in management of the difficult paediatric airway. *Can J Anaesth* 1987; **34**: 606–8.

103. Wrigley SR, Black AE, Sidhu VS. A fiberoptic laryngoscope for paediatric anaesthesia; a study to evaluate the usse of the 2.2 mm Olympus (LF-P) intubating fiberscope. *Anaesthesia* 1995; **50**: 709–12.

104. Gordon MD, ed. Burn care protocols: anchoring endotracheal tubes on patients with facial burns. *J Burn Care Rehabil* 1987; **8**: 233–7.

105. McCall VE, Fischer CG, Schomaker E, Young VM. Laryngeal mask airway use in children with acute burns: intraoperative airway management. *Paediatr Anaesth* 1999; **9**: 515–20.

106. Sheridan RL, Prelack KM, Petras LM, Szyfelbein SK, Tompkins RG. Intraoperative reflectance oximetry in burn patients. *J Clin Monit* 1995; **11**(1): 32–4.

107. Bainbridge LC, Simmons HM, Elliot D. The use of automatic blood pressure monitors in the burned patient. *Br J Plast Surg* 1990; **43**(3): 322–4.

108. Talke P, Nichols RJ, Traber DL. Does measurement of systolic blood pressure with a pulse oximeter correlate with conventional methods? *J Clin Monit* 1990; **6**: 5–9.

109. Murray WB, Foster PA. The peripheral pulse wave: information overlooked. *J Clin Monit* 1996; **12**: 365–77.

110. Tavernier B, Makhotine O, Lebuffe G, Dupont J, Scherpereel P. Systolic pressure variation as a guide to fluid therapy in patients with sepsis-induced hypotension. *Anesthesiology* 1998; **89**: 1313–21.

111. Perel A. Assessing fluid responsiveness by the systolic pressure variation in mechanically ventilated patients. *Anesthesiology* 1998; **89**: 1309–10.

112. Slogoff S, Keats AS, Arlund C. On the safety of radial artery cannulation. *Anesthesiology* 1983; **59**: 42–7.

113. Bedford RF. Radial arterial function following percutaneous cannulation with 18-and 20-gauge catheters. *Anesthesiology* 1977; **47**: 37–9.

114. Thomas F, Burke JP, Parker J, et al. The risk of infection related to radial versus femoral sites for arterial catheterization. *Crit Care Med* 1983; **11**: 807–12.

115. Gurman GM, Kriemerman S. Cannulation of big arteries in critically ill patients. *Crit Care Med* 1985; **13**: 217–20.

116. Purdue GF, Hunt JL. Vascular access through the femoral vessels: indications and complications. *J Burn Care Rehabil* 1986; **7**: 448–50.

117. Cilley RE. Arterial access in infants and children. *Semin Pediatr Surg* 1992; **3**: 174–80.

118. Norwood SH, Cormier B, McMahon NG, Moss A, Moore V. Prospective study of catheter-related infection during prolonged arterial catheterization. *Crit Care Med* 1988; **16**: 836–9.

119. Frezza EE, Mezghebe H. Indications and complications of arterial catheter use in surgical or medical intensive care units: analysis of 4932 patients. *Am Surg* 1998; **64**: 127–31.

120. Kocis KC, Vermilion RP, Callow LB, Kulik TJ, Ludomirsky A, Bove EL. Complications of femoral artery cannulation for perioperative monitoring in children. *J Thorac Cardiovasc Surg* 1996; **112**: 1399–400.

121. Graves PW, Davis AL, Maggi JC, Nussbaum E. Femoral artery cannulation for monitoring in critically ill children: prospective study. *Crit Care Med* 1990; **18**: 1363–6.

122. Randolph AG, Cook DJ, Gonzales CA, Andrew M. Benefit of heparin in peripheral venous and arterial catheters: systematic review and meta-analysis of randomized clinical trials. *Br Med J* 1998; **316**: 969–75.

123. Sheridan RL, Weber JM, Tompkins RG. Femoral arterial catheterization in pediatric burn patients. *Burns* 1994; **20**: 451–2.

124. Franken EA, Girod D, Sequeirs FW, Smith WL, Hurwitz R, Smith JA. Femoral artery spasm in children: catheter size is the principal cause. *Am J Rad* 1982; **138**: 295–8.

125. Smith-Wright DL, Green TP, Lock JE, Egar MI, Fuhrman BP. Complication of vascular catheterization in critically ill children. *Crit Care Med* 1984; **12**: 1015–17.

126. Sellden H, Nilsson K, Eksrom-Jodal B. Radial arterial catheters in children and neonates: a prospective study. *Crit Care Med* 1987; **15**: 1106–9.

127. Miyasaka K, Edmonds JF, Conn AW. Complication of radial artery lines in the paediatric patient. *Canad Anaesth Soc J* 1976; **23**: 9–14.

128. Soderstom CA, Wasserman DH, Dunham CM, Caplan ES, Cowley RA. Superiority of the femoral artery for monitoring. *Am J Surg* 1982; **144**: 309–12.

129. Saint S, Matthay MA. Risk reduction in the intensive care unit. *Am J Med* 1998; **105**: 515–23.

130. Hagley MT, Marin B, Gast P, Traeger SM. Infectious and mechanical complications of central venous catheters placed by percutaneous venipuncture and over guidewire. *Crit Care Med* 1192; **20**: 1426–30.

131. Stenzel JP, Green TP, Fuhrman BP, Carlson PE, Marchessault RP. Percutaneous femoral venous catheterizations: a prospective study of complications. *J Pediatr* 1989; **114**: 411–15.

132. Trottier SJ, Veremakis C, O'Brien J, Auer AI. Femoral deep vein thrombosis associated with central venous catheterization: results from a prospective, randomized trial. *Crit Care Med* 1995; **23**: 52–9.

133. Venkataraman ST, Thompson AE, Orr RA. Femoral vascular catheterization in critically ill infants and children. *Clin Ped* 1997; **311**: 310–19.

134. Purdue GF, Hunt JL. Pulmonary emboli in burned patients. *J Trauma* 1988; **28**: 218–20.

135. Goldstein AM, Weber JM, Sheridan RL. Femoral venous access is safe in burned children: an analysis of 224 catheters. *J Pediatr* 1997; **130**: 442–6.

136. Kanter RK, Zimmerman JJ, Strauss RH, Stoeckel KA. Central venous catheter insertion femoral vein: safety and effectiveness for the pediatric patient. *Pediatrics* 1986; **77**: 842–7.

137. Murr MM, Rosenquist MD, Lewis RW, Heinle JA, Kealey GP. A prospective safety study of femoral vein versus nonfemoral vein catheterization in patients with burns. *J Burn Care Rehabil* 1991; **12**: 576–8.

138. Still JM, Law E, Thiruvaiyaru D, Belcher K, Donker K. Central line-related sepsis in acute burn patients. *Am Surg* 1998; **64**: 165–70.

139. Kealey GP, Chang P, Heinle J, Rosenquist MD, Lewis RW. Prospective comparison of two management strategies of central venous catheters in burns patients. *J Trauma* 1995; **38**: 344–9.

140. Lesseva M. Central venous catheter-related bacteremia in burn patients. *Scand J Infect Dis* 1998; **30**: 585–9.

141. Cobb DK, High KP, Sawyer RG, et al. A controlled trial of scheduled replacement of central venous and pulmonary artery catheters. *N Engl J Med* 1992; **327**: 1062–8.

142. Snyder RH, Archer FJ, Endy T, et al. Catheter infection: a comparison of two catheter maintenance techniques. *Ann Surg* 1988; **208**: 651–3.

143. Eyer S, Brummitt C, Crossley K, Siegel R, Cerra F. Catheter-related sepsis:

prospective, randomized study of three methods of long-term catheter maintenance. *Crit Care Med* 1990; **18**: 1073–9.

144. Sheridan RL, Weber JM, Peterson HF, Tompkins RG. Central venous catheter sepsis with weekly catheter change in paediatric burn patients: an analysis of 221 catheters. *Burns* 1995; **21**: 127–9.

145. Stenzel JP, Green TP, Fuhrman BP, Carlson PE, Marchessault RP. Percutaneous central venous catherization in a pediatric intensive care unit: a survival analysis of complications. *Crit Care Med* 1989; **17**: 984–8.

146. Garrison RN, Wilson MA. Intravenous and central catheter infections. *Surg Clin N Am* 1994; **74**: 557–70.

147. American Society of Anesthesiologists. *Recommendations for Infection Control for the Practice of Anesthesiology. Prevention of Infection During Insertion and Maintenance of Central Venous Catheters.* ASA, 1997.

148. Ahmed Z, Mohyuddin Z. Complications associated with different insertion techniques for Hickman catheters. *Postgrad Med J* 1998; **868**: 104–7.

149. Pearson ML. Guideline for prevention of intravascular device-related infections. The Hospital Infection Control Practices Advisory Committee. *Am J Infect Control* 1996; **24**: 262–93.

150. Thornton J, Todd NJ, Webster NR. Central venous line sepsis in the intensive care unit. *Anaesthesia* 1996; **51**: 1018–20.

151. Idris AH, Melker RJ. High-flow sheaths for pediatric fluid resuscitation: a comparison of flow rates with standard pediatric catheters. *Pediatr Emerg Care* 1992; **8**: 119–22.

152. Hodge D, Delgado-Paredes C, Fleisher G. Central and peripheral catheter flow rates in 'pediatric' dogs. *Ann Emerg Med* 1986; **15**: 1151–4.

153. de la Roche MR, Gauthier L. Rapid transfusion of packed red blood cells: effects of dilution, pressure, and catheter size. *Ann Emerg Med* 1993; **22**: 1551–5.

154. Millikan JA, Cain TL, Hansbrough J. Rapid volume replacement for hypovolemic shock: a comparison of techniques and equipment. *J Trauma* 1984; **24**: 428–31.

155. Dutky PA, Stevens SL, Maull KI. Factors affecting fluid resuscitation with large-bore introducer catheters. *J Trauma* 1989; **29**: 856–60.

156. Beebe DS, Beck D, Belani KG. Comparison of the flow rates of central venous catheters designed for rapid transfusion in infants and small children. *Paedr Anaes* 1995; **5**: 35–9.

157. White PF, Way WL, Trevor AJ. Ketamine – its pharmacology and therapeutic uses. *Anesthesiology* 1982; **56**: 119–36.

158. Layon AJ, Vetter TR, Hanna PG, Bingham HG. An anesthetic technique to fabricate a pressure mask for controlling scar formation from facial burns. *J Burn Care Rehabil* 1991; **12**: 349–52.

159. Maldini B. Ketamine anesthesia in children with acute burns and scalds. *Acta Anaesthesiol Scand* 1996; **40**: 1108–111.

160. Irving GA, Butt AD. Anaesthesia for burns in children: a review of procedures practiced at Red Cross War Memorial Children's Hospital, Cape Town. *Burns* 1994; **20**: 241–3.

161. Mann R, Heimbach DM, Engrav LH, Foy H. Changes in transfusion practices in burn patients. *J Trauma* 1994; **37**: 220–2.

162. Sittig KM, Deitch EA. Blood transfusions: for the thermally injured or for the doctor? *J Trauma* 1994; **36**: 369–72.

163. American Society of Anesthesiologists Practice Guidelines for blood component therapy: A report by the American Society of Anesthesiologists Task Force on Blood Component Therapy. *Anesthesiology* 1996; **84**: 732–47.

164. Smoot EC III. Modified use of extremity tourniquets for burn wound debridement. *J Burn Care Rehabil* 1996; **17**: 334–7.

165. Missavage AE, Bush RL, Kien ND, Reilly DA. The effect of clysed and topical epinephrine on intraoperative catecholamine levels. *J Trauma* 1998; **45**: 1074–8.

166. Barret JP, Dziewulski P, Wolf SE, Desai MH, Nichols RJ II, Herndon DN. Effect of topical and subcutaneous epinephrine in combination with topical thrombin in blood loss during immediate near-total burn wound excision in pediatric burned patients. *Burns* 1999; **25**: 509–13.

167. Barret JP, Desai MH, Herndon DN. Massive transfusion of reconstituted whole blood is well tolerated in pediatric burn surgery. *J Trauma* 1999; **47**: 526–8.

168. Dzik WH, Kirkley SA. Citrate toxicity during massive blood transfusion. *Transfus Med Rev* 1988; **2**: 76–94.

169. Graves TA, Cioffi WG, Mason AD Jr, McManus WF, Pruitt BA Jr. Relationship of transfusion and infection in a burn population. *J Trauma* 1989; **29**: 948–52.

Chapter 14

The skin bank
Robert L McCauley

Introduction

Early excision and coverage of the burn wound has increasingly become the standard of care for burned patients, with primary closure of the burn wound using split-thickness skin grafts being the ultimate goal. In patients with massive thermal injury, temporary coverage with skin donated by another person (allograft or homograft) is essential.[1] Although tissue transplantation was described in the seventeenth century, the development of the US Navy Skin Bank in Bethesda, Maryland in 1949 signified the emergence of modern day skin banking.[2]

Historical development

Transplantation of skin was adopted as a clinical method for wound closure soon after Reverdin's introduction of split-thickness skin grafts in 1869.[3] Girdner reported the first clinical use of allografts in 1881 by harvesting a suicide victim's skin to use for closure of a burn wound. Although a large part of the skin graft initially took, during the second and third weeks 'erysipelatous inflammation' resulted, probably indicating rejection.[4] Similar

investigations were performed simultaneously by Wolfe and Thiersch.[5,6]

In 1938, Bettman reported the successful use of allografts in two children with more than 60% total body surface area (TBSA) burn.[7] In 1944, Webster reported that the refrigeration of autograft skin in a Vaseline gauze, wrapped in a saline sponge and stored 3 weeks at 4–7°C, still resulted in a successful 'take' of the graft.[8] The routine use of allograft skin did not occur until the early 1950s when Brown and Fryer reported its use in extensive burns as a biological dressing.[9] At that time, allograft was introduced as routine therapy for burn patients at the Brooke Army Medical Center in San Antonio, Texas. In 1966, Zaroff reported his 10-year experience with the use of allografts. The benefits listed below are classic and represent the benefits of allograft use as both a physiologic and mechanical barrier:[10]

- reduction in water, electrolyte, and protein loss;
- reduction in energy requirements secondary to the attainment of a closed wound;
- reduction in wound infection rates;
- reduction in pain;
- conservation of autografts; and
- improved general welfare and psychological outlook of the patient.

In 1966, Morris et al. reported the beneficial effects of allografts in healing infected ulcers and other heavily contaminated wounds as a 'physiologic primary closure'.[11] As a result of those reports, research into the mechanisms of wound healing began in an attempt to elucidate the reasons why allografts were superior to conventional dressings. In 1958, Eade reported reduction in the number of bacteria under biological dressings.[12] Woods subsequently reported that phagocytes within a wound used the fibrin network established between the allograft and the wound to trap and phagocytose bacteria without the production of opsonins or antibody.[13] Further investigations by O'Donoghue and Zarem demonstrated that both fresh and preserved skin allograft stimulated neovascularization.[14] Shuck et al., using the Vietnam war experience, extended the use of allografts to difficult nonburn traumatic wounds with great benefit.[15] The effects of allografts in reducing bacteria and promoting healing have proven to be beneficial.

Tissue preservation

Clearly, an essential component in the use of allograft is the ability to store the tissue for use at a later time. In 1903, Wentscher experimented with the transplantation of a human skin graft stored in a refrigerator for from 3 to 14 days.[16] Alexis Carrel appears to have been the first investigator to address the problems surrounding storage methods and length of time for storage of human tissues.[17]

Although it appears that refrigerated skin grafts were successfully employed in the early 1900s, the routine banking of human tissue was delayed until reliable refrigeration methods became available in the 1930s. The development of the first blood bank at Cook County Hospital in 1937 provided the necessary security for the development and use of banked allograft skin. In 1944, Webster and Mathews reported the successful use of banked allograft skin after 3–8 weeks of refrigeration.[8,18] In 1945, Strumia and Hodge reported the successful use of frozen allograft stored in citrated plasma at –15°C for 1–16 days.[19] Controversy was created when Baxter and Entin demonstrated that skin exposed to dry ice was killed by ice crystal formation.[20] In 1949, Polge et al. noted that glycerol in a saline solution allowed frozen sperm to be thawed and remain viable.[21] Several investigators subsequently documented the survival of mammalian skin in the presence of glycerol under freezing conditions.[22] In 1956, Taylor et al. documented that glycerol reduced ice crystal formation in tissues with freezing.[23] It was not until 1964 that Lehr et al. reported that freezing of rat skin in a glycerol solution led to a successful 'take' when thawed and reapplied.[24] These experimental studies were repeated by Cochrane using a controlled freezing technique with liquid nitrogen storage of rat skin autograft at –100°C in 15% glycerol. A successful 'take' of the autograft was documented after 10 days of freezing with rapid rewarming.[25] In 1968, Cochrane reported the first successful clinical use of frozen skin autografts.[26] Subsequently, the burn units at Massachusetts General Hospital and the US Navy Skin Bank established methods for the storage of frozen skin. Although the development of various methods for tissue preservation evolved rapidly, each has specific indications and roles in a skin bank.

Hypothermia

Hypothermia involves the storage of allograft for future use in nutrient media at temperatures of 2–8°C.[27] It is believed that temperature reduction decreases oxygen consumption of viable cells secondary to a slowing of the metabolic rate. Hypothermia is intended for use only on a short-term basis, usually 14 days before the integrity of the allograft is called into question. To date, however, very little information exists as to the reduction in viability of the allograft and subsequent 'take' on patients within a 2-week period. Lehr et al. documented the survival of rat autograft skin for 10 days after simple refrigeration.[24]

Cryopreservation

A controlled rate for freezing of allograft is essential when the preservation of cell viability is crucial. Cryopreservation accomplishes this goal by the controlled freezing of tissue, typically 0.5–5.0°C/min in a cryoprotectant solution.[28] This method is usually computer controlled with liquid nitrogen as the coolant. Storage at –196°C in liquid nitrogen is standard for long-term maintenance. May and DeClements have shown that allograft treated with a cryoprotectant and placed in liquid nitrogen will retain 85% viability for 1 year.[29]

Rewarming

There is significant evidence to support the belief that cell viability is affected by the rate at which skin is rewarmed. More specifically, rapid rewarming at a rate of 50–70°C/min is essential to maintain cell viability.[28] Thus, for cryopreserved tissue, tempera-ture changes from –196°C to 0°C must occur in 3–4 minutes. In 1980, May and DeClements provided significant evidence to show that the flat packaging of skin allograft was 10 times more efficient in the rapid rewarming rate when compared to allograft stored in the rolled form.[30] These investigations also pointed out that flat packaging allowed more efficient storage of allograft skin, and thereby, increased efficiency and decreased liquid nitrogen requirements.

Regional skin banks and their governance

Regional skin banks have been established throughout the United States as a means to supply the increasing need for allograft skin as well as to provide a mechanism for the donation of cadaveric skin. Most skin banks have evolved into tissue banks with the harvesting of skin, but also cornea, various internal organs, heart valves, veins, and bone. Currently there are 250–300 tissue banks in the United States. About 100 of these banks are eye banks only and the remainder provide bone, skin, ligaments, cartilages, tendons, and other musculoskeletal transplants.[31] It is estimated that 30–35- tissue banks procure, process, and distribute skin from cadaveric donors. Although the amount of allograft skin used annually is unknown, May et al. estimated 6000 square feet annually among 19 skin banks in 1983.[32] In 1984, the Skin Council of the American Association of Tissue Banks (AATB) estimated the national yearly need for allograft skin to be 32 000 square feet.[33] These tissue banks supply large numbers of allograft tissue to local, regional, and national health care facilities. Consequently, this prompted the establishment of commercial tissue processing organizations. In 1989, the National Organ Transplantation Act (PL 98–507) was passed to prohibit the sale of human organs and tissues. Presently, two organizations heave emerged as leaders in the field of tissue banking. The AATB and the South Eastern Organ Procurement Foundation (SEOPF) have adopted guidelines and standards for tissue banking to ensure quality control of processed human tissue.[34]

In 1984, the AATB published Standards for Tissue Banking to ensure that all activities related to the collection, processing, storage, and distribution of human organs and tissue for medical use are carried out in a safe and professional manner. The standards set by the Skin Council of the AATB specifically outline the necessary protocols required for the establishment of a safe and ethical skin bank. In 1986, AATB developed a program of inspection and accreditation to insure compliance with the processes of retrieval and distribution of human tissue.[3,35]

The SEOPF was founded in 1969 with a primary focus on the transplantation of internal organs, especially kidneys. The SEOPF established the Tissue Banking Committee to provide a means of networking its scarce resources. The subsequent publication of Guidelines and Standards for Excision, Preparation, Storage and Distribution of Human Tissue Allografts for Transplantation in 1988 established guidelines for the technical and ethical standards of procurement, storage, and distribution of tissue similar to those designed by the AATB.[36]

More recently the Food and Drug Administration (FDA) issued specific guidelines for quality control of tissue bank specimens which echo preciously established guidelines set up by AATB.[37] In 1993, the FDA regulations recognized that although compliance with AATB's standards for the banking of various tissues should provide assurances of safety, the need for improved quality control in the future was apparent. Recently, the AATB has taken these major steps to upgrade its standards and, thus, to monitor compliance by accredited banks:[31]

- more rigid and precise testing requirements for potentially transmissible diseases;
- strengthening of the accreditation program by adding a trained, experienced, full-time staff;
- completion of the AATB Technical Manual to include detailed and responsible avenues for the provision of safe and effective tissue grafts.

Components of a Skin Bank

Since the development of an ability to store allograft skin, thousands of burn victims and patients with nonburn traumatic wounds have benefited. In most parts of the United States, legislation has been passed which enables hospitals to develop a mechanism whereby families of potential donors are informed of their opportunity to donate. According to the Uniform Anatomical Gift Act (UAGA), the recovery of organs and tissues from a deceased individual requires the consent of the next of kin, in order of priority, unless the deceased carries a properly signed and witnessed Uniform Donor Card. The UAGA outlines an order of priority for such a consent as follows: (1) spouse, (2) adult son or daughter, (3) either parent, (4) an adult brother or sister, (5) a guardian of the deceased other than guardian *ad litem*, and (6) any other person authorized or under obligation to dispose of the body.[31] In Philadelphia, the consent rate for requested skin donation from the 7% of acceptable donors was found to be 30%. Thus, skin donations were only obtained from 2% of all deaths screened.[38] The concept of skin donation can be difficult for relatives to understand and requires full explanations in order to alleviate fears of mutilation and disfigurement of the deceased at the time of open casket style funeral services.

Donor Referral

The establishment of a donor referral base is essential for the growth and development of a skin bank. Most hospitals have a centralized referral system for the dispersal of information related to donor procurement. This referral system may operate out of a hospital's emergency room or may be formalized into a decedent affairs department at a particular institution. In many areas, in-services are provided to these institutions by various organ procurement organizations (OPOs) which also serve to coordinate the harvesting of various organs and tissues for later use. Contracts between such OPOs and various hospitals are not uncommon. Consequently, skin banks usually are contacted by the OPO, although contracts between hospitals and skin banks do no exist.

Donor Selection

The establishment of a donor referral pattern ultimately necessitates the need for a routine screening process, which identifies any disease process and can eliminate a potential donor from being accepted. This is to insure that all procured skin is safe for transplantation. The suitability of any individual for tissue donation is based on medical and social history, clinical status, physical examination, and blood tests.

A general donor criteria worksheet is specifically designed to assess logistical issues such as legal consent for donation, location of the body, and time of death as well as medical history. The United States Public Health Service (USPHS) lists criteria for the exclusion of high-risk donors (**Table 14.1**). The USPHS criteria for unsuitable donors include men who have had sex with men since 1977, men and women who have exchanged sex for money or drugs since 1977, past or present intravenous drug abusers, certain hemophiliacs, and all sexual partners in the last 12 months of all persons in these categories. Also included are persons who in the past 12 months have had syphilis, gonorrhea, or have been exposed to known or potentially HIV-infected blood.[31] To date, more than 3 000 000 tissue transplants have been carried out since the identification of AIDS. AATB records indicate that only two donors' tissues have been associated with documented transmission of the human immunodeficiency virus.[31] Once the basic criteria are met, skin-specific criteria are then utilized to complete the screening process. Potential donors should be between 14 and 75 years of age; however, potential donors above or below this range should be evaluated for size, skin conditions, and state of health. Skin donor specific criteria include the absence of collagen vascular diseases, skin infections, acute burns, dermatitis, toxic exposure to chemicals, tattoos within 3 months or excessive skin trauma, obesity, or malnourishment.

Table 14.1 AATB guidelines for donor exclusion (revised November 1993)

Infection or sepsis by history, physical examination, and laboratory testing
History of intravenous drug use
History of neoplasm
History of hepatitis, syphilis, sow virus infection, AIDS, AIDS-related complex or high risk of AIDS
History of autoimmune disease
Positive serologic tests
Toxic substance in potentially toxic amounts in tissues to be collected
Evidence of serious illness of unknown cause
Death from unknown cause

Skin removal, processing, and cryopreservation

The recovery of skin from cadaveric donors is only instituted once donor selection, screening, and proper consent forms have been completed. All necessary arrangements for the time and location of the procurement are made by contacting the appropriate personnel and the procurement site. The tissue bank coordinator usually arranges for a procurement team to perform the recovery. The timing for the retrieval of skin should insure tissue quality and avoid delay of funeral service. Skin from cadaveric donors should be retrieved within 12 hours following the time of death if the donor is unrefrigerated and within 24 hours if the donor is refrigerated. No procedures are utilized which may interfere with investigations of a coroner or medical examiner. All donor skin is procured in an aseptic manner.

The initiation of the skin procurement process begins with an assessment of the donor. This is performed with gloves and protective garb. The body is properly identified and the overall appearance and condition of the body is observed as part of the final step in donor screening. Visual inspection of the skin is completed, and bruises, lacerations, abrasions, tattoos, dermatitis, acne, other skin lesions, or unusual marks are documented. The coordinator then makes a final decision to accept or decline the donation. It the donor is rejected, all of the appropriate personnel are notified. If the donor is accepted, the procedure table is cleansed with alcohol and the body placed onto the table, with the arms positioned such that they do not interface with draping or procurement. A head block is used to elevate the head so as to prevent or decrease periorbital swelling or bleeding. A puncture site is prepped with alcohol and at least 10 ml of blood are obtained from the donor. The femoral vein is the preferred site. The tubes are labeled by a unique donor number, placed in a biohazard zip-lock bag, and packed into an ice cooler.

In order to obtain usable skin donations, a donor must be prepared and the procedure must be carefully followed. The donor's hair is covered with a bouffant head cover and the body rinsed with tap water to remove any debris. Using clean washcloths or lap sponges, the donor is given a chlorhexidine bath and all hair is shaved from the nipple line down to the feet and from one side to the other side down the front of the body. The back is shaved from the shoulders to the feet. All hair and chlorhexidine are rinsed from the body and the table with clean water. The body is then prepped with iodophor from the shoulders on the back, down the trunk and continuing along both legs to the toes. The iodophor is then rinsed with alcohol, in a unidirectional manner and in a caudal direction. The procurement team then washes and dons sterile attire; and the donor is draped in a sterile fashion. The procurement team requires a 'circulator' and one or two 'scrub' technicians. Prior to the removal of skin, each area is moistened with saline sterile dermatome set at 0.010 inches and proper thickness of the skin strip is assessed. The depth gauge is then adjusted as needed. The depth of the cut is continually assessed throughout the procedure as different parts of the body require different settings.

After completely harvesting the skin from one side of the body, all skin strips are rinsed with sterile saline and placed in sterile jars with sterile RPMI-1640 media, 300 ml media for every square foot of skin. The jars are then placed into a cooler. The body is turned over; and the process is repeated. Clean-up includes: the discarding of all used, disposable items; washing of all instruments and donor with clean water; replacement of identification tags; and coverage of the body. Further duties include: completion of on-site retrieval documentation; cleaning of the tables, counters, cabinets, sinks, and floors; removal and proper disposal of all gowns, caps, masks, gloves, shoe cover, etc.; and finally, notification to the facility personnel that the procedure has been completed. Once the procurement team arrives at the skin bank, donor check-in procedures are essential in order to insure proper preservation of skin allograft and disposition of paperwork, serology, and culture laboratory tests. Serum of each donor is tested for anti-HIV-1/2, anti-HCV, anti-HTLV-1, HB$_s$Ag, and anti-HB$_c$, and RPR. Testing of cadaveric samples for HIV-1, HIV-2, and hepatitis B should be performed using test kits specifically labeled for screening of cadaveric blood specimens.[39] Under sterile conditions, skin samples are aseptically collected and tested for aerobic and anaerobic bacteria as well as yeast and fungi. Skin and blood samples are then stored in a separate refrigerator for 'UNPROCESSED – NOT CLEAR' tissues. The donor is entered into the donor log and assigned the next consecutive number. Once microbiology surveys and serology tests

have cleared, allograft skin is processed and packaged according to AATB Standards and Technical Manual Guidelines.

Tissues are processed and packaged individually so that there is no chance of cross-contamination between donors. Usually, two technicians verify that only one donor is being processed. Only skin from donors with negative serologies and microbiology is processed. Processing is carried out under sterile conditions in a biological safety cabinet. Tissue edges are trimmed and blocked according to preestablished standards in equal measurements of 0.25 square feet. If skin is to be meshed, the prepared skin (dermal side down) is placed on 4-inch wide gauze which extends 2 inches beyond each skin edge and folded. Skin must be frozen within 10 days of procurement using a control rate freezer and cryoprotectant.

Future considerations

Skin banking in the United States is in a state of flux. The FDA has issued regulations to strengthen federal oversight of tissue transplantation. The participation of AATB in the congressional considerations of new legislation is crucial. While it is apparent that the FDA requirements will build on AATB standards, AATB continues to strive in upgrading its own standards and requirements for tissue distribution.

Although all major tissue banks are either AATB accredited or pursuing accreditation to date, no program is in place to mandate compulsory registration of tissue banks, nor compliance with accepted donor screening criteria, procurement procedures, or processing methods for that tissue. In addition, the ability to track the distribution of tissue from donor to recipient must form an integral part of any system designed to regulate tissue banking. Uniform inspection procedures and scheduled recertification of tissue banks should address quality assurance issues. Presently, the AATB estimates that 90% of skin grafts distributed in the USA last year were produced by AATB accredited banks. However, it appears that only through mandated legislation at a national level will this compliance reach 100%.

References

1. Baxter CR, Marvin JA, Curreri PW. Early management of thermal burns. *Postgrad Med* 1974; 55: 131.
2. Tier WC, Sell KW. United States Navy Skin Bank. *Plast Reconstr Surg* 1968; 41: 543–8.
3. Reverdin JL. *Greffe Epidermique*. Bull de la Sol Imperiale de Chir de Paris. 1869; 493–511.
4. Girdner JH. Skin grafting with grafts from a dead subject. *Med Record NY* 1888; 20: 119–20.
5. Wolf JR. A new method of performing plastic operation. *Br Med J* 1875; 2: 360–5.
6. Thiersch JC. On skin grafting. *Verhandl 2nd Deutsch Ges Chir* 1886; 15: 17–20.
7. Bettman AG. Homogenous thiersch grafting as a life saving measure. *Am J Surg* 1938; 39: 156–62.
8. Webster JP. Refrigerated skin grafts. *Ann Surg* 1944; 120: 431–9.
9. Brown JB, Fryer MP, Randall P, Lu M. Post mortem homografts as 'biological dressings' for extensive burns and debrided areas. *Ann Surg* 1953; 138: 618–23.
10. Zaroff LI, Mills W, Duckett JW, Switzer WE, Moncrief JA. *Surgery* 1966; 59: 368–72.
11. Morris PJ, Bondac C, Burke JF. The use of frequently changed skin allografts to promote healing in the non-healing infected ulcer. *Surgery* 1966; 60: 13–19.
12. Eade GG. The relationship between granulation tissue, bacteria and skin grafts in burn patients. *Plast Reconstr Surg* 1958; 22: 42–55.
13. Woods WB. Phagocytosis with particular reference to encapsulated bacteria. *Bact Rev* 1960; 224: 41.
14. O'Donaghue MN, Zarem HA. Stimulation of neurovascularization. Comparative efficacy of fresh and preserved skin grafts in burn patients. *Plast Reconstr Surg* 1958; 22: 42–55.

15. Shuck JM, Pruitt BA, Moncrief JA. Homograft skin for wound coverage. *Arch Surg* 1969; **98**: 472–8.
16. Perry VP. A review of skin preservation cryobiology. 1966; **3(2)**: 109–30.
17. Carrel A. The preservation of tissues and its application to surgery. *JAMA* 1912; **59**: 523–7.
18. Mathews D. Storage of skin for autogenous grafts. *Lancet* 1945; **1**: 775.
19. Strumia MM, Hodge CC. Frozen human skin grafts. *Ann Surg* 1945; **121**: 860–5.
20. Baxter H, Entin ME. Experimental and clinical studies of reduced temperatures in injury and repair in man. III. Direct effect of cooling and freezing on various elements of the human skin. *Plast Reconstr Surg* 1948; **3**: 303–34.
21. Polge C, Smith VA, Parkes AS. Revival of spermatozoa after UV factors and dehydration at low temperatures. *Nature* 1949; **164**: 66.
22. Billingham RE, Medawer PB. The freezing, drying and storage of mammalian skin. *J Exp Biol* 1952; **29**: 454–68.
23. Taylor AC. Survival of rat skin and changes in hair pigmentation following freezing. *J Exp Zool* 1949; **110**: 77–112.
24. Lehr HB, Berggren RB, Lotke PA, Coriell LL. Permanent survival of preserved skin autograft. *Surgery* 1964; **56(4)**: 742–96.
25. Bondac CC, Burke JF. Clinical experience with viable frozen human skin and a frozen skin bank. *Ann Surg* 1971; **174(3)**: 371–82.
26. Cochrane ET. The low temperature storage of skin. A preliminary report. *Br J Plast Surg* 1966; 118–25.
27. Southard JH, Belzer FO. *Organ Preservation: Principles of Organ Transplantation.* Philadelphia: WB Saunders, 1989; **10**: 195.
28. American Association of Tissue Banks. *Technical Manual for Tissue Banking.* Arlington, VA: AATB, 1987.
29. May SR, DeClement FA. Skin banking. Part II. Low contamination cadaveric dermal allograft for temporary burn wound coverage. *J Burn Care Rehabil* 1981; **1**: 64–76.
30. May SR, DeClement FA. Skin banking methodology. Evaluations of packaging format, cooling and warming rates and storage efficiency. *Cryobiology* 1980; **17**: 33–45.
31. American Association of Tissue Banks. *Information Alert.* Arlington, VA: AATB, 1993; **3(6)**: 1–8.
32. May SR, Still JM, Atkinson WB. Recent developments in skin banking in the clinical uses of cryopreserved skin. *Med Assoc GA* 1984; **73**: 233–57.
33. Standards Committee of the Skin Council of the American Association of Tissue Banks. Guidelines for the banking of skin tissues. *Am Assoc Tissue Banks Newsletter* 1979; **3**: 5–8.
34. Leslie HW, Bottenfeid S. Donation banking and transplantation of allograft tissues. *Nurs Clin ANM* 1989; **24(4)**: 891–905.
35. American Association of Tissue Banks. *Standards for Tissue Banking.* Arlington, Virginia: AATB, 1998.
36. Southeastern Organ Procurement Foundation. *Guidelines and Standards for Excision, Preparation, Storage and Distribution of Human Tissue Allografts for Transplantation.* Richmond, VA: SEOPF, 1988.
37. Real ES and Regulations. *Federal Register* July 29, 1997 (62 FR 40429).
38. May SR, DeClements FA. Skin banking. Part 1. Procurement of transplantable cadaveric allograft for burn wound coverage. *J Bum Care Rehabil* 1981; **2**: 7–23.
39. FDA. Guidance for Industry: Availability of Licensed Donor Screening Tests Labeled for Use with Cadaveric Blood Specimens. *AATB Bulletin,* June 23, 2000.

Chapter 15

Alternative wound coverings
Robert L Sheridan, Ronald G Tompkins

Introduction

Serious short-term and long-term problems occur when the epidermal and dermal layers of the skin are destroyed. The short-term problems, which can be life-threatening, include the loss of protein-rich fluid and the invasion of bacteria and other microbes. These essential barrier functions are provided by the epidermis which consists of keratinocytes attached to an underlying basement membrane. The dermal layer provides for the durable and pliable characteristics of skin, which are so vital to proper skin function and cosmesis. When available, the replacement material of choice is the patient's own (autologous) skin as shown in an algorithm describing the decision process to treat acute burns. In smaller injuries, this can be accomplished by split-thickness sheet autograft (**Figure 15.1**). However in larger injuries, meshed autologous skin grafts are required.

Physiologic considerations

Skin is a truly amazing organ, rarely properly appreciated until it is missing. To date, all attempts to replace it, either temporarily or permanently, have been highly imperfect. As those with serious burns survive in increasing numbers, the absence of effective skin replacements is increasingly a hindrance to progress in burn care.

Structure and Function of the Skin

Skin, the body's largest organ, is incredibly complex. Functionally there are two layers with a highly specialized and effective bonding mechanism. Numerous appendages traverse the skin and a rich and reactive capillary network provides nutrient flow while con-

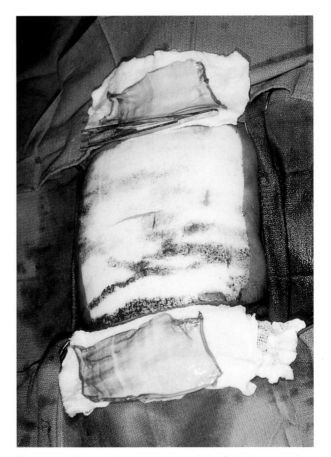

Fig. 15.1 The replacement material of choice remains the patient's own (autologous) skin.

trolling temperature. The epidermis, consisting of the strata basale, spinosum, granulosum, and corneum, provides a vapor and bacterial barrier. The dermis provides strength and elasticity. The thin epidermal layer is constantly refreshing itself from its basal layer, with new keratinocytes undergoing terminal differentiation over approximately 4 weeks to anuclear keratin-filled cells that make up the stratum corneum, which provides much of the barrier function of the epidermis. The basal layer of the epidermis is firmly attached to the dermis by a complex bonding mechanism containing collagen types IV and VII. When this bond fails, serious morbidity results, as demonstrated by the disease processes of toxic epidermal necrolysis[1] and epidermolysis bullosa[2] (**Figure 15.2**).

Consequences of Loss of Barrier Function

Loss of substantial areas of the epidermal barrier has immediate and profound adverse physiologic effects. Direct and evaporative fluid losses are immediately seen. If wounds are large, this quickly leads to dehydration and shock. Protein losses are also substantial, leading to loss of colloid oncotic pressure and secondary edema. Microrganisms have unimpeded access to the microcirculation with resulting systemic infection. Deep tissues become desiccated with secondary cell death and progression of wound depth. Dry

wounds will not epithelialize as readily. It is clearly important for the burn surgeon to have prompt biologic closure of wounds as an important early objective.

Although it is an imperfect replacement, autologous split-thickness skin is closest to being the ideal skin substitute (**Table 15.1**). Because of the paucity of autologous donor skin available in patients with massive burn injuries, both the short-term and long-term problems of skin loss must be solved by alternative wound closure materials. Alternative materials can be used for either wound coverage which will be temporary or for permanent wound closure. Currently, allogenic (cadaver) skin is the most commonly used alternative wound closure material. Many studies are underway, however, to develop materials that might substitute for the allografts and to contribute to permanent wound closure. This is an exciting and fast-paced area of research which is likely to profoundly impact the care of patients with serious burns. The objective of this chapter is to review the currently available alternative skin closure materials, both temporary and permanent.

Table 15.1 The perfect skin substitute – autologous split-thickness skin

- Prevents water loss
- Barrier to bacteria
- Inexpensive
- Long shelf life
- Can be applied in one operation
- Does not become hypertrophic
- Flexible
- Conforms to irregular wound surfaces
- Can be used 'off the shelf'
- Does not require refrigeration
- Cannot transmit viral diseases
- Does not incite inflammatory response
- Durable
- Easy to secure
- Grows with a child

Temporary skin substitutes

Temporary skin substitutes provide transient physiologic wound closure, thereby helping to control pain, absorb wound exudate, and prevent wound desiccation. They are clinically useful in several settings in burn care:

- as a dressing on donor sites to facilitate pain control and epithelialization from skin appendages;
- as a dressing on clean superficial wounds for the same reasons;
- to provide temporary physiologic closure of deep dermal and full-thickness wounds after excision while awaiting autografting or healing of underlying widely meshed autografts; and
- as a 'test' graft in questionable wound beds.

Their principal utility is provision of temporary physiologic closure of wounds which implies protection from mechanical trauma, vapor transmission characteristics similar to skin, and a physical barrier to bacteria. These membranes create a moist wound environment with a low bacterial density.

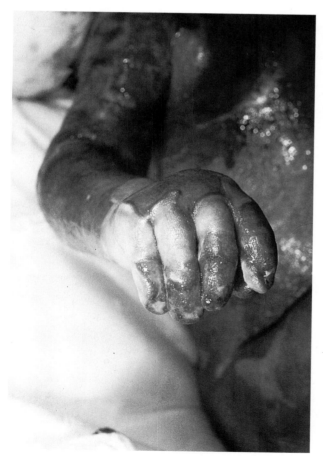

Fig. 15.2 The basal layer of the epidermis is firmly attached to the dermis by a complex bonding mechanism containing collagen types IV and VII. When this bond fails, serious morbidity results, as demonstrated here by the disease processes of dystrophic epidermolysis bullosa.

Human Allograft

Human allograft is generally used as a split-thickness graft after being procured from organ donors. When used in a viable fresh or cryopreserved state, it vascularizes and remains the 'gold standard' of temporary wound closures.[3–5] It can be refrigerated for up to 7 days, but can be stored for extended periods when cryopreserved. It is also used in a nonviable state after preservation in glycerol or after lyophilization; however, most existing data describe results when it is used in a viable state. Viable split-thickness allograft provides durable biologic cover until it is rejected by the host, usually within 3 or 4 weeks. Prolongation of allograft survival, through the use of antirejection drugs, has been advocated,[6] but is not generally practiced for fear that antirejection drugs will increase the risk of infection.[7]

Human skin allografts are generally placed into frozen storage awaiting the return of numerous laboratory tests allowing one to safely exclude the possibility of viral disease transmission. When modern screening techniques are followed, the risk of viral disease transmission is exceedingly small. Allograft is also effectively used in combination with meshed autograft in patients with large burns, the interstices of the meshed graft being immediately closed by the overlying unexpanded allograft, possibly reducing metabolic stress and local wound inflammation (**Figure 15.3**).

Human Amnion

Human amniotic membrane is used in many parts of the world as a temporary dressing for clean superficial wounds such as partial-thickness burns, donor sites, and freshly excised burns awaiting donor site availability.[8,9] Amniotic membrane is generally procured fresh and used after brief refrigerated storage.[10,11] It can also be used in a nonviable state after preservation with glycerol. It has been treated with silver to facilitate control of bacterial overgrowth.[12] Amnion does not vascularize[13] but still can provide effective temporary wound closure.[13] The principal concern with amnion is the difficulty in screening the material for viral diseases unless preservation methods can eliminate potential viral contamination. Without the ability to screen the material in this way, the risks of disease transmission must be balanced against the clinical need and the known characteristics of the donor.

Allogenic Epithelial Sheets

In many centers, particularly in Europe, sheets of allogenic and autogenous epithelium are used to dress partial-thickness wounds or to cover the interstices of meshed split-thickness autografts.[14,15] These are generally applied as thin sheets placed on a gauze carrier for ease of handling. Cell suspensions in fibrin sealant have also been trailed. The concept is that the sheets will both prevent desiccation of underlying wounds and that the release of unknown growth stimulating substances by the cells as they die will stimulate native wound healing.[16] The concept is attractive, but controlled data are not available, particularly as regards any impact on long-term outcomes.

Xenografts

Although various animal skins have been used for many years to provide temporary coverage of wounds,[17] only porcine xenograft is widely used today (**Figure 15.4**).[18] Porcine xenograft is commonly distributed as a reconstituted product consisting of homogenized porcine dermis which is fashioned into sheets and meshed.[19] Split-

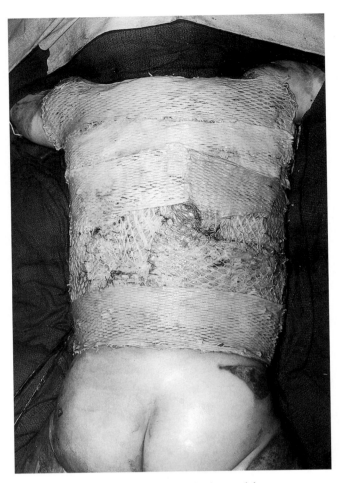

Fig. 15.3 Allograft is also effectively used in combination with meshed autograft in patients with large burns, the interstices of the meshed graft being immediately closed by the overlying unexpanded allograft, possibly reducing metabolic stress and local wound inflammation.

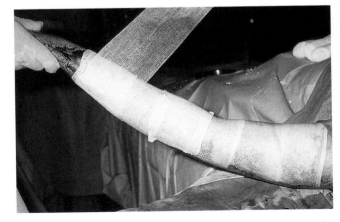

Fig. 15.4 Although various animal skins have been used for many years to provide temporary coverage of wounds, only porcine xenograft is widely used today.

thickness porcine skin is also used fresh, after brief refrigeration, after cryopreservation, or after glycerol preservation. It effectively provides temporary coverage of clean wounds such as superficial second degree burns and donor sites[20] and has been used in patients with toxic epidermal necrolysis.[1,21] Porcine xenograft has been combined with silver to suppress wound colonization.[22,23] Porcine xenograft does not vascularize, but it will adhere to a clean superficial wound and can provide excellent pain control while the underlying wound heals.

Synthetic Membranes

A number of semipermeable membrane dressings can provide a vapor and bacterial barrier and control pain while the underlying superficial wound or donor sites heal. These typically consist of a single semipermeable layer that provides a mechanical barrier to bacteria and has physiologic vapor transmission characteristics.[24,25] Biobrane™ (Dow-Hickham, Sugarland, TX) is a two-layer membrane constructed of an inner layer of nylon mesh that allows fibrovascular ingrowth and an outer layer of silastic that serves as a vapor and bacterial barrier.[26] It is widely used to provide temporary closure of superficial burns and donor sites. All synthetic membranes are occlusive and can foster infection if placed over contaminated wounds, especially in the presence of necrotic tissue.[27] Appropriate monitoring is essential to their proper use.

Hydrocolloid dressings are generally designed with a three-layer structure: a porous, gently adherent inner layer; a methyl cellulose absorbent middle layer; and a semipermeable outer layer. They foster a moist wound environment while absorbing exudate. A moist wound environment has been found to favor wound healing.[28] A variety of pastes and powders made from hydrocolloid materials are also widely available. These can be applied to superficial or deeper chronic wounds to absorb wound exudate while maintaining a moist wound environment.

Combined Allogenic and Synthetic Membranes

Epidermal growth factor, transforming growth factor-β, insulin-like growth factor (IGF), platelet-derived growth factors (PDGF), fibroblast growth factors, and other mediators play an important role in wound healing.[29,30] To provide some of these substances topically to wounds, investigators have placed both viable and nonviable allogenic cell types into temporary wound dressings.[31] These cells persist for no more than 14 days, but it is hoped that factors secreted by the allogeneic cells, or released upon their death and dissolution, will enhance wound healing. These membranes are generally regulated as both devices and biologics.

An allogeneic dermal–epidermal device that used a collagen lattice to culture both cell types was shown effective in an athymic mouse model[32–34] and then went into clinical trials. Although it has not been demonstrated to have a clinical role in burn patients, the device is being explored for utility in chronic ulcers of the lower extremity.[35–39] Dow-Hickam's Biobrane™ has been used as a scaffold to support the growth of allogenic fibroblasts. This device is currently undergoing evaluation as an adjunct to the management of dermal burns.[40–44] Viral transfection can be employed to modify keratinocytes so that they overexpress PDGF, human growth hormone, IGF-1, and other growth factors,[45] and it is possible that such cells might be employed as components of wound membranes over the next few years.[46] Although stimulation of wound healing by topical application of mixed growth factors in this fashion is an intriguing concept, convincing evidence of the concept's general validity is awaited.

Permanent skin substitutes

Realization of a practical permanent skin substitute will revolutionize the care of patients with burns and other difficult wounds. The perfect substitute is described in **Table 15.1**, but has yet to be approached by any currently available device. However, there are a number of imperfect or partial skin substitutes available at the present time that are valuable in particular clinical settings and may be the forerunners of this hypothetical ideal.

Epidermal Cells

For over 20 years it has been possible to culture vast numbers of epithelial cells from a small skin biopsy,[47,48] and this has led to the widespread clinical use of cultured epithelial grafts to cover burn wounds. Epithelial cells are procured from a full-thickness skin biopsy, the cells being separated with trypsin. The resulting epithelial cell suspension is cultured in medium containing fetal calf serum, insulin, transferrin, hydrocortisone, epidermal growth factor, and cholera toxin, overlying a layer of murine fibroblasts that have been treated with a nonlethal dose of radiation that prevents them from multiplying. Colonies of epithelial cells expand into broad sheets of undifferentiated epithelial cells. These cells are separated from the culture vessel with trypsin and taken to secondary culture using the same techniques until confluent thin sheets of undifferentiated cells are obtained. The resulting sheets are removed from the dishes after treatment with dipsase, which digests the proteins attaching the epithelial cells to the dish. The sheets of epithelial cells are attached to a petrolatum gauze carrier to ease handling.

When epithelial cultures were first used in patients with large burns it was hoped that they would provide the definitive answer to the clinical problem of the massive wound.[49–51] With more frequent use of epithelial grafts, specific liabilities have become apparent including suboptimal engraftment rates and long-term durability.[52,53] However, when faced with a very large wound and minimal donor sites, epithelial cell wound closure is a useful adjunct to split-thickness autograft, their liabilities and expense becoming more acceptable as wound size increases.

Many of the imperfections associated with epithelial cell wound closure may be attributed to the absence of a dermal element. Epithelial grafts are now commercially available. Application is generally most successful in wounds from which vascularized allograft has been removed. Despite scattered cases, application of cultured epithelial grafts onto synthetic dermal analogs has not been shown effective.

Dermal Analogs

Virtually all of the characteristics of normal skin that are not related to barrier function are provided by the dermis. These characteristics include flexibility, strength, heat dissipation and conservation, lubrication, and sensation. The first dermal substitute used clinically was 'artificial skin', also called Integra™ (Integra LifeSciences Corporation, Plainsboro, NJ, USA); it has been recently approved by the US Food and Drug Administration for use in life-threatening burns. This material was developed in the early 1980s by a biomaterials research team from the

Massachusetts General Hospital and Massachusetts Institute of Technology.[54] The research team, lead by surgeon John Burke from the Massachusetts General Hospital and materials scientist Ionnas Yannas from the Massachusetts Institute of Technology, had the goal of developing a wound covering that would both provide a temporary vapor and bacterial while providing a scaffold for later dermal regeneration. The material was intended to be placed on excised burn wounds and is now approved for clinical use. Its use for other indications is being explored. The inner layer of this material is a 2 mm thick combination of fibers of collagen isolated from bovine tissue and the glycosaminoglycan chondroitin-6-sulfate. This 2 mm thick inner layer has a 70–200 μm pore size that allows fibrovascular ingrowth, after which it is designed to slowly biodegrade.[55,56] To manufacture the device, glycosaminoglycan and collagen fibers are precipitated and then freeze-dried and cross-linked by glutaraldehyde. The outer layer of the membrane is 0.009-inch (0.23 mm) thick polysiloxane polymer with vapor transmission characteristics similar to normal epithelium. This membrane is intended to be placed on freshly excised full-thickness burns and the outer silicone membrane replaced with an ultra-thin epithelial autograft 2–3 weeks later (**Figure 15.5**).[57] Clinical reports in patients with large burns have been generally favorable,[58–60] although submembrane infection must be watched for. Post-marketing trials of Integra™ are in progress.

Another currently available device designed as a dermal replacement is cryopreserved allogenic dermis. This material is intended to be combined with a thin epithelial autograft at the time of initial wound closure. It is marketed as AlloDerm® (LifeCell Corporation, The Woodlands, TX, USA).[61,62] Split-thickness allograft skin is obtained from cadaver donors through tissue banks after proper screening for transmissible diseases. Using hypertonic saline, the epithelial elements of the grafts are removed and the remaining dermis is treated in a detergent to inactivate any viruses and the device is freeze-dried. The process is intended to provide a nonantigenic dermal scaffold, leaving basement membrane proteins (particularly laminin and type IV and VII collagen) intact. The material is rehydrated immediately prior to placement on wounds with overlying ultra-thin epithelial autograft (**Figure 15.6**). Clinical experi-

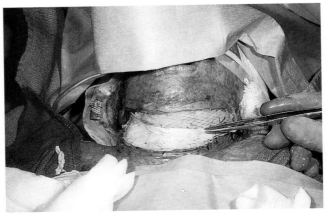

Fig. 15.6 AlloDerm® is rehydrated immediately prior to placement on wounds with overlying ultra-thin epithelial autograft.

ence with this material in burn surgery is limited, but early experiences have been favorable.[63,64]

Generating a dermal replacement through the prior use of human split-thickness allograft is another strategy with significant clinical support. This has been done on occasion for many years by surgeons who 'leave behind' remnants of vascularized allograft dermis when replacing allograft with thin split-thickness autografts in patients with large injuries. This has been modified for use with cultured epithelial grafts, such that the cultured epithelial cells are placed on wounds closed initially with vascularized allograft. Once allograft has vascularized, the allogeneic epithelial cells are removed by dermabrasion or tangential excision, purposefully leaving behind a vascularized but theoretically nonantigenic allogenic dermal layer.[65–67] The method has been favorably reported,[68,69] but has not been universally adopted. Perhaps the epithelial excision either leaves behind nests of antigenic epithelial cells if too superficial or removes the epidermal–dermal attachment structures if too deep.

Composite Substitutes

Ideally, a skin replacement technique would provide immediate replacement of both dermal and epidermal layers. Combining epithelial cells with a dermal analog in the laboratory seems logical. A completely biologic composite skin substitute, culturing human fibroblasts in a collagen-glycosaminoglycan membrane, and then growing keratinocytes upon this, has been under development for some years.[70,71] This composite membrane has been successful in a nude mouse model,[72] but engraftment was suboptimal in a small clinical series.[73] This potentially exciting technology continues to be refined in laboratory and clinical investigations.[74] A similar project, in which autogenic epithelial cells are cultured onto allogenic dermis, is underway.[75] This device was also successful in a small animal model, and is in early clinical pilot trials. It remains to be seen if either technique will lead to a reliable and durable permanent skin replacement.

The future of alternative wound coverings

We are likely to see significant improvements in skin substitute technologies, both temporary and permanent, over the next few

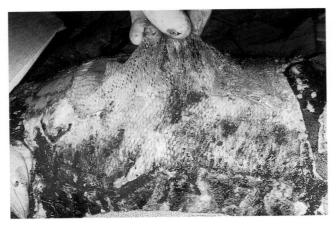

Fig. 15.5 Integra™ is intended to be placed on freshly excised full-thickness burns and the outer silicone membrane replaced with an ultra-thin epithelial autograft 2–3 weeks later.

years. In temporary wound coverings, not only are improved synthetics and improved skin banking techniques probable but we may see temporary dressings containing growth factor secreting allogenic tissues that stimulate native wound healing. Genetic modification of keratinocytes is now possible. These cells have been engineered to overexpress PDGF, human growth hormone, IGF-1, and other growth factors.[45] It is likely that they will be trialled in animal models and human wounds over the next few years.[46] If they prove efficacious, their application to healing burns and donor sites, through incorporation in temporary dressings, may become possible. It might be further possible to combine autogenous cells with modified allogenic cells such that the resulting chimeric graft benefits from transient overexpression of critical growth factors during the early stages of engraftment.

As we become increasingly successful at salvaging the lives of those with large burns, our need for a durable and reliable permanent skin substitute becomes increasingly acute. This material is needed both to truncate the acute illness through earlier wound closure and to facilitate timely and effective burn reconstruction. Just what form that substitute will take is not clear. Most likely, it would seem to be an *in vitro* combination of autologous keratinocytes and possibly fibroblasts and/or endothelial cells with a dermal analog. Whatever form the successful replacement takes, it is certain to profoundly impact the field of burn care.

References

1. Heimbach DM, Engrav LH, Marvin JA, Harnar TJ, Grube BJ. Toxic epidermal necrolysis. A step forward in treatment [published erratum appears in *JAMA* 1987; 258(14): 1894]. *JAMA* 1987; **257**: 2171–5.
2. Fine JD, Johnson LB, Cronce D, *et al.* Intracytoplasmic retention of type VII collagen and dominant dystrophic epidermolysis bullosa: reversal of defect following cessation of or marked improvement in disease activity. *J Invest Dermatol* 1993; **101**: 232–6.
3. Bondoc CC, Burke JF. Clinical experience with viable frozen human skin and a frozen skin bank. *Ann Surg* 1971; **174**: 371–82.
4. Herndon DN. Perspectives in the use of allograft. *J Burn Care Rehabil* 1997; **18**: S6.
5. May SR, Still JM Jr, Atkinson WB. Recent developments in skin banking and the clinical uses of cryopreserved skin. [Review]. *J Med Assoc GA.* 1957; **73**: 233–6.
6. Burke JF, May JW Jr, Albright N, Quinby WC, Russell PS. Temporary skin transplantation and immunosuppression for extensive burns. *N Engl J Med* 1974; **290**: 269–71.
7. Bale JF Jr, Kealey GP, Ebelhack CL, Platz CE, Goeken JA. Cytomegalovirus infection in a cyclosporine-treated burn patient: case report. *J Trauma* 1992; **32**: 263–7.
8. Ramakrishnan KM, Jayaraman V. Management of partial-thickness burn wounds by amniotic membrane: a cost-effective treatment in developing countries. *Burns* 1997; **23(Suppl 1)**: S33–6.
9. Subrahmanyam M. Amniotic membrane as a cover for microskin grafts. *Br J Plast Surg* 1995; **48**: 477–8.
10. Ganatra MA, Durrani KM. Method of obtaining and preparation of fresh human amniotic membrane for clinical use. *J Pakistan Med Assoc* 1996; **46**: 126–8.
11. Thomson PD, Parks DH. Monitoring, banking, and clinical use of amnion as a burn wound dressing. *Ann Plast Surg* 1981; **7**: 354–6.
12. Haberal M, Oner Z, Bayraktar U, Bilgin N. The use of silver nitrate-incorporated amniotic membrane as a temporary dressing. *Burns Thermal Injury* 1987; **13**: 159–63.
13. Quinby WC Jr, Hoover HC, Scheflan M, Walters PT, Slavin SA, Bondoc CC. Clinical trials of amniotic membranes in burn wound care. *Plast Reconstr Surg* 1982; **70**: 711–17.
14. Braye F, Oddou L, Bertin-Maghit M, *et al.* Widely meshed autograft associated with cultured autologous epithelium for the treatment of major burns in children: report of 12 cases. *Eur J Pediatr Surg* 2000; **10**: 35–40.
15. Horch RE, Corbei O, Formanek-Corbei B, Brand-Saberi B, Vanscheidt W, Stark GB. Reconstitution of basement membrane after 'sandwich-technique' skin grafting for severe burns demonstrated by immunohistochemistry. *J Burn Care Rehabil* 2000; **19**: 189–202.
16. Phillips TJ, Gilchrest BA. Cultured epidermal allografts as biological wound dressings. *Prog Clin Biol Res* 2000; **365**: 77–94.
17. Song IC, Bromberg BE, Mohn MP, Koehnlein E. Heterografts as biological dressings for large skin wounds. *Surgery* 1966; **59**: 576–83.
18. Elliott RA Jr, Hoehn JG. Use of commercial porcine skin for wound dressings. *Plast Reconstr Surg* 1973; **52**: 401–5.
19. Ersek RA, Hachen HJ. Porcine xenografts in the treatment of pressure ulcers. *Ann Plast Surg* 1980; **5**: 464–70.
20. Chatterjee DS. A controlled comparative study of the use of porcine xenograft in the treatment of partial thickness skin loss in an occupational health centre. *Curr Med Res Opin* 1978; **5**: 726–33.
21. Marvin JA, Heimbach DM, Engrav LH, Harnar TJ. Improved treatment of the Stevens-Johnson syndrome. *Arch Surg* 1984; **119**: 601–5.
22. Ersek RA, Navarro JA. Maximizing wound healing with silver-impregnated porcine xenograft. *Todays OR Nurse* 1990; **12**: 4–9.
23. Ersek RA, Denton DR. Silver-impregnated porcine xenografts for treatment of meshed autografts. *Ann Plast Surg* 1984; **13**: 482–7.
24. Salisbury RE, Wilmore DW, Silverstein P, Pruitt BA Jr. Biological dressings for skin graft donor sites. *Arch Surg* 1973; **106**: 705–6.
25. Salisbury RE, Carnes RW, Enterline D. Biological dressings and evaporative water loss from burn wounds. *Ann Plast Surg* 1980; **5**: 270–2.
26. Demling RH. Burns. *N Engl J Med* 1985; **313**: 1389–98.
27. Bacha EA, Sheridan RL, Donohue GA, Tompkins RG. Staphylococcal toxic shock syndrome in a paediatric burn unit. *Burns* 1994; **20**: 499–502.
28. Vanstraelen P. Comparison of calcium sodium alginate (KALTOSTAT) and porcine xenograft (E-Z DERM) in the healing of split-thickness skin graft donor sites. *Burns* 1992; **18**: 145–8.
29. Greenhalgh DG. The role of growth factors in wound healing. [Review]. *J Trauma* 1996; **41**: 159–67.
30. Bennett NT, Schultz GS. Growth factors and wound healing: biochemical properties of growth factors and their receptors. [Review]. *Am J Surg* 1993; **165**: 728–37.
31. Teepe RG, Koch R, Haeseker B. Randomized trial comparing cryopreserved cultured epidermal allografts with tulle-gras in the treatment of split-thickness skin graft donor sites. *J Trauma* 1993; **35**: 850–4.
32. Bell E, Ehrlich HP, Buttle DJ, Nakatsuji T. Living tissue formed *in vitro* and accepted as skin-equivalent tissue of full thickness. *Science* 1981; **211**: 1052–4.
33. Nolte CJ, Oleson MA, Hansbrough JF, Morgan J, Greenleaf G, Wilkins L. Ultrastructural features of composite skin cultures grafted onto athymic mice. *J Anat* 1994; **185**: 325–33.
34. Hansbrough JF, Morgan J, Greenleaf G, Parikh M, Nolte C, Wilkins L. Evaluation of graftskin composite grafts on full-thickness wounds on athymic mice. *J Burn Care Rehabil* 1994; **15**: 346–53.
35. Gentzkow GD, Iwasaki SD, Hershon KS, *et al.* Use of dermagraft, a cultured human dermis, to treat diabetic foot ulcers [see comments]. *Diabetes Care* 1996; **19**: 350–4.
36. Sacks MS, Chuong CJ, Petroll WM, Kwan M, Halberstadt C. Collagen fiber architecture of a cultured dermal tissue. *J Biomechan Engin* 1997; **119**: 124–7.
37. Economou TP, Rosenquist MD, Lewis RW II, Kealey GP. An experimental study to determine the effects of Dermagraft on skin graft viability in the presence of bacterial wound contamination. *J Burn Care Rehabil* 1995; **16**: 27–30.
38. Falanga V, Sabolinski M. A bilayered living skin construct (APLIGRAF) accelerates complete closure of hard-to-heal venous ulcers. *Wound Repair Regen* 2000; **7**: 201–7.
39. Wickware P. Progress from a fragile start. *Nature* 2000; **403**: 466.
40. Hansbrough JF, Morgan J, Greenleaf G, Underwood J. Development of a temporary living skin replacement composed of human neonatal fibroblasts cultured in Biobrane, a synthetic dressing material. *Surgery* 1994; **115**: 633–44.
41. Hansbrough J. Dermagraft-TC for partial-thickness burns: a clinical evaluation. *J Burn Care Rehabil* 1997; **18**: S25–8.
42. Parente ST. Estimating the economic cost offsets of using Dermagraft-TC as an alternative to cadaver allograft in the treatment of graftable burns. *J Burn Care Rehabil* 1997; **18**: S18–24.
43. Spielvogel RL. A histological study of Dermagraft-TC in patients' burn wounds. *J Burn Care Rehabil* 1997; **18**: S16–18.
44. Purdue GF. Dermagraft-TC pivotal efficacy and safety study. *J Burn Care Rehabil* 1997; **18**: S13–14.
45. Morgan JR, Barrandon Y, Green H, Mulligan RC. Expression of an exogenous growth hormone gene by transplantable human epidermal cells. *Science* 1987; **237**: 1476–9.
46. Morgan JR, Yarmush ML. Bioengineered skin substitutes. *Sci Med* 1997; July/August: 6–15.
47. Rheinwald JG, Green H. Serial cultivation of strains of human epidermal keratinocytes: the formation of keratinizing colonies from single cells. *Cell* 1975; **6**: 331–43.

48. Green H, Kehinde O, Thomas J. Growth of cultured human epidermal cells into multiple epithelia suitable for grafting. *Proc Natl Acad Sci USA* 1979; **76**: 5665–8.

49. Green H. Cultured cells for the treatment of disease. [Review]. *Sci Am* 1991; **265**: 96–102.

50. Gallico GG III, O'Connor NE, Compton CC, Kehinde O, Green H. Permanent coverage of large burn wounds with autologous cultured human epithelium. *N Engl J Med* 1984; **311**: 448–51.

51. Gallico GG III, O'Connor NE, Compton CC, Remensnyder JP, Kehinde O, Green H. Cultured epithelial autografts for giant congenital nevi [see comments]. *Plast Reconstr Surg* 1989; **84**: 1–9.

52. Sheridan RL, Tompkins RG. Cultured autologous epithelium in patients with burns of ninety percent or more of the body surface. *J Trauma* 1995; **38**: 48–50.

53. Rue LW III, Cioffi WG, McManus WF, Pruitt BA Jr. Wound closure and outcome in extensively burned patients treated with cultured autologous keratinocytes. *J Trauma* 1993; **34**: 662–7.

54. Tompkins RG, Burke JF. Progress in burn treatment and the use of artificial skin. [Review]. *World J Surg* 1990; **14**: 819–24.

55. Yannas IV, Burke JF, Warpehoski M, *et al.* Prompt, long-term functional replacement of skin. *Trans Am Soc Artif Intern Organs* 1981; **27**: 19–23.

56. Yannas IV, Burke JF, Orgill DP, Skrabut EM. Wound tissue can utilize a polymeric template to synthesize a functional extension of skin. *Science* 1982; **215**: 174–6.

57. Tompkins RG, Hilton JF, Burke JF, *et al.* Increased survival after massive thermal injuries in adults: preliminary report using artificial skin. *Crit Care Med* 1989; **17**: 734–40.

58. Scalea TM, Simon HM, Duncan AO, *et al.* Geriatric blunt multiple trauma: improved survival with early invasive monitoring. *J Trauma* 1990; **30**: 129–34; discussion 134–6.

59. Sheridan RL, Heggerty M, Tompkins RG, Burke JF. Artificial skin in massive burns – results at ten years. *Eur J Plast Surg* 1994; **17**: 91–3.

60. Heimbach D, Luterman A, Burke J, *et al.* Artificial dermis for major burns. A multi-center randomized clinical trial. *Ann Surg* 1988; **208**: 313–20.

61. Wainwright DJ. Use of an acellular allograft dermal matrix (Alloderm) in the management of full-thickness burns. *Burns* 1995; **21**: 243–8.

62. Wainwright D, Madden M, Luterman A, *et al.* Clinical evaluation of an acellular allograft dermal matrix in full-thickness burns. *J Burn Care Rehabil* 1996; **17**: 124–36.

63. Sheridan RL, Choucair RJ. Acellular allograft dermis does not hinder initial engraftment in burn resurfacing and reconstruction. *J Burn Care Rehabil.* 1997; **18**: 496–9.

64. Sheridan RL, Choucair RJ. Acellular allodermis in burn surgery: 1-year results of a pilot trial. *J Burn Care Rehabil* 1998; **19**: 528–30.

65. Langdon RC, Cuono CB, Birchall N, *et al.* Reconstitution of structure and cell function in human skin grafts derived from cryopreserved allogeneic dermis and autologous cultured keratinocytes. *J Invest Dermatol* 1988; **91**: 478–85.

66. Cuono CB, Langdon R, Birchall N, Barttelbort S, McGuire J. Composite autologous-allogeneic skin replacement: development and clinical application. *Plast Reconstr Surg* 1987; **80**: 626–37.

67. Cuono C, Langdon R, McGuire J. Use of cultured epidermal autografts and dermal allografts as skin replacement after burn injury. *Lancet* 1986; **1**: 1123–4.

68. Hickerson WL, Compton C, Fletchall S, Smith LR. Cultured epidermal autografts and allodermis combination for permanent burn wound coverage. *Burns* 1994; **20** (Suppl 1): S52–5; discussion S55–6.

69. Compton CC, Hickerson W, Nadire K, Press W. Acceleration of skin regeneration from cultured epithelial autografts by transplantation to homograft dermis. *J Burn Care Rehabil* 1993; **14**: 653–62.

70. Boyce ST, Christianson DJ, Hansbrough JF. Structure of a collagen-GAG dermal skin substitute optimized for cultured human epidermal keratinocytes. *J Biomed Materials Res* 1988; **22**: 939–57.

71. Boyce ST, Hansbrough JF. Biologic attachment, growth, and differentiation of cultured human epidermal keratinocytes on a graftable collagen and chondroitin-6-sulfate substrate. *Surgery* 1988; **103**: 421–31.

72. Cooper ML, Hansbrough JF. Use of a composite skin graft composed of cultured human keratinocytes and fibroblasts and a collagen-GAG matrix to cover full-thickness wounds on athymic mice. *Surgery* 1991; **109**: 198–207.

73. Hansbrough JF, Boyce ST, Cooper ML, Foreman TJ. Burn wound closure with cultured autologous keratinocytes and fibroblasts attached to a collagen-glycosaminoglycan substrate. *JAMA* 1989; **262**: 2125–30.

74. Hansbrough JF, Morgan JL, Greenleaf GE, Bartel R. Composite grafts of human keratinocytes grown on a polyglactin mesh-cultured fibroblast dermal substitute function as a bilayer skin replacement in full-thickness wounds on athymic mice. *J Burn Care Rehabil* 1993; **14**: 485–94.

75. Sheridan RL, Morgan JR. Initial clinical experience with an autologous composite skin substitute. *J Burn Care Rehabil* 2000; **21**: S214.

Inhalation injury

Chapter 16

The pathophysiology of inhalation injury

Daniel L Traber, David N Herndon, Kazutaka Soejima

injured patients.[3,4] Although that may still be true today, many new things have been learned that have reduced the morbidity and mortality in burned patients who have sustained a concomitant inhalation injury.[5] While some have reported little progress has been made in reducing the mortality associated with inhalation injury,[6] others have noted significant progress,[5] improved techniques for ventilating the patient,[7] more aggressive fluid therapy,[8,9] and better techniques for trachea bronchial toilet. Better understanding of the pathophysiology caused by cutaneous burn and smoke to the lung will lead to even further advances in the treatment of the lesions.

Toxic smoke compounds

Approximately 80% of fire-related deaths occur, not from burn injury to the airway, but from inhalation of the toxic products of combustion.[10] Many of these compounds may act synergistically to increase mortality. This is especially true for carbon monoxide and hydrogen cyanide[11,12] where a synergistic effect has been found to increase tissue hypoxia and acidosis,[11] and may also decrease cerebral oxygen consumption and metabolism.[13] Incapacitation of potential victims may be potentiated by the blinding and irritating effects of smoke as well as by the decreasing oxygen concentration that occurs with combustion and results in progressive hypoxia. The extent of inhalation damage produced depends on the ignition source and temperature generated as well as the concentration and solubility of the toxic gases generated. It is thus imperative to obtain knowledge of both the source of the fire and the combustion products generated when treating a fire victim (**Table 16.1**).

Carbon monoxide toxicity

Carbon monoxide (CO) toxicity remains one of the most frequent immediate causes of death in smoke-induced inhalation injury; it must be suspected in every fire victim and treated promptly. Inhalation of a 0.1% carbon monoxide mixture may result in generation of a carboxyhemoglobin level as high as 50%. In fact, carbon monoxide has an affinity for hemoglobin that is 200–250 times that of oxygen; therefore, it readily combines with it resulting in a decrease in oxyhemoglobin saturation, leading to anoxia and death. The oxygen–hemoglobin dissociation curve loses its sigmoid shape and is shifted to the left, thus further impairing tissue oxygen availability.[12] Competitive inhibition with cytochrome oxidase enzyme systems, most notably cytochrome P-450, results in an inability of cellular systems to utilize oxygen.[14] Lower concentrations of CO may also impair decision-making and psychomotor responses.[15]

Symptoms and Signs

Diagnosis may be difficult and few symptoms generally occur when the carboxyhemoglobin level is less than 10%.[15] Toxic symp-

Introduction

It has been over a decade since the authors published their first manuscript on inhalation injury.[1,2] In the review article published the next year it was reported that that inhalation injury was a main, if not *the* main, factor responsible for mortality in thermally

Table 16.1 Origin of selected toxic compounds other than CO or CO₂ (From Prien and Traber[12].)		
Material	Source	Decomposition products
Cellulose	Wood, paper, cotton, jute	Aldehydes, acrolein
Wool, silk	Clothing, fabric, blankets, furniture	Hydrogen cyanide, ammonia, hydrogen sulfide
Rubber	Tires	Sulfur dioxide, hydrogen sulfide
PVC	Upholstery, wire/pipe coating, wall, floor, furniture coverings	Hydrogen chloride, phosgene
Polyurethane	Insulation, upholstery material	Hydrogen cyanide, isocyanates, ammonia, acrylonitriles
Polyester	Clothing, fabric	Hydrogen chloride
Polypropylene	Upholstery, carpeting	Acrolein
Polyacrylonitrile	Appliances, engineering plastics	Hydrogen cyanide
Polyamide	Carpeting, clothing	Hydrogen cyanide, ammonia
Melamine resins	Household and kitchen goods	Hydrogen cyanide, ammonia, formaldehyde
Acrylics	Aircraft windows, textiles, wall coverings	Acrolein

toms become manifest at levels greater than 20% and death may occur at levels greater than 60% (**Table 16.2**). Diagnosis may be facilitated by use of on-site portable breath analyzers or by direct measurement of the carboxyhemoglobin level in a venous or arterial blood sample. However, as high oxygen concentrations are usually administered to the victim in transit to hospital, and there is also some delay from cessation of exposure to measurement of the level, tests may thus not reflect the true extent of exposure.[16] Carter et al. have found a close correlation between carboxyhemoglobin levels and the incidence of inhalation injury.[17] They devised a nomogram whereby the level of carboxyhemoglobin at the time of injury could be estimated. The carboxyhemoglobin is determined, and the time elapsed estimated. In animal studies, the authors have found a close correlation between the duration of smoke exposure and carboxyhemoglobin levels.[18]

Table 16.2 Symptoms and signs at various concentrations of carboxyhemoglobin[43,127]	
CO-Hb%	Signs and symptoms
0–10	None
10–20	Tightness over forehead, slight headache, dilation of cutaneous blood vessels
20–30	Headache and throbbing in the temples
30–40	Severe headache, weakness, dizziness, dimness of vision, nausea, vomiting, collapse
40–50	As above; greater possibility of collapse, syncope, increased pulse and respiratory rate
50–60	Syncope, increased pulse and respiratory rate, coma, intermittent convulsions, Cheyne–Stokes respirations
60–70	Coma, intermittent convulsions, depressed cardiac and respiratory function, possible death
70–80	Weak pulse, slow respirations, death within hours
80–90	Death in less than 1 hour
90–100	Death within minutes

Treatment

The half-life of carboxyhemoglobin is 250 minutes in room air, to 40–60 minutes in a person breathing 100% oxygen; therefore all fire victims should commence 100% oxygen while in transit to hospital.[19] This allows delivery of an inspired oxygen concentration of 50–60%, which is usually adequate. If, however, loss of consciousness, cyanosis, or an inability to maintain the airway is present, then endotracheal intubation, which will allow delivery of 100% oxygen to the patient, may be necessary.

Hyperbaric oxygen therapy may be necessary if the carboxyhemoglobin level exceeds 25% or if significant clinical toxicity is present. Administration of three atmospheres of pressure will further reduce the carboxyhemoglobin half-life to 30 minutes.[20,21] Carbon monoxide may cause xanthine dehydrase to convert to xanthine oxidase;[22] the latter is associated with the formation of oxygen free radicals and tissue damage.[23] Treatment with hyperbaric oxygen will convert the xanthine oxidase back to its less toxic dehydrogenase. If neurological impairment persists, this treatment may be repeated.[21] Finally, as many as 10% of survivors may demonstrate a 'pseudorecovery' associated with neurological or mental deterioration some months after an initial recovery.[15] Hyperbaric oxygen may reduce these neurological problems.[24]

Hydrogen cyanide toxicity

Hydrogen cyanide is produced in fires involving nitrogen-containing polymers and may produce a rapid and lethal incapacitation of a victim at the fire source, with death occurring later either from cyanide or carbon monoxide toxicity or from burn-related pathology.[25] Toxicity is produced by inhibition of cellular oxygenation with resultant tissue anoxia, which is caused by reversible inhibition of cytochrome oxidase (Fe^{3+}) by cyanide.[16]

Symptoms and Signs

Diagnosis at the fire scene may be difficult and should be suspected in a patient with an underlying lactic acidosis that is not rapidly responsive to oxygen therapy.[17,26] Concentrations greater than 20 ppm are considered dangerous (**Table 16.3**). A distinctive odor of bitter almonds may initially arouse suspicion of cyanide toxicity in a fire victim. Symptoms may progress rapidly, and include lethargy, nausea, headache, weakness, and coma. Cardiovascular symptoms include acute electrocardiograph S-T segment elevation, which may mimic an acute myocardial infarction.[27] Cyanide increases ventilation through carotid body and peripheral chemoreceptor stimulation; this may augment toxicity in the early stages. Death is later caused by respiratory center paralysis (>100 ppm). Hydrogen cyanide is found routinely in low levels blood of healthy individuals at levels of 0.02 µg/ml in nonsmokers and 0.04 µg/ml in smokers. Toxicity occurs at a level of 0.1 µg/ml, and at 1.0 µg/ml death is likely.[28]

Table 16.3 Hydrogen cyanide concentrations in air and associated symptoms in humans[9,127]

HCN concentration (ppm)	Symptoms
0.2–5.0	Threshold of odor
10	TLV-MAC
18–36	Slight symptoms (headache) after several hours
45–54	Tolerated for 0.5–1 hour without difficulty
100	Death in 1 hour
110–135	Fatal in 0.5–1 hour
181	Fatal in 10 minutes
280	Immediately fatal

Treatment

Controversy surrounds the management of hydrogen cyanide poisoning, as treatment may in itself be hazardous. Such treatment may, however, be considered in a hypoxic or an unconscious victim. Oxygen therapy has been found beneficial, though hyperbaric oxygen is not recommended.[27,28] Nitrate administration results in oxidation of hemoglobin to methemoglobin, which then competes with cytochrome oxidase for cyanide.[12] Methemoglobin, however, decreases oxygen transport capacity and may thus worsen the prognosis if administered.[29] Sodium thiosulfate administration, in the presence of the mitochondrial enzyme rhodanese, results in the transfer of sulfur to the cyanide ion, forming thiocyanate. Toxicity is minimal other than an osmotic diuretic action, which in itself may be beneficial. Onset of action, however, is quite slow.[12] Chelating agents, which form a complex with cyanide, thus increasing its renal excretion, may also be administered. Cobalt EDTA is relatively toxic and may cause cardiovascular instability and anaphylaxis; therefore, hydroxocobalamin may be preferable as it is nontoxic apart from causing occasional urticarial reactions.[12,27] In summary, suitable treatment at the fire site involves intravenous administration of sodium thiosulfate (125–250 mg/kg) and hydroxocobalamin (4 g). One hundred percent oxygen should also be given.

Other degradation products

Other degradation products may also contribute substantially to the morbidity and mortality in a burn victim. Hydrogen chloride is produced by polyvinyl chloride degradation and causes severe respiratory tract damage and pulmonary edema. Nitrogen oxides may cause pulmonary edema and a chemical pneumonitis and may contribute to cardiovascular depression and acidosis. Aldehydes, such as acrolein and acetaldehyde, which are found in wood and kerosene, may further contribute towards pulmonary edema and respiratory irritability. The most important aspect of management of acute inhalation toxicology involves the prompt removal of victims from the fire site to minimize further exposure to toxic combustion products which may initially 'stun' and render them unable to escape from the fire, and eventually may cause toxicity as discussed above. Prompt administration of oxygen, maintenance of the basic ABCs of airway, breathing and circulation, and rapid hospitalization are then of paramount importance. Finally, a high index of suspicion and a thorough knowledge of the appropriate management of the smoke inhalation victim is essential in assuring a good prognosis.

Injury to the oropharynx

Much of the pathophysiology that occurs with inhalation injury is related to edema formation, which is the result of an increased transvascular fluid flux. Before a discussion of the changes following inhalation injury, a review of the forces responsible for the variables of the Starling–Landis equation[30,31] should be reviewed:

$$J_v = K_f[(P_c - P_{if}) - \sigma(COP_p - COP_{if})]$$

This equation describes the physical forces and physiologic mechanisms that govern fluid transfer between vascular and extravascular compartments. J_v, the transvascular fluid flux, is equal to lymph flow during equilibrium states. As transvascular fluid flux increases, interstitial volume also increases (edema formation) until a new equilibrium with lymph flow occurs. K_f is the filtration coefficient, an index of the total number of pores that are filtering. The number of pores could increase if a larger area of the microcirculation were perfused or if there were more pores per given area of the microcirculation. These pores are the same size as water and electrolytes, as opposed to the larger pores associated with protein. P_c and P_{if} are the hydrostatic pressures in the microcirculation and interstitial space, respectively. The reflection coefficient, σ, is an index of microvascular permeability to protein. If σ is 1, the membrane is impermeable to protein; when σ is 0, the membrane is completely permeable to protein. COP_p and COP_{if} are the oncotic or colloid osmotic pressures in the plasma and interstitial spaces, respectively.

The damage seen in the oropharynx following inhalation injury is the same as that seen with thermal injury in other areas of the body. The heat denatures protein that, in turn, activates complement.[32,33] Complement activation causes the release of histamine.[32,34] Histamine then causes the formation of xanthine oxidase,[35] an enzyme involved in the breakdown of uric acid to urea. One of the stages in this degradation process is the formation of hypoxanthine from xanthine. During this conversion, oxygen free radicals are released.[36,37] Oxygen free radicals cause edema formation through increasing permeability to protein and increasing the microvascular pressure. The latter is the result of inhibiting the formation of nitric oxide. Eicosanoids are also released,[38,39] which, along with oxygen free radicals, attract polymorphonuclear cells to the area. The attraction then amplifies the release of oxygen radicals, proteases, and other materials into burned areas.

The massive edema occurring in the soft tissue of the oropharynx following burns involves most of the variables in the Starling equation (**Figure 16.1**). There is a large increase in microvascular hydrostatic pressure,[43] a decrease in interstitial hydrostatic pressure,[41] a fall in the reflection coefficient,[40] and an increase in interstitial oncotic pressure.[42,43] The usual treatment for burn resuscitation calls for the administration of large amounts of crystalloid solutions, which has the effect of reducing the plasma oncotic pressure.[44,45] This reduction not only affects the oncotic pressure gradient in the microcirculation but also has been reported to increase the filtration coefficient.[46,47] The result of this almost complete breakdown in control of the microvascular function and the insult of fluid administration is massive edema. This is probably nowhere more apparent than in soft tissues of the face and oropharynx. The danger to the patient is extreme. The edema may obstruct the airway, not only making it laborious or impossible to

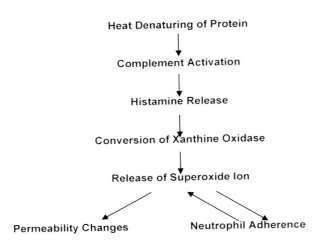

Heat Denaturing of Protein

↓

Complement Activation

↓

Histamine Release

↓

Conversion of Xanthine Oxidase

↓

Release of Superoxide Ion

Permeability Changes   Neutrophil Adherence

Fig. 16.1 Mechanism for edema formation in the oropharynx.

breathe but also making it difficult for the anesthesiologist to intubate the patient. To avoid this problem, many units prophylactically intubate patients who have evidence of thermal injury to the upper airway on admission. However, intubation in itself may present problems. The tube may further damage injured areas, especially the larynx.[48] It may be time to reconsider some of these practices. Perhaps some consideration should be given to fluid resuscitation with colloids, which can prevent some of this soft tissue edema and reduce the volume of fluids required for resuscitation.[49,50]

Tracheobronchial areas

Victims of fire accidents, especially those who are injured in enclosed areas, sustain chemical injury to their respiratory tract as a result of breathing toxic gases associated with the incomplete combustion of the burning materials, especially acrolein and formaldehyde.[51–53] Actual thermal injury to the airway is rare. The heat capacity of air is low, and the upper airway is very efficient at warming and cooling the inspiratory gases. Consequently, flames must almost come into direct contact with the airway to induce injury.[54] There are some instances in which hot particles might be inhaled. There are also reports of individuals with steam inhalation. In these cases, there is direct thermal injury to the airway. In most of these cases, damage to the bronchi and trachea are the result of chemical injury.

With chemical damage to the airway, there are two almost instantaneous happenings: ciliated epithelial cells separate from the basement membrane[55,56] and there is an almost immediate dilation of the systemic circulation to the lung and the bronchial circulation.[57,58] These latter changes appear mainly in the mucosal areas and can be detected by laser Doppler technique.[59] Shortly after this has occurred, edema can be visually detected in the trachea.[2] The edema is also evident histologically[2,60] and by gravimetric techniques.[58,61] The edema is associated with permeability to larger molecular weight substances.[60,62] The rapid occurrence of these changes to the airway and their universal presence after some insufflation into the bronchial areas should make it relatively easy to diagnose inhalation injury by bronchoscopy.[3,63,64] The degree of

increased airway blood flow does not appear to be related to the extent of smoke exposure. Rather, the dilation appears to be an all-or-nothing phenomenon. Longer duration of exposure appears to correlate with more areas of the airway showing greater increases in blood flow. The hyperemia associated with greater injury spreads down the bronchial tree with greater duration of exposure to smoke.[61]

The early inflammatory changes that occur in the airway are followed by a period of diffuse exudate formation.[65] There are copious quantities of these materials from both patients[66] and animals subjected to inhalation injury. The protein composition of this material suggests that it is an ultrafiltrate of the lung lymph.[62,65] This transudate can induce a bronchoconstriction. The material contains thromboxane (TX) B_2, the stable metabolite of a potent smooth muscle constrictor, TXA_2.[2,67] Thus, the period of airway injury that extends for the following 12–24 hours is associated with bronchoconstriction and an elevation in airway resistance.[68–70] Unlike many other forms of airway inflammatory diseases, inhalation injury also demonstrates narrowing of the large airways. The mucosa of the airway can hold a large amount of edema, which can produce marked narrowing of the airway.

As the time after injury increases, the exudative materials coalesce to form fibrin casts. These materials can induce an almost complete occlusion of the airway[2,71–73] and can obstruct the smallest of the airways. As a result of the destruction of the epithelium and the presence of these airway casts, which function as culture media, there is a greater susceptibility of the airway to infection, often leading to pneumonia, sepsis, and death. During the recovery period, there is first the formation of pseudomembrane in the airways. This is followed by a squamous cell metaplasia.[74] Healing may take place as late as 18 days after injury.[75] There is a high incidence of permanent airway damage, including airway stenosis and granuloma scar formation of the trachea.[63] It is sometimes difficult to determine if these long-term effects are the result of the injury or the cure.

Mediation of the changes in bronchial blood flow

Following inhalation injury, there is a marked, almost immediate, 20-fold increase in bronchial blood flow.[57,58,60] These changes in blood flow are also associated with changes in vascular permeability,[60] which are so rapid and apparent that they are used to diagnose inhalation injury. There have been numerous attempts to identify the mediators responsible for the increased bronchial artery blood flow and microvascular permeability, which occur with smoke inhalation. Since histamine is associated with vasodilatation, and edema formation with burn injury, the effects of H_1 and H_2 histaminergic blockade in inhalation injury in sheep were investigated. Neither the H_1 blocker diphenhydramine nor the H_2 receptor antagonist ranitidine affected the response.[76] In previous studies, we have identified the fact that prostacyclin was increased in the blood and lymph following inhalation injury.[65] Because this material is a vasodilator, the cyclooxygenase inhibitor ibuprofen was investigated to determine if it would affect the bronchial hyperemia seen with inhalation injury in sheep. Again, there was no noticeable effect on bronchial artery blood flow following smoke inhalation.[77] Therefore, it appears that neither histamine nor prostanoids are putative mediators of bronchial hyperemia.

As a result of the inability of the antihistamines and antiprostanoids to affect the increase in bronchial blood flow seen with the insufflation of smoke, other possible mediators were evaluated. The most obvious of these was to consider a neural source for the effect. Because the vagosympathetic trunk is virtually the only source of innervation of the vasculature of the lung, the first studies performed were to determine the effects of blocking this neural trunk with a local anesthetic. These studies were performed in acute preparations. The animals that received the local anesthetic had a markedly reduced elevation in bronchial blood flow in response to inhalation injury.[78] Many of the motor fibers that innervate the bronchial microvasculature, and are vasodilatory, are parasympathetic and thus release acetylcholine. Consequently, the effect of atropine on the elevated bronchial blood flow seen with inhalation injury was determined. The sheep that received the anticholinergic compound had an elevation in blood flow that was virtually identical with the untreated animals exposed to smoke. Thus, the increase in blood flow is not mediated by acetylcholine.

Martling et al. reported that the majority of the bronchial circulatory vasodilatation induced by vagal stimulation in the pig was mediated by sensory nerves;[79] these are neuropeptide-containing nerve fibers.[80] The fact that these fibers are capsaicin-sensitive, that is, they could be desensitized by the administration of capsaicin,[81] a material isolated from peppers, led to the determination of how the airway blood flow response of the sheep to smoke inhalation could be affected by capsaicin desensitization. In addition, the bronchial vasodilatation induced by the inhalation of cigarette smoke was prevented by the administration of capsaicin.[79] Lundberg et al. also reported that permeability was elevated by cigarette smoke, an effect that was blocked by the administration of capsaicin.[82] Preliminary data demonstrate that the changes in airway blood flow noted with inhalation injury can be reduced by pretreatment with capsaicin.[83]

Some of the bronchial hyperemia noted with smoke inhalation may be mediated hematogenously. Experiments were carried out in which the trachea and right lung were injured with smoke, while the left lung was being ventilated with air. The usual hyperemia and edema were observed in the smoke-insufflated airway.[84] These changes occurred almost immediately as measured by both laser Doppler and radioactive microsphere techniques.[59,85] The air-insufflated lung did not demonstrate a change in bronchial blood flow immediately, but by 24 hours after the contralateral right lung and trachea had been injured, the small airways of the left lung began to show an increase in blood flow. Because the normal sequence of blood flow change in the smoke-injured lung is from trachea down, this hyperemic spread from the small airway up is evidence of a spread of injury from the pulmonary system.[86]

Recent investigations have demonstrated that there is constant release of nitric oxide (NO) from airway vascular endothelium to modulate bronchial circulation, which plays a part in the regulation of temperature and water contents of inspired air.[87,88] The augmented airway blood flow associated with inflammation has been suggested to be influenced by NO. Alving et al. reported that bronchial and pulmonary vascular dilation in anesthetized pigs was attenuated during inhalation of cigarette smoke when the nonspecific NO synthase inhibitor N^G-nitro-L-arginine (L-NNA) was infused into the animals.[89] Recently, induction of inducible NO synthase (iNOS) by administration of mercaptoethylguanidine (MEG), and subsequent increased production of NO, played an important role in the significant increase in airway blood flow fol-

lowing smoke inhalation. The airway blood flow was measured using the microsphere technique. In the iNOS-inhibited animals, the increase in airway blood flow after smoke inhalation injury was significantly attenuated;[90] thus, the inducible form of NO synthase appears to play a role in the response.

Pulmonary microvascular changes

Following inhalation injury, there is evidence of microvascular changes in the pulmonary microvasculature. There is a profound increase in lung lymph flow.[2,67] Extravascular lung water as measured by the thermal dilution technique is elevated.[91] Postmortem histological and gravimetric analysis of the lung reveals an increased water content.[2,67] These increases in extravascular fluid formation are proportional to the duration of smoke exposure.[18] These pulmonary microvascular changes are obviously related to alterations of the parameters of the Starling equation.

Pulmonary artery pressure and pulmonary vascular resistance increase between 4 and 12 hours after inhalation injury.[57,92,93] Pulmonary capillary pressure, measured by the technique of Holloway et al.,[94] also rises approximately 24 hours after smoke inhalation injury.[92] This technique estimates the pulmonary microvascular pressure as a function of the decay in pulmonary arterial pressure after the balloon on the pulmonary artery catheter has been inflated. In association with the changes in pressure, there is also an elevation in microvascular resistance. The resistance rises on both sides of the microvasculature but is increased to a greater extent on the venular side of the pulmonary circuit. Simultaneously with these changes in resistance and pressure, permeability to protein was evaluated as measuring the reflection coefficient.[95] This variable was reduced, suggesting a marked elevation in pulmonary microvascular permeability to protein after inhalation injury;[96] the filtration coefficient was calculated and this index of permeability to small molecules was also elevated. These changes in pulmonary microvascular pressure are obviously important in the formation of edema; however, changes in vascular permeability appear to be of much greater importance, especially during the first 24 hours after injury.[96]

Mediation of the pulmonary microvascular changes

There is a change in lung lymph flow after inhalation injury. This phenomenon differs from that seen in the tracheal areas, as it occurs over a 4-hour latency period after the airway exposure to smoke, suggesting that it is a mediated phenomenon. After inhalation injury there was a marked reduction in the reflection coefficient and an elevation in filtration coefficient.[96] This demonstrates an elevation in permeability both to proteins and to low molecular weight materials. Further, the relative contributions of permeability and capillary pressure on transvascular fluid flux were calculated as described above. Capillary permeability was responsible for the majority of the edema found during the first 24 hours. During the next 24 hours, permeability and the lung lymph flow begin to return toward the baseline value, and microvascular pressure appears to be responsible for the majority of the lymph flow changes noted at 48 hours after smoke insufflation.[96]

Lung parenchymal pathology is associated with the deposition of neutrophils in the pulmonary microvasculature.[2,91,97] The extravascular lung water and wet/dry ratio are increased,[18,91] and lipid peroxidation[98] and histological changes occur in the lung.[99] Hypoxic pulmonary vasoconstriction is impaired,[100,101] and the Pao_2/Fio_2 ratio falls.[18] Many of these pathological changes can be reversed by the administration of oxygen free radical scavengers, suggesting that leukocytes mediate production of reactive oxygen intermediates.[102,103] These changes in microvascular fluid flux occur with the elevation of polymorphonuclear cells in the lung, as evidenced by histology and bronchoalveolar lavage and the release of materials associated with the polymorphonuclear cells, such as proteases and oxygen free radicals (**Figure 16.2**).[18,65,67] High concentrations of conjugated dienes have been found in the lung lymph and pulmonary tissues, suggesting the lung as a source of these materials.[104–106] Consistent with these observations, the pathology associated with smoke insufflation can also be prevented by depleting the sheep of neutrophils.[104] The adherence of these cells in the microcirculation of the lung can be markedly reduced by the administration of an antibody to L-selectin.[87,107] The selectins are a family of compounds that are involved with the initial adherence of leukocytes in the microcirculation.[108]

The levels of NO_2^-/NO_3^- (NOx), intermediate and end products of NO oxidation, were serially measured in plasma and lung lymph after inhalation injury by a chemiluminescence assay (**Figure 16.1**). The result revealed that plasma NOx did not increase significantly, but that lung lymph NOx did, beginning from 18 hours after injury. iNOS inhibition significantly attenuated the degree of lung edema and concentrations of conjugated dienes in the pulmonary tissue after smoke inhalation injury. These data suggest that NO from iNOS may be produced mainly in the pulmonary tissue and is a major source of edema formation and oxidative tissue injury seen with smoke inhalation injury. The role of the polymorphonuclear cell as the vector of the cytotoxins responsible for pulmonary microvascular permeability changes has likewise been supported by a finding that the proteolytic enzymes, lipid peroxidation, and lung lymph flow changes are markedly reduced when the polymorphonuclear cells are depleted using nitrogen mustard.[104] The changes in lung lymph flow seen with smoke inhalation may also be obtunded by administration of antiproteases[109] and oxygen free radical scavengers.[110] We have also demonstrated that the administration of superoxide dismutase will prevent the reduction in reflection coefficient seen with smoke inhalation.[111] Both proteases and oxygen free radicals have been shown to be released by polymorphonuclear leukocytes.[112,113]

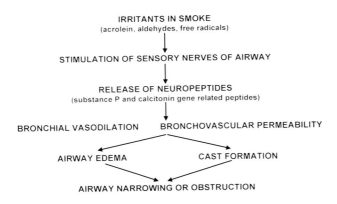

Fig. 16.2 Sequence of airway pathology following smoke inhalation.

Role of the bronchial circulation in mediating the pulmonary parenchymal injury

The delayed onset of the changes in transvascular fluid flux in the pulmonary bed suggests the release of mediators from other areas. It is certainly difficult to conceive of materials in the smoke traveling from the oral pharynx to the alveoli. Certainly these materials come into contact with the airway circulation. The changes in bronchial blood flow and the denudation of the tracheobronchial basement membrane are phenomena that occur almost instantaneously with smoke insufflation.[53,57] Consequently, this airway injury must in some way guide polymorphonuclear cells to the parenchyma. The mechanisms by which cytokines might reach the pulmonary parenchyma from the airway may be related to the unique anatomy of the bronchial circulation. Systemic drainage from the intrapulmonary bronchi has been demonstrated to drain into the pulmonary circulation at the precapillary level.[114,115] Consequently, chemotactic materials released in the airway could traverse this network and present themselves to the pulmonary microvasculature to attract polymorphonuclear cells; this results in adherence to the microvasculature, transepithelial migration, and the release of their cytotoxins.

Several experiments physiologically support a bronchopulmonary portal system. Using their dog model with acrolein inhalation injury, Hales and his group demonstrated an elevation in extravascular lung water using both the thermal technique and a gravimetric determination.[60,116] In animals with ligated bronchial arteries, this effect was markedly reduced.[60] Similar experiments have been performed in chronically instrumented sheep. The sheep is unique from other animal species, having only a single bronchial artery, which supplies from 50% to 80% of the systemic circulation to the bronchial areas.[117] Occlusion of this vessel with a pneumatic device resulted in a reduction in both lung lymph flow and extravascular lung water, determined by the gravimetric technique.[118]

Recently, a technique to evaluate the role of the bronchial circulation in the parenchymal changes which are induced by inhalation injury has been developed. Pneumatic occluders are placed on the pulmonary arteries and veins of the left lung.[119] When these vessels are occluded, the left lung is isolated from the pulmonary circuit. The blood entering into this lung pouch, then, is the bronchial venous drainage. The flow rate into this pouch is similar to that previously reported for the bronchial blood flow to the left lung. This blood flow into the isolated lung vascular pouch increases markedly with smoke inhalation. The occlusion of the bronchial artery causes a near 70% reduction in the blood flow into the pouch. This is in close agreement with previous studies regarding the contribution of the bronchial artery to the total airway blood flow.[58,117] Following inhalation injury, there is a marked increase in bronchial blood draining into the pouch. Occlusion of the bronchial artery reduces the blood flow into the pouch by 70% after inhalation injury. This is in agreement with our previous finding after bronchial artery occlusion.[58] These data are consistent with the hypothesis that the bronchial venous drainage enters into the pulmonary circuit. With injury to the airway, mediators would be released into the bronchial venous blood and be delivered directly into the pulmonary microvasculature. Also, the data of the changes in the concentration of NOx in plasma and lung lymph described above support that bronchial blood flow empties into the

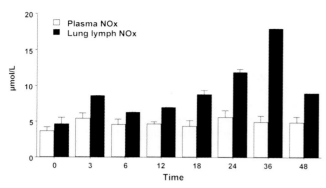

Fig. 16.3 Changes in NOx following smoke inhalation injury.

pulmonary circulation at the precapillary level, since the lung lymph NOx, but not plasma NOx, significantly increased after smoke inhalation injury (**Figure 16.3**).

Experiments have also been performed in which one lung was insufflated with smoke, while the contralateral lung was insufflated with air. If the smoke exposure was limited to the intrapulmonary airways, the injury was localized to the ipsilateral lung.[106,120] On the other hand, when the smoke damage included the trachea and bronchi (extrapulmonary airway), then the contralateral air-insufflated lung likewise demonstrated injury.[106] The changes in airway blood flow were also investigated using radioactive microspheres. With time, blood flow changes in the lung that was insufflated with smoke showed the greatest intensity in the upper airway, with a gradient down to the smaller airways.[58,61] These changes in blood flow occurred almost instantaneously. Previous studies have shown that there was no increase in blood flow in areas above the cuffs of the endotracheal tube that were not in direct contact with smoke.[58] This suggests that airway blood flow is locally regulated. The rapid inactivation of NO in the blood may explain the localized vascular regulation. On the other hand, the blood flow changes to the air-insufflated lung occurred after a latency period and had greater intensity in the smaller airways.[86] This suggests a

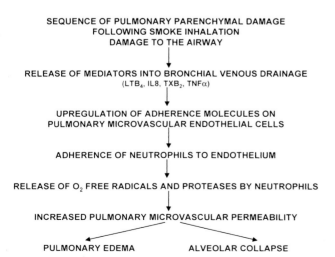

Fig. 16.4 Sequence of pulmonary parenchymal damage following smoke inhalation damage to the airway.

hematogenous origin for the mediators of vasodilatation. The venous drainage from the extra pulmonary airway enters into the azygous vein and thus the right atrium.[114] Mediators, therefore, released from these airways outside the lung would enter into the right heart and be distributed to both lungs. Bronchopulmonary pathophysiology is a fertile area for further investigation (**Figure 16.4**).

Hypoxia after smoke inhalation

The progressive decline in oxygenation seen with smoke inhalation injury results partially from the loss of pulmonary vascular regulation called hypoxic pulmonary vasoconstriction (HPV).[100] This homeostatic mechanism prevents the ventilation–perfusion mismatching by vasoconstriction of pulmonary vessels of poorly ventilated area and diversion of blood to better-ventilated regions of the lung.[121] In the early phase after smoke inhalation, it is believed that HPV remains.[100] It is then blunted by progression of the lung tissue damage from injured airway, while simultaneously there is deterioration in oxygenation. Apparently, 24 hours is required for the injury to spread from the airway to the lung parenchyma and thereby blunt HPV. Recently, iNOS-NO has played a major role in the loss of HPV after smoke inhalation injury. In animals that had sustained an inhalation injury, a specific inhibitor of iNOS prevented the fall in Pao_2/Fio_2 seen in similarly injured animals that were not treated.[96] Inhalation injury was associated with the expression for the iNOS message and protein.[122]

Changes in the systemic organs induced by smoke inhalation

With burn injury and other forms of trauma, mortality is usually the result of multiple organ system failure.[123,124] The contribution made by acute lung injury to this phenomenon has, in the past, been considered the result of reduced oxygenation. With improved techniques of artificial restoration of arterial oxygenation saturation, it has now become obvious that other factors are involved. It has been recognized that persons who have suffered combined thermal and smoke inhalation injury require more fluid for resuscitation to nonpathogenic cardiovascular status than individuals with thermal injury alone.[125,126] This phenomenon has been studied by cannulation of a lymphatic which drains the soft tissues of the skin on the lateral surface of sheep.[127] With inhalation injury, there was a twofold increase in the flow from this vessel.[128,129] With thermal injury, this flow was much greater, reaching some 3–5 times the baseline levels.[129] When smoke inhalation was combined with thermal injury, again, the soft tissue lymphatic showed a severalfold increase in flow. A similar finding was made by Lalonde *et al.*.[130] These changes in peripheral microvascular fluid flux occur with a concomitant elevation in plasma lipid peroxidation products, suggesting that they may be the result of the release of oxygen free radicals. The etiology of the formation of these cytotoxins is unknown.

It has been reported that the lung releases peptidoleukotrienes following inhalation injury.[131] A similar finding was reported by Hales and his group,[132] who reported that there is a systemic vasoconstriction with inhalation injury and that this systemic vasoconstriction could be reversed by administration of a peptidoleukotriene antagonist. It has also been reported that there is an elevation in systemic vascular resistance with inhalation injury,[93] and a selective vasoconstriction in the distribution of the cephalic mesenteric artery of sheep following inhalation injury was demonstrated.[133] This vasoconstriction lasts about 4 hours and is followed by reperfusion. Consequently, damage to the systemic circulation may be the result of an ischemia-reperfusion phenomenon. Lung injury is also seen with systemic reperfusion injury.[134] Reperfusion phenomena are mediated by the action of xanthine oxidase.[37] An effect of the xanthine oxidase inhibitor allopurinol on the lung response to smoke inhalation could not be demonstrated.[135] The observation period was limited to 24 hours and it is possible that the reperfusion might have had an effect in later time periods. Further study is warranted in this area of investigation.

In association with these systemic vascular resistance changes, there was a fall in myocardial contractility.[93,136] It was natural to assume that this fall in contractility was the result of ischemia reperfusion in the coronary bed as a result of the elevated carbon monoxide levels seen after inhalation injury. The animals with inhalation injury were compared to sheep insufflated with carbon monoxide to an equivalent level of carboxyhemoglobin. Only the animals given smoke showed a reduction in myocardial contractility.[93]

Systemic pathophysiology has also been noted with acid aspiration.[137] Aspiration resulted in the disposition of polymorphonuclear cells in the several systemic organs, including the heart. The depositions of these cells were associated with an increase in the wet/dry weight ratio. These results were mediated by leukotrienes and thromboxane,[138] which is in agreement with the results of Quinn, who demonstrated a vasoconstriction and its reversal of systemic vascular resistance changes after insufflating sheep with artificial smoke.[132] A thromboxane inhibitor will reverse the changes in systemic vascular resistance and myocardial contractility seen with smoke inhalation.[139] In addition, the changes in lung lymph flow in these animals were not as marked. There is, therefore, a great deal of promise in future trials with thromboxane inhibitors.

The effect of iNOS inhibition on the cardiac dysfunction seen with smoke inhalation injury and/or burn injury was investigated. In smoke inhalation injury alone, cardiac function tended to be improved by iNOS inhibition, although there was no statistically significant difference from the nontreatment animals. In the animals subjected to combined smoke inhalation and burn injury, the cardiac dysfunction consisted of two phases; the later phase was significantly improved by iNOS inhibition. These data suggest that NO from iNOS also plays a role in the pathophysiology in this injury.

Heparin

Because the casts found in the airways of individuals contained fibrin, heparin was nebulized into the airway after inhalation injury. The nebulization was found not only to reduce the number of casts in the airway but also to reduce the changes in transvascular fluid flux.[102,110] Selectin adherence molecules are involved in the deposition of polymorphonuclear neutrophils in the pulmonary microcirculation.[87] Heparin has been shown to prevent the binding of the selectin molecules.[140] Consequently, heparin may show promise in the clinical area. Taking this into consideration, studies were performed in a patient population. In an open label clinical trial, heparin was found to reduce many of the moribund aspects

of inhalation injury, such as reintubation, atelectasis, and the mortality of patients with inhalation injury compared to cohorts studied simultaneously that were not treated.[141] Recently, other investigators have reported that heparin would reduce the inflammation in a classical model of airway inflammation aerosolized ovalbumin in the guinea pig.[142] This finding has focused renewed interest in the use of heparin and other glucose aminoglycans in airway inflammation.[143] There has also been a recent report that coating contact lenses with heparin would reduce eye inflammation.[144] Using histological techniques, the degree of airway occlusion by cast formation in chronically instrumented sheep after inhalation injury was evaluated. The number of casts was remarkably reduced by nebulization of heparin into the airway (**Figure 16.5**). The Pao_2/Fio_2 values were higher and the pulmonary shunt fraction lower in the animals treated with heparin. Of interest, these same animals had a tendency to have lower levels of nitrate/nitrite in the circulation, suggesting that heparin was also reducing the formation of NO in these injured animals. These recent findings suggest that further clinical trials with heparin should be carried out.

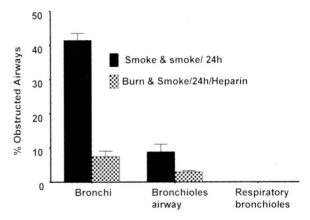

Fig. 16.5 Airway casts after burns & inhalation injury.

Clinical trials

Despite the skills that have been developed in ventilatory management of the patient with inhalation injury, many patients cannot be managed with the ventilator and need extracorporeal oxygenation (ECMO). Conventional ECMO was effective in reducing the morbidity and mortality of inhalation injury.[145,146] The logistics of such a procedure and its associated risks to the burn patient have caused the authors to consider other forms of extracorporeal pulmonary support. An extracorporeal arteriovenous carbon dioxide removal device was developed and tested in an ovine model of burn and smoke inhalation injury;[147] this device was found to reduce ventilatory days and survival of these animals.[148] The use of these devices still requires the use of heparin. Consequently, some of the efficacy of the use of extracorporeal pulmonary support must also be related to the use of heparin. Multicenter clinical trials are presently underway utilizing this device in the treatment of burned children with inhalation injury.

References

1. Herndon DN, Adams T Jr, Traber LD, Traber DL. Inhalation injury and positive pressure ventilation in a sheep model. *Circ Shock* 1984; **12**: 107–13.
2. Herndon DN, Traber DL, Niehaus GD, Linares HA, Traber LD. The pathophysiology of smoke inhalation injury in a sheep model. *J Trauma* 1984; **24**: 1044–51.
3. Herndon DN, Thompson PB, Traber DL. Pulmonary injury in burned patients. *Crit Care Clin* 1985; **1**: 79–96.
4. Thompson PB, Herndon DN, Traber DL, Abston S. Effect on mortality of inhalation injury. *J Trauma* 1986; **26**: 163–5.
5. Rue LW, Cioffi WG, Mason AD Jr, McManus WF, Pruitt BA Jr. Improved survival of burned patients with inhalation injury. *Arch Surg* 1993; **128**: 772–8.
6. Sobel JB, Goldfarb IW, Slater H, Hammell EJ. Inhalation injury: a decade without progress. *J Burn Care Rehabil* 1992; **13**: 573–5.
7. Cioffi WG Jr, Rue LW, Graves TA, McManus WF, Mason AD Jr, Pruitt BA Jr. Prophylactic use of high-frequency percussive ventilation in patients with inhalation injury. *Ann Surg* 1991; **213**: 575–80.
8. Herndon DN, Traber DL, Traber LD. The effect of resuscitation on inhalation injury. *Surgery* 1986; **100**: 248–51.
9. Hughes KR, Armstrong RF, Brough MD, Parkhouse N. Fluid requirements of patients with burns and inhalation injuries in an intensive care unit. *Intensive Care Med* 1989; **15**: 464–6.
10. Birky MM, Clarke FB. Inhalation of toxic products from fires. *Bull NY Acad Med* 1981; **57**: 997–1013.
11. Moore SJ, Ho IK, Hume AS. Severe hypoxia produced by concomitant intoxication with sublethal doses of carbon monoxide and cyanide. *Toxicol Appl Pharmacol* 1991; **109**: 412–20.
12. Prien T, Traber DL. Toxic smoke compounds and inhalation injury – a review. *Burns Incl Therm Inj* 1988; **14**: 451–60.
13. Pitt BR, Radford EP, Gurtner GH, Traystman RJ. Interaction of carbon monoxide and cyanide on cerebral circulation and metabolism. *Arch Environ Health* 1979; **34**: 345–9.
14. Goldbaum LR, Orellano T, Dergal E. Mechanism of the toxic action of carbon monoxide. *Ann Clin Lab Sci* 1976; **6**: 372–6.
15. Einhorn IN. Physiological and toxicological aspects of smoke produced during the combustion of polymeric materials. *Environ Health Perspect* 1975; **11**: 163–89.
16. Charnock EL, Meehan JJ. Postburn respiratory injuries in children. *Pediatr Clin N Am* 1980; **27**: 661–76.
17. Clark CJ, Campbell D, Reid WH. Blood carboxyhaemoglobin and cyanide levels in fire survivors. *Lancet* 1981; **1**: 1332–5.
18. Kimura R, Traber LD, Herndon DN, Linares HA, Lübbesmeyer HJ, Traber DL. Increasing duration of smoke exposure induces more severe lung injury in sheep. *J Appl Physiol* 1988; **64**: 1107–13.
19. Crapo RO. Smoke-inhalation injuries. *JAMA* 1981; **246**: 1694–6.
20. Hart GB, Strauss MB, Lennon PA, Whitcraft D. III. Treatment of smoke inhalation by hyperbaric oxygen. *J Emerg Med* 1985; **3**: 211–15.
21. Myers RA, Snyder SK, Linberg S, Cowley RA. Value of hyperbaric oxygen in suspected carbon monoxide poisoning. *JAMA* 1981; **246**: 2478–80.
22. Thom SR. Dehydrogenase conversion to oxidase and lipid peroxidation in brain after carbon monoxide poisoning. *J Appl Physiol* 1992; **73**: 1584–9.
23. McCord JM. Oxygen-derived radicals: a link between reperfusion injury and inflammation. *Fed Proc* 1987; **46**: 2402–6.
24. Thom SR. Functional inhibition of leukocyte B2 integrins by hyperbaric oxygen in carbon monoxide-mediated brain injury in rats. *Toxicol Appl Pharmacol* 1993; **123**: 248–56.
25. Purser DA, Grimshaw P, Berrill KR. Intoxication by cyanide in fires: a study in monkeys using polyacrylonitrile. *Arch Environ Health* 1984; **39**: 394–400.
26. Baud FJ, Barriot P, Toffis V, *et al.* Elevated blood cyanide concentrations in victims of smoke inhalation. *N Engl J Med* 1991; **325**: 1761–6.
27. Smith PW, Crane R, Sanders DC, Abbott JK, Endocott B. Effects of exposure to carbon monoxide and hydrogen cyanide In: *Physiological and Toxological Aspects of Combustion Products*, Washington DC: National Academy of Science, 1976: 75–78.
28. Becker CE. The role of cyanide in fires. *Vet Hum Toxicol* 1985; **27**: 487–90.
29. Moore SJ, Norris JC, Walsh DA, Hume AS. Antidotal use of methemoglobin forming cyanide antagonists in concurrent carbon monoxide/cyanide intoxication. *J Pharmacol Exp Ther* 1987; **242**: 70–3.
30. Landis EM, Pappenheimer JR. Exchange of substances through the capillary walls. In: Hamilton WF, Dow P, eds. *Handbook of Physiology*, Section 2, Vol. 2, Baltimore, MD: Williams & Wilkins, 1963: 961–1034.
31. Starling EH. On the absorption of fluids from the connective tissue spaces. *J Physiol (Lond)* 1896; **19**: 312–26.
32. Friedl HP, Till GO, Trentz O, Ward PA. Roles of histamine, complement and xanthine oxidase in thermal injury of skin. *Am J Pathol* 1989; **135**: 203–17.
33. Oldham KT, Guice KS, Till GO, Ward PA. Activation of complement by hydroxyl radical in thermal injury. *Surgery* 1988; **104**: 272–9.
34. Ward PA, Till GO. Pathophysiologic events related to thermal injury of skin. *J Trauma* 1990; **30**: S75–9.
35. Schlayer HJ, Laaff H, Peters T, *et al.* Involvement of tumor necrosis factor in endotoxin-triggered neutrophil adherence to sinusoidal endothelial cells of mouse liver and its modulation in acute phase. *J Hepatol* 1988; **7**: 239–49.
36. Granger D, Rutili G, McCord J. Superoxide radicals in feline intestinal ischemia. *Gastroenterology* 1981; **81**: 22–9.
37. Granger DN, McCord JM, Parks DA, Hollwarth ME. Xanthine oxidase inhibitors attenuate ischemia-induced vascular permeability changes in the cat intestine. *Gastroenterology* 1986; **90**: 80–4.
38. Demling RH, LaLonde C. Topical ibuprofen decreases early postburn edema. *Surgery* 1987; **102**: 857–61.
39. Herndon DN, Abston S, Stein MD. Increased thromboxane B2 levels in the plasma of burned and septic burned patients. *Surg Gynecol Obstet* 1984; **159**: 210–13.
40. Pitt RM, Parker JC, Jurkovich GJ, Taylor AE, Curreri PW. Analysis of altered capillary pressure and permeability after thermal injury. *J Surg Res* 1987; **42**: 693–702.
41. Lund T, Wiig H, Reed RK. Acute postburn edema: role of strongly negative interstitial fluid pressure. *Am J Physiol* 1988; **255**: H1069–74.
42. Lund T, Reed RK. Microvascular fluid exchange following thermal skin injury in the rat: changes in extravascular colloid osmotic pressure, albumin mass, and water content. *Circ Shock* 1986; **20**: 91–104.
43. Pitkanen J, Lund T, Aanderud L, Reed RK. Transcapillary colloid osmotic pressures in injured and non-injured skin of seriously burned patients. *Burns Incl Therm Inj* 1987; **13**: 198–203.
44. Onarheim H, Reed RK. Thermal skin injury: effect of fluid therapy on the transcapillary colloid osmotic gradient. *J Surg Res* 1991; **50**: 272–8.
45. Zetterstrom H, Arturson G. Plasma oncotic pressure and plasma protein concentration in patients following thermal injury. *Acta Anaesthesiol Scand* 1980; **24**: 288–94.
46. Conhaim RL, Harms BA. A simplified two-pore filtration model explains the effects of hypoproteinemia on lung and soft tissue lymph flux in awake sheep. *Microvasc Res* 1992; **44**: 14–26.
47. Sheng ZY, Tung YL. Neutrophil chemiluminescence in burned patients. *J Trauma* 1987; **27**: 587–95.
48. Calhoun KH, Deskin RW, Garza C, *et al.* Long-term airway sequelae in a pediatric burn population. *Laryngoscope* 1988; **98**: 721–5.
49. Demling RH, Kramer GC, Gunther R, Nerlich M. Effect of nonprotein colloid on postburn edema formation in soft tissues and lung. *Surgery* 1984; **95**: 593–602.
50. Honeycutt D, Traber L, Toole D, Herndon D, Traber D. Colloid resuscitation of ovine burn shock. *Circ Shock* 1991; **31**: 72.
51. Dost FN. Acute toxicology of components of vegetation smoke. *Rev Environ Contam Toxicol* 1991; **119**: 1–46.
52. Morikawa T. Acrolein, formaldehyde, and volatile fatty acids from smoldering combustion. *J Combust Toxicol* 1976; **3**: 135–51.
53. Zikria BA, Ferrer JM, Floch HF. The chemical factors contributing to pulmonary damage in 'smoke poisoning'. *Surgery* 1972; **71**: 704–9.
54. Moritz AR, Henriques FC, McLean R. The effect of inhaled heat on the air passages and lungs: An experimental investigation. *Am J Pathol* 1945; **21**: 311–26.
55. Abdi S, Evans MJ, Cox RA, Lubbesmeyer H, Herndon DN, Traber DL. Inhalation injury to tracheal epithelium in an ovine model of cotton smoke exposure. Early phase (30 minutes). *Am Rev Respir Dis* 1990; **142**: 1436–9.
56. Barrow RE, Wang CZ, Cox RA, Evans MJ. Cellular sequence of tracheal repair in sheep after smoke inhalation injury. *Lung* 1992; **170**: 331–8.
57. Abdi S, Herndon D, Mcguire J, Traber L, Traber DL. Time course of alterations in lung lymph and bronchial blood flows after inhalation injury. *J Burn Care Rehabil* 1990; **11**: 510–15.
58. Stothert JC Jr, Ashley KD, Kramer GC, *et al.* Intrapulmonary distribution of bronchial blood flow after moderate smoke inhalation. *J Appl Physiol* 1990; **69**: 1734–9.
59. Loick HM, Traber LD, Hurst C, Herndon DN, Traber DL. Endoscopic laser flowmetry: a valid method for detection and quantitative analysis of inhalation injury. *J Burn Care Rehabil* 1991; **12**: 313–18.
60. Hales CA, Barkin P, Jung W, Quinn D, Lamborghini D, Burke J. Bronchial artery ligation modifies pulmonary edema after exposure to smoke with acrolein. *J Appl Physiol* 1989; **67**: 1001–6.
61. Ashley KD, Stothert JC Jr, Traber DL, Traber LD, Kramer G, Herndon D. Airway blood flow following light and heavy smoke inhalation injury. *Surg Forum* 1990; **41**: 293–5.
62. Barrow RE, Morris SE, Basadre JO, Herndon DN. Selective permeability changes in the lungs and airways of sheep after toxic smoke inhalation. *J Appl Physiol* 1990; **68**: 2165–70.

63. Lund T, Goodwin CW, McManus WF, Shirani KZ, Stallings RJ, Mason AD Jr, Pruitt BA Jr. Upper airway sequelae in burn patients requiring endotracheal intubation or tracheostomy. *Ann Surg* 1985; **201**: 374–82.

64. Moylan JA, Adib K, Birnbaum M. Fiberoptic bronchoscopy following thermal injury. *Surg Gynecol Obstet* 1975; **140**: 541–3.

65. Herndon DN, Traber LD, Linares H, *et al.* Etiology of the pulmonary pathophysiology associated with inhalation injury. *Resuscitation* 1986; **14**: 43–59.

66. Mathru M, Venus B, Rao T, Matsuda T. Noncardiac pulmonary edema precipitated by tracheal intubation in patients with Injury. *Crit Care Med* 1983; **11**: 804–6.

67. Traber DL, Herndon DN, Stein MD, Traber LD, Flynn JT, Niehaus GD. The pulmonary lesion of smoke inhalation in an ovine model. *Circ Shock* 1986; **18**: 311–23.

68. Petroff PA, Hander EW, Clayton WH, Pruitt BA Jr. Pulmonary function studies after smoke inhalation. *Am J Surg* 1976; **132**: 346–51.

69. Prien T, Traber DL, Richardson JA, Traber LD. Early effects of inhalation injury on lung mechanics and pulmonary perfusion. *Intens Care Med* 1988; **14**: 25–9.

70. Stenton SC, Kelly CA, Walters EH, Hendrick DJ. Induction of bronchial hyperresponsiveness following smoke inhalation injury. *Br J Dis Chest* 1988; **82**: 436–8.

71. Lippton H, Goff J, Hyman A. Effects of endothelin in the systemic and renal vascular beds *in vivo*. *Eur J Pharmacol* 1988; **155**: 197–9.

72. Pruitt BA Jr, Erickson DR, Morris A. Progressive pulmonary insufficiency and other pulmonary complications of thermal injury. *J Trauma* 1975; **15**: 369–79.

73. Traber DL, Linares HA, Herndon DN, Prien T. The pathophysiology of inhalation injury – a review. *Burns Incl Therm Inj* 1988; **14**: 357–64.

74. Toor AH, Tomashefski JF, Kleinerman J. Respiratory tract pathology in patients with severe burns. *Hum Pathol* 1990; **21**: 1212–20.

75. Wang CZ, Evans MJ, Cox RA, *et al.* Morphologic changes in basal cells during repair of tracheal epithelium. *Am J Pathol* 1992; **141**: 753–9.

76. Traber LD, Herndon DN, Abdi S, Traber DL. Histamine does not mediate the increase in bronchial blood flow during inhalation injury. *FASEB J* 1990; **4**: A575.

77. Abdi S, Traber LD, Herndon DN, Traber DL. Ibuprofen does not attenuate the increase in bronchial blood flow after inhalation injury. *Am Rev Respir Dis* 1991; **143**: A785.

78. Abdi S, Maguire JP, Herndon DN, Traber LD, Traber DL. Lidocaine attenuates bronchial artery response to inhalation trauma. *Crit Care Med* 1990; **18**: S200.

79. Martling CR, Matran R, Alving K, Lacroix JS, Lundberg JM. Vagal vasodilatory mechanisms in the pig bronchial circulation preferentially involves sensory nerves. *Neurosci Lett* 1989; **96**: 306–11.

80. Martling CR, Matran R, Alving K, Hokfelt T, Lundberg JM. Innervation of lower airways and neuropeptide effects on bronchial and vascular tone in the pig. *Cell Tissue Res* 1990; **260**: 223–33.

81. Matran R, Alving K, Martling CR, Lacroix JS, Lundberg JM. Effects of neuropeptides and capsaicin on tracheobronchial blood flow of the pig. *Acta Physiol Scand* 1989; **135**: 335–42.

82. Lundberg JM, Martling CR, Saria A, Folkers K, Rosell S. Cigarette smoke-induced airway oedema due to activation of capsaicin-sensitive vagal afferents and substance P release. *Neuroscience* 1983; **10**: 1361–8.

83. Traber LD, Herndon DN, Turner J, Sant'Ambrogio G, Traber DL. Peptide mediation of the bronchial blood flow elevation following inhalation injury. *Circ Shock* 1990; **31**: 13.

84. Prien T, Traber LD, Herndon DN, Stothert JC Jr, Lübbesmeyer HJ, Traber DL. Pulmonary edema with smoke inhalation, undetected by indicator-dilution technique. *J Appl Physiol* 1987; **63**: 907–11.

85. Loick HM, Traber LD, Theissen JL, Flynn J, Traber DL. Effect of thromboxane receptor blockade following inhalation injury in sheep. *Anesthesiology* 1991; **75**: A224.

86. Loick HM, Traber LD, Stothert JC Jr, Herndon DN, Traber DL. Smoke inhalation causes an increase in bronchial blood flow and edema in primarily uninjured lung areas. *FASEB J* 1992; **6**: A1818.

87. Kim YD, Kwon OC, Song SY, *et al.* Distribution of nitric oxide in the nasal mucosa of the rat: a histochemical study. *Auris Nasus Larynx* 1997; **24**: 373–8.

88. Sasaki F, Pare P, Ernest D, *et al.* Endogenous nitric oxide influences acetylcholine-induced bronchovascular dilation in sheep. *J Appl Physiol* 1995; **78**: 539–45.

89. Alving K, Fornhem C, Lundberg JM. Pulmonary effects of endogenous and exogenous nitric oxide in the pig: relation to cigarette smoke inhalation. *Br J Pharmacol* 1993; **110**: 739–46.

90. Soejima K, McGuire R, Snyder N, *et al.* The effect of inducible nitric oxide synthase (iNOS) inhibition on smoke inhalation injury in sheep. *Shock* 2000; **13**: 261–6.

91. Traber DL, Schlag G, Redl H, Traber LD. Pulmonary edema and compliance changes following smoke inhalation. *J Burn Care Rehabil* 1985; **6**: 490–4.

92. Isago T, Fujioka K, Traber LD, Herndon DN, Traber DL. Derived pulmonary capillary pressure changes after smoke inhalation in sheep. *Crit Care Med* 1991; **19**: 1407–13.

93. Sugi K, Theissen JL, Traber LD, Herndon DN, Traber DL. Impact of carbon monoxide on cardiopulmonary dysfunction after smoke inhalation injury. *Circ Res* 1990; **66**: 69–75.

94. Holloway H, Perry M, Downey J, Parker J, Taylor A. Estimation of effective pulmonary capillary pressure in intact lungs. *J Appl Physiol* 1983; **54(3)**: 846–51.

95. Isago T, Traber LD, Herndon DN, Abdi S, Fujioka K, Traber DL. Determination of pulmonary microvascular reflection coefficient in sheep by venous occlusion. *J Appl Physiol* 1990; **69**: 2311–16.

96. Isago T, Noshima S, Traber LD, Herndon DN, Traber DL. Analysis of pulmonary microvascular permeability after smoke inhalation. *J Appl Physiol* 1991; **71**: 1403–8.

97. Linares HA, Herndon DN, Traber DL, Traber LD. Experimental inhalation injury: histopathological evaluation. *Annu Meet ABA* 1983; **15**: 90–1.

98. Loick HM, Traber LD, Tokyay R, *et al.* Thromboxane receptor blockade with BM 13,177 following toxic airway damage by smoke inhalation in sheep. *Eur J Pharmacol* 1993; **248**: 75–83.

99. Linares HA, Herndon DN, Traber DL. Sequence of morphologic events in experimental smoke inhalation. *J Burn Care Rehabil* 1989; **10**: 27–37.

100. Theissen JL, Herndon DN, Traber LD, Linares HA, Traber DL. Smoke inhalation and pulmonary blood flow. *Prog Resp Res* 1990; **26**: 77–84.

101. Theissen JL, Prien T, Maguire J, *et al.* Respiratory and hemodynamic sequelae of unilateral inhalation injury of the lung. *Anaesthesist* 1989; **38**: 531–5.

102. Kimura R, Mlcak R, Richardson J, *et al.* Treatment of smoke-induced pulmonary injury with nebulized dimethylsulfoxide. *Circ Shock* 1988; **25**: 333–41.

103. Nguyen TT, Cox CS Jr, Herndon DN, *et al.* Effects of manganese superoxide dismutase on lung fluid balance after smoke inhalation. *J Appl Physiol* 1995; **78**: 2161–8.

104. Basadre JO, Sugi K, Traber DL, Traber LD, Niehaus GD, Herndon DN. The effect of leukocyte depletion on smoke inhalation injury in sheep. *Surgery* 1988; **104**: 208–15.

105. Isago T, Traber LD, Herndon DN, Traber DL. Pulmonary capillary pressure changes following smoke inhalation in sheep. *Anesthesiology* 1990; **73**: A1234.

106. Loick HM, Traber LD, Tokyay R, Linares HA, Prien T, Traber DL. Mechanical alteration of blood flow in smoked and unsmoked lung areas after inhalation injury. *J Appl Physiol* 1992; **72**: 1692–700.

107. Schenarts PJ, Schmalstieg FC, Hawkins H, Bone HG, Traber LD, Traber DL. Effects of an L-selectin antibody on the pulmonary and systemic manifestations of severe smoke inhalation injuries in sheep. *J Burn Care Rehabil* 2000; **21**: 229–40.

108. Lasky LA. Selectins: interpreters of cell-specific carbohydrate information during inflammation. [Review]. *Science* 1992; **258**: 964–9.

109. Niehaus GD, Kimura R, Traber LD, Herndon DN, Flynn JT, Traber DL. Administration of a synthetic antiprotease reduces smoke-induced lung injury. *J Appl Physiol* 1990; **69**: 694–9.

110. Brown M, Desai M, Traber LD, Herndon DN, Traber DL. Dimethylsulfoxide with heparin in the treatment of smoke inhalation injury. *J Burn Care Rehabil* 1988; **9**: 22–5.

111. Nguyen TT, Herndon DN, Cox CS, *et al.* Effect of manganous superoxide dismutase on lung fluid balance after smoke inhalation injury. *Proc Am Burn Assoc* 1993; **25**: 31.

112. Carlin G, Arfors KE. Peroxidation of liposomes promoted by human polymorphonuclear leucocytes. *J Free Radic Biol Med* 1985; **1**: 437–42.

113. Guice KS, Oldham KT, Caty MG, Johnson KJ, Ward PA. Neutrophil-dependent, oxygen-radical mediated lung injury associated with acute pancreatitis. *Ann Surg* 1989; **210**: 740–7.

114. Charan NB, Turk GM, Dhand R. Gross and subgross anatomy of bronchial circulation in sheep. *J Appl Physiol* 1984; **57**: 658–64.

115. Lakshminarayan S, Kowalski TF, Kirk W, Graham MM, Butler J. The drainage routes of the bronchial blood flow in anesthetized dogs. *Respir Physiol* 1990; **82**: 65–73.

116. Hales CA, Barkin PW, Jung W, *et al.* Synthetic smoke with acrolein but not HCl produces pulmonary edema. *J Appl Physiol* 1988; **64**: 1121–33.

117. Magno MG, Fishman AP. Origin, distribution, and blood flow of bronchial circulation in anesthetized sheep. *J Appl Physiol* 1982; **53**: 272–9.

118. Abdi S, Herndon DN, Traber LD, *et al.* Lung edema formation following inhalation injury: role of the bronchial blood flow. *J Appl Physiol* 1991; **71**: 727–34.

119. Hinder F, Nakazawa H, Matsumoto N, Traber LD, Herndon DN, Traber DL. Separation of the bronchial circulation from the pulmonary in a left lung pouch model. *Am Rev Respir Dis* 1993; **147**: A657.

120. Prien T, Linares HA, Traber LD, Herndon DN, Traber DL. Lack of hematogenous

mediated pulmonary injury with smoke inhalation. *J Burn Care Rehabil* 1988; **9**: 462–6.

121. Cutaia M, Rounds S. Hypoxic pulmonary vasoconstriction. Physiologic significance, mechanism, and clinical relevance. [Review]. *Chest* 1990; **97**: 706–18.

122. Soejima K, Traber LD, Schmalstieg FC, *et al.* Role of nitric oxide in vascular permeability after burns and smoke inhalation combined injury. *Am J Respir Crit Care Med* 2000 (in press).

123. Cerra FB. The multiple organ failure syndrome. *Hosp Pract [Off]* 1990; **25**: 169–76.

124. Dinarello CA. The proinflammatory cytokines interleukin-1 and tumor necrosis factor and treatment of the septic shock syndrome. *J Infect Dis* 1991; **163**: 1177–84.

125. Herndon DN, Barrow RE, Traber DL, Rutan TC, Rutan RL, Abston S. Extravascular lung water changes following smoke inhalation and massive burn injury. *Surgery* 1987; **102**: 341–9.

126. Navar PD, Saffle JR, Warden GD. Effect of inhalation injury on fluid resuscitation requirements after thermal injury. *Am J Surg* 1985; **150**: 716–20.

127. Demling RH, Smith M, Gunther R, Wandzilak T, Pederson NC. Use of a chronic prefemoral lymphatic fistula for monitoring systemic capillary integrity in unanesthetized sheep. *J Surg Res* 1981; **31**: 136–44.

128. Demling RH, LaLonde C. Moderate smoke inhalation produces decreased oxygen delivery, increased oxygen demands, and systemic but not lung parenchymal lipid peroxidation. *Surgery* 1990; **108**: 544–52.

129. Montero K, Lübbesmeyer HJ, Traber DL, Kimura R, Traber LD, Herndon DN. Inhalation injury increases systemic microvascular permeability. *Surg Forum* 1987; **38**: 303–5.

130. LaLonde C, Knox J, Youn YK, Demling R. Burn edema is accentuated by a moderate smoke inhalation injury in sheep. *Surgery* 1992; **112**: 908–17.

131. Traber DL, Sugi K, Flynn JT, Traber LD. Leukotrienes and lung response to inhalation injury. *FASEB J* 1989; **3**: A695.

132. Quinn DA, Robinson D, Jung W, Hales CA. Role of sulfidopeptide leukotrienes in synthetic smoke inhalation injury in sheep. *J Appl Physiol* 1990; **68**: 1962–9.

133. Morris SE, Navaratnam N, Townsend CM Jr, Herndon DN. Bacterial translocation and mesenteric blood flow in a large animal model after cutaneous thermal and smoke inhalation injury. *Surg Forum* 1988; **39**: 189–90.

134. Lundberg JM, Saira A. Bronchial smooth muscle contraction induced by stimulation of capsaicin-sensitive sensory neurons. *Acta Physiol Scand* 1982; **116**: 473–6.

135. Ahn SY, Sugi K, Talke P, *et al.* Effects of allopurinol on smoke inhalation in the ovine model. *J Appl Physiol* 1990; **68**: 228–34.

136. Newald J, Sugi K, Vogl C, Krosl P, Traber DL, Schlag G. Evaluation of heart performance during septic shock in sheep. *Prog Clin Biol Res* 1989; **308**: 237–45.

137. Goldman G, Welbourn R, Kobzik L, Valeri CR, Shepro D, Hechtman HB. Tumor necrosis factor-alpha mediates acid aspiration-induced systemic organ injury. *Ann Surg* 1990; **212**: 513–19.

138. Goldman G, Welbourn R, Kobzik L, Valeri CR, Shepro D, Hechtman HB. Synergism between leukotriene B4 and thromboxane A2 in mediating acid-aspiration injury. *Surgery* 1992; **111**: 55–61.

139. Noshima S, Fujioka K, Isago T, Traber LD, Herndon DN, Traber DL. The effect of a thromboxane synthetase inhibitor, OKY-046, on cardiopulmonary function after smoke inhalation injury. *FASEB J* 1991; **5**: A371.

140. Nelson RM, Cecconi O, Roberts WG, Aruffo A, Linhardt RJ, Bevilacqua MP. Heparin oligosaccharides bind L-and P-selectin and inhibit acute inflammation. *Blood* 1993; **82**: 3253–8.

141. Desai MH, Mlcak R, Richardson J, Nichols R, Herndon DN. Reduction in mortality in pediatric patients with inhalation injury with aerosolized heparin/acetylcystine therapy. *J Burn Care Rehabil* 1998; **19**: 210–12.

142. Wang QL, Shang XY, Zhang SL, *et al.* Effects of inhaled low molecular weight heparin on airway allergic inflammation in aerosol-ovalbumin-sensitized guinea pigs. *Jpn J Pharmacol* 2000; **82**: 326–30.

143. Trocme SD, Li H. Effect of heparin-surface-modified intraocular lenses on postoperative inflammation after phacoemulsification: a randomized trial in a United States patient population. Heparin-Surface-Modified Lens Study Group. *Ophthalmology* 2000; **107**: 1031–7.

144. Perretti M, Page CP. Heparin and inflammation: a new use for an old GAG? [comment]. *Gut* 2000; **47**: 14–15.

145. Brown M, Traber DL, Herndon DN, Oldham KT, Traber LD. The use of venovenous extracorporeal membrane oxygenation in sheep receiving severe smoke inhalation injury. *Burns Incl Therm Inj* 1987; **13**: 34–8.

146. Zwischenberger JB, Cox CS, Minifee PK, *et al.* Pathophysiology of ovine smoke inhalation injury treated with extracorporeal membrane oxygenation. *Chest* 1993; **103**: 1582–6.

147. Brunston RL, Zwischenberger JB, Tao WK, Cardenas VJ, Bidani A. Total arteriovenous CO$_2$ removal – simplifying extracorporeal support for respiratory failure. *Ann Thorac Surg* 1997; **64**: 1599–604.

148. Tao WK, Brunston RL, Bidani A, *et al.* Significant reduction in minute ventilation and peak inspiratory pressures with arteriovenous CO$_2$ removal during severe respiratory failure. *Crit Care Med* 1997; **25**: 689–95.

Chapter 17

Diagnosis and treatment of inhalation injury

John C Fitzpatrick, William G Cioffi Jr

Introduction

The two most critical injuries caused by fires are cutaneous burns and inhalation injury. The multitude of respiratory complications caused by smoke inhalation, cutaneous burns, and their treatment epitomizes the clinical challenge that confronts burn care providers today. Of 1256 patients treated at the US Army Institute of Surgical Research from 1985 to 1990, 330 (26%) sustained a significant inhalation injury,[1] with 97 of those 330 patients (29.4%) succumbing to their injuries. A similar study of 1447 patients from a civilian burn center demonstrated a 20% incidence of inhalation injury in their population, with a 31% mortality rate.[2]

Inhalation injury is an acute respiratory tract insult caused by steam or toxic inhalants such as fumes, gases, and mists. Fumes are various irritants or cytotoxic chemicals adherent to small particles dispersed in air. Mists consist of aerosolized irritant or cytotoxic liquids. Smoke is a combination of fumes, gases, mists, and hot air. Inhalation injury may occur without cutaneous burn injury, though the two injuries usually occur together. Inhalation injury is notable both for its in homogeneous distribution within a patient and its variable severity between patients. The physiocochemical properties of the causative agent, the amount of smoke inhaled, and pre-existing diseases that might lower a patient's immunological resistance determine the site and degree of injury. Despite increasing clinical interest in the problem of inhalation injury over the past few decades, the pathophysiology of inhalation injury remains poorly understood and there have been few improvements in treatment. Inhalation injury continues to be one of the most serious associated injuries complicating the care of thermally injured patients. Prevention or early diagnosis and treatment of associated life-threatening complications are necessary to decrease its associated morbidity and mortality.

Inhalation injury can occur in any of the three anatomic regions of the respiratory tract: the supraglottic, tracheobronchial (major airways), and lung parenchymal regions. The site of injury determines the patient's diagnostic and therapeutic needs. Supraglottic injuries occur by both thermal and chemical means, and may be so severe that upper airway obstruction quickly occurs. The presence of a supraglottic injury is not a reliable indicator of the presence or absence of more distal pulmonary injuries. Tracheobronchial and parenchymal injuries constitute the majority of injuries that require prolonged treatment.

Several forms of pulmonary dysfunction may result from the complex pathophysiologic reactions to inhalation injury. Hypoxia, V_A/Q mismatching, increased airway resistance, increased alveolar epithelial permeability, decreased pulmonary compliance, and increased pulmonary vascular resistance can result from the initial release of vasoactive substances from the damaged epithelium. Immediately after an inhalation injury occurs, these changes probably result from edema formation (at least partly mediated by activated neutrophils) and the release of smooth muscle constrictors such as thromboxane A_2, C_{3a}, and C_{5a}. The contribution of neutrophil activation to this process is highlighted by recent animal studies demonstrating amelioration of lung injury, increased oxygenation, decreased epithelial permeability, and an improvement in alveolar liquid clearance with the use of Sulfo Lewis C[3] (a ligand binding to E-selectins, inhibiting neutrophil rolling adhesion) and anti-interleukin-8 antibody[4] (inhibiting neutrophil chemotaxis). The tracheobronchial mucociliary apparatus, which is responsible for clearing foreign material from the respiratory tract, is damaged and nonfunctional. Further epithelial injury results from the toxic inhalants that are present and no longer being removed. Sloughed necrotic epithelium, serous exudate, blood cells, and mucus form casts that may cause atelectasis and exacerbate both V_A/Q mismatching and hypoxia. Air trapping, which occurs distal to obstructions caused by casts, results in volutrauma. Alternatively, total occlusion of the airways by casts will produce atelectasis and increase the risk of pneumonia.[5] At the cellular level, smoke-exposed macrophages have a decreased ability to phagocytize opsonized bacteria and adhere to solid substratum. The respiratory burst of alveolar macrophages has been shown to increase with increased production of tumor necrosis factor (TNF)-α and superoxide radicals in response to phorbol myristate acetate, an effect not seen in matched peripheral blood polymorphonuclear cells.[6,7]

Patients with inhalation injury frequently develop respiratory failure and require mechanical ventilatory support. Decreased compliance and increased airway resistance may lead to elevated airway pressures and barotrauma, a sometimes unavoidable complication of the use of positive pressure ventilation. Mean airway pressures exceeding the mucosal capillary perfusion pressure may result in ischemia of the already damaged tracheobronchial mucosa, compounding the initial epithelial insult. Overdistention of the normal alveoli leads to alveolar interstitial edema that aggravates the extent of atelectasis, the decrement in compliance, and the increased V_A/Q mismatch caused by the initial injury. Increasing amounts of mucosal slough, interstitial edema, and decreasing compliance lead to further elevation in ventilatory pressures and worsening barotrauma, as well as the likelihood of the development of pneumonia. Multiple organ system failure may develop as a result of perpetuation or exacerbation of the inflammatory process.

Diagnosis

A high index of suspicion for inhalation injury is essential to avoid missed injuries. A history of closed-space smoke exposure is common among these patients, as is concurrent cutaneous burn injury. Many patients are intoxicated at the time of admission to the hospital and will admit to ethanol or drug use immediately before the time of injury. Most will present with some combination of the symptoms and signs listed in **Table 17.1**.

The physical findings of inhalation injury that cause the greatest concern are hoarseness and stridor. Patients with these findings have a partial airway obstruction, usually secondary to edema, and are at substantial risk of complete airway obstruction. These patients should be intubated immediately to maintain airway patency and avoid catastrophic airway obstruction. Disorientation, obtundation, and coma commonly indicate significant exposure to carbon monoxide (CO) or the presence of an associated closed head injury. Patients with a suggestion of cranial trauma by history or physical examination will require cervical spine precautions when being moved. Their initial evaluation, as well as the evaluation of those patients with initially elevated carboxyhemoglobin (COHb) levels that do not clinically improve as their COHb levels return to normal, should include both cervical spine films and cranial computed tomography to rule out cervical or intracranial trauma.

Carbon monoxide exposure is common among patients with inhalation injury and is responsible for the death of many victims at the scene of a fire. The diagnosis is made by direct measurement of the blood COHb level using a co-oximeter. CO displaces

oxygen from the four binding sites available on the hemoglobin molecule and has a much greater affinity for these sites than oxygen. Displacement of oxygen from the binding sites decreases the oxygen-carrying capacity of blood in a linear manner and results in inadequate oxygen delivery to the tissues. Measurements of arterial oxygen tension and noninvasive hemoglobin saturation monitoring do not reflect the percentage of COHb present, and in fact may be expected to be normal despite lethal COHb levels in the fire victim.

Although the majority (56%) of patients with inhalation injury will present with some combination (usually three or more)[8] of history and physical findings indicative of inhalation injury, the specificity and sometimes the sensitivity of these findings are poor. The inability of clinicians to depend on historical details and physical findings to identify patients with inhalation injury requires the use of fiberoptic bronchoscopy and occasionally intravenous xenon-133 ventilation scanning to establish the diagnosis. The use of fiberoptic bronchoscopy also allows immediate institution of therapy if severe inhalation injury or impending airway obstruction is diagnosed. Nasotracheal intubation may be conveniently performed under direct visualization over the bronchoscope if the bronchoscope is placed through an appropriately sized endotracheal tube before the procedure.

Fiberoptic bronchoscopy permits the clinician to perform a detailed examination of the supraglottic area and identify patients with marked edema who are at risk for acute airway obstruction requiring immediate endotracheal intubation to maintain airway patency. Careful examination of the major airways allows the diagnosis of tracheobronchial inhalation injury to be made based on the presence of infraglottic soot or early inflammatory changes of the tracheal mucosa (hyperemia, edema, superficial mucosal sloughing, and ulceration). These changes are often present before arterial blood gas abnormalities, deteriorating pulmonary function tests, or respiratory failure signal the presence of inhalation injury. The best examination is obtained in patients who are euvolemic and normotensive. Hypotensive and hypovolemic patients sometimes do not demonstrate hyperemia and edema, and sloughing or ulceration may not be present during the first few hours following injury. Under ideal conditions, accuracy of the examination approaches 100%. Normally, accuracy is approximately 87%.[9]

The technique for performing fiberoptic bronchoscopy in patients suspected of having an inhalation injury is the same as that used during standard diagnostic bronchoscopy for other diseases. Meticulous attention to the need for good topical supraglottic and infraglottic anesthesia makes the examination tolerable for the patient. When adequate local anesthesia has been achieved in a cooperative patient, intravenous sedation is rarely necessary. Spray bottles of lidocaine or similar agents are particularly useful in anesthetizing the supraglottic area. For anesthesia of the glottis and infraglottic area, 0.5 or 1% injectable plain lidocaine may be instilled through the biopsy channel of the bronchoscope in 3–5 ml aliquots. The use of video endoscopy equipment, especially in teaching institutions, allows observers to learn proper bronchoscopic technique and the gross pathologic appearance of the injury. In any institution, it allows support personnel to anticipate the needs of the endoscopist, thus directly benefiting the patient.

When experienced personnel perform bronchoscopy in appropriately monitored settings, complications are rare. Excellent large retrospective[10,11] and prospective[12] studies of the risk of bron-

Table 17.1 Symptoms and signs suggesting possible inhalation injury	
Symptoms	**Signs**
Lacrimation	Conjunctivitis
Severe, brassy cough	Carbonaceous sputum
Hoarseness	Facial burns
Shortness of breath	Singed basal vibrissae
Anxiety	Stridor
Wheezing	Bronchorrhea
Dyspnea	
Disorientation	
Obtundation	
Coma	

choscopy have indicated that the incidence of major complications, such as death (0.01–0.1%), pneumonia (0.01–0.6%), pneumothorax (0.2–0.4%), hypoxia (0.2%), cardiac arrhythmia (0.6–0.9%), and nausea or vomiting (0.2%) is small. Many of the minor risks of bronchoscopy, such as hemoptysis, are related to the use of brushes and biopsy forceps and rarely occur during bronchoscopy for the diagnosis of inhalation injury. The risks of bronchoscopy are sufficiently small compared to the risks of delayed treatment or the risks of iatrogenic complications for patients without injury who might erroneously receive mechanical ventilation.

Intravenous xenon-133 ventilation–perfusion scanning is a means of identifying regions of complete or incomplete small airway obstruction secondary to inhalation injury. After injection of the radionuclide, serial scans demonstrate respiratory exchange and excretion of xenon by the lungs. Areas retaining isotope for more than 90 seconds are presumed to have segmental airway obstruction secondary to inhalation injury. False-positive examinations may occur in patients with a prior history of chronic obstructive pulmonary disease, or those patients who have a chemical tracheobronchitis, pneumonia from aspiration of gastric contents, or a preexisting respiratory tract infection or pneumonia before smoke exposure. Although not as frequently performed as bronchoscopy, xenon-133 scanning is still useful as a complementary examination, particularly if clinical suspicion is high but bronchoscopic examination fails to confirm that inhalation injury has occurred. The combination of bronchoscopy and xenon-133 scanning is 93% accurate in the diagnosis of smoke inhalation injury.

Pulmonary function tests are useful for long-term follow-up of inhalation injury. Unfortunately, they are not as useful in making an early diagnosis of inhalation injury because they are effort-dependent. It is also frequently difficult to obtain reliable and reproducible results in the acute setting. Pain, weakness, dyspnea, or narcotic administration may adversely affect the patient's ability to comply with testing and thus complicate the interpretation of the results. Despite these concerns, pulmonary function tests are useful for their negative predictive value (94–100%)[13] and low cost when triaging large numbers of victims for identification of those who may require additional diagnostic procedures. Normal pulmonary function tests essentially rule out the possibility of significant inhalation injury. The FEV_1/FVC ratio is a sensitive early marker for airway obstruction. In patients able to comply with testing, the magnitude of decrement in this ratio in comparison to the predicted normal value correlates well with the severity of injury. Flow–volume and pressure–volume loops also have utility during long-term follow-up for assessing lung compliance in patients with restrictive fibrosis or extensive thoracic cage skin grafts and changes in chest wall compliance.

Management

Although there are many causes of inhalation injury, initial therapy consists of a few common-sense measures to stabilize the patient and confirm the diagnosis. With the exception of specific treatments for poisonings, treatment is supportive. Careful and repeated evaluation of therapeutic interventions is necessary to prevent iatrogenic injuries (barotrauma, suction catheter trauma) that perpetuate the inflammatory process and prevent healing. Conservative approaches to the management of inhalation injury

emphasize the use of measures to avoid intubation and positive pressure ventilation. If ventilatory support is necessary, permissive hypercapnia and borderline adequacy of oxygenation is preferable to attain arbitrarily 'normal' blood gases at the cost of inflicting barotrauma and volutrauma. Lung protective strategies are essential to decrease further iatrogenic lung injury.

Initial stabilization follows the standard principles of management of trauma and burn patients. First, the patient must be removed from the hazardous area by individuals sufficiently knowledgeable and appropriately equipped to prevent further injury to either the patient or to themselves. For patients sustaining both cutaneous burns and inhalation injury, the rescuer must ensure that the burning process is stopped. A patent airway must be maintained. In most patients, airway obstruction develops gradually, but if obstruction is present when the patient is first evaluated it must be relieved immediately by oropharyngeal sweep, oropharyngeal or nasopharyngeal airway, or airway intubation by endotracheal tube or (rarely) cricothyroidotomy. While adequate ventilation and circulation are being obtained, supplemental 100% oxygen should be administered as the patient is being transported to the nearest appropriate medical facility. Intravenous access should be secured and appropriate fluid resuscitation initiated.

The patient should be assessed for other life-threatening injuries while a pertinent history is obtained and a physical examination is expeditiously performed (**Table 17.2**). Baseline laboratory studies should be obtained, including arterial blood gases, a chest roentgenogram, and an electrocardiogram. Although the study results may be normal early after an inhalation injury has occurred, they serve as a useful baseline against which subsequent studies may be compared. Direct inspection of the airway by fiberoptic bronchoscopy should be performed if the patient is breathing spontaneously and has a history of smoke exposure and symptoms or signs suggesting possible inhalation injury (see **Table 17.1**), or in any patient requiring ventilatory assistance to confirm or refute the presence of inhalation injury. Early intubation under semiurgent circumstances to protect the airway is preferable to waiting until airway obstruction is so severe that intubation under emergency circumstances becomes necessary. Upper airway edema normally progresses to maximal edema and peak airway narrowing at approximately 24 hours post-injury. If edema is not present on admission, a period of observation in an intensive care unit is warranted.

Most patients sustaining an inhalation injury will also have sustained a cutaneous thermal injury. The presence of a thermal injury requires appropriate fluid resuscitation to avoid hypovolemic shock, renal failure, and death in the early postburn period. The endpoint of resuscitation is not changed by the presence of an inhala-

Table 17.2 Important injury site characteristics and transport details
- Type of materials and fuels ignited
- Type of toxic inhalant
- Closed space versus open space exposure
- Duration of exposure
- Use of supplemental oxygen
- Transport time to hospital
- Mental status
- Evidence of intoxication

tion injury. Urine output of 30–50 ml/h in adults or 0.5–1 ml/kg/h in children weighing 30 kg or less is the best indication that appropriate fluid resuscitation is being administered. It is common for patients with both inhalation injury and cutaneous thermal injury to require more resuscitation fluid than patients with cutaneous thermal injury alone. Several retrospective clinical reviews[14–18] have shown that coexisting thermal injury and inhalation injury increase fluid resuscitation requirements of patients with cutaneous thermal injury, particularly in the first 24 hours by 40–75% (range 13.5–110%) compared to patients without inhalation injury. A prospective animal study demonstrated that inadequate fluid resuscitation following smoke inhalation injury was detrimental.[19] A group of sheep resuscitated with intravenous fluid infused at a normal maintenance rate following severe smoke inhalation injury experienced significantly increased lung lymph flow, elevated lymph to plasma oncotic pressure, decreased arterial oxygen pressure (Pao_2), decreased cardiac output, and increased mortality (100% vs. 30%) compared to a group of sheep with an identical smoke inhalation injury resuscitated with intravenous fluid infused at twice the normal maintenance rate. The data indicate that limiting fluid resuscitation 'to protect the lung' may actually lead to increased extravascular lung water, hypoxia, and decrements in lung function, along with the risks of inadequate tissue perfusion, renal failure, and possible death from hypovolemic shock.

For patients exposed only to simple asphyxiants (carbon dioxide, helium, methane, nitrogen), no evidence of supraglottic or tracheobronchial mucosal injury will be found and only supportive care is necessary. Serial neurologic examinations should be performed with all deficits carefully documented to allow for objective assessment of the patient's prognosis. If the anoxic period was short and no permanent neurologic damage occurred, recovery can be expected.

For patients with inhalation injury secondary to CO exposure, it is important to establish the COHb level on admission, both to estimate length of treatment for CO exposure and for calculation of the peak COHb level, which in animal models has been shown to correlate with the presence of inhalation injury.[20] It should be noted, however, that a low or normal COHb level does not rule out the presence of inhalation injury. Patients should receive 100% oxygen until their COHb level is less than 10%. The elimination half-life ($t_{1/2}$) for COHb depends on oxygen tension. The $t_{1/2}$ for COHb at sea level is 250 minutes while breathing room air (20.8% oxygen), 40–50 minutes breathing 100% oxygen,[21,22] and 27 minutes breathing 100% oxygen at two atmospheres pressure.[23]

There is much controversy regarding the indications for, and efficacy of, hyperbaric oxygen administration. Some proponents recommend the use of hyperbaric oxygen to prevent certain neurologic complications (blindness, deafness, psychosis, and Parkinson's disease) reputedly due to CO poisoning, though the correlation of those changes with COHb levels is poor.[24,25] Physiologic monitoring of patients in hyperbaric chambers is difficult due to the risk of fire and the effect of pressure on solid-state electrical components. Small chambers isolate the patient from physicians and nursing staff; large chambers require exposure of physicians and nursing staff to the risks of 'diving' with the patient. One study reported severe complications related to hyperbaric treatment (cardiac arrest, seizures, and cardiac arrhythmia) in seven of 10 patients.[26] The question remains whether the potential benefits of hyperbaric oxygen outweigh the documented risks. At this time, with the exception of symptomatic patients (coma, seizures, respiratory failure) with very high COHb levels for whom the benefits may outweigh the risks, hyperbaric oxygen should be restricted to randomized prospective trials to determine the efficacy of this therapy for specific groups of patients.

Specific therapy for cyanide poisoning in patients with inhalation injury is also controversial, as there is no consensus on the incidence of clinically important cyanide exposure. Proponents of therapy point out the increased incidence of fires involving polyurethanes, which produce large amounts of hydrogen cyanide (HCN). Opponents cite the lack of correlation between cyanide levels and mortality in fire victims. For adequately resuscitated patients with unexplained severe metabolic acidosis, tachycardia, tachypnea, elevated central venous oxygen content and normal arterial oxygen content, treatment should be considered. Cyanide uncouples oxidative phosphorylation by binding to mitochondrial cytochrome $a–a_3$. The goal of therapy is to create a sink of ferric iron that will trap the cyanide until it can be converted to thiocyanate through the actions of the hepatic enzyme rhodanase. The most convenient sink is hemoglobin. Administration of amyl and sodium nitrite, which converts the ferrous iron in heme to the ferric form, accelerates the formation of cyanhemoglobin. Both agents are potent vasodilators, however, which limits their use to normotensive or hypertensive patients. Sodium thiosulfate is administered to ensure that sufficient sulfur substrate is available to rhodanase for conversion of cyanate (CN^-) to thiocyanate (SCN^-), which is excreted by the kidney.

Except for therapy to counteract the effects of specific toxins as described, the care of patients with inhalation injury is supportive. Despite the lack of specific interventions, assiduous supportive care is essential to decrease the morbidity and mortality resulting both from complications of the initial injury and iatrogenic injury caused by necessary treatment. **Table 17.3** illustrates treatment algorithms for patients with mild, moderate, and severe inhalation injury. Once a secure airway has been established and the patient has been placed on supplemental oxygen, priority should be given to minimizing airway edema, maintaining pulmonary toilet, relieving mechanical restriction of chest wall motion, and treating bronchospasm to reduce the patient's work of breathing and reduce the need for mechanical ventilation. Elevation of the head of the bed to 30° helps to decrease airway edema and minimize pressure from abdominal contents that limits diaphragmatic excursion. If the patient has cutaneous burns, appropriate resuscitation must be carried out regardless of the presence of inhalation injury and the possibility that resulting airway edema may necessitate intubation. Respiratory failure is much easier to treat and much less morbid than persistent hypovolemic shock and renal failure. Circumferential full-thickness burns of the thorax that mechanically limit chest wall excursion require escharotomies placed in the anterior axillary lines bilaterally and connected by a transverse incision at the costal margin. These escharotomies may allow some patients to avoid the need for mechanical ventilatory support. In those requiring ventilatory support, escharotomies help to minimize pressure generated during ventilator cycles, thus avoiding iatrogenic barotrauma.

Airway clearance techniques are an essential component of respiratory management of patients with smoke inhalation injury. Therapeutic coughing, chest physiotherapy, early ambulation, airway suctioning, and pharmacologic agents may all be effective

Table 17.3 Treatment algorithms for pathophysiologic events resulting from mild, moderate, and severe inhalation injury

Problem	Diagnosis/treatment	Seen in
Hypoxia	Supplemental oxygen	All injuries
Reactive bronchorrhea, copious secretions	Incentive spirometry, chest physiotherapy, nasotracheal suctioning	All injuries
Inspissated secretions	Humidification, nasotracheal suctioning	Moderate and severe injuries
Wheezing	Diagnostic bronchoscopy to distinguish endobronchial obstruction (plugging) from bronchospasm and edema	Moderate and severe injuries
Plugging (inspissated mucus or mucosal slough)	Humidification, therapeutic bronchoscopy as needed, aerosolized heparin	Moderate and severe injuries
Bronchospasm	Nebulized β_2-agonists; if ineffective, then intravenous aminophylline	Moderate and severe injuries
Respiratory failure	Intubation, mechanical ventilation, permissive hypercapnia, tracheostomy if failure is prolonged (>14 days)	Severe inhalation injury

in mobilizing and removing retained secretions. Secretions that the patient cannot clear spontaneously may accrete and from life-threatening airway obstructions; they may also cause atelectasis, V_A/Q mismatch, and contribute to the development of pneumonia.

For several reasons (altered mental status, the presence of endotracheal or tracheostomy tubes) the ability to cough may be impaired and stimulation may be necessary to clear secretions. Stimulation may be provided by tracheal suctioning or by giving a large tidal volume breath using a manual resuscitation bag and, if possible, by providing chest percussion simultaneously. Chest physiotherapy and bronchial drainage may also be useful, but these are frequently limited by confounding factors such as the location of skin grafts and donor sites. The use of an internal pneumatic percussion device obviates some of these difficulties.

Tracheobronchial suctioning is important to remove debris that cannot be cleared by patients with an incapacitated mucociliary apparatus and ineffective cough. Adequate humidification of inspired gas is essential to help limit inspissation of mucus in the injured airways. The patient should be placed in Fowler's position and ventilated with 100% oxygen before suctioning is performed. Suctioning should not be performed for more than 15 seconds (and less in children) to minimize the occurrence of transient hypoxia, excessive vagal stimulation, and bradycardia. Adequate preoxygenation and short suctioning times have been shown to decrease or eliminate hypoxic episodes during pulmonary toilet.

Despite adequate humidification, inspissation of secretions still occurs in many patients with severe inhalation injury. In experimental ovine models of inhalation injury, heparin administered either systemically[27] or by nebulizer[28] prevented or decreased the formation of tracheobronchial casts. Both methods produced significant reductions in minute ventilation, peak inspiratory pressure, and positive end-expiratory pressure (PEEP). Both methods should reduce the risk of barotrauma associated with mechanical ventilation. Since heparin delivery by nebulizer has not caused systemic anticoagulation in patient trials, this method of administration should remain the treatment of choice if heparin therapy is indicated. Further validation of this approach has been reported in a pediatric trial of combined heparin and acetylcysteine administration via nebulizer. Pao_2/Fio_2 ratios improved, and reintubations and mortality decreased compared to controls.[29]

Wheezing may be caused by several mechanisms such as endobronchial obstruction from sloughed mucosa, bronchospasm, or mucosal edema. The disparate pathophysiologic mechanisms require fundamentally different treatments, and prophylactic therapies (e.g. prophylactic bronchodilator therapy) are of little value. If wheezing occurs and endobronchial obstruction from mucosal slough is ruled out, a trial of standard β_2-agonists may decrease bronchospasm. β_2-Agonists relax bronchial smooth muscle and stimulate mucociliary clearance. If this therapy is not successful, intravenous aminophylline should be instituted and blood levels carefully monitored to avoid potential cardiac and central nervous system toxicities. Wheezing from mucosal edema may be minimized by appropriate fluid administration during resuscitation and elevation of the head of the bed. In prospective clinical trials,[30,31] steroids have not been shown to be of benefit in altering morbidity or mortality after inhalation injury, and they may be associated with a higher rate of infection-related complications. Therefore, they should be avoided unless the patient was steroid-dependent before injury or has persistent bronchospasm unresponsive to other therapy.

When all other techniques fail to remove secretions, the use of fiberoptic bronchoscopy has proven effective. In addition to its diagnostic function, bronchoscopy has important therapeutic applications. Inspissated secretions, particularly when hardened by the presence of blood to form casts, may prove resistant to all simpler methods of removal from the tracheobronchial tree. Bronchoscopy allows instrumentation of the airway under direct vision and enables meticulous pulmonary toilet to be maintained in patients with severe inhalation injury. Despite all efforts to support unassisted ventilation, patients with moderate or severe inhalation injury may develop respiratory failure and require mechanical ventilatory support. Some patients have preexisting obstructive pulmonary diseases (e.g. emphysema or chronic bronchitis) that make it difficult to adequately mobilize the increased volume of secretions caused by the inhalation injury. Other patients may have cardiovascular insufficiency and be unable to tolerate the volume of fluid required for resuscitation. Some may not be able to achieve and maintain the large minute ventilation required to clear the excess carbon dioxide (CO_2) produced by the hypermetabolic response to burn injury. Regardless of the cause, when tachypnea and recruitment of accessory muscles of respiration are noted, the probability of respiratory failure must be considered and plans made to initiate mechanical ventilatory support. Objective data should be collected at this time, not only to document the diagnosis of respiratory failure, but also to provide a baseline that can be used for serial assessment of the efficacy of therapy. Common indices indicative of respiratory failure include respiratory rate greater than 30 breaths/min, hypoxemia (Pao_2 <70 mmHg), hypercapnia ($Paco_2$>50 mmHg), vital capacity less than 4 ml/kg, dead space/tidal volume ventilation ratio (V_D/V_T)>0.6 and a Pao_2/Fio_2 ratio less than 200.

The intent of mechanical ventilation is to provide adequate ventilatory support to meet the patient's needs without exacerbating the existing pulmonary lesions or causing barotrauma. Airway resistance is increased in airways narrowed by edema. Thus, airway pressures must be increased to maintain sufficient flow to support minute ventilation. In patients with severe inhalation injury who require mechanical ventilation, it is unnecessary and unwise to ventilate the patient to attain an arbitrarily 'normal' blood gas due to the high mean airway pressures that may be required. High mean airway pressures decrease tracheobronchial mucosal capillary blood flow, resulting in mucosal ischemia. Elevated levels of carbon dioxide are surprisingly well tolerated, if the pH can be maintained above 7.25. Thus, the slightly acidic (pH_a = 7.30–7.32) environment associated with permissive hypercapnia can be expected to minimize the mean airway pressure required for ventilation. Similarly, 'normal' levels of Pao_2 may require high levels of PEEP, resulting in high mean airway pressures. Oxygen saturations greater than 93% or Pao_2 > 70 mmHg are sufficient to maintain an adequate oxygen concentration gradient in peripheral tissues. To keep airway pressures to a minimum, ventilator settings should be adjusted to slightly higher rates (15–20 breaths/min) and smaller tidal volumes (6 ml/kg) with the addition of physiologic PEEP (5 cmH$_2$O) to prevent small airway closure, alveolar collapse, and resulting high airway and alveolar opening pressures. Lung protective strategies have recently been shown to decrease morbidity and mortality in adult respiratory distress syndrome (ARDS) patients randomized to conventional or low tidal volumes.

Experimental evidence reported by Cioffi et al.[32] showed that in a baboon model of moderate smoke inhalation injury, the barotrauma index (rate × pressure product) was significantly increased during conventional ventilation compared to high-frequency flow interruption ventilation, while both attained adequate ventilation and oxygenation. There was also significantly more parenchymal injury in the group treated with conventional ventilation compared to the high-frequency flow interruption group. Data collected in three retrospective studies[1,33,34] indicate that optimal ventilation and survival in adults may be attained with high-frequency flow interruption ventilation compared to conventional (volume-limited) ventilation and that significant decreases in the incidence of pneumonia and mortality in patients with inhalation injury have been noted when high-frequency percussive ventilation rather than conventional ventilation was used. Recent retrospective studies of pediatric patients have demonstrated a significant decrease in the incidence of pneumonia, improved P/F ratios (arterial oxygen partial pressure/fractional inspired oxygen concentration ratio), and work of breathing for patients receiving high-frequency flow interruption ventilation compared to controls receiving conventional

ventilation.[35,36] This form of ventilatory support represents one method to protect the lung with inhalation injury. Conventional ventilator strategies may be effective if meticulous attention is paid to minimizing tidal volumes.

If prolonged ventilatory failure is expected due to severe inhalation injury, preexisting pulmonary disease, or difficulty in maintaining pulmonary toilet (secondary to small airway size or to complications of inhalation injury such as pneumonia), the risks and benefits of tracheostomy should be considered. Early tracheostomy, performed for airway management rather than endotracheal intubation, has been shown to have a 6% operative complication rate and a 30% long-term complication rate.[31] Long-term endotracheal intubation has similar long-term complications and is also uncomfortable for the patient. Endotracheal tubes are limited to those that will fit easily through the larynx and, in patients with small airways, the small tube size may cause significant resistance to air flow, resulting in increased work of breathing and higher pressure during mechanical ventilatory cycles to achieve adequate air exchange. Pulmonary toilet is also more difficult to maintain through small-diameter endotracheal tubes and residual debris and secretions can cause life-threatening airway obstruction. The multitude of considerations regarding tracheostomy requires that the decision be individualized for each patient. Indiscriminant use of any single rule regarding the type of injury or time of endotracheal intubation is inadequate for selecting patients who will benefit from this procedure.

After the patient's clinical condition has reached sustained improvement in ventilatory indices and decreased bronchorrhea, ventilatory support should be carefully weaned by gradual reductions in inspired oxygen concentration, PEEP, and ventilator rate until patients can independently support their own ventilatory needs. Weaning cannot be forced and patience is important, especially when preexisting disease or prolonged periods of ventilatory assistance and pharmacologic neuromuscular blockade complicate the process. Patients should be capable of supporting their own ventilatory needs when they are hemodynamically stable and no longer tachypneic (respiratory rate less than 30 breaths/min), acidotic (pH_a>7.35), hypoxic (Pao_2>70 with Fio_2<0.40 and Pao_2/Fio_2>300) or weak (vital capacity greater than 10 ml/kg and V_D/V_T<0.6). Following weaning and extubation or disconnection of the tracheostomy, the patient should be provided with humidified supplemental oxygen (Fio_2 not greater than 0.4) and carefully observed for evidence of recurrent ventilatory failure necessitating resumption of mechanical ventilatory support.

Complications

Early Complications

Early complications of inhalation injury are usually mechanical or infectious. Rapid recognition of these complications is essential so that appropriate treatment may be started, thus minimizing the potential for morbidity and added mortality. Mechanical complications are typically manifestations of barotrauma or patient care procedures. Barotrauma represents a spectrum of iatrogenic injuries caused by mechanical ventilation, and it most commonly presents as a pneumothorax, pneumomediastinum, subcutaneous emphysema, or pneumoperitoneum. The patient at risk for barotrauma is one who requires high mean airway pressure to maintain alveolar recruitment, and thus this patient is at risk for sustaining persistent tracheobronchial mucosal ischemia. Continued ischemia prevents healing of the already damaged tracheal mucosa and may contribute to the continued release of inflammatory mediators. Occasionally, barotrauma may occur as the result of vigorous coughing in the unintubated patient and usually presents as a spontaneous pneumothorax.

Infectious complications such as tracheobronchitis or pneumonia have their own well-defined morbidity and mortality.[37] The injured trachea is known to be at risk for infection,[38,39] and respiratory tract infection has been shown to be the most common complication following inhalation injury.[40] The incidence of pneumonia appears to be constant (38%) in patients with inhalation injury, as reported in two different patient cohorts from the same institution (1980–1984 and 1985–1990), although the mortality rate in these patients was noted to decrease from 46.6% to 29.4% over the same period.[1] There are several determinants that predispose patients with inhalation injury to pulmonary infections, but the most significant risk factor (aside from the inhalation injury itself) is colonization of the airway secondary to endotracheal intubation, aspiration, and oropharyngeal colonization with pathogenic organisms.[41] Many of the natural airway defenses that help to prevent infection are bypassed in intubated patients. The source of most pathogenic organisms causing nosocomial infection is the patient. Oropharyngeal and burn wound colonization, usually with the patient's own skin and gastrointestinal tract flora, are the primary repositories of these bacteria. Improvements in outcome in burn patients with pneumonia appear to be related to increased survival in those patients with mild inhalation injury and increased survival in patients placed on high-frequency flow interruption ventilation compared to those receiving conventional ventilation.[1]

Establishing a diagnosis of tracheobronchitis or pneumonia can be extraordinarily difficult due to the presence of inhalation injury and bacterial colonization of the airway. The diagnosis rests on the presence of fever, leukocytosis, and productive cough as well as organisms and white blood cells on Gram's stain of sputum preparations. In addition, parenchymal infiltrates must be present on the chest roentgenogram to make the diagnosis of pneumonia. Inhalation injury without a superimposed infection is characterized by the presence of white blood cells on Gram's stain sputum preparations, productive cough, fever, leukocytosis (especially if there is an associated cutaneous burn), and patchy perivascular and peribronchial infiltrates on chest roentgenogram. Upper respiratory tract colonization with organisms abnormal for that site – such as Gram-negative bacilli and *Staphylococcus aureus* – is also common, thus not supporting the diagnosis of pneumonia. The diagnosis is best made when the criteria above are present (greater than 20 white blood cells and organisms on a Gram's stain sputum preparation), and there has been a substantial change in the quantity and purulence of the patient's sputum, a change in the fever pattern, a need for an increase in the amount of ventilatory support, a change in the pattern of infiltrates on chest roentgenogram, or a decline in the patients' clinical condition without another identifiable source. Unfortunately, techniques such as bronchoalveolar lavage or protected brush specimens have not been helpful in increasing the sensitivity and specificity of the diagnosis of pneumonia.

Treatment consists of empiric intravenous antibiotic therapy based on the results of the Gram's stain sputum preparation and regularly obtained surveillance cultures until the specific sputum culture and antibiotic sensitivity results are available to allow refinement of the antibiotic therapy. Prospective randomized trials of prophylactic antibiotic therapy[30,42] have shown that prophylactic antibiotics do not change the incidence, morbidity, or mortality of pneumonia but do hasten the emergence of resistant flora. Therapy should be administered for an appropriate length of time (usually 10–14 days for common pulmonary pathogens), and both clinical indices and serial Gram's stain sputum preparation results should be followed during treatment to verify the clinical effectiveness of administered treatment. When appropriate, serum antibiotic levels should be monitored to ensure that effective, but not toxic, quantities of antibiotic are being administered. Meticulous pulmonary toilet is also necessary to minimize pooling of secretions and prevent atelectasis, which may serve as sources of continued infection.

Questions have been posed recently as to whether the incidence of nosocomial pneumonia in thermally injured patients with inhalation injury is affected by the method of stress ulcer prophylaxis being used. In a prospective study[43] of 96 thermally injured patients (49 with inhalation injury) randomized to receive either sucralfate or acid neutralizing treatment (H_2 blocker and antacid), the sputum colonization rate and the overall incidence, type, and time to diagnosis of pneumonia was unaffected by the method of prophylaxis, although a significantly greater number of patients receiving sucralfate developed pneumonia while intubated. The group receiving sucralfate also was noted to have three episodes of clinically apparent upper gastrointestinal bleeding (none in the acid-neutralizing group); this difference did not reach significance. Thus, in thermally injured patients it appears that the method of stress ulcer prophylaxis does not affect the occurrence of nosocomial pneumonia.

Late Complications

Late complications of inhalation injury may be related to mechanical damage or the consequences of an uncontrolled inflammatory process. These complications are not as easily treated as the early complications of inhalation injury, and prevention is often the only effective therapy.

Mechanical complications occur most often as the result of iatrogenic injury from an endotracheal tube or tracheostomy tube cuff. Tube cuffs may cause erosion of the tracheal cartilages, allowing tracheal wall collapse from negative airway pressures during inspiration (tracheomalacia). Injury to the tracheal epithelium may eventually result in fibrosis and stenosis of the trachea (subglottic stenosis) as the wound contracts. Erosion into adjacent structures (innominate artery or esophagus) may result in exsanguinating hemorrhage or severe mediastinitis. These injuries are difficult to diagnose and often develop slowly, and are thus undiscovered until after the patient's acute care has been completed and rehabilitation has begun. Tube instability, high cuff pressures (>20 cmH$_2$O) and duration of intubation all contribute to airway damage. These injuries are difficult to treat satisfactorily once they occur, emphasizing the importance of prevention (e.g. stabilization of the tube, careful maintenance of the cuff pressure at the minimum required for an appropriate seal not exceeding 20 cmH$_2$O, and expedient extubation or conversion to a tracheostomy in patients requiring prolonged ventilatory support) and vigilance as the most important mechanisms to avoid these complications.

Inflammatory complications (bronchiectasis and bronchial stenosis) probably occur as a result of neutrophil activation in the area of airway damaged by inhalation injury. Activated neutrophils produce both proteases and oxygen radicals that may cause severe damage to the already injured bronchial mucosa and extracellular matrix. Although most proteases are produced by neutrophils, other cells, including alveolar macrophages, mast cells, basophils, eosinophils, and fibroblasts all may participate in protease secretion. Oxidants secreted by neutrophils are known to inhibit the function of α_1-antitrypsin, an important inhibitor of proteases such as neutrophil elastase, collagenase, cathepsins, and gelatinase.[44] Normal host defense mechanisms protecting mucosal integrity (antiproteases and antioxidants) have been shown to function poorly after inhalation injury.[45] Uncontrolled degradation of extracellular matrix proteins may lead to acute lung diseases such as ARDS and chronic lung diseases such as emphysema and bronchiectasis. Damage of both smoke-injured and normal tissues by proteases and oxidants may lead to persistent escalation of the inflammatory response[46] which prevents healing and worsens pulmonary function and may result in an inability to ventilate the patient, multisystem organ failure, and death.

Future directions

At this time, care of the patient with inhalation injury is supportive, with an emphasis on prevention and early recognition of complications. Efforts to minimize barotrauma are important to decrease the incidence of the side-effects of mechanical ventilation. Further research into the pathogenesis of inhalation injury may lead to the development of specific therapies to minimize the insult and to prevent the exaggerated inflammatory sequelae that can cause considerable morbidity and mortality.

Reduction of Barotrauma

Modification of conventional ventilator therapy to include high-frequency positive pressure ventilation has resulted in favorable trends in the incidence of pneumonia and mortality rates. In a study of patients with severe inhalation injury requiring mechanical ventilation, high-frequency percussive ventilation was found to permit adequate ventilation and oxygenation of patients who had failed conventional ventilation.[5] The utility of this mode of ventilation appears to be its ability to recruit damaged collapsed alveoli and maintain these alveoli in an open state during expiration. Maintaining alveolar recruitment at low mean airway pressures helps prevent or minimize barotrauma from high airway pressures and overdistention of normal alveoli, and allows improved distribution of ventilation. Other methods of ventilation such as hybrid or total liquid ventilation are being evaluated to determine their role in the treatment of inhalation injury. Liquid ventilation, although promising in early animal studies, has not been efficacious in human trials. Extracorporeal membrane oxygenation,[47,48] arteriovenous carbon dioxide removal,[49,50] and intravascular membrane oxygenation[51] have all been used to provide ventilation in extreme cases of respiratory failure, but so far these have had limited clinical applicability. The most promising of these appears to be arteriovenous carbon dioxide removal. Because of the success in animal trials, clinical trials are now underway.

Prospective Therapies

Identification of the pathogenetic mechanisms that amplify the initial mucosal damage caused by smoke exposure and produce pulmonary and systemic dysfunction may permit the development of specific therapies to prevent progressive systemic inflammation. The pathophysiologic responses to inhalation injury are complex, overlapping, and redundant. Almost certainly, control of the inflammatory response will require coordination of several therapies rather than one omnipotent therapy. Current work in the field of lung injury centers on the following areas: mechanisms of neutrophil recruitment and activation, modulation of lipid peroxidation, extracellular proteases and oxygen radicals, the role of deficient surfactant function, prevention of tracheobronchial cast formation, reduction of pulmonary hypertension, and the role of numerous inflammatory mediators (TNF, IL-1, IL-8, prostaglandins, phospholipase A_2, eicosanoids, and leukotrienes) in propagation of local injury.

Numerous cells residing in the lung can produce chemotactic and activating substances, notably alveolar macrophages (TNF, IL-1, IL-8, platelet activating factor, platelet-derived growth factor), endothelial cells (IL-1[52] and IL-8[53]) and possibly epithelial cells (IL-8[54] and leukotrienes[55]). Many of these substances are also being investigated for their contributions to the pathogenesis of ARDS and multiorgan system failure. Identification of the roles of these substances in amplification of the initial injury response, such as selectins[3] and IL-8,[4] will provide an excellent opportunity to intervene and modulate the inflammatory cascade before injury of normal lung, progression of respiratory dysfunction and the development of multiorgan system dysfunction occurs.

Extracellular proteases and oxidants are the direct mediators of neutrophil-induced injury. Protease inhibitors, such as α_1-antitrypsin and α_2-macroglobulin, are the primary antiproteases present in the lung under normal circumstances. Extensive neutrophil activation and release of large amounts of oxidant species result in inactivation of antiproteases. Therapy that increases the quantity of free radical scavengers and functional antiproteases, or controls the synthesis and secretion of oxygen radicals and proteases, may be effective in preventing secondary injury to normal lung. Experimentally free radical scavengers such as dimethylsulfoxide[28,56] have been shown to improve survival (in one study) and decrease microvascular permeability as measured by lung lymph flow and lung wet to dry weight ratios after inhalation injury in an ovine model. Pentoxifylline[57] has been demonstrated to reduce significantly the degree of leukocytosis, absolute polymorphonuclear cell counts, total protein content of bronchoalveolar lavage fluid, and lung wet to dry weight ratios following inhalation injury. In addition, pulmonary compliance, respiratory index (a measure of oxygenation efficiency), V_A/Q mismatching, pulmonary capillary wedge pressure, and pulmonary vascular resistance were all significantly improved following administration of pentoxifylline. In contrast, a study investigating the effects of nitric oxide[58] insufflation after inhalation injury found improvement in pulmonary vascular resistance without apparent effect on the magnitude of inflammation, and little improvement in V_A/Q mismatching or pulmonary gas exchange. Human trials have been equally disappointing. In an ovine model of inhalation injury, the administration of a platelet activating factor antagonist decreased leukocytosis and lipid peroxidation.[59] Recently, lazaroids have been shown to decrease lipid peroxidation and free radical production, and appeared to decrease the histologic severity of smoke inhalation injury in a rabbit model.[60,61] Another study has implicated activation of cytosolic phospholipase A_2 as a mediator of local lung injury.[62] Clinical studies will be necessary to document whether these various agents will influence morbidity and mortality favorably in patients with inhalation injury.

Deficient surfactant function has been demonstrated in many animal models of lung injury as well as in studies of ARDS patients.[63] The deficiency results from inactivation of existing surfactant by lipid peroxidation and apoprotein cleavage, as well as decreased surfactant production by type II pneumocytes. Inactivation of surfactant results in loss of hysteresis in the lung, encourages alveolar collapse, markedly increases peak and mean airway pressure, worsens V_A/Q mismatch, increases extravascular lung water, and greatly decreases ventilatory efficiency.[64] Clinical trials assessing the efficacy of exogenous surfactant administration are ongoing.

In experimental models of inhalation injury heparin has proved effective, alone[27] and in combination with dimethylsulfoxide,[28,56] in reducing the amount of airway obstruction in damaged airways caused by casts formed by sloughed epithelial cells and protein-rich exudate. Significant reductions in minute ventilation, peak inspiratory pressure, and PEEP were also noted that should reduce the risk of barotrauma during mechanical ventilation.

The first major improvement in the treatment of burn injury came with the recognition of the importance of fluid resuscitation to prevent shock and renal failure. The use of topical antibiotics to control burn wound infection and prevent invasive burn wound sepsis led to the next significant reduction in morbidity and mortality of burn patients. Although progress has been made in the treatment of inhalation injury, the pathophysiology of the injury is still incompletely defined. A better understanding of pathogenetic mechanisms may lead to the development of therapeutic agents and treatment regimens that will modulate the cascades of humoral mediators of organ dysfunction and reduce the associated morbidity and mortality.

References

1. Rue LW III, Cioffi WG Jr, Mason AD Jr, et al. Improved survival of burned patients with inhalation injury. *Arch Surg* 1993; **128**: 772–80.
2. Smith DL, Cairns BA, Ramadan F, et al. Effect of inhalation injury, burn size, and age on mortality: a study of 1447 consecutive burn patients. *J Trauma* 1994; **37**: 655–9.
3. Tasaki O, Mozingo DW, Ishihara S, et al. Effect of Sulfo Lewis C on smoke inhalation injury in an ovine model. *Crit Care Med* 1998; **26(7)**: 1238–43.
4. Laffon M, Pittet JF, Modelska K, et al. Interleukin-8 mediates injury from smoke inhalation to both the lung endothelial and the alveolar epithelial barriers in rabbits. *Am J Respir Crit Care Med* 1999; **160**: 1443–9.
5. Cioffi WG Jr, Graves TA, McManus WF, et al. High-frequency percussive ventilation in patients with inhalation injury. *J Trauma* 1989; **29**: 350–4.
6. Bidani A, Wang CZ, Heming TA. Cotton smoke inhalation primes alveolar macrophages for tumor necrosis factor-production and suppresses macrophage antimicrobial activities. *Lung* 1998; **176**: 325–36.
7. Bidani A, Hawkins HK, Wang CZ, Heming TA. Dose dependence and time course of smoke inhalation injury in a rabbit model. *Lung* 1999; **177**: 111–22.
8. Clark WR, Bonaventura M, Myers W. Smoke inhalation and airway management at a regional burnt unit: 1974–1983, part I: diagnosis and consequences of smoke inhalation. *J Burn Care Rehabil* 1989; **10**: 52–62.
9. Agee RN, Long JM, Hunt JL, et al. Use of [133]xenon in early diagnosis of inhalation injury. *J Trauma* 1976; **16**: 218–24.
10. Suratt PM, Smiddy JF, Gruber B. Deaths and complications associated with fiberoptic bronchoscopy. *Chest* 1976; **69**: 747–51.
11. Credle WF Jr, Smiddy JF, Elliott RC. Complications of fiberoptic bronchoscopy. *Am Rev Respir Dis* 1974; **109**: 67–72.
12. Pereira W Jr, Kovnat DM, Snider GL. A prospective cooperative study of complications following flexible fiberoptic bronchoscopy. *Chest* 1978; **73**: 813–16.
13. Haponik EF. Clinical and functional assessment. In: Haponik EF, Munster AM, eds. *Respiratory Injury: Smoke Inhalation and Burns.* New York: McGraw-Hill, 1990: 171.
14. Scheulen JJ, Munster AM. The Parkland formula in patients with burns and inhalation injury. *J Trauma* 1982; **22**: 869–71.
15. Navar PD, Saffle JR, Warden GD. Effect of inhalation injury on fluid resuscitation requirements after thermal injury. *Am J Surg* 1985; **150**: 716–20.
16. Lu W. Clinical analysis of fluid resuscitation in severe burned patients with or without inhalation injury. *Chung-Hua Cheng Hsing Shao Shang Wai Ko Tsa Chih (Chinese Journal of Plastic Surgery Burns)* 1992; **8**: 116–18.
17. Hughes KR, Armstrong RF, Brough MD, et al. Fluid requirements of patients with burns and inhalation injuries in an intensive care unit. *Intensive Care Med* 1989; **15**: 464–6.
18. Herndon DN, Barrow RE, Linares HA, et al. Inhalation injury in burned patients: effects and treatment. *Burns Incl Therm Inj* 1988; **14**: 349–56.
19. Herndon DN, Traber DL, Traber LD. The effect of resuscitation on inhalation injury. *Surgery* 1986; **100**: 248–51.
20. Shimazu T, Yukioka T, Hubbard GB, et al. A dose-responsive model of smoke inhalation injury. *Ann Surg* 1988; **206**: 89–98.
21. Fein A, Leff A, Hopewell PC. Pathophysiology and management of the complications resulting from fire and the inhaled products of combustion: review of the literature. *Crit Care Med* 1980; **8**: 94–8.
22. Boutros AR, Hoyt JL. Management of carbon monoxide poisoning in the absence of hyperbaric oxygen chamber. *Crit Care Med* 1976; **4**: 144–7.
23. Smith G, Ledingham IM, Sharp GR, et al. Treatment of coal-gas poisoning with oxygen at 2 atmospheres pressure. *Lancet* 1962; **1**: 816–19.
24. Mathieu D, Nolf M, Durocher A, et al. Acute carbon monoxide poisoning: risk of late sequelae and treatment with hyperbaric oxygen. *J Toxicol Clin Toxicol* 1985; **23**: 315–24.
25. Norkool DM, Kirkpatrick JN. Treatment of acute carbon monoxide poisoning with hyperbaric oxygen: a review of 115 cases. *Ann Emerg Med* 1985; **14**: 1168–71.
26. Grube BJ, Marvin JA, Heimbach DM. Therapeutic hyperbaric oxygen: Help or hindrance in burn patients with carbon monoxide poisoning? *J Burn Care Rehabil* 1988; **9**: 249–52.
27. Cox CS Jr, Zwischenberger JB, Traber DL, Traber LD, Haque AK, Herndon DN. Heparin improves oxygenation and minimizes barotrauma after severe smoke inhalation in an ovine model. *Surg Gynecol Obstet* 1993; **176**: 339–49.
28. Brown M, Desai M, Traber LD, Herndon DN, Traber DL. Dimethylsulfoxide with heparin in the treatment of smoke inhalation injury. *J Burn Care Rehabil* 1988; **9**: 22–5.
29. Desai MH, Mlcak R, Richardson J, et al. Reduction in mortality in pediatric patients with inhalation injury with aerosolized heparin/acetylcysteine therapy. *J Burn Care Rehabil* 1998; **19**: 210–12.
30. Levine BA, Petroff PA, Slade CL. Prospective trials of dexamethasone and aerosolized gentamicin in the treatment of inhalation injury in the burned patient. *J Trauma* 1978; **18**: 188–93.
31. Moylan JA, Alexander LG Jr. Diagnosis and treatment of inhalation injury. *World J Surg* 1978; **2**: 185–91.
32. Cioffi WG, deLemos RA, Coalson JJ, et al. Decreased pulmonary damage in primates with inhalation injury treated with high-frequency ventilation. *Ann Surg* 1993; **218**: 328–37.
33. Cioffi WG Jr, Rue LW III, Graves TA, et al. Prophylactic use of high-frequency percussive ventilation in patients with inhalation injury. *Ann Surg* 1991; **213**: 575–82.
34. Lentz CW, Peterson HD. Smoke inhalation is a multilevel insult to the pulmonary system. *Curr Opin Pulm Med* 1997; **3**: 221–6.
35. Mlcak R, Cortiella J, Desai M, Herndon D. Lung compliance, airway resistance and work of breathing in children after inhalation injury. *J Burn Care Rehabil* 1997; **18(6)**: 531–4.
36. Cortiella J, Mlcak R, Herndon D. High frequency percussive ventilation in pediatric patients with inhalation injury. *J Burn Care Rehabil* 1999; **20(3)**: 232–5.
37. Shirani KZ, Pruitt BA Jr, Mason AD. The influence of inhalation injury and pneumonia on burn mortality. *Ann Surg* 1987; **205**: 82–7.
38. Demarest GB, Hudson LD, Altman LC. Impaired alveolar macrophage chemotaxis in patients with acute smoke inhalation. *Am Rev Respir Dis* 1979; **119**: 279–86.
39. Loke J, Paul E, Virgulto JA, et al. Rabbit lung after acute smoke inhalation: cellular responses and scanning electron microscopy. *Arch Surg* 1984; **119**: 956–9.
40. Pruitt BA Jr, Erickson DR, Morris A. Progressive pulmonary insufficiency and other pulmonary complications of thermal injury. *J Trauma* 1975; **15**: 369–79.
41. Sears SD. Pulmonary infections in the burn patient and their management. In: Haponik EF, Munster AM, eds. *Respiratory Injury: Smoke Inhalation and Burns.* New York: McGraw-Hill, 1990: 226.
42. Klastersky J, Bogaerts AM, Noterman J, et al. Infections caused by *Providencia* bacilli. *Scand J Infect Dis* 1974; **6**: 153–8.

43 Cioffi WG Jr, McManus AT, Rue LW III, *et al*. Comparison of acid neutralizing and non-acid neutralizing stress ulcer prophylaxis in thermally injured patients. *J Trauma* 1994; **36**: 541–7.

44 Ossanna PJ, Test ST, Matheson NR, *et al*. Oxidative regulation of neutrophil elastase alpha-1-protease inhibitor interactions. *J Clin Invest* 1986; **77**: 1939–51.

45 Gadek JE, Fells GA, Zimmerman RL, *et al*. Antielastases of the human alveolar structures. *J Clin Invest* 1981; **68**: 889–98.

46 Henson PM, Johnston RB. Tissue injury in inflammation: oxidants, proteinases and cationic proteins. *J Clin Invest* 1987; **79**: 669–74.

47 O'Toole G, Peek G, Jaffe W, *et al*. Extracorporeal membrane oxygenation in the treatment of inhalation injuries. *Burns* 1998; **24**: 562–5.

48 Pierre EJ, Zwischenberger JB, Angel C, *et al*. Extracorporeal membrane oxygenation in the treatment of respiratory failure in pediatric patients with burns. *J Burn Care Rehabil* 1998; **19(2)**: 131–4.

49 Brunston RL, Tao W, Bidani A, *et al*. Prolonged hemodynamic stability during arteriovenous carbon dioxide removal for severe respiratory failure. *J Thorac Cardiovasc Surg* 1997; **114**: 1107–14.

50 Brunston RL, Zwischenberger JB, Tao W, *et al*. Total arteriovenous CO$_2$ removal: simplifying extracorporeal support for respiratory failure. *Ann Thorac Surg* 1997; **64**: 1599–605.

51 Zwischenberger JB, Tao W, Bidani A. Intravascular membrane oxygenator and carbon dioxide removal devices: a review of performance and improvements. *ASAIO J* 1999; **45**: 41–6.

52 Libby P, Ordovas JM, Auger KR, *et al*. Endotoxin and tumor necrosis factor induce interleukin-1 gene expression in adult human vascular endothelial cells. *Am J Pathol* 1986; **124**: 179–85.

53 Strieter RM, Kunkel SL, Showell HJ, *et al*. Endothelial cell gene expression of a neutrophil chemotactic factor by TNF-alpha, LPS and IL-1. *Science* 1989; **243**: 1467–9.

54 Standiford TJ, Kunkel SL, Basha MA, *et al*. Human alveolar macrophage induced gene expression of neutrophil chemotactic factor/interleukin-8 from pulmonary epithelial cells. *Clin Res* 1990; **38**: 139A.

55 Butler GB, Adler KB, Evan JN, *et al*. Modulation of rabbit airway smooth muscle responsiveness by respiratory epithelium. *Am Rev Respir Dis* 1987; **135**: 1099–104.

56 Kimura R, Traber LD, Herndon DN, *et al*. Treatment of smoke-induced pulmonary injury with nebulized dimethylsulfoxide. *Circ Shock* 1988; **25**: 333–41.

57 Ogura H, Cioffi WG Jr, Okerberg CV, *et al*. The effects of pentoxifylline on pulmonary function following smoke inhalation. *J Surg Res* 1994; **56**: 242–50.

58 Ogura H, Cioffi WG Jr, Jordan BS, *et al*. The effect of inhaled nitric oxide on smoke inhalation injury in an ovine model. *J Trauma* 1994; **37**: 893–8.

59 Ikeuchi H, Sakano T, Sanchez J, *et al*. The effects of platelet-activating factor (PAF) and a PAF antagonist (CV-3988) on smoke inhalation injury in an ovine model. *J Trauma* 1992; **32**: 344–50.

60 Wang S, Lantz RC, Robledo RF, *et al*. Early alterations of lung injury following acute smoke exposure and 21-aminosteroid treatment. *Tox Pathol* 1999; **27(3)**: 334–41.

61 Wang S, Lantz RC, Vermeulen MW, *et al*. Functional alterations of alveolar macrophages subjected to smoke exposure and antioxidant lazaroids. *Tox Ind Health* 1999; **15**: 464–9.

62 Fukuda T, Kim DK, Chin M, *et al*. Increased group IV cytosolic phospholipase A$_2$ activity in lungs of sheep after smoke inhalation injury. *Am J Physiol* 1999; **277 (Lung Cell. Mol. Physiol. 21)**: L533–42.

63 Spragg RG, Smith RM. Biology of acute lung injury. In: Crystal RG, West JB, eds. *Lung Injury*. New York: Raven Press, 1992: 252.

64 Clark WR Jr, Nieman GF. Smoke inhalation. *Burns Incl Therm Inj* 1988; **6**: 473–94.

Chapter 18

Respiratory care
Ronald P Mlcak
David N Herndon

Introduction

The multitude of respiratory complications caused by smoke inhalation, thermal burns, and their treatment epitomize the clinical challenges which confront respiratory care practitioners. Smoke inhalation injury and its sequelae impose demands upon the respiratory care practitioners who play a central role in its clinical management. These demands may range from intubation and resuscitation of victims in the emergency room to assistance with diagnostic bronchoscopies, to performance of pulmonary function studies, monitoring of arterial blood gases, airway maintenance,

chest physiotherapy, and mechanical ventilator management.[1] Additional demands are placed upon the respiratory care practitioner in the rehabilitation phase in determining disability or limitations diagnosed by pulmonary function studies or cardiopulmonary stress testing. In some countries outside the United States, the duties of the respiratory care practitioner are augmented by a combination of physicians, nurses, and physiotherapists. It is imperative that a well-organized, protocol-driven approach to burn care be utilized so that improvements can be made, and the morbidity and mortality associated with inhalation injury can be reduced. This chapter provides an overview of the common hands-on approaches to the treatment of inhalation injury, with emphasis on mucociliary clearance techniques, pharmacologic adjuncts, mechanical ventilation, infection control, and the late complications associated with inhalation injury.

Bronchial hygiene therapy

Airway clearance techniques are an essential component of respiratory management of patients with smoke inhalation. Bronchial hygiene therapy is a term used to describe several of the modalities intended to accomplish this goal. Therapeutic coughing, chest physiotherapy, early ambulation, airway suctioning, therapeutic bronchoscopy, and pharmacologic agents have been effective in the removal of retained secretions.

Therapeutic Coughing

Therapeutic coughing functions to promote airway clearance of excess mucus and fibrin cast in the tracheal bronchial tree. The impairment of the cough mechanism will result in retained secretions, bronchial obstruction, atelectasis, and/or pneumonia. A cough may be either a reflex or a voluntary action. The mechanisms of a cough include:

- a deep inspiration;
- the closure of the glottis;
- contraction of the muscles of the chest wall, abdomen, and pelvic floor;
- opening of the glottis; and
- a rapid expulsive exhalation phase.

During a cough, alveolar, pleural, and subglottic pressures may rise as much as 200 cmH$_2$O. A failure of the cough mechanism may be due to an impairment of any step in the sequences described. When this occurs, it is necessary to perform techniques which are used to improve the cough.

Series of three coughs

The patient is asked to start a small breath and small cough, then a bigger breath and harder cough, and finally a really deep breath and hard cough. This technique is especially effective for postoperative patients who tend to splint from pain.[2]

Tracheal tickle

The therapist places the index and middle finger flat in the sternal notch and gently massages inward in a circular fashion over the trachea. This is most effective in obtunded patients or in patients coming out of anesthesia.[2]

Cough stimulation

Patients with artificial airways cannot cough normally since a tube is either between the vocal cords (endotracheal) or below the cords (tracheostomy). Adequate pressure cannot be built up without approximation of the cords. These patients may have a cough stimulated by inflating the cuff on the tube, giving a large, rapid inspiration by a manual resuscitation bag, holding the breath for 1–2 seconds, and rapidly allowing the bag to release and exhalation to ensue. This technique is normally performed by two persons and is made more effective by one therapist performing vibration and chest compressions from the time of the inspiratory hold, all during exhalation.[2] Coughing and deep breathing is encouraged every hour to aid in removing retained secretions.

Chest Physiotherapy

Chest physiotherapy has come to mean gravity-assisted bronchial drainage with chest percussion and vibrations. Studies have shown that a combination of techniques are effective in secretion removal.[3–6]

Bronchial drainage/positioning

Bronchial drainage/positioning is a therapeutic modality that uses gravity-assisted positioning designed to improve pulmonary hygiene in patients with inhalation injury or retained secretions. There are 12 basic positions in which patients can be placed for postural drainage. Due to skin grafts, donor sites, and the use of air fluid beds, clinical judgment dictates that most of these positions are not practical. In fact, positioning in the Trendelenburg and various other positions may acutely worsen hypoxemia. Evidence has shown that a patient's arterial oxygenation may fall during positioning.[7] To accomplish the same goal it is common practice, in intensive care units, to turn patients side to side every 2 hours so as to aid in mobilizing secretions (**Figure 18.1**).

Percussion

Percussion aids in the removal of secretions from the tracheal bronchial tree. Percussion is done by cupping the hand so as to allow a cushion of air to come between the percussor's hand and the patient. If this is done properly, a popping sound will be heard when the patient is percussed. There should be a towel between the patient and the percussor's hand in order to prevent irritation of the skin.[8] Percussion is applied over the surface landmarks of the bronchial segments that are being drained. The hands rhythmically and alternately strike the chest wall. Incisions, skin grafts, and bony prominences should be avoided during percussion (**Figure 18.2**).

Vibration/shaking

Vibration/shaking is a shaking movement used to move loosened secretions to larger airways so that they can be coughed up or removed by suctioning. Vibration involves rapid shaking of the chest wall during exhalation. The percussor vibrates the thoracic cage by placing both hands over the percussed areas and vibrating into the patient, isometrically contracting or tensing the muscles of their arms and shoulders. Mechanical vibrations have been reported to produce good clinical results. Gentle mechanical vibration may be indicated for patients who cannot tolerate manual percussion (**Figure 18.3**). Chest physiotherapy techniques should be used every 2–4 hours for patients with retained secretions. Therapy should continue until breath sounds improve.

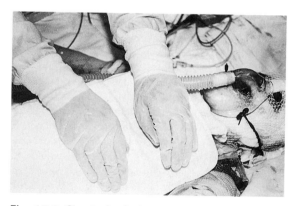

Fig. 18.2 Chest physiotherapy techniques.

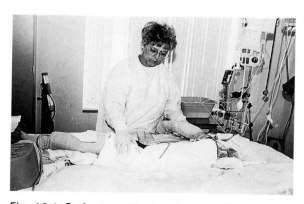

Fig. 18.1 Patient positioning for secretion mobilization.

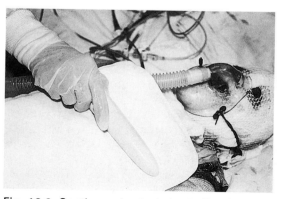

Fig. 18.3 Gentle mechanical chest vibrations.

Early Ambulation

Early ambulation is another effective means of preventing respiratory complications. With appropriate use of analgesics, even patients on continuous ventilatory support can be gotten out of bed and into a chair (**Figure 18.4**). The rocking chair (**Figure 18.5**) has several beneficial effects:

- the patient can breathe with regions of the lungs which are normally hyperventilated;
- muscular strength and tone are preserved;
- contractions are prevented and exercise tolerance is maintained.[9]

Airway Suctioning

Airway suctioning is another method of clearing an airway. Normal bronchial hygiene is usually accomplished by the mucociliary escalator process. When these methods are not effective in maintaining a clear airway, tracheobronchial suctioning is indicated.[10–13] Nasotracheal suctioning is intended to remove from the trachea accumulated secretions and other foreign material which cannot be removed by the patient's spontaneous cough or less invasive procedures. Nasotracheal suctioning has been used to avoid intubation which was solely intended for the removal of secretions. Nasotracheal suctioning refers to the insertion of a suction catheter through the nasal passages and pharynx into the trachea in order to aspirate secretions or foreign material. The first step in this process is to hyperoxygenate the patient with 100% oxygen. The patient should be positioned in the Fowler's position and the catheter slowly advanced through the nares to a point just above the larynx. The therapist or nurse then listens for air sounds at the proximal end of the catheter. When airflow is felt to be strongest and respiratory sounds are loudest, the tip of the catheter is immediately above the epiglottis. On inspiration, the catheter is advanced into the trachea. After the vocal cords have been passed, a few deep breaths are allowed and the patient is reoxygenated. Suction is begun while the catheter is slowly withdrawn from the trachea. The patient should not be suctioned for more than 15 seconds without being reoxygenated. Suctioning is not without potential hazards.[14,15] Complications include irritation of the nasotracheal mucosa with bleeding, abrupt drops in P_{O_2}, vagal stimulation, and bradycardia. Preoxygenating and limiting suction time have been shown to decrease or eliminate the fall in the P_{O_2}.[12–14]

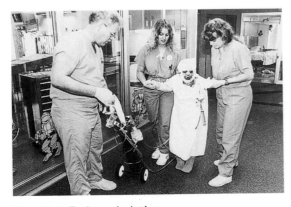

Fig. 18.4 Early ambulation.

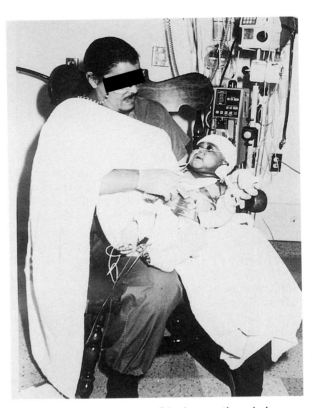

Fig. 18.5 Patient up out of bed, secretions being mobilized by rocking, and chest physiotherapy techniques.

Therapeutic Bronchoscopy

When all other techniques fail to remove secretions, the use of the fiberoptic bronchoscope has proven to be of benefit. In addition to its diagnostic functions, bronchoscopy retains important therapeutic applications. Copious secretions encountered in patients with inhalation injury may require repeated bronchoscopic procedures when more conservative methods are unsuccessful. The modern fiberoptic bronchoscope is small in diameter, flexible, and has a steerable tip that can be maneuvered into the fourth- or fifth-order bronchi for examination or specimen removal.

Pharmacologic Adjuncts

Bronchodilators

Bronchodilators can be helpful in some cases. Inhalation injury to the lower airways results in a chemical tracheobronchitis which can produce wheezing and bronchospasms. This is especially true for patients with preexisting reactive airway diseases. Most drugs used in the management of bronchospasms are believed to act on the biochemical mechanism which controls bronchial muscle tone. Aerosolized sympathomimetics are effective in two ways: they result in bronchial muscle relaxation and they stimulate mucociliary clearance. The newer bronchodilators are more effective and have fewer side-effects than the older generation drugs. Some of the newer compounds used in the United States are worthy of note. First, metaproterenol is available in cartridge inhalers, as a liquid to be aerosolized, as an oral medication in tablets, or as a syrup. The recommended oral dose is 10–20 mg every 6–8 hours; as an inhaled bronchodilator, 1–2 puffs every 3–4 hours. Its duration of action as an inhaled bronchodilator is 1–5 hours.[16]

Albuterol can also be administered orally, parenterally, and by aerosol. Albuterol is available in a metered cartridge inhaler and its standard dose is 1–2 puffs three to four times daily. Aerosolized albuterol has a duration of action of approximately 4–6 hours.[17]

Racemic epinephrine is used as an aerosolized topical vasoconstrictor, bronchodilator, and secretion bond breaker. The vasoconstrictive action of racemic epinephrine is useful in reducing mucosal and submucosal edema within the walls of the pulmonary airways. A secondary bronchodilator action serves to reduce potential spasm of the smooth muscles of the terminal bronchioles. Water, employed as a diluent for racemic epinephrine, serves to lower both adhesive and cohesive forces of the retained endobronchial secretions, thus serving as a bond-breaking vehicle. Racemic epinephrine has also been used for the treatment of post-extubation stridor.[18] Its mode of action is thought to be related to the vasoconstrictive activity, with the resultant decrease in mucosal edema. Aerosolized treatments may be given every 2 hours as long as the heart rate is not increased.

Hypertonic saline offers a theoretically more effective form of mucokinetic therapy. The deposition of hypertonic droplets on the respiratory mucosa results in the osmotic attraction of fluids from the mucosal blood vessels and tissues into the airway. Thus a 'bronchorrhea' is induced, and the watery solution helps to dilute down the respiratory tract secretions and to increase their bulk, thereby augmenting expectoration. Furthermore, there is evidence that hypertonic saline has a direct effect on the mucoprotein DNA complexes, and by reducing the cohesive intramolecular forces, the salt helps reduce the viscous properties of the mucoid fluid.[19] Excessive use of hypertonic saline is not recommended because irritation can occur in the respiratory tract, absorption can occur, and burn patients who cannot tolerate the sodium load may develop edema.

Finally, aerosolized acetylcysteine is a powerful mucolytic agent in use in respiratory care. Acetylcysteine contains a thiol group; the free sulfhydryl radical of this group is a strong reducing agent which ruptures the disulfide bonds that serve to give stability to the mucoprotein network of molecules in mucus. Agents that break down these disulfide bonds produce the most effective mucolysis.[20] Acetylcysteine is an irritant to the respiratory tract. It can cause mucosal changes, and it may induce bronchospasm. For this reason, patients are evaluated for signs of bronchospasm, and a bronchodilator may be added if necessary. Acetylcysteine has proven to be effective in combination with aerosolized heparin for the treatment of inhalation injury in animal studies.[21]

Heparin/acetylcysteine combinations have been used as scavengers for the oxygen free radicals produced when alveolar macrophages are activated either directly by chemicals in smoke or by one or more of the compounds in the arachidonic cascade.[22] Animal studies have shown an increased *P/F* ratio, decreased peak inspiratory pressures, and a decreased amount of fibrin cast formation with heparin/acetylcystine combinations.[23] In a retrospective review, Desai *et al.* have shown that the use of heparin/N-acetylcysteine is effective in pediatric patients with inhalation injury.[24] Results indicate a significant decrease in the reintubation rates, incidence of atelectasis, and improved mortality for patients treated with heparin/N-acetylcysteine therapy. Therefore a standard treatment for patients with inhalation injury

might include 5000–10 000 units of heparin and 3 ml normal saline nebulized every 4 hours, alternating with 3–5 ml of 20% acetylcysteine for 7 days. This insures that the patient receives an aerosolized treatment every 2 hours. Baseline and daily clotting studies are recommended for the entire length of the aerosolized treatments.

A prospective randomized study on the use of nebulized heparin for the treatment of inhalation injury is necessary to validify the continued used of this mode of therapy. A multicenter study is being developed that will evaluate the effectiveness of therapy and answer some of the questions regarding the mechanism of action, safety, and affects on lung function.

Mechanical ventilation

Over the past 30 years, and especially over the past decade, there has been an increase in new ventilatory techniques which present alternatives for the treatment of patients with smoke inhalation. Unfortunately, although the number of options available to the clinician has appeared to increase exponentially, well-controlled clinical trials defining the specific role for each of the modes of ventilation and comparing them to other modes of ventilation have not been forthcoming. Based upon current available data, the recommendations from the American College of Chest Physicians consensus conference on mechanical ventilation generally serve as guidelines.[25] The general consensus concludes:

- The clinician should choose a ventilator mode that has been shown to be capable of supporting oxygenation and ventilation and that the clinician has experience in using.
- An acceptable oxygen saturation should be targeted.
- Based primarily on animal data, a plateau pressure of greater than 35 cmH$_2$O is cause for concern. With clinical conditions that are associated with a decreased chest wall compliance, plateau pressures greater than 35 cmH$_2$O may be acceptable.
- To accomplish the goal of limiting plateau pressures, P_{CO_2} values should be permitted to rise (permissive hypercapnia) unless other contraindications exist that demand a more normal P_{CO_2} or pH.
- Positive end-expiratory pressure (PEEP) is useful in supporting oxygenation. An appropriate level of PEEP may be helpful in preventing lung damage. The level of PEEP required should be established by empirical trials and reevaluated on a regular basis.
- Large tidal volumes (12–15 ml/kg) with PEEP may be needed to improve oxygenation when the use of protective ventilatory strategies become ineffective. Peak flow rates should be adjusted as needed to satisfy patient inspiratory needs.[25]

A new multicenter study by the Acute Respiratory Distress Syndrome Network of the National Heart, Lung, and Blood Institute is the first large randomized study comparing high versus low tidal volumes for patients with ARDS.[47] The trial compared traditional ventilation treatment, which involved an initial tidal volume of 12 ml/kg of predicted body weight, and an airway pressure measured of 50 cmH$_2$O or less, to ventilation with a lower tidal volume, which involved an initial tidal volume of 6 ml/kg of predicted body weight and a plateau pressure of 30 cmH$_2$O or less.

The volume–assist-control mode was used for the ventilation study. The trial was stopped after the enrollment of 861 patients because mortality was lower in the group treated with lower tidal volumes than in the group treated with traditional tidal volumes, and the number of days without ventilator use during the first 28 days after randomization was greater in this group.[47]

This study was the first large randomized investigation documenting a decrease in mortality with the use of lower tidal volumes for the treatment of patients with ARDS. In light of this new evidence, the tidal volumes used when initiating mechanical ventilation should be 6–8 ml/kg of predicted body weight. If the patient becomes obstructed with fibrin cast and presents with an acute increase in P_{CO_2} and decrease in P_{ao_2}, the clinician should first provide aggressive pulmonary toilet, then consider changing over to volume ventilation with higher tidal volumes. If ventilation continues to worsen, tidal volumes of 12–15 ml/kg may be needed to provide adequate mechanical ventilation.

Modes of Ventilation

Control mode

In the control mode of ventilation, the ventilator cycles automatically at a rate selected by the operator. The adjustment is usually made by a knob calibrated in breaths/min. The ventilator will cycle regardless of the patient need or desire for a breath, but guarantees a minimum level of minute ventilation in the apneic, sedated. or paralysed patient. The control mode of ventilation is often utilized in patients with ARDS because of the high peak pressures needed to achieve adequate chest expansion. The major disadvantage with this mode is that the patient cannot cycle the ventilator and thus the minute ventilation must be set appropriately.

Assist-control mode

In the assist-control mode of ventilation, in which every breath is supported by the ventilator, a backup control rate is set; however, the patient may choose any rate above the set rate. Using this mode of ventilation, the tidal volume, inspiratory flow rate, flow waveform, sensitivity, and control rate are set.[26–28] Advantages are that assist-control ventilation combines the security of controlled ventilation with the possibility of synchronizing the breathing pattern of the patient and ventilator, and it ensures ventilatory support during each breath. Disadvantages are as follows:

- Excessive patient work occurs in case of inadequate peak flow or sensitivity settings, especially if the ventilator drive of the patient is increased.[26–28]
- It is sometimes poorly tolerated in awake, nonsedated subjects and can require sedation to insure synchrony of patient and machine.
- It can cause respiratory alkalosis.
- It may worsen air trapping with patients with chronic obstructed lung disease.[24]

Synchronized intermittent mandatory ventilation

Synchronized intermittent mandatory ventilation (SIMV) combines a preset number of ventilator-delivered mandatory breaths of present tidal volume with the facility for intermittent patient-generated spontaneous breaths.[29,30]
Advantages are as follows:

- The patient is able to perform a variable amount of respiratory work and yet there is the security of a preset mandatory level of ventilation.
- SIMV allows for a variation in level of partial ventilatory support from near total ventilatory support to spontaneous breathing.
- It can be used as a weaning tool.

Disadvantages are:

- Hyperventilation with respiratory alkalosis.
- Excessive work of breathing due to the presence of a poorly responsive demand valve, suboptimal ventilatory circuits, or inappropriate flow delivery could occur.
- In each case, extra work is imposed on the patient during spontaneous breaths.

Pressure control mode

In pressure-controlled ventilation all breaths are time- or patient-triggered, pressure-limited, and time-cycled. The ventilator provides a constant pressure of air to the patient during inspiration. The length of inspiration, the pressure level, and the back-up rate are set by the operator. Tidal volume is based upon the compliance and resistance of the patient's lungs, the ventilator system, as well as on the preset pressure. Pressure control ventilation has become a frequently used mode of ventilation for the treatment of ARDS.

Pressure support ventilation

Pressure support ventilation (PSV) is a pressure-targeted, flow-cycled, mode of ventilation in which each breath must be patient-triggered. It is used both as a mode of ventilation during stable ventilatory support periods and as a weaning method.[30–34] It is primarily designed to assist spontaneous breathing and therefore the patient must have an intact respiratory drive.
Advantages are:

- It is generally regarded as a comfortable mode of ventilation for most patients.
- Pressure support reduces the work of breathing.
- It can be used to overcome the airway resistance caused by the endotracheal tube.
- Pressure support may be useful in patients who are difficult to wean.

Disadvantages are:

- The tidal volume is not controlled and is dependent on respiratory mechanics, cycling frequency, and synchrony between the patient and ventilator.
- Pressure support may be poorly tolerated in some patients with high airway resistances because of the preset high initial flow rates.

Alternate Modes of Ventilation

During the last decade, a new concept has emerged regarding acute lung injury. In severe cases of ARDS, only a small part of the lung parenchyma remains accessible to gas delivered by mechanical ventilation.[35,36] As a consequence, tidal volumes of 10 ml/kg or more may overexpand and injure the remaining normally aerated lung parenchyma and could worsen the prognosis of severe acute respiratory failure by extending nonspecific alveolar damage. High airway pressures may result in overdistension and local hyperventilation of more compliant parts of the diseased lung. Overdistension of lungs in animals has produced diffuse alveolar damage.[37-39] This is the reason why alternative modes of ventilation, all based on a reduction of end-inspiratory airway pressures and/or tidal volumes delivered to the patient, have been developed and are used by many clinicians caring for patients with severe forms of acute or chronic respiratory failure. Two alternative modes of ventilation – high-frequency percussive ventilation (HFPV) and inverse ratio ventilation (IRV) – will be discussed.

High-frequency ventilation

High-frequency ventilation (HFV) is the administration of small tidal volumes of 1–3 ml/kg at high frequencies of 100–3000 cpm.[40] Because it is a mode of ventilation based on a marked reduction in tidal volumes and airway pressures, it has the greatest potential for reducing pulmonary barotrauma. There are a number of different types of high-frequency ventilation techniques. The two most common are HFPV and high-frequency jet ventilation (HFJV).

High-frequency jet ventilation is the only high-frequency mode routinely used to ventilate patients with ARDS, mainly in Europe.[25] Comparative data concerning the advantages of HFJV over conventional ventilation are limited. There is no agreement, however, that HFJV is better than conventional mechanical ventilation in ARDS.[41]

High-frequency percussive ventilation is a new technique that has shown some promise in the ventilation of patients with inhalation injury.[42-44] Clinical studies indicate that this mode of ventilation may aid in reducing pulmonary barotrauma.[42,43] In a retrospective study, Cortiella et al., have shown a decrease incidence of pneumonia, peak inspiratory pressure, and an improved P/F ratio in children ventilated with the use of HFPV as compared to controls.[45]

In the first prospective randomized study on HFPV, Mlcak et al. have shown a significant decrease in the peak inspiratory pressures needed to ventilated pediatric patients with inhalation injury.[46] No significant differences were found for incidence of pneumonia, P/F ratios or mortality.

Based upon clinical experience, the following guidelines are given for initial set up of the HFPV in children (**Table 18.1**). The pulsatile flow (PIP) rate should set at 20 cmH$_2$O. The pulse frequency (high rate) should be set between 500 and 600. The low respiratory rate should be set at about 15–20. Oscillatory PEEP levels should be initially set at about 3 cmH$_2$O, and demand PEEP set on 2 cmH$_2$O. Ventilator settings are adjusted based upon the patient's clinical condition and blood gas values. To improve oxygenation, the ventilator can be set up in a more diffusive mode

(increased pulse frequency) and, to eliminate carbon dioxide, the ventilator can be set up in a more convective mode (decreased pulse frequency). With this mode of ventilation, subtidal volumes are delivered in a progressive stepwise fashion until a preset oscillatory equilibrium is reached and exhalation is passive.

Clinicians must be familiar with the technique used and its possible limitations. There must be adequate humidification of the respiratory gases or severe necrotizing tracheobronchitis can occur. Special delivery devices for providing adequate humidification during HFV are required.

Inverse ratio ventilation

Inverse ratio ventilation (IRV) is the use of an inspiratory/expiratory (I:E) ratio greater than 1:1. The rationale behind this is to maintain a high mean airway pressure and to hold peak alveolar pressure within a safe range. The second theoretical concept underlying IRV is the prolongation of inspiration to allow for recruitment of lung units with a long time constant. Deep sedation and/or paralysis is nearly always required with this mode of ventilation. At this time there is no conclusive scientific data comparing IRV to conventional mechanical ventilation in patients with inhalation injury.

Typical Ventilator Settings Required

A large multicentered study by the NHLBI evaluated the use of volume ventilation with low versus high tidal volume on ARDS. This study documented a decreased incidence of mortality in patients with ARDS who were ventilated with small tidal volumes.[47] Based upon this study, it has become clinically accepted practice to use small tidal volumes when initially setting up mechanical ventilation (**Table 18.2**).

Tidal volumes

In volume-cycled ventilation, a machine-delivered tidal volume is set to be consistent with adequate gas exchange and patient comfort. The tidal volume selected for burned patients normally varies between 6 and 8 ml/kg of predicted body weight. Numerous factors, such as lung/thorax compliance, system resistance, compressible volume loss, oxygenation, ventilation, and barotrauma are considered when volumes are selected.[46] Of critical importance is the avoidance of overdistension. This can generally be accomplished by insuring that peak airway and alveolar pressures do not exceed a maximum target. Many would agree that a peak alveolar pressure greater than 35 cmH$_2$O in adults raises concern regarding the development of barotrauma and ventilator-induced lung injury increases.[49,50] The clinician must always look at the patient to insure adequate chest expansion with the setting of the tidal volume. Expired tidal volumes should be

Table 18.1 High-frequency percussive ventilation set-up guidelines	
Variable	Settings
Pulsatile flow rate (PIP)	20 cmH$_2$O
Pulse frequency (high rate)	500–600
Low respiratory rate	15–20
I : E ratio	1:1 or 2:1
Oscillatory PEEP	3 cmH$_2$O
Demand PEEP	2 cmH$_2$O

Table 18.2 Traditional mechanical ventilation guidelines in children	
Variable	Settings
Tidal volumes	6–8 ml/kg
Respiratory rate	12–45 breaths/min
Plateau pressures	<30 cmH$_2$O
I : E ratio	1:1–1:3
Flow rate	40–100 l/min
PEEP	7.5 cmH$_2$O

measured for accuracy at the connection between the patient's wye and the artificial airway. This insures that the volume selected reaches the patient and is not lost in the compressible volume of the ventilator tubing.

The range of tidal volumes will vary depending on the disease process, with some diseases requiring maximum tidal volumes and others needing less. Severe interstitial diseases such as pneumonia and ARDS may require a tidal volume of 12–15 ml/kg to adequately inflate the lungs and improve gas exchange if protective ventilatory strategies are become inadequate. However, the acceptable range of 6–8 ml/kg allows the clinician to make more precise adjustments in volume, as needed by the patient.

Respiratory rate

Setting of the mandatory ventilator respiratory rate is dependent on the mode of ventilation selected, the delivered tidal volume, dead space to tidal volume ratio, metabolic rate, targeted P_{CO_2} levels, and level of spontaneous ventilation. With adults, set mandatory rate normally varies between 4 and 20 breaths/min, with most clinically stable patients requiring mandatory rates in the 8–12 range.[48] In patients with inhalation injury, mandatory rates exceeding 20 per minute may be necessary, depending on the desired expired volume and targeted P_{CO_2}. It is important to have targeted arterial blood gas values set to aid the clinical team in proper management (**Table 18.3**) Along with the P_{CO_2}, pH, and patient comfort, the primary variable controlling the selection of the respiratory rate is the development of air trapping and auto PEEP.[51]

Table 18.3 Arterial blood gas goals	
Variable	Goal
pH	7.25–7.45
P_{O_2}	55–80 mmHg or Sao_2 of 88–95%
P_{CO_2}	35–55 mmHg (permissive hypercapnia can be used as long as pH >7.25)

The respiratory rates of children and infants all need to be set substantially higher than those of adults. For pediatrics, the respiratory rate can be set at from 12 to 45, depending on the disease state and the level of targeted P_{CO_2} one wishes to achieve. Slower respiratory rates are useful in the patient with obstructed airways because slower rates allow more time for exhalation and emptying of hyperinflated areas.

Arterial blood gases should be checked after the patient has been on the ventilator for approximately 20 minutes and the respiratory rate adjusted accordingly.

Flow rates

The selection of peak inspiratory flow rate during volume ventilation is primarily determined by the level of spontaneous inspiratory effort. In patients triggering volume breaths, patient effort, work of breathing, and patient ventilator synchrony depend on the selection of peak inspiratory flow.[27] Peak inspiratory flows should ideally match patient peak inspiratory demands. This normally requires peak flows to be set at 40–100 l/min, depending on expired volume and the inspiratory demand.[25]

Inspiratory/expiratory (I:E) ratio

The time allowed for the inspiratory and expiratory phases of mechanical ventilation is commonly referred to as the inspiratory/expiratory (I:E) ratio. The inspiratory part of the ratio includes the time to deliver the tidal volume before the exhalation valve opens and exhalation begins. The expiratory part of the ratio includes the time necessary for the tidal volume to exit through the exhalation valve before the next inspiration begins. The inspiratory time should be long enough to deliver the tidal volume at flow rates that will not result in turbulence and high peak airway pressures. The usual I:E ratio is 1:1–1:3.[52]

In severe lung disease, it is acceptable to prolong the inspiratory time to allow for better distribution of gas and enhance oxygen diffusion. When a longer inspiratory time is required, careful attention should be given to sufficient expiration to avoid stacking of breaths and impeding venous return. Prolonged inspiratory time creates a more laminar flow, which helps to keep the peak pressures lower. Fast inspiratory times are tolerated in patients with severe airway obstruction. The fast inspiratory time allows for a longer expiratory phase, which may help to decrease the amount of overinflation.

Inspired oxygen concentration

As a starting point, and until the level of hypoxemia is determined, a patient placed on a ventilator should receive an oxygen concentration of 100%. The concentration should be systematically lowered as soon as arterial blood gases dictate. In general, as a result of the concerns regarding the effects of high oxygen concentration on lung injury, the lowest acceptable oxygen level should be selected as soon as possible. In patients who are difficult to oxygenate, oxygen concentrations can be minimized by optimizing PEEP and mean airway pressures and selecting a minimally acceptable oxygen saturation.[53]

Positive end-expiratory pressure

Positive end-expiratory pressure (PEEP) is applied to recruit lung volumes, elevate mean airway pressure, and improve oxygenation.[54] The level of PEEP used varies with the disease process. PEEP levels should start at 5 cmH₂O and be increased in 2.5-cm increments. Increasing levels of PEEP, in conjunction with a prolonged inspiratory time, aids in oxygenation and allows for the safe level of oxygen to be used. The use of pressure–volume curves to determine the best PEEP level has been recommended to aid in overstretching the alveoli. This technique has certain limitations and is difficult to perform in the clinical setting. The use of PEEP trials can determine the best PEEP without causing a decrease in cardiac output.

Usually a minimum of 5 cmH₂O of PEEP will be indicated for use during mechanical ventilation since tracheal intubation holds the larynx constantly open, which leads to alveolar collapse and a reduction in the functional residual capacity.

Optimal PEEP is the level of end-expiratory pressure that results in the lowering of intrapulmonary shunting, significant improvement in arterial oxygenation, and only a small change in cardiac output, arteriovenous oxygen content differences, or mixed venous oxygen tension.

Extubation Criteria

Standard extubation criteria include a wide variety of physiologic indices that have been proposed to guide the process of discontinuing ventilatory support. Traditional indices include:

- Pao_2/Fio_2 ratio of greater than 250.
- Maximum inspiratory pressure of greater than 60 cmH$_2$O.
- Vital capacity of at least 15–20 ml/kg.
- Tidal volume of at least 5–7 ml/kg.
- Maximum voluntary ventilation of at least twice the minute volume.[55–58]

In general, these indices evaluate a patient's ability to sustain spontaneous ventilation. They do not assess a patient's ability to protect the upper airway. For this reason, traditional indices often fail to reflect the true clinical picture of a patient with an inhalation injury. For a complete evaluation prior to extubation, bronchoscopic examination will aid in determining if the airway edema has decreased enough to attempt extubation. Prior to a scheduled extubation it is recommended that reintubation equipment be set up and that the person doing the extubation be experienced in emergency intubations.

If the patient demonstrates signs of inspiratory stridor, the use of racemic epinephrine by aerosol has been effective in reducing the mucosal edema and may prevent the patient from being reintubated.

Infection control of respiratory equipment

Infections are the leading cause of mortality in burned patients. Pneumonia has become one of the most frequent life-threatening infections and is an important determinant of survival.[57] The majority of pneumonias are nosocomial, occurring in the burned patient after 72 hours of hospitalization, and are often associated with either an inhalation injury or endotracheal intubation with exposure to respiratory care equipment, or both.[62–64] One of the most important risk factors predisposing to pneumonia in burned patients is endotracheal intubation.[65,66] The incidence of pneumonia developing is estimated to be five times higher for intubated than nonintubated patients, and tracheostomy increases this risk even higher.[67] Exposure to respiratory care equipment adds an increased risk of pneumonia above and beyond the risk associated with endotracheal intubation.[68,69] After the use of nebulization equipment in respiratory care became popular, several epidemics of nosocomial pneumonia were reported.[70] The risk of pneumonia from mechanical ventilators was significant but decreased with a better understanding of the necessity to decontaminate respiratory equipment.[71,72]

Intubated patients receiving respiratory care may be at an increased risk of pneumonia because of coincidental exposure to other procedures such as suctioning and bronchoscopy. Respiratory care equipment, if not properly cared for, may provide a source of extraneous organisms that can contaminate the patient's respiratory tract.

The potential role of respiratory care equipment in providing reservoirs for organisms that are capable of infecting the lungs is well established. This problem, particularly pertaining to reservoir devices and medications, has been recognized for a number of years, and effective control strategies have been developed. Most hospitals maintain a bacteriological monitoring system, and significant contamination by this route is not likely.[73] Contamination of the compressed gases used to operate respiratory care devices is uncommon, principally because of the desiccation of gases and the inability of most bacterial species to survive such harsh treatment. Nebulization equipment delivers a fine-particle aerosol and, if contaminated, the aerosol droplets may contain bacteria. Humidification equipment provides water vapor but does not deliver a large quantity of water in particulate form. In fact, humidifiers generally remove bacteria from airstreams, because the bacteria are physically trapped in the fluid phase and are not vaporized.

Bag-mask units have been shown to allow the persistence of infectious organisms and the subsequent infection of other patients on whom the equipment has been later used.[74]

Ventilator circuits are inevitably contaminated by the patient's own respiratory tract flora during exhalation and coughing, and the fluid that collects in this tubing is thereby contaminated. Allowing such a collection of tubing condensate to drain back into a reservoir nebulizer can provide ample time for bacteria multiplication. Towards the end of the changeover time for ventilator circuits, the patient will receive a large inhalation exposure to bacteria.

Generally, as long as equipment is sterile when placed in service, changing equipment more often than at 24-hour intervals is not necessary.[75] **Table 18.4** demonstrates the time period generally acceptable for equipment changeover as well as the appropriate method of disinfection or sterilization of the product. Whenever possible, disposable respiratory equipment is preferred for use in the burn intensive care unit, since it is frequently contaminated with blood, body fluids, and secretions. For hospitals where disposable equipment is not an option, the following types of disinfection of sterilization techniques should be employed (**Table 18.5**).

Table 18.4 Common methods of disinfection and sterilization

Method	Equipment	Advantages	Disadvantages
Autoclaving	Linens, surgical instruments, laryngoscope handles	Inexpensive, fast, nontoxic	Damages heat- and moisture-sensitive equipment
Acid glutaraldehyde	Rubber, plastic, metals	Sterilizes in 1 hour, disinfects	Forms toxic residues, in 20 minutes, lasts 28 days contact dermatitis, recontamination can occur
Alkaline glutaraldehyde	Rubber, plastic, metals	Sterilizes in 10 hours, disinfects in 10 minutes, lasts 14 days	Toxic residues, recontamination can occur, contact dermatitis
Gas sterilization	All items moisture or heat sensitive	Effectively sterilizes prewrapped materials	Expensive, time consuming, aeration is needed to remove toxic residues
Boiling	Home care items	Inexpensive, simple	Time-consuming, does not produce sterility, damages sensitive equipment

Table 18.5 Decontamination procedures

Reusable equipment	Changes time	Soap and water clean	Disinfectant spray	Liquid disinfectant	ETO	Steam autoclave
Nebulizers	8–12 h	Disassemble	–	–	+	–
Ultrasonic nebulizer	Between patients	Wipe down, clean filters	+	Reusable filter	–	–
Portable spirometers	After PT use	–	Wipe with 70% alcohol	–	+	–
Ventilators	After PT	Fan filters	Cascade and unit	–	–	–
Bag-mask units	After PT use	–	–	–	+	–
Fiberoptic bronchoscopes	After each	+	–	+	+	–

ETO = ethylene oxide, – = non-applicable, + = applicable.

Disinfection and Sterilizing Techniques

Handwashing

Handwashing is generally considered the single most important procedure for preventing nosocomial infections. Regardless of whatever benefits are accrued by cleaning or sterilization, they are negated if the simple process of handwashing is overlooked. The recommended handwashing procedures depend on the purpose of washing. In most situations, a vigorous brief washing with soap under a strong running water is adequate to remove transient flora. Generally, simple handwashing with soap is performed before and after contact with patients and whenever the hands are soiled.

Antimicrobial handwashing procedures are indicated before all invasive procedures, during the care of patients in strict, respiratory, or enteric isolation, before entering intensive care units. The most commonly used agents are 70% isopropyl alcohol, iodophors, and chlorhexidine. Scrub regimens such as the povidone–iodine surgical scrub are appropriate for these areas.[76] For mechanical removal of microbes, the three key methods are scrubbing, filtration, and sedimentation. In respiratory care, mechanical scrubbing and filtration processes are commonly employed, whereas sedimentation has little current application. The most common nonmechanical physical agent used in the process of sterilization and disinfection is the application of heat.

Scrubbing

Scrubbing is the basic process for disinfection and sterilization. In practice it is both mechanical and chemical. The physical act removes many microbes and is often augmented by soap, water, and antimicrobial agents. Unless the microbes are of extreme virulence, contaminated respiratory care equipment is first disassembled and scrubbed so that dirt, debris, and extraneous materials are removed. This step is paramount if the later disinfection or sterilization processes are to be effective.[77]

Filtration

Filtration of bacteria is accomplished by passing a liquid or gas through a material whose pores are small enough to retain the microbes. In that liquid and gases are difficult to disinfect or sterilize, most commonly either is accomplished through the process of filtration.[77] Filters interposed between the ventilator and breathing circuits effectively eliminate contaminants from the driving gas and prevent retrograde contamination. These filters should be changed according to manufacturer's specifications.

Boiling

Boiling is an old method for sanitation and low-level disinfection. At sea level, the minimal level of exposure should be 30 minutes, with the time period adjusted upward 5 minutes per 1000 feet elevation above sea level. The efficiency of this process in killing spores can be increased by the addition of sodium bicarbonate sufficient to make a 2% solution or the addition of sodium hydroxide so as to make a 0.1% solution. With the addition of these chemicals, bacterial spores are destroyed in 10–30 minutes.[77]

Pasteurization

Pasteurization is an inexpensive and environmentally safe method of disinfection that has gained popularity for respiratory care equipment. The process employs a mild heat to destroy vegetative pathogens. With the current concerns for environmental safety, pasteurization offers a low-cost, nontoxic alternative to glutaraldehyde or ethylene oxide in areas where disinfection alone is sufficient. Not all respiratory care equipment can be pasteurized; the heat and moisture causes some plastic devices to become deformed, and rubber products such as anesthesia masks and ventilator reservoir bags may deteriorate due to the process.[77]

Autoclaving

Autoclaving is the application of steam and pressure to accomplish sterilization. Steam under two atmospheres of pressure has a temperature of 121°C. With this temperature and pressure, virtually all spores are killed within 15 minutes. The moisture enhances the conduction of heat and the rate of killing. With autoclaving the microorganisms are destroyed by disruption of the cell membrane, the coagulation of the cell protoplasm, or both. Autoclaving is the most commonly used effective form of sterilization and is preferred unless the material is injured by temperature or pressure. This is problematic for respiratory care, because much of the equipment is rubber or plastic, which cannot withstand the process.

Chemical Agents for Sterilization/Disinfection

Disinfectants act to kill microorganisms by several methods:

- oxidating microbial cells;
- hydrolyzing;
- combining with microbial proteins to form salts;
- coagulating the proteins of microbial cells;
- denaturing enzymes; or
- modifying cell wall permeability.[77]

Aldehydes

Aldehydes contain some of the most commonly used antimicrobials in respiratory care practice. These agents achieve their antimicrobial action through the alkylation of enzymes.

The cidal action of glutaraldehyde is accomplished by disruption of the lipoproteins in the cell membrane and cytoplasm of vegetative bacterial forms. This reaction between the chemical glutaraldehyde and cell proteins is dependent on both time and contact. Items to be disinfected must be free of material that would inhibit contact, and adequate contact time is needed for the chemical reaction to be complete.

Alkaline glutaraldehyde, buffered by a 0.3% bicarbonate agent, is used as a 2% solution. Once activated with the buffering agent, it is fully potent for approximately 14 days. This solution is bactericidal, virucidal, and tuberculocidal within 10 minutes and produces sterilization when applied for 10–20 hours. Equipment disinfected or sterilized with glutaraldehyde should be thoroughly rinsed and dried prior to use, because any residue would be irritating to mucous membranes.

Glutaraldehyde solutions are commonly used for the cold disinfection or sterilization of respiratory care equipment and have a large degree of safety. These solutions can be used to disinfect bronchoscopes as well as many of the current respiratory supplies.

Alcohols

Alcohols, especially ethylene and isopropyl alcohol, are perhaps the most commonly used disinfectants. Alcohols, as a chemical family, have many desirable characteristics needed in disinfectants. They are generally bactericidal and accomplish their bactericidal activity by damaging the cell wall membrane. They also have the ability to denature proteins, particularly enzymes called dehydrogenases. For alcohol to coagulate microbial proteins, water must be present. For this reason, 70% has been considered the critical dilution for alcohol, with a rapid loss of bactericidal activity with dilutions less than 50%. Both ethyl and isopropyl alcohols are rapidly effective against vegetative bacteria and tubercle bacilli but are not sporicidal.

Ethylene oxide

Ethylene oxide is a gas with a broad range of antimicrobial action. It is thought to destroy the microorganism by alkylating cellular constitutes. It kills both spores and bacteria, and has become a very popular method for sterilizing much of the heat- and moisture-sensitive respiratory care equipment. The gas is extremely penetrating and does not require high temperatures for activation. Sterilization of equipment is usually accomplished under conditions of 30–50% relative humidity and at temperatures of 50–60°C.[77]

To avoid contact irritation from ethylene oxide, it is necessary that the residue gas be removed after sterilization is complete. Without the use of an aeration chamber, materials such as neoprene rubber and polyvinyl chloride require extended aeration times of up to 7 days.

To be sure that the current infection control practice is effective in each institution, use of random microbiological cultures should be done whenever a problem is suspected or to test the reliability of the disinfection or sterilization techniques.

Late complications of inhalation injury

Tracheal Stenosis

Tracheal complications are commonly seen and consist of tracheitis, tracheal ulcerations, and granuloma formation. The location of the stenosis is almost invariably subglottic and occurs at the site of the cuff of the endotracheal or tracheostomy tube.[78] Several problems arising after extubation represent sequelae of laryngeal or tracheal injury incurred during the period of incubation. While tracheal stenosis or tracheomalacia are usually mild and asymptomatic, in some patients they can present as severe fixed or dynamic upper airway obstructions. These conditions can require surgical correction. In the management of intubated patients, such complications should be mostly preventable by meticulous attention to the tracheostomy or endotracheal tube cuff. Inflation of the cuff should be to the minimal pressure level consistent with preventing a leak in the ventilator at end inspiration.

Obstructive/Restrictive Disease

Chronic airway disease is a relatively rare reported sequel of inhalation injury and its supportive treatment. Spirometry is a useful screening tool for airway obstruction. Reports in the literature for adults indicate that lung function returns to normal after inhalation injury.[79,80] However, Mlcak et al. reported pulmonary function changes following inhalation injury for up to 10 years post-injury in children.[81] Fortunately, most pulmonary function abnormalities will persist for only months following lung parenchymal injury. In the great majority of cases, eventual resolution of both symptoms and physiologic abnormalities will occur. During the resolution phase, serial measurement of airflow obstruction should be obtained.[82] Desai et al. demonstrated that physiologic insults that occur as a result of thermal injury may limit exercise endurance in children.[83] Data from exercise stress testing showed evidence of a respiratory limitation to exercise. This was confirmed by a decrease in the maximal heart rate, decrease in the maximal oxygen consumption, and increased respiratory rate. In the cases of persistent severe respiratory symptoms, the severity of the impairment should be documented and the patient evaluated for a pulmonary rehabilitation program.

Conclusion

Inhalation injury and associated major burns provide a challenge for health care workers who provide direct hands-on care. The technical and physiologic problems which complicate the respiratory management of these patients require a practical knowledge of the possible sources of nosocomial infections. Patients with inhalation injury frequently require the use of respiratory care equipment that, if not properly cared for, can aid in the spread of infections. Important priorities for reducing the risk of infections include: an aggressive bronchial hygiene therapy program, the adherence to established infection control practices, the use of universal precautions during procedures, meticulous cleaning of respiratory care equipment, as well as routine epidemiologic surveillance of the established infection control practices within each institution.

References

1. Haponik E. Smoke inhalation injury: some priorities for respiratory care professionals. *Resp Care* 1992; 37: 609.

2. Frownfelter D. *Chest Physical Therapy and Pulmonary Rehabilitation*. 2nd edn. Chicago: Year Book Medical, 1987.

3. Ivarez SE, Peterson M, Lansford BR. Respiratory treatments of the adult patients with spinal cord injury. *Phys Ther* 1981; **61**: 1738.

4. Chopra SK, Taplin GV, Simmons DH. Effects of hydration and physical therapy on tracheal transport velocity. *Am Rev Respir Dis* 1974; **115**: 1009–14.

5. Marini JJ, Person DJ, Hudson LD. A prospective comparison of fiberoptic bronchoscopy and respiratory therapy. *Am Rev Respir Dis* 1979; **119**: 971–8.

6. Oldenburg FA, Dolovich MB, Montgomery JM, *et al.* Effects of postural drainage, exercise and cough on mucus clearance in chronic bronchitis. *Am Rev Respir Dis* 1979; **12**: 730–47.

7. Remolina C, Khan AV, Santiago TV. Positional hypoxemia in unilateral lung disease. *N Engl J Med* 1981; **304**: 522–5.

8. Soria C, Walthall W, Price H. *Breathing and Pulmonary Hygiene Techniques: Pulmonary Rehabilitation*. Oxford: Butterworth Publishers, 1984: 860.

9. Caldwell S, Sullivan K. *Respiratory Care – A Guide to Clinical Practice*. Philadelphia: J B Lippincott, 1977: 91.

10. Albanese AJ, Toplitz AD. A hassle free guide to suctioning a tracheostomy. *RN* 1982; **24**: 29.

11. Landa JF, Kwoka M, Chapman G, Bioto M. Effects of suctioning on mucociliary transport. *Chest* 1980; **77**: 202–7.

12. McFadden R. Decreasing respiratory compromise during infant suctioning. *Am J Nurs* 1981; **12**: 2158–61.

13. Wanner A. Nasopharyngeal airway: a facilitated access to the trachea. *Ann Intern Med* 1971; **75**: 592–5.

14. Brandstater B, Maullem M. Atelectasis following trachea suctioning in infants. *Anesthesiology* 1979; **31**: 294–7.

15. Roper PC, Vonwiller JB, Fisk GL, *et al.* Lobar atelectasis after nasotracheal intubation in infants. *Aust Pediat J* 1982; **12**: 272–5.

16. Yee A, Connors G, Cress D. *Pharmacology and the Respiratory Patient, Pulmonary Rehabilitation*. Oxford: Butterworth Publishers, 1984: 125.

17. Whitbet TL, Manion CV. Cardiac and pulmonary effects of albuterol and isoproterenol. *Chest* 1978; **74**: 251–5.

18. Zimet I. Pharmacology of drugs used in respiratory therapy. *Respiratory Care – A Guide to Clinical Practice*. Philadelphia: J B Lippincott Co, 1977: 473.

19. Lieberman J, Kurnick NB. Influence of deoxyribonucleic acid content on the proteolysis of sputum and pus. *Nature* 1962; **196**: 988.

20. Hirsh SR, Zastrow JE, Kory RC. Sputum liquification agents: a comprehensive in vitro study. *J Lab Clin Med* 1969; **74**: 346.

21. Brown M, Desai MH, Mlcak R, *et al.* Dimethylsulfoxide with heparin in the treatment of smoke inhalation injury. *J Burn Care Rehabil* 1988; **9(1)**: 22.

22. Desai MH, Mlcak R, Brown M, *et al.* Reduction of smoke injury with DMSO and heparin treatment. *Surg Form* 1985; **36**: 103.

23. Desai MH, Brown M, MLcak R, *et al.* Nebulization treatment of smoke inhalation injury in sheep model with DMSO, heparin combinations and acetylcysteine. *Crit Care Med* 1986; **14**: 321.

24. Desai MH, Mlcak R, Nichols R, Herndon DN. Reduction in mortality in pediatric patients with inhalation injury with aerosolized heparin/N-acetylcysteine therapy. *J Burn Care Rehabil* 1998; **19(3)**: 210–12.

25. Slutsky A. American College of Chest Physicians Consensus Conference, Mechanical Ventilation. *Chest* 1993; **104**: 1833–59.

26. Marini JJ, Capps JS, Culver BH. The inspiratory work of breathing during assisted mechanical ventilation. *Chest* 1985; **87**: 612–18.

27. Marini JJ, Rodriquez RM, Lamb V. The inspiratory workload of patient initiated mechanical ventilation. *Am Rev Respir Dis* 1986; **134**: 902–4.

28. Ward ME, Corbeil C, Gibbons MW, *et al.* Optimization of respiratory muscle relaxation during mechanical ventilation. *Anesthesiology* 1988; **69**: 29–35.

29. Downs JB, Klein EF, Desautels D, *et al.* Intermittent mandatory ventilation: a new approach to weaning patients. *Chest* 1973; **64**: 331–5.

30. Weisman IH, Rinaldo JE, Rodgers RM, *et al.* Intermittent mandatory ventilation. *Am Rev Respir Dis* 1983; **127**: 641–7.

31. Hirsch C, Kacmareck RM, Stanek K. Work of breathing during CPAP and PSV imposed by the new generation mechanical ventilators. *Resp Care* 1991; **36**: 815–28.

32. Macintyre NR. Respiratory function during pressure support ventilation. *Chest* 1986; **89**: 677–83.

33. Brochard L, Harf A, Lorino H. Inspiratory pressure support prevents diaphragmatic fatique during weaning from mechanical ventilation. *Am Rev Respir Dis* 1989; **139**: 513–21.

34. Fiastro JF, Habib MP, Quan SF. Pressure support compensates for inspiratory work due to endotracheal tubes. *Chest* 1988; **93**: 499–505.

35. Brochard L, Rau F, Lorino H, *et al.* Inspiratory pressure support compensates for the additional work of breathing caused by the endotracheal tube. *Anesthesiology* 1991; **75**: 739–45.

36. Hickling KG. Ventilatory management of ARDS: can it affect outcome? *Intensive Care Med* 1990; **9**: 239–50.

37. Gattinoni L, Pesenti A, Avalli L, *et al.* Pressure volume curve of total respiratory system in acute respiratory failure. *Am Rev Respir Dis* 1987; **136**: 730–60.

38. Dreyfuss D, Soler P, Basset G, *et al.* High inflation pressures, pulmonary edema, respective effects of high airway pressure, high tidal volume and PEEP. *Am Rev Respir Dis* 1988; **137**: 1159–64.

39. Kolobow T, Moretti MP, Fumagalli R, *et al.* Severe impairment of lung function induced by high peak airway pressure during mechanical ventilation. *Am Rev Respir Dis* 1987; **135**: 312–15.

40. Froese AB, Bryan AC, High frequency ventilation. *Am Rev Respir Dis* 1987; **135**: 1363–74.

41. Fusciardi J, Rouby JJ, Barakat T, *et al.* Hemodynamic effects of high frequency jet ventilation in patients with and without shock. *Anesthesiology* 1986; **65**: 485–91.

42. Cioffi W, Graves T, McManus W, *et al.* High-frequency percussive ventilation in patients with inhalation injury. *J Trauma* 1989; **29**: 350–4.

43. Cioffi W, Rue LW III, Graves T, *et al.* Prophylactic use of high-frequency percussive ventilation in patients with inhalation injury. *Ann Surg* 1991; **213**: 575–81.

44. Mlcak R, Cortiella J, Desai MH, Herndon DN. Lung compliance, airway resistance, and work of breathing in children after inhalation injury. *J Burn Care Rehabil* 1997; **18(6)**: 531–4.

45. Cortiella J, Mlcak R, Herndon DN. High frequency percussive ventilation in pediatric patients with inhalation injury. *J Burn Care Rehabil* 1999; **20(3)**: 232–5.

46. Mlcak R, Desai MH, Herndon DN. A prospective randomized study of high frequency percussive ventilation compared to conventional mechanical ventilation in pediatric patients with inhalation injury. *J Burn Care Rehabil* 2000; **21(1)**.

47. The Acute Respiratory Distress Syndrome Network. Ventilation with lower tidal volumes as compared with traditional tidal volumes for acute lung injury and the acute respiratory distress syndrome. *N Engl J Med* 2000; **342(18)**: 1301–8.

48. Kacmarek RM, Vengas J. Mechanical ventilatory rates and tidal volumes. *Resp Care* 1987; **32**: 466–78.

49. Hickling KG, Henderson SJ, Jackson R. Low mortality associated with low volume, pressure limited ventilation with permissive hypercapnia in severe adult respiratory distress syndrome. *Intensive Care Med* 1990; **16**: 372–7.

50. Marini JJ. New approaches to the ventilatory management of the adult respiratory distress syndrome. *J Crit Care* 1992; **87**: 256–7.

51. Pepe PE, Marini JJ. Occult positive pressure in mechanically ventilated patients with airflow obstruction. *Am Rev Respir Dis* 1982; **126**: 166–70.

52. Kacmareck RM. Management of the patient mechanical ventilator system. In: Pierson DJ, Kacmareck RM, eds. *Foundations of Respiratory Care*. New York: Churchill Livingstone, 1992: 973–97.

53. Stroller JK, Kacmareck RM. Ventilatory strategies in the managment of the adult respiratory distress syndrome. *Clin Chest Med* 1990; **11**: 755–72.

54. Suter PM, Fairley HB, Isenberg MD. Optimum end-expiratory airway pressure in patients with acute respiratory failure. *N Engl J Med* 1975; **292**: 284–9.

55. Sahn SA, Lakshminarayan S. Bedside criteria for discontinuation of mechanical ventilation. *Chest* 1973; **63**: 1002–5.

56. Tahvanainen J, Salmenpera M, Nikki P. Extubation criteria after weaning from IMV and CPAP. *Crit Care Med* 1983; **11**: 702–7.

57. Herndon DN, Lange F, Thompson P, *et al.* Pulmonary injury in burned patients. *Surg Clin N Am* 1987; **67**: 31.

58. Demling RH. Improved survival after major burns. *J Trauma* 1983; **23**: 179.

59. Luterman A, Dacso CC, Curreri WP. Infections in burned patients. *Am J Med* 1986; **81(A)**: 45.

60. Pruitt BA Jr. The diagnosis and treatment of infection in the burned patient. *Burns* 1984; **11**: 79.

61. Pruitt BA Jr, Flemma RJ, DiVincenti FC, *et al.* Pulmonary complications in burned patients. *J Thorac Cardiovasc Surg* 1970; **59**: 7.

62. Foley DF, Concrief JA, Mason AD. Pathology of the lungs in fatally burned patients. *Ann Surg* 1968; **167**: 251.

63. Moylan JA, Chan C. Inhalation injury – an increased problem. *Ann Surg* 1978; **188**: 34.

64. Craven DE, Kunches LM, Kilinsky V, *et al.* Risk factors for pneumonia and fatalities in patients receiving controlled mechanical ventilation. *Am Rev Respir Dis* 1986; **133**: 792.

65. Garibaldi RA, Britt MR, Coleman ML, *et al.* Risk factors for postoperative pneumonias. *Am J Med* 1984; **70**: 677.

66. Pennington JE. Hospital acquired pneumonias. In: Wenzel RP, ed. *Prevention and Control of Nosocomial Infections*. Baltimore: Williams & Wilkins, 1987: 321–4.

67. Centers for Disease Control National Nosocomial Infection Study Report. Annual Summary 1983. *MMWR* 1983; **33(259)**: 935.

68. Schwartz SN, Dowling JN, Ben Youic C, *et al.* Sources of Gram-negative bacilli colonizing the trachea of intubated patients. *J Infect Dis* 1978; **138**: 227.

69. Pierce AK, Edmonson EB, McGee G, *et al.* An analysis of factors predisposing to Gram-negative bacillary necrotizing pneumonia. *Am Rev Respir Dis* 1966; **94**: 309.

70. Ringros RE, McKown B, Felton FG, *et al.* A hospital outbreak of *Serratia marcescens* associated with ultrasonic equipment. *Ann Intern Med* 1968; **69**: 719.

71. Simmons BP, Wong ES. CDC guidelines for the prevention and control of nosocomial infections. *Am J Infect Control* 1983; **11**: 230.

72. Rhame F. The inanimate environment. In: Bennett JV, Bracham PS, eds. *Hospital Infections.* Boston: Little Brown, 1986: 223–50.

73. Cross AS, Roupe B. Role of respiratory assistance devices in endemic nosocomial pneumonia. *Am J Med* 1981; **70**: 681–5.

74. Johanson WG. *Resp Care* 1982; **27**: 445–52.

75. Lareau SC, Ryan KJ, Diener CF. The relationship between frequency of ventilator circuit changes and infection hazard. *Am Rev Respir Dis* 1978; **118**: 493–6.

76. Garner JS, Faverno MS. CDC guidelines for the prevention and control of nosocomial infections. *Am J Infect Control* 1986; **14**: 110–29.

77. Edge RS. *Infection Control, Respiratory Care Practice.* Chicago: Year Book Medical, 1988: 574.

78. Munster AM, Wong LA. *Miscellaneous Pulmonary Complications in Respiratory Injury,* New York: McGraw-Hill, 1990: 326.

79. Demling RH. Smoke inhalation injury. *Postgrad Med* 1987; **82**: 63.

80. Cahalane M, Demling RH. Early respiratory abnormalities from smoke inhalation. *JAMA* 1984; **251**: 771.

81. Mlcak R, Desai MH, Robinson E, *et al.* Inhalation injury and lung function in children – a decade later. *J Burn Care Rehabil* 2000; **21(1)**.

82. Colic GL. Long term respiratory complications of inhalation injury. In: *Respiratory Injury, Smoke Inhalation and Burns.* New York: McGraw-Hill, 1990: 342.

83. Desai MH, Mlcak R, Robinson E. Does inhalation injury limit exercise endurance in children convalescing from thermal injury. *J Burn Care Rehabil* 1993; **14**: 16–20.

Response to injury

Chapter 19

The systemic inflammatory response syndrome

Edward R Sherwood
Daniel L Traber

Introduction

Burn patients with or without inhalation injury commonly exhibit a clinical picture produced by systemic inflammation. The phrase 'systemic inflammatory response syndrome (SIRS)' has been introduced to designate the signs and symptoms of patients suffering from such a condition. SIRS has a continuum of severity ranging from the presence of tachycardia, tachypnea, fever, and leukocytosis, to refractory hypotension and, in its most severe from, shock and multiple organ system dysfunction. In thermally injured patients, the most common causes of SIRS is the burn itself. Sepsis, SIRS with the presence of infection or bacteremia, is also a common occurrence. Sepsis is a major complication in burn patients and a significant factor in the high morbidity and mortality seen in these patients. Starting from a local infection at the burn wound or an infected catheter tip, the spread of bacteria and their toxins, or of fungi might further potentiate the already activated immune system. Pathological alterations of metabolic, cardiovascular, gastrointestinal, and coagulation systems occur as a result of the hyperactive immune system. Paradoxically, a state of immunosuppression often follows or co-exists with SIRS. The counter antiinflammatory response syndrome (CARS) appears to be an adaptive mechanism designed to limit the injurious effects of systemic inflammation. However, this response may also render the host more susceptible to systemic infection due to impaired antimicrobial immunity. Both cellular and humoral mechanisms are involved in these disease processes and have been extensively studied in various burn and sepsis models. This chapter will review current understanding of SIRS and the associated immunological, cardiovascular, and pulmonary dysfunction that occurs following trauma and thermal injury.

Definition of SIRS

The phrase systemic inflammatory response syndrome (SIRS) was recommended by the American College of Chest Physicians/ Society for Critical Care Medicine (ACCP/SCCM) consensus conference in 1992 to describe a systemic inflammatory process, independent of its cause.[1] The proposal was based on clinical and experimental results indicating that a variety of conditions, both infectious and noninfectious (i.e. burns, ischemia–reperfusion injury, multiple trauma, pancreatitis), induce a similar host response. Two or more of the following conditions must be fulfilled for the diagnosis of SIRS to be made:

- body temperature >38°C or <36°C;
- heart rate >90 beats/min;
- respiratory rate >20/min or $P\mathrm{aco_2}$ <32 mmHg;
- leukocyte count >12 000/μl, <4000/μL, or >10% immature (band) forms.

All of these pathophysiologic changes must occur as an acute alteration from baseline in the absence of other known causes for them such as chemotherapy-induced neutropenia and leukopenia. This definition is very sensitive and its clinical and prognostic significance has not been conclusively demonstrated. Most of the SIRS criteria are also addressed in other scoring systems of injury-induced physiologic derangement such as the Acute Physiology and Chronic Health Evaluation (APACHE), Mortality Probability Model (MPM), and Simplified Acute Physiology Severity (SAPS) systems. Several investigators have criticized the definition of SIRS as being too sensitive and encompassing the majority of ICU patients and certainly the vast majority of patients suffering extensive thermal injury.[2,3] In addition, these definitions are difficult to apply to children. Some of the criteria, particularly those for heart rate and respiratory rate, fall within the normal physiologic range for young children. The initial definition of SIRS did not address the continuum of disease severity as was defined for sepsis. Specifically, sepsis was defined by the same criteria as SIRS in patients with demonstrable infection. In addition to the criteria defined for sepsis above, severe sepsis included the additional derangements of organ dysfunction, hypotension, and hypoperfusion. Evidence of hypoperfusion included, but was not limited to, lactic acidosis, oliguria, and altered mental status. Septic shock, the most severe form of sepsis, was characterized by hypotension and hypoperfusion in patients who were adequately volume resuscitated. Muckart and Bhagwangee,[2] in an effort to define a continuum of severity for SIRS, later proposed the categories of severe SIRS and sterile shock. These conditions were defined by the same criteria as severe sepsis and septic shock in the absence of demonstrable infection. In its most severe form, SIRS can induce organ injury and subsequent multiple organ dysfunction syndrome (MODS) and multiple organ system failure (MOSF).

Several studies have been conducted with the goal of determining the prognostic value of the SIRS designation. In the acute setting, SIRS has been demonstrated in the majority of critically injured patients and the intensity of the response correlates directly with the severity of injury.[3,4] The presence of SIRS within the first 24 hours after severe injury has not served as a predictor of mortality in trauma or burn patients in some studies.[3,4] However, the presence of sterile or septic shock is an important predictor of poor outcome, particularly when associated with multiple system organ dysfunction (MSOD).[2] In addition, the presence of more than two of the SIRS criteria in the setting of acute injury has correlated with increased morbidity and mortality.[5,6] A study by Rangel-Frausto and colleagues[6] showed that trauma patients who did not meet SIRS criteria had a mortality rate of 3% compared with 6% mortality in those with two SIRS markers. Patients with three or four SIRS criteria had mortality rates of 10 and 17%, respectively, while those with culture-negative shock had a 46% death rate. Haga and colleagues[7] have shown that the persistence of SIRS for more than 3 days in surgical patients is a harbinger of complications and is associated with increased morbidity. Talmor and colleagues[4] reported that persistence of SIRS to the second postoperative day in high-risk surgical patients correlated with an increased incidence of MSOD. Additional studies have shown that persistence of SIRS criteria for more than 3 days in trauma and burn patients is associated with worse outcome.[8,9] Therefore, three important factors appear to determine the effect of SIRS on the host. The first factor is the severity of the initial inflammatory response. This response is proportional to the severity of injury. Specifically, the presence of shock or MSOD within the first 24 hours after injury bears a poor prognosis. The second determinant is the persistence of SIRS beyond the first days of injury. Specifically, prolongation of SIRS beyond the second day after

severe trauma or thermal injury is associated with an increased complication rate. Factors that appear to be important in decreasing the incidence of a prolonged inflammatory state include adequate fluid resuscitation within the first 24 hours of injury, aggressive excision of necrotic tissue, and enteral feeding;[8-10] a further factor is the adaptive capacity of the host. Results of several studies have shown that extremes of age, either old or young, and the presence of coexisting disease will diminish the adaptive capacity of the host and predict a worse prognosis for any given severity of injury.[10,11] The definition of SIRS comprises the clinical signs of the pathophysiologic alterations of systemic inflammation and should be viewed as a continuum of severity. In the remainder of this chapter, the pathophysiology of the systemic inflammatory response will be reviewed.

The initiating event

The crucial pathophysiologic event that precipitates systemic inflammation is tissue damage. This can occur both as a result of the direct injury to tissues from mechanical or thermal trauma as well as cellular injury induced by mediators of ischemia–reperfusion injury such as oxygen free radicals. Injury results in the acute release of proinflammatory cytokines. If injury is severe, such as in extensive thermal injury, a profound release of cytokines occurs, resulting in the induction of a systemic inflammatory reaction. The ability of the host to adapt to this systemic inflammatory response is dependent on the magnitude of the response, the duration of the response, and the adaptive capacity of the host. Factors that have been implicated in prolongation of SIRS include underresuscitation in the acute phase following thermal injury, persistent or intermittent infection, ongoing tissue necrosis, and translocation of endotoxin across the bowel.[11,12] For analysis of mechanisms and their importance in the development of SIRS, one must consider several factors. The immune system is a complicated network. Soluble mediators secreted by immune and vascular endothelial cells regulate many immune functions and serve as means of communication between different parts of the system. Mediators are involved in the regulation of their own release as well as in the production and secretion of other mediators. Therefore, experimental intervention in order to study the effects of one mediator will necessarily affect the whole network. The existence of a network also explains why administration of a specific mediator might trigger systemic inflammation. Therapeutic intervention at different steps might be successful in the prevention of SIRS if the mediator plays a pivotal role in the development of the systemic inflammatory response. However, interventions aimed at neutralizing single mediators of SIRS such as tumor necrosis factor α (TNFα), interleukin-1 (IL-1), and platelet activating factor have not been successful in clinical trials.

Cytokine and non-cytokine mediators of SIRS

Several proinflammatory cytokines, chemokines, and non-cytokine inflammatory mediators play a role in the pathogenesis of SIRS. Cytokines comprise a broad group of polypeptides with varied functions within the immune response (**Table 19.1**). The classical mediator of systemic inflammation is TNFα. TNFα is released primarily by macrophages within minutes of local or systemic injury and modulates a variety of immunologic and metabolic events.[13] At

Table 19.1 Cytokine and chemokine mediators of systemic inflammation

Cytokine	Polypeptide size	Cell source	Cell target	Primary effects
Tumor necrosis factor α (TNFα)	17 kDa	Monocytes, macrophages, T lymphocytes	(a) Neutrophil	Activation (inflammation)
			(b) Endothelial cell	Activation (inflammation/coagulation) Release of vasodilators (NO)
			(c) Hypothalamus	Fever
			(d) Liver	Acute phase response
			(e) Muscle, fat	Catabolism
			(f) Heart	Myocardial suppression
			(g) Macrophages	Release of cytokines, Inflammation
			(h) T lymphocytes	Inflammation
			(i) Various tissues	Apoptosis?
Interleukin-1 (IL-1)	17 kDa	Monocytes, macrophages	(a) T cells	Activation (inflammation)
			(b) Endothelial cell	Activation (inflammation/coagulation) Release of vasodilators (NO)
			(c) Liver	Acute phase response
			(d) hypothalamus	Fever
			(e) muscle, fat	Catabolism
Interleukin-6 (IL-6)	26 kDa	Monocytes, macrophages, T cells, endothelial cells	(a) Liver	Acute phase response
			(b) B cells	Activation
Interleukin-8 (IL-8)	10 kDa	Monocytes, macrophages, endothelial cells	Neutrophils	Chemotaxis, activation
Interferon γ (IFN-γ)	21–24 kDa	T cells, NK cells	Macrophages	Activation (inflammation)
Interleukin-12 (IL-12)	70 kDa	Macrophages	T cells, B cells NK cells	Activation, differentiation
Interleukin-18		Macrophages	T cells, NK cells	Activation, differentiation

sites of local infection or inflammation, TNFα initiates an immune response that activates antimicrobial defense mechanisms and, once the infection is eradicated, tissue repair. It is a potent activator of neutrophils and mononuclear phagocytes, and also serves as a growth factor for fibroblasts and as an angiogenesis factor. However, systemic release of TNFα can precipitate a destructive cascade of events that can result in tissue injury, organ dysfunction and, potentially, death. Among the systemic effects of TNFα are the induction of fever, stimulation of acute phase protein secretion by the liver, activation of the coagulation cascade, myocardial suppression, induction of systemic vasodilators with resultant hypotension, catabolism, and hypoglycemia.[13,14] Numerous studies have shown that administration of TNFα to experimental animals will mimic the systemic inflammatory response observed in sepsis and after severe injury. Another important effect of TNFα is its ability to induce apoptosis of a variety of cell types.[15] TNF-induced apoptosis may be one mechanism by which it induces tissue injury at high systemic concentrations.

Tumor necrosis factor α is also a potent stimulus for the release of other inflammatory mediators, particularly IL-1 and IL-6. Interleukin-1 is released primarily by mononuclear phagocytes and its physiologic effects are essentially identical to those of TNFα.[16] However, important differences between the functions of IL-1 and TNFα exist. Most notably, IL-1 does not induce tissue injury or apoptotic cell death by itself but can potentiate the injurious effects of TNFα. The IL-1 family of proteins, including IL-18, are the only group of cytokines for which known natural antagonists have been identified. The IL-1 receptor antagonists (IL-1ra) bind to the IL-1 receptor but do not induce receptor activation.[16] These proteins appear to function as competitive inhibitors of IL-1 action.

Interleukin-6 is another protein that is commonly increased in the circulation of patients with SIRS.[16] This protein is secreted by macrophages, endothelial cells, and fibroblasts. Interleukin-6 itself does not induce tissue injury but its presence in the circulation has been associated with poor outcome in trauma patients, probably because it is a marker of ongoing inflammation. The primary effect of IL-6 is to induce secretion of acute phase proteins from the liver as well as serve as a growth and differentiation factor for B lymphocytes.

Interferon γ (IFN-γ) is a cytokine involved in the amplification of the acute inflammatory response, particularly the stimulation of cytokine secretion, phagocytosis, and respiratory burst activity by macrophages.[17,18] Interferon γ is secreted primarily by T lymphocytes and natural killer (NK) cells in response to antigen presentation as well as macrophage-derived cytokines such as IL-12 and IL-18. The primary effect of IFN-γ is to amplify the inflammatory response of macrophages. In response to IFN-γ, the phagocytic and respiratory burst activity of macrophages are increased, secretion of inflammatory mediators such as TNFα and IL-1 are enhanced, and antigen presentation is potentiated by upregulation of class II major histocompatability complex. Blockade of IFN-γ production or function has been shown to markedly decrease the deleterious inflammatory effects induced by bacterial endotoxin.[19] Therefore, IFN-γ is believed to be an important factor in the amplification of SIRS.

Chemokines are a family of proteins that function primarily as chemotactic factors for leukocytes (**Table 19.2**). Interleukin-8 is the most widely studied chemokine in the setting of sepsis and SIRS; it is a potent chemoattractant for neutrophils and is a major factor in recruiting neutrophils to inflammatory foci. Several studies have shown that IL-8 plays a role, particularly in the lung, in mediating tissue injury in the setting of trauma and burn injury.[20] It is likely that that other chemokines also play a role in inflammatory injury. A recent study demonstrated increased circulating levels of macrophage inflammatory protein (MIP) 1α in patients with SIRS.[21]

A central feature in the upregulation of many of the soluble mediators described above is the transcription factor nuclear factor-κB (NF-κB).[22] NF-κB is comprised of a family of proteins including p50 (NF-κB1), p65 (RelA), C-Rel, and p52 (NF-κB2) that combine to form homo- or heterodimers and ultimately function to regulate the transcription of a variety of cytokine, chemokine, adhesion molecule, and enzyme genes involved in SIRS (**Table 19.3**). NF-κB is constitutively expressed in many cell types and sequestered in the cytoplasm of cells in a functionally inactive form bound to the protein inhibitory κB (IκB). The binding of TNFα or IL-1β to their receptors activates a signal transduction cascade, which results in the activation of NF-κB-inducing kinase (NIK) and, subsequently, inhibitory κB kinase (IKK). IKK phosphorylates IκB, resulting in ubiquitinization and degradation of IκB by the 26S proteosome. Degradation of IκB frees NF-κB and allows it to migrate into the nucleus where it binds to specific sites in the promoter region of a variety of SIRS-associated gene products and modulates their expression (**Figure 19.1**). Increased activation of NF-κB has been associated with poor outcome in some studies. Activation of NF-κB in peripheral blood monocytes correlated with increased mortality in septic patients, and alveolar

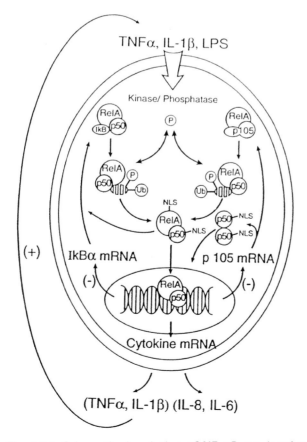

Fig. 19.1 Schematic description of NF-κB regulated pro-inflammatory gene transcription.

Table 19.2 Classification of chemokines

Chemokine type	Target cell
α Chemokines	
IL-8	Neutrophils
GROα (mouse equivalent is GRO/KC)	Neutrophils
GROβ (mouse equivalent is GRO/KC)	Neutrophils
GROγ (mouse equivalent is GRO/KC)	Neutrophils
ENA-78	Neutrophils
LDGF-PBP	Neutrophils, fibroblasts
GCP-2	Neutrophils
PF4	Fibroblasts
Mig	T lymphocytes
IP-10	T lymphocytes
I-TAC	T lymphocytes
SDF-1α/β	T lymphocytes
β Chemokines	
MIP-1α	Monocyte/macrophages, T lymph, B cells, NK cells, basophils
MIP-1β	Same as above
MDC	Monocyte, T lymphocytes
TECK	Macrophages, T lymphocytes
TARC	T lymphocytes
RANTES	Monocyte/macrophages, T lymph, NK cells, basophils
HCC-1	Monocytes
HCC-4	Monocytes, lymphocytes
DC-CK-1	T lymphocytes
MIP-3α	T lymphocytes
MIP-3β	T lymphocytes
MCP-1	T lymphocytes, monocytes
MCP-2	Same
MCP-3	Same
MCP-4	Same
Eotaxin	Eosinophils
Other chemokines	
Lymphotacin	T lymphocytes, NK cells
Fractalkine	T lymphocytes, monocytes

Table 19.3 Proinflammatory molecules regulated by NF-κB

Cytokines	Enzymes
TNFα	COX-2
TNFβ	iNOS
IL-1β	
IL-6	Chemokines
IL-12	IL-8
IL-2	Gro α,β,γ
IFN-β	MCP-1
	RANTES
Colony-stimulating factors	Adhesion molecules
G-CSF	ICAM-1
GM-CSF	E-selectin
	V-CAM

macrophages from patients with adult respiratory distress syndrome (ARDS) exhibited greater nuclear NF-κB levels than critically ill patients without ARDS.[23,24]

Several non-cytokine factors have been implicated in the pathogenesis of SIRS. Platelet activating factor (PAF) is a phospholipid autocoid released by endothelial cells that regulates the release of cytokines and amplifies the proinflammatory response. It appears to be an important factor in the adhesion of neutrophils to endothelial cells. The prolonged presence of PAF in the serum of patients with SIRS has correlated with poor outcome.[25] Eicosanoids are arachadonic acid metabolites that regulate many aspects of the immune response. Leukotrienes (LTC$_4$–LTE$_4$) induce contraction of endothelial cells and encourage capillary leakage.[26] Thromboxane A$_2$, a macrophage and platelet-derived factor, promotes platelet aggregation, vasoconstriction and, potentially, tissue thrombosis.[27]

The complement cascade is comprised of more than 30 proteins that interact in a complex fashion to mediate inflammation and direct lysis of microbes and other cells. However, in SIRS, excessive complement activation appears to cause significant cellular injury in the host. Products of the complement cascade, most notably C3a and C5a, are potent activators of inflammation and leukocyte chemotaxis.[28] C3a and C5a also directly activate neutrophils and promote release of reactive oxygen intermediates and proteases. Excessive release of these factors can result in significant tissue injury. The membrane attack complex (MAC) is the terminal component of the complement cascade. MAC results from the aggregation of the complement components C5–C9 on biological membranes. The accumulation of MAC on cell surfaces can result in significant tissue and cellular injury and may be a major factor in the pathogenesis of MSOD.

Several other factors such as nitric oxide, selectins, tissue factor, and thrombin play important roles in the hemodynamic response, alterations in capillary permeability, and activation of the coagulation cascade that occur with SIRS and will be discussed in more detail later in this chapter.

Circulating cytokines as markers of SIRS and predictors of outcome

Numerous studies have been undertaken with the goal of using plasma cytokine levels as diagnostic and prognostic markers in patients with SIRS. This approach seems logical based on the observation that circulating cytokines have been observed in several clinical studies of trauma, sepsis, and thermal injury. Given its central role in the activation and regulation of the proinflammatory response, TNFα has been studied extensively as a plasma marker of SIRS. The results have been inconsistent. Martin and colleagues[29] showed that TNFα levels were markedly elevated in patients with septic shock and correlated with fatal outcome. However, their results also showed that trauma patients did not exhibit the same marked elevations in circulating TNFα nor did circulating TNFα concentrations correlate with increased mortality in trauma patients. In some published studies, measurement of circulating TNFα levels in burn patients has not provided a useful marker of outcome.[30–32] Overall, plasma TNFα levels have been variable and inconsistent and have not correlated with mortality or the development of MODS. However, a study by Zhang and co-workers[33] in 25 patients with greater than 30% total body surface area (TBSA) burns demonstrated marked increases in plasma TNFα levels in burned patients and a significant correlation between TNFα concentration and shock, MODS, and death. These findings support the results of Marano et al.[34] who showed a significant correlation between circulating TNFα concentration and mortality in burned patients. Therefore, taken together, these results show that the value of TNFα as a marker of ongoing inflammation as well as an indicator of morbidity and mortality in the setting of burn injury remains to be established.

TNFα interacts with two known cell surface receptors designated tumor necrosis factor receptor (TNFR)-I and TNFR-II. TNFR-I, also known as TNF-R55 or p55, is expressed on a variety of cells and its activation mediates most of the activities of TNFα, including induction of apoptosis. Activation of TNFR-II (TNF-R75 or p75) results in cellular proliferation and activation. During inflammatory states, TNFR are released from cells and may serve as antagonists of TNFα. Several investigators have characterized surface-bound and soluble TNFR (sTNFR) in sepsis and trauma.[33,35,36] Hubl and colleagues[35] showed that surface TNFR-I were upregulated while TNFR-II were downregulated in patients with SIRS. Increased TNFR-I correlated with increased body temperature but not with survival. SIRS patients with decreased surface TNFR-II had a trend toward increased mortality. A study by Zhang and co-workers[33] showed a higher incidence of shock, MODS, and mortality in burn patients with increased plasma sTNFR-I and sTNFR-II levels. Presterl et al.[36] showed a correlation between sTNFR and APACHE III scores, as well as the incidence of shock and mortality in septic patients. Overall, in the studies published to date, the presence of high levels of circulating sTNFR is a poor prognostic indicator.

Another family of proteins that has been extensively analyzed as markers of SIRS is IL-1 and IL-1 receptor antagonist (IL-1ra). In burn patients, low IL-1β levels have correlated with mortality in two independent studies.[32,33] Plasma IL-1ra levels have been shown to correlate with body surface area burned, extent of third degree burn, and the presence of inhalational injury.[32,37] In addition, ratios of IL-1ra to IL-1β in plasma of greater than 4:1 correlate with increased mortality in burned patients.[33] These finding support the notion that IL-1β plays an important role in the adaptive capacity of the host after thermal injury.

Of the cytokine markers studied to date, elevated levels of IL-6 appear to be one of the more consistent markers of poor outcome in burn, trauma, and septic patients. One of the primary known functions of IL-6 is induction of acute phase proteins such as C-reactive protein (CRP) by the liver. In some studies, CRP has been shown to parallel IL-6 as a marker of increased mortality.[38] Although IL-6 itself does not have any known direct injurious effects, it apparently serves as a consistent marker of ongoing inflammation. Elevated plasma IL-6 levels have correlated with increased mortality in experimental and clinical studies of thermal injury, sepsis, trauma, and hemorrhagic shock.[36,39,40] A study by Taniguchi and colleagues[40] showed that an increased ratio of IL-6 to the immunosuppressive cytokine IL-10 was a predictor of poor outcome in patients with SIRS.

In trauma and burn patients it is often difficult to differentiate whether SIRS is a result of the injury itself or due to superimposed infection. Most of the clinical signs of infection, such as fever and leukocytosis are, by definition, present in SIRS. Considerable attention has been placed on identifying indirect markers of systemic infection. The identification of circulating markers of infection that can be rapidly assessed and serve as reliable markers of the presence of infection has important implications. First, it is important clinically to identify patients with systemic infection in order to initiate antibiotic therapy in a timely fashion. Secondly, blood cultures are the gold standard for diagnosis of systemic infections. Although blood cultures provide important information regarding the presence of infection and the identity of the infecting organism, it can often take several days to obtain reliable results, and the presence of negative cultures does not assure the absence of infection. Therefore, efforts have been made to identify other markers of systemic infection. The two markers that have been most consistently elevated in patients with infection are procalcitonin and C-reactive protein (CRP). Several recent studies have shown that increased plasma levels of procalcitonin is a sensitive marker of systemic infection.[41–43] Likewise, increased circulating CRP has been shown to be a sensitive marker of infection.[44,45] Both of these markers have been shown to be more reliable than clinical signs in the diagnosis of infection in high-risk surgical and trauma patients.

Overall, several markers of inflammation and infection have been identified in burn and trauma patients. Some of these markers have been shown to be consistent indicators of high-risk patients. However, cytokine and non-cytokine markers of inflammation are not used routinely in the laboratory evaluation of burned patients. With further research and demonstration of the reliability of these markers, they may become an accepted part of clinical practice. In addition, technology is evolving to measure these markers in a rapid and cost-effective manner. The combination of these factors may allow blood cytokine markers to become a component of patient management in the future.

Anti-inflammatory therapy for SIRS

Despite our increased understanding of the role of inflammatory mediators in the pathologenesis of SIRS, most anti-inflammatory drug regimens have had little success in the treatment of this problem. Neutralizing approaches to several inflammatory mediators have been studied. All of these studies have demonstrated, at best, marginal improvement in septic morbidity and mortality. One of the most widely studied approaches for the treatment of SIRS is the use of monoclonal antibodies to TNFα. Several multicenter, prospective, clinical trials have been undertaken in septic patients using several different antibodies to TNFα.[46–52] These studies did not demonstrate improved outcome in patients receiving anti-TNFα compared to placebo. One recent study evaluated the efficacy of a chimeric antibody to TNF in patients with severe sepsis.[52] Circulating levels of TNFα as well as a variety of other inflammatory mediators were assessed. Although circulating levels of TNFα were transiently decreased, anti-TNFα therapy did not result in reduction of circulating levels of other inflammatory mediators such as IL-1β, IL-1ra, sTNFR, or IL-6. In addition, evidence of systemic inflammation was not decreased and overall mortality was not improved in anti-TNFα-treated patients. Similarly, the use of sTNFR as a strategy to neutralize the systemic effects of TNFα and decrease sepsis-associated morbidity and mortality have been unsuccessful.[53,54] Other anti-inflammatory approaches that have been studied and found to be largely ineffective include the use of IL-1ra,[55–57] anti-bradykinin,[58] PAFra,[59,60] and ibuprofen.[61,62]

Because of the relative ineffectiveness of anti-inflammatory therapy aimed at neutralizing single mediators, more broad-based strategies were developed with the goal of neutralizing, removing, or inhibiting the production of several inflammatory mediators. Hemofiltration was one approach that received considerable attention. Several studies have shown that hemofiltration will increase the clearance of inflammatory mediators, particularly IL-6, from blood in patients with sepsis.[63–65] However, none of these studies has demonstrated a significant reduction in IL-6 plasma levels. A study by Kellum and colleagues[65] showed that continuous venovenous hemofiltration (CVVH) reduced plasma TNFα concentrations by 13%, while the use of continuous venovenous hemodialysis (CVVHD) resulted in a 32% increase in circulating TNFα levels. Overall, the use of hemofiltration has been largely ineffective in removing significant amounts of inflammatory mediators from the blood of patients with sepsis and there is currently no evidence that this approach will decrease morbidity and mortality.

The use of glucocorticoids in the treatment of sepsis has been proposed for more than 30 years. Two meta-analyses[66,67] of studies using high-dose glucocorticoids in the treatment of sepsis were published in 1995 and later summarized by Zeni and colleagues.[68] Overall, the use of glucocorticoids to treat sepsis and septic shock has not been beneficial. In many studies, the use of glucocorticoids in septic patients was associated with increased mortality. In burned patients, there is no evidence that administration of glucocorticoids provides effective treatment for systemic inflammation.

Reasons for the lack of efficacy of these agents are likely to be multifactorial. Firstly, the inflammatory response to injury and sepsis is mediated by a complex array of mediators that are largely interrelated. Therefore, blocking or neutralization of a single mediator is not likely to have a marked effect on the overall response. Secondly, the same mediators that are important in inducing tissue injury also play an important role in antimicrobial immunity. Blockade of these mediators may leave the host more susceptible to subsequent infection. Thirdly, many of the mediators, particularly TNFα and IL-1β, are released within minutes of injury and mobilize the inflammatory cascade shortly thereafter. Therefore, by the time that signs of SIRS or sepsis are apparent, many of the injurious effects of the inflammatory response have already been set into motion, making therapy ineffective. A recent emphasis has been placed on the identification of late mediators of inflammatory injury. This search has been prompted by the observation that SIRS and sepsis-associated death occur days after the peak effect of inflammatory cytokines. One potential late mediator that has recently been identified is high-mobility group protein-1 (HMG-1).[69] HMG-1 is released by macrophages up to 8 hours after LPS challenge and persists in the circulation for days. Administration of anti-HMG-1 in mice has been shown to improve survival. Conversely, systemic administration of HMG-1 to mice is lethal. Whether HMG-1 plays an important role in inflammatory injury in humans remains to be determined. However, the concept of late mediators of inflammatory tissue injury may improve our understanding of the pathophysiology of SIRS.

As discussed earlier in this chapter, factors that appear to be important in limiting the extent of SIRS and, in many cases, decreasing the incidence of shock and MSOD, are aggressive fluid resuscitation, excision of necrotic tissue, and adequate nutritional support.[11] There is controversy regarding the ideal fluid for volume resuscitation in trauma and burn patients. However, recent studies show that hypertonic saline has beneficial effects in modulating the SIRS-associated immunological cascade as well as restoring hemodynamic parameters and microcirculatory flow. The effect of hypertonic saline on immune function has largely centered around attenuation of post-injury immunosuppression. Recent studies have shown that resuscitation with hypertonic saline will improve macrophage and T cell function as well as increase resistance to infection in experimental models or trauma and hemorrhage.[70–72] Proper nutritional support is also an important factor in the treatment of severely injured patients. Enteral feeding formulas supplemented with glutamine, arginine, omega-3 fatty acids, and nucleotides have been shown to improve outcome in trauma patients.[73,74] Overall, trauma patients receiving immune-enhancing diets have been shown to have fewer infectious complications.

The hemodynamic response

The full clinical picture of systemic inflammation after thermal injury, multiple trauma, or sepsis includes a hyperdynamic circulation. It is characterized by a low systemic vascular resistance, which requires a high cardiac output to maintain mean arterial pressure. This fall in resistance is not the result of an increase in metabolic rate. The oxygen extraction of the tissues remains the same. Blood is thus flowing to tissues which are not metabolically active. Patients who are not well resuscitated or whose heart function is compromised may not be able to increase their cardiac output to the extent needed to maintain arterial pressure during states of extensive vasodilatation and, thus, might go into shock. A reduced vascular responsiveness to vasoconstrictors finally prevents successful pharmacologic intervention and patients might die in irreversible shock. The time period from insult until the hyperdynamic response develops can vary between hours after a septic insult or days after multiple trauma. It has been hypothesized that the development of the hyperdynamic state might be dependent on the presence of endotoxin or bacteria in the blood. An intravenous bolus injection of 4 ng/kg endotoxin into healthy volunteers mimics some aspects of the hemodynamic response seen in patients.[75,76] The low systemic vascular resistance and the elevated cardiac output can also be induced in animal models by continuous infusion of low dose endotoxin[77] or bacteria.[78] Studies in conscious sheep revealed that the hemodynamic response to continuous low dose endotoxin can be divided into three parts.[79] The first two phases might be missed under clinical conditions most of the time due to their short duration (<3 h).

Phase 1

Systemic vascular resistance and pulmonary vascular resistance increase markedly both upon intermittent administration of endotoxin[80] or during its continuous infusion into conscious sheep.[81] This reaction occurred within 30 minutes to 1 hour of the endotoxin administration and was attributed to the release of the potent vasoconstrictor thromboxane (TX) A_2. Lymph and plasma levels of TXB_2, the stable metabolite of the eicosanoid TXA_2, were found

elevated 1 and 4 hours after challenge of sheep with 1 μg/kg endotoxin.[82] Cyclooxygenase[83] and thromboxane synthetase inhibition diminished the hypertensive response.[82] Thromboxane synthetase inhibition was equally effective in preventing the marked pulmonary vasoconstriction after burn injury in pigs.[84] The high pulmonary vascular resistance during phase 1 of endotoxemia has been demonstrated to compromise myocardial function of the right heart in terms of a low ejection fraction and an increase in end-systolic diameter.[85,86] Administration of the thromboxane synthetase inhibitor OKY046 blocked these early changes in right heart function.[85]

The early systemic vasoconstriction did not occur equally throughout the vasculature. Blood flow through the superior mesenteric artery was particularly reduced.[87] Vasoconstriction of the splanchnic vessels has been associated with the release of so-called myocardial depressant factors[88] and with bacterial translocation.[87] The coincidence of markedly decreased mesenteric blood flow and bacterial translocation has also been demonstrated after burn injury[89] and multiple trauma associated with a state of circulatory shock.[90] Moreover, hypoperfusion, particularly of the ileal mucosa, was still noted during the hyperdynamic phase in a *murine* sepsis model, when blood flow to most of the splanchnic area was not decreased.[91] Bacterial translocation has been hypothesized to be one of the major factors maintaining systemic inflammation.

Phase 2

This portion of the response, between 3 and 4 hours after the endotoxin infusion has been started, is characterized more by pulmonary permeability changes (see below) than by hemodynamic alterations. In the hyperdynamic sheep model, the pulmonary artery pressure is mildly elevated and cardiac output demonstrates the lowest values throughout the experiment. The underlying mechanisms of this response are not yet clear. Many mediators of the immune system have been released by that time including TNFα, IL-6, PAF, and peptidoleukotrienes.[92] This might indicate that these mediators are proximal elements of the mediator cascades. Although investigations into the release of many of these cytokines are few as a result of the limitations of respective assays, TNFα has been shown to be increased in both phase 1 and 2 of the response in sheep[92,93] and volunteers.[95,96] Moreover, the vasoconstrictor endothelin is elevated in the chronic sheep model of endotoxemia at that time,[97] as well as the vasodilator atrial natriuretic peptide.[98,99] Endothelin has also been correlated with reductions in cardiac output in septic humans.[100] The hemodynamic changes in phase 2 are most likely the result of the action of the mediator cocktail.

Phase 3

Continuous infusion of endotoxin into sheep and pigs resulted in a hyperdynamic circulation.[81,94,101] Beside a low systemic vascular resistance and a high cardiac output with a slightly decreased mean arterial pressure the hyperdynamic response is further characterized by hyporesponsiveness of isolated vessels to vasoconstrictors[102] and an increased pulmonary shunt fraction in the presence of a reduced pulmonary hypoxic vasoconstriction.[81,103,104] The high cardiac output is due to an increase in heart rate in the presence of depressed myocardial contractility.[105,106]

Nitric Oxide

The endothelial-derived relaxing factor, recently identified as nitric oxide (NO), has been implicated as a mediator in this reaction. NO can be synthesized from its precursor L-arginine by two different enzymes. The calcium-dependent constitutive nitric oxide synthase (NOS) is responsible for the basal release of NO, which seems to play an important role for the regulation of vascular tone under physiologic conditions. *In vitro* data suggest that this enzyme might become inactivated early after administration of endotoxin, thus accounting for some of the vasoconstrictive phenomena seen in phases 1 and 2.[107] Dependent on the species, cells producing the inducible NOS include macrophages, vascular smooth muscle cells, and vascular endothelium upon stimulation by endotoxin, TNFα, interleukin-1, or α-interferon.[108] On the other hand, it has recently been reported that the human macrophage cannot form NO under these circumstances.[109,110]

NO is a lipophilic gas which can easily enter vascular smooth muscle cells where it stimulates the soluble guanylate cyclase[111,112] to synthesize cyclic guanosine monophosphate (cGMP). High levels of cGMP stimulate cells to lower their intracellular Ca^{2+} concentration. This leads to vascular dilatation and hyporesponsiveness to vasoconstrictors. Administration of a NOS inhibitor to septic humans[113,114] and to endotoxemic sheep[81] increases their vascular resistance and restores their responsiveness to vasoconstrictors. It was assumed that the hemodynamic abnormalities mediated by NO formed via the inducible NOS. However, plasma concentrations of nitrite/nitrate and nitrosylated proteins were not elevated during *ovine* endotoxemia. Species specificity was also indicated by the finding that human macrophages do not produce the inducible form of NOS. However, the inducible form of the enzyme seems to be present in human hepatocytes. Elevated nitrite levels were reported in one study evaluating septic newborns.[115] There are currently no convincing data available with regard to high nitrite levels in adult humans with SIRS. Ochoa found somewhat elevated nitrite concentrations in some septic patients, but failed to demonstrate them in septic trauma patients.[116] At this point it can neither be concluded nor can it be excluded that NO mediates the hyperdynamic response during systemic inflammation.

Guanylate Cyclase

The second messenger cGMP appears to play an important role in the vasodilation seen with sepsis. There have been reports of cGMP elevations in plasma of septic patients[117] and endotoxic rats.[118] cGMP was elevated in tissues removed from our animals following a continuous infusion of endotoxin.[119] The guanylate cyclase occurs in a soluble and in a particulate form.[120] The particulate form is activated by atrial natriuretic peptide (ANP).[121,122] The soluble form has a heme group that is activated by NO. This reaction is inhibited by methylene blue and hemoglobin.[123] There is a high probability that ANP is the source of the stimulation of guanylate cyclase during sepsis and endotoxemia, because the cGMP formed in some of the experiments was not inhibited by methylene blue or L-arginine analogs.

Atrial Natriuretic Peptide

We have reported a marked elevation in ANP after the injection of endotoxin into sheep.[98,99] We have also examined our chronic sheep models and found that the increase in plasma levels of ANP was sustained with the continuous infusion of endotoxin or bacteria.

ANP has also been shown to be elevated in septic humans.[117,121] In the rat study reported above, in which the plasma levels of cGMP remained elevated despite administration of an NOS inhibitor, a marked increase in plasma levels of ANP was found.[118] ANP elevates smooth muscle cGMP[125,127] through stimulation of particulate or membrane guanylate cyclase, which is not affected by methylene blue,[120,121] and thereby produces vasodilation. ANP is released from the right atrium and might be the material responsible for the cGMP elevation that was seen in animal models of sepsis and humans with septicemia. Brigham's group has shown that cGMP levels were higher in the lung lymph than in the plasma, and higher in plasma from arterial than mixed venous blood, suggesting a thoracic origin for the second messenger.[128]

The Kallikrein–Kinin System

The kallikrein–kinin system, which includes several vasoactive substances, has been shown to be activated during endotoxemia in humans[129] and in sheep.[130] However, administration of a bradykinin antagonist did not change the cardiovascular or microvascular response to endotoxin in chronically instrumented sheep.[130] Therefore, activation of this mediator cascade seems rather to be an epiphenomenon of endotoxemia.

Changes in permeability

Endothelial Permeability

Endotoxemia increases microvascular permeability both in the systemic[131] and in the pulmonary circulation.[132] The lung is the organ most commonly compromised during processes that lead to systemic inflammation. Edema formation due to an increase in microvascular permeability is a hallmark of the acute lung injury. The factors that determine the transvascular fluid flux are summarized in the Starling–Landis equation:[133,134]

$$J_v = K_f[(P_{mv} - P_i) - \sigma(\pi_{mv} - \pi_i)]$$

where J_v is the transvascular fluid flux, K_f is the filtration coefficient (measure of the endothelial permeability to small solutes and water as well as of the permeability surface area), P_{mv} is the microvascular hydrostatic pressure, P_i is the interstitial hydrostatic pressure, σ is the osmotic reflection coefficient to protein, π_{mv} is the microvascular oncotic pressure, and π_i is the interstitial oncotic pressure.

A model has been developed in sheep that allows the determination of the variables included in the Starling equation. The lymph flow draining from the efferent vessel of the caudal mediastinal lymph node has been used as a measure of the transvascular fluid flux. Using this model, changes in lymph flow and lymph protein flux were evaluated during sepsis and endotoxemia. Again, the changes in pulmonary endothelial permeability can be divided into three phases.

Phase 1

Several investigators studied lymph flow and lymph protein flux after administration of bacteria or short-time infusion of 1–2 µg/kg of endotoxin in sheep. Two phases of permeability change could be distinguished in these models.[135] During phase 1 there was a high microvascular hydrostatic pressure as defined by the Gaar equation.[136] It was associated with an increase in lung lymph flow, while the lymph protein concentration was low. It was concluded that the high microvascular hydrostatic pressure was responsible for the early increase in transvascular fluid flux. As mentioned above, TXA$_2$ had been found to be responsible for the vasoconstriction occurring during phase 1 of the response to endotoxin. Therefore, it is not surprising that administration of the thromboxane synthetase inhibitor OKY046 prevented the rise in lymph flow during phase 1.[82] This effect was also noted after blockage of the cyclooxygenase by ibuprofen.[83] Early edema formation after burns at the site of the injury might be due to a different mechanism. Recent data suggest that a marked fall in interstitial hydrostatic pressure might occur in the injured tissue, which can explain the immediate onset of edema formation after thermal injury.[137,138] These changes might be the result of an inhibition of the fibroblast β$_1$-integrin attachment to collagen.

Phase 2

During phase 2 lymph flow continues to be high. However, the lymph protein concentration rises considerably[135] and the pulmonary artery pressure is only mildly elevated. The oncotic pressure gradient between microvasculature and interstitial space is reduced during that period.[139] Together these data suggest that the permeability of the pulmonary endothelium to protein increases in phase 2. In fact, the reflection coefficient for total protein fell from 0.73 to 0.58, with respective changes of the reflection coefficients for albumin (0.66 to 0.5), IgG (0.76 to 0.64), and IgM (0.91 to 0.83) after 4 hours of *Escherichia coli* sepsis in sheep.[140] Confirmation of this hypothesis is still pending in models of endotoxemia, but it has been generally accepted that the changes in pulmonary transvascular fluid flux in phase 2 represent changes in microvascular permeability. The mechanisms of the increased microvascular permeability are still under discussion.

Endothelial cells play an important role in the development of vascular permeability. It has been hypothesized that endothelial cells can contract upon stimulation.[141] As a result, the intercellular gaps might increase in number and/or size, establishing the so-called capillary leak syndrome. The development of the protein-rich high permeability edema can be ameliorated if substances are administered that raise the endothelial cell content of cyclic adenosine or guanosine monophosphate.[142,143] Endothelial cells do not merely serve as targets during systemic inflammation. They actively contribute to the ongoing inflammatory process. Their role in the inflammatory reaction has been estimated so highly that even the term 'endothelial inflammation' has been used to describe it. The endothelial cell can be stimulated by endotoxin, TNFα, or interleukin-1 to express E-selectin, an adhesion molecule.[144] E-selectin on the surface of endothelial cells interacts with the corresponding L-selectin complex on PMNs to facilitate rolling of these cells along the endothelium.[145] Moreover, endothelial cells secrete the proinflammatory cytokine IL-1,[146] which activates PMNs.

Conflicting data exist regarding the role of PMNs in SIRS. PMNs are usually found at the site of tissue injury, to which they migrate following a concentration gradient of chemotactic stimuli. Upon stimulation, PMNs roll along endothelial cells, and in a further step, after interaction of the PMN CD11/18 integrin with its ligand, the intercellular adhesion molecule (ICAM-1), the PMN can emigrate from the vessel into the interstitial space. Antibodies against the common CD18 β chain showed beneficial effects in an animal model of sepsis-induced lung injury.[147] On the other hand, patients who are deficient in CD18 have abundant PMNs in their alveolar spaces. In addition, the monoclonal antibody 60.3 was ineffective in completely blocking the migration of PMNs into the lung in a number of conditions.[148] We have recently reported that in chronic endotoxemia there were few PMNs in the lung but numerous macrophages.[149] Activated PMNs and macrophages secrete oxygen free radicals and proteases, which is part of their defense mechanism against bacteria. Administration of oxygen free radical scavengers and antiproteases proved to be useful in diminishing edema accumulation after endotoxin.[150,151] However, proteases and oxygen radicals are also released by macrophages, which are already present in the tissue and by monocytes that can immigrate. Animals were depleted of their granulocytes by anti-PMN antiserum[152] or by treatment with nitrogen mustard.[153] This did not prevent the changes in microvascular permeability following the administration of endotoxin. Moreover, patients deficient in PMNs would still develop the adult respiratory distress syndrome associated with sepsis.[154,155] On the other hand, treatment of sheep or goats with hydroxyurea, which is another compound used to deplete granulocytes, was effective and diminished the fluid accumulation in the lung.[156] However, urea scavenges free radicals that might explain its efficacy.[157] As the inflammatory response becomes chronic, many mediators have been released and more than one mechanism might be assumed to be responsible for the capillary leak.

Many studies were performed to evaluate the role of metabolites of the arachidonic acid for the increase in permeability. Administration of the thromboxane synthetase inhibitor OKY046 did not only reduce transvascular fluid flux in phase 1, but it was also effective in phase 2 after a bolus of endotoxin.[82] Nevertheless, this does not mean that TXA$_2$ itself had induced the increase in permeability. Indication has been reported that TXB$_2$, previously assumed to be an inactive metabolite of TXA$_2$, might cause lung damage.[158] Moreover, thromboxane synthetase blockage by OKY046 reduced the plasma-conjugated dienes, which are peroxidation products of oxygen free radicals.[82] Granulocyte chemiluminescence was elevated 4 hours after administration of 1.5 µg/kg of endotoxin to chronically instrumented sheep indicating the production of oxygen free radicals.[159] Oxygen free radicals can increase microvascular permeability both by activation of endothelial cell contraction[160] and by damaging the endothelial cell membrane. OKY046 has been demonstrated to reverse other forms of oxygen free radical induced lung injury.[161,162] On the other hand, inhibition of the cyclooxygenase did not affect transvascular fluid flux during phase 2, even if TXA$_2$ is a cyclooxygenase metabolite.[83] This discrepancy is still unexplained; however, prostacyclin is elevated after endotoxin administration and this material has many actions that counter the actions of thromboxane. Administration of a cyclooxygenase inhibitor will prevent the release of this salutary eicosanoid.

Microvascular damage during systemic inflammation might also be regarded as ischemia/reperfusion injury, particularly when it was preceded by a period of intestinal hypoperfusion. Xanthine oxidase-generated oxygen free radicals have been reported to mediate changes in microvascular and epithelial permeability.[163] Endotoxin-induced ileal and cecal permeability was associated with an increased xanthine oxidase activity and inhibition of xanthine oxidase by allopurinol has been shown to reduce intestinal mucosal damage.[164,165] Circulating xanthine oxidase after ischemia/reperfusion injury in rats was associated with pulmonary retention of PMNs and pulmonary capillary leak, which was diminished by pretreatment with allopurinol.[166] Intravenous injection of purified xanthine oxidase, however, induced pulmonary retention of PMNs without increasing microvascular permeability. Therefore, a final evaluation of the role of xanthine oxidase in ischemia/reperfusion induced permeability changes are not yet possible.

TNFα is one of the early mediators in systemic inflammation. It has been reported to be elevated during sepsis and endotoxemia, after hemorrhagic shock or thermal injury. It is considered as one of the most important mediators in the cascade because it has the potential to stimulate or enhance most of the steps in the inflammatory response. Moreover, administration of human recombinant TNFα reproduced most of the effects of endotoxemia, including the alterations in pulmonary microvascular permeability in the chronic sheep model.[167,168] However, it has been questioned whether the *ovine* response to human TNFα was only related to the cytokine,[79] because contamination of the recombinant material with endotoxin is not uncommon.

TNFα also induces the secretion of PAF, which is a further early mediator of the systemic inflammation. PAF causes an increase in lung lymph flow and permeability to protein when it is infused into conscious sheep.[169] Administration of a PAF antagonist abolished the cardiopulmonary response that occurs during phase 1 and attenuated it during phase 2.[170] However, PAF had no direct effect on endothelial cells.[169] This suggests that it probably increased microvascular permeability through other mechanisms such as its priming effect on PMNs.[171]

Phase 3

The hyperdynamic cardiovascular response is associated with profound changes in pulmonary transvascular fluid flux in the *ovine* model of continuous endotoxemia.[101,132] The lymph protein concentration gradually decreased after phase 2 and after 24 hours of endotoxemia the reflection coefficient to protein was at baseline level, while the lymph flow was still high. Microvascular hydrostatic pressure, evaluated by Holloway's technique, was not significantly different from baseline.[172] The elevated transvascular fluid flux was attributed to a high filtration coefficient. An increase both in perfused surface area and in pore numbers might have contributed to the change in filtration. Repeated injections of endotoxin also decreased subsequent lung lymph production in response to endotoxin.[173] These changes in lung lymph flow were associated with elevations in endothelin[97,172] and atrial natriuretic peptide. However, further studies must determine if these factors affect the pulmonary microvascular changes during the late phases of sepsis and multiple organ failure.

Increased Epithelial Permeability

Permeability changes during systemic inflammation are not restricted to the endothelium. Loss of epithelial barrier function has been noted both in the lung and in the intestine. Administration of 2–4 ng/kg endotoxin to healthy human volunteers increased their alveolar epithelial permeability to the inhaled 492 Da molecule [^{99m}Tc] diethylenetriamine pentacetate (DTPA) 3 hours after endotoxin had been given.[76] Human volunteers demonstrated a higher intestinal epithelial permeability to mannitol/lactulose.[174] Bacterial translocation occurred both during endotoxemia,[87] thermal injury,[84] and multiple trauma with hemorrhagic shock.[175] This might well be interpreted as a loss of intestinal barrier function. Nevertheless, one must bear in mind that epithelial permeability to

molecules like lactulose/mannitol and bacterial translocation do not necessarily relate to each other. The epithelium could also be injured by ischemia reperfusion that occurs in all of these situations.[176]

The hypercoagulatory response

Disseminated intravascular coagulation (DIC) is a serious complication of systemic inflammation. During hemorrhagic shock or sepsis, widespread activation of the coagulation systems as well as decreased fibrinolysis and levels of inhibitors of the contact and coagulation systems might all contribute to the development of DIC. DIC is due to local thrombosis of the microcirculation as opposed to microembolism. Endotoxin has been reported to play a decisive role in burn-induced coagulopathy.[177] Endothelial fibrin deposits could be demonstrated in the *ovine* lung ultrastructure *in vivo*, 6 hours after intravenous administration of a bolus of endotoxin. Endotoxin stimulates the production of an endothelium-dependent procoagulant tissue factor (thromboplastin).[178] Thromboplastin is a substrate both for the extrinsic (factor VII) and the intrinsic pathway (factor XII) of blood coagulation. Endotoxin can also damage endothelial cells directly or indirectly by mediators like TNFα, which are released in response to endotoxin. The damaged cells release tissue thromboplastin and, in addition, the exposed collagen can then further enhance activation of factor XII. Moreover, endotoxin induces endothelial cell secretion of a fast-acting inhibitor of the plasminogen activator[179] and it decreases the endothelial expression of thrombomodulin,[180] which plays an important role for the activation of the anticoagulatory protein C. In addition to its direct effects, endotoxin can influence the coagulation system by its induction of mediators like TNFα and IL-1. Both cytokines have been shown to exert procoagulant activity themselves.[146,181] The resultant principal mediator of coagulation through the different pathways is thrombin. Administration of thrombin induced intravascular coagulation *in vivo* (sheep and dogs).[182] Moreover, the coagulation cascade seems to interfere with endothelial permeability, because thrombin also increased the pulmonary microvascular permeability to protein.[184,184] So far, multiple coagulation factor abnormalities have already been documented both in septic patients[185] and in human volunteers treated with endotoxin.[186] The mechanisms by which the complex failure of the blood coagulation system is initiated are not yet completely understood.

The two-hit hypothesis

It has been known in cellular immunology for several years that monocytes and macrophages can undergo several steps during the activation process. For instance, the lymphokine γ-interferon might act as the first signal and prime macrophages. The cells respond with a number of changes, including an increase in the transcription rate of mRNA for TNFα. Nevertheless, no TNFα is produced. If a second stimulus like endotoxin is provided in even a small dose, the macrophages are triggered to become fully activated and to secrete large amounts of TNFα. The same effect can be induced if a very high dose of endotoxin is administered. Recently, several studies focused on organ injury by systemic inflammatory processes indicate that a phenomenon comparable to the cellular events described above can occur and involve the whole body.[187] Dehring *et al.* found a more persistent pulmonary hypertension and an exaggerated hyperdynamic response to bacteremia in sheep when a week-old thermal injury preceded the bacterial challenge.[188] In a rat model of intestinal ischemia–reperfusion injury and endotoxemia, lung albumin leak and mortality rate increased only if both injuries occurred.[189] Combined administration of low doses of endotoxin and TNFα to rats resulted in the similar hypotensive and metabolic effect as a highly lethal dose of either compound.[190] These findings are in keeping with the fact that multiple organ damage usually develops over a prolonged period of time during which several insults might occur. It also emphasizes why it is so important to prevent any subsequent ischemia or host response in general, particularly in patients in whom systemic inflammation is already present.

Summary

Burn injury, associated ischemia–reperfusion injury, the presence of necrotic tissue, or a septic episode might function as the initiating event of SIRS. The host response to this insult might be a localized inflammation or, if the stimulus surpasses a certain threshold, a systemic inflammatory response might occur. After a limited injury, the local tissue perfusion will increase and mediators released by macrophages and endothelial cells attract monocytes and polymorphonuclear neutrophils to the area. These cells, as well as the vascular endothelium, are stimulated to express adhesion molecules and their interaction enables the inflammatory cells to leave the vascular lumen and to enter the interstitial space. Once there, activated cells of the immune system will secrete proteolytic enzymes and oxygen radicals, phagocytize and digest bacteria and necrotic tissue, and thereby defend the organism. A side-effect of this reaction is that healthy tissue will be affected by the immune attack and will be damaged. As long as the inflammatory response is localized and feedback mechanisms are effective, tissue repair will follow tissue injury as recovery ensues. When the immune system becomes extensively activated and the inflammatory mechanisms escape local control, the whole body can seriously become involved in a systemic inflammatory response. A vicious circle might evolve in which the cytotoxicity of the immune cells might contribute to early organ dysfunction. Widespread increase in microvascular permeability will lead to interstitial edema and thereby impair oxygen diffusion to the tissue. Blood flow also becomes maldistributed due to a loss of vasoregulative function and as a result of widespread microthrombosis. Oxygenated blood does not reach the capillary bed. Moreover, oxygen utilization is impaired. The resultant hypoxic cell damage further promotes organ dysfunction. One important difference between localized and systemic inflammation is that the early dysfunction of the intestine might itself sustain the inflammatory reaction. Extensive studies have provided evidence that during a state of systemic inflammation the barrier properties of the intestine seem to fail. Similar changes might also occur in the airway barrier to bacteria. Subsequently, enternal bacteria traverse these barriers in a process called bacterial translocation. These bacteria can be cultured from the blood where they might act as potent stimuli for both the immune system and endothelial cells.

References

1. Bone RC, Balk RA, Cerra FB, et al. Definitions for sepsis and organ failure and guidelines for the use of innovative therapies in sepsis. The ACCP/SCCM Consensus Conference Committee. American College of Chest Physicians/Society of Critical Care Medicine. Chest 1992; 101: 1644–55.

2. Muckart D, Bhagwangee S. American College of Chest Physicians/Society of Critical Care Medicine Consensus Conference. Definitions of systemic inflammatory response syndrome and allied disorders in relation to critically injured patients. Crit Care Med 1997; 25: 1789–94.

3. Pittet D, Rangel-Frausto S, Li N, et al. Systemic inflammatory response syndrome, sepsis, severe sepsis and septic shock: incidence, morbidities and outcomes in surgical ICU patients. Intensive Care Med 1995; 21: 302–9.

4. Talmor M, Hydo L, Barie P. Relationship of systemic inflammatory response syndrome to organ dysfunction, length of stay and mortality in critical surgical illness. Arch Surg 1999; 134: 81–7.

5. Asayama K, Aikawa N. Evaluation of systemic inflammatory response syndrome criteria as a predictor of mortality in emergency patients transported by ambulance. Keio J Med 1998; 47: 19–27.

6. Rangel-Frausto M, Pittet D, Costigen M, Hwang T, Davis C, Wenzel R. The natural history of the systemic inflammatory response syndrome (SIRS): a prospective study. JAMA 1995; 273: 117–23.

7. Haga Y, Beppu T, Doi K, et al. Systemic inflammatory response syndrome and organ dysfunction following gastrointestinal surgery. Crit Care Med 1997; 25: 1994–2000.

8. Sheridan R, Ryan C, Yin L, Hurley J, Tompkins R. Death in the burn unit: sterile multiple organ failure. Burns 1998; 24: 307–11.

9. Gando S, Nanzaki S, Kemmotsu O. Disseminated intravascular coagulation and sustained systemic inflammatory syndrome predict organ dysfunctions after trauma: Application of clinical decision analysis. Ann Surg 1999; 229: 121–7.

10. Still J, Law E, Belcher K, Thiruvaiyaru D. A regional medical center's experience with burns of the elderly. J Burn Care Rehabil 1999; 20: 218–23.

11. Wolf S, Rose J, Desai M, Mileski J, Barrow R, Herndon D. Mortality determinants in massive pediatric burns. An analysis of 103 children with > or = 80% TBSA burns (> or = 70% full thickness). Ann Surg 1997; 225: 554–65.

12. Kelly J, O'Sullivan C, O'Riordain M, et al. Is circulating endotoxin the trigger for systemic inflammatory response syndrome seen after injury? Ann Surg 1997; 225: 530–43.

13. Spooner C, Markowitz N, Saravolatz L. The role of tumor necrosis factor in sepsis. Clin Immunol Immunopathol 1992; 62: S11–17.

14. Torre-Amione G, Bozkurt B, Deswal A, Mann D. An overview of tumor necrosis factor and the failing human heart. Curr Opin Cardiol 1999; 14: 206–10.

15. Voss M, Cotton M. Mechanisms and clinical implications of apoptosis. Hosp Med 1998; 59: 924–30.

16. Van der Poll T, van Deventer S. Cytokines and anticytokines in the pathogenesis of sepsis. Infect Dis Clin N Am 1999; 13: 403–26.

17. Tominaga K, Yoshimoto T, Torigoe K, et al. IL-1 synergizes with IL-18 or IL-1β for IFN-γ production from human T cells. Int Immunol 2000; 12: 151–60.

18. Heinzel F. The role IFN-γ in the pathology of experimental endotoxemia. J Immunol 1990; 145: 2920–4.

19. Doherty G, Lange J, Langstein H, et al. Evidence for IFN-γ as a mediator of lethality of endotoxin and tumor necrosis factor alpha. J Immunol 1992; 144: 1666–70.

20. Laffon M, Pittet J, Modelska K, Matthay M, Young D. Interleukin-8 mediates injury from smoke inhalation to both the lung endothelial and alveolar epithelial barriers in rabbits. Am J Respir Crit Care Med 1999; 160: 1443–9.

21. Stoiser B, Knapp S, Thalhammer F, et al. Time course of immunological markers in patients with the systemic inflammatory response syndrome: evaluation of sCD14, sVCAM-1, sELAM-1, MIP-1α and TGF-β2. Eur J Clin Invest 1998; 28: 672–78.

22. Christman J, Lancaster L, Blackwell T. Nuclear factor κB: A pivotal role in the systemic inflammatory response syndrome and a new target for therapy. Intensive Care Med 1998; 24: 1131–8.

23. Bohrer H, Qui F, Zimmerman T, et al. Role of NF-κB in the mortality of sepsis. J Clin Invest 1997; 100: 972–85.

24. Schwartz M, Moore E, Moore F, et al. Nuclear factor-kappaB is activated in alveolar macrophages from patients with adult respiratory distress syndrome. Crit Care Med 1996; 24: 1285–92.

25. Graham R, Stephens C, Silvester W, et al. Plasma degradation of platelet activating factor in severely ill patients with clinical sepsis. Crit Care Med 1994; 22: 204–12.

26. Quinn JV, Slotman GJ. Platelet-activating factor and arachidonic acid metabolites mediate tumor necrosis factor and eicosanoid kinetics and cardiopulmonary dysfunction during bacteremic shock. Crit Care Med 1999; 27(11): 2485–94.

27. Heller A, Koch T, Schmeck J, van Ackern K. Lipid mediators in inflammatory disorders. Drugs 1998; 55(4): 487–96.

28. Czermak BJ, Sarma V, Pierson CL, et al. Protective effects of C5a blockade in sepsis. Nature Med 1999; 5(7): 788–92.

29. Martin C, Boisson C, Haccoun M, Thomachot L, Mege J. Patterns of cytokine evolution (tumor necrosis factor-α and interleukin-6) after septic shock, hemorrhagic shock, and severe trauma. *Crit Care Med* 1997; **25**: 1813–19.

30. Cannon J, Friedberg J, Gelfand J, Tompkins R, Burke J, Dinarello C. Circulating interleukin-1β and tumor necrosis factor-α concentrations after burn injury in humans. *Crit Care Med* 1992; **20**: 1414–19.

31. Vindenes H, Ulvestad E, Bjerknes R. Concentrations of cytokines in plasma of patients with large burns: their relation to time after injury, burn size, inflammatory variables, infection and outcome. *Eur J Surg* 1998; **164**: 647–56.

32. Drost A, Burleson D, Cioffi W, Jordan B, Mason A, Pruitt B. Plasma cytokines following thermal injury and their relationship with mortality, burn size and time postburn. *J Trauma* 1993; **35**: 335–9.

33. Zhang B, Huang Y, Chen Y, Yang Y, Hao Z, Xie S. Plasma tumor necrosis factor-α, its soluble receptors and interleukin-1β levels in critically burned patients. *Burns* 1998; **24**: 599–603.

34. Marano M, Fong Y, Moldawer L, et al. Serum cachectin/tumor necrosis factor in critically ill patients with burns correlates with infection and mortality. *Surg Gynecol Obstet* 1990; **170**: 32–8.

35. Hubl W, Wolfbauer G, Streicher J, et al. Differential expression of tumor necrosis factor receptor subtypes on leukocytes in systemic inflammatory response syndrome. *Crit Care Med* 1999; **27**: 319–24.

36. Presterl E, Staudinger T, Pettermann M, et al. Cytokine profile and correlation to APACHE III and MPM II scores in patients with sepsis. *Am J Resp Crit Care Med* 1997; **156**: 825–32.

37. Mandrup-Poulsen T, Wogensen L, Jensen M, et al. Circulating interleukin-1 receptor antagonist concentrations are increased in adult patients with thermal injury. *Crit Care Med* 1995; **23**: 26–33.

38. Neely A, Hoover D, Holder I, Cross A. Circulating levels of tumor necrosis factor, interleukin-6 and proteolytic activity in a murine model of burn and infection. *Burns* 1996; **7**: 524–30.

39. Aosasa S, Ono S, Mochizuki H, et al. Activation of monocytes and endothelial cells depends on the severity of surgical stress. *World J Surg* 2000; **24**: 10–16.

40. Taniguchi T, Koido Y, Aiboshi J, Yamashita T, Suzaki S, Kurokawa A. Change in the ratio of interleukin-6 to interleukin-10 predicts a poor outcome in patients with systemic inflammatory response syndrome. *Crit Care Med* 1999; **27**: 1262–4.

41. Braithwaite S. Procalcitonin: new insights on regulation and origin. *Crit Care Med* 2000; **28(2)**: 586–8.

42. Nijsten MW, Olinga P, The TH, et al. Procalcitonin behaves as a fast responding acute phase protein *in vivo* and *in vitro*. *Crit Care Med* 2000; **28(2)**: 458–61.

43. Brunkhorst FM, Eberhard OK, Brunkhorst R. Discrimination of infectious and noninfectious causes of early acute respiratory distress syndrome by procalcitonin. *Crit Care Med* 1999; **27(10)**: 2172–6.

44. Miller P, Munn D, Meridith JW, Chang MC. Systemic inflammatory response syndrome in the trauma intensive care unit: who is infected? *J Trauma* 1999; **47(6)**: 1004–8.

45. Clyne B, Olshaker JS. The C-reactive protein. *J Emerg Med* 1999; **17(6)**: 1019–25.

46. Abraham E, Anzueto A, Gutierrez G, et al. Double-blind randomized controlled trial of monoclonal antibody to human tumor necrosis factor in treatment of septic shock. *Lancet* 1998; **351**: 929–33.

47. Abraham E, Wunderlink R, Silverman H, et al. Efficacy and safety of monoclonal antibody to human tumor necrosis factor alpha in patients with sepsis syndrome: a randomized, controlled, double-blind, multicenter trial. TNF-alpha Mab sepsis study group. *JAMA* 1995; **273**: 934–41.

48. Cohen J, Carlet J. INTERSEPT: An international, multicenter, placebo-controlled trial of monoclonal antibody to human tumor necrosis factor-alpha in patients with sepsis. International sepsis trial study group. *Crit Care Med* 1996; **24**: 1431–40.

49. Dhainaut J, Vincent J, Richard C, et al. CPD571, a humanized antibody to human tumor necrosis factor-alpha: safety, pharmacokinetics, immune response, and the influence of the antibody on cytokine concentrations in patients with septic shock. CPD571 Sepsis Study Group. *Crit Care Med* 1995; **23**: 1461–9.

50. Fisher C, Opal S, Dhainaut J, et al. Influence of an anti-tumor necrosis factor monoclonal antibody on cytokine levels in patients with sepsis. The CB0006 Sepsis Syndrome Study Group. *Crit Care Med* 1993; **21**: 318–27.

51. Rheinhart K, Wiegand-Lohnert C, Grimminger F, et al. Assessment of the safety and efficacy of the monoclonal anti-tumor necrosis factor antibody-fragment, MAK 195F, in patients with sepsis and septic shock: a multicenter, randomized, placebo-controlled, dose-ranging study. *Crit Care Med* 1996; **24**: 733–42.

52. Clark M, Plank L, Connolly A, et al. Effect of a chimeric antibody to tumor necrosis factor-alpha on cytokine and physiologic responses in patients with severe sepsis: a randomized clinical trial. *Crit Care Med* 1998; **17**: 36–8.

53. Abraham E, Glauser M, Butler T, et al. P55 tumor necrosis factor receptor fusion protein in the treatment of patients with severe sepsis and septic shock. Ro45-2081 study group. *JAMA* 1997; **277**: 1531–8.

54. Fisher C, Agosti J, Opal S, et al. Treatment of septic shock with the tumor necrosis factor receptor:Fc fusion protein. *N Engl J Med* 1977; **334**: 1697–702.

55. Fisher C, Dhainaut J, Opal S, et al. Recombinant human interleukin-1 receptor antagonist in the treatment of patients with sepsis syndrome. Phase III rhIL-1ra sepsis syndrome study group. *JAMA* 1994; **271**: 1836–43.

56. Fisher C, Slotman G, Opal S, et al. Initial evaluation of human recombinant interleukin-1 receptor antagonist in the treatment of sepsis syndrome: a randomized, open-label, placebo-controlled, multicenter trial. *Crit Care Med* 1994; **22**: 12–21.

57. Opal S, Fisher C, Dhainaut F. Confirmatory interleukin-1 receptor antagonist trial in severe sepsis: a phase III, randomized, double-blind, placebo-controlled, multicenter trial. *Crit Care Med* 1997; **25**: 1115–24.

58. Fein A, Bernard G, Criner G, et al. Treatment of severe systemic inflammatory response syndrome and sepsis with a novel bradykinin antagonist, deltibant (CP-0127): results of a randomized, double-blind, placebo-controlled trial. CP-0127 SIRS and sepsis study group. *JAMA* 1997; **277**: 482–7.

59. Dhainaut J, Tenaillon A, Hemmer M, et al. Confirmatory platelet-activating factor receptor antagonist trial in patients with severe gram-negative bacterial sepsis: a phase III, randomized, double-blind, placebo-controlled, multicenter trial. *Crit Care Med* 1998; **26**: 1963–71.

60. Dhainaut J, Tenaillon A, Le Tulzo Y, et al. Platelet activating factor receptor antagonist BN 52021 in the treatment of severe sepsis. A randomized, double-blind, placebo-controlled, multicenter clinical trial. *Crit Care Med* 1994; **22**: 1720–8.

61. Bernard G, Wheeler A, Russell J, et al. The effects of ibuprofen on the physiology and survival of patients with sepsis. The ibuprofen in sepsis study group. *N Engl J Med* 1997; **336**: 912–18.

62. Haupt M, Jastremski M, Clemmer T, et al. Effect of ibuprofen in patients with severe sepsis: a randomized, double-blind, multicenter trial. *Crit Care Med* 1991; **19**: 1339–47.

63. Sander A, Armbruster W, Sander B, Daul AE, Lange R, Peters J. Hemofiltration increases IL-6 clearance in early systemic inflammatory response syndrome but does not alter IL-6 and TNF alpha plasma concentrations. *Intensive Care Med* 1997; **23(8)**: 878–84.

64. Braun N, Rosenfeld S, Giolai M, et al. Effect of continuous hemodiafiltration on IL-6, TNF-alpha, C3a, and TCC in patients with SIRS/septic shock using two different membranes. *Contrib Nephrol* 1995; **116**: 89–98.

65. Kellum JA, Johnson JP, Kramer D, Palevsky P, Brady JJ, Pinsky MR. Diffusive vs. convective therapy: effects on mediators of inflammation in patient with severe systemic inflammatory response syndrome. *Crit Care Med* 1998; **26(12)**: 1995–2000.

66. Cronin L, Cook DJ, Carlet J, et al. Corticosteroid treatment for sepsis: a critical appraisal and meta-analysis of the literature. *Crit Care Med* 1995; **23(8)**: 1430–9.

67. Lefering R, Neugebauer EA. Steroid controversy in sepsis and septic shock: a meta-analysis. *Crit Care Med* 1995; **23(7)**: 1294–303.

68. Zeni F, Freeman B, Natanson C. Anti-inflammatory therapies to treat sepsis and septic shock: a reassessment. *Crit Care Med* 1997; **25(7)**: 1095–100.

69. Wang H, Bloom O, Zhang M, et al. HMG-1 as a late mediator of endotoxin lethality in mice. *Science* 1999; **285**: 248–51.

70. Junger WG, Coimbra R, Liu FC, et al. Hypertonic saline resuscitation: a tool to modulate immune function in trauma patients? *Shock* 1997; **8(4)**: 235–41.

71. Junger WG, Hoyt DB, Hamreus M, et al. Hypertonic saline activates protein tyrosine kinases and mitogen-activated protein kinase p38 in T-cells. *J Trauma* 1997; **42(3)**: 437–43.

72. Junger WG, Liu FC, Loomis WH, Hoyt DB. Hypertonic saline enhances cellular immune function. *Circ Shock* 1994; **42(4)**: 190–6.

73. Beale RJ, Bryg DJ, Bihari DJ. Immunonutrition in the critically ill: a systematic review of clinical outcome. *Crit Care Med* 1999; **27(12)**: 2799–805.

74. Napolitano LM, Faist E, Wichmann MW, Coimbra R. Immune dysfunction in trauma. *Surg Clin N Am* 1999; **79(6)**: 1385–416.

75. Suffredini AF, Fromm RE, Parker MM, et al. The cardiovascular response of normal humans to the administration of endotoxin. *N Engl J Med* 1989; **321**: 280–7.

76. Suffredini AF, Shelhamer JH, Neumann RD, Brenner M, Baltaro RJ, Parrillo JE. Pulmonary and oxygen transport effects of intravenously administered endotoxin in normal humans. *Am Rev Respir Dis* 1992; **145**: 1398–403.

77. Traber DL, Redl H, Schlag G, et al. Cardiopulmonary responses to continuous administration of endotoxin. *Am J Physiol* 1988; **254**: H833–9.

78. Dehring D, Lingnau W, McGuire R, Traber LD, Traber DL. L-NAME transiently reverses hyperdynamic status during continuous infusion of *Pseudomonas aeroginosa*. *Circ Shock* 1993; **39**: 49.

79. Traber DL. Models of endotoxemia in sheep. In: Schlag G, Redl H, Traber DL, eds.

Pathophysiology of Shock Sepsis and Organ Failure. New York: Springer Verlag, 1993: 194–9.

80. Godsoe A, Kimura R, Herndon D, et al. Cardiopulmonary changes with intermittent endotoxin administration in sheep. *Circ Shock* 1988; **25**: 61–74.

81. Meyer J, Traber LD, Nelson S, et al. Reversal of hyperdynamic response to continuous endotoxin administration by inhibition of NO synthesis. *J Appl Physiol* 1992; **73**: 324–28.

82. Fujioka K, Sugi K, Isago T, et al. Thromboxane synthase inhibition and cardiopulmonary function during endotoxemia in sheep. *J Appl Physiol* 1991; **71**: 1376–81.

83. Adams TJ, Traber DL. The effects of a prostaglandin synthetase inhibitor, ibuprofen, on the cardiopulmonary response to endotoxin in sheep. *Circ Shock* 1982; **9**: 481–9.

84. Tokyay R, Loick HM, Traber DL, Heggers JP, Herndon DN. Effects of thromboxane synthetase inhibition on postburn mesenteric vascular resistance and the rate of bacterial translocation in a chronic porcine model. *Surg Gynecol Obstet* 1992; **174**: 125–32.

85. Redl G, Abdi S, Nichols RJ, et al. The effects of a selective thromboxane synthetase inhibitor on the response of the right heart to endotoxin in sheep. *Crit Care Med* 1991; **19**: 1294–302.

86. Redl G, Newald J, Schlag G, Traber LD, Traber DL. Cardiac function in an ovine model of endotoxemia. *Circ Shock* 1991; **35**: 31–6.

87. Navaratnam RL, Morris SE, Traber DL, et al. Endotoxin (LPS) increases mesenteric vascular resistance (MVR) and bacterial translocation (BT). *J Trauma* 1990; **30**: 1104–13.

88. Lefer AM. Interaction between myocardial depressant factor and vasoactive mediators with ischemia and shock. *Am J Physiol* 1987; **252**: R193–R205.

89. Morris SE, Navaratnam N, Herndon DN. A comparison of effects of thermal injury and smoke inhalation on bacterial translocation. *J Trauma* 1990; **30**: 639–43.

90. Schlag G, Redl H, Davies J, Dinges HP, Radmore K. Aspects of the mechanisms of bacterial translocation in a hypovolemic-traumatic shock mode in baboons. *Circ Shock* 1991; **34**: 26–7.

91. Xu D, Qi L, Guillory D, Cruz N, Berg R, Deitch EA. Mechanisms of endotoxin-induced intestinal injury in a hyperdynamic model of sepsis. *J Trauma* 1993; **34**: 676–82.

92. Koltai M, Hosford D, Braquet PG. Platelet-activating factor in septic shock. *New Horizons* 1993; **1**: 87–95.

93. Traber DL. Endotoxin: the causative factor of mediator release during sepsis. In: Schlag G, Redl H, eds. *Progress in Clinical and Biological Research.* New York: Alan R. Liss, 1987: 377–92.

94. Sloane PJ, Elsasser TH, Spath JA, Albertine KH, Gee MH. Plasma tumor necrosis factor-alpha during long-term endotoxemia in awake sheep. *J Appl Physiol* 1992; **73**: 1831–7.

95. Martich GD, Danner RL, Ceska M, Suffredini AF. Detection of interleukin 8 and tumor necrosis factor in normal humans after intravenous endotoxin: the effect of antiinflammatory agents. *J Exp Med* 1991; **173**: 1021–4.

96. Michie HR, Manogue KR, Spriggs DR, et al. Detection of circulating tumor necrosis factor after endotoxin administration. *N Engl J Med* 1988; **318**: 1481–6.

97. Morel DR, Pittet JF, Gunning K, Hemsen A, Lacroix JS, Lundberg JM. Time course of plasma and pulmonary lymph endothelin-like immunoreactivity during sustained endotoxaemia in chronically instrumented sheep. *Clin Sci* 1991; **81**: 357–65.

98. Redl G, Woodson L, Traber LD, et al. Mechanism of immunoreactive atrial natriuretic factor release in an ovine model of endotoxemia. *Circ Shock* 1992; **38**: 34–41.

99. Lübbesmeyer HJ, Woodson L, Traber LD, Flynn JT, Herndon DN, Traber DL. Immunoreactive atrial natriuretic factor is increased in ovine model of endotoxemia. *Am J Physiol* 1988; **254**: R567–71.

100. Pittet JF, Morel DR, Hemsen A, et al. Elevated plasma endothelin-1 concentrations are associated with the severity of illness in patients with sepsis. *Ann Surg* 1991; **213**: 261–4.

101. Morel DR, Lacroix JS, Hemsen A, Steinig DA, Pittet JF, Lundberg JM. Increased plasma and pulmonary lymph levels of endothelin during endotoxin shock. *Eur J Pharmacol* 1989; **167**: 427–8.

102. Nelson S, Stewart RH, Traber L, Traber D. Endotoxin-induced alterations in contractility of isolated blood vessels from sheep. *Am J Physiol* 1991; **260**: H1790–94.

103. Theissen JL, Loick HM, Curry BB, Traber LD, Herndon DN, Traber DL. Time course of hypoxic pulmonary vasoconstriction after endotoxin infusion in unanesthetized sheep. *J Appl Physiol* 1991; **70**: 2120–5.

104. Meyer J, Lentz CW, Stothert JC, Traber LD, Herndon DN, Traber DL. Effects of nitric oxide synthesis inhibition in hyperdynamic endotoxemia. *Crit Care Med* 1993; **22**: 306–12.

105. Sugi K, Newald J, Traber LD, et al. Cardiac dysfunction after acute endotoxin administration in conscious sheep. *Am J Physiol* 1991; **260**: H1474–81.

106. Noshima S, Noda H, Herndon DN, Traber LD, Traber DL. Left ventricular performance during continuous endotoxin-induced hyperdynamic endotoxemia in sheep. *J Appl Physiol* 1993; **74**: 1528–33.

107. Myers PR, Wright TF, Tanner MA, Adams HR. EDRF and nitric oxide production in cultured endothelial cells: direct inhibition by E. coli endotoxin. *Am J Physiol* 1992; **262**: H710–18.

108. Vallance P, Moncada S. Role of endogenous nitric oxide in septic shock. *New Horizons* 1993; **1**: 77–86.

109. Sakai N, Milstien S. Availability of tetrahydrobiopterin is not a factor in the inability to detect nitric oxide production by human macrophages. *Biochem Biophys Res Commun* 1993; **193**: 378–83.

110. Schneemann M, Schoedon G, Hofer S, Blau N, Guerrero L, Schaffner A. Nitric oxide synthase is not a constituent of the antimicrobial armature of human mononuclear phagocytes. *J Infect Dis* 1993; **167**: 1358–63.

111. Moncada S. The first Robert Furchgott lecture: from endothelium-dependent relaxation to the L-arginine:NO pathway. *Blood Vessels* 1991; **27**: 208–17.

112. Furchgott RF. The 1989 Ulf von Euler lecture. Studies on endothelium-dependent vasodilation and the endothelium-derived relaxing factor. *Acta Physiol Scand* 1991; **139**: 257–70.

113. Petros A, Bennett D, Vallance P. Effect of nitric oxide synthase inhibitors on hypotension in patients with septic shock. *Lancet* 1991; **338**: 1557–8.

114. Geroulanos S, Schilling J, Cakmakci M, Jung HH, Largiader F. Inhibition of NO synthesis in septic shock. *Lancet* 1992; **339**: 435.

115. Shi Y, Li H-Q, Shen C-K, et al. Plasma nitric oxide levels in newborn infants with sepsis. *J Pediatr* 1993; **123**: 435–8.

116. Ochoa JB, Udekwu AO, Billiar TR, et al. Nitrogen oxide levels in patients after trauma and during sepsis. *Ann Surg* 1991; **214**: 621–6.

117. Schneider F, Lutun P, Couchot A, Bilbault P, Tempe JD. Plasma cyclic guanosine 3′–5′ monophosphate concentrations and low vascular resistance in human septic shock. *Intensive Care Med* 1993; **19**: 99–104.

118. Schuller F, Fleming I, Stoclet JC, Gray GA. Effect of endotoxin on circulating cyclic GMP in the rat. *Eur J Pharmacol* 1992; **212**: 93–6.

119. Nelson SH, Dehring DJ, Erhardt JS, Traber L, Traber D. Regional variation in content of c-GMP and associated vascular reactivity in bacteremia. *Circ Shock* 1993; **39**: 54.

120. Martin W, White DG, Henderson AH. Endothelium-derived relaxing factor and atriopeptin II elevate cyclic GMP levels in pig aortic endothelial cells. *Br J Pharmacol* 1988; **93**: 229–39.

121. Cherner JA, Singh G, Naik L. Atrial natriuretic factor activates membrane-bound guanylate cyclase of chief cells. *Life Sci* 1990; **47**: 669–77.

122. Goy MF. Activation of membrane guanylate cyclase by an invertebrate peptide hormone. *J Biol Chem* 1990; **265**: 20220–7.

123. Boulanger C, Schini VB, Moncada S, Vanhoutte PM. Stimulation of cyclic GMP production in cultured endothelial cells of the pig by bradykinin, adenosine diphosphate, calcium ionophore A23187 and nitric oxide. *Br J Pharmacol* 1990; **101**: 152–6.

124. Mitaka C, Nagura T, Sakanishi N, Tsunoda Y, Toyooka H. Plasma alpha-atrial natriuretic peptide concentrations in acute respiratory failure associated with sepsis: preliminary study. *Crit Care Med* 1990; **18**: 1201–3.

125. Leitman DC, Agnost VL, Catalano RM, et al. Atrial natriuretic peptide, oxytocin, and vasopressin increase guanosine 3′,5′-monophosphate in LLC-PK1 kidney epithelial cells. *Endocrinology* 1988; **122**: 1478–85.

126. Gerzer R, Heim JM, Schutte B, Weil J. Cellular mechanisms of action of atrial natriuretic factor. *Klin Wochenschr* 1987; **65 (Suppl 8)**: 109–14.

127. Garbers DL. The guanylyl cyclase receptor family. *New Biol* 1990; **2**: 499–504.

128. Snapper JR, Brigham KL, Heflin AC, Bomboy JDJ, Graber SE. Effects of endotoxemia on cyclic nucleotides in the unanesthetized sheep. *J Lab Clin Med* 1983; **102**: 240–9.

129. DeLa Cadena RA, Suffredini AF, Page JD, et al. Activation of the kallikrein-kinin system after endotoxin administration to normal human volunteers. *Blood* 1993; **81**: 3313–17.

130. Mann R, Woodson LC, Traber LD, Herndon DN, Traber DL. Role of bradykinin in ovine endotoxemia. *Circ Shock* 1991; **34**: 224–30.

131. Matsuda T, Eccleston CA, Rubinstein I, Rennard SI, Joyner WL. Antioxidants attenuate endotoxin-induced microvascular leakage of macromolecules *in vivo*. *Am J Physiol* 1991; **70**: 1483–9.

132. Nakazawa H, Noda H, Noshima S, et al. Pulmonary transvascular fluid flux and cardiovascular function in sheep with chronic sepsis. *J Appl Physiol* 1993; **75**: 2521–8.

133. Landis EM, Pappenheimer JR. Exchange of substances through the capillary walls. In: Hamilton WF, Dow P, eds. *Handbook of Physiology*, Section 2, Vol. 2. Baltimore, MD: Williams & Wilkins, 1963: 961–1034.

134. Starling EH. On the absorption of fluids from the connective tissue spaces. *J Physiol (Lond)* 1896; **19**: 312–26.

135. Brigham KL, Bowers R, Haynes J. Increased sheep lung vascular permeability caused by *Escherichia coli* endotoxin. *Circ Res* 1979; **45**: 292–7.

136. Gaar KA, Taylor AE, Owens LJ, Guyton AC. Effect of capillary pressure and plasma protein on development of pulmonary edema. *Am J Physiol* 1967; **213**: 79–82.

137. Lund T, Wiig H, Reed RK, Aukland K. A 'new' mechanism for oedema generation: strongly negative interstitial fluid pressure causes rapid fluid flow into thermally injured skin. *Acta Physiol Scand* 1987; **129**: 433–5.

138. Lund T, Wiig H, Reed RK. Acute postburn edema: role of strongly negative interstitial fluid pressure. *Am J Physiol* 1988; **255**: H1069–74.

139. Traber DL, Herndon DN, Fujioka K, Traber LD. Permeability changes during experimental endotoxemia and sepsis. In: Schlag G, Redl H, Siegel JH, Traber DL, eds. *Shock, Sepsis, and Organ Failure: Second Wiggers Bernard conference*, New York: Springer-Verlag, 1991: 425–47.

140. Smith L, Andreasson S, Thoren Tolling K, Rippe B, Risberg B. Sepsis in sheep reduces pulmonary microvascular sieving capacity. *J Appl Physiol* 1987; **62**: 1422–9.

141. Oliver JA. Endothelium-derived relaxing factor contributes to the regulation of endothelial permeability. *J Cell Physiol* 1992; **151**: 506–11.

142. Farrukh IS, Gurtner GH, Michael JR. Pharmacological modification of pulmonary vascular injury: possible role of cAMP. *J Appl Physiol* 1987; **62**: 47–54.

143. Kurose I, Kubes P, Wolf R, et al. Inhibition of nitric oxide production. Mechanisms of vascular albumin leakage. *Circ Res* 1993; **73**: 164–71.

144. Leeuwenberg FM, Jeunhomme TMA, Buurman WA. Induction of an activation antigen on human endothelial cells *in vitro*. *Eur J Immunol* 1989; **19**: 715–20.

145. Lasky LA. Selectins: interpreters of cell-specific carbohydrate information during inflammation. *Science* 1992; **258**: 964–9.

146. Nawroth PP, Stern DM. Modulation of endothelial cell hemostatic properties by tumor necrosis factor. *J Exp Med* 1986; **163**: 740–5.

147. Walsh CJ, Carey D, Cook DJ, Bechard DE, Fowler AA, Sugerman HJ. Anti-CD18 antibody attenuates neutropenia and alveolar capillary-membrane injury during gram-negative sepsis. *Surgery* 1991; **110**: 205–12.

148. Doerschuk CM, Winn RK, Coxson HO, Harlan JM. CD18-dependent and -independent mechanisms of neutrophil emigration in the pulmonary and systemic microcirculation of rabbits. *J Immunol* 1990; **144**: 2327–33.

149. Wang CZ, Herndon DN, Traber LD, et al. Pulmonary inflammatory cell response to sustained endotoxin administration. *J Appl Physiol* 1993 (in press)

150. Traber DL. Anti-proteases in endotoxemia. In: Schlag G, Redl H, eds. *Progress in Clinical and Biological Research*. New York: Alan R. Liss, 1987: 149–57.

151. Seekamp A, LaLonde C, Zhu DG, Demling R. Catalase prevents prostanoid release and lung lipid peroxidation after endotoxemia in sheep. *J Appl Physiol* 1988; **65**: 1210–16.

152. Basadre JO, Singh H, Herndon DN, et al. Effect of antibody-mediated neutropenia on the cardiopulmonary response to endotoxemia. *J Surg Res* 1988; **45**: 266–75.

153. Winn R, Maunder R, Chi E, Harlan J. Neutrophil depletion does not prevent lung edema after endotoxin infusion in goats. *J Appl Physiol* 1987; **62**: 116–21.

154. Maunder RJ, Hackman RC, Riff E, Albert RK, Springmeyer SC, Occurrence of the adult respiratory distress syndrome in neutropenic patients. *Am Rev Respir Dis* 1986; **133**: 313–16.

155. Laufe MD, Simon RH, Flint A, Keller JB. Adult respiratory distress syndrome in neutropenic patients. *Am J Med* 1986; **80**: 1022–6.

156. Heflin ACJ, Brigham KL. Prevention by granulocyte depletion of increased vascular permeability of sheep lung following endotoxemia. *J Clin Invest* 1981; **68**: 1253–60.

157. Klausner JM, Paterson IS, Goldman G, et al. Interleukin-2-induced lung injury is mediated by oxygen free radicals. *Surgery* 1991; **109**: 169–75.

158. Goldman G, Welbourn R, Klausner JM, Valeri CR, Shepro D, Hechtman HB. Thromboxane mediates diapedesis after ischemia by activation of neutrophil adhesion receptors interacting with basally expressed intercellular adhesion molecule-1. *Circ Res* 1991; **68**: 1013–19.

159. Traber DL, Schlag G, Redl H, Strohmair W, Traber LD. Pulmonary microvascular changes during hyperdynamic sepsis in an ovine model. *Circ Shock* 1987; **22**: 185–93.

160. Miller FN, Sims DE. Contractile elements in the regulation of macromolecular permeability. *Fed Proc* 1986; **45**: 84–8.

161. Paterson IS, Klausner JM, Goldman G, et al. Thromboxane mediates the ischemia-induced neutrophil oxidative burst. *Surgery* 1989; **106**: 224–9.

162. Turker RK, Aksulu HE, Ercan ZS, Aslan S. Thromboxane A2 inhibitors and iloprost prevent angiotensin II-induced oedema in the isolated perfused rat lung. *Arch Int Pharmacodyn Ther* 1987; **287**: 323–9.

163. Deitch EA, Taylor M, Grisham M, Ma L, Bridges W, Berg R. Endotoxin induces bacterial translocation, and increases xanthine oxidase activity. *J Trauma* 1989; **29**: 1679–83.

164. Deitch EA, Ma L, Ma WJ, et al. Inhibition of endotoxin-induced bacterial translocation, in mice. *J Clin Invest* 1989; **84**: 36–42.

165. Deitch EA, Specian RD, Berg RD. Endotoxin-induced bacterial translocation and mucosal permeability: role of xanthine oxidase, complement activation, and macrophage products. *Crit Care Med* 1991; **19**: 785–91.

166. Terada LS, Dormish JJ, Shanley PF, Leff JA, Anderson BO, Repine JE. Circulating xanthine oxidase mediates lung neutrophil sequestration after intestinal ischemia-reperfusion. *Am J Physiol* 1992; **263**: L394–L401.

167. Redl H, Schlag G, Lamche H. TNF- and LPS-induced changes of lung vascular permeability: studies in unanesthetised sheep. *Circ Shock* 1990; **31**: 183–92.

168. Johnson J, Meyrick B, Jesmok G, Brigham KL. Human recombinant tumor necrosis factor alpha infusion mimics endotoxemia in awake sheep. *J Appl Physiol* 1989; **66**: 1448–54.

169. Burhop KE, Garcia JG, Selig WM, et al. Platelet-activating factor increases lung vascular permeability to protein. *J Appl Physiol* 1986; **61**: 2210–17.

170. Sessler CN, Glauser FL, Davis D, Fowler AA. Effects of platelet-activating factor antagonist SRI 63–441 on endotoxemia in sheep. *J Appl Physiol* 1988; **65**: 2624–631.

171. Vercellotti GM, Yin HQ, Gustavson KS, Nelson RD, Jacob HS. Platelet activating factor primes neutrophil responses to agonists: role in promoting neutrophil-mediated endothelial damage. *Blood* 1988; **71**: 1100–7.

172. Holloway H, Perry M, Downey J, Parker J, Taylor A. Estimation of effective pulmonary capillary pressure in intact lungs. *J Appl Physiol* 1983; **54(3)**: 846–51.

173. Mann R, Traber LD, Herndon DN, Traber DL. Prior infusion of endotoxin dininishes the pulmonary response to bolus administration of lipopolysaccharide (LPS). *Int J Radiat Oncol Biol Phys* 1988; **20**: 138.

174. O'Dwyer ST, Michie HR, Ziegler TR, Revhaug A, Smith RJ, Wilmore DW. A single dose of endotoxin increases intestinal permeability in healthy humans. *Arch Surg* 1988; **123**: 1459–64.

175. Roumen RM, Hendriks T, Wevers RA, Goris JA. Intestinal permeability after severe trauma and hemorrhagic shock is increased without relation to septic complications. *Arch Surg* 1993; **128**: 453–7.

176. Zeigler ST, Traber DL, Herndon DN. Bacterial translocation in burns. In: Schlag G, Redl H, eds. *Pathophysiology of Shock, Sepsis, and Organ Failure*. New York: Springer-Verlag, 1993: 300–13.

177. Schlag G, Redl H, Hallstrom S. The cell in shock: the origin of multiple organ failure. *Resuscitation* 1991; **21**: 137–80.

178. Schorer AE, Rick PD, Swaim WR, Moldow CF. Structural features of endotoxin required for stimulation of endothelial cell tissue factor production. Exposure of preformed tissue factor after oxidant-mediated endothelial cell injury. *J Lab Clin Med* 1985; **106**: 38–42.

179. Colluci M, Paramo JA, Collen D. Generation in plasma of a fast-acting inhibitor of plasminogen activator in response to endotoxin stimulation. *J Clin Invest* 1985; **75**: 818–24.

180. Moore KL, Andreoli SP, Esmon NL, Esmon CT, Bang NU. Endotoxin enhances tissue factor and suppresses thrombomodulin expression of human vascular endothelium *in vitro*. *J Clin Invest* 1987; **79**: 124–30.

181. Beutler B, Cerami A. Cachectin: more than a tumor necrosis factor. *N Engl J Med* 1987; **316**: 379–85.

182. Malik AB, Horgan MJ. Mechanisms of thrombin-induced lung vascular injury and edema. *Am Rev Respir Dis* 1987; **136**: 467–70.

183. Lo SK, Perlman MB, Niehaus GD, Malik AB. Thrombin-induced alterations in lung fluid balance in awake sheep. *J Appl Physiol* 1985; **58**: 1421–7.

184. Malik AB, Lo SK, Bizios R. Thrombin-induced alterations in endothelial permeability. *Ann NY Acad Sci* 1986; **485**: 293–309.

185. Bone RC. Modulators of coagulation. A critical appraisal of their role in sepsis. *Arch Intern Med* 1992; **152**: 1381–9.

186. Martich GD, Boujoukos AJ, Suffredini AF. Response of man to endotoxin. *Immunobiology* 1993; **187**: 403–16.

187. Anderson BO, Harken AH. Multiple organ failure: inflammatory priming and activation sequences promote autologous tissue injury. *J Trauma* 1990; **30**: S44–9.

188. Dehring DJ, Lubbesmeyer HJ, Fader RC, Traber LD, Traber DL. Exaggerated cardiopulmonary response after bacteremia in sheep with week-old thermal injury. *Crit Care Med* 1993; **21**: 888–93.

189. Koike K, Moore FA, Moore EE, Poggetti RS, Tuder RM, Banerjee A. Endotoxin after gut ischemia/reperfusion causes irreversible lung injury. *J Surg Res* 1992; **52**: 656–62.

190. Ciancio MJ, Hunt J, Jones SB, Filkins JP. Comparative and interactive in vivo effects of tumor necrosis factor alpha and endotoxin. *Circ Shock* 1991; **33**: 108–20.

Chapter 20

Metabolic support of the burned patient

Jeffrey R Saffle

Marsha Hildreth

Introduction

The metabolic consequences of major burn injury are profound, and constitute a major challenge to effective burn treatment. Metabolic rates of burn patients can be twice that of a normal person, and cause tremendous wasting of lean body mass within a few weeks of injury. Failure to satisfy these increased energy and protein requirements results in impaired wound healing, cellular dysfunction, decreased resistance to infection, and ultimately death. Provision of early and aggressive nutritional support throughout the postburn period can reduce mortality and complications, optimize wound healing, and minimize the devastating effects of hypermetabolism and subsequent catabolism. The purpose of this chapter is to provide practical guidelines for the assessment of the nutritional needs of burn patients, and for the provision of aggressive nutritional support.

The hypermetabolism of burn injury

Over 70 years ago, Cuthbertson documented that traumatic injury was associated with increased energy utilization, and accelerated metabolism of protein and losses of body nitrogen.[1,2] In the 1970s, clinicians documented that burn patients exhibited the most severe hypermetabolism of any patient group, with energy expenditure from 60 to 100% above normal following a major burn, and con-

comitant catabolism of body protein stores.[3,4] These studies also demonstrated the so-called 'ebb and flow' response, which characterizes the metabolic response to injury, in which an initial, transient (12–24 hour) reduction in metabolic rate is followed by a gradual, crescendo–decrescendo curve of sustained and severe hypermetabolism that can persist for weeks. This response is illustrated in **Figure 20.1**.

Early attempts to nourish burn patients with oral feeding were largely unsuccessful. Altered mental status, ileus and gastrointestinal dysfunction, and inhalation injury often precluded significant oral intake. Even patients who could eat were rarely able to tolerate the amount of nutrition necessary for adequate support. As a consequence, patients with major burns predictably incurred weight loss of 20% or greater within the first few weeks of injury,[5,6] with associated immune compromise and delayed wound healing. This often proved to be a fatal degree of inanition, as patients succumbed to respiratory failure, pneumonia, and systemic infection (**Figure 20.2**).

Mediators of Hypermetabolism

The hypermetabolism seen after burn injury is a consequence of the hormonal changes which accompany severe trauma.[7,8] As initially described by Wilmore,[4] Long,[3] and others,[6] burn trauma produces major increases in the catabolic hormones epinephrine, cortisol, and glucagon. The result is greatly accelerated gluconeogenesis,

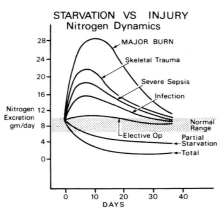

Fig. 20.1 This is a classic illustration of nitrogen excretion following injury compared to starvation and other conditions. Burn injury evokes the most pronounced catabolism of any clinical condition, with nitrogen excretion exceeding 25 g/day (150 g of protein, almost a half-pound of lean body mass!). From Long *et al.*[3]

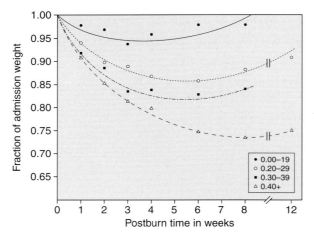

Fig. 20.2 Weight loss following burn injury. Dramatic losses of lean body mass are documented within a week or two of injury, and progress continuously in the absence of effective nutritional support. By 4–6 weeks postburn, patients with major burns have lost 15% of lean body mass or more, a fatal degree of inanition. From Wilmore.[6]

glycogenolysis, and muscle proteolysis.[9] Though plasma insulin levels are not depressed in this setting, catabolic hormones make insulin less able to act as a counter-regulatory hormone. As a result, blood sugar levels are increased, and protein synthesis, lipogenesis, and glycogenesis are inhibited. Growth hormone, another anabolic hormone, is similarly antagonized and less effective.

The clinical consequence of these hormonal changes is a markedly increased metabolic rate, with skeletal muscle serving as the preferred fuel. In contrast to starvation, in which lipolysis and ketosis provide energy and protect muscle reserves, burn injury limits the ability of the body to utilize fat as an energy source. As a result, lipids have limited 'protein-sparing' effect. Instead, a diet composed largely of carbohydrates is required to reduce protein

catabolism, and even glucose is limited in its ability to prevent protein wasting.[10]

Although these hormonal changes complicate attempts to provide nutritional support, they also provide mechanisms which can potentially be manipulated to reduce hypermetabolism, and improve nutrition in burn patients. Hormonal manipulation of the metabolic response to injury, discussed below, is a new field which shows some promise for improving the care of patients in the future.

Modern Burn Care and Metabolic Requirements

Current techniques of caring for burn patients probably have not altered the *nature* of burn-induced hypermetabolism, but abundant evidence suggests that the *magnitude* of energy expenditure and protein catabolism are reduced among patients treated in today's burn centers. The widespread use of indirect calorimetry to measure energy expenditure has led to a number of reports documenting metabolic rates significantly less than those observed by Wilmore,[4] Long,[3] and others.[6] Though still increased, energy requirements are now more likely to approximate 120–150% of normal, rather than the 160–200% previously observed.[11–14]

Several commonly used treatments are known to affect patients' energy expenditure. Environmental stress adds significantly to metabolic rate: maintaining a high ambient temperature and relative humidity may reduce caloric requirements by up to 20%;[4] this should be a standard policy in all burn centers. Local and systemic infection also aggravate hypermetabolism; better antibiotics and aggressive burn wound excision have significantly reduced the incidence of burn wound sepsis, and probably also reduced energy requirements for many patients. Although surgical procedures have never been shown directly to reduce energy expenditure,[15] covering burn wounds with autografts, allografts, or synthetic skin substitutes almost certainly shortens the duration of hypermetabolism, leading to improved energy balance over the course of treatment. Other therapies, including the use of mechanical ventilators and chemical paralysis, also reduce energy requirements.[16] Nonetheless, both temporal and patient-specific variations in energy expenditure make it difficult to predict requirements for individual patients.

Assessment of nutritional needs

Nutritional support is a vital component of successful burn care. All members of the burn team must recognize the importance of nutrition, be familiar with the basics of nutritional monitoring and therapy, and work toward the success of nutritional treatment. To optimize nutritional therapy, each burn center should develop a protocol for nutritional support that involves all disciplines, and standardizes the assessment, initiation, and monitoring of nutritional support for all patients.

Initial Assessment

Many patients suffering from systemic disease such as cancer and AIDS may initially present with serious nutritional depletion which presents a major threat to patient survival, and requires careful assessment and treatment before the underlying disease can be addressed. A number of assessment techniques have been proposed for use, ranging from careful clinical histories (which may be as accurate as more elaborate tests[17]) to assessment of serum proteins, anthropometric measurements, tests of immune function, etc.

Unfortunately, or perhaps fortunately, such an assessment is of little value in the treatment of the acutely burned patient, for several reasons. First, burn injury itself induces major abnormalities in almost every parameter of nutritional status, which cannot be differentiated from the effects of pre-existing nutritional depletion: swelling and burn eschar preclude accurate anthropometric measurements; serum proteins are altered quickly and significantly following major burns; and, immune function is similarly disturbed. Secondly, the metabolic consequences of burn injury are so severe that they overshadow any pre-existing problems. Satisfying ongoing requirements in such patients is more important than compensating for underlying deficiencies. Thirdly, burn patients require the same aggressive nutritional support regardless of their preburn status; attempting to 'catch up' by providing excess calories and/or protein is ineffective, and likely to contribute to liver enzyme abnormalities, CO_2 retention, and azotemia (see Overfeeding, below). For all these reasons, nutritional support of the burn patient is aimed at satisfying *burn-specific* abnormalities and requirements. To do so, obtain as accurate measurements of height and weight as possible at the time of admission.

Formulas for Estimating Caloric Requirements

Recognition of the need to provide nutritional support has led to a wide variety and number of published regimens for providing nutrients in the early postburn period.[18] One of the most popular formulas is that developed by Curreri *et al.*[19] Though this formula has been widely (and successfully) used, its accuracy is open to question. In developing the formula, Curreri's group examined only nine patients, too few to obtain an accurate sampling of metabolic requirements. Moreover, the formula was derived by calculating backwards to estimate how many calories would have been needed to make up for patients' lost weight. As discussed below, this is a dubious assumption at best.

Formulas for adult nutrition are reviewed in **Table 20.1**.[19–22] As this demonstrates, these formulas vary greatly in their estimation of the calories required to nourish specific patients. All these formulas suffer from inherent limitations. As noted above, modern techniques of burn treatment have resulted in a blunting of the hypermetabolic response to burn injury. Older formulas, such as Curreri's, probably overestimate energy requirements significantly.[11] Patients vary significantly in their metabolic responses and even individual patients experience significant daily fluctuations in metabolic rate in response to activity, medications, and environmental changes. Static formulas ignore these variables, as well as the more gradual rise and fall of postburn energy expenditure presented previously. Formulas are likely to result in overfeeding early and late in the postburn course, and may underfeed patients during periods of peak energy utilization.[11]

Pediatric formulas

Considerable attention has been paid to developing formulas to estimate energy requirements of children. Commonly used formulas are presented in **Table 20.2**.[23–27] Separate formulas are presented for children of different ages, which is appropriate. Even with this accommodation, however, it can be seen that different formulas predict very different caloric requirements for the same patients.

Indirect Calorimetry

Very early studies of the response to injury relied on measurement of metabolic rate by *direct* calorimetry, i.e. the amount of heat generated by patients, a cumbersome and difficult technique that was not applicable to clinical care. Over the past 50 years, improvements in the techniques and equipment for performance of *indirect* calorimetry have allowed the measurement of energy expenditure to be moved from the laboratory to the bedside, and made possible the routine assessment of metabolic rate by clinicians.

Indirect calorimetry (IC) utilizes the relationship between consumption of inhaled oxygen and the generation of energy. Modern IC devices contain sensors which measure inhaled and exhaled concentrations of oxygen and carbon dioxide and the minute volume of expired gas (VE). This permits calculation of oxygen consumption (VO_2) and carbon dioxide production (VCO_2), which

Table 20.1 Commonly used formulas for estimating caloric requirements in adult burn patients			
Formula name	Formula	Daily caloric estimate (kcal), 25-year-old male (80 kg; BSA = 2.0 m²) with 60% TBSA burn	Comment
Harris–Benedict[22]	Basal energy expenditure: Men: 66.5 + (13.8)W + (5)H–(6.76)A Women: 655 + (9.6)W + (1.85)H–(4.68)A **Adjust for stress by multiplying BEE by a factor of 1.2–2.0**	Basal rate = 1915 If factor is 1.2 = 2299 If factor is 1.5 = 2872 If factor is 2.0 = 3830	The Harris–Benedict formula is an accepted standard for estimating *basal* energy expenditure (BEE). For burn patients, multiplying BEE by an arbitrary factor introduces significant inaccuracy. A factor of 1.2–1.5 should be sufficient for all but the largest burn injuries
Curreri formula[19]	Age 16–59: (25)W + (40)TBSA Age 60: (20)W + (65)TBSA	4400	This widely used formula probably overestimates energy requirements significantly. A modification for elderly patients is included
Davies and Lilijedahl[20]	(20)W + (70) TBSA	5800	This formula will grossly overestimate energy requirements for patients with very large injuries
RDA[21]	37(W)	2960	'One size fits all' is convenient, but inaccurate for most patients, particularly the elderly and obese

For all formulas: W = weight in kilograms; H = height in centimeters; A = age in years; TBSA = burn size (percent total body surface area).

Table 20.2 Commonly used formulas for estimating caloric requirements in pediatric burn patients

Formula name	Age	Formula	Daily caloric estimate (kcal) for patients with 40% TBSA burn			
			11-month-old, 10 kg BSA = 0.5 m²	3-year-old, 12 kg BSA = 0.6 m²	10-year-old, 30 kg BSA = 1.1 m²	14-year-old, 60 kg BSA = 1.6 m²
Recommended dietary allowances (RDA)[24]	0–6 months	108 × (W)				
	6 months–1 year	98 × (W)	980			
	1–3 years	102 × (W)		1224		
	4–10 years	90 × (W)			2700	
	11–14 years					
	(male)	55 × (W)				3300
	(female)	47 × (W)				
Curreri Junior[23]	<1 year	(RDA + 15 kcal/TBSA)	1580			
	1–3 years	(RDA + 25 kcal/TBSA)		2224		
	4–15 years	(RDA + 40 kcal/TBSA)			4300	4900
Galveston Infant[26]	0–1 year	2100 kcal/m² + 1000 kcal/m² burn	1250			
Galveston Revised[25]	1–11 years	1800 kcal/m² + 1300 kcal/m² burn		1392	2552	
Galveston Adolescent[27]	12 years	1500 kcal/m² + 1500 kcal/m² burn				3360

For all formulas: W = weight in kilograms; H = height in centimeters; A = age in years; BSA = body surface area; TBSA = burn size (percent total body surface area).

can be used to calculate metabolic rate.[28,29] Measurements are made by a tight-fitting face mask or hood which fits over the head, or by direct connection to the ventilator in mechanically ventilated patients. Measurements have been shown to be reliable and reproducible over a wide range of metabolic rates and FIO_2.

Indirect calorimetry is also useful in detecting significant under- or overfeeding, through calculation of the respiratory quotient (RQ), defined as the ratio of oxygen consumption to CO_2 production (VO_2/VCO_2).[30] The body's metabolism of specific substrates affects this ratio, which gives the clinician information about metabolic supply and demand. For example, utilization of fat as a primary energy source, which characterizes starvation, results in an RQ of 0.7 or less.[31] Normal metabolism of mixed substrates (carbohydrate, fat, and protein) produces an RQ of 0.75–0.90, while the synthesis of fat from carbohydrate, which typifies overfeeding, results in an RQ of 1.0 or greater. This increased production of CO_2 in overfed states can contribute to respiratory distress and failure to wean from ventilatory support; the finding of an RQ approaching or exceeding 1.0 is an indication to reduce feedings, particularly carbohydrates.[32]

Use of IC is widely recommended for use in estimating caloric requirements for burn patients, and to detect and prevent significant under- or overfeeding through measurement of RQ.[33,34] To maximize the usefulness of IC, and 'tailor' nutritional support to match utilization, IC measurements should be performed 2–3 times weekly. Oxygen consumption is usually measured in the early morning, with patients at bed rest. Fluctuations in energy utilization associated with activity must be factored into nutritional support, and are usually estimated by increasing measured metabolic rate by 10–20%.[35]

Despite the theoretical advantages of IC-based nutritional support, and the limitation inherent in static formulas, the superiority of IC has not been proven clinically. Many patients have been suc-

cessfully nourished using the Curreri and others formulas. It is unknown how closely nutritional support must be 'matched' to energy requirements; minor episodes of over- and underfeeding are probably both unavoidable and frequent, and do not appear to affect outcome significantly. In a randomized study, Saffle et al., found no differences in outcomes among patients fed according to the Curreri formula, compared to patients whose nutrition was guided by IC.[36] This may reflect the inaccuracies inherent in any method of estimating nutritional needs, as well as the practical problems associated with actually delivering the calculated number of calories to critically ill patients. Thus, it is probably safe to conclude that either formulas or IC measurements can be used to nourish burn patients. Far more important than the method selected for nutritional assessment is the continued awareness by the burn team of the critical importance of providing a regimen of aggressive nutritional support to patients throughout their course of treatment.

Specific nutrient requirements

Carbohydrates

The major source of calories for thermally injured patients should be carbohydrates. Glucose is the preferred fuel for healing wounds and accessory metabolic pathways to provide glucose, including the alanine and Cori cycles, are activated. This can sometimes result in mild elevations of lactic acid in burn patients, even in the absence of shock or sepsis.

The major complication of feeding burn patients carbohydrate diets is glucose intolerance. Though plasma insulin levels are not decreased in burn patients – in fact, they are usually increased – they are overshadowed by elevations of glucagon and cortisol, producing relative glucose intolerance, the so-called 'diabetes of injury'.[37] In addition, even patients with relatively normal glucose tolerance may have caloric requirements that exceed the body's ability to assimilate glucose, which is estimated at approximately 7 g/kg/day (2240 kcal for an 80-kg man).[38] Patients often require significant amounts of supplemental insulin to improve glucose absorption, but refractory hyperglycemia can occur despite insulin administration, and force reduction or even discontinuation of nutrition until blood sugar can be brought under control. Providing a limited amount of dietary fat reduces requirements for carbohydrates, and can improve glucose tolerance significantly.

Protein

The hormonal environment that accompanies burn injury greatly increases proteolysis, and provision of carbohydrate and fat calories is only partially successful in reducing protein catabolism. Increased quantities of protein must be supplied, both to satisfy ongoing demands and to provide amino acids for wound healing, synthesis of enzymes, immunocompetence, and other functions. Protein should not be administered primarily as an energy source; calculated energy requirements must be supplied as *nonprotein* calories.

Protein catabolism in burn patients can exceed 150 g/day, or almost a half-pound of skeletal muscle. Attempting to satisfy these requirements by feeding protein does not necessarily reduce breakdown of endogenous protein stores;[39] it facilitates protein synthesis, and reduces net negative nitrogen balance. Evidence demonstrates that provision of supranormal quantities of dietary protein is associated with improved outcomes in burn patients. In 1980, Alexander *et al.* fed a group of seriously burned children with isocaloric diets containing different amounts of protein.[40] Children who received 23% of their intake as protein had significantly better immune function, less bacteremia, and improved survival, compared to a group who received 17% protein diets. Cunningham's group found that wound healing and recovery were enhanced in burned children with provision of diets containing 2.5 g/kg/day protein.[41] Matsuda *et al*, found that patients with increasingly large burns require progressively more protein to attain nitrogen balance; patients with burns in excess of 10% total body

surface area (TBSA) required a nonprotein calorie:nitrogen ratio of 100:1 or less.[42] Numerous other studies have documented similar findings.[36,43]

Current recommendations call for 1.5–2.0 g protein/kg body weight/day for adult burn patients, and up to 3.0 g/kg/day in children.[33,44] With provision of sufficient nonprotein calories, this should result in a calorie:nitrogen ratio of 100:1 or less (see **Table 20.3** for a list of commonly used enteral products). Measurement of nitrogen balance, and visceral protein markers, may be helpful in assessing the adequacy of nutritional support (see below).

Arginine

Some specific amino acids appear to play significant roles in postburn metabolism. Among these is arginine, which is known to stimulate T lymphocytes and enhance natural killer cell function, and to stimulate synthesis of nitric oxide, which is important in communication and host resistance to infection.[45–47] Data from Barbul and others have suggested that the addition of supplemental arginine to enteral diets is associated with improved immune responsiveness and wound healing.[48,49] Improved survival was demonstrated in burned guinea pigs given arginine-enhanced diets.[50] Arginine is one component of so-called 'immune enhancing diets' discussed below.

Glutamine

Glutamine serves as a primary fuel for enterocytes. As such, it may play an important role in maintaining the integrity of the small intestine, including the preservation of gut-associated immune function.[51–53] Glutamine supplementation was associated with some benefits when used to enhance total parenteral nutrition (TPN) in neutropenic cancer patients,[54] and appeared to be of benefit in patients maintained on prolonged TPN.[55] The effect of glutamine in postburn hypermetabolism has not been well described.

Branched-chain amino acids

The branched-chain amino acids (BCAAs) – leucine, isoleucine, and valine – have been postulated to spare endogenous muscle

Table 20.3 Composition of commercially-available enteral nutrition products

Brand Name	ml	g	(% kcal)	g	(% kcal)	Cal:N₂	g	(% kcal)	ω-3 FFAs	Vit A (IU)	Vit C (mg)	Iron (mg)	Zn (mg)
Immune-enhancing and stress formulas													
Impact™ (Novartis)	1000	130	53	56	22	71:1	28	25	43%	3350	80	12	15
Immun-Aid™ (McGaw)	1000	120	48	80	32	53:1	22	20	32%	2665	60	9	25
Replete™ (Nestle)	1000	113	45	62	25	75:1	34	30	25%	4000	340	18	24
TraumaCal™ (Mead-Johnson)	667	95	38	55	22	91:1	45	40	14%	1667	99	5.9	9.9
Maintenance diets													
Isocal HN™ (Mead-Johnson)	94	117	46	42	17	125:1	43	37	N/A	3962	236	14	16
Osmolite HN™	94	136	54	42	17	125:1	33	29	17%	3575	217	13	17
Pediatric formulas													
Compleat™ (Novartis)	1000	126	50	38	15	139:1	39	35	N/A	3300	96	13	12
Pediasure™ (Abbot Labs)	1000	110	44	30	12	185:1	50	44	9%	2570	100	14	12

Contents per 1000 calories of feeding — CHO's / Micronutrients | Protein | Fat

Abbreviations: CHO = carbohydrates; kcal = kilocalories; g = grams; % kcal = percentage of total kilocalories; Cal:N₂ = ratio of nonprotein calories to nitrogen; ω-3 FFAs = omega-3 free fatty acids; IU = international units. Adapted from *Enteral Product Reference Guide*, Deerfield IL: Nestle Clinical Nutrition, 1999.

catabolism by stimulating protein synthesis, and by serving as energy substrates. In clinical trials in trauma and ICU patients, BCAA-enriched nutrition has been associated with improved nitrogen balance, but has had no effect on survival.[56,57] In both animal and clinical studies in burn injury, BCAA-enriched feedings have not been shown to produce significant improvements in outcome, protein synthesis, or immune function.[58,59]

Requirements and Uses of Fat

A certain (small) quantity of fat is an essential component of nutritional support. Essential fatty acid deficiency is a well-documented complication of patients given long-term TPN.[7] Modern TPN formulas contain a significant amount of lipid for this reason. In addition, providing a substantial proportion of fat calories improves glucose tolerance, and lessens the chance of elevated CO_2 production. However, the hormonal environment of the burn patient suppresses lipolysis, and limits the extent to which lipids can be utilized for energy. For this reason, most authorities recommend that fat comprise no more than about 30–35% of nonprotein calories, or about 1 g/kg/day of intravenous lipids in TPN[7] (see **Table 20.3**).

Some recent evidence suggests that it may be desirable to give less fat. Mochizuki et al. found an adverse effect on immune function in burned guinea pigs when diets contained more than 15% lipids.[60] Limited clinical research supports this finding,[61] leading some authorities to recommend low-fat diets for use in burn patients. However, most commercially available nutritional supplements contain 25–35% of calories as fat. Patients given TPN can be given fat as little as once or twice per week, though this will require increasing glucose calories, and aggravating glucose intolerance.

The composition of administered fat may be even more important than the quantity. Most lipids contain primarily omega-6 free fatty acids (ω-6 FFAs) such as linoleic acid. These fatty acids are metabolized largely through synthesis of arachidonic acid, a pre-cursor of proinflammatory cytokines such as prostaglandin E_2. Lipids such as fish oil contain a high proportion of ω-3 FFAs, and reduced amounts of ω-6 FFAs. In several studies, diets high in fish oil are associated with reduced production of arachidonic acid metabolites, improved immune response, and possibly improved outcomes. Alexander et al. showed that burned guinea pigs fed a diet high in fish oil had less weight loss, better cell-mediated immune response, and higher serum transferrin than animals fed a diet containing primarily linoleic acid.[62] Omega-3 fatty acids are a major component of 'immune-enhancing diets', and may be of benefit in the nutritional management of burn patients (see below).

Micronutrients: Vitamins and Trace Elements

In addition to the major nutrients, metabolism and excretion of many so-called 'micronutrients', vitamins, and trace elements which are important in wound healing and immunity are also greatly affected by burn injury.[63] These compounds have not been evaluated extensively in burn patients, though depressed serum levels of some compounds have been demonstrated after burn injury. Limited data suggest that supplementation of some substances (vitamin A, vitamin C) may be beneficial, **Table 20.4** contains a list of the most important micronutrients, their recommended daily allowances (RDAs), and the contents of several commonly used enteral formulas.

A complete listing of micronutrients and their functions is beyond the scope of this chapter; excellent reviews are available.[63-65] A few of the most important compounds are described below.

■ **Vitamin A:** vitamin A is an important factor in wound healing and epithelial growth. It functions as a circulating antioxidant, and helps in preventing free radical damage after burn injury. Decreased levels of vitamin A and C have been demonstrated after burn injury.[66] Vitamin A

Table 20.4 Micronutrient requirements, and composition of commercially available products

	Vit A (μg RE)	Vit C (mg)	Vit E (mg α-TE)	Vit D (μg)	Vit K (μg)	Folate (μg)	Iron (mg)	Calcium (mg)	Phosphorus (mg)	Zinc (mg)	Selenium (μg)
Recommended daily allowances (by age)[21]											
<1 year	375	30	4	5	10	80	10	270	275	5	15
1–3 yrs	400	40	6	5	15	150	10	500	460	10	20
4–10 yrs	600	45	7	5	20	200	10	800	500	10	20
Adults	1000	60	8–10	5	40–80	400	10–15	1300	700	15	40–70
Recommended supplementation[67,]*											
<3 years	1500	500								110	
>3 years	3000	1000								220	
Quantities in commercial products (per 1000 kcal)											
Impact™	1005	80	60	6.8	67	400	12	800	800	15	100
Replete™	1200	340	60	10	50	540	18	1000	1000	24	100
TraumaCal™	500	99	25	3.3	85	133	6	500	500	10	N/A
Osmolite HN™	1072	217	33	7.2	58	429	13.2	717	717	17	51
Compleat Pediatric™	990	96	22	12	38	350	13	1000	1000	12	52
Pediasure™	771	100	23	13	38	370	14	970	800	12	23
Cernevit-12™	1050	125	11.2	5	0	414	–	–	–	–	–
(Liquid vitamin supplement for enteral nutrition)											

Abbreviations and conversions: Vit = vitamin; IU = international units; mg = milligrams; μg = micrograms. To convert from, the following factors were used [X]: Vit D: 1 μg = 40 IU; Vit A: 0.3 (IU) = 1 μg RE (retinol equivalent); Vit E: 1 IU = 1 mg α-TE (alpha-tocopherol). Data extrapolated from *Enteral Product Reference Guide*, Deerfield, IL: Nestle Clinical Nutrition, 1999.
* Note that these recommendations are in addition to an adult or children's multivitamin given daily.

supplementation has been recommended for burn patients;[67] however, toxicity of vitamin A can also occur.

- **Vitamin C:** ascorbic acid is necessary for normal synthesis and crosslinking of collagen and is thus essential for wound healing. In addition, it functions as a circulating antioxidant. Some data support a beneficial role for vitamin C supplementation in burn patients, and toxicity does not appear to be a clinical problem.[64] Supplementation of up to 1000 mg/day in burn patients has been recommended.[67] This dose is approximately 20 times the recommended dietary allowance (RDA) for adults.[21]
- **Iron:** iron plays an essential role in oxygen-carrying proteins (hemoglobin and myoglobin), and also acts as a cofactor for a number of important enzymes. Burn patients are prone to iron deficiency, partially due to blood loss, but it should also be remembered that blood transfusions deliver a significant amount of iron.
- **Zinc:** zinc is required for the function of many metalloenzymes. Several aspects of wound healing appear to be affected by the availability of zinc, including DNA and RNA replication, and lymphocyte function. Zinc deficiency has been documented during the first several days after burn injury.[68] Supplementation of up to 220 mg/day (15 times RDA) has been recommended.[67]
- **Selenium:** selenium is important in the function of lymphocytes, and hence, in cell-mediated immunity. Selenium is lost through the skin after burn injury; selenium deficiency in burn patients has been documented.[69]

A survey by Shippee *et al.* in 1987 found that many burn centers provide some supplementation of trace elements, though both indications and specific doses varied among units.[70] Current reviews of nutrition in burn patients recommend supplementing at least the micronutrients listed above, and perhaps others.[8]

In attempting to provide supplemental vitamins and minerals, remember that many commercially available tube feedings contain substantial quantities of these micronutrients (**Table 20.4**). For example, feeding an adult patient 2500 kcal of Replete™ would provide 3000 mg vitamin A and 850 mg vitamin C, which are well in excess of RDA values, and approximate the recommendations for supplementation listed by Mayes *et al.*[67] The addition of a daily multivitamin tablet, or liquid multivitamins to tube feedings or TPN, will provide far more than RDA for most of these micronutrients. It is unclear whether additional supplementation is of value in clinical care of burn patients. Remember also that in the early days of TPN, micronutrient solutions were unavailable; instead, clinicians gave patients on TPN weekly blood transfusions to provide these substances. While this cannot be advocated today, it remains true that many burn patients do receive transfusions, which contain significant amounts iron, chromium, and other nutrients.

Formulas for Enteral Nutrition

Successful enteral nutrition has been provided with very simple concoctions of milk, eggs, and other nutrients.[18] Patients with gastrostomy tubes can be successfully nourished with low-cost blenderized diets for long periods. However, commercially prepared enteral formulas offer several advantages for nourishing burn patients. They are nutritionally complete, sterile, and carefully composed to contain appropriate quantities of all necessary nutrients. Canned enteral diets are thin liquids that can be infused through narrow feeding tubes with minimal clogging. Most are reasonably inexpensive, though some specialized formulas can be quite costly. **Table 20.3** lists the nutrient composition of a number of popular, commercial enteral formulas. Remember that a bewildering array of additional products are available, including fiber-containing diets, elemental diets, dietary supplements, and specialized diets for patients with renal failure, hepatic failure, glucose intolerance, etc. The burn center dietician should be involved in evaluating and selecting the products used to feed each patient.

Formulas for TPN

Solutions for TPN must be composed of elemental components that do not require digestion. Dextrose is usually the main calorie source, and the large quantities required result in hypertonic solutions that must be infused through central venous catheters. Protein is supplied as elemental amino acids, usually in set proportions, although custom solutions can be prepared. Because of its instability in solution, glutamine is not a component of TPN, a potential disadvantage. In recent years, lipid emulsions have been perfected for intravenous use, and lipids should comprise a significant proportion of TPN solution.

The exact composition of TPN must be ordered by the burn physician. While this is time-consuming, it permits exact tailoring of the solution to individual patient needs. **Table 20.5** is an example of a protocol for ordering and administering TPN used at the University of Utah. It illustrates an order for TPN using standard components (70% dextrose, 15% amino acids, and 20% lipid emulsion). The physician can also choose to order customized TPN; in addition to major nutrients, electrolytes, vitamins, and minerals can be custom-ordered, or standard 'packages' can be used. Medications such as insulin and H_2 blockers can be added as well.

Methods of nutritional support

Route of Nutrition: Parenteral versus Enteral

Total parenteral nutrition is defined as the administration of complete nutrition support by the intravenous route. Although the provision of nutrients by vein has only been possible for a few decades, it is ironic that the development of TPN in the 1960s and 1970s led the way to the era of modern nutritional support, and actually predated many enteral nutritional techniques.[71] At the peak of its popularity, it was estimated that 550 000 hospitalized patients were treated yearly, at a cost of over 3 billion dollars.[72] This included burn patients, for whom TPN was widely advocated.[18,73,74]

More recently, development of safe and effective techniques for enteral nutrition – delivery of nutrients directly into the gastrointestinal tract – has led to the widespread replacement of TPN by enteral techniques. Enteral nutrition has a number of both theoretical and practical advantages over TPN. First, enteral nutrition provides nourishment for the bowel itself, thus maintaining the integrity of bowel mucosa, which may result in a decreased incidence of bacterial translocation and sepsis, and preservation of important gut-associated immune function.[75–78] In addition, administration of TPN appears to be associated with increased secretion of tumor necrosis factor (TNF), a 'proinflammatory' cytokine associated with many aspects of multiple organ failure, and other inflammatory mediators.[79]

In clinical trials, early and aggressive enteral nutrition has been

Table 20.5 A protocol for administration of TPN in burn patients (Adapted from the *Adult Parenteral Nutrition Orders, University of Utah*)

Step One: Calculated required energy and protein needs

Example: 25-year-old man, 80 kg in weight. Body surface area = 2.2 m².

1. Indirect calorimetry indicates energy expenditure of 2400 kcal/24 hours. To account for fluctuations in energy expenditure, increase measured value by 20% (480 kcal); total = 2880 nonprotein kcal/day

2. Estimate protein requirements at 2.0 g/kg/day = 160 g protein

Step Two: Order TPN solution

1. *Carbohydrates:* Carbohydrates are supplied as 70% dextrose (D70), which contains 2.4 kcal/ml. To give 75% of nonprotein calories as dextrose, calculate:

$$[(2880 \text{ total kcal}) \times (0.75 \text{ calories as dextrose})] \div 2.4 \text{ kcal/ml} = 900 \text{ ml D70}$$

2. *Fat:* The remainder of nonprotein calories will be given as lipid emulsion. This is commonly available as 10% (1.0 kcal/ml) or 20% (2.0 kcal/ml) solution. To give 25% of nonprotein calories as lipid, calculate:

$$[(2880 \text{ total kcal}) \times (0.25 \text{ calories as lipid})] \div 2.0 \text{ kcal/ml} = 360 \text{ ml } 20\% \text{ lipid emulsion}$$

3. *Protein:* Protein is supplied as crystalline amino acid solutions at a concentration of 10% (0.1 g/ml) or 15% (0.15 g/ml). To give 160 g of protein, calculate:

$$(160 \text{ g protein}) \div 0.15 \text{ g/ml} = 1067 \text{ ml of } 15\% \text{ amino acid solution}$$

4. Total volume = 900 ml D70 + 360 ml lipids + 1067 ml amino acids = 2327 ml.

5. *Add electrolytes:* These can be ordered as customized additions in any quantity, but a standard electrolyte 'package' contains (per liter of TPN):
   Sodium chloride: 35 mEq
   Potassium phosphate: 15 mmol (22 mEq potassium)
   Magnesium sulfate: 8 mEq
   Calcium gluconate: 5 mEq

6. *Add vitamins:* A standard vitamin 'package' contains approximately 100% of recommended dietary allowances of vitamins A, C, D, E, and B_{12}, pyridoxine, thiamine, riboflavin, niacin, pantothenic acid, folate, and biotin

7. *Add trace elements:* A standard 'package' contains:
   Zinc: 2.5 mg
   Copper: 1.0 mg
   Mn: 0.25 mg
   Chromium: 10 µg

8. *Add additional water, and calculate infusion rate:* If patients require additional fluid, water can be added to the TPN solution as desired. If no additional water is required, then the goal rate for infusion is 2327 ml ÷ 24 hours = 97 ml/h

Step Three: Protocol for administration

1. Begin infusion at 20 ml/h via central vein

2. Increase rate every 4–6 hours by 10–20 ml/h until rate of 120 ml/h is achieved

Step Four: Begin monitoring on nutritional support

Blood glucose:

1. As infusion is initiated, measure blood glucose every 4 hours. If glucose Is 200 mg/dl, consider administration of exogenous insulin by 'sliding scale'

2. After goal rate is achieved, measure blood glucose every 6 hours

Daily: Serum electrolytes, blood urea nitrogen, creatinine

Twice weekly:

1. Hepatic enzymes (lactate dehydrogenase, alkaline phosphatase, total bilirubin, transaminases)

2. 24-hour urine for nitrogen balance

3. Serum transferrin or prealbumin

4. Serum phosphorus, magnesium, and calcium

associated with a decreased frequency of infectious complications in trauma and ICU patients.[80–82] In burn patients, Herndon *et al.* demonstrated that TPN supplementation of enteral nutrition did not improve infectious outcomes or immune function, and was actually associated with increased mortality.[83,84]

In addition to maintaining gut integrity, enteral nutrition provides 'first-pass' delivery of nutrients to the liver, which facilitates their utilization, and reduces complications such as hyperglycemia and hyperosmolarity. TPN requires central venous access, with the inherent risk of life-threatening complications, including pneumo/hemothorax, bacteremia, endocarditis, air embolism, etc. Lastly, but by no means unimportant, TPN solutions are a great deal more costly than enteral formulas, require more expensive delivery systems, and more frequent monitoring of glucose and other blood chemistries. For all these reasons, *enteral nutrition should be considered the route of choice for the nutritional support of all burn patients with functioning (or even partially functioning) gastrointestinal tracts.*

Early Enteral Feeding

Recent research has evaluated the potential value of beginning enteral nutrition as early as possible following injury in patients suffering trauma and burns. In 1984, Mochizuki *et al.* published data demonstrating that immediate enteral feeding following burn injury in guinea pigs was well tolerated, and was associated with improved maintenance of small bowel mass, and reduction in post-burn hypermetabolism to levels approximating normal.[85] Other studies in animals and humans have not demonstrated a significant amelioration of the hypermetabolic response with early enteral nutrition.[86,87] However, it appears clear that enteral feedings can be started safely within hours of burn injury, and that doing so will likely improve nitrogen balance and overall nutrition.[88] This concept is supported by similar data in trauma and surgery patients.[89] With gradual increases in infusion rates, tube feedings are usually well tolerated, even during the first day postburn. In addition, tube feedings administered through nasal-jejunal tubes need not be stopped hours before surgery, and can even be given during surgical procedures, without increased risk of aspiration or other complications. Such a policy significantly reduces interruptions in feedings, assures adequate nutrition for patients who may have to undergo multiple operations, and may reduce the incidence of infectious complications.[90] For all these reasons, tube feedings should be started as soon as practically possibly following injury, and certainly within 48 hours. To enhance success, begin feedings at rate of 20–40 ml/h (as little as 5 ml/h in infants), and try to reach the therapeutic goal rate within 24 hours. Unless they are likely to eat within 3–4 days, patients with relatively small burns should not be given a chance to fail with an oral diet. Even 3–5 days of starvation can produce significant muscle wasting and immune compromise, which will be difficult to compensate for later.

Gastric versus Intestinal Feeding

It remains unclear whether there are any physiologic differences between enteral feedings given into the small bowel compared to the stomach, though there are several practical considerations. One advantage of gastric feedings is the ability to place large-diameter nasogastric tubes blindly, facilitating early feeding and reducing problems with clogging. Blenderized diets, and other 'low-tech' (and low-cost) supplements can be used via this route. Intermittent bolus feedings can also be given into the stomach, reducing nursing time and the expense and inconvenience of continuous infusion pumps. A major disadvantage is the tendency of the stomach to develop ileus, both immediately postburn and accompanying episodes of sepsis or stress. Clinicians who employ gastric feeds must remember to check residuals frequently, and to hold feedings if they appear to be backing up in the stomach. Frequent or prolonged intolerance of gastric feedings is a relative indication to switch to small intestinal feeding, which is much less prone to be affected by ileus.

Intestinal feeding requires placement of a feeding tube beyond the pylorus; while this is sometimes successful with blind placement, the technique requires at least an abdominal X-ray to confirm tube position. Many facilities prefer fluoroscopic placement of tubes by radiologists, which usually means transporting patients out of the burn unit. Naso-enteric tubes are smaller and more comfortable, but they clog rather easily, and are also prone to becoming dislodged, and migrating into the stomach. While aspiration is theoretically more likely with gastric feedings, no clear data have documented a reduced rate of aspiration using naso-enteric feeds,[91] and aspiration remains a risk for either technique. The choice of route for enteral feedings remains largely a matter of individual preference. Either method can be used effectively when incorporated into a systematic regimen for nutritional support.

Developing a Program of Nutritional Support

Effective nutritional support can be provided most effectively by developing a comprehensive protocol, which involves all members of the burn team and defines their roles and responsibilities.

The level of support required by various patients differs greatly. A simple algorithm for determining the level of nutritional support is displayed in **Figure 20.3**. Apply such an algorithm proactively, without waiting for problems to develop; all patients should have their nutritional requirements evaluated, and even patients who appear to be doing well should have regular and formal assessment of the adequacy of their nutritional support. Use the simplest and most physiologic method to provide nutrition, but re-evaluate patients frequently to assure that they are achieving nutritional goals, and to determine if support can be simplified, or if escalation of support is required.

Patients with relatively small injuries (20–25% TBSA), who are not intubated, will generally be able to eat, though it may take several days following injury for initial ileus and nausea to resolve completely. In this circumstance you can permit a few days of inadequate nutrition if it appears the patient will soon be able to eat. Patients who are failing to progress with oral intake, who require major surgery, or who develop complications, will benefit from the early institution of more formal nutritional support. Use enteral nutrition whenever possible, and reserve TPN for patients with concomitant abdominal trauma, refractory ileus, or other complications that render their GI tracts unusable. Patients given TPN should be re-assessed frequently for evidence of GI function; patients who cannot tolerate all their nutrition enterally should be given low-rate 'trophic' feeds if at all possible. These help preserve small bowel integrity and function, and facilitate gradually increasing enteral nutrition (and decreasing TPN) as the bowel recovers. By the same token, try to permit some oral intake in patients given enteral nutrition. Oral intake, even sips of liquid, is of great psychological benefit to patients, and encourages them to wean from tube feedings quickly as recovery progresses.

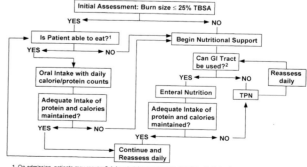

1. On admission, patients may require 3-4 days to tolerate adequate oral intake. Patients who require longer should be considered for nutritional support.

2. Patients should be given some enteral nutrition even if they still require TPN for the balance of nutritional support.

Fig. 20.3 An algorithm for determining the route of nutritional support for burn patients (see text).

Two groups of patients require special considerations in planning and implementing nutritional support: infants, and the elderly.

Infants

Though little research has defined the optimal nutritional mixture for infants, many of the high-protein formulas used in adults contain solute loads which are too high for infants to tolerate. For that reason, infant formulas are more dilute, with a concentration of 20 or 24 kcal/ounce (0.66–0.8 kcal/ml). By age 2–3, children can tolerate more concentrated solutions; some popular pediatric formulas are included in **Table 20.3**. Similarly, TPN solutions should be more dilute in young children; their relatively high fluid requirements enable them to tolerate such formulas without difficulty.

The elderly

Elderly patients may also require specialized nutritional formulas. Older patients are particularly prone to glucose intolerance, and their metabolic rates do not rise as significantly with burn injury as do those of younger adults. Both of these factors predispose the elderly to hyperglycemia. Reliance on static formulas to estimate nutritional needs is likely to produce significant overfeeding, and worsen this problem. Protein catabolism is similarly reduced in older adults, who develop reduced renal function with aging. These patients require less protein, and may benefit from use of a standard maintenance tube feeding rather than a high-protein 'stress' formula. Examples of such formulas are included in **Table 20.3**.

Monitoring and complications

Monitoring of Nutritional Support

An important aspect of any comprehensive program of nutrition support in burn patients is ongoing monitoring of the adequacy and success of the regimen used. A host of sophisticated tests of nutritional status have been used in various clinical situations. As mentioned previously, however, the physiologic changes produced by burn injury make most of them difficult or impossible to interpret. *Careful assessment of clinical status*, including vital signs, respiratory status, muscle mass, and wound healing, remains the most important aspect of nutritional monitoring. The tests described below are probably most useful for identifying trends in nutritional status with serial results obtained over time.

Body weight

Body weight is a basic parameter of patient well-being, and should be measured regularly. However, you must recognize that weight is often misleading in burn patients. Initial fluid resuscitation can routinely add 20–30 kilograms to patients' weights, and much greater increases are not unusual. Theoretically, this accumulated fluid will dissipate in a few days with the onset of diuresis, but this time course may be much longer, particularly for patients' resuscitation with very large volumes.[92] As this progresses, loss of lean body mass may occur simultaneously, so that patients can suffer significant inanition and still weigh more than at the time of admission. In addition, fluid shifts in response to infections, ventilator support, and other stresses, coupled with the fluid retention produced by hypoproteinemia, and elevations in aldosterone and antidiuretic hormone, lead to wide fluctuations in weight that have little to do with nutritional status. Even weeks after injury, patients may have elevations in total body water, and have almost always lost more lean body mass than is apparent from weight alone.[93,94] In following weights, try to recognize long-term trends more than daily variations.

Nitrogen balance

Providing sufficient protein intake is a major goal of nutritional support. Because burn patients differ so widely in their protein requirements, some ongoing monitor of this parameter is very desirable. In addition to serum protein measurements (described below), a widely-used test is the routine assessment of nitrogen balance. Measurements should be obtained at least twice weekly, and require accurate 24-hour collections of urine for determination of urea nitrogen, and concomitant recording of nitrogen intake. Nitrogen balance (N_2bal) is then calculated by the following formula:[95]

$$N_2\text{bal} = N_2I - [1.25 \times (UUN + 4)]$$

$$\text{where } N_2I = \text{24-hour nitrogen intake}$$

This formula contains two constants which may introduce significant error in nitrogen balance calculations. Urinary urea nitrogen (UUN) is increased by 4 (2 is used for children less than 4 years old, and 3 for children 4–10 years) to estimate total urinary nitrogen (TUN). However, TUN may exceed this value in burn patients,[96] leading to underestimation of nitrogen losses. Direct measurement of TUN could eliminate this problem, but is not routinely available in clinical laboratories. In this formula, UUN is also multiplied by 1.25 to estimate the loss of protein-rich exudate from burn wounds, which can vary widely, and may be significant in patients with large burns. Actual losses which exceed this can again lead to an overly optimistic estimation of the adequacy of protein intake.

Attainment of positive or even neutral nitrogen may not always be possible. Inactivity causes muscle wasting and increased nitrogen excretion. In the early postburn period, patients are often bedridden, and may even be sedated or chemically paralyzed; in the absence of muscle activity, positive nitrogen balance may be impossible to achieve, as increasing levels of protein intake only result in increased nitrogen excretion. Fluctuations in daily protein intake, which are common, also make nitrogen balance data hard to interpret.

Serum proteins

The acute response to burn injury shifts metabolic pathways away from maintenance of some visceral proteins.[97] Albumin, while an important indicator of *chronic* nutritional status, is of much less value in assessing *acute* nutritional changes. In burn patients, serum albumin levels are both immediately and chronically depressed, and even the most successful nutritional support will not be reflected in rising albumin levels for long periods, partially because of the protein's excessively long half-life. Some clinicians administer supplemental albumin, to improve colloid oncotic pressure and control edema; however, this has not been shown to affect clinical or nutritional outcomes, including the occurrence of diarrhea.[98,99]

Some other, 'acute-phase' proteins may be more usable markers of nutrition. Of these, prealbumin (or transthyretin) has been utilized frequently.[95] Prealbumin has a short half-life, making it more responsive to changes in acute nutritional status.[97] Even this protein, however, demonstrates fluctuations during the early postburn course; while levels appear to correlate with susceptibility to infection, it is unclear how closely they reflect ongoing nutritional status, including protein intake.[33,100] Serum transferrin, retinol-binding protein, and others, have also been used in this setting. While several studies have shown correlation between these proteins and changes in nutritional status, it remains unclear how sensitive and/or specific these changes are.[40,97,101] In addition, some of these proteins require specialized assays which may be exorbitantly expensive, or not routinely available. Protein markers, if used, should be interpreted in the context of patients' clinical condition and assessment, and evaluated serially over time.

Immune function

Abnormalities of many aspects of the immune system, and resulting increased susceptibility to infection, is a major consequence of malnutrition. A number of studies have documented immune deficiency in malnourished patients who have improved with provision of adequate nutrition. In addition, several markers of immune competence have been advocated for use in nutritional assessment. These include total lymphocyte count,[37] and measurement of delayed-type hypersensitivity (DTH) to common antigens injected into the dermis.[102,103] As with other tests, however, results of these studies must be interpreted carefully in burn patients. Acute thermal injury is profoundly immunosuppressive itself; and while maintenance of normal immune response, or its return to normal, imply successful nutritional support, continued anergy can be produced by infection, old age, or other complicating factors, and cannot by itself be taken as evidence of inadequate nutrition.

Summary

As the above suggests, no single laboratory test is universally applicable or entirely reliable for nutritional monitoring of burn patients. A survey by Williamson of nutrition practices in burn centers[104] indicated that the most commonly used parameters were body weight (46 of 46 centers; 100%), serum albumin (93%), nitrogen balance (70%), transferrin (41%), and prealbumin (26%). In establishing a nutrition protocol, it remains essential to follow clinical course and wound healing, and it is probably reasonable to monitor at least body weight, and one or two indices of protein status, such as nitrogen balance, transferrin, or prealbumin. Other tests probably do not add much additional information, and can be reserved for research studies.

Other parameters

While not specific markers of nutritional status, a number of other parameters should be followed routinely in all patients receiving nutritional support. Burn injury is associated with accelerated evaporative water losses, so hydrational status should be monitored closely. Electrolyte abnormalities, and depressed levels of phosphorus, magnesium, and calcium are also common, and should be assessed regularly. Liver function abnormalities can result from overfeeding, but can also indicate other serious conditions which complicate burn treatment, including hepatitis and acute acalculous cholecystitis. The large protein loads required by burn patients result in increased urinary excretion of nitrogenous wastes, and predispose to elevations of blood urea nitrogen. **Table 20.5** illustrates a protocol for administration of TPN to a burn patient, including the recommended monitoring of nutritional status.

Overfeeding

While almost any disorder of fluid and electrolyte balance, or homeostasis of specific nutrients, can occur with prolonged nutritional support, one of the most frequent complications of modern nutrition is overfeeding. Success in providing nutrition to burn patients can be hard to achieve; often patients suffer some degree of inanition in the early postburn period, a time when ileus and nausea can interfere with successful enteral nutrition, and hyperglycemia can complicate administration of TPN. By the time minor problems are corrected, metabolic rate may be decreasing. The temptation to 'catch up' by continuing nutrition at a high rate can be difficult to resist. Significant overfeeding, especially for long periods, can produce three major complications:

Increased production of CO_2

As mentioned previously, overfeeding carbohydrates results in fat synthesis and increased CO_2 production. In many patients this may be unimportant, but patients with underlying respiratory compromise may demonstrate tachypnea, respiratory distress, or difficulty weaning from ventilatory support. This problem can be particularly severe with administration of large glucose loads in TPN.[105,106] Regular monitoring of metabolic rate with indirect calorimetry will readily detect this problem. Treatment should consist of reducing the level of total nutritional support to match measured values, or reducing glucose administration by giving a higher percentage of calories as fat, or both. If it is possible to switch patients on TPN to enteral nutrition, this may be helpful as well.

Fatty liver

Excess carbohydrate administration leads to deposition of fat in the liver parenchyma.[107] Some degree of hepatic enzyme elevation is common in burn patients, and this may be more pronounced in patients on TPN. Enzymes may display either a hepatocellular or cholestatic picture. Monitor liver enzymes regularly, and attempt to reduce feedings if enzymes become elevated above 2–3 times normal. Pronounced elevations can suggest other disorders (hepatitis, acalculous cholecystitis, etc.).

Azotemia

The large amounts of protein required by burn patients can lead to elevation of blood urea nitrogen (BUN), particularly if dehydration occurs.[106] Acute renal failure is one of the most dreaded complications of sepsis, with a persistently high mortality rate.[108] Fluid intake, urine output, and blood chemistries should be monitored frequently in burn patients who require nutritional support. An increase in BUN in excess of 30% above baseline suggests relative dehydration or overfeeding of protein, particularly if nitrogen balance is positive. Reduce the amount of protein being given. However, if values continue to increase, suspect acute renal injury. Even in established renal failure, patients continue to require large amounts of protein. Protein restriction should be avoided, even if doing so commits the patient to hemodialysis.

Complications of Enteral Nutrition

Technical complications

Placement of enteral feeding tubes is easier and less dangerous than the central venous access required for TPN. Nonetheless, serious complications can occur, particularly if feedings are started before tube position is verified. Tubes placed blindly through the nose can be advanced into the trachea or bronchi, or even perforate the lung; administering feedings through such tubes can produce serious pneumonia, empyema, or even death. Some authors have advocated the routine placement of gastrostomy or jejunostomy tubes in trauma patients who require initial laparotomy.[7] This circumstance rarely occurs in burn patients, but if laparotomy is indicated, surgically placed feeding tubes can be used. These tubes are associated with risks of dislodgement, leakage, and bowel perforation.

Feeding-related complications

As noted previously, aspiration of tube feedings is a risk of any enteral feeding regimen, and may occur more frequently than is apparent on clinical exam. Check gastric residuals regularly in all patients given gastric feeds; this can be done in patients with jejunal tubes as well, if they require NG tubes for gastric decompression. The sudden finding of high residuals in these patients may suggest that the feeding tube has pulled back into the stomach (or the NG tube has migrated through the pylorus). Confirm tube placement with an abdominal X-ray. If patients receiving enteral feedings develop nausea, abdominal pain, or distension, consider holding or reducing feedings.

Bowel necrosis and perforation

A number of recent reports have documented bowel necrosis and perforation as a complication of enteral nutrition in the critically ill, including burn patients.[109–111] Though this is thankfully a rare complication, it is believed that continued administration of tube feedings in the face of decreased bowel motility causes distension, interfering with intestinal blood supply. Bacterial overgrowth of stagnant, glucose-containing tube feedings, and overzealous administration of narcotics and antidiarrheal agents may also contribute to this complication.[7,110] Perform a careful clinical examination of all patients daily. Fever, leukocytosis, tachycardia, and abdominal distension may precede frank peritonitis. Abdominal CT scanning can confirm perforation. Perform immediate laparotomy with resection of necrotic bowel in any patient suspected of having this complication. Mortality rates approximate 50%.[111]

Diarrhea

Tube feedings frequently cause diarrhea, which can be a minor problem, or a major source of patient discomfort, morbidity, fluid and electrolyte imbalance, and other complications Often the cause is multifactorial.[112] The high glucose loads of tube feedings may contribute to diarrhea, though diluting feedings has not proved helpful in treatment. Medications given enterally, including antacids, phosphates, antibiotics, and other supplements contribute to diarrhea as well. Infectious causes include cytomegalovirus infection,[113] and pseudomembranous colitis caused by *Clostridium difficile*.[114] A prospective study by Gottschlich *et al.* found an association between the concentration of fat in tube feedings and the incidence of diarrhea;[115] a subsequent study showed a reduction in the incidence of diarrhea in a group of children fed a diet low in fat, and supplemented with glutamine, arginine, and vitamins (see 'Immune-enhancing diets', below).[115] Because the gut's tolerance of tube feedings is limited, diarrhea is a frequent complication of overfeeding that can be controlled by reducing infusion rate.

A variety of compounds have been suggested for treatment of diarrhea, including opiates (Imodium™, Lomotil™, Paregoric, etc.), bulk agents (Metamucil™), and others. Some clinicians advocate the use of fiber-containing tube feedings to reduce this complication. Fiber is a normal component of nutrition, and its presence may help prevent bacterial overgrowth and stasis.[116] However, these compounds may favor intestinal stasis and bowel necrosis.[110] In addition, adding such agents to tube feedings may clog small-diameter tubes, and prove a real nuisance for nursing staff. In our experience, attempts to control diarrhea with medications are often either ineffective, or lead to constipation and distension. Infectious diarrheas may be worsened significantly by slowing intestinal transit. Most diarrhea is self-limited, and does not require pharmacologic therapy. Try altering the tube formula, stopping enteral medications, reducing the infusion rate, or simply waiting a day or two. If diarrhea is unresponsive to simple treatments, specific drug therapy may be indicated. Also consider more serious contributing factors, including infectious diarrhea, sepsis,[117] or intestinal ischemia. It may be necessary to hold feedings temporarily to permit refractory diarrhea to resolve, then restart them gradually.

Complications of Parenteral Nutrition

Technical complications of TPN

Technical complications are those associated with line placement and maintenance. These complications are infrequent, but they can be life-threatening, and demand close attention to protocols for line care. Complications can occur at the time of line placement, and include pneumothorax, hemothorax, pericardial tamponade, hydrothorax, and catheter misplacement. These complications can also occur later in the course of TPN therapy if lines erode through venous structures. Indwelling central venous lines can cause hemorrhage or air embolism if disconnected inadvertently. In addition, central lines are prone to the development of serious infections, including catheter sepsis, septic thrombophlebitis, and even endocarditis; not surprisingly, these infectious complications are more common when catheters are placed through cutaneous burn wounds.[118] Central lines used for TPN are particularly prone to infectious problems, and risk is increased if lines are left in place for long periods, and if they are used for multiple purposes (blood draws, hemodynamic monitoring, antibiotics, maintenance fluids, etc.). Consider changing central venous catheters, especially TPN lines, in any patients with persistent, unexplained fevers, or other evidence of infection.

Metabolic complications of TPN

Metabolic complications of TPN are sometimes the most severe, and can be difficult to treat. Almost any disorder of electrolyte or vitamin deficiency or excess can be seen following TPN, but the most common include:

- *Hyperglycemia* occurs almost invariably to some extent following TPN administration. This can be a particular problem in burn patients, who require large caloric loads, and who are predisposed to hyperglycemia due to elevated catecholamine levels. Monitor blood sugar levels carefully during TPN administration See **Table 20.5** for an example of a monitoring protocol.

- *Fluid imbalance.* Fluid overload can result from the administration of large volumes of TPN. Poorly nourished patients may tolerate a sudden bolus of sodium and water poorly, leading to edema formation and fluid overload. In contrast, untreated hyperglycemia can cause an osmotic diuresis, leading to volume depletion. Monitor fluid balance carefully, particularly when beginning TPN.
- *Hyperosmolarity* can result when large volumes of hypertonic glucose solutions are given too quickly. This can be potentiated by hyperglycemia, hypernatremia, and underlying dehydration.
- *Hypokalemia* can be associated with TPN administration, as potassium is taken up during anabolism, or lost in the urine from obligatory diuresis produced by hyperglycemia.
- *Hypophosphatemia* occurs frequently with initiation of TPN. Phosphorus is utilized for protein synthesis, and available phosphorus is often consumed within 48 hours of starting TPN. Unless phosphorus is replaced with the TPN mixture, a variety of systemic effects can occur, including weakness, numbness, red cell dysfunction, seizures, and cardiomyopathy. Phosphate is included in 'standard' electrolytes for TPN (**Table 20.5**), but additional supplementation may be required.
- *Fatty acid deficiency.* Though rarely seen today, essential fatty acid deficiency is a serious complication of prolonged TPN, resulting in intestinal malabsorption and diarrhea, hair loss, poor wound healing (particularly cutaneous wounds such as burns), thrombocytopenia, and anemia. Giving lipid emulsions are infrequently as once or twice per week will eliminate this problem.

Future directions in burn nutrition

Immune-Enhancing Diets

Even the earliest efforts to nourish burn patients sought to define an 'ideal' nutritional mixture for nutritional support. Recognition of the need for large amounts of protein led to early diets supplemented with eggs or milk.[18] Modern efforts have utilized knowledge of the biochemical alterations that accompany burns, and focused on the use of components that appear to improve immune function and wound healing. These components, reviewed above, include glutamine, arginine, ω-3 FFAs, and others. A variety of mixtures supplemented with these ingredients have been developed for clinical use, group under the term 'immune-enhancing diets' (IEDs).

In an early study, Gottschlich *et al.* evaluated three dietary regimens in a group of children with severe burns. One group was given a prototype, custom-made 'modular tube feeding' (MTF) diet, containing ω-3 FFAs, arginine, histidine, and vitamins A and C. Patients fed the MTF diet had significantly fewer wound infections, shorter lengths of hospitalization, and a trend toward improved survival, compared to two control groups fed commercially-available tube feedings (TraumaCal™ and Osmolite™).[119]

A number of subsequent studies have evaluated IEDs in a variety of clinical settings; most have demonstrated improvements in

biochemical markets of immunity and wound healing, and/or clinical parameters, including infection rates, incidence of multiple organ failure, or hospital stay.[120–123] This topic has been the subject of recently published reviews and meta-analyses, which conclude that evidence supports a beneficial effect of IEDs on the incidence of infections and length of hospital stay in patients with trauma and critical illness.[124–126] No effect on mortality has been documented, however.

Although evidence is accumulating in support of clinical efficacy of IEDs, many of the studies performed to date have significant flaws. In early studies, patients fed IEDs received significantly more calories or protein than 'control' patients,[120] though subsequent studies comparing isocaloric, isonitrogenous diets have tended to validate their findings.[122] Some studies demonstrated benefits only in selected subgroups of patients, or fed patients for very short periods of time. In addition, little information has been obtained on the use of available IEDs in burn patients. Saffle *et al.* conducted a randomized, controlled trial of a highly publicized IED (Impact™) with another commercially available, high-protein 'stress' solution (Replete™).[127] They found no differences in major outcome variables. One criticism of this study is that both solutions contained significant amounts of ω-3 FFAs, though they differed in their contents of vitamin A, arginine, and RNA (both feedings also contained significantly more fat than the modular tube feeding of Gottschlich *et al.*). In addition, previous reviews found no benefit to IEDs in reducing incidence of pneumonia,[126] which is a frequent and serious problem for burn patients, particularly those suffering inhalation injury. Finally, it should be remembered that the high volume of feedings required by burn patients may mean that a satisfactory *dose* of some immune-enhancing nutrients are delivered even with the use of conventional, non-'immune enhancing' diets. The entire issue of IEDs is further confounded by the fact that the effects of individual components have not been evaluated in human trials. It remains unknown which, if any, of the components of IEDs produce the beneficial effects sometimes observed, or if specific components might even be harmful to patients.

At present, use of IEDs in nourishing burn patients is not widespread. While the efficacy of these specialized formulas is under investigation, it is clear that some aspects of 'burn-specific' nutrition have been clearly demonstrated, and should be utilized in caring for all burn patients.

Hormonal Manipulation of Burn Hypermetabolism

As stated previously, the metabolic response to burn injury is produced by increased levels of several catabolic hormones, including catecholamines, cortisol, and glucagon. Awareness of these influences has led investigators to attempt to reduce hypermetabolism and protein wasting by manipulating this hormonal environment in a variety of ways, including blocking catecholamines with propranolol, administering agents with counter-regulatory effects (insulin, insulin-like growth factor-1 [IGF-1]), or use of anabolic hormones such as growth hormone, testosterone, or synthetic anabolic agents such as oxandrolone.[128,129] Although some of these methods show promise for widespread clinical use, it must be remembered that the hormonal milieu which accompanies burn injury is extremely complex and incompletely understood. Additional research will be needed to confirm the efficacy and safety of these techniques.

β-Blockade

Several recent studies have evaluated the effect of administration of supplemental propranolol, a β-antagonist, on the hypermetabolism of burn injury. Herndon *et al.* have demonstrated consistent reductions in heart rate and cardiac work following intravenous or oral propranolol.[130–132] Metabolic rate was not reduced in these studies, but modest reductions in resting metabolic expenditure has been shown with propranolol administration by other authors.[133] Propranolol appeared to reduce lipolysis in this setting, but short-term administration did not change, or perhaps increased, proteolysis.[130] Recently, however, this group has demonstrated that more prolonged administration of β-blockers enhanced measured net muscle synthesis in burned extremities using stable isotope techniques.[128]

Growth hormone

Growth hormone is an anabolic hormone that antagonizes the effects of catecholamines and cortisol. Secretion of growth hormone is depressed following burn injury.[134] Studies in burn and ICU patients of the effect of exogenous recombinant human growth hormone (rHGH) demonstrated modest reductions in nitrogen excretion, improved healing of skin graft donor sites, and reduced length of hospital stay, compared to control groups.[135–137] In children, growth hormone therapy produced decreased synthesis of C-reactive protein, a marker of enhanced inflammation and sepsis,[138] and increased synthesis of retinol-binding protein, and albumin, with no increase in mortality or serious side-effects.[139] In two small, non-randomized clinical trials in burned adults, administration of rHGH was associated with significantly improved survival.[140,141] Other studies have not demonstrated this finding, possibly because mortality rates in control groups were already very low. In contrast, a recent report of two large controlled trials from Europe found a twofold increase in mortality in ICU patients given rHGH.[142] Demling postulated that this finding arose from the transient increase in proinflammatory response caused by growth hormone, which could be harmful to elderly ICU patients, but would probably not affect burn patients, whose inflammation is already maximally stimulated.[143] Growth hormone has been used in the treatment of a wide range of catabolic illnesses, including respiratory failure,[144] AIDS,[145] trauma,[146,147] and others, with apparent benefits. Nonetheless, this widely divergent experience underscores the limitation of our understanding of the inflammatory and metabolic responses to acute injury, and the potential dangers of attempting to manipulate them. Widespread adoption of the use of growth hormone and other metabolic mediators in clinical burn care will need to await confirmation of safety and efficacy in large, multicenter trials.

Insulin/insulin-like growth factor-I

Growth hormone appears to exert some of its effect on metabolic rate through stimulation of IGF-I, which does not produce the hyperglycemia seen with administration of rHGH. Levels of IGF-I are decreased in burn patients,[148,149] and are restored following administration of rHGH.[150] In animal and clinical studies, administration of IGF-I is associated with reductions in metabolic rate and depletion of lean body mass, and improved weight gain.[151,152] Insulin itself appears to have similar beneficial effects on protein metabolism and wound healing. In two small clinical studies, infusions of low-dose supplemental insulin in burn patients produced increased muscle protein synthesis and slightly improved healing of skin graft donor sites.[153,154]

Synthetic anabolic hormones

Androgens, including testosterone, are another class of anabolic hormones which are suppressed in burn patients.[155] Testosterone and similar agents have been used in a variety of settings to enhance muscle mass and strength. Oral analogs, including the drug oxandrolone, prolong bioavailability and reduce costs and difficulty of administration.[129] In a prospective, randomized trial in patients with major burns, Demling found that administration of either oxandrolone, 20 mg/day, or HGH 0.1 mg/kg/day, was associated with significantly reduced weight loss, improved nitrogen balance, and accelerated healing of donor sites, compared to control patients. Use of HGH was associated with significant hyperglycemia, which was not seen with oxandrolone.[156] In a second randomized, controlled study, the same group confirmed these metabolic effects of oxandrolone, and again noted no significant complications associated with use of this agent.[157] In a study of convalescing burn patients, administration of oxandrolone produced increased weight gain and improved physical function compared to control patients.[158]

The manipulation of hypermetabolism is obviously an area of great current interest. Recently, the group from Shriners Hospital in Galveston summarized their experience with several controlled trials anabolic agents – including propranolol, rHGH, IGF-I, and oxandrolone, alone or in various combinations. They demonstrated consistent reduction of negative nitrogen balance in these studies, using stable-isotope assessment of net protein balance in burned extremities. They commented that 'most sub-populations of the severely burned do receive significant clinical gain from anabolic treatment.' At present, it remains a matter of opinion whether sufficient information is available to justify utilization of any of these therapies in general clinical practice, and exactly which patients should receive these treatments. In the years ahead, this field may represent the next major advance in the metabolic therapy of thermally injured patients.

References

1. Cuthbertson D. The disturbance of metabolism produced by bony and nonbody injury with notes of certain abnormal conditions of bone. *Biochem J* 1930; **24**: 1244–63.
2. Cuthbertson D, Zagreb H. The metabolic response to injury and its nutritional implications: retrospect and prospect. *JPEN* 1979; **3**: 108–29.
3. Long C, Schaffel N, Geiger C, et al. Metabolic response to injury and illness: estimation of energy and protein needs from indirect calorimetry and nitrogen balance. *JPEN* 1979; **3**: 452–6.
4. Wilmore D, Long J, Mason A, et al. Catecholamines: mediators of the hypermetabolic response to thermal injury. *Ann Surg* 1974; **180**: 653–68.
5. Newsome T, Mason A, Pruitt B. Weight loss following thermal injury. *Ann Surg* 1973; **178**: 215–7.
6. Wilmore D. Nutrition and metabolism following thermal injury. *Clin Plas Surg* 1974; **1**: 603–19.
7. Kudsk K, Brown R. Nutritional support. In: Mattox K, Feliciano D, Moore E, eds. *Trauma*. McGraw-Hill: New York, 2000: 1369–405.
8. Demling R, Seigne P. Metabolic management of patients with severe burns. *World J Surg* 2000; **24**: 673–80.
9. Bessey P, Jiang Z, Johnson D, Smith R, Wilmore D. Posttraumatic skeletal muscle proteolysis: the role of the hormonal environment. *World J Surg* 1989; **13**: 465–70.
10. Long C, Kinney J, Geiger J. Nonsuppressibility of gluconeogenesis by glucose in septic patients. *Metabolism* 1976; **25**: 193.
11. Saffle J, Medine E, Raymond J, et al. Use of indirect calorimetry in the nutritional management of burn patients. *J Trauma* 1985; **25**: 32–9.

12. Turner W, Ireton C. Hunt J, Purdue G. Predicting energy expenditures in burn patients. *J Trauma* 1985; **25**: 11–16.

13. Hildreth M, Herndon D, Desai M, Boremeling L. Current treatment reduces calories required to maintain weight in pediatric patients with burns. *J Burn Care Rehabil* 1990; **11**: 405–9.

14. Ireton D, Turner W, Hunt J, *et al.* Evaluation of energy expenditures in burn patients. *J Am Diet Assoc* 1986; **86**: 331–3.

15. Rutan T, Herndon D, VanOsten T, Abston S. Metabolic rate alterations in early excision and grafting versus conservative treatment. *J Trauma* 1986; **26**: 140–6.

16. Barton R, Craft W, Saffle J. Chemical paralysis reduces energy expenditure in mechanically ventilated trauma patients. *J Burn Care Rehabil* 1997; **18**: 461–8.

17. Baker J, Detsky A, Wesson D, *et al.* Nutritional assessment: a comparison of clinical judgement and objective measurements. *N Engl J Med* 1982; **306**: 969–72.

18. Ireton-Jones C, Gottschlich M. The evolution of nutrition support in burns. *J Burn Care Rehabil* 1993; **14**: 272–80.

19. Curreri P, Richmond D, Marvin J, Baxter C. Dietary requirements of patients with major burns. *J Am Diet Assoc* 1974; **65**: 415–17.

20. Davies J, Liljedahl S. Metabolic consequences of an extensive burn. In: Polk H, ed. *Contemporary Burn Management.* Boston: Little Brown, 1971: 151–69.

21. *Recommended Dietary Allowances*, 10 ed. Washington, DC: National Academy of Sciences, 1989.

22. Harris J, Benedict F. *A Biometric Study of Basal Metabolism in Man.* Washington, DC: Carnegie Institute of Washington, 1919.

23. Day T, Dean P, Adams M, *et al.* Nutritional requirements of the burned child: The Curreri Junior formula. *Proc Am Burn Assoc* 1986; **18**: 86.

24. Food and Nutrition Board. *National Research Council Recommended Dietary Allowances.* Washington, DC: National Academy of Sciences, 1980.

25. Hildreth M, Herndon D, Desai M, *et al.* Current treatment reduces calories required to maintain weight in pediatric patients with burns. *J Burn Care Rehabil* 1990; **11**: 405–9.

26. Hildreth M, Herndon D, Desai M, *et al.* Caloric requirements of patients with burns under one years of age. *J Burn Care Rehabil* 1993; **14**: 108–12.

27. Hildreth M, Herndon D, Desai M, *et al.* Caloric needs of adolescent patients with burns. *J Burn Care Rehabil* 1989; **10**: 523–6.

28. Burszstein S, Glaser P, Trichet B, *et al.* Utilization of protein, carboydrate, and fat in fasting and postabsorptive subjects. *Am J Clin Nutr* 1980; **33**: 998–1001.

29. Weir J. New methods for calculating metabolic rate with special reference to protein metabolism. *J Physiol* 1949; **109**: 1–9.

30. Ireton-Jones C, Turner W. The use of respiratory quotient to determine the efficacy of nutrition support regimens. *J Am Diet Assoc* 1987; **87**: 1880–3.

31. Shaw-Delanty S, Elwyn D, Askanazi J, *et al.* Resting energy expenditure in injured, septic, and malnourished adult patients on intravenous diets. *Clin Nutr* 1990; **9**: 305–12.

32. Hester D, Lawson K. Suggested guidelines for use by dietitians in the interpretation of indirect calorimetry data. *J Am Diet Assoc* 1989; **89**: 100–1.

33. Peck M. Practice guidelines for burn care: nutritional support. *J Burn Care Rehabil* 2001; (in press).

34. Gottschlich M, Alexander J, Bower R. Enteral nutrition in patients with burns or trauma. In: Rombeau J, Cladwell M, eds. *Enternal and Tube Feeding.* Philadelphia: WB, Saunders, 1984: 306–24.

35. Swinamer D, Phang P, Jones R, *et al.* Twenty-four hour energy expenditure in critically ill Patients. *Crit Care Med* 1987; **15**: 637–41.

36. Saffle J, Larson C, Sullivan J. A randomized trial of indirect calorimetry-based feedings in thermal injury. *J Trauma* 1990; **30**: 776–83.

37. Mayes T, Gottschlich M, Burns. In: Matarese L, Gottschlich M, eds. *Contemporary Nutrition Support Practice: A Clinical Guide.* Philadelphia: WB Saunders, 1998: 590–607.

38. Wolfe R, Allsop J, Burke J. Glucose metabolism in man: responses to intravenous glucose infusion. *Metabolism* 1979; **28**: 210–17.

39. Wolfe R, Goodenough R, Burke J, Wolfe M. Response of proteins and urea kinetics in burn patients to different levels of protein intake. *Ann Surg* 1983; **197**: 163–71.

40. Alexander J, MacMillan B, Stinnet J, *et al.* Beneficial effects of aggressive protein feeding in severely burned children. *Ann Surg* 1980; **192**: 505–17.

41. Cunningham J, Lydon M, Russell W. Calorie and protein provision for recovery from severe burns in infants and young children. *Am J Clin Nutr* 1990; **51**: 553–7.

42. Matsuda T, Kagan R, Hanumadass M, Jonasson O. The importance of burn wound size in determining the optimal calorie: nitrogen ratio. *Surgery* 1983; **94**: 562–8.

43. Prelack K, Cunningham J, Sheridan R, Tompkins R. Energy and protein provisions for thermally injured children revisited: an outcome-based approach for determining requirements. *J Burn Care Rehabil*, 1997; **18**: 177–81.

44. Waymack J, Herndon D. Nutritional support of the burned patient. *World J Surg* 1992; **16**: 80–6.

45. Hishikawa K, Nakaki T, Tsuda M, *et al.* Effect of systemic L-arginine administration on hemodynamics and nitric oxide release in man. *Jpn Heart J* 1992; **33**: 41–8.

46. Kirk S, Barbul A. Role of arginine in trauma, sepsis, and immunity. *JPEN* 1990; **14**: 226S.

47. Kirk S, Barbul A. Role of arginine in trauma, sepsis, and immunity. *JPEN* 1990; **14**: 226S.

48. Barbul A, Sisto D, Wasserkrug H, *et al.* Arginine stimulates lymphocyte immune response in healthy human beings. *Surgery* 1981; **90**: 244–8.

49. Barbul A, Larzarrow S, Efron O. Arginine enhances wound healing and lymphocyte immune response in humans. *Surgery* 1990; **108**: 331–5.

50. Saito H, Trocki O, Wang S, *et al.* Metabolic and immune effects of dietary arginine supplementation after burn. *Arch Surg* 1987; **122**: 785–9.

51. Souba W. Glutamine: a key substrate for the splanchnic bed. *Ann Rev Nutr* 1991; **11**: 285–9.

52. Barton R. Nutrition support in critical illness. *Nutr Clin Pract* 1994; **9**: 127–31.

53. Alverdy J. Effects of glutamine-supplemented diets on immunology of the gut. *JPEN* 1990; **14**: 109S–13S.

54. Ziegler T, Young L, Benfell K, *et al.* Clinical and metabolic efficacy of glutamine supplemented parenteral nutrition after bone marrow transplantation: a randomized, double-blind controlled trial. *Ann Int Med* 1992; **116**: 821–30.

55. Hwang T, O'Dwyer S, Smith R, *et al.* Preservation of small bowel mucosa using glutamine-enriched parenteral nutrition. *Surg Forum* 1980; **37**: 56–8.

56. Cerra F, Mazuski J, Chute E, *et al.* Branched-chain metabolic support: a prospective, randomized, double-blind trial in surgical stress. *Ann Surg* 1984; **199**: 286–91.

57. Cerra F, Hirsch J, Mullen K, *et al.* The effect of stress level, amino acid formula, and nitrogen dose on nitrogen retention in traumatic and septic stress. *Ann Surg* 1987; **205**: 282–7.

58. Mochizuki H, Trocki O, Dominioni L, Alexander J. Effect of a diet rich in branched chain amino acids on severly burned guinea pigs. *J Trauma* 1986; **26**: 1077–85.

59. Yu Y, Wagner D, Walesreswki J, Burke J, Young V. A kinetic study of leucine metabolism in severely burned patients. Comparison between conventional and branched-chain amino acid enriched nutritional therapy. *Ann Surg* 1988; **207**: 421–90.

60. Mochizuki H, Trocki O, Dominioni L, *et al.* Optimal lipid content for enteral diets following thermal injury. *JPEN* 1984; **8**: 638–46.

61. Garrel D, Razi M, Lariviere R. Improved clinical status and length of care with low-fat nutrition support in burn patients. *JPEN* 1995; **19**: 482–91.

62. Alexander J, Saito H, Trocki O, Ogle C. The importance of lipid type in the diet after burn injury. *Ann Surg* 1986; **204**: 1–8.

63. Gamliel Z, DeBiasse M, Demling R. Essential microminerals and their response to burn injury. *J Burn Care Rehabil* 1996; **17**: 264–72.

64. Gottschlich M, Warden G. Vitamin supplementation in the patient with burns. *J Burn Care Rehabil* 1990; **11**: 275–9.

65. Caldwell M, Kennedy-Caldwell C, Micronutrients and enteral nutrition. In: Rombeau J, Caldwell M, eds. *Enteral and Tube Feeding.* Philadelphia: WB Saunders, 1984: 84–126.

66. Rock C, Dechert R, Khilnani R, Parker R, Rodriguez J. Carotenoids and antioxidant vitamins in patients after burn injury. *J Burn Care Rehabil* 1997; **18**: 269–78.

67. Mayes T, Gottschlich M, Warden G. Clinical nutrition protocols for continuous quality improvement in the outcomes of patients with burns. *J Burn Care Rehabil* 1997; **18**: 365–8.

68. Selmanpakoglu ACC, Sayal A, Isimer A. Trace element (Al, Se, Zn, Cu) levels in serum, urine, and tissues of burn patients. *Burns* 1994; **20**: 99–103.

69. Hunt D, Lane H, Beesinger D, *et al.* Selenium depletion in burn patients. *JPEN* 1984; **8**: 695–9.

70. Shippee R, Wilson S, King N. Trace mineral supplementation of burn patients: a national survey. *J Am Diet Assoc* 1987; **87**: 300–3.

71. Dudrick S, Wilmore D, Vars H, *et al.* Long-term parenteral nutrition with growth, development, and positive nitrogen balance. *Surgery* 1968; **64**: 134–9.

72. Steinberg E, Anderson G. Implications of medicare's prospective payment system for specialized nutrition services: the 'Hopkins' report. *Nutr Clin Pract* 1986; **1**: 12–28.

73. Popp M, Law E, MacMillan B. Parenteral nutrition in the burned child: a study of twenty-six patients. *Ann Surg* 1974; **179**: 219–25.

74. Wilmore D, Moylan J, Helmkamp G, *et al.* Clinical evaluation of a 10% intravenous fat emulsion for parenteral nutrition in thermally injured patients. *Ann Surg* 1973; **178**: 503–13.

75. Alverdy J, Aoys E, Moss G. Total parenteral nutrition promotes bacterial translocation from the gut. *Surgery* 1988; **104**: 185–90.

76. Eastwood G. Small bowel morphology and epithelial proliferation in intravenously alimented rabbits. *Surgery* 1977; **82**: 13–20.

77. Rombeau J, Barot L. Enteral nutritional therapy. *Surg Clin N Am* 1981; **61**: 605–20.

78. Saito H, Trocki O, Alexander J, *et al*. The effect of route of nutrient administration on the nutritional state, catabolic hormone secretion and gut mucosal integrity after burn injury. *JPEN* 1987; **11**: 1–7.

79. Fong Y, Marano M, Barber E, *et al*. Total parenteral nutrition and bowel rest modify the metabolic response to endotoxin in humans. *Ann Surg* 1989; **210**: 449–54.

80. Kudsk K, Croce M, Fabian T, *et al*. Enternal vs. parenteral feeding: effects on septic morbidity following blunt and penetrating abdominal trauma. *Ann Surg* 1992; **215**: 503–8.

81. Moore F, Fliciano D, Andrassy R, *et al*. TEN vs. TPN following major abdominal trauma – reduced septic morbidity. *J Trauma* 1989; **29**.

82. Border J, Hassett J, LaDuca J, *et al*. The gut origin septic states in blunt multiple trauma (ISS = 40) in the ICU. *Ann Surg* 1987; **206**: 427–32.

83. Herndon D, Barrow R, Stein M, *et al*. Increased mortality with intravenous supplemental feeding in severely burned patients. *J Burn Care Rehabil* 1989; **10**: 309–13.

84. Herndon D, Stein M, Rutan T, *et al*. Failure of TPN supplementation to improve liver function, immunity, and mortality in thermally injured patients. *J Trauma* 1987; **27**: 195–204.

85. Mochizuki H, Trocki O, Dominioni L, *et al*. Mechanism of prevention of postburn hypermetabolism and catabolism by early enteral feeding. *Ann Surg* 1984; **200**: 297–310.

86. Wood R, Caldwell F, Bowser-Wallace B. The effect of early feeding on postburn hypermetabolism. *J Trauma* 1988; **28**: 177–83.

87. Chiarelli A, Enzi G, Casadei A, *et al*. Very early nutrition supplementation in burned patients. *Am J Clin Nutr* 1990; **51**: 1035–9.

88. McDonald W, Sharp D, Deitch E. Immediate enternal feeding in burn patients is safe and effective. *Ann Surg* 1991; **213**: 177–83.

89. Moore E, Jones T. Benefits of immediate jejunostomy feeding after major abdominal trauma – a prospective, randomized study. *J Trauma* 1988; **26**: 874–81.

90. Jenkins M, Gottschlich M, Mayes T, *et al*. Enteral feeding during operative procedures. *J Burn Care Rehabil* 1994; **15**: 199–295.

91. Kearns P, Chin D, Mueller L, *et al*. The incidence of ventilator-associated pneumonia and success in nutrient delivery with gastric vs. small intestinal feeding: a randomized clinical trial. *Crit Care Med* 2000; **28**: 1742–6.

92. Gump F, Kinney J. Energy balance and weight loss in burned patients. *Arch Surg* 1971; **103**: 442–8.

93. Streat S, Beddoe A, Hill G. Aggressive nutritional support does not prevent protein loss despite fat gain in septic intensive care patients. *J Trauma* 1987; **27**: 262–6.

94. Zdolsek H, Lindahl O, Augquist K, Sjoberg F. Non-invasive assessment of intercompartmental fluid shifts in burn victims. *Burns* 1998; **24**: 233–40.

95. Rodriguez D. Nutrition in patients with severe burns: state of the art. *J Burn Care Rehabil* 1996; **17**: 62–70.

96. Konstantinides F, Radmer W, Becker W, *et al*. Inaccuracy of nitrogen balance determinations in thermal injury with calculated total urinary nitrogen. *J Burn Care Rehabil* 1992; **13**: 254–60.

97. Rettmer R, Williamson J, Labbe R, Heimbach D. Laboratory monitoring of nutrition status in burn patients. *Clin Chem* 1992; **38**: 334–7.

98. Gottschlich M, Warden G, Michel M, *et al*. Diarrhea in tube-fed burn patients: incidence, etiology, nutritional impact, and prevention. *JPEN* 1988; **12**: 338–45.

99. Greenhalgh D, Housinger T, Kagan R, *et al*. Maintenance of serum albumin levels in pediatric burn patients: a prospective randomized trial. *J Trauma* 1995; **39**: 67–73.

100. Cynober L, Prugnaud O, Lioret H, *et al*. Serum transthyretin levels in patients with burn injury. *Surgery* 1991; **109**: 640–4.

101. Manelli J, Badetii C, Botti G, Golstein M. A reference standard for plasma proteins is required for nutritional assessment of adult burn patients. *Burns* 1998; **24**: 337–45.

102. Meakins J, Pietsch J, Bubenik O. Delayed hypersensitivity: indicator of acquired failure of host defenses in sepsis and trauma. *Ann Surg* 1977; **186**: 241–50.

103. Pietsch J, Meakins J. Delayed hypersensitivity response: application in clinical surgery. *Surgery* 1977; **82**: 349–55.

104. Williamson J. Actual burn nutrition care practices: a national survey (Part II). *J Burn Care Rehabil* 1989; **10**: 185–94.

105. Askanazi J, Rosenbaum S, Hyman A, *et al*. Respiratory changes induced by the large glucose loads of total parenteral nutrition. *JAMA* 1980; **243**: 1444–7.

106. Iapichino G, Radrizzani D. Parenteral nutrition. In: Webb A, *et al*., eds. *Oxford Textbook of Critical Care*. New York: Oxford University Press, 1999: 398–401.

107. Lowry S, Brennan M. Abnormal liver function during parenteral nutrition: relation to infusion excess. *J Surg Res* 1979; **26**: 300–7.

108. Grant W, Eyre G, Morris S, Saffle J. Acute renal failure in thermally-injured patients: a retrospective 15-years study. *J Burn Care Rehabil*, 2001 (in press).

109. Kowal-Vern A, McGill V, Gamelli R. Ischemic necrotic bowel disease in thermal injury. *Arch Surg* 1997; **132**: 440–3.

110. Scaife C, Saffle J, Morris S. Intestinal obstruction secondary to enteral feedings in burn trauma patients. *Proceedings of the Western Trauma Association*, Crested Butte, CO, February 1999.

111. Marvin R, McKinley B, McQuiggan M, Cocanour C, Moore F. Nonocclusive blowel necrosis occurring in critically ill trauma patients receiving enteral nutrition manifests no reliable clinical signs for early detection. *Am J Surg* 2000; **179**: 7–12.

112. Eisenberg P. Causes of diarrhea in tube-fed patients: a comprehensive approach to diagnosis and management. *Nutr Clin Pract* 1993; **8**: 119–23.

113. Kealey G, Aguiar J, Lewis R, *et al*. Cadaver skin allografts and transmission of human cytomegaolvirus to burn patients. *J Am Coll Surg* 1996; **182**: 201–5.

114. Grube B, Heimbach C, Marvin J. *Clostridium difficile* diarrhea in critically ill burn patients. *Arch Surg* 1987; **122**: 655–61.

115. Gottschlich M, Warden G, Michel M, *et al*. Diarrhea in tube-fed burn patients: incidence, etiology, nutritional impact, and prevention. *JPEN* 1988; **12**: 338–45.

116. Frankenfeld D, Beyer P. Dietary fiber and bowel function in tube-fed patients. *J Am Diet Assoc* 1991; **91**: 590–6.

117. Wolf S, Jeschke M, Rose J, Desai M, Herndon D. Enteral feeding intolerance: an indicator of sepsis-associated mortality in burned children. *Arch Surg* 1997; **132**: 1310–13.

118. Gottschlich M, Warden G. Parenteral nutrition in the burned patients. In: Fischer J, ed. *Total Parenteral Nutrition*, 2nd edn. Boston: Little Brown, 1991.

119. Gottschlich M, Jenkins M, Warden G, *et al*. Differential effects of three enteral dietary regimens on selected outcome variables in burn patients. *JPEN* 1990; **14**: 225–36.

120. Moore F, Moore E, Kudsk K, *et al*. Clinical benefits of an immune-enhancing diet for ealy post-injury feeding. *J Trauma* 1994; **27**: 607.

121. Bower R, Cerra F, Bershadshy B, *et al*. Early enteral administration of a formula (Impact™) supplemented with arginine, nucleotides, and fish oil in intensive care unit patients: results of a multicenter, prospective, randomized clinical trial. *Crit Care Med* 1995; **23**: 436.

122. Kudsk K, Minard G, Croce M, *et al*. A randomized trial of isonitrogenous enteral diets following severe trauma: an immune-enhancing diet reduces septic complications. *Ann Surg* 1996; **224**: 531.

123. Daly J, Lieberman M, Godlfine J, *et al*. Enteral nutrition with supplemental arginine, RNA, and omega-3 fatty acids in patients after operation: immunologic, metabolic, and clinical outcome. *Surgery* 1992; **112**: 56.

124. Beale R, Bryg D, Bihari D. Immunonutrition in the critically ill: a systematic review of clinical outcome. *Crit Care Med* 1999; **27**: 2729–2805.

125. Barton R. Immune-enhancing enteral formulas: are they beneficial in critically-ill patients? *Nutr Clin Pract* 1997; **12**: 61–2.

126. Heys S, Walker L, Smith I, Eremin O. Enteral nutritional supplementation with key nutrients in patients with critical illness and cancer: a meta-analysis of randomized controlled trials. *Ann Surg* 1999; **229**: 467–77.

127. Saffle J, Wiebke G, Jennings K, Morris S, Barton R. Randomized trial of immune-enhancing enteral nutrition in burn patients. *J Trauma* 1997; **42**: 793–802.

128. Hart D, Wolf S, Chinkes D, *et al*. Determinants of catabolism after severe burn. *Ann Surg* 2000; **232**: 455–65.

129. Demling R, Signe P. Metabolic management of patients with severe burns. *World J Surg* 2000; **24**: 673–80.

130. Herndon D, Barrow R, Rutan T, *et al*. Effect of propranolol administration on hemodynamic and metabolic responses of burned pediatric patients. *Ann Surg* 1988; **208**: 484–92.

131. Baron P, Barrow R, Pierre E, Herndon D. Prolonged use of propranolol safely decreases cardiac work in burned children. *J Burn Care Rehabil* 1997; **18**: 223–7.

132. Minifee P, Barrow R, Abston S, Desai M, Herndon D. Improved myocardial oxygen utilization following propranolol infusion in adolescents with postburn hypermetabolism. *J Pediatr Surg* 1989; **24**: 806–10.

133. Breitenstein E, Chiolero R, Jequier E, *et al*. Effects of beta-blockade on energy metabolism following burns. *Burns* 1990; **16**: 259–64.

134. Jeffries M, Vance M. Growth hormone and cortisol secretion in patients with burn injury. *J Burn Care Rehabil* 1992; **13**: 391–5.

135. Ziegler T, Young L, Ferrari-Baiviera E, Demling R, Wilmore D. Use of human growth hormone combined with nutritional support in a critical care unit. *JPEN* 1990; **14**: 574–81.

136. Herndon D, Barrow R, Kunkel K, Broemling L, Rutan R. Effects of recombinant human growth hormone on donor site healing in severely burned children. *Ann Surg* 1990; **212**: 424–9.

137. Gilpin D, Barrow R, Rutan R, Broemling L, Herndon D. Recombinant human

growth hormone accelerates wound healing in children with large cutaneous burns. *Ann Surg* 1994; **220**: 19–24.

138. Neely A, Smith W, Warden G. Efficacy of a rise in C-reactive protein serum levels as an early indicator of sepsis in burned children. *J Burn Care Rehabil* 1998; **19**: 102–5.

139. Jeschke M, Barrow R, Herndon D. Recombinant human growth hormone treatment in pediatric burn patients and its role during the hepatic acute phase response. *Crit Care Med* 2000; **28**: 1578–84.

140. Knox J, Demling R, Wilmore D, Sarraf P, Santos A. Increased survival after major thermal injury: the effect of growth hormone therapy in adults. *J Trauma* 1995; **39**: 526–30.

141. Singh F, Prasad R, Chari P, Dash R. Effect of growth hormone therapy in burn patients on conservative treatment. *Burns* 1998; **24**: 733–9.

142. Talala J, Ruokonen E, Webster N, *et al.* Increased mortality associated with growth hormone treatment in critically ill adults. *N Engl J Med* 1999; **341**: 785–92.

143. Demling R. Growth hormone therapy in critically ill patients. *N Engl J Med* 1999; **341**: 837–9.

144. Knox J, Wilmore D, Demling R, Sarraf P, Santos A. Use of growth hormone for postoperative respiratory failure. *Am J Surg* 1996; **171**: 576–80.

145. Mulligan K, Tai V, Schambelan M. Use of growth hormone and other anabolic agents in AIDS wasting. *JPEN* 1999; **23**: S202–9.

146. Behrman S, Kudsk K, Brown R, *et al.* The effect of growth hormone on nutritional markers in enterally fed immobilized trauma patients. *JPEN* 1995; **19**: 41–6.

147. Petersen S, Holaday N, Jeevanandam M. Enhancement of protein synthesis efficiency in parenteral fed trauma victims by adjuvant recombinant human growth hormone. *J Trauma* 1994; **36**: 726–32.

148. Strock L, Singh H, Abdullah A, Miller J, Herndon D. The effect of insulin-like growth factor I on postburn hypermetabolism. *Surgery* 1990; **108**: 161–4.

149. Moller S, Jensen M, Swensson P, Skakkeback N. Insulin-like growth factor I in burn patients. *Burns* 1991; **17**: 278–81.

150. Kimbrough T, Shernan S, Ziegler T, Scheltinga M, Wilmore D. Insulin-like growth factor I response is comparable following intravenous and subcutaneous administration of growth hormone. *J Sug Res* 1991; **51**: 472–6.

151. Meyer N, Barrow R, Herndon D. Combined insulin-like growth factor I and growth hormone improves weight gain and wound healing in burned rats. *J Trauma* 1996; **41**: 1008–12.

152. Cioffi W, Gore D, Rue L, *et al.* Insulin-like growth factor I lowers protein oxidation in patients with thermal injury. *Ann Surg* 1994; **220**: 310–16.

153. Ferrando A, Chinkes D, Wolfe S, *et al.* A submaximal dose of insulin promotes net skeletal muscle protein synthesis in patients with severe burns. *Ann Surg* 1999; **229**: 11–18.

154. Pierre E, Barrow R, Hawkins H, *et al.* Effects of insulin on wound healing. *J Trauma* 1998; **44**: 342–5.

155. Plymate S, Vaughan G, Mason A, Pruitt B. Central hypogonadism in burned men. *Hormone Res* 1987; **27**: 152–8.

156. Demling R. Comparison of the anabolic effects and complications of human growth hormone and the testosterone analog, oxandrolone, after severe burn injury. *Burns* 1999; **25**: 215–21.

157. Demling R, Orgill D. The anticatabolic and wound healing effects of the testosterone analog oxandrolone after severe burn injury. *J Crit Care* 2000; **15**: 12–17.

158. Demling R, DeSanti L. Oxandrolone, an anabolic steroid, significantly increases the rate of weight gain in the recovery phase after major burns. *J Trauma* 1997; **43**: 47–51.

Chapter 21

The hepatic response to a thermal injury

Marc G Jeschke

- *Blood*: diagnosis of function and damage;
- *Ultrasonography*: diagnosis of morphological changes and blood flow (duplex);
- *Computed tomography (CT)*: morphological lesions (with the use of vascular enhancement);
- *Magnetic resonance imaging (MRI)*: vascular lesions or intrahepatic focal lesions;
- *Scintigrams*: dynamic measures;
- *Angiography*: vascular patterns for the diagnosis of morphologic changes; and
- *Needle biopsy of the liver*: pathologic diagnosis.

Liver Damage and Morphological Changes

After a thermal injury a variable degree of liver injury is present, usually related to the severity of the thermal injury. Fatty changes, a very common finding, are reversible *per se* and their significance depends on the cause and severity of accumulation (**Figure 21.1**).[5] However, autopsies of burned children have shown that fatty liver infiltration is associated with increased bacterial translocation, liver failure, and endotoxemia, thus delineating the crucial role of the liver during the postburn response (unpublished observations).

Immediately after burn, the damage of the liver may be associated with an increased hepatic edema formation. Liver weight and liver/body weight significantly increased 2–7 days after burn when compared to controls. Hepatic protein concentration was significantly decreased in burned rats, suggesting that the liver weight gain is due to increased edema formation rather than increases in the number of hepatocytes or protein levels. An increase in edema

Liver morphology and blood flow

Liver Function Tests and Diagnostic Tools

Liver function tests evaluate liver activity by assessing the degree of functional impairment. They do not provide a pathologic diagnosis, and the extreme functional reserve of the organ occasionally produces normal results in the face of significant lesions. Many of these tests do not measure a specific function of the liver, and other organ systems may be implicated. False-positive results for each of the tests are found in about 10% of hospital controls. False-negative tests also occur in about 10% of most tests.[1-5] Diagnostic tools are:

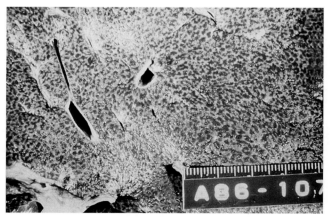

Fig. 21.1 Histological section of a fatty liver after thermal injury at autopsy. The liver appears to be yellow and enriched with fat.

formation may lead to cell damage, with the release of the hepatic enzymes (**Table 21.1**).[6]

Enzymes

The three enzymes that achieve abnormal serum levels in hepatic disease, and that have been studied widely, are alkaline phosphatase, serum glutamic oxaloacetic transaminase (SGOT), and serum glutamic pyruvic transaminase (SGPT). SGOT is present in the liver, myocardium, skeletal muscles, kidney, and pancreas. Cellular damage in any of the above-mentioned tissues results in elevation of the serum level. In reference to the liver, the most marked increases accompany acute cellular damage regardless of cause, and extremely high levels are noted in patients with hepatitis. SGOT is only moderately increased in cirrhosis and biliary obstruction. SGPT is more particularly applicable to the evaluation of liver disease, since the hepatic content greatly exceeds myocardial concentration. Elevations accompany acute hepatocellular damage. Lactic acid dehydrogenase (LDH) levels may also be elevated. Serum alkaline phosphatase (ALP) is found in many tissues, including the liver, bile ducts, intestines, bones, kidneys, placenta, and white blood cells. It provides an elevation of the patency of the bile channels at all levels, both intrahepatic and extrahepatic. Elevation is demonstrated in 94% of patients with obstruction of the extrahepatic biliary tract due to neoplasm, and 76% of those in whom the obstruction is caused by calculi. Intrahepatic biliary obstruction and cholestasis also cause a rise in the enzyme level. In the presence of space-occupying lesions such as metastases, primary hepatic carcinoma, and abscesses, the alkaline phosphate level is also increased. The overall correlation between metastatic carcinoma of the liver and an elevated enzyme level is as high as 92%. Sixty percent of patients with primary hepatic carcinoma also demonstrate a significant increase. ALP is also elevated in several nonhepatic disease states, such as bone tumor, pregnancy, and growth.

Liver damage has been associated with increased hepatocyte cell death.[6] In general, cell death occurs by two distinctly different mechanisms: programmed cell death (apoptosis) or necrosis.[7] Apoptosis is characterized by cell shrinkage, DNA fragmentation, membrane blebbing, and phagocytosis of the apoptotic cell fragments by neighboring cells or extrusion into the lumen of the bowel without inflammation. This is in contrast to necrosis, which involves cellular swelling, random DNA fragmentation, lysosomal activation, membrane breakdown, and extrusion of cellular contents into the interstitium. Membrane breakdown and cellular content release induce inflammation with the migration of inflammatory cells and release of proinflammatory cytokines and free radicals, which leads to further tissue breakdown. Pathological studies found that about 10–15% of thermally injured patients have liver necrosis at autopsy.[8,9] The necrosis is generally focal or zonal, central or paracentral, sometimes microfocal, and related to burn shock and sepsis. The morphological differences between apoptosis and necrosis are used to differentiate the two processes.

A cutaneous thermal injury induces liver cell apoptosis.[6] This increase in hepatic programmed cell death is compensated by an increase in hepatic cell proliferation, suggesting that the liver attempts to maintain homeostasis (**Figure 21.2a,b**). Despite the attempt to compensate increased apoptosis by increased hepatocyte proliferation, the liver cannot regain hepatic mass and protein concentration; a significant decrease was found in hepatic protein concentration in burned rats. It has been shown that a cutaneous burn induces small bowel epithelial cell apoptosis.[10] In the same study the authors showed that small bowel epithelial cell proliferation was not increased, leading to a loss of mucosal cells and hence mucosal mass.[10] Similar findings were demonstrated in the heart.[11] Burn-induced cardiocyte apoptosis; however, cardiocyte proliferation remained unchanged, causing cardiac impairment and dysfunction.[11]

The mechanisms whereby a cutaneous burn induces programmed cell death in hepatocytes are not defined. Studies suggested that, in general, hypoperfusion and ischemia–reperfusion are associated to promote apoptosis.[12–14] After a thermal injury it has been shown that the blood flow to the bowel decreases by nearly 60% of baseline and stays decreased for approximately 4 hours.[15] It can be surmised that the hepatic blood flow also decreases, thus causing programmed cell death. In addition, proinflammatory cytokines such as interleukin (IL)-1 and tumor necrosis factor α (TNFα) have been described to be an apoptotic signal.[16,17] We have shown in our burn model that, after a thermal injury, serum and hepatic concentration of proinflammatory cytokines such as IL-1α/β, IL-6, and TNFα are increased.[18] We therefore suggest that two possible mechanisms are involved in increased hepatocyte apoptosis: decreased splanchnic blood flow and elevation of proinflammatory cytokines, initiating intracellular signaling mechanisms. Signals which may be involved encompass many signals that play an important role during the acute phase response (see below).

Therapeutic possibilities could be the administration of anabolic growth factors, such as growth hormone (GH), insulin-like growth factor (IGF)-I or hepatocyte growth factor (HGF), all of which have been shown to be anti-apoptotic.[18–21] In exerting anti-apoptotic effect, these growth factors could improve hepatic morphology, function, and thus homeostasis after a thermal injury.

Biliary Formation

Bile secretion is an active process, relatively independent of total liver blood flow, except in conditions of shock. Bile is formed at two sites: (1) the canalicular membrane of the hepatocyte; and (2)

Table 21.1 Liver weight, liver weight/100 g body weight, and liver protein content for control and burned rats							
	Control days postburn				Burn days postburn			
	1 (*n* = 5)	2 (*n* = 5)	5 (*n* = 5)	7 (*n* = 5)	1 (*n* = 14)	2 (*n* = 14)	5 (*n* = 14)	7 (*n* = 14)
Liver weight (g)	13.0 ± 0.9	12.4 ± 0.8	13.2 ± 0.3	13.1 ± 0.4	13.1 ± 0.5	15.3 ± 0.7*	13.6 ± 0.4	13.6 ± 0.5
Liver/body weight (%)	3.4 ± 0.1	3.4 ± 0.3	3.8 ± 0.2	3.9 ± 0.2	3.5 ± 0.1	4.1 ± 0.1*	3.6 ± 0.1	3.7 ± 0.1
Liver protein content (mg/ml)	0.98 ± 0.01	0.97 ± 0.01	1.04 ± 0.02	1.0 ± 0.01	0.88 ± 0.02*	0.90 ± 0.02*	0.92 ± 0.01*	0.88 ± 0.01*

Data presented as means ± SEM. *Significant difference vs. control at corresponding day, $p < 0.05$.

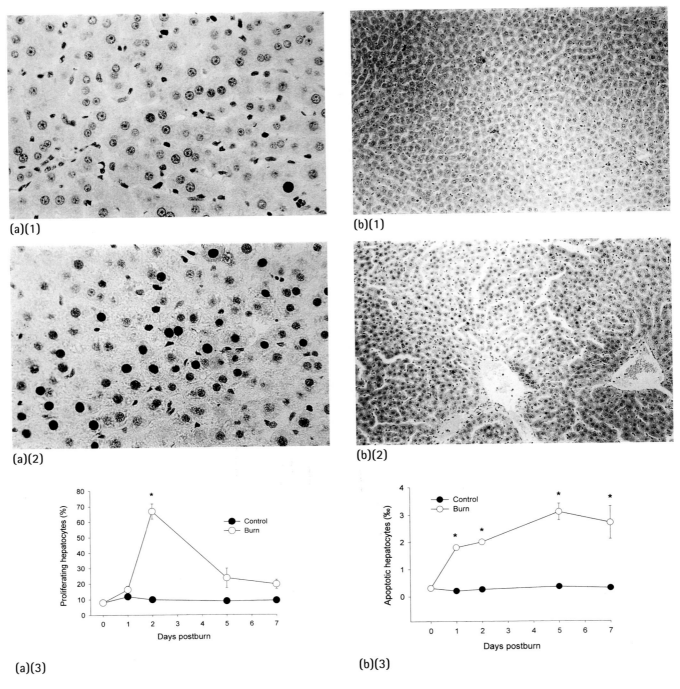

(a)(1)

(b)(1)

(a)(2)

(b)(2)

(a)(3)

(b)(3)

Fig. 21.2 (a) (1) Representative section of the liver of a control rat 2 days after the sham–burn. Few hepatocytes were identified (dark staining) as proliferating, PCNA positive. Magnification × 100. (2) Representative section of the liver of a burned rat (60% TBSA) 2 days after burn. Several hepatocytes were identified (dark staining) as proliferating, PCNA positive. Magnification × 100. (3) Percent of proliferating cells measured by PCNA. *Significant difference between burn and control, p < 0.05. Data presented as means ± SEM. (Burned animals $n = 7$ and controls $n = 2$ per time point.) (b) (1) Representative section of the liver in a control rat 24 hours after sham–burn. Few cells were identified (dark staining) as apoptotic, TUNEL positive. Magnification × 40. (2) Representative section of the liver in a rat 24 hours after burn (60% TBSA). Several cells were identified (dark staining) as apoptotic, TUNEL positive. Magnification × 40. (3) Apoptotic cells measured by TUNEL assay 1, 2, 5, and 7 days after burn expressed as positive apoptotic hepatocytes per 1000 hepatocytes. Burned rats had significantly higher rates of hepatocyte apoptosis when compared to controls. Data presented as means ± SEM. (Burned animals $n = 7$ and controls $n = 2$ per time point.*) Significant difference between burn and control, $p < 0.05$.

the bile ductules or ducts. Total unstimulated bile flow in a 70 kg man has been estimated at 0.41–0.43 ml/min. Eighty percent of the total daily production of bile (approximately 1500 ml) is secreted by hepatocytes, and 20% is secreted by the bile duct epithelial cells. The principal organic compounds in bile are the conjugated bile acids, cholesterol, phospholipid, and protein. As bile passes through the biliary ductules or ducts it is modified by secretion or absorption of epithelial cells. The highest cells in the biliary ductules have functions and architecture in common with both hepatocytes and ductular cells, and are called cholangiocytes. The best characterized hormone to stimulate bile secretion is secretin. The bile is then being secreted into the gallbladder, whose only function is to concentrate and store bile during fasting. Approximately 90% of the water in gallbladder bile is absorbed in 4 hours. Cholecystokinin appears to be the principal physiologic stimulator of gallbladder concentration. Cholinergic stimulation causes contraction of the gallbladder and relaxation of the sphincter of Oddi, which means that bile is secreted into the intestine. Most of the bile salt is being absorbed into the enterohepatic circulation. The liver extracts the bile acids and transports them back to the canalicular membrane where they are resecreted back into the biliary system. Total bile pool size in humans is 2–5 g and undergoes this circulation 2–3 times per meal and 6–10 times a day, depending on the dietary habit. In addition, 0.2–0.6 g are lost in the stool per day, and this quantity is replaced by newly synthesized bile acids.[3]

Bilirubin is a breakdown product of heme and is almost completely excreted in the bile. With hepatocellular disease or extrahepatic biliary obstruction, free bilirubin may accumulate in blood and tissues. Approximately 75% of bilirubin is derived from senescent red blood cells. Bilirubin circulates bound to albumin, which protects tissue from its toxicity. It is rapidly removed from the plasma by the liver through a carrier transport system. In the hepatocyte, bilirubin is conjugated with glucuronide and secreted in bile. Conjugated bilirubin may form a covalent bound with albumin, so-called delta bilirubin. In the intestine, bilirubin is reduced by bacteria to mesobilirubin and stercobilirubin, collectively termed urobilinogen. These are both excreted in the stool. A part of urobilinogen is oxidized to urobilin, which is brown pigment and gives stool its normal colour.

In trauma and sepsis, intrahepatic cholestasis occurs frequently. It appears to be an important pathophysiologic factor and occurs without demonstrable extrahepatic obstruction. This phenomenon has been described in association with a number of processes, such as hypoxia, drug toxicity, or total parenteral nutrition.[22] The mechanisms of intrahepatic cholestasis seem to be associated with an impairment of basolateral and canicular hepatocyte transport of bile acids and organic anions.[23] This is most likely due to decreased transporter protein and RNA expression, thus leading to increased bile. Intrahepatic cholestasis, which is one of the prime manifestations of hepatocellular injury, was present in 26% in a clinical study.[9] All of these were concurrent with sepsis. The cellular damage observed in sepsis is most likely the result of decreased hepatic blood flow rather than direct cellular damage.[24]

Energy, Carbohydrate, Insulin, and Lipid Metabolism
(see Chapter 27, Modulation of the Hypermetabolic Response after Burn Injury)
Most of the body's metabolic needs are regulated in some way by the liver. The liver expends approximately 20% of the body's energy and consumes 20–25% of the total utilized oxygen, which is due to the remarkable hepatic architecture and the blood supply. The hepatocellular organelles in plasma membranes permit specific functions and, at the same time, interrelate with an extracellular matrix, which facilitates metabolic exchange between blood and hepatocytes.[2] The liver does not only conduct a large number of functions but also manufactures many substances which serve other organs or tissues. The liver collects such substrates to meet the fuel requirements of other tissues in response to multiple metabolic signals. It is the only organ producing acetoacetate for use by muscle, brain, and kidney, but not itself. The energy-related functions of the liver are regulated by hormones, other agonists, and substrates coming to and from the liver.

The liver has a central role in energy metabolism: as a glucose source, it supports energy requirements of the central nervous system and red blood cells. During the fed state, results of intestinal carbohydrates digestion (glucose: 80%; galactose and fructose: 20%) are delivered to the liver. The latter two are rapidly converted into glucose. Glucose absorbed by the hepatocyte is converted directly into glycogen for storage up to a maximum 65 g of glycogen per kilogram of liver mass. Excess glucose is converted to fat. Glycogen is also produced by muscle, but this is not available for use by any other tissues. During the fasting state, this glycogen is the primary source of glucose. However, after 48 hours of fasting, liver glycogen is exhausted, and proteins mobilized primarily from muscle, mainly alanine, are converted by the liver to glucose. Lactate by anaerobic metabolism is metabolized only in the liver. Ordinarily glucose is converted to pyruvate and subsequently back into glucose. This shuttling of glucose and lactate between liver and peripheral tissue is carried out in the Cori cycle. The brain does not participate in the cycle, and a continuous source of glucose for the brain must come at the expense of muscle proteins.

In liver disease, the metabolism of glucose is often deranged. Frequently, in patients with cirrhosis, the portal-systemic shunting causes decreased exposure of portal blood to the hepatocytes, producing an abnormal result of the oral glucose tolerance test (OGTT). Hypoglycemia is rare in chronic liver disease as the synthetic capacity of hepatocytes is preserved until late in the disorder. In fulminate hepatic failure, however, there is extensive loss of hepatocyte mass and function, and hypoglycemia supervenes as gluconeogenesis fails.

Glycogenesis, glycogen storage, glycogenolysis, and the conversion of galactose into glucose all represent hepatic functions. Hypoglycemia is a rare accompaniment of extensive hepatic disease, but the amelioration of diabetes in patients with hemochromatosis is considered an indication of neoplastic change. The more common effect of hepatic disease is the deficiency of glycogenesis of resulting hyperglycemia. An hepatic enzyme system is responsible for the conversion of galactose into glucose, and abnormal galactose tolerance tests are seen in hepatitis and active cirrhosis. In rare instances a familial deficiency in this enzyme system accounts for spontaneous galactosemia accompanied by an obstructive type of jaundice that appears after the first week, and subsides when lactose is removed from the diet.

There are three sources of free fatty acids available to the liver: fat absorbed from the gut, fat liberated from adipocytes in response lipolysis, and fatty acids synthesized from carbohydrates and amino acids. These fatty acids are etherified with glycerol to form triglyceride. The export of triglycerides is dependent on the synthesis of very low density lipoproteins. In cases of excess supply of fatty acid, there is lipid accumulation in the liver because there is an imbalance of triglyceride relative to very low density lipoproteins. This is seen in obesity, corticosteroid use, pregnancy, diabetes, and total parenteral nutrition. Simple protein malnutrition or protein-calorie imbalance may also result in fatty change of liver, based on decreased export of triglycerides, because of limited supply of precursors for hepatic synthesis of lipoproteins.

Synthesis of both the phospholipid and cholesterol takes place in the liver, and the latter serves as a standard for the determination of lipid metabolism. The liver is the major organ involved in the synthesis, esterification, and excretion of cholesterol. In the presence of parenchymal damage, both the total cholesterol and the percentage of esterified fraction decreased. Biliary obstruction results in the rise in cholesterol, and the most pronounced elevations are noted in the primary biliary cirrhosis and the cholangiolitis accompanying toxic reactions to the phenothiazine derivatives.[3,4]

Vitamin Metabolism

The liver has many important roles of uptake, storage, and mobilization of vitamins. Most important are the fat-soluble vitamins A, E, D, and K. The absorption of these is dependent on bile salts. The vitamins appear in the thoracic duct 2–6 hours after oral administration. Vitamin A is exclusively stored in the liver, and excess ingestion of vitamin A may be associated with significant liver injury. A role for storage of vitamin A in the Ito cells has been suggested. The initial step in vitamin D activation occurs in the liver, where vitamin D_3 is converted to 25-hydroxycholecalciferol. Of particular surgical significance was the discovery of vitamin K, which is essential for the γ-carboxylation of the vitamin K-dependent coagulation factors II, VII, IX, and X. These factors are inactive without γ-carboxylation.[3,4] Vitamins play an important role in wound healing, energy, metabolism, inflammation, and antioxidants. Postburn hypermetabolism causes a vitamin deficiency requiring substitution.[25]

- There are decreased vitamin A levels in burn patients. This may be due to a reduction of retinol-binding protein (RBP, see Proteins), which is a vitamin A transporter. Vitamin A has been shown to enhance wound healing; thus, its substitution is important for dermal wound repair.
- Vitamin E encompasses antioxidant properties, and in animal experiments its administration has been shown to reduce lung injury. After a thermal injury, its concentration is decreased; thus, its substitution is suggested.
- Vitamin D, with its crucial function in the ossear cascade,

is also decreased after burn injury; however, its substitution has not been proven.

- Thiamin and riboflavin are vitamins that affect energy and protein metabolism and wound healing, both of which are decreased after trauma. Thiamin serves as a co-factor in the Krebs cycle and for the oxidation of glucose; thus, its needs is related to the energy intake. Thiamin is further necessary for the lysyl oxidase function to form collagen. Riboflavin is involved as a co-enzyme in oxidation–reduction reactions; it is decreased after burn and an increased need for burn victims has been shown.[25]
- Folic acid is depleted after a burn and can lead to impaired synthesis of DNA and RNA. Inadequate supplies of vitamin B_{12} and the indispensable amino acid methionine impair folate utilization. Thus, a deficiency of either of these nutrients can produce signs of folate deficiency.
- Complex with vitamins B_6 and B_{12} serve as co-enzymes in the energy and protein metabolic process. Vitamin B_6 is involved in amino acid metabolism, while vitamin B_{12} is involved in the catabolism of odd-chain long fatty acids. Both should be substituted in the form of a multivitamin complex, as both are decreased in the postburn hypermetabolic response.
- Vitamin C plays an important role during the postburn hypermetabolic response. During that period, oxygen free radicals such as superoxide, peroxide, and hydroxyl may cause increased postburn vascular permeability.

  Administration of vitamin C, a free radical scavenger, has thus been suggested to be beneficial in terms of reducing microvascular permeability and required fluid volume. In recent studies, vitamin C has been described as enhancing wound healing in skin, bones, and other tissues.

Table 21.2 gives a therapeutic guideline for vitamin substitution.[26]

Coagulation and Clotting Factors

The liver produces multiple coagulation factors, which can be altered or be defective in the state of liver disease. In the state of jaundice, vitamin K resorption is decreased, resulting in a decreased synthesis of prothrombin. When the liver is severely damaged, as in hepatocellular dysfunction, prothrombin is not synthesized at all. The diagnosis of pathologic prothrombin synthesis is made by the prothrombin time. Decreases in factors V, VII, IX, and fibrinogen also have been noted in hepatic disease.[4] Homeostasis of clotting is complex and has been recently investigated in thermally injured patients.[26] Thrombotic and fibrinolytic mechanisms are activated after burn, and the extent of activation is

Table 21.2 Medication guideline for vitamin and mineral supplementation[26]			
Vitamins and minerals	0–2 years	2–12 years	> 12 years
Multivitamin	Poly Vi Sol 1 ml	Poly Vi Sol 1 ml	Vi Deylin 5 ml or Theragran
Ascorbic acid	250 mg QD	250 mg QD	500 mg QD
Folic acid	1 mg QMWF	1 mg QMWF	1 mg QMWF
Vitamin A	2500 U	5000 U	10 000 U
Vitamin E	5 mg	5 mg	10 mg
Zinc sulfate	55 mg	110 mg	220 mg
Elemental iron	< 30 kg dose = 2 mg/kg/dose PO TID		
	> 30 kg dose = 65 mg PO TID or FeSO$_4$ 325 mg PO TID		

increased with the severity of the thermal injury. Most homeostatic markers fall during the early shock phase of burns owing to dilutional effects, loss, and degradation of plasma proteins. Clotting factors return to normal levels after the aggressive resuscitation period. Later in the postburn course, thrombogenicity has been suggested to be increased due to a decrease in antithrombin III, protein C, and protein S levels. Fibrinolysis activation occurs via increases in tissue plasminogen activation factor, thus leading to an increased risk of thrombosis. The hypercoagulable state places many thermally injured patients at risk for disseminated intravascular coagulation (DIC), which has been described post mortem in 30% of examined cases. Heparin has been administered as a prophylaxis for deep venous thrombosis and thus for the onset of DIC (Fraxiparin 0.5 ml subcutaneous). If needed, fresh frozen plasma is therapeutically administered to improve coagulation.

Hepatic acute phase response

Proteins

The acute phase response comprises a cascade of events initiated to prevent tissue damage and to activate repair processes. Activated phagocytic cells, fibroblasts, and endothelial cells which release proinflammatory cytokines initiated the acute phase response, leading to systemic phase reactions in the following:

- the hypothalamus, which leads to fever;
- the pituitary–adrenal axis, which releases steroid hormones;
- the liver, which causes the synthesis and secretion of acute phase proteins;
- the bone marrow, promulgating further hematopoietic responses; and
- the immune system, which allows both the activation of the reticuloendothelial system and the stimulation of lymphocytes.

A crucial step in this cascade of reactions involves the interaction between the site of injury and the liver, which is the principal organ responsible for producing acute phase proteins and modulating the systemic inflammatory response.

After major trauma, such as a severe burn, hepatic protein synthesis shifts from hepatic constitutive proteins, such as albumin, prealbumin, transferrin, and retinol-binding protein, to acute phase proteins.[1–6] Acute phase proteins are divided into type I acute phase proteins and type II acute phase proteins.[6] The upregulation of acute phase proteins represents a redirection of the liver in order to fulfil immune functions, coagulation, and wound healing processes (**Figure 21.3**).[2,3,7,8]

In contrast to acute phase proteins, constitutive hepatic proteins are down regulated.[27–31] After a thermal injury, albumin and transferrin decrease by 50–70% below normal levels.[28–31] Studies have shown that two mechanisms are responsible for the decrease of constitutive hepatic proteins:

- the liver reprioritizes its protein synthesis from constitutive hepatic proteins to acute phase proteins; this has been shown in many studies in which the mRNA synthesis for constitutive hepatic proteins is decreased;
- capillary leakage and the loss of these proteins into the massive extravascular space and burn wound.

Albumin and transferrin, however, have important physiologic functions as they serve as transporter proteins and contribute to osmotic pressure and plasma pH.[28,29] Their downregulation after trauma has been described as potentially harmful and the synthesis of these proteins has been used as a predictor of mortality, nutritional status, and severity of stress, as well as an indicator of improved recovery.[29,32–34] As albumin could be drastically decreased after burn injury, human albumin was administered to maintain albumin levels at 2.5 mg/dl. Other studies have suggested that albumin substitution should not occur.

The therapeutic guideline at our institute is as follows: serum albumin is measured daily at 4:30 a.m. If serum albumin concentrations are less than 2.0 g/dl, albumin is supplemented based upon age and body weight to maintain colloid osmotic pressure at 2.0 g/dl. Children <2 years of age and <20 kg body weight receive 6.25 g/day exogenous albumin over 6 hours; children 2–9 years old weighing >20 kg but <40 kg receive 12.5 g/day over 6 hours; and children 10–18 years old weighing >40 kg receive 25 g/day. Total albumin infused, albumin infused per day, and grams of albumin infused per meter square burn are recorded.

Mediators of the Acute Phase Response

Mediators of the acute phase response are cytokines. Type I acute phase proteins, such as haptoglobin and α_1-acid glycoprotein, are mediated by IL-1-like cytokines (IL-1α/β, TNFα/β); and type II acute phase proteins, such as α_2-macroglobulin and fibrinogen, are mediated by IL-6-like cytokines (IL-6, IL-11).[27] In several studies, the biphasic time course of proinflammatory cytokines have been demonstrated. Immediately after burn, IL-1, IL-6, IL-8, and TNFα increase 2–10-fold above normal levels, decrease slightly after approximately 12 hours, increase again, and then start to decrease. Animal and human studies demonstrated that cytokines can either approach normal levels within 2 days after trauma or can be elevated up to 2 weeks after thermal injury. Cytokine elevation has been shown to be dependent upon the extend of the burn and concomitant injuries.

The signal cascade of cytokines is the following: the cytokines bind to their receptors, activate intracellular signals by tyrosine phosphorylation, for the type I acute phase response c-jun/c-fos, hepatic nuclear factor-kappa B (NF-κB), or the CCAAT/enhancer-binding-proteins (C/EBPs).[35–47] The intracellular signal cascade for type II has been shown to be a tyrosine phosphorylation and activation of intracellular tyrosine kinases (JAKs), latent cytoplasmic transcription factors, STAT1, STAT3, and STAT5 (signal transducer and activator of transcription), or mitogen-activated protein (MAP).[27,35–47] These signals activate transcription, translation, and expression of acute phase proteins. In particular, IL-6 has been speculated to be the main mediating cytokine. IL-6 activates glycoprotein 130 (gp 130) and the JAK-kinases (JAK-1), leading to activation of STAT1 and STAT3 translocating to the nucleus. Intranuclearly, the genes for acute phase proteins are turned on (**Figure 21.4**).

The aim of the acute phase response is to protect the body from further damage, and the aim will be achieved when all elements of the acute phase response coalesce in a balanced fashion. However, a prolonged increase in proinflammatory cytokines and acute phase proteins has been shown to be associated with a hypercatabolic state, increased risk of sepsis, multi organ failure, morbidity, and mortality.[32–34] Therefore, an important therapeutic approach to improve trauma mortality may be the modulation of the acute phase response by decreasing acute phase proteins and proinflam-

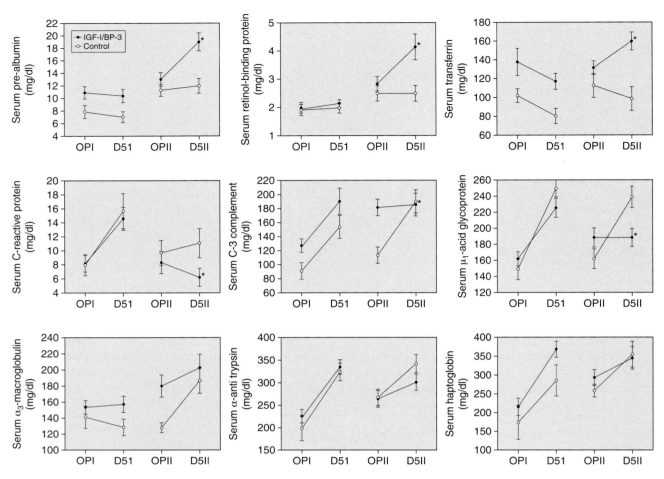

Fig. 21.3 Serum constitutive hepatic proteins (upper line), type I acute phase proteins (middle line), and type II acute phase proteins after thermal injury. The figures depict a clinical study in which the complex IGF-I/BP-3 was determined. All pediatric patients received after saline (control) from OP I to D 5 I. After this first control period patients received either IGF-I/BP-3 or saline OP II to D 5 II. Upper line: all constitutive hepatic proteins were decreased after burn (periods I and II). IGF-I/BP-3 increased constitutive hepatic proteins during the second study period, as saline did not. Normal levels: prealbumin: 25–45 mg/dl; retinol-binding protein: 3–6 mg/dl; transferrin: 203–430 mg/dl. Middle line: all type I acute phase proteins are increased after thermal injury during the control and the study period. IGF-I/BP-3 decreased type I acute phase proteins when compared to controls. Normal levels: C-reactive protein: <5 mg/dl; C-3 complement: 50–90 mg/dl; α_1-acid glycoprotein: 55–140 mg/dl. Lower line: type II acute phase proteins are also increased after burn and stay elevated. IGF-I/BP-3 had no effect on type II acute phase proteins when compared with controls. Normal levels: α_2-macroglobulin: 100–150 mg/dl; α-antitrypsin: 150–250 mg/dl; haptoglobin: 50–300 mg/dl. Values are presented as means ± SEM. *Significant between IGF-I/BP-3 and controls, $p < 0.05$.

matory cytokines and increasing constitutive hepatic proteins.[32–35] The use of antibodies against proinflammatory cytokines such as TNFα, IL-1β, or their receptors showed promising results *in vitro* and in animal models by increasing survival rates in the state of septicemia.[48–50] However, when these approaches entered clinical trials it became evident that these promising animal data could not be found in humans. One possibility is that the anti-inflammatory agents used failed to control the exaggerated synthesis of proinflammatory cytokines because they focused on only one pathway or mediator in the inflammatory cascade, leading to a compensation through other pathways.[51,52] Another cause of the failure may have been that the anti-inflammatory cascade did not undergo

intensive studies. Only recently have investigations speculated about the importance of a balance between pro- and anti-inflammatory agents.[53,54] Two studies demonstrated that nonsurvivors with pancreatitis had decreased IL-6: IL-10 ratios when compared with survivors.[53,54] The relevance of cytokine ratios in the pathogenesis and the prediction of trauma, sepsis, and shock still needs to be defined; however, individual effects have been investigated. A prolonged and increased inflammatory response contributes to multi organ failure and mortality.[32–34] The over-expression of proinflammatory cytokines, such as IL-1, IL-6, and TNFα inhibit the GH–IGF-1 axis and increase the hypermetabolic response, resulting in increased morbidity and mortality.[55–57]

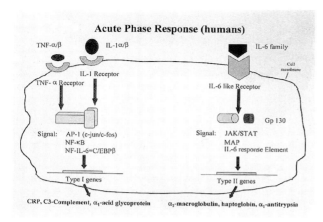

Acute Phase Response (humans)

Fig. 21.4 Signal cascade of the hepatic acute phase response.

In contrast to proinflammatory cytokines, anti-inflammatory cytokines appear to have protective characteristics. Interleukin-2 and interferon-γ (IFN-γ) are signals in the TH-1 response and play a critical role in initiating and maintaining cellular immune responses, in the defense against intracellular pathogens.[58] Interleukin-4 and IL-10 are TH-2 cytokines, characterized by production of B-cell activating cytokines.[58] TH-2 responses enhance the production of antibodies, which are crucial for the humoral immune response, e.g. in preventing disseminated infections. Administration of IL-10 can protect against lethal doses of endotoxin in mice, and decreases the release of endotoxin-induced IL-6 and IL-1.[33,59,60] Thus, IL-10 administration may ameliorate the endotoxemic shock and may improve survival. The effect of anti-inflammatory cytokines in burns still need to be defined.

Current research is focusing on new mediators and their modulation. Wang and Tracey showed that hypermobility-shift group protein-1 (HMG-1) is a late mediator responsible for lethality in the state of septicemia.[61] They suggest that blocking HMG-1 may be a new approach to improve survival. Another group showed that macrophage inhibitory factor (MIF) plays a crucial role in the proinflammatory cascade and its attenuation may also improve survival after massive trauma.[62] Despite the research focusing on attenuating the proinflammatory acute phase response, the optimal treatment for severely injured trauma patients needs to be defined. Our group has been studying the effect of growth factors, such as GH, HGF, IGF-I, IGF-I in combination with its principal binding protein-3 (IGF-I/BP-3) on the hepatic acute phase response, and cytokine expression as a physiologic approach to attenuate the proinflammatory cascade.[18–21]

Growth Factors

Our group has investigated the effect of growth factors such as GH, HGF, IGF-I, IGF-I/BP-3 on the hepatic acute phase response. The hypothesis was that physiologic anabolic agents would improve constitutive hepatic protein synthesis and thus equilibrate the pro- to anti-inflammatory hepatic response. It was shown that the growth factors tested all had different effects on hepatic cytokine and protein synthesis.[18–21]

Recombinant Human Growth Hormone

The effect of recombinant human growth hormone (rhGH) on the hepatic acute phase response has been tested in animal models and pediatric burn patients.[18,19,63] Data show in burned children that GH modulated the acute phase response by decreasing both serum TNFα and IL-1β. Decreases in serum TNFα and IL-1β were associated with decreased type I acute phase proteins serum amyloid A (SAA) and C-reactive protein (CRP). rhGH did not affect either IL-6 concentration or its dependent acute phase proteins haptoglobin, α_1-antitrypsin, or α_2-macroglobulin. The mechanisms by which rhGH modulates the acute phase response are not entirely defined; however, it has been demonstrated that rhGH binds to its cell surface receptor (GHR) and leads to tyrosine phosphorylation of CCAAT/enhancer-binding-proteins (C/EBPs), the AP-1 family of transcription factors, intracellular tyrosine kinases (JAKs), octamer-binding-proteins, and STATs.[41,43,47,64–68] These signal transcription factors translocate to the nucleus where they can interact with specific DNA sequences to modulate the gene expression of c-fos/c-jun and NF-κB, which regulate the expression of constitutive hepatic and acute phase proteins.[69,70] Interestingly, cytokines regulate constitutive hepatic and acute phase protein expression through a similar cascade.[27] IL-I-like cytokines bind to their receptors, leading to activation/phosphorylation, which results in activation of cellular signals AP-1, NF-κB, and C/EBPβ.[27] The stimulation of these signals leads to activation of the transcription and translation of type I acute phase protein genes. Given the fact that rhGH decreases IL-I-like cytokines, it is unknown whether rhGH decreases type I acute phase proteins through direct down-regulation of AP-1, NF-κB, or C/EBPβ, or through modulation of the IL-I-like cytokine expression, which decreases both these cellular signals and type I acute phase proteins.[43,69,70]

RrhGH administration increased endogenous albumin levels, reducing the amount of required exogenous substitution to maintain normal serum albumin levels. Similar to acute phase proteins, the mechanisms by which rhGH increases endogenous albumin concentrations are unknown; however, rhGH might exert this effect through activation of C/EBPα.[43,72] C/EBPα is a transactivator of liver-specific genes, such as albumin. Its mRNA concentration decreases during trauma and stress, and can be considered as a negative regulated acute phase gene.[41–43,72–74] Recently, C/EBPα mRNA levels, which are decreased after trauma, were shown to increase with rhGH,[43] thus indicating that a stimulation of the α isoform may lead to a stimulation of constitutive hepatic proteins, such as albumin and retinol-binding protein.[43]

Despite the advantages seen with rhGH administration Takala *et al.* reported increased mortalities in septic adult patients;[75] therefore, based on Takala's data, rhGH should not be given in septic patients or patients with multi organ failure (MOF). Another side-effect of rhGH that has been recently delineated is an increase in hepatic triglyceride concentration and development of a fatty liver.[18,76] RrhGH administration over 10 days increased hepatic triglyceride concentration by nearly 50% in burned rats.[18] The mechanisms have been discussed in clinical studies, where the authors speculated that rhGH increased peripheral lipolysis and, owing to a lack of transporter proteins (LDL, HDL), triglycerides accumulate in the liver.[76] It has been demonstrated in pediatric burn patients that rhGH increased free fatty acid concentration when compared to placebo, indicating that rhGH stimulates peripheral lipolysis and, subsequently, free fatty acid concentration.[63]

In summary, rhGH modulates the acute phase response by affecting proinflammatory IL-1-like cytokine expression followed by decreased type I acute phase proteins and increasing constitutive hepatic proteins. No effect on IL-6-like cytokines and type II acute phase proteins could be demonstrated. Although the acute phase response is a contributor to mortality after trauma, rhGH administration does not appear to cause an increase in mortality in severely burned children as described by Takala et al., as rhGH does not cause an increased and prolonged acute phase response.[75]

Hepatocyte Growth Factor

Hepatocyte growth factor (HGF) has been shown to accelerate hepatic regeneration and improve hepatic function in rats after trauma.[77] HGF and its receptor c-met (HGFR) are known to modulate the acute phase response in primary hepatocyte cultures.[78] HGF stimulates in vitro synthesis of constitutive hepatic proteins and decreases the synthesis of acute phase proteins.[78,79] Within 30–60 minutes of injury, plasma HGF is elevated, presumably sending a strong mitogenic signal to the hepatocytes, which are already primed by IL-6, TNFα, or insulin.[80] The cause of plasma HGF increase is currently unknown; however, it has been postulated to be due either to increased production of HGF in extrahepatic organs, such as lung, spleen, kidney, or gut, or to a decrease in hepatic HGF excretion.[80,81] Rapid increase in HGF stimulates hepatocyte mitogenesis, motogenesis, and DNA synthesis.[80] HGF administered to normal rats only stimulates a small number of hepatocytes to enter the DNA synthesis cycle, indicating that hepatocytes in normal livers are not ready to respond to mitogenic signals without the priming events that switch them into a responsive mode.[80]

We have shown that HGF administration stimulates constitutive hepatic proteins after burn injury in vivo.[20] In fact, serum transferrin reached normal levels 7 days after injury with HGF treatment, whereas in saline-treated animals serum transferrin remained low. Serum albumin levels decreased; however, beginning at day 2 after burn, HGF attenuated this drop in serum albumin. The exact mechanisms by which HGF stimulates constitutive hepatic proteins are unknown, though HGF is capable of stimulating the synthesis of C/EBPα, which regulates constitutive hepatic proteins.[67]

In contrast to recent in vitro studies, where the authors demonstrated that HGF decreased acute phase proteins, we showed in vivo that HGF increased serum α_2-macroglobulin (type II acute phase protein), with no effect on α_1-acid glycoprotein and haptoglobin (type I acute phase proteins).[78,79] Type II acute phase proteins are mediated through IL-6-like cytokines, including cytokines such as IL-6 and IL-11.[27] IL-6 secreted by Kupffer cells in the liver is capable of regulating the synthesis of transcription factors that have response elements in the 5'-flanking region of the HGF gene that may be potentially utilized in inducing HGF gene expression at the transcriptional level.[80,82–84] Therefore, IL-6 appears likely to substantially and quickly upregulate HGF mRNA and HGF mRNA receptor expression.[82] However, the interaction between HGF and IL-6 in vitro has been shown to be complex and controversial.[78,83,86] In our study, we demonstrated that administration of rhHGF stimulated serum IL-6, along with an increase in its dependent type II acute phase protein, serum α_2-macroglobulin and TNFα.[20] TNFα is another important mediator during the acute

phase response, which has been shown to modulate type I acute phase proteins and to stimulate IL-6, HGF, and HGF-receptor gene expression.[77,80,82,85,86] TNFα is a proinflammatory cytokine, associated with increased catabolic activity and mortality.[87] However, a recent study suggested that increased TNFα concentrations after liver injury play an important role in the early signaling pathways of liver regeneration.[80] In support of this hypothesis, we found that serum and hepatic gene expression for TNFα was significantly elevated with HGF. This finding suggests that HGF stimulates IL-6, TNFα, and type II acute phase proteins. Increased TNFα could not be shown to contribute to any detectable adverse side-effects; however, one may speculate that body weight loss may be due to elevated TNFα.

HGF exerted beneficial effects after thermal injury by increasing liver weight, liver weight/100 g body weight, and higher total hepatic protein content compared to rats receiving saline.[20] HGF, furthermore, demonstrated no increase in liver triglyceride content, a phenomenon associated with thermal injury.[19,76] These findings are most likely due to the strong mitogenic effect of HGF on hepatocytes.

HGF has been shown to have some beneficial effects and be a potential therapeutic agent. More studies need to be done before this growth factor can be applied in patients.

Insulin–like Growth Factor–I in Combination with its Principal Binding Protein–3

Insulin-like growth factor-I is a 7.7-kDa single-chain polypeptide of 70 amino acids with sequence hormology to proinsulin.[88] In the system, 95–99% of IGF-I is bound and transported with one of its six binding proteins IGFBP 1–6.[89] The majority of IGF-I is bound to IGFBP-3. Administration of the IGF-I/BP-3 complex as a therapeutic agent provides several advantages over the administration of IGF-I alone, because when IGF-I is already bound to IGFBP-3, it rapidly transforms into a ternary complex. This complex confers decreased serum clearance and allows the delivery of significantly larger amounts of IGF-I without inducing hypoglycemia and electrolyte imbalances. In general, IGF-I has been shown to improve cell recovery, wound healing, peripheral muscle protein synthesis, and gut and immune function after thermal injury.[90–92] Recent evidence suggests that IGF-I is instrumental in the early phases of liver regeneration after trauma and modulates the hepatic acute phase response in burned rats.[21]

As administration of IGF-I in therapeutic dosages causes adverse side-effects, a new complex has been recently developed, in which IGF-I is bound to its principal binding protein-3 (IGFBP-3) in a 1:1 molar ratio. This complex has been shown to be safe and efficacious.[21] Thus, the effect of IGF-I/BP-3 was investigated in thermally injured pediatric patients.[93] IGF-I in combination with IGFBP-3 decreased proinflammatory cytokines IL-1β and TNFα, with subsequent decreases in type I acute phase proteins CRP, complement C-3, and α_1-acid glycoprotein.[93] An increase in IL-6 or type II acute phase proteins was observed, suggesting that IGF-I effectively decreased IL-1β and TNFα without compensatory elevation of IL-6 and type II acute phase proteins. Decreased acute phase protein and proinflammatory cytokine concentration was associated with increased synthesis of constitutive hepatic proteins, such as prealbumin, retinol-binding protein, and transferrin.[93]

IGF-I appears to have anti-apoptotic, pro-mitogenic effects on multiple cell lines, such as hepatocytes, small bowel epithelial cells, and hematopoietic progenitor cells.[94–96] Therefore, IGF-I seems to affect extra- and intracellular signaling pathways. Recent studies demonstrated that IGF-I decreases the C/EBPβ subtype, which increases after trauma and regulates cytokine and protein synthesis.[73] In contrast, IGF-I increases the C/EBPα subtype, which decreases after trauma and regulates constitutive hepatic protein synthesis.[46] Furthermore, IGF-I has been shown to affect NF-κB, which controls the transcriptional regulation of many proinflammatory cytokines and acute phase proteins containing the NF-κB response elements in their promoter region.[27,37,39] NF-κB has also been shown as one of the most potent anti-apoptotic transcription factors in several organs. It has been demonstrated recently that IGF-I increases hepatic NF-κB concentration and decreases hepatocyte apoptosis after trauma.[96] IGF-I further affects nitric oxide, JAK/STAT, Gp 130, and many more transcription and translation factors.[45,46] This suggests that IGF-I plays a major role after trauma by maintaining organ homeostasis and function.

In thermally injured children, rhIGF-I in combination with its principal binding protein modulates the hepatic acute phase response by decreasing proinflammatory cytokines IL-1β and TNFα, followed by a decrease in type I acute phase proteins. IGF-I/BP-3 had no effect on IL-6 and type II acute phase proteins. Decreases in acute phase protein and proinflammatory cytokine synthesis were associated with increases in constitutive hepatic protein synthesis. Attenuating the hepatic acute phase response with IGF-I/BP-3 modulated the hypermetabolic response, which may prevent multi organ failure and improve clinical outcome after a thermal injury without any detectable adverse side-effects. Data shown would make IGF-I/BP-3 an ideal therapeutic agent; however, our group recently found that IGF-I/BP-3 increased the risk for peripheral neuropathies, thus limiting the use of this agent (unpublished observations). There are many therapeutic approaches to improve the hepatic acute phase response. The optimal agent has yet to be defined.

Enzymes

Liver enzymes, such as aspartate aminotransferase (AST) and alanine aminotransferase (ALT), are the most sensitive indicators of hepatocyte injury. Both AST and ALT are present normally in low concentrations. However, with cellular injury or changes in cell membrane permeability, these enzymes leak into circulation. Of the two, ALT is the more sensitive and specific test for hepatocyte injury, as AST can be also elevated in the state of cardiac arrest or muscle injury. Serum glutamate dehydrogenase (GLDH) is also a marker and is elevated in the state of severe hepatic damage. Serum alkaline phosphatase (ALP) provides an elevation of the patency of the bile channels at all levels, intrahepatic and extrahepatic. Elevation is demonstrated in patients with obstruction of the extrahepatic biliary tract or caliculi. In general, serum levels are elevated in hepatobiliary disease.[97]

As mentioned earlier, liver damage occurs after a thermal injury. The elevation of hepatic enzymes correlates with the severity and extent of the hepatic injury. Small hepatic injury leads predominantly to elevation of ALT, and to only a slight elevation of AST; the so-called de Ritis ratio is GOT/GPT <1. In a state of severe hepatic damage, mitochondrial-bound enzymes are strongly elevated and the de Ritis ratio is GOT/GPT >1 (**Table 21.3**).[97]

Thermal injury causes liver damage by edema formation, hypoperfusion, proinflammatory cytokines or other cell death signals with the release of the hepatic enzymes. It has been shown that serum AST, ALT, and ALKP are elevated between 50 and 200% when compared with normal levels (**Figure 21.5**). Serum AST and ALT peaked during the first day postburn, and ALKP during the second day postburn. During hepatic regeneration, all enzymes returned to baseline between 5 and 7 days postburn. If liver

Table 21.3 Localization of hepatic enzymes and their function in hepatic damage diagnosis[97]

Enzyme	Localization Cytoplasma	Mitochondrial	Liver specific
AST	+	+	No: heart, muscle
ALT	+	–	Yes
GLDH	–	+	Yes
ALKP	Combination of several isoenzymes		No: bone, growth, pregnancy, etc.

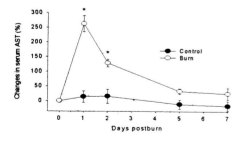

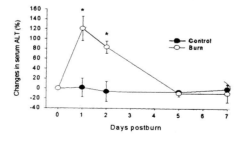

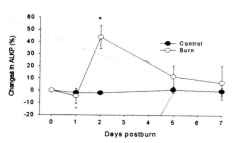

Fig. 21.5 Serum AST (a), ALT (b), and ALKP (c) levels were determined in controls and thermally injured rats. Serum AST and ALT increased during the first day after burn, whereas ALKP increased 2 days after burn when compared with controls. Data presented as means ± SEM. *Significant difference between burn and controls, $p < 0.05$.

damage persists, enzymes stay elevated. There is no need for therapeutic intervention to decrease elevated enzymes. Enzymes can only be used as markers and the effect of therapeutics can be studied.

Summary

The liver plays a crucial role in the aftermath of a thermal injury. The synthesis of constitutive hepatic proteins, acute phase proteins, cytokines, and other mediators makes it a determining factor for survival. A new approach for improving hepatic function maybe the use of anabolic, anti-inflammatory agents.

References

1. Moll KJ. *Anatomie. Leber*. München: Jungjohann Verlag, 366–75.
2. Winkeltau G, Kraas E. Leber. In: Schumpelick V, Bleese NM, Mommsen U, eds. *Chirurgie*. Stuttgart: Enke Verlag, 658–75.
3. Schwarz, *Principles of Surgery*.
4. Küttler T. *Biochemie*. München: Jungjohann Verlag, 240–65.
5. Linares HA. Autopsy findings in burned children. In: Carvajal HF, Parks DH, eds. *Burns in Children*. Chicago: Year Book Medical, 1988.
6. Jeschke MG, Low JFA, Spies M, Vita R, Barrow RE, Herndon DN. Liver mitosis, apoptosis, NF-κB expression and liver morphology after a thermal injury. *Am J Pathol* 2000 (submitted).
7. Steller H. Mechanisms and genes of cellular suicide. *Science* 1995; 267: 1445–9.
8. Teplitz C. The pathology of burns and the fundamental of burn wound sepsis. In: Artz CL, Moncrief JA, Pruitt BA, eds. *Burns: A Team Approach*. Philadelphia: WB Saunders, 1979: 45.
9. Linares HA. Sepsis, disseminated intravascular coagulation and multi organ failure: catastrophic events in severe burns. In: Schlag G, Redl H, Siegl JH, Traber DL, eds. *Shock, Sepsis, and Organ Failure*. Berlin: Springer Verlag, 1991: 370–98.
10. Wolf SE, Ikeda H, Matin S, *et al*. Cutaneous burn increases apoptosis in the gut epithelium of mice. *J Am Coll Surg* 1999; 188: 10–16.
11. Lightfoot E Jr, Horton JW, Maass DW, White DJ, McFarland RD, Lipsky PE. Major burn trauma in rats promotes cardiac and gastrointestinal apoptosis. *Shock* 1999; 11: 29–34.
12. Baron P, Traber DL, Traber LD, *et al*. Gut failure and translocation following burn and sepsis. *J Surg Res* 1994; 57: 197–204.
13. Ikeda H, Suzuki Y, Suzuki M, *et al*. Apoptosis is a major mode of cell death caused by ischemia and ischemia/reperfusion injury to the rat intestinal epithelium. *Gut* 1998; 42: 530–7.
14. Noda T, Iwakiri R, Fujimoto R, Matsuo S, Aw TY. Programmed cell death induced by ischemia-reperfusion in rat intestinal mucosa. *Am J Physiol* 1998; 274: G270–6.
15. Ramzy PI, Irrtun O, Wolf SE, Thompson JC, Herndon DN. Decreased blood flow is associated with increased small bowel epithelial cell apoptosis after burns. *J Am Coll Surg* 2000 (in press).
16. Beg AA, Finco TS, Nantermet PV, Baldwin AS Jr. Tumor necrosis factor and interleukin-1 lead to phosphorylation and loss of I kappa B alpha: a mechanism for NF-kappa B activation. *Mol Cell Biol* 1993; 13: 3301–10.
17. Bellas RE, FitzGerald MJ, Fausto N, Sonenshein GE. Inhibition of NF-kappa B activity induces apoptosis in murine hepatocytes. *Am J Pathol* 1997; 151: 891–6.
18. Jeschke MG, Herndon DN, Wolf SE, *et al*. Recombinant human growth hormone alters acute phase reactant proteins, cytokine expression and liver morphology in burned rats. *J Surg Res* 1999; 83: 122–9.
19. Jeschke MG, Wolf SE, DebRoy MA, Herndon DN. The combination of growth hormone with hepatocyte growth factor alters the acute phase response. *Shock* 1999; 12: 181–7.
20. Jeschke MG, Herndon DN, Wolf SE, *et al*. Hepatocyte growth factor (HGF) modulates the hepatic acute phase response in thermally injured rats. *Crit Care Med* 2000; 28: 504–510.
21. Jeschke MG, Herndon DN, Barrow RE. Insulin-like growth factor-I plus insulin-like growth factor binding protein-3 affects the hepatic acute phase response and hepatic morphology in thermally injured rats. *Ann Surg* 2000; 231: 408–16.
22. Cano N, Gerolami A. Intrahepatic cholestasis during total parenteral nutrition. *Lancet* 1983; 1: 985.
23. Bolder U, Ton-nu HT, Schteingart CD, Frick E, Hofmann AF. Hepatocyte transport of bile acids and organic anions in endotoxemic rats: impaired uptake and secretion. *Gastroenterology* 1997; 112: 214–25.
24. Hurd T, Lysz T, Dikdan G, McGee J, *et al*. Hepatic cellular dysfunction in sepsis: an ischemic phenomenon? *Curr Surg* 1988; 45: 114–19.
25. Manning AJ, Meyer N, Klein GL. Vitamin and trace element homeostasis following burn injury. In: Herndon DN, ed. *Total Burn Care*. Philadelphia: WB Saunders, 251–5.
26. Wolf SE, Sanford A. Daily work. In: Wolf SE, Herndon DN, eds. *Handbook of Burn Care*. Austin, TX: Landes Bioscience, 122.
27. Moshage H. Cytokines and the hepatic acute phase response. *J Pathol* 1997; 181: 257–66.
28. Fey G, Gauldie J. The acute phase response of the liver in inflammation. In: Popper H, Schaffner F, eds. *Progress in Liver Disease*. Philadelphia: WB, Saunders, 1990: 89–116.
29. Rotheschild MA, Oratz M, Schreiber SS. Serum albumin. *Hepatology* 1988; 8: 385–401.
30. Hiyama DT, Von Allmen D, Rosenblum L, Ogle CK, Hasselgren PO, Fischer JE. Synthesis of albumin and acute-phase proteins in perfused liver after burn injury in rats. *J Burn Care Rehabil* 1991; 12: 1–6.
31. Gilpin DA, Hsieh CC, Kunninger DT, Herndon DN, Papaconstantinou J. Regulation of the acute phase response genes alpha 1-acid glycoprotein and alpha 1-antitrypsin correlates with sensitivity to thermal injury. *Surgery* 1996; 119(6): 664–73.
32. Livingston DH, Mosenthal AC, Deitch EA. Sepsis and multiple organ dysfunction syndrome: a clinical-mechanistic overview. *New Horizons* 1995; 3: 276–87.
33. Selzman CH, Shames BD, Miller SA, *et al*. Therapeutic implications of interleukin-10 in surgical disease. *Shock* 1998; 10: 309–18.
34. De Maio A, de Mooney ML, Matesic LE, Paidas CN, Reeves RH. Genetic component in the inflammatory response induced by bacterial lipopolysaccharide. *Shock* 1998; 10: 319–23.
35. Yin MJ, Yamamoto Y, Gaynor RB. The anti-inflammatory agents aspirin and salicylate inhibit the activity of I (kappa) B kinase-beta. *Nature* 1998; 6706: 77–80.
36. Shakhov AN, Collart MA, Vassalli P, Nedospasov SA, Jongeneel CV. Kappa B-type enhances are involved in lipopolysaccharide-mediated transcriptional activation of the tumor necrosis factor alpha gene in primary macrophages. *J Exp Med* 1990; 171: 35–47.
37. Siebenlist U, Franzoso G, Brown K. Structure, regulation and function of NF-κB. *Ann Rev Cell Biol* 1994; 10: 405–55.
38. Yao J, Mackman N, Edgington TS, Fan ST. Lipopolysaccharide induction of tumor necrosis factor alpha promoter in human monocyte cells: regulation by Erg-1, c-jun, and NF-κB transcription factors. *J Biol Chem* 1997; 272: 17795–801.
39. Dinarello CA. Biologic basis for interleukin-1 in disease. *Blood* 1996; 87: 2095–147.
40. Kishimoto T, Taga T, Akira S. Cytokine signal transduction. *Cell* 1994; 76: 325–8.
41. Gilpin DA, Hsieh CC, Kuninger DT, Herndon DN, Papaconstantinou J. Effect of thermal injury on the expression of transcription factors that regulate acute phase response genes: the response of C/EBPα, C/EBPβ, and C/EBPδ to thermal injury. *Surgery* 1996; 119: 674–83.
42. Alam T, An MR, Papaconstantinou J. Differential expression of three C/EBP isoforms in multiple tissues during the acute phase response. *J Biol Chem* 1992; 267: 5021–4.
43. Jarrar D, Herndon DN, Wolf SE, Papaconstantinou J. Growth hormone treatment after burn affects expression of C/EBPs, regulators of the acute phase response *J Burn Care Rehabil* 1998; 19: S163.
44. Umayahara Y, Ji C, Centrella M, Rotwein P, McCarthy TL. CCAAT/enhancer-binding protein delta activates insulin-like growth factor-I gene transcription in osteoblasts. Identification of a novel cyclic AMP signaling pathway in bone. *J Biol Chem* 1997; 272: 31793–800.
45. Nolten LA, Steenbergh PH, Sussenbach JS. Hepatocyte nuclear factor 1 alpha activates promoter 1 of the human insulin-like growth factor I gene via two distinct binding sites. *Mol Endocrinol* 1995; 9: 1488–99.
46. Nolten LA, van Schaik FM, Steenbergh PH, Sussenbach JS. Expression of the insulin-like growth I gene is stimulated by the liver-enriched transcription factors C/EBP alpha and LAP. *Mol Endocrinol* 1994; 8: 1636–45.
47. Thomas MJ, Gronowski AM, Berry SA, *et al*. Growth hormone rapidly activates rat serine protease inhibitor 2.1 gene transcription and induces a DNA-binding activity distinct from those of STAT1, -3, and -4. *Mol Cell Biol* 1995; 15: 12–18.
48. Tracey KJ, Fong Y, Hesse DG, *et al*. Anti-cachectin/TNF monoclonal antibodies prevent septic shock during lethal bacteraemia. *Nature* 1987; 330: 662–4.
49. Beutler B, Milsark IW, Cerami AC. Passive immunization against cachectin/tumor necrosis factor protects mice from lethal effect of endotoxin. *Science* 1985; 229: 869–71.
50. Alexander HR, Doherty GM, Buresh CM. A recombinant human receptor antagonist to interleukin 1 improves survival after lethal endotoxemia in mice. *J Exp Med* 1991; 173: 1029–32.
51. Pruitt JH, Copeland EM, Moldawer LL. Interleukin-1 and interleukin-1

antagonism in sepsis systemic inflammatory response syndrome and septic shock. *Shock* 1995; **3**: 235–51.

52. Williams G, Giroir B. Regulation of cytokine gene expression: tumor-necrosis factor, interleukin-1, and the emerging biology of cytokine receptors. *New Horizons* 1995; **2**: 276–87.

53. Taniguchi T, Koido Y, Aiboshi J, Yamashita T, Suzaki S, Kurokawa A. Change in the ratio of interleukin-6 to interleukin-10 predicts a poor outcome in patients with systemic inflammatory response syndrome. *Crit Care Med* 1999; **27**: 1262–4.

54. Simovic MO, Bonham MJ, Abu-Zidan FM, Windsor JA. Anti-inflammatory cytokine response and clinical outcome in acute pancreatitis. *Crit Care Med* 1999; **27**: 2662–5.

55. Thissen JP, Verniers J. Inhibition by interleukin-1β and tumor necrosis factor-α of the insulin-like growth factor I messenger ribonucleic acid response to growth hormone in rat hepatocyte primary culture. *Endocrinology* 1997; **138**: 1078–84.

56. Lang CH, Fan J, Cooney R, Vary TC. IL-1 receptor antagonist attenuates sepsis-induced alterations in the IGF system and protein synthesis. *Am J Physiol* 1996; **270**: E430–7.

57. Delhanty PJ. Interleukin-1 beta suppresses growth hormone-induced acid-labile subunit mRNA levels and secretion in primary hepatocytes. *Biochem Biophys Res Com* 1998; **243**: 269–72.

58. Salgame P, Abrams JS, Clayberger C, et al. Differing lymphokine profiles of functional subsets of human CD4 and CD8 T cell clones. *Science* 1991; **254**: 279–82.

59. de Waal Malefyt R, Abrams J, Bennett B. Interleukin 10 (IL-10) inhibits cytokine synthesis by human monocytes: an autoregulation role of IL-10 produced by monocytes. *J Exp Med* 1991; **174**: 1209–20.

60. Kusske AM, Rongione AJ, Reber HA. Cytokines and acute pancreatitis. *Gastroenterology* 1996; **110**: 639–42.

61. Wang T, Tracey KJ. HMG-1 a late mediator of endotoxin lethality. *Science* 1999; **285**: 248–50.

62. Calandra T, Echtenacher B, Le Roy D, et al. Protection from septic shock by neutralization of macrophage migration inhibitory factor. *Nature Med* 2000; **2**: 164–70.

63. Jeschke MG, Barrow RE, Herndon DN. Recombinant human growth hormone (rhGH) treatment in pediatric burn patients and its role during the acute phase response. *Crit Care Med* 2000; **28**: 1578–84.

64. Postel-Vinay MC, Finidori J. Growth hormone receptor: structure and signal transduction. *Eur J Endocrinol* 1995; **133**: 654–9.

65. Waxman DJ, Zhao S, Choi HK. Interaction of a novel sex-dependent, growth hormone-regulated liver nuclear factor with CYP2C12 promoter. *J Biol Chem* 1996; **271**: 29978–87.

66. Kelly PA, Diane J, Postel-Vinay MC. The prolactin/growth hormone receptor family. *Endocr Rev* 1991; **12**: 235–51.

67. Seth A, Gonzalez FA, Gupta S. Signal transduction within the nucleus by mitogen-activated protein kinase. *J Biol Chem* 1992; **267**: 24796–804.

68. Han Y, Leaman DW, Watling D. Participation of JAK and STAT proteins in growth hormone-induced signaling. *J Biol Chem* 1996; **271**: 5947–52.

69. Haeffner A, Thieblemont N, Deas O. Inhibitory effect of growth hormone on TNF-α secretion and nuclear factor-kappa B translocation in lipopolysaccharide-stimulated human monocytes. *J Immunol* 1997; **158**: 1310–14.

70. Sumantran VN, Tsai ML, Schwartz J. Growth hormone induces c-fos and c-jun expression in cells with varying requirements for differentiation. *Endocrinology* 1992; **130**: 2016–24.

71. Clarkson RW, Chen CM, Harrison S. Early responses of trans-activating factors to growth hormone in preadipocytes: differential regulation of CCAAT enhancer-binding protein-beta (C/EBP beta) and C/EBP delta. *Mol Endocrinol* 1995; **9**: 108–20.

72. Schwander JC, Hauri C, Zapf J. Synthesis and secretion of insulin-like growth factor and its binding protein by the perfused rat liver: dependence on growth hormone status. *Endocrinology* 1983; **113**: 297–305.

73. Alam T, An MR, Mifflin RC. Trans-activation of the α1-acid glycoprotein gene acute phase response element by multiple isoforms of C/EBP and glucocorticoid receptor. *J Biol Chem* 1993; **268**: 15681–8.

74. Xia ZF, Coolbaugh MI, Kuninger DT, et al. Regulation of the acute phase response genes alpha₁-acid glycoprotein and alpha₁-antitrypsin correlates with sensitivity to thermal injury. *Surgery* 1996; **119**: 664–73.

75. Takala J, Ruokonen E, Webster N, et al. Increased mortality associated with growth hormone treatment in critically ill adults. *N Engl J Med* 1999; **341**: 785–92.

76. Aarsland A, Chinkes D, Wolfe RR. Beta-blockade lowers peripheral lipolysis in burn patients receiving growth hormone. Rate of hepatic very low density lipoprotein triglyceride secretions remains unchanged. *Ann Surg* 1996; **223**: 777–89.

77. Ishii T, Sato M, Sudo K. Hepatocyte growth factor stimulates liver regeneration and elevates blood protein level in normal and partially hepatectomized rats. *J Biochem* 1995; **117**: 1105–12.

78. Guillén MI, Gomez-Lechon MJ, Nakamura T. The hepatocyte growth factor regulates the synthesis of acute-phase proteins in human hepatocytes: divergent effect on interleukin-6 stimulated genes. *Hepatology* 1996; **23**: 1345–52.

79. Pierzchalski P, Nakamura T, Takehara T. Modulation of acute phase protein synthesis in cultured rat hepatocytes by human recombinant hepatocyte growth factor. *Growth Factors* 1992; **7**: 161–5.

80. Michalopoulos GK, DeFrances MC. Liver regeneration. *Science* 1997; **276**: 60–6.

81. Michalopoulos GK, Appasamy R. Metabolism of HGF-SF and its role in liver regeneration. *EXS* 1993; **65**: 275–83.

82. Zarnegar R. Regulation of HGF and HGFR gene expression. In: Goldberg ID, Rosen EM, eds. *Epithelial–Mesenchymal Interactions in Cancer*. Basel: Birkhauser Verlag, 1995.

83. Ohira H, Miyata M, Kuroda M. Interleukin-6 induces proliferation of rat hepatocytes *in vivo*. *J Hepatol* 1996; **25**: 941–7.

84. Chen-Kiang S, Hsu W, Natkunman Y. Nuclear signaling by interleukin-6. *Curr Opin Immunol* 1993; **5**: 124–8.

85. Castell JV, Gomez-Lechon MJ, David M. Interleukin 6 is the major regulator of acute phase protein synthesis in adult human hepatocytes. *FEBS Lett* 1989; **242**: 237–9.

86. Rai RM, Zhang JX, Clemens MG. Gadolinium chloride alters the acinar distribution of phagocytosis and balance between pro- and anti-inflammatory cytokines. *Shock* 1996; **6**: 243–7.

87. Frost RA, Lang CH, Gelato MC. Transient exposure of human myeloblasts to tumor necrosis factor-α inhibits serum and insulin-like growth factor-I stimulated protein synthesis. *Endo* 1997; **138**: 4153–9.

88. Humbel RE. Insulin-like growth factor-I and factor-II. *Eur J Biochem* 1990; **190**: 445–62.

89. Baxter RC. Circulating levels and molecular distribution of the acid-labile (alpha) subunit of the high molecular weight insulin-like growth factor-binding protein complex. *J Clin Endocrinol Metab* 1990; **70**: 1347–53.

90. Huang KF, Chung DH, Herndon DN. Insulin-like growth factor-1 (IGF-I) reduces gut atrophy and bacterial translocation after severe burn injury. *Arch Surg* 1993; **128**: 47–54.

91. Strock LL, Singh H. Abdullah A. The effect of insulin-like growth factor-1 on postburn hypermetabolism. *Surgery* 1990; **108**: 161–4.

92. Steenfos HH. Growth factors and wound healing. *Scand J Plast Reconstr Hand Surg* 1994; **28**: 95–105.

93. Jeschke MG, Barrow RE, Herndon DN. IGF-I/IGFBP-3 attenuates the pro-inflammatory acute phase response in severely burned children. *Ann Surg* 2000; **231(2)**: 246–52.

94. Pugazhenti S, Miller E, Sable C, et al. Insulin-like growth factor-I induces bcl-2 promoter through the transcription factor camp response element-binding protein. *J Biol Chem* 1999; **274**: 27529–35.

95. Delaney CL, Cheng HL, Feldman EL. Insulin-like growth factor-I prevents caspase-mediated apoptosis in Schwann cells. *J Neurobiol* 1999; **41**: 540–8.

96. Jeschke MG, Herndon DN, Vita R, Traber DL, Barrow RE. Insulin-like growth factor-I in combination with insulin-like growth factor binding protein-3 affects hepatocyte apoptosis through nitric oxide and NF-κB. *Ann Surg* 2000 (submitted for publication).

97. Herold G. Lebererkrankungen. In: Herold G, ed. *Innere Medizin*. Köln: Herold Verlag, 2000; 411–60.

Chapter 22 Effects of burn injury on bone and mineral metabolism

Gordon L Klein

David N Herndon

The effects of burn injury on homeostasis of three critical minerals (calcium, phosphorus, and magnesium) have not been studied in great detail. These three minerals play key roles in metabolism and also are stored in bone, a tissue that is significantly affected by burn injury. This chapter covers the roles of calcium (Ca), phosphorus (P), and magnesium (Mg) in normal body metabolism, the homeostasis of these three elements, what is known about the alterations in Ca, P, and Mg homeostasis by burn injury with suggestions for corrective therapy, and what is known about the effects of burn injury on bone turnover.

Metabolic functions of calcium, phosphorus, and magnesium

All three of these minerals play important roles in intracellular and extracellular metabolism.

Calcium

Ca plays a major role in neuromuscular impulse propagation and membrane depolarization and, consequently, in muscle contractil-ity. Ca may also serve as a second messenger, mediating the secretory release of peptides such as amylase, insulin, and aldosterone via intracellular pathways utilizing calmodulin, an intracellular calcium receptor protein, or protein kinase C. From the standpoint of extracellular metabolism, Ca serves as a co-factor in blood coagulation, specifically in the conversion of prothrombin to thrombin and the activation of several factors in the coagulation cascade. Ca also contributes to plasma membrane stability by binding to phospholipids.[1–3]

Phosphorus

P plays a major role in intracellular energy metabolism. P, in the form of phosphate esters, is a constituent of purine nucleotides, an important source of intracellular energy. Phosphorylation of various metabolic intermediate products is also the means of intracellular energy transfer. In the form of phospholipids, P is also a major structural component of cell membranes.[1]

Magnesium

Mg, primarily stored in mitochondria, is a vital co-factor for the function of enzymes involved in the transfer of phosphate groups; and thus, it is important for all reactions which require adenosine triphosphate (ATP) and in reactions involving replication, transcription, and translation of nucleic acids.[1] Extracellular Mg is important in plasma membrane excitability.

Homeostasis of calcium, phosphorus, and magnesium

Calcium

Absorption of Ca is generally well regulated by the body. With high Ca intake, absorption can be as low as 20%, while with low Ca intake, absorption can reach 70%.[4] The mechanism for this regulation is shown in **Figure 22.1**. With high Ca intake, there is a transient hypercalcemia followed by a suppression of parathyroid hormone (PTH) secretion, and consequently a suppression of PTH-stimulated renal conversion of 25-hydroxyvitamin D, the chief circulating form of the vitamin, to calcitriol, or 1,25-dihydroxyvitamin D. With low Ca intake, the reverse occurs. There is a transient reduction in serum Ca concentration, followed by a rapid, within 5 minutes, rise in PTH secretion. PTH will, under normal circumstances, stimulate bone resorption and increase renal tubular Ca reabsorption in order to raise serum Ca concentration. Furthermore, it stimulates the renal enzyme 25-hydroxyvitamin D-1-α hydroxylase to convert 25-hydroxyvitamin D to calcitriol. Calcitriol then binds to intestinal epithelial cells and increases transcellular Ca absorption by altering cell membrane phospholipid and by facilitating the intracellular passage of the absorbed Ca by stimulating the cellular synthesis of *calcium binding proteins*. Thus, the efficiency of Ca absorption is improved.

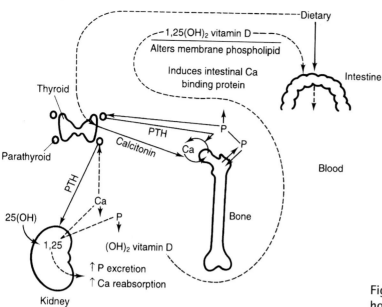

Fig. 22.1 Diagram of actions involved in calcium homeostasis.

Ca, given intravenously, bypasses the intestinal control mechanism and suppresses PTH production by the parathyroids as well as production of calcitriol by the kidney. The bone stores 99% of the body's Ca.[1]

Phosphorus

In contrast to Ca, the intestine plays no significant regulatory role in P absorption. Approximately 80% of dietary phosphate is absorbed. Homeostatic control appears to rest primarily within the kidney.[5,6] The regulatory mechanisms are unknown, but they are most likely PTH-independent.[5,6] Thus, the renal excretory rate of phosphate will primarily regulate the serum P concentration and maintain it within a normal range. The bone stores approximately 90% of the body's phosphate.

Magnesium

Approximately 60% of the body's Mg is stored in the skeleton,[7] although not at sites where matrix is calcified. Mg absorption, like P, varies directly with dietary intake with about 40% of an average daily load being absorbed.[8] The relationship between Ca and Mg absorption is described as inverse, but the mechanism of this is unclear. Renal excretion is the main route of Mg elimination and it may vary with serum Mg concentration.[9] Thus, hypermagnesemia and hypercalcemia inhibit renal tubular reabsorption of Mg while hypomagnesemia and PTH increase Mg reabsorption.[9]

Effect of burn injury on calcium, phosphorus, and magnesium homeostasis

The effects of burn injury on mineral homeostasis have not been studied in great detail. Data from the studies at the University of Texas Medical Branch and the Shriners Burns Hospital in Galveston most recently describe some of the newer developments in this area.

A study of children burned ≥30% total body surface area (TBSA) demonstrated that serial measurements of blood ionized Ca were a mean of 5% below the lower limits of normal.[10] These levels were associated with serum levels of PTH that were too low for the ionized Ca concentration in the blood, indicative that these patients were hypoparathyroid following acute burn injury. Furthermore, administration of a standard amount of PTH failed to produce the expected increases in urinary cyclic AMP and phosphate excretion,[10] providing evidence for PTH resistance in these patients. Mg depletion, encountered in all of the patients studied,[10,11] is known to impair secretion of PTH in response to hypocalcemia, and to result in resistance to PTH infusion. A recent study at our hospital indicates that aggressive parenteral Mg supplementation will replete approximately 50% of burn victims. However, Mg repletion failed to improve the hypoparathyroidism.[11] Therefore, the cause of the postburn hypoparathyroidism remains unknown. Recent data obtained from animal studies show that there may be an upregulation of the parathyroid gland Ca-sensing receptor, which is associated in humans with decreased circulating Ca levels necessary to suppress PTH secretion.[12] This phenomenon is known as a *reduced set point* for Ca suppression of PTH secretion.

In data collected from 11 adult patients in the burn unit between December 1989 and January 1992,[13] low serum concentrations of ionized Ca, P, and Mg were far more common than high serum levels of these minerals. Six patients had low serum concentrations of ionized Ca, three of them manifesting the hypocalcemia during the first 48 hours postburn. Four of these patients were hypophosphatemic; this was most prevalent on day 7 postburn. Five of the patients were hypomagnesemic, with this finding most likely to be present on day 3 postburn. In contrast, only one patient demonstrated hypercalcemia, and one hyperphosphatemia. No one was hypermagnesemic. In each case, the elevated serum level of either ionized Ca or P was transient. The studies in adults are not yet as detailed as the studies in children have been in this regard.

Hypocalcemia cannot be diagnosed from determinations of total serum Ca concentration, due to the variability of serum albumin concentrations postburn. Determination of serum-ionized Ca concentration should be encouraged, if available, for a more accurate diagnosis. Several possible mechanisms for hypocalcemia have been proposed. One is a shift of Ca from the extracellular to the intracellular compartment, as has been suggested by the accumulation of Ca in the erythrocyte of the burn patient,[14] a manifestation of what is termed the 'sick cell' syndrome. Alternative hypotheses include increased urinary calcium excretion, which has been documented to occur in burned children,[15] but is consistent with the documented hypoparathyroidism.[10] Losses of Ca in tissue exudate could also theoretically contribute to hypocalcemia. While it has been argued that the amount of Ca in wound exudate is probably insufficient to entirely account for postburn hypocalcemia,[16] there are not enough studies that actually measure Ca content of the burn wound exudate.

While fecal Ca losses can be high in burn patients,[16] and the large amount of endogenous corticosteroids produced by burn injury may impair intestinal Ca absorption,[17] there is no evidence to suggest that hypocalcemia is caused by corticosteroid-induced impairment of intestinal reabsorption of Ca secreted into the intestinal lumen. Other proposed mechanisms include reduced bone turnover.[13,18] The possibility of the reduced set point for calcium suppression of PTH secretion as a contributor to postburn hypocalcemia, while preliminary,[12] is an attractive hypothesis.

Possible explanations for postburn hypophosphatemia include intracellular accumulation of phosphate, inadequate phosphate intake, excessive urinary phosphate excretion, not likely in view of the documented hypoparathyroidism, or phosphate loss into the extravascular fluid. In a review of the subject, Dolecek[16] found increased urinary phosphate excretion only during the third and fourth weeks postburn in adults, while hypophosphatemia was documented to occur earlier. Thus, it is possible that the increased urinary phosphate excretion, seen later postburn, is more a function of increased tissue breakdown and filtered load than of inappropriate or excessive urinary phosphate losses. There is little documentation of inadequate phosphate intake following burns. Burn victims at our institution have been documented to take in a minimum of 1.6 g phosphate per day in enteral feedings alone.[13] Loss of significant phosphate in the extravascular fluid, excessive secretion of phosphate into the intestine with failure to reabsorb, and intracellular accumulation are all theoretically possible explanations for hypophosphatemia, but remain unproven. Similarly,

the cause of hypomagnesemia occurring postburn is unknown, although excessive urinary and fecal losses have been reported in adults,[16] and excessive losses in the burn wound have also been described.[19]

Rationale for therapy

Because of their importance in the maintenance of bodily metabolic processes, low serum levels of ionized Ca, P, and Mg should be treated (**Figure 22.2**). Hypocalcemia, especially in the immediate postburn period during the resuscitation effort, can potentiate abnormalities of cardiac muscle produced by hyperkalemia[20] and cause unresponsiveness to repletion in shock.[20] If a patient is not hypocalcemic, there is insufficient evidence of benefit following provision of parenteral Ca during resuscitation[21–23] unless the patient has hyperkalemia, hypomagnesemia, or Ca channel blocker toxicity.[24] Similarly, while caution should be exercised during massive transfusion with citrate-containing blood, Ca therapy may not be necessary if the patient is normocalcemic and if hepatic and renal function are only minimally impaired. The liver will clear citrate, which may transiently chelate Ca, at a rate of 1 unit of blood transfused every 5 minutes.[25] Only when clinical and electrocardiographic evidence suggests hypocalcemia, should treatment be initiated. Ca infusions, when given, should be administered slowly, since rapid replacement of Ca has resulted in cardiac arrhythmias.[20,25]

Hypophosphatemia may result in tissue hypoxemia due to increased hemoglobin affinity for oxygen and decreased tissue ATP, metabolic encephalopathy, hemolysis, shortened platelet survival time, myalgias, weakness, and possible impairment of myocardial contractility.[26] Hypomagnesemia, or Mg depletion with normal serum Mg, can blunt the effect of parathyroid hormone secreted in response to hypocalcemia on target organs and can impair the secretion of parathyroid hormone itself.[27] Mg deficiency can also cause generalized convulsions, muscle tremors, and weakness.[27]

Recommended treatment of hypocalcemia

Acute symptomatic hypocalcemia should be treated with intravenous Ca. In adults, 90–180 mg of elemental Ca over 5–10 min-

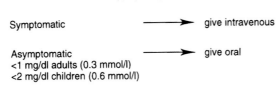

Fig. 22.2 Algorithm for the management of low levels of ionized calcium, phosphorus, or magnesium that may occur postburn.

utes is given so as to reverse twitching. In infants or children, Ca chloride in a 20 mg/kg dose or Ca gluconate in a 200–500 mg/kg/dose in four divided doses is suggested.[27,28] Caution should attend the use of parenteral chloride since it may cause phlebitis and/or acidosis. While hypocalcemia is asymptomatic and patients can tolerate enteral feedings, milk and/or infant formula can provide as much as 3 g/day of bioavailable Ca.[13] If, as we and others have found, hypocalcemia can occur despite enteral provision of such a large quantity of Ca, intermittent parenteral administration of Ca salts will be necessary. While the amounts given to each patient must be determined individually, as an example of what may be needed, six of our recent patients with burns exceeding 40% TBSA received 0.9–15 g of 10% calcium gluconate per day over the first 5 weeks following burn injury. Treatment was given an average of twice daily on approximately 75% of the days during those 5 weeks.

Symptomatic hypophosphatemia requires parenteral treatment with a starting dose of 2 mg/kg infused over 6 hours and treatment continued until serum P concentrations exceed 1.0 mg/dl (0.3 mmol/l).[26] Infants and children with symptomatic hypophosphatemia should receive 5–10 mg/kg infused over 6 hours, followed by 15–45 mg/kg given by infusion over 24 hours or until the serum P concentration rises above 2.0 mg/dl (0.6 mmol/l).[29]

Our adult patients who tolerated enteral feedings and consumed an average of 1.6 g/day of phosphate should have consumed enough to treat asymptomatic hypophosphatemia.[13] Hypophosphatemia has not been reported to be prolonged in burn patients; however, in such cases where this may occur, parenteral supplementation would be necessary.

Adults who have signs or symptoms of Mg deficiency with serum Mg concentration below 1.5 mEq/l (1.8 mg/dl or 0.8 mmol/l) usually require parenteral therapy. A 24-hour infusion of 48 mEq/l (58 mg/dl or 24 mmol/l) may be the treatment of choice.[27,30] For those who have convulsions or arrhythmias in association with hypomagnesemia, intravenous administration of 8–16 mEq (10–19 mg, 4–8 mmol) over 5–10 minutes may be necessary. This bolus would then be followed by the parenteral infusion mentioned above. For children, routine combined administration of enteral and parenteral Mg of 12–14 mg/kg/day (4.9–5.8 mmol/kg/day or 9.8–10.6 mEq/kg/day) has resulted in normalization of serum Mg in nearly all children studied, but repletion of only 50% of the severely burned children at our institution.[11] For treatment of symptomatic hypomagnesemia in children, Mg sulfate can be given parenterally 20–40 mEq (25–50 mg, 10–20 mmol) per dose followed by a 24-hour infusion of 25–50 mEq (30–60 mg, 12–25 mmol)/kg not exceeding 830 mEq (1 g, 450 mmol) per 24 hours.[29,30] If there is any impairment of renal function, the dose of Mg should be reduced by 50%. While enteral infusion should serve to maintain normal serum Mg concentration, parenteral administration of Mg is also indicated for those patients who cannot tolerate enteral feedings. Parenteral administration of 8 mEq (10 mg, 4 mmol) Mg per day should be given to *adults* to maintain normal serum Mg levels.[27,29] For maintenance of serum Mg levels in the normal range in *children* exclusively by the parenteral route, the intravenous infusion rate stated above should be used. In the patients reported above,[11] daily infusions of 123 mg–1.45 g of elemental Mg as Mg sulfates were given to support serum Mg concentrations.

Bone

The main Ca storage depot in the body is bone. Both linear growth and bone remodeling are adversely affected by burn injury. Linear growth at the epiphysis of the long bones usually occurs by means of proliferation of cartilage cells with production of extracellular matrix; these chondrocytes and matrix undergo a series of biochemical changes which lead to the appearance of ossification centers, which appear as single expanding foci. As these ossifications expand, cartilaginous tissue is replaced by bone in a vascular supply system, which provides for the delivery of nutrients, hormones, and growth factors.

It has been reported by Rutan and Herndon[31] that linear growth velocity is retarded in children with severe burns. The mechanism for this effect of burn injury is unknown, but it has been established that the rate of growth does return to normal.[31] The effects of burn injury on bone remodeling are profound and long-lasting. In a study of 12 adult patients with burns of greater than 50% TBSA, there was a marked reduction in bone formation.[13] In children the findings are more dramatic. Iliac crest bone biopsies from 18 children burned over 40% TBSA revealed even more markedly depressed bone formation,[18] and a cross-sectional study of children undergoing biopsy a mean of 5 years after suffering a similar-sized burn injury revealed that fully 50% of them had persistent decreased bone formation.[32] To put these findings in perspective, it is necessary to discuss the normal process of bone remodeling.

Bone remodeling is a continuous process of breakdown of calcified bone matrix by osteoclasts and formation of new bone matrix by osteoblasts and the mineralization of that matrix by calcium and phosphate forming a mature crystal lattice of calcium phosphate hydroxyapatite. One remodeling cycle takes about 4 months in an adult. Bone resorption and formation are normally biochemically and, perhaps mechanically, linked. All the details of this linkage are not known, but, as an example, parathyroid hormone receptors have been identified on osteoblasts but have so far not been identified on osteoclasts.[33] Thus, parathyroid hormone can increase the number of osteoblasts on bone surfaces in both humans[34] and animals.[35] Therefore, osteoblasts, which are bone-forming cells, must serve as an intermediary in the process of parathyroid hormone-mediated bone resorption. The reduced bone formation after burn injury was first identified on bone biopsies in adults between 9 weeks and 9 months postburn.[13] By administering tetracycline to the patients in two doses separated by 2 weeks, we found that the newly mineralized bone surface taking up tetracycline was markedly reduced in burned patients compared to age- and sex-matched controls.[13] In contrast, the distance between the two tetracycline fluorescent labels in the bone was not significantly reduced. The distance between the tetracycline bands represents the *mineral apposition rate*, and is an index of osteoblast function. The mineral apposition rate when multiplied by the percentage of bone surface taking up tetracycline is the *bone formation rate*,[36] and is an index of osteoblast number as well as function. Thus, in adult burn patients, bone formation is reduced possibly due to a reduced number of osteoblasts rather than to reduced osteoblast function. Consistent with these findings is the reduced amount of osteoid or unmineralized bone matrix, a product of osteoblasts. There is no evidence in the adult that bone formation is similarly reduced or is significantly increased. Therefore, there appears to be a dissociation of bone formation and bone resorption. In children, the situation is actually worse. There is no separation between tetracycline labels,[18] indicating that osteoblast function as well as osteoblast number may be impaired. Furthermore, in children, biochemical markers of both bone formation and bone resorption are reduced,[18] suggesting the lower bone turnover that is seen with hypoparathyroidism,[10] which has been identified in these patients.

The consequences of the reduced bone formation include chronically diminished bone mineral density of the lumbar spine.[15,18] This results in an increased fracture risk[15] and possible reduction in *peak bone mass*.[15] A reduction in peak bone mass would put a burned child at risk to develop adult-onset osteoporosis. Cross-sectional studies of bone mineral density of the lumbar spine were performed using dual-energy X-ray absorptiometry (DEXA) in 68 children:[15] 16 were burned between 15 and 36% TBSA, 22 were burned over 40% TBSA and studied within 8 weeks of their burn, and 30, also with burns over 40% TBSA, were studied a mean of 5 years after burn injury. The bone density z-scores (standard deviation scores) were less than −1 in 60% of the severely burned patients and less than −2 in 27% of the same group, with no difference between those studied within 8 weeks and those studied a mean of 5 years following burn injury; z-scores were not as low for those receiving moderate burns. These data suggest that the reduced bone density in the severely burned children compared to age-related normal children is prolonged[15] and that there is no significant improvement of bone density over time. Longitudinal studies are currently in progress in order to better define the issues causing the prolonged reduction in bone density.

There are several potential contributing factors to this pathology, including the production of proinflammatory cytokines, especially interleukins(IL)-1β and IL-6;[18] immobilization, which induces bone resorption and decreases formation;[37] and increased endogenous glucocorticoid production,[18] which may have direct toxicity to osteoblasts. Another possible contributing factor is aluminum loading, which can cause reduced bone formation in uremic patients[38] and in those receiving total parenteral nutrition.[39] Aluminum loading in adult burn patients would be most significant if the contaminated products bypassed the normal intestinal, cutaneous, and pulmonary barriers to aluminum entry into the blood. The main sources would be albumin[40,41] and Ca gluconate.[41–43] However, it is highly unlikely that aluminum loading constitutes the primary cause of this pathology in adults because similar histomorphometric abnormalities were found in the biopsies of adult patients without detectable bone aluminum.[13] Furthermore, no aluminum was detected in the bones of burned children who had a much greater depression of bone formation than the burned adults.[18] In addition, bed rest may contribute to decreased bone formation.[44,45]

Attempts to improve bone formation, thereby preventing bone loss, following burn injury are in the early stages of study. Attempts to use high-dose recombinant human growth hormone (rHGH), 0.2 mg/kg/day subcutaneously during the course of hospitalization for the acute burn injury, led to a rise in circulating levels of insulin-like growth factor I (IGF-I). However, serum levels of osteocalcin, a vitamin D- and vitamin K-dependent peptide produced by osteoblasts and which serves as an index of bone formation, remained low following a 6-week period of treatment. The failure of rHGH to improve bone formation despite producing a rise in circulating IGF-1 may be attributable to GH-independent high circulating levels of IGF-binding protein-4 (IGFBP-4), a binding protein that can block access of IGF-1 to local tissue receptors. Similarly, circulating levels of IGFBP-5, a binding protein that can help bind IGF-1 to hydroxyapatite matrix of bone is initially low following a burn, rising to normal by time of hospital discharge.[46] However, preliminary data obtained from the administration of rHGH to children at a dose of 0.05 mg/kg/day from hospital discharge to 1 year postburn suggest that there is a significant improvement in both bone mineral content and bone size.[47] Other potential therapies, such as oxandrolone, an orally administered anabolic agent that has been shown to reduce postburn weight loss and nitrogen wasting,[48] are currently under study.

References

1. Broadus AE. Mineral balance and homeostasis. In: Favus MJ, ed. *Primer on the Metabolic Bone Diseases and Disorders of Mineral Metabolism*, 4th edn. Philadelphia: Lippincott, Williams and Wilkins, 1999: 74–9.
2. Joff GA, Rosenberg RB. Physiology of hemostasis, the fluid phase. In: Nathan DG, Oski FA, eds. *Hematology of Infancy and Childhood*. Philadelphia: WB Saunders, 1993: 1534–60.
3. Rasmussen H. The calcium messenger system. *N Engl J Med* 1986; **314**: 1094–101.
4. Neer RM. Calcium and inorganic phosphate homeostasis. In: DeGroot LJ, ed. *Endocrinology*. Philadelphia: WB Saunders, 1989; 927–53.
5. Klein GL, Coburn JW. Parenteral nutrition: effect on bone and mineral homeostasis. *Annu Rev Nutr* 1991; **11**: 93–119.
6. Portale AA, Halloran BP, Murphy MM, Morriss RC Jr. Oral intake of phosphorus can determine the serum concentration of 1,25-dihydroxyvitamin D by determining production rate in humans. *J Clin Invest* 1986; **77**: 7–12.
7. Silverberg SJ. The distribution and balance of calcium, magnesium and phosphorus. In: Favus MJ, ed. *Primer on the Metabolic Bone Diseases and Disorders of Mineral Metabolism*. Kelseyville, CA: American Society for Bone and Mineral Research, 1990: 32–6.
8. Lemann J Jr, Favus MJ. The intestinal absorption of calcium, magnesium, and phosphate. In: Favus MJ, ed. *Primer on the Metabolic Bone Diseases and Disorders of Mineral Metabolism*, 4th edn. Philadelphia: Lippincott, Williams and Wilkins, 1999: 63–6.
9. Bushinsky DA, Calcium, magnesium, and phosphorus: renal handling and urinary excretion. In: Favus MJ ed. *Primer on the Metabolic Bone Diseases and Disorders of Mineral Metabolism*, 4th edn. Philadelphia: Lippincott, Williams and Wilkins. 1999: 67–73.
10. Klein GL, Nicolai M, Langman CB, Cuneo BF, Sailer DE, Herndon DN. Dysregulation of calcium homeostasis after severe burn injury in children: possible role of magnesium depletion. *J Pediatr* 1997; **131**: 246–51.
11. Klein GL, Langman CB, Herndon DN. Persistent hypoparathyroidism following magnesium repletion of burn-injured children. *Pediatr Nephrol* 2000; **14**: 301–4.
12. Murphey ED, Chattopadhyay N, Bai M, *et al.* Burn-associated upregulation of the parathyroid calcium-sensing receptor in sheep: a possible contributor to postburn hypocalcemia. *Critical Care Medicine*, 2000; **28**: 3885–90.
13. Klein GL, Herndon DN, Rutan TC, *et al.* Bone disease in burn patients. *J Bone Miner Res* 1993; **8**: 337–45.
14. Baar S. The effect of thermal injury on the loss of calcium from calcium loaded cells: its relationship to red cell function and patient survival. *Clin Chem Acta* 1982; **126**: 25–39.
15. Klein GL, Herndon DN, Langman CB, *et al.* Long-term reduction in bone mass following severe burn injury in children. *J Pediatr* 1995; **126**: 252–6.
16. Dolecek R. Calcium-active hormones and postburn low-calcium syndrome. In: Dolecek R, Brizio-Moltens L, Moltens A, Traber D. eds. *Endocrinology of Thermal Trauma: Pathophysiologic Mechanisms and Clinical Interpretation*. Philadelphia, Lea and Febiger, 1990: 216–37.
17. Hahn TJ, Halstead LR, Teitelbaum SI, Hahn BH. Altered mineral metabolism in glucocorticoid induced osteopenia: effect of 25-hydroxyvitamin D administration. *J Clin Invest* 1979; **64**: 655–65.
18. Klein GL, Herndon DN, Goodman WG, *et al.* Histomorphometric and biochemical characterization of bone following acute severe burns in children. *Bone* 1995; **17**: 455–60.
19. Berger MM, Rothen C, Cavadini C, Chiolero RL. Exudative mineral losses after serious burns: a clue to the alterations of magnesium and phosphate metabolism. *Am J Clin Nutr* 1997; **65**: 1473–81.
20. British Committee for Standardization in Haematology Blood Transfusion Task

Force. Guidelines for transfusion for massive blood loss. *Clin Lab Haematol* 1988; **10**: 265–73.

21. Stueven H, Thompson BM, Aprahamian C, *et al.* Use of calcium in pre-hospital cardiac arrest. *Ann Emerg Med* 1983; **12**: 136–9.

22. Stueven HA, Thompson BM, Aprahamian C, Tonsfeldt DJ. Calcium chloride, reassessment of use in asystole. *Ann Emerg Med* 1984; **13**: 820–2.

23. Harrison EE, Amey BD. Use of calcium in electromechanical dissociation. *Ann Emerg Med* 1984; **13**: 844–5.

24. Harinan RJ, Mangiardi LM, McAllister RG, Surawicz B, Shabetal R, Kishida H. Reversal of cardiovascular effects of verapamil by calcium and sodium. Differences between electrophysiologic and hemodynamic response. *Circulation* 1979; **59**: 797–804.

25. Dzik WH, Kirkley SA. Citrate toxicity during massive blood transfusion. *Transfusion Med Rev* 1988; **2**: 76–94.

26. Hruska KA, Lederer E. Hyperphosphatemia and hypophosphatemia In: Favus MJ, ed. *Primer on the Metabolic Bone Diseases and Disorders of Mineral Metabolism*, 4th edn., Philadelphia: Lippincott, Williams and Wilkins, 1999: 245–53.

27. Rude RK. Magnesium depletion and hypermagnesemia. In: Favus MJ, ed. *Primer on the Metabolic Bone Disease and Disorders of Mineral Metabolism*, 4th edn. Philadelphia: Lippincott, Williams and Wilkins, 1999: 241–4.

28. Shane E. Hypocalcemia: pathogenesis, differential diagnosis, and management. In: Favus MJ, ed. *Primer on the Metabolic Bone Diseases and Disorders of Mineral Metabolism*, 4th edn. Philadelphia: Lippincott, Williams and Wilkins, 1999: 223–5.

29. Carpenter TO. Neonatal hypocalcemia. In: Favus MJ, ed. *Primer on the Metabolic Bone Diseases and Disorders of Mineral Metabolism*, 4th edn. Philadelphia: Lippincott, Williams and Wilkins, 1999: 235–7.

30. Greene MG. In: *The Harriet Lane Handbook*. St. Louis, MO: Mosby-Yearbook, 1991: 150–244.

31. Rutan RL, Herndon DN. Growth delay in post-burn pediatric patients. *Arch Surg* 1990; **125**: 392–5.

32. Klein GL, Wolf SE, Goodman WG, Phillips WA, Herndon DN. The management of acute bone loss in severe catabolism due to burn injury. *Hormone Res* 1997; **48**(suppl 5): 83–7.

33. Simmons DJ, Seitz PK, Kidder LS, *et al.* Partial characterization of marrow stromal cells. *Calcif Tissue Int* 1991; **48**: 326–34.

34. Parisien M, Charhon SA, Arlot M, *et al.* Evidence for a toxic effect of aluminum on osteoblasts: a histomorphometric study in hemodialysis patients with aplastic bone disease. *J Bone Miner Res* 1988; **3**: 259–67.

35. Rodriguez M, Felsenfeld AJ, Llach F. Aluminum administration in the rat separately affects the osteoblast and bone mineralization. *J Bone Miner Res* 1990; **5**: 59–67.

36. Parfitt AM, Drezner MK, Glorieux FH, *et al.* Bone histomorphometry: standardization of nomenclature symbols and units. Report of the ASBMR Histomorphometry Nomenclature Committee. *J Bone Miner Res* 1987; **2**: 595–610.

37. Ishimi Y, Miyausa C, Jin CH, *et al.* IL-6 is produced by osteoblasts and induces bone resorption. *J Immunol* 1990; **145**: 3297–303.

38. Ott SM, Maloney NA, Coburn JW, Alfrey AC, Sherrard DJ. The prevalence of bone aluminum deposition in renal osteodystrophy and its relation to the response to calcitriol therapy. *N Engl J Med* 1982; **307**: 709–13.

39. Ott SM, Maloney NA, Klein GL, *et al.* Aluminum is associated with low bone formation in patients receiving chronic parenteral nutrition. *Ann Intern Med* 1983; **98**: 910–14.

40. Milliner DS, Shinaberger JH, Shuman P, Coburn JW. Inadvertent aluminum administration during plasma exchange due to aluminum contamination of albumin replacement solutions. *N Engl J Med* 1985; **312**: 165–7.

41. Sedman AB, Klein GL, Merritt RJ, *et al.* Evidence of aluminum loading in infants receiving intravenous therapy. *N Engl J Med* 1985; **312**: 1337–43.

42. Koo WWK, Kaplan LA, Horn J, *et al.* Aluminum in parenteral nutrition solutions – sources and possible alternatives. *J Parenter Enter Nutr* 1986; **10**: 591–5.

43. Klein GL, Herndon DN, Rutan TC, Barnett JL, Miller NL, Alfrey AC. Risk of aluminum loading in burn patients and ways to reduce it. *J Burn Care Rehabil* 1994; **15**: 354–8.

44. Arnaud SB, Sherrard DJ, Maloney NA, *et al.* Effects of one-week head-down tilt bed rest on bone formation with calcium endocrine system. *Aviat Space Environ Med* 1992; **63**: 14–20.

45. Leukens S, Arnaud SB, Taylor AK, Baylink DJ. Immobilization causes an acute and sustained increase in markers of bone resorption (abstract). *Clin Res* 1990; **38**: 123A.

46. Klein GL, Wolf SE, Langman CB, *et al.* Effect of therapy with recombinant human growth hormone on insulin-like growth factor system components and serum levels of biochemical markers of bone formation in children following severe burn injury. *J Clin Endocrinol Metab* 1998; **83**: 21–4.

47. Hart DW, Wolf SE, Klein GL, *et al.* Attenuation of post-traumatic muscle catabolism and osteopenia by long-term growth hormone therapy (abstract); submitted to the annual meeting of the Southern Surgical Association 2000 *Ann Surg* 2000; **233**: In Press.

48. Demling RH. Comparison of the anabolic effects and complications of human growth hormone and the testosterone analog, oxandrolone, after severe burn injury. *Burns* 1999; **25**: 215–21.

Chapter 23

Vitamin and trace element homeostasis following severe burn injury

Gordon L Klein

Introduction

Despite all the known metabolic consequences of burn injury, including the improvements in our understanding of protein and carbohydrate metabolism and of calcium and magnesium metabolism postburn, there remains very little understood about the effects of burn injury on trace element and vitamin homeostasis and postburn requirements. The limited research that has been done has concentrated on homeostasis of trace elements and vitamins after burn injury, wound healing in relation to trace elements, vitamins, and the antioxidant properties of various of the trace elements and vitamins. We will examine each of these aspects in the context of available data.

Homeostasis of trace elements and vitamins and role in burns

There is concern regarding trace element loss after burn injury. The major trace elements studied are zinc and copper, although a limited amount of work has also been done on selenium status postburn.

Several groups have reported low serum concentrations of zinc and copper, as well as albumin and ceruloplasmin, their associated binding proteins.[1-6] Urine and skin are considered major routes of excessive loss of these elements.[3,5,7] Thus, Cunningham et al.[5] and Boosalis et al.[8] found that patients with moderate to severe burns had excessive urinary zinc excretion associated with reduced plasma zinc levels, especially the plasma subfraction bound to albumin.[5] Zinc supplementation by means of total parenteral nutrition resulted in hyperzincuria, although not as pronounced as if zinc supplementation were given orally.[5,8] In contrast, increased urinary copper excretion was not found despite parenteral delivery of supplemental copper, although both plasma copper and ceruloplasmin were reduced. Only one study documented an increase in urinary copper excretion.[1] Thus it would appear as if, while there is a consensus that plasma copper and zinc concentrations fall postburn, urinary zinc losses may play a role but excessive urinary copper excretion is probably not of consequence.

With regard to cutaneous losses of zinc, Berger et al.[7] found that the losses through wound exudate greatly exceeded excretory losses over the first week postburn. Guo et al.[1] also detected elevated quantities of zinc in wound exudate. The other explanation offered for the uniformly reported fall in plasma zinc levels postburn is the redistribution of zinc within the body. In a study in which rats given ^{65}Zn received a 20% total body surface area (TBSA) burn, van Rij et al.[9] reported that there was a rapid uptake of ^{65}Zn by spleen, kidney, wound, and, particularly, liver, while there was a decrease in ^{65}Zn in brain, muscle, and, particularly, bone. Zinc-binding protein was demonstrated in the liver cytosol, suggesting that there is a flow of zinc to the liver at the expense of plasma, bone, and even wound after burn injury. It was also found by Cunningham et al.[5] that zinc supplementation exacerbates the urinary zinc excretion, suggesting that the body cannot take up the supplemental zinc, and perhaps suggesting that rather than zinc depletion, zinc redistribution is largely responsible for the low plasma levels. With regard to copper, it is clear that reduced plasma copper concentrations are associated with reduced circulating levels of ceruloplasmin.[2,6] Even though ceruloplasmin is an acute phase reactant stimulated by proinflammatory cytokines such as interleukin-1,[10] which is known to be elevated in the postburn inflammatory state,[11,12] there is also evidence that ceruloplasmin, in addition to copper, can be lost in the burn wound exudate. Cunningham et al.[2] reported a strong relationship between the size of the open wound and the amount of circulating ceruloplasmin. Gosling et al.[4] reported that hypocupremia in severe burns was inversely correlated with burn surface area, in contrast to circulating zinc levels, which showed no such correlation. Furthermore, ceruloplasmin, like albumin, may be extravasated from the intravascular compartment and carry the copper with it.

Loss of zinc and copper after burn injury are of potential significance due to the important roles of each as antioxidants, especially as components of the enzyme superoxide dismutase, and the additional roles of zinc in wound healing, collagen cross-linking, which may affect skeletal calcification,[11] and immune function.[13] Clearly, further studies will be required to elucidate the mechanism of hypocupremia and hypozincemia inasmuch as the available evidence would suggest that the etiologies may be different, and thus the management of these conditions may also need to be different.

Another trace element that acts as an antioxidant is selenium. In 1984, Hunt et al.[14] reported that plasma and erythrocyte selenium concentrations were reduced after burn injury, as was urinary selenium excretion. Boosalis et al.[15] confirmed these findings in 1986 and suggested that urinary selenium loss was not the chief explanation for the postburn selenium deficiency. They postulated that there may be an antagonistic relationship between selenium and the silver that is administered to the burn wounds. A trace element reported to be elevated after burn injury is aluminum. Klein et al.[16] reported elevated serum aluminum concentration in adults suffering severe burn injury (≥40% TBSA), even finding some aluminum deposition in the bones of burn patients as few as 8 days postburn.[17] While aluminum is toxic to bone and is a known inhibitor of bone formation,[17] it is clearly not the only contributor to postburn osteopenia and increased fracture risk. Nonetheless, the sources of aluminum contamination in burn treatment have been published[18] and attempts to minimize aluminum loading in these patients may hasten their skeletal recovery from burn injury.

Studies of the homeostasis of vitamins following burn injury are sparse. Rettmer et al.[19] performed functional testing for thiamin, riboflavin, and pyridoxine in burn patients and found them all to be normal. However, many adult burn victims are alcoholic and will require the standard thiamin supplementation of 50 mg/day. In a study of serum vitamin K levels in severely burned pediatric patients, Jenkins et al.[20] reported that 91% of the 48 children studied demonstrated circulating vitamin K levels below expected norms. These low levels were correlated with days of antibiotic therapy, percentage body surface area excised, and administration of blood products. However, there was no relationship between serum vitamin K concentration and prothrombin time. Therefore, it is not certain if the low circulating levels of vitamin K are clinically significant. It should be pointed out, however, that osteocalcin, a protein produced by osteoblasts, is a vitamin K-dependent gamma carboxylated protein that is used as a standard index of new bone formation. Osteocalcin is documented to be low in burned children during the same time period covered by the study of Jenkins et al.,[20] i.e. the first 4 weeks postburn. Thus, the possibility remains open that low circulating vitamin K levels may contribute to low osteocalcin in the serum, although bone formation has been documented to be low by other studies as well (see Chapter 22).

Serum levels of other vitamins have also been measured within 2–3 weeks postburn. These were vitamin A (retinol), vitamin E (α tocopherol), and vitamin C (ascorbic acid). Nguyen et al.[21] reported low serum vitamin E levels during the first 14 days postburn as part of a study examining peroxidation products following thermal injury. Similar findings were noted by Rock et al.,[22] not only for vitamin E but also for vitamins A and C. However, serum levels of all these vitamins improved with enteral supplementation.

Circulating levels of vitamin D (Klein GL and Langman CB, unpublished data) have been low but so has vitamin D-binding protein.[17] Serum calcitriol (1,25(OH)$_2$-vitamin D) levels have been slightly low, but calcitriol, the metabolically active form of vitamin D, is bound to albumin in serum. Therefore, in light of the postburn hypoproteinemia, it is difficult to assess the significance of the marginally low levels of circulating vitamin D. However, preliminary data suggest that burn patients do develop vitamin D deficiency after they are discharged from the hospital due to the recommendation that they minimize their exposure to sunlight.[23]

Effect of therapy on wound healing, fluid requirements, and the immune response

Despite the well-known role that zinc plays in wound healing, relatively little is known of the effects of zinc depletion postburn on healing of the burn wound. A recent in vivo study in rats by Li et al.[24] indicated that dietary zinc supplementation by itself may not be sufficient to improve wound healing. However, zinc applied directly to the experimental wound may accelerate healing. This subject is very difficult to evaluate, however, because of the evolving nature of wound management, including artificial skin, antibiotic therapy, and surgical intervention. There has also been a report suggesting that nicotinamide may increase capillary density and rapidity of wound healing in rats.[25]

With regard to other potentially beneficial effects of supplementation with trace elements of vitamins, there are conflicting studies regarding whether administration of ascorbic acid alters the volume of fluid required for initial burn resuscitation.[26-28] In a recent study from Japan by Tanaka and colleagues,[26] infusion of ascorbic acid during the initial 24 hours postburn in adults burned over 30% TBSA lessened the amount of fluid required to maintain heart rate and blood pressure and cut by 50% the amount of body weight gain. This is consistent with an earlier report by Nelson et al.,[27] who found that guinea pigs given large quantities of dietary ascorbic acid after burn injury had improved weight gain and reduced metabolic rates compared to controls. In contrast, a study involving infusion of ascorbic acid into dogs given graded scald burns of the paw failed to reduce paw weight gain.[28] However, this study was limited to a local burn injury involving the paw and did not take into account other systemic factors that might affect body fluid accumulation after a more extensive burn. In addition, a report by Chen and colleagues[29] showed that pretreatment of rats and mice with 1,25-dihydroxyvitamin D (calcitriol) lessens fat pad edema and pulmonary vascular permeability. However, this has limited practical value in that data are not available reporting the similar efficacy of postburn treatment with calcitriol.

Contradictory reports have been published with regard to the effects of vitamin E on the immune response. Kuroiwa et al.[30] failed to demonstrate a difference in lymphocyte response to phytohemagglutinin or in ear thickness response to 2,4-dinitrofluorobenzene in guinea pigs after a 30% burn and vitamin E supplements ranging from 0 to 100 mg/kg/day. Those receiving vitamin E supplements were less anemic than those that did not. In contrast, Haberal et al.[31] showed in patients with a ≥20% partial-or full-thickness burn injury, vitamin E supplementation for 3 days resulted in an increased number of circulating T cells compared to normal and in contrast to burn patients who did not receive vitamin E. In agreement with Kuroiwa et al.,[30] Berger and colleagues[32] studying severely burned adults reported that supplementation of these patients 30 days postburn with zinc, copper, and selenium for 8 days failed to alter lymphocyte proliferation to mitogens. The number of pulmonary infections in the supplemented group decreased, resulting in a shorter hospital stay when data were normalized for burn size.

In summary, there is much to learn regarding the homeostasis of trace elements and vitamins in response to burn injury and how changes affect wound healing, fluid resuscitation requirements, the immune response, and skeletal recovery. This area remains wide open to advances that could potentially hasten recovery and improve the quality of life for victims of severe burn injury.

References

1. Guo Z, Li L, Zhao L. Changes in contents of Zn, Cu, Fe, Ca, Mg in serum, urine and blister fluid after burn surgery. *Chung Hua Cheng Hsing Shao, Shang, Wai, Ko Tsa Chih* 2000; 13: 195–8.
2. Cunningham JJ, Lydon MK, Emerson R, Harmatz PR. Low ceruloplasmin levels during recovery from major burn injury: influence of open wound size and copper supplementation. *Nutrition* 2000; 12: 83–8.
3. Selmanpakoglu AN, Cetin C, Sayal A, Isimer A. Trace element (Al, Se, Zn, Cu) levels in serum, urine and tissues of burn patients. *Burns* 1994 20: 99–103.
4. Gosling P, Rothe HM, Sheehan TM, Hubbard LD. Serum copper and zinc concentrations in patients with burns in relation to burn surface area. *J Burn Care Rehabil* 1995 16: 481–6.
5. Cunningham JJ, Lydon MK, Briggs SE, DeCheke M. Zinc and copper status of severely burned children during TPN. *J Am Coll Nutr* 1991; 10: 57–62.
6. Shewmake KB, Talbert GE, Bowser-Wallace BH, Caldwell FT Jr, Cone JB. Alterations in plasma copper, zinc, and ceruloplasmin levels in patients with thermal trauma. *J Burn Care Rehabil* 1988; 9: 13–17.
7. Berger MM, Cavadini C, Bart A, et al. Cutaneous copper and zinc losses in burns. *Burns* 1992; 18: 373–80.
8. Boosalis MG, Solem LD, Cerra FB, et al. Increased urinary zinc excretion after thermal injury. *J Lab Clin Med* 1991; 118: 538–45.
9. van Rij AM, Hall MT, Bray JT, Pories WJ. Zinc as an integral component of the metabolic response to trauma. *Surg Gynecol Obstet* 1981; 153: 677–82.
10. Daffada AA, Young SP. Coordinated regulation of ceruloplasmin and metallothionein mRNA by interleukin-1 and copper in HepG2 cells. *FEBS Lett* 1999; 457: 214–18.
11. Klein GL, Herndon DN, Goodman WG, et al. Histomorphometric and biochemical characterization of bone following acute severe burns in children. *Bone* 1995; 17: 455–460.
12. Kupper TJ, Deitch EA, Baker CC, Wong W. The human burn wound as a primary source of interleukin-1 activity. *Surgery* 1986; 100: 409–15.
13. Keen CL, Gershwin ME. Zinc deficiency and immune function. *Annu Rev Nutr* 1990; 10: 415–31.
14. Hunt DR, Lane HW, Beesinger D, et al. Selenium depletion in burn patients. *J Parenter Enteral Nutr* 1984; 8: 695–9.
15. Boosalis MG, Solem LD, Ahrenholz DH, McCall JT, McClain CJ. Serum and urinary selenium levels in thermal injury. *Burns Incl Therm Inj* 1986; 12: 236–40.
16. Klein GL, Herndon DN, Rutan TC, Miller NL, Alfrey AC. Elevated serum aluminum levels in severely burned patients receiving large quantities of albumin. *J Burn Care Rehabil* 1990; 11: 526–30.
17. Klein GL, Herndon DN, Rutan TC, et al. Bone disease in burn patients. *J Bone Miner Res* 1993; 8: 337–45.
18. Klein GL, Herndon DN, Rutan TC, Barnett JR, Miller NL, Alfrey AC. Risk of aluminum accumulation in burn patients and ways to reduce it. *J Burn Care Rehabil* 1994; 15: 354–8.
19. Rettmer RL, Williamson JC, Labbe RF, Heimbach DM. Laboratory monitoring of nutritional status in burn patients. *Clin Chem* 1992; 38: 334–7.
20. Jenkins ME, Gottschlich MM, Kopcha R, Khoury J, Warden GD. A prospective analysis of serum vitamin K in severely burned pediatric patients. *J Burn Care Rehabil* 1998; 19: 75–81.
21. Nguyen TT, Cox CS, Traber DL, et al. Free radical activity and loss of plasma antioxidants, vitamin E, and sulfhydryl groups in patients with burns: the 1993 Moyer Award. *J Burn Care Rehabil* 1993; 14: 602–9.
22. Rock CL, Dechert RE, Khilnani R, Parker RS, Rodriguez JL. Carotenoids and antioxidant vitamins in patients after burn injury. *J Burn Care Rehabil* 1997; 18: 269–78.
23. Klein GL, Langman CB, Herndon DN. Late-onset vitamin D depletion following burn injury: a possible factor in post-burn osteopenia (abstract). *J Bone Miner Res* 2000; 15(Suppl 1): 5358.
24. Li L, Guo Z, Zhao L. Effects of supplement Zn on levels of Zn in serum, growth hormone and hydroxyproline. *Chung Hua Cheng Hsing Shao Shang Wai Ko Tsa Chih* 1998; 14: 425–8.
25. Smith YR, Klitzman B, Ellis MN, Kull FC Jr. The effect of nicotinamide on microvascular density and thermal injury in rats. *J Surg Res* 1989; 47: 465–9.
26. Tanaka H. Matsuda T, Miyagantani Y, Yukioka T, Matsuda H, Shimazaki S. Reduction of resuscitation fluid volumes in severely burned patients using ascorbic acid administration: a randomized, prospective study. *Arch Surg* 2000; 135: 326–31.
27. Nelson JL, Alexander JW, Jacobs PA, Ing RD, Ogle CK. Metabolic and immune effects of enteral ascorbic acid after burn trauma *Burns* 1992; 18: 92–7.
28. Aliabadi-Wahle S, Gilman DA, Dabrowski GP, Choe EU, Flint LM, Ferrara JJ. Postburn vitamin C infusions do not alter early postburn edema formation. *J Burn Care Rehabil* 1999; 20: 7–14.
29. Chen SF, Ruan YJ. 1 alpha, 25-dihydroxyvitamin D3 decreases scalding-and-platelet-activating factor-induced high vascular permeability and tissue oedema. *Pharmacol Toxicol* 1995; 76: 365–7.
30. Kuroiwa K, Nelson JL, Boyce ST, Alexander JW, Ogle CK, Inoue S. Metabolic and immune effect of vitamin E supplementation after burn. *J Parenter Enteral Nutr* 1991; 15: 22–6.
31. Haberal M, Hamaloglu E, Bora S, Oner G, Bilgin N. The effects of vitamin E on immune regulation after thermal injury. *Burns Incl Therm Inj* 1988; 14: 388–93.
32. Berger MM, Cavadini C, Chiolero R, Guinchard S, Krupp S, Dirren H. Influence of large intakes of trace elements on recovery after major burns. *Nutrition* 1994; 10: 327–34.

Chapter 24

Hypophosphatemia

David W Mozingo

Arthur D Mason Jr

a possible deficiency in the high-energy phosphate compounds essential for cellular metabolism. Thermal injury induces a precipitous decrease in serum phosphate concentration that reaches its nadir between the second and fifth postburn days. This phenomenon has been recognized for quite some time[2] and was recently confirmed by the authors in a large series of burn patients.[3] Despite aggressive phosphorus supplementation, normal levels of serum phosphorus are rarely reached prior to the tenth postburn day (**Figure 24.1**). Of 550 patients studied, 175 had serum phosphorus concentrations below 2.0 mg/dl, and of these 49 were below 1.0 mg/dl, with the lower limit of normal serum phosphorus being 3.0 mg/dl. Such hypophosphatemia is not exclusive to thermal injury, having been described following multiple trauma,[4] head injury,[5] and elective surgery.[6] The exact mechanism by which thermal injury or severe stress induces hypophosphatemia is unknown. Several events associated with burn injury, however, affect phosphorus metabolism, and these may combine to produce hypophosphatemia.

Etiology of postburn hypophosphatemia

Many of the pathophysiologic changes and therapeutic interventions that occur during the first postburn week influence serum phosphorus concentration (**Table 24.1**). Hypophosphatemia does not necessarily imply phosphorus depletion; in the case of burn injury, most patients are healthy prior to injury and presumably have normal phosphorus stores. Nor do simple calculations of phosphate balance explain the dramatic decrease in serum levels;

Certain humoral and metabolic responses to thermal and mechanical trauma that maintain homeostasis and prevent cellular dysfunction also produce alterations in electrolyte balance. An example is renal retention of sodium during the resuscitative phase of burn injury, which alters sodium balance in the course of preserving intravascular volume. Despite the markedly increased cardiac output and renal plasma flow that occur in the subsequent flow phase, a decrease in blood volume persists and results in sustained elevation of plasma renin activity, secretion of antidiuretic hormone, and sodium retention.[1] Conversely, the severe hypophosphatemia that often follows major injury occurs concomitantly with a 50–100% increase in resting energy expenditure, leading to

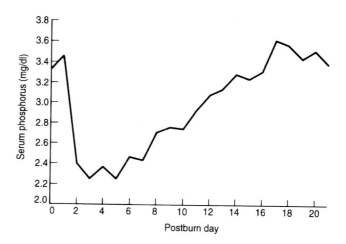

Fig. 24.1 Serum phosphorus levels abruptly decline with a nadir between postburn days 2 and 5. The data were obtained from 550 consecutive burn patients admitted to the US Army Institute of Surgical Research.

---

*The opinions or assertions contained herein are the private views of the authors and are not to be construed as official or as reflecting the views of the Department of the Army or the Department of Defense.

Table 24.1 Possible causes of postburn hypophosphatemia

Fluid resuscitation
- Volume loading
- Lactate administration

Carbohydrate administration
- Enteral alimentation
- Parenteral hyperalimentation
- 5% Dextrose

Elevated catecholamines
Phosphate-binding antacids/sucralfate
Acid–base disturbance
Electrolyte imbalance
- Hypokalemia
- Hypomagnesemia
- Hypocalcemia

Carbonic anhydrase inhibition (mafenide acetate)

simultaneous reduction of urinary phosphate excretion is observed, suggesting an extrarenal mechanism. The fractional excretion of phosphate, however, increases during the early period of diuresis following burn injury (postburn days 2–4), potentially contributing to the decline in serum levels. The pathophysiologic events and therapeutic interventions discussed below are associated with hypophosphatemia in other disease states and in certain experimental animal models, but the extent of their contributions to the postburn decrease in serum phosphorus has not been critically evaluated and is, at present, undefined.

Stress response

In the early postburn period, the classic 'fight or flight' response occurs, with elevation of plasma catecholamines, glucose, glucagon, and cortisol. Exogenous epinephrine administration has been associated with the development of hypophosphatemia, and the profound catecholamine release accompanying thermal injury may contribute to the early decrease in serum phosphorus. The mechanism by which this occurs is uncertain but may be a consequence of the accompanying hyperglycemia, resulting in a redistribution of phosphorus from the extracellular to the intracellular compartment (see section on Metabolic Support). In acute clinical states of glucagon excess, tubular reabsorption of phosphate is impaired in both the proximal and distal nephron, leading one to expect renal phosphate wastage.[7] Since urinary excretion of phosphate is usually decreased in the early post-injury period, the importance of hyperglucagonemia remains uncertain. Administration of pharmacologic doses of glucocorticoids enhances phosphorus excretion and impairs phosphate absorption by the gut and reabsorption by the kidney. Whether or not the adrenocortical response significantly contributes to the hypophosphatemia after burn injury is not known.

Resuscitation and topical therapy

Administration of large doses of sodium lactate for initial burn resuscitation may decrease the serum phosphorus concentration by several mechanisms.[8] Lactate is converted to glucose in the liver, a process requiring high-energy phosphate availability. Additionally, though it does not usually occur clinically, metabolic alkalosis induced by lactate infusion may result in depression of

serum phosphorus concentration. Alkalosis is associated with an increase in glycolysis that promotes transfer of phosphorus to the intracellular space. During resuscitation, alkalemia is uncommon and patients are more likely to manifest a mild metabolic acidosis, which is compensated by hyperventilation, resulting in a normal or mildly alkaline blood pH. Acidosis markedly inhibits renal phosphate reabsorption, resulting in phosphaturia. The contribution of this mechanism to postburn hypophosphatemia is probably minor; early renal phosphate wastage is not observed, perhaps being obscured by diminished glomerular filtration early in burn injury. In addition, the p-carboxy metabolite of mafenide acetate strongly inhibits carbonic anhydrase. Such inhibition diminishes proximal tubular reabsorption of phosphate and probably occurs following topical burn wound treatment with mafenide, but the magnitude of the effect is unknown.

Expansion of the extracellular fluid volume is also associated with inhibition of proximal tubular phosphate reabsorption. A tight coupling exists between sodium and phosphate transport across the renal epithelial cell. In patients with burns, mobilization and excretion of the large edema volume usually begins by the second postburn day and continues throughout the next week to 10 days. In contrast to the relative paucity of phosphate excretion during the first 24 hours after injury, when glomerular filtration is markedly reduced, a modest loss of phosphate may occur with diuresis of the edema fluid. In fact, the diuretic phase is associated with an increase in the fractional excretion of phosphate despite a concomitant reduction in the serum phosphate concentration.[9] Phosphorus excretion during the natriuretic phase of early burn injury is consistent with the tight coupling observed in other diuretic states.

Ulcer prophylaxis

Effective prophylaxis against Curling's ulcers with H_2-antagonists and antacid buffering has been a mainstay of burn care for the past two decades. Significant degrees of hypophosphatemia and phosphate depletion occur during continuous or chronic administration of phosphate-binding agents containing magnesium, calcium, and aluminum. These agents bind not only dietary phosphate but also phosphate secreted into the intestinal lumen, often resulting in a net negative phosphate balance. The severity of such hypophosphatemia clearly depends on the dose of phosphate-binding agents, dietary phosphorus intake, and pre-existing phosphate balance. To reduce alimentary scavenging of dietary and secreted phosphate, buffering with antacids containing aluminum phosphate salts (Al_2PO_4), which do not bind any additional phosphate, may be utilized. Sucralfate, which is also effective in preventing upper gastrointestinal stress ulceration following thermal injury is not a buffering agent, but as a complex salt of aluminum hydroxide, is capable of binding phosphate. Its administration has also been associated with the development of hypophosphatemia in critically ill patients.[10]

Hyperventilation

Respiratory alkalosis is often present during the first week postburn and may be enhanced by anxiety or pain, and even by the inhibition of carbonic anhydrase induced by mafenide acetate burn cream. As fluid resuscitation progresses, respiratory rate and tidal volume progressively increase, resulting in minute ventilation that may be twice normal. Mild hyperventilation induces only a slight decline of serum phosphorus levels; prolonged, intense hyperventilation, however, may result in serum phosphorus values less than 1.0 mg/dl.[11] During respiratory alkalosis, phosphorus virtually disappears from the urine, eliminating renal losses as the causative mechanism. Respiratory alkalosis induces a rapid movement of carbon dioxide from the intracellular to the extracellular space. Intracellular pH increases, activating glycolysis and increasing the formation of intracellular phosphorylated carbohydrate compounds. The readily diffusible inorganic phosphate pool supplies the required phosphorus, and serum phosphorus concentrations consequently fall abruptly. The extent to which this mechanism contributes to postburn hypophosphatemia is uncertain.

Metabolic support

Administration of carbohydrates may play a major role in the development of postburn hypophosphatemia. Infusion of glucose solutions or oral intake of carbohydrates produces mild hypophosphatemia in healthy individuals. This decrease in serum phosphate is associated with an increase of inorganic phosphate, ATP, and glucose 6-phosphate in muscle cells. The mechanism by which such carbohydrate administration induces hypophosphatemia is somewhat speculative. Experience with phosphate-deficient total parenteral nutrition and subsequent development of hypophosphatemia has provided some insight into the etiology.[12,13] As carbohydrates are absorbed, insulin secretion increases, shifting phosphorus from the extracellular to the intracellular space. If phosphate reserve is low, ATP is poorly regenerated since hypophosphatemia inhibits glucose 3-phosphate dehydrogenase. Inorganic phosphates in the intracellular pool become further diminished because of incorporation, initially as newly synthesized ATP, but eventually as triose phosphates when the ATP is consumed in the hexokinase reaction. Glucose utilization by red blood cells requires ATP at the hexokinase and phosphofructokinase steps, but regeneration of ATP does not occur during phosphate deficiency or acute hypophosphatemia due to a block at the glucose 3-phosphate dehydrogenase step. In states of phosphate depletion, the scant phosphate that enters the red blood cell is incorporated into 1,3-diphosphoglycerate, but most is diverted to 2,3-diphosphoglycerate, also preventing complete glycolysis to regain the ATP consumed.

In thermally injured patients, infusion of dextrose-containing solutions usually begins 24 hours postburn, and enteral nutrition, in which most of the calories are supplied as carbohydrates, is initiated within several days of injury. These interventions are temporally correlated with the rapid descent of serum phosphorus concentrations. In other clinical states, severe hypophosphatemia following the initiation of enteral or parenteral nutrition is most commonly associated with the feeding of patients with advanced protein–calorie malnutrition. When total body phosphorus is depleted by starvation, serum phosphorus levels usually remain normal, but carbohydrate administration produces a rapid marked decline in serum phosphorus concentration. If untreated, this may result in multisystem organ dysfunction, respiratory and cardiac failure, or death. Thermally injured patients are usually well nourished prior to burn injury and the clinical scenario of refeeding

hypophosphatemia may not apply to them. Similar findings, however, have been described recently in previously well-nourished surgical intensive care unit patients in whom the initiation of isotonic enteral feedings resulted in a decrease of serum phosphorus from normal levels to approximately 1 mg/dl, a level that is considered to be dangerously low and to require prompt supplementation.[14,15] In addition, the authors have recently reported that hypophosphatemia in thermally injured patients is exacerbated by the initiation of enteral feeding and occurs regardless of the postburn day when feeding is initiated.[3] This further reduction of serum phosphorus during the first postburn week, when levels are already low, may be particularly hazardous and speaks for aggressive phosphorus supplementation prior to and during the initiation of enteral alimentation.

Wound healing

In patients recovering from thermal injury, the burn wound itself may act as a significant phosphorus sink. Despite the overall catabolism accompanying major injury and loss of lean body mass, healing burn wounds and skin grafts are anabolic and require phosphorus for normal repair. In addition, the continued loss of fluid and protein through the burn wound surface is a potential source of unquantified phosphorus loss and may contribute to hypophosphatemia.[16]

Acute phase response and sepsis

Burn injury is characterized by an abrupt increase in acute phase proteins as patients enter the hypermetabolic phase of burn injury. These same responses are similar to those observed in the sepsis syndrome. Recently, the development of hypophosphatemia has been characterized in patients with the acute phase response syndrome.[17] Similar findings have been documented in patients with sepsis and infection, and correlation to increase in levels of cytokines such as tumor necrosis factor alpha and interleukin-6 has been made.[18] Similar findings were observed in patients with a variety of infectious diseases, and correlation of high levels of C-reactive protein and white blood cell count was made with the magnitude of hypophosphatemia.[19] Though these reports did not include burn injured patients, one may infer that activation of the inflammatory cascades such as occurs in major thermal injury may contribute to the development of hypophosphatemia.

Other electrolytes

Disorders of electrolyte balance may contribute to the development of hypophosphatemia. Experimental magnesium deficiency in animals may lead to phosphaturia and phosphorus deficiency, but intentional magnesium deficiency in man results in no change or a slight rise in serum phosphate.[20,21] In chronic alcoholics, however, hypomagnesemia and hypophosphatemia are coexistent. Hypokalemia, which is also exacerbated by magnesium deficiency, may result in phosphate wasting and hypophosphatemia. The mechanism is uncertain, but may be related to coexistent metabolic alkalosis, diuretic use, or the underlying illness. Changes in calcium and phosphate homeostasis, and in the regulating hormones calcitonin and parathyroid hormone, have been described after thermal injury.[22] Coincident with the early depression of serum phosphorus, the fraction of ionized calcium was shown to decrease and remain low, but within the normal range, for the 14 postburn days studied. Urinary calcium output was low, about 4.5 mmol/day, and urinary phosphate output was as high as 30 mmol/day, despite a low serum phosphorus. Serum calcitonin levels were significantly elevated for up to 2 weeks post-injury, whereas parathyroid hormone remained within the normal range. The magnitude of the contribution of the classic regulating hormones of calcium and phosphorus homeostasis to the observed decrease in serum phosphorus after severe injury is not known with certainty. Catecholamines and glucagon are known to induce an increase in calcitonin secretion, and the administration of pharmacologic doses of calcitonin results in phosphaturia. A direct effect of calcitonin on phosphate transport in the nephron has been demonstrated. In those burn patients, it was notable that ionized calcium decreased slightly though still within the normal range, despite very high levels of calcitonin and normal parathyroid hormone concentrations. A slight, though statistically significant, increase in parathyroid hormone was observed around the fourth postburn day and may be related, albeit indirectly through calcium regulation, to the observed postburn decrease in serum phosphorus concentration.

Summary

Clearly, multiple factors influence the serum phosphorus level following burn injury. Fluid resuscitation and subsequent mobilization of interstitial edema fluids, catecholamine excess, respiratory alkalosis, the use of phosphate-binding antacids or sucralfate, hypokalemia, hypomagnesemia, and the initiation of enteral nutrition have all been associated with hypophosphatemia in other illnesses and experimental models. All or most of these factors may be encountered in the early treatment of burn patients and the contribution and relative importance of individual factors to the depression of serum phosphorus is difficult to analyze. Most likely, carbohydrate administration, respiratory alkalosis, and diuresis of edema fluid are the more important etiologic factors contributing to hypophosphatemia in the early postburn course.

Consequences of hypophosphatemia

The clinical manifestations of hypophosphatemia (**Table 24.2**) are mainly those of organ system hypofunction. These responses have been defined through clinical observation and laboratory studies in circumstances in which hypophosphatemia occurred as a relatively isolated event. Phosphorus supplementation has been reported to reverse these abnormalities, suggesting a cause and effect relationship. Hypofunction of organ systems associated with phosphorus depletion has been attributed to a lack of available inorganic phosphate for synthesis of high-energy phosphorus compounds; breakdown of stored ATP occurs, and the inorganic phosphate is diverted to other intracellular pathways. Organ system dysfunction after thermal injury is characterized by early hypofunction and later hyperfunction of most organ systems. Whether hypophosphatemia contributes significantly to the early postburn depression of function that occurs in multiple organs is not known. Clearly, some of the clinical manifestations shown in **Table 24.2** are commonly observed in thermally injured patients, while others are not usually associated with such injury. Most patients reported to have had complications of hypophosphatemia have also had a

Table 24.2 Clinical manifestations of hypophosphatemia
CNS:
■ Lethargy, malaise, neuropathy, seizures, coma
Cardiovascular:
■ Impaired cardiovascular contractility
■ Decreased response to pressor agents
■ Hypotension
■ Acute cardiac decompensation
Pulmonary:
■ Tachypnea
■ Decreased vital capacity
■ Respiratory failure
Gastrointestinal:
■ Anorexia, dysphagia
Renal:
■ Glycosuria, calciuria, magnesuria, renal tubular acidosis
Musculoskeletal:
■ Weakness, myalgia, arthralgia, rhabdomyolysis

coexistent and severe illness. It is important to remember that prior cellular injury has been prerequisite in most instances in which hypophosphatemia has been implicated as a cause of organ system dysfunction. The following discussions of organ system abnormalities should be interpreted in light of the specific circumstances under which the observations were made.

Cardiac Dysfunction

Although the early depression of cardiac function following burn injury has been attributed to an initial decrease in circulating blood volume, the search for intrinsic myocardial depression after burn injury and for mediators of such depression continues. In experimental studies and in clinical material, a correlation between hypophosphatemia and cardiac decompensation has been reported. Cardiac output, measured by bolus thermodilution, was impaired in seven critically ill hypophosphatemic patients and improved significantly with phosphorus supplementation.[4] In one experimental study, myocardial contractility was impaired by phosphorus deficiency and reversed by phosphorus repletion, suggesting that phosphorus deficiency may be a cause of heart failure in certain clinical conditions.[23] Hypophosphatemic cardiac depression has been described as occurring in 28.8% of surgical intensive care patients.[24] Despite these reports, there appears to be little evidence that hypophosphatemic cardiomyopathy is a frequently encountered clinical entity; most patients in whom this mechanism is invoked have already had a number of other causes for myocardial dysfunction.[25]

Neuromuscular Dysfunction

Varying degrees of areflexic paralysis, paresthesias, sensory loss, weakness, and respiratory insufficiency have been reported to be associated with acute hypophosphatemia, usually induced with feeding malnourished patients.[12] A reduction in available ATP to support respiratory muscle contraction has been suggested as a mechanism for acute respiratory failure, and diaphragmatic contractility has been reported to improve with phosphorus repletion in mechanically ventilated hypophosphatemic patients.[26] Profound generalized muscle weakness associated with isolated phosphorus depletion has been observed in both clinical and laboratory studies.[27,28] In a study of hypophosphatemia and muscle phosphate metabolism in patients with burns or mechanical trauma, no direct correlation was demonstrated between the serum phosphorus concentration and the high-energy phosphate content of muscle cells; all these patients, however, were receiving phosphorus supplementation during the study.[29] If acute hypophosphatemia is superimposed on pre-existing cellular injury, potentially reversible muscle cell dysfunction may extend to irreversible necrosis.[30] Several authors have reported severe rhabdomyolysis associated with severe hypophosphatemia following burns and major trauma.[31,32] This spectacular clinical event is rare but may occur to a lesser, subclinical, extent in critically ill patients.[30,33] Hypophosphatemia as the underlying etiology may often be dismissed since muscle cell destruction results in release of phosphate and elevation of serum phosphorus. In the absence of significant hemochromogenuria, the diagnosis may not even be suspected. Further investigation is required to determine whether this 'asymptomatic' rhabdomyolysis is, in fact, an important clinical entity, or merely an obligate manifestation of critical illness.

Hematologic Dysfunction

When untreated, severe hypophosphatemia may lead to red blood cell dysfunction by alterations in cell shape, survival, and physiologic function. Lack of high-energy phosphate results in a decrease in erythrocyte 2,3-diphosphoglycerate and subsequent leftward shift of the dissociation curve, with a consequent risk of tissue hypoxia.[7] Clinical hypophosphatemia, with or without previous phosphate depletion, results in reduced production of 2,3-diphosphoglycerate, erythrocyte ATP, and other phosphorylated intermediates of red blood cell glycolysis. In a variety of experimental and clinical situations including burn injury and mechanical trauma, red blood cell 2,3-diphosphoglycerate has been shown to be reduced in the presence of hypophosphatemia.[34,35] In thermally injured patients it has been demonstrated that postburn disturbance of red cell phosphate metabolism may be prevented by administration of phosphorus in the early postburn course.[35] Hypophosphatemia has also been associated with decreased red cell survival and decreased red cell deformability, with impaired capillary transit and the potential for further deficiency of tissue oxygenation.

White blood cell dysfunction also has been observed as a result of hypophosphatemia induced by the initiation of phosphate-free parenteral nutrition and was associated with depressed chemotactic, phagocytic, and bactericidal activity of granulocytes.[35] A reduction in granulocyte ATP content was also documented and amelioration of these white blood cell abnormalities was coincident with phosphorus repletion. Any correlation between these observations and an increased risk of infection remains speculative for hypophosphatemic patients in general and burn patients in particular.

Summary

Though it is clear that organ system dysfunction may be a manifestation of severe untreated hypophosphatemia, the relationship between these specific abnormalities and those observed in either the hypodynamic or the hyperdynamic phases of burn injury remains unclear. Clinical experience dictates that even when severe hypophosphatemia is avoided, the scenario of early organ system hypofunction and later hyperfunction persists. This is not to say that the marked hypophosphatemia observed following burn injury is part and parcel to the disease process, without bearing on the postburn physiologic response, but that thus far, the pathophysiologic milieu following thermal injury has not permitted definition of the contribution of hypophosphatemia to the overall postburn response. Until cause and effect relationships are defined through ongoing research, aggressive phosphorus repletion should be approached cautiously following thermal injury. Such therapy does, however, clearly ameliorate red blood cell 2,3-diphosphoglycerate depletion, which, in and of itself, supports treatment.

Prevention and treatment of hypophosphatemia

An unequivocal recommendation to treat hypophosphatemia in thermally injured patients should be supported by evidence that the treatment is of benefit. Such evidence is somewhat lacking in thermally injured patients, but in many analogous instances of hypophosphatemia from other causes, a direct benefit has been ascribed to repletion.

Serum phosphorus levels should be measured daily during the early phase of burn care and intravenous phosphate repletion initiated when levels drop below 2.0 mg/dl (**Figure 24.2**). Most of the severe adverse effects of hypophosphatemia occur with concentrations below 1.0 mg/dl, and this replacement strategy should prevent the development of clinically significant hypophosphatemia. Correction of severe hypophosphatemia with serum phosphorus levels less than 1.0 mg/dl requires intravenous replacement, usually with solutions of sodium or potassium phosphate containing 0.16 mmol/kg body weight (5 mg/kg body weight) of elemental phosphorus over 6 hours. The dose may be halved for patients with serum phosphorus levels between 1.0 and 2.0 mg/dl.[36] Following completion of the infusion, a repeat serum phosphorus determination should be obtained, and further treatment based on the post-infusion plasma concentration. A potential hazard associated with intravenous administration of phosphate salts is hyperphosphatemia, which may induce metastatic deposition of calcium phosphate salts and hypocalcemia. Additionally, when potassium phosphate salts are used, care must be taken to avoid excessive or too rapid administration of potassium. Phosphorus replacement should be carefully monitored and proceed with great caution in patients with impaired renal function or evidence of soft tissue injury or necrosis.

Prevention of hypophosphatemia may be facilitated by beginning oral phosphorus replacement prior to interventions such as the initiation of either enteral or parenteral carbohydrate administration, gastric acid neutralization with phosphate-binding antacids or sucralfate, and the administration of diuretics. The nadir of serum phosphorus concentration typically occurs between 3 and 5 days postburn, during the period of edema mobilization, and the need to initiate phosphorus supplementation should be anticipated in this interval. Additionally, to temper the gastrointestinal losses due to administration of phosphate-binding antacids, substitution of, or alternation with, antacids containing aluminum phosphate should be considered.

For mild asymptomatic hypophosphatemia or for prophylaxis when worsening of hypophosphatemia is expected, oral supplementation with any of several available formulations is recommended. Such oral regimens have been shown to be cost-effective.[37] Five milliliters of Phospho-Soda, containing 4.2

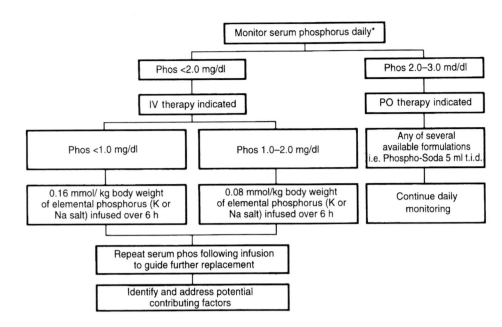

Fig. 24.2 The use of this algorithm permits prompt detection and timely correction of hypophosphatemia following burn injury.

mmol/ml of elemental phosphorus, is commonly administered three times daily. Correction of other electrolyte abnormalities, most notably hypomagnesemia, hypocalcemia, and hypokalemia, as well as maintenance of acid–base normality, may prevent further renal phosphate losses and maintain the extracellular phosphate pool. After the tenth postburn day, the phosphorus delivered in standard liquid enteral formulas and hospital diets is usually sufficient to maintain serum phosphorus levels above 3.0 mg/dl.

Summary

Thermal injury induces a precipitous decrease in serum phosphate concentration that reaches its nadir between the second and fifth postburn days. This phenomenon has been recognized for some time, but interest in the problem has been limited. The organ system dysfunctions induced by hypophosphatemia are in many ways similar to certain of the pathophysiologic changes observed following burn injury. The contribution of hypophosphatemia to these manifestations remains undefined. Wound fluid losses, increased circulating catecholamines, intracellular phosphate redistribution and increased fractional excretion of urinary phosphate, as well as iatrogenic induction of hypophosphatemia through various therapeutic interventions, have been implicated as contributing to postburn hypophosphatemia. Frequent serum phosphate measurement and prompt phosphorus replacement when hypophosphatemia is recognized should minimize any sequelae of this potentially deleterious electrolyte deficiency.

References

1. Cioffi WG, Vaughan GM, Heironimus JD, Jordan BS, Mason AD Jr, Pruitt BA Jr. Dissociation of blood volume and flow in regulation of salt and water balance in burn patients. *Ann Surg* 1991; **214**(3): 213–18.
2. Nordstrom H, Lennquist S, Lindell B, Sjoberg HE. Hypophosphataemia in severe burns. *Acta Chir Scand* 1977; **143**: 395–9.
3. Mozingo DW, Cioffi WG, Mason AD Jr, Milner EA, McManus WF, Pruitt BA Jr. Initiation of continuous enteral feeding induces hypophosphatemia in thermally injured patients. *Proceedings of the 35th World Congress of Surgery/International Society of Surgery/International Surgical Week, 22–27 August 1993.*
4. O'Connor LR, Weeler WS, Bethune JE. Effects of hypophosphatemia on myocardial performance in man. *N Engl J Med* 1977; **297**: 901.
5. Polderman KH, Bloemers FW, Peerdeman SM, Girbes AR. Hypomagnesemia and hypophosphatemia at admission in patients with severe head injury. *Crit Care Med* 2000; **28**(6): 2022–5.
6. England PC, Duari M, Tweedle DET, Jones A, Gowland E. Postoperative hypophosphatemia. *Br J Surg* 1979; **66**: 340.
7. Lau K. Phosphate disorders. In: Kokko JP, Tannen RL, eds. *Fluids and Eletrolytes*. Philadelphia, PA: WB Saunders, 1986: 398–471.
8. Knochel JP. The pathophysiology and clinical characteristics of severe hypophosphatemia. *Arch Intern Med* 1977; **137**: 203–20.
9. Lennquist S, Lindell B, Nordstrom H, Sjoberg HE. Hypophosphatemia in severe burns a prospective study. *Acta Chir Scand* 1979; **145**: 1–6.
10. Miller SJ, Simpson J. Medication-nutrient interactions: hypophosphatemia associated with sucralfate in the intensive care unit. *Nutr Clin Pract* 1991; **6**: 199–201.
11. Mostellar ME, Tuttle EP Jr. The effects of alkylosis on plasma concentration and urinary excretion of inorganic phosphate in man. *J Clin Invest* 1964; **43**: 138–49.
12. Solomon SM, Kirby DF. The refeeding syndrome: a review. *J Parenter Enter Nutr* 1990; **14**(1): 90–7.
13. Sheldon GF, Grzyb S. Phosphate depletion and repletion: relation to parenteral nutrition and oxygen transport. *Ann Surg* 1975; **182**(6): 683–9.
14. Hayek ME, Eisenberg PG. Severe hypophosphatemia following the institution of enteral feedings. *Arch Surg* 1989; **124**: 1325–8.
15. Marik PE, Bedigian MK. Refeeding hypophosphatemia in critically ill patients in an intensive care unit. A prospective study. *Arch Surg* 1996; **131**(10): 1043–7.
16. Berger MM, Rothen C, Cavadini C, Chiolero RL. Exudative mineral losses after serious burns: a clue to the alteration of magnesium and phosphate metabolism. *Am J Clin Nutr* 1997; **65**(5): 1473–81.
17. da Cunah DF, dos Santos VM, Monterio JP, de Carvalho da Cunha SF. Hypophosphatemia in acute-phase response syndrome patients. Preliminary data. *Miner Electrolyte Metab* 1998; **24**(5): 337–40.
18. Barak V, Schwartz A, Kalickman I, Nisman B, Gurman G, Shoenfeld Y. Prevalence of hypophosphatemia in sepsis and infection: the role of cytokines. *Am J Med* 1998; **104**(1): 40–7.
19. Haglin L, Burman LA, Nilsson M. High prevalence of hypophosphatemia amongst patients with infectious diseases. A retrospective study. *J Intern Med* 1999; **246**(1): 45–52.
20. Whang R, Welt LG. Observations in experimental magnesium depletion. *J Clin Invest* 1963; **42**: 305–13.
21. Shils ME. Experimental human magnesium depletion. *Medicine* 1969; **48**: 61–82.
22. Loven L, Nordstrom H, Lennquist S. Changes in calcium and phosphate and their regulating hormones in patients with severe burn injuries. *Scand J Plast Reconstr Surg* 1984; **18**: 49–53.
23. Fuller TJ, Nichols WW, Brenner BJ, Peterson JC. Reversible depression in

myocardial performance in dogs with experimental phosphorus deficiency. *J Clin Invest* 1978; **62**: 1194–2000.

24. Zazzo JF, Troche G, Ruel P, Maintenant J. High incidence of hypophosphatemia in surgical intensive care patients: efficacy of phosphorus therapy on myocardial function. *Intensive Care Med* 1995; **21(10)**: 826–31.

25. Knochel JP. The clinical status of hypophosphatemia. *N Engl J Med* 1985; **313(7)**: 447–9.

26. Aubier M, Murciano D, Lecocguic Y, *et al.* Effect of hypophosphatemia on diaphragmatic contractility in patients with acute respiratory failure. *N Engl J Med* 1985; **313**: 420–4.

27. Lotz M, Nay R, Bartter FC. Osteomalacia and debility resulting from phosphorus depletion. *Trans Assoc Am Physicians* 1964; **77**: 281–95.

28. Lotz M, Zisman E, Bartter FC. Evidence for a phosphorus depletion syndrome in man. *N Engl J Med* 1968; **278**: 409.

29. Loven L, Lennquist S, Liljedahl SO. Hypophosphataemia and muscle phosphate metabolism in severely injured patients. *Acta Chir Scand* 1983; **149**: 743–9.

30. Knochel JP, Barcenas C, Cotton JR, Fuller TJ, Haller R, Carter NW. Hypophosphatemia and rhabdomyolysis. *J Clin Invest* 1978; **62**: 1240–6.

31. Guechot J, Cynober L, Lioret N, Betourne C, Saizy R, Giboudeau J. Rhabdomyolysis and acute renal failure in a patient with thermal injury. *Intensive Care Med* 1986; **12**: 159–60.

32. Pfeifer PM. Acute rhabdomyolysis following surgery for burns. *Anaesthesia* 1986; **41**: 614–69.

33. Singhal PC, Kumar A, Desroches L, Gibbons N, Mattana J. Prevalence and predictors of rhabdomyolysis in patients with hypophosphatemia. *Am J Med* 1992; **92**: 458–64.

34. Loven L, Anderson E, Larsson J, Lennquist S. Muscular high-energy phosphates and red-cell 2.3-DPG in post-traumatic hypophosphataemia. *Acta Chir Scand* 1983; **149**: 735–41.

35. Loven L, Larsson L, Nordstrom H, Lennquist S. Serum phosphate and 2,3-diphosphoglycerate in severely burned patients after phosphate supplementation. *J Trauma* 1986; **26(4)**: 348–52.

36. Perreault MM, Ostrop NJ, Tierney MG. Efficacy and safety of intravenous phosphate replacement in critically ill patients. *Ann Pharmacother* 1997; **31(6)**: 683–8.

37. Mathews JJ, Aleen RF, Gamelli RL. Cost reduction strategies in burn nutrition services: adjustment dietary treatment of patients with hyponatremia and hypophosphatemia. *J Burn Care Rehabil* 1999; **20(1 Pt 1)**: 80–4.

38. Craddock PR, Yawata Y, VanSanten L, Gilberstadt S, Silvis S, Jacob HS. Acquired phagocyte dysfunction: a complication of the hypophosphatemia of parenteral hyperalimentation. *N Engl J Med* 1974; **290(25)**: 1403–7.

Chapter 25

The immunological response and strategies for intervention

Andrew M Munster

The heightened susceptibility of burn patients to infection has been noted for over 30 years. By the mid-1960s, in both burned humans and experimental animals, alterations in immunoglobulin kinetics, phagocytic function, neutrophil function, and in the humoral response to primary and recall antigens has been documented. Skin testing for delayed hypersensitivity had been performed and pro-

longation of allograft survival demonstrated. These early historical developments and original work are described in a number of early reviews.[1,2] A review published in the mid-1970s on this subject already contained over 200 references.[3] More recently, extensive new reviews of work in the areas of mechanisms of immunological suppression, the role of inflammatory mediators, and the influence of hormonal milieu have become available.[4–7]

Perhaps the most dramatic change in the last 5 years, that is, since the publication of the first edition of this book, has occurred in our understanding of the graded or ubiquitous role of these reactions, and the importance of the anatomical or regional locations where they occur. The acute phase reaction basically begins to be measurable following relatively small physical and psychological stresses, and reaches its maximum in patients with major burns and complex multi-trauma (for comprehensive review, see Gabay and Kushner[8]). Since regulation of the acute phase response is stimulated by many of the inflammatory cytokines produced by local macrophages and monocytes at the site of injury, *local* induction may well match or exceed *systemic* induction in its importance to the host.

It is widely recognized that the immunological status of the burned patient has a measurable impact on outcome in terms of survival, death, and major morbidity. This can be documented using almost any *in vivo* or *in vitro* test of immune function which happens to be convenient; many of them correlate very well with prognosis (references 9, 10, reviewed in reference 11). Nutritional support of the burned patient is considered in detail in Chapter 23, but nutritional support is clearly essential for adequate immune function. This evolving field is well reviewed in a recent publication in which three papers are particularly recommended for overview.[12–14]

The story of cutaneous burn toxin has been with us for 40 years, and throughout, toxin has had its champions and its detractors. Most recently, using modern immunological techniques, it has been shown that the biological effects of cutaneous burn toxin are indeed separable from endotoxin and affect the cytokine cascade.[16,17] Nevertheless, the precise biological role of burn toxin remains elusive. By contrast, there is now little disagreement that the burn wound remains a serious source of suppressive activity and that early removal of the burned tissue and wound coverage is an essential part of the immunological care of the burned patient.[18–20] Experimentally, early burn wound excision restores antibody synthesis to bacterial antigen,[21] and restores cytotoxic T-cell function.[22] An exciting recent finding concerns the ability of cerium nitrate as a topical agent to mimic the effect of surgical excision of the wound by lowering tumor necrosis factor-α (TNFα) levels in the serum.[23]

Perhaps the greatest difficulty in attempting to decipher the body's response to injury is the complex interrelationship of the cytokine cascade, the arachidonic acid cascade, and the neuroendocrine axis. The multiple feedback loops and regulatory systems are only just now beginning to be elucidated and the very complexity of the system has defeated the optimism of many workers for the early achievement of simple interventions. These networks have been recently reviewed[24-26] and make interesting reading for individuals wishing to delve into the subject more deeply.

Terminology is evolving rapidly. To help with the reading of this chapter, an algorithm follows (**Table 25.1**) and a short glossary of important cytokine and receptor nomenclature (**Table 25.2**). In addition, there is now a family of so-called chemokines; these are held to among the oldest and most basic responses to injury and their principal function is to bring inflammatory cells to the needed site. A number of interleukins induce chemokine production. There are now over 50 chemokines, reviewed in reference 27.

The host response to thermal injury

The Arachidonic Acid Cascade

The major product of the arachidonic acid cascade following thermal injury is prostaglandin E_2 (PGE$_2$). Originally, because of evidence that endotoxin-mediated immunosuppression could be blocked by indomethacin, it was thought that the induction of PGE$_2$ production by macrophages was mediated by endotoxin.[28] While this has been partially substantiated, there is also evidence that PGE$_2$ exerts its suppressive effect principally by inhibition of lymphocyte interleukin (IL)-2 production and T-cell activation.[29] In addition, PGE$_2$ appears to downregulate IL-6 secretion.[30] The induction of the arachidonic acid cascade itself is complex, apparently dependent on at least two pathways, one calcium channel dependent and one calcium independent.[31] There are massive increases of another arachidonic acid derivative, thromboxane B$_2$ (TXB$_2$), in the plasma of burned patients, particularly immediately postburn and during septic episode.[32] 6-Keto-PGF$_{1\alpha}$ levels are unchanged following burn injury, this being a stable metabolite of prostacyclin (PGI$_2$), suggesting that there is a postburn alteration in the arachidonic acid pathway in favor of the PGE$_2$ series and TXB$_2$. In view of the immunosuppressive effects of PGE$_2$, and the physiologic actions of TXB$_2$, which include vasoconstriction, leukocyte and platelet aggregation, and membrane destabilization, these two products must be considered key in the immediate effects of thermal injury. Leukotriene B$_4$, another arachidonic acid product (**Table 25.3**), is a potent neutrophil chemotactic factor, and is produced following thermal injury.

The Cytokine Cascade

Following injury, induction of a number of cytokines rapidly occurs: the best studies of these are for tumor necrosis factor, IL-1, and IL-6. Burned patients are no different from other injured patients in the timetable of induction of the cytokines. TNFα is detectable early during the period of burn shock; at that time, the levels cannot be correlated with prognosis. By contrast, the maximum TNFα level over the whole clinical course is of prognostic significance.[33] Because endotoxin injuries have very comparable abilities to induce a cytokine cascade, considerable effort has been made to attempt to separate these two mechanisms. Both TNF and endotoxin can cause neutrophil activation, but the pathways appear to be different in that anti-TNF antibody blocks TNF-mediated neutrophil activation but does not inhibit endotoxin-mediated neutrophil activation.[34] Patients with high TNF levels

Table 25.1 Major time-related responses to injury		
Initial (1–2 hours)	**Subsequent (48 hours)**	**Late**
Cytokine induction	Coagulation changes	Sepsis
Activation of AA cascade	Substrate utilization changes	MSOF
Hormonal changes	Lymphocyte, macrophage and neutrophil alterations	Toxic metabolite release
Translocation		

Table 25.2 Some key cytokines and membrane receptors	
Name	**Function (partial list)**
Interleukin-1 (IL-1)	Mitogenic, stimulates granulocytes, T- and B-cell proliferation, fever, acute phase proteins
Interleukin-2 (IL-2)	Mitogenic, activates macrophages, T- and B-cell activation, fever
Tumor necrosis factor (TNF)	Mitogenic, activates macrophages, stimulates granulocytes, T-cells, fever
Interleukin-6 (IL-6)	Mitogenic, stimulates T- and B-cells, induces acute phase response
Interleukin-8 (IL-8)	Granulocyte activation and migration
	Interleukin 12 (IL-12) induces expression of T-helper cell phenotype
	Interleukin-10 (IL-10) downregulates T-helper cell activity
	Interleukin-4, -8 and -13 (IL-4, -8, and -13) induce chemokine production in a variety of cells.
Transforming growth factor (TGF)	Mitogenic, inhibits T- and B-cells, stimulates cell growth and angiogenesis
CD4	T-cell marker, MHC Class II coreceptor
CD8	T-cell marker, non-NK suppressor cell
CD11	Adhesion molecule (many subtypes)
CD14	Myeloid differentiation antigen, LPB–LPS complex binding
CD18	β Chain of epithelial cell receptor
CD21	Complement receptor
CD23	B-cell activation marker
CD25	NK, T-, and B-cell activation marker
CD69	Early T- and B-cell activation marker
CD71	Ubiquitous leukocyte activation marker

(over 540 pg/ml) have a very poor prognosis, although the absolute level of TNF does not correlate with burn size.[35] These changes are not restricted to the area of injury, an important principle: for example, IL-6 is induced in unburned skin following experimental burns.[36]

There are further intriguing physiologic actions of TNF which are only now being fully researched. Repeated exposure to endotoxin results in progressively reduced secretions of TNF, and thereby provides a possible mode for endotoxin tolerance. A similar effect is seen if experimental endotoxin-sensitive mice are first treated with dexamethasone.[37,38] Further, it appears that the peak production of TNFα in monocytes occurs concomitantly with massive production of PGE$_2$.[39] Induction of TNFα of the membrane-associated type is associated with a very high mortality rate and may provide a clue into the role of TNF in the mediation of systemic inflammatory syndrome.[40]

Because the physiologic effects of TNF are almost indistinguishable from endotoxin, the induction of TNF has been held responsible for the clinical effects of endotoxemia; the induction and secretion of TNF has become a reasonable target for interventional modalities for sepsis. This will be considered later in this chapter.

Much of the work on the interleukins has been done in trauma rather than burned patients, and some of the data need to be extrapolated. Specifically with regard to IL-1, after the initial induction of IL-1, synthesis is significantly impaired for several days after injury.[41] By contrast, there appears to be an upregulated local production of IL-1 and IL-6 in inflammatory sites, thus inducing polymorphonuclear neutrophil chemoattraction.[42]

Interleukin-2 has been identified as a key cytokine in the mediation of the cellular immune response. In a series of burned patients, initial IL-1 production was initially significantly elevated and then returned to normal, but patients with large burns had significantly suppressed production of IL-2 which correlated with the length of time from injury.[43] The kinetics of IL-2 secretion are interesting and of potential importance in postburn immunosuppression. Following lymphocyte activation, there is increased expression of IL-2 receptors (IL-2R) on the surface of the T-cell which is then rapidly shed into the serum, resulting in elevated serum IL-2R levels following burn injury. This phenomenon could have two implications: either the free IL-2R now competes with ligands which would activate cell surface IL-2R, or diminished receptor expression on the surface, following a burst of lymphocyte activity, renders the cell relatively inactive and reduces further IL-2 secretion.[44–48]

Investigations of IL-8 after burn injury are in their infancy, but because of the importance of pulmonary production of IL-8 following adult respiratory distress syndrome (ARDS), it is an interleukin of potential importance in burned patients.[49]

Interleukin-6 is an interesting cytokine which is probably the most studied of all the immunoregulatory cytokines following injury and stress. It is a ubiquitous cytokine which is produced by a variety of cells and is detected in increased concentrations in blood or tissues following disturbances in physiologic homeostasis of any kind, including psychological stressors.[50] Presumably the most important role of IL-6 following burn injury is the induction of phase reactants, some of which include antibacterial products such as fibronectin.[51] The induction of IL-6 in burn patients is very rapid, is followed by induction of acute phase proteins,[52] and can be closely correlated with prognosis in severe burns.[53] Interestingly, although the induction of PGE$_2$ production parallels that of IL-6 induction in the macrophage, and PGE$_2$ downregulates IL-1 production, it has no effect on blocking the induction of IL-6.[54] Experimentally, the synthesis of acute phase proteins will persist for several days following induction even after the removal of the original stimulant.[55] In addition to the correlation of IL-6 levels with acute phase reactants, these levels can also be correlated with the clinical parameters of inflammation and injury.[56] It has been known for some time that cell activation can be inhibited by high levels of IL-6, and that TGFβ elevates macrophage PGE$_2$ production.[57] Recently, evidence has been produced that the immunosuppressive activity of high concentrations of IL-6 are mediated by the activation of TGFβ.[58]

A recent observation of potentially great significance has been reported. T-cell phenotypes were correlated with signature production of cytokines, with the finding that following major burns there is a shift towards the production of T-2 type cytokines. These are compensatory anti-inflammatory cytokines such as IL-4; interventions would clearly need to differentiate between acting against T-1 or T-2 type cytokines.[59]

The role of IL-10 remains controversial. There is elevated production of IL-10 postburn which can be correlated with septic episodes, and, in animals models, survival in a burn/cecal puncture model can be improved with early anti-IL-10 therapy; IL-10 knock-out mice survive burn injury as well as the controls.[60,61]

Cell-mediated immunity

T Cells

Early observations of suppression on cell-mediated immunity using technology available in the 1960s and 1970s documented delays in allograft rejection, impairment in mitogenic and antigenic responsiveness of lymphocytes, burn size related suppression of graft versus host reactivity, suppression of delayed cutaneous sensitivity tests, and diminution in both peripheral lymphocyte numbers and thoracic duct lymphocyte concentration (see reviews quoted earlier). The introduction of immunofluorescent labeling and the characterization of lymphocyte subpopulations led to the description of alterations in the various populations of lymphocytes in peripheral blood and tissue. Currently, there is general agreement that the functional capacity of thymic-dependent lymphocytes (T cells) to perform their normal physiologic responses is impaired; there is enormous controversy as to whether this failure is due to an intracellular defect related to thermal injury, the result of 'overuse', or indirectly the result of downregulation by the cytokine cascade or other products of the inflammatory reaction.

Initially, it was suggested that the immunosuppression of burn injury may be related to an imbalance between suppressor and helper cells.[62] Analysis of peripheral blood in the hands of several groups appeared to show support for this hypothesis.[63–65] More recent evidence supports the theory that, rather than an absolute reduction in CD4 and an increase in CD8 cells, there may be a redistribution of lymphocyte traffic. Suppression in the numbers of the total lymphocyte population is the only consistent overall change.[66–68] There is evidence, however, that suppressive cytokine products rather than suppressor cells may be in evidence early post-injury,[59] a finding confirmed by a new technique of intracellular cytokine measurement.[69] Further, not only is there lymphocyte traffic between central lymphocyte stores and the peripheral blood after thermal injury but the responsiveness of these lymphocyte populations also varies according to site; for example, splenic lymphocytes of experimentally burned animals remain most profoundly depressed in response to antigenic stimulation compared with the peripheral blood and other organs.[70] In addition, in peripheral blood, the appearance of 'activation' antigens on CD4 and CD8 cells (HLA-DR, IL-2R, and transferrin receptor) is significantly depressed as early as 1 day postburn.[71] This finding has not been universally confirmed, as other workers have reported an increase in activation receptors CD25, CD69, and CD71 in the peripheral blood of adult burned patients.[72]

Addition of recombinant IL-2 does not appear to reverse the suppression of the appearance of surface markers such as IL-2R in burned patients,[73] although it does not improve the response of NK cells to stimulation.[74] The appearance of free IL-2R in serum has already been alluded to.[39] Another intriguing observation is that peripheral lymphocyte membrane fluidity, usually affected in the stressed state by increased cortisol levels in the blood, is altered in burned patients, which could be part of the explanation of postburn immune suppression.[75] Perhaps the most convincing evidence of T-cell failure following a high level of activation is the temporal coexistence in the same samples of high serum IL-2 levels, low cellular expression of IL-2Ra, and high free soluble IL-2R levels.[76] Recent evidence also links T-cell dysfunction with macrophages, related to increased sensitivity to cyclic AMP and leading to an uncoupling of cell surface receptors from protein C activation.[77]

In summary, following major thermal injury, there is a partition of lymphocyte compartments with an overall suppression of the total lymphocyte population and strong activation of helper T cells and proinflammatory T-4 products, which quickly yields to activation of T-8 lymphocytes and induction of the antiinflammatory T-8 cytokines. Following continued activation, and perhaps because of some other still not completely understood physiologic alteration in intracellular or membrane physiology, there is sustained failure of responsiveness of T cells to normal physiologic stimuli which is of clinical consequence. It is also worth mentioning that these findings, although heightened in burn patients, are not unique, but can be brought on by any form of stress, even mental and psychosocial.[78,79] In experimental preparations, at least some of the observed suppression can be alleviated by early removal of the burn wound,[80] thereby creating one further argument for the prompt closure of the burn wound.

Macrophages

Suppression of the ability of the reticuloendothelial system to take up particulate material was among the original observations of burn immunology made in the 1960s (see review in reference 1) and has been recently confirmed.[81] In the more recent report, however, there was a differentially increased uptake of colloid in alveolar macrophages compared with other organs, perhaps indicating alveolar macrophage activation. Macrophages and monocytes appear to be activated in a fashion similar to lymphocytes following thermal injury. A popular way of measuring macrophage activation is the serum neopterin level, which is increased following thermal injury.[82,83] This activation is confirmed by increased expression of the monocyte cell surface antigen C3b and iC3b.[84] At the same time, there is a reduction of HLA-DR, HLA-DQ, and

HLA-DP expression by monocytes, and these class II antigens are obligatory for many cell-mediated immunological processes, thereby implying a possible loss of monocyte function following thermal injury.[85] Indeed, monocyte expression of HLA-DR is decreased after a burn injury, and this decrease appears to be mediated by IL-10.[86] Not only does macrophage function appear to be altered, but products of macrophages are capable of suppressing mitogenic responsiveness in normal lymphocytes[87] and the macrophage/monocyte is among the principal cell types which secrete immunoregulatory cytokines.

C3 production by burned patients' macrophages is suppressed, but the synthetic ability for key cytokines such as IL-6 which, as mentioned,[53] is massively increased, is difficult to assess because so many other cells produce cytokines.[88] In multiple injury and septic patients, elevation of neopterin secretion is accompanied by severe impairment of IL-1 and IL-8 synthesis, but IL-6 synthesis remains high. It is likely that a similar set of circumstances prevails in the burned patient as well.[41] In experimental septic preparations, to which burned patients and burned animals usually bear a striking similarity, there is specific activation of alveolar macrophages which produce superoxide anions, A-glucuronidase, and arachidonic metabolites directly leading to lung injury.[89]

In summary, the macrophage/monocyte axis, which is biologically much more multifaceted than the lymphocyte, undergoes activation following thermal injury. This activation is differentiated both by product and by site. Proinflammatory cytokines are produced as a short burst, probably inhibited by a feedback loop, at which time there is a decreased receptor expression. The activation includes the lung, and may provide the background for the development of the ARDS seen in burned patients.

B Cells

The function of bone marrow-derived thymocytes or B cells following thermal injury is less well documented than that of macrophages or T cells and particularly confusing because the B cell population is subject to many messenger and environmental influences which are altered as a result of thermal injury. When B cells endocytose and degrade foreign antigens, the fragments of that antigen are expressed on the B cell surface in noncovalent association with class II major histocompatibility complex (MHC) molecules, which serve as recognition complex for CD4 helper T-cells. As has been already mentioned[85] the expression of this MHC complex is impaired and, therefore, some diminution of B cell function can be expected as a result of diminished recognition of antigenic presentation.[90] Some of this suppression may be prostaglandin-mediated: in a burn-mouse model, PGE_2 suppressed all B cell functions except IgG production, and some of these effects could be restored by indomethacin.[39,91] Under the influence of stress-induced corticosteroid circulation, there is a relative increase of circulating B cells compared with T cells in peripheral blood.[92] Spontaneous and cytokine (IL-4 and IL-2)-induced expression of the activation antigen CD23 is significantly reduced during the second to fifth week postburn.[93] At the same time, the release of the proteolytic cleavage product, sCD23, which represents B cell growth and differentiation, is also reduced.[94] On the other hand, IL-6 is a polyclonal B cell activator and, therefore, could be expected to induce widespread B cell activation following thermal injury.[95]

If the products of B cell activation, namely the immunoglobulins, are measured *in vivo*, the results are somewhat difficult to interpret because of the increased catabolism of protein and the leakage through the burn wound. This will be discussed later. In summary, the B cell population is subject to the same nonspecific activation as the rest of the lymphocyte population, and in addition, the products are quickly degraded by other mechanisms to where overall physiologic function is seriously impaired.

Neutrophils

Work on neutrophil dysfunction following thermal injury has been reviewed in previous references,[1-3] as well as in a more recent review of neutrophil disorders following injury.[96] Fc receptor expression is decreased,[97] intracellular killing capacity is depressed (this is a differential suppression, more for some organisms than others),[98] and this is accompanied by a brief increase in neutrophil respiratory burst response.[71] This dysfunction seems to be related to a failure of initial alkalization of the phagolysosome,[99] and subsequent kinetics of acidification are also altered.[100] This is an oxygen-independent bactericidal mechanism, depression of which would impair the capacity of the neutrophil for intracellular killing following thermal injury. Some of this impairment may result from the external environment, as with other immunocytes, because it has been shown that PGE elevates intracellular cyclic-3′, 5′-adenosine monophosphate (cAMP) content in polymorphonuclear cells which can be restored by cyclooxygenase blockade.[101] Expression of CD16 (FcR, Fc IgG receptor) and CD11 (adhesion molecule) on neutrophils is impaired after major injury; and this reduction appears to be directly related to the appearance of bacteremia or pneumonia.[102] These changes in adhesion molecule expression, which is closely related to chemotaxis,[103] may play a part in the failure of delivery of neutrophils in adequate numbers to the local site of a burn.[104] Recently, it has also been found that there is a defect in actin polymerization in burn patients' neutrophils, a basic mechanism of chemotaxis, which may also contribute to a failure of motility.[105] There is an impairment in leukotriene generation (LTB_4, 20-OH-LTB_4, 20-COOH-LTB_4) from the polymorphs of severely burned patients.[106] This appears to be based on the availability, or lack of availability, of the metabolizable substrate-free arachidonic acid. Because leukotriene B_4 is also a potent neutrophil chemotactic agent, this may further contribute to the failure of neutrophil function.

The apoptosis of neutrophils appears to have some part in mediator-induced tissue damage in burns, particularly in the lung.[107] Interestingly, burn patients' plasma has a protective effect against this process, which has now been ascribed to granulocyte–macrophage colony-stimulating factor (GM-CSF).[108,109] An interesting recent report addresses the increased permeability of endothelium induced by burn-activated neutrophils, which may account for a new mechanism of tissue damage.[110]

Basophil granulocytes participate in the dysfunction of other immunologically active cells. Anti-IgE-induced basophil histamine release in burned patients is reduced immediately, while the calcium-ionosphere release of histamine does not fail until the second day postburn.[111] As with other cells, the baseline granulocyte oxidative activity in burn neutrophils is increased.[112] Induction of neutrophil activation probably takes several different stimulants, but it is known that tumor necrosis factor and endotoxin can both activate neutrophils;[34] IL-6 is also a potent inducer of superoxide production by the neutrophil.[113]

The neuroendocrine axis and postburn immunity

The role of opioids in immunity has recently been reviewed.[114] The induction of opioid-induced suppression has been defined for natural killer cells, CD4 and CD8 cells, and the receptor types have been characterized.[115] Clearly, the interrelationship of the neuroendocrine axis and the immune system is key in the stressed burned patient, but the full implications of this axis are only now beginning to be explored. It has been reported that plasma β-endorphins return to normal rapidly after 36 hours postburn. Morphine stimulates neutrophil oxygen consumption.[117]

There is an emerging concept that local injury and the events that follow is mediated by the neuroendocrine axis and that it may be shared by different types of noxious insults. In this scenario, injury to sensory nerves causes the release of substance P, which is a proinflammatory neuropeptide binding to a neurokinin receptor on local macrophages. This hypothesis is strongly supported by a number of experimental findings, such as the production of IL-6 both by skin cells and recirculating inflammatory cells following injury and the similarity of these changes to inflammatory changes mediated by an immune reaction, e.g. toxic epidermonecrolysis, or even in another organ like the pancreas.[118-120] The relationship between opioids and immune changes following thermal injury remains a fertile field for further research.

Endotoxin

Complete discussion of the biological effects of endotoxin is beyond the scope of this chapter, but because the pathophysiology of endotoxemia is interwoven with the immunological response of the burned patient and, in particular, with the cytokine cascade, a brief consideration of endotoxemia is necessary. In this discussion, the terms 'endotoxin' and 'lipopolysaccharide' (LPS) will be used interchangeably.

Endotoxemia in the burned patient has two principal sources: translocation from the gastrointestinal tract and the burn wound. Of course, any septic focus can give rise to endotoxemia. It is well documented that thermal injury increases intestinal permeability, leading to translocation in both experimental animals and man.[121-123] Because endotoxin itself increases intestinal permeability,[124] a vicious cycle may well be set up. Endotoxemia is related to burn size[125] and, further in the postburn course, the level of endotoxin in the plasma is related to prognosis.[126]

The response of cytokine gene regulation to endotoxin is both dose- and time-independent. Extremely low concentrations of endotoxin (0.001 ng/ml) will induce IL-8 mRNA. With concentrations of 0.01 ng/ml, IL-1β and TNFα mRNA are activated. The cytokine mRNA for IL-1α, IL-6, and GM-CSF are activated only with higher doses of endotoxin and after a longer exposure time.[127] Human monocytes treated with bacterial lipopolysaccharide also release PGE_2 and TXB.[128] Hematologic changes which follow endotoxemia are probably mediated by TNF and IL-1, and include lymphopenia and neutrophilia.[129] Endotoxin induces a polymorphonuclear leukocyte infiltration factor in human macrophages.[130] *Pseudomonas* causes induction of histamines and leukotrienes from mast cells and granulocytes.[131] Interferon-γ is induced, a reaction dependent on the presence of macrophages and IL-2.[132] Different types of endotoxins from different organisms have a different potency and a different timetable in the induction of cytokines.[133] The exact correlation between the clinical action of the lipopolysaccharides and the induction of cytokines is controversial. There are many differences in the induction kinetics in various experimental settings; and it is likely that lipopolysaccharides produce a number of effects independent of the cytokine cascade, more particularly TNF.[134]

Complicating the effect of the endotoxin-induced arachidonic acid and cytokine cascade is the fact that there are a number of natural host antagonists to endotoxin in blood and in the tissues, the best studied of which is lipopolysaccharide-binding protein (LBP).[135] In addition to lipoprotein-binding factor, there are a number of other polysaccharide LPS binders in plasma, complement, tissue factor, endothelial-produced agents such as ELAM and ICAM, and the products of coagulation which can all interfere with the measurable level of endotoxin in plasma.[136] Much attention has been paid recently to the CD14 receptor of monocytes and macrophages. CD14 is the receptor for the LPS–LPS binding protein complex which activates the response to endotoxin, although there is recent evidence that a second receptor may be involved.[137] In burn patients, the same induction followed by activity, receptor expression, and soluble receptor shedding seems to happen for CD14 as it does for IL-2R. It has been reported that soluble CD14 serum levels are observed in conjunction with clinical signs of septicemia.[138] In addition to the appearance of CD14 on macrophages, this receptor is also found on neutrophils and activation of the binding site can induce neutrophils without the need for other cytokines.[139] The injection of lipopolysaccharides into normal human subjects manifests the same alterations in lymphocyte traffic and behavior that has often been documented in burn patients, principally marked by a severe lymphopenia[140] and suppression of lymphocyte proliferation in response to PHA and PWM, apparently a macrophage-dependent effect, but no suppression and PGE_2 or TXB_2 production.[141] Whether the endotoxin (or thermal injury)-induced immunosuppression of lymphocytes is mediated by suppressor cells, as yet unidentified suppressor factors, cytokine or PGE_2, is not yet clear.

Experimentally, in the absence of postburn complications or interventions, translocation-generated endotoxemia is cleared by 96 hours postburn.[142] If for any reason endotoxemia persists, the much studied clinical effects of endotoxin can begin to be seen; this includes the cardiovascular response[143] as well as the overwhelming of the Kupffer cell sequestration of LPS in the liver with a resultant spill over to the lung,[144] where surfactant synthesis will be suppressed[145] and alveolar macrophages and neutrophils induced.[146] There is evidence that the mechanism of pulmonary failure in acute endotoxemia and chronic endotoxemia may be different, with chronic endotoxemia leading to activation of the arachidonic acid cascade locally in the lung.[147] The exact contribution to pulmonary failure by the burn injury itself and by the subsequent endotoxemia is not clear, but they may be supplementing each other.[148]

LPS is also capable of inducing opiate production.[149] An important recent addition to our knowledge of endotoxemia has been the observation that different types of antibiotics result in different quantities of endotoxin released from gram-negative organisms. This may well be relevant to burned patients because of the frequency of broad-spectrum antibiotic therapy for these patients. On this point, much more information will be needed.[150]

Humoral Immunity

Original investigations into humoral immunity following thermal injury can be found in previously referenced reviews. Briefly, there is marked diminution of serum IgG concentration, total and all subclasses, and these levels return to normal between 10 and 14 days postburn. Extremely low levels of IgG on admission (300–400 mg%) are predictors of a poor prognosis. IgM and IgA levels appear to be relatively unaffected. There are also perturbations of complement metabolism, including depletion of various serum components. Most of these changes have been ascribed to a combination of leakage through the burn wound, protein catabolism, and a relative diminution in synthesis.

There is a mild impairment of C3 production and release by burned patients' macrophages *in vitro*.[88] Both the classical and the alternative pathways are depleted, but the alternative pathway is more profoundly perturbed.[151] Complement inactivation by heat appears to ameliorate cell-mediated immunosuppression (CMI), suggesting that at least in part some of the impairment of the CMI postburn may be due to a complement-associated mechanism.[152] The results of investigations of immunoglobulin production by cultured B cells have been controversial. Following blunt trauma, there is some suppression of immunoglobulin production, but the suppression can be restored by a variety of lymphokines, suggesting that there is not a basic decrease in B-lymphocyte function.[153,154] By contrast, in thermal injury, immunoglobulin synthesis may be normal to supernormal[155] or vary depending on the origin of the cells.[156] In summary, it would seem that the defective immunoglobulin production following major injury, including thermal injury, is probably a factor of macrophage/lymphocyte interaction rather than a failure of intrinsic activity by B cells.[157,158]

An additional group of humoral factors which have been investigated following thermal injury are those concerned with granulopoiesis which will be considered more fully in another chapter.

In brief, there seems to be an impairment of the production of GCSF and of GM-CSF.[159] A number of plasma components which can be considered nutritional in nature have been investigated for their effect on immunity after thermal injury, and one in particular, glutamine, has been reported to make a major contribution to immune reactivity after thermal injury. Diminished glutamine concentrations in blood suppress lymphocyte transformation and, by implication, lymphocyte function.[160]

Reports have been made on the favorable influence of selective gut decontamination on cell-mediated immunity[161] and on T-4/8 ratios;[162] clinical experience, unfortunately, indicates that immunoenhancing nutrition is no more effective than regular high-protein nutrition in achieving desirable outcomes.[15]

Finally, mention must be made of unidentified or partially identified immunosuppressive factors in burn serum and in burn subeschar tissue fluid. Mention has already been made of cutaneous burn toxin and the current status of research in this area.[17] A small molecular weight immunosuppressive peptide has been found in blood which is capable of suppressing neutrophil chemotaxis and T cell blastogenesis, and, to a lesser extent, B cell blastogenesis.[163,164] Immunosuppressive material exists in subeschar tissue fluid, perhaps by seepage from the serum.[165] There are undoubtedly other products following thermal injury as a result of breakdown, polymerization, or other biological processes which are immunosuppressive and which remain unidentified.

Toxic metabolites

A discussion of toxic intracellular metabolites, such as superoxide anion and hydroxyl ion generation, are beyond the scope of this chapter and are more fully discussed in other chapters in this book. The subject is mentioned only because the generation of toxic metabolites in cells have a dual importance following thermal injury: first, as the final common pathway for cell damage induced by both the cytokine pathway and by endotoxemia, and secondly, as the active mode of destruction of microorganisms by phagocytic cells. In this respect, it is worth mentioning that there is a suppression of superoxide anion production in polymorphs following thermal injury.[166] It would also appear that the generation of superoxide anion in some tissues, particularly the liver, following endotoxemia, is an earlier event than was previously thought.[167]

Autoimmune phenomena

Burned patients produce autoimmune antibodies to a large variety of tissues, which have been extensively investigated.[168,169] At one time, it was thought that the presence of autoantibodies was significant in the induction of suppressive phenomena following thermal injury. Indeed, the control of endotoxemia with polymyxin B, which reduces the effect of suppressor T cells following burns, results in a modest increase in detectable autoimmune antibodies to various tissues.[170] In neither burned patients nor controls does actual titer of autoantibodies reach levels regarded as clinically significant, and no clinical correlation between postburn pathology and autoimmunity has ever been convincingly demonstrated. There are several 'downregulatory' mechanisms in place following thermal injury, including anti-idiotype mechanisms, the suppressor cell network, and prostaglandins; so it is possible that the presence of autoantibodies plays some part in the induction of downregulatory response.[171]

Intervention

Overview

Search for enhancement of the host defense is as old as research in burn immunology itself. It has been appropriately termed the 'Search for the Holy Grail'.[172] The subject has been recently reviewed;[173] indeed, an entire symposium was devoted to the topic recently.[174] It is appropriate to point out, before going into detail, that improvements in the general surgical care of the burned patient have played a major role improving the immunological status of the host, similar to other surgical patients.[175] In particular, early excision of the burn wound with wound coverage,[176–178] plasma exchange therapy,[179] improvements in resuscitation and oxygen delivery,[180] and advances in nutrition[181,182] have played a major role in immunological support of the burned patient. As with all recent advances, a degree of caution is appropriate: for instance, overnutrition can do damage.[183]

The difficulties in evaluating new agents for intervention are enormous. The clinical picture of inflammation and of sepsis is very similar, as it should be, considering that the two induce similar biological cascades. The mortality of thermal injury is rapidly reaching an almost irreducible minimum such that the mortality rate, as an endpoint, will be difficult to influence further, and, therefore, secondary endpoints will have to be used in clinical trials. These and other difficulties have been well outlined in an excellent recent review.[184] We would recommend enthusiastically to future investigators who desire to use intervention for the improvement of the immunological status of burn patients to develop or use one of the detailed scales available for measurement of the septic response.[185]

Active and passive vaccination

Early attempts at active and passive vaccination of burned patients (Feller, 1964; Sachs, 1970; Alexander, 1969–74; Jones, 1973, 1977, 1978) have been summarized in a recent review.[186] These attempts were based on the dominance of *Pseudomonas* as a burn pathogen at the time, against which, because of the low number of immunotypes, it is relatively easy to prepare vaccines. With the advent of other gram-negative organisms and finally gram-positive organisms as pathogens, specific vaccination became more difficult. Other studies were beset by difficulties of inadequate or retrospective controls, concurrent advances in other areas on burn therapy, over which there was not adequate control, and the increasing cost of developing human vaccines. Even polyvalent *Pseudomonas* vaccine appears to produce an inadequate IgG_1 and IgG_2 subclass response in patients with thermal injury, throwing some doubts on the possible benefits of active immunization.[187]

The advent of commercial preparations of intravenous immunoglobulin produced an era of renewed enthusiasm for passive vaccination, since older studies[1] have clearly shown that low immunoglobulin concentration postburn, particularly that of IgG, is of poor prognostic significance. Unfortunately, none of the human trials of intravenous immunoglobulin in burned patients was able to demonstrate improvement in survival although there were occasional improvements in *in vitro* findings.[188–191]

There is currently a federal hyperimmune immunological trial (FHIT) in progress, the results of which are not yet available at this time of writing, which may shed further light on the potential utility of passive vaccination.[192] Decrease of serum fibronectin concentration in burned patients has also been documented, and it parallels a decrease in serum opsonizing function.[193] Although definitive studies in burned patients are not available, in severe trauma patients with septic complications the passive administration of fibronectin has failed to improve outcome.[194] While the results of these trials are disappointing, they are not surprising when one considers the multifactorial defects in the host defense. Basically, it is unlikely that any therapy which solely improves antibody concentration would be effective if phagocytic defects, intracellular killing defects, alterations in antigenic recognition and presentation, and cellular chemotaxis and migration went untreated.

Cell-Mediated Immunity and Neutrophils

Use of immunostimulants to treat human disease began with the use of Coley's toxin, a group of mixed bacterial toxins used to treat cancer early in the century. Cancer research has provided most of the data on immunostimulation of host resistance, but research on infection, trauma, and burns has benefited from this work as well. The source of the stimulatory substances can be classified roughly into four categories:

1. fungal glycans – which enhance macrophage microbicidal activity and induce monokine release (an example of this is glucan);
2. detoxified forms of endotoxin which will be dealt with further in this chapter;
3. active components of the mycobacterial cell wall such as used in Freund's adjuvant, the most recent example of this being MDP or muramyl dipeptide; and
4. a number of other agents which stimulate interferon induction and natural killer cells.

In addition, maturation products of normal T cells such as thymic extracts have also provided active substances. Further products have become available thanks to recombinant technology. Currently, there are several such products licensed for use not only in both Europe and the United States but also in Japan. Thymic extracts are actively used in Europe, in both cancer and infection control. Thymic peptide, thymopentin (TP-5) is licenced for use in Italy and Germany at this time of writing. These adjuvants work by their ability to activate one of the two CD4 T cell populations, either TH1 or TH2, which controls the major features of specific immune responses.[195,196]

A number of these agents have been investigated in human or animal burn settings. Thymopentin (TP-5) has been most extensively examined in experimental animal models in the United States and in clinical situations in Europe, both in burns and in trauma.[197–202] Reported improvements include an improvement in antigen cocktail induced lymphocyte proliferation, improved DCH responses, opsonization, improved peripheral lymphocyte traffic, and improved survival. In experimental situations, TP-5 decreases PGE_2 production, and this may be its mode of action. At this time, there are no large prospective randomized studies available, which suggest that TP-5 should be added to the routine armamentarium in the management of major burns. The same statement may be applied to all other adjuvants or immunomodulators which have been licensed to this point.

Granulocyte colony-stimulating factor (G-CSF) has been explored in burned patients and appears to have beneficial effects in burned and burn-infected animals. Clinical trials are currently ongoing both with G-CSF and granulocyte–macrophage colony-stimulating factor (GM-CSF) in burned patients; the results are awaited with interest.[203,204]

An intriguing approach to downregulate tissue destruction by neutrophils is by interference with the β_2-integrin system by recombinant antibodies. The oxidative burst of neutrophils is an adherence-dependent phenomenon which can be blocked by antibodies directed against the α- or β-chain of the MAC-1 integrin. While this has not been attempted in burns, there are preclinical studies available in the treatment of septic shock.[205] An exciting new class of compounds, the pyridinyl imidazoles, recently described, inhibit cytokine biosynthesis. One of these compounds, FR 167653, specifically inhibits IL-1β and TNFα production.[206] Antioxidant treatment has been reported to improve the burn-suppressed contact hypersensitivity reaction and graft-versus-host reaction, both reliable measures of cell-mediated immunity, in a rat model.[207]

Arachidonic Acid Cascade, Cytokine Cascade

A discussion of interventions aimed at modulation of the arachidonic acid cascade and cytokine cascade must necessarily extend outside the area of thermal injury, for most of the experimental work in this area is in the treatment of sepsis and trauma rather than pure burn models.

Administration of ibuprofen to block prostanoid production in septic animals has been generally beneficial. In dogs, ibuprofen prevents TNF-mediated septic responses.[208] In an unanesthetized sheep model, ibuprofen improves lung microvascular permeability and the systemic vascular response.[209] In a septic porcine model, ibuprofen improves lung compliance and parameters of pulmonary function.[210] In burn models, however, the contribution of prostanoid blockade has been somewhat less convincing. Decreased bacterial translocation following burns can be achieved by prostaglandin analogs (misoprostol, enisoprost) which improve survival.[211] Other workers were unable to reverse the postburn suppression of murine lymphocyte and neutrophil function with prostaglandin blockade by either indomethacin or ibuprofen.[212] In a septic mouse model, prostanoid blockade actually increased mortality.[213]

An extensive multicenter ibuprofen trial for intensive care patients showed reduction in urinary TXB_2 dimer excretion and some favorable some impact on the clinical sepsis syndrome, but no definitive reduction in overall mortality rate.[214] Polyclonal anti-PGE serum can mitigate the suppressive effect on burns and sepsis in a mouse peritoneal macrophage model.[215]

Much research has been done in the field of TNF blockade; unfortunately, almost none of this work has been published in the burn field. There were early reports showing that recombinant human TNF protects animals against death in a septic model.[216,217] Antibodies against TNF reduce IL-1 and IL-6 induction;[218] in experimental models, suppression of TNF production by a TNF inhibitor (pentoxifylline, PTX) results in a decrease in LPS toxicity.[219] Antibody to TNF also prevents hemorrhage-induced suppression of Kupffer cell function[220] and endotoxin-induced shock and lethality in a rat model.[217] TNFα can also be antagonized by a TNFR immunoadhesin[221] and by the passive administration of soluble human TNF receptor, presumably by competitive inhibition and receptor blockade of macrophage induction.[222] In a baboon model, humanized anti-TNFα antibody protected against the lethal effect of *E. coli*-induced shock.[223]

Although this early work looks most encouraging, the lack of information in the burn model will mandate that a great deal more work be done before suppression of TNF production can be accepted as a valid therapeutic modality.

Interleukin-1 blockade is currently undergoing clinical trials with some promising early results in phase III trials.[224,225] In a murine burn wound sepsis model, IL-1 administration resulted in improved survival and diminished positive blood cultures.[226] Intervention using other cytokines and cytokine blockades remains controversial. Interferon-γ showed some promise in a prospective trial in the reduction of major septic complications.[227] There is also evidence that suppression of interferon-γ production as well as IL-6 production is of benefit in the septic response.[228–230] There is evidence, by contrast, that IL-6 may be a marker of inflammation rather than an inductive part of the inflammatory cascade, for recombinant IL-6 has strong anti-inflammatory effects.[231] In experimental endotoxin shock in the rat, a leukotriene antagonist has been shown to be of value;[232] in burned patients, the impaired expression of the IL-2 receptor can be reversed by exogenous recombinant IL-2.[233] Interleukin-10 is a strong anti-inflammatory cytokine which downregulates IL-1, IL-6, and TNFα *in vitro* and can protect mice against lethal intraperitoneal injection of endotoxin.[234]

Favorable results have been reported in various animal models by IL-8 and IL-12, and antimacrophage inflammatory protein.[235–237] Nonspecific immunoenhancement by lymphocyte culture products, either human or animal, have been shown to be beneficial in *Pseudomonas*-challenged animal models in several older reports.[238,239] Unfortunately, the precise nature of the stimulants has not been identified, nor have the data using whole lymphocyte extracts been precisely reproduced in any model of cytokine administration. Platelet-activating factor (PAF) receptor antagonist can also improve survival and downregulate PGB$_2$ and PGE$_2$ release.[240] Finally, the interaction of the neuroendocrine–cytokine axis has been addressed in preliminary fashion. In both septic and burn models, naloxone, a morphine antagonist, appears to attenuate some of the immunosuppressive effects of burn and sepsis.[241,242]

Endotoxin

Production and administration of lipopolysaccharide antagonists is the oldest and most popular experimental technique to modulate the effects of gram-negative sepsis and to support the host. An excellent recent review is recommended for detailed analysis of the structure of lipopolysaccharide and the preparation of antagonists.[243] Anti-LPS agents can be classified into several categories. Chemical compounds which inhibit the biological actions of LPS include polymyxin B, a polycationic antibiotic which stoichiometrically neutralizes the effects of LPS both *in vitro* and *in vivo* by binding directly to the anionic lipid A portion of LPS. Next, there are the structurally based lipid A antagonists which either bind to some portion of the lipopolysaccharide molecule or its precursors such as lipid X, or provide competitive inhibition by blocking a receptor site or sites. Constitutive serum proteins such as lipopolysaccharide-binding protein can be administered.

Bacterial/permeability-increasing protein antagonizes LPS. All *in vitro* test systems for the effects of such neutralizing agents show either decreased expression of membrane receptors, such as CD18 or CD14, or, alternatively, downregulation of cytokine production induced by LPS. For instance, HA-1A antibody, *in vitro*, reduces the production of tumor necrosis factor and IL-6.[244]

In vivo evaluation of these substances is far more difficult. Several clinical trials have been conducted for the testing of monoclonal anti-endotoxin antibodies. E5 antibody administration improved patients with clinical signs of organ failure.[245] Animal experiments have been somewhat more controversial, including actual decrease of survival in a recently published canine model.[246] In human trials, successful treatment of gram-negative bacteremia and septic shock have been reported;[247] but the methodology of these clinical studies has been questioned.[248] The mechanism of action of anti-endotoxin antibodies is not known. Anti-LPS monoclonal antibodies inhibit the synthesis of TNF messenger RNA *in vitro*,[249] enhance bacterial and endotoxin clearance,[250] and bind to specific epitopes within the deep core region of LPS.[251] Monoclonal antibodies also reduce endotoxin-induced vascular permeability.[252] In one report, reduction in septic shock and death was obtained by use of an anti-endotoxin core glycolipid preparation.[253] In a more recent report, however, core-lipopolysaccharide hyperimmune globulin was not effective in reducing the incidence of gram-negative systemic complications, while intravenous immunoglobulin was.[254] Another study of surgical patients with and without septic shock noted that patients in septic shock and patients who died showed serum levels of anti-lipopolysaccharide antibody.[255]

Polymyxin B has been quite a popular experimental drug in controlling endotoxemia, and has had both animal and clinical trials following thermal injury. Polymyxin B can act by extracorporeal absorption, by hemoperfusion and fiber absorption, or by direct administration.[256–259] Polymyxin B administered intravenously to burn patients has been reported to reverse the unfavorable T4:T8 ratio, improve natural killer cell function and its responsiveness to exogenous IL-2, and reduce serum endotoxin concentration.[260] Intravenous polymyxin has been used to reduce translocational endotoxemia in a group of burned patients with successful reduction of serum endotoxin concentrations; however, in the early postburn stage, no downregulation of cytokine induction and no reduction in clinical septic parameters was seen.[261] Absorption of gram-negative bacteria and their products, attempted and abandoned in the past, is being revisited.[262] Other techniques under current experimental trial include the use of LPS-binding protein,[263] human growth hormone,[264] leumedin and bradykinin antagonists,[265] and the use of cytokine downregulation using radical spin trapping.[266] Unfortunately, there is continuing evidence that there is little correlation between the induction of proinflammatory cytokines and plasma LPS.[267] Indeed, even the addition of ibuprofen to polymyxin B to patients with major burns has no major beneficial effects.[268]

Toxic Metabolites

There is a dearth of information on the effect of intervention in the prevention of injury by toxic metabolites following thermal injury. The generation of toxic metabolites as a final common pathway to tissue injury has been recently reviewed[269] and this section will merely update some research of particular interest and note what work is available in thermal injury models.

Polymyxin B, in addition to having the anti-endotoxin effect just discussed, is also capable of inhibiting superoxide anion release in polymorphs by inhibition of protein kinase C.[270] Nitric oxide has recently become of interest as a superoxide quencher.[271] One of the mechanisms of cell damage in immunocytes is apparent upregulation of calcium transport across membranes, with an increased intracellular calcium concentration. Calcium channel blockers have been shown to have immunoprotective effects with preservation of antigen presentation function and IL-1 synthesis after hemorrhage.[272] As mentioned previously, some attention has been given to the effect of cyclic nitrones as antioxidants following endotoxemia. Synthetic antioxidants can now be manufactured which are of greater potency than α-phenyl *N-tert*-butyl nitrone (PBN).[273]

Lipid peroxidation has been studied in some detail in the burn model. Lipid peroxidation persists for 3–5 days post-injury in the presence of a sterile burn wound.[274] Fluid resuscitation with deferoxamine, an iron chelator, prevents hydroxyl radical release and prevents systemic burn-induced oxidant injury in the sheep burn model.[275] Intraperitoneal injection of lipid peroxidation products from burned rats enhances humoral immunity.[276] Two practical difficulties lie in the way of effective intervention using antagonists to toxic radicals following burn injury. First is the extremely short half-life of most standard superoxide scavengers. Secondly, the apparent evidence that, although toxic radical release does not occur reasonably early following the cause of injury, biologically significant release is a preterminal event which would be difficult to reverse. Clearly, much more research on this subject is needed before the final conclusions are reached.

Combination Therapy

Most workers agree that combination therapy has to be the wave of the future, given the extraordinary complexity of the response to endotoxin, the cytokine cascade, and the feedback loops of the cytokine network. In nonburned patients, several combinations have been attempted. Cytokine therapy in combination with ibuprofen[277] in cancer patients, the combination of indomethacin and thymopentin in major surgical patients,[278] and the combination of antibiotics with cytokines in hemorrhagic shock and infection rat models[279] appear to provide enhanced effectiveness.

In burn models, the combination of IL-1 with indomethacin has shown increased survivals[280] as well as IL-2 activated LAK cells, although this is not truly 'combination therapy'.[281] G-CSF and gentamicin have been combined.[282] Experience with the combination of antibiotics and immunoglobulin or anti-endotoxin therapy is mixed. In one recent report, antibiotic therapy with passive immunization with intravenous Ig resulted in a reduction of mortality and a reduction of hospitalization time[283] but in another study the combination of IgG and T$_4$ showed no improvement,[284] nor did the combination of polymyxin B with IgG.[285] The interaction of IL-10 and IL-4 appears to have some salutary effect.[286]

This discussion wouldn't be complete without mention of the recent attention paid, and rightly so, to immunological events surrounding the scarring process which follows burn injury. Patients with proliferative scars have a much greater production of IL-1, IL-6 TNFα, and TNFβ$_2$ than controls.[287] Elevated anticollagen IgG as well as IgE are also correlated with hypertrophic scarring.[288] Since it is believed that local IL-6 production may induce metalloproteinase which has a profound effect on wound healing,[289] it is clear than injury and healing represent a biochemical continuum which promises to be a fruitful area for future research.

Conclusions

Immunology has come of age to the point where a reasonably clear understanding of the timetable of immunological alterations now exists. Following injury, there is immediate activation of the arachidonic acid cascade and the cytokine cascade, together with early translocation of bacteria and endotoxin. Major metabolic, hormonal, and cellular alterations begin within 24–48 hours. After 3–4 days, there is a second peak of endotoxemia which appears to reinduce the cytokine and arachidonic acid cascade. The triggering of toxic metabolites occurs early but is probably not of biological significance until several days after the injury, following the induction of earlier changes. It is clear that there will be no single agent which can alter this course of events; rather, a combination of two to three agents aimed at the interruption of several of the sequences described above at various points in time will be indicated. The influence of intervention in the inflammatory cascade on wound healing and epithelialization is not yet clearly understood, but is becoming the subject of intensive research.

In summary, the difficulties of performing excellent clinical studies have only recently become appreciated. It should be re-emphasized that thermal injury has reached a relatively low mortality in most developed countries. Death of the patient as an endpoint for interventions, although obviously essential, becomes a statistical nightmare unless very large multicenter trials involving thousands of patients are recruited. Therefore, investigators must look at secondary endpoints, and pay closer attention to the evaluation of septic complications on some kind of precise quantifiable scale,: length of stay, cost of therapy, and similar outcomes. Finally, many of the therapies discussed in this chapter are extremely costly. Cost-effectiveness studies must be conducted in parallel with safety and efficacy studies if new proposed regimens are to take their place successfully in the armamentarium of burn therapy.

Summary

Much progress has been made in the last 20 years in our understanding of the intricacies of the host defect created by thermal injury. The arachidonic acid cascade is triggered early, as is the induction of the inflammatory cytokine cascade. Alterations occur in the function of lymphocytes, macrophages, and neutrophils. Bacteria and bacterial products translocate. The net result of these complex changes following thermal injury is twofold: first, they interfere with the biological efficiency of the host in fighting invading pathogens, and secondly, there is a cell damage and death from the inflammatory cascade itself, probably by the way of the formation of toxic intracellular metabolites as the final common pathway.

Because of the complexity of these changes, which are only now beginning to be understood, early optimism for successful intervention has not been borne out. There are a number of promising leads for therapy, but it has become apparent that therapeutic modalities will have to be developed which address each of the major immunological alterations following thermal injury, and that there will not be a single accent which can reverse the observed changes for the benefit of the host.

References

1. Munster AM. Alterations of the host defense mechanism in burns. *Surg Clin North Am* 1970; **50**: 1217–25.
2. Rapaport FT, Miligram F, Kano K, *et al.* Immunologic sequelae of thermal injury. *Ann NY Acad Sci* 1968; **150**: 1004–8.
3. Munster AM. Immune response in burns and injuries. In: Seligson D, ed. *Handbook of Clinical Laboratory Science.* Boca Raton: CRC Press, 1978: 375–93.
4. Calvano SE. Hormonal mediation of immune dysfunction following thermal and traumatic injury. In: Gullinard JI, Fauci AS, eds. *Advances in Host Defense Mechanisms*, Vol 6. New York: Raven Press, 1986.
5. Alexander JW. Mechanism of immunologic suppression in burn injury. *J Trauma* 1990; **30**: S70–5.
6. Konig W, Schluter B, Scheffer J, Koller M. Microbial pathogenicity and host defense in burned patients – the role of inflammatory mediators. *Infection* 1992; **2**: S128–34.
7. Heideman M, Bengtsson A. The immunologic response to thermal injury. *World J Surg* 1992; **16(1)**: 53–6.
8. Gabay C, Kushner I. Acute-phase proteins and other systemic responses to inflammation. *New Engl J Med* 1999; **340**: 448–54.
9. Imhoff M, Gahr RH, Hoffman P. Delayed cutaneous hypersensitivity after multiple injury and severe burn. *Ann Ital Chir* 1990; **61(5)**: 525–8.
10. Munster AM, Winchurch RA, Birmingham WJ, Keeling P. Longitudinal assay of lymphocyte responsiveness in patients with major burns. *Ann Surg* 1980; **192**: 772–5.
11. Peck MD, Alexander JW. The use of immunologic tests to predict outcome in surgical patients. *Nutrition* 1990; **6**: 16–19.
12. Bach FH. Cell-mediated immunity. Its basis and analysis. *Nutrition* 1990; **6**: 2–4.

13. Wells CL, Jechorek RP, Erlandsen SL, et al. The effect of dietary glutamine and dietary RNA on ileal flora, histology, and bacterial translocation in mice. Nutrition 1990; 6: 70–5.

14. Kinsella JE, Lokesh B, Broughton S, Whelan J. Dietary polyunsaturated fatty acids and eicosanoids: potential effects on the modulation of inflammatory and immune cells: an overview. Nutrition 1990; 6: 24–44.

15. Saffle JR, Wiebke G, Jennings K, Morris SE, Barton RG. Randomized trial of immune-enhancing enteral nutrition in burn patients. J Trauma 1997; 42(5): 793–800.

16. Monge G, Sparkes BG, Allgower M, Schoenenberger GA. Influence of burn-induced lipid-protein complex on IL1 secretion by PBMC in vitro. Burns 1991; 17(4): 269–75.

17. Sparkes BG, Gyorkos JW, Gorczynski RM, Brock AJ. Comparison of endotoxins and cutaneous burn toxin as immunosuppressants. Burns 1990; 16: 123–6.

18. Deitch EA, Lu Q, Xu DZ, Special RD. Effect of local and systemic burn microenvironment on neutrophil activation as assessed by complement receptor expression and morphology. J Trauma 1990; 30(3): 259–68.

19. Stratta RJ, Saffle JR, Ninnemann JL, et al. The effect of surgical excision and grafting procedures on postburn lymphocyte suppression. J Trauma 1985; 25: 46–52.

20. Lazarou SA, Barbul A, Wasserkrug HL, Efron G. The wound is a possible source of posttraumatic immunosuppression. Arch Surg 1989; 124: 1429–31.

21. Yamamoto H, Siltharm S, DeSerres S, Hulman CS, Meyer AA. Immediate burn wound excision restores antibody synthesis to bacterial antigen. J Surg Res 1996; 63: 157–62.

22. Hultman CS, Yamamoto H, deSerres S, Frelinger JA, Meyer AA. Early but not late burn wound excision partially restores viral specific T-lymphocyte cytotoxicity. J Trauma 1997; 43: 441–7.

23. Devecci M, Eski M, Sengezer M, Kisa U. Effects of cerium nitrate bathing and prompt wound excision on IL-6 and TNF-alpha levels in burned rats. Burns 2000; 26: 41–5.

24. Wilmore D. Hypermetabolic response to burn injury. J Trauma 1990; 30: S4–S6.

25. Fong Y, Moldawer LL, Shires GT, Lowry SF. The biologic characteristics of cytokines and their implication in surgical injury. Surg Gynecol Obstet 1990; 170: 363–78.

26. Santos AA, Schltinga MR, Lynch E, et al. Elaboration of interleukin-1 receptor antagonism is not attenuated by glucocorticoids after endotoxemia. Arch Surg 1993; 128: 138–44.

27. Mantovani A. The chemokine system: redundancy for robust outputs. Immunol Today 1999; 20: 254–7.

28. Ninnemann JL, Stockland AE, Condie JT. Induction of prostaglandin synthesis-dependent suppressor cells with endotoxin: occurrence in patients with thermal injuries. J Clin Immunol 1983; 3(2): 42–50.

29. Grbic JT, Mannick JA, Gough DB, Rodrick ML. The role of prostaglandin E, in immune suppression following injury. Ann Surg 1991; 214: 253–63.

30. Callery MP, Kamei T, Mangino MJ, Flye MW. Interleukin-6 (IL-6) production by endotoxin (LPS)-stimulated Kupffer cells is regulated by prostaglandin E. J Surg Res 1990; 48(6): 523–7.

31. Hoffman T, Lizzio EF, Suissa J, et al. Dual stimulation of phospholipase activity in human monocytes: role of calcium-dependent and calcium-independent pathways in arachidonic acid release and eicosanoid formation. J Immunol 1988, 140: 3912–18.

32. Herndon DN, Abston S, Stein MD. Increased thromboxane B_2 levels in the plasma of burned and septic burned patients. Surg Gynecol Obstet 1984; 159: 210–13.

33. Endo S, Inada K, Yamada Y, et al. Plasma tumor necrosis factors (TNF-α) levels in patients with burns. Burns 1993; 19: 124–7.

34. Moore FD, Socher SH, Davis C. Tumor necrosis factor and endotoxin can cause neutrophil activation through separate pathways. Arch Surg 1991; 126: 70–3.

35. Marano MA, Fong Y, Moldawer LL, et al. Serum cachectin/tumor necrosis factor in critically ill patients with burns correlates with infection and mortality. Surg Gynecol Obstet 1990; 170: 32–8.

36. Kawakami M, Kaneko N, Anada H, Terai C, Okada Y. Measurement of interleukin-6, interleukin-10, and tumor necrosis factor-alpha levels in tissues and plasma after thermal injury in mice. Surgery 1997; 121: 440–8.

37. Sanchez-Cantu L, Rode HN, Christou NV. Endotoxin tolerance is associated with reduced secretion of tumor necrosis factor. Arch Surg 1989; 124: 1432–6.

38. Beutler B, Krochin N, Milsark IW, et al. Control of cachectin (tumor necrosis factor) synthesis: mechanisms of endotoxin resistance. Science 1986; 232: 977–80.

39. Takayama TK, Miller C, Szabo G. Elevated tumor necrosis factor production concomitant to elevated prostaglandin E, production by trauma patients' monocytes. Arch Surg 1990; 125: 29–35.

40. Furse RK, Kodys K, Zhu D, Miller-Graziano CL. Increased monocyte TNF-alpha message stability contributes to trauma patients' increased TNF production. J Leukoc Biol 1997; 62: 524–34.

41. Faist E, Storck M, Hultner L, et al. Functional analysis of monocyte activity through synthesis patterns of proinflammatory cytokines and neopterin in patients in surgical intensive care. Surgery 1992; 112: 562–72.

42. Tellado JM, Christou NV. Increased polymorphonuclear neutrophil delivery to inflammatory lesions in anergic patients is medicated via interleukin-1 and interleukin-6. Surg Forum 1990; 41: 99–100.

43. Wood JJ, Rodrick ML, O'Mahony JB, et al. Inadequate interleukin-2 production: a fundamental immunological deficiency in patients with major burns. Ann Surg 1984; 200: 311–20.

44. Teodorczyk-Injeyan JA, Sparkes BG, Mills GB, Peters WJ. Soluble interleukin 2-receptor alpha secretion is related to altered interleukin 2 production in thermally injured patients. Burns 1991; 17(4): 290–5.

45. Teodorczyk-Injeyan JA, Sparkes BG, Peters WJ. Serum interleukin-2 receptor as a possible mediator of immunosuppression after burn injury. J Burn Care Rehabil 1989; 10(2): 112–18.

46. Teodorczyk-Injeyan JA, Sparkes BG, Lalani S, et al. IL-2 regulation of soluble EL-2 receptor levels following thermal injury. Clin Exp Immunol 1992; 90(1): 36–42.

47. Teodorczyk-Injeyan JA, Sparkes BG, Mills GB, et al. Increase of serum interleukin 2 receptor level in thermally injured patients. Clin Exp Immunol 1989; 51(2): 202–15.

48. Xiao, G-X, Chopra RK, Adler WH, Munster AM, Winchurch RA. Altered expression of lymphocyte IL-2 receptors in burned patients. J Trauma 1992; 33: 74–82.

49. Rodriguez JL, Miller CG, De Forge LE, et al. Local production of interleukin-8 is associated with nosocomial pneumonia. J Trauma 1992; 33: 74–82.

50. Zhou D, Kusnecov A, Shurin M, et al. Exposure to physical and psychological stressors elevates plasma levels of IL-6: relationship to the activation of hypothalamic-pituitary-adrenal axis. Endocrinology 1993; 133(6): 2523–30.

51. Lanser ME, Brown GE. Control of hepatocyte fibronectin secretion by interleukin-6. Surg Res Commun 1989; 5: 32.

52. Nijsten MWN, DeGroot ER, TenDuis HJ, et al. Serum levels of interleukin-6 and acute phase responses. Lancet 1987; 2: 921.

53. Zhou D, Munster AM, Winchurch RA. Inhibitory effects of interleukin 6 on immunity: possible implications in burn patients. Arch Surg 1992; 127: 65–9.

54. Miller C, Szabo G, Kodys K. Elevated IL-6 production by immunosuppressed trauma patients' monocytes (MO). J Leuk Biol 1989; 46: 323.

55. Mazuski JE, Ortiz Towle HC, Cerra FB. Withdrawal of inflammatory mediator does not abrogate a sustained hepatic acute phase response. Presented at the meeting of the Surgical Infection Society, Denver, 1989.

56. Nijsten MW, Hack CE, Helle M, et al. Interleukin-6 and its relation to the humoral immune response and clinical parameters in burned patients. Surgery 1991; 109(6): 761–7.

57. Miller-Graziano CL, Szabo G, Griffey K, et al. Role of elevated monocyte transforming growth factor beta (TNF-β) production in posttrauma immunosuppression. J Clin Immunol 1991; 11: 95–102.

58. Zhou D, Munster A, Winchurch RA. Pathologic concentrations of interleukin 6 inhibit T cell responses via induction of activation of TGF-β. FASEB J 1991; 5: 2582–5.

59. Zedler S, Bone RC, Baue AE, von Donnersmarck GH. T-cell reactivity and its predictive role in immunosuppression after burns. Crit Care Med 1999; 27: 66–72.

60. Lyons A, Goebel A, Mannick JA, Lederer JA. Protective effects of early interleukin-10 antagonism on injury-induced immune dysfuction. Arch Surg 1999; 134: 1317–23.

61. Kavanagh EK, Kell MR, Goebel A, Soberg CC, Mannick JA, Lederer JA. Interleukin 10 is not essential for survival or for modulating T-cell fuction after injury. Surgery 1999; 126: 456–62.

62. Munster AM. Post-traumatic immunosuppression is due to activation of suppressor T-cells. Lancet 1976; 1: 1329–30.

63. Kupper TS, Green DR. Immunoregulation after thermal injury: sequential appearance of I-J+, LY-1, T suppressor inducer cells and LY-2 T suppressor effector cells following thermal trauma in mice. J Immunol 1984; 133: 3047–53.

64. Hansbrough JF, Bender EM, Zapata-Sirvent R, Anderson J. Altered helper and suppressor lymphocyte populations in surgical patients: a measure of postoperative immunosuppression. Am J Surg 1984; 148: 303–7.

65. Rioja LF, Alonso P, de Haro J, de la Cruz J. Prognostic value of the CD4/CD8 lymphocyte ration in moderately burned patients. Burns 1993; 19(3): 198–201.

66. O'Mahony JB, Wood J, Rodrick ML, Mannick JA. Changes in T lymphocyte subsets following injury: assessment by flow cytometry and relationship to sepsis. Ann Surg 1985; 202: 580–6.

67. Burleson DG, Mason AD, Pruitt BA. Lymphoid subpopulation changes after thermal injury and thermal injury with infection in an experimental model. Ann Surg 1988; 207: 208–12.

68. Organ BC, Antonacci AC, Chiao J, *et al.* Changes in lymphocyte number and phenotype in seven lymphoid compartments after thermal injury. *Ann Surg* 1988; **210**: 78–89.

69. Zedler S, Faist E, Ostermeier B, von Donnersmark GH, Schildberg FW. Postburn constitutional changes in T-cell reactivity occur in CD8+ rather than CD4+ cells. *J Trauma* 1997; **42(5)**: 872–80.

70. Deitch EA, Xu D, Qi L. Different lymphocyte compartments respond differently to mitogenic stimulation after thermal injury. *Ann Surg* 1990; **211**: 72–7.

71. Maldonado MD, Venturoli A, Franco A, Nunez-Roldan A. Specific changes in peripheral blood lymphocyte phenotype from burn patients: probable origin of the thermal injury-related lymphocytopenia. *Burns* 1991; **17**: 188–92.

72. Zapata-Sirvent RL, Hansbrough JF. Temporal analysis of human leukocyte surface antigen expression and neutrophil respiratory burst activity after thermal injury. *Burns* 1993; **19(1)**: 5–11.

73. Gadd MA, Hansbrough JF, Hoyt DB, Ozkan N. Defective T-cell surface antigen expression after mitogen stimulation: an index of lymphocyte dysfunction after controlled murine injury. *Ann Surg* 1989; **29**: 112–18.

74. Bender BS, Winchurch RA, Thupari JN, *et al.* Depressed natural killer cell function in thermally injured adults: successful in vivo and in vitro immunomodulation and the role of endotoxin. *Clin Exp Immunol* 1988; **71**: 120–5.

75. Tolentino MV, Sarasua MM, Hill OA, *et al.* Peripheral lymphocyte membrane fluidity after thermal injury. *J Burn Care Rehabil* 1991; **12(6)**: 498–504.

76. Teodorczyk-Injeyan JA, Sparkes BG, Mills GB, Peters WJ. Immunosuppression follows systemic T lymphocyte activation in the burn patient. *Clin Exp Immunol* 1991; **85(3)**: 515–18.

77. Schwacha MG, Ayala A, Cioffi WG, Bland KI, Chaudry IH. Role of protein kinase C in cyclic AMP-mediated suppression of T-lymphocyte activation following burn injury. *Biochim Biophys Acta* 1999; **1455**: 45–53.

78. Marsland AL, Graham RE, Bachen EA, *et al.* Fitness as a predictor of cellular immune response to mental stress. Presented at the meeting for Research Perspectives in Psychoneuroimmunology IV, Boulder, Colorado, 1993.

79. Shelby J, Sullivan J, Groussman M, Gray R, Saffle J. Severe burn injury: effects on psychologic and immunologic function in noninjured close relatives. *J Burn Care Rehabil* 1992; **13(1)**: 58–63.

80. Hansbrough JF, Zapata-Sirvent R, Hoyt D. Postburn immune suppression: an inflammatory response to the burn wound? *J Trauma* 1990; **30**: 671–5.

81. Trop M, Schiffrin EJ, Carter EA. Role of skin in the burn-induced reduction of reticuloendothelial phagocytic activity in rats. *Burns* 1990; **16**: 57–9.

82. Cooper KD, Oberheiman L, Hamilton TA, *et al.* Neopterin as parameter of cell-mediated immunity response in thermally injured patients. *Burns* 1992; **18(2)**: 113–16.

83. Balogh D, Lammer H, Komberger E, *et al.* Neopterin plasma levels in burn patients. *Burns* 1992; **18(3)**: 185–8.

84. Moore FD Jr, Davis CF. Monocyte activation after burns and endotoxemia. *J Surg Res* 1989; **46(4)**: 350–4.

85. Gibbons RA, Martinez OM, Lim RC, *et al.* Reduction in HLA-DR, HLA-DQ and HLA-DP expression by Leu-M3 + cells. *Clin Exp Immunol* 1989; **75(3)**: 371–5.

86. Sachse C, Prigge M, Cramer G, Pallua N, Henkel E. Association between human leucocyte antigen (HLA)-DR expression on blood monocytes and increased plasma level of interleukin-10 in patients with severe burns. *Clin Chem Lab Med* 1999; **37**: 193–8.

87. Yang L, Hsu B. The roles of macrophage (M phi) and PGE-2 in postburn immunosuppression. *Burns* 1992; **18(2)**: 132–6.

88. Ogle CK, Johnson C, Guo X, *et al.* Production and release of C3 cultured monocytes/macrophages isolated from burned, trauma, and septic patients. *J Trauma* 1992; **29**: 189–94.

89. Tomomochi G, Masayoshi A, Hidehiko S, Motonijchi T. Characteristics of alveolar macrophages in experimental septic lung. *J Leukoc Biol* 1992; **52**: 236–43.

90. Noelle RJ, Snow EC. T helper cell-dependent B cell activation. *FASEB J* 1991; **5**: 2770–6.

91. Yamamoto H, Siltharm S, deSerres S, Hultman CS, Meyer AA. Effect of cyclooxygenase inhibition on in vitro B-cell function after burn injury. *J Trauma* 1996; **41**: 612–19.

92. Kagan RJ, Bratescu A, Jonasson O, *et al.* The relationship between the percentage of circulating B cells, corticosteroid levels, and other immunologic parameters in thermally injured patients. *J Trauma* 1989; **29**: 208–13.

93. Schluter B, Konig W, Koller M, *et al.* Differential regulation of T- and B-lymphocyte activation in severely burned patients. *J Trauma* 1991; **31**: 239–46.

94. Schluter B, Konig W, Koller M, *et al.* Studies on B-lymphocyte dysfunctions in severely burned patients. *J Trauma* 1990; **30**: 1380–9.

95. Miller-Graziano CL, Szabo G, Kodys K, Griffey K. Aberrations in post-trauma monocyte (MO) subpopulation: role in septic shock syndrome. *J Trauma* 1990; **30**: S86–96.

96. Solomkin JS. Neutrophil disorders in burn injury: complement, cytokines, and organ injury. *J Trauma* 1990; **30**: S80–5.

97. Jeyapaul J, Mehta LN, Arora S, Antia NH. Fc and complement receptor integrity of polymorphonuclear (PMN) cells following thermal injury. *Burns* 1984; **10**: 387–95.

98. Ogle CK, Alexander W, Nagy H, *et al.* A long-term study and correlation of lymphocyte and neutrophil function in the patient with burns. *J Burn Care Rehabil* 1990; **11**: 105–11.

99. Bjerknes R, Vindenes H, Pitkanen J, *et al.* Altered polymorphonuclear neutrophilic granulocyte functions in patients with large burns. *J Trauma* 1989; **29(6)**: 847–55.

100. Bjerknes R, Vindenes H. Neutrophil dysfunction after thermal injury, alteration of phagolysosomal acidification in patients with large burns. *Burns* 1989; **15(2)**: 77–81.

101. Bjomson AB, Knippenberg RW, Bjomson HS. Bactericidal defect of neutrophils in a guinea pig model of thermal injury is related to elevation of intracellular cyclic-3′,5′-adenosine monophosphate. *J Immunol* 1989; **143**: 2609–16.

102. Babcock GF, Alexander JW, Warden GD. Flow cytometric analysis of neutrophil subsets in thermally injured patients developing infection. *Clin Exp Immunol* 1990; **54(1)**: 117–25.

103. Deitch EA. The relationship between thermal injury and neutrophil membrane functions as measured by chemotaxis, adherence and spreading. *Burns* 1984; **10**: 264–70.

104. Tchervenkov JI, Latter DA, Psychogios J, Christou NV. Altered leukocyte delivery to specific and nonspecific inflammatory skin lesions following burn injury. *J Trauma* 1988; **25**: 582–8.

105. Hasslen SR, Ahrenholz DH, Solem LD, Nelson RD. Actin polymerization contributes to neutrophil chemotactic dysfunction following thermal injury. *J Leukoc Biol* 1992; **52**: 495–500.

106. Killer M, Konig W, Brom J, *et al.* Studies on the mechanisms of granulocyte dysfunctions in severely burned patients – evidence for altered leukotriene generation. *J Trauma* 1989; **29**: 435–45.

107. Arbak S, Ercan F, Hudag CG, *et al.* Acute lung Injury following thermal insult to the skin: a light and transmission electron microscopial study. *Acta Histochem* 1999; **101**: 255–62, .

108. Goodman ER, Stricker P, Velavicius M, *et al. Arch Surg* 1999; **134**: 1049–54.

109. Chitnis D, Dickerson C, Munster AM, Winchurch RA. Inhibition of apoptosis in polymorphonuclear neutrophils from burn patients. *J Leucocyte Biol* 1996; **59**: 835–9.

110. Nwariaku F, Hallihil N, Wright JK, *et al.* Burn-activated neutrophils (NP) and TNF-alpha alter endothelial cell (EC) actin cytoskeleton and enhance monolayer permeability. Material presented to the 61st Annual Meeting, Society of University Surgeons, Toronto, 11 February 2000.

111. Bergmann U, Konig W, Gross-Weege W, *et al.* Basophil releasability in severely burned patients. *J Trauma* 1990; **30(11)**: 1372–9.

112. Cioffi WG Jr, Burleson DG, Jordan BS, Mason AD Jr, Pruitt BA Jr. Granulocyte oxidate activity after thermal injury. *Surgery* 1992; **112(5)**: 860–5.

113. Mullen P, Windsor A, Walsh C, *et al.* Tumor necrosis factor (TNF-α) and interleukin-6 (IL-6) regulate neutrophil (PMN) function selectively. Presented at the meeting of the Association for Academic Surgeons, Montreal, 18–21 November 1992.

114. Carr DJ. The role of endogenous opioids and their receptors in the immune system. *Proc Soc Exp Biol Med* 1991; **198**: 710–20.

115. Weber RJ. Neutral and peripheral mechanisms involved in opioid regulation of immune function. Presented at the meeting for Research Perspectives in Psychoneuroimmunology IV, Boulder, Colorado, 1993.

116. Elliot D, Everitt AS, Gault D, *et al.* The role of endorphins in septicaemic shock: a pilot study in burned patients. *Burns* 1985; **11**: 387–92.

117. Deitch EA, Xu D, Bridges RM. Opioids modulate human neutrophil and lymphocyte function: thermal injury alters plasma B-endorphin levels. *Surgery* 1988; **104**: 41–8.

118. Paquet P, Pierard GE. Interleukin-6 and the skin. *Int Arch Allergy Immunol* 1996; **109**: 308–17.

119. Paquet P, Pierard GE. Soluble fractions of TNF alpha, IL-6, and their receptors in toxic epidermal necrolysis: a comparison with second degree burns. *Int J Mol Med* 1998; **1**: 459–62.

120. Maa J, Grady EF, Yoshimi SK, *et al.* Neurokikin-1 receptor activation promotes polymorphonuclear leucocyte infiltration in acute pancreatitis. Material presented at the 61st Annual Meeting, Society of University Surgeons, Toronto, 11 February 2000.

121. Carter EA, Tompkins RG, Schiffrin E, Burke IF. Cutaneous thermal injury alters macromolecular permeability of rat small intestine. *Surgery* 1990; **107**: 335–41.

122. LeeVoyer T, Cioffi WG, Pratt L, *et al.* Alterations in intestinal permeability after thermal injury. *Arch Surg* 1992; **127**: 26–30.

123. Deitch EA. Intestinal permeability is increased in burn patients shortly after injury. *Surgery* 1990; **107**: 411–16.

124. O'Dwyer ST, Michie HR, Ziegler TR, et al. A single dose of endotoxin increases intestinal permeability in healthy humans. Arch Surg 1988; 123: 1459–64.

125. Winchurch RA. Thupari JN, Munster AM. Endotoxemia in burn patients: levels of circulating endotoxins are related to burn size. Surgery 1987; 102: 808–12.

126. Endo S. Inada K, Kikuchi M, et al. Are plasma endotoxin levels related to burn size and prognosis? Burns 1992; 18: 486–9.

127. Zhong W. Hand T, Burke P, Forse RA. Human macrophage cytokine gene regulation to endotoxin is both dose and time dependent. Surg Inf Soc Prog 1992; 12: 38.

128. Nichols FC, Garrison SW, Davis HW. Prostaglandin E and thromboxane B₂ release from human monocytes treated with bacterial lipopolysaccharide. J Leukoc Biol 1988; 44: 376–84.

129. Ulich TR, del Castillo J, Ni RX, Bikhazi N. Hematologic interactions of endotoxin, tumor necrosis factor alpha (TNF-α), interleukin-1, and adrenal hormones and the hematologic effects of TNF-α in Corynebacterium parvum-primed rats. J Leukoc Biol 1989; 45: 546–57.

130. Megyeri P, Issekutz TB, Issekutz AC. An endotoxin-induced factor distinct from interleukin-1 and tumor necrosis factor produced by the THP-1 human macrophage line stimulates polymorphonuclear leukocyte infiltration in vivo. J Leukoc Biol 1990; 47: 70–8.

131. Bergmann U, Scheffer J, Koller M, et al. Induction of inflammatory mediators (histamine and leukotrienes) from rat peritoneal mast cells and human granulocytes by Pseudomonas aeruginosa strains from burn patients. Infect Immun 1989; 57(7): 2187–95.

132. Blanchard DK. Djeu JY, Klein TW, et al. Interferon-γ induction by lipopolysaccharide: dependence on interleukin-2 and macrophages. J Immunol 1986; 136: 963–70.

133. deGroote MA, Martin MA, Denesen P, et al. Plasma tumor necrosis factor alone does not explain the lethal effect of lipopolysaccharide. Arch Surg 1991; 126: 231–5.

134. Sanchez-Cantu L, Rode HN, Yun TJ, Christou NV. Tumor necrosis factor alone does not explain the lethal effect of lipopolysaccharide. Arch Surg 1991; 126: 231–5.

135. Tobias PS, Mathison JC, Ulevitch RJ. A family of lipopolysaccharide binding proteins involved in responses to gram-negative sepsis. J Biol Chem 1988; 263(27): 13479–81.

136. Taylor FB Jr. Presented at the Seminar on Advances in Prevention and Treatment of Endotoxemia and Sepsis, Philadelphia, 22–23 June 1992.

137. Birkenmaier C, Hong Y, Hom J. Modulation of the endotoxin receptor CD 14 in septic patients. J Trauma 1992; 32: 473–9.

138. Kruger C, Schutt C, Obertacke U, et al. Serum CD14 levels in polytraumatized and severely burned patients. Clin Exp Immunol 1991; 85(2): 297–301.

139. Weingarten R, Sklar LA, Mathison JC, et al. Interactions of lipopolysaccharide with neutrophils in blood via CD14. J Leukoc Biot 1993; 53: 518–24.

140. Richardson RP, Rhyne CD, Fong Y, et al. Peripheral blood leukocyte kinetics following in vivo lipopolysaccharide (LPS) administration to normal human subjects. Ann Surg 1989; 210: 239–45.

141. Ogle CK, Arita H, Nagy H, et al. The immunosuppressive effects of the in vivo administration of endotoxin as influenced by macrophages. J Trauma 1999; 29: 1015–20.

142. Tokyay R, Zeigler ST, Heggers JP, et al. Effects of anesthesia, surgery fluid resuscitation, and endotoxin administration on postburn bacterial translocation. J Trauma 1991; 31: 1376–9.

143. Suffredini AF, Fromm RE, Parker MM, et al. The cardiovascular response of normal humans to the administration of endotoxin. N Engl J Med 1989; 321: 280–7.

144. Callery MP, Mangino M 3, Kamei T, Flye MW. Organ interactions in sepsis: host defense and the hepatic-pulmonary macrophage axis. Arch Surg 1991; 126(1): 28–32.

145. Li JJ, Sanders RL, McAdam KPWJ, et al. Endotoxin suppresses surfactant synthesis in cultured rat lung cells. J Trauma 1989; 29: 180–8.

146. Maier RV, Hannel GB, Pohlman TH. Endotoxin requirements for alveolar macrophage stimulation. J Trauma 1990; 30: S49–S57.

147. Dean P, Yagi K, Naunheim K, Baudendistal L. Chronic endotoxin induced lung injury. Presented at the meeting of the Association for Academic Surgeons, Louisville, 15–18 November 1989.

148. Demling RH, LaLonde C. Effect of a body burn on endotoxin induced lipid peroxidation: comparison with physiologic and histologic changes. Surgery 1990; 107: 669–76.

149. Yirmiya R, Ovadia H, Rosen H, et al. Behavioral effects of LPS: involvement of endogenous opioids. Presented at the meeting for Research Perspectives in Psychoneuroimmunology IV, Boulder, Colorado, 1993.

150. Jackson JJ, Kropp H. O-Lactam antibiotic-induced release of free endotoxin: in vitro comparison of penicillin-binding protein (PBP) 2-specific imipenem and PBP 3-specific ceftazidime. J Infect Dis 1992; 165: 1033–41.

151. Gelfand JA, Donelan M, Burke JF. Preferential activation and depletion of the alternative complement pathway by burn injury. Ann Surg 1983; 198: 58–62.

152. Ferrara JJ, Dyess DL, Luterman A, et al. In vitro effects of complement inactivation upon burn-associated cell-mediated immunosuppression. Am Surgeon 1990; 56(9): 571–4.

153. Teodorczyk-Injeyan JA, Sparkes BG, Girotti MJ. Induced immunologloglobulin secretion by T-cell replacing products from blunt trauma patients. J Trauma 1982; 33: 171–8.

154. Ertel W, Faist E, Nestle C, et al. Dynamics of immunologloglobulin synthesis after major trauma. Arch Surg 1989; 124: 1437–42.

155. Shorr RM, Ershler WB, Gamelli RL. Immunoglobulin production in burned patients. J Trauma 1984; 24: 319–22.

156. Kawakami M, de Serres S, Meyer AA. Immunoglobulin synthesis by cultured lymphocytes from spleen and mesenteric lymph nodes after thermal injury. J Burn Care Rehabil 1991; 12: 474–81.

157. Teodorczyk-Injeyan JA, Sparkes BG, Peters WJ. Regulation of IgM production in thermally injured patients. Burns 1989; 15: 241–7.

158. Faist E, Eziel W, Baker CC, Heberer G. Terminal B-cell maturation and immunoglobulin (Ig) synthesis in vitro in patients with major injury. J Trauma 1989; 29: 2–9.

159. Peterson V, Hansbrough J, Buerk C, et al. Regulation of granulopoiesis following severe thermal injury. J Trauma 1983; 23: 1923.

160. Parry-Billings M, Evans J, Calder PC, Newsholme EA. Does glutamine contribute to immunosuppression after major burns? Lancet 1990; 336: 523–5.

161. Yao YM, Lu LR, Yu Y, et al. Influence of selective decontamination of the digestive tract on cell-mediated immune function and bacteria/endotoxin translocation in thermally injured rats. J Trauma 1997; 42: 1073–9.

162. Yao Y, Sheng Z, Yu Z. The relationship between abnormalities of cell-mediated immunity and gut origin endotoxemia in a rat model of thermal injury. Chung Hua Cheng Hsing Shao Shang Wai Ko Tsa Chih 1997; 13: 255–8.

163. Ozkan AN, Hoyt DB, Tompkins S, et al. Inununosuppressive effects of a trauma-induced suppressor active peptide. J Trauma 1988; 28: 589–92.

164. Ninnemann JL, Ozkan AN. Definition of a burn injury-induced immunosuppressive serum component. J Trauma 1985; 25: 113–17.

165. Dyess DL, Ferrara JJ, Lutennan A, Curteri PW. Subeschar tissue fluid: a source of cell-mediated immune suppression in victims of severe thermal injury. J Burn Care Rehabil 1991; 12(2): 101–5.

166. Bjomson AB, Somers SD, Knippenberg RW, Bjomson HS. Circulating factors contribute to elevation of intracellular cyclic-3′, 5′-adenosine monophosphate and depression of superoxide anion production in polymorphonuclear leukocytes following thermal injury. J Leukoc Biol 1992; 52: 407–14.

167. Bautista AP, Meszaros K, Bojta J, Spitzer JJ. Superoxide anion generation in the liver during the early stage of endotoxemia in rats. J Leukoc Biol 1990; 48: 123–8.

168. Ablin RJ, Holder IA. Immunologic sequelae of thermal injury: I. Frequency and relationship of epithelial antibodies to extent of burn. Immunol Immunopathol 1976; 5: 195–207.

169. Leguit P Jr, Feitkamp TEW, van Rossum AL, et al. Immunological studies in burn patients: HI. Autoimmune phenomena. Int Arch Allergy 1973; 45: 392–404.

170. Moran KT, Anholt GT, O'Reilly TJ, Thupari JN. Autoantibody formation in burn patients after inhibition of suppressor T cell activity with polymyxin B. J Burn Care Rehabil 1989; 10: 213–15.

171. Katz DR. Immunosuppression as a physiological homeostatic mechanism. Immunol Today 1984; 5(4): 96–7.

172. Polk HC Jr. The enhancement of host defenses against infection: search for the holy grail? Surgery 1986; 99: 1–6.

173. Munster AM. Control of infection following major burns: the immunological approach. In: Imbach P, ed. Immunotherapy with Intravenous Immunoglobulins. London: Academic Press, 1991.

174. Faist TE, Ninneman J, Green D, eds. Symposium: Immune Consequences of Trauma, Shock and Sepsis. Berlin: Springer Verlag, 1989.

175. Meakins JL. Surgeons, surgery, and immunomodulation. Arch Surg 1991; 126: 494–8.

176. Hansbrough JF, Zapata-Sirvent RL, Peterson VM. Immunomodulation following burn injury. Surg Clin N Am 1987; 67: 69–92.

177. Demling RH, LaLonde C. Early burn excision attenuates the postburn lung and systemic response to endotoxin. Surgery 1990; 108: 28–35.

178. Stratta RH, Warden GD, Ninneman JL, et al. Immunologic parameters in burned patients: effect of therapeutic interventions. J Trauma 1986; 26: 7–17.

179. Warden GD, Stratta RJ, Saffle JR, et al. Plasma exchange therapy in patients failing to resuscitate from burn shock. J Trauma 1983; 23: 945–51.

180. Benhaim P, Hunt TK. Natural resistance to infection: leukocyte functions. J Burn Care Rehabil 1992; 13: 287–92.

181. Alexander JW, Gottschlich MM. Nutritional immunomodulation in burn patients. Crit Care Med 1990; 18: S149–53.

182. Gerinenis AE, Achillcos OA, Stavropoulos-Giokas C, *et al*. The effect of very early enteral tube feeding on the humoral immunity of burned children. *Ann Medit Burns Club* 1992; 5: 69–72.

183. Herndon DN, Stein MD, Rutan TC, *et al*. Failure of TPN supplement to improve liver function immunity and mortality in thermally injured patients. *J Trauma* 1987; 27: 195–204.

184. Bone RC. A critical evaluation of new agents for the treatment of sepsis. *JAMA* 1991; 266: 1686–91.

185. Meek M, Munster AM, Winchurch RA. Dickerson C. The Baltimore Sepsis Scale: measurement of sepsis in burn patients using a new scoring system. *J Burn Care Rehabil* 1991; 12: 564–8.

186. Munster AM. Infections in burns. In: Morell A, Nydegger VE, eds. *Clinical Use of Intravenous Immunoglobulins*. London: Academic Press, 1986.

187. Frame JD, Everitt AS. Pilot study into the IgG, and IgG, subclass response to polyvalent pseudomonas vaccine in burned adults. *Burns* 1989; 15(3): 167–70.

188. Waymack JP, Jenkins ME, Alexander JW, *et al*. A prospective trial of prophylactic intravenous immune globulin for the prevention of infections in severely burned patients. *Burns* 1989; 5: 71–6.

189. Frame JD, Everitt AS, Gordon PWN, Hackett ME. IgG subclass response to gamma globulin administration in burned children. *Burns* 1990; 16: 437–40.

190. Burleson DG, Mason AD, McManus AT, Pruitt BA Jr. Lymphocyte phenotype and function changes in burn patients after intravenous IgG therapy. *Arch Surg* 1988; 123: 1379–82.

191. Munster AM, Moran KT, Thupari J, Allo M, Winchurch RA. Prophylactic intravenous immunoglobulin replacement in high-risk burn patients. *J Burn Care Rehabil* 1987; 8: 376–80.

192. Cross AS. Use of hyperimmune immunoglobulin. Presented at the Seminar on Advances in Prevention and Treatment of Endotoxemia and Sepsis, Philadelphia, 17–18 June 1993.

193. Dobke MK, Pearson G, Roberts C, *et al*. Effect of circulating fibronectin on stimulation of leukocyte oxygen consumption and serum opsonizing function in burned patients. *J Trauma* 1983; 23: 882–9.

194. Mansberger AR, Doran JE, Treat R, *et al*. The influence of fibronectin administration on the incidence of sepsis and septic mortality in severely injured patients. *Ann Surg* 1989; 210: 297–307.

195. Audibert FM, Lise LD. Adjuvants: current status, clinical perspectives and future prospects. *Immunol Today* 1993; 14: 281–4.

196. Hadden JW. Immunostimulants. *Immunol Today* 1993; 14: 275–80.

197. Hamilton G, *et al*. Thymopentin (TP5) in the treatment of the postburn and postoperative immunodeficiency syndrome. *Prog Clin Biol Res* 1989; 308: 995–9.

198. Waymack JP, Miskell P, Gonce SJ, Alexander JW. Effect of two new immunomodulators on normal and burn injury neutrophils and macrophages. *J Burn Care Rehab* 1987; 8: 9–14.

199. Visenti P. Extensive burn patients: immunological problems. *Ann Medit Burns Club* 1989; 2: 185.

200. Faist E, Ertel W, Salmen B, *et al*. The immune-enhancing effect of perioperative thymopentin administration in elderly patients undergoing major surgery. *Arch Surg* 1988; 123: 1449–53.

201. Donati L, Lazzarin A, Signorini M, *et al*. Preliminary clinical experiences with the use of immunomodulators in burns. *J Trauma* 1983; 23: 816–31.

202. Stinnett JD, Loose LD, Miskell P, *et al*. Synthetic immunomodulators for prevention of fatal infections in a burned guinea pig model. *Ann Surg* 1983; 198: 53–7.

203. Sartorelli KH, Silver GM, Gamelli RL. The effect of granulocyte colony-stimulating factor (G-CSF) upon burn-induced defective neutrophil chemotaxis. *J Trauma* 1991; 31: 523–30.

204. Mooney DP, Gamelli RL, O'Reilly M, *et al*. Recombinant human granulocyte colony-stimulating factor and pseudomonas burn wound sepsis. *Arch Surg* 1988; 123: 1353–7.

205. Rusche JR. Preclinical studies with anti-integrin monoclonal antibodies for treatment of septic shock. Presented at the Seminar on Advances in Prevention and Treatment of Endotoxemia and Sepsis, Philadelphia, 22–23 June 1992.

206. Kawano T, Ogushi F, Tanik, *et al*. Comparison of suppressive effects of a new antiinflammatory compound, FR 167653, on production of PGE2 and inflammatory cytokines, human monocytes, and alveolar macrophages in response to endotoxin. *J Leucocyte Biol* 1999; 65: 80–6.

207. Cetinkale O, Senel O, Bulan R. The effect of antioxidant therapy on cell-mediated immunity following burn injury in an animal model. *Burns* 1999; 25: 113–18.

208. Evans DA, Jacobs DO, Revhaug A, Wilmore DW. The effects of tumor necrosis factor and their selective inhibition by ibuprofen. *Ann Surg* 1989; 209: 312–20.

209. Demling RH, LaLonde C, Pequet Goad MD. Effect of ibuprofen on the pulmonary and systemic response to repeated doses of endotoxin. *Surgery* 1989; 105: 421–9.

210. Byme K, Carey D, Sielaff TD, *et al*. Ibuprofen prevents deterioration in static transpulmonary compliance and transalveolar protein flux in septic porcine acute lung injury. *J Trauma* 1991; 31: 155–66.

211. Fukushima R, Giamotti L, Alexander W, Pyles T. The degree of bacterial translocation is a determinant factor for mortality after burn injury and is improved by prostaglandin analogs. *Ann Surg* 1992, 216: 438–45.

212. Gadd MA, Hansbrough JF. Postburn suppression of murine lymphocyte and neutrophil functions is not reversed by prostaglandin blockade. *J Surg Res* 1990; 48: 84–90.

213. Waymack JP, Guzman RF, Mason AD Jr, Pruitt BA Jr. Effect of prostaglandin E in multiple experimental models. VII: Effect on resistance to sepsis. *Burns* 1990; 16: 9–12.

214. Bernard GR. Sepsis syndrome: current practice and new therapy. Presented at the Seminar on Advances in Prevention and Treatment of Endotoxemia and Sepsis, Philadelphia, 17–18 June 1993.

215. Gamelli R, He LK, Liu LH. Macrophage mediated suppression of granulocyte and macrophage growth after burn wound infection reversal by means of anti-PGE2. *J Burn Care Rehab* 2000; 21: 64–9.

216. Sheppard BC, Fraker DL, Norton JA. Prevention and treatment of endotoxin and sepsis lethality with recombinant human tumor necrosis factor. *Surgery* 1989; 106: 156–62.

217. Alexander HR, Langstein HN, Doherty GM, *et al*. Human recombinant tumor necrosis factor (hrTNF) protection against endotoxin-induced shock and lethality in the rat. *Surg Forum* 1990; 41: 103–5.

218. Fong Y, Tracey KJ, Moldawer LL, *et al*. Antibodies to cachectin/tumor necrosis factor reduce interleukin 1B and interleukin 6 appearance during lethal bacteremia. *J Exp Med* 1989; 170: 1627–33.

219. Doherty GM, Jensen JC, Alexander HA, *et al*. Pentoxifylline (FTX) suppression of tumor necrosis factor gene transcription. *Surgery* 1991; 110(2): 192–8.

220. Ertel W, Morrison MH, Ayala A, *et al*. Passive immunization against cachectin (TNF-α) prevents hemorrhage-induced suppression of Kupffer cell functions. *Surg Forum* 1990; 41: 91–30.

221. Ashkenazi A. Results with TNF receptor immunoadhesins for the treatment of sepsis. Presented at the Seminar on Advances in Prevention and Treatment of Endotoxemia and Sepsis, Philadelphia, 22–23 June 1992.

222. Mohler DS, Torrance RV, Widmer MB. Therapeutic potential of soluble cytokine receptors in septic shock. Presented at the seminar on Advances in Prevention and Treatment of Endotoxemia and Sepsis, Philadelphia, 22–23 June 1992.

223. Bodmer M. Pre-clinical evaluation of CDP571, a humanized antiTNFα antibody. Presented at the Seminar on Advances in Prevention and Treatment of Endotoxemia and Sepsis, Philadelphia, 22–23 June 1992.

224. Opal SM. Experience with interleukin-1 receptor antagonist in the treatment of sepsis. Presented at the Seminar on Advances in Prevention and Treatment of Endotoxemia and Sepsis, Philadelphia, 17–18 June 1993.

225. Pribble J. Interleukin-1 receptor antagonist for the treatment of sepsis syndrome. Presented at the Seminar on Advances in Prevention and Treatment of Endotoxemia and Sepsis, Philadelphia, 22–23 June 1992.

226. Silver GM, Gamelli RL, O'Reilly M, Herbert JC. The effect of interleukin 1 on survival in a murine model of burn wound sepsis. *Arch Surg* 1990; 125: 922–5.

227. Polk HC Jr, Cheadle WG, Livingston DH, *et al*. A randomized prospective clinical trial to determine the efficacy of interferon-gamma in severely injured patients. *Am J Surg* 1992; 163: 191–6.

228. Redmond HP, Chavin KD, Bromberg JS, Daly JM. Inhibition of macrophage-activating cytokines is beneficial in the acute septic response. *Ann Surg* 1991; 214: 502–9.

229. Lee JD, Swisher SG, Minehart EH, *et al*. Interleukin-4: a potent inhibitor of IL-6, TNF-α, IFN-γ, and IL-1β production. *Surg Forum* 1990; 41: 441–4.

230. Yim JH, Tewari A, Pearce MK, *et al*. Monoclonal antibody against murine interleukin-6 prevents lethal effects of *Escherichia coli* sepsis and tumor necrosis factor challenge in mice, *Surg Forum* 1990; 41: 114–17.

231. Barton BE. The anti-inflammatory effect of interleukin 6. Presented at the Seminar on Advances in Prevention and Treatment of Endotoxemia and Sepsis, Philadelphia, 17–18 June 1993.

232. Etemadi A, Tempel GE, Farah BA, *et al*. Beneficial effects of a leukotriene antagonist on endotoxin-induced acute hemodynamic alterations. *Circ Shock* 1987; 22(1): 55–63.

233. Teodorczyk-Injeyan JA, Sparkes BG, Mills GB, *et al*. Impaired expression of interleukin 2 receptor (IL-2R) in the immunosuppressed burned patient: reversal by exogenous IL2. *J Trauma* 1987; 27: 180–6.

234. Howard M, Muchameul T, Andrade S, Menon S. Interleukin 10 protects mice from lethal endotoxemia. *J Exp Med* 1993; 177: 1205–8.

235. Laffon M, Pittet JF, Modelska K, Matthay MA Young DM. Interleukin 8 mediates injury from smoke inhalation to both the lung endothelial and the alveolar epithelial barrier in rabbits. *Am J Respir Crit Care Med* 1999; 160: 1441–2.

236. O'Suilleabhain C, O'Sullivan ST, Kelly JL, Lederer J, Mannick JA, Riodrick ML.

Interleukin-12 treatment restores normal resistance to bacterial challenge after burn injury. *Surgery* 1996; **120**: 290–6.

237. Piccolo MT, Wang Y, Sannomiya P, *et al.* Chemotactic mediator requirements in lung injury following skin burns in rats. *Exp Mol Pathol* 1999; **66**: 220–6.

238. Miller AS, Meredith JW, Meredith JH, *et al.* Immuno-enhancement in the thermally injured guinea pig. *J Burn Care Rehabil* 1985; **6**: 358–62.

239. Munster AM, Leary AG. Treatment of pseudomonas sepsis in the rat with lymphocyte culture products. *Surg Forum* 1974; **25**: 33–4.

240. Fletcher JR, DiSimone AG, Earnest MA. Platelet activating factor receptor antagonist improves survival and attenuates eicosanoid release in severe endotoxemia. *Ann Surg* 1990; **211**: 312–16.

241. Hinshaw LB, Archer LT, Beller BK, *et al.* Evaluation of naloxone therapy for *E. coli* sepsis in the baboon. *Arch Surg* 1988; **123**: 700–4.

242. Hendrickson M, Shelby J, Sullivan JJ, Saffle JR. Naloxone inhibits the in vivo immunosuppressive effects of morphine and thermal injury in mice. *J Burn Care Rehabil* 1989; **10**: 494–8.

243. Lynn WA, Golenbock DT. Lipopolysaccharide antagonists. *Immunol Today* 1992; **13**: 271–6.

244. Magee GD, Hoper M, Halliday MI, *et al.* An in vitro study of the effect of centoxin on the production of tumor necrosis factor and interleukin-6 by normal human mononuclear cells. Presented at the meeting of the Surgical Infection Society, 1992.

245. Wedel NI. Update on the use of E5, an anti-endotoxin monoclonal antibody, in the treatment of gram-negative sepsis. Presented at the Seminar on Advances in Prevention and Treatment of Endotoxemia and Sepsis, Philadelphia, 22–23 June 1992.

246. Quezado ZMN, Natanson C, Ailing DW, *et al.* A controlled trial of HA-1A in a canine model of gram-negative septic shock. *JAMA* 1993; **269**: 2221–7.

247. Ziegler EF, Fisher CJ Jr, Sprung CL, *et al.* Treatment of gram-negative bacteremia and septic shock with HA-IA human monoclonal antibody against endotoxin. *N Engl J Med* 1991; **324**: 429–36.

248. Warren HS, Danner RL, Munford RS. Sounding board: anti-endotoxin monoclonal antibodies. *N Engl J Med* 1992; **326**: 1153–8.

249. Battafarano RJ, Burd RS, Cody CS, Kellogg TA. Anti-lipopolysaccaharide monoclonal antibodies inhibit macrophage TNF messenger RNA synthesis *in vitro. J Surg Res* 1993; **54(4)**: 342–8.

250. Burd RS, Cody CS, Raymond CS, Dunn DL. Anti-endotoxin monoclonal antibodies protect by enhancing bacterial and endotoxin clearance. *Arch Surg* 1993; **128**: 145–51.

251. Cody CS, Burd RS, Mayoral JL, Dunn DL. Protective antilipopolysaccharide monoclonal antibodies inhibit tumor necrosis factor production. *J Surg Res* 1992; **52(4)**: 314–19.

252. Rubin RM, Noland J, Rosenbaum JT. Monoclonal antibodies directed against endotoxin reduce endotoxin-induced vascular permeability. *Clin Res* 1989; **36**: 147A.

253. Baumgartner JD, Glauser MP, McCutchan JA, *et al.* Prevention of gram negative shock and death in surgical patients by antibody to endotoxin core glycolipid. *Lancet* 1985; **2**: 59–63.

254. Cometta A, Baumgartner J-D, Lee ML, *et al.* Prophylactic intravenous administration of standard immune globulin as compared with core-lipopolysaccharide immune globulin in patients at high risk of postsurgical infection. *N Engl J Med* 1992; **327**: 234–40.

255. Nys M, Damas P, Joassin L, Lamy M. Sequential anti-core glycolipid immunoglobulin antibody activities in patients with and without septic shock and their relation to outcome. *Ann Surg* 1993; **217**: 300–6.

256. Staubach KH, Kooistra A, Kujath P, *et al.* Extracorporeal absorption of endotoxin by a new polymyxin B detoxification column in pigs with endotoxin shock. Presented at the meeting of the Surgical Infection Society, 1992.

257. Hanasawa K, Tani T, Kodama M. New approach to endotoxic and septic shock by means of polymyxin B immobilized fiber. *Surg Gynecol Obstet* 1989; **168**: 323–31.

258. Crowley BM, O'Riodain G, Ellwanger K, Collins KH. Antiendotoxin therapy improves survival in a model of thermal injury and sepsis. *Surg Forum* 1990; **41**: 72–4.

259. Cheadle WG, Hanasawa K, Gaflinaro RN, *et al.* Endotoxin filtration and immune stimulation improve survival from Gram-negative sepsis. *Surgery* 1991; **110**: 785–92.

260. Munster AM, Winchurch RA, Thupari JN, Ernst CB. Reversal of postburn immunosuppression with low-dose polymyxin B. *J Trauma* 1986; **26**: 995–8.

261. Munster AM, Meek M, Dickerson C, Winchurch RA. Translocation: true pathology of phenomenology. *Ann Surg* 1993; **218**: 321–7.

262. Nedeliaeva AV, Levin GY The influence of enterosorption on endotoxemia in burn illness. *Ann Medit Burns Club* 1992; **5**: 236–9.

263. Coffadin SB, Mauel J, Gallay P, *et al.* Enhancement of murine macrophage binding of and response to bacterial lipopolysaccharide (LPS) by LPS-binding protein. *J Leukoc Biol* 1992; **52**: 363–8.

264. Gottardis M, Benzer A, Koller W, Luger TJ. Improvement of septic syndrome after administration of recombinant human growth hormone (rhGH). *J Trauma* 1991; **31**: 81–6.

265. Noronha-Blob L. Leumedins and bradykinin receptor antagonists. Presented at the Seminar on Advances in Prevention and Treatment of Endotoxemia and Sepsis, Philadelphia, 17–18 June 1993.

266. Pogrebniak HW, Merino MJ, Hahn SM, *et al.* Spin trap salvage from endotoxemia: the role of cytokine down-regulation. *Surgery* 1992; **112**: 130–9.

267. Kelly JL, O'Sullivan C, O'Riordain D, *et al.* Is circulating endotoxin the trigger for the systemic inflammatory response syndrome seen after injury? *Ann Surg* 1997; **225(5)**: 530–41.

268. Smith-Meek MA, Munster AM, Dickerson C, Winchurh RA. Ibuprofen increases endotoxemia but downregulates the cytokine cascade in burn patients. Presented at the American Burn Association, Orlando, Florida, March 1999.

269. Reilly PM, Schiller HJ, Bulkley GB. Pharmacologic approach to tissue injury mediated by free radicals and other reactive oxygen metabolites. *Am J Surg* 1991; **161**: 488–503.

270. Aida Y, Pabst MJ, Rademacher JM, *et al.* Effects of polymyxin B on superoxide anion release and priming in human polymorphonuclear leukocytes. *J Leukoc Biol* 1990; **47**: 283.

271. Lefer AM. Endothelial preserving agents in endotoxin shock. Presented at the Seminar on Advances in Prevention and Treatment of Endotoxemia and Sepsis, Philadelphia, 17–18 June 1993.

272. Ertel W, Meldrum DR, Morrison MH, Ayala A. Immonoprotective effect of a calcium channel blocker on macrophage antigen presentation function, major histocompatibility class 11 antigen expression, and interleukin-1β synthesis after hemorrhage. *Surgery* 1990; **108**: 154–60.

273. Ertel W, Meldrum DR, Morrison MH, Ayala A. Immonoprotective effect of a calcium channel blocker on macrophage antigen presentation function, major histocompatibility class 11 antigen expression, and interleukin-1β synthesis after hemorrhage. *Surgery* 1990; **108**: 154–60.

274. Demling RH, Lalonde C. Identification and modifications of the pulmonary and biochemical changes caused by a skin burn. *J Trauma* 1990; **30**: S57–S62.

275. Demling RH, Lalonde C, Knox J, *et al.* Fluid resuscitation with deferoxamine prevents systemic burn-induced oxidant injury. *J Trauma* 1990; **30**: 918.

276. Thomson PD, Till GO, Prasad JK, Smith DJ Jr. Enhancement of humoral immunity by heterologous lipid peroxidation products resulting from burn injury. *J Burn Care Rehabil* 1991; **12**: 38–40.

277. Mackensen A, Galanos C, Andreesen R, Engelhardt R. Cytokines in cancer patients treated with endotoxin in combination with ibuprofen. *J Leukoc Biol* 1989; **46**: 326.

278. Faist E, Markewitz A, Fuchs D, *et al.* Immunomodulatory therapy with thymopentin and indomethacin: successful restoration of interleukin-2 synthesis in patients undergoing major surgery. *Ann Surg* 1991; **214**: 264–75.

279. Malangani MA, Lingston DR, Sonnenfeld G, Polk HC. Interferon gamma and tumor necrosis factor alpha. *Arch Surg* 1990; **125**: 444–6.

280. O'Riordain MG, Collins KH, Pitlz M, *et al.* Modulation of macrophage hyperactivity improves survival in a burn-sepsis model. *Arch Surg* 1992; **127**: 152–8.

281. Mendez MV, Molloy RG, O'Riordain DS, *et al.* Lymphokine activated killer cells enhance IL-2 prevention of sepsis-related death in a murine model of thermal injury. *J Surg Res* 1993; **54(6)**: 565–70.

282. Silver GM, *et al.* The beneficial effect of granulocyte colony stimulating factor (G-CSF) in combination with gentamicin on survival after *Pseudomonas* infection. *Surgery* 1989; **106**: 452–6.

283. Oliva RG, Sica I. Intravenous immunoglobulin in severely burned patients: five years of successful experience. *Ann Medit Burns Club* 1993; **6**: 20–4.

284. Missavage AE, Vaughan GM, McManus AT, *et al.* Alteration of host resistance in burned soldiers: therapy with IgG and T4 in burn patients. *Annual Research Progress Report for Fiscal Year 1987*, US Army Institute of Surgical Research, pp 188–99.

285. Munster AM, Winchurch RA. Unpublished data, 1987.

286. Ayala A, Lehmans DL, Herdar CD, Chaudry IH. Mechanism of enhanced susceptibility to sepsis following hemorrhage: interleukin 10 suppression of T-cell responses is mediated by eicosanoid-induced IL4 release. Presented to the 14th Annual Meeting of the Surgical Infection Society, Toronto, 28–30 April 1994.

287. Polo M, Ko F, Busillo F, Cruse W, Krizek TJ, Robson MC. Cytokine production in patients with hypertrophic burn scars. *J Burn Care Rehabil* 1997; **18**: 477–82.

288. Smith CJ, Payne VM, Scott SM, Luterman A. Immunoglobulin E levels and anticollagen antibodies in patients with postburn hypertrophic scars. *J Burn Care Rehab* 1997; **18**: 411–16.

289. Pajulo OT, Pulkki KJ, Alanen MS, *et al.* Correlation between interleukin-6 and matrix metalloproteinase-9 in early wound healing in children. *Wound Repair Regen* 1999; **7**: 453–7.

Chapter 26a

Hematologic, hematopoietic, and acute phase response

Ravi Shankar, Craig S Amin

Richard L Gamelli

Introduction

Although our ability to care for major burns has improved over the last two decades, mortality due to septic complications still remains a major threat to the survival of severely injured patients. General physiological and cellular changes that occur immediately following burn injury are not only important for the initial survival of the injured patients but act as triggers for initiating the inflammatory response. Much of our recently acquired understanding of the pathophysiology of burn injury has come from advances in the molecular and cellular biology of inflammation. Well-regulated inflammation to any given insult including burn trauma is an essential part of the healing process. The inflammatory reaction allows the recruitment of leukocytes, antibodies, and other serum proteins to the site of injury with the direct result of initiating the wound healing process.[1,2] Furthermore, these events serve to localize and eradicate microbial infection.[3] While controlled inflammation is an essential part of the 'healing process', uncontrolled 'whole body inflammation', often seen during prolonged hospitalization of severely injured burn patients, represents a generalized systemic response to trauma.[4,5]

One of the major components of the burn trauma-induced negative immune environment is the loss of balance in both leukocyte and erythrocyte production and functions. How severe thermal injury precipitates these hematologic and hematopoietic changes and the implications these changes have for understanding the underlying biology and the treatment of burn patients is the primary focus of this chapter. Within this framework, we discuss recent advances in the cellular and molecular biology that have helped shed new insights into burn biology. In particular, we outline the cellular and molecular mechanisms that are responsible for the dysregulated hematopoiesis and hematologic changes that occur following severe burn injury. Lastly, we will describe how hematopoietic transcription factors can potentially play a role in the hematopoietic changes observed following severe thermal injury.

Red blood cells and erythropoiesis

Almost all hematologic parameters are significantly affected by severe burns with a characteristic biphasic response. Following burns that are greater than 10% total body surface area (TBSA), anemia is frequently present.[6,7] The extent of anemia due to erythrocyte loss is directly proportional to the extent of the initial injury. It is estimated that patients with 15–40% full-thickness burn lose approximately 12% of their red cells within 6 hours of the injury, and as much as 18% in 24 hours.[7] Patients with severe burns continue to loose red blood cells at the rate of 1–2% per day until the burn wound is healed, primarily as a result of blood loss through multiple surgical procedures and repeated blood draws for various hematologic and biochemical tests.[6,8–10]

Several factors could explain the onset of anemia in burn patients. First, acute red blood cell destruction occurs as a direct result of thermal injury. Secondly, extensive burns induce the formation of thrombi within the capillaries, arterioles, and venules due to the activation of complement and coagulation cascades.[11] In general, for burn wounds with similar depth, large burns elicit greater prothrombogenic effect than smaller burns. Additionally, the loss of red blood cell mass can arise from burn-induced intrinsic and extrinsic alterations to the erythrocytes. Previous studies have shown that thermal energy damages the normal morphology of red blood cells not only at the site of burn wound but within the peripheral circulation.[12,13] In addition, systemically released oxygen free radicals and proteases from the inflammatory cells can also damage the integrity of red blood cell membrane.[13] It is hypothesized that the burn wound triggers the release of these biological mediators that compromise the integrity of red blood cell membranes to induce osmotic fragility and loss of membrane deformability. These changes in red blood cell membrane property manifest themselves as increased spherocytosis, membrane disruption, and vesiculation of erythrocytes and are apparent within a short time following severe thermal injury.[14,15] If these cell membrane defects continue it may lead to red cell lysis and an increase in acute hemoglobinuria.[14,16]

Paradoxically, despite the initial and continued loss of red blood cells following burns, erythrocytosis and an increase in hematocrit are often observed in the acute phase of burn injury.[16,17] The primary reason for this observed effect is loss of plasma volume into extracellular space following thermal injury.[18,19] Nevertheless, the long-term postburn period is characterized by diminished red cell production. Under normal conditions, the loss of blood would stimulate the bone marrow to produce more erythrocytes. A major factor in the induction of bone marrow erythropoiesis or red blood cell production is the availability of the growth factor erythropoietin. Interestingly, despite the high circulating levels of erythropoietin, burn patients remain anemic. The inherent defect appears to be the inability of erythroid progenitor cells in the bone marrow to respond adequately to erythropoietin.[10,20–22] A possible explanation for this hyporesponsiveness is the high circulating levels of cytokines such as tumor necrosis factor-α (TNFα) and interleukin-1 (IL-1), which are often seen in severe burns. These cytokines can retard erythropoiesis by disrupting the physiologic regulation between erythropoietin and hemoglobin levels in erythroid progenitor cells.[23]

In addition, burn patients may have reduced serum iron levels due to substantial loss of blood and repeated surgical procedures for purposes of skin grafting and debridement of the burn wound.[8,10,20] This apparent reduction in serum iron levels may act as an impediment to hemoglobin synthesis and hence erythropoiesis. However, serum iron levels are unlikely to be the sole cause of burn-induced anemia, particularly among patients receiving blood transfusions during their course of burn care. Other potential explanations exist for burn-induced anemia. For example, bone marrow's unresponsiveness to erythropoietin can stem from a yet unidentified serum factor termed erythropoietin inhibitory factor that inhibits erythropoietin's action on erythroid progenitor cells.[10,20,22,24] Recently, glucocorticoids have been shown to play an important role in stress-induced erythropoiesis.[25] In burn patients and in animal models of thermal injury, high circulating levels of glucocorticoids occur with simultaneous anemia, which suggests the potential for signaling defects in erythroid differentiation in severe thermal injury. Hence, the anemia that is observed following burns results from several factors that cause increased red blood cell destruction and decreased production of mature red blood cells within the bone marrow.

Platelets and coagulation cascade in burns

Thermal injury causes marked reduction in circulating platelet levels during the acute phase of resuscitation of burn patients, primarily due to the consumption of platelets during the formation of systemic microthrombi.[26–28] Although microthrombi formation within the immediate vicinity of burn injury is essential for maintaining the integrity of the microvasculature surrounding the burn wound, generalized systemic microthrombi formation leads to reduced organ perfusion and failure. In addition, dilutional effects of extensive fluid resuscitation may also contribute to an apparent reduction in platelet counts.[26] Thrombocytopenia that is observed in burn patients during the first week following the injury is believed to be due to the diminished half-lives of platelets in cir-

culation.[27] The thrombocytopenic phase is subsequently followed by a period of increased platelet production or bone marrow megakaryocytopoiesis during the 2–3 weeks following the initial injury that results in either a return to normal levels or to overt thrombocytosis.[29] However, in some burn patients, thrombocytopenia persists and is often considered a poor prognostic indicator.[30] In addition, an apparent thrombocytosis may be observed among patients with critical burn injuries who develop intravascular hemolysis.[29] Thrombocytosis in these instances are due to inadvertent counting of fragmented red cells and red cell microvesicles as platelets in an automated counter. Therefore, in severe burns, the clinician should be aware of the possibility of spurious platelet counts in the presence of intravascular hemolysis.

In addition to the observed changes in the platelet numbers, there are significant differences in concentrations of coagulation proteins following thermal injury. The interplay amongst antithrombotic, prothrombotic cellular interactions, and fibrinolytic processes within the vasculature intricately control the homeostatic regulation of coagulation. In physiology, fluidity of blood is maintained by morphological integrity of the endothelium lining the blood vessels and normal levels of prothrombotic and antithrombotic factors that are well regulated and remain for the most part in their quiescent state. In burn patients, however, both the thrombotic and fibrinolytic pathways are triggered directly in proportion to the extent of the injury.[31–33] During the shock phase of the burns there is a general reduction in the levels of coagulation proteins.[31] Dilutional effects due to fluid resuscitation during this period and the loss of plasma proteins to the interstitium could partially explain the decrease in plasma concentrations of many coagulation proteins. This phase, however, appears to be transient in most patients as clotting factors return to normal levels a week after the postburn shock.[26] Many patients suffering from major burn injuries present with a hypercoagulable state later in the postburn course.[31] Prior clinical studies indicate that the antithrombotic factors such as antithrombin III, protein S, and protein C levels are decreased in burn patients.[26,31] Administration of antithrombin III to burn patients has been shown to be beneficial in both reversing the thrombogenicity and overall patient recovery.[32,33]

Additionally, fibrinolytic pathways are activated due to the increased levels of tissue plasminogen activator protein.[31] The combination of diminished levels of antithrombotic proteins and activation of fibrinolytic activities predisposes burn patients to thrombosis. Several additional factors could also contribute to the thrombotic state in severely injured burn patients. Among these are the releases of tissue phospholipids and tissue factor, activation of complement cascade, tissue ischemia, and the presence of sepsis.[26,30,31,34] As a result, patients are at increased risk for developing disseminated intravascular coagulation (DIC) in all major organ systems, and DIC may play a role in the development of multiorgan dysfunction and/or failure. It has been reported from postmortem studies that 30% of severely burned patients exhibit pathological findings of DIC with extensive microthrombi accumulation in all major organ systems.[35] Clinical scenarios in which DIC is a component of the acute burn phase typically occur in patients with massive burns, delayed presentation, hypotension, acidosis, and/or hypothermia. When evidence for DIC is observed later in the burn course of a patient, it is usually a manifestation of a septic process. In DIC, fragmented red cells with the morphological changes tend to increase the viscosity of blood, further compromising organ perfusion and organ failure beyond that of their post-injury response.[31] Hence, clinical signs for DIC should be closely monitored in burn patients as possible sequelae in order to prevent multiorgan failure. If thermally injured patients manifest severe shock disproportionate to the apparent loss of blood, DIC is the most likely cause and should be suspected. Other clues of DIC include bleeding around venipuncture sites and around intravascular cannula. Furthermore, patients should frequently also be monitored for coagulation parameters. Standard laboratory values in patients with suspected DIC include prolonged prothrombin time (PT) and activated partial thromboplastin time (APTT), increased levels of fibrinogen degradation products, and decreased platelet counts and fibrinogen levels. Therefore, the treatment modalities for DIC are geared toward maintaining hemostatic parameters with replacement therapy.

Acute phase proteins

The body's normal reaction towards any injury including burns is to initiate natural defense mechanisms that are activated as a part of antimicrobial host defense and includes synthesis and release of the acute phase protein.[36] Acute phase response manifests itself through leukocytosis, fever, increased vascular permeability, increases in metabolic responses and stimulation of nonspecific host defense.[37,38] The acute phase proteins are a set of proteins that mediate these effects and therefore play a role in protecting cells and tissues from further cellular injury and restoring homeostasis[38] (Table 26.1). Acute phase proteins serve as mediators of the inflammatory process, function as transport proteins, and participate in burn wound healing.[39,40] In response to burn injury, an acute phase response is initiated which results in the activation of coagulation and complement cascades, activation of granulocytes and monocyte/macrophages as well as platelets.[26–28,41,42] Simultaneously, endothelial cells and fibroblasts are also activated.[43] The net result of this orchestrated activation is the production of proinflammatory cytokines such as IL-6, IL-1, and TNFα that precipitates the acute phase response.[36,44,45] The acute phase response stimulates the hypothalamus, which leads to pyrexia.[46] It also activates the pituitary–adrenal axis to release steroid hormones. More importantly, it induces the liver to synthesize and release acute phase proteins

capable of exerting pleiotropic effects on many tissues.[38] During an acute illness or a significant injury such as a burn injury, enhanced production of acute phase proteins serves to stimulate the healing process and is sustained by the proinflammatory cytokines.[40] However, prolongation of the acute phase response and the unabated production of acute phase proteins are potentially detrimental to patients and can lead to hypermetabolism, multiple organ failure, and death.[45,47–49] Furthermore, the scenario is complicated by the fact that the increase in acute phase proteins is sustained at the expense of constitutive hepatic proteins, thus fueling the detrimental effects.[49–51]

In burn patients and in animal models of thermal injury, increases in several acute phase proteins have been demonstrated.[40,52–57] In particular, increases in C-reactive protein, serum amyloid A, α_1-acid glycoprotein, α_1-antitrypsin, fibrinogen, haptoglogulin, ceruloplasmin, and α_1-chymotrypsin have been reported following burns, while levels of albumin, transferrin, and α_1-lipoprotein decrease.[38,58–60] Generally, the greater the size of the burn, the greater is the change in acute phase proteins. It has been shown that even minor thermal burns can lead to alterations in acute phase protein.[42,61,62] The kinetics of induction of acute phase proteins closely parallels the burn shock for the first 24–48 hours and is driven by IL-1, IL-6, and TNFα levels, with IL-6 having the most direct effect on the stimulation of acute phase proteins. Moreover, IL-6 may be considered an amplification system for the production of acute phase proteins.[59] IL-6 directly stimulates the production of C-reactive proteins, ceruloplasmin, haptoglobins, fibrinogen α_1-antitrypsin, and α_1-acid glycoprotein on the one hand and depresses the synthesis of hepatic constitutive proteins such as albumin, fibronectin, and transferrin on the other.[38,60] While IL-6 is the prime mediator of acute phase response, TNFα and IL-1 play a subsidiary role through their ability to stimulate IL-6 production.[58,60] Thus when in balance, the concerted actions of the cytokines help to heal the burn wound and maintain homeostasis; however, if this balance is tilted the very same paradigm can become the driving force of dyshomeostasis with deleterious consequences.

Aside from its role as a regulator of acute phase protein production, IL-6 is also considered an indicator of the survival outcome in burn patients.[61,63] Clinical data indicate that survivors of extensive burns have high levels of IL-6 and acute phase proteins that may be

Table 26.1 Status of acute phase protein response following thermal injury

Acute phase protein	Levels	Functions
C-reactive protein	Increased	Opsonin, complement activation, and immune modulation
Serum amyloid A	Increased	Leukocyte chemotaxis and phagocytosis
α_1-antitrypsin	Increased	Protease inhibitor of elastase and trypsin
α_1-antichymotrypsin	Increased	Inhibits chymotrypsin
α_1-acid glycoprotein	Increased	Immunomodulator, potential wound healing properties, decreases albumin clearance from circulation, transport protein, steroid binding
α_1-antiplasmin	Increased	Protease inhibitor of fibrinolysis
Ceruloplasmin	Increased	Copper transport protein, potential antioxidant properties
Haptoglobin	Increased	Hemoglobin scavenger
Fibrinogen	Increased	Mediate coagulation
C_1 inhibitor	Increased	Complement inactivation opsonization
Complement-C_3	Increased	Complement activation
α_2-macroglobulin	Decreased	Transports zinc, panproteinase inhibitor, binds growth factors and cytokines and targets them toward particular cells
α_1-lipoprotein	Decreased	Transport protein
Transferrin	Decreased	Iron transport

important for patient survival and represent a potential target for treatment efficacy and better patient outcome. Nonsurvivors have been shown to have an even more marked increase in IL-6 levels.[64,65] The difference between the survivors and nonsurvivors appears to be the ability to respond to IL-6 levels by adequate production of acute phase proteins.[63] Typically, nonsurviving burn patients fail to produce sufficient acute phase proteins despite high levels of IL-6.[64,65] Hence, it is thought that relative levels of IL-6 may serve as a prognostic marker for survival in burn patients. Additionally, prostaglandins, activated complement factors, cortisol, neuroendocrine, and other hormones have been implicated in the activation of acute phase proteins.[66] Future studies on the role of cytokines in the regulation and functions of acute phase proteins will add insights into their role as protective physiological mediators.

Since the proinflammatory cytokines may lead to the overproduction of acute phase proteins, several clinical trials have been undertaken to attenuate the rise in proinflammatory cytokines and acute phase proteins but with little success.[43,47,67,68] Failures of these trials clearly indicate that such anti-cytokine monotherapies are not useful in controlling the prolonged acute phase response. However, other therapeutic modalities aimed at simultaneously enhancing the constitutive production of hepatic proteins (e.g. albumin, fibronectin) while inhibiting acute phase protein expression have been shown to be beneficial both in animal models of thermal injury and in burn patients.[40,51–53,56,69,70] Administration of growth hormone to thermally injured rats with 40% TBSA burns have been shown to decrease α_1 acid glycoprotein mRNA expression and protein levels while reversing the decline in albumin production.[53] In severely burned pediatric patients, administration of recombinant human growth hormone (GH) was able to decrease the production of acute phase protein and serum TNFα and IL-1β levels without any effect on IL-6.[69] Such a treatment protocol, however, did not influence the rate of mortality in these studies. Since recombinant GH exerts some of its effects through its ability to stimulate insulin-like growth factor 1 (IGF-1), administration of a combination of IGF-1 and IGF binding protein 3 was attempted as a therapeutic modality to control acute phase response in severely burned children.[52] Similar to rGH administration, infusion of IGF-1/IGFBP3 decreased IL-1β and TNFα levels as well as type I acute phase protein production in burn patients, while increasing constitutive hepatic protein production. Interestingly, administration of cholesterol containing cationic liposomes used in gene delivery systems have been shown to attenuate the acute phase response in thermally injured rats.[71] These results highlight that this delivery system may has some additional beneficial effect if chosen as a delivery system in gene therapy experiments against thermal injury and severe trauma. Given the deleterious effect of unabated and prolonged acute phase response following severe burns, continued improvements in therapeutic modalities aimed at regulating this response may prove yet another tool in the care of burn patients.

Leukocytes and burn injury

Leukocytes function primarily as sentinels of our host defense. Their purpose in health as well as following burn injury is to search and destroy potentially harmful invasions of microbes. The umbrella term 'leukocytes' includes T- and B-lymphocytes, NK-cells, polymorphonuclear neutrophilic granulocytes (PMN), and monocyte/macrophages. A balanced activation of these cells is important for robust host-defense. Inappropriate activation of these leukocytes, especially the PMN and macrophages, can lead to tissue destruction and systemic inflammation with dire consequences to the burn patient. Over-activation of PMN and macrophages has been implicated in the development of adult respiratory distress syndrome (ARDS) and multiorgan failure.[43,72–76,77]

Similar to the red blood cell response, leukocyte response to major burn injury is bimodal and temporally linked. In the first 24–48 hours following burns, both leukocytosis and granulocytosis are observed that are dependent on the size of the burn wound, the larger burns giving rise to a greater degree of leukocytosis.[78] The initial leukocytosis is attributable to two major factors. The acute plasma volume loss due to thermal burns and demargination of mature neutrophils from peripheral blood vessels and the rapid release of bone marrow reserves accounts for the observed early leukocytosis. Following this initial period of leukocytosis, burn patients are either in a state of leukopenia or leukocytosis. The postburn period that includes fluid resuscitation and microvascular leakage accounts for loss of peripheral leukocytes and their accumulation at the burn wound and distal sites. Leukopenia is also frequently seen in burn patients whose burn wounds are treated with silver sulfadiazine topical application.[79] The extent of leukopenia is directly proportional to the extent of application, and hence on the extent of burn injury. The mechanism underlying this drug-induced leukopenia is yet to be elucidated although direct bone marrow and cellular toxicity may play a role.[79] In general, leukopenia is self-limiting and does not require discontinuation of silver sulfadiazine treatment.

Leukopenia and granulocytopenia are often seen in burn patients with severe superimposed sepsis, especially those with Gram-negative bacterial sepsis.[41,80,81] In the early 1970s, Newsome and Eurenius demonstrated that the initial granulocytosis was due to demargination of PMN from the blood vessels and through accelerated release of bone marrow stores in their rat model of thermal injury.[82] This granulocytosis, however, was transient and was followed by robust bone marrow response in an attempt to replenish granulocyte stores.[83–85] If the burn injury is complicated by sepsis, granulocytopenia is not an infrequent finding.[86,87] Granulocytopenia under these conditions appears to be due to bone marrow failure.[83,86–88] McEuen demonstrated a significant inhibition of granulocyte colony forming units in the bone marrow of burn septic rats.[86] In addition, serum from burn septic animals retarded the granulocyte colony-formation when added to bone marrow cells from normal nonseptic animals.[84] In septic animals and in burn patients with sepsis, the observed granulocytopenia is unlikely to be due to lack of available colony-stimulating factor. Granulocyte colony-stimulating factor (G-CSF) is the mandatory growth factor responsible for the proliferation and differentiation of bone marrow granulocyte progenitors into mature granulocytes.[89,90] In thermal injury and sepsis, the activation of macrophages, endothelial cells, and fibroblast by bacterial products and cytokines such as TNFα and IL-1 lead to increased production of G-CSF. This scenario is very similar to that seen with erythropoietin levels following thermal injury. Administration of recombinant G-CSF to burn septic animals prior to the initiation of septic insult has been shown to improve the survival rate of the burn septic mice.[91–93] However, administration of G-CSF 24 hours after the onset of septic insult had little effect on their survival.[94,95] The use of G-CSF in burn patients has typically been seen in severely burned patients with refractive neutropenia, in particular with active HIV disease.

In addition to changes in the kinetics of the production, the PMN exhibit qualitative functional changes in both burn patients and in animal models of burn injury.[96–99] In major burns, PMN exhibit depressed chemotaxis and phagocytosis.[100–102] Quantitative chemotaxis studies across a region of burn wound demonstrated a reduction in chemotactic potential in burned animals compared to the uninjured animals.[103] Their ability to produce superoxide in response to stimuli such as FMLP and TNFα are also compromised.[104,105] Furthermore, burn superimposed with bacterial infection led to substantial loss of ability for phagocytosis.[106–108] For example, isolated neutrophils of burn patients were shown to be defective in intracellular killing of *Pseudomonas aeruginosa* and the impairment in phagocytosis and intracellular killing are further exacerbated in burn patients with sepsis.[109,110] These alterations in the production and function of PMN provide additional evidence for the depressed immune status in severely burned patients.

While neutropenia may be common in severe burns and septic complications, monocytosis has been reported both in animal models of thermal injury and in burn patients.[81,111,112] Results of patient studies involving thermal injury and sepsis demonstrated marked monocytosis with a dramatic increase (3–5-fold) associated with sepsis.[111,113] The relevance of the burn-induced monocytosis is borne by the observation that attenuation of monocytosis as well as blunted macrophage activation results in improved survival following thermal injury and sepsis.[114] Similar to PMN, monocyte/macrophages functions are influenced considerably by thermal injury. While monocyte/macrophages are activated in severe thermal injury and sepsis and are considered central to the pathophysiology of SIRS response, the monocyte/macrophage overactivation is not a uniform phenomenon. The elegant work of Miller-Grazziano and Faist clearly demonstrated that subsets of monocyte/macrophages were present under injury conditions including burn trauma, and that some groups of cells are hyperreactive while others are hyporeactive to stimulation.[115,116] Whether the phenotypic differences arise in circulation and in tissues as the result of local environmental conditions dictated by the cytokine milieu or whether these subsets arise as a result of altered monocytopoietic developmental program within the bone marrow or both is not known. However, Ogle et al. have demonstrated that thermal injury stimulates TNFα, IL-1, and PGE$_2$ production by *in vitro* bone marrow-derived macrophages in comparison to non-burn-derived bone marrow macrophages.[117,118] This study makes an argument that thermal injury can stimulate the development of functionally different monocytes within the bone marrow.

Aside from alterations in PMN and monocyte/macrophage functions, patients with severe burns often suffer from suppressed cell-mediated immunity due to impairment in T cell functions.[119,120] Although impairment in cell-mediated immunity has been implied by the observations of delay in skin allografts rejection, suppression of graft versus host response, and skin hypersensitivity reactions in burn patients, the role for T cells has been established through advances in molecular and cell biological techniques.[121–123] *In vitro* functional studies with T cells isolated from burn patients and in animal models have provided conclusive evidence of T cell abnormalities in burn patients. The various alterations that have been reported include an overall suppression of circulating T lymphocytes, decreased mitogenesis in response to concanavalin A or pokeweed mitogens, reduced antigenic stimulation or activation, and redistribution of T lymphocytes within peripheral blood and tissue compartments.[119,124–127] T lymphocytes are divided into T$_{helper}$ and T$_{suppressor}$ populations based on expression of lymphokine profiles, cell surface receptors, and ability to effect functions of NK cells, T$_{cytotoxic}$, and B lymphocytes. In recent years strong evidence has emerged to support the hypothesis that burn injury-induced immune suppression is in part mediated by a shift in T$_{helper}$ and T$_{suppressor}$ populations as assessed by their functional activities and cytokine profiles.[120,122] The initial response to significant burns is the activation of T$_{helper}$ cells as assayed by IL-2R, HLA-2R, and transferrin receptor markers.[128,129] *In vitro* functional assays reveal that the initial activation of T cells leads to inability to respond to mitogenic and/or antigenic stimulation. The addition of IL-2 fails to restore T cell anergy and fails to relieve the suppression of IL-2R in burn patients.[130] These data indicate that thermal injury leads to dysregulation of T cell signal transduction pathways or activation of genes that are normally inactive. In addition, thermal injury triggers the apoptotic pathway in T cells.[131,132] The exact mechanisms that initiate T lymphocyte apoptosis are still unclear. However, Fas ligand, TNFα, and IL-2 mediated pathways have been implicated in T lymphocyte cell death.[133,134] Furthermore, macrophage activation products such as PGE$_2$ and tumor transforming growth factor-β (TGFβ) can also contribute T cell suppression.

The other arm of lymphocytes, the B lymphocytes, also undergo functional changes. There is profound reduction of immuglobin levels following thermal injury. All classes of immunoglobulins are reduced; however, IgG levels display the greatest reduction, with concentration reaching as low as 300–400% mg/dl.[135–138] The rapid drop in immunoglobulins is attributed to plasma leakage, increased protein turnover, and decreased IgG synthesis by the B cells. The initial drop in immunoglobulins slowly returns to near normal levels within the 2-week period after thermal injury.[122] There are reports of nonspecific B cell activation by burn toxins and antigen-dependent mechanisms. The expression of major histocompatability complex (MHC) glycoproteins is reduced upon thermal injury. It is postulated that the ability of B lymphocytes to form antigen–MHC complexes is diminished upon phagocytosis of antigens by the B lymphocytes.[139] Additionally, the display of self-antigens by the B lymphocytes could contribute to antigen-dependent cell death of T lymphocytes and T cell anergy.[119,122] Previous work has shown that CD23 expression on activated B cells is abrogated in response to thermal injury.[140] Additionally, IL-7 levels rise during the 1-week postburn period and could account for the decreased proliferative capacity of mature B lymphocytes. Taken together, these data indicate that the functional alterations in B cells induced by thermal injury could further exacerbate the immune suppression in these patients.

Hematopoiesis and burns

Hematologic changes seen in severely burned patients are reflections of the extent of tissue necrosis, shifts in fluid balance, and the result of repeated surgical interventions. Bone marrow hematopoiesis responds to this demand by replacing or providing additional blood cells to the circulation. Robust hematopoietic response with a balanced production of the different elements of leukocytes is required for adequate immune response and host defense in burn patients. In order to understand the dynamic response of the bone marrow to the burn injury, an elementary understanding of hematopoiesis itself is essential. Hematopoiesis is a dynamic orchestration of cellular events that follows a series of tightly coupled proliferation and differentiation signals. Within this paradigm, the pluripotent hematopoietic stem cells (HSCs) give rise to erythrocytes, megakaryocytes, mature T cells and B cells, and cells of myeloid lineage such as neutrophils, basophils, eosinophils, and monocyte/macrophages (**Figure 26.1**). The process of hematopoiesis requires interactions between the pluripotent hematopoietic stem or committed progenitor cells and the stromal microenvironment.[141] Among other functions, the stromal environment acts as source of cytokines for regulated

hematopoiesis.[141] The proliferation and differentiation of HSCs/progenitor cells into specific terminally differentiated blood cells is dependent on the actions of both the lineage-specific early-acting and late-acting cytokines.[142] While stem cell factor and IL-3 are examples of the former, erythropoietin, granulocyte–macrophage colony-stimulating factor (GM-CSF), G-CSF, macrophage colony-stimulating factor (M-CSF or CSF-1), and thrombopoietin belong to the latter group.[90,143]

Throughout life, the hematopoietic stem cell has the ability for self-renewal that insures abundant numbers of cells are present for commitment towards lineage-specific cells in response to certain conditions. For example, it has shown that during acute bacterial

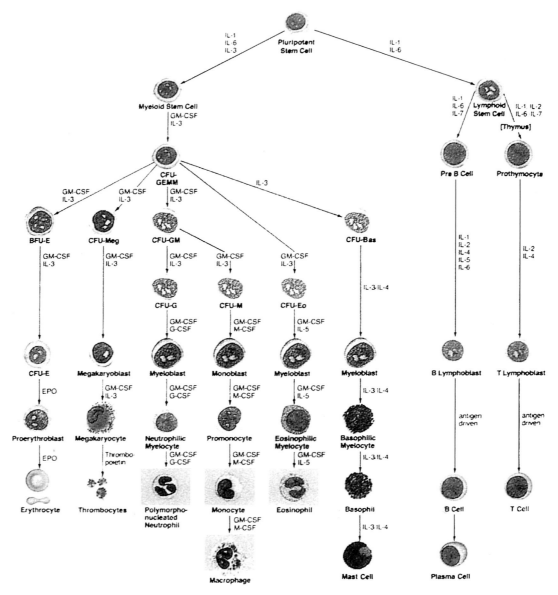

Fig. 26.1 **Hematopoietic commitment paradigm: regulation by cytokines.** GM-CSF, granulocyte–macrophage colony-stimulating factor; G-CSF, granulocyte colony-stimulating factor; M-CSF, monocyte colony-stimulating factor; CFU-GEEM, colony-forming unit-granulocyte, erythroid, monocyte/macrophage, megakaryocyte; BFU-E, burst forming unit-erythroid; EPO, erythropoietin; CFU-G, colony forming unit-granulocyte; CFU-M, colony forming unit-monocyte; CFU-GM, colony forming unit-granulocyte, monocyte/macrophage; CFU-Eo, colony forming unit-eosinophil; CFU-Meg, colony forming unit-megakaryocyte. (Reprinted with permission from Sandoz Pharmaceuticals Corporation.)

infection, an expansion of granulocytes predominates that is attributed to increases within the stem cell compartment.[144,145] Additionally, a small percentage of the total stem cell pool that circulates in peripheral blood is activated in response to the local cytokine environment. The current consensus is that HSCs give rise to the multipotential CFU-GEMM cell, granulocyte-erythrocyte-monocyte-megakaryocyte and the lymphoid stem cell. Although the actual existence of the lymphoid stem cell has not been definitive, it is hypothesized that this stem cell gives rise to mature T- and B cells.[146] The CFU-GEMM cell in the presence of steel factor or stem cell factor, IL-3, and GM-CSF can develop into the myeloid-restricted bipotential cell CFU-GM, which can form either granulocytes or monocyte-macrophages depending upon the presence of G-CSF or M-CSF.[147] The terminally differentiated granulocytes in the bone marrow reserves are recruited into the circulation during periods of bacterial infection, stress, and thermal injury. Additionally, monocytes can either circulate in the peripheral blood or migrate into sites of inflammation and infection and become tissue macrophages in response to the local cytokine milieu.

Much of the knowledge on how hematopoiesis is modulated by thermal injury and sepsis has been gained primarily through the use of animal models. The only pertinent information on burn patients is the demonstration of a reduction in the circulating stem cells in severely burned patients.[148] Animal models of thermal injury, however, continue to provide significant information on the status of bone marrow hematopoiesis during thermal injury. These models have allowed us to probe the role of hematopoiesis in the overall pathophysiology of thermal injury and sepsis. For example, animal models of thermal injury have demonstrated that the initial granulocytosis observed is due to peripheral demargination and release of nondividing granulocyte from bone marrow reserves, which stimulates an increase in the bone marrow CFU-G growth.[82] By contrast, in the same animal model, burn superimposed with *P. aeruginosa* infection led to significant decrease in CFU-G colonies.[149] Moreover, the serum from burn-infected animals inhibited the formation of CFU-G colonies from normal bone marrow cells.[150] These observations pointed to a primary defect in bone marrow granulocyte production or myelopoiesis. Despite these observations, until recently, data on the potential mechanisms for the altered myelopoiesis have been lacking.[151]

Although Eurenius and McEuen were able to demonstrate that the granulocytopenia observed in their rat model of thermal injury and sepsis was due to the failure of bone marrow hematopoiesis, Gamelli and his co-workers paved the way for much of our current understanding of the hematopoietic changes that occur following thermal injury. They were the first ones to compare the size of burn wound and superimposed localized *P. aeruginosa* infection to inflammatory mediators.[87,152] Using these criteria, they demonstrated that mice exhibited peripheral leukopenia and lymphopenia on day 1 postburn and returned to normal values in 8 and 12 days.[87] Mice also exhibited diminished bone marrow and splenic cellularity following thermal injury that increased in a time-dependent manner.[87] In addition, *in vitro* clonogenic assays showed that burn injury led to an initial depression of bone marrow and splenic cellularity. This initial decrease was followed by a consistent bone marrow and splenic hypercellularity.[87] The bone marrow and splenic mitotic index positively correlated with the cellularity. In addition, the number of bone marrow and splenic CFU-GM cells was consistently elevated beginning days 4–12 postburn. The

increased CFU-GM production within the bone marrow and splenic compartment were threefold and 100-fold, respectively.

In direct contrast to thermal injury alone, the superimposition of sepsis dramatically altered the bone marrow myelopoietic responses. When mice were subjected to scald burn injury followed by a septic challenge with *P. aeruginosa* inoculation at the burn wound site, a marked reduction (~50%) in CFU-GM growth was observed 3 days after the initial injury.[152] Interestingly, the introduction of endotoxin into normal or burned mice led to a similar decrease in CFU-GM proliferation as observed in infected burn mice.[152] Under these conditions, the total colony-stimulating activity (CSA) was also reduced in burn-infected animals, suggesting either the levels of CSFs were low or the serum contained a potent inhibitor of colony growth.[152]

In severe thermal injury and sepsis, however, the circulating levels of the myelopoietic growth factors such as G-CSF and M-CSF are elevated. Therefore the logical hypothesis was that the burn sera contained a potent inhibitor for clonal growth of bone marrow cells. Based on the literature evidence, PGE$_2$ appeared to be a logical choice for this clonal growth inhibitory substance. Prostaglandins of the E-series (PGE$_1$ and PGE$_2$) but not the prostaglandins of the F-series (PGF$_1\alpha$ and PGF$_2\alpha$) have been shown to inhibit profoundly CFC-proliferation *in vitro*.[153] In addition, Pelus and his co-workers have demonstrated that administration of PGE$_2$ to cyclophosphamide-treated or intact mice resulted in significant suppression of myelopoiesis.[154] Pelus went on to show that inhibition of prostaglandin biosynthesis through administration of indomethacin, a cyclooxygenase inhibitor, reversed the clonal inhibitory effect of IL-1β administration.[155] Extending these observations to their murine model of thermal injury and sepsis, Gamelli *et al.* were able to show that administration of indomethacin could reverse burn sepsis or burn endotoxin-induced suppression in CFU-GM growth and improve survival of the septic animals.[152] While these studies directly implicated prostaglandin metabolites in burn sepsis-induced bone marrow myeloid suppression, further studies confirmed that PGE$_2$ is the primary mediator of this myelosuppression. Thermal injury and sepsis activate macrophages to produce PGE$_2$ through the induction of the enzyme cyclooxygenase-2 (COX-2).[156] Recently, administration of a specific COX-2 inhibitor, NS-398, has been shown to both inhibit PGE$_2$ production of endotoxin-treated macrophages to improve the survival rate of burn septic animals compared to controls, and to restore absolute neutrophil counts and CFU-GM's proliferative capacity.[151] Similar results were also reported with the treatment of burn septic mice with a PGE$_2$ receptor antagonist SC-19220.[157] Thus, these results have helped establish a significant role for PGE$_2$ in burn-induced myelosuppression and paved the way for new treatment modalities for burn injury and sepsis.

Although PGE$_2$ has been established as a mediator of bone marrow myelosuppression in thermal injury and sepsis, until recently, no attempt has been made to explain the cellular mechanism for this myelosuppression (**Figure 26.2**). Using the same murine model of scald burn injury, Shoup *et al.*[151] characterized the specific stages in granulopoiesis that are altered upon burn sepsis. The specific granulocytic cell surface marker, GR-1 was employed to document the stage of bone marrow myeloid maturation arrest in the injured animals. The expression of GR-1 also designated as Ly-6C, progressively increases with granulocytic maturation. The lowest levels of GR-1 expression are found in myeloblasts and the

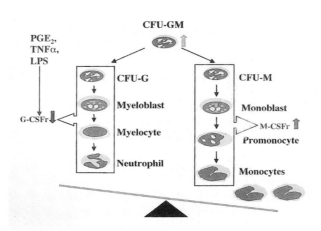

Fig. 26.2 Reprioritization of myeloid commitment following thermal injury and sepsis. PGE₂, Prostagladin E₂; TNFα, tumor necrosis factor-α; LPS, lipopolysaccharide/endotoxin; CFU-GM colony forming unit-granulocyte, monocyte; CFU-M, colony forming unit-monocyte; CFU-G, colony forming unit-granulocyte; G-CSFr, G-CSF receptor; M-CSFr, M-CSF receptor (*c-fms*).

highest levels in neutrophils, with promyelocytes and myelocytes expressing intermediate levels of the antigen.[158,159] Hence, the strength of GR-1 expression allowed these investigators to follow the developmental stages of granulocytopoiesis in sham, burn, and burn septic mice. Their results revealed that burn infection gave rise to an increased number of cells in the compartment comprising immature granulopoietic cells compared to sham or burn mice. Furthermore, there was a concomitant decrease in the compartment comprising the mature granulocyte population. Using another granulocyte marker, myeloperoxidase, whose mRNA expression is restricted up to promyelocytes, they demonstrated that burn sepsis resulted in an accumulation of promyelocyte, suggesting the possibility of myeloid maturation arrest at this stage of granulopoietic development. They could further demonstrate in burn sepsis that myelosuppression was accompanied by an attenuation of G-CSF receptor mRNA expression and G-CSF-stimulated proliferation of bone marrow cells, thereby providing a mechanistic explanation for the observed myelosuppression in thermal injury and sepsis.

Despite these data on the mechanisms regulating granulopoietic development during thermal injury and sepsis, very little information is available on the development of monocytes or monocytopoiesis in the bone marrow under the same conditions. Myelopoiesis is a developmental paradigm responsible for the production of granulocytes and monocytes within the bone marrow. The common myeloid committed progenitor for these lineages is the bipotential progenitor CFU-GM.[160] The CFU-GM cells under the influence of GM-CSF and M-CSF give rise to committed CFU-M progenitors and progressively differentiate into mature monocytes. The mature monocytes are released into peripheral circulation and can differentiate into tissue macrophages upon entry into tissue.[161,162] Although monocyte/macrophage activation and the resultant dysregulated cytokine milieu are considered central players in the development of systemic inflammation in severe burns and sepsis, the status of monocyte production by the bone marrow has been largely neglected. In fact, thermal injury has been

shown to be associated with increased CFU-GM levels.[85,87] Patients suffering from acute peritonitis and various acute infections have also been shown to possess elevated circulating levels of CFU-GM in their blood.[163] Furthermore, increased monocytopoiesis has been documented in animal models with bacterial infections.[81,112] Recently, Santangelo *et al.* have specifically addressed this issue of the status of monocytopoiesis during thermal injury and sepsis.[149] These investigators took advantage of the recent development of monoclonal antibodies against monocyte developmental antigens ERMP-12 and ERMP-20.[164,165] While ERMP-12 antigen is predominantly expressed in CFU-M cells, ERMP-20 antigen is expressed primarily in monoblasts and promonocytes.[165] Through flowcytometric analysis (FACS) of ERMP-12 and ERMP-20 antigen expression, a significant increase was shown in the early monocyte progenitors expressing both ERMP-12 and ERMP-20 antigens in both burn and burn septic animals compared to sham-treated animals. The burn sepsis group also showed a significant increase in the late monocyte progenitors compared to the sham and burn group. These increases in monocytopoiesis were also reflected in the peripheral blood counts. Thermal injury and sepsis stimulated absolute monocytosis and a concomitant reduction in absolute neutrophil counts in circulation. Interestingly, the creation of a localized infection without systemic involvement did not result in any changes in absolute monocyte or granulocyte counts.

This study also demonstrated that M-CSF-responsive colony growth of the total bone marrow cells, as well as ERMP-12-enriched bone marrow cells, was significantly increased in thermal injury and sepsis compared to the sham group. Similar increases were also seen with GM-CSF. Of interest, G-CSF-responsive colony growth was severely depressed in thermal injury and sepsis. More importantly, they were able to provide a mechanistic explanation for the enhanced monocytopoiesis in thermal injury and sepsis through the documentation of increased M-CSF receptor expression on ERMP12+/RMP–20+ enriched bone marrow cells. These studies provided a novel observation that the acute expansion of CFU-GM compartment caused a shift in the production of the myeloid lineage toward monocytopoiesis and away from granulocytopoiesis. The observed shift led to overproduction of monocytes with concurrent underproduction of granulocytes that could be due to increased M-CSF receptor expression on monocytic lineage cells and a downregulation of G-CSF receptor expression on the cells of the granulocytic lineage. Both the increased susceptibility to infections and the maintenance of systemic inflammatory response syndrome (SIRS) can be explained in part by the shift in myelopoiesis during severe burn injury and sepsis. Thus, these studies highlight the importance of understanding the pathophysiology of burn injury through concerted regulation of related cellular events and pave the way to newer rational therapies.

This thought process is supported by the observation that blocking PGE₂'s actions could reverse the preferential shift in myelopoiesis observed during the course of experimental thermal injury.[151,157] Administration of a PGE₂ receptor antagonist, SC-19220, that specifically blocks cellular interactions of PGE₂ without affecting synthesis or activation of other prostaglandins to burn septic animals restored the balance between monocytopoiesis and granulocytopoiesis toward near normal levels. Measurement of circulating neutrophil and monocyte counts also mirrored the bone marrow myelopoietic changes. More importantly, the administration of SC-19220 improved overall survival of burn septic mice.

Aside from the hematopoietic colony-stimulating factors other pro- and anti-inflammatory cytokines that are often elevated in burn patients can also modulate hematopoiesis. Interleukin-6, which plays a central role in the acute phase response of burn injury is also a potent stimulator of early progenitor cell proliferation without inducing differentiation.[166] Furthermore, IL-6 is a powerful mitogen for megakaryocytes and committed myeloid cells.[167-169] It also synergizes with IL-3 and GM-CSF to modulate multiple lineages within the hematopoietic hierarchy.[90,142,143] Thus, increased IL-6 production in severely burned patients could serve to stimulate hematopoiesis so that adequate number of leukocytes and platelets could be produced to meet the increased demands placed on the body. Similarly, TNFα can also modulate myelopoiesis through its capacity to downregulate G-CSF receptor expression on granulocytic cells.[170,171] TGFβ is another cytokine that can influence hematopoiesis through its ability to suppress early hematopoietic precursor growth.[172-174] Therefore, depending on the severity of the burn injury and the presence or absence of other complicating factors such as sepsis, these and other pleiotropic cytokines in the burn milieu can significantly influence the hematopoietic commitment patterns.

In addition to thermal injury and infection, stress response of the burn injury can also profoundly influence myelopoiesis. It is established that immune and hematopoietic systems are under physiologic regulation by neuroendocrine modulation. Conversely, the cytokine and hematopoietic products can alter functions of nervous system and endocrine organs. The ability of sympathetic activation to influence not only the cardiovascular and metabolic functions of the body following severe thermal injury but also its effects on the regulation of myelopoiesis are discussed elsewhere in this book.

Putative Role for Hematopoietic Transcription Factors in Thermal Injury

Recent advances in molecular and cellular biology have begun to describe the importance of the multi-tier control of pathophysiological changes that occur as a response to any injury state. The initial injury and the resultant changes in metabolic and cardiovascular responses trigger alterations in hematologic parameters, which in turn initiate the appropriate hematopoietic commitment programs. Ultimately, specific sequential and temporal gene expression patterns dictate the hematopoietic commitment. Inherent in this concept of physiological regulation is the hierarchy of genes that control proliferation, developmental fate, and functions of hematopoietic progenitor cells. These genetic processes are governed though modulations in the rate of gene transcription which are accomplished through the binding of DNA-binding proteins or transcription factors to specific regions on a gene.[175] The goal of this molecular scheme appears to be the regulation of the quantity and the duration of synthesis of any given protein.

Transcription factors are nuclear proteins that act as dominant control points in the conversion of a gene to a functional protein.[175] Since many key proteins are turned over rapidly to meet the changing needs of the tissues, a complex system of cell signaling architecture, with the final common pathway of gene transcription, must exist to produce bioactive proteins on demand. To regulate exquisitely the rate of protein synthesis, genes need to be quickly transcribed into RNA within the nucleus, transported to the cytoplasm, and proteins synthesized from the RNA templates. Since cells

respond to several signals simultaneously, and many ligand–cell interactions stimulate similar proximal signals, a tighter control of transcriptional initiation must exist for the proper orchestration of cellular responses. The complexity of physiology with coordination of cellular functions at multiple organ levels that is encountered in humans necessitates complex transcriptional mechanisms that can be tuned up or down by binding of specific DNA-binding proteins to multiple DNA elements upstream of the transcription initiation site. Transcription factors fill this role.

The lineage-restricted proliferation and differentiation program in hematopoiesis is achieved through switching on and off specific sets of genes in a temporal manner in response to cell signals. Since thermal injury and sepsis are accompanied by hematologic and hematopoietic changes that determine the overall pathophysiological response of burn patients, it is reasonable to assume that transcriptional regulation of hematopoietic developmental genes plays a significant role. Although, at present, there is little direct evidence for the role of hematopoietic transcription factors in the pathophysiology of burn injury, considerable evidence does exist to support their pivotal role in hemtaopoietic commitment.[176-178] Therefore a brief understanding of the relevant transcription factors is essential to continuing research endeavors in burn biology. Much of our current knowledge of hematopoietic transcription factors has come from diverse fields such as hematology-oncology, immunology, mammalian virology, and signal transduction. Many concepts have been found by studying the molecular controls of normal and aberrant hematopoiesis of leukemias, *in vitro* cell clonal assays, and various hematopoietic cell lines. The gene knock-out technology has also aided in ascertaining the functional roles of characterized genes in hematopoiesis. Biological processes in cells involve changes in gene expression that manifest as altered function or cellular response. Basically, alterations in expression of a certain gene can arise from modulating its level (transcription) or changes in mRNA stability and translation (post-transcriptional mechanisms). In this section, we will review a set of transcription factors that have been shown to be essential for the normal development of many elements of hemtaopoietic lineage.

tal-1/SCL

The *tal-1/SCL* gene encodes a bHLH (basic helix-loop-helix) protein that was originally identified at chromosomal breakpoint in a human acute T cell leukemia.[179,180] *tal-1/SCL* is a master gene required for formation of hematopoietic stem cells that eventually develop into lineage-specific blood cells.[181] Previous studies have revealed that the early hematopoietic stem cells (CD34[+]/c-kit[+]/Sca[+] cells) express the *tal-1/SCL* gene.[181-183] T cell leukemia, a clonal cell line with the potential to differentiate into myeloid and lymphoid lineages, was shown to express tal-1/SCL protein.[180,181] In addition, mature erythrocytes, megakaryocytes, mast cells, and endothelial cells also express tal-1/SCL.[181] These data indicate that the *tal-1/SCL* gene may play a required role in a later stage of maturation of committed progenitors. Homozygous *tal-1/SCL* gene knockout mice provided definitive evidence for its role in hematopoiesis. The homozygous *tal-1/SCL* gene deletion was embryonic lethal and the mice died *in utero*.[181,184] These mice exhibited a failure in blood formation and their yolk sac contained no detectable blood elements and lacked *in vitro* clonogenic potential.[181] These results were further confirmed by the inability of the tal-1/SCL knockout embryonic stem (ES) cells to develop into any hematopoietic lineages.[181]

GATA Family

Another set of transcription factors that are essential in hematopoiesis belong to the GATA family of proteins. The GATA transcription factors are a family of related zinc-finger DNA-binding proteins. These transcription activators bind to the canonical GATA sequence motif found in the cis-regulatory regions of many hematopoietic genes. The proteins have differential expression patterns and activate a unique set of target genes in their restricted cells. GATA-1, GATA-2, and GATA-3 proteins represent the predominant proteins that play pivotal roles in hematopoiesis. It was reported that GATA-2 is involved with proliferation or self-renewal of early hematopoietic stem cells. Mice engineered with homozygous deletion of *GATA-2* gene display severe hematopoietic defects. The GATA-2 knockout mice survive to E10–11, harbor a small number of red blood cells at that stage, undergo anemic crisis, and eventually die.[185] *In vitro* clonogenic assays revealed drastic reduction in the number of erythroid progenitors and substantial loss of mature erythroid and mast cell precursors. The GATA-2 knockout ES cells are unable to contribute to myeloid and lymphoid lineages when introduced into RAG-2 –/– blastocysts to create GATA-2 –/– and RAG-2 –/– chimeric mice.[181, 185] GATA-1, the other important member of this family, is expressed in erythroid, eosinophil, megakaryocyte, and mast cell progenitors.[186,187] GATA-1 appears to be critical for survival and differentiation of erythroid progenitors. Mice lacking GATA-1 protein display normal hematopoiesis, except for the erythroid lineage.[188] *In vitro* differentiation assay with the GATA-1-deficient ES cells demonstrated differentiation up to the proerythroblast stage of erythropoiesis with eventual apoptosis of the arrested cells.[181,188] Interestingly, there seems to be interrelated complex regulation among the GATA family of transcription factors. During erythroid differentiation, GATA-1 levels increase and GATA-2 expression is downregulated.[181] Moreover, this interplay is absent in GATA-1-deficient ES cells that display high levels of GATA-2 during *in vitro* erythroid differentiation assays.[181,186,189] Aside from its role on erythroid differentiation GATA-1 appears to have a negative regulatory role in myeloid differentiation. Increased expression of GATA-1 has been shown to negatively modulate PU.1 expression and thus suppress myeloid commitment.[178,190] Since burn injury is commonly associated with a downregulation of erythropoiesis despite increased levels of endogenous erythropoietin, studies specifically designed to correlate the strength of GATA-1 expression in progenitor cells to the status of erythropoiesis will provide novel and mechanistic information on the pathophysiology of anemia in burn injury. Lastly, mice lacking GATA-3 fail to develop normal fetal liver hematopoiesis, lack all hematopoietic lineages, except the megakaryocytic cells, and succumb to embryonic lethal hemorrhage.[181]

PU.1

The PU.1 proto-oncogene encodes a member of the ets family of DNA-binding proteins. It was originally cloned as a sequence-specific DNA-binding protein that was found to be homologous to the *spi-1* oncogene.[191] The *spi-1* oncogene was isolated from erythroblastic leukemia cells transformed by spleen focus forming virus (SFFV).[191] The PU.1 transcription factor contains an amino-terminal glutamine/aspartic acid-rich region (TAD) followed by PEST domain and a carboxy-terminal ets DNA-binding domain.[192] PU.1 possesses transcription activation potential that requires other coactivators for full transactivation.[193] PU.1 expression is found in

monocytic, granulocytic, and B lymphoid cells.[194] Two different PU.1 knockout mice reveal the absence of monocytes, B cells, and greatly reduced neutrophil production.[195,196] Moreover, these neutrophils are unable to express some markers of fully differentiated neutrophils.[196,197] Curiously, of the two PU.1 knockout mouse models available, in one the mice die around 1–3 days before birth,[196] while in the other PU.1-deficient mice die a few days after birth.[195] Embryonic stem cells from PU.1-deficient mice can differentiate into immature myeloid progenitors in the presence of IL-3 and G-CSF cytokines. Additionally, these PU.1 hematopoietic progenitors express low levels of mRNA for the GM-CSF, G-CSF, and M-CSF receptors.[197,198] The primitive hematopoietic progenitors are unable to differentiate into M-CSF and G-CSF responsive progenitors after introduction of M-CSF-R or G-CSF-R genes.[181,198] Nevertheless, exogenous PU.1 expression in the PU.1-deficient hematopoietic progenitors restores myeloid differentiation. Therefore, multiple lines of evidence implicate PU.1's central role in commitment to myeloid lineage and terminal differentiation of monocytes, granulocytes, and B cells.

c-Myb

c-myb proto-oncogene belongs to the basic helix-turn-helix (bHTH) family of DNA-binding proteins.[199] c-Myb protein contains an LZ motif that mediates homotypic and heterotypic protein interactions.[200] Multiple serines are located within the amino-terminal and carboxy-terminal regions of c-Myb protein that affect its DNA-binding activity and negative regulatory domain.[201–203] Studies have shown that c-myb expression is restricted to myeloid, erythroid, and immature lymphoid cells.[204–206] Collaborative data from *c-myb* knockout mice reveal the absence of all hematopoietic lineage, except within the megakaryocytic compartment. Interestingly, *c-myb* knockout mice exhibited normal yolk sac hematopoiesis, while liver hematopoiesis was greatly compromised and these mice die *in utero* at E14–15.[207] Detailed analysis of hematopoietic lineages revealed that functional granulocytes and monocytes were present, but they harbored 10–20-fold reduction in mature cells compared to normal mice. It is hypothesized that c-Myb functions to control quantitative effects rather than differentiation *per se* during hematopoiesis. It was also noted that c-Myb levels decrease during differentiation of hematopoietic progenitors and enforced c-Myb expression promotes proliferation and blocks hematopoietic differentiation.[181,204,205] Hence, c-Myb plays a critical role in controlling proliferation of immature hematopoietic progenitors and its physiological downregulation is required for commitment towards lineage-specific differentiation.

C/EBPs

CCAAT/enhancer binding proteins (C/EBPs) are transcription factors that bind to core cis-regulatory sequence of CCAAT found in many regulated genes. C/EBPα was the original transcription factor described as a basic leucine zipper (bLZ) DNA-binding protein in hepatocytes and adipocytes.[208] Subsequently, *C/EBPα* expression was observed in hematopoietic cells.[209] Interestingly, CEBP family of transcription factors, including *CEBPα* have been shown to be elevated following thermal injury.[210] Although their expression is implicated in the acute phase response, the role of CEBPs in the regulation of hematopoiesis during thermal injury and sepsis is yet to be delineated. Other members of this family include *C/EBPβ*, *C/EBPδ*, *C/EBPε*, and GADD153/CHOP proteins. These C/EBPs are able to homodimerize and heterodimerize with each other via the leucine zipper regions.[211] Expression studies showed that *C/EBPα* is present in monocytes, eosinophils, and neutrophils.[209,212] Moreover, human myeloid precursors and immature myeloid cell line, 32 DC13, express high levels of *C/EBPα* that decreased upon G-CSF induced differentiation.[213,214] *C/EBPα* was shown to possess transcriptional activation domain involved with the upregulation of mRNAs of certain neutrophil genes such as G-CSF-R, lactoferrin, and collagenase. *C/EBPα* gene knockout mice are deficient in neutrophils and eosinophils, but harbor functional lymphocytes and monocytes.[215] Fetal liver cells formed M-CSF- and GM-CSF-responsive colonies, but G-CSF-induced colonies were not obtained. Hence, these studies formulate that *C/EBPα* is essential for neutrophil differentiation, but was not essential for monocytic differentiation.[215] Conversely, during neutrophil differentiation of myeloid cell line, 32 DC13, *C/EBPβ* levels increase.[209] Recently, data from the *C/EBPβ*-deficient mice revealed that hematopoiesis proceeds normally, but defects in macrophage activation and decreased B lymphocytes were observed.[216–218] Additionally, *C/EBPε* gene knockout mice exhibited abnormal neutrophilic function and deficiencies in certain key enzymes.[219] Otherwise, the mice appeared to have intact hematopoietic tissues. The preceding studies demonstrate the important regulatory function of the C/EBPs transcription factors in myelopoiesis.

c-Myc/MAD/Mxi-1

c-myc proto-oncogene is part of the bHLHLZ (basic helix-loop-helix leucine zipper) family of transcription factors.[220] c-Myc binds to canonical CANNTG DNA motifs located in many proliferative or cell cycle-regulated genes.[221] c-Myc has three transcriptional activation domains in the amino terminus and a carboxy-terminal with sequence-specific basic region and helix-loop-helix leucine zipper domains that mediate protein–protein interactions.[220] c-Myc is required for cellular proliferation and its downregulation is essential for differentiation of many cell types.[205,220,222,223] Max is another bHLHLZ protein partner of c-Myc and this heterodimeric complex is essential for cognate DNA binding and transactivation of target genes.[224,225] Another set of genes that belong to *c-myc* family are *MAD*, *Mxi-1*, *Mxi-3*, and *Mxi-4* genes. The most important ones in hematopoiesis are *MAD* and *Mxi-1*.[226,227] MAD and Mxi-1 proteins can heterodimerize with Max to form heterodimers that unlike Myc–Max can repress transcription at the same cognate DNA sites bound by c-Myc–Max heterodimers. Hence, within a given cell, there is a dynamic equilibrium of c-Myc–Max and MAD–Max complexes that compete for the same binding sites and the predominant complex determines whether proliferation or differentiation ensues.[225,228] During *in vitro* and *in vivo* hematopoietic differentiation, MAD/Mxi-1 levels increase, while *c-myc* expression is downregulated.[226,229,230] Recently, it was reported that *MAD* null mice have defects in myelopoiesis as demonstrated by delayed cell cycle exit during granulocytic differentiation.[231] In summary, c-Myc/MAD's roles in regulating the onset of proliferation versus differentiation are crucial for hematopoietic development.

Hox Genes

The *Hox* genes encode homeo-box containing transcription factors that are involved in neural development, organogenesis, and segmental development of brachial and mesoderm layers.[232] The homeo domain common to these proteins is a sequence-specific helix-turn-helix DNA-binding motif. The role of the various *Hox* genes has been examined in hematopoietic development.[233] The *Hox* genes identified in this process are *HoxA9*, *HoxA5*, *HoxA10*, *HoxB4*, and *HoxB7*.[233,234] In myeloid development, *HoxA9* and *HoxA10* are expressed at highest levels in immature progenitors, but are downregulated during differentiation.[235] *HoxA10* null mice exhibit increased levels of peripheral monocytes and neutrophils with other apparent abnormality. Conversely, *HoxA9* knockout mice had decreased number of granulocytes and attenuation in G-CSF responsiveness.[235] A recent study on *HoxA5* gene expression using antisense oligos demonstrated inhibition of neutrophil and monocytic differentiation.[236] It was hypothesized that *HoxA5* functions in early myeloid progenitors before commitment. Lastly, it was reported that *HoxB7* and *Hlx* genes might be involved in terminal differentiation or maturation of granulocytic cells.[237,238] The overall importance of the Hox gene family is well established in that they seem to control progression of immature myeloid precursors into mature granulocytes.

Hematologic and acute phase response: treatment strategies

Patients suffering 15% or greater body surface area burns undergo significant alterations in their circulatory status. The blood and its constituent elements must be supported, with the primary goal in the initial management phase being support of intravascular volume. A patient suffering 40% surface area burn would be subjected to a 40–50% reduction in circulating volume if not resuscitated. If the volume of resuscitation fluid is insufficient to meet the patient's needs then hemo-concentration will develop. This further interferes with perfusion of blood in a non-Newtonian fluid and with progressive increases in hemoglobin concentration, there is a disproportionate change in the blood's viscosity and resistance to flow through the circulatory bed. By maintaining plasma volume and supporting circulatory volume, perfusion will be enhanced with restoration of the rheological properties of the blood.

Patients suffering significant extent of body burns will experience some progressive decreases in their hemoglobin and hematocrit values over the first several days of hospitalization.[10,20,22,24] This, in part, is related to the reduction in red cell mass, due to the changes in red cell characteristics and erythropoietic response. Additionally, with expansion in plasma volume following successful resuscitation, there may be an element of dilution. Further reductions in hemoglobin and hematocrit concentrations are also the consequences of repeated blood sampling and blood loss related to wound manipulation. The performance of escharotomies can be associated with significant blood loss from thrombosed vessels that bleed once tissue turgor is reduced following eschar release. The characteristics of the burn wound can also contribute to ongoing hematologic loss. Patients with deep partial-thickness wounds with their associated damaged capillary bed can serve as sites for ongoing hematologic instability.

The optimum hematocrit for patients suffering extensive burn injuries is a matter of opinion. Many experts suggest maintaining hematocrit values of 25% or greater. In doing so, a considerable number of transfusions are likely to be required as attempts at replacement with iron and erythropoietin are typically not overly successful in patients with major body surface area injuries. Many patients can tolerate hematocrit less than 25%, and young and healthy individuals whose wounds are closed will tolerate hematocrit in the 18–22% range with a mild tachycardia and no impairment in wound healing or physiologic response. The optimum hematocrit for the individual burn patient should be adjusted to their clinical status and their co-morbid conditions. Elderly patients with significant underlying cardiac disease should be supported more aggressively with maintenance of their hemoglobin and hematocrit values above the 30%. Strategies should be invoked throughout the patient's care and surgical interventions to limit blood loss. The use of tourniquets, vasoconstrictive agents, tumesence with burn eschar excision, and fibrin sealants provide opportunities to limit operative blood loss. Additionally, the use of hemo-dilution with auto-transfusion represents another approach that can be used to limit the need for transfusions, particularly in patients who will not accept transfusions.[239] Blood volume replacement must be closely followed during the course of surgery to avoid hypotensive episodes and the development of systemic acidosis which will further compromise the patient's hemostatic capacity and exacerbate bleeding. Attention to the patient's coagulation parameters and platelet numbers are important to avoid the development of coagulopathic complications due to dilutional coagulopathy. Patients receiving intensive broad-spectrum antibiotic therapy must be carefully monitored for the development of vitamin K dependent coagulopathy. This must be corrected with the replacement of vitamin K as well as coagulation factor component therapy.

The goal of nutritional support in patients with burn injuries is to replete lean body mass and to facilitate restoration of visceral proteins. Hypoalbuminia is a near universal response to significant burn injury. The benefit of albumin replacement therapy and how it impacts outcomes is a matter of opinion. In today's environment of cost containment, the challenge to the clinician is to provide care that is evidence based. A recent analysis by the Cochrane Injuries Group has suggested that there is no indication for the use of albumin in the management of critically ill patients.[70,240] Whether burn patients fall outside this recommendation remains controversial.

The response of the formed elements of the blood following burn injuries has been reviewed in great detail previously in this chapter. The impact of various interventions may also compound the pathologic response induced by the burn injury. Patients receiving heparin for the maintenance of various vascular devices may experience heparin-induced thrombocytopenia. It has been our practice for the last decade to not use heparin flushes to maintain intravascular catheters. With this approach we have had no increase in complications related to line occlusion or embolic events and no incidences of heparin-induced thrombocytopenia. Changes in leukocyte numbers occur as part of the response to injury and can be further compounded by responses to drug therapy and/or septic events. Rapid diagnosis and effective therapy of infections should be done. In patients who developed profound neutropenia, current clinical experience suggests that exogenous administration of recombinant human G-CSFs is effective in supporting increases in circulating neutrophil numbers.

Following burn injury there are dilutional reductions and depletion of coagulation factors. However, after the early burn phase, the predominated tendency for burn patients is to be hypercoagulable. A reduction in antithrombin III levels is associated with an increased propensity for microvascular thrombosis. Limited clinical trials have been performed in which there appears to be a therapeutic effect for the administration of antithrombin III in the early postburn phases. The studies that have been reported suggest that there is a relative preservation of burn wound vascularity and an enhancement in the healing process. There is also some suggestion that there may be a benefit to other microvascular beds such as in the lung with preservation of pulmonary function. These studies are preliminary and provide intriguing observations that need to be confirmed in larger multicenter trials. Burn patients with intravascular devices are at risk for the development of thrombotic complications with limb ischemia as can occur with femoral arterial lines. Also, the presence of a large-bore femoral venous catheter has been reported to be associated with up to a 30% incidence of deep vein thrombosis. The risk of pulmonary emboli is a recognized risk in burn patients. Preservation of circulatory volume and aggressive and early ambulation are important strategies to limit deep vein thrombotic complications and pulmonary emboli. The risk of thromboembolic complications can extend into the rehabilitation phase in patients with large burns.

Conclusion

Burn-induced changes in hematopoiesis and the induction of the acute phase response are components of the body's reaction to injury. With an extensive degree of injury, or when complications develop, the physiologic limits of this system are exceeded. The blood and its constituent elements must provide tissue nutrition, and maintain host defenses and hemostasis. Modern day burn care allows the clinician to limit the impact of injury and provide access to various components in the form of replacement therapy. Further, understanding the basic pathobiology that results with thermal injury will provide additional opportunities to support this cell system and its response to injury with the goal of improved patient outcome.

References

1. DiPietro LA. Wound healing: the role of the macrophage and other immune cells. *Shock* 1995; 4: 233.
2. DiPietro LA, Burdick M, Low QE, Kunkel SL, Strieter RM. MIP-1a as a critical macrophage chemoattractant in wound repair. *J Clin Invest* 1998; 101: 1693–8.
3. Munster AM. Alterations of the host defense mechanism in burns. *Surg Clin North Am* 1970; 50: 1217–25.
4. Stratta RJ, Warden GD, Ninnemann JL, Saffle JR. Immunologic parameters in burned patients: effect of therapeutic interventions. *J Trauma* 1986; 26: 7–17.
5. Winkelstein A. What are the immunological alterations induced by burn injury? *J Trauma* 1984; 24: S72–83.
6. Loebl EC, Baxter CR, Curreri PW. The mechanism of erythrocyte destruction in the early post-burn period. *Ann Surg* 1973; 178: 681–6.
7. Topley E, Jackson DM, Cason JS, Davies JWL. Assessment of red blood cell loss in the first two days after severe burns. *Ann Surg* 1962; 155: 581–90.
8. Birdsell DC, Birch JR. Anemia following thermal burns: a survey of 109 children. *Can J Surg* 1971; 14: 345–50.
9. Desai MH, Herndon DN, Broemeling L, Barrow RE, Nichols RJ Jr, Rutan RL. Early burn wound excision significantly reduces blood loss. *Ann Surg* 1990; 211: 753–9; discussion 759–62.
10. Deitch EA, Sittig KM. A serial study of the erythropoietic response to thermal injury. *Ann Surg* 1993; 217: 293–9.
11. Robb HJ. Dynamics of the microcirculation during a burn. *Arch Surg* 1967; 94: 776–80.
12. Kimber RJ, Lander H. The effect of heat on human red cell morphology, fragility and subsequent survival in vivo. *J Lab Clin Med* 1964; 64: 922–33.
13. Heatherill RJ, Till GO, Burner LH, Ward PA. Thermal injury, intravascular hemolysis, and toxic oxygen products. *J Clin Invest* 1986; 78: 629–36.
14. Endoh Y, Kawakami M, Orringer EP, Peterson HD, Meyer AA. Causes and time

course of acute hemolysis after burn injury in the rat. *J Burn Care Rehabil* 1992; **13**: 203–9.

15. Kawakami M, Endoh Y, Orringer EP, Meyer AA. Improvements in rheologic properties of blood by fluid resuscitation after burn injury in rats. *J Burn Care Rehabil* 1992; **13**: 316–22.

16. Dacie JV, Lewis, SM. Laboratory methods used in the investigation of hemolytic anaemia II. Hereditary haemolytic anaemias. In: *Practical Haematology*, 5th edn. Edinburgh: Churchill Livingstone, 1975: 202–35.

17. Wallner SF, Vautrin R. The anemia of thermal injury: mechanism of inhibition of erythropoiesis. *Proc Soc Exp Biol Med* 1986 **181**: 144–50.

18. Wolfe RR. Review: acute versus chronic response to burn injury. *Circ Shock* 1981; **8**: 105–15.

19. Shoemaker WC, Vladeck BC, Bassin R, *et al*. Burn pathophysiology in man. I. Sequential hemodynamic alterations. *J Surg Res* 1973; **14**: 64–73.

20. Andes WA, Rogers PW, Beason JW, Pruitt BA Jr. The erythropoietin response to the anemia of thermal injury. *J Lab Clin Med* 1976; **88**: 584–92.

21. Erslev AJ. Erythrokinetics. In: Williams WS, Beutley E, Lichtman MD, eds. *Erythrokinetics*. New York: McGraw-Hill, 1990: 424–32.

22. Wallner SF, Warren GH. The haematopoietic response to burning: an autopsy study. *Burns Incl Therm Inj* 1985; **12**: 22–7.

23. Jelkmann W, Wolff M, Fandrey J. Modulation of the production of erythropoietin by cytokines: in vitro studies and their clinical implications. *Contrib Nephrol* 1990; **87**: 68–77.

24. Wallner SF, Vautrin RM, Buerk C, Robinson WA, Peterson VM. The anemia of thermal injury: studies of erythropoiesis in vitro. *J Trauma* 1982; **22**: 774–80.

25. Bauer A, Tronche F, Wessely O, *et al*. The glucocorticoid receptor is required for stress erythropoiesis. *Genes Dev* 1999; **13**: 2996–3002.

26. Bartlett RH, Fong SW, Marrujo G, Hardeman T, Anderson W. Coagulation and platelet changes after thermal injury in man. *Burns* 1981; **7**: 370–7.

27. Eurenius K, Mortensen PF, Meserol PM, Curreri PW. Platelet and megakaryocyte kinetics following thermal injury. *J Lab Clin Med* 1971; **79**: 147–57.

28. Eurenius K, Rossi TD, McEuen DD, Arnold J, McManus WF. Blood coagulation in burn injury. *Proc Soc Exp Biol Med* 1974; **147**: 878–82.

29. Lawrence C, Atac B. Hematologic changes in massive burn injury. *Crit Care Med* 1992; **20**: 1284–8.

30. Housinger TA, Brinkerhoff C, Warden GD. The relationship between platelet count, sepsis, and survival in pediatric burn patients. *Arch Surg* 1993; **128**: 65–6; discussion 66–7.

31. Kowal-Vern A, Gamelli RL, Walenga JM, Hoppensteadt D, Sharp-Pucci M, Schumacher HR. The effect of burn wound size on hemostasis: a correlation of the hemostatic changes to the clinical state. *J Trauma* 1992; **33**: 50–6; discussion 56–7.

32. Kowal-Vern A, McGill V, Walenga JM, Gamelli RL. Antithrombin III concentrate in the acute phase of thermal injury. *Burns* 2000; **26**: 97–101.

33. Kowal-Vern A, McGill V, Walenga JM, Gamelli RL. Antithrombin (H) concentrate infusions are safe and effective in patients with thermal injuries. *J Burn Care Rehabil* 2000; **21**: 115–27.

34. Heideman M. The effect of thermal injury on hemodynamic, respiratory, and hematologic variables in relation to complement activation. *J Trauma* 1979; **19**: 239–47.

35. Wells S, Sissons M, Hasleton PS. Quantitation of pulmonary megakaryocytes and fibrin thrombi in patients dying from burns. *Histopathology* 1984; **8**: 517–27.

36. Suffredini AF, Fantuzzi G, Badolato R, Oppenheim JJ, O'Grady NP. New insights into the biology of the acute phase response. *J Clin Immunol* 1999; **19**: 203–14.

37. Baumann H, Gauldie J. The acute phase response [see comments]. *Immunol Today* 1994; **15**: 74–80.

38. Kushner I. The phenomenon of the acute phase response. *Ann NY Acad Sci* 1982; **389**: 39–48.

39. Tilg H, Dinarello CA, Mier JW. IL-6 and APPs: anti-inflammatory and immunosuppressive mediators. *Immunol Today* 1997; **18**: 428–32.

40. Jeschke MG, Herndon DN, Wolf SE, DebRoy MA, Rai J, Lichtenbelt BJ, Barrow RE. Recombinant human growth hormone alters acute phase reactant proteins, cytokine expression, and liver morphology in burned rats. *J Surg Res* 1999; **83**: 122–9.

41. Emerson WA, Leve PD, Krevans JR. Hematologic changes in septicemia. *Johns Hopkins Med J* 1970; **126**: 69–76.

42. Xia ZF, Coolbaugh MI, He F, Herndon DN, Papaconstantinou J. The effects of burn injury on the acute phase response. *J Trauma* 1992; **32**: 245–50; discussion 250–1.

43. Schlag G, Redl H. Mediators of injury and inflammation. *World J Surg* 1996; **20**: 406–10.

44. Dinarello CA. Interleukin-1 and the pathogenesis of the acute-phase response. *N Engl J Med* 1984; **311**: 1413–18.

45. Guirao X, Lowry SF. Biologic control of injury and inflammation: much more than too little or too late. *World J Surg* 1996; **20**: 437–46.

46. Turchik JB, Bornstein DL. Role of the central nervous system in acute-phase responses to leukocytic pyrogen. *Infect Immun* 1980; **30**: 439–44.

47. Ertel W, Friedl HP, Trentz O. Multiple organ dysfunction syndrome (MODS) following multiple trauma: rationale and concept of therapeutic approach. *Eur J Pediatr Surg* 1994; **4**: 243–8.

48. Ching N, Grossi CE, Angers J, Zurawinsky HS, Jham G, Mills CB, Nealon TF Jr. The outcome of surgical treatment as related to the response of the serum albumin level to nutritional support. *Surg Gynecol Obstet* 1980; **151**: 199–202.

49. Brown RO, Bradley JE, Bekemeyer WB, Luther RW. Effect of albumin supplementation during parenteral nutrition on hospital morbidity. *Crit Care Med* 1988; **16**: 1177–82.

50. Moshage H. Cytokines and the hepatic acute phase response. *J Pathol* 1997; **181**: 257–66.

51. Jeschke MG, Herndon DN, Barrow RE. Insulin-like growth factor I in combination with insulin-like growth factor binding protein 3 affects the hepatic acute phase response and hepatic morphology in thermally injured rats. *Ann Surg* 2000; **231**: 408–16.

52. Jeschke MG, Barrow RE, Herndon DN. Insulinlike growth factor I plus insulinlike growth factor binding protein 3 attenuates the proinflammatory acute phase response in severely burned children. *Ann Surg* 2000; **231**: 246–52.

53. Jarrar D, Wolf SE, Jeschke MG, *et al*. Growth hormone attenuates the acute-phase response to thermal injury. *Arch Surg* 1997; **132**: 1171–5; discussion 1175–6.

54. Pos O, van der Stelt ME, Wolbink GJ, Nijsten MW, van der Tempel GL, van Dijk W. Changes in the serum concentration and the glycosylation of human alpha 1-acid glycoprotein and alpha 1-protease inhibitor in severely burned persons: relation to interleukin-6 levels. *Clin Exp Immunol* 1990; **82**: 579–82.

55. Sevaljevic L, Glibetic M, Poznanovic G, Savic J, Petrovic M. Effect of lethal scald on the mechanisms of acute-phase protein synthesis in rat liver. *Circ Shock* 1991; **33**: 98–107.

56. Jeschke MG, Herndon DN, Wolf SE, *et al*. Hepatocyte growth factor modulates the hepatic acute-phase response in thermally injured rats. *Crit Care Med* 2000; **28**: 504–10.

57. Sevaljevic L, Ivanovic-Matic S, Petrovic M, Glibetic M, Pantelic D, Poznanovic G. Regulation of plasma acute-phase protein and albumin levels in the liver of scalded rats. *Biochem J* 1989; **258**: 663–8.

58. Fey GH, Fuller GM. Regulation of acute phase gene expression by inflammatory mediators. *Mol Biol Med* 1987; **4**: 323–38.

59. Heinrich PC, Castell JV, Andus T. Interleukin-6 and the acute phase response. *Biochem J* 1990; **265**: 621–36.

60. Nijsten MW, Hack CE, Helle M, ten Duis HJ, Klasen HJ, Aarden LA. Interleukin-6 and its relation to the humoral response and clinical parameters in burned patients. *Surgery* 1991; **109**: 761–7.

61. Dickson PW, Bannister D, Schreiber G. Minor burns lead to major changes in synthesis rates of plasma proteins in the liver. *J Trauma* 1987; **27**: 283–6.

62. Schluter B, Konig B, Bergmann U, Muller FE, Konig W. Interleukin 6 – a potential mediator of lethal sepsis after major thermal trauma: evidence for increased IL-6 production by peripheral blood mononuclear cells. *J Trauma* 1991; **31**: 1663–70.

63. Biffl WL, Moore EE, Moore FA, Peterson VM. Interleukin-6 in the injured patient. Marker of injury or mediator of inflammation? *Ann Surg* 1996; **224**: 647–64.

64. Ueyama M, Maruyama I, Osame M, Sawada Y. Marked increase in plasma interleukin 6 in burn patients. *J Lab Clin Med* 1992; **120**: 693–8.

65. Guo Y, Dickerson C, Chrest FJ, Adler WH, Munster AM, Winchurch RA. Increased levels of circulating interleukin 6 in burn patients. *Clin Immunol Immunopathol* 1990; **54**: 361–71.

66. Li JJ, Sanders RL, McAdam KP, *et al*. Impact of C-reactive protein (CRP) on surfactant function. *J Trauma* 1989; **29**: 1690–7.

67. Livingston DH, Mosenthal AC, Deitch EA. Sepsis and multiple organ dysfunction syndrome: a clinical-mechanistic overview. *New Horiz* 1995; **3**: 257–66.

68. Pruitt JH, Copeland EM III, Moldawer LL. Interleukin-1 and interleukin-1 antagonism in sepsis, systemic inflammatory response syndrome, and septic shock [editorial]. *Shock* 1995; **3**: 235–51.

69. Jeschke MG, Barrow RE, Herndon DN. Recombinant human growth hormone treatment in pediatric burn patients and its role during the hepatic acute phase response. *Crit Care Med* 2000; **28**: 1578–84.

70. Bunn F, Lefebvre C, Li Wan Po A, Li L, Roberts I, Schierhout G. Human albumin solution for resuscitation and volume expansion in critically ill patients. The Albumin Reviewers. *Cochrane Database Syst Rev* 2000; **2**.

71. Jeschke MG, Barrow RE, Hawkins HK, Tao Z, Perez-Polo JR, Herndon DN. Biodistribution and feasibility of non-viral IGF-I gene transfers in thermally injured skin. *Lab Invest* 2000; **80**: 151–8.

72. Goris RJ. MODS/SIRS: result of an overwhelming inflammatory response? [see comments]. *World J Surg* 1996; **20**: 418–21.

73. Border JR. Hypothesis: sepsis, multiple systems organ failure, and the macrophage [editorial]. *Arch Surg* 1988; **123**: 285–6.

74. Weiss SJ. Tissue destruction by neutrophils [see comments]. *N Engl J Med* 1989; **320**: 365–76.

75. Peterson VM, Rundus CH, Reinoehl PJ, Schroeter SR, McCall CA, Bartle EJ. The myelopoietic effects of a *Serratia marcescens*-derived biologic response modifier in a mouse model of thermal injury. *Surgery* 1992; **111**: 447–54.

76. Henson PM, Johnston RB Jr. Tissue injury in inflammation. Oxidants, proteinases, and cationic proteins. *J Clin Invest* 1987; **79**: 669–74.

77. Callery MP, Kamei T, Mangino MJ, Flye MW. Organ interactions in sepsis. Host defense and the hepatic-pulmonary macrophage axis. *Arch Surg* 1991; **126**: 28–32.

78. Eriksson E, Straube RC, Robson MC. White blood cell consumption in the microcirculation after a major burn. *J Trauma* 1979; **19**: 94–7.

79. Gamelli RL, Paxton TP, O'Reilly M. Bone marrow toxicity by silver sulfadiazine. *Surg Gynecol Obstet* 1993; **177**: 115–20.

80. Wolach B, Coates TD, Hugli TE, Baehner RL, Boxer LA. Plasma lactoferrin reflects granulocyte activation via complement in burn patients. *J Lab Clin Med* 1984; **103**: 284–93.

81. Peterson V, Hansbrough J, Buerk C, *et al.* Regulation of granulopoiesis following severe thermal injury. *J Trauma* 1983; **23**: 19–24.

82. Eurenius K, Brouse RO. Granulocyte kinetics after thermal injury. *Am J Clin Pathol* 1973; **60**: 337–42.

83. Asko-Seljavaara S. Granulocyte kinetics in burned mice. Inhibition of granulocyte studied in vivo and in vitro. *Scand J Plast Reconstr Surg* 1974; **8**: 185–91.

84. Asko-Seljavaara S. Inhibition of bone marrow cell proliferation in burned mice. An in vitro study of the effect of fluid replacement and burn serum on bone marrow cell growth. *Scand J Plast Reconstr Surg* 1974; **8**: 192–7.

85. Huang WH, Wu JZ, Hu ZX, *et al.* Bone marrow granulopoietic response to scalds and would infection in mice. *Burns Incl Therm Inj* 1988; **14**: 292–6.

86. McEuen DD, Ogawa M, Eurenius K. Myelopoiesis in the infected burn. *J Lab Clin Med* 1977; **89**: 540–3.

87. Gamelli RL, Hebert JC, Foster RS Jr. Effect of burn injury on granulocyte and macrophage production. *J Trauma* 1985; **25**: 615–19.

88. Maestroni GJ. Catecholaminergic regulation of hematopoiesis in mice [letter; comment]. *Blood* 1998; **92**: 2971; discussion 2972–3.

89. Broxmeyer HE, Williams DE. Actions of hematopoietic colony-stimulating factors in vivo and in vitro. *Pathol Immunopathol Res* 1987; **6**: 207–20.

90. Metcalf D. The hemopoietic regulators – an embarrassment of riches. *Bioessays* 1992; **14**: 799–805.

91. Gamelli RL, He LK, Liu H. Recombinant human granulocyte colony-stimulating factor treatment improves macrophage suppression of granulocyte and macrophage growth after burn and burn wound infection. *J Trauma* 1995; **39**: 1141–6; discussion 1146–7.

92. Sartorelli KH, Silver GM, Gamelli RL. The effect of granulocyte colony-stimulating factor (G-CSF) upon burn-induced defective neutrophil chemotaxis. *J Trauma* 1991; **31**: 523–9; discussion 529–30.

93. Silver GM, Gamelli RL, O'Reilly M. The beneficial effect of granulocyte colony-stimulating factor (G-CSF) in combination with gentamicin on survival after Pseudomonas burn wound infection. *Surgery* 1989; **106**: 452–5; discussion 455–6.

94. Smith WS, Sumnicht GE, Sharpe RW, Samuelson D, Millard FE. Granulocyte colony-stimulating factor versus placebo in addition to penicillin G in a randomized blinded study of gram-negative pneumonia sepsis: analysis of survival and multisystem organ failure. *Blood* 1995; **86**: 1301–9.

95. Toda H, Murata A, Matsuura N, *et al.* Therapeutic efficacy of granulocyte colony stimulating factor against rat cecal ligation and puncture model. *Stem Cells* 1993; **11**: 228–34.

96. Grogan JB, Miller RC. Impaired function of polymorphonuclear leukocytes in patients with burns and other trauma. *Surg Gynecol Obstet* 1973; **137**: 784–8.

97. Solomkin JS. Neutrophil disorders in burn injury: complement, cytokines, and organ injury. *J Trauma* 1990; **30**: S80–5.

98. el-Falaky MH, Abdel-Hafez A, Houtah AH. Phagocytic activity of polymorphonuclear leucocytes in burns. *Burns Incl Therm Inj* 1985; **11**: 185–91.

99. Braquet M, Lavaud P, Dormont D, *et al.* Leukocytic functions in burn-injured patients. *Prostaglandins* 1985; **29**: 747–64.

100. Bjerknes R, Vindenes H, Pitkanen J, Ninnemann J, Laerum OD, Abyholm F. Altered polymorphonuclear neutrophilic granulocyte functions in patients with large burns. *J Trauma* 1989; **29**: 847–55.

101. Solomkin JS, Nelson RD, Chenoweth DE, Solem LD, Simmons RL. Regulation of neutrophil migratory function in burn injury by complement activation products. *Ann Surg* 1984; **200**: 742–6.

102. Solomkin JS, Cotta LA, Brodt JK, Hurst JW, Ogle CK. Neutrophil dysfunction in sepsis. III. Degranulation as a mechanism for nonspecific deactivation. *J Surg Res* 1984; **36**: 407–12.

103. Tchervenkov JI, Latter DA, Psychogios J, Christou NV. Altered leukocyte delivery to specific and nonspecific inflammatory skin lesions following burn injury. *J Trauma* 1988; **28**: 582–8.

104. Sayeed MM. Neutrophil signaling alteration: an adverse inflammatory response after burn shock. *Medicina* 1998; **58**: 386–92.

105. Bjornson AB, Somers SD, Knippenberg RW, Bjornson HS. Circulating factors contribute to elevation of intracellular cyclic-3′,5′-adenosine monophosphate and depression of superoxide anion production in polymorphonuclear leukocytes following thermal injury. *J Leukoc Biol* 1992; **52**: 407–14.

106. Duque RE, Phan SH, Hudson JL, Till GO, Ward PA. Functional defects in phagocytic cells following thermal injury. Application of flow cytometric analysis. *Am J Pathol* 1985; **118**: 116–27.

107. Bjerknes R, Vindenes H. Neutrophil dysfunction after thermal injury: alteration of phagolysosomal acidification in patients with large burns. *Burns* 1989; **15**: 77–81.

108. Bjerknes R, Vindenes H, Laerum OD. Altered neutrophil functions in patients with large burns. *Blood Cells* 1990; **16**: 127–41.

109. Bjornson AB, Knippenberg RW, Bjornson HS. Bactericidal defect of neutrophils in a guinea pig model of thermal injury is related to elevation of intracellular cyclic-3′,5′-adenosine monophosphate. *J Immunol* 1989; **143**: 2609–16.

110. Mooney DP, Gamelli RL, O'Reilly M, Hebert JC. Recombinant human granulocyte colony-stimulating factor and Pseudomonas burn wound sepsis. *Arch Surg* 1988; **123**: 1353–7.

111. Volenec FJ, Wood GW, Mani MM, Robinson DW, Humphrey LJ. Mononuclear cell analysis of peripheral blood from burn patients. *J Trauma* 1979; **19**: 86–93.

112. Wallner S, Vautrin R, Murphy J, Anderson S, Peterson V. The haematopoietic response to burning: studies in an animal model. *Burns Incl Therm Inj* 1984; **10**: 236–51.

113. Moore FD Jr, Davis CF. Monocyte activation after burns and endotoxemia. *J Surg Res* 1989; **46**: 350–4.

114. O'Riordain MG, Collins KH, Pilz M, Saporoschetz IB, Mannick JA, Rodrick ML. Modulation of macrophage hyperactivity improves survival in a burn-sepsis model. *Arch Surg* 1992; **127**: 152–7; discussion 157–8.

115. Miller-Graziano CL, Szabo G, Kodys K, Griffey K. Aberrations in post-trauma monocyte (MO) subpopulation: role in septic shock syndrome. *J Trauma* 1990; **30**: S86–96.

116. Miller-Graziano CL, Szabo G, Griffey K, Mehta B, Kodys K, Catalano D. Role of elevated monocyte transforming growth factor beta (TGF beta) production in posttrauma immunosuppression. *J Clin Immunol* 1991; **11**: 95–102.

117. Ogle CK, Guo X, Wu JZ, Ogle JD. Production of cytokines and PGE2 and cytotoxicity of stimulated bone marrow macrophages after thermal injury and cytotoxicity of stimulated U-937 macrophages. *Inflammation* 1993; **17**: 583–94.

118. Ogle CK, Guo X, Alexander JW, Fukushima R, Ogle JD. The activation of bone marrow macrophages 24 hours after thermal injury. *Arch Surg* 1993; **128**: 96–100; discussion 100–1.

119. Sparkes BG. Immunological responses to thermal injury. *Burns* 1997; **23**: 106–13.

120. Hansbrough JF, Bender EM, Zapata-Sirvent R, Anderson J. Altered helper and suppressor lymphocyte populations in surgical patients. A measure of postoperative immunosuppression. *Am J Surg* 1984; **148**: 303–7.

121. Munster AM, Eurenius K, Katz RM, Canales L, Foley FD, Mortensen RF. Cell-mediated immunity after thermal injury. *Ann Surg* 1973; **177**: 139–43.

122. Munster AM. Alteration of the immune system in burns and implications for therapy. *Eur J Pediatr Surg* 1994; **4**: 231–42.

123. Rapaport FT, Milgrom F, Kano K, *et al.* Immunologic sequelae of thermal injury. *Ann NY Acad Sci* 1968; **150**: 1004–8.

124. Organ BC, Antonacci AC, Chiao J, *et al.* Changes in lymphocyte number and phenotype in seven lymphoid compartments after thermal injury. *Ann Surg* 1989; **210**: 78–89.

125. O'Mahony JB, Wood JJ, Rodrick ML, Mannick JA. Changes in T lymphocyte subsets following injury. Assessment by flow cytometry and relationship to sepsis. *Ann Surg* 1985; **202**: 580–6.

126. Kupper TS, Green DR. Immunoregulation after thermal injury: sequential appearance of I-J+, Ly-1 T suppressor inducer cells and Ly-2 T suppressor effector cells following thermal trauma in mice. *J Immunol* 1984; **133**: 3047–53.

127. Munster AM. Post-traumatic immunosuppression is due to activation of suppressor T cells. *Lancet* 1976; **1**: 1329–30.

128. Hansbrough JF, Zapata-Sirvent R, Hoyt D. Postburn immune suppression: an inflammatory response to the burn wound? *J Trauma* 1990; **30**: 671–4; discussion 674–5.

129. Maldonado MD, Venturoli A, Franco A, Nunez-Roldan A. Specific changes in peripheral blood lymphocyte phenotype from burn patients. Probable origin of the thermal injury-related lymphocytopenia. *Burns* 1991; **17**: 188–92.

130. Gadd MA, Hansbrough JF, Hoyt DB, Ozkan N. Defective T-cell surface antigen

expression after mitogen stimulation. An index of lymphocyte dysfunction after controlled murine injury. *Ann Surg* 1989; 209: 112–18.

131. Tenen DG, Hromas R, Licht JD, Zhang DE. Transcription factors, normal myeloid development, and leukemia. *Blood* 1997; 90: 489–519.

132. Teodorczyk-Injeyan JA, Cembrzynska-Nowak M, Lalani S, Peters WJ, Mills GB. Immune deficiency following thermal trauma is associated with apoptotic cell death. *J Clin Immunol* 1995; 15: 318–28.

133. Golstein P, Ojcius DM, Young JD. Cell death mechanisms and the immune system. *Immunol Rev* 1991; 121: 29–65.

134. Mountz JD, Zhou T, Wu J, Wang W, Su X, Cheng J. Regulation of apoptosis in immune cells. *J Clin Immunol* 1995; 15: 1–16.

135. Arturson G, Hogman CF, Johansson SG, Killander J. Changes in immunoglobulin levels in severely burned patients. *Lancet* 1969; 1: 546–8.

136. Kohn J, Cort DF. Immunoglobulins in burned patients. *Lancet* 1969; 1: 836–7.

137. Munster AM, Hoagland HC. Serum immunoglobulin patterns after burns. *Surg Forum* 1969; 20: 76–7.

138. Ritzmann SE, Larson DL, McClung C, Abston S, Falls D, Goldman AS. Immunoglobulin levels in burned patients. *Lancet* 1969; 1: 1152–3.

139. Noelle RJ, Snow EC. T helper cell-dependent B cell activation. *Faseb J* 1991; 5: 2770–6.

140. Schluter B, Konig W, Koller M, Erbs G, Muller FE. Differential regulation of T- and B-lymphocyte activation in severely burned patients. *J Trauma* 1991; 31: 239–46.

141. Dexter TM. Introduction to the haemopoietic system. *Cancer Surv* 1990; 9: 1–5.

142. Testa NG, Dexter TM. Cell lineages in haemopoiesis: comments on their regulation. *Semin Immunol* 1990; 2: 167–72.

143. Metcalf D. Cellular hematopoiesis in the twentieth century. *Semin Hematol* 1999; 36: 5–12.

144. Heyworth CM, Vallance SJ, Whetton AD, Dexter TM. The biochemistry and biology of the myeloid haemopoietic cell growth factors. *J Cell Sci Suppl* 1990; 13: 57–74.

145. Cheers C, Haigh AM, Kelso A, Metcalf D, Stanley ER, Young AM. Production of colony-stimulating factors (CSFs) during infection: separate determinations of macrophage-, granulocyte-, granulocyte-macrophage-, and multi-CSFs. *Infect Immun* 1988; 56: 247–51.

146. Kondo M, Weissman IL, Akashi K. Identification of clonogenic common lymphoid progenitors in mouse bone marrow. *Cell* 1997; 91: 661–72.

147. Kozutsumi H. Special education. *Oncologist* 1996; 1: 116–18.

148. Peterson VM, Robinson WA, Wallner SF, Rundus C, Hansbrough JF. Granulocyte stem cells are decreased in humans with fatal burns. *J Trauma* 1985; 25: 413–18.

149. Santangelo S, Gamelli RL, Shankar R. Myeloid commitment shifts toward monocytopoiesis following thermal injury and sepsis. *Ann Surg* 2001; 233: 97–106.

150. McEuen DD, Gerber GC, Blair P, Eurenius K. Granulocyte function and *Pseudomonas* burn wound infection. *Infect Immun* 1976; 14: 399–402.

151. Shoup M, He LK, Liu H, Shankar R, Gamelli R. Cyclooxygenase-2 inhibitor NS-398 improves survival and restores leukocyte counts in burn infection. *J Trauma* 1998; 45: 215–20; discussion 220–1.

152. Gamelli RL, He LK, Liu H. Marrow granulocyte-macrophage progenitor cell response to burn injury as modified by endotoxin and indomethacin. *J Trauma* 1994; 37: 339–46.

153. Gentile PS, Pelus LM. In vivo modulation of myelopoiesis by prostaglandin E2. IV. Prostaglandin E2 induction of myelopoietic inhibitory activity. *J Immunol* 1988; 141: 2714–20.

154. Pelus LM. Modulation of myelopoiesis by prostaglandin E2: demonstration of a novel mechanism of action in vivo. *Immunol Res* 1989; 8: 176–84.

155. Pelus LM. Blockade of prostaglandin biosynthesis in intact mice dramatically augments the expansion of committed myeloid progenitor cells (colony-forming units-granulocyte, macrophage) after acute administration of recombinant human IL-1 alpha. *J Immunol* 1989; 143: 4171–9.

156. Hahn EL, Tai HH, He LK, Gamelli RL. Burn injury with infection alters prostaglandin E2 synthesis and metabolism. *J Trauma* 1999; 47: 1052–7; discussion 1057–9.

157. Santangelo S, Shoup M, Gamelli RL, Shankar R. Prostaglandin E2 receptor antagonist (SC-19220) treatment restores the balance to bone marrow myelopoiesis after burn sepsis. *J Trauma* 2000; 48: 826–30; discussion 830–1.

158. Fleming TJ, Fleming ML, Malek TR. Selective expression of Ly-6G on myeloid lineage cells in mouse bone marrow. RB6-8C5 mAb to granulocyte-differentiation antigen (Gr-1) detects members of the Ly-6 family. *J Immunol* 1993; 151: 2399–408.

159. Hestdal K, Ruscetti FW, Ihle JN, et al. Characterization and regulation of RB6-8C5 antigen expression on murine bone marrow cells. *J Immunol* 1991; 147: 22–8.

160. Akashi K, Traver D, Miyamoto T, Weissman IL. A clonogenic common myeloid progenitor that gives rise to all myeloid lineages. *Nature* 2000; 404: 193–7.

161. Van Furth R, Diesselhoff-den Dulk MC, Mattie H. Quantitative study on the production and kinetics of mononuclear phagocytes during an acute inflammatory reaction. *J Exp Med* 1973; 138: 1314–30.

162. Dexter TM, Coutinho LH, Spooncer E, et al. Stromal cells in haemopoiesis. *CIBA Found Symp* 1990; 148: 76–86.

163. Selig C, Nothdurft W. Cytokines and progenitor cells of granulocytopoiesis in peripheral blood of patients with bacterial infections. *Infect Immun* 1995; 63: 104–9.

164. Leenen PJ, Melis M, Slieker WA, Van Ewijk W. Murine macrophage precursor characterization. II. Monoclonal antibodies against macrophage precursor antigens. *Eur J Immunol* 1990; 20: 27–34.

165. de Bruijn MF, Slieker WA, van der Loo JC, Voerman JS, van Ewijk W, Leenen PJ. Distinct mouse bone marrow macrophage precursors identified by differential expression of ER-MP12 and ER-MP20 antigens. *Eur J Immunol* 1994; 24: 2279–84.

166. Ikebuchi K, Wong GG, Clark SC, Ihle JN, Hirai Y, Ogawa M. Interleukin 6 enhancement of interleukin 3-dependent proliferation of multipotential hemopoietic progenitors. *Proc Natl Acad Sci USA* 1987; 84: 9035–9.

167. Lazzari L, Henschler R, Lecchi L, Rebulla P, Mertelsmann R, Sirchia G. Interleukin-6 and interleukin-11 act synergistically with thrombopoietin and stem cell factor to modulate ex vivo expansion of human CD41+ and CD61+ megakaryocytic cells. *Haematologica* 2000; 85: 25–30.

168. Sui X, Tsuji K, Ebihara Y, et al. Soluble interleukin-6 (IL-6) receptor with IL-6 stimulates megakaryopoiesis from human CD34(+) cells through glycoprotein (gp) 130 signaling. *Blood* 1999; 93: 2525–32.

169. Metcalf D. Actions and interactions of G-CSF, LIF, and IL-6 on normal and leukemic murine cells. *Leukemia* 1989; 3: 349–55.

170. Nicola NA, Vadas MA, Lopez AF. Down-modulation of receptors for granulocyte colony-stimulating factor on human neutrophils by granulocyte-activating agents. *J Cell Physiol* 1986; 128: 501–9.

171. Walker F, Nicola NA, Metcalf D, Burgess AW. Hierarchical down-modulation of hemopoietic growth factor receptors. *Cell* 1985; 43: 269–76.

172. Fogli M, Carlo-Stella C, Curti A, et al. Transforming growth factor beta3 inhibits chronic myelogenous leukemia hematopoiesis by inducing Fas-independent apoptosis. *Exp Hematol* 2000; 28: 775–83.

173. Batard P, Monier MN, Fortunel N, et al. TGF-(beta) 1 maintains hematopoietic immaturity by a reversible negative control of cell cycle and induces CD34 antigen up-modulation. *J Cell Sci* 2000; 113: 383–90.

174. Cashman JD, Clark-Lewis I, Eaves AC, Eaves CJ. Differentiation stage-specific regulation of primitive human hematopoietic progenitor cycling by exogenous and endogenous inhibitors in an in vivo model. *Blood* 1999; 94: 3722–9.

175. Macfarlane WM. Demystified ... Transcription. *Mol Pathol* 2000; 53: 1–7.

176. Ward AC, Loeb DM, Soede-Bobok AA, Touw IP, Friedman AD. Regulation of granulopoiesis by transcription factors and cytokine signals. *Leukemia* 2000; 14: 973–90.

177. Guerriero A, Langmuir PB, Spain LM, Scott EW. PU.1 is required for myeloid-derived but not lymphoid-derived dendritic cells. *Blood* 2000; 95: 879–85.

178. Nerlov C, Querfurth E, Kulessa H, Graf T. GATA-1 interacts with the myeloid PU.1 transcription factor and represses PU.1-dependent transcription. *Blood* 2000; 95: 2543–51.

179. Finger LR, Kagan J, Christopher G, et al. Involvement of the TCL5 gene on human chromosome 1 in T-cell leukemia and melanoma. *Proc Natl Acad Sci USA* 1989; 86: 5039–43.

180. Xia Y, Brown L, Yang CY, et al. TAL2, a helix-loop-helix gene activated by the (7;9)(q34;q32) translocation in human T-cell leukemia. *Proc Natl Acad Sci USA* 1991; 88: 11416–20.

181. Shivdasani RA, Orkin SH. The transcriptional control of hematopoiesis [see comments]. *Blood* 1996; 87: 4025–39.

182. Mouthon MA, Bernard O, Mitjavila MT, Romeo PH, Vainchenker W, Mathieu-Mahul D. Expression of tal-1 and GATA-binding proteins during human hematopoiesis. *Blood* 1993; 81: 647–55.

183. Begley CG, Aplan PD, Denning SM, Haynes BF, Waldmann TA, Kirsch IR. The gene SCL is expressed during early hematopoiesis and encodes a differentiation-related DNA-binding motif. *Proc Natl Acad Sci USA* 1989; 86: 10128–32.

184. Robb L, Lyons I, Li R, et al. Absence of yolk sac hematopoiesis from mice with a targeted disruption of the scl gene. *Proc Natl Acad Sci USA* 1995; 92: 7075–9.

185. Tsai FY, Keller G, Kuo FC, et al. An early haematopoietic defect in mice lacking the transcription factor GATA-2. *Nature* 1994; 371: 221–6.

186. Orkin SH. GATA-binding transcription factors in hematopoietic cells. *Blood* 1992; 80: 575–81.

187. Visvader JE, Elefanty AG, Strasser A, Adams JM. GATA-1 but not SCL induces megakaryocytic differentiation in an early myeloid line. *Embo J* 1992; 11: 4557–64.

188. Weiss MJ, Keller G, Orkin SH. Novel insights into erythroid development

revealed through in vitro differentiation of GATA-1 embryonic stem cells. *Genes Dev* 1994; 8: 1184–97.

189. Simon MC, Pevny L, Wiles MV, Keller G, Costantini F, Orkin SH. Rescue of erythroid development in gene targeted GATA-1-mouse embryonic stem cells. *Nat Genet* 1992; 1: 92–8.

190. Zhang P, Behre G, Pan J, et al. Negative cross-talk between hematopoietic regulators: GATA proteins repress PU.1. *Proc Natl Acad Sci USA* 1999; 96: 8705–10.

191. Klemsz MJ, McKercher SR, Celada A, Van Beveren C, Maki RA. The macrophage and B cell-specific transcription factor PU.1 is related to the ets oncogene [see comments]. *Cell* 1990; 61: 113–24.

192. Ray-Gallet D, Mao C, Tavitian A, Moreau-Gachelin F. DNA binding specificities of Spi-1/PU.1 and Spi-B transcription factors and identification of a Spi-1/Spi-B binding site in the c-fes/c-fps promoter. *Oncogene* 1995; 11: 303–13.

193. Klemsz MJ, Maki RA. Activation of transcription by PU.1 requires both acidic and glutamine domains. *Mol Cell Biol* 1996; 16: 390–7.

194. Chen HM, Zhang P, Voso MT, et al. Neutrophils and monocytes express high levels of PU.1 (Spi-1) but not Spi-B. *Blood* 1995; 85: 2918–28.

195. McKercher SR, Torbett BE, Anderson KL, et al. Targeted disruption of the PU.1 gene results in multiple hematopoietic abnormalities. *Embo J* 1996; 15: 5647–58.

196. Scott EW, Simon MC, Anastasi J, Singh H. Requirement of transcription factor PU.1 in the development of multiple hematopoietic lineages. *Science* 1994; 265: 1573–7.

197. Anderson KL, Smith KA, Conners K, McKercher SR, Maki RA, Torbett BE. Myeloid development is selectively disrupted in PU.1 null mice. *Blood* 1998; 91: 3702–10.

198. DeKoter RP, Walsh JC, Singh H. PU.1 regulates both cytokine-dependent proliferation and differentiation of granulocyte/macrophage progenitors. *Embo J* 1998; 17: 4456–68.

199. Biedenkapp H, Borgmeyer U, Sippel AE, Klempnauer KH. Viral myb oncogene encodes a sequence-specific DNA-binding activity. *Nature* 1988; 335: 835–7.

200. Klempnauer KH, Sippel AE. The highly conserved amino-terminal region of the protein encoded by the v-myb oncogene functions as a DNA-binding domain. *Embo J* 1987; 6: 2719–25.

201. Ramsay RG, Morrice N, Van Eeden P, et al. Regulation of c-Myb through protein phosphorylation and leucine zipper interactions. *Oncogene* 1995; 11: 2113–20.

202. Sakura H, Kanei-Ishii C, Nagase T, Nakagoshi H, Gonda TJ, Ishii S. Delineation of three functional domains of the transcriptional activator encoded by the c-myb protooncogene. *Proc Natl Acad Sci USA* 1989; 86: 5758–62.

203. Weston K, Bishop JM. Transcriptional activation by the v-myb oncogene and its cellular progenitor, c-myb. *Cell* 1989; 58: 85–93.

204. Ess KC, Witte DP, Bascomb CP, Aronow BJ. Diverse developing mouse lineages exhibit high-level c-Myb expression in immature cells and loss of expression upon differentiation. *Oncogene* 1999; 18: 1103–11.

205. Gonda TJ, Metcalf D. Expression of myb, myc and fos proto-oncogenes during the differentiation of a murine myeloid leukaemia. *Nature* 1984; 310: 249–51.

206. Sheiness D, Gardinier M. Expression of a proto-oncogene (proto-myb) in hemopoietic tissues of mice. *Mol Cell Biol* 1984; 4: 1206–12.

207. Mucenski ML, McLain K, Kier AB, et al. A functional c-myb gene is required for normal murine fetal hepatic hematopoiesis. *Cell* 1991; 65: 677–89.

208. Friedman AD, Landschulz WH, McKnight SL. CCAAT/enhancer binding protein activates the promoter of the serum albumin gene in cultured hepatoma cells. *Genes Dev* 1989; 3: 1314–22.

209. Scott LM, Civin CI, Rorth P, Friedman AD. A novel temporal expression pattern of three C/EBP family members in differentiating myelomonocytic cells. *Blood* 1992; 80: 1725–35.

210. Gilpin DA, Hsieh CC, Kuninger DT, Herndon DN, Papaconstantinou J. Effect of thermal injury on the expression of transcription factors that regulate acute phase response genes: the response of C/EBP alpha, C/EBP beta, and C/EBP delta to thermal injury. *Surgery* 1996; 119: 674–83.

211. Landschulz WH, Johnson PF, McKnight SL. The DNA binding domain of the rat liver nuclear protein C/EBP is bipartite. *Science* 1989; 243: 1681–8.

212. Nerlov C, McNagny KM, Doderlein G, Kowenz-Leutz E, Graf T. Distinct C/EBP functions are required for eosinophil lineage commitment and maturation. *Genes Dev* 1998; 12: 2413–23.

213. Radomska HS, Huettner CS, Zhang P, Cheng T, Scadden DT, Tenen DG. CCAAT/enhancer binding protein alpha is a regulatory switch sufficient for induction of granulocytic development from bipotential myeloid progenitors. *Mol Cell Biol* 1998; 18: 4301–14.

214. Wang X, Scott E, Sawyers CL, Friedman AD. C/EBPalpha bypasses granulocyte colony-stimulating factor signals to rapidly induce PU.1 gene expression, stimulate granulocytic differentiation, and limit proliferation in 32D cl3 myeloblasts. *Blood* 1999; 94: 560–71.

215. Zhang DE, Zhang P, Wang ND, Hetherington CJ, Darlington GJ, Tenen DG.

Absence of granulocyte colony-stimulating factor signaling and neutrophil development in CCAAT enhancer binding protein alpha-deficient mice. *Proc Natl Acad Sci USA* 1997; 94: 569–74.

216. Screpanti I, Romani L, Musiani P, et al. Lymphoproliferative disorder and imbalanced T-helper response in C/EBP beta-deficient mice [published erratum appears in *Embo J* 1995 Jul 17;14(14):3596]. *Embo J* 1995; 14: 1932–41.

217. Tanaka T, Akira S, Yoshida K, et al. Targeted disruption of the NF-IL6 gene discloses its essential role in bacteria killing and tumor cytotoxicity by macrophages. *Cell* 1995; 80: 353–61.

218. Chen X, Liu W, Ambrosino C, et al. Impaired generation of bone marrow B lymphocytes in mice deficient in C/EBPbeta. *Blood* 1997; 90: 156–64.

219. Antonson P, Stellan B, Yamanaka R, Xanthopoulos KG. A novel human CCAAT/enhancer binding protein gene, C/EBPepsilon, is expressed in cells of lymphoid and myeloid lineages and is localized on chromosome 14q11.2 close to the T-cell receptor alpha/delta locus. *Genomics* 1996; 35: 30–8.

220. Cole MD. The myc oncogene: its role in transformation and differentiation. *Annu Rev Genet* 1986; 20: 361–84.

221. Blackwell TK, Kretzner L, Blackwood EM, Eisenman RN, Weintraub H. Sequence-specific DNA binding by the c-Myc protein. *Science* 1990; 250: 1149–51.

222. Baumbach WR, Stanley ER, Cole MD. Induction of clonal monocyte/macrophage tumors in vivo by a mouse c-myc retrovirus: evidence for secondary transforming events. *Curr Top Microbiol Immunol* 1986; 132: 23–32.

223. Delgado MD, Lerga A, Canelles M, Gomez-Casares MT, Leon J. Differential regulation of Max and role of c-Myc during erythroid and myelomonocytic differentiation of K562 cells. *Oncogene* 1995; 10: 1659–65.

224. Blackwood EM, Eisenman RN. Max: a helix-loop-helix zipper protein that forms a sequence-specific DNA-binding complex with Myc. *Science* 1991; 251: 1211–17.

225. Amin C, Wagner AJ, Hay N. Sequence-specific transcriptional activation by Myc and repression by Max. *Mol Cell Biol* 1993; 13: 383–90.

226. Ayer DE, Eisenman RN. A switch from Myc: Max to Mad:Max heterocomplexes accompanies monocyte/macrophage differentiation. *Genes Dev* 1993; 7: 2110–19.

227. Zervos AS, Gyuris J, Brent R. Mxi1, a protein that specifically interacts with Max to bind Myc-Max recognition sites [published erratum appears in *Cell* 1994 Oct 21;79(2):following 388]. *Cell* 1993; 72: 223–32.

228. Kretzner L, Blackwood EM, Eisenman RN. Transcriptional activities of the Myc and Max proteins in mammalian cells. *Curr Top Microbiol Immunol* 1992; 182: 435–43.

229. Cultraro CM, Bino T, Segal S. Regulated expression and function of the c-Myc antagonist, Mad1, during a molecular switch from proliferation to differentiation. *Curr Top Microbiol Immunol* 1997; 224: 149–58.

230. Larsson LG, Pettersson M, Oberg F, Nilsson K, Luscher B. Expression of mad, mxi1, max and c-myc during induced differentiation of hematopoietic cells: opposite regulation of mad and c-myc. *Oncogene* 1994; 9: 1247–52.

231. Foley KP, McArthur GA, Queva C, Hurlin PJ, Soriano P, Eisenman RN. Targeted disruption of the MYC antagonist MAD1 inhibits cell cycle exit during granulocyte differentiation. *Embo J* 1998; 17: 774–85.

232. McGinnis W, Garber RL, Wirz J, Kuroiwa A, Gehring WJ. A homologous protein-coding sequence in Drosophila homeotic genes and its conservation in other metazoans. *Cell* 1984; 37: 403–8.

233. Lawrence HJ, Largman C. Homeobox genes in normal hematopoiesis and leukemia. *Blood* 1992; 80: 2445–53.

234. Helgason CD, Sauvageau G, Lawrence HJ, Largman C, Humphries RK. Overexpression of HOXB4 enhances the hematopoietic potential of embryonic stem cells differentiated in vitro. *Blood* 1996; 87: 2740–9.

235. Lawrence HJ, Helgason CD, Sauvageau G, et al. Mice bearing a targeted interruption of the homeobox gene HOXA9 have defects in myeloid, erythroid, and lymphoid hematopoiesis. *Blood* 1997; 89: 1922–30.

236. Fuller JF, McAdara J, Yaron Y, Sakaguchi M, Fraser JK, Gasson JC. Characterization of HOX gene expression during myelopoiesis: role of HOX A5 in lineage commitment and maturation. *Blood* 1999; 93: 3391–400.

237. Lill MC, Fuller JF, Herzig R, Crooks GM, Gasson JC. The role of the homeobox gene, HOX B7, in human myelomonocytic differentiation. *Blood* 1995 85: 692–7.

238. Allen JD, Adams JM. Enforced expression of Hlx homeobox gene prompts myeloid cell maturation and altered adherence properties of T cells. *Blood* 1993; 81: 3242–51.

239. McGill V, Kowal-Vern A, Gamelli RL. A conservative thermal injury treatment protocol for the appropriate Jehovah's Witness candidate. *J Burn Care Rehabil* 1997; 18: 133–8.

240. Offringa M. Excess mortality after human albumin administration in critically ill patients. Clinical and pathophysiological evidence suggests albumin is harmful [editorial; comment] [see comments]. *Br Med J* 1998; 317: 223–4.

Chapter 26b

Significance of the adrenal and sympathetic response to burn injury

Stephen B Jones, Kumudika I de Silva
Ravi Shankar, Richard L Gamelli

Introduction

The physiological importance of the adrenal gland is most often associated with the release of epinephrine and glucocorticoids in response to cognitive stress widely recognized as the 'fight or flight' response. Such responses involving the hypothalamic–pituitary–adrenal axis begin with the hypothalamic release of corticotropin releasing hormone (CRH) that mediates the release of adrenocorticotrophic hormone (ACTH) from the pituitary that in turn stimulates cortisol synthesis and release from the adrenal cortex. Hypothalamic stimulation also initiates epinephrine and norepinephrine release from the adrenal medulla as well as the release of sympathetic neurotransmitter norepinephrine from adrenergic nerve terminals throughout the body. The action of these hormones and neurotransmitters is traditionally thought to serve in a compensatory manner, facilitating heightened mental awareness along with metabolic and cardiovascular activity that supports rapid increases in muscular work.

Thermal injury, like other forms of trauma as well as infectious challenge, is a noncognitive stimulus but also results in an elevated hormone/neurotransmitter milieu similar in magnitude to that of the cognitive 'fight or flight' response.[1,2] However, there are important characteristics of the injury response that contrast with the fight or flight response. These include prolonged hormone/neurotransmitter elevation, the absence of increased muscle work limiting metabolic demand, and the presence of massive tissue injury. Additional hormone/neurotransmitter responses may also be evoked by surgical debridement of burn wounds and skin grafting procedures. The second surge of stress hormones complicates the severe metabolic derangements and compromised immune capacity that is characteristic of the burn course during the initial 7–10 days following injury.

Regardless of the cognitive or noncognitive nature of stress hormone stimulation, events that increase corticosteroids and catecholamines represent a stress response but may or may not involve pathology. Traumatic injury, however, clearly initiates an initial stress response with a magnitude that is proportional to the severity of injury. Under these conditions, hormone/neurotransmitter release seems to promote survival. Although such a benefit may be difficult to see in human injury, experimental animal models have provided some insights. Animals that lack stress hormones or suffer from impaired release or where hormone action is pharmacologically blocked often die of an otherwise survivable event. Similarly, overwhelming traumatic injury in man may result in stress hormone release that is detrimental to survival. Whereas this may also be difficult to document in burn patients, animal studies have demonstrated that exogenous administration of high amounts of stress hormones is detrimental.

Two historical perspectives are important to consider regarding stress and the trauma of burn injury. First is the concept described by Cuthbertson,[3] where the initial response to thermal injury is considered an 'ebb' phase characterized by reduced metabolism and tissue perfusion. Within days there is a transition to a 'flow' phase typified by increased resting energy expenditure and hypermetabolism with supportive cardiovascular function. Changes in endocrine hormone levels are important for these acute catabolic alterations. The concepts of 'stress' and release of 'stress hormones' widely used today, were clarified by the classic work of Selye.[4] His notion of stress responses include an initial 'alarm reaction' of fairly short duration with high levels of stress hormones followed by a 'resistance phase' described as a prolonged period during which there is compensation to maintain homeostasis during continued stress. Selye's final stage of 'exhaustion' is where compensation could not be maintained and death rapidly follows. The acute initial period of high stress hormone release encompasses both Cuthbertson's 'ebb' phase and Selye's 'alarm reaction' and the 'flow phase'[3] has similar features of 'resistance phase'.[4] These compensatory changes promote increased energy expenditure and support cardiovascular function; however, in patients with severe injury the same compensatory changes result in depletion of energy reserves, extensive muscle wasting, and immune suppression, all of which are hallmarks of postburn sequelae. This compensatory pattern is described as a hypermetabolic state with patients displaying elevated resting metabolic rates for several weeks to months following injury.[5-7] The extent of the hypermetabolic response is dependent upon the extent and depth of burn injury, septic complications, and surgical interventions. Although the well-conceived concepts of 'ebb and flow' and generalized phases of stress help to conceptualize what is happening during recovery from uncomplicated thermal injury, questions related to the magnitude of stress hormone responses and beneficial versus detrimental actions in the recovery from severe thermal injury remain unanswered.

During the last 50 years great strides have been made in the care of burn patients using various treatment modalities in an attempt to exploit some of the concepts described above. Examples include: rapid fluid resuscitation to stabilize cardiovascular function and reduce the stimulus for continued sympathetic drive; nutritional support to meet metabolic demands and to support homeostasis during healing; elevated environmental temperatures and occlusive dressings to lessen the metabolic demands, reduce metabolic rate and cardiac output, and to optimize wound healing. Aside from the regulation of metabolic and cardiovascular function, neuro-immune interactions may be important in mediating the marked alterations in immune function that often follow severe injury. In this chapter we have chosen to present the adrenomedullary—neurotransmitter activation and actions as separate from the adrenocortical activation and actions to clarify specific responses as we currently understand them. To this end, the current chapter will review the magnitude and time course of the stress hormone/neurotransmitter responses to thermal injury as well as how the action of these substances may be integrated. How these responses may be beneficial or detrimental during the course of recovery will also be addressed. Given the cadre of pharmacologic antagonists and agonists available to the clinician, taking a mechanistic approach to understanding adrenal hormones and neurotransmitter involvement in the pathophysiology of severe thermal injury is critical to further advance the successful treatment of these patients.

Part I – Sympathetic activation following burn trauma: release of catecholamines

Although clinical observations suggested the activation of sympathetic nerves in response to thermal injury,[8-10] direct evidence for such activation was not fully appreciated until the simultaneous publication of papers by both American and Swedish groups that documented these responses.[11,12] These landmark studies described marked elevations in 24-hour urinary levels of norepinephrine and epinephrine in burn patients using a bioassay system. Despite considerable variation both within individuals and between patients, the increases in urinary norepinephrine and epinephrine were proportional to the severity (size) of the injury, were highest within the first 3 days postburn, and in many cases remained elevated for several weeks. Furthermore, these studies also suggested that subse-

quent surgical interventions and the onset of sepsis and septic shock such as hypotension or serious infections, caused catecholamine secretion to increase again. Since these early reports of urinary catecholamines, as measured by bioassay techniques, many studies have confirmed the initial sympathetic responses in burn patients using fluorometric, HPLC/electrochemical, or radioenzymatic techniques in plasma and urine samples.[13-16] However, documentation of the striking prolongation of sympathetic activation extending from 5 to 35 weeks following thermal injury[12] has not been repeated using newer analytical techniques. With improvements in critical care medicine and management of burn patients during the last 40 years, prolonged sympathetic activity may not occur during extended recovery. In contrast, elevations in catecholamines may still occur but cardiovascular, nutritional, and immune-related interventions, as part of the treatment regimen, may ameliorate the extent or impact of the hormone response. Nonetheless, in the light of the strong evidence for sympathetic activation consequent to thermal injury, the compensatory or possible decompensatory consequences are important to consider.

In response to thermal injury there are acute responses in what Cuthbertson[3] described as an 'ebb' phase and long-term responses that support a 'flow' phase. Cardiovascular adjustments to thermal injury appear to be critical for survival following burn trauma and with initial reductions in cardiac output sympathetic responses are rapidly brought into play as reviewed by Carleton.[17] Initial sympathetic activation contributes to the dramatic increases in peripheral vascular resistance that preserves mean arterial pressure but typically limits perfusion to the kidney and splanchnic beds. Although the mechanisms for the reduction in cardiac output are not completely understood, they are in part related to the sudden loss of vascular volume as a result of fluid transudation of plasma from the wound and from non-wound vascular sites.[18,19] Movement of fluids from the vascular to interstitial spaces are compounded by the loss of plasma proteins through the incompetent capillary beds that normally act to retain ions by Donnan equilibrium.[20] Such apparent hypovolemia would initially decrease blood pressure and baroreceptor afferent nerve activity with resultant increases in efferent sympathetic nerve activity. The resultant increase in peripheral vasoconstriction and consequent increase in peripheral vascular resistance are mediated in part by nerve-stimulated release of norepinephrine but also to a significant degree by both angiotensin II (AII) and arginine vasopressin.[14,21] Since arginine vasopressin (AVP) has been shown to directly depress myocardial function in the isolated heart and this depression can be reversed pharmacologically, AVP may contribute to myocardial depression following burn injury.[22]

Myocardial depression following thermal injury can be manifest as decreased cardiac output due to decreases in vascular volume, reductions in diastolic compliance, as well as decreases in myocardial contractility. Various 'myocardial depressant factors' have also been described for many years without specific detailed identification of the actual substances. Such deficits in contractility are compounded by the increases in aortic pressure afterload that is the consequence of increased peripheral vascular resistance and, in total, contribute to the observed reductions in cardiac output. Although diastolic dysfunction has been demonstrated in patients following thermal injury, evidence for decreases in contractility are largely based on animal studies with little evidence that this occurs in patients. Consequent to decreased ventricular performance and potential intrinsic myocardial dysfunction, sympathetic drive would be important to maintain ventricular function of the non-compromised muscle upon recovery from thermal injury. However, partial β-adrenergic blockade has been successfully used in pediatric burn patients without severe compromise in cardiovascular function.[23] Such treatment did not change cardiac index, but significantly decreased heart rate, left ventricular stroke work index, stroke volume index, and rate–pressure product. Adult burn patients have also been treated with β-blockade but cardiovascular measurements are not available.[24]

Cardiovascular disturbances might be predicted to be the dominant signal initiating a generalized sympathetic response but the persistence of such sympathetic activation after hemodynamic stabilization suggests that afferent stimulation from other sources may initiate as well as maintain this response. Hemodynamic stabilization in burn patients typically requires 1–2 days after fluid resuscitation and is followed by the 'flow phase' of recovery characterized by low peripheral vascular resistance, elevated cardiac output, increased peripheral blood flow, and increased metabolism.[25] The marked decrease in peripheral vascular resistance most likely drives this hyperdynamic phase by decreasing cardiac afterload, increasing cardiac preload and thus, increasing cardiac output. There is abundant evidence that mediators of neural, humoral, and metabolic origin are involved in driving the decrease in vascular resistance following thermal injury but, which ones are dominant and details of the time sequence of release are not well-defined. Specific adrenergic agonists such as epinephrine may be involved through actions on vascular β-adrenergic receptors that mediate vasodilation[26] and the specific importance of β_2-adrenergic receptors in vasodilation has recently been demonstrated using knockout mice.[27] The situation is complicated in the burn patient by the increase in nerve-stimulated release of norepinephrine, which has the potential to mediate vasoconstriction. However, there is evidence that the local distribution of adrenergic receptors mediating either vasodilation or vasoconstriction will determine the effect of circulating epinephrine and nerve-stimulated norepinephrine release on peripheral vascular resistance.[28] In addition, increased tissue metabolism has been recognized for many years to produce metabolites that mediate increased blood flow by decreasing vascular resistance.[29] With markedly increased metabolism in major burns, these metabolites along with catecholamines, nitric oxide,[30] and atrial natriuretic peptide[14] may contribute to the observed decreased vascular resistance.

Typically, decreases in tissue perfusion leading to compromised organ function only occur in patients with complications related to septic events or severe metabolic acidosis. Most often in thermally injured patients there is a modest decrease in mean arterial blood pressure that is not indicative of hypoperfusion and is left untreated. Where decreases in peripheral vascular resistance become dominant with marked decreases in mean arterial pressure, pressor agents may be required to maintain adequate tissue perfusion and norepinephrine is the drug of choice providing both vasoconstrictor and inotropic effects. Clinical use of vasoconstrictor and intropic agents is essential to counter low tissue perfusion during periods of altered hemodynamic function often seen with the onset of sepsis in burn patients.

In this regard it is interesting to note the recent work by Macarthur et al.[31] suggesting that the inactivation of catecholamines by superoxide anions contributes to the observed hypotension of septic shock. Treatment of rats with superoxide dismutase not only abrogated the endotoxin-induced hypotension but also elevated circulating levels of catecholamines. These findings suggest that compensatory sympathetic activation to counteract hypotension may be blunted by inactivation of catecholamines by the extracellular milieu in sepsis. Similar deactivation of catecholamines may take place in burn patients with septic complications, thereby reducing the availability of endogenous norepinephrine to maintain normal blood pressure and organ perfusion. In routine clinical management of critically ill burn patients, exogenous norepinephrine is routinely administered to correct life-threatening hypotension.

Following the initial insult of thermal injury the 'ebb' or immediate phase of recovery is characterized by decreased body temperature and decreased oxygen consumption that is accompanied with progressively elevated lactate levels and developing hyperglycemia.[32,33] The same period of recovery involves intense sympathetic stimulation, suggesting the involvement of adrenergic mechanisms mediated by adenylyl cyclase and cAMP in the mobilization of liver glycogen to glucose.[34] Developing hypermetabolism that follows 1–2 days later in the 'flow' phase can also be attributed to adrenergic influences[15,35] but does not involve increased glucose mobilization and utilization since adrenergic blockade increases rather than decreases glucose production and clearance under these hypermetabolic conditions.[36] The experimental studies of Wolfe and Durkot[36] suggest that adrenergic drive following thermal injury facilitates lipolysis, driving increased fatty acid oxidation. These results are based on changes observed following adrenergic blockade with propranolol and further clarify that the observed increase in glucose production and clearance under such conditions reflects a shift to carbohydrate utilization in the absence of mobilized lipid. Examination of the importance of adrenergic drive on lipid metabolism following thermal injury was extended to human patients through the use of stable isotopic studies as well as adrenergic antagonists.[37–39] These results not only indicate that lipolysis following thermal injury is mediated by β_2-adrenergic receptors but suggest increased triglyceride-fatty acid cycling with resultant heat production.

The initial description of the sustained hypermetabolic response to thermal injury[40] prompted studies to examine the role of thyroid function and catecholamines in mediating this response. Although abnormal thyroid function was not involved in the response,[40,41] Wilmore developed experimental paradigms supportive of the role of catecholamines in the hypermetabolic response to thermal injury.[15] Evidence for the positive correlation of increased plasma catecholamines and whole-body oxygen consumption following thermal injury,[15] as well as the demonstration that adrenergic blockade lowers the thermal injury-induced increase in metabolic rate and cardiac output to control levels in animal models directly support this contention.[15,36] However, experimental findings using the rat suggested that the adrenal medulla is essential for high rates of heat production following thermal injury but is not responsible for the primary drive of the hypermetabolic response.[42,43] These conclusions are further supported by experiments examining hypothalamic temperature regulation that suggest an upward shift in the set or operating temperature following thermal injury. The net result of this shift is increased metabolism at room temperature. Animals with hypothalamic lesions did not increase metabolism following thermal injury and were chronically hypothermic[44] not unlike experiments where the adrenal medulla was removed prior to thermal injury.[42] These results are consistent with clinical observations in burn patients, in whom reductions in heat loss were achieved with occlusive dressings and elevated environmental temperatures causing decreased metabolic rate and catecholamine secretion.[13,45] Taken together, these findings suggest that in burn patients, catecholamines are important components of the hypermetabolic response but act through temperature regulatory mechanisms. Regardless of the specific mechanisms involved, maintaining elevated environmental temperatures reduces the metabolic demands of the burn patient, resulting in decreased oxygen consumption and cardiac output.

An important and all too frequent complication of severe thermal injury is infection that frequently leads to sepsis, septic shock, multiple organ failure, and death. The development of septic complications can decrease predicted survivability by up to 50%.[46] As with thermal injury, infection results in marked sympathetic responses that are well-characterized in both experimental and clinical settings. Whereas experimental paradigms of sepsis have used plasma catecholamines, nerve recordings, and norepinephrine turnover to assess sympathetic activation,[47–52] human studies have primarily focused on changes in plasma catecholamines.[1] Similar to thermal injury, sympathetic responses also appear to be proportional to the degree of insult, based on experiments using incremental doses of bacterial endotoxin.[48] Furthermore, animal models of septic peritonitis suggest that initial sympathetic activation as measured by elevated levels of plasma norepinephrine and norepinephrine turnover persist for many hours.[49,50] Burn patients are most susceptible to infection during the second week of their hospitalization when the sympathetic response as reflected by urinary and plasma catecholamines has moderated but is still elevated.[13,14,16] Although the onset of bacterial infection and developing sepsis would be expected to cause marked increases in plasma catecholamines above that due to burn alone, longitudinal studies charting the course of plasma catecholamines following thermal injury leading into infection and progressing into septic shock are not available. While the consequences of secondary insults following the initial injury are important to consider, unfortunately no information is available comparing plasma catecholamine changes with burn and burn plus sepsis.

Sympathetic Influences on Immune Function (Table 26b.1)

Over the last 15 years our understanding of the interactions between neural and immune cell systems has greatly advanced. The present review is particularly concerned with the relationship between sympathetic nerves and immune cell functions that would provide insight relative to the host response of thermally injured patients. For the activation of sympathetic nerves to influence immune responses, evidence of sympathetic innervation in peripheral immune structures, namely the lymphoid organs, is important to consider. Existing anatomical evidence is based on immunohistochemical techniques to visualize tyrosine hydroxylase, the rate-limiting step in the biosynthesis of norepinephrine. These studies clearly indicate a substantial innervation of all primary (thymus and bone marrow) and secondary (spleen and lymph nodes) lymphoid organs.[53–57] Furthermore, they also show sympathetic innervation in the immune cell compartment of the spleen (the white pulp), the periarterial lymphoid sheath, marginal zone and marginal sinus areas, as well as in the splenic capsule and trabecu-

Table 26b.1 Influence of catecholamines on cardiovascular, metabolic and immune response to thermal injury

Physiologic Variable	Sympathetic Mediated change following burn injury
Resting metabolic rate	Increase[35] Increase[36] Increase[15] Increase (in vitro)[264]
Proteolysis	No change (urea production)[39] No change (protein oxidation)[35] Decrease[23]
Glucose production and oxidation	Decrease secondary to increase in lipid catabolism[36,265] No change[35]
Glycogenolysis	Increase (indirect evidence via cAMP)[34]
Gluconeogenesis	Increase (indirect evidence via cAMP)[34]
Lipolysis	Increase[39] Increase[35] Increase[36] Increase[38]
Cardiac output	Increase[36] Increase[39]
Peripheral vascular resistance	Unknown
Heart rate	Increase[23] Increase[39]
T cell number and function	Unknown
B cell number and function	Unknown
Neutrophil number and function	Unknown
Monocyte number and function	Increase (indirect – clonogenic potential)[144]

Citation of studies from the current literature, suggesting that sympathetic activation is involved in changing the above physiologic variables following thermal injury.

lae.[58–62] Sympathetic nerve terminals have been described in direct apposition to T cells, interdigitating dendritic cells and B cells using electron microscopic techniques.[61] The proximity of nerve terminals to immune cells may be critical in achieving the necessary local concentrations of neurotransmitters at the neuro–immune junctions to modulate immune functions. In fact, the neuro–immune junction is estimated at 6 nm[62] in comparison to 20 nm in typical CNS junctions. Therefore, a high enough neurotransmitter concentration could be realized across these small junctions to impact on resident immune cells.

Anatomical evidence of sympathetic innervation of the immune system is complemented by evidence for nerve-stimulated release of norepinephrine neurotransmitter in both spleen and bone marrow.[63] Whereas evidence in spleen has been recognized for many years and has been assessed in a variety of ways, norepinephrine release in bone marrow has only been recently described using norepinephrine turnover techniques based on radiotracer methods involving *in vivo* experimental paradigms.[63] In contrast, exocytosis of norepinephrine from lymph nodes has not been demonstrated. To complete the criteria for the physiologic importance of functional innervation, nerve-stimulated release of norepinephrine within lymphoid organs must increase at the appropriate time to influence the immune response and norepinephrine modulation of immune responses must be demonstrated.

β-adrenergic receptors, particularly β-2 subtypes, are known to be expressed on a number of different immune cells including activated and resting B cells, naïve CD4+ T cells, T-helper (Th1) cell clones and newly generated Th1 cells, but they are not expressed in newly-generated Th2 cells.[64–67] Furthermore, there is significant evidence that norepinephrine can modulate the function of CD4+ T cells, which in turn can modulate antibody production of B cells.[68] In addition, norepinephrine can directly influence B cell antibody production depending upon the time of exposure following activation.[69,70] The physiologic importance of these *in vitro* findings are supported by a series of *in vivo* experiments involving severe combined immune deficient (*scid*) mice depleted of norepinephrine prior to reconstitution with antigen-specific Th2 and B cells. These experiments demonstrate that norepinephrine is necessary for maintaining a normal level of antibody production *in vivo*.[64] Furthermore, other recent whole animal experiments, also involving *scid* mice, provide evidence that the immune response itself stimulates the release of norepinephrine from adrenergic nerve terminals in bone marrow and spleen, that in turn can influence antibody production by B cells.[71] Although these findings fall far short of direct application to immune cell function following thermal injury they suggest the important potential of sympathetic activation in mediating immune responses.

In addition to neural influences on T and B cell function, there are direct effects on myeloid cell function particularly with respect to lipopolysaccharide (LPS)-stimulated cytokine production. The most striking example of neural influences on macrophage function was demonstrated by the work of Spengler *et al.*[72] who concluded that α-adrenergic stimulation increased TNFα release whereas β-adrenergic stimulation decreased such release in response to LPS. They provided further evidence to suggest that extracellular stores of catecholamines in macrophages are capable of modulating TNFα release. Furthermore, sympathetic inhibition of TNFα release initiated by LPS has been suggested to occur in whole animal preparations although adrenergic actions on macrophages were indirect.[73–78] More direct evidence of adrenergic inhibition of LPS-stimulated TNFα production has involved whole blood.[78–83] Apart from adrenergic inhibition of LPS-stimulated TNFα release in isolated macrophages[84–87] similar inhibition of LPS-stimulated TNFα production has also been demonstrated in human mast cells,[88] microglial cells[89] astrocytes,[90] and cytotoxic T lymphocytes.[91] In contrast to adrenergic stimulation of TNFα release, experiments with isolated atria,[92,93] myenteric plexus[94] and brain tissue[95] have demonstrated that TNFα can negatively impact the release of norepinephrine.

Adrenergic influences on the expression and release of interleukin-6 (IL-6) has been suggested by a number of studies demonstrating increases in plasma IL-6 in response to direct or indirect stimulation.[96–98] Adrenergic enhancement of IL-6 responses to LPS has also been demonstrated *in vivo*[73,75] as well as in *ex vivo* paradigms using isolated liver.[87] In isolated cell systems, adrenergic

stimulation enhances LPS-induced IL-6 response.[99,100] Catecholamines in combination with IL-1β stimulate IL-6 release from rat C6 glioma cells and vasoactive intestinal polypeptide (VIP) has been reported to synergize with norepinephrine to induce IL-6 release in astrocytes.[101,102] In addition, adrenergic agonists have been shown to mediate IL-6 release in brown adipocytes, pituicytes, hepatocytes, astrocytes and thymic epithelial cells.[101,103–107]

In contrast, Nakamura *et al.*[90] reported that catecholamines decreased the IL-6 response to LPS and van der Poll *et al.*[82] demonstrated that norepinephrine inhibits the LPS-induced IL-6 response in whole blood. Other evidence for adrenergic suppression of IL-6 responses has been suggested by the work of Straub.[108–110] Using isolated splenic tissue preparation, electrically stimulated release of norepinephrine appears to inhibit IL-6 production induced by LPS or bacteria. These authors suggest that adrenergic inhibition of IL-6 is reduced under conditions simulating infection where cytokine mediation of the inflammatory response is compensatory in eradicating the bacterial load. It is apparent from these studies that catecholamines can exert a negative or a positive influence on proinflammatory cytokines, especially IL-6. However, when these different modulatory functions come into play and what role(s) they play in the pathophysiology of burn injury are unexplored.

Although the exact mechanisms of the negative modulation of proinflammatory cytokines by catecholamines are poorly understood, it may be achieved through the ability of catecholamines to induce the anti-inflammatory cytokine IL-10.[75,79,111–113] Whole animal studies involving assessment of circulating levels of IL-10[75] as well as studies of human whole blood and mononuclear cells stimulated with LPS in the presence of adrenergic agonists[78,79,112] support this premise. In addition, experimental neurotrauma results in increased IL-10 consequent to endogenous adrenergic stimulation in the absence of LPS or other evidence of infectious challenge.[114] The only experimental evidence suggesting an attenuation of IL-10 with adrenergic stimulation involved a macrophage cell line (RAW 264.7).[115]

Evidence that elevations of IL-10 can be blocked with inhibition of protein kinase A[112,116] is consistent with adrenergic mediation of changes in TNFα and IL-6 and suggest that activation of protein kinase A is important in mediating these adrenergic modulations of cytokine release. More specifically, the recent work of Platzer *et al.*[113] suggests that catecholamines in monocytic cells directly stimulate the IL-10 promoter/enhancer and provide evidence that a cAMP response element was the major target of the cAMP/protein kinase A pathway. Taken together, these findings suggest that sympathetic stimulation as a consequence of traumatic injury or infectious challenge may serve in a compensatory manner to blunt excessively high production and release of inflammatory cytokines. However, given the very limited exploration of this concept with experimental injury and sepsis, such beneficial actions of catecholamine–cytokine interactions remain speculative.

Adrenergic Stimulation of Bacterial Growth

Since the identification of mammalian hormone and neurotransmitter receptors in bacterial cells there has been considerable interest in defining a role for such signaling molecules in bacterial cells. As a consequence during the last 10 years support has emerged for the concept that release of norepinephrine within intestinal tissue promotes the growth of bacteria within the gut.[117–119] Initial experiments demonstrated the growth-promoting action of catecholamines *in vitro* using several different bacterial species and provided evidence that these compounds were not acting as nutritional substrates. Since growth-stimulating effects of norepinephrine were not blocked by adrenergic blocking agents, adrenergic receptors do not appear to be involved.[120,121] Further observations suggest that norepinephrine may act within an 8-hour period to induce bacterial growth during which time stimulation of growth factors can promote bacterial growth.[122,123] Norepinephrine-stimulated bacterial growth has also been shown to produce Shiga-like enterotoxins from enterohemorrhagic strains of *E. coli*. Furthermore, norepinephrine promotes the expression of K99⁺ pilus adhesin, a virulence factor known to play a critical role in the attachment of these bacteria to the intestinal wall which initiates the infective process.[124,125] Although these studies utilize very high concentrations of norepinephrine compared to the observed plasma concentrations following thermal injury, bacteria *in vivo* may be exposed to high norepinephrine concentrations if such bacteria are in close proximity to the nerve terminal synapse. A related concern is the lack of information regarding the actual norepinephrine concentration within the culture media throughout the incubation period. Whereas rapidly growing bacterial cultures may generate an acid environment in which catecholamines are quite stable, initial growth conditions containing low bacterial counts and minimal nutrients may promote rapid deterioration of norepinephrine. However, high initial norepinephrine concentrations in cultures may counteract such unfavorable conditions but in turn would provide misleading dose–response information.

The intense sympathetic innervation of the gut and associated structures has been recognized for many years with well-defined nerve terminals located primarily along blood vessels but without evidence of neurotransmitter release into the intestinal lumen. Furthermore, there is considerable evidence that once released from nerve terminals, most norepinephrine is taken back into the same terminals by uptake 1 (active) or 2 (passive) mechanisms, metabolized into a non-active form or diffuses through tissues to reach blood vessels to become part of the circulation.[126] Thus, even though intestinal bacterial growth has the potential to be enhanced by the neurotransmitter norepinephrine, transport of the norepinephrine into the intestinal lumen would seem problematic. However, since massive catecholamine release is such a consistent component of burn patients, especially those with superimposed sepsis, the hypothesis that bacterial growth can be enhanced by norepinephrine is very appealing.

Important *in vivo* findings strengthen this concept by demonstrating that cecal bacterial growth increases dramatically following massive *in vivo* release of norepinephrine and that passage of bacteria through the gut enhance their growth response to norepinephrine. In the first case[117] mice were treated with 6-hydroxydopamine, a neurotoxin that displaces norepinephrine from adrenergic nerve terminals causing a transient but massive sympathetic reaction. At 24 hours post treatment, cecal bacterial growth was elevated 3–4 degrees of magnitude compared to vehicle-treated controls but bacterial growth returned to control levels by 14 days. In the second study,[127] an attenuated strain of *Salmonella typhimurium* was administered to rhesus monkeys, whereupon isolated fecal bacterial cultures from these animals displayed increased *in vitro* growth response to norepinephrine. To elucidate whether this hypothesis has a role in the pathophysiology of thermal injury with sepsis, future studies must build on experimental paradigms of thermal injury to demonstrate that endogenous norepinephrine enhances bacterial growth leading to sepsis.

Evidence For Norepinephrine Regulation of Myelopoiesis in Experimental Thermal Injury with Sepsis

Patients with severe burn trauma often display significant impairment in cell-mediated immunity involving defective neutrophil chemotaxis, phagocytosis, and superoxide production.[128–131] Patients with sepsis and systemic inflammatory response may also present with monocytosis and neutropenia.[132,133] While neutropenia and defective neutrophil functions may compromise host defense, monocytosis has the potential to fuel excessive cytokine production through increased availability of circulating and tissue monocyte/macrophages. For the past several years our laboratory has been investigating bone marrow function following thermal injury with sepsis to understand mechanisms that govern leukocyte production and how they might contribute to the observed defects in leukocyte functions. Since adrenergic mechanisms as described above are involved in a variety of host-defense functions[134–137] we have begun to consider the possibility that sympathetic activation may in some way contribute to the immunological components of the pathophysiology of thermal injury with sepsis. Several key factors suggest the possibility that the observed changes in myelopoiesis may be in part mediated by sympathetic nerve activation associated with thermal injury. First, adrenergic signaling has been shown to function in regulation and control of hematopoiesis.[138,139] Maestroni[139] has demonstrated not only the presence of adrenergic receptors on bone marrow immune cells but also that adrenergic agonists stimulate lymphopoiesis while attenuating myelopoiesis. These findings are further strengthened by experiments in animal models demonstrating adrenergic agents can modulate lympho- and myelopoiesis.[140–143] A second major finding is the demonstration that sympathetic activation within the bone marrow compartment results in nerve-stimulated release of norepinephrine that could reach high concentrations in close proximity to proliferating immune cells. We have recently reported a significant increase in bone marrow norepinephrine release in response to either cold exposure or bacteria through the use of traditional pulse-chase experiments.[63] More recently, we have extended these measurements to our murine model of thermal injury with sepsis and demonstrated increased bone marrow norepinephrine release in response to thermal injury with sepsis.[144]

Taken together these findings argue for a relationship between sympathetic activation and alterations in bone marrow production of leukocytes that may lead to development of opportunistic bacterial infection. Whereas experimental evidence suggests adrenergic regulation of myelopoiesis under normal conditions, evidence demonstrating cause–effect relationships between the two injury states has never been examined. Therefore, we hypothesized that immune alterations induced by thermal injury with infection are mediated at least in part by sympathetic modulation of myelopoiesis in bone marrow consequent to the trauma of thermal injury.

Previous studies of potential mechanisms that could account for immunosuppression of patients with severe burns have focused primarily on functional alterations in circulating and tissue leukocytes.[145–151] In contrast, our focus has been on the bone marrow responses following thermal injury with sepsis as it is a major source of leukocytes both in the circulation and tissues. Using a well-established murine model of thermal injury (15% TBSA) and *Pseudomonas aeruginosa* sepsis (1000 CFU at the wound site) we have previously demonstrated a shift in myeloid commitment toward monocytopoiesis and away from granulocytopoiesis.[152,153]

Since we have also demonstrated increased nerve-stimulated release of norepinephrine following thermal injury with sepsis, we tested the premise that such neural stimulation was modulating myeloid function under such conditions by manipulating the peripheral stores of norepinephrine prior to injury. Peripheral norepinephrine levels were reduced by using 6-hydroxydopamine (6-OHDA) and then animals were subjected to thermal injury with sepsis. Following thermal injury and sepsis, femoral bone marrow cells from mice with reduced norepinephrine demonstrated a significant decrease in monocytopoetic potential compared to mice with intact bone marrow norepinephrine stores subjected to the same experimental conditions.[144] This abrogated monocytopoietic potential following injury consequent to reduced norepinephrine suggests that injury-induced sympathetic responses may have marked effects on bone marrow progenitor cells and may significantly alter leukocyte production following traumatic injury.

The influence of norepinephrine on bone marrow monocyte production was also assessed following thermal injury with sepsis by determining the presence of developmental cell surface markers ER-MP12 and 20 using flow cytometry. While ER-MP12 is an antibody to early monocyte progenitors and represents predominantly CFU-M, progressively more ER-MP20 antigen is expressed from the CFU-M stage onwards but disappears after the monocytic stage.[154] By following the distribution pattern of the expression of these two antigens on bone marrow cells the phenotypic separation and identification of bone marrow monocyte precursors have been demonstrated.[155] Results of bone marrow cell staining using such markers in animals with intact norepinephrine stores suggests that under control (sham) conditions there is a substantial population of the immature monocyte progenitors which decrease with thermal injury with sepsis. Furthermore, there is a substantial population of cells in the intermediate stage of development and this population increases with thermal injury and increases even more following thermal injury with sepsis. In contrast, norepinephrine-depleted animals subjected to the same protocols present an entirely different distribution pattern of monocyte progenitors using these markers. The norepinephrine-depleted sham group has very few cells in the immature and intermediate compartments, with most cells staining for the mature monocyte progenitor cells. Thermal injury in norepinephrine-depleted animals resulted in further increases in mature monocyte progenitors. Taken together these results suggest that monocyte maturation pathways may be greatly influenced by the presence of norepinephrine.

Both these findings in monocyte maturation and monocytopoietic potential with reduced bone marrow norepinephrine take on added significance in light of altered lethality of animals in these same experimental paradigms. Animals with reduced tissue norepinephrine levels as a result of 6-OHDA were subjected to thermal injury with sepsis and then followed for 12 days and compared to vehicle-treated animals subjected to the same protocol. Results indicate an 18% mortality at day 3 in norepinephrine-depleted mice compared to 44% mortality in vehicle-treated mice. More dramatic, however, are the 10 of 16 total mice treated with 6-

OHDA that survived the thermal injury with sepsis after 7 days. Thermal injury alone did not result in any mortality. Norepinephrine-depleted mice surviving thermal injury with sepsis were monitored for 5 days beyond the time when all of the vehicle-treated mice had died. This 62% survival with norepinephrine depletion compared with no survivors beyond day 7 in the non-treated group suggest that norepinephrine reductions in some way facilitate a positive outcome to thermal injury with sepsis.

These results are the first evidence of a modulation of bone marrow myelopoiesis by sympathetic activation following thermal injury with sepsis. Based on the reduction of tissue norepinephrine stores prior to thermal injury that significantly attenuates the elevated monocytopoetic potential of bone marrow cells, there is also a dramatic increase in survival of burn-septic animals. The reductions in monocytopoetic potential and improved survival are consistent with the widely accepted concept that increased availability and activation of monocyte/macrophage following thermal injury and sepsis promote systemic inflammatory responses, sepsis, and multiple organ failure. Linking the increases in bone marrow norepinephrine release and bone marrow monocytopoiesis define a previously unknown role for norepinephrine in the pathophysiology of injury and sepsis. Recognizing the relationship between sympathetic nerves and regulation of myelopoietic function by linking the increases in bone marrow norepinephrine release and bone marrow monocytopoiesis under injury conditions is the most significant aspect of this work and sheds new light on the importance of sympathetic activation in bone marrow myelopoiesis.

Although the murine animal model in the present study involves essential clinical features of thermal injury with infection there may be important limitations. Whereas the murine animal model involves immediate infection following thermal injury, burn patients typically develop septic complications in the second week of their hospitalization. This does not, however, change the interpretation that the present work is important new evidence that links increased sympathetic activation in bone marrow and increased myelopoietic potential following thermal injury with sepsis. In understanding the pathophysiology of injury states, the present results dictate a new conceptual framework in which to consider immune responses that occur in response to injury. This new frame of reference implies that immune responses following injury should be considered in regard to the potential action of sympathetic neurotransmitters on cellular events including the bone marrow compartment.

Part II – Adrenal cortical steroids following burn trauma: release of glucocorticoids

Whereas the acute 'ebb' phase of recovery from thermal injury is mainly dependent upon re-establishment of cardiovascular function following circulatory disruption, the 'flow' phase is considered to be dependent upon an adequate metabolic response. These responses are mediated in part by adrenal cortical steroids, of which cortisol is the dominant glucocorticoid hormone. Elevation of glucocorticoids occurs in response to most forms of trauma,[156] including burn injury, with rapid increases in blood and urine levels.[8,157] During the first 2 weeks following burn injury, the extent of elevation of total plasma cortisol concentration is proportional to the severity of the injury.[158] Early studies observed that glucocorticoid levels were excessively high in severely burned patients and remained high in nonsurviving patients.[157,159] In burn patients where recovery is likely, plasma glucocorticoid levels are moderately elevated or are in the upper normal range and can persist for up to 36 days[158,160] and return to normal as healing progresses.[157] In contrast, patients with severe injury (90% TBSA) have markedly lower levels of glucocorticoid concentration, suggesting that they are unable to mount an adequate response.[158]

Glucocorticoids circulate in the body bound to cortisol-binding protein (CBG) or transcortin, as an inactive complex. Only 1–10% of total plasma cortisol circulates unbound and it is this free fraction that is responsible for the biological activity of glucocorticoids. Burn injury results in a shift in the equilibrium between unbound cortisol and total cortisol towards an elevation in the unbound fraction.[158] Serum CBG as well as CBG-binding capacity are low in burn injury, severe infection, and septic shock.[158,161,162] In burn patients, CBG levels have been shown to decrease markedly, with lowest values occurring 48 hours after injury.[163] Even a minor burn such as 3% TBSA results in the reduction of serum CBG levels by 30%,[164] which return to normal levels 1–2 weeks later. The net effect of the decrease in CBG levels following thermal injury may not only result in increased free levels of cortisol but also in the amount of excreted cortisol which is reflected in high urinary corticosteroid levels in burn patients. Additional explanations for the increased levels of corticosteroids in burn patients may be due to the direct inhibitory effect of corticosteroids on the biosynthesis of CBG.[165–167] Furthermore, the proinflammatory cytokine IL-6 which is known to be elevated following massive burns has also been implicated in reducing CBG synthesis. Human hepatoma-derived cells (HepG2) respond to IL-6 by decreasing CBG protein and mRNA.[168]

The hypothalamic–pituitary–adrenal axis displays a biphasic pattern during the course of critical illness. In the initial phase, excessive cortisol levels are associated with elevated levels of ACTH. In the second phase, which occurs 3–5 days after the initial injury, ACTH levels decline while cortisol remains elevated.[2,169] There is some evidence to suggest that cortisol elevation with decreased ACTH may be driven by endothelin or atrial natriuretic peptide/hormone (ANP/H). Vermes et al.[169] demonstrated that both plasma endothelin and ANP levels were significantly elevated for 8 days following hospitalization in severely ill patients with sepsis or trauma. In addition, infusion of ANP in humans has been shown to block CRH-stimulated secretion of ACTH and cortisol,[170] while endothelin-1 and endothelin-3 enhance secretion of steroid hormones from the adrenal cortex.[171] Furthermore, endothelin-3 has been reported to elevate ACTH and corticosterone levels in rats[172] while endothelin-1 results in elevated ACTH in humans.[173] Based on this information, Vermes et al.[169] suggest that endothelin may be responsible for stimulating steroid secretion while ANP's action on the hypothalamic–pituitary axis may suppress ACTH secretion, thus explaining the paradoxical increase in cortisol with concomitant low ACTH levels in severely stressed patients.

Release of C_{19} Steroids

Dehydroepiandrosterone sulfate (DHEAS), a weak androgen, is the major androgen product of the human adrenal cortex. Despite the increase in cortisol secretion by the adrenals in burn patients, there is a distinct decrease in serum DHEAS levels.[174] This is due to a reduction in the synthesis and secretion rather than an effect of enhanced metabolism or excretion.[175] While serum DHEAS levels

decrease gradually, testosterone and androstenedione levels decrease abruptly. In some burn patients, subnormal testosterone levels persist for 3–18 months following the burn injury whereas cortisol levels return to normal earlier.[175] The decrease in testosterone secretion may be due to a direct effect of excessive cortisol levels on the testis.[176,177]

It appears that synthesis of C_{19} steroids by the adrenals and testes is compromised as a result of enhanced production of the C_{21}-steroids such as cortisol. Aldosterone levels are also subnormal despite elevated plasma renin activity. This suggests a shift of pregnenolone metabolism away from mineralocorticoid and adrenal androgen pathways towards the glucocorticoid pathway.[174] The low level of DHEAS may also contribute to the suppressed state of the immune system in burn patients and will be discussed later.

Influence On Metabolic Pathways (Table 26b.2)

High energy expenditure and hyperglycemia are hallmarks of thermal injury. The heavy demand for energy is due to the

Table 26b.2 Influence of glucocorticoids on metabolic and immune response to thermal injury

Physiologic variable	Glucocorticoid-mediated change following burn injury
Resting energy expenditure	Increased[5–7]
Oxygen consumption	Increased[266,267]
Primary fuel	Lipids, glucose[214]
Proteolysis	Increased in skeletal muscle[188,189,191,192,268]
Acute phase protein synthesis	Increased[168,269,270]
Nitrogen excretion	Increased[267]
Glycogenolysis	Increased via effect on glucagon[184,186]
Gluconeogenesis	Increased[180,181,269]
Lipolysis	Increased[215]
Ketone body formation	Normal[217]
Triglyceride level	Increased[217,269]
Thymic changes	Involution[236]
T cell population	Decreased[235,271]
T cell proliferation	Inhibited[237,238,270]
B cell population	Not conclusive from current data
Neutrophil population	Increased[240,271,272]
chemotaxis	Suppressed[240]
demargination	Increased[240,243]
bactericidal activity	Suppressed[244]
Monocyte population	Increased transiently with corticosteroids but decreased in burn patients[133,272,273]
chemotaxis	Suppressed[241]
bactericidal activity	Suppressed[241,274]
Bone formation	Decreased[223]

Citation of studies from the current literature suggesting that glucocorticoid release is involved in changing the above physiologic variables following thermal injury.

increase in essential functions such as the synthesis of proteins required for wound healing and the synthesis of acute phase proteins and inflammatory mediators. In addition, severe burns exert a burden on the metabolism to generate heat which in part compensates for the loss through the wound site. Part of the elevation in resting energy expenditure in burn patients is due to the increase in substrate cycling. This occurs when enzymes catalyzing opposing reactions of the same pathway are active simultaneously: for example, the conversion of glucose to glucose-6-phosphate and back to glucose. The demand for energy is increased in order to resynthesize ATP used in this and similar reactions. In burn patients the rates of glucose production and glycolysis as well as lipolysis and reesterification of triglycerides are elevated.[37] This cycling of substrates generates heat due to the hydrolysis of high-energy phosphate bonds in ATP, thus contributing to thermogenesis as well as increased energy requirement in burn patients. Keeping burn patients thermally comfortable lowers the metabolic rate and thus the demand for energy can also be lowered.[178] Increased glucocorticoid levels during severe burns can orchestrate multiple metabolic pathways to meet this energy demand. In order to understand how glucocorticoids may influence major metabolic pathways following thermal injury to facilitate the hypermetabolic state, in this section we will review the effects of glucocorticoids on glucose, protein, and fatty acid metabolism as they pertain to thermal injury.

Glucocorticoids and Glucose Metabolism

Glucocorticoids can contribute to hyperglycemia, which persists for several days, by enhancing endogenous production of glucose in the liver.[7,179–181] In burn injury, elevated glucose levels are predominantly sustained through gluconeogenesis and impaired glucose utilization. Increased levels of plasma lactate produced by peripheral tissues following thermal injury, as documented by Wolfe et al.,[182] is an essential substrate for gluconeogenesis by the liver. Recent evidence further confirms that thermal injury causes metabolic adaptations to enhance gluconeogenesis. Burn injury causes intrinsic alterations in the liver, which increases the flow of pyruvate to oxaloacetate at the expense of non-tricarboxylic acid cycle sources.[183] Mobilization of glucose stored as glycogen and skeletal muscle amino acids as substrates for gluconeogenesis requires glucagon secretion,[184,185] which is stimulated by glucocorticoids.[184,186] In addition to gluconeogenesis, insulin resistance can also play a role in sustaining high circulating levels of glucose in burn patients. For example, glucose utilization is impaired in burn patients who do not respond to insulin infusion.[7]

Glucocorticoids and Protein Metabolism

In severe burn injury protein catabolism is a part of the hypermetabolic state resulting in negative nitrogen balance. Cuthbertson's landmark studies[187] were the first to suggest the important concept that nitrogen loss is a whole-body response rather than a local burn-wound response. The increase in proteolysis seen in burn injury is, at least partly, mediated by glucocorticoids. In humans[188] and in animal models,[189] administration of glucocorticoids enhances muscle proteolysis. Further, burn injury-induced muscle proteolysis can be inhibited by a glucocorticoid receptor antagonist.[190] Amino acids mobilized from peripheral tissues are transported to the liver, where unlike in other tissues, cortisol stimulates protein synthesis. The increased hepatic protein synthesis in

response to cortisol can drive the new synthesis of gluconeogenic enzymes and acute phase proteins in response to injury.

Specific mechanisms involved in burn-mediated alterations in protein metabolism following thermal injury are not known. However, some information could be gleaned from studies on other states of excessive catabolism. In conditions such as metabolic acidosis, adrenalectomy halts muscle proteolysis and does not increase expression of components of the ubiquitin-proteasome pathway.[191,192] These effects can be reversed by dexamethasone administration. Further support for this premise is provided by in vitro studies, which show that dexamethasone-induced increases in proteolytic degradation in myocytes can be abolished by the glucocorticoid receptor inhibitor RU486.[193] Ding and coworkers[194] suggest that partial inhibition of the ubiquitin-proteasome pathway may be beneficial in enhanced catabolic states. Taken together these data suggest that interaction of glucocorticoids and the ATP-requiring ubiquitin-proteosome system may play an important role in burn-induced proteolysis.[194–199]

Another important aspect of protein catabolism following thermal injury is the generation of gluconeogenic amino acids. In fact, following thermal injury plasma levels of alanine are increased.[200] Nitrogen produced as a result of transaminating alanine to the gluconeogenic intermediate pyruvate is converted into glutamine and then to urea for excretion by the liver. Glutamine is one of the major participants in the translocation of amino acids from peripheral tissues to the liver for nitrogen excretion. Expression of the enzyme responsible for synthesis of this amino acid, glutamine synthase, is increased to compensate for the glutamine depletion in peripheral tissues. Following burn injury, glutamine synthase mRNA is increased first in the lung and later in muscle.[201] This is further supported by the observation that adrenalectomy partially decreases burn injury-induced glutamine synthase mRNA.[201] This is a tissue-specific response as no such effect is seen in the kidney or liver. There is evidence to suggest that glucocorticoids may augment glutamine synthesis. In lung and muscle tissues glucocorticoid administration increases glutamine production.[202] Mobilization of protein from peripheral tissues is also indicated by the increase in phenylalanine in the blood of burn patients.[200] Phenylalanine is the only amino acid that is not degraded by peripheral tissue and hence accumulates in the circulation when uptake by the liver is compromised.

The hypermetabolic and catabolic states seen in thermal injury remain long after the burn wound is completely healed.[5–7,203,204] In a recent study by Hart et al.[203] stable isotopic methodology and gas chromatography–mass spectrometry analysis were used to measure muscle kinetics in burned children. Reduction in protein catabolism and enhancement of lean body mass were only seen 9–12 months after the initial injury.[203] This suggests that treatment to alter growth deficiency must be prolonged long after early wound healing is complete.

Other more indirect effects of glucocorticoids on glucose levels in thermal injury include modulation of IGF-1, an important mediator of GH action.[205,206] Marked depression of all components of the IGF-1 complex are seen in burn injury.[207–211] Elevated glucocorticoid levels in burn patients may contribute to the suppression of the acid labile subunit (ALS) of the IGF-1 complex. Treatment of rats with dexamethasone results in low levels of serum ALS as well as liver ALS mRNA.[212,213]

In addition to the use of amino acids released from peripheral tissue to increase endogenous glucose production, body fat is the major source of energy in traumatic situations.[214] Free fatty acids are released from adipose tissue to be used as an alternate source of fuel during times of crisis, as is the case in thermal injury. Cortisol stimulates lipolysis,[215] enabling the release of free fatty acids. In burned children and adults increased lipolysis is reflected in the elevated plasma levels of palmitic and oleic acid.[38,216,217]

Influence on Bone Metabolism

Aside from combating the increased demand for energy, glucocorticoids also affect bone development, which has profound effects in children. Abnormal bone metabolism in burn injury has been demonstrated in animals and humans.[218,219] In children, the reduction in bone mineral density persists for at least 5 years after severe burn injury (>40% TBSA) and results in permanent retardation of linear growth.[220,221] The reasons for loss of bone mineral density include increased production of endogenous glucocorticoids, the inflammatory response, immobilization, aluminium loading, and production of cytokines such as IL-1 and IL-6 that facilitate bone resorption.[222]

Glucocorticoids have potent effects on bone formation and resorption, resulting in loss of bone mass. Weinstein and co-workers[223] investigated the long-term (equivalent to 3–4 human years) effects of glucocorticoids on bone metabolism in an animal model and reported a reduction in osteoclastogenesis causing reduced bone turnover and a reduction in osteoblastogenesis resulting in reduced bone formation. Enhanced osteoclast and osteoblast apoptosis was observed in mice subjected to long-term glucocorticoid administration as well as in patients with glucocorticoid-induced osteoporosis.[223] This depletion in the bone cell population limits the number of cells that can synthesize matrix proteins. In addition, glucocorticoids directly downregulate expression of type I collagen and upregulate expression of collagenase-3 in chondrocytes.[224] On the other hand, IGF-1 enhances expression of type I collagen and suppresses the expression of collagenase-3.[225] Thus the massive increase in glucocorticoids and the corresponding decrease in IGF-1 in burn injury has the ability to profoundly alter bone and cartilage formation.

The mechanisms by which glucocorticoids mediate bone resorption are not clear. One possible mechanism is that glucocorticoids increase osteoclast apoptosis.[226] Glucocorticoids may also mediate bone resorption by its dual capacity to initially inhibit osteoclast synthesis but later stimulate osteoclast synthesis coupled with an increase in bone resorption.[227] Yet another mechanism by which cortisol may influence bone resorption is by suppression of IGF-1- or GH-induced chondrocyte proliferation.[228] The anti-proliferative effect of glucocorticoids may be mediated through downregulation of the GH receptor and binding affinity as well as suppression of the local production of IGF-1 by these cells. These effects illustrate probable mechanisms by which glucocorticoids may impair the growth stimulatory effects of GH.

Influence on Immune Suppression

Severely burned patients are susceptible to opportunistic infections and sepsis is a major cause of death associated with burn injury. Immune suppression occurs soon after burn injury, perhaps to prevent over-responsiveness. This however, leaves the patient extremely vulnerable to bacterial infection through a number of routes. Patients can be infected through the wound site and by translocation of gut bacteria.[229] Surgery and other life-supporting procedures such as nutritional supplementation and ventilation are also fertile sources of infection. The glucocorticoid response to thermal injury appears to play an important role in immune dysfunction with impairment of both specific and nonspecific defenses. Corticosteroids reduce lymphocyte, eosinophil, and basophil numbers, alter lymphocyte subpopulations, depress immunoglobulin production by B cells, and suppress neutrophil and monocyte/macrophage activity.

Acute thymic involution[230,231] and a reduction of the total T cell population occurs soon after burn injury.[231–233] During initial thymic involution in an animal model there is marked depression of CD4+CD8+ lymphocytes. CD4−CD8− cell numbers are also reduced with recovery in the ensuing thymic regeneration phase during the next 2 weeks. Thymic involution is a common response to various types of stress and trauma.[234] In humans, the depression of T lymphocytes is reflected by reduction of both CD4+ as well as CD8+ cell numbers.[232] In an animal model[231] CD4+ CD8− cells are reported to be more sensitive to the effects of thermal injury than CD4−CD8+ cells. CD4+CD8− cell numbers remain constantly depressed during a 2-week period following burn injury, whereas CD4−CD8+ cell numbers are variable and can even be increased in comparison to control animals not subjected to thermal injury.

Thymic changes following exogenous administration of glucocorticoids are similar to that seen in burn injury[235,236] in that exogenous hypercortisolism in noninjury states or that following burn injury is associated with decreasing CD4+CD8+ and elevating CD4−CD8− thymocytes.[230] The reduction of CD4+CD8+ cell numbers during the first 24 hours after thermal injury is due to glucocorticoid-mediated apoptosis since burn injury-induced thymocyte apoptosis is suppressed by adrenalectomy or administration of a glucocorticoid receptor antagonist (RU486).[230] Other factors contributing to lymphocyte dysfunction and immunosuppression resulting from elevated corticosteroid levels may include the ability to directly inhibit T cell proliferation, IL-2 production,[237,238] as well as the ability to alter lymphocyte membrane fluidity.[239]

Apart from these effects on lymphocytes, glucocorticoids also enhance susceptibility to infections by altering monocyte and neutrophil functions at several stages. Movement of circulating inflammatory cells to the site of infection is suppressed by the ability of glucocorticoids to reduce the cellular response to chemotactic stimuli,[240–242] diminish neutrophil adherence,[243] and induce a shift from marginal to circulating cells.[240] Glucocorticoids also suppress bactericidal activity of monocytes[241] and neutrophils,[244] perhaps through impairment of lysosomal function.[245]

Although severe burns are associated with alterations in B cell production and function, there is considerable inconsistency in the status of literature concerning B cell biology.[246–251] For example, in rats subjected to 30% burn injury, splenic lymphocytes respond poorly to LPS and immunoglobulin synthesis is reduced in comparison to control animals.[252] Others have found an increase in circulating B cells early after burn injury.[251,253] Interestingly, administration of methylprednisolone to normal volunteers for 2–4 weeks also reduces serum immunoglobulin levels.[254] Changes in the B cell population parallel changes in urine 17-hydroxysterol levels and increase in stress hormones in the early stages of burn injury may result in the release of B cells from lymphoid organs.

Aside from glucocorticoids, adrenal androgens such as DHEA-

SO_4, also have profound influence on immune responses. In fact, a role for DHEAS as a potent modulator of the immune response is now well established.[255-258] DHEAS which has immunosuppressive properties on Th1 helper cells, are low during severe illness.[174] *In vitro* treatment of human T cells with DHEAS increases IL-2 production (which is required for clonal expansion) and IL-2 mRNA synthesis.[258] It is interesting to note that this effect was seen only in $CD4^+CD8^-$ and not in $CD4^-CD8^+$ cells. DHEAS-treated cells were also able to mediate a more potent cytotoxic effect than cells without DHEAS treatment.

Yet another factor that profoundly influences the immune status and adrenal steroid secretion in burn patients is the neurotransmitter dopamine. Dopamine is often used in the treatment of critically ill patients because of its vasopressor, renal vasodilating, and cardiac inotropic properties. However, several studies indicate that dopamine treatment may undermine an already depressed immune system. This effect appears to act via the suppression of prolactin release from the anterior pituitary. Dopamine suppresses serum prolactin and DHEAS levels but not cortisol concentration.[259,260] *In vitro*, prolactin has a synergistic effect on ACTH-induced DHEAS secretion by human adrenal cells.[261] Thus it is possible that the dopamine-induced suppression of prolactin is responsible for lowering DHEAS levels and therefore suppression of the T cell proliferative response. The *in vitro* proliferative response of T cells from patients on dopamine therapy is diminished[259] and cells treated with DHEAS mediate a more potent T cell cytotoxic effect.[258] Dopamine levels are elevated under conditions of severe physical stress and chronic illness.[262,263] This may partly be responsible for the anergic state of the immune system during severe stress.

The present review affirms that catecholamines and adrenal steroid hormones are integral parts of the physiologic response to thermal injury that are thought to support recovery through compensatory cardiovascular, metabolic, and immunologic changes. Although adrenergic mechanisms are important for their ability to influence intracellular signaling pathways their role as modulators of gene expression is still being explored. On the other hand, while much is known about the modulation of gene expression by glucocorticoids very little is known about their modulation of gene expression consequent to severe thermal injury or other forms of trauma. Future studies hold great promise of providing important new information in these areas as to how these bioactive compounds may influence responses to thermal injury and how such information can lead to the development of new treatment modalities.

References

1. Benedict CR, Grahame-Smith DG. Plasma noradrenaline and adrenaline concentrations and dopamine-beta-hydroxylase activity in patients with shock due to septicaemia, trauma and haemorrhage. *Q J Med* 1978; **47**: 1–20.
2. Murton SA, Tan ST, Prickett TC, Frampton C, Donald RA. Hormone responses to stress in patients with major burns. *Br J Plast Surg* 1998; **51**: 388–392.
3. Cuthbertson D. Post-shock metabolic response. *Lancet* 1942; **1**: 433–436.
4. Selye HA. Syndrome produced by diverse nocuous agents. *Nature* 1936; **138**: 32–33.
5. Soroff HS, Pearson E, Artz C. An estimation of nitrogen requirements for equilibrium in burned patients. *Surg Gynecol Obstet* 1961; **2**: 159.
6. Cunningham JJ, Hegarty MT, Meara PA, Burke JF. Measured and predicted calorie requirements of adults during recovery from severe burn trauma. *Am J Clin Nutr* 1989; **49**: 404–408.
7. Khorram-Sefat R, Behrendt W, Heiden A, Hettich R. Long-term measurements of energy expenditure in severe burn injury. *World J Surg* 1999; **23**: 115–122.
8. Evans EI, Butterfield WJH. The stress response in the severely burned. *Ann Surg* 1951; 588.
9. Moore FD. Adaptation of supportive treatment to needs of the surgical patient. *JAMA* 1949; 646.
10. Taylor FHL, Levenson SM, Adams MA. Abnormal carbohydrate metabolism in human thermal burns. *N Engl J Med* 1944; 437.
11. Birke G, Duner H, Liljedahl SO, Pernow B, Plantin LO, Troell L. Histamine. Catecholamines and adrenocortical steroids in burns. *Acta Chir Scand* 1957; 87–98.
12. Goodall M, Stone C, Haynes BW. Urinary output of adrenaline and noradrenaline in severe thermal burns. *Ann Surg* 1957; **145**: 479–487.
13. Birke G, Carlson LA, Euler USv, Liljedahl SO, Plantin LO. Studies on burns. XII. Lipid metabolism, catecholamine excretion, basal metabolic rate, and water loss during treatment of burns with warm dry air. *Acta Chir Scand* 1972; **138**: 321–333.
14. Crum RL, Dominic W, Hansbrough JF, Shackford SR, Brown MR. Cardiovascular and neurohumoral responses following burn injury. *Arch Surg* 1990; **125**: 1065–1069.
15. Wilmore DW, Long JM, Mason AD, Jr., Skreen RW, Pruitt BA, Jr. Catecholamines: mediator of the hypermetabolic response to thermal injury. *Ann Surg* 1974; **180**: 653–669.
16. Becker RA, Vaughan GM, Goodwin CW, Jr., Ziegler MG, Harrison TS, Mason AD, Jr., Pruitt BA. Plasma norepinephrine, epinephrine, and thyroid hormone interactions in severely burned patients. *Arch Surg* 1980; **115**: 439–443.
17. Carleton SC Cardiac problems associated with burns. *Cardiol Clin* 1995; **13**: 257–262.
18. Michie D, Goldsmith R, Mason A. Hemodynamics of the immediate post-burn period. *J Trauma* 1963; **3**: 111–119.
19. Pruitt BA, Jr. Current treatment of thermal injury. *South Med J* 1971; **64**: 657–662.
20. Ganrot K, Jacabsson S, Rothman U. Transcapillary passage of plasma proteins in experimental burns. *Acta Physiol Scand* 1974; 497–501.
21. Carvajal HF, Reinhart JA, Traber DL. Renal and cardiovascular functional response to thermal injury in dogs subjected to sympathetic blockade. *Circ Shock* 1976; 287–298.
22. Boyle WAd, Segel LD. Direct cardiac effects of vasopressin and their reversal by a vascular antagonist. *Am J Physiol* 1986; **251**: H734–741.
23. Herndon DN, Barrow RE, Rutan TC, Minifee P, Jahoor F, Wolfe RR. Effect of propranolol administration on hemodynamic and metabolic responses of burned pediatric patients. *Ann Surg* 1988; **208**: 484–492.
24. Honeycutt D, Barrow R, Herndon D. Cold stress response in patients with severe burns after beta-blockade. *J Burn Care Rehabil* 1992; **13**: 181–186.
25. Szabo K. Cardiac support in burned patients with heart disease. *Acta Chir Plast* 1989; **31**: 22–34.
26. Bevan J, Pegram B, Prehn J, Winquist R. β-adrenergic receptor-mediated vasodilation. In: Vanhoutte P, Leusen I, eds *Mechanisms in Vasodilatation* New York: S Karger, 1977: 258–265.
27. Chruscinski AJ, Rohrer DK, Schauble E, Desai KH, Bernstein D, Kobika BK. Targeted disruption of the beta2 adrenergic receptor gene. *J Biol Chem* 1999; **274**: 16694–16700.
28. Jacob G, Costa F, Shannon J, Robertson D, Biaggioni I. Dissociation between neural and vascular responses to sympathetic stimulation: contribution of local adrenergic receptor function. *Hypertension* 2000; **35**: 76–81.
29. Sheperd J. Circulation to skeletal muscle. In: Geiger S, Sheperd J, Abboud F, eds. *Handbook of Physiology. Section 2: The Cardiovascular System* Maryland: American Physiological Society, 1983: 319–370.
30. Kilbourn RG, Traber DL, Szabo C. Nitric oxide and shock. *Dis Mon* 1997; **43**: 277–348.
31. Macarthur H, Westfall TC, Riley DP, Misko TP, Salvemini D. Inactivation of catecholamines by superoxide gives new insights on the pathogenesis of septic shock. *Proc Natl Acad Sci USA* 2000; **97**: 9753–9758.
32. Wolfe RR, Miller HI. Cardiovascular and metabolic responses during burn shock in the guinea pig. *Am J Physiol* 1976; **231**: 892–7.
33. Wolfe RR, Miller HI, Elahi D, Spitzer JJ. Effect of burn injury on glucose turnover in guinea pigs. *Surg Gynecol Obstet* 1977; **144**: 359–364.
34. Arturson G. Metabolic changes and nutrition in children with severe burns. *Prog Pediatr Surg* 1981; **14**: 81–109.
35. Breitenstein E, Chiolero RL, Jequier E, Dayer P, Krupp S, Schutz Y. Effects of beta-blockade on energy metabolism following burns. *Burns* 1990; **16**: 259–264.
36. Wolfe RR, Durkot MJ. Evaluation of the role of the sympathetic nervous system in the response of substrate kinetics and oxidation to burn injury. *Circ Shock* 1982; **9**: 395–406.

37. Wolfe RR, Herndon DN, Jahoor F, Miyoshi H, Wolfe M. Effect of severe burn injury on substrate cycling by glucose and fatty acids. *N Engl J Med* 1987; **317**: 403–408.

38. Wolfe RR, Herndon DN, Peters EJ, Jahoor F, Desai MH, Holland OB. Regulation of lipolysis in severely burned children. *Ann Surg* 1987; **206**: 214–221.

39. Herndon DN, Nguyen TT, Wolfe RR, Maggi SP, Biolo G, Muller M, Barrow RE. Lipolysis in burned patients is stimulated by the beta 2-receptor for catecholamines. *Arch Surg* 1994; **129**: 1301–1304; discussion 1304–1305.

40. Cope O, Nardi G, Ouijano M, Rovit R, Stanbury J, Wright A. Metabolic rate and thyroid function following acute thermal trauma in man. *Ann Surg* 1953; **137**: 165–174.

41. Caldwell FT, Jr., Ostermann H, Sower N, Moyer C. Metabolic response to thermal trauma of normal and thyroprivic rats at three environmental temperatures. *Ann Surg* 1959; **150**: 976–988.

42. Caldwell FT, Jr. Energy metabolism following thermal burns. *Arch Surg* 1976; **111**: 181–185.

43. Chance WT, Nelson JL, Foley-Nelson T, Kim MW, Fischer JE. The relationship of burn-induced hypermetabolism to central and peripheral catecholamines. *J Trauma* 1989; **29**: 306–312.

44. Caldwell FT, Jr., Graves DB, Wallace BH, Moore DB, Crabtree JH. Alteration in temperature regulation induced by burn injury in the rat. *J Burn Care Rehabil* 1989; **10**: 486–493.

45. Neely WA, Petro AB, Holloman GH, Jr., Rushton FW, Jr., Turner MD, Hardy JD. Researches on the cause of burn hypermetabolism. *Ann Surg* 1974; **179**: 291–294.

46. Shirani KZ, Pruitt BA, Jr., Mason AD, Jr. The influence of inhalation injury and pneumonia on burn mortality. *Ann Surg* 1987; **205**: 82–87.

47. Jones SB, Westfall MV, Sayeed MM. Plasma catecholamines during *E. coli* bacteremia in conscious rats. *Am J Physiol* 1988; **254**: R470–477.

48. Jones SB, Romano FD. Dose- and time-dependent changes in plasma catecholamines in response to endotoxin in conscious rats. *Circ Shock* 1989; **28**: 59–68.

49. Kovarik MF, Jones SB, Romano FD. Plasma catecholamines following cecal ligation and puncture in the rat. *Circ Shock* 1987; **22**: 281–290.

50. Jones SB, Kovarik MF, Romano FD. Cardiac and splenic norepinephrine turnover during septic peritonitis. *Am J Physiol* 1986; **250**: 892–897.

51. Zhou ZZ, Jones SB. Involvement of central vs. peripheral mechanisms in mediating sympathoadrenal activation in endotoxic rats. *Am J Physiol* 1993; **265**: R683–688.

52. Zhou ZZ, Wurster RD, Jones SB. Arterial baroreflexes are not essential in mediating sympathoadrenal activation in conscious endotoxic rats. *J Auton Nerv Syst* 1992; **39**: 1–12.

53. Reilly FD, McCuskey PA, Miller ML, McCuskey RS, Meineke HA. Innervation of the periarteriolar lymphatic sheath of the spleen. *Tissue Cell* 1979; **11**: 121–126.

54. Williams JM, Felten DL. Sympathetic innervation of murine thymus and spleen: a comparative histofluorescence study. *Anat Rec* 1981; **199**: 531–542.

55. Van Oosterhout AJ, Nijkamp FP. Anterior hypothalamic lesions prevent the endotoxin-induced reduction of beta-adrenoceptor number in guinea pig lung. *Brain Res* 1984; **302**: 277–280.

56. Felten SY, Felten DL, Bellinger DL, Carlson SL, Ackerman KD, Madden KS, Olschowka JA, Livnat S. Noradrenergic sympathetic innervation of lymphoid organs. *Prog Allergy* 1988; **43**: 14–36.

57. Calvo W. The innervation of the bone marrow in laboratory animals. *J Anatomy* 1968; **123**: 315–328.

58. Felten DL, Felten SY, Carlson SL, Olschowka JA, Livnat S. Noradrenergic and peptidergic innervation of lymphoid tissue. *J Immunol* 1985; **135**: 755s–765s.

59. Livnat S, Felten SY, Carlson SL, Bellinger DL, Felten DL. Involvement of peripheral and central catecholamine systems in neural-immune interactions. *J Neuroimmunol* 1985; **10**: 5–30.

60. Ackerman KD, Felten SY, Bellinger DL, Felten DL. Noradrenergic sympathetic innervation of the spleen: III. Development of innervation in the rat spleen. *J Neurosci Res* 1987; **18**: 49–54.

61. Felten DL, Ackerman KD, Wiegand SJ, Felten SY. Noradrenergic sympathetic innervation of the spleen: I. Nerve fibers associate with lymphocytes and macrophages in specific compartments of the splenic white pulp. *J Neurosci Res* 1987; **18**: 28–36.

62. Felten SY, Olschowka J. Noradrenergic sympathetic innervation of the spleen: II. Tyrosine hydroxylase (TH)-positive nerve terminals form synaptic like contacts on lymphocytes in the splenic white pulp. *J Neurosci Res* 1987; **18**: 37–48.

63. Tang Y, Shankar R, Gamelli R, Jones S. Dynamic norepinephrine alterations in bone marrow: evidence of functional innervation. *J Neuroimmunol* 1999; **96**: 182–189.

64. Kohm AP, Sanders VM. Suppression of antigen-specific Th2 cell-dependent IgM and IgG1 production following norepinephrine depletion in vivo. *J Immunol* 1999; **162**: 5299–5308.

65. Sanders VM, Baker RA, Ramer-Quinn DS, Kasprowicz DJ, Fuchs BA, Street NE. Differential expression of the beta2-adrenergic receptor by Th1 and Th2 clones: implications for cytokine production and B cell help. *J Immunol* 1997; **158**: 4200–4210.

66. Ramer-Quinn DS, Baker RA, Sanders VM. Activated T helper 1 and T helper 2 cells differentially express the beta-2-adrenergic receptor: a mechanism for selective modulation of T helper 1 cell cytokine production. *J Immunol* 1997; **159**: 4857–4867.

67. Sanders VM. The role of adrenoceptor-mediated signals in the modulation of lymphocyte function. *Adv Neuroimmunol* 1995; **5**: 283–298.

68. Swanson M, Lee W, Sanders VM. INF-g production by Th1 cells generated from naive CD4⁺ T cell exposed to norepinephrine. *J Immunol* 2000. (In Press).

69. Kasprowicz DJ, Kohm AP, Berton MT, Chruscinski AJ, Sharpe A, Sanders, VM. Stimulation of the B cell receptor, CD86 (B7-2), and the beta 2- adrenergic receptor intrinsically modulates the level of IgG1 and IgE produced per B cell. *J Immunol* 2000; **165**: 680–690.

70. Melmon KL, Bourne HR, Weinstein Y, Shearer GM, Kram J, Bauminger S. Hemolytic plaque formation by leukocytes in vitro. Control by vasoactive hormones. *J Clin Invest* 1974; **53**: 13–21.

71. Kohm AP, Tang Y, Sanders VM, Jones SB. Activation of antigen-specific CD4+ Th2 cells and B cells in vivo increases norepinephrine release in the spleen and bone marrow. *J Immunol* 2000; **165**: 725–733.

72. Spengler RN, Chensue SW, Giacherio DA, Blenk N, Kunkel SL. Endogenous norepinephrine regulates tumor necrosis factor-alpha production from macrophages in vitro. *J Immunol* 1994; **152**: 3024–3031.

73. Hasko G, Elenkov IJ, Kvetan V, Vizi ES. Differential effect of selective block of alpha 2-adrenoreceptors on plasma levels of tumour necrosis factor-alpha, interleukin-6 and corticosterone induced by bacterial lipopolysaccharide in mice. *J Endocrinol* 1995; **144**: 457–462.

74. Monastra G, Secchi EF. Beta-adrenergic receptors mediate in vivo the adrenaline inhibition of lipopolysaccharide-induced tumor necrosis factor release. *Immunol Lett* 1993; **38**: 127–130.

75. Szabo C, Hasko G, Zingarelli B, Nemeth ZH, Salzman AL, Kvetan V, Pastores SM, Vizi ES. Isoproterenol regulates tumour necrosis factor, interleukin-10, interleukin-6 and nitric oxide production and protects against the development of vascular hyporeactivity in endotoxaemia. *Immunology* 1997; **90**: 95–100.

76. Szelenyi J, Kiss JP, Vizi ES. Differential involvement of sympathetic nervous system and immune system in the modulation of TNF-alpha production by alpha2- and beta-adrenoceptors in mice. *J Neuroimmunol* 2000; **103**: 34–40.

77. Beno DW, Kimura RE. Nonstressed rat model of acute endotoxemia that unmasks the endotoxin-induced TNF-alpha response. *Am J Physiol* 1999; **276**: H671–678.

78. van der Poll T, Coyle SM, Barbosa K, Braxton CC, Lowry SF. Epinephrine inhibits tumor necrosis factor-alpha and potentiates interleukin 10 production during human endotoxemia. *J Clin Invest* 1996; **97**: 713–719.

79. Bergmann M, Gornikiewicz A, Sautner T, Waldmann E, Weber T, Mittlbock M, Roth E, Fugger R. Attenuation of catecholamine-induced immunosuppression in whole blood from patients with sepsis. *Shock* 1999; **12**: 421–427.

80. Guirao X, Kumar A, Katz J, Smith M, Lin E, Keogh C, Calvano SE, Lowry SF. Catecholamines increase monocyte TNF receptors and inhibit TNF through beta 2-adrenoreceptor activation. *Am J Physiol* 1997; **273**: E1203–1208.

81. Severn A, Rapson NT, Hunter CA, Liew FY. Regulation of tumor necrosis factor production by adrenaline and beta-adrenergic agonists. *J Immunol* 1992; **148**: 3441–3445.

82. van der Poll T, Jansen J, Endert E, Sauerwein HP, van Deventer SJ. Noradrenaline inhibits lipopolysaccharide-induced tumor necrosis factor and interleukin 6 production in human whole blood. *Infect Immun* 1994; **62**: 2046–2050.

83. Yoshimura T, Kurita C, Nagao T, Usami E, Nakao T, Watanabe S, Kobayashi J, Yamazaki F, Tanaka H, Inagaki N, Nagai H. Inhibition of tumor necrosis factor-alpha and interleukin-1-beta production by beta-adrenoceptor agonists from lipopolysaccharide-stimulated human peripheral blood mononuclear cells. *Pharmacology* 1997; **54**: 144–152.

84. Chou RC, Stinson MW, Noble BK, Spengler RN. Beta-adrenergic receptor regulation of macrophage-derived tumor necrosis factor-alpha production from rats with experimental arthritis. *J Neuroimmunol* 1996; **67**: 7–16.

85. Hu XX, Goldmuntz EA, Brosnan CF. The effect of norepinephrine on endotoxin-mediated macrophage activation. *J Neuroimmunol* 1991; **31**: 35–42.

86. Ignatowski TA, Spengler RN. Regulation of macrophage-derived tumor necrosis factor production by modification of adrenergic receptor sensitivity. *J Neuroimmunol* 1995; **61**: 61–70.

87. Liao J, Keiser JA, Scales WE, Kunkel SL, Kluger MJ. Role of epinephrine in TNF and IL-6 production from isolated perfused rat liver. *Am J Physiol* 1995; **268**: R896–R901.

88. Bissonnette EY, Befus AD. Anti-inflammatory effect of beta 2-agonists:

inhibition of TNF-alpha release from human mast cells. *J Allergy Clin Immunol* 1997; **100**: 825–831.

89. Hetier E, Ayala J, Bousseau A, Prochiantz A. Modulation of interleukin-1 and tumor necrosis factor expression by beta-adrenergic agonists in mouse ameboid microglial cells. *Exp Brain Res* 1991; **86**: 407–413.

90. Nakamura A, Johns EJ, Imaizumi A, Abe T, Kohsaka T. Regulation of tumour necrosis factor and interleukin-6 gene transcription by beta2-adrenoceptor in the rat astrocytes. *J Neuroimmunol* 1998; **88**: 144–153.

91. Kalinichenko VV, Mokyr MB, Graf LH, Jr. Cohen RL, Chambers DA. Norepinephrine-mediated inhibition of antitumor cytotoxic T lymphocyte generation involves a beta-adrenergic receptor mechanism and decreased TNF-alpha gene expression. *J Immunol* 1999; **163**: 2492–2499.

92. Abadie C, Foucart S, Page P, Nadeau R. Interleukin-1 beta and tumor necrosis factor-alpha inhibit the release of [3H]-noradrenaline from isolated human atrial appendages. *Naunyn Schmiedebergs Arch Pharmacol* 1997; **355**: 384–389.

93. Foucart S, Abadie C. Interleukin-1 beta and tumor necrosis factor-alpha inhibit the release of [3H]-noradrenaline from mice isolated atria. *Naunyn Schmiedebergs Arch Pharmacol* 1996; **354**: 1–6.

94. Hurst SM, Collins SM. Mechanism underlying tumor necrosis factor-alpha suppression of norepinephrine release from rat myenteric plexus. *Am J Physiol* 1994; **266**: G1123–1129.

95. Ignatowski TA, Noble BK, Wright JR, Gorfien JL, Heffner RR, Spengler RN. Neuronal-associated tumor necrosis factor (TNF alpha): its role in noradrenergic functioning and modification of its expression following antidepressant drug administration. *J Neuroimmunol* 1997; **79**: 84–90.

96. DeRijk RH, Boelen A, Tilders FJ, Berkenbosch F. Induction of plasma interleukin-6 by circulating adrenaline in the rat. *Psychoneuroendocrinology* 1994; **19**: 155–163.

97. van Gool J, van Vugt H, Helle M, Aarden LA. The relation among stress, adrenalin, interleukin 6 and acute phase proteins in the rat. *Clin Immunol Immunopathol* 1990; **57**: 200–210.

98. Takaki A, Huang QH, Somogyvari-Vigh A, Arimura A. Immobilization stress may increase plasma interleukin-6 via central and peripheral catecholamines. *Neuroimmunomodulation* 1994; **1**: 335–342.

99. Gornikiewicz A, Sautner T, Brostjan C, Schmierer B, Fugger R, Roth E, Muhlbacher F, Bergmann M. Catecholamines up-regulate lipopolysaccharide-induced IL-6 production in human microvascular endothelial cells. *Faseb J* 2000; **14**: 1093–1100.

100. von Patay B, Loppnow H, Feindt J, Kurz B, Mentlein R. Catecholamines and lipopolysaccharide synergistically induce the release of interleukin-6 from thymic epithelial cells. *J Neuroimmunol* 1998; **86**: 182–189.

101. Maimone D, Cioni C, Rosa S, Macchia G, Aloisi F, Annunziata P. Norepinephrine and vasoactive intestinal peptide induce IL-6 secretion by astrocytes: synergism with IL-1 beta and TNF alpha. *J Neuroimmunol* 1993; **47**: 73–81.

102. Zumwalt JW, Thunstrom BJ, Spangelo BL. Interleukin-1beta and catecholamines synergistically stimulate interleukin-6 release from rat C6 glioma cells in vitro: a potential role for lysophosphatidylcholine. *Endocrinology* 1999; **140**: 888–896.

103. Burysek L, Houstek J. beta-Adrenergic stimulation of interleukin-1 alpha and interleukin-6 expression in mouse brown adipocytes. *FEBS Lett* 1997; **411**: 83–86.

104. Christensen JD, Hansen EW, Frederiksen C, Molris M, Moesby L. Adrenaline influences the release of interleukin-6 from murine pituicytes: role of beta2-adrenoceptors. *Eur J Pharmacol* 1999; **378**: 143–148.

105. Jung BD, Kimura K, Kitamura H, Makonodo K, Okita K, Kawasaki M, Saito M. Norepinephrine stimulates interleukin-6 mRNA expression in primary cultured rat hepatocytes. *J Biochem (Tokyo)* 2000; **127**: 205–209.

106. Norris JG, Benveniste EN. Interleukin-6 production by astrocytes: induction by the neurotransmitter norepinephrine. *J Neuroimmunol* 1993; **45**: 137–145.

107. von Patay B, Kurz B, Mentlein R. Effect of transmitters and co-transmitters of the sympathetic nervous system on interleukin-6 synthesis in thymic epithelial cells. *Neuroimmunomodulation* 1999; **6**: 45–50.

108. Straub RH, Herrmann M, Frauenholz T, Berkmiller G, Lang B, Scholmerich J, Falk W. Neuroimmune control of interleukin-6 secretion in the murine spleen. Differential beta-adrenergic effects of electrically released endogenous norepinephrine under various endotoxin conditions. *J Neuroimmunol* 1996; **71**: 37–43.

109. Straub RH, Hermann M, Berkmiller G, Frauenholz T, Lang B, Scholmerich J, Falk W. Neuronal regulation of interleukin 6 secretion in murine spleen: adrenergic and opioidergic control. *J Neurochem* 1997; **68**: 1633–1639.

110. Straub RH, Linde HJ, Mannel DN, Scholmerich J, Falk W. A bacteria-induced switch of sympathetic effector mechanisms augments local inhibition of TNF-alpha and IL-6 secretion in the spleen. *Faseb J* 2000; **14**: 1380–1384.

111. Zhong W, Chavali S, Forse R. IL-10 is the major mediator of the protection against lethality by b$_2$-adrenergic receptor agonist terbutaline in endotoxic mice. *Surg Forum* 1996; **47**: 87–89.

112. Siegmund B, Eigler A, Hartmann G, Hacker U, Endres S. Adrenaline enhances LPS-induced IL-10 synthesis: evidence for protein kinase A-mediated pathway. *Int J Immunopharmacol* 1998; **20**: 57–69.

113. Platzer C, Docke W, Volk H, Prosch S. Catecholamines trigger IL-10 release in acute systemic stress reaction by direct stimulation of its promoter/enhancer activity in monocytic cells. *J Neuroimmunol* 2000; **105**: 31–38.

114. Woiciechowsky C, Asadullah K, Nestler D, Eberhardt B, Platzer C, Schoning B, Glockner F, Lanksch WR, Volk HD, Docke WD. Sympathetic activation triggers systemic interleukin-10 release in immunodepression induced by brain injury [see comments]. *Nat Med* 1998; **4**: 808–813.

115. Hasko G, Nemeth ZH, Szabo C, Zsilla G, Salzman AL, Vizi ES. Isoproterenol inhibits II-10, TNF-alpha, and nitric oxide production in RAW 264.7 macrophages. *Brain Res Bull* 1998; **45**: 183–187.

116. Suberville S, Bellocq A, Fouqueray B, Philippe C, Lantz O, Perez J, Baud L. Regulation of interleukin-10 production by beta-adrenergic agonists. *Eur J Immunol* 1996; **26**: 2601–2605.

117. Lyte M, Bailey MT. Neuroendocrine-bacterial interactions in a neurotoxin-induced model of trauma. *J Surg Res* 1997; **70**: 195–201.

118. Lyte M. The role of catecholamines in gram-negative sepsis. *Med Hypotheses* 1992; **37**: 255–258.

119. Lyte M. The role of microbial endocrinology in infectious disease. *J Endocrinol* 1993; **137**: 343–345.

120. Lyte M, Ernst S, Driemeyer J, Baissa B. Strain-specific enhancement of splenic T cell mitogenesis and macrophage phagocytosis following peripheral axotomy. *J Neuroimmunol* 1991; **31**: 1–8.

121. Lyte M, Ernst S. Alpha and beta adrenergic receptor involvement in catecholamine-induced growth of gram-negative bacteria. *Biochem Biophys Res Commun* 1993; **190**: 447–452.

122. Freestone PP, Haigh RD, Williams PH, Lyte M. Stimulation of bacterial growth by heat-stable, norepinephrine-induced autoinducers. *FEMS Microbiol Lett* 1999; **172**: 53–60.

123. Lyte M, Frank CD, Green BT. Production of an autoinducer of growth by norepinephrine cultured *Escherichia coli* O157:H7. *FEMS Microbiol Lett* 1996; **139**: 155–159.

124. Lyte M, Arulanandam BP, Frank CD. Production of Shiga-like toxins by *Escherichia coli* O157:H7 can be influenced by the neuroendocrine hormone norepinephrine. *J Lab Clin Med* 1996; **128**: 392–398.

125. Lyte M, Erickson AK, Arulanandam BP, Frank CD, Crawford MA, Francis DH. Norepinephrine-induced expression of the K99 pilus adhesin of enterotoxigenic *Escherichia coli. Biochem Biophys Res Commun* 1997; **232**: 682–686.

126. Iverson L. Neuronal and extraneuronal catecholamine uptake mechanisms. In: Usdin E, Synder S, eds. *Frontiers in Catecholamine Research.* London: Pergamon, 1973: 403–408.

127. Bailey MT, Karaszewski JW, Lubach GR, Coe CL, Lyte M. In vivo adaptation of attenuated *Salmonella typhimurium* results in increased growth upon exposure to norepinephrine. *Physiol Behav* 1999; **67**: 359–364.

128. Sartorelli KH, Silver GM, Gamelli RL. The effect of granulocyte colony-stimulating factor (G-CSF) upon burn-induced defective neutrophil chemotaxis. *J Trauma* 1991; **31**: 523–529; discussion 529–530.

129. Solomkin JS. Neutrophil disorders in burn injury: complement, cytokines, and organ injury. *J Trauma* 1990; **30**: S80–85.

130. Warden GD, Mason AD, Jr., Pruitt BA, Jr. Evaluation of leukocyte chemotaxis in vitro in thermally injured patients. *J Clin Invest* 1974; **54**: 1001–1004.

131. Duque RE, Phan SH, Hudson JL, Till GO, Ward PA. Functional defects in phagocytic cells following thermal injury. Application of flow cytometric analysis. *Am J Pathol* 1985; **118**: 116–127.

132. Peterson V, Hansbrough J, Buerk C, Rundus C, Wallner S, Smith H, Robinson WA. Regulation of granulopoiesis following severe thermal injury. *J Trauma* 1983; **23**: 19–24.

133. Volenec FJ, Wood GW, Mani MM, Robinson DW, Humphrey LJ. Mononuclear cell analysis of peripheral blood from burn patients. *J Trauma* 1979; **19**: 86–93.

134. Besedovsky HO, del Rey A. Immune-neuro-endocrine interactions: facts and hypotheses. *Endocr Rev* 1996; **17**: 64–102.

135. Madden KS, Sanders VM, Felten DL. Catecholamine influences and sympathetic neural modulation of immune responsiveness. *Annu Rev Pharmacol Toxicol* 1995; **35**: 417–448.

136. Madden KS, Moynihan JA, Brenner GJ, Felten SY, Felten DL, Livnat S. Sympathetic nervous system modulation of the immune system. III. Alterations in T and B cell proliferation and differentiation in vitro following chemical sympathectomy. *J Neuroimmunol* 1994; **49**: 77–87.

137. Madden KS, Felten SY, Felten DL, Hardy CA, Livnat S. Sympathetic nervous system modulation of the immune system. II. Induction of lymphocyte proliferation and migration in vivo by chemical sympathectomy. *J Neuroimmunol* 1994; **49**: 67–75.

138. Maestroni GJ. Adrenergic regulation of haematopoiesis. *Pharmacol Res* 1995; 32: 249–253.

139. Maestroni GJ, Conti A. Modulation of hematopoiesis via alpha 1-adrenergic receptors on bone marrow cells. *Exp Hematol* 1994; 22: 313–320.

140. Dresch C, Minc J, Poirier O, Bouvet D. Effect of beta adrenergic agonists and beta blocking agents on hemopoiesis in human bone marrow. *Biomedicine* 1981; 34: 93–98.

141. Dresch C, Minc J, Mary JY. In vivo protection of normal mouse hematopoiesis by a beta 2 blocking agent during S-phase chemotherapy. *Cancer Res* 1984; 44: 493–497.

142. Togni M, Maestroni GJ. Hematopoietic rescue in mice via a1-adrenoceptors on bone marrow B cell precursors. *International Journal of Oncology* 1996; 313–318.

143. Maestroni GJ, Conti A, Pedrinis E. Effect of adrenergic agents on hematopoiesis after syngeneic bone marrow transplantation in mice. *Blood* 1992; 80: 1178–1182.

144. Tang Y, Shankar R, Gamboa M, Desai S, Gamelli RL, Jones SB. Norepinephrine modulates myelopoiesis following experimental thermal injury with sepsis. *Annals of Surgery* 2000; 233: 266–275.

145. Miller-Graziano CL, Fink M, Wu JY, Szabo G, Kodys K. Mechanisms of altered monocyte prostaglandin E2 production in severely injured patients. *Arch Surg* 1988; 123: 293–299.

146. Faist E. The mechanisms of host defense dysfunction following shock and trauma. *Curr Top Microbiol Immunol* 1996; 216: 259–274.

147. Miller CL, Baker CC. Changes in lymphocyte activity after thermal injury. The role of suppressor cells. *J Clin Invest* 1979; 63: 202–210.

148. Faist E, Schinkel C, Zimmer S, Kremer JP, Von Donnersmarck GH, Schildberg FW. Inadequate interleukin-2 synthesis and interleukin-2 messenger expression following thermal and mechanical trauma in humans is caused by defective transmembrane signalling. *J Trauma* 1993; 34: 846–853; discussion 853–854.

149. Ayala A, Chaudry IH. Immune dysfunction in murine polymicrobial sepsis: mediators, macrophages, lymphocytes and apoptosis. *Shock* 1996; 6: S27–38.

150. Miller-Graziano CL, Szabo G, Kodys K, Griffey K. Aberrations in post-trauma monocyte (MO) subpopulation: role in septic shock syndrome. *J Trauma* 1990; 30: S86–96.

151. Miller-Graziano CL, Zhu D, Kodys K. Differential induction of human monocyte transforming growth factor beta 1 production and its regulation by interleukin 4. *J Clin Immunol* 1994; 14: 61–72.

152. Shoup M, Weisenberger JM, Wang JL, Pyle JM, Gamelli RL, Shankar R. Mechanisms of neutropenia involving myeloid maturation arrest in burn sepsis. *Ann Surg* 1998; 228: 112–122.

153. Santangelo S, Gamelli R, Shankar R. Myeloid commitment shifts toward monocytopoiesis following thermal injury and sepsis. *Ann Surg* 2000; 233: 97–106.

154. Leenen PJ, Melis M, Slieker WA, Van Ewijk W. Murine macrophage precursor characterization. II. Monoclonal antibodies against macrophage precursor antigens. *Eur J Immunol* 1990; 20: 27–34.

155. de Bruijn MF, Slieker WA, van der Loo JC, Voerman JS, van Ewijk W, Leenen PJ. Distinct mouse bone marrow macrophage precursors identified by differential expression of ER-MP12 and ER-MP20 antigens. *Eur J Immunol* 1994; 24: 2279–2284.

156. Moore FD. Recent progress in hormone research. In: Pincus G, ed. *Hormones and Stress.* New York: Academic Press, 1957: 511.

157. Hume DM, Nelson DH, Miller DW. Blood and urinary 17-hydroxycorticosteroids in patients with severe burns. *Ann Surg* 1956; 143: 316–329.

158. Wise L, Margraf HW, Ballinger WF. Adrenal cortical function in severe burns. *Arch Surg* 1972; 105: 213–220.

159. Moore FD. *Metabolic Care of the Surgical Patient.* Philadelphia: WB Saunders Co, 1959: 511.

160. Bane JW, McCaa RE, McCaa CS, Read VH, Turney WH, Turner MD. The pattern of aldosterone and cortisone blood levels in thermal burn patients. *J Trauma* 1974; 14: 605–611.

161. Pugeat M, Bonneton A, Perrot D, Rocle-Nicolas B, Lejeune H, Grenot C, Dechaud H, Brebant C, Motin J, Cuilleron CY. Decreased immunoreactivity and binding activity of corticosteroid-binding globulin in serum in septic shock. *Clin Chem* 1989; 35: 1675–1679.

162. Mortensen RF, Johnson AA, Eurenius K. Serum corticosteroid binding following thermal injury. *Proc Soc Exp Biol Med* 1972; 139: 877–882.

163. Garrel DR. Corticosteroid-binding globulin during inflammation and burn injury: nutritional modulation and clinical implications. *Horm Res* 1996; 45: 245–251.

164. Garrel DR, Zhang L, Zhao XF, Hammond GL. Effect of burn injury on corticosteroid-binding globulin levels in plasma and wound fluid. *Wound Rep Reg* 1993; 1: 10–14.

165. Feldman D, Mondon CE, Horner JA, Weiser JN. Glucocorticoid and estrogen regulation of corticosteroid-binding globulin production by rat liver. *Am J Physiol* 1979; 237: E493–499.

166. Smith CL, Hammond GL. Hormonal regulation of corticosteroid-binding globulin biosynthesis in the male rat. *Endocrinology* 1992; 130: 2245–2251.

167. Frairia R, Agrimonti F, Fortunati N, Fazzari A, Gennari P, Berta L. Influence of naturally occurring and synthetic glucocorticoids on corticosteroid-binding globulin-steroid interaction in human peripheral plasma. *Ann NY Acad Sci* 1988; 538: 287–303.

168. Emptoz-Bonneton A, Crave JC, LeJeune H, Brebant C, Pugeat M. Corticosteroid-binding globulin synthesis regulation by cytokines and glucocorticoids in human hepatoblastoma-derived (HepG2) cells [see comments]. *J Clin Endocrinol Metab* 1997; 82: 3758–3762.

169. Vermes I, Beishuizen A, Hampsink RM, Haanen C. Dissociation of plasma adrenocorticotropin and cortisol levels in critically ill patients: possible role of endothelin and atrial natriuretic hormone [see comments]. *J Clin Endocrinol Metab* 1995; 80: 1238–1242.

170. Kellner M, Wiedemann K, Holsboer F. Atrial natriuretic factor inhibits the CRH-stimulated secretion of ACTH and cortisol in man. *Life Sci* 1992; 50: 1835–1842.

171. Hinson JP, Vinson GP, Kapas S, Teja R. The role of endothelin in the control of adrenocortical function: stimulation of endothelin release by ACTH and the effects of endothelin-1 and endothelin-3 on steroidogenesis in rat and human adrenocortical cells. *J Endocrinol* 1991; 128: 275–280.

172. Hirai M, Miyabo S, Ooya E, Miyanaga K, Aoyagi N, Kimura K, Kishida S, Nakai T. Endothelin-3 stimulates the hypothalamic-pituitary-adrenal axis. *Life Sci* 1991; 48: 2359–2363.

173. Vierhapper H, Hollenstein U, Roden M, Nowotny P. Effect of endothelin-1 in man – impact on basal and stimulated concentrations of luteinizing hormone, follicle-stimulating hormone, thyrotropin, growth hormone, corticotropin, and prolactin. *Metabolism* 1993; 42: 902–906.

174. Parker CR, Jr., Baxter CR. Divergence in adrenal steroid secretory pattern after thermal injury in adult patients. *J Trauma* 1985; 25: 508–510.

175. Lephart ED, Baxter CR, Parker CR, Jr. Effect of burn trauma on adrenal and testicular steroid hormone production. *J Clin Endocrinol Metab* 1987; 64: 842–848.

176. Doerr P, Prike KM. Cortisol-induced suppression of plasma testosterone in normal adult males. *J Clin Endocrinol Metab* 1976; 43: 622–629.

177. Welsh TH, Jr., Bambino TH, Hsueh AJ. Mechanism of glucocorticoid-induced suppression of testicular androgen biosynthesis in vitro. *Biol Reprod* 1982; 27: 1138–1146.

178. Wallace BH, Caldwell FT, Jr., Cone JB. The interrelationships between wound management, thermal stress, energy metabolism, and temperature profiles of patients with burns. *J Burn Care Rehabil* 1994; 15: 499–508.

179. Allison SP, Hinton P, Chamberlain MJ. Intravenous glucose-tolerance, insulin, and free-fatty-acid levels in burned patients. *Lancet* 1968; 2: 1113–1116.

180. Plager JE, Matsui N. An in vitro demonstration of the anti-insulin action of cortisol on glucose metabolism. *Endocrinol* 1966; 78: 1154–1158.

181. Wolfe RR, Durkot MJ, Allsop JR, Burke JF. Glucose metabolism in severely burned patients. *Metabolism* 1979; 28: 1031–1039.

182. Wolfe RR, Miller HI, Spitzer JJ. Glucose and lactate kinetics in burn shock. *Am J Physiol* 1977; 232: E415–418.

183. Yarmush DM, MacDonald AD, Foy BD, Berthiaume F, Tompkins RG, Yarmush ML. Cutaneous burn injury alters relative tricarboxylic acid cycle fluxes in rat liver. *J Burn Care Rehabil* 1999; 20: 292–302.

184. Shuck JM, Eaton P, Shuck LW, Wachtel TL, Schade DS. Dynamics of insulin and glucagon secretions in severely burned patients. *J Trauma* 1977; 17: 706–713.

185. Vaughan GM, Becker RA, Unger RH, Ziegler MG, Siler-Khodr TM, Pruitt BA, Jr., Mason AD, Jr. Nonthyroidal control of metabolism after burn injury: possible role of glucagon. *Metabolism* 1985; 34: 637–641.

186. Marco J, Calle C, Roman D, Diaz-Fierros M, Villanueva ML, Valverde I. Hyperglucagonism induced by glucocorticoid treatment in man. *N Engl J Med* 1973; 288: 128–131.

187. Cuthbertson DP. Observations on disturbance of metabolism produced by injury to the limbs. *Qjm* 1932; 25: 233–246.

188. Darmaun D, Matthews DE, Bier DM. Physiological hypercortisolemia increases proteolysis, glutamine, and alanine production. *Am J Physiol* 1988; 255: E366–373.

189. Kayali AG, Young VR, Goodman MN. Sensitivity of myofibrillar proteins to glucocorticoid-induced muscle proteolysis. *Am J Physiol* 1987; 252: E621–626.

190. Fang CH, James HJ, Ogle C, Fischer JE, Hasselgren PO. Influence of burn injury on protein metabolism in different types of skeletal muscle and the role of glucocorticoids. *J Am Coll Surg* 1995; 180: 33–42.

191. May RC, Kelly RA, Mitch WE. Metabolic acidosis stimulates protein degradation in rat muscle by a glucocorticoid-dependent mechanism. *J Clin Invest* 1986; 77: 614–621.

192. Price SR, England BK, Bailey JL, Van Vreede K, Mitch WE. Acidosis and

glucocorticoids concomitantly increase ubiquitin and proteasome subunit mRNAs in rat muscle. *Am J Physiol* 1994; **267**: C955–960.

193. Isozaki U, Mitch WE, England BK, Price SR. Protein degradation and increased mRNAs encoding proteins of the ubiquitin-proteasome proteolytic pathway in BC3H1 myocytes require an interaction between glucocorticoids and acidification. *Proc Natl Acad Sci USA* 1996; **93**: 1967–1971.

194. Ding X, Price SR, Bailey JL, Mitch WE. Cellular mechanisms controlling protein degradation in catabolic states. *Miner Electrolyte Metab* 1997; **23**: 194–197.

195. Mitch WE, Medina R, Grieber S, May RC, England BK, Price SR, Bailey JL, Goldberg AL. Metabolic acidosis stimulates muscle protein degradation by activating the adenosine triphosphate-dependent pathway involving ubiquitin and proteasomes. *J Clin Invest* 1994; **93**: 2127–2133.

196. Wing SS, Goldberg AL. Glucocorticoids activate the ATP-ubiquitin-dependent proteolytic system in skeletal muscle during fasting. *Am J Physiol* 1993; **264**: E668–676.

197. Bailey JL, Wang X, England BK, Price SR, Ding X, Mitch WE. The acidosis of chronic renal failure activates muscle proteolysis in rats by augmenting transcription of genes encoding proteins of the ATP-dependent ubiquitin-proteasome pathway. *J Clin Invest* 1996; **97**: 1447–1453.

198. Medina R, Wing SS, Goldberg AL. Increase in levels of polyubiquitin and proteasome mRNA in skeletal muscle during starvation and denervation atrophy. *Biochem J* 1995; **307**: 631–637.

199. Price SR, Bailey JL, Wang X, Jurkovitz C, England BK, Ding X, Phillips LS, Mitch WE. Muscle wasting in insulinopenic rats results from activation of the ATP-dependent, ubiquitin-proteasome proteolytic pathway by a mechanism including gene transcription. *J Clin Invest* 1996; **98**: 1703–1708.

200. Aulick LH, Wilmore DW. Increased peripheral amino acid release following burn injury. *Surgery* 1979; **85**: 560–565.

201. Abcouwer SF, Lohmann R, Bode BP, Lustig RJ, Souba WW. Induction of glutamine synthetase expression after major burn injury is tissue specific and temporally variable. *J Trauma* 1997; **42**: 421–427; discussion 427–428.

202. Abcouwer SF, Bode BP, Souba WW. Glucocorticoids regulate rat glutamine synthetase expression in a tissue-specific manner. *J Surg Res* 1995; **59**: 59–65.

203. Hart DW, Wolf SE, Mlcak R, Chinkes DL, Ramzy PI, Obeng MK, Ferrando AA, Wolfe RR, Herndon DN. Persistence of muscle catabolism after severe burn. *Surgery* 2000; **128**: 312–319.

204. Milner EA, Cioffi WG, Mason AD, McManus WF, Pruitt BA, Jr. A longitudinal study of resting energy expenditure in thermally injured patients. *J Trauma* 1994; **37**: 167–170.

205. Rosen CJ, Pollak M. Circulating IGF-1: New perspectives for a new century. *Trends Endocrinol Metab* 1999; **10**: 136–141.

206. Casanueva FF. Physiology of growth hormone secretion and action. *Endocrinol Metab Clin North Am* 1992; **21**: 483–517.

207. Bereket A, Wilson TA, Blethen SL, Sakurai Y, Herndon DN, Wolfe RR, Lang CH. Regulation of the acid-labile subunit of the insulin-like growth factor ternary complex in patients with insulin-dependent diabetes mellitus and severe burns. *Clin Endocrinol (Oxf)* 1996; **44**: 525–532.

208. Ghahary A, Fu S, Shen YJ, Shankowsky HA, Tredget EE. Differential effects of thermal injury on circulating insulin-like growth factor binding proteins in burn patients. *Mol Cell Biochem* 1994; **135**: 171–180.

209. Abribat T, Brazeau P, Davignon I, Garrel DR. Insulin-like growth factor-I blood levels in severely burned patients: effects of time post injury, age of patient and severity of burn. *Clin Endocrinol (Oxf)* 1993; **39**: 583–589.

210. Moller S, Jensen M, Svensson P, Skakkebaek NE. Insulin-like growth factor 1 (IGF-1) in burn patients. *Burns* 1991; **17**: 279–281.

211. Davies SC, Wass JA, Ross RJ, Cotterill AM, Buchanan CR, Coulson VJ, Holly JM. The induction of a specific protease for insulin-like growth factor binding protein-3 in the circulation during severe illness. *J Endocrinol* 1991; **130**: 469–473.

212. Dai J, Baxter RC. Regulation in vivo of the acid-labile subunit of the rat serum insulin-like growth factor-binding protein complex. *Endocrinology* 1994; **135**: 2335–2341.

213. Dai J, Scott CD, Baxter RC. Regulation of the acid-labile subunit of the insulin-like growth factor complex in cultured rat hepatocytes. *Endocrinology* 1994; **135**: 1066–1072.

214. Al Shamma GA, Goll CC, Baird TB, Broom J, Nicholas GA, Richards JR. Changes in body composition after thermal injury in the rat. *Br J Nutr* 1979; **42**: 267–275.

215. Fain SN, Scow RO, Chernick SS. Effects of glucocorticoids on metabolism of adipose tissue in vitro. *J Biol Chem* 1963; **238**: 54–58.

216. Galster AD, Bier DM, Cryer PE, Monafo WW. Plasma palmitate turnover in subjects with thermal injury. *J Trauma* 1984; **24**: 938–945.

217. Harris RL, Frenkel RA, Cottam GL, Baxter CR. Lipid mobilization and metabolism after thermal trauma. *J Trauma* 1982; **22**: 194–198.

218. Klein GL, Herndon DN, Rutan TC, Sherrard DJ, Coburn JW, Langman CB, Thomas ML, Haddad JG Jr., Cooper CW, Miller NL, *et al*. Bone disease in burn patients. *J Bone Miner Res* 1993; **8**: 337–345.

219. Schaffler MB, Li XJ, Jee WS, Ho SW, Stern PJ. Skeletal tissue responses to thermal injury: an experimental study. *Bone* 1988; **9**: 397–406.

220. Klein GL, Herndon DN, Langman CB, Rutan TC, Young WE, Pembleton G, Nusynowitz M, Barnett JL, Broemeling LD, Sailer DE, *et al*. Long-term reduction in bone mass after severe burn injury in children. *J Pediatr* 1995; **126**: 252–256.

221. Rutan RL, Herndon DN. Growth delay in postburn pediatric patients. *Arch Surg* 1990; **125**: 392–395.

222. Klein GL, Wolf SE, Goodman WG, Phillips WA, Herndon DN. The management of acute bone loss in severe catabolism due to burn injury. *Horm Res* 1997; **48**: 83–87.

223. Weinstein RS, Jilka RL, Parfitt AM, Manolagas SC. Inhibition of osteoblastogenesis and promotion of apoptosis of osteoblasts and osteocytes by glucocorticoids. Potential mechanisms of their deleterious effects on bone. *J Clin Invest* 1998; **102**: 274–282.

224. Canalis E. Clinical review 83: Mechanisms of glucocorticoid action in bone: implications to glucocorticoid-induced osteoporosis. *J Clin Endocrinol Metab* 1996; **81**: 3441–3447.

225. Canalis E, Rydziel S, Delany AM, Varghese S, Jeffrey JJ. Insulin-like growth factors inhibit interstitial collagenase synthesis in bone cell cultures. *Endocrinology* 1995; **136**: 1348–1354.

226. Dempster DW, Moonga BS, Stein LS, Horbert WR, Antakly T. Glucocorticoids inhibit bone resorption by isolated rat osteoclasts by enhancing apoptosis. *J Endocrinol* 1997; **154**: 397–406.

227. Manelli I, Giustina I. Glucocorticoid-induced osteoporosis. *Trends Endocrinol Metab* 2000; **11**: 79–85.

228. Jux C, Leiber K, Hugel U, Blum W, Ohlsson C, Klaus G, Mehls O. Dexamethasone impairs growth hormone (GH)-stimulated growth by suppression of local insulin-like growth factor (IGF)-I production and expression of GH- and IGF-I-receptor in cultured rat chondrocytes [see comments]. *Endocrinology* 1998; **139**: 3296–3305.

229. Herndon DN, Zeigler ST. Bacterial translocation after thermal injury. *Crit Care Med* 1993; **21**: S50–54.

230. Nakanishi T, Nishi Y, Sato EF, Ishii M, Hamada T, Inoue M. Thermal injury induces thymocyte apoptosis in the rat. *J Trauma* 1998; **44**: 143–148.

231. Colic M, Mitrovic S, Dujic A. Thymic response to thermal injury in mice: I. Alterations of thymocyte subsets studied by flow cytometry and immunohistochemistry. *Burns* 1989; **15**: 155–161.

232. Maldonado MD, Venturoli A, Franco A, Nunez-Roldan A. Specific changes in peripheral blood lymphocyte phenotype from burn patients. Probable origin of the thermal injury-related lymphocytopenia. *Burns* 1991; **17**: 188–192.

233. Organ BC, Antonacci AC, Chiao J, Kumar A, de Riesthal HF, Yuan L, Black D, Calvano SE. Changes in lymphocyte number and phenotype in seven lymphoid compartments after thermal injury. *Ann Surg* 1989; **210**: 78–89.

234. Selye H. Thymus and adrenals in the response of organism to injuries and intoxications. *Br J Exp Pathol* 1936; **17**.

235. Blomgren H, Andersson B. Characteristics of the immunocompetant cells in the mouse thymus: Cell population changes during cortisone-induced atrophy and subsequent regeneration. *J Immunol* 1971; **1**: 545–560.

236. Cowan WK, Sorenson DG. Electron microscopic observations of acute thymic involution produced by hydrocortisone. *Lab Invest* 1964; **13**: 353–370.

237. Gillis S, Crabtree GR, Smith KA. Glucocorticoid-induced inhibition of T cell growth factor production. I. The effect on mitogen-induced lymphocyte proliferation. *J Immunol* 1979; **123**: 1624–1631.

238. Taniguchi T. Regulation of cytokine gene expression. *Annu Rev Immunol* 1988; **6**: 439–464.

239. Tolentino MV, Sarasua MM, Hill OA, Wentworth DB, Franceschi D, Fratianne RB. Peripheral lymphocyte membrane fluidity after thermal injury. *J Burn Care Rehabil* 1991; **12**: 498–504.

240. Dale DC, Fauci AS, Wolff SM. Alternate-day prednisone. Leukocyte kinetics and susceptibility to infections. *N Engl J Med* 1974; **291**: 1154–1158.

241. Rinehart JJ, Balcerzak SP, Sagone AL, LoBuglio AF. Effects of corticosteroids on human monocyte function. *J Clin Invest* 1974; **54**: 1337–1343.

242. Ward PA. The chemosuppression of chemotaxis. *J Exp Med* 1966; **124**: 209–226.

243. MacGregor RR, Spagnuolo PJ, Lentnek AL. Inhibition of granulocyte adherence by ethanol, prednisone, and aspirin, measured with an assay system. *N Engl J Med* 1974; **291**: 642–646.

244. Mandell GL, Rubin W, Hook EW. The effect of an NADH oxidase inhibitor (hydrocortisone) on polymorphonuclear leukocyte bactericidal activity. *J Clin Invest* 1970; **49**: 1381–1388.

245. Hibbs JB, Jr. Heterocytolysis by macrophages activated by bacillus Calmette-Guerin: lysosome exocytosis into tumor cells. *Science* 1974; **184**: 468–471.

246. Arturson G, Hogman CF, Johansson SG, Killander J. Changes in immunoglobulin levels in severely burned patients. *Lancet* 1969; **1**: 546–548.

247. Bjornson AB, Altemeier WA, Bjornson HS. Changes in humoral components of host defense following burn trauma. *Ann Surg* 1977; **186**: 88–96.

248. Kawakami M, Meyer AA, deSerres S, Peterson HD. Effects of acute ethanol ingestion and burn injury on serum immunoglobulin. *J Burn Care Rehabil* 1990; **11**: 395–399.

249. Kohn J, Cort DF. Immunoglobulins in burned patients. *Lancet* 1969; **1**: 836–837.

250. Munster AM, Hoagland HC, Pruitt BA, Jr. The effect of thermal injury on serum immunoglobulins. *Ann Surg* 1970; **172**: 965–969.

251. Kagan RJ, Bratescu A, Jonasson O, Matsuda T, Teodorescu M. The relationship between the percentage of circulating B cells, corticosteroid levels, and other immunologic parameters in thermally injured patients. *J Trauma* 1989; **29**: 208–213.

252. Kawakami M, deSerres S, Meyer AA. Immunoglobulin synthesis by cultured lymphocytes from spleen and mesenteric lymph nodes after thermal injury. *J Burn Care Rehabil* 1991; **12**: 474–481.

253. Sakai H, Daniels JC, Beathard GA, Lewis SR, Lynch JB, Ritzmann SE. Mixed lymphocyte culture reaction in patients with acute thermal burns. *J Trauma* 1974; **14**: 53–57.

254. Butler WT, Rossen RD. Effects of corticosteroids on immunity in man. I. Decreased serum IgG concentration caused by 3 or 5 days of high doses of methylprednisolone. *J Clin Invest* 1973; **52**: 2629–2640.

255. Araneo BA, Shelby J, Li GZ, Ku W, Daynes RA. Administration of dehydroepiandrosterone to burned mice preserves normal immunologic competence. *Arch Surg* 1993; **128**: 318–325.

256. Blauer KL, Poth M, Rogers WM, Bernton EW. Dehydroepiandrosterone antagonizes the suppressive effects of dexamethasone on lymphocyte proliferation. *Endocrinology* 1991; **129**: 3174–3179.

257. Daynes RA, Meikle AW, Araneo BA. Locally active steroid hormones may facilitate compartmentalization of immunity by regulating the types of lymphokines produced by helper T cells. *Res Immunol* 1991; **142**: 40–45.

258. Suzuki T, Suzuki N, Daynes RA, Engleman EG. Dehydroepiandrosterone enhances IL2 production and cytotoxic effector function of human T cells. *Clin Immunol Immunopathol* 1991; **61**: 202–211.

259. Devins SS, Miller A, Herndon BL, O'Toole L, Reisz G. Effects of dopamine on T-lymphocyte proliferative responses and serum prolactin concentrations in critically ill patients. *Crit Care Med* 1992; **20**: 1644–1649.

260. Van den Berghe G, de Zegher F, Wouters P, Schetz M, Verwaest C, Ferdinande P, Lauwers P. Dehydroepiandrosterone sulphate in critical illness: effect of dopamine. *Clin Endocrinol (Oxf)* 1995; **43**: 457–463.

261. Higuchi K, Nawata H, Maki T, Higashizima M, Kato K, Ibayashi H. Prolactin has a direct effect on adrenal androgen secretion. *J Clin Endocrinol Metab* 1984; **59**: 714–718.

262. Van Loon GR, Schwartz L, Sole MJ. Plasma dopamine responses to standing and exercise in man. *Life Sci* 1979; **24**: 2273–2277.

263. Viquerat CE, Daly P, Swedberg K, Evers C, Curran D, Parmley WW, Chatterjee K. Endogenous catecholamine levels in chronic heart failure. Relation to the severity of hemodynamic abnormalities. *Am J Med* 1985; **78**: 455–460.

264. Wang XM, Yang L, Chen KM. Catecholamines: important factors in the increase of oxidative phosphorylation coupling in rat-liver mitochondria during the early phase of burn injury. *Burns* 1993; **19**: 110–112.

265. Durkot MJ, Wolfe RR. Effects of adrenergic blockade on glucose kinetics in septic and burned guinea pigs. *Am J Physiol* 1981; **241**: R222–227.

266. Wilmore DW, Aulick LH, Mason AD, Pruitt BA Jr. Influence of the burn wound on local and systemic responses to injury. *Ann Surg* 1977; **186**: 444–458.

267. Bessey PQ, Watters JM, Aoki TT, Wilmore DW. Combined hormonal infusion simulates the metabolic response to injury. *Ann Surg* 1984; **200**: 264–281.

268. Batstone GF, Levick PL, Spurr E, Shakespeare PG, George SL, Ward CM. Changes in acute phase reactants and disturbances in metabolism after burn injury. *Burns Incl Therm Inj* 1983; **9**: 234–239.

269. Batstone GF, Alberti KGMM, Hinks L, Smythe P. Metabolic studies in subjects following thermal injury. *Burns* 1976; **2**: 207–225.

270. Sevaljevic L, Petrovic M, Bogojevic D, Savic J, Pantelic D. Acute-phase response to scalding: changes in serum properties and acute-phase protein concentrations. *Circ Shock* 1989; **28**: 293–307.

271. Calvano SE, Albert JD, Legaspi A, Organ BC, Tracey KJ, Lowry SF, Shires GT, Antonacci AC. Comparison of numerical and phenotypic leukocyte changes during constant hydrocortisone infusion in normal humans with those in thermally injured patients. *Surg Gynecol Obstet* 1987; **164**: 509–520.

272. Webel ML, Ritts RE, Jr., Taswell HF, Danadio JV, Jr., Woods JE. Cellular immunity after intravenous administration of methylprednisolone. *J Lab Clin Med* 1974; **83**: 383–392.

273. Wallner S, Vautrin R, Murphy J, Anderson S, Peterson V. The haematopoietic response to burning: studies in an animal model. *Burns Incl Therm Inj* 1984; **10**: 236–251.

274. Rinehart JJ, Sagone AL, Balcerzak SP, Ackerman GA, LoBuglio AF. Effects of corticosteroid therapy on human monocyte function. *N Engl J Med* 1975; **292**: 236–241.

Chapter 27

Modulation of the hypermetabolic response after burn

Marcus Spies, Michael J Muller

David N Herndon

The hypermetabolic response to burn trauma

The stress response to burn injury is similar to any critical illness or severe trauma only differing by its severity and duration. Burn patients experience an 'ebb' phase immediately after injury lasting 2 or 3 days during which their metabolic rate and cardiac output are decreased.[1-3] Following the 'ebb' phase, patients pass through a 'flow' or hypermetabolic phase. The hypermetabolic response after major burn is characterized by a hyperdynamic circulatory response[4] with increased body temperature,[5] oxygen and glucose consumption,[6,7] CO_2 production,[7] glycogenolysis,[8] proteolysis,[9,10] lipolysis,[11,12] and futile substrate cycling.[13] This response begins on the fifth day post-injury and continues up to 9 months postburn (**Figure 27.1**),[14] causing erosion of lean body mass,[9] muscle weakness,[10] immunodepression,[15] and poor wound healing.[16]

In no other disease or trauma is the hypermetabolic response as severe as it is following a thermal injury. While patients with peritonitis may have metabolic rates elevated from 5% to 25%, and severely multiple traumatized patients 30–75% above normal, severely burned patients with a body surface area burned greater than 40% may have metabolic requirements twice normal.[1,2] The increased metabolic requirements in patients with major burns can cause a major tissue breakdown leading to nitrogen loss and a potentially lethal depletion of essential protein stores.[17] The resting metabolic rates in burn patients increase in a curvilinear fashion ranging from near normal for burn less than 10% total body surface area (TBSA) to twice normal over 40% TBSA burned.[18] This

response is temperature-sensitive but not temperature-dependent. It may be attenuated but not completely abolished by environmental heating. However, environmental temperatures greater than skin temperatures do not reduce metabolic rates in patients with greater than 40% TBSA burns. Largely burned individuals strive to maintain skin and core body temperature at approximately 1–2°C above normal.[18,19]

The stress response to trauma is also influenced by the nervous

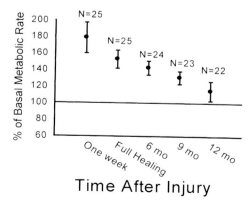

Fig. 27.1 Resting energy expenditure. Measured energy expenditure (indirect calorimetry) in percentage of basal metabolic rate as predicted by the Harris–Benedict equation (adapted from Hart *et al.*[14]).

system. Several mechanisms of activation are involved. The limbic system is activated by fear, emotion, by thalamic relay of peripheral nociceptive stimuli.[20] Cardiovascular and respiratory reflexes regulated by the brain stem are altered by hypoxemia, hypercapnia, and hypotension.[21,22] Inflammatory mediators such as bacterial endotoxin and various cytokines, such as interleukin-1 and tumor necrosis factor-α (TNFα), stimulate the hypothalamus directly.[23-27] They reset thermoregulation setpoint and alter endocrine function.[28,29]

The hormonal response to trauma

Catecholamines involved in the hypermetabolic response to burn injury are released from sympathetic nerve ends (norepinephrine) and the adrenal medulla (epinephrine).[18,23] Catecholamine production following thermal injury is under hypothalamic control.[30] Norepinephrine levels are raised 2- to 10-fold in proportion to burn size.[31] A close correlation exists between the increase in plasma catecholamines and metabolic rate.[32,33] Catecholamine levels remain elevated until wound repair is complete. Cortisol facilitates the action of catecholamines.[34] Catecholamines act via α, β-1, and β-2 adrenoreceptors. Epinephrine accelerates hepatic gluconeogenesis, hepatic glycogenolysis, adipocyte lipolysis (via β-1 adrenoreceptors) and muscle proteolysis with the intent to increase the substrate availability for gluconeogenesis and maintain blood glucose levels.

Insulin levels usually are normal or elevated after burn injury. However, stress hormone-induced insulin resistance counteracts most anabolic effects, such as hypoglycemia, lipogenesis, glycogenesis, increased protein synthesis, and decreased gluconeogenesis.[35]

Paradoxically, glucagon levels are elevated following burn despite a decreased glucagon secretion due to insulin and hyperglycemia.[36] Glucagon secretion is stimulated by elevated catecholamines, glucocorticoids, and hypoglycemia.[37,38] Increased sympathetic nervous activity and elevated catecholamine levels stimulate and maintain glucagon release despite hyperglycemia and hyperinsulinemia. Furthermore, infusion of tumor necrosis factor in animal models results in increased glucagon levels without changes to insulin or catecholamine levels.[39]

Glucocorticosteroid substitution is crucial for the survival of adrenal- or pituitary-deficient patients in critical illness. Cortisol production can rise up to 10-fold in severely burned patients. Following burn injury, the circadian rhythm of plasma cortisol levels is disrupted.[40] Although adrenocorticotrophic hormone (ACTH) levels increase proportional to burn-size, the ACTH–cortisol relationship during trauma is difficult to interpret because of ACTH pulsatile production and short half-life. ACTH is primarily released by the hypothalamic corticotrophin-releasing hormone (CRH), but antidiuretic hormone (ADH) and interleukin-1 (IL-1) are also ACTH secretagogues. ACTH plasma levels are elevated in the initial days after burn injury but then return to normal but lose circadian rhythm.[41] ACTH plasma levels after major burns often do not correlate with cortisol levels.[42]

Cortisol, glucagon, and the catecholamines are characterized as counter-regulatory, anti-insulin, or stress hormones. After injury they all are elevated and have synergistic effects.[43] Cortisol stimulates gluconeogenesis, increases proteolysis and alanine synthesis, sensitizes adipocytes to the action of lipolytic hormones (cate-

cholamines), and has an anti-inflammatory action. It causes insulin resistance. Cortisol facilitates the action of catecholamines and helps maintain cardiovascular stability during stress.[34,44] It synergizes with catecholamines and glucagon to divert glucose utilization from skeletal muscle to central organs such as the brain. As a group, the stress hormones cause hyperglycemia. Glucagon increases intrahepatic cyclic adenine monophosphate (cAMP) levels and promotes gluconeogenesis, glycogenolysis, lipolysis, and ketogenesis in the liver. Catecholamines cause increased glycogenolysis, hepatic gluconeogenesis, and gluconeogenic precursor mobilization, promote lipolysis, peripheral insulin resistance, and inhibit insulin release.[35] Glucagon and catecholamines synergize to promote gluconeogenesis. If they are infused together into normal subjects, gluconeogenesis is more prolonged than if they are infused alone[43] and combined infusion simulates the metabolic response to injury.[45]

The mechanisms of synergy of cortisol, glucagon, and catecholamines are varied. Cortisol may induce inhibition of catechol O-methyltransferase and block re-uptake of catecholamines by the sympathetic nerve ends.[46] Cortisol also increases β-adrenergic receptor messenger RNA and so may increase the total number of β-receptors, making catecholamines as adrenoreceptor agonists even more effective.[47] Together with glucagon-induced increased intracellular cyclic AMP levels by a non-β-receptor mechanism, this leads to increased systemic glucose availability.

However, not only stress hormones affect the hypermetabolic response after trauma. Follicle-stimulating hormone (FSH) and luteinizing hormone (LH) regulated by hypothalamic luteinizing hormone-releasing hormone (LHRH) are altered with injury. FSH levels are decreased in males and females after burn and sensitively indicate the degree of burn trauma.[41,48] LH levels remain below normal following burn injury.[49] Despite 17-β-estradiol reaching high levels as during ovulation amenorrhea is common in female burn patients.[48] Progesterone levels after burn are decreased in premenopausal women and lack the rise usually seen in the secretory phase of the menstrual cycle. As also males show high to very high 17-β-estradiol levels after burn, this is in both sexes most likely due to synthesis in the adrenal gland. Adrenal androgens such as dehydroepiandrosterone sulfate (DHEA-S) and dehydroepiandrosterone (DHEA) levels are low postburn.[50] It has been postulated that low levels of DHEA and DHEA-S cause the pentose phosphate pathway to become more active and produce more NADPH which is required in the myeloperoxidase system of leukocytes.[51,52] Decreased testosterone production in males after burn injury is burn-size dependent[53,54] and is associated with histologic changes in the male gonads: interstitial atrophy, absence of spermatogenic and Leydig cells, and hyalinization of the basement membranes of the seminiferous tubules.[55] Hypospermia is common but spontaneous recovery can be expected.

Prolactin levels increase after burn injury in both men and women, but to a greater extent and for a longer time in women.[41] Hyperprolactinemia causes impotence in men and in women prevents pregnancy during lactation. Postburn impotence is common and can be longlasting.

Metabolic response

In addition to the increased total caloric requirements in severely burned patients, alterations in the oxidation of specific substrates occur. This includes changes in intracellular substrate oxidation, the availability of energy substrates, and their influence on each other.

Glucose and Insulin Production

Glucose kinetics in severely burned patients are almost always abnormal. Glucose utilization in burned patients is almost entirely through inefficient anaerobic mechanisms as characterized by increased lactate production,[56] which accounts for increased glucose consumption. Glucose production, particularly from alanine,[8] is elevated in almost all patients with severe burn.[57,58] The increased gluconeogenesis from amino acids renders these amino acids unavailable for reincorporation into body protein. Nitrogen is excreted, primarily in urea, thus contributing to the progressive depletion of body protein stores.

Plasma insulin levels usually remain normal or slightly elevated in burn patients.[58] The fact, that the basal rate of glucose production is elevated despite normal or elevated plasma insulin levels, indicates hepatic insulin resistance, since under normal conditions elevated serum insulin would lower the rate of glucose production.[59] Furthermore, the plasma glucose concentration is frequently increased, which would normally directly inhibit glucose production.

Protein and amino acid metabolism

Major trauma, burns, and sepsis often lead to a rapid net catabolism of body protein, as well as a redistribution of the nitrogen pool within the body. The rate of protein breakdown in critical illness is increased in comparison to normal individuals who are fed comparable amounts of protein and calories.[60] Muscle protein breakdown is accelerated to satisfy the increase in protein synthetic activity required for the rapid production of 'acute-phase' proteins in the liver, promotion of wound healing, and increased immunologic activity. The increased muscle protein breakdown results in an increased efflux of amino acids, including gluconeogenic amino acids. Alanine, in particular is released from the muscle and is cleared from the plasma in the liver, where it is converted to glucose. It has been proposed that the availability of alanine directly influences the rate of glucose production.[61] The high rate of glucose production and thus glucose uptake drives the rate of peripheral release of alanine. In addition, glutamine, which is also released by peripheral muscle, may be directly used as fuel in the gut and by white blood cells. The magnitude of the net catabolism of muscle may be so pronounced in severely burned patients that maintenance of lean body mass is an unrealistic goal. Nonetheless, provision of dietary protein and amino acids is essential for minimizing net protein catabolism. There is, however, a limit to the extent to which increased protein intake can ameliorate net protein catabolism in a previously well nourished trauma patient. Protein intake of more than 1.5 g protein/kg/day has not demonstrated any additional benefit.[60] Therefore, dietary provision of 1.2–1.5 protein/kg/day seems reasonable in adults. Due to higher than normal protein requirements, a higher protein intake of 2 g/kg/day is recommended in children. An additional increase of protein intake above this level to up to 3 g/kg/day in unburned children failed to have any additional advantage.[62] Formulations enriched with branched-chain amino acids to supply nitrogen for the production

of alanine from pyruvate, have been promoted, but clinical trials failed to show a significant advantage in most critically ill patients. Glutamine has been considered a conditionally essential amino acid in trauma. Muscle-free glutamine levels decrease during injury, and most likely serve as a reservoir to fulfill the requirement of immunocompetent cells after trauma.[63,64] Although intracellular glutamine has been proposed as a key regulator of protein synthesis, exogenous administration of glutamine has not shown a beneficial effect and the body seems to depend on the *de novo* synthesis of glutamine.[65] Other amino acids, such as arginine and histidine, have been promoted as 'unique pharmacological effectors'; however, convincing experimental evidence of their benefit in humans is not yet available.

Lipid metabolism

In normal humans, lipids constitute more than 80% of stored fuel reserves. Fat stores, along with very small carbohydrate stores, can be almost completely depleted without detriment to the individual. Conversely, the use of protein reserves is limited, because even moderate depletion can adversely affect an organism exposed to stress by reducing structural protein reserves.[66] When an individual must rely on endogenous fuel supplies to meet energy requirements, lipids are physiologically the preferred source. Most tissues can readily use fatty acids as substrates for energy metabolism. The use of fatty acids by these tissues preserves limited carbohydrate stores for use by central nervous tissue and red blood cells. A theoretically optimal 'stress' response would involve the mobilization and use of fat. The rate of free fatty acids (FFA) mobilization exceeds by far the rate of oxidation as an energy substrate. In severely burned patients, over 70% of released fatty acids are re-esterified into triglyceride (TG) predominantly in the liver. The rate of TG synthesis is determined by delivery of FFA to the liver. The normal cycle between TG and FFA involves synthesis of TG in proportion to hepatic FFA uptake and secretion into the plasma as very-low-density lipoprotein (VLDL)-TG.[67] The VLDL-TG then are returned for storage to adipose tissue. In critically ill patients, the export of VLDL-TG from the liver seems to be limited by decreased formation of VLDL-TG, potentially as a result of impaired apo-B protein synthesis. This leads to fat accumulation in the liver even in the absence of significant hepatic fatty acid synthesis. The amount of fat deposition in the liver of critically ill patients is directly related to the severity of illness and unrelated to the nature of the nutritional support.[68] The hormonal response associated with stress and characterized by increased epinephrine, cortisol, and glucagon levels with low insulin levels would favor the mobilization of lipid from storage depots.[11,12] Other factors, however, may simultaneously suppress the mobilization or use of fat.

Modulation of the hypermetabolic response

Influence of Environmental Changes

The metabolic rate is increased after burn injury by nearly 50%[69] when burn size is greater than 20–30% TBSA and even greater in larger burns or if burn wound sepsis is present. If the burn size is greater than 40% TBSA, hypermetabolism can be attenuated by increasing the ambient temperature from 25°C to 33°C.[70] It was noted that those who failed to respond to lower ambient temperatures by increasing metabolic rate and catecholamine production were more likely to succumb to their injuries. When allowed to select their own environmental temperature, burn patients chose ambient temperatures of 31.5±0.7°C.[71] This is the temperature range that minimizes the metabolic expenditure required to maintain core temperatures 1–2°C higher than normal.[72] Clearly, patients treated by closed techniques with dressings and bandages tolerate slightly lower ambient temperatures, probably about 28°C. Shivering evokes an enormous increase in energy expenditure and should be avoided. Blockade of evaporative water loss with water-impermeable membranes does not prevent hypermetabolism.[73] However, when evaporative water loss occurs, it should be accompanied by environmental heating to minimize hypermetabolism.[74] The heat of water evaporation is 0.576 kcal/ml, and water loss can be as high as 200 ml/m² body surface area burn/h; and if the energy of evaporation does not come from the environment, it must be produced by the patient.[75] This simple but very effective means of modulating postburn hypermetabolism can be achieved with patient-controlled temperature regulation of air conditioning or infra-red heaters[18] altered at the patient's request.[76,77] While increasing ambient temperature will attenuate hypermetabolism and increase patient comfort, the underlying altered metabolic state with thermogenic futile substrate cycling will continue and requires additional nutrition support.

Nutritional modulation

A 30% weight loss has been observed in patients with moderate sized burns, in spite of maximal oral intake. Wound healing is limited and mortality increased when weight losses exceed 20% of preburn weights. Tissue breakdown may liberate as much as 30 g nitrogen/day.[78] This can be limited by adequate dietary carbohydrate.[70] A patient's appetite seldom exceeds their preburn levels and voluntary eating almost never meets protein or caloric requirements in any but those with small burns. This observation led to parenteral supplementation of nutrition, but this was shown not to improve mortality or indices of immunity.[79,80] This may be the result of a negative effect on the immune system by parenteral nutrition.[81] Immediate enteral nutrition can be safely administered and may limit postburn hypermetabolism[82,83] by preserving intestinal mucosal integrity, thereby limiting bacterial translocation.[84–86]

When the metabolic response after burn injury was assessed using stable isotope infusions of leucine, valine, lysine, and urea in the acute, flow, convalescent, and recovery phases, increased protein breakdown was present during the acute, flow, and convalescent phases. The rate of urea production (RQ urea), used as an indirect measure of net protein catabolism, was significantly increased during the flow phase only, suggesting that protein breakdown was adequately normalized in the acute and convalescent phases by elevations in protein synthesis but not in the flow phase[87]. The switch from net protein catabolism to net protein anabolism in convalescence occurs in spite of an elevated protein breakdown rate.

Modulation of protein dynamics has included increased provision of protein, supplementation of branched-chain amino acids, and supplementation of arginine. When children with large burns (60% or greater TBSA) were fed either 16.5% or 23% of their caloric intake as proteins, neither achieved the desired level of calories with the 23% protein group taking significantly fewer calories (87% vs 77%). Furthermore, the higher protein group received less intravenous hyperalimentation and fewer glucose infusions. As well, the higher protein group showed better indices of immunity,[74] higher protein levels, fewer bacteremic days, and improved survival.[88] Severely burned adults (70% TBSA) have also been studied with differential protein intake and stable isotope infusions of leucine, α-ketoisocaproic acid, and urea. Protein intake of 1.4 g/kg/day showed balance between protein synthesis and catabolism. When protein intake was increased to 2.2 g protein/kg/day, the isotopic methods did not indicate a further benefit in net protein synthesis, although the absolute rates of protein synthesis and catabolism were stimulated. Urinary nitrogen losses, on the other hand, indicated a significant improvement in net protein synthesis with higher protein intake. Further, the underlying alterations in protein metabolism consequent to the burn persisted, regardless of the level of protein intake[89] as the levels of protein intake had no effect on endogenous leucine production or intracellular leucine oxidation. When the daily protein intake was increased to nearly 3 g/kg, no further changes in the rate of muscle protein synthesis could be detected. Protein synthesis in skin, however, showed a significant increase. Thus, while this high protein diet may enhance wound healing, it seems of little additional benefit to severely burned patients.[90]

Branched-chain amino acid-enriched nutritional therapy was shown not to alter leucine kinetics when compared to conventional intact protein formulation in severely burned adults in a crossover study using stable isotope infusions of leucine. Nitrogen balance measurements were not statistically different between the study periods and the major consequence of increased intake of leucine from the branched-chain amino acid formula was an enhanced rate of leucine oxidation. Although evidence suggests benefit for surgical patients, branched-chain amino acid formulas do not appear to offer any advantages over intact protein.[91] Intact protein was also shown to enhance nitrogen retention and maintain body weight better than free amino acids when fed enterally to burned guinea pigs.[92]

In general, the caloric requirements must mainly be met by the carbohydrate component of the nutrition formula. Carbohydrates stimulate endogenous insulin production, which has beneficial effects in muscle and the burn wound.[93,94] During postburn hypermetabolism, glucose seems to be the preferred cellular fuel.[95] In a recent study on severely burned children, it was shown that a high carbohydrate diet significantly improves protein net balance by decreasing muscle protein breakdown without effecting protein synthesis compared to a high fat diet.[96] This effect can be explained by the stimulation of endogenous insulin secretion. Recently it was shown that peripheral lipolysis and not de novo synthesis in the liver is the major source of fat transported via VLDL after burn;[97] thus high fat diets might add a detrimental fat load to the liver after severe burn injury. The cause of fat deposition in the liver postburn is more likely due to peripheral lipolysis than de novo fatty acid synthesis in the liver.[98] These findings suggest that a diet that delivers nonprotein calories in the form of carbohydrates is preferred. However, essential fatty acid supplementation is required to avoid a deficiency.

Omega-3 (ω-3) fatty acids, such as in fish oil, lead to production of prostaglandin E₃ (PGE₃), an immuno-inert substance. Most dietary fats in enteral feeding formulas are linoleic acids, which lead to production of immunosuppressive PGE₆. Recently, a linoleic acid restricted, tube feeding formulation of high protein, enriched with ω-3 fatty acids, arginine, cysteine, histidine, vitamin A, zinc, and ascorbic acid, was compared to two other standard formulations. Trends towards decreased wound infection, shorter length of hospital stay, reduced incidence of diarrhea, lower serum triglycerides, reduced numbers of infectious episodes, and improved preservation of muscle mass were apparent. Increased patient numbers with adjustment for burn size and age in the analysis may demonstrate this formulation to be effective in modulating the immune response to burn injury.[99] It has also been shown that postoperative enteral nutrition with supplemental arginine, RNA, and ω-3 fatty acids significantly improved immunologic, metabolic, and clinical outcomes in patients with upper abdominal malignancies who were undergoing major elective surgery.[100]

Enteral feeding, applied as soon as possible, consisting of about 20% protein, 70% carbohydrate, with the remainder as low linoleic fats, will help prevent weight loss. Polymeric diets are preferable to the more expensive elemental diets. Quantities required can be estimated by the feeding formulas described elsewhere. It must be stressed that if expense or availability preclude use of more sophisticated feeds, cow's milk has been used extensively to good effect.

Hormonal modulation

Following major trauma, the control of body metabolism shifts from the thyroid axis to that of the sympathetic adrenal axis. Free thyronine (T_4) and free 3, 5, 3′ tri-iodothyronine (T_3) serum levels decrease while reverse T_3, an inactive metabolite, increases.[101] Plasma norepinephrine and epinephrine are correlated negatively with T_3 while plasma catechol levels are correlated positively with T_3 levels. An attempt to modulate this relationship by T_3 treatment resulted in decreased levels of T_4 and norepinephrine but did not change epinephrine levels.[101] The hypermetabolic syndrome of low tri-iodothyronine levels after burn is similar to other states of critical illness and is also known as the sick euthyroid syndrome.[102] The thyroid remains responsive to TSH, whose levels are also diminished.

Animal studies have revealed that adrenalectomy limits the increase in metabolic rate after burns, but that thyroidectomy does not[103] (**Table 27.1**).

Table 27.1 Oxygen consumption of Rats with 50% TBSA scald burn[103]

	Oxygen consumption		
	Non-burned (mg/g/h)	Burned (mg/g/h)	Increase (%)
Control	0.84 ± 0.10	1.16 ± 0.02*	38%
Thyroidectomized	0.54 ± 0.10	0.80 ± 0.08*	48%
Adrenalectomized	0.85 ± 0.20	0.98 ± 0.02	15%

* Significantly different $p<0.05$.
Data presented as mean±SEM.

Pinealectomy performed before a burn in hamsters did not prevent liver-induced depression of serum T_4 or testosterone.[104] Neither T_3 treatment in burn patients nor T_4 treatment in trauma patients improved survival and may well be disadvantageous by inhibiting T_4 secretion,[105–107] a notion supported by decreased survival in an animal model of sepsis.[108]

While thyroid hormone therapy has not been shown to improve survival and absence of a thyroid does not prevent postburn hyper-metabolism, thyroxine therapy may improve wound healing following burn. Guinea pigs were thyroidectomized prior to a 50% TBSA scald burn and treated with different doses of L-thyroxine. Oxygen consumption, as an index of metabolic rate, was measured at 32°C. Wound healing was significantly improved at an intermediate dose but was retarded at a higher dose[109] (**Table 27.2**).

Table 27.2 Thyroidectomized guinea pigs treated with different doses of L-thyroxine after 50% TBSA burn[109]

	Dose (μg/kg)	O_2 consumption burn/control (%)	Wound healing (days)
Nonthyroidectomized	0	53	93
Thyroidectomized	15	44	86
	30	34	63*
	60	41	105
	120	32	138

* Significantly different $p<0.05$.
Data presented as mean±SEM.

The quality of scar was improved by T_3 treatment of rats with deep dermal burns. Histologic examination showed better-organized collagen bundles, fewer retraction spaces, and smoother scars in the T_3-treated group.[110] Thyroid hormone modulation of the postburn response may improve the quality of survival by limiting unsightly scars.

Growth factors and cytokines

Cytokines, particularly interleukin 1 (IL-1), interleukin 6 (IL-6), and tumor necrosis factor (TNF), are the principal chemical messengers responsible for many of the events occurring at both the wound and systemically in distal tissues. Cytokines were originally considered to be regulatory chemicals secreted by cells of the immune system, and growth factors were seen as chemicals originating from inflammatory and reparative tissues. Now, the differences between growth factors, peptide hormones, and cytokines are no longer distinct. In this chapter, growth factors and cytokines are considered together and may be defined as any naturally occurring substance having a combination of mitogenic, angiogenic, activating, or chemotactic properties on the cell of origin and/or on other cells.[111] Many of these growth factors are released from damaged tissues at the wound site where they exert local and systemic effects.

Disruption of the vascular endothelium by wounding exposes blood cells to collagen, which precipitates a cascade of events ultimately leading to blood clotting, inflammation, and repair. Platelet degranulation, endothelial damage, and leukocytes contribute to a pool of growth factors and cytokines at the wound site, which subsequently regulate enzymatic degradation, phagocytosis, chemotaxis, angiogenesis, and re-epithelialization.[112] Re-epithelialization, the migration of proliferating epithelial cells from the wound edges, provides a protective roof over the wound under which repair can proceed away from abrasive forces, dehydration, and the risk of infection. The wound site contains factors from multiple sources. Growth factors and cytokines produced locally at the wound site spill over into the circulation where they are carried to distal organs or tissues and stimulate the production of other mediators, growth factors, and cytokines distally. By disseminating these distal tissue mediators into the circulation, more target tissues become involved by a cascading mechanism (**Figure 27.2**). It is this mechanism by which cytokines also activate the hepatic acute phase response. Predominantly, IL-1 and TNFα induce type I acute phase reactant production, whereas IL-6 activates synthesis of type II acute phase proteins. This shift of protein synthesis in the liver results in a reduction in constitutive protein production, such as albumin, pre-albumin, and transferrin.[113,114]

Growth factors bind to specific cell surface receptors, which transmit messages to the cell nucleus directing it to upregulate or downregulate synthesis of a specific secretory protein. Typically these receptors consist of three domains: an extracellular, a transmembrane, and an intracellular domain. The union of the extracellular domain with its ligand produces a conformational change in the extracellular domain with subsequent transmembrane activation (**Figure 27.3**). The activation of each receptor is unique; for example, some receptors require the binding of two sites on the same ligand molecule before transmembrane activation occurs. Other receptors require interaction between two neighboring receptor/ligand complexes before transmembrane transmission occurs. Another feature is cross-reactivity between growth factors for a given receptor due to structural homology between ligand proteins. This feature of sharing exists between the receptors of many factors. Although each receptor/ligand reaction is unique, there are many common features, and the growth hormone receptor and its ligand is a good example.

The growth hormone/growth hormone binding protein complex

Growth hormone (GH) binds to specific receptor molecules on the cell surface. Recent studies suggest that the binding of growth factors to their receptors occurs as a result of conformational diversity with relatively little change in the amino acid sequence.[115] The GH peptide is an asymmetrical molecule of 191 amino acids containing four helices and supporting two receptor-binding sites. Topographical examination shows that the shapes of these binding sites on the hormone molecule are quite different.[115] Growth hormone binds two separate surface receptors and forms a dimeric complex GH-GHBP$_2$. The binding site in the extracellular portion of the GH receptor consists of cysteine-rich areas.[115,116] There are marked similarities in the structure of the GH receptor extracellular domain and those of several other growth factors.[117] Cytokine/growth factor receptors may be divided into two classes, 1 and 2, based on homology between their extracellular domains. Members of the class 1 receptor family include receptors for GH, prolactin, erythropoietin, IL-3, IL-6, IL-7, IL-4, and the granulocyte and granulocyte–macrophage colony-stimulating factors (G-CSF, GM-CSF).[117–119]

The cytokine/growth factor molecules IL-6, GH, prolactin, erythropoietin, G-CSF, and myelomonocyte growth factor (MGF), which bind to class 1 receptors, share structural similarities. By the interaction of accessory proteins, which bind to specific sites on the ligand, a stronger ligand/ receptor union may be created. In this manner, cytokines, which differ in their primary structure but have

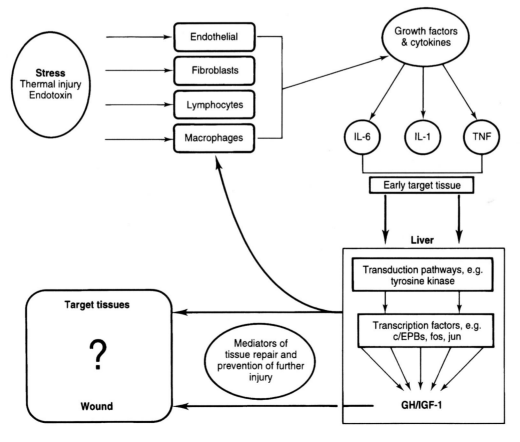

Fig. 27.2 Stress induces the release of inflammatory mediators from cells such as macrophages, lymphocytes, fibroblasts, and endothelial cells. These mediators are thought to be disseminated via the circulation to distal tissues, such as the liver, where they induce families of stress response genes. The protein products of these genes (e.g. growth hormone (GH) and insulin–like growth factor–1 (IGF–1)) regulate the processes of wound repair and prevention of further injury in target tissues, such as the wound and other organs.

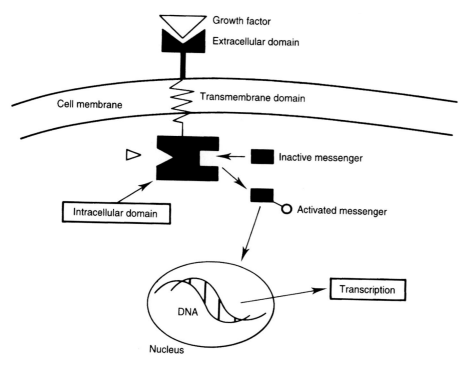

Fig. 27.3 Many growth factors and cytokines produce cell activation by binding to specific cell surface receptors. In doing this, the signal from the cytokine is passed via an intercellular cascade in order to reach the nucleus where protein synthesis is initiated. Reprinted with permission from Herndon DN, Hayward PG. Rutan RL, Barrow RE. Growth hormones and factors in surgical patients. In: Cameron JL, ed. *Advances in Surgery*, Vol. 25, Chicago: Mosby Yearbook, Inc., 1991, pp. 65–97.

similarities in secondary structure, may be able to bind to several different cell surface receptors. For example, human GH may bind to prolactin receptors. If the growth factor is present in sufficient concentration, weak binding may also have an intracellular effect. More permanent and high-affinity binding would only occur if the accessory protein recognizes specific features on the ligand. There may be an 'evolutionary conserved interaction between homologous receptors and structurally similar cytokines'.[117] The structure of the GH-GHBP$_2$ complex is known and is easy to relate to the proposed model. Growth hormone can bind to both prolactin and GH receptors, indicating a degree of cross-reactivity.[120] The ability of GH to bind to both prolactin and GH receptors may be altered by changing certain amino acid residues in specific areas of the GH molecule.[121] These facts help to provide further evidence for links within the cytokine/growth factor family. The significance of these structural similarities between different peptide ligands and the extracellular receptor domains is that a single growth factor may elicit several different responses, inhibitory or stimulatory, depending upon interactions with other factors and the cellular environment into which it is released. In addition, the phases of phagocytosis, re-epithelialization, and angiogenesis are timed and regulated by the factors which predominate at any particular time as well as on the presence and intensity of surface receptors on the target tissues which, in turn, will vary with the state of cellular differentiation. Several growth factors have been shown to be of particular importance in wound healing: platelet derived growth factor (PDGF), fibroblast growth factor (FGF), transforming growth factors (TGFs), and epidermal growth factor (EGF).

Platelet derived growth factor

Platelet derived growth factor is a glycoprotein dimer consisting of two chains, α and β, which have a 60% homology between their amino acid sequences. The PDGF dimer can exist in one of three forms AA (α,α), BB (β,β), and AB (α,β).[122] The dimers exert their effect by binding to specific surface receptors. There are two types of receptor, α and β. All three dimeric PDGF molecules bind to the α-receptor, but only PDGF (BB) binds to the β-receptor. Platelet derived growth factor and the factors EGF, TGF, and FGF, all activate the same signal transduction pathway, starting with the enzyme tyrosine kinase, within the cytoplasm in order to convey messages to the nucleus.[123] Sources of PDGF include degranulated platelets, vascular endothelium, and macrophages.[124] PDGF is thought to play a role in regulating other factors. For example, PDGF can induce the production of KC, the rodent homologue of human melanocyte growth stimulatory activity (MGSA),[125] a member of the IL-8 family of intercrine cytokines. MGSA is known to downregulate collagen synthesis in tissue culture and to have chemotactic qualities, which are features of obvious importance in wound healing. Platelet derived growth factor is itself chemotactic for fibroblasts and inflammatory cells. Clinical studies using topically applied PDGF show enhanced healing of chronic ulcers and nonhealing wounds.[126] Collagen synthesis is also effected by PDGF. The mechanism of action at membrane, cytoplasmic, and nuclear levels, as well as which isoform is optimal, are questions which are still to be determined.

Fibroblast growth factor

The FGF family consists of seven proteins, all with some degree of structural homology.[127,128] The proteins each have their own cell surface receptors; but as with PDGF, there is cross-reactivity between factors. One receptor binds several FGF factors, but with differing affinities for each. The FGF family helps to control angiogenesis through its stimulatory action on vascular endothelium. FGF-2, from damaged endothelium and macrophages is thought to have an autocrine feedback upon the vascular lining;[128] and this stimulates growth of the endothelial cells. Fibroblast growth factors are also mitogenic for fibroblasts and keratinocytes.[127]

Transforming growth factor

Transforming growth factor-β exists in three forms TGF (1, 2 and 3) and is located within platelet granules.[129,130] TGF-β (1) is a dimer of two identical chains and remains in an inactive complex while linked to a glycoprotein, TGF-binding protein. Release and activation of TGF occur upon exposure of the complex to extremes of physiological pH, which are conditions found in wounds. *In vivo* animal studies confirm the usefulness of TGF at enhancing wound healing and tensile strength.[131]

Epidermal growth factor

Transforming growth factor and EGF share a 30% amino acid sequence homology.[132,133] Both factors have been found in wounds. *In vivo* animal studies indicate that EGF is necessary for collagen formation, epithelialization, and granulation tissue formation; and this suggests that it has an effect on epithelial and fibroblast cells. Clinical studies in which TGF and EGF were topically applied to burn wounds, independently, showed an enhancement in epithelialization with TGF being more effective than EGF.[110] Epidermal growth factor has also been shown to be of benefit in other areas of wound healing, including venous stasis and corneal ulcers.[134,135]

Topical growth factor application

There is diversity and cross-reactivity between growth factors regarding structure, receptors, and subsequent actions. Clinical studies suggest the benefit of topical factors; however, many obstacles surround such a course, not least of which are the methods used in assessing the efficiency of the factor. Unintentional bias and the subjective nature of many assessment techniques make comparisons between studies and factors difficult. The massive production of proteolytic enzymes by neutrophils in wounds may inactivate growth factors. The degree to which this occurs depends on the number and activity of the leukocytes present. The effect of growth factors is entirely dependent on the variable state of receptivity of the wound itself.

An ideal growth factor would be tremendously valuable in the field of burn surgery where large wounds must be closed and kept free of infection. Unfortunately these two simple aims create a dilemma. Wounds heal best if kept moist, warm, and undisturbed, yet burn wounds contain multiple endogenous bacteria which may flourish under certain conditions, and which may, either by becoming pathogenic themselves or by creating conditions, through local pH changes, favor the growth of other pathogens. Obviously this sequence of events is undesirable and can result in wound infection and systemic sepsis. The application of topical antibacterial agents, frequent dressing changes, improved resuscitation, and early wound excision have vastly reduced infective complications and mortality. Unfortunately, the requirements for prevention of infection and those optimal for wound healing do not completely coincide. Dressing changes abrade epithelializing surfaces and soak up tissue fluid rich in the very growth factors desired for heal-

ing. In addition, some topical antimicrobial agents inhibit re-epithelialization. The incorporation of growth factors along with topical antibiotics is a possibility as is the direct application of a growth 'cocktail', (possibly of PDGF, FGF, and EGF) onto a skin-grafted area. This 'ideal' growth factor should have the qualities listed in **Table 27.3**. It should be nontoxic both locally at the wound site in terms of allergy or systemically if absorbed. Secondly, there should be no potential drug interactions between the growth factor or its carrier and constituents of dressing materials or topical agents used for wound debridement. No systemically administered drug should cross-react with or interact with the factor. The growth factor should be inexpensive, readily available, and in a form easy to prepare, apply, and, if necessary, remove (water-soluble) without lengthy preparation. The half-life of the agent at the wound site must be sufficiently long for it to have histological benefit. Burn wounds produce considerable tissue fluid. Even after grafting, tissue fluid loss is substantial. Topical factor preparations should be of physiological pH with no tendency to create osmotic gradients and electrolyte disturbances, a feature of particular importance in young children. Substantial tissue fluid production at the wound site can dilute topical growth factors and carry them into absorbent dressings, thereby reducing their effectiveness. Tissue fluid can also interfere with wound penetration by the factor. Any topical agent should be stable so that the number of applications required to maintain a therapeutic range are kept to a minimum. Unfortunately maintenance of uniform rates of diffusion, and therefore, concentration are virtually impossible to standardize. The development of *in vivo* gene transfer using viral vectors, particle-mediated transfer, microseeding, or liposomal gene transfer have introduced new therapeutic applications of growth factors.[136-138] The integration of growth factor genes in to local wound fibroblasts or keratinocytes leads to auto- or paracrine secretion of these growth factors. When adequate growth factor is produced, enhanced wound healing is possible.[152,154] Although many studies are very encouraging in this area, there remain many difficulties to overcome in achieving uniformity for assessing 'wound healing' and in standardizing regimens for the application of these agents.

Table 27.3 Qualities of the ideal topical growth factor application

- Nontoxic
- Inexpensive
- Easily applied and removed if needed
- Long half-life when in contact with the wound
- Wide therapeutic range
- Good tissue penetration
- Long shelf life
- No interactions with dressing materials

The growth hormone/insulin–like growth factor axis

Growth hormone and insulin-like growth factor (IGF-1) levels are often decreased following burn injury.[139-141] These decreased levels of anabolic growth factors may play a role in the recently reported deficit in transmembrane amino acid transport observed in burned patients.[142] The principal cause of net protein catabolism during flow phase postburn is an accelerated rate of breakdown with a concomitant failure to increase synthesis sufficiently to compensate.[142–145] A variation in transport rates could limit the availability of intracellular amino acids for synthesis. It is well established that growth hormone is a potent anabolic agent and can induce stimulation of net protein synthesis directly or indirectly through the action of IGF-1[144–148] and growth hormone; and IGF-1 has been shown to increase transmembrane amino acid transport *in vitro*.[149] Growth hormone's effects include increased appetite, decreased nitrogen losses, increased retention of nitrogen and potassium, weight gain, more rapid wound healing, increased oxygen utilization, and decreased respiratory quotient.[150,151] These effects are in addition to its well-known linear growth-promoting effect.

GH promotes protein synthesis by increasing the cellular uptake of amino acids and accelerating nucleic acid translation and transcription, thereby enhancing cell proliferation. Fatty acids are released from the hydrolysis of fat for conversion to acetyl Co-A, an essential energy-producing molecule for the tricarboxylic acid cycle. Through the preferential use of adipose tissue for energy production, there is a decrease in body fat with the result that protein is spared from catabolism.[152] GH treatment of obese dieters allows lean body mass conservation at the expense of adipose stores.[153] GH also decreases cellular uptake of glucose, thereby exacerbating or precipitating hyperglycemia, which then triggers insulin release.[154] There is decreased sensitivity to insulin at the cellular level; and this causes increased insulin resistance and hyperglycemia.

Growth hormone when given to GH-deficient children promotes active growth and rapidly improves nitrogen balance and increases muscle mass.[155] When a rat diaphragm is exposed to pharmacological doses of GH, the rates of both amino acid transport and protein synthesis increase.[156] GH seems to have a more marked anabolic action in those whose protein balance is catabolic. No improvement in muscle mass or strength has been detected in young adults undergoing exercise training; while nontrained subjects show improved net protein balance through an increased rate of whole-body protein synthesis with no change in protein degradation.[157] Further, the protein catabolic effect of prednisone, a glucocorticoid, is prevented by the concomitant administration of GH.[158]

GH anabolic action appears to be primarily mediated by an increase of protein synthesis. Brachial artery infusion of GH in both normal and postoperative patients reveals a direct effect of GH on skeletal muscle.[159,160] GH also acts to stimulate insulin-like growth factor synthesis. GH administration increases IGF-1 blood concentration via increased IGF-1 production by the liver.[161] GH also increases IGF-1 production in other tissues, such as skeletal muscle and cartilage, where IGF-1 may exert an autocrine/paracrine action. The efficacy of growth hormone in treating critically ill patients has been questioned from two prospective, double-blind, randomized placebo-controlled multicenter trials, in which the mortality rate of critically ill adults receiving 0.1 mg/kg/day rhGH was 39% and 44%, respectively, compared to 20% and 18% with placebo.[162] In the survivors, the length of intensive care, hospital stay, mechanical ventilation were prolonged. Most deaths were related to multiorgan dysfunction, septic shock, or uncontrolled infection, suggesting a possible immune modulating effect.[129] Growth hormone may exert anti- as well as proinflammatory effects, suggesting an effect on immune function in hypermetabolic patients depending on the underlying clinical situation.[163–168] These findings could not be reproduced in pediatric

burn patients. In a controlled study in 263 pediatric burn patients, no increase in septic complications or organ dysfunction could be observed.[169] The mortality rate was 2% in both GH-treatment group (0.2 mg/kg/day) and placebo. In a randomized, prospective, double-blinded study on 28 severely burned children receiving either 0.2 mg/kg/day rhGH or placebo, no increase in mortality (8% vs 7%) or sepsis (20% vs 26%) could be shown. Serum IGF-1 and IGFBP-3 levels increased with rhGH treatment, while serum TNFα and IL-1β levels, as well as acute phase proteins (CRP and serum amyloid-A) were decreased.[170] In 54 adult burn patients, Knox et al. showed a decrease in mortality from 37% for placebo controls to 11% for patients receiving 0.1 mg/kg/day rhGH from 37% in placebo controls.[171] In another study of adult burn patients receiving standard conservative treatment there was a 8% mortality rate with rhGH (0.167 mg/kg/day) compared to 44.5% for those receiving placebo.[172]

Systemic growth hormone effects in burn injury

While the beneficial metabolic effects of growth hormone in burns have been known for some time,[173–176] the wound healing potential of GH has only recently been investigated. An extensive prospective randomized, double-blinded clinical trial has examined the basic mechanisms of protein anabolism, hyperglycemia, and wound healing in massively burned children and adolescents.

GH (0.2 mg/kg/day) increased protein turnover with increases in both protein synthesis and breakdown, but with synthesis exceeding breakdown in a group of severely burned (70% TBSA) hypermetabolic adolescents.[177] This resulted in a net reduction in protein loss of 50% compared to controls. Whole body and isolated limb assessments were performed using N^{15} lysine stable isotope technique. GH treatment raised leg blood flow significantly. This increase in peripheral blood flow did not cause an increase in cardiac index, which was raised equally in both groups to twice the normal range. Urinary nitrogen excretion was also decreased.

GH causes hyperglycemia in burned patients by induction of insulin resistance and inhibition of glucose uptake relative to the availability of insulin. This was examined in a group of severely burned adolescents receiving GH (0.2 mg/kg/day) or placebo in blinded fashion.[178] All were hypermetabolic at 140% predicted resting energy expenditure. A euglycemic hyperinsulinemic clamp was performed. Growth hormone administration was also shown to significantly reduce glucose uptake and inhibit glucose oxidation compared to the placebo patients. Glucose utilization (percentage glucose uptake oxidized) in both patient groups remained similar. This implies that GH induces an insulin resistance by inhibiting glucose transport. As counter-regulation, plasma levels of insulin then increase to maintain euglycemia. Clinically, about one-third of patients treated with GH require therapeutic insulin for 2–3 days, after which time borderline hyperglycemia persists but not at a level requiring insulin.

Further examination of this effect revealed increases in levels of stress hormones in a group of severely burned older children who had early morning blood samples collected during their hyperdynamic, hypermetabolic postburn phase[179] (**Tables 27.4** and **27.5**).

GH significantly elevated plasma levels of catecholamines, glucagon, and insulin above the already elevated levels found in severely burned patients. Catecholamines and glucagon are typically considered to be catabolic hormones and mediators of the

Table 27.4 Patient characteristics[179]					
	n	Age (years)	TBSA (%)	REE/predicted	Heart Rate (bpm)
Placebo	8	11 ± 1	67 ± 6	1.3 ± 0.2	136 ± 7
GH	6	9 ± 2	71 ± 9	1.3 ± 0.1	149 ± 7

Table 27.5 Hormonal and metabolic parameters with rhGH treatment[179]		
	Controls $n = 8$	GH $n = 6$
GH (normal: < 8 mg/ml)	2.3 ± 0.3	30.4 ± 19.9*
IGF-1 (normal: 22–138 U/ml)	56 ± 15	168 ± 24*
Free fatty acids (normal: 0.19–0.90 mEq/l)	0.59 ± 0.04	0.74 ± 0.01*
Glucose (normal: 60–115 mg/dl)	129 ± 13	133 ± 16
Insulin (normal: 5–25 uU/ml)	25 ± 3	33 ± 3*
Total catecholamines (normal: 120–450 pg/ml)	1117 ± 137	1817 ± 177*
Glucagon (normal: 50–200 pg/ml)	158 ± 22	215 ± 18*
Cortisol (normal: 7–27 mg/dl)	21.3 ± 1.6	28.4 ± 5.4

* Significantly different $p < 0.05$.
Data presented as mean ± SEM.

postburn catabolic response. An increase in these mediators might have been expected to increase the hypermetabolic response and its associated protein catabolism; however, as has already been shown, protein anabolism, not catabolism, is induced by GH in burn. As insulin infusion has been shown to significantly increase plasma catecholamine levels, it was felt that GH-induced insulin resistance led to hyperinsulinemia and then to subsequent elevation of catecholamine levels.[180] In turn, catecholamines or growth hormone or both can stimulate glucagon release, even though they are not the primary stimulus for glucagon release.[181] The reversal of the insulin: glucagon ratio, typically seen in burned patients, was maintained in the GH-treated group. The increase in free fatty acid levels was not surprising, as both catecholamines and GH serve to stimulate lipolysis and release free fatty acids into the circulation. It is significant that metabolic rate/resting energy expenditure was not increased by these hormonal changes as would be expected if the increases in the stress hormone levels were clinically significant.

Systemic metabolic changes can improve the burn patient's ability to react to different stress during acute hospital course. Enhanced host-nonspecific resistance against bacterial infection has been demonstrated.[182,183] Takagi *et al.* showed that treating burned mice with 4 mg/kg rhGH before exposure to lethal amounts of herpes simplex virus type 1 could significantly reduce mortality.[184] In this study, GH was shown to restore the burn suppressed IFN-γ response, reduce burn-induced suppressor macrophages, and increase the production of cytostatic macrophages.[185] suggest-

ing, that GH induces an immunoregulatory effect important for survival in burn patients.

Wound healing effects of growth hormone

Skin is a target tissue for GH, either indirectly via circulating IGF-1 or directly by GH interaction with specific receptors on the surface of epidermal and dermal cells.[186,187] Direct effects of GH on cultured human skin fibroblasts have been demonstrated and include increased IGF-1 and IGF-binding protein production and increased thymidine uptake.[188,189] Animal studies have shown that biosynthetic GH increased the collagen content and the tensile strength of skin and granulation tissue.[190–192] A significant increase in skin thickness was noted when 12 healthy men, aged 61–81 years, who had subnormal IGF-1 levels, were treated with subcutaneous injections of biosynthetic GH three times per week.[193] Incisional wounds in the skin of rats show increased strength after biosynthetic growth hormone treatment, even if malnourished.[194–196]

GH treatment of the severely burned improves wound healing dramatically if the dose is sufficient. A pilot study showed no protein anabolic benefit at 0.03 mg/day or 0.06 mg/kg/day in adult burn patients.[197] GH at a dose of 0.1 mg/kg/day did not raise serum levels sufficiently, or for a long enough time, to improve wound healing in severely burned children (**Figure 27.4**). Using a dose of

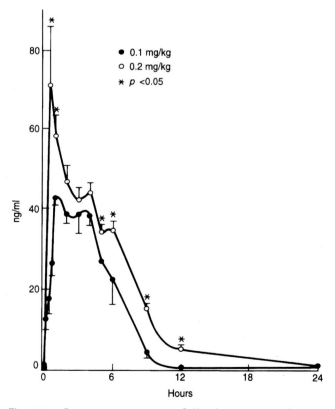

Fig. 27.4 Dose–response curve following parenteral administration of recombinant human growth hormone. Reprinted with permission from Herndon *et al.* Effect of recombinant human growth hormone on donor site healing in severely burned children. *Annals of Surgery* 1990; 212(4): 424–31.[198]

0.2 mg/kg/day in a prospective, randomized, placebo-controlled trial has shown accelerated skin graft donor site wound healing by 25% in children with a mean burn size of 60% TBSA. This means that these massively burned children could be taken to the operating room for further skin grafting about 2 days earlier if treated with GH. The use of GH significantly decreased the overall time to total burn wound closure and, consequently, length of hospital stay. GH was shown to reduce the healing times of the initial donor site compared to the placebo group, as well as that of the second and third donor site; however, the patient numbers for the third donor site group were small. When adjusted for percentage of total body surface area burned (% TBSA), the treated group took 0.54 ± 0.04 days/% TBSA (mean ± SD) and the placebo group took 0.80 ± 0.09 days/% TBSA to achieve total wound closure. This decreased total wound closure time for a patient with the average burn size in the study group of 60% TBSA from 46 to 32 days[198] (**Table 27.6**).

Table 27.6 Donor site healing times (days)[198]			
	First harvest	Second harvest	Third harvest
Placebo	9.0 ± 0.4	9.0 ± 0.7	8.0 ± 1.0
GH(0.2 mg/kg/day)	7.0 ± 0.5*	6.0 ± 0.4*	6.0 ± 1.0

* Significantly different $p <0.05$.
Data presented as mean ± SEM.

Electronmicroscopical and immunohistochemical studies correlated these clinical findings with increased basal lamina formation at the dermo–epidermal junction. Basal lamina covering the dermo–epidermal junction increased from 26% ± 11% to 68% ± 16% with rhGH, while immunostaining for IGF-1 receptor, laminin, collagen type IV and VII, and cytokeratin 14 was increased (**Figure 27.5**).[199]

No antibodies to rhGH were exhibited during treatment. Insulin given therapeutically, and, therefore, the hyperglycemia for which it was given, did not affect the rate of healing. Over 100 children have now been treated with rhGH, including a number who were not included in the prospective trial due to extremes of age or late presentation. Infants, less than 2 years of age, showed the same beneficial effects of rhGH as those who are older, without adverse effect. Patients presenting 2 or 3 weeks after injury, who were all in poor condition and looked cachectic from sepsis, hypermetabolism, or inadequate nutrition were noted to have donor site healing times of about 7 days (**Table 27.7**). This is remarkable in patients so nutritionally and metabolically disadvantaged.[200]

Burned adults, when treated with rhGH in a double-blind, randomized study, also showed a 2-day decrease in the length of time for split-thickness donor sites to heal.[201] The effect of GH on burned patients is profound and beneficial. Insulin resistance is induced, but glucose utilization does not change. Protein anabolism is induced in spite of further elevation of the levels of

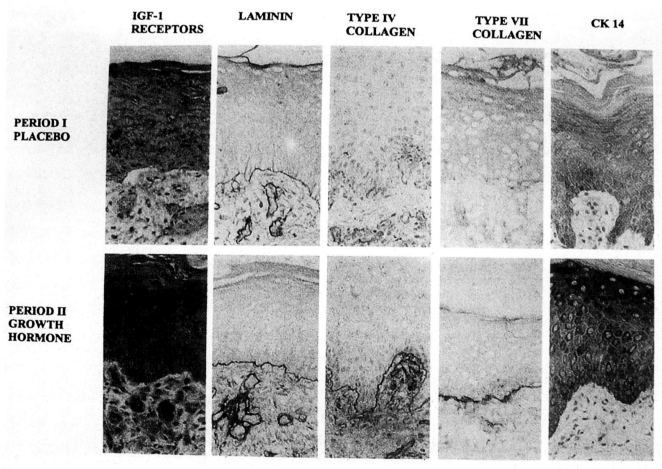

| | IGF-1 RECEPTORS | LAMININ | TYPE IV COLLAGEN | TYPE VII COLLAGEN | CK 14 |

PERIOD I PLACEBO

PERIOD II GROWTH HORMONE

Fig. 27.5 Immunohistochemical staining of healed donor site. (Reproduced with permission from Herndon DN, *et al*.[199])

Table 27.7 Donor site healing times of infants and late presenters[200]

	n	Age (years)	TBSA burn (%)	Healing time (days)
GH < 2 years	9	1.4 ± 0.2	56 ± 5	6.0 ± 0.4*
GH late	6	5.2 ± 1.2	57 ± 7	6.0 ± 0.7*
Control	26	8.4 ± 0.9	67 ± 3	8.5 ± 0.5

* Significantly different p <0.05.
Data presented as mean ± SEM.

catabolic hormones. Improved donor site wound healing is so marked that it is visible without special assessment techniques (**Figure 27.6**).

Another postburn response in children is growth retardation. Severe delays in both height and weight growth have been demonstrated in pediatric patients who had sustained greater than a 40% TBSA burn. This growth delay persisted for as long as 3 years post-injury without any 'catch-up' growth experienced.[202] Major illnesses have been demonstrated to produce a profound change in growth. Growth changes can be transient, disappearing with the resolution of the illness, or permanent, such as with intrinsic defects of endocrine function or with pathologic states, like chronic renal failure. In other serious medical conditions, once resolution is achieved, the patient experiences a period of explosive growth and is able to return to comparable peer-group growth patterns. This 'catch-up' growth spurt has been observed in other severe trauma conditions.[203] This does not occur in pediatric burn patients who do not exhibit such a growth spurt. Nail and hair

growth are attenuated during the catabolic phase of burn response and evidence is mounting that a bony lesion exists which is of an aplastic nature.[204,205] The exact mechanism of this growth retardation is unknown. Adequate nutrition is required for normal growth. It may be that these patients continue to expend energy stores on the damaged integument, thus leaving few resources for growth. A recent study on severely burned children receiving rhGH during their acute hospitalization showed a marked improvement in their rate of linear growth between 6 months and 2 years post-injury compared to placebo-treated controls.[206] Similar effects could be demonstrated in a group of growth-retarded children with chronic steroid therapy for juvenile chronic arthritis.[207] In severe burns, bone formation has been found markedly reduced.[208] Pediatric burn patients treated with 0.2 mg/kg/day rhGH showed an increase of IGF-1 and IGFBP-3 of 229% and 187%, respectively, compared to placebo. Serum osteocalcin remained below normal levels, while type I procollagen propeptide levels rose to low normal levels. The inhibitory IGF-binding protein 4, however, was markedly elevated, suggesting a mechanism by which improved bone formation may be prevented despite of increased IGF-1 and IGFBP-3 levels.[209]

Growth hormone has many uses in patients who are catabolic, malnourished, or have received severe trauma such as burn.[210,211] Its more widespread availability and application will benefit many,[212] and ultimately reduce costs. Growth hormone use in an American pediatric burn center with bed costs of US$1600 per day has achieved an 18% cost saving for severely burned (60% TBSA) children.[213]

Insulin–like growth factor-1

Growth hormone acts both directly and indirectly via IGF-1 production in the liver and elsewhere.[214,215] IGF-1 serum levels are decreased in burn patients.[216] This is consistent with the observation that hepatic IGF-1 secretion is directly impaired despite normal pituitary GH secretion in many disease states, and, that simultaneous use of GH and IGF-1 gives enhanced anabolic effects in normal humans.[217]

Growth hormone given to septic patients failed to increase IGF-1 levels. Also, the IGF-1 response to GH treatment is attenuated with increasing severity of trauma or burn.[218,219] These facts have led to speculation that IGF alone or in combination with GH, may achieve better results in malnourished, septic burn patients. Early animal work has been most encouraging.

When 1 mg/day of IGF-1 was administered via osmotic pumps implanted subcutaneously to 50% scald-burned rats, circulating IGF-1 levels were significantly decreased in untreated animals compared to unburned controls while rhIGF-1-treated animals showed IGF-1 levels which were restored to levels similar to unburned controls.[220] The metabolic rates (estimated by oxygen consumption) of burned animals treated with IGF-1 were comparable to those of the unburned control group, while placebo treated burned rats had significantly elevated metabolic rates. That is, postburn hypermetabolism was completely obviated. Using the same model, small intestinal mucosal DNA and protein content, gut mucosal weight, splenic weight, and body weight were increased with 3 mg/kg/day IGF-1. Additionally, the IGF-1-treated rats had a decrease in the usual postburn hyperglycemia, a positive nitrogen balance, and increased weight gain for 5 days.

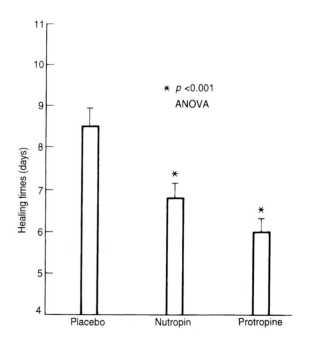

Fig. 27.6 Differences in donor site healing time following treatment with Protropin, Nutropin, and placebo. Reprinted with permission from Gilpin *et al.*[200]

The incidence of bacterial translocation to the mesenteric lymph nodes was reduced from 90% to 30% as gut mucosal function was improved.[221] IGF-1 (3 mg/g/day) given by continuous infusion to 50% scald burn rats attenuated body weight loss, corrected the burn-induced decrease in hepatic adenosine triphosphate concentration, prevented burn-induced decrease in hepatic ketone body levels, and prevented the fever-induced impairment in hepatic redox potential.[222] Inhaled, aerosolized barrier IGF-1 accelerated epithelial repair of smoke-injured trachea in sheep.[223]

This animal work promised to lead to an additional and safer way of influencing the GH-IGF-1 axis avoiding GH-related morbidity, especially hyperglycemia, by using the growth hormone mediator IGF-1. Although IGF-1 treatment with 12 µg/h and 20 µg/h resulted in net anabolic effects, this treatment was associated with severe hypoglycemia, electrolyte imbalances, edema, neuropathies, and cardiac arrest.[224–226] This promoted the search for a safer application form of IGF-1. When IGF-1 is administered in equimolar ratio with its principal binding protein-3, the availability and function of IGF-1 is strictly regulated.[227] This application form, IGF-1/IGFBP-3, showed no clinical side effects in initial studies. In recent studies in pediatric and adult burn patients IGF-1/IGFBP-3 in doses of 1–4 mg/kg/day resulted in anabolic stimulation by improving net protein balance and increasing muscle protein fractional synthetic rates, without hypo- or hyperglycemia, or electrolyte imbalances.[228,229] In the same pediatric patient population IGF-1/IGFBP-3 showed a marked influence on the systemic acute phase response. Treatment with IGF-1/IGFBP-3 (1.0–4.0 mg/kg/day) resulted in increased hepatic production of constitutive serum proteins (prealbumin, retinol-binding protein, and transferrin) and decreased levels of IL-1β and TNFα stimulated type I acute phase proteins (C-reactive protein, α1-acid glycoprotein, complement C-3). However, changes were seen in the IL-6-mediated type II acute phase response. This could be correlated to decreased IL-1β and TNFα serum levels, and unchanged IL-6 serum levels, indicating a potential mechanism for the IGF-1/IGFBP-3 effects.[230]

The use of IGF-1 as topical wound healing stimulant has been addressed before. Systemic application showed improved anabolism and wound healing with combined IGF-1 and GH treatment.[231]

β-adrenergic-receptor agents

The hyperdynamic circulatory response to burn injury, stimulated by 10-fold increases in catecholamines, plays a significant role in increasing energy expenditure. Tachycardia of 120–150 beats/min is often sustained for many weeks in massively burned patients. Cardiac dysfunction commonly contributes to mortality with myocarditis, cardiomyopathy, and focal myocardial ischemia often found at autopsy.[232,233] These findings are similar to those found in patients who succumb to other catechol excess states such as pheochromocytoma. Adrenergic blockade had been used with success in pathologic hypercatecholamine states and thyrotoxicosis by decreasing myocardial workload, whole-body irritability, and tremulousness.[234] Total catecholamine absence in 60% burned rats, induced by either adrenalectomy or chronic reserpine administration, certainly decreased hypermetabolism but also increased mortality.[235]

Catecholamines also stimulate lipolysis in burned patients.[236,237]

Acute administration of β-blocking agents precipitously decreases the rate of release or appearance of free fatty acids (FFA) in plasma, indicating the important role which pre-existing sympathetic activity plays in the mobilization of FFA. Chronic catecholamine blockade could, therefore, indirectly increase protein catabolism, since FFA is the primary endogenous energy substrate. The concern that adrenergic blockade could have a detrimental metabolic effect has been amplified by the notion that catecholamines may have a direct protein anabolic effect.[238–240] Wilmore examined adrenergic blockade in exposed patients with α, β, and combined α and β blockade.[70] Alpha blockade alone did not change metabolic rate; however, significant decreases were seen with combined α and β blockade and with β blockade alone. The decrease in metabolic rate was associated with a decrease in pulse rate, blood pressure, minute ventilation, and free fatty acids. Larger than normal doses were required to obtain adequate blockade. In the same study, a significant correlation between increasing urinary catecholamine excretion and an increasing metabolic rate was induced by cold stress. Four nonresponders to cold stress, who showed a paradoxical decrease in metabolic rate, later succumbed. Consequently, adrenergic blockade which interferes with cold stress response (catecholamine-induced calorigenic response) would seem best avoided.

A number of more recent and extensive studies have shown that limited β blockade can be safely used in severely burned patients. Propranolol, 2 mg/kg/day, was given intravenously to 18 patients for 5 days with burns of 70 ± 30% TBSA.[241] Heart rate was decreased by 20%, left ventricular work index by 22%, and rate pressure product by 36%. Plasma glucose, free fatty acids, triglyceride, and insulin levels remained unchanged. Propranolol concentrations were approximately ten times the blood levels normally required for effective β blockade at 700 ± 500 mg/ml. Catecholamine levels were not affected by nonselective β blockade; however, blood urea nitrogen was elevated in the treated group. Stable isotope infusions of urea were performed in both the fed and fasted state. Rate of urea production (Ra) was increased 1- to 5-fold in the treated group.

A group of six septic patients, age 17 ± 3 years, with burns 82 ± 11% TBSA, were given propranolol under continuous hemodynamic monitoring with a Swan–Ganz catheter.[242] Pressure-work index and rate pressure product were significantly decreased with both 0.5 and 1.0 mg/kg. Cardiac index, oxygen delivery index, and oxygen consumption were improved without adversely affecting overall oxygen delivery or total body oxygen consumption. The ability of patients treated with propranolol at this dose, 1–2 mg/kg/day necessary to achieve the desired 25% decrease in heart rate, to respond appropriately to cold stress and isoproterenol challenge was undiminished.[243] In a more recent study, the long-term efficacy of propranolol was demonstrated on severely burned children (>40% TBSA) at dosages between 0.5 and 1.0 mg/kg every 8 hours to achieve 10–20% decrease in heart rate. In both septic and nonseptic patients propranolol significantly decreased heart rate and rate pressure product (between 10 and 20%) compared to values prior to propranolol. No significant changes in mean arterial blood pressure, plasma urea nitrogen, creatinine, or glucose levels was noted. Further, no hypotension, arrhythmias, peripheral ischemia, hypothermia, azotemia, hyper- or hypoglycemia, or bronchospasm was noted.[244]

Selective β-1 blockade with metoprolol has been compared with β-1, β-2, nonselective blockade using propranolol. At a dose of 0.5 mg/kg/day, metoprolol decreased heart rate by 18% and rate pressure product by 15%. Equivalent effects were achieved by adjusting the dose of propranolol. Stable isotope infusions of leucine, urea, and glycerol were used to assess protein and lipid metabolism. This technique showed that metoprolol had no effect on protein or lipid metabolism, while propranolol showed a decrease in lipolysis (Ra Glycerol) and no change in urea production.[245] In a study, in which severely burned children were given rhGH or rhGH/propranolol (titrated to achieve a 20% decrease in heart rate) free fatty acid release by peripheral tissue was decreased with rhGH/propranolol. The rate of fatty acid secretion as VLDL-TG from the liver was maintained. Thus, the persistent peripheral lipolysis and deficiency in hepatic VLDL-TG secretion in burned patients may be attenuated by nonselective β-blockade.[97] Long-term β-blockade with propranolol given orally to severely burned children resulted in lower heart rates and REE compared to values before treatment and matched controls. In propranolol-treated patients muscle protein net balance improved by 82% compared to pretreatment baseline values and decreased by 27% in untreated controls.[246] Additionally, lean body mass was maintained by propranolol treatment compared to a 9% loss in controls.[246]

Selective β-1 blockade is a metabolically inert, cardiovascularly safe means of limiting the postburn hyperdynamic cardiovascular response. Therefore, metoprolol would appear to be the drug of choice for the often-encountered problem of burn-induced hypertension.[247] Tremulousness, irritability, and marked tachycardia are almost universal among those with large burns; and β blockade is indicated for these patients.

Selective β-2 adrenergic receptor agonists have known protein anabolic effects. Clenbuterol, a totally selective β-2 agonist, has structural similarities to epinephrine and is well known to promote protein anabolism in normal animals via β-2 adrenergic receptor activation.[248] Postsurgical rats and burned rats showed increased muscle mass and body weight with clenbuterol, and showed with evidence that hypermetabolism was also increased.[249,250]

In 30% burned rats given a dorsal incision and clenbuterol, 2 mg/kg/day, by continuous infusion, muscle and body mass were increased after both 14 and 21 days.[251] Non-temperature dependent hypermetabolism occurred which was not aggravated by clenbuterol. Clenbuterol induced increased wound breaking strength in a free-feeding group. This effect was obviated by nutritional matching (pair feeding), indicating that substrate availability is essential for clenbuterol to show effect. Beta blockade with metoprolol combined with selective β-2 stimulation with clenbuterol or salbutamol may offer stressed patients induction of protein anabolism, enhanced wound healing, and decreased myocardial strain at reasonable cost.

Anabolic steroids

Another class of anabolic agents are the steroid hormones. These have not been as extensively tested in burned patients as the above-mentioned anabolic agents. Animals studies and in patient groups, however, have shown improvements in the post-stress metabolic response. Particularly attractive is the combination with anabolic proteins due to their different binding characteristics and potential synergistic effects. Substances in this group include oxandrolone, testosterone, and dehydroepiandrosterone sulfate.

Steroid hormones rely on translocation into the nucleus, where they can modulate transcription events. Healthy, adult males given 200 mg testosterone intramuscularly, showed a 2-fold increase in muscle protein synthesis. This effect was not caused by changes in the inward transport of amino acids, but by increases in the protein synthetic rate through more efficient reutilization of the intracellular amino acids.[252] Currently, the systemic side-effects of testosterone has restricted its clinical use in burn care.

Oxandrolone, a synthetic testosterone analogue with potent anabolic effects, shows only minimal androgenic side-effects. Oxandrolone can be administered orally, which is more attractive to clinicians and patients compared to frequent GH or testosterone injections. This anabolic steroid has been used as adjunctive therapy to promote weight gain in chronically ill and debilitated patients. Oxandrolone has been shown to improve weight gain in patients with AIDS-wasting myopathy[253] and has been used in the treatment of children with growth disorders.[254,255] In a recent study, short-term oral oxandrolone (5 days at 15 mg/day), when given to six healthy young adult males increased muscle protein synthesis, whereas protein breakdown remained unchanged. In this study, the uptake of amino acids remained unchanged, whereas outward transport of amino acids decreased, indicating an improved cellular reutilization of amino acids. Additional RT-PCR showed significant increases in androgen receptor mRNA in the skeletal muscle, thus suggesting a potential mechanism of action.[256] When used in burn patients with 30–50% TBSA burns, oxandrolone improved weight gain.[257] In a randomized double-blinded placebo control trial, severely burned adult patients with 40–70% TBSA burns received oxandrolone at 20 mg/day. These treated patients showed a significant improvement in weight gain during a 3-week study period without major liver dysfunction or other complications. Additionally, a standardized donor site healed in 9 ± 2 versus 13 ± 3 days for placebo.[258] In severely malnourished burned children oxandrolone reversed the decrease in muscle protein net balance compared to controls. This was thought to be due to improved protein metabolism and an increased protein synthetic efficiency (**Figure 27.7**).[259] Thus the therapeutic application of oxandrolone seems very promising.

Hormone antagonists

Alternative approaches to modulate the post-traumatic hypermetabolic response involve agents that antagonize known mediators of hypermetabolism and protein catabolism such as glucocorticoids and cytokine blocking agents. Agents affecting glucocorticoid synthesis (ketoconazole) or glucocorticoid receptor blockers (mifepristone) seem effective not only for their anticatabolic effects but also for their beneficial effects on immune function.

Modulators of inflammation

The inflammatory response to skin burn is the release of mediators such as cytokines, histamine, and thromboxane, which produce distant organ inflammation as a result of lipid peroxidation. Oxidants are produced by activated neutrophils, free metal ions, increased xanthine oxidase activity, and increased arachidonic acid metabolism. Allopurinol, a xanthine oxidase inhibitor, has prevented lipid peroxidation in a sheep burn model.[260] Ibuprofen, a cyclooxygenase inhibitor, also inhibits oxidant release from neu-

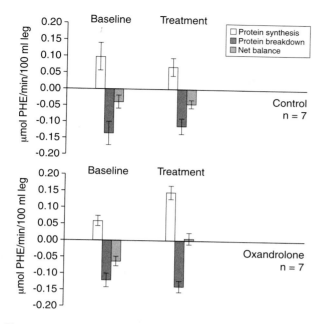

Fig. 27.7 Calculation for muscle protein synthesis, protein breakdown, and net protein balance. Data presented as mean±SEM (adapted from Hart et al.[259]).

trophils and decreases lipid peroxidation in the lungs.[261] Ibuprofen has been shown to decrease hypermetabolism in the 50% burn rat model.[262] Flurbiprofen, a topical anti-inflammatory agent, similarly prevents free oxygen radical release from neutrophils. When applied to the skin burn, flurbiprofen attenuated the postburn hypermetabolic state similar to that seen with total excision and complete wound closure.[235]

Summary

The degree of hypermetabolism, which develops prior to complete burn wound closure, can be influenced by environmental warming, infection control, and by the use of topical or systemic agents which affect free oxygen radical release and the inflammatory cascades. As the hypermetabolic response persists well beyond complete wound closure, the persisting effects of catabolism can only be limited by immediate and adequate enteral nutrition supplemented with protein, ω-3 fatty acids, arginine, and glutamine. Hormonal or pharmacological intervention with growth factors, β-adrenoreceptor agents and other anabolic agents are also suspected to speed wound closure and to reverse the protein catabolism associated with hypermetabolism. In combining these therapeutic modalities with early surgical treatment of the burn wound, mortality and morbidity of burn victims has been significantly improved.

References

1. Kinney JM, Long CL, Gump FE, et al. Tissue composition of weight loss in surgical patients: I. Elective operations. Ann Surg 1968; 168: 459.
2. Long CL, Spencer JL, Kinney JM, et al. Carbohydrate metabolism in man: effect of elective operations and major injury. J Appl Physiol 1971; 31: 110.
3. Campbell RM, Cuthbertson DP. Effect of environmental temperature on the metabolic response to injury. Nature 1966; 210: 206–208.
4. Asch MJ, Feldman RJ, Walker HL, et al. Systemic and pulmonary hemodynamic changes accompanying thermal injury. Ann Surg 1973; 178: 218–221.
5. Wilmore DW, Mason AD, Johnson DW, Pruitt BA. Effects of ambient temperature on heat production and heat loss in burn patients. J Appl Physiol 1975; 38: 593–597.
6. Reiss W, Pearson E, Artz CP. The metabolic response to burns. J Clin Invest 1956; 35: 62.
7. Turner WW, Ireton CS, Hunt JL, Baxter CR. Predicting energy expenditures in burned patients. J Trauma 1985; 259: 11–16.
8. Jahoor F, Herndon DN, Wolfe RR. Role of insulin and glucagon in the response of glucose and alanine kinetics in burn-injured patients. J Clin Invest 1986; 78: 807–814.
9. Newsome T, Mason AD, Pruitt BA. Weight loss following thermal injury. Ann Surg 1973; 178: 215–220.
10. Bessey PQ, Jiang ZM, Johnson DJ, et al. Posttraumatic skeletal muscle proteolysis: the role of the hormonal environment. World J Surg 1989; 13: 465–470.
11. Wolfe RR, Herndon DN, Jahoor F, et al. Effect of severe burn injury on substrate cycling by glucose and fatty acids. N Engl J Med 1987; 317: 403–408.
12. Wolfe RR, Herndon DN, Peters EJ, et al. Regulation of lipolysis in severely burned children. Ann Surg 1987; 206: 214–221.
13. Newsholme EA, Crabtree B. Substrate cycles in metabolic regulation and in heat generation. Biochemical Society Symposium 1976; 41: 61–109.
14. Hart DW, Wolf SE, Mlcak R, et al. Persistence of muscle catabolism after severe burn. Surgery 2000; 128: 312–319.
15. Yurt RW, McManus AT, Mason AD, Pruitt BA. Increased susceptibility to infection related to extent of burn injury. Arch Surg 1984; 119: 183–188.
16. Clark MA, Plank LD, Hill GL. Wound healing associated with severe surgical illness. World J Surg 2000; 24: 648–654.
17. Sorhoff HS, Pearson E, Artz CP. An estimation of nitrogen requirements for equilibrium in burn patients. Surg Gynecol Obstet 1961; 112: 159.
18. Wilmore DW, Long JM, Skreen RW, et al. Studies of the effect of variations of temperature and humidity on energy demands of the burned soldier in a controlled metabolic room. Ft. Sam Houston, U.S. Army Institute of Surgical Research, Annual Report 1973, Report Control Symbol MEDDH-288 (R).
19. Herndon DN, Wilmore DW, Mason AD, et al. Development and analysis of a small animal model simulating the human postburn hypermetabolic response. J Surg Res 1978; 25: 394.
20. Hume DM, Egdahl RH. The importance of the brain in the endocrine response to injury. Ann Surg 1959; 150: 697–712.
21. Auichbau SV, Malyafuna EI, Pashalenka AN, et al. Reflexes from carotid bodies upon the adrenals. Arch Int Pharma Ther 1969; 129: 156–165.
22. Gann DS, Egdahl RH. Responses of adrenal corticosteroid secretion to hypotension and hypovolemia. J Clin Invest 1965; 44: 1–7.
23. Egdahl RH. The differential response of the adrenal cortex and medulla to bacterial endotoxin. J Clin Invest 1959; 38: 1120–1125.
24. Kupper TS, Deitch EA, Baker CC, Wong WC. The human burn wound as a primary source of interleukin-1 activity. Surgery 1986; 100: 409–415.
25. Beutler B, Cerami A. Cachectin: more than a tumor necrosis factor. N Engl J Med 1987; 316: 379–385.
26. Dinarello CA, et al. Tumor necrosis factor (cachectin) is an endogenous pyrogen and induces production of interleukin 1. J Exp Med 1986; 163: 1433–1450.
27. Michie HR, Wilmore DW. Sepsis, signals, and surgical sequelae: a hypothesis. Arch Surg 1990; 125: 531–536.
28. Dinarello CA, Conno JG, Wolff SM. New concepts on pathogenesis of fever. Rev Infect Dis 1988; 10: 168–189.
29. Morimoto A, Murakami N, Nakamori T, Watanabe T. Multiple control of fever production in the central nervous system of rabbits. J Physiol 1988; 397: 269–280.
30. Wilmore DW, Orcutt TW, Mason AD Jr., Pruitt BA. Alterations in hypothalamic function following thermal injury. J Trauma 1975; 15: 697–703.
31. Becker RA, Vaughan GM, Goodwin CW Jr, et al. Plasma norepinephrine, epinephrine and thyroid hormone interactions in severely burned patients. Arch Surg 1980; 115: 439–443.
32. Wilmore DW, Long JM, Mason AD, et al. Catecholamines: mediator of the hypermetabolic response to thermal injury. Ann Surg 1974; 180: 653–669.
33. Vaughan GM, Becker RA, Allen JP, et al. Cortisol and corticotrophin in burned patients. J Trauma 1982; 22: 263–273.
34. Ganong WF. The stress response: a dynamic overview. Hosp Pract (Off Ed) 1988; 23: 155–158, 161–162, 167.
35. Deibert DC, DeFronzo RA. Epinephrine-induced insulin resistance in man. J Clin Invest 1980; 65: 717–721.
36. Wilmore DW, Lindsey CA, Moylan JA, et al. Hyperglucagonemia after burns. Lancet 1974; 1: 73–75.

37. Wise JK, Hendler R, Felig P. Influence of glucocorticoids on glucagon secretion and plasma amino acid concentrations in man. *J Clin Invest* 1973; **52**: 2774–2782.

38. Unger RH, Orci L. Glucagon and the A cell: physiology and pathophysiology. *N Engl J Med* 1981; **304**: 1518–1524.

39. Sakurai Y, Zhang X-J, Wolfe RR. Short-term effects of tumor necrosis factor on energy and substrate metabolism in dogs. *J Clin Invest* 1993; **91**: 2437–2445.

40. Molteni A, Warpeha RL, Brizio-Molteni L, *et al.* Circadian rhythms of serum aldosterone, cortisol and plasma renin activity in burn injuries. *Ann Clin Lab Sci* 1979; **9**: 518–523.

41. Brizio-Molteni L, Molteni A, Warpeha RL, *et al.* Prolactin, corticotropin, and gonadotropin concentrations following thermal injury in adults. *J Trauma* 1984; **24**: 1–7.

42. Dolecek R, Adamkova M, Sotornikova T, *et al.* Endocrine response after burn. *Scand J Plast Reconstr Surg* 1979; **13**: 9–16.

43. Shamoon H, Hendler R, Sherwin RS. Synergistic interactions among anti-insulin hormones in the pathogenesis of stress hyperglycemia in humans. *J Clin Endocrinol Metab* 1981; **52**: 1235–1241.

44. Weissman C. The metabolic response to stress: an overview and update. *Anesthesiology* 1990; **73**: 308–327.

45. Bessey PQ, Watters JM, Aoki TT, Wilmore DW. Combined hormonal infusion simulates the metabolic response to injury. *Ann Surg* 1984; **200**: 260–282.

46. Kalsner S. Mechanism of hydrocortisone potentiation of responses to epinephrine and norepinephrine in rabbit aorta. *Circ Res* 1969; **24**: 383–395.

47. Fraser CM, Potter PC, Chung FZ, *et al.* Glucocorticoid regulation of human lung beta-adrenergic receptor density occurs at the level of gene transcription. *Fed Proc* 1987; **46**: 1463.

48. Diem E, Schmid R, Schneider WHF, Spona J. The influence of burn trauma on the hypothalamus pituitary axis in normal female subjects. *Scand J Plast Reconstr Surg* 1979; **13**: 17–20.

49. Dolecek R, Zavada M, Adamkova M, *et al.* Endocrine response in burned subjects: insulin, somatotrophin, renin, angiotensin-II, ACTH and LH. *Burns* 1974; **1**: 43–46.

50. Lephart ED, Baxter CR, Parker CR Jr. Effect of burn trauma on adrenal and testicular steroid hormone production. *J Clin Endocrinol Metab* 1987; **64**: 842–848.

51. Sanka J. Dehydroepiandrosterone: metabolic effects. *Acta Univ Carol (Med Monogr)* 1976; **71**: 146–171.

52. Schmidt KH, Bruchelt G, Koslowski L. Granulocyte function: current knowledge and methods of assessment. *J Burn Care Rehabil* 1985; **6**: 261–269.

53. Vogel AV, Peake GT, Rada RT. Pituitary–testicular axis dysfunction in burned men. *J Clin Endocrinal Metab* 1985; **60**: 658–665.

54. Dolecek R, Adamkova M, Sotarnikova T, *et al.* Endocrine response after burn. *Scand J Plast Reconstr Surg* 1979; **13**: 12–16.

55. Cuppage FE, Brizio-Molteni L, Molteni A, *et al.* Aspects of systemic pathologic changes after thermal trauma. In: Dolecek R, Brizio-Molteni L, Molteni A, *et al.* (eds) *Endocrinology of Thermal Trauma.* Philadelphia, PA: Lea & Fiebiger. 1990: 383–384.

56. Wilmore DW, Aulick LH, Pruitt BA. Influence of the burn wound on local and systemic response to injury. *Ann Surg* 1977; **186**: 4.

57. Herndon DN, Barrow RE, Rutan TC, *et al.* Effect of propranolol administration on hemodynamic and metabolic responses of burned pediatric patients. *Ann Surg* 1988; **208**: 484–492.

58. Wolfe RR, Durkot MJ, Allsop JR, *et al.* Glucose metabolism in severely burned patients. *Metabolism* 1979; **28**: 1031–1039.

59. Wolfe RR, Shaw JH, Jahoor F, *et al.* Response to glucose infusion in humans: role of the changes in insulin concentration. *Am J Physiol* 1986; **250**: E306–311.

60. Wolfe RR, Goodenough RD, Burke JF, *et al.* Response of protein and urea kinetics in burn patients to different levels of protein intake. *Ann Surg* 1983; **197**: 163–171.

61. Blackburn GL, Maini BS, Pierce EC. Nutrition in the critically ill patient. *Anesthesiology* 1977; **47**: 181–194.

62. Patterson BW, Nguyen T, Pierre E, *et al.* Urea and protein metabolism in burned children: effect of dietary protein intake. *Metabolism* 1997; **46**: 573–578.

63. Gamrin L, Essen P, Forsberg AM, *et al.* A descriptive study of skeletal muscle metabolism in critically ill patients: free amino acids, energy rich phosphates, protein, nucleic acids, fat, water, and electrolytes. *Crit Care Med* 1996; **24**: 575–583.

64. Ogle CK, Ogle JD, Mao JM, *et al.* Effect of glutamine on phagocytosis and bacterial killing by normal and pediatric burn patient neutrophils. *JPEN* 1994; **18**: 128–133.

65. Ferrando AA, Chinkes DL, Wolf SE, *et al.* Acute dichloroacetate administration increases skeletal muscle free glutamine concentrations after burn injury. *Ann Surg* 1998; **2**: 249–256.

66. Wolfe RR, Jahoor F, Herndon DN, *et al.* The glucose alanine cycle: origin of control. *JPEN* 1985; **9**: 107 (Abstr).

67. Wolfe RR, Shaw JH, Durkat MJ. Effects of sepsis on VLDL kinetics: responses in basal state and during glucose infusion. *Am J Physiol* 1985; **248**: E432–440.

68. Wolfe BM, Walker BK, Shaul DB, *et al.* Effect of total parenteral nutrition on hepatic histology. *Arch Surg* 1988; **123**: 1084–1090.

69. Rutan T, Herndon DN, Van Osten T, Abston S. Metabolic rate alterations in early excision and grafting versus conservative treatment. *J Trauma* 1986; **26**: 140–142.

70. Wilmore DW, Long JM, Mason AD, *et al.* Catecholamines: mediator of the hypermetabolic response to thermal injury. *Ann Surg* 1974; **180**: 653–669.

71. Wilmore DW, Long JM, Skreen RW, *et al.* Studies of the effect of variations of temperature and humidity on energy demands of the burned soldier in a controlled metabolic room. Ft. Sam Houston, U.S. Army Institute of Surgical Research, Annual Report 1973, Report Control Symbol MEDDH-288 (R).

72. Aulich LH, Hander EH, Wilmore DW, *et al.* The relative significance of thermal and metabolic demands on burn hypermetabolism. *J Trauma* 1979; **19**: 559–566.

73. Zawacki BE, Spitzer KW, Mason AD Jr. Does increased evaporative water loss cause hypermetabolism in burn patients. *Ann Surg* 1970; **171**: 236–240.

74. Neely AW, Petra AB, Holloman GH, *et al.* Research on the cause of burn hypermetabolism. *Ann Surg* 1974; **179**: 290–294.

75. Barr PO, Birke G, Liljedahl SO, *et al.* Oxygen consumption and water loss during treatment of burns with warm dry air. *Lancet* 1968; **1**: 164–168.

76. Wilmore DW, Mason AD, Jr., Johnson DW, *et al.* Effect of ambient temperature on heat production and heat loss in burn patients. *J Appl Physiol* 1975; **38**: 593–597.

77. Danielsson U, Arturson G, Wennberg L. The elimination of hypermetabolism in burned patients. *Burns* 2: 110–114.

78. Sonhoff HS, Pearson E, Artz CP. An estimation of nitrogen requirements for equilibrium in burn patients. *Surg Gynecol Obstet* 1961; **112**: 159.

79. Herndon DN, Stein MD, Rutan TC, *et al.* Failure of TPN supplementation to improve liver function, immunity, and mortality in thermally injured patients. *J Trauma* 1987; **27**: 195–204.

80. Herndon DN, Barrow RE, Stein M, *et al.* Increased mortality with intravenous supplemental feeding in severely burned patients. *J Burn Care Rehabil* 1989; **10**: 309–313.

81. Moore FA, Feliciano DV, Andrassy RJ, *et al.* Early enteral feeding, compared with parenteral, reduces post operative septic complications: the results of a meta-analysis. *Ann Surg* 1992; **216**: 172–183.

82. McDonald WS, Sharp CW, Deitch EA. Immediate enteral feeding in burn patients is safe and effective. *Ann Surg* 1991; **213**: 177–183.

83. Mochizuki H, Trocki O, Dominioni L, *et al.* Mechanism of prevention of postburn hypermetabolism and catabolism by early enteral feeding. *Ann Surg* 1984; **200**: 297–310.

84. Mochizuki H, Trocki O, Dominioni L, *et al.* Reduction of postburn hypermetabolism by early enteral feedings. *Curr Surg* 1985; **42**: 121–125.

85. Herndon DN, Ziegler ST. Bacterial translocation after thermal injury. *Crit Care Med* 1993; **21**: S50–S54.

86. Saito H, Trocki O, Alexander JW, *et al.* The effect of route of nutrient administration on the nutritional state, catabolic hormone secretion, and gut mucosal integrity after burn injury. *JPEN* 1987; **11**: 1–7.

87. Jahoor F, Desai M, Herndon DN, Wolfe RR. Dynamics of the protein metabolic response to a burn injury. *Metabolism* 1988; **37**: 330–337.

88. Alexander JW, MacMillan BG, Stinnett JD, *et al.* Beneficial effects of aggressive protein feeding in severely burned children. *Ann Surg* 1980; **192**: 505–517.

89. Wolfe RR, Goodenough RD, Burke JF, Wolfe MH. Response of protein and urea kinetics in burn patients to different levels of protein intake. *Ann Surg* 1983; **197**: 163–171.

90. Patterson BW, Nguyen T, Pierre E, *et al.* Urea and protein metabolism in burned children: effect of dietary protein intake. *Metabolism* 1997; **46**: 573–578.

91. Yu Y-M, Wagner DA, Walesreswski JC, *et al.* A kinetic study of leucine metabolism in severely burned patients: comparison between a conventional and branched chain amino acid-enriched nutritional therapy. *Ann Surg* 1988; **207**: 421–429.

92. Trocki O, Mochizuri H, Dominioni L, Alexander JW. Intact protein versus free amino acids in the nutritional support of thermally injured animals. *J Pen* 1986; **10(2)**: 139–145.

93. Pierre EJ, Barro RE, Hawkins HL, Nguyen TT, Sakurai Y, Desai M, Wolfe RR, Herndon DN. Effects of Insulin on wound healing. *J Trauma* 1998; **44**: 342–345.

94. Ferrando AA, Chinkes DL, Wolf SE, Matin S, Herndon DN, Wolfe RR. A submaximal dose of insulin promotes net skeletal protein synthesis in patients with severe burns. *Ann Surg* 1999; **1**: 11–18.

95. Gore DC, Wolfe RR, Wolf SE, Herndon DN. Glucose kinetics and plasma concentrations in severely burned adults. *J Trauma* 1999 in press.

96. Hart DW, Wolf SE, Zhang XJ, Chinkes DL, Buffalo MC, Matin SI, DebRoy MA,

Wolfe RR, Herndon DN. Efficacy of high carbohydrate diet in catabolic illness. *Crit Care Med* submitted.

97. Aarsland A, Chinkes D, Wolfe RR, Barrow RE, Nelson SO, Pierre EJ, Herndon DN. Beta blockade lowers peripheral lipolysis in burn patients receiving growth hormone. Rate of hepatic very low density lipoptriceride synthesis secretion remains unchanged. *Ann Surg* 1996; 223: 777–789.

98. Wolf SE, Barrow RE, Herndon DN. Growth hormone and IGF-1 therapy in the hypercatabolic patient. *Clin Endo Metab* 1996; 10: 447–463.

99 Gottschlich MM, Jenkins M, Warden GD, *et al*. Differential effects of three enteral dietary regimens on selected outcome variables in burn patients. *JPEN* 1990; 14(3): 225–236.

100. Daly JM, Lieberman MD, Goudfine J, *et al*. Enteral nutrition with supplemental arginine, RNA, and omega-3 fatty acids in patients after operation: immunologic, metabolic, and clinical outcome. *Surgery* 1992; 112: 56–67.

101. Becker RA, Vaughan GM, Goodwin CW, *et al*. Interactions of thyroid hormones and catecholamines in severely burned patients. *Rev Inf Des* 1983; 5(55): S908–S913.

102. Aun F, Medeiros-Neto GA, Younes RN, Birogini D, Ramos de Oliveira M. The effect of major trauma on the pathways of thyroid hormone metabolism. *J Trauma* 1983; 23(12): 1048–1050.

103. Herndon DN, Wilmore DW, Mason AD, Pruitt BA. Humoral mediators of non-temperature dependent hypermetabolism in 50% burned adult rats. *Surg Forum* 1977; 28: 37–39.

104. Vaughan GM, Shirani KZ, Vaugnology and MK, Pruitt BA, Mason AD. Hormonal changes in burned hamsters. *Endocrinology* 1985; 117(3): 1090–1095.

105. Brent GA, Hershman JM. Thyroxine therapy in patients with severe non thyroidal illnesses and low serum thyroidine concentration. *J Clin Endocrinal Metabol* 1986; 63(1): 1–8.

106. Becker RA, Vaughan GM, Ziegler MG, *et al*. Hypermetabolic low tricoelathyranine syndrome of burn injury. 1982; 10(12): 870–875.

107. Becker RA, Vaughan GM, Goodwin CW, *et al*. Plasma norepinephrine, epinephrine and thyroid hormone interactions in severely burned patients. *Arch Surg* 1980; 115: 439–443.

108. Little S. Effect of thyroid hormone supplementation on survival after bacterial infection. *Endocrinology* 1985; 117(4): 1431–1435.

109. Herndon DN, Wilmore DW, Mason AD, Curreri PW. Increased rates of wound healing in burned guinea pigs treated with L-thyronine. *Surg Forum* 1979; 95–97.

110. Mehregan AH, Zamick P. The effect of triioela thyronine in healing of deep chemical burns and marginal scars of skin grafts. A histologic study. *J Cutan Path* 1974; 1: 113–116.

111. Herndon DN, Nguyen TT, Gilpin DA. Growth factors: local and systemic. *Arch Surg* 1993; 128(11): 1227–1233.

112. Martin PM, Wooley JH, McCluskey J. Growth factors and cutaneous wound repair. *Prog Growth Factor Res* 1992; 4: 25–44.

113. Moshage H. Cytokines and the hepatic acute phase response. *J Pathol* 1997; 181: 257–268.

114. Hiyama DT, Von Allmen D, Rosenblum L, *et al*. Synthesis of albumin and acute phase proteins in perfused liver after burn injury in rats. *J Burn Care Rehab* 1991; 12: 1.

115. Vos AM, Ultsch M, Kossiakoff AA. Human growth hormone and extracellular domain of its receptor: crystal structure of the complex. *Science* 1992; 255: 306–312.

116. Fuh G, Mulkerrin MG, Bass S, McFarland N, Brochier M, Bourell JH, *et al*. The human growth hormone receptor. *J Biol Chem* 1990; 265(6): 3111–3115.

117. Bazan JF. Haemopoietic receptors and helical cytokines. *Immonol Today* 1990; 11(10): 350–354.

118. Bazan JF. A novel family of growth factor receptors: a common binding domain in the growth hormone, prolactin, erythropoietin and IL-6, receptors and the p751 L-2 receptor-chain. *Biochem Biopsy Res Commun* 1989; 164(2): 788–795.

119. Bazan JF. Structural design and molecular evolution of a cytokine receptor superfamily. *Proc Natl Acad Sci* 1990; 87: 6934–6938.

120. Leung DW, Spencer SA, Cachianes G, Hammonds RG, Collins C, Henzel WJ, *et al*. Growth hormone receptor and serum binding protein: purification, cloning and expression. *Nature* 1987; 330: 537–543.

121. Cunningham BC, Wells JA. Rational design of receptor-specific variants of human growth hormone. *Proc Natl Acad Sci* 1991; 88: 3407–3411.

122. Hammacher A, Hellman U, Johnson A, *et al*. A major part of PDGF purified from human platelets is a heterodimer of one A chain and one B chain. *J Biol Chem* 1986; 263: 16493–16498.

123. Ullrich A, Schlessinger J. Signal transduction by receptors with tyrosine kinase activity. *Cell* 1990; 61: 203–212.

124. Ross R, Glomset JA, Kariya B, Harker L. A platelet dependent serum factor that stimulates the proliferation of arterial smooth muscle cells in vitro. *Proc Natl Acad Sci USA* 1974; 71: 1207–1210.

125. Kawahara RS, Deng Z-W, Deuel TF. Glucocorticoid inhibit the transcriptional induction of JE, a platelet derived growth factor inducible gene. *J Biol Chem* 1991; 266: 13261–13266.

126. Robson MC, Phillips LG, Thomason A, Robson LE, Pierce GF. Platelet derived growth factor BB for the treatment of chronic pressure ulcers. *Lancet* 1992; 339: 23–25.

127. Schweigerer L, Neufield G, Friedman J, *et al*. Capillary endothelial cells express basic fibroblast growth factor, a mitogen that promoted their own growth. *Nature* 1987; 325: 257–259.

128. Folkman J, Klagsbrun M. Angiogenic factors. *Science* 1987; 235: 442–447.

129. Assoian RK, Sporn MB. Type-beta transforming growth factor in human platelets: release during platelet degranulation and action on vascular smooth muscle cells. *J Biol Chem* 1986; 102: 1217–1223.

130. Mustoe TA, Pierce GF, Thomason A, Gramates P, Sporn MB, Deuel TF. Accelerated healing of incisional wounds in rats induced by transforming growth factor. *Science* 1987; 237: 1333–1336.

131. Quaglino D, Nanney LB, Ditesheim JA, Davidson JM. Transforming growth factor beta stimulates wound healing and modulates extracellular matrix gene expression in pig skin: incisional wound model. *J Invest Dermatol* 1991; 97: 34–42.

132. Derynk R. Transforming growth factor. *Cell* 1988; 54: 593–595.

133. McGrath MH. Peptide growth factors and wound healing. *Clin Plastic Surg* 1990; 17: 421–432.

134. Falanga V, Eaglstein WH, Bucalo B, Katz MH, Harris B, Carson P. Topical use of human recombinant epidermal growth factor (h-EGF) in venous ulcers. *J Dermat Surg Oncol* 1992; 18: 604–606.

135. Brown GL, Curtsinger L, Jurkiewicz *et al*. Stimulation of healing of chronic wounds by epidermal growth factors. *Plast Reconstr Surg* 1991; 88: 189–194.

136. Vogt PM, Thompson S, Andree C, *et al*. Genetically modified keratinocytes transplanted to wounds reconstitute epidermis. *Proc Natl Acad Sci USA* 1994; 91: 9307–9311.

137. Eriksson E, Yao F, Svensjo T, *et al*. In vivo gene transfer to skin and wound by microseeding. *J Surg Res* 1998; 78: 85–91.

138. Jeschke MG, Barrow RE, Hawkins HK *et al*. IGF-I gene transfer in thermally injured rats. *Gene Therapy* 1999; 6: 1015–1020.

139. Jeffries MK, Vance ML. Growth hormone and cortisol secretion in patients with burn injury. *J Burn Care Rehabil* 1992; 13: 391–395.

140. Abribat T, Brazeau P, Davignon I, Garrel DR. Insulin-like growth factor-I blood levels in severely burned patients: effects of time post injury, age of patient and severity of burn. *Cline Endocrine* 1993; 39: 583–589.

141. Moller S, Jensen M, Svensson P, Skakkebaek H. Insulin-like growth factor-1 (IGF-1) in burn patients. *Burns* 1991; 17(4): 279–281.

142. Tessari P, Inchiostro S, Biolo G, Trevisan R, Fantin G, Marescotti MC, Iori E, Tiengo A, Crepaldi G. Differential effects of hyperinsulinemia and hyperaminoacidemia on leucine-carbon metabolism in vivo. *J Clin Invest* 1987; 79: 1062–1069.

143. Gelfand RA, Glichman MG, Castellino P, Louard RJ, DeFronzo RA. Measurement of L-^{14}C-leucine kinetics in splanchnic and leg tissues in humans. *Diabetes* 1988; 37: 1365–1372.

144. Wolfe RR, Jahoor F, Hartl WH. Protein and amino acid metabolism after injury. *Diabetes/Metabolism Revs* 1989; 5: 149–164.

145. Finkelstein JW, Roffward HP, Boyer RM, Kream J, Hellman L. Age-related change in the twenty-four hour spontaneous secretion of growth hormone. *J Clin Endocrin Metabol* 1972; 35: 5: 665–670.

146. Soroff HS, Rozin RR, Mooty J, *et al*. Role of human growth hormone in the response to trauma: metabolic effects following burns. *Ann Surg* 1967; 166(5): 739–752.

147. Liljadahl SO, Gemzell CA, Plantin LO, Birke G. Effect of human growth hormone in patients with severe burns. *Acta Chir Scand* 1961; 122: 1–4.

148. McManson JM, Smith RJ, Wilmore DW. Growth hormone stimulates protein synthesis during hypocaloric parenteral nutrition. *Ann Surg* 1988; 208: 136–149.

149. Shorwell MA, Kilbeg MS, Oxender DL. The regulation of neutral amino acid transport in mammalian cells. *Biochem Biophys Acta* 1983; 737: 267–284.

150. Roe CF, Kinky J. The influence of human growth hormone on energy sources in convalescence. *Surg Forum* 1962; 13: 369–371.

151. MacGorman LR, Rizza R, Gerich JE. Physiological concentrations of growth hormone exert insulin like and insulin antagonistic effect on both hepatic and extra hepatic tissues in man. *J Clin Endocrinol Metab* 1981; 53: 556–559.

152. vanVliet G, Bosson D, Craen M, *et al*. Comparative study of the lipolytic potencies of pituitary-derived and biosynthetic human growth hormone in hypopituitary children. *J Clin Endocrinol Metab* 1987; 65: 876.

153. Clemmons DR, Snyder DK, Williams R, *et al*. Growth hormone administration conserves lean body mass during dietary restriction in obese subjects. *J Clin Endocrinol Metab* 1987; 64: 878.

154. Young FG. Insulin and insulin antagonists. *Endocrinology* 1963; 73: 654.

155. Tanner JM, Hughes CPR, Whitehouse RH. Comparative rapidity of response of height, limb muscle and limb fat to treatment with human growth hormone in patients with and without growth hormone deficiency. *Acta Endocrinol* 1977; **84**: 681–696.

156. Kostyo JL. Rapid effects of growth hormone on amino acid transport and protein synthesis. *Ann NY Acad Sci* 1968; **148**: 389–407.

157. Yarasheski KE, Campbell JA, Rennie MK, *et al.* Effect of strength training and growth hormone administration on whole-body and skeletal muscle leucine metabolism. *Med Sci Sports Exerc* 1990; **22**: 505A.

158. Horber FF, Haymond MW. Human growth hormone prevents the protein catabolic side effects of prednisone in humans. *J Clin Invest* 1990; **86**: 265–272.

159. Fryburg DA, Gelfand RA, Barrett EJ. Growth hormone acutely stimulates forearm muscle protein synthesis in normal humans. *Am J Physiol* 1991; **260** (Endocrinol Metab 23): E499–E504.

160. Mjaawand M, Unneberg K, Larsson J, Nilsson L, Revhaug A. Growth hormone after abdominal surgery attenuated forearm glutamine, alanine, 3-methyhistidine and total amino acid effluxes in patients receiving total parenteral nutrition. *Ann Surg* 1993; **217**(4): 413–422.

161. Daughaday WH, Hall K, Salmon WD, Jr, *et al.* Letter to the editor: On the nomenclature of the somatomedins and insulin-like growth factors. *J Clin Endocrinol Metab* 1987; **65**: 1075–1076.

162. Takala J, Ruokonen E, Webster NR, *et al.* Increased mortality associated with growth hormone treatment in critically ill adults. *New Eng J Med* 1999; **341**: 785–792.

163. Warwick-Davies J, Lowrie DB, Cole PJ. Growth hormone is a human macrophage activating factor: priming of human monocytes for enhanced release of H_2O_2. *J Immunol* 1995; **154**: 1909–1918.

164. Edwards CK III, Lorence RM, Dunham DM, *et al.* Hypophysectomy inhibits the synthesis of tumor necrosis factor (alpha) by rat macrophages: partial restoration by exogenous growth hormone or interferon (gamma). *Endocrinology* 1991; **128**: 989–996.

165. Kappel M, Hansen MB, Diamant M, Pedersen BK. In vitro effects of human growth hormone on the proliferative responses and cytokine production of blood mononuclear cells. *Horm Metab Res* 1994; **26**: 612–614.

166. Elsasser TH, Fayer R, Rumsey TS, Hartnell GF. Recombinant bovine somatotropin blunts plasma tumour necrosis factor-(alpha), cortisol, and thromboxane-B2 responses to endotoxin in vivo. *Endocrinology* 1994; **134**: 1082–1088.

167. Inoue T, Saito H, Fukushima R, *et al.* Growth hormone and insulinlike growth factor I enhance host defense in a murine sepsis model. *Arch Surg* 1995; **130**: 1115–1122.

168. Liao W, Rudling M, Angelin B. Growth hormone potentiates the in vivo biological activities of endotoxin in the rat. *Eur J Clin Invest* 1996; **26**: 254–258.

169. Ramirez RJ, Wolf SE, Barrow RE, Herndon DN. Growth hormone treatment in pediatric burns: a safe therapeutic approach. *Ann Surg* 1998; **228**: 439–448.

170. Jeschke MG, Barrow RE, Herndon DN. Recombinant human growth hormone treatment in pediatric burn patients and its role during the hepatic acute phase response. *Crit Care Med* 2000; **28**: 1578–1584.

171. Knox J, Demling R, Wilmore D, Sarraf P, Santos A. Increased survival after major thermal injury: the effect of growth hormone therapy in adults. *J Trauma* 1995; **39**: 526–532.

172. Singh KP, Prassad R, Chari PS, Dash RJ. Effect of growth hormone therapy in burn patients on conservative treatment. *Burns* 1998; **24**: 733–738.

173. Soroff HS, Rozin RR, Mooty J, *et al.* Role of human growth hormone in the response to trauma: metabolic effects following burns. *Ann Surg* 1967; **166**: 739–752.

174. Liljadahl SO, Gemzell CA, Plantin LO, *et al.* Effect of human growth hormone in patients with severe burns. *Acta Chir Scand* 1961; **122**: 1–4.

175. Wilmore DW, Moyland JA Jr, Bristow BF, Mason AD, Pruitt BA. Anabolic effects of growth hormone and high caloric feedings following thermal injury. *Surg Gynecol Obstet* 1974; **138**: 875–884.

176. Soroff HS, Pearson E, Green NL, Artz CP. The effect of growth hormone on nitrogen balance at various levels of intake in burned patients. *Surg Gynecol Obstet* 1960; **111**(3): 259–273.

177. Gore DC, Honeycutt D, Jahoor F, Wohfer R, Herndon DN. Effect of exogenous growth hormone on whole-body and isolated limb protein kinetics in burned patients. *Arch Surg* 1991; **126**: 38–43.

178. Gore DC, Honeycutt D, Jahoor F, Rutan T, Wolfe RR, Herndon DN. Effect of exogenous growth hormone on glucose utilization in burn patients. *J Surg Res* 1991; **51**: 518–523.

179. Fleming RYD, Rutan RI, Jahoor F, Barrow RE, Wolfe RR, Herndon DN. Effect of recombinant human growth hormone on catabolic hormones and free fatty acids following thermal injury. *J Trauma* 1992; **32**: 698–703.

180. Rowe JW, Young JB, Minaker KL, *et al.* Effect of insulin and glucose infusions on sympathetic nervous system activity in normal man. *Diabetes* 1981; **30**: 219–225.

181. Thompson JC, Marx M. *Gastrointestinal Hormones Curr Probl Surg* 1984; 7–80.

182. Edwards CK, Ghiasuddin SM, Yunger LM, Lorence RM, Arkins S, Dantzer R, Kelley KW. In vivo administration of recombinant growth hormone or gamma interferon activates macrophages: enhanced resistance to experimental *Salmonella typhimurium* infections is correlated with generation of reactive oxygen intermediates. *Infect Immunol* 1992; **60**: 2514.

183. Inoue T, Saito H, Fukushima R, Inaba T, Lin M, Fakatsu K, Muto T. Growth hormone and insulin-like growth factor-1 enhance host defense in a murine sepsis model. *Arch Surg* 1995; **130**: 1115.

184. Takagi K, Suzuki F, Barrow RE, Wolf SE, Kobayashi M, Herndon DN. Growth hormone improves the resistance of thermally injured mice infected with herpes simplex virus type 1, *J Trauma* 1998; **44**: 517–522.

185. Takagi K, Suzuki F, Barrow RE, Wolf SE, Kobayashi M, Herndon DN. Growth hormone improves immune function and survival in burned mice infected with herpes simplex virus type 1. *J Surg Res* 1997; **69**: 166–170.

186. Gabrilove JL, Schwartz A, Churg J. Effect of hormones on the skin in endocrinologic disorders. *J Clin Endocrinol Metab* 1962; **22**: 688–692.

187. Tavakkol A, Elder JT, Griffiths CEM, *et al.* Expression of growth hormone receptor, insulin-like growth factor 1 (IGF-1) and IGF-1 receptor mRNA and proteins in human skin. *J Invest Dermatol* 1992; **99**: 343–349.

188. Conover CA, Liu F, Powell D, *et al.* Insulin-like growth factor binding proteins from cultured human fibroblasts. Characterization and hormonal regulation. *J Clin Invest* 1989; **83**: 852–859.

189. Cook JJ, Haynes KM, Werther GA. Mitogenic effects of growth hormone in cultured human fibroblasts. Evidence for action via local insulin-like growth factor I production. *J Clin Invest* 1988; **81**: 206–212.

190. Jorgensen PH, Andreassen TT, Jorgensen KD. Growth hormone influences collagen deposition and mechanical strength of intact rat skin. A dose-response study. *Acta Endocrinol (Copenh)* 1989; **120**: 767–772.

191. Jorgensen PH, Andreassen TT. A dose-response study of the effects of biosynthetic human growth hormone on formation and strength of granulation tissue. *Endocrinology* 1987; **121**: 1637–1641.

192. Jorgensen PH, Andreassen TT. The influence of biosynthetic human growth hormone on biomechanical properties and collagen formation in granulation tissue. *Horm Metab Res* 1988; **20**: 490–493.

193. Rudman A, Feller AG, Nagraj HS. Effect of human growth hormone in men over 60 years old. *N Engl J Med* 1990; **323**: 1–6.

194. Jorgensen PH, Andreassen TT. The influence of biosynthetic human growth hormone on biomechanical properties of rat skin incisional wounds. *Acta Chir Scand* 1988; **154**: 623–626.

195. Zaizen Y, Ford EG, Costin G, Atkinson JB. The effect of perioperative exogenous growth hormone on wound bursting strength in normal and malnourished rats. *J Pediatr Surg* 1990; **25**: 70–74.

196. Atkinson JB, Kosi M, Srikanth MS, *et al.* Growth hormone reverses impaired wound healing in protein-malnourished rats treated with corticosteroids. *J Pediatr Surg* 1992; **27**: 1026–1028.

197. Belcher HJCR, Mercer D, Judkins KC, *et al.* Biosynthetic growth hormone in burned patients: a pilot study. *Burns* 1989; **15**: 99–107.

198. Herndon DN, Barrow RE, Kunkel KR, Broemeling L, Rutan RL. Effects of recombinant human growth hormone on donor-site healing in severely burned children. *Ann Surg* 1990; **212**(4): 424–431.

199. Herndon DN, Hawkins HK, Nguyen TT, Pierre E, Cox R, Barrow RE. Characterization of growth hormone enhanced donor site healing in patients with large cutaneous burns. *Ann Surg* 1995; **221** (6): 649–659.

200. Gilpin DA, Barrow RE, Rutan RL, Broemeling BSN, Herndon DN. Recombinant human growth hormone accelerates wound healing in children with large cutaneous burns. *Ann Surg* 1994; **220**(1): 19–24.

201. Sherman SK, Demling RH, Lalonde C, *et al.* Growth hormone enhances re-epithelialization of human split thickness skin graft donor sites. *Surg Forum* 1989; **40**: 37–39.

202. Rutan RI, Herndon DN. Growth delay in postburn pediatric patients. *Arch Surg* 1990; **125**(3): 392–395.

203. Prader A. Catch-up growth. *Postgrad Med J* 1978; **54**(suppl): 133–146.

204. Bruno LP, Stern PJ, Wyrick JD. Skeletal changes after burn injuries in an animal model. *J Burn Care Rehabil* 1988; **9**: 148–151.

205. Klein GL, Herndon DN, Rutan TC, *et al.* Bone disease in burn patients. *J Bone Miner Res* 1993; **8**: 337–345.

206. Low JF, Herndon DN, Barrow RE. Growth hormone ameliorates growth delay in burned children: a 3 year follow-up study. *Lancet* 1999; **354**: 1789.

207. Touati G, Prieur AM, Ruiz JC, Noel M, Czernichow P. Beneficial effects of one-year growth hormone adminstration to children with juvenile chronic arthritis on chronic steroid therapy. I. Effects on growth velocity and body composition. *J Clin Endocrinol Metab* 1998; **83**: 403–409.

208. Klein GI, Herndon DN, Langman CB, *et al.* Long-term reduction in bone mass following severe burn injury in children. *J Pediatr* 1995; **126**: 252–256.

209. Klein GL, Wolf SE, Langman CB, Rosen CJ, Mohan S, Keenan BS, Matin S, Stedffen C, Nicolai M, Sailer DE, Herndon DN. Effect of therapy with recombinant human growth hormone on insulin-like growth factor system components and serum levels of biochemical markers of bone formation in children after burn injury. *J Clin Endocrinolo Metab* 1998; **83**: 21–24.

210. Voerman HJ, Strack RVS, Groeneveld ABJ, et al. Effects of recombinant human growth hormone in patients with severe sepsis. *Ann Surg* 1992; **216(6)**: 648–655.

211. Byrne TA, Morrissey TB, Gatzen C, et al. Anabolic therpay with growth hormone accelerates protein gain in surgical patients requiring nutritional rehabilitation. *Ann Surg* 1993; **218(4)**: 400–418.

212. Muller MJ, Gilpin DA, Biolo G, Herndon DN. Biosynthetic human growth hormone: current and potential applications in amino acids in cancer and critical illness. In: Latifi R Landers RG, eds. *Amino Acids in Cancer and Critical Illness* 1994.

213. Rutan R, Herndon DN. Justification for the use of growth hormone in a pediatric burn center. *Proceedings American Burn Assoc* 1994; Orlando, Fla.

214. Chwans WJ, Bistrian BR. Role of erogenous growth hormone and insulin-like growth factor 1 in malnutrition and acute metabolic stress: a hypothesis. *Critical Care Med* 1991; **19(10)**: 1317–1322.

215. Boulivare SD, Tamborlane WV, Matthews LS, Sherwin RS. Diverse effects of insulin-like growth factor 1 on glucose lipid and amino acid metabolism. *Am J Physiol* 1992; 262 (Endocrinol Metab 25): E130–E133.

216. Moller S, Jensen M, Svensson P, Skakkebæk NE. Insulin-like growth-factor-1 (IGF-1) in burn patients. *Burns* 1991; **17(4)**: 279–281.

217. Kupfer SR, Underwood LE, Baxter RC, Clemmons DR. Enhancement of the anabolic effects of growth hormone and insulin-like growth factor 1 by use of both agents simultaneously. *J Clin Invest* 1993; **91**: 391–396.

218. Dahn MS, Lange MP, Jacobs LA. Insulin-like growth factor-1 production is inhibited in human sepsis. *Arch Surg* 1988; **123**: 1409–1414.

219. Kimbrough TD, Shernan S, Ziegler TR, et al. Insulin-growth factor-1 response is comparable following intravenous and subcutaneous administration of growth hormone. *J Surg Res* 1991; **51**: 472–476.

220. Strock LL, Singh H, Abdullah A, et al. The effect of insulin-like growth factor-1 on postburn hypermetabolism. *Surgery* 1990; **108(2)**: 161–164.

221. Huang KF, Chung DH, Herndon DN. Insulin-like growth factor-1 (IGF-1) reduces gut atrophy and bacterial translocation after severe burn injury. *Arch Surg* 1993; **128**: 47–54.

222. Dong Y-L, Huang KF, Xia ZF, Chung DH, Yan TZ, Herndon DN, Waymack JP. Impact of erogenous insulin-like growth factor-1 on hepatic energy metabolism in burn injury. *Arch Surg* 1993; **128(6)**: 703–708.

223. Barrow RE, Wang CZ, Evans MJ, Herndon DN. Growth factors accelerate epithelial repair in sheep trachea. *Lung* 1993; **171**: 335–344.

224. Lieberman SA, Butterfield GE, Harrison D, Hoffman AR. Anabolic effects of recombinant human insulin-like growth factor-1 in cachectic patients with acquired immunodeficiency syndrome. *J Clin Endocrin Metab* 1994; **78**: 404–410.

225. Cioffi WG, Gore DC, Rue LW, et al. Insulin-like growth factor-I lowers protein oxidation in patients with thermal injury. *Ann Surg* 1994; **220**: 310–319.

226. Bondy CA, Underwood LE, Clemmoms DR, et al. Clinical uses of insulin-like growth factor-I. *Ann Intern Med* 1994; **120**: 593–601.

227. Clemmons DR. Insulin-like growth factor binding proteins and their role in controlling IGF actions. *Cytokine Growth Factor Rev* 1997; **8**: 45–62.

228. Herndon DN, Ramzy PI, DebRoy MA, Zheng M, Ferrando AA, Chinkes DL, Barret JP, Wolfe RR, Wolf SE. Muscle protein catabolism after severe burn: effects of IGF-1/IGFBP-3 treatment. *Ann Surg* 1999; **229**: 713–722.

229. DebRoy MA, Wolf SE, Zhang XJ, Chinkes DL, Ferrando AA, Wolfe RR, Herndon DN. Anabolic effects of insulin-like growth factor in combination with insulin-like growth factor binding protein-3 in severely burned adults. *J Trauma* 1999; **47**: 904–911.

230. Jeschke MG, Barrow RE, Herndon DN. Insulin-like growth factor I plus insulin like growth factor binding protein-3 attenuates the proinflammatory acute phase response in severely burned children. *Ann Surg* 2000; **231**: 246–252.

231. Meyer NA, Barrow RE, Herndon DN. Combined Insulin-like growth factor-1 and growth hormone improves weight loss and wound healing in burned rats. *J Trauma* 1996; **41**: 1008–1012.

232. Linares HA. Autopsy findings in burned children. In Carvajal HF, Parks DH, (eds). *Pediatric Burn Management. Burns in Children*. Chicago, IL: Yearbook Medical Publishers, 1988: 298–299.

233. Joshi VV. Effects of burns on the heart. *JAMA* 1970; **211(13)**: 2130–2134.

234. Gelfand RA, Hutchinson-Williams KA, Bonde AA, et al. Catabolic effects of thyroid hormone excess: the contribution of adrenergic activity to hypermetabolism and protein breakdown. *Metabolism* 1987; **36(6)**: 562–569.

235. Herndon DN. Mediators of metabolism. *J Trauma* 1981; **21**: 701–705.

236. Wolfe RR, Herndon DN, Peters EJ, et al. Regulation of lipolysis in severely burned children. *Ann Surg* 1987; **290(2)**: 214–221.

237. Wolfe RR, Durkot MJ. Evaluation of the role of the sympathetic nervous system in the response of substrate kinetics and oxidation to burn injury. *Circ Shock* 1982; **9**: 395–406.

238. Garber AJ, Karl IE, Kipnis DM. Alanine and glutamine synthesis and release from skeletal muscle. IV. B-adrenergic inhibition of amino acid release. *J Biol Chem* 1976; **251**: 851–857.

239. Miles JM, Nissen SL, Gerich JE, Haymond MW. Effects of epinephrine infusion on leucine and alanine kinetics in humans. *Am J Physiology* 1984; **247**: E166–172.

240. Keller U, Kraenzlin W, Stauffacher W, Arnaud M. B-adrenergic stimulation results in diminished protein breakdown, decreased amino acid oxidation and increased protein synthesis in man. *JPEN* 1987; **11(suppl)**: 7S. Abstract.

241. Herndon DN, Barrow RE, Rutan TC, et al. Effect of propranolol administration on hemodynamic and metabolic responses of burned pediatric patients. *Ann Surg* 1988; **208**: 484–492.

242. Minifee PK, Barrow RE, Abston S, et al. Improved myocardial oxygen utilization following propranolol infusion in adolescents with postburn hypermetabolism. *J Paed Surg* 1989; **24**: 806–811.

243. Honeycutt D, Barrow R, Herndon DN. Cold stress response in patients with severe burns after beta-blockade. *J Burn Care Rehabil* 1992; **13(2)**: 181–186.

244. Baron PW, Barrow RE, Pierre EJ, Herndon DN. Prolonged use of propranolol safely decreases cardiac work in burned children. *J Burn Care Rehabil* 1997; **18**: 223–227.

245. Herndon DN, Nguyen TT, Wolfe RR, et al. Lipolysis in burned patients with severe burns after beta-blockade. *J Burn Care Rehabil* 1992; **13**: 1301–1305.

246. Hart DW, Wolf SE, Chinkes DL, et al. Reversal of catabolism after severe burn: the effects of long-term β-blockade. (Submitted to *NEJM*)

247. Popp MB, Silverstein EB, Srivastaver LS, et al. A pathophysiologic study of the hypertension associated with burn injury in children. *Ann Surg* 1981; **193(6)**: 817–824.

248. Choo JJ, Horan MA, Little RA, et al. Anabolic effects of clenbuterol on skeletal muscle are mediated by beta-2 adrenoreceptor activation. *Am J Physiol* 1992; **263(Endocrinol Metab 26)**: E50–E56.

249. Carter WJ, Dang ASQ, Faas FG, et al. Effects of clenbuterol on skeletal mass, body composition and recovery from surgical stress in senescent rats. *Metabolism* 1991; **40**: 855–860.

250. Chance WT, Von Allmen D, Benson D, et al. Clenbuterol decreases catabolism and increases hypermetabolism in burned rats. *J Trauma* 1991; **31**: 365–370.

251. Hollyoak MA, Muller MJ, Meyer NA, et al. Beneficial wound healing at metabolic effects of clenbuterol in burned and non-burned rats. *J Burn Care Rehabil* 1995; **16**: 233–240.

252. Ferrando AA, Tipton KD, Doyle D, et al. Testosterone injection stimulates net protein synthesis but not tissue amino acid transport. *Am J Physiol* 1998; **275**: E864–871.

253. Berger JR, Pall L, Hall CD, et al. Oxandrolone in AIDS-wasting myopathy. *AIDS* 1996; **10**: 1657–1662.

254. Wilson DM, McCauley E, Brown DR, Dudley R. Oxandrolone therapy in constitutionally delayed growth and puberty. Bio-Technology General Corporation Cooperative Study Group. *Pediatrics* 1995; **96**: 1095–1100.

255. Rosenfeld RG, Attie KM, Frane J, et al. Growth hormone therapy of Turner's syndrome: beneficial effect on adult height. *J Pediatrics* 1998; **132**: 319–324.

256. Sheffiled-Moore M, Urban RJ, Wolf SE, et al. Short-term oxandrolone administration stimulates net muscle protein synthesis in young men. *J Clin Endocrinol Metab* 1999; **84**: 2705–2711.

257. Demling RH, DeSanti L. Oxandrolone, an anabolic steroid, significantly increases the rate of weight gain in the recovery phase after major burns. *J Trauma* 1997; **43**: 47–51.

258. Demling RH, Orgill DP. The anticatabolic and wound healing effects of the testosterone analog oxandrolone after severe burn injury. *J Crit Care* 2000; **15**: 12–17.

259. Hart DW, Wolf SE, Ramzy PI, Chinkes DL, et al. Anabolic effects of oxandrolone after severe burn. *Ann Surg* 2001; **233**: 556–64.

260. Demling RH, Lalonde C. Early postburn lipid peroxidation: effect of ibuprofen and allopurinol. *Surgery* 1990; **107**: 85–93.

261. Jin LJ, Lalonde C, Demling RH. Lung dysfunction after thermal injury in relation to prostanoid and oxygen radical release. *J Appl Physiol* 1986; **61**: 103–112.

262. Demling RH, Lalonde C. Identification and modifications of the pulmonary and systemic inflammatory and biochemical changes caused by a skin burn. *J Trauma* 1990; **30**: S57–S62.

Chapter 28

Etiology and prevention of multisystem organ failure
Robert L Sheridan, Ronald G Tompkins

Multiple system organ failure remains a principal cause of death after major operative procedures and/or severe trauma. – D.E. Fry[1]

Introduction

Despite its common occurrence in critically ill burn patients, our understanding of the multisystem organ failure syndrome remains fragmented and incomplete. The cascade of organ dysfunctions which typify the multisystem organ failure syndrome is driven by an unregulated inflammatory state, often, but not always, associated with uncontrolled infection.[1] Other potential 'engines' driving this cascade of organ dysfunctions are an impaired gastrointestinal barrier,[2,3] the open burn wound,[4] and inadequate delivery of oxygen to peripheral tissues.[5] The line between organ dysfunction and failure is admittedly unclear, but a set of organ-specific definitions of failure (**Table 28.1**) is helpful and has been developed.[6] Approximately 15% of patients admitted to surgical intensive care units have multisystem organ failure,[7] and perhaps 8% of burn patients ultimately develop the syndrome.[8]

The sequence of failures often follows a predictable course, although the cascade can be modified by various treatments, such as the prophylactic use of H_2 receptor blockers. In burn patients, two cascades have been described.[8] An early cascade characterized by resuscitation failure, adult respiratory distress syndrome, hemodynamic failure, renal failure, liver failure, gut failure, and infection, and a late cascade typified by pulmonary failure,

Table 28.1 Organ-specific definitions of failure (OSF)

If the patient had one or more of the following during a 24-hour period (regardless of the values), OSF existed on that day

Cardiovascular failure (presence of *one or more* of the following):
 Heart rate ≤ 54 beats/min
 Mean arterial blood pressure ≤ 49 mmHg
 Occurrence of ventricular tachycardia and/or ventricular fibrillation
 Serum pH ≤7.24 with a Pa_{CO_2} of ≤ 49 mmHg

Respiratory failure (presence of *one or more* of the following):
 Respiratory rate ≤5 beats/min or ≥40 beats/min
 Pa_{CO_2} ≥ 50 mmHg
 Aa_{DO_2} ≥ 350 mmHg (Aa_{DO_2} = 713 F_{IO_2} – Pa_{CO_2} – Pa_{O_2})
 Dependent on ventilator on the fourth day of OSF, e.g. *not* applicable for the initial 72 hours of OSF

Renal failure (presence of *one or more* of the following):*
 Urine output ≤ 479 ml/24 h or ≤ 159 ml/8 h
 Serum BUN ≥ 100 mg/dl
 Serum creatinine ≥ 3.5 mg/dl

Hematologic failure (presence of *one or more* of the following):
 WBC ≤ 1000 mm³
 Platelets ≤ 20 000 mm³
 Hematocrit ≤ 20%

Neurological failure
 Glasgow Coma Score ≤ 6 (in absence of sedation at any one point in day)
 Glasgow Coma Score: sum of best eye opening, best verbal, and best motor responses. Scoring of responses as follows: (points)
  Eye – Open: spontaneously (4), to verbal command (3), to pain (2), no response (1)
  Motor – Obeys verbal command (6); response to painful stimuli: localizes pain (5), flexion-withdrawal (4), decorticate rigidity (3), decerebrate rigidity (2); no response (1); movement without any control (4)
  Verbal – Oriented and converses (5), disoriented and converses (4), inappropriate words (3), incomprehensible sounds (2), no response (1). If intubated, use clinical judgment for verbal responses as follows: patient generally unresponsive (1), patient's ability to converse in question (3), patient appears able to converse (5)

*Excluding patients on chronic dialysis before hospital admission.
Reproduced from Knaus *et al.*[6] with permission.

hemodynamic instability, renal failure, gut failure, and liver failure. Frequently, vasomotor failure and death is seen at the end of both cascades. Mortality increases with increasing numbers of failed organ systems. When three organs have failed, mortality has been reported as 100%, although survival is sometimes seen in patients with even more failed organ systems.[9] An understanding of the progression of the syndrome aids in prognostication and facilitates decisions regarding termination of futile efforts.[10,11] The management of specific organ failures will be presented in the next chapter. The purpose of this chapter is to discuss the etiology and prevention of the syndrome.

Etiology

The etiology of multisystem organ failure remains a mystery under intense investigation. All patients seem to share characteristics associated with an uncontrolled inflammatory state, and there are several proposed 'engines' which drive this uncontrolled inflammation, including sepsis, the open burn wound, the gut, and hypoperfusion.

Sepsis is clearly the most common initiator of the syndrome, and was recognized early on as the primary cause.[1] One single overwhelming infection is not required, as small repetitive infections may initiate the cascade,[12] perhaps by priming immune cells making them react more intensely to each subsequent stimulus.[12] It was recognized later that many patients with multisystem organ failure did not have infection,[13] and this led the search for other 'engines'. Endotoxin liberated from the walls of gram-negative bacteria is a major, but not the only, intermediary,[14] as gram-positive bacteria cause similar aberrations in oxygen transport and hemodynamics,[15] via similar cascades of mediators.[16]

In burn patients the wound may also be a source of the inflammatory mediators leading to multiple organ failure. Certainly, an infected wound will do this, but wound sepsis is decreasing in incidence with the advent of early burn wound excision[17] and most infectious deaths in burn patients today are caused by pneumonia rather than wound sepsis.[18] Complete wound closure, without donor sites, decreases oxygen consumption[19] and presumably ameliorates the inflammatory response to the open wound. Incomplete wound closure does not have this effect.[20] Increased levels of circulating mediators such as interleukin-6 (IL-6), IL-8, and tumor necrosis factor (TNF) have been shown to originate from the burn wound[21] and contribute to the hypermetabolic and inflammatory state seen in burn patients. Interleukin-8 has been demonstrated to be upregulated in the lung after burn injury[21] and the stimulus for this upregulation, which is associated with pulmonary dysfunction, may come from the wound.[21]

Intensive recent work has demonstrated the importance of gut barrier function and the relation of gut barrier failure to the development of multisystem organ failure.[22] Normal barrier function prevents the movement of bacteria and their products from the gut lumen into the portal and lymphatic circulations. Bacterial densities range from near 0 in the stomach, to 10^4–10^5 in the distal small bowel, to 10^{11}–10^{12}/g of stool in the normal colon.[23] That the normal gut can carry this bacterial load, without the frequent occurrence of gram-negative infection, is a tribute to normal barrier function. Although not seen immediately after trauma,[24] several insults have been shown to result in increased translocation of bacteria and their products into the portal and lymphatic circulations. Hemorrhagic shock,[25] endotoxin administration,[26] burns,[27] and burn wound sepsis[28] have each been shown to result in increased translocation of bacteria from the gut. Gut permeability to macro-

molecules, such as endotoxin, has been shown to increase with increasing burn wound size using polyethylene glycol 3350 as a tracer.[29] Smaller molecules, with lactulose as the tracer, have also been shown to pass more readily through the gastrointestinal membrane after injury.[30] The exact mechanism by which bacteria and their products pass through the gastrointestinal barrier is not clear. Both intra- and transcellular processes may be involved.[31,32] The consequences of loss of the gastrointestinal barrier are profound. Translocating whole bacteria can be a direct source of sepsis or can activate Kupffer cells[2,3] and promulgate an inflammatory response in conjunction with bacterial products such as endotoxin.

Cellular dysfunction, caused by inadequate oxidative metabolism secondary to hypoperfusion, is another potential 'engine' resulting in multisystem organ failure. In ischemia–reperfusion models, oxygen radicals are generated, resulting in peroxidation of cell membrane lipids and accumulation of activated neutrophils,[33] with progressive cellular and whole-organ dysfunction. It has been proposed that critically ill patients suffer from supply-dependent oxygen consumption because of defects in cellular oxygen extraction and utilization.[34,35] This results in inadequate aerobic metabolism unless supranormal levels of oxygen are supplied.[36] The reality of this proposal is still actively debated.[37,38] Certainly, a grossly inadequate amount of oxygen available to cells dependent on aerobic metabolism can lead to cellular dysfunction, and this may be followed by organ failures.[5] Maintaining oxygen delivery at at least normal, and possibly supranormal, levels should help maintain cellular homeostasis and minimize the risk of multiple organ failure.[39] Although the requirement for a supranormal level of tissue oxygenation in critical illness is controversial and our ability to predict organ-specific oxygen delivery and consumption from whole-body data is poor,[40] careful attention to whole-body hemodynamics is an integral part of the management of any critically ill patient.

Common ground: mediators

Sepsis, open burn wounds, impaired gut barrier function, and hypoperfusion are all associated with multiorgan failure. The similarity in the response to these differing events implies that there is some common ground. These processes all probably impact on individual organs via a number of mediators, whose complex interactions are still very poorly understood,[41] but are being unraveled by investigators using blocking antibodies, soluble receptors, and receptor antagonists.[42] At this point, these mediators, including endotoxin, arachidonic acid metabolites, cytokines, platelet activating factor, activated neutrophils and adherence molecules, nitric oxide, complement, and oxygen free radicals will be reviewed briefly.

Endotoxin, a lipopolysaccharide component of gram-negative bacterial cell walls, induces many of the symptoms associated with sepsis including fever, hypotension, the release of acute phase proteins, and the production of multiple cytokines including TNF and IL-1.[43] Endotoxin also activates complement,[44] causes activation of the coagulation cascade,[45] and results in the release of platelet activating factor.[46] Potential sources of endotoxin include both gram-negative bacteria in foci of infection and gram-negative bacteria within the gut when the gut barrier fails.

Arachidonic acid makes up approximately 20% of cell membranes, is released from these membranes in response to a multitude of stimuli which activate phospholipases A_2 and C, and is then metabolized by one of two major enzyme systems (**Figure 28.1**).

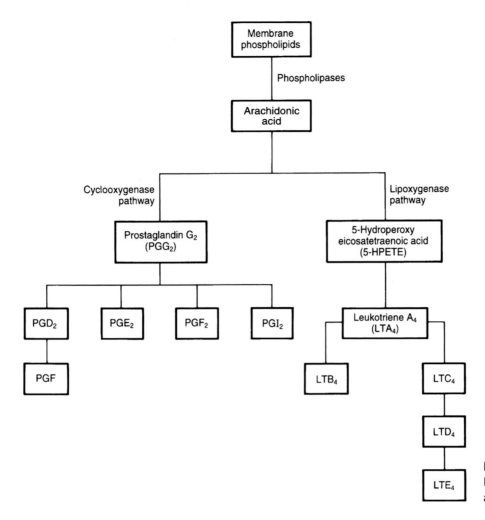

Fig. 28.1 The cyclooxygenase and lipoxygenase pathways of arachidonic acid metabolism.

The cyclooxygenase pathway results in production of prostaglandins and thromboxanes, and the lipoxygenase pathway results in the production of leukotrienes.[47] The prostaglandins and leukotrienes interact with other mediators in a complex fashion, and are later degraded by enzyme systems, which are dispersed throughout the body.[48]

Arachidonic acid, which is metabolized via the cyclooxygenase pathway, results in the formation of prostaglandins and thromboxanes. Prostacyclin inhibits platelet aggregation, thrombis formation, and gastric secretion.[49] Thromboxane A_2 (TXA_2) causes platelet aggregation, has profound vasoconstricting effects on both the splanchnic and pulmonary microvasculature, causes bronchoconstriction, and increased membrane permeability.[50] It is studied via its longer lived but inactive metabolite, TXB_2. Aspirin has its physiologic effects by inhibiting thromboxane synthetase.[51]

Arachidonic acid metabolized via the lipoxygenase pathway results in the formation of leukotrienes. There are two types based on their metabolism after the action of 5-lipooxygenase, leukotrienes (LT) C_4, D_4, and E_4 (the sulfidopeptide group) and LTB_4.[52] Leukotrienes are generated in response to multiple stimuli by several cell types including neutrophils, macrophages, and monocytes.[53] Vessel walls are also capable of generating leukotrienes.[54] Leukotrienes C_4, D_4, and E_4 have variable actions on vascular tone depending on the presence or absence of other mediators such as cyclooxygenase product.[55] In addition to their variable effects in redirecting blood flow, LTC_4, LTD_4, and LTE_4 also increase vascular permeability,[56] and have been described to be elevated immediately prior to the development of pulmonary failure.[57] The major effect of LTB_4 is an enhancement of neutrophil chemotaxis.[58] Thus, leukotrienes as a group may be involved in the edema formation and pulmonary and systemic vascular changes that are seen in the multisystem organ failure syndrome.

Cytokines are regulatory proteins that are secreted by immune cells and have multiple paracrine and endocrine effects. There are six major classes[59] including interleukins, TNF, interferons, colony-stimulating factors, chemotactic factors, and growth factors. Those which have been most extensively characterized are IL-1, IL-6, and TNF.

Interleukin-1 and IL-6 are elevated in septic states, and high levels are associated with a fatal outcome[60] and predict systemic infection.[61] Interleukin-1β causes hypotension and decreased systemic vascular resistance, which may be synergistic with the effects of TNF.[62] Even better characterized is TNF, the administration of which causes hypotension, cardiac depression, and pulmonary dysfunction in animals.[63–65] When administered to humans, TNF causes fever, hypotension, decreased systemic vascular resistance, increased protein turnover, elevation of stress hormone levels,[66,67] and activation of the coagulation cascade.[68]

Platelet activating factor is a nonprotein phospholipid, which is secreted by many cells including platelets, endothelial cells, and inflammatory cells,[69] and is a major mediator of the pulmonary[70] and hemodynamic[71] effects of endotoxin. The major effects of platelet activating factor are vasodilation, cardiac depression, and enhancement of capillary leak. Its complex interactions with other mediators are still poorly understood.

Although tissue injury can occur in the absence of neutrophils,[72] the inflammatory process results in local accumulation of activated inflammatory cells which release various local toxins such as oxygen radicals, proteases, eicosanoids, platelet activating factor, and other substances. When unregulated, such accumulations of activated cells can cause tissue injury.[73] The initial attachment of neutrophils to the vascular endothelium at an inflammatory site is facilitated by the interaction of adherence molecules on the neutrophil and endothelial cell surfaces.[74]

These neutrophil adherence receptors are induced by numerous stimuli but, interestingly, are reduced after major thermal and non-thermal injury,[75] perhaps explaining in part the increased incidence of infection in such patients. The importance of this adherence mechanism can be seen in patients who are deficient in one of the integrin class of neutrophil adherence receptors, CD-18, who suffer from frequent bacterial infections.[76] The biology of the transmembrane polypeptides that govern these complex cell-to-cell interactions is an active area of research[77] and holds promise for therapeutic interventions in the future.

Oxygen radicals, such as hydrogen peroxide and superoxide anion, are released by activated neutrophils in response to a variety of stimuli.[78] They are also released when xanthine oxidase is activated after reperfusion in ischemia–reperfusion models. These highly reactive products cause cell membrane dysfunction, increased vascular permeability, and release of eicosanoids.

Nitric oxide, released when citrulline is formed from arginine (**Figure 28.2**), was only identified as an endothelial product in the middle 1980s.[79] Its half-life is only a few seconds, as it is quickly oxidized, but it has profound local microvascular effects. Nitric oxide synthesis is stimulated by various cytokines, endotoxin, thrombin, and by injury to the vascular endothelium. It is a potent vasodilator,[80] but its actions vary depending on the vascular bed and presence of other mediators.[81] Nitric oxide is one of the major mediators of the hypotensive response to sepsis.[82,83]

Antigen–antibody complexes activate the complement cascade, and complement fragments thus generated can interact with other cytokines to promulgate the inflammatory response.[84] Diminished levels of a natural inhibitor of C5a have been demonstrated in patients with adult respiratory distress syndrome (ARDS)[85] and administration of anti-C5a antibody diminishes hypotension in an animal model of endotoxemia.[86] Complement fragments may be involved in the development of burn wound edema.[87]

Obviously, our understanding of the incredibly complex cellular and subcellular biology, of which multisystem organ failure is but one manifestation, is poorly understood at the present time. This dim understanding highlights the important role that prevention plays in managing the syndrome.

Prevention of multisystem organ failure

Once established, multisystem organ failure is very difficult to reverse, emphasizing the importance of prevention.[88] Prevention is based on our crude knowledge of the 'engines' that drive the process – sepsis, the gut, the wound, and inadequate perfusion (**Table 28.2**). Dealing with these issues is far more practical than dealing with an incompletely understood complex web of mediators. Also, this complex cascade evolved in numerous species over thousands of generations and interference in the network may do more harm than good. The discussion that follows will address prevention of sepsis via proper wound management and attention to unusual causes of sepsis, support of the gut, and prevention of inadequate oxygen delivery. Subsequently, the potential role of nutritional and specific immunomodulators will be addressed.

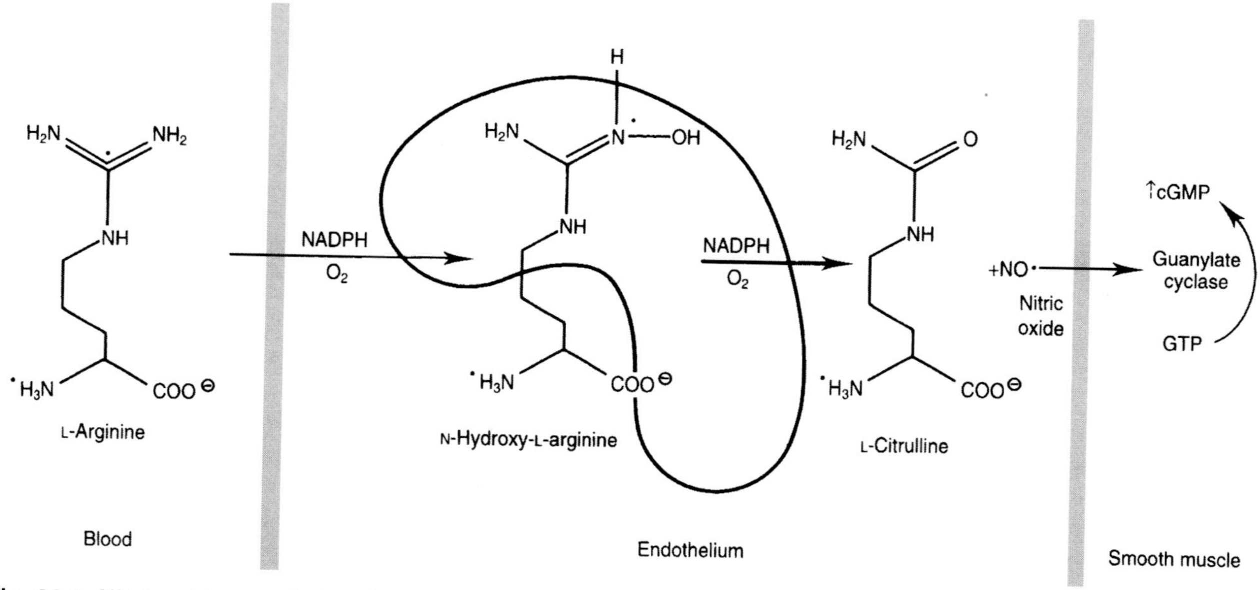

Fig. 28.2 Nitric oxide metabolism (from Cobb *et al.*[189] with permission).

Table 28.2 Multiple organ failure etiology and established preventive measures	
Etiology	Prevention
Sepsis	Early excision and biologic closure of deep wounds
	Anticipation and early treatment of occult septic foci
Gut barrier failure	Optimize whole-body hemodynamics
	+/– Early enteral feedings
Inadequate organ perfusion	Optimize whole-body hemodynamics
	+/– Enhanced oxygen delivery

Prevention of sepsis

In the burn patient, prevention of multisystem organ failure is greatly facilitated by prevention of wound sepsis via an aggressive surgical approach to deep wounds. The increasing survival of burn patients has paralleled the evolution of this approach to the burn wound.[89–91] Not only is overt wound sepsis prevented by early removal of devitalized tissue, but multiple smaller septic insults are also prevented, as manipulation of heavily colonized burn wounds is a frequent source of transcient bacteremia.[92,93] Such multiple occult bacteremias occurring during frequent manipulation of heavily colonized wounds could contribute to the development of multisystem organ failure by priming immune cells, making them react more intensively to each subsequent insult.[12] The role of perioperative antibiotics in minimizing bacteremias in the perioperative period has yet to be defined clearly. However, they are clearly beneficial in patients with injuries greater than 60% of body surface and in any other patient in whom the probability of bacteremia with wound manipulation is felt to be high.[94] Appropriate perioperative antibiotics are guided by surface cultures. Burn patients are prone to a large number of unusual and often occult infectious complications[95] which can result in sepsis and potentially contribute to the development of multiorgan failure. Rapid diagnoses and treatment are facilitated by a high index of suspicion.

Intravascular infections such as suppurative thrombophlebitis and endocarditis typically present in burn patients with fever and bacteremia without localizing signs. Burn patients with endocarditis develop a new murmur in only 9% of cases,[96] and only 10% have been reported to present antemortem.[97] Of those with septic thrombophlebitis, 68% have no localizing signs and present with fever and positive blood cultures only.[98] The diagnoses is made in patients without localizing signs only by thorough examination of all sites of prior cannulation, with surgical exposure of any suspicious sites and complete excision of any involved veins.[99] Vigilant care and scheduled replacement of intravascular devices will minimize the occurrence of catheter-related sepsis. Occult intracompartmental sepsis can also present with fever and bacteremia without localizing signs, and is diagnosed only by careful examination and exploration of suspicious compartments.[100]

Pneumonia, seen in approximately 35% of patients with inhalation injury, adds between 20 and 60% to the expected mortality of burn patients.[101] Although a difficult diagnosis to make in critically ill patients, pneumonia should be vigilantly anticipated and aggressively treated with appropriate endobronchial toilet and specific antibiotics. The incidence of nosocomial pneumonia increases with longer durations of intubation,[102] emphasizing the importance of judicious use of mechanical ventilation.

Suppurative sinusitis is being recognized with increasing frequency in the intensive care unit, and may be more frequent in patients who are nasotracheally intubated.[103] Diagnosis may require examination and culture of material obtained by antral puncture, in addition to plain radiographs and computed tomography. Although there is some controversy about the role of the nasotracheal tube in causing sinusitis,[104] treatment involves removing all nasotracheal devices, topical decongestants, and appropriate antibiotics. Surgical drainage is reserved for recalcitrant cases.

Acalculous cholecystitis often presents with generalized sepsis without localizing signs in the burn patient, and, like intravascular infection, is a very difficult diagnosis to make.[105] Recently, bedside placement of percutaneous cholecystostomy tubes under ultrasonic guidance has become an option in the management of suspected cholecystitis in critically ill patients.[106] This technique allows an accurate diagnoses to be made and the condition to be temporarily treated in patients too unstable for immediate operation.

Sepsis accounts for at least half of cases of multisystem organ failure. In perhaps no other area can the vigilance of the burn team have a greater impact in multisystem organ failure prevention than in the early detection and aggressive treatment of occult septic foci.

Support of the gut

Bacteria and their products released when the gut barrier fails may fuel the multiorgan failure syndrome. Gut mucosal integrity suffers when mesenteric flow is inadequate and gut blood flow is decreased after burn injury, a response exacerbated by the release of TXA_2.[107] Thus, support of splanchnic blood flow is an important aspect of multisystem organ failure prevention,[108] and this is best done by careful attention to whole-body hemodynamics. There is no substitute for a carefully monitored burn resuscitation.

The enterocyte may be better supported by intraluminal, rather than parenteral feedings, as gut deprived of intraluminal feedings develops mucosal atrophy.[109] Early enteral feedings are tolerated in the burn patients,[110] and may reduce the magnitude of the hypermetabolic response to the injury.[111] Parenteral feedings do not prevent gut mucosal atrophy as well as isocaloric and isonitrogenous intraluminal feeds,[112] although convincing human data are not available to support the clinical significance of this point.

The value of specific nutrients to support the enterocyte is far less clear than the value of providing adequate mesenteric blood flow and perhaps intraluminal nutrition. However, this is an exciting and active area of research. Glutamine, a nonessential amino acid, is the preferred fuel of the small bowel enterocyte[113] as well as other rapidly dividing cells. Sepsis has been shown to decrease glutamine uptake by the small bowel enterocyte, which may result in barrier failure,[114] and the addition of glutamine to the nutritional regimen has been theorized to improve barrier function. Glutamine is not a component of commercial parenteral nutritional formulae because of its short shelf life, although the dipeptide is well tolerated parenterally, and has a longer shelf life.[115] Although supplemental glutamine may improve protein balance in surgical patients,[115] and may partially reverse gut atrophy,[116] it has not been shown to improve gut barrier function when given parenterally.[117]

The role of specific nutrients in support of the large intestinal mucosa is less clear, but butyrate, a fatty acid liberated by fiber fermentation, is a favored fuel of the colonic mucosal cell.[118] Enteral pectin may help support the colonic mucosa,[119] but the value of such support in the hypermetabolic burn patient is as yet unclear.

A decontaminated gut lumen might diminish the impact of gastrointestinal barrier failure. Attempts have been made to access the impact of selective decontamination of the gut[120] and coating enteric bacteria to inhibit their ability to attach to the intestinal mucosa and translocate.[121] Although there is a suggestion that the rate of pneumonia may be decreased by such maneuvers, there is no apparent impact on mortality.

Support of the gut in an effort to prevent multisystem organ failure is certain to have real value. Maintenance of adequate mesenteric perfusion via careful attention to whole-body hemodynamics is crucial. There is some data to support the contention that enteral feedings have beneficial effects on outcome in injured patients when compared with parenteral feedings, possibly via an enhancement of gastrointestinal barrier integrity.[122] However, these data require confirmation prior to general application. Data supporting the administration of specific mucosal substrates or gut decontamination are less convincing, but further research in these important areas may show such benefit.

Insuring adequate oxygen delivery

The normal intracellular partial pressure of oxygen is 0.5 mmHg, and this small amount of midochrondial oxygen allows for the aerobic generation of most of the cell's adenosine triphosphate (ATP). When cells have to adapt to a lower oxygen tension, ATP generation continues at a lower rate by anaerobic channels,[123] possibly triggered by the build-up of adenosine diphosphate (ADP). As outlined by Gutierrez, the anaerobic reactions which generate ATP are glycolysis, the creatine kinase reaction, and the adenylate kinase reaction.[123] Glycolysis describes the conversion of glucose to lactate with the generation of two ATP molecules. The creatine kinase reaction is the breakdown of the high-energy phosphate storage molecule, phosphocreatine, with the generation of ATP and creatine. The adenylate kinase reaction describes the combination of nucleotides to form ATP and AMP which, although generating ATP, depletes the cells of adenine nucleotides. In conjunction with this conversion to anaerobic ATP generation, the intracellular concentration of hydrogen ion increases, the amount of adenine nucleotides within the cell decreases, and intracellular calcium levels increase with decreased function of the ATP-driven sodium–calcium pump.[124] There also may be an increase in the liberation of intracellular oxygen free radicals with the activation of xanthine oxidase.[125] If low oxygen tensions continue, membrane phospholipids may be degraded by the combined effects of elevated calcium, oxygen free radicals, and the decreased synthetic capabilities coincident with decreased levels of ATP.[126] These effects may be magnified if there is also systemic sepsis as cellular oxygen extraction may be impaired. That such cellular hypoxic dysfunction is involved in the development of organ dysfunction is implied by the fact that cocarboxylase, which enhances ATP generation by ischemic cells, ameliorates some of the metabolic and hemodynamic consequences of endotoxic shock in an animal model.[127]

An understanding of progressive cell destruction and dysfunction which is caused by low intracellular oxygen tensions, coupled with the perception of oxygen extraction abnormalities associated with sepsis, has led to an intense interest in the delivery of supranormal amounts of oxygen to prevent organ dysfunction, as clinical data suggest that inadequate oxygen delivery is associated with the development of multisystem organ failure.[128] Clinically, it is somewhat cumbersome to measure and follow oxygen delivery, and other markers of the adequacy of tissue oxygenation have been tried, including the use of lactate and the lactate/pyruvate ratio, base deficit, mixed venus oxygen tension and pH, and gut tonometry. However, none of these secondary markers of oxygen delivery have proven to be as reliable as the direct determination of oxygen delivery and consumption by the reverse Fick technique.

Normal physiologic oxygen supply dependency is different than the pathologic supply dependency seen in septic states. In this circumstance, supranormal oxygen delivery is said to be required, as extraction is decreased.[129] The exact reasons for this pathologic supply dependency are unclear, but may involve microcirculatory shunting or aberrations of intracellular physiology. It has been proposed that the purposeful delivery of supranormal amounts of oxygen is associated with a decreased incidence of multiple organ failure and increased survival.[130] The reality of the proposal is still controversial, with data showing no increase in oxygen consumption with transfusion of critically ill children[131] and the absence of a consumption plateau in patients with ARDS.[132] Also, regional blood flow is poorly predicted by whole-body oxygen delivery and consumption data[133] implying that whole-body delivery and consumption data may be of no value even if pathologic supply dependency was real. Normally, oxygen consumption is approximately 25% of oxygen delivery, and delivery can be maximized by optimizing the hemoglobin, partial pressure of oxygen, and cardiac output, which are the major determinants of oxygen delivery, although total flow may be more important than the blood's oxygen-carrying capacity.[134]

Inadequate oxygen delivery clearly leads to organ dysfunction. At a minimum, the clinician should insure that injured patients are resuscitated to the conventional clinical endpoints of appropriate urine output, skin perfusion, blood pressure, and sensorium. In selected critically ill patients, invasive monitoring is justified to document oxygen delivery and consumption, extraction ratio, and the possible presence of supply dependency in which circumstance supranormal levels of oxygen delivery with plateau of oxygen consumption is an appropriate resuscitation endpoint.

The potential role of nutritional and specific immunomodulators

The holy grail of those who study the complex biology of the multisystem organ failure syndrome is an ability to modulate the common pathways that lead to organ dysfunction and death. The three general approaches to this goal are nutritional, nonspecific, and specific immunomodulation.

Nutritional immunomodulation

Three categories of substances show some promise as potential nutritional immunomodulators in burn patients: long-chain fatty acids; arginine, glutamine, and branched-chain amino acids; and nucleotides. Short- and medium-chain fatty acids are commonly utilized for energy, whereas long-chain fatty acids are important constituents of cell membranes and can profoundly influence cell function.[135] Omega-3 long-chain fatty acids play a particularly important role in the membranes of immunocompetent cells.[136] There is animal data suggesting that supplementation of the diet with ω-3 fatty acids may improve immune function after burn injury;[137] however, there is no clear clinical data yet available to support the routine administration of ω-3 fatty acids as a dietary supplement in injured patients.

The potential immunostimulating effects of specific amino acids, particularly arginine, glutamine, and the branched-chain amino acids leucine, isoleucine, and valine, is an active area of research. Arginine is a nonessential amino acid with important functions in the urea cycle and in the generation of nitric oxide.[138] It also may have important effects in insuring immune cell competence.[139,140] Although there are some animal data suggesting improved immunocompetence and outcome after burn with supplementation of arginine,[141–143] human data are not yet adequate to support its routine administration to burn patients. Glutamine, the most common amino acid in the body, and a preferred fuel of rapidly dividing cells, may be conditionally essential in hypermetabolic patients,[113,114] and its administration has been proposed as a method to support the gut barrier thereby abrogating the consequences of barrier failure. Early human data suggest that administration of supplemental glutamine may improve amino acid protein economy in stressed surgical patients,[115] but there are inadequate data as yet to support the routine administration of glutamine as an immune stimulant.

The branched-chain amino acids leucine, isoleucine, and valine are important energy sources in stressed surgical patients. Although there was an early enthusiasm for the supplemental administration of these substrates, subsequent data have suggested that the supplemental administration of branched-chain amino acids does not benefit stressed surgical patients.[144]

Based on limited animal and human data it has been suggested that the administration of adenine nucleotides may have beneficial effects on immune function in stressed patients.[145] Again, at the present time there is inadequate human data to support the routine use of supplemental nucleotides.

The concept of nutritional immunomodulation via supplementation of specific substances is exciting. However, despite preliminary human studies suggesting a beneficial effect of supplemental arginine and ω-3 fatty acids,[146] with additional nucleotides,[145] and glutamine[115] there do not yet exist adequate data to support nutritional immunomodulation as a routine maneuver in the management of burned patients.

Nonspecific and specific immunomodulation

It seems intuitively unlikely that there exists a magic immunomodulating bullet that will prevent the development of multisystem organ failure in critically ill surgical patients, particularly if sepsis is uncontrolled, the integrity of the gut barrier is compromised, burn wounds are unaddressed, or patients are inadequately supported hemodynamically. However, such efforts have tremendous potential to facilitate our understanding of cellular and subcellular biology and may, in time, provide a clinical dividend. Efforts at nonspecific immunomodulation have included the use of

steroids,[147] immunoglobulin G,[148] and naloxone[149] with no significant impact on patient outcomes. With the exception of steroids for those with suspected adrenal insufficiency[150] and naloxone for those with opiate intoxication, there is no role for these substances in critically ill burn patients.

Although there have been efforts to absorb lipopolysaccharide,[151] and to prevent endotoxemia with prophylactic polymyxin B in burn patients,[152] the greatest efforts at specific immunomodulation have been applied to the development of anti-endotoxin antibodies. The earliest clinical efforts used human serum with anti-J5 activity and demonstrated an enhanced survival in patients with gram-negative septic shock.[153] Later, two monoclonal IgMs were developed, and human trials were completed. The first was anti-E5, a murine monoclonal antibody. Clinical trials suggested a benefit in septic patients without refractory shock.[154] Large numbers of treated patients developed antibodies to the murine monoclonal, and although these patients were not retreated, attention turned more toward a human product. A subsequent effort with this murine monoclonal did not show statistically significant improvements in outcome.[155]

HA-1A, a human monoclonal IgM, was trailed in a large multicenter effort without statistically significant improvement in outcome, except in a subgroup of patients that had gram-negative bacteremia and shock.[156] Multiple confounding factors made these marginally beneficial results suspect, leaving the ultimate utility of HA-1A still unclear.

Anti-endotoxin monoclonal therapy, which may have potential to be beneficial if significantly refined, has also been criticized for its expense. It is estimated that it would cost $24 100 per year of life saved should this technology be used widely.[157] Integrating such advanced and expensive technology into common practice poses tremendous practical problems, and is therefore very unlikely to happen soon when one considers its lack of clear efficacy and high expense.

Significant efforts have also been made toward modifying the actions of arachidonic acid metabolites or eicosanoids, both cyclooxygenase and lipoxygenase products. Numerous animal models of sepsis and endotoxemia exist, and cyclooxygenase pathway blockade with nonsteroidal anti-inflammatory agents has demonstrated improved survival,[158,159] improved pulmonary hemodynamics,[160] and improved mesenteric blood flow.[161] There has been little work documenting outcome improvement in human patients, but it has been suggested that nonsteroidal anti-inflammatory agents improve symptoms associated with endotoxin infusion in normal volunteers[162] and septic patients,[163] and may improve immune function after surgical trauma.[164] In an animal model, infusion of the vasodilating arachidonic acid metabolite, prostacyclin, ameliorates the pulmonary dysfunction associated with endotoxin infusion.[165] Less work has been done with lipoxygenase pathway inhibitors. Survival is enhanced in a murine model of endotoxin infusion with lipoxygenase pathway blockade.[166] Endotoxin-associated pulmonary dysfunction is diminished in sheep[167] and pigs[168] when this pathway is blocked. The ultimate role of lipoxygenase blockade in human remains uninvestigated.

Cytokines are difficult to measure accurately and their complex interactions are poorly understood. The production of IL-1 receptor antagonist is increased in human endotoxemia,[169] and, in an animal model, its administration enhances survival.[170] However, infusion of IL-1 may improve immune function in humans.[171]

Clearly our understanding of the complex functions of this cytokine are inadequate to allow intelligent intervention.

Tumor necrosis factor is produced by macrophages and other inflammatory cells when stimulated by endotoxin.[172] In animal models, the physiologic effects of both endotoxin infusion and Gram-negative sepsis[173,174] are attenuated by TNF blockade with monoclonal antibodies. Circulating levels of TNF are high immediately after sepsis begins and then fall, implying that only anti-TNF pretreatment would be beneficial.[175] However, even anti-TNF administration prior to experimental sepsis[176] and endotoxemia[177] has variable effects, at best, on survival. Again, our incomplete understanding precludes effective intervention.

Interference with the effects of platelet activating factor (PAF) has been shown to decrease neutrophil priming by human burn serum,[178] to improve endotoxin-induced pulmonary dysfunction,[179] to decrease eicosanoid release,[180] and to attenuate thromboxane release and improve survival[181] in various animal models of endotoxemia. These exciting initial results, and the availability of several blockers and receptor antagonists, portend a future use for PAF modification.

Efforts to modulate both the adherence and function of inflammatory cells is an exciting area of research, as activated neutrophils clearly play an important role in the development of multiple organ failure. Blockade of neutrophil adhesion receptors with monoclonal antibodies enhances survival in animal models of endotoxic and hemorrhagic shock.[182,183] Again, our basic understanding is not yet adequate to intelligently modify such important processes.

Oxygen free radicals generated by activated neutrophils or xanthine oxidase may oxidize membrane lipids, forming lipid peroxides, resulting in membrane dysfunction.[184] Native antioxidant systems do exist, but can be overwhelmed. Circulating levels of vitamin E, a natural antioxidant, are low in patients with ARDS.[185] Efforts to modify oxidant activity have included blockade of free radical generation, addition of free radical scavengers, augmentation of host antioxidant defenses, and prevention of amplification of tissue damage by neutrophils.[184] Particularly exciting are free radical scavengers such as superoxide dismutase[186] and spin-trapping nitrones[187] which improve survival in animal models of endotoxic and hemorrhagic shock. But, despite such encouraging initial animal work, such therapy is not yet appropriate in human patients.

The continuous synthesis of nitric oxide (**Figure 28.2**) plays an important role in the regulation of pulmonary and systemic vascular tone in sepsis[188] and this presents potential opportunities for intervention.[189] Aerosolized nitric oxide has been shown to be useful in reversing the pulmonary hypertension associated with ARDS[190] and nitric oxide synthesis blockade may improve the hypotension[191] and renal dysfunction[192] associated with sepsis. However, its complex interactions with other cytokines and variable effects on different vascular beds render any nitric oxide-based interventions investigational at the present time.

Most patients who die in the burn unit after surviving resuscitation succumb to multiple organ failure.[193] Although modification of the cascade of events leading to multiorgan failure at the cellular and subcellular level is an enticing possibility, our fragmented understanding of these processes mitigates against such therapy in human patients at the present time. That TNF enhances the ability of neutrophils to kill invading bacteria[194] and of rats to survive Gram-negative sepsis;[195] that cyclooxygenase inhibition increases

TNF production after burn;[196] that PGE$_2$ is important in renal autoregulation;[197] and that cytokine levels do not predict survival as well as conventional variables[198] makes one loathe to interfere in such complex, and poorly understood processes. Vigilant clinical care in the intensive care unit, with the prevention of sepsis, proper management of burn wounds, support of the gut barrier, and careful attention to whole-body hemodynamics is a much more fruitful area in which a vigilant clinician can make a difference.

References

1. Fry DE, Pearlstein L, Fulton RL, Polk HC Jr. Multiple system organ failure. The role of uncontrolled infection. *Arch Surg* 1980; **115**: 136–40.
2. Biffi WL, Moore EE, Moore FA, Carl VS, Kim FJ, Franciose RJ. Interleukin-6 potentiates neutrophil priming with platelet-activating factor. *Arch Surg* 1994; **129(11)**: 1131–6.
3. Saadia R, Schein M, McFarlane C, Boffard KD. Gut barrier function and the surgeon. *Br J Surg* 1990; **77**: 487–92.
4. Echinard CE, Sajdel-Sulkowska E, Burke PA, Burke JF. The beneficial effect of early excision on clinical response and thymic activity after burn injury. *J Trauma* 1982; **22**: 560–5.
5. Schumacker PT, Samsel RW. Oxygen delivery and uptake by peripheral tissues: physiology and pathophysiology. *Crit Care Clin* 1989; **5**: 255–69.
6. Knaus WA, Droper EA, Wagner DP, Zimmerman JE. Prognosis in acute organ-system failure. *Ann Surg* 1985; **202**: 685–93.
7. Knaus WA, Draper EA, Wagner DP, Zimmerman JE. APACHE II: a severity of disease classification system. *Crit Care Med* 1985; **13**: 818–29.
8. Goodwin CW. Multiple organ failure: clinical overview of the syndrome. *J Trauma* 1990; **30**: s163–5.
9. Huanag YS, Yang ZC, Liu XS, *et al*. Serial experimental and clinical studies on the pathogenesis of multiple organ dysfunction syndrome (MODS) in severe burns. *Burns* 1998; **24(8)**: 706–16.
10. Meisel A, Jernigan JC, Younger SJ. Prosecutors and end-of-life decision making. *Arch Intern Med* 1999; **159(10)**: 1089–95.
11. Meisel A. Legal myths about terminating life support. *Arch Intern Med* 1991; **151**: 1497–502.
12. Meakins JL. Etiology of multiple organ failure. *J Trauma* 1990; **30**: S165–8.
13. Bone RC, Fisher CJ Jr, Clemmer TP, Slotman GJ, Metz CA, Balk RA. Sepsis syndrome: a valid clinical entity. *Crit Care Med* 1989; **17**: 389–93.
14. Suffredini AF, Fromm RE, Parker MM, *et al*. The cardiovascular response of normal humans to the administration of endotoxin. *N Engl J Med* 1989; **321**: 280–7.
15. Ahmed AJ, Kruse JA, Haupt MT, Chandrasekar PH, Carlson RW. Hemodynamic responses to Gram-positive versus Gram-negative sepsis in critically ill patients with and without circulatory shock. *Crit Care Med* 1991; **19**: 1520–5.
16. Wakabayashi G, Gelfand JA, Jung WK, Connolly RJ, Burke JF, Dinarello CA. *Staphylococcus epidermidis* induces complement activation, tumor necrosis factor and interleukin-1, a shock-like state and tissue injury in rabbits without endotoxemia. Comparison to *Escherichia coli*. *J Clin Invest* 1991; **87**: 1925–35.
17. Merrell SW, Saffle JR, Larson CM, Sullivan JJ. The declining incidence of fatal sepsis following thermal injury. *J Trauma* 1989; **29**: 1362–6.
18. Peck MD, Heimbach DM. Does early excision of burn wounds change the pattern of mortality? *J Burn Care Rehabil* 1989; **10**: 7–10.
19. Lalonde C, Demling RH. The effect of complete burn wound excision and closure on postburn oxygen consumption. *Surgery* 1987; **102**: 862–8.
20. Demling RH, Lalonde C. Effect of partial burn excision and closure on postburn oxygen consumption. *Surgery* 1988; **104**: 846–52.
21. Rodriguez JL, Miller CG, Garner WL, *et al*. Correlation of the local and systemic cytokine response with clinical outcome following thermal injury. *J Trauma* 1993; **34**: 684–94.
22. Deitch EA. The role of intestinal barrier failure and bacterial translocation in the development of systemic infection and multiple organ failure. *Arch Surg* 1990; **125**: 403–4.
23. Schaedler RW, Goldstein F. Bacterial populations of the gut in health and disease; basic microbiologic aspects. In: Brochus HL, Beck JE, Haubrich WS, *et al*, eds. *Gastroenterology*. Philadelphia: WB Saunders, 1976: 147–9.
24. Peitzman AB, Udekwu AO, Ochoa J, Smith S. Bacterial translocation in trauma patients. *J Trauma* 1991; **31**: 1083–6.
25. Baker JW, Deitch EA, Li M, Berg RD, Specian RD. Hemorrhagic shock induces bacterial translocation from the gut. *J Trauma* 1988; **28**: 896–906.
26. Deitch EA, Berg R. Specian R. Endotoxin promotes the translocation of bacteria from the gut. *Arch Surg* 1987; **122**: 185–90.

27. Deitch EA, Winterton J, Berg R. Thermal injury promotes bacterial translocation from the gastrointestinal tract in mice with impaired T-cell-mediated immunity. *Arch Surg* 1986; **121**: 97–101.

28. Jones WG, Minei JP, Barber AE, *et al.* Bacterial translocation and intestinal atrophy after thermal injury and burn wound sepsis. *Ann Surg* 1990; **211**: 399–405.

29. Ryan CM, Yarmush ML, Burke JF, Tompkins RG. Increased gut permeability early after burns correlates with the extent of burn injury. *Crit Care Med* 1992; **20**: 1508–12.

30. Deitch EA. Intestinal permeability is increased in burn patients shortly after injury. *Surgery* 1990; **107**: 411–506.

31. Fink MP. Gastrointestinal mucosal injury in experimental models of shock, trauma, and sepsis. *Crit Care Med* 1991; **19**: 627–41.

32. Alexander JW, Boyce ST, Babcock GF, *et al.* The process of microbial translocation. *Ann Surg* 1990; **212**: 496–510.

33. Schoenberg MH, Beger HG. Reperfusion injury after intestinal ischemia. *Crit Care Med* 1993; **21**: 1376–86.

34. Bihari D, Smithies M, Gimson A, Tinker J. The effects of vasodilation with prostacyclin on oxygen delivery and uptake in critically ill patients. *N Engl J Med* 1987; **317**: 397–403.

35. Kaufman BS, Rackow EC, Falk JL. The relationship between oxygen delivery and consumption during fluid resuscitation of hypovolemic and septic shock. *Chest* 1984; **85**: 336–40.

36. Cain SM, Curtis SE. Experimental models of pathologic oxygen supply dependency. *Crit Care Med* 1991; **19**: 603–12.

37. Barone JE, Lowenfels AB. Maximization of oxygen delivery: a plea for moderation. *J Trauma* 1992; **33**: 651–3.

38. Hotchkiss RS, Karl IE. Reevaluation of the role of cellular hypoxia and bioenergetic failure in sepsis. *JAMA* 1992; **267**: 1503–10.

39. Shoemaker WC, Kram HB, Appel PL, Fleming AW. The efficacy of central venous and pulmonary artery catheters and therapy based upon them in reducing mortality and morbidity. *Arch Surg* 1990; **125**: 1332–7.

40. Ruokonen E, Takala J, Kari A. Regional blood flow and oxygen transport in patients with low cardiac output syndrome after cardiac surgery. *Crit Care Med* 1993; **21**: 1304–13.

41. Cerra FB. The systemic septic response: concepts of pathogenesis. *J Trauma* 1990; **30**: S169–S174.

42. Dinarello CA. The proinflammatory cytokines interleukin-1 and tumor necrosis factor and treatment of the septic shock syndrome. *J Infect Dis* 1991; **163**: 1177–84.

43. Fukushima R, Alexander JW, Gianotti L, Pyles T, Ogle CK. Bacterial translocation-related mortality may be associated with neutrophil-mediated organ damage. *Shock* 1995; **3**(5): 323–8.

44. Morrison DC, Kline LF. Activation of the classical and the properdin pathways of complement by bacterial lipopolysaccharides (LPS). *J Immunol* 1977; **118**: 362–8.

45. Morrison DC, Ulevitch RJ. The effects of bacterial endotoxins on host mediation systems. A review. *Am J Pathol* 1978; **93**: 526–617.

46. Chang SW, Fedderson CO, Henson PM, Voelkel NF. Platelet-activating factor mediates hemodynamic changes and lung injury in endotoxin-treated rats. *J Clin Invest* 1987; **79**: 1498–1509.

47. Ramwell PW, Leovey EM, Sintetos AL. Regulation of arachidonic acid cascade. *Biol Reprod* 1977; **16**: 70–87.

48. Henderson WR Jr. Eicosanoids and lung inflammation. *Am Rev Respir Dis* 1987; **135**: 1176–85.

49. Whittle BJ, Moncada S. Pharmacological interactions between prostacyclin and thromboxanes. *Br Med Bull* 1983; **39**: 232–8.

50. Ogletree ML. Overview of physiological and pathophysiological effects of thromboxane A2. *Fed Proc* 1987; **46**: 133–8.

51. Fitzgerald GA, Reilly IA, Pedersen AK. The biochemical pharmacology of thromboxane synthase inhibition in man. *Circulation* 1985; **72**: 1194–201.

52. Sprague RS, Stephenson AH, Dahms TE, Lonigro AJ. Proposed role for leukotrienes in the pathophysiology of multiple systems organ failure. *Crit Care Clin* 1989; **5**: 315–29.

53. Lewis RA, Austen KF. The biologically active leukotrienes. Biosynthesis, metabolism, receptors, functions, and pharmacology. *J Clin Invest* 1984; **73**: 889–97.

54. Feinmark SJ. Cooperative synthesis of leukotrienes by leukocytes and vascular cells. *Ann NY Acad Sci* 1988; **524**: 122–32.

55. Pfister RR, Haddox JL, Sommers CL. Injection of chemoattractants into normal cornea: a model of inflammation after alkali injury. *Invest Ophthalmol Vis Sci* 1998; **39**(9): 1744–50.

56. Hedqvist P, Dahlen SE, Bjork J. Pulmonary and vascular actions of leukotrienes. *Adv Prostaglandin Thromboxane Leukot Res* 1982; **9**: 187–200.

57. Davis JM, Meyer JD, Barie PS, *et al.* Elevated production of neutrophil leukotriene B$_4$ precedes pulmonary failure in critically ill surgical patients. *Surg Gynecol Obstet* 1990; **170**: 495–500.

58. Goetzl EJ, Pickett WC. The human PMN leukocyte chemotactic activity of complex hydroxy-eicosatetraenoic acids (HETEs). *J Immunol* 1980; **125**: 1789–91.

59. Arai KI, Lee F, Miyajima A, Miyatake S, Arai N, Yokota T. Cytokines: coordinators of immune and inflammatory responses. *Annu Rev Biochem* 1990; **59**: 783–836.

60. Waage A, Brandtzaeg P, Halstensen A, Kierulf P, Espevik T. The complex pattern of cytokines in serum from patients with meningococcal septic shock. Association between interleukin-6, interleukin-1, and fatal outcome. *J Exp Med* 1989; **169**: 333–8.

61. Fassbender K, Pargger H, Muller W, Zimmerli W. Interleukin-6 and acute-phase protein concentrations in surgical intensive care unit patients: diagnostic signs in nosocomial infection. *Crit Care Med* 1993; **21**: 1175–80.

62. Okusawa S, Gelfand J, Ikejima T, Connolly RJ, Dinarello CA. Interleukin-1 induces a shock-like state in rabbits. Synergism with tumor necrosis factor and the effect of cyclooxygenase inhibition. *J Clin Invest* 1988; **81**: 1162–72.

63. Zhange B, Huang YH, Chen Y, Yang Y, Hao ZL, Xie SL. Plasma tumor necrosis factor-alpha, its soluble receptors and interleukin-1beta levels in critically burned patients. *Burns* 1998; **24**(7): 599–603.

64. Hollenberg SM, Cunnion RE, Parrillo JE. The effect of tumor necrosis factor on vascular smooth muscle. In vitro studies using rat aortic rings. *Chest* 1991; **100**: 1133–7.

65. Heard SO, Perkins MW, Fink MP. Tumor necrosis factor-a causes myocardial depression in guinea pigs. *Crit Care Med* 1992; **20**: 523–7.

66. Warren RS, Starnes HF Jr, Gabrilove JL, Oettgen HF, Brennan MF. The acute metabolic effects of tumor necrosis factor administration in humans. *Arch Surg* 1987; **122**: 1396–400.

67. Michie HR, Spriggs DR, Manogue KR, *et al.* Tumor necrosis factor and endotoxin induce similar metabolic responses in human beings. *Surgery* 1988; **104**: 280–6.

68. van der Poll T, Buller HR, ten Cate H, *et al.* Activation of coagulation after administration of tumor necrosis factor to normal subjects. *N Engl J Med* 1990; **322**: 1622–7.

69. Anderson BO, Bensard DD, Harken AH. The role of platelet activating factor and its antagonists in shock, sepsis and multiple organ failure. *Surg Gynecol Obstet* 1991; **172**: 415–24.

70. Rabinovici R, Esser KM, Lysko PG, *et al.* Priming by platelet-activating factor of endotoxin-induced lung injury and cardiovascular shock. *Circ Res* 1991; **69**: 12–25.

71. Qi M, Jones SB. Contribution of platelet activating factor to hemodynamic and sympathetic responses to bacterial endotoxin in conscious rats. *Circ Shock* 1990; **32**: 153–63.

72. Yonemaru M, Hatherill JR, Hoffmann H, Zheng H, Ishii K, Raffin TA. Pentoxifylline does not attenuate acute lung injury in the absence of granulocytes. *J Appl Physiol* 1991; **71**: 342–51.

73. Weiss SJ. Tissue destruction by neutrophils. *N Engl J Med* 1989; **320**: 365–76.

74. Horgan MJ, Ge M, Gu J, Rothlein R, Malik AB. Role of ICAM-1 in neutrophil-mediated lung vascular injury after occlusion and reperfusion. *Am J Physiol* 1991; **261**: H1578–H1584.

75. White-Owen C, Alexander JW, Babcock GF. Reduced expression of neutrophil CD11b and CD16 after severe traumatic injury. *J Surg Res* 1992; **52**: 22–6.

76. Anderson DC, Springer TA. Leukocyte adhesion deficiency: an inherited defect in the Mac-1, LFA-1, and p150, 95 glycoproteins. *Annu Rev Med* 1987; **38**: 175–94.

77. Benton LD, Khan M, Greco RS. Integrins, adhesion molecules, and surgical research. *Surg Gynecol Obstet* 1993; **177**: 311–27.

78. Bautista AP, Shuler A, Spolarics Z, Spitzer JJ. Tumor necrosis factor-a stimulates superoxide anion generation by perfused rat liver and Kupffer cells. *Am J Physiol* 1991; **261**: G891–G895.

79. Palmer RM, Ferrige AG, Moncada S. Nitric oxide release accounts for the biological activity of endothelium-derived relaxing factor. *Nature* 1987; **327**: 524–6.

80. Moncada S, Palmer RM, Higgs EA. Nitric oxide physiology, pathophysiology, and pharmacology. *Pharmacol Rev* 1991; **43**: 109–42.

81. Bernard C, Szekely B, Philip I, Wollman E, Payen D, Tedgui A. Activated macrophages depress the contractility of rabbit carotids via an L-arginine/nitric oxide-dependent effector mechanism. Connection with amplified cytokine release. *J Clin Invest* 1992; **89**: 851–60.

82. Nava E, Palmer RM, Moncada S. Inhibition of nitric oxide synthesis in septic shock: how much is beneficial? *Lancet* 1991; **338**: 1555–7.

83. Ochoa JB, Udekwu AO, Billiar TR, *et al.* Nitrogen oxide levels in patients after trauma and during sepsis. *Ann Surg* 1991; **214**: 621–6.

84. Hosea S, Brown E, Hammer C, Frank M. Role of complement activation in a model of adult respiratory distress syndrome. *J Clin Invest* 1980; **66**: 375–82.

85. Allen JN, Pacht ER, Gadek JE, Davis WB. Acute eosinophilic pneumonia as a

reversible cause of noninfectious respiratory failure. *N Engl J Med* 1989; **321**: 569–74.

86. Smedegard G, Cui LX, Hugli TE. Endotoxin-induced shock in the rat. A role for C5a. *Am J Pathol* 1989; **135**: 489–97.

87. Friedl HP, Till GO, Trentz O, Ward PA. Roles of histamine, complement and xanthine oxidase in thermal injury of skin. *Am J Pathol* 1989; **135**: 203–17.

88. Livingston DH. Management of the surgical patients with multiple system organ failure. *Am J Surg* 1993; **165**: 8S–13S.

89. Tompkins RG, Burke JF, Schoenfeld DA, *et al*. Prompt eschar excision: a treatment system contributing to reduced burn mortality. A statistical evaluation of burn care at the Massachusetts General Hospital (1974–1984). *Ann Surg* 1986; **204**: 272–81.

90. Sheridan RL, Remensnyder JP, Schnitzer JJ, Schulz JT, Ryan CM, Tompkins RG. Current expectations for survival in pediatric burns. *Arch Pediatr Adolesc Med* 2000; **154(3)**: 245–9.

91. Herndon DN, Barrow RE, Rutan RL, Rutan TC, Desai MH, Abston S. A comparison of conservative versus early excision. Therapies in severely burned patients. *Ann Surg* 1989; **209**: 547–52.

92. Sasaki TM, Welch GW, Herndon DN, Kaplan JZ, Lindberg RB, Pruitt BA Jr. Burn wound manipulation-induced bacteremia. *J Trauma* 1979; **19**: 46–8.

93. Beard CH, Ribeiro CD, Jones DM. The bacteraemia associated with burns surgery. *Br J Surg* 1975; **62**: 638–41.

94. Piel P, Scarnati S, Goldfarb IW, Slater H. Antibiotic prophylaxis in patients undergoing burn wound excision. *J Burn Care Rehabil* 1985; **6**: 422–4.

95. Luterman A, Dacso CC, Curreri PW. Infections in burn patients. *Am J Med* 1986; **81(1A)**: 45–52.

96. Baskin TW, Rosenthal A, Pruitt BA. Acute bacterial endocarditis: a silent source of sepsis in the burn patient. *Ann Surg* 1976; **184**: 618–21.

97. Srivastava RF, MacMillan BG. Cardiac infection in acute burned patients. *Burns* 1979; **6**: 48–54.

98. Pruitt BA Jr, Stein JM, Foley FD, Moncrief JA, O'Neil JA Jr. Intravenous therapy in burn patients. Suppurative thrombophlebitis and other life threatening complications. *Arch Surg* 1970; **100**: 399–404.

99. Pruitt BA Jr, McManus WF, Kim SH, Treat RC. Diagnosis and treatment of cannula-related intravenous sepsis in burn patients. *Ann Surg* 1980; **191**: 546–54.

100. Sheridan RL, Tompkins RG, McManus WF, Pruitt BA Jr. Intracompartmental sepsis in burn patients. *J Trauma* (In press).

101. Shirani KZ, Pruitt BA, Jr., Mason AD Jr. The influence of inhalation injury and pneumonia on burn mortality. *Ann Surg* 1987; **205**: 82–7.

102. Langer M, Mosconi P, Cigada M, Mandelli M. Long-term respiratory support and risk of pneumonia in critically ill patients. *Am Rev Respir Dis* 1989; **140**: 302–5.

103. Deutschman CS, Wilton P, Sinow J, Dibbell D Jr, Konstantinides FN, Cerra FB. Paranasal sinusitis associated with nasotracheal intubation: a frequently unrecognized and treatable source of sepsis. *Crit Care Med* 1986; **14**: 111–14.

104. Halzapfel L, Shervet S, Madinier G, *et al*. Influence of long-term oro- or nasotracheal intubation on nosocomial maxillary sinusitis and pneumonia: results of a prospective, randomized, clinical trial. *Crit Care Med* 1993; **21**: 1132–8.

105. Slater H, Goldfarb IW. Acute septic cholecystitis in patients with burn injuries. *J Burn Care Rehabil* 1989; **10**: 445–7.

106. Vauthey JN, Lerut J, Martini M, Becker C, Gertsch P, Blumgart LH. Indications and limitations of percutaneous cholecystostomy for acute cholecystitis. *Surg Gynecol Obstet* 1993; **176**: 49–54.

107. Herndon DN, Zeigler ST. Bacterial translocation after thermal injury. *Crit Care Med* 1993; **21**: S50–4.

108. Wilmore DW, Smith RJ, O'Dwyer ST, Jacobs DO, Ziegler TR, Wang XD. The gut: a central organ after surgical stress. *Surgery* 1988; **104**: 917–23.

109. Johnson LR, Copeland EM, Dudrick SJ, Lichtenberger LM, Castro GA. Structural and hormonal alterations in the gastrointestinal tract of parenterally fed rats. *Gastroenterology* 1975; **68**: 1177–83.

110. McDonald WS, Sharp CW, Deitch EA. Immediate enteral feeding in burn patients is safe and effective. *Ann Surg* 1991; **213**: 177–83.

111. Saito H, Trocki O, Alexander JW, Kopcha R, Heyd T, Joffee SN. The effect of route of nutrient administration on the nutritional status, catabolic hormone secretion, and gut mucosal integrity after burn injury. *JPEN* 1987; **11**: 1–7.

112. Levine GM, Deren JJ, Steiger E, Zinno R. Role of oral intake in maintenance of gut mass and disaccharide activity. *Gastroenterology* 1974; **67**: 975–82.

113. Souba WW, Smith RJ, Wilmore DW. Glutamine metabolism by the intestinal tract. *JPEN* 1985; **9**: 608–17.

114. Souba WW, Herskowitz K, Klimberg VS, *et al*. The effects of sepsis and endotoxemia on gut glutamine metabolism. *Ann Surg* 1990; **211**: 543–9.

115. Stehle P, Zander J, Merts N, *et al*. Effect of parenteral glutamine peptide supplements on muscle glutamine loss and nitrogen balance after major surgery. *Lancet* 1989; **1**: 231–3.

116. Platell C, McCauley R, McCulloch R, Hall J. The influence of parenteral glutamine and branched-chain amino acids on total parenteral nutrition-induced atrophy on the gut. *JPEN* 1993; **17**: 348–54.

117. Spaeth G, Gottwald T, Haas W, Holmes M. Glutamine peptide does not improve gut barrier function and mucosal integrity in total parenteral nutrition. *JPEN* 1993; **17**: 317–23.

118. Roediger WE. Utilization of nutrients by isolated epithelial cells of the rat colon. *Gastroenterology* 1982; **83**: 424–9.

119. Koruda MJ, Rollandelli RH, Settle RG, Saul SH, Rombeau JL. The effect of pectin-supplemented elemental diet on intestinal adaptation to massive small bowel resection. *JPEN* 1986; **10**: 343–50.

120. Gastinne H, Wolff M, Delatour F, Faurisson F, Chevret S. A controlled trial in intensive care units of selective decontamination of the digestive tract with nonabsorbable antibiotics. The French Study Group on Selective Decontamination of the Digestive Tract. *N Engl J Med* 1992; **326**: 594–9.

121. Wang X, Andersson R, Soltesz V, Guo W, Bergmark S. Water-soluble ethylhydroxyethyl cellulose prevents bacterial translocation induced by major liver resection in the rat. *Ann Surg* 1993; **217**: 155–67.

122. Moore FA, Moore EE, Jones TN, McCroskey BL, Petersen VM. TEN versus TPN following major abdominal trauma–reduced septic morbidity. *J Trauma* 1989; **29**: 916–22.

123. Gutierrez G. Cellular energy metabolism during hypoxia. *Crit Care Med* 1991; **19**: 619–26.

124. Dixon IM, Elyolfson DA, Ohalla NS. Sarcolemmal Na^+–Ca^{2+} exchange activity in hearts subjected to hypoxia reoxygenation. *Am J Physiol* 1987; **253**: H1026–34.

125. Granger DN. Role of xanthine oxidase and granulocytes in ischemia-reperfusion injury. *Am J Physiol* 1988; **255**: H1269–75.

126. Das DK, Engelman RM, Rousou JA, Breyer RH, Otani H, Lemeshow S. Role of membrane phospholipids in myocardial injury induced by ischemia and reperfusion. *Am J Physiol* 1986; **251**: H71–9.

127. Lindenbaum GA, Larrieu AJ, Carroll SF, Kapusnick RA. Effect of cocarboxylase in dogs subjected to experimental septic shock. *Crit Care Med* 1989; **17**: 1036–40.

128. Shoemaker WC, Appel PL, Kram HB. Role of oxygen debt in the development of organ failure sepsis, and death in high risk surgical patients. *Chest* 1992; **102**: 208–15.

129. Cain SM. Supply dependancy of oxygen uptake in ARDS: myth or reality? *Am J Med Sci* 1984; **288**: 119–24.

130. Shoemaker WC, Appel PL, Kram HB, Waxman K, Lee TS. Prospective trial of supranormal values of survivors as therapeutic goals in high risk surgical patients. *Chest* 1988; **94**: 1176–86.

131. Mink RB, Pollack MM. Effect of blood transfusion on oxygen consumption in pediatric septic shock. *Crit Care Med* 1990; **18**: 1087–91.

132. Clarke C, Edwards JD, Nightingale P, Mortimer AJ, Morris J. Persistence of supply dependency of oxygen uptake at high levels of delivery in adult respiratory distress syndrome. *Crit Care Med* 1991; **19**: 497–502.

133. Ruokonen E, Takala J, Kori A, Saxen H, Mertsala J, Hansen ED. Regional blood flow and oxygen transport in septic shock. *Crit Care Med* 1993; **21**: 1296–303.

134. Lorente JA, Landin L, DePablo R, Renes E, Rodrigues-Diez R, Liste D. Effects of blood transfusion on oxygen transport variables in severe sepsis. *Crit Care Med* 1993; **21**: 1312–31.

135. Kinsella JE, Lokesh B, Broughton S, Whelan J. Dietary polyunsaturated fatty acids and eicosanoids: potential effects on the modulation of inflammatory and immune cells: an overview. *Nutrition* 1990; **6**: 24–44.

136. Barton RG, Wells CL, Carlson A, Singh R, Sullivan JJ, Cerra FB. Dietary omega-3 fatty acids decrease mortality and Kupffer cell prostaglandin E_2 production in a rat model of chronic sepsis. *J Trauma* 1991; **31**: 768–73.

137. Alexander JW, Saito H, Trocki O, Ogle CK. The importance of lipid type in the diet after burn injury. *Ann Surg* 1986; **204**: 1–8.

138. Daly JM, Reynolds J, Thom A, *et al*. Immune and metabolic effects of arginine in the surgical patient. *Ann Surg* 1988; **208**: 512–23.

139. Reynolds JV, Daly JM, Zhang S, *et al*. Immunomodulatory mechanisms of arginine. *Surgery* 1988; **104**: 142–51.

140. Barbul A, Wasserkrug HL, Seifter E, Rettura G, Levenson SM, Efron G. Immunostimulatory effects of arginine in normal and injured rats. *J Surg Res* 1980; **29**: 228–35.

141. Madden HP, Breslin RJ, Wasserkrug HL, Efron G, Barbul A. Stimulation of T cell immunity by arginine enhances survival in peritonitis. *J Surg Res* 1988; **44**: 658–63.

142. Barbul A, Wasserkrug HL, Yoshimura N, Tao R, Efron G. High arginine levels in intravenous hyperalimentation abrogate post-traumatic immune suppression. *J Surg Res* 1984; **36**: 620–4.

143. Saito H, Trocki O, Wang SL, Gonce SJ, Jaffe SN, Alexander JW. Metabolic and immune effects of dietary arginine supplementation after burn. *Arch Surg* 1987; **122**: 784–9.

144. Yu YM, Wagner DA, Walesreswski JC, Burke JF, Young VR. A kinetic study of leucine metabolism in severely burned patients. Comparison between a

conventional and a branched-chain amino acid-enriched nutritional therapy. *Ann Surg* 1988; **207**: 421–9.

145. Daly JM, Lieberman MD, Goldfine J, *et al*. Enteral nutrition with supplemental arginine, RNA, and omega₃-fatty acids in patients after operation: immunologic, metabolic, and clinical outcome. *Surgery* 1992; **112**: 56–67.

146. Gottschlich MM, Jenkins M, Warden GD, *et al*. Differential effects of three enteral dietary regimens on selected outcome variables in burn patients. *JPEN* 1990; **14**: 225–36.

147. Bone RC, Fisher CJ, Jr, Clemmer TP, Slotman GJ, Metz CA, Balk RA. A controlled clinical trial of high-dose methylprednisolone in the treatment of severe sepsis and septic shock. *N Engl J Med* 1987; **317**: 653–8

148. Dominioni L, Dionigi R, Zanello M, *et al*. Effects of high-dose IgG on survival of surgical patients with sepsis scores of 20 or greater. *Arch Surg* 1991; **126**: 236–40.

149. Hackshaw KV, Parker GA, Roberts JW. Naloxone in septic shock. *Crit Care Med* 1990; **18**: 47–51.

150. Sheridan RL, Ryan CM, Tompkins RG. Acute adrenal insufficiency in the burn intensive care unit. *Burns* 1993; **19**: 63–6.

151. McCune S, Short BL, Miller MK, Lotze A, Anderson KD. Extracorporeal membrane oxygenation therapy in neonates with septic shock. *J Pediatr Surg* 1990; **25**: 479–82.

152. Munster AM, Xiao GX, Guo Y, Wong LA. Control of endotoxemia in burn patients by use of polymyxin B. *J Burn Care Rehabil* 1989; **10**: 327–30.

153. Ziegler EJ, McCutchan JA, Fierer J, *et al*. Treatment of gram-negative bacteremia and shock with human antiserum to a mutant *Escherichia coli*. *N Engl J Med* 1982; **307**: 1225–30.

154. Greenman RL, Schein RM, Martin MA, *et al*. A controlled clinical trial of E5 murine monoclonal IgM antibody to endotoxin in the treatment of gram-negative sepsis. *JAMA* 1991; **266**: 1097–102.

155. Wentzel RP. Anti-endotoxin monoclonal antibodies – a second look [editorial; comment]. *N Engl J Med* 1992; **326**: 1151–3.

156. Zeigler EJ, Fisher CJ Jr, Sprung CL, *et al*. Treatment of gram-negative bacteremia and septic shock with HA-1A human monoclonal antibody against endotoxin. A randomized, double blind, placebo-controlled trial. *N Engl J Med* 1991; **324**: 429–36.

157. Shulman KA, Glick HA, Ruben H, Eisenberg JM. Cost-effectiveness of HA-1A a monoclonal antibody for gram-negative sepsis. Economic assessment of a new therapeutic agent. *JAMA* 1991; **266**: 3466–71.

158. Wise WC, Cook JA, Eller T, Halushka PV. Ibuprofen improves survival from endotoxic shock in the rat. *J Pharmacol Exp Ther* 1980; **215**: 160–4.

159. Fletcher JR, Ramwell PW. Indomethacin treatment following baboon endotoxin shock improves survival. *Adv Shock Res* 1980; **4**: 103–11.

160. Adams T Jr, Traber DL. The effects of a prostaglandin synthetase inhibitor, ibuprofen, on the cardiopulmonary response to endotoxin in sheep. *Circ Shock* 1982; **9**: 481–9.

161. Temple GE, Cook JA, Wise WC, Halushka PV, Corral D. Improvement in organ blood flow by inhibition of thromboxane synthetase during experimental endotoxic shock in the rat. *J Cardiovasc Pharmacol* 1986; **8**: 514–19.

162. Revhaug A, Michie HR, Manson JM, *et al*. Inhibition of cyclo-oxygenase attenuates the metabolic response to endotoxin in humans. *Arch Surg* 1988; **123**: 162–70.

163. Bernard GR, Reines HD, Halushka PV, *et al*. Prostacyclin and thromboxane A₂ formation is increased in human sepsis syndrome. Effects of cyclooxygenase inhibition. *Am Rev Respir Dis* 1991; **144**: 1095–101.

164. Faist E, Ertel W, Cohnert T, Huber P, Inthorn D, Heberer G. Immunoprotective effects of cyclooxygenase inhibition in patients with major surgical trauma. *J Trauma* 1990; **30**: 8–17.

165. Demling RH, Smith M, Gunther R, Gee M, Flynn J. The effect of prostacyclin infusion on endotoxin-induced lung injury. *Surgery* 1981; **89**: 257–63.

166. Matera G, Cook JA, Hennigar RA, *et al*. Beneficial effects of a 5-lipooxygenase inhibitor in endotoxic shock in the rat. *J Pharmacol Exp Ther* 1988; **247**: 363–71.

167. Coggeshall JW, Christman BW, Lefferts PL, *et al*. Effect of inhibition of 5-lipooxygenase metabolism of arachidonic acid on response to endotoxemia in sheep. *J Appl Physiol* 1988; **65**: 1351–9.

168. Fink MP, Kruithoff KL, Antonsson JB, Wang H, Rothschild HR. Delayed treatment with an LTD₄/E₄ antagonist limits pulmonary edema in endotoxic pigs. *Am J Physiol* 1991; **260**: R1007–R1013.

169. Granowitz EV, Santos AA, Poutsiaka DD, *et al*. Production of interleukin-1 receptor antagonist during experimental endotoxaemia. *Lancet* 1991; **338**: 1423–4.

170. Ohlsson K, Bjork P, Bergenfeldt M, Hageman R, Thompson RC. Interleukin-1 receptor antagonist reduces mortality from endotoxin shock. *Nature* 1990; **348**: 550–2.

171. Watters JM, Bessey PQ, Dinarello CA, Wolff SM, Wilmore DW. The induction of interleukin-1 in humans and its metabolic effects. *Surgery* 1985; **98**: 298–305.

172. Beutler BA, Milsark IW, Cerami A. Cachectin/tumor necrosis factor: production, distribution, metabolic fate in vivo. *J Immunol* 1985; **135**: 3972–7.

173. Tracey KJ, Fong Y, Hesse DG, *et al*. Anti-cachectin/TNF monoclonal antibodies prevent septic shock during lethal bacteremia. *Nature* 1987; **330**: 662–4.

174. Hinshaw LB, Tekamp-Olson P, Chang AC, *et al*. Survival of primates in LD₁₀₀ septic shock following therapy with antibody to tumor necrosis factor. *Circ Shock* 1990; **30**: 279–92.

175. Marks JD, Marks CB, Luce JM, *et al*. Plasma tumor necrosis factor in patients with septic shock. Mortality rate, incidence of adult respiratory distress syndrome, and effects of methylprednisolone administration. *Am Rev Respir Dis* 1990; **141**: 94–7.

176. Franks AK, Kujawa KI, Yaffe LJ. Experimental elimination of tumor necrosis factor in low-dose endotoxin models has variable effects on survival. *Infect Immun* 1991; **59**: 2609–14.

177. Eskandari MK, Bolgos G, Miller C, Nguyen DT, DeForge LE, Remick DG. Anti-tumor necrosis factor antibody therapy fails to prevent lethality after cecal ligation and puncture or endotoxemia. *J Immunol* 1992; **148**: 2724–30.

178. Pitman JM, 3d, Thurman GW, Anderson BO, *et al*. WEB2170, a specific platelet-activating factor antagonist, attenuates neutrophil priming by human serum after clinical burn injury: the 1991 Moyer Award. *J Burn Care Rehabil* 1991; **12**: 411–509.

179. Chang S-W, Fernyak S, Voelkel NF. Beneficial effect of a platelet-activating factor antagonist, WEB 2086, on endotoxin-induced lung injury. *Am J Physiol* 1990; **258**: H153–H158.

180. Fletcher JR, DiSimone AG, Earnest MA. Platelet activating factor receptor antagonist improves survival and attenuates eicosanoid release in severe endotoxemia. *Ann Surg* 1990; **211**: 312–406.

181. Moore JM, Earnest MA, DiSimone AG, Abumrad NN, Fletcher JR. A PAF receptor antagonist, BN 52021, attenuates thromboxane release and improves survival in lethal canine endotoxemia. *Circ Shock* 1991; **35**: 53–9.

182. Eichacker PQ, Farese A, Hoffman WD, *et al*. Leukocyte CD1 1b/18 antigen-directed monoclonal antibody improves early survival and decreases hypoxemia in dogs challenged with tumor necrosis factor. *Am Rev Respir Dis* 1992; **145**: 1023–9.

183. Vedder NB, Winn RK, Rice CI, Chi EY, Arfors KE, Harlan JM. A monoclonal antibody to the adherence-promoting leukocyte glycoprotein, CD18, reduces organ injury and improves survival from hemorrhagic shock and resuscitation in rabbits. *J Clin Invest* 1988; **81**: 939–44.

184. Schiller HJ, Reilly PM, Bulkley GB. Tissue perfusion in critical illnesses. Antioxidant therapy. *Crit Care Med* 1993; **21**: S92–S102.

185. Richard C, Lemonnier F, Thibault M, Couturier M, Auzepy P. Vitamin E deficiency and lipoperoxidation during adult respiratory distress syndrome. *Crit Care Med* 1990; **18**: 4–9.

186. Rhee P, Waxman K, Clark L, Tominaga G, Soliman MH. Superoxide dismutase polyethylene glycol improves survival in hemorrhagic shock. *Am Surg* 1991; **57**: 747–50.

187. Novelli GP. Oxygen radicals in experimental shock: effects of spin-trapping nitrones in ameliorating shock pathophysiology. *Crit Care Med* 1992; **20**: 499–507.

188. Lovente JA, Landin L, DePablo R, Renes E, Liste D. L-arginnine pathway in the sepsis syndrome. *Crit Care Med* 1993; **21**: 1261–3.

189. Cobb JP, Cunnian RE, Donner RL. Nitric oxide as a target for therapy in septic shock. *Crit Care Med* 1993; **21**: 1261–3.

190. Pepke-Zaba J, Higenbottam TW, Dinh-Xuan AT, Stone D, Wallwork J. Inhaled nitric oxide as a cause of selective pulmonary vasodilatation in pulmonary hypertension. *Lancet* 1991; **338**: 1173–4.

191. Nava E, Palmer RM, Moncada S. Inhibition of nitric oxide synthesis in septic shock: how much is beneficial. *Lancet* 1991; **338**: 1555–7.

192. Lieberthal W, McGarry AE, Sheils J, Valeri CR. Nitric oxide inhibition in rats improves blood pressure and renal function during hypovolemic shock. *Am J Physiol* 1991; **261**: F868–F872.

193. Saffle JR, Sullivan JJ, Tuohig GM, Larson CM. Multiple organ failure in patients with thermal injury. *Crit Care Med* 1993; **21**: 1673–83.

194. Shalaby MR, Aggarwal BB, Rinderknecht E, Svedersky LP, Finkle BS, Palladino MA Jr. Activation of human polymorphonuclear neutrophil functions by interferon-gamma and tumor necrosis factors. *J Immunol* 1985; **135**: 2069–73.

195. Alexander HR, Sheppard BC, Jensen JC, *et al*. Treatment with recombinant human tumor necrosis factor-alpha protects rats against the lethality, hypotension, and hypothermia of gram-negative sepsis. *J Clin Invest* 1991; **88**: 34–9.

196. Dong YL, Herndon DN, Yan TZ, Waymack JP. Blockade of prostaglandin products augments macrophage and neutrophil tumor necrosis factor synthesis in burn injury. *J Surg Res* 1993; **54**: 480–5.

197. Schael GL, Fink MP, Chernow B, Ahmed S, Parrillo JE. Renal hemodynamics and prostaglandin E₂ excretion in a nonhuman primate model of septic shock. *Crit Care Med* 1990; **18**: 52–9.

198. Calandra T, Baumgartner JD, Grau GE, *et al*. Prognostic values of tumor necrosis factor/cachectin, interleukin-1, interferon-a, and interferon-c in the serum of patients with septic shock. *J Infect Dis* 1990; **161**: 982–7.

Chapter 29

Renal failure in burn patients

Yotaro Shinozawa

Naoki Aikawa

Introduction

Acute renal failure is one of the major complications of burns and is accompanied by a high mortality rate. Most renal failure occurs either immediately after the injury or at a later period when sepsis develops. Owing to recent advances in cardiovascular management, acute renal failure has become a much less frequent complication than in the past; renal failure itself is no longer life-threatening because hemodialysis is available. The renal failure occurring in extensively burned patients, however, is usually associated with failure or dysfunction of other organs in a form of multiple organ dysfunction syndrome, which has adverse influence on the prognosis. Acute renal failure occurring immediately after burns is mostly due to reduced cardiac output, which is mainly caused by fluid loss. It is usually reversible.

Renal failure in burned patients

In an experimental shock model,[1] it was demonstrated that acute renal failure developing 2 hours after scalding is associated with a marked reduction in glomerular filtration rate (GFR) and almost complete reabsorption in the normally functioning distal tubule. Under such circumstances, the reduced GFR depends not only on decreased blood pressure but on the regulation of the filtration rate via tubuloglomerular feedback. Proximal tubular damage and organic and/or nonorganic glomerular damage develop when acute renal failure becomes irreversible.[2]

Acute renal failure occurring in the second week or later is sometimes irreversible. This may be the result of renal damage in the early period. In most cases of acute renal failure developing in patients surviving beyond 48 hours after burns, the patients are polyuric.[3] A primary glomerular impairment,[4] osmolar regulatory disturbance[5] due to the lack of an osmolar gradient in the papilla of the renal medulla, and impairment of tubuloglomerular feedback mechanisms have been hypothesized. Proximal tubular dysfunction causes a modest 'downstream' solute diuresis in spite of intact distal exchange function. A reduction in GFR, low urinary sodium concentration, and high urinary potassium concentration are present, and a consequent nonresorbable solutes load causes osmotic diuresis.[3] Polyuria in acute renal failure is also believed to reflect inadequate response to aldosterone in the distal tubule.[2]

Etiologic factors in renal failure

The major etiologic factors in the development of early acute renal failure after burns are hypovolemia and a decrease in cardiac output. The resultant decrease in renal blood flow is primarily responsible for the oliguria seen immediately after burns. Two major mechanisms are involved in the pathophysiological changes in the kidneys; filtration failure and tubular dysfunction caused by various factors and interacting with each other (**Figure 29.1**).[6]

Fluid Shifts and Hypovolemia

In burn patients, increased vascular permeability causes extensive fluid shifts manifested as both local and generalized edema. This results in hypovolemia and centralization of circulation, inducing oliguria early after burns. Sodium retention in collagen fibers and sodium–potassium pump impairment also participate in giving rise

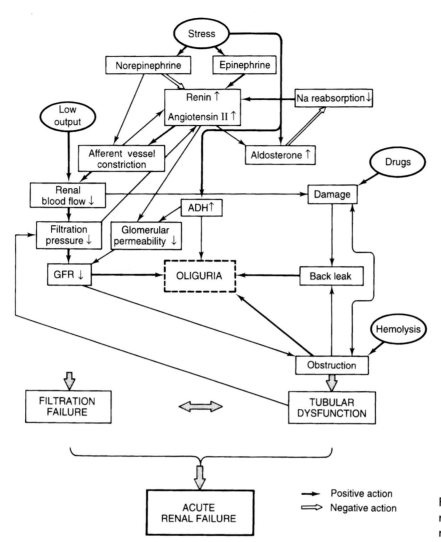

Fig. 29.1 Etiologic factors and mechanisms in the development of acute renal failure in the early postburn period.

Positive action
Negative action

to generalized edema. Excess free water given in this period lowers the tonicity of plasma, which also results in renal edema, followed by acute renal failure.[7]

Myocardial Depression

Besides the decreased circulatory volume and plasma tonicity, myocardial depression, due to a presumed myocardial depressant factor, tumor necrosis factor and/or oxygen free radicals, serves to reduce renal flow and is followed by tubular necrosis.

Stress-related Hormones

Burn stress and the associated circulatory derangement induce elevated levels of catecholamines, angiotensin II, aldosterone, and vasopressin. These hormonal changes cause vasoconstriction and fluid retention as well as alteration of regional blood flow, especially in the kidney. On the other hand, plasma atrial natriuretic polypeptide (ANP) levels are elevated for sustained periods after burns. ANP counterbalances the actions of the stress-related hormones through vasodilatation and natriuresis.[6] Excessively high levels of stress-related hormones and/or impairment of ANP secretion may participate in reduced renal function.

Inflammatory Mediators

Besides the hormonal mediators mentioned above, many mediators including cytokines (TNF, IL-1, etc.), eicosanoids (prostaglandins [PGs], thromboxane, leukotrienes), and platelet-aggregating (activating) factor (PAF) are produced or released in the early postburn period. They act variably to increase vascular permeability and to induce tissue damage. These mediators are also involved in the development of disseminated intravascular coagulation (DIC), in which microthrombi are formed in the capillaries of the glomeruli and renal tubule. Vasodilator PGE_2 is a specific PG in the kidney and works to counteract the above vasoconstrictor substances, but its production is inhibited in the early phase of burns. Similar inflammatory changes occur when a burn patient develops sepsis in the late period.

Denatured Proteins (Pigmenturia)

Free hemoglobin released from degraded red blood cells by heat is conjugated by haptoglobin and transferred to the liver. When a large amount of free hemoglobin is produced in extensive third degree burns, unconjugated free hemoglobin passes through the glomeruli and is excreted in the urine. This could cause degenerative changes in the tubule cells, occlusion of the renal tubules by the formation of hemoglobin casts, and eventually renal failure, especially when combined with dehydration, acidosis, shock or endotoxemia.[8,9] The free hemoglobin absorbed by tubular epithelium is degraded into globin and heme; the latter may induce tubular damage by generating oxygen free radicals via iron ion.

Increased serum myoglobin has also been reported in patients with destroyed muscle in deep thermal injury, electrical injury, distal ischemia due to persistent hypotension or sustained compression, high fever, and drug-induced myolysis.[10] These proteins can be etiologic factors of acute renal failure in the first 1–2 days after injury.

Nephrotoxic Agents

Antibiotics, such as aminoglycoside and certain cephalosporins, are known to be nephrotoxic. Acute or chronic intoxication with alcohol, barbiturates, chlorpromazine, toluene, and paint thinner have been reported as possible associated agents inducing renal failure in burned patients. In some of these patients, early resuscitation therapy was delayed.[11]

Respiratory Dysfunction

Associated respiratory dysfunction adversely affects renal function because of reduced oxygen supply to the kidney. Reduced cardiac output caused by mechanical ventilation with continuous positive airway pressure modes decreases renal flow.

Incidence of renal failure

Ten to thirty percent of burn patients are reported to suffer renal failure, depending on the criteria used to define renal failure and on the patient population.[3] Generally, the more severely burned the patients are, the higher the incidence of renal failure is. Even in severely burned patients, the incidence of renal failure ranges from 1.3 to 38%.[2] In a report on 1785 children with 67+/–5% total body surface area (TBSA) burns, only four developed acute renal failure. All of the cases of renal failure occurring more than 1 week after burn were associated with sepsis.[12] Of 328 adult patients with 48% (13–95%) TBSA burns, 48 (14.6%) developed acute renal failure (AFR). In 15 (31%) of these patients, AFR developed within the first 5 days after the burn, while the other 33 (69%) patients developed AFR more than 5 days after the burn. The patients with late ARF had sepsis as a complication more frequently than the patients with early renal failure. Thirty-eight (79%) of the 48 patients had inhalation injuries and 10 (21%) patients did not.[13]

Prognosis

The prognosis of burn patients with acute renal failure is usually unfavorable. Mortality rates of 73–100% have been reported.[2] The survival rate of patients with renal failure (defined as serum creatinine levels above 2.5 mg/dl) was 30%; this was lower than the survival rate of 75% in patients having normal renal function, although the former patients were older and more severely burned than the latter.[14] In patients in whom serum creatine increased to a level greater than 1.5 mg/dl above initial values in the absence of shock,[15] the mortality rate was 72.7%, which was much higher than among patients without renal dysfunction (16.6%). Moreover, in patients with multiple organ failure, the mortality rate was 88% among patients with acute renal failure, the criteria for which was C_{H_2O}>–0.5 ml/min, blood urea nitrogen level >50 mg/dl and serum creatinine level >2.0 mg/dl.[15] Of 1404 adult patients with more than 30% TBSA burns, 76 (5.4%) developed ARF, and fluid resuscitation was commenced in the 67 (88%) patients who died 4.4 +/–2.1 hours after the burn, compared with 1.7 +/–1.0 hours after the burn in the survivors.[16]

Diagnosis of acute renal failure

Urinary output is the key parameter in evaluating both renal function and the patient's circulatory state. Generally, a urine volume of 0.8–1.0 ml/kg/h reflects adequate perfusion pressure. In an oliguric state, however, it must be determined whether the reduced urine volume is due to functional renal (or prerenal) failure or due to organic (or renal) failure (**Table 29.1**). Prolonged functional renal failure is often observed before organic failure develops. In nonoliguric renal failure, urine volume is of no value in the diagnosis. Urine and serum osmolality and electrolyte concentrations are useful in the differential diagnosis (**Table 29.2**).

Prevention of renal failure

Circulatory Stabilization

Adequate fluid therapy is crucial in maintaining renal function. In extensively burned patients, fluid formulas, such as the Parkland

Table 29.1 Differential diagnosis of acute renal failure

	Functional (Prerenal)	Organic (Renal)
U_{osm} (mosmol/l)	>500	<350
U_{osm}/P_{osm}	>2	<1.2
U_{Na} (mEq/l)	<20	>40
FE_{Na} (%)	<1	>3
C_{H_2O} (ml/min)	<–1.0	–0.5~0
U_{cr}/P_{cr}	>40	<20

U_{osm}, urine osmolality; P_{osm}, plasma osmolality; U_{Na}, urine sodium; FE_{Na}, fractional excretion of filtered sodium, $FE_{Na}=(U_{Na}/P_{Na})/(U_{cr}/P_{cr})$; C_{H_2O}, free water clearance, $C_{H_2O}=UV(1-U_{osm}/P_{osm})$; UV, urine volume; U_{cr}, urine creatinine; P_{cr}, plasma creatinine.

Table 29.2 Differential diagnosis of oliguric and nonoliguric renal failure

	Oliguric	Nonoliguric
Urine volume (ml/day)	<400~500	500<
Serum K (mEq/l)	Increased	Normal range
Serum creatinine (mg/dl)	Increased	Gradually increased
Furosemide test*	No response	Response
U_{Na} (mEq/l)	40–80	Various
C_{H_2O} (ml/min)	–0.25~0.25	–0.25~0.25
FE_{Na} (%)	>3	>3
C_{cr} (ml/min)	<5	5~30

'Response' to the furosemide test means doubled urine volume in 2 hours, compared with the urine volume (UV) during the 2 hours before administration 40–200 mg of furosemide or 40 ml/h urinary excretion by diuretics; U_{Na}, urine sodium; C_{H_2O}, free water clearance, $C_{H_2O}=UV(1-U_{osm}/P_{osm})$; FE_{Na}, fractional excretion of filtered sodium, $FE_{Na}=(U_{Na}/P_{Na})/(U_{cr}/P_{cr})$; C_{cr}, creatinine clearance, $C_{cr}=UV \times U_{cr}/P_{cr} \times 1.48/m^2$.

formula, are just general guidelines; the argument as to what kind of fluid to use has not been settled. Thus, initial fluid resuscitation should be carried out according to the individualized fluid resuscitation program in order to maintain optimal ranges of the various hemodynamic parameters.[17] Monitoring by Swan–Ganz catheterization and thermodilution cardiac output determination is useful in the circulatory management of severely burned patients.[18] Particularly in extensive third degree burns or in-patients with inhalation injury, more fluid than the calculated volume[19] is needed in order to maintain circulatory status. Albumin infusion increased plasma volume by 37% and normalized elevated basal levels of aldosterone and plasma renin activity, but it decreased the GFR by 32% without any significant change in urine output, sodium excretion, or effective renal plasma flow.[20] Dopamine, 3–5 μg/kg/min, for dilatation of renal blood vessels is useful in oliguric burn patients who have received adequate fluid therapy. When cardiac output is reduced in spite of full fluid resuscitation, higher doses of dopamine (5–12 μg/kg/min) and dobutamine (5–12 μg/kg/min) are used.

Monitoring Renal Functions

Early diagnosis of renal failure is very important. To evaluate renal failure, monitoring glomerular and tubular function, persistent proteinuria, and urinary tubule enzymes are recommended in addition to taking measurements of urine volume, blood urea nitrogen, and serum creatinine.

Creatinine clearance reflects the GFR, and is useful in evaluating the prognosis in renal dysfunction. Increased serum concentrations of β_2-microglobulin reflect a decreased GFR. Free water clearance (C_{H_2O}) is a useful parameter for the early diagnosis of renal failure. C_{H_2O} falls to nearly zero before organic renal failure is established. Fractional excretion of filtered sodium (FE_{Na}) is another parameter reflecting tubular function, but it is not useful in evaluating renal function in burn patients. In spite of normal tubular function, FE_{Na} becomes abnormally high when a large amount of sodium is administered in the early postburn phase and when the sequestered sodium is excreted in the urine in the late phase. Temporarily increased FE_{Na}, immediately after a burn and on postburn days 2–4, has been reported in patients with burn >30% TBSA who did not develop renal failure.[21]

Glomerular dysfunction is associated with increased renal excretion of higher molecular weight proteins, and tubular dysfunction is associated with increased excretion of lower molecular weight proteins (<60 000 daltons) due to tubular impairment of reabsorption and/or degradation of these proteins. In some burn patients, a transient glomerular lesion may cause albuminuria immediately after the burn, followed by increased excretion of higher molecular weight proteins, such as α1-acid glycoprotein, α1-antichymotrypsin and γ-glutamyltransferase (GT), around 5 days after the burn.[22] There is no correlation, however, between proteinuria and the development of renal dysfunction.

Urinary α-glucosidase is specific for the epithelium of the proximal renal tubule. Its elevation above a level of 1.5 unit/l indicates proximal renal tubule injury. Urinary N-acetyl-β-D-glucosaminidase (NAG) is not exclusive for lesions of the proximal renal tubule. Increased urinary β_2-microglobulin suggests proximal renal tubular damage. These enzymes were elevated even in burn patients who were not suffering from acute renal failure, but who finally died.[2] The excretion of β_2-microglobulin, coinciding with the max-

imal liberation of tissue breakdown products, increases 2–3 weeks postburn when sepsis develops, and it is correlated with the extent and depth of the burn.[23]

Haptoglobin Administration

Haptoglobin combines specifically with free hemoglobin, forming a conjugate, which is metabolized in the liver. In extensive third degree burns, haptoglobin administration is useful in preventing or decreasing hemoglobinuria[8] (**Figure 29.2**). It was approved for clinical use in Japan in 1985, but not yet in the United States. Haptoglobin preparations must be administered immediately after burns when hemoglobulinemia is anticipated or trace hemoglobulinemia is detected. Alkalinizing urine by administering sodium bicarbonate and increasing urine output by massive fluid loading or diuretics prevent hemoglobin precipitation in the tubules, but may not prevent the possible toxic effects of hemoglobin on tubular cells.[6]

Other Measures to Prevent Renal Failure

Correction of hypoxia and acidosis are important measures in preventing the development of renal failure.[24] Anticoagulation therapy, such as antithrombin III and heparin, is indicated in the hypercoagulatory state. More importantly, early excision of deep second degree and third degree burns followed by immediate grafting, decreases the incidence of renal failure, which develops in sepsis.

Management of renal failure

Fluid Balance

If a hemofiltration device, such as hemodialysis, is not indicated, then urine volume, insensible water loss, and gastrointestinal fluid loss must be determined. Fluid overload should be avoided in order to prevent pulmonary edema and heart failure. In burn patients with extensive raw surfaces, fluid loss through the wound is not accurately assessed. Central venous pressure and/or pulmonary capillary wedge pressure monitoring is recommended.[18]

Diuretics

Diuretics are indicated in prerenal oliguria but not in established organic renal failure. Intravenous furosemide (20–80 mg/day) is given to maintain urine output when oliguria continues in spite of adequate fluid replacement. The required minimum urine volume (UV) necessary to prevent an increase in blood urea nitrogen or creatinine is calculated using the following formula:

$UV = P_{urea}/U_{urea} \times 10$ (l/day) to maintain urea clearance at 10 l/day.
$UV = P_{cr}/U_{cr} \times 30$ (l/day) to maintain creatinine clearance at 30 l/day.

Management of Hyperkalemia

Serum potassium levels above 6.0 mEq/l and/or abnormal ECG (tenting of the T wave, flattening of the P wave, and widened QRS complex) are indications of the need for immediate treatment. Intravenous administration of 500 ml of 10% dextrose with 20 units of regular insulin will lower the serum potassium level by approximately 2 mEq/l. When metabolic acidosis is present, elevating pH by intravenous sodium bicarbonate also lowers the serum potassium concentration. Until the serum potassium levels

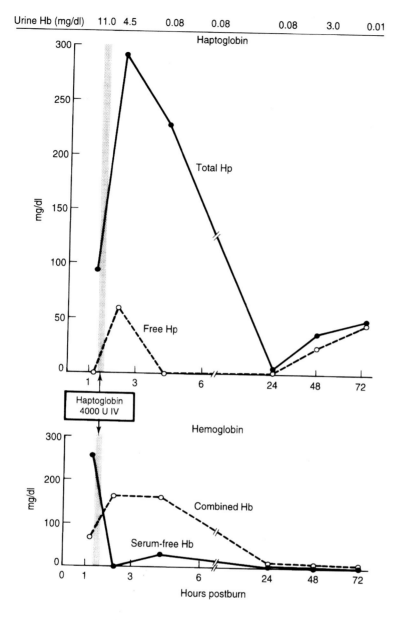

Fig. 29.2 Changes in serum haptoglobin (Hp) and hemoglobin (Hb) in a 60-year-old man with 58% TBSA full-thickness burn. Free Hp increased following Hp infusion.

are reduced, calcium chloride is given intravenously in order to counteract the cardiac abnormalities due to hyperkalemia. In less critical settings, ion-exchange resins (sodium polystyrene sulfonate: Kayexalate[R]) are administered by mouth or by retention enema.

Hemodialysis

Early and frequent hemodialysis (HD) is recommended. The criteria for the introduction of HD to treat acute renal failure in burn patients are listed in **Table 29.3**. Although HD is most effective in the management of renal failure, it is sometimes difficult to ensure stable circulation. Also, in extensive burns, bleeding through burns may be a problem due to the use of anticoagulants. In hypotensive patients, albumin or blood should be transfused prior to HD. To remove excess water and circulating toxic substances other than creatinine and urea, continuous hemofiltration may be combined with HD.[25] In burn patients, the blood access site must be chosen as

far away from the burn site as possible. Peritoneal dialysis has little value in the treatment of acute renal failure in burns.

Nutritional Support

In burned patients, energy requirements are high, and adequate nutritional support is critical to the outcome. Renal failure itself does not increase the metabolic rate, but the stress causing renal failure may induce a hypermetabolic state. Energy requirements can be assessed by indirect calorimetry (IC). When IC is not available,

Table 29.3 Criteria for HD
BUN > 70 mg/dl
Creatinine > 5 mg/dl
K > 6 mEq/l
Base excess ≤ 15-mEq/l
Pulmonary edema
Systemic signs of uremia

a daily energy supply of (23–26) kcal/kg × (1.5–2.0) should be given.[26] The major substrate is glucose, and 30% of the energy is provided as lipid products. As for the nitrogen administration, amino acids, 0.5–1.0 g/kg/day, balanced with essential amino acids and nonessential amino acids, is recommended. When urea nitrogen (calculated by increased nitrogen in the body, urinary nitrogen loss, and nitrogen loss into the dialysis water) is 10 g/day or more, then more than 1.0 g/kg/day of amino acids, rich in branched-chain amino acids, should be administered. Nutritional support requires much carrier water to be infused; if more than 1000 ml/day of water is administered into anuric patients, then continuous hemofiltration is applied in order to remove the excess water.

References

1. Loew D, Meng K. Acute renal failure in experimental shock due to scalding. *Kidney Int* 1976; **10**: S81–S85.
2. Schiavon M, DiLandro D, Baldo M, *et al.* A study of renal damage in seriously burned patients. *Burns* 1988; **14**: 107–114.
3. Planas M, Wachtel T, Frank G, *et al.* Characterization of acute renal failure in the burned patient. *Arch Int Med* 1982; **142**: 2087–2091.
4. Sevitt S. Renal function after burning. *J Clin Pathol* 1965; **18**: 572–578.
5. Eklund J. Studies on renal function in burns: II. Early signs of impaired renal function in lethal burns. *Acta Chir Scand* 1970; **136**: 735–740.
6. Aikawa N, Wakabayashi G, Ueda M, *et al.* Regulation of renal function in thermal injury. *J Trauma* 1990; **30**: S174–S178.
7. Hauben DJ. Invited comment on acute renal failure in burned patients. *Burns* 1988; **14**: 113–114.
8. Aikawa N, Ishibiki K, Okusawa S, *et al.* Use of haptoglobin to prevent renal damage due to hemolysis in extensive third-degree burns. *J Burn Care Rehabil* 1984; **5**: 20–24.
9. Yoshioka T, Sugimoto T, Ukai T, *et al.* Haptoglobin therapy for possible prevention of renal failure following thermal injury: a clinical study. *J Trauma* 1985; **25**: 281–287.
10. Cynober L, Guechot J, Lioret N, *et al.* Rhabdomyolysis and acute renal failure in a patient with thermal injury. *Int Care Med* 1986; **12**: 159–160.
11. Sawada Y, Momma S, Takamizawa A, *et al.* Survival from acute renal failure after severe burns. *Burns* 1984; **11**: 143–147.
12. Tweddell JS, Waymack JP, Warden GD, *et al.* Hematuria in the burned child. *J Pediatr Surg* 1987; **22**: 899–903.
13. Holm C, Horbrand E, von Donnersmarck GH, *et al.* Acute renal failure in severely burned patients. *Burns* 1999; **25**: 171–178.
14. Vanholder R, Bogaerde JVD, Vogelaers D, *et al.* Renal function in burns. *Acta Anaesth Belg* 1987; **38**: 367–371.
15. Aikawa N, Shinozawa Y, Ishibiki K, *et al.* Clinical analysis of multiple organ failure in burned patients. *Burns* 1987; **13**: 103–109.
16. Chrysopoulo MT, Jeschke MG, Dziewulski P, *et al.* Acute renal dysfunction in severely burned adults. *J Trauma-Injury Infection and Crit Care* 1999; **46**: 141–144.
17. Aikawa N, Ishibiki K, Naito C *et al.* Individualized fluid resuscitation based on haemodynamic monitoring in the management of extensive burns. *Burns* 1982; **8**: 249–255.
18. Aikawa N, Martyn JAJ and Burke JF. Pulmonary artery catherization and thermodilution cardiac output determination in the management of critically burned patients. *Am J Surg* 1978; **135**: 811–817.
19. Herndon DN, Barrow RE, Traber DL, *et al.* Extravascular lung water changes following smoke inhalation and massive burn injury. *Surg* 1987; **102**: 341–349.
20. Gore DC, Dalton JM and Gehr TW. Colloid infusions reduce glomerular filtration in resuscitated burn victims. *J Trauma Inj Infect Crit Care* 1996; **40**: 356–360.
21. Naito C, Aikawa N, Yamamoto S, *et al.* FENa test in burned patients. *Jpn J Burn Injury* 1981; **6**: 187–192.
22. Shakespeare PG, Coombes EJ, Hambleton J, *et al.* Proteinuria after burn injury. *Ann Clin Biochem* 1981; **18**: 353–360.
23. Barison AS, Graziani MG, Rigotti G, *et al.* B$_2$-microglobulins and renal dysfunction in burned patients. *Burns* 1988; **14**: 369–372.
24. Walsh MB, Miller SL, Kagen LJ. Myoglobinemia in severely burned patients; Correlations with severity and survival. *J Trauma* 1982; **22**: 6–10.
25. Leblanc M, Thibeault Y, Ouerin S. Continuous haemofiltration and haemodiafiltration for acute renal failure in severely burned patients. *Burns* 1997; **23**: 160–165.
26. Wesson DE, Mitch WE, Wilmore DW. Nutritional considerations in the treatment of acute renal failure. In: Brenner BM, Lazarus JM, eds. *Acute Renal Failure*, Philadelphia: WB Saunders, 1983.

Chapter 30

Critical care in the severely burned: organ support and management of complications

Steven E Wolf, Donald S Prough, David N Herndon

Introduction

Over 1.2 million people are burned in the United States every year, most of whom have minor injuries and treated in the out-patient setting. However, approximately 50 000 burns per year in the USA are moderate to severe and require hospitalization for appropriate treatment. Most of these will require critical care for at least part of their hospitalization, and some will require it for months. Of burn patients treated in hospitals, over 5000 die from complications related to the burn.[1] Burn deaths generally occur in a bimodal distribution, either immediately after the injury or weeks later due to multiple organ failure, a pattern similar to all trauma-related deaths.[2]

Morbidity and mortality from burns are decreasing in incidence. Recent reports revealed a 50% decline for burn-related deaths and hospital admissions in the USA over the last 20 years.[1] This rate of decline was similar in sample statistics for all burns receiving medical care above a reportable level of severity. The declines were likely from prevention efforts causing a decreased number of patients with potentially fatal burns, and improved critical care and wound management of those still sustaining severe burns.[3] In 1949, Bull and Fisher reported 50% mortality rates for children aged 0–14 with burns of 49% of the total body surface area (TBSA), 46% TBSA for patients aged 15–44, 27% TBSA for those aged between 45 and 64, and 10% TBSA for those 65 and older.[4] These dismal statistics have improved, with the latest studies reporting a 50% mortality for 98% TBSA burns in children 14 and under, and 75% TBSA burns in other young age groups.[5,6] Therefore, a healthy young patient with almost any size burn should be expected to live using modern wound treatment and critical care techniques.

Burned patients die of two general causes, 'burn shock' resulting in early deaths, and multiple organ failure and sepsis, leading to late deaths. With the advent of vigorous fluid resuscitation protocols in the severely burned, irreversible burn shock has been replaced by sepsis and subsequent multiple organ failure as the leading cause of death associated with burns. Many burned patients who develop sepsis and organ failure do not die precipitously, however, and it is these patients who require what is termed as *critical care*, which is performed in specialized units containing the equipment, supplies, and personnel required for intensive monitoring and life-sustaining organ support until the patient can recover.

Critical illness in burned patients has typically been equated to sepsis. In our pediatric burn population with massive burns over 80% TBSA, 17.5% of the children developed sepsis defined by bacteremia.[7] The mortality rate in the whole group was 33%, most of whom succumbed to multiple organ failure. Some of the patients who died were bacteremic and 'septic', but the majority were not. These findings highlight the observation that the development of severe critical illness and multiple organ failure is often associated with infectious sepsis, but it is by no means required to develop this syndrome. What is required is an inflammatory focus, which in severe burns is the massive skin injury that requires inflammation to heal.

It has been postulated that the progression of patients to multiple organ failure exists in a continuum with the systemic inflammatory response syndrome (SIRS).[8] Nearly all burn patients meet the criteria for SIRS as defined by the consensus conference of the American College of Chest Physicians and the Society of Critical Care Medicine.[9] It is therefore not surprising that severe critical illness and multiple organ failure are common in burned patients.

Patients who develop dysfunction of various organs, such as the cardiopulmonary system, renal system, and gastrointestinal system can be supported to maintain homeostasis until the organs repair themselves, or a chronic support system can be established. This support is provided in intensive care units (critical care units) designed specifically to treat the severely burned. Critical care may be defined loosely as the process of high-frequency physiologic monitoring coupled with short response times for pharmacologic, ventilatory, and procedural interventions.[10] This chapter will describe the organization of specialized burn intensive care units (BICUs), including requirements for personnel and equipment.

The techniques used in BICUs will be described, then organ specific management will be addressed.

Burn intensive care unit organization

Physical Plant

Optimally, a BICU should exist within a designated burn center in conjunction with a recognized trauma center, thus providing the capability to treat thermal and non-thermal injuries. This unit, however, need not be physically located in the same space as that designated for non-burned trauma patients. In fact, the requirements for the care of wounds in burned patients necessitates additional equipment such as shower tables and overhead warmers, and thus separate space dedicated to the severely burned is optimal. This space may be located in a separate hospital with established guidelines for transfer to the facility.[11]

The number of beds required in the unit may be calculated for the incidence of moderate to severe burns in the referral area, which in the USA is approximately 20 per 100 000 people per year. The Committee on Trauma of the American College of Surgeons recommends that 100 or more patients should be admitted to this facility yearly, with an average daily census of three or more patients to maintain sufficient experience and acceptable access to specialized care.[11]

Most moderate to severe burns requiring admission will require intensive monitoring for at least the day of admission during the resuscitative phase. Thereafter, approximately 20% will require prolonged cardiopulmonary monitoring for inhalation injury, burn shock, cardiopulmonary compromise, renal dysfunction, and the development of SIRS and multiple organ dysfunction syndrome (MODS). In these severely burned patients, the average length of stay in the BICU is approximately 1 day per % TBSA burned, including readmission for delayed complications. Using an average of 25 days admission for a severely burned patient and 2 days for those not so severely injured, this will require approximately 130–150 BICU inpatient days per 100 000 population. An eight-bed BICU can then serve a population of 1 000 000 sufficiently. Space provided should be at least 3000 ft², including patient beds and support space for nursing/charting areas, office space, wound care areas, and storage.

Personnel

A BICU functions best using a team approach between surgeons/intensivists, nurses, laboratory support staff, respiratory therapists, occupational and physical therapists, mental health professionals, dietitians, and pharmacists (**Table 30.1**). The unit should have a designated medical director, who is a burn surgeon, to coordinate and supervise personnel, quality management, and resource utilization. The burn surgeon will usually work with other qualified surgical staff to provide sufficient care for the patients. It is recommended that medical directors and each of their associates be well versed in critical care techniques, and care for at least 50 patients per year to maintain skills.[11] In teaching hospitals, two to three residents should be assigned to the eight-bed unit described above. A coverage schedule should be devised to provide 24-hour prompt coverage.

Nursing personnel should consist of a nurse manager with at least 2 years of intensive care and acute burn care experience, and 6 months of management responsibilities. The rest of the nursing

Table 30.1 Assigned burn unit personnel

Experienced burn surgeons (Burn Unit Director and qualified surgeons)
Dedicated nursing personnel
Physical and occupational therapists
Social workers
Dietitians
Pharmacists
Respiratory therapists
Psychiatrists and clinical psychologists
Prosthetists

staff in the BICU should have documented competencies specific to the care of burned patients, including critical care and wound care.[11] Owing to the high intensity of burn intensive care, at least three full-time equivalents are required per ICU bed to provide sufficient 24-hour care. Additional personnel are required for respiratory care, occupational and physical therapy, and other support. A dedicated respiratory therapist for the burn unit is optimal.

Owing to the nature of critical illness in burned patients, complications may arise for which management could be best treated by specialists not generally in the field of burn care (**Table 30.2**). For these reasons, these specialists should be available for consultation should the need arise.

Equipment

The equipment that must be present or available in the BICU are those items which are common for all ICUs, and some which are specialized to the BICU (**Table 30.3**). Each BICU bed must be

Table 30.2 Consultants for the BICU

General Surgery	Pediatrics
Plastic Surgery	Psychiatry
Anesthesiology	Cardiology
Cardiothoracic Surgery	Gastroenterology
Neurosurgery	Hematology
Obstetrics/Gynecology	Pulmonology
Ophthalmology	Nephrology
Orthopedic Surgery	Neurology
Otolaryngology	Pathology
Urology	Infectious Disease
Radiology	

Table 30.3 Equipment for a fully equipped BICU

Standard
- Monitors (heart rate, electrocardiography, blood pressure, cardiac output, oxygen saturation, temperature
- Scales
- Ventilators
- ACLS cardiac cart
- Laboratory support (blood gas analysis, hematology, chemistry, microbiology

Specialty
- Fiberoptic bronchoscopes
- Fiberoptic gastroscopes/colonoscopes
- Dialysis equipment (peritoneal dialysis and hemodialysis)
- Portable plain radiography
- Computed tomography/fluoroscopy/angiography
- Indirect calorimetry

equipped with monitors to measure heart rate, continuous electro-cardiography, noninvasive blood pressure, invasive arterial and venous blood pressures, and right heart cardiac output using either dye dilution or thermal dilution techniques. Continuous arterial blood oxygen saturation measurement is also required, while continuous mixed venous saturation monitoring is optional. Equipment to measure weight and body temperature should also be standard. Oxygen availability and at least two vacuum pumps must be present for each bed.

Ventilatory equipment too must be available for all beds. A number of types of ventilators is optimal, including servo-type ventilators and percussion type ventilators. An emergency cardiac cart containing Advanced Cardiac Life Support (ACLS) medications and a battery-powered electrocardiograph/defibrillator must be present on the unit should the need arise. Infusion pumps to deliver continuous medications and intravenous/intra-arterial fluids must also be readily available. A laboratory providing blood gas analysis, hematology, and blood chemistry must be located on site. Microbiologic support to complete frequent, routine bacterial cultures should also be present.

Specialty equipment to be available include various sizes of fiberoptic bronchoscopes for the diagnosis and treatment of pulmonary disorders, including personnel versed in these techniques. Fiberoptic gastroscopes and colonoscopes for gastrointestinal complications are also necessary. For renal insufficiency, equipment to provide for peritoneal dialysis and both intermittent and continuous hemodialysis and hemofiltration should be available. Portable radiographic equipment for standard chest/abdominal/extremity radiographs must be imminently available. Equipment for computed tomography, fluoroscopy, and angiography should be available in other parts of the hospital. Indirect calorimeters to measure metabolic rate are preferable. Overhead warmers and central heating with individualized ambient temperature controls must be available for each room.

Hemodynamic monitoring in the burn intensive care unit

All burned patients follow an anticipated course of recovery, which is 'monitored' in the ICU by measuring physiologic parameters. Experienced clinicians assess these physiologic measures in a repeated and sequential fashion to discern when potential interventions may be initiated to improve outcomes. Oftentimes, no intervention will be required, as the patient is following the anticipated course. At other times, this is not the case and procedural or pharmacologic intervention is necessary. Physiologic monitoring is then used further to determine the adequacy of the interventions. The following is a survey of monitoring techniques used in the BICU.

Cardiovascular Monitoring

Arterial lines
Hemodynamic monitoring is directed at assessing the results of resuscitation and maintaining organ and tissue perfusion. Currently used measures are only estimates of tissue perfusion, as the measurement of oxygen and nutrient transfer to cells cannot be made directly at the bedside. Instead, global physiologic measures of central pressures serve as the principal guides.

Measurement of arterial blood pressure is the mainstay for the assessment of tissue perfusion. In critical illness, this measurement can be made using cuff sphyngmomamometers; however, in practice this technique is not useful because the measurement is episodic, and placement of these cuffs on burned extremities is problematic. In addition, blood pressure can be increased in the extremity from the inflation and deflation of the cuff.[12] Diastolic pressures can also be elevated in the elderly and obese.[13,14] Instead, continuous monitoring for hemodynamic instability through the use of intra-arterial catheters is generally done. Lines are typically placed in either the radial or femoral artery. The radial artery is the preferred site for most critically ill patients, because of safety with the dual arterial supply to the hand should a complication occur. However, it has been shown recently that radial artery catheters are inaccurate in the measurement of central blood pressure when vasopressors are used,[15] and are notoriously inaccurate in children because of greater vascular reactivity.[16] For these reasons, we recommend femoral arterial blood pressure measurement in burned patients.

In arterial catheters, systolic, diastolic, and mean arterial pressures should be displayed continuously on the monitor screen. Either systolic or mean arterial pressure can be used to determine adequacy of pressure, although recently, a mean arterial pressure of greater than 70 mmHg has been considered a more accurate description of tissue perfusion. The mean pressure is a more accurate description of central arterial pressure, because as the arterial pressure wave traverses proximally to distally, the systolic pressure gradually increases, while the diastolic pressure decreases. The mean pressure determined by integrating areas under the curve, however, remains constant.[17] The adequacy of the waveform must also be determined, with a diminished waveform indicative of catheter dampening, requiring catheter replacement. Care must be taken to ensure that the diminished waveform is not true hypotension, which can be determined using a manual or cycling sphyngmomamometer placed on the arm or leg. Exaggerated waveforms with an elevated systolic pressure and additional peaks in the waveform (generally only two are found) may be a phenomena referred to as 'catheter whipping', which is the result of excessive movement of the catheter within the artery. Typically, this problem is self-limited, but care must be taken not to interpret typically normal systolic blood pressure values with evidence of catheter whipping as normal, as the effect generally overestimates pressures.

Complications associated with arterial catheters include distal ischemia associated with vasospasm and thromboembolism, catheter infection, and arterial damage/pseudoaneurysm during insertion and removal. Although these complications are uncommon, the results can be devastating. Physical evidence of ischemia in the distal hand or foot should prompt removal of the catheter and elevation of the extremity. If improvement in ischemic symptoms is not seen in 1–2 hours, angiography should be considered. Should thromboembolism be found, the clot can be removed with operative embolectomy or clot lysis at the discretion of the treating physician. If during angiography, extensive arterial damage is found with ischemia, operative repair will be necessary.

Evidence of catheter infection evidenced by purulence and surrounding erythema should instigate removal of the catheter which will often suffice. With continued evidence of infection, antibiotics and incision and drainage of the site should be entertained. Great caution must be exercised if an incision is made over the catheter site to avoid arterial bleeding. If a pseudoaneurysm is encountered after arterial catheterization and removal without signs of distal ischemia, compression with a vascular ultrasound device until no further flow is seen in the pseudoaneurysm will often alleviate the problem without operative intervention.[18]

Pulmonary artery catheters

Pulmonary artery catheters placed percutaneously through a central vein (internal jugular, subclavian, or femoral vein) and 'floated' into the pulmonary artery through the right heart, have been used extensively in hemodynamic monitoring in ICUs. By measuring the back pressure through the distal catheter tip 'wedged' into an end-pulmonary branch, an estimate of left atrial pressure can be measured. In addition, dyes or isotonic solutions injected into a proximal port can be used to determine cardiac output from the right heart. These data are used to estimate preload delivery to the heart, cardiac contractility, and afterload against which the heart must pump, which then directs therapy at restoration of hemodynamics. These catheters are used in ICUs under conditions of unexplained shock, hypoxemia, renal failure, and monitoring of high-risk patients.

Pulmonary artery catheters, while used widely in critical care settings, have come under scrutiny lately from reports indicating no benefit with their use. A recent study of 5735 critically ill adults in medical and surgical ICUs showed an increase in mortality and use of resources when pulmonary artery catheters were used. Most of these patients had medical conditions. The authors of this report suggested that their results should prompt a critical evaluation of the use of pulmonary artery catheters under all conditions.[19] An accompanying editorial went so far as to suggest an FDA mandated moratorium on pulmonary artery catheters until further data were forthcoming.[20] While this suggestion may be somewhat draconian, it should certainly cause the clinician to question whether using a pulmonary catheter would be of benefit in the particular situation.

Several reports exist in the literature regarding the use of pulmonary artery catheters in burned patients, most in regards to parameters of resuscitation immediately after the injury. The first report in 1978 on pulmonary artery catheterization in 39 patients concluded that pulmonary wedge pressure was a more reliable indicator of circulating volume than central venous pressures. These authors also noted a consistent depression in myocardial function in the early phase of injury.[21] Other authors have noted similar findings in terms of heart dysfunction using pulmonary artery catheters in children. They concluded that routine use of pulmonary artery catheters is useful in directing therapy during resuscitation, including modifying resuscitation volumes and the use of inotropes.[22] A recent report indicated that use of values generated from the pulmonary artery catheter during resuscitation to hyperdynamic endpoints improved survival in severely burned patients.[23] Furthermore, they found that if patients were unable to reach the hyperdynamic parameters measured by the pulmonary artery catheter, they were more likely to die.[24] These studies used historical controls, and their conclusions must be held in this light. In spite of the above findings, pulmonary artery catheters are rarely used during resuscitation in most burn centers,[25,26] and their use is primarily limited to patients with identified hemodynamic problems.

As mentioned above, the values derived from the pulmonary artery catheter can be used to drive heart function to supranormal levels with intravascular volume and inotropic support under defined protocols to improve oxygen consumption and presumably improve outcomes.[27] While this approach received enthusiasm after the initial report, other studies have not found any benefit with the use of pulmonary artery catheters in the critically ill, and some have in found it to be detrimental.[28,29] The only study in burns is mentioned above, which found improved survival using the technique.[24] Regardless, no well designed prospective trial investigating whether pulmonary artery catheter-guided supraphysiologic resuscitation parameters improve outcomes has been performed in burns, and this practice cannot be widely espoused.

Newly designed pulmonary artery catheters with sensors providing additional data have been used in critically ill patients other than burns. One of these catheters contains an oxygen saturation monitor on its tip, allowing the continuous measure of mixed venous oxygen saturation. The potential benefits of such a measure would be to give earlier notice of cardiogenic compromise, and allow for a more direct measure of whole body resuscitation. Problems with calibration and position sensitivity, however, have limited its use. Another of these catheters has an implanted rapid response thermistor, and when combined with a electrocardiographic lead measuring P-R interval on a beat-to-beat basis can give a reasonable estimate of right heart ejection fraction and thus heart function on a frequent basis.[30] Another variant of this is a catheter with an implanted heating filament and sensor that uses thermodilution to measure cardiac output every 30 seconds. The accuracy of both these catheters has been verified in clinical studies, but neither has been widely accepted for use.[31]

Base deficit

The base deficit is a value calculated using the Henderson–Hasselbach equation based on the relationship between pH, pCO_2, and serum bicarbonate:

$$pH = 6.1 + \log (HCO_3)/(pCO_2)(0.03)$$

The base deficit is the stoichiometric equivalent of base required to return the pH to 7.40. Base deficit is routinely calculated on blood gas analysis, and provides the best estimate of the degree of tissue anoxia and shock at the whole body level, particularly in hemorrhagic shock.[32] A rising base deficit indicates increasing metabolic acidosis, and may stratify mortality in patients after major trauma.[33] The same can be said for the use of base deficit in burn resuscitation.[7,32,34] These studies were able to show a correlation of higher base deficit and increased mortality, and some have suggested this value is a better monitor of resuscitation than the time honored monitors of urine output and arterial blood pressure.[35] Despite its utility as an indicator of shock, base deficit is a non-specific indicator of metabolic acidosis, and may be elevated with alcohol, cocaine, and methamphetamine use. Interpretation may be difficult under these circumstances.[10,36]

Transesophageal echocardiography

Transesophageal echocardiography has been used for a number of years as an intraoperative monitor in high-risk cardiovascular patients. It has not been used extensively in other critically ill patients because of the lack of available expertise and paucity of equipment. Since this device can be used as a diagnostic tool for the evaluation of hemodynamic function, it serves to reason that it could be used as a monitor in critically ill severely burned patients. A recent report documented the use of transesophageal echocardiography in resuscitation of a child with a 30% TBSA burn, which was successful.[37] Another more remote study used transesophageal echocardiography to measure cardiac function after burn, revealing the typical depression in left ventricular function documented using other means.[38] No study has been done to date investigating whether transesophageal echocardiography is of benefit in monitoring hemodynamics in burned subjects.

Mechanical ventilation

The use of mechanical ventilation is central to the function of the BICU. Burned patients are at risk for airway compromise necessitating endotracheal intubation and mechanical ventilation for a number of reasons. Inhalation of smoke causing damage to the upper airway, development of massive whole-body edema restricting the airway, and hypoxia occur relatively frequently during the initial resuscitation, all of which may require endotracheal intubation and mechanical ventilation. Thereafter, acute lung injury and acute respiratory distress syndrome may intervene, necessitating pulmonary support with ventilators. This section will deal briefly with indications for intubation, common ventilator strategies, and monitoring of mechanical ventilation.

Indications for Intubation

Intubation entails passing an endotracheal tube from either the nose or the mouth through the pharynx into the trachea. This tube is then connected to a mechanical ventilator to cause inspiration and passive exhalation through the lungs. Indications for intubation in burned patients are in general to improve oxygenation and ventilation, or to maintain gas exchange during clinical conditions expected to compromise the airway. These indications are as follows (see also **Table 30.4**):

- Respiratory distress indicated by:
  - tachypnea
  - hypoxia
- Impending need for airway maintenance:
  - Initial management of smoke inhalation injury
  - Expected massive whole body edema after resuscitation for a major burn.

Ventilatory Modes

The complexity of mechanical ventilators has increased dramatically since the first generation of volume cycle ventilators used in the 1960s. The development of positive end-expiratory pressure (PEEP) to maintain functional residual capacity was followed by development of modes using partial ventilatory support, such as intermittent mandatory ventilation in the 1970s. Efficient

Table 30.4 Clinical indications for intubation	
Criteria	Value
Pa_{O_2} (mmHg)	<60
Pa_{CO_2} (mmHg)	>50 (acutely)
P/F ratio	<200
Respiratory/ventilatory failure	Impending
Upper airway edema	Severe

microprocessors were then developed that permitted modes of ventilation such as pressure support ventilation, time-cycled pressure control ventilation, and inverse ratio ventilation. Most recently, new processors have been used to combine modes of ventilation, such as pressure support and time-cycled pressure control ventilation, to some success. However, even with these new developments, the function of mechanical ventilators remains identical to those first used. Whether these new ventilators have had any appreciable effect on mortality remains to be fully elucidated.[10]

The principle difference in mechanical ventilation from spontaneous ventilation that each of us does every minute of the day, is the effect of positive pressure as opposed to normal physiologic negative pressure. The use of positive pressure improves gas exchange by recruiting alveoli and increasing functional residual capacity (i.e. the number and volume of open alveoli at the end of expiration), thus improving ventilation perfusion mismatching and decreasing intrapulmonary shunting of blood past nonventilated lung areas. Adverse effects of positive pressure ventilation lie in its propensity to produce trauma to the airways (barotrauma) and its effects on intrathoracic pressure which can impede venous return to the heart and decrease cardiac output.

Control and Assist Control Ventilation

The volume control modes are volume-cycled settings that deliver a preset tidal volume at a minimum respiratory rate and inspiratory flow rate regardless of the patient's own respiratory efforts (**Figure 30.1**). Of the two, the control mode will not trigger with patient effort. This mode is typically very uncomfortable for patients because it will not respond to their efforts, and should not be under general use. The assist control mode differs in that a breath will be delivered upon patient effort to open a flow valve, at which time the ventilator will fire, allowing the patient to control his or her own ventilatory rate with a preset minimum rate as a back-up. This mode is typically used in heavily sedated patients who cannot generate enough tidal volume under pressure support modes or intermittent mandatory ventilation mode, or in those patients that the clinician wishes to minimize the work of breathing. It must be noted, however, that the work of breathing can be increased dramatically in patients with excessive ventilator triggering.

Increasing the minimum number of breaths to match the patient's effort can minimize this effect.[40]

Intermittent Mandatory Ventilation

Intermittent mandatory ventilation (IMV) was developed to allow spontaneous ventilation interspersed with volume-cycled mechanical ventilation. It was developed initially as a method to wean patients from the ventilator by depending more and more on patient effort for ventilation. The addition of a synchronized mode (SIMV) to avoid placing a mechanical breath on top of a spontaneous patient breath greatly improved this mode of ventilation. This mode has the advantage of maintaining some patient work in breathing to preserve respiratory strength when mechanical ventilation is required, and as a weaning tool to progressively increase patient effort while decreasing mechanical support in preparation for discontinuing mechanical ventilation. This method can be problematic in patients with low pulmonary compliance, and the IMV mode may not allow for sufficient spontaneous tidal volumes due to extremely limited inspiratory capacity.[10] The addition of pressure support to augment spontaneous ventilatory efforts can be used (**Figure 30.2**).

Pressure Support Ventilation

Pressure support ventilation is a patient-triggered, pressure-limited, flow-cycled ventilatory mode (**Figure 30.3**). Each pressure support breath is triggered by patient effort, at which time a valve opens producing a high flow, pressure-limited ventilatory-assisted breath. The breath ends when the patient's inspiratory demand falls below a preset limit, allowing spontaneous respiration and complete patient control. It also differs from the other modes in that it is flow-cycled as opposed to volume- or pressure-cycled. Because this mode is triggered and completed entirely from patient response, it cannot be used in patients with decreased respiratory drive, such as paralyzed patients and those who are heavily sedated. This mode has a number of advantages because of improved synchrony with patient effort. It can be used to provide full ventilatory support by dialing in a pressure such that an adequate tidal volume is delivered. It can also be used effectively during weaning by decreasing the pressure incrementally to allow

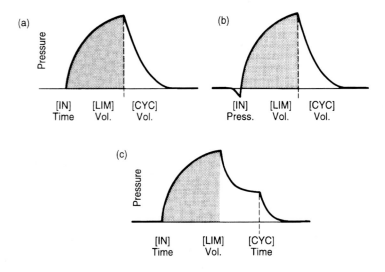

(a)   (b)   (c)

Fig. 30.1 Airway pressure curves illustrating the three mechanical functions: IN, initiation of the cycle; LIM, the preset limit (i.e. pressure or volume) imposed on the positive pressure cycle; CYC, the function (i.e. time or volume) ending the cycle. Each mechanical function is governed by one of four physical factors: volume, pressure, flow, and time. (a) a time initiated, volume limited mode. (b) a pressure initiated (sub–baseline pressure produced by the patients' effort to breathe), volume limited mode. (c) a time initiated, volume limited, time cycled mode that extends inspiration beyond the time that the volume is delivered. A plateau is reached after flow has stopped but before the ventilator cycles into exhalation. Reprinted with permission from Shapiro et al.[39]

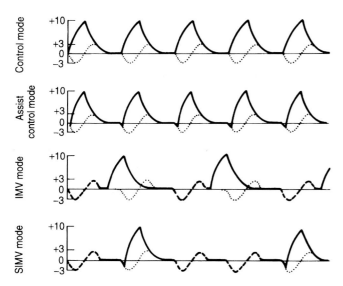

Fig. 30.2 Airway pressure tracings of four volume cycled modes. The thick solid lines represent ventilator breaths. The thick dotted lines are spontaneous breaths. The thin dotted lines illustrate the spontaneous breathing pattern in the absence of ventilator breaths. IMV, intermittent mandatory ventilation; SIMV, synchronized intermittent mandatory ventilation. Reprinted with permission from Shapiro et al.[39]

for progressively greater patient effort. Caution must be exercised when decreasing ventilatory support such that a sufficient tidal volume is still delivered to maintain adequate ventilation.

Time-Cycled Pressure Control Ventilation

Volume-cycled ventilation delivers a set volume of air regardless of the pressure required. In the case of poor lung compliance, such as in ARDS, this mode could lead to excessively high ventilatory pressures leading to significant airway injury. For this reason, time-cycled pressure control ventilation was developed that delivers inspiration at a given flow rate to a preset pressure. The breath is terminated at a set cycle time, not on the basis of volume of flow

as is the case with volume-cycled ventilation. Therefore, pressure control has the advantage of limiting peak inspiratory pressures despite changes in compliance. It also has the disadvantage of a variable tidal volume during dynamic changes in lung compliance, which can lead to inadequate or excessive minute ventilation if compliance worsens or improves respectively. This puts the onus on the clinician to monitor changes in compliance and make appropriate changes in the preset pressure to compensate. This is not required in the volume-cycled mode. Another disadvantage is that this mode is not as well tolerated by awake patients as other modes, and often requires conscious sedation.

Inverse Ratio Ventilation

Inverse ratio ventilation is a mode of ventilation which is designed to improve oxygenation at a given level of inspired oxygen. Conventional ventilation uses the times of inspiration and expiration in a ratio of 1:4 or 1:2, giving a longer time for expiration, which is generally a passive process. Inverse ratio ventilation reverses this ratio to give a longer inspiratory time (1:1 or 2:1) by using rapid inspiratory flow rates and decelerating flow patterns during the inspiratory phase. The effect of inverse ratio ventilation is to increase mean airway pressures and thus recruit alveoli in an effect similar to PEEP. Secondly, in severe lung disease, ventilation in the lung is unequal due to peribronchial narrowing. Thus, some underventilated alveoli that are actually open are not able to exchange gases efficiently, increasing the intrapulmonary shunt and decreasing arterial oxygenation. Inverse ratio ventilation can improve this by selective air-trapping, or intrinsic PEEP, in these compromised air spaces. Inverse ratio ventilation can be done either in a volume-cycled or time-cycled pressure ventilation mode, but it is most commonly used with pressure controlled ventilation to decrease peak airway pressures.

The beneficial effects of inverse ratio ventilation are questioned. It may be that the same effect can be gained by just increasing peak airway pressures with PEEP or peak inspiratory pressures. In fact, studies have showed no benefit of inverse ratio ventilation compared to conventional volume ventilation in terms of oxygenation.[41,42] These studies did show some slight improvements in ventilation (Pa_{CO_2}). Other studies have shown that functional residual capacity is indeed not improved with inverse ratio ventilation, and in fact is detrimental to cardiac function because of increased

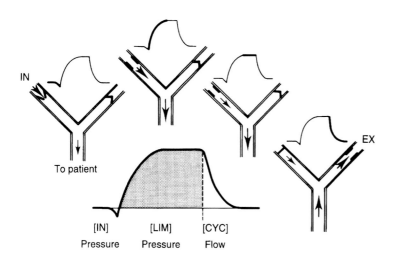

[IN]   [LIM]   [CYC]
Pressure   Pressure   Flow

Fig. 30.3 Schematic illustration of pressure support ventilation. IN, initiation by spontaneous breath; LIM limit (pressure); CYC, cycle (derived from decreasing inspiratory flow); EX, expiration. Reprinted with permission from Shapiro et al.[39]

intrathoracic pressures.[43,44] For these reasons, inverse ratio ventilation cannot be recommended except in the setting of ARDS refractory to other therapies.

High Frequency Percussive Ventilation

High frequency percussive ventilation is a new mode of ventilation which combines features of conventional ventilation with jet ventilation. A standard pressure controlled breath is superimposed on a high frequency (200–600 breaths/min) delivery of breaths, providing for a percussive element to standard pressure control ventilation (10–30 breaths/min). The purported advantages are to loosen airway exudate and casts for better pulmonary toilet, and to provide adequate gas exchange at lower airway pressures. This method of ventilation has been tested primarily in burned patients with inhalation injury, and was first reported in 1989.[45] In this study, high frequency percussive ventilation was used as a salvage therapy in patients with inhalation injury and as primary therapy in another group. Improvements in oxygenation and a lower rate of pneumonia were seen. Another study by these authors documented an improvement in mortality in burned patients with inhalation injury treated with high frequency percussive ventilation compared to historical controls.[45,46] More recent studies have shown significant decreases in the work of breathing, and lower inspiratory pressures in addition to improvements in oxygenation and the rate of pneumonia.[47,48] This method of ventilation seems to be particularly efficacious in the treatment of inhalation injury, and should be given consideration as the standard of care.

Inhaled Nitric Oxide

Nitric oxide is a short-lived gaseous product of endothelial cells that is a powerful local vasodilator.[49] Because it is a gas, this product can be delivered through the endotracheal tube to be delivered to areas of ventilated lung where it can provide localized pulmonary vasodilation. Thus, areas of ventilated lung can receive more blood flow to decrease intrapulmonary shunting and improve oxygenation. This compound has been used extensively in neonates and children[50] with hypoxemic respiratory failure with beneficial effect.[51] It has also been used in ventilated burned children to improve oxygenation.[52,53] Although nitric oxide therapy has received considerable attention as a potential therapeutic option in severe pulmonary disease, no reports to date have documented improved mortality in spite of improvements in oxygenation. For this reason, its use cannot be recommended outside of a clinical trial.

Limiting Barotrauma

All ventilator modes deliver some level of barotrauma because they use nonphysiologic positive pressure. This barotrauma has been implicated as a major cause of morbidity in ventilated patients, and it is conceivable that limiting barotrauma by using lower airway pressures may decrease some of this morbidity. Many reports have been published that are both proactive and contrary to the use of pressure-limited ventilation as compared to conventional volume-cycled techniques. Almost all these trials showed no effect of pressure-limited ventilation,[54-56] which is accomplished by giving lower tidal volumes more frequently to maintain minute ventilation, and to accept a higher Paco$_2$ value and lower arterial pH, which is termed permissive hypercapnia. Criticisms of these trials lie in their low enrollment and lack of

power to show differences. A recent large multicenter trial, however, documented improved survival and decreased ventilator days in patients treated with a well-defined protocol designed to limit barotrauma. In fact, this study was stopped early by the data safety committee because of the benefits incurred to the treated group.[57] Suspected reasons for the improvements seen in this trial which were not detected in others, is the number of subjects enrolled as well as the defined protocol which limited peak airway pressures to less than 30 cm H$_2$O. It serves to reason, therefore, that pressure limited ventilation strategies are of benefit in burned patients as well, although the merits have not been tested in this population.

Weaning from Mechanical Ventilation

Regardless of the mode of ventilation, almost all patients surviving the initial insult requiring mechanical ventilation will arrive at a stage to be weaned off the ventilator. Clinicians continue to debate the advantages of weaning patients with various forms of mechanical ventilation. Some clinicians prefer to use pressure support ventilation (PSV) with or without SIMV because of the ease with which the level can gradually be reduced. Others maintain that intermittent trials with abrupt cessation of ventilator support while maintaining endotracheal intubation ('t-tube trials') results in more rapid weaning (**Figure 30.4**).[58] It must be noted that weaning from ventilation depends upon the rate at which the patient recovers from the condition causing mechanical ventilation and the aggression of the clinician driving the weaning process. In practice, either method of weaning from the ventilator (gradual weaning with pressure support or intermittent t-tube trials) will be successful. What will certainly prolong the process is random changes in ventilation parameters without a directed plan.

Monitoring of Mechanical Ventilation

For patients on mechanical ventilation, the normal physiologic regulation of ventilation and oxygenation are often impaired by sedatives and paralytics required for the presence of the endotracheal tube, or due the pathophysiologic condition requiring mechanical ventilation. For these reasons, monitoring of ventilation and oxygenation by the clinician is required.

Ventilation

Arterial CO$_2$ tension remains the most accurate means of assessing ventilation. This is typically measured on blood gas analysis. After assessment of the pCO$_2$, ventilatory settings to adjust minute ventilation can then be made to reach the desired level. Another method that has received attention of late is expiratory end-tidal CO$_2$ monitoring through infrared measurement of CO$_2$. This technique allows for continuous on line determination end-tidal CO$_2$, which is an estimate of arterial Paco$_2$. For end-tidal CO$_2$ to equate with Paco$_2$, an assumption of a low alveolar–arterial gradient must be made. In patients with healthy lungs, this gradient is only 2–3 mmHg. In certain trauma patients, particularly those with head injuries, the gradient remains low, and may be used for continuous Paco$_2$ monitoring. However, in other critically ill patients, the alveolar–arterial gradient may be in a state of flux, calling into question values received from an end-tidal CO$_2$ monitor. Factors affecting the alveolar–arterial gradient include cardiac output, airway dead space, airway resistance, and metabolic rate. Each of these may change in a severely burned patient, particularly those with inhalation injury. For these reasons, end-tidal CO$_2$ monitoring

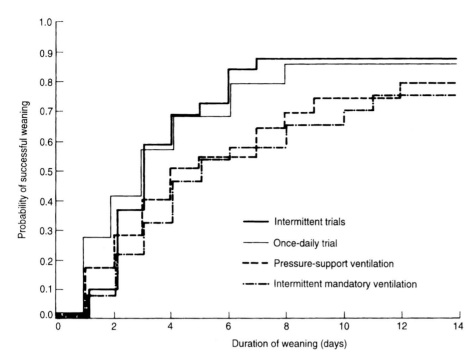

Fig. 30.4 The probability of successful weaning with intermittent mandatory ventilation, pressure support ventilation, intermittent trials of spontaneous breathing, and once-daily trials of spontaneous breathing (Kaplan–Meier curves). After adjustments for baseline characteristics (Cox proportional hazards model), the rate of successful weaning with a once-daily trial of spontaneous breathing was 2.83 times higher than that with intermittent mandatory ventilation (p < 0.006) and 2.05 times higher than that with pressure support ventilation (p < 0.04). Reprinted with permission from Esteban et al.[58]

is not recommended in burned patients for the estimation of $P\text{aco}_2$.

In general, $P\text{aco}_2$ varies indirectly with minute ventilation, and thus, this value must be considered when making ventilator adjustments to alter $P\text{aco}_2$. Minute ventilation is equal to tidal volume multiplied by respiratory rate. Therefore, $P\text{aco}_2$ can be adjusted downward by either increasing tidal volume or respiratory rate. In general, respiratory rate should be set at between 10 and 20 breaths and tidal volume at 6 and 10 ml/kg for the initial settings. Adjustments can then be made in minute ventilation to optimize $P\text{aco}_2$, which is usually 40 mmHg. When making these adjustments, it should be noted that the respiratory rate cannot be increased above 40 breaths/min, and tidal volume should be minimized to avert barotrauma.

When peak airway pressures are greater than 30 mmHg, the ventilated lung is relatively noncompliant indicative of acute respiratory distress syndrome or pulmonary edema. In this situation, 'permissive hypercapnia' is a strategy that may be used to decrease barotrauma. This strategy seeks to limit peak airway pressures by decreasing minute ventilation to allow for respiratory acidosis ($P\text{aco}_2 > 45$ mmHg, arterial pH < 7.30). This strategy was used to some extent in the trial investigating the efficacy of pressure limited ventilation on improving outcomes in critically ill ventilated patients.[56]

Oxygenation

As with the determination of the adequacy of ventilation, oxygenation has been classically determined using the partial pressure of O_2 in arterial blood. In general, a pO_2 value of 60 mmHg has been considered sufficient. Another frequently used monitor is pulse oximetry, which is an optical measurement of oxygenated hemoglobin in pulsatile vessels. Using differences in absorption of red and infrared light, the percentage of oxygenated hemoglobin in the arteries can be calculated. Shortcomings of this technique lie in the disregard for methemoglobin and carboxyhemoglobin, which

can be present in patients with smoke inhalation injury. Otherwise, this is a very accurate technique for the determination of oxygen content in arterial blood, as 97% of oxygen is carried to the tissues via hemoglobin. This assertion has been corroborated by *in vitro* studies,[59] which showed the accuracy of pulse oximetry to within 2–3% of oxyhemoglobin levels. The major limitations to this technique lie in the insensitivity to changes in pulmonary gas exchange. Because of the shape of the oxyhemoglobin dissociation curve, when the $S\text{ao}_2$ exceeds 90% and the $P\text{ao}_2$ is greater than 60 mmHg, the curve is flat and changes in $P\text{ao}_2$ can change considerably with little change in $S\text{ao}_2$. Regardless, it is assumed that an $S\text{ao}_2$ value greater than 92% is indicative of adequate oxygenation.

Initial ventilator settings to assure adequate oxygenation are usually 40% oxygen in the inspired gas with 5 mmHg PEEP. This amount of PEEP is used to mimic the normal physiologic pressures in nonintubated subjects. When oxygenation begins to decline, initial maneuvers are to increase the fractional inspired oxygen ($F\text{io}_2$) to greater than 40% and possibly to 100%. Concentrations of oxygen greater than 60% are considered toxic to airway epithelium, and other means to increase oxygenation should be employed. This should consist initially of increasing the level of PEEP incrementally until the desired level of oxygenation is reached while keeping the $F\text{io}_2$ to less than 60%. Once a level of 15–20 mmHg of PEEP is reached, other means of increasing oxygenation will need to be employed. These consist of inverse ratio ventilation, high frequency percussive ventilation, inhaled nitric oxide, etc. which are described above.

Organ system failure and management

Etiology and Pathophysiology

As stated earlier, it has been hypothesized that organ dysfunction commonly seen in the critically ill exists in a continuum with SIRS. Certain patients with SIRS will go on to develop multiple organ dysfunction syndrome (MODS), which is characterized by nonfatal signs of organ system dysfunction, such as renal insufficiency or ventilator dependence. A subset of these patients will go on to develop frank organ failure, termed multiple system organ failure (MSOF), which often leads to death (**Figure 30.5**).[8,9] What is required for the development of SIRS is inflammation, which in the severely burned emanates primarily from the burn wound. Factors associated with progression from the systemic inflammatory response syndrome to multiple organ failure are not well explained, although *some* of the responsible mechanisms in *some* patients are recognized. Occasionally, failure of the gut barrier with penetration of organisms into the systemic circulation may incite a similar reaction.[60] However, this phenomena has only been demonstrated in animal models, and it remains to be seen if this is a cause of human disease.

A number of theories have been developed to explain the progression to multiple organ failure[61] (**Table 30.5**). One of these is the infection theory that incriminates uncontrolled infection as the major cause. In the severely burned patient, these infectious sources most likely emanate from invasive wound infection, or from lung infections (pneumonias). As organisms proliferate out of control, endotoxins are liberated from Gram-negative bacterial walls, and exotoxins from Gram-positive and Gram-negative bacteria are released.[62] Their release causes the initiation of a cascade of inflammatory mediators called cytokines, as well as the recruitment of inflammatory cells that can result, if unchecked, in organ damage and progression toward organ failure. Cytokines are a group of signaling proteins produced by a variety of cells that are thought to be important for host defense, wound healing and other essential host functions. Although, cytokines in low physiologic concentrations preserve homeostasis, excessive production may lead to widespread tissue injury and organ dysfunction. Four of these cytokines, tumor necrosis factor alpha (TNFα), interleukin 1 beta (IL-1β), interleukin 6 (IL-6) and interleukin 8 (IL-8) have been most strongly associated with sepsis and multiple organ failure. The primary detraction to this theory is that many patients, including burned patients, can develop multiple organ failure without identified infection.[63] It seems that inflammation from the presence of necrotic tissue and open wounds can incite a similar inflammatory mediator response to that seen with endotoxin. The mechanism by which this occurs, however, is not well understood. Regardless, it is known that a cascade of systemic events is set in motion either by invasive organisms or from open wounds that initiates the systemic inflammatory syndrome which may progress to multiple organ failure.

Another theory is that implicating macrophages and their activity in the development of multiple organ failure. Macrophages activated by inflammation release excessive levels of cytokines and inflammatory mediators into the systemic circulation which cause end organ damage, and incite further inflammation and macrophage activation. Elevated circulating and bronchoalveolar fluid cytokine levels have been associated with increased risk for SIRS/MODS;[64] however, trials investigating the efficacy of cytokine blockade in patients with multiple organ failure have not improved survival rate in very large studies.

Yet another theory implicates prolonged tissue hypoxia and the generation of toxic free-radicals during reperfusion as the primary mediator of end-organ damage. Deficits in resuscitation then would lead to areas of the microcirculation throughout the body that receive inadequate nutrients, and shift to anaerobic metabolism and formation of superoxides from ATP metabolites. The effects of the toxic products of oxygen free radical formation are only now being elucidated. From *in vitro* models and *in vivo* animal models, we know that tissues that initially were in shock and are then reperfused produce oxygen free radicals that are known to damage a number of cellular metabolism processes. This process occurs throughout the body during burn resuscitation, but the significance of these free radicals in human burn injury is unknown. It was found that free radical scavengers such as superoxide dismutase improve survival in animal models; however, these results are not established in patients.[65] Oxygen free radicals oxidize membrane lipids, resulting in cellular dysfunction. Endogenous natural antioxidants, such as vitamins C and E, are low in patients with burns, suggesting that therapeutic interventions may be beneficial.[66] Serum nitrate levels correlate well with multiple organ failure scores in critically ill patients, implying a role for this constellation of events in SIRS/MODS.[67]

The role of vascular endothelium and leukocyte interactions to cause the changes seen in multiple organ failure has also been suggested. Cytokines and oxidants can convert endothelial cells to a proinflammatory state with upregulation of adhesion molecule expression, leading to leukocyte adherence and neutrophil-mediated tissue damage. Inhibition of this association with monoclonal antibodies has been shown to reduce tissue damage and organ injury in animal models of hemorrhagic shock, and was shown to attenuate skin injury when used during burn resuscitation.[68] The relevance of this model to the generation and maintenance of organ failure is yet to be established.

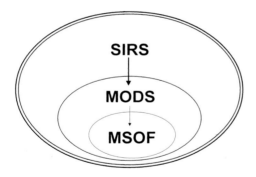

Fig. 30.5 Progression to multiple organ failure. All severely burned patients have the systemic inflammatory response syndrome (SIRS). A subset of these will develop signs and symptoms of multiple organ dysfunction (MODS). Still fewer will go on to develop multiple system organ failure (MSOF).

Table 30.5 Theories for the development of multiple organ failure
Infectious causes
Macrophage theory
Microcirculatory hypothesis
Endothelial–leukocyte interactions
Gut hypothesis
Two-hit theory

The last two theories revolve around the role of the gut in the generation of organ failure, and the 'two-hit' theory of multiple organ failure. For years, investigators have implicated the gut as the 'engine' of organ failure, which is associated with loss of gut barrier function and translocation of enteric bacteria and their toxic metabolites. Bacterial translocation has been shown to occur repeatedly in animal models after burn,[60,69,70] as well as in humans.[71] These bacteria and their products then activate the inflammatory cells described above, culminating in organ failure. The relevance of gut mediated bacterial translocation to human disease, however, has been hotly debated. No clear studies have shown whether bacterial translocation is the cause of SIRS/MODS, probably because as of yet, investigators have been unable to control bacterial translocation effectively during shock in humans, thus a cause and effect relationship cannot be established. The 'two-hit' theory ascribes a summation of insults to the development of organ failure. Each of the insults alone is inadequate to cause the response, but one or more of these insults can 'prime' the inflammatory response system such that another normally insignificant injury causes the release of toxic mediators that end in multiple organ failure.

Prevention

This brief outline of the potential pathophysiology and causes of burn-induced critical illness and multiple organ failure demonstrates the complexity of the problem. Since different cascade systems are involved in the pathogenesis, it is so far impossible to pinpoint a single mediator that initiates the event. Thus, since the mechanisms of progression are not well known and thus specific treatments cannot be accurately devised, it seems that prevention is likely the best solution. The current recommendations are to prevent the development of organ dysfunction, and to provide optimal support to avoid conditions which promote the onset.

Course of Organ Failure

Even with the best efforts at prevention, the presence of the systemic inflammatory syndrome that is ubiquitous in burn patients may progress to organ failure. Experience with the severely burned dictates that virtually all burned patients will display the signs and symptoms of SIRS, including tachycardia, tachypnea, increased white blood cell count, etc. Thereafter, various organ systems may begin to show signs of dysfunction. Generally, these will begin in the renal and/or pulmonary systems and progress through the liver, gut, hematologic system, and central nervous system in a systematic fashion. The development of multiple organ failure does not preclude mortality, however, and efforts to support the organs until they heal is justified.

Renal system

Pathophysiology

Acute renal failure (ARF) is a potentially lethal complication of burns. Despite substantial technical developments in dialysis to replace the function of the kidneys, mortality meets or exceeds 50% for all critically ill patients who develop acute renal failure.[72,73] Interestingly, mortality associated with ARF requiring dialysis in the critically ill has not improved significantly for over 30 years. The same can be said for renal failure requiring dialysis in the severely burned specifically.[74] The causes of death in these critically ill patients is not uremia because of advances in dialysis, but primarily sepsis and cardiovascular and pulmonary dysfunction.[75]

With the advent of early aggressive resuscitation after burn, the incidence of renal failure coincident with the initial phases of recovery has diminished significantly in severely burned patients.[74] However, a second period of risk for the development of renal failure 2–14 days after resuscitation is still present, which is probably related to the development of infectious sepsis.

Acute renal failure, also referred to as acute tubular necrosis (ATN), is characterized by deterioration of renal function over a period of hours to days, resulting in the failure of the kidney to excrete nitrogenous waste products and to maintain fluid and electrolyte homeostasis.[76] It may be caused by a number of factors interfering with glomerular filtration and tubular resorption. In burned patients, the causes can be generally narrowed to renal hypoperfusion, or nephrotoxic insults from pharmacologic treatments (e.g. aminoglycosides or intravenous contrast agents) or sepsis (**Figure 30.6**).

Ischemic renal failure is the more common of the two causes, and is induced by hypoperfusion from an imbalance between vasoconstrictive and vasodilatory factors acting on the small renal vessels during low flow states. Decreased flow to the renal cells directly alters endothelial cell function, decreasing the production of and response to vasodilatory substances.[78] The renal medulla is the most sensitive portion of the kidney to hypoxia, and the damage is initially to the renal tubular cells. The outer medulla and proximal tubules have high oxygen requirements, and the resulting ischemia causes swelling of tubular and endothelial cells with necrosis, apoptosis, and inflammation evident on histologic examination.[79] These changes lead to further vascular congestion and decreased blood flow, leading to more cell loss and further decrements in renal function.[80]

Structural changes in the tubular cells include loss of polarity and the integrity of the tight junctions.[81,82] Integrins are redistributed to the apical surface, resulting in live and dead cells sloughing into the tubular lumen, causing cast formation.[83] The casts then cause increased intratubular pressure and reduced glomerular filtration rate. Loss of epithelial cell barrier and the tight junctions between viable cells causes back-leakage of the glomerular filtrate, further reducing the effective glomerular filtration rate. Arg-Gly-Asp peptides which prevent adhesion between cells in the tubular lumen and thus decrease cast formation prevent increases in proximal tubular pressure and mitigate ischemic renal failure in experimental animals.[83]

After the initiating event, tubular function and the glomerular filtration rate decrease to reduce urine production. The progression of ARF is commonly divided into three phases: initiation, maintenance, and recovery,[72] and can be oliguric (urine output <400 ml/day) or nonoliguric (urine output >400 ml/day) in nature. Patients with nonoliguric ARF have a better prognosis that those with oliguric renal failure, probably due in large measure to the decreased severity of the insult and the fact that many have drug-associated nephrotoxicity or interstitial nephritis.[76,84,85] The percentage of critically ill patients with ARF who require dialysis ranges from 20 to 60%. Among the subgroup who survive initial dialysis, less than 25% require long-term dialysis, demonstrating the potential reversibility of the syndrome.[86,87]

Once ARF is established, pharmacologic improvement of renal blood flow will not reverse the injury. Agents such as dopamine,

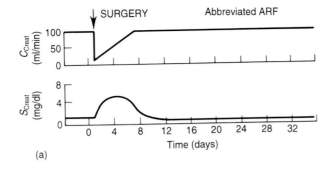

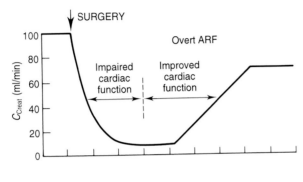

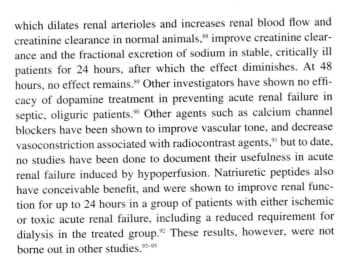

(a)

(b)

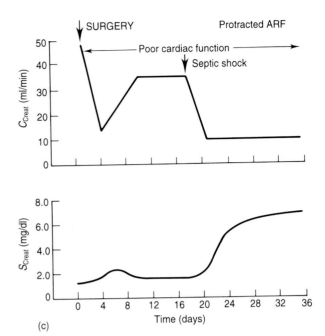

(c)

Fig. 30.6 Three patterns of hemodynamically mediated acute renal failure (ARF) occur after major burn.
(a) Abbreviated ARF consists of an acute reduction in creatinine clearance (C_{cr}) with prompt recovery. Serum creatinine (S_{cr}) may increase even as C_{cr} is recovering.
(b) Overt ARF consists of concurrent mirror image increases in C_{cr} and S_{cr} in association with compromised cardiac function followed by recovery. (c) Protracted ARF develops as a consequence of prolonged hemodynamic compromise often complicated by systemic sepsis. Reproduced with permission from Myers and Moran.[77]

which dilates renal arterioles and increases renal blood flow and creatinine clearance in normal animals,[88] improve creatinine clearance and the fractional excretion of sodium in stable, critically ill patients for 24 hours, after which the effect diminishes. At 48 hours, no effect remains.[89] Other investigators have shown no efficacy of dopamine treatment in preventing acute renal failure in septic, oliguric patients.[90] Other agents such as calcium channel blockers have been shown to improve vascular tone, and decrease vasoconstriction associated with radiocontrast agents,[91] but to date, no studies have been done to document their usefulness in acute renal failure induced by hypoperfusion. Natriuretic peptides also have conceivable benefit, and were shown to improve renal function for up to 24 hours in a group of patients with either ischemic or toxic acute renal failure, including a reduced requirement for dialysis in the treated group.[92] These results, however, were not borne out in other studies.[93–95]

Diuretic therapies, such as mannitol and loop diuretics, have been used extensively in patients with acute renal failure to increase urine flow, and protect the kidney from further ischemic damage. Mannitol can decrease cellular swelling in the proximal

tubule and increase intratubular flow, thus potentially decreasing intratubular obstruction and further renal dysfunction. Mannitol is recommended along with vigorous volume replacement and sodium bicarbonate for the treatment of early myoglobinuric acute renal failure.[96] Loop diuretics also increase intratubular flow rates, and can convert an oliguric state to a nonoliguric state, thus making clinical management of renal failure easier. Although nonoliguric renal failure is generally associated with a lower mortality rate,[85,86] there is no evidence that conversion from an oliguric to a nonoliguric state improves mortality. It is likely that those patients who respond to diuretics have less severe renal damage at the outset of treatment, thus the outcomes are better.

Treatment

The initial care of patients with ARF is focused on reversing the underlying cause, and correcting fluid and electrolyte imbalances. Renal failure is heralded by a decrease in urinary output. Volumes of urine less than 1 ml/kg/h may indicate the onset of ARF. This failure may be due to prerenal causes, which is typically decreased renal blood flow from hypoperfusion, or intrinsic renal causes, which are associated with medications or sepsis. Differentiation between these etiologies can be made with laboratory examinations (**Table 30.6**). Prerenal etiologies are associated with concentrated urine (urine osmolarity >400 mosmol/kg), decreased urinary sodium concentrations, and decreased fractional excretion of sodium. Intrinsic renal causes will be associated with more dilute urine with higher sodium concentrations. These tests should be performed before diuretics are used, as this treatment will increase urinary sodium and decrease urine osmolality even in prerenal conditions. In general, urine osmolarity and urinary sodium concentrations are primarily used for these determinations because of the ease of measurement.

Should these tests reveal a prerenal cause, volume replacement should ensue to prevent further renal ischemia. The physical exam and invasive monitoring if deemed appropriate should guide this volume replacement. The decision to administer or remove fluids may prove difficult, however, since both strategies have detrimental consequences if followed inappropriately. Although volume replacement is ineffective in restoring renal function once tubular necrosis is established, it remains our most effective prophylactic strategy,[97] and is generally the place to start with the onset of renal failure.

Once renal failure begins, serum creatinine will begin to increase with the decrease in glomerular filtration. However, up to 70% of renal function must be lost prior to significant increases in serum creatinine concentrations, making its use as a screening examination for renal failure suspect. Increases in serum creatinine may also be masked by increased plasma volume associated with aggressive volume resuscitation. Because renal failure is treated best by prevention with early detection, the use of a clinical measure of glomerular filtration rate, such as creatinine clearance (C_{cr}), may be of greater clinical utility early in the course of failure. Creatinine clearance can be measured effectively over short-time periods (2-hour collections), with the only caveat for an overestimation of glomerular filtration rate when compared to inulin.[98] Nonetheless, serial measurements to examine changes in creatinine clearance will improve monitoring for acute renal failure.

After assuring adequate volume status, every effort should be made to prevent other causes of renal injury. All nephrotoxins should be discontinued or avoided. Hyperkalemia that may develop can be treated with resins, glucose and insulin, and sodium bicarbonate in the presence of metabolic acidosis. Medications eliminated through the kidney should be adjusted.[76] Once the diagnosis of ARF is established, consideration can be given for diuretic therapy, especially if it is determined that the patient is volume overloaded. Decreasing the volume of fluid given can also alleviate fluid overload in burned patients. These patients have increased insensible losses from the wounds which can be roughly calculated

at 3750 ml/m² TBSA wound plus 1500 ml/m² TBSA total. Decreasing the infused volume of intravenous fluids and enteral feedings below the expected insensate losses may alleviate some fluid overload problems. Decreasing potassium administration in the enteral feedings and giving oral bicarbonate solutions can minimize electrolyte abnormalities. Almost invariably, severely burned patients require exogenous potassium because of the heightened aldosterone response which results in potassium wasting, therefore hyperkalemia is rare even with some renal insufficiency.

Intermittent dialysis remains the standard replacement therapy for severe ARF. The indications for dialysis are fluid overload or electrolyte abnormalities not amenable to other treatments. In recent years, continuous hemodialysis has emerged as yet another option for replacement therapy for critically ill patients.[99] The advantage of continuous treatment over intermittent include more precise fluid and metabolic control, decreased hemodynamic stability, and the enhanced ability to remove injurious cytokines.[100] Disadvantages include the need for anticoagulation and heightened surveillance. Bleeding problems are particularly prevalent in burned patients during anticoagulation.[101] Trials to date have not shown any benefit of continuous hemodialysis over traditional intermittent dialysis.[102]

Peritoneal dialysis is another option for acute renal failure in burned patients with severe acute renal failure.[103] Catheters can be placed at the bedside with near continuous exchanges to improve electrolyte and volume overload problems. The capital required for this treatment is minimal. Hypertonic solutions are used to treat fluid overload, and the concentrations of potassium and bicarbonate are modified to produce the desired results. The dwell time is usually 30 minutes followed by drainage for 30 minutes. This treatment can be repeated in cycles until the problem is resolved. For maintenance, 4–6 such cycles a day with prolonged dwell times (1 hour) is usually sufficient during the acute phase.

After beginning dialysis, renal function may return, especially in those patients that maintain some urine output. Therefore, patients requiring such treatment may not require life-long dialysis. It is a clinical observation that whatever urine output was present will decrease once dialysis is begun, but it may return in several days to weeks once the acute process of closing the burn wound nears completion.

Pulmonary system

Mechanical ventilation in the severely burned generally takes place for three reasons: airway control during the resuscitative phase, airway management for smoke inhalation, and for the development of acute lung injury and ARDS. The first is for airway control early in the course with the development of massive whole-body edema associated with the great resuscitative volumes required to maintain euvolemia. In this situation, the need for mechanical ventilation is not due to lung failure, *per se*, but instead to maintain the airway until the whole-body edema resolves. Once this occurs, usually 2–3 days into the course, extubation can be accomplished. Ventilator management during this phase is routine. The second primary reason for mechanical ventilation is for airway management early in the course of smoke inhalation. Another chapter in the book will deal specifically with this issue. The third is the development of hypoxemia. Severe burns are known to be

Table 30.6 Laboratory tests to distinguish prerenal from intrinsic renal failure		
Examination	Prerenal	Intrinsic Renal
Urine osmolarity (mosmol/kg)	>400	<400
Urinary sodium (mEq/dl)	<20	>40
FE_{NA} (%)*	<1	>2

* FE_{Na}, fractional excretion of sodium, calculated as $(U/P_{Na}/U/P_{Cr}) \times 100$, where U is urinary concentration, and P is plasma concentration. Na is sodium and Cr is creatinine.

associated with hypoxemia and the development of acute lung injury (ALI) and its more severe counterpart, ARDS. The clinical manifestations are dyspnea, severe hypoxemia, and decreased lung compliance with radiographic evidence of diffuse bilateral pulmonary infiltrates (**Figure 30.7**). These conditions exist as a continuum from ALI, which is a mild form, to its most severe form, which is dense ARDS. These conditions have been defined by the American–European Consensus Conference Committee, and are listed on **Table 30.7**. These definitions are relatively simple, and are used in other critically ill populations. The rest of the discussion will be related to ALI and ARDS.

Epidemiology and Pathophysiology

ALI and ARDS occur as a result of injury to the lung, which can be direct through smoke inhalation or pneumonia, or indirect through mediators associated with sepsis. Until recently, most studies of ALI and ARDS reported mortality rates between 40 and 60%.[104–106] The majority of deaths were attributable to sepsis or multiorgan dysfunction.

Recently, two reports suggest that mortality in ARDS has been decreasing, with a group from Seattle reporting a 67% decrease in mortality for 1987–1993 compared to a period from 1983 to 1987. Another group in the United Kingdom reported a 50% decline in mortality over a similar time period. Explanations include more effective treatment of sepsis, changes in methods of mechanical ventilation, and improved support of the critically ill. No reports of improved mortality have been forthcoming in the severely burned with ARDS.

ALI and ARDS occur because of damage to the endothelium and lung epithelium. It is speculated that the products of inflammation, such as cytokines, endotoxin, complement, and coagulation system products, induce the changes that are characteristic of ALI and ARDS. The acute phase of ALI is characterized by influx of protein-rich edema fluid into the air spaces as a consequence of increased permeability of the alveolar–capillary barrier.[107] The importance of endothelial injury and increased vascular permeability to the formation of pulmonary edema is well established.[104] Epithelial injury is also of great importance. In fact, the degree of alveolar epithelial injury is an important predictor of outcome.[108]

The normal alveolar epithelium is composed of two cell types. Flat type I cells make up 90% of the alveolar surface, and these cells are easily injured. Cuboidal type II cells make up the remaining 10%, and are more resistant to injury. Type I cells function to move gases from the interstitium to the alveoli. Type II cells function to produce surfactant, participate in ion transfer and fluid movement, and proliferate/differentiate to type I cells after injury.

Loss of epithelial integrity has a number of consequences. Under normal conditions, the epithelial barrier is much less permeable than the endothelial barrier,[109] therefore its loss contributes to alveolar flooding. Also, loss of type II cells disrupts epithelial fluid transport, impairing the removal of edema from the alveolar space. Lastly, loss of type II cells reduces the turnover and production of surfactant, causing a loss of surface tension in the alveoli and contributing to alveolar collapse.

Neutrophils are likely to play a role in the pathogenesis of ALI. Histologic studies of lung specimens obtained early in the course demonstrate marked accumulation of neutrophils in the alveolar fluid.[110] These neutrophils can be recovered from bronchoalveolar lavage fluid from affected patients,[108] demonstrating a clear association between neutrophil accumulation and lung injury. However, it must be stated that ALI and ARDS develop in patients with profound neutropenia,[112] and some animals models of ARDS are neutrophil independent, intimating that neutrophils may be nothing more than bystanders in the inflammatory process.

The effects of ventilator injury on the development and progression of ALI and ARDS are just now coming to light. Previous studies focused on the potential damaging effects of high oxygen concentrations on lung epithelium.[113] Recent evidence suggests that mechanical ventilation at high pressures can injure the lung,[114] causing increased pulmonary edema in the uninjured lung and enhanced edema in the injured lung.[115–117] Alveolar overdistention and cyclic opening and closing of alveoli associated with high ventilatory pressures is also potentially damaging to the lung.[118]

After the development of ALI and ARDS, some patients have a rapid recovery over a few days.[108,119] Others progress to fibrotic lung injury, which is observed as early as 5–7 days into the course of the disease.[107,110,117] The alveolar space becomes filled with mesenchymal cells, extracellular proteins, and new blood vessels.[121] The finding of fibrosis on histologic analysis correlates with increased mortality.[122]

In the nonfatal cases of ARDS, the lung heals by proliferation of type II epithelial cells, which begin to cover the denuded basement membrane and differentiate into type I epithelial cells, thus restoring normal alveolar architecture and increasing the fluid-transport capacity of the alveolar epithelium.[123] This proliferation is controlled by keratinocyte growth factor and hepatocyte growth factors.[104] Alveolar edema is resolved by active transport of sodium from the distal airspace into the interstitium by intact alveoli.[124] Soluble protein is removed primarily by diffusion between alveolar cells, and

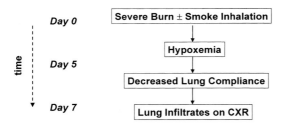

Fig. 30.7 Typical timeline for progression to ARDS. Patients are typically intubated for airway compromise and operative intervention. At day 4 or 5 after severe burn, oxygenation will deteriorate, requiring higher inspired concentrations of oxygen. These measures will soon fail with the introduction of decreased lung compliance requiring higher inspired airway pressures. Only then will infiltrates begin to appear on the chest x-ray (CXR).

Table 30.7 Definitions of Acute Lung Injury and Acute Respiratory Distress Syndrome
Acute onset
Bilateral infiltrates on chest radiography
Pulmonary artery wedge pressure <18
Acute lung injury (ALI) if Pao_2/Fio_2 is <30 but >200
Acute respiratory distress syndrome (ARDS) if Pao_2/Fio_2 is <200

insoluble protein is eliminated by endocytosis and transcytosis by alveolar epithelial cells and phagocytosis by macrophages.[125]

The severely burned are unique among patients that develop ALI and ARDS. Because direct injury to the lung from smoke inhalation is common, oftentimes patients will present with respiratory insufficiency and relative hypoxia caused by increased capillary permeability, ciliary dysfunction, and interstitial edema associated with the chemical injury of smoke. A few days later, the damaged and necrotic respiratory mucosa begins to slough, causing bronchial plugging and atelectasis, further worsening the clinical condition. However, it is not usually until 4–6 days into the course of injury that severe hypoxemia and ARDS develop in burned patients, a scenario not unlike other types of patients who develop ALI and ARDS, such as after abdominal sepsis or multiple blunt trauma. It serves to reason that smoke inhalation is associated with the development of ARDS, but perhaps this association is related to the inflammation associated with the injury in addition to that rendered by the burn wound. It may be, then, that smoke inhalation and ALI/ARDS are two separate conditions which are inter-related. Regardless, the treatment for both remains primarily supportive until the processes resolve.

Treatment

The treatment of ALI and ARDS is largely supportive until the healing processes described above can be accomplished. A careful search for potential underlying causes should ensue, including attention to potentially treatable causes such as intra-abdominal infections, pneumonia, line sepsis, and invasive burn wound infection. An improved understanding of the pathogenesis of ALI has lead to the assessment of several novel treatment strategies,[104] including changes in mechanical ventilation strategies, fluid management, surfactant therapy, nitric oxide treatments, and anti-inflammatory strategies.

Potential treatments

The most appropriate method of mechanical ventilation for ALI and ARDS has been controversial for some time. Older strategies recommended supraphysiologic tidal volumes of 12–15 ml/kg, which as stated previously may contribute to further alveolar damage. This was recognized in the 1970s, which led to studies of extracorporeal membrane oxygenation to reduce tidal volumes to 8 ml/kg. However, this strategy failed to decrease mortality.[126] Similar studies have been performed in severely burned patients, with no effect on mortality.[127] Recently, a National Institutes of Health (NIH) study group reported a 22% decline in mortality in patients with ALI and ARDS treated with tidal volumes of 6 ml/kg compared to those treated with conventional volumes of 12 ml/kg. In this study, peak airway pressures could not exceed 30 cm water in the lower tidal volume group, and a detailed protocol was used to adjust the fraction of inspired oxygen and PEEP.[57] These results were different from two previous smaller studies showing no improvement with pressure-limited ventilation.[56,128] Potential reasons for the discrepancy between the NIH study and the others are as follows: the NIH study had the lowest tidal volume of the three studies, respiratory acidosis was allowed in the NIH study with sodium bicarbonate treatment if necessary to maintain homeostasis, and the NIH study had more patients, thus may have been more sufficiently powered to show differences between treatment groups.[104]

Positive end-expiratory pressure has clearly been shown to benefit patients with ALI and ARDS;[129,130] however, the most optimum level has been controversial. The best documented effect of PEEP is to increase functional residual capacity,[127] or the number of open alveoli at the end of expiration.[131] However, the use of prophylactic PEEP therapy in patients at risk for ALI showed no benefit for the treatment group compared to controls.[132]

A more recent study of PEEP therapy aimed at raising the level of PEEP above the lower inflection point on pressure–volume curves to prevent alveolar closure in addition to low tidal volumes and pressure controlled inverse ratio ventilation showed improved mortality compared to a control group managed with conventional ventilation.[133] Drawbacks to this study were the unusually high mortality (71%) in the control group, and improvements in mortality for the treatment group compared to controls could only be determined at hospital day 28, which was not appreciated at hospital discharge.[104] Nonetheless, the potentials for benefit of this therapy have warranted further studies, which are underway.

Surfactant therapy has been suggested for patients with ALI and ARDS, which should decrease alveolar surface tension, and maintain open alveoli. This therapy was proved effective in neonates with respiratory distress;[134] however, a study done in adults with ARDS showed no effect on oxygenation, duration of mechanical ventilation, or survival.[135] Newer preparations of surfactant with recombinant proteins and new approaches to instillation such as bronchoalveolar lavage and tracheal administration are being evaluated in clinical trials.[104]

Inhaled nitric oxide is an effective pulmonary vasodilator with effects localized to ventilated areas of the lung, thus directing more blood to the functional areas of the lung. The conceivable effect, then, is to diminish the fraction of blood shunted through the lungs without oxygenation, thus improving pulmonary venous oxygenation. Observational studies suggest that inhaled nitric oxide might be beneficial in the treatment of ARDS by improving oxygenation without increased ventilatory pressures and reducing barotrauma. However, randomized trials testing this hypothesis have been disappointing. In a recent study, inhaled nitric oxide therapy did not reduce mortality or decrease the duration of mechanical ventilation. Improvements in oxygenation were seen; however, the effects were not sustained.[136] Treatment with less selective pulmonary vasodilators such as sodium nitroprusside,[137] hydralazine,[138] alprostadil (prostaglandin E_1),[139] and epoprostenol (prostacyclin)[140] have not been shown to be beneficial.[104]

Glucocorticoids have been used in the treatment of ARDS because of the inflammatory nature of the disease. However, these agents were not shown to be of any benefit when given at the onset of the condition.[141] More recently, glucocorticoids have been used in the later fibrosing phases of the disease to good effect.[142,143] Preliminary studies in a small population have shown improved oxygenation, decreased ventilator dependence, and decreased mortality with no increased risk of sepsis in nonburned patients.[144] This type of therapy may be treacherous in burned patients at risk for invasive burn wound infection, but might be considered upon complete burn wound closure.

Cardiovascular system

Principles

Treatment of cardiovascular responses after burn requires an understanding of cardiovascular physiology and the effects of treatment. One of the hallmarks of serious illness is the direct link between cardiac performance and patient performance. The four determinants of cardiac function and thus tissue perfusion of blood at the whole body level are the following:

- Ventricular preload or end-diastolic muscle fiber length;
- Myocardial contractility or strength of the heart muscle;
- Ventricular afterload, of the degree of resistance against which the heart must pump; and
- Heart rate and rhythm.

A thorough comprehension of the effects of each of these components on heart function is required in order to initiate effective treatments for burned patients with cardiovascular abnormalities.

Preload

Preload is defined as the force that stretches the cardiac muscle prior to contraction. This force is composed of volume that fills the heart from venous return. Because of the molecular arrangement of actin and myosin in muscle, the more the muscle is stretched with incoming venous volume, the further it will contract.[145] This is best demonstrated on a Frank–Starling curve (**Figure 30.8**) which was first described by Otto Frank in a frog heart preparation in 1884; Ernest Starling extended this observation in the mammalian heart in 1914. The relationship demonstrated in the Frank–Starling curve justifies the use of preload augmentation by volume resuscitation to increase cardiac performance. However, when the end-diastolic volume becomes excessive cardiac function can decrease, probably by overstretch of the muscle fibers such that the contractile fibers are pulled past each other, thus reducing the contact required for contractile force. The preload required to decrease cardiac function in experimental settings is in excess of 60 mmHg, which is rarely encountered in patients.

Preload is measured clinically by either central venous pressure or by pulmonary artery wedge pressure obtained with a pulmonary artery catheter. Of these, the pulmonary artery wedge pressure is the best estimate since it assesses the left side of the heart.

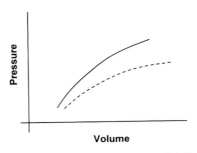

Fig. 30.8 Frank–Starling Curve. The solid line depicts the pressure–volume relationship of the heart, showing that as pressure to the heart (preload) increases, the volume pumped by the heart increases. Immediately after burn, contractility diminishes, shifting the curve downward (dashed line). It still must be noted that with this change, the volume pumped by the heart still increases with increased pressure (preload), validating the use of increased atrial pressure as a means of increasing cardiac output after severe burn.

Cardiac Contractility

The force with which the heart contracts is referred to as cardiac contractility. It is directly related to the number of fibers contracting, and will be diminished in patients with vascular occlusive disease of the myocardium who lose muscle fibers from infarction and ischemia, and in burned patients during the acute resuscitation.[146] Calculating the left ventricular stroke work from pulmonary artery catheter derived values provides the best estimate of cardiac contractility, and can be calculated with the following formula:

$$LVSW = SV \, (MAP - PCWP) \times 0.0136$$

where LVSW is left ventricular stroke work, SV is the stroke volume (cardiac index ÷ heart rate), MAP is mean arterial pressure, and PCWP is pulmonary capillary wedge pressure.

Afterload

Afterload is the force that impedes or opposes ventricular contraction. This force is equivalent to the tension developed across the wall of the ventricle during systole. Afterload is measured clinically by arterial resistance as an estimate of arterial compliance. Arterial resistance is measured as the difference between inflow pressure (mean arterial) and outflow pressure (venous) divided by the flow rate (cardiac output):

$$SVR = (MAP - CVP)/CO$$

where SVR is systemic vascular resistance, MAP is mean arterial pressure, CVP is central venous pressure, and CO is cardiac output.

Heart Rate and Rhythm

For the heart to function properly, the electrical conduction system must be intact, so as to provide rhythmic efficient contractions to develop sufficient force to propel blood through the circulatory system. For example, if the heart rate approaches 200 beats/min, the heart will not have time to fill completely, thus decreasing myocardial fiber stretch and decreasing heart function. Also, if frequent premature ventricular contractions are present, the heart will not perform as well for similar reasons. Heart rate and rhythm are monitored continuously as a routine in all critically ill patients using electrocardiography.

Effects of Burn on Cardiac Performance

Severe burns affect cardiac performance in a number of ways. The first is to reduce preload to the heart through volume loss into the burned and nonburned tissues. It is for this reason that volumes predicted by resuscitation formulas must be used to maintain blood pressure and maintain hemodynamics. In addition, severe burn induces myocardial depression[21,147] characterized by a decrease in tension development and velocities of contraction and relaxation.[148] Cardiac output is then reduced. These effects are most evident early in the course of injury; however, they are followed shortly thereafter by a hyperdynamic phase of increased cardiac output caused primarily by a decrease in afterload through vasodilation and an increase in heart rate. Deficits in myocardial contractility are for the most part maintained.

Hemodynamic Therapy: Preload Augmentation

When hypotension or other signs of inadequate cardiac function (i.e. decreased urine output) are encountered, the usual response is to augment preload by increasing intravascular volume. This is a sound physiologic approach based on the Frank–Starling principle, and should be the first therapy for any patient in shock. Intravascular volume can be increased with either crystalloid or colloid to increase the central venous pressure and pulmonary capillary wedge pressure to a value between 10 and 20 mmHg. The adequacy of this therapy can be monitored by the restoration of arterial blood pressure, a decrease in tachycardia, and a urine output greater than 0.5 ml/kg/h.

Some caution must be exercised when augmenting preload for hemodynamic benefit in burned patients. Excessive volume administration may lead to significant fluid overload with the development of peripheral and pulmonary edema. These changes can lead to conversion of partial-thickness burns to full-thickness injuries in the periphery, and can cause significant respiratory problems. Judicious use of fluid administration after hemodynamics are restored with spontaneous diuresis will usually alleviate this problem, however, at times pharmacologic diuresis will be required.

Hemodynamic Therapy: Inotropes

If volume replacement is insufficient to improve hemodynamics in burned patients in shock, inotropes may be required. These inotropes generally consist of adrenergic receptor agonists, although phosphodiesterase inhibitors that increase intracellular cAMP levels to increase myocyte CA^{++} levels or digoxin that acts to increase myocyte Ca^{++} levels by inhibiting the Na+/K+ pump can also be used to improve myocardial contractility.

Dopamine is a commonly used inotropic agent which has both α-adrenergic and β-adrenergic properties. The α effects are seen primarily at higher doses (10–20 µg/kg/min), while the β effects are seen at all doses. Therefore, dopamine can be thought of as an 'inoconstrictor', because it has both intropic and vasoconstrictive properties. Other inotropes in this class include epinephrine and norepinephrine. One caveat to the use of these inoconstrictors is that myocardial oxygen consumption increases, which may affect areas of the heart that are ischemic.

At low doses, dopamine also produces splanchnic and renal vasodilation through specific dopamine receptors. It is thought that these vasodilatory effects can be used to optimize renal function through antagonism of α-receptor induced vasoconstriction. However, this practice has recently been questioned. Dopamine has also been used in burned patients to increase left ventricular stroke work during myocardial depression seen during resuscitation.[21]

Dobutamine is another commonly used inotrope which has effects limited to β-adrenergic stimulation, thus cardiac contractility is increased without vasoconstriction. The effect is to improve cardiac output generally without specific splanchnic or renal effects.

Agents with primary effects on the α-adrenergic receptor can be used to induce vasoconstriction and increase blood pressure. These agents consist of norepinephrine and phenylephrine, and can be used effectively during septic shock or neurogenic shock to increase vascular tone. In burned patients, it is felt that these agents will cause vasoconstriction of the skin circulation and the splanchnic circulation to preserve blood flow to major organs such as the heart and brain. This redistribution in blood flow can cause conversion of partial-thickness skin injuries to full-thickness and result in ischemic injury to the gut. The use of specific vasoconstrictors must be weighed against these effects.

Effects of β-Blockade on Cardiac Performance After Severe Burn

One of the responses to severe burn is a dramatic increase in catecholamine production that has been linked to a number of metabolic abnormalities, including increased resting energy expenditure,[149] muscle catabolism, and altered thermoregulation.[150] The effects of this sustained catecholamine surge on the cardiac system are to increase heart rate and therefore myocardial work. Propranolol, as a nonspecific β-blocker, has been used to decrease heart rate and myocardial work in severe burns.[151–154] Propranolol can be given through both the intravenous and oral routes to equal effect on heart rate and myocardial work without detrimental effect on cardiac output[153] or response to stress.[155] Propranolol administration also decreases peripheral lipolysis[156] and muscle catabolism,[157] which are additional beneficial effects. Consideration should be given to further trials with the use of propranolol to improve outcomes in burned patients.

Gastrointestinal system

Pathophysiologic Changes in the Gut After Cutaneous Burn

The gastrointestinal response to burn is highlighted by mucosal atrophy,[158–160] changes in digestive absorption,[161] and increased intestinal permeability.[70,162,163] Atrophy of the small bowel mucosa occurs within 12 hours of injury in proportion to the burn size,[160] and is related to increased epithelial cell death by apoptosis.[164] The cytoskeleton of the mucosal brush border undergoes atrophic changes associated with vesiculation of microvilli and disruption of the terminal web actin filaments. These findings were most pronounced 18 hours after injury,[69] which suggests changes in the cytoskeleton, such as those associated with cell death by apoptosis, are processes involved in the changed gut mucosa. Burn also causes reduced uptake of glucose and amino acids,[165] decreased absorption of fatty acids, and reduction in brush border lipase activity.[161] These changes peak in the first several hours after burn, and return to normal at 48–72 hours after injury, a timing that parallels mucosal atrophy.

Intestinal permeability to macromolecules that are normally repelled by an intact mucosal barrier, increase after burn.[60,166] Intestinal permeability to polyethylene glycol 3350, lactulose, and mannitol increases after injury, which correlates to the extent of the burn.[69,159] Gut permeability increases even further when burn wounds become infected.[167] A study using fluorescent dextrans showed that larger molecules appeared to cross the mucosa between the cells, while the smaller molecules traversed the mucosa through the epithelial cells, presumably by pinocytosis and vesiculation.[168]

Changes in gut blood flow are related to changes in permeability (**Figure 30.9**).[169] Intestinal blood flow was shown to decrease in non-resuscitated animals, a change that was associated with increased gut permeability at 5 hours after burn.[170] This effect was abolished at 24 hours. Systolic hypotension has been shown to occur in the first hours after burn in animals with a 40% TBSA full-thickness injury. These animals showed an inverse correlation between blood flow and permeability to intact *Candida albicans*.[171]

Clinical Changes in the Gut after Burn

Given the changes in the gut to burn described above, it is common to see some evidence of gut dysfunction after burn evidenced by

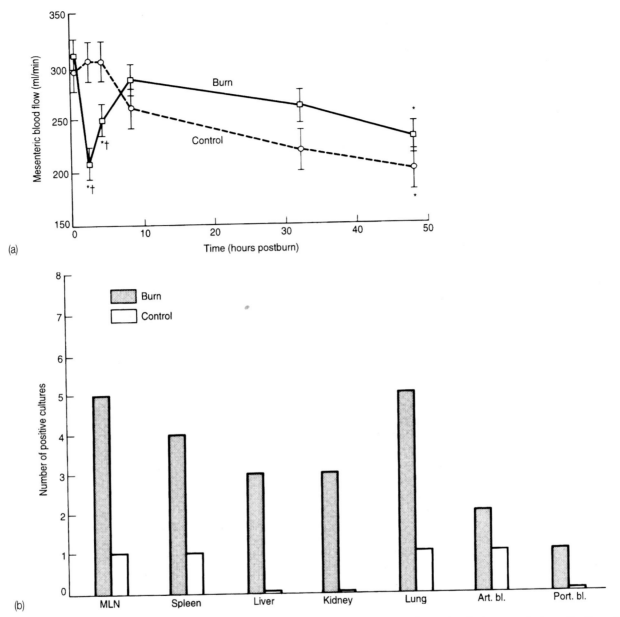

Fig. 30.9 (a) after a severe burn in pigs, superior mesenteric blood flow (solid line) decreased abruptly then recovered with resuscitation. *$P \leq 0.05$ vs. baseline, †$P \leq 0.05$ vs. unburned controls (dotted line). (b) bacterial tissue culture results from mesenteric lymph nodes (MLN), spleen, liver, kidney, lung, arterial blood (art. bl.), and portal blood (port. bl.) after sham injury (open bars) and severe burn (solid bars). Reprinted with permission from Tokyay et al.[169]

feeding intolerance,[172] and mucosal ulceration and bleeding particularly in the stomach and duodenum. Enteral feeding is one of the most important means of providing nutrition to burned patients and has led to a decrease in mortality,[173] but at times the gut will not cooperate. Reduced motility and ileus are common, at times requiring parenteral nutrition to meet caloric needs. At the present time, there is no specific treatment for burn induced ileus, but it seems that early enteral feeding will prevent some of these potential complications (see Chapter 20 for complete recommendations).[6]

Stress ulceration of the stomach and duodenum, on the other

hand, can be prevented effectively with antacid therapy. In the 1970s stress ulceration leading to life threatening hemorrhage was common. The mechanism of injury is related to an imbalance between protective factors such as mucus production, protective prostaglandin output and bicarbonate secretion, and injurious factors such as decreased blood flow and acid production. Gastric ulcers develop in the watershed zones between capillary beds which are worsened by gastric acid-induced injury.

Antacid therapies and early enteral feeding have dramatically decreased the incidence of gastrointestinal ulceration and life threatening hemorrhage after severe burn,[174–177] such that this complication is very rare in modern burn units. A number of types of therapies including gastric antacids, cimetidine, ranitidine, and sucralfate have been tested in various combinations or alone, all of which are equally effective. Some have even suggested that early enteral nutrition alone is sufficient.[177] A recent survey of critical care physicians was found to use histamine-2 antagonists such as ranitidine most commonly for stress ulceration prophylaxis, followed by sucralfate.[178] Regardless, it can be concluded that some type of prophylaxis against gastrointestinal hemorrhage is required in the severely burned, and will be very effective in preventing this complication.

Summary

Improved critical care of the severely burned has decreased mortality over the past two to three decades. This has been in part through the development of specialized units for care for burned patients which are equipped with the personnel and equipment to deliver state of the art care. Better understanding of the processes of critical illness and multiple organ failure has led to effective prevention strategies and treatment modalities. Further advances in the understanding of mechanisms of the progression from the SIRS to multiple organ failure will engender new breakthroughs that can be expected to further improve the outcomes of burned patients.

References

1. Brigham PA, McLoughlin E. Burn incidence and medical care in the United States: estimates, trends, and data sources. *J Burn Care Rehabil* 1996; **17**: 95–107.
2. Wolf SE, Herndon DN. Burns. In: Townsend CM, ed. Sabiston's Textbook of Surgery, 15th edn 2000.
3. Sarhadi NS, Murray GD, Reid WH. Trends in burn admission in Scotland during 1970–92. *Burns* 1995; **21**: 612–15.
4. Bull JP, Fisher AJ. A study in mortality in a burn unit: standards for the evaluation for alternative methods of treatment. *Ann Surg* 1949; **130**: 160–73.
5. Herndon DN, Gore DC, Cole M, *et al.* Determinants of mortality in pediatric patients with greater than 70% full thickness total body surface area treated by early excision and grafting. *J Trauma* 1987; **27**: 208–12.
6. McDonald WS, Sharp CW, Deitch EA. Immediate enteral feeding is safe and effective. *Ann Surg* 1991; **213**: 177–83.
7. Wolf SE, Rose JK, Desai MH, Mileski JH, Barrow RE, Herndon DN. Mortality determinants in massive pediatric burns: an analysis of 103 children with greater than 80% TBSA burns (70% full-thickness). *Ann Surg* 1997; **225**: 554–69.
8. Baue AE, Durham R, Faist E. Systemic inflammatory response syndrome (SIRS), multiple organ dysfunction syndrome (MODS), multiple organ failure (MOF): are we winning the battle? *Shock* 1998; **10(2)**: 79–89.
9. Muckart DJ, Bhagwanjee S. American College of Chest Physicians/Society of Critical Care Medicine Consensus Conference definitions of the systemic inflammatory response syndrome and allied disorders in relation to critically injured patients. *Crit Care Med* 1997; **25**: 1789–95.
10. MacKersie RC, Campbell AR, Cammarano WB. Principles of Critical Care. In: Feliciano D, Moore FD, Mattox KD, eds. *Trauma*. Philadelphia: WB Saunders, 2000; 1231–65.
11. Committee on Trauma American College of Surgeons. Guidelines for the operation of burn units. In: Resources for the optimal care of the injured patient, 1999; 55–62.
12. Bruner JMR, Krewis LJ, Kunsman JM, Sherman AP. Comparison of direct and indirect methods of measuring arterial blood pressure. *Med Instr* 1981; **15**: 11–21.
13. Hla KM, Vokaty KA, Feussner JR. Overestimation of diastolic blood pressure in the elderly. *J Am Geriatr Soc* 1985; **33**: 659–63.
14. Linfors EW, Feussner JR, Blessing CL. Spurious hypertension in the obese patient: effect of sphyngmomamometer cuff size on prevalence of hypertension. *Arch Intern Med* 1984; **144**: 1482–85.
15. Dorman T, Breslow MJ, Lipsett PA, *et al.* Radial artery pressure monitoring

16. underestimates central arterial pressure during vasopressor therapy in critically ill surgical patients. *Crit Care Med* 1998; **26**: 1646–49.
16. Park MK, Robotham JL, German VF. Systolic amplification in pedal arteries of children. *Crit Care Med* 2000; **11**: 286–89.
17. O'Rourke MF, Yaginuma T. Wave reflections and the arterial pulse. *Arch Intern Med* 1984; **144**: 366–71.
18. Chatterjee T, Do DD, Mahler F, Meier B. A prospective randomized evaluation of nonsurgical closure of femoral pseudoaneurysm by compression device with and without ultrasound guidance. *Catheter Cardiovasc Interv* 1999; **47**: 304–09.
19. Connors AF, Speroff T, Dawson NV, *et al.* The effectiveness of right heart catheterization in the initial care of critically ill patients. *JAMA* 1996; **276**: 889–97.
20. Dalen JE, Bone RC. Is it time to pull the pulmonary artery catheter? *JAMA* 1996; **276**: 916–19.
21. Aikawa N, Martyn JA, Burke JF. Pulmonary artery catheterization and thermodilution cardiac output determination in the management of critically burned patients. *Am J Surg* 1978; **135**: 811–17.
22. Reynolds EM, Ryan DP, Sheridan RL, Doody DP. Left ventricular failure complicating severe pediatric burn injuries. *J Pediatr Surg* 1995; **30**: 264–69.
23. Schiller WR, Bay RC, Garren RL, Parker I, Sagraves SG. Hyperdynamic resuscitation improves survival in patients with life-threatening burns. *J Burn Care Rehabil* 1997; **18**: 10–16.
24. Schiller WR, Bay RC, Mclachlan JG, Sagraves SG. Survival in major burn injuries is predicted by early response to Swan-Ganz-guided resuscitation. *Am J Surg* 1995; **170**: 696–99.
25. Holm C, Melcer B, Horbrand F, Worl H, von Donnersmarck GH, Muhlbauer W. Intrathoracic blood volume as an end point in resuscitation of the severely burned: an observational study of 24 patients. *J Trauma* 2000; **48**: 728–34.
26. Mansfield MD, Kinsella J. Use of invasive cardiovascular monitoring in patients with burns greater than 30 per cent body surface area: a survey of 251 centres. *Burns* 1996; **22**: 549–51.
27. Shoemaker WC, Appel PL, Kram HB, Waxman K, Lee TS. Prospective trial of supranormal values of survivors as therapeutic goals in high-risk surgical patients. *Chest* 1988; **94**: 1176–86.
28. Gattinoni L, Brazzi L, Pelosi P, *et al.* A trial of goal-oriented hemodynamic therapy in critically ill patients. SvO2 Collaborative Group. *N Engl J Med* 1995; **333**: 1025–32.
29. Hayes MA, Timmins AC, Yau EH, Palazzo M, Hinds CJ, Watson D. Elevation of systemic oxygen delivery in the treatment of critically ill patients. *N Engl J Med* 1994; **330**: 1717–22.
30. Vincent JL, Thirion M, Brimioulle S, Lejeune P, Kahn RJ. Thermodilution measurement of right ventricular ejection fraction with a modified pulmonary artery catheter. *Intensive Care Med* 1986; **12**: 33–38.
31. Haller M, Zollner C, Briegel J, Forst H. Evaluation of a new continuous thermodilution cardiac output monitor in critically ill patients: a prospective criterion standard study. *Crit Care Med* 1995; **23**: 860–66.
32. Davis JW, Kaups KL, Parks SN. Base deficit is superior to pH in evaluating clearance of acidosis after traumatic shock. *J Trauma* 1998; **44**: 114–18.
33. Rutherford EJ, Morris JA Jr, Reed GW, Hall KS. Base deficit stratifies mortality and determines therapy. *J Trauma* 1992; **33**: 417–23.
34. Kaups KL, Davis JW, Dominic WJ. Base deficit as an indicator or resuscitation needs in patients with burn injuries. *J Burn Care Rehabil* 1998; **19**: 346–48.
35. Jeng JC, Lee K, Jablonski K, Jordan MH. Serum lactate and base deficit suggest inadequate resuscitation of patients with burn injuries: application of a point-of-care laboratory instrument. *J Burn Care Rehabil* 1997; **18**: 402–05.
36. Davis JW, Kaups KL, Parks SN. Effect of alcohol on the utility of base deficit in trauma. *J Trauma* 1997; **43**: 507–10.
37. Gueugniaud PY, David JS, Petit P. Early hemodynamic variations assessed by an echo-Doppler aortic blood flow device in a severely burned infant: correlation with the circulating cytokines. *Pediatr Emerg Care* 1998; **14**: 282–84.
38. Kuwagata Y, Sugimoto H, Yoshioka T, Sugimoto T. Left ventricular performance in patients with thermal injury or multiple trauma: a clinical study with echocardiography. *J Trauma* 1992; **32**: 158–64.
39. Shapiro BA, Lacmak RM, Care RD, *et al.* Clinical application of respiratory care. St Louis, MO: Mosby Year Book, 1991.
40. Hinson JR, Marini JJ. Principles of mechanical ventilator use in respiratory failure. *Ann Rev Med* 1992; **43**: 341–55.
41. Lessard MR, Guerot E, Lorino H, Lemaire F, Brochard L. Effects of pressure-controlled with different I:E ratios versus volume-controlled ventilation on respiratory mechanics, gas exchange, and hemodynamics in patients with adult respiratory distress syndrome. *Anesthesiology* 1994; **80**: 983–91.
42. Zavala E, Ferrer M, Polese G, *et al.* Effect of inverse I:E ratio ventilation on pulmonary gas exchange in acute respiratory distress syndrome. *Anesthesiology* 1998; **88**: 35–42.

43. Ludwigs U, Klingstedt C, Baehrendtz S, Hedenstierna G. A comparison of pressure- and volume-controlled ventilation at different inspiratory to expiratory ratios. *Acta Anaesthesiol Scand* 1997; **41**: 71–77.

44. Mercat A, Graini L, Teboul JL, Lenique F, Richard C. Cardiorespiratory effects of pressure-controlled ventilation with and without inverse ratio in the adult respiratory distress syndrome. *Chest* 1993; **104**: 871–75.

45. Cioffi WG, Graves TA, McManus WF, Pruitt BA Jr. High-frequency percussive ventilation in patients with inhalation injury. *J Trauma* 1989; **29**: 350–54.

46. Cioffi WG Jr, Rue LW III, Graves TA, et al. Prophylactic use of high-frequency percussive ventilation in patients with inhalation injury. *Ann Surg* 1991; **213**: 575–80.

47. Cortiella J, Mlcak R, Herndon D. High frequency percussive ventilation in pediatric patients with inhalation injury. *J Burn Care Rehabil* 1999; **20**: 232–35.

48. Mlcak R, Cortiella J, Desai M, Herndon D. Lung compliance, airway resistance, and work of breathing in children after inhalation injury. *J Burn Care Rehabil* 1997; **18**: 531–34.

49. Palmer RM, Ferrige AG, Moncada S. Nitric oxide release accounts for the biological activity of endothelium-derived relaxing factor. *Nature* 1987; **327**: 524–26.

50. Ream RS, Hauver JF, Lynch RE, Kountzman B, Gale GB, Mink RB. Low-dose inhaled nitric oxide improves the oxygenation and ventilation of infants and children with acute, hypoxemic respiratory failure. *Crit Care Med* 1999; **27**: 989–96.

51. Roberts JD, Polaner DM, Lang P, Zapol WM. Inhaled nitric oxide in persistent pulmonary hypertension of the newborn. *Lancet* 1992; **340**: 818–19.

52. Sheridan RL, Zapol WM, Ritz RH, Tompkins RG. Low-dose inhaled nitric oxide in acutely burned children with profound respiratory failure. *Surgery* 1999; **126**: 856–62.

53. Sheridan RL, Hurford WE, Kacmarek RM, Ritz RH, Yin LM, Ryan CM, Tompkins RG. Inhaled nitric oxide in burn patients with respiratory failure. *J Trauma* 1997; **42**: 629–34.

54. Brower RG, Shanholtz CB, Fessler HE, et al. Prospective, randomized, controlled clinical trial comparing traditional versus reduced tidal volume ventilation in acute respiratory distress syndrome patients. *Crit Care Med* 1999; **27**: 1492–98.

55. Brochard L, Roudot-Thoraval F, Roupie E, et al. Tidal volume reduction for prevention of ventilator-induced lung injury in acute respiratory distress syndrome. The Multicenter Trial Group on Tidal Volume reduction in ARDS. *Am J Respir Crit Care Med* 1998; **158**: 1831–38.

56. Stewart TE, Meade MO, Cook DJ, et al. Evaluation of a ventilation strategy to prevent barotrauma in patients at high risk of acute respiratory distress syndrome. *N Eng J Med* 1998; **338**: 355–61.

57. The Acute Respiratory Distress Syndrome Network. Ventilation with lower tidal volumes as compared with traditional tidal volumes for acute lung injury and acute respiratory distress syndrome. *N Eng J Med* 2000; **342**: 1301–08.

58. Esteban A, Frutos F, Tobin MJ, et al. A comparison of four methods of weaning patients from mechanical ventilation. *N Eng J Med* 1995; **332**: 345–50.

59. Tremper KK, Barker SJ. Pulse oximetry. *Anesthesiology* 1989; **70**: 98–108.

60. Deitch EA, Ma L, Ma JW, Berg RD. Lethal burn induced bacterial translocation: role of genetic resistance. *J Trauma* 1989; **29**: 1480–87.

61. Deitch EA, Goodman ER. Prevention of multiple organ failure. *Surgical Clinics of North America* 1999; **79**: 1471–88.

62. Tanaka H, Mituo T, Yukioka T, Matsuda H, Shimazaki S, Igarashi H. Comparison of hemodynamic changes resulting from toxic shock syndrome toxin-1-producing *Staphylococcus aureus* sepsis and endotoxin-producing gramnegative rod sepsis in patients with severe burns. *J Burn Care Rehabil* 1995; **16**: 616–21.

63. Sprung CL. Definitions of sepsis – have we reached a consensus? [editorial]. *Crit Care Med* 1991; **19**: 849–51.

64. Goodman ER, Kleinstein E, Fusco AM, et al. Role of interleukin 8 in the genesis of acute respiratory distress syndrome through an effect on neutrophil apoptosis. *Arch Surg* 1998; **133**: 1234–39.

65. Rhee P, Waxman K, Clark L, Tominaga G, Soliman MH. Superoxide dismutase polyethylene glycol improves survival in hemorrhagic shock. *Am Surg* 1991; **57**: 747–50.

66. Schiller HJ, Reilly PM, Bulkley GB. Tissue perfusion in critical illnesses. Antioxidant therapy. *Crit Care Med* 1993; **21**: S92–102.

67. Groeneveld PH, Kwappenberg KM, Langermans JA, Nibbering PH, Curtis L. Nitric oxide (NO) production correlates with renal insufficiency and multiple organ dysfunction syndrome in severe sepsis. *Intensive Care Med* 1996; **22**: 1197–202.

68. Mileski WJ, Winn RK, Vedder NB, Pohlman TH, Harlan JM, Rice CL. Inhibition of CD18-dependent neutrophil adherence reduces organ injury after hemorrhagic shock in primates. *Surgery* 1990; **108**: 206–12.

69. Ezzell RM, Carter EA, Yarmush ML, Tompkins RG. Thermal injury-induced changes in the rat intestine brush border cytoskeleton. *Surgery* 1993; **114**: 591–97.

70. Carter EA, Gonnella A, Tompkins RG. Increased transcellular permeability of rat small intestine after thermal injury. *Burns* 1992; **18**: 117–20.

71. Deitch EA. Intestinal permeability is increased in burn patients shortly after injury. *Surgery* 1990; **107**: 411–16.

72. Wilkes BM, Mailloux LU. Acute renal failure: pathogenesis and prevention. *Am J Med* 1986; **80**: 1129–36.

73. Chertow GM, Christiansen CL, Cleary PD, Munro C, Lazarus JM. Prognostic stratification in critically ill patients with acute renal failure requiring dialysis. *Arch Intern Med* 1995; **155**: 1505–11.

74. Jeschke MG, Wolf SE, Barrow RE, Herndon DN. Mortality in burned children with acute renal failure. *Arch Surg* 1998; **134**: 752–56.

75. Woodrow G, Turney JH. Cause of death in acute renal failure. *Nephrol Dial Transplant* 1992; 230–34.

76. Thadhani R, Pascual M, Bonventre JV. Acute renal failure. *N Eng J Med* 1996; **334**: 1448–60.

77. Myers BD, Moran SM. Hemodynamically mediated acute renal failure. *N Eng J Med* **314**: 97–105.

78. Conger JD, Robinette JB, Hammond WS. Differences in vascular reactivity in models of ischemic acute renal failure. *Kidney Int* 1991; **39**: 1087–97.

79. Mason JC, Joeris B, Welsch J, Kris W. Vascular congestion in ischemic renal failure: the role of cell swelling. *Miner Electrolyte Metab* 1989; **15**: 114–24.

80. Vetterlein F, Petho A, Schmidt G. Distribution of capillary blood flow in rat kidney during post-ischemic renal failure. *Am J Physiol* 1986; **251**: H510–H519.

81. Kellerman PS, Clark RA, Hoilien CA, Linas SL, Molitoris BA. Role of microfilaments in maintenance of proximal tubule structural and functional integrity. *Am J Physiol* 1990; **259**: F279–F285.

82. Fish EM, Molitoris BA. Alterations in epithelial polarity and the pathogenesis of disease states. *N Eng J Med* 1994; **330**: 1580–88.

83. Goligorsky MS, DiBona GF. Pathogenic role of Arg-Gly-Asp recognizing integrins in acute renal failure. *Proc Natl Acad Sci USA* 1993; **90**: 5700–04.

84. Dixon BS, Anderson RJ. Nonoliguric acute renal failure. *Am J Kidney Dis* 1985; **6**: 71–80.

85. Corwin HL, Teplick RS, Schrieber MJ, Coggins CH. Prediction of outcome in renal failure. *Am J Nephrol* 1987; **7**: 8–12.

86. Liano F, Garcia-Martin F, Gallego A, et al. Easy and early prognosis in acute tubular necrosis: a forward analysis of 228 cases. *J. Nephron* 1989; **8**: 307–13.

87. Pascual J, Orofino L, Liano F, Marcen R, Orte L, Ortuno J. Prognosis of acute renal failure among elderly patients. *J Am Geriat Soc* 1990; **38**: 25–30.

88. Lindner A, Cutler RE, Goodman G. Synergism of dopamine plus furosemide in preventing acute renal failure in the dog. *Kidney Int* 1979; **16**: 158–66.

89. Ichai C, Passeron C, Carles M, Bouregba M, Grimaud D. Prolonged low-dose dopamine infusion induces a transient improvement in renal function in hemodynamically stable, critically ill patients: a single-blind, prospective, controlled study. *Crit Care Med* 2000; **28**: 1329–35.

90. Marik PE, Iglesias J. Low-dose dopamine does not prevent acute renal failure in patients with septic shock and oliguria. NORASEPT II Study Investigators. *Am J Med* 1999; **107**: 387–90.

91. Neumayer HH, Junge W, Kufner A, Wenning A. Prevention of radiocontrast media induced nephrotoxicity by the calcium channel blocker nitrendipine: a prospective randomized clinical trial. *Nephrol Dial Transplant* 1989; **4**: 1030–36.

92. Rahman SN, Kim GE, Mathew AS, et al. Effects of atrial natriuretic peptide in clinical acute renal failure. *Kidney Int* 1994; **45**: 1731–38.

93. Sands JM, Neylan JF, Olson RA, O'Brien DP, Whelchel JD, Mitch WE. Atrial natriuretic factor does not improve outcome of cadaveric renal transplantation. *J Am Soc Nephrol* 1991; **1**: 1081–86.

94. Meyer M, Pfarr E, Schirmer G, et al. Therapeutic use of the natriuretic peptide ularitide in acute renal failure. *Ren Fail* 1999; **21**: 85–100.

95. Shilliday I, Allison ME. Diuretics in renal failure. *Ren Fail* 1994; **1**: 3–17.

96. Better OS, Stein JH. Early management of shock and prophylaxis of acute renal failure in traumatic rhabdomyolysis. *N Eng J Med* 1990; **322**: 825–29.

97. Conger JD. Interventions in clinical acute renal failure: what are the data? *Am J Kidney Dis* 1995; **26**: 565–76.

98. Kim K, Onesti G, Ramirez O. Creatinine clearance in renal disease: a reappraisal. *BMJ* 1969; **4**: 11–18.

99. Bellomo R, Parkin G, Love J, Boyce N. A prospective comparative study of continuous arteriovenous hemofiltration and continuous venovenous hemodiafiltration in critically ill patients. *Am J Kidney Dis* 1993; **21**: 400–04.

100. Bellomo R, Tipping P, Boyne N. Continous veno-venous hemofiltration with dialysis removes cytokines from the circulation of septic patients. *Crit Care Med* 1993; **21**: 522–26.

101. Leblanc M, Thibeault Y, Querin S. Continuous haemofiltration and haemodiafiltration for acute renal failure in severely burned patients. *Burns* 1997; **23**: 160–65.

102. Swartz RD, Messana JM, Orzol S, Port FK. Comparing continuous hemofiltration

with hemodialysis in patients with severe acute renal failure. *Am J Kidney Dis* 1999; **34**: 424–32.

103. Pomeranz A, Reichenberg Y, Schurr D, Drukker A. Acute renal failure in a burn patient: the advantages of continuous peritoneal dialysis. *Burns Incl Therm Inj* 1985 Jun; **11**(5): 367–70

104. Ware LB, Matthay MA. The acute respiratory distress syndrome. *N Eng J Med* 2000; **342**: 1334–49.

105. Doyle RL, Szaflarski N, Modin GW, Wiener-Kronish JP, Matthay MA. Identification of patients with acute lung injury: predictors of mortality. *Am J Respir Crit Care Med* 1995; **152**: 1818–24.

106. Suchyta MR, Clemmer TP, Elliot CG, Orme JF Jr, Weaver LK. The adult respiratory distress syndrome: a report of survival and modifying factors. *Chest* 1992; **101**: 1074–79.

107. Pugin J, Verghese G, Widmer MC, Matthay MA. The alveolar space is the site of intense inflammatory and profibrotic reactions in the early phase of acute respiratory distress syndrome. *Crit Care Med* 1999; **27**: 304–12.

108. Ware LB, Matthay MA. Maximal alveolar epithelial fluid clearance in clinical acute lung injury: an excellent predictor of survival and the duration of mechanical ventilation. *Am J Respir Crit Care Med* 1999; **159**: Suppl: A694. abstract.

109. Wiener-Kronish JP, Albertine KH, Matthay MA. Differential responses of the endothelial and epithelial barriers of the lung in sheep to Escherichia coli endotoxin. *J Clin Invest* 1999; **88**: 864–75.

110. Bachofen M, Weibel ER. Structural alterations of lung arenchyma in the adult respiratory distress syndrome. *Clin Chest Med* 1982; **3**: 35–56.

111. Pittet JF, MacKersie RC, Martin TR, Matthay MA. Biological markers of acute lung injury: prognostic and pathogenic significance. *Am J Respir Crit Care Med* 1997; **155**: 1187–205.

112. Laufe MD, Simon RH, Flint A, Keller JB. Adult respiratory distress syndrome in neutropenic patients. *Am J Med* 1986; **80**: 1022–26.

113. Pratt PC, Vollmer RT, Shelburne JD, Crapo JD. Pulmonary morphology in a multihospital collaborative extracorporeal membrane oxygenation project. *Am J Physiol* 1979; 191–214.

114. Webb HH, Tierney DF. Experimental pulmonary edema due to intermittent positive pressure ventilation with high inflation pressures: protection by positive end-expiratory pressure. *Am Rev Respir Dis* 1974; **110**: 556–65.

115. Dreyfuss D, Soler P, Basset G, Saumon G. High inflation pressure pulmonary edema: respective effects of high airway pressure, high tidal volume, and positive end-expiratory pressure. *Am Rev Respir Dis* 2000; **137**: 1159–64.

116. Parker JC, Townsley MI, Rippe B, Taylor AE, Thigpen J. Increased microvascular permeability in dog lungs due to high peak airway pressures. *J Appl Physiol* 1984; **57**: 1809–16.

117. Corbridge TC, Wood LDH, Crawford GP, Chudoba MJ, Yanos J, Sznajder JI. Adverse effects of large tidal volumes and low PEEP in canine acid aspiration. *Am Rev Respir Dis* 1990; **142**: 311–15.

118. Slutsky AS, Tremblay LN. Multiple system organ failure: is mechanical ventilation a contributing factor? *Am J Respir Crit Care Med* 1998; **157**: 1721–25.

119. Ware LB, Golden JA, Finkbeiner WE, Matthay MA. Alveolar epithelial fluid transport capacity in reperfusion lung injury after lung transplantation. *Am J Respir Crit Care Med* 1999; **159**: 980–88.

120. Anderson DR, Thielen K. Correlative study of adult respiratory distress syndrome by light, scanning, and transmission electrom microscopy. *Ultrastruct Pathol* 1992; **16**: 615–28.

121. Fukuda Y, Ishizaki M, Masuda Y, Kimura G, Kawanami O, Masugi Y. The role of intraalveolar fibrosis in the process of pulmonary structural remodeling in patients with diffuse alveolar damage. *Am J Pathol* 1992; **126**: 171–82.

122. Martin C, Papazian L, Payan MJ, Saux P, Gouin F. Pulmonary fibrosis correlates with outcome in adult respiratory distress syndrome: a study in mechanically ventilated patients. *Chest* 1995; **107**: 196–200.

123. Folkesson HG, Nitenberg G, Oliver BL, Jayr C, Albertine KH, Matthay MA. Upregulation of alveolar epithelial fluid transport after subacute lung injury in rate from bleomycin. *Am J Physiol* 1998; **275**: L478–L490.

124. Matthay MA, Folkesson HG, Verkman AS. Salt and water transport across alveolar and distal airway epithelia in the adult lung. *Am J Physiol* 1996; **270**: L487–L503.

125. Folkesson HG, Matthay MA, Westrom BR, Kim KJ, Karlsson BW, Hastings RH. Alveolar epithelial clearance of protein. *J Appl Physiol* 1996; **80**: 1431–35.

126. Morris AH, Wallace CJ, Menlove RL, *et al.* Randomized clinical trial of pressure-controlled inverse ratio ventilation and extracorporeal CO2 removal for adult respiratory distress syndrome. *Am J Respir Crit Care Med* 2000; **149**: 295–305.

127. Pierre EJ, Zwischenberger JB, Angel C, *et al.* Extracorporeal membrane oxygenation in the treatment of respiratory failure in pediatric patients with burns. *J Burn Care Rehabil* 1998; **19**: 131–34.

128. Brochard L, Roudot-Thoraval F, Roupie E, *et al.* Tidal volume reduction for

129. Petty TL, Ashbaugh DG. The adult respiratory distress syndrome: clinical features, factors influencing prognosis and principles of management. *Chest* 1971; **60**: 233–39.

130. Falke KJ, Pontappidan H, Kumar A, Leith DE, Geffin B, Laver MB. Ventilation with end-expiratory pressure in acute lung disease. *J Clin Invest* 1972; **51**: 2315–23.

131. Gattinoni L, Presenti A, Bombino M, *et al.* Relationships between lung computed tomographic density, gas exchange, and PEEP in acute respiratory failure. *Anesthesiology* 1988; **69**: 824–32.

132. Pepe PE, Hudson LD, Carrico CJ. Early application of positive end expiratory pressure in patients at risk from adult respiratory distress syndrome. *N Eng J Med* 1984; **311**: 281–86.

133. Amato MB, Barbas CS, Medeiros DM, *et al.* Effect of a protective ventilation strategy on mortality in acute respiratory distress syndrome. *N Eng J Med* 1998; **338**: 347–54.

134. Long W, Thompson T, Sundell H, Schumacher R, Volberg F, Guthrie R. Effects of two rescue doses of a synthetic surfactant on mortality rate and survival without bronchopulmonary dysplasia in 700 to 1350 gram infants with respiratory distress syndrome. *J Pediatr* 1991; **118**: 595–605.

135. Anzueto A, Baughman RP, Guntupalli KK, *et al.* Aerosolized surfactant in adults with sepsis induced acute respiratory distress syndrome. *N Eng J Med* 1996; **334**: 1417–21.

136. Dellinger RP, Zimmerman JL, Taylor RW, *et al.* Effects of inhaled nitric oxide in patients with acute respiratory failure: results of a randomized phase II trial. *Crit Care Med* 1998; **26**: 15–23.

137. Prewitt RM, Wood LDH. Effect of sodium nitroprusside on cardiovascular function and pulmonary shunt in canine oleic acid pulmonary edema. *Anesthesiology* 1981; **55**: 537–41.

138. Bishop MJ, Kennard S, Artman LD, Cheney FW. Hydralazine does not inhibit canine hypoxic pulmonary vasoconstriction. *Am Rev Respir Dis* 1983; **128**: 998–1001.

139. Abraham E, Baughman R, Fletcher E, *et al.* Liposomal prostaglandin E1 (TLC C-53) in acute respiratory distress syndrome: a controlled, randomized, double-blind, multicenter trial. *Crit Care Med* 1999; **27**: 1478–85.

140. Radermacher P, Snatak B, Wust HJ, Tarnow J, Falke KJ. Prostacyclin for the treatment of pulmonary hypertension in the adult respiratory distress syndrome: effects on pulmonary capillary pressure and perfusion-ventilation distributions. *Anesthesiology* 1990; **72**: 238–44.

141. Bernard GR, Luce JM, Sprung CL, *et al.* High-dose corticosteroids in patients with adult respiratory distress syndrome. *N Eng J Med* 1987; **317**: 1565–70.

142. Meduri GU, Belenchia JM, Estes RJ, Wunderink RG, el Torky M, Leeper KV, Jr. Fibroproliferative phase of ARDS. Clinical findings and effects of corticosteroids. *Chest* 1991; **100**: 943–52.

143. Meduri GU, Chinn AJ, Leeper KV, *et al.* Corticosteroid rescue treatment of progressive fibroproliferation in late ARDS. Patterns of response and predictors of outcome. *Chest* 1994; **105**: 1516–27.

144. Meduri GU, Headley AS, Golden E, *et al.* Effect of prolonged methylprednisolone therapy in unresolving acute respiratory distress syndrome: a randomized controlled trial. *JAMA* 1998; **280**: 159–65.

145. Braunwald E, Sonnenblick EH, Ross J. Mechanisms of cardiac contraction and relaxation. In: Braunwald E, ed. *Heart Disease A Textbook of Cardiovascular Medicine*, 3rd edn 1988; Philadelphia: WB Saunders.

146. Suzuki K, Nishina M, Ogino R, Kohama A. Left ventricular contractility and diastolic properties in anesthetized dogs after severe burns. *Am J Physiol* 1991; **260**: H1433–H1442.

147. Agarwal N, Petro J, Salisbury RE. Physiologic profile monitoring in burned patients. *J Trauma* 1983; **23**: 577–83.

148. Cioffi WG, DeMeules JE, Gamelli RL. The effects of burn injury and fluid resuscitation on cardiac function in vitro. *J Trauma* 1986; **26**: 638–42.

149. Breitenstein E, Chiolero RL, Jequier E, Dayer P, Krupp S, Schutz Y. Effects of beta-blockade on energy metabolism following burns. *Burns* 1990; **16**: 259–64.

150. Wilmore DW, Long JM, Mason AD, Skreen RW, Pruitt BA. Catecholamines: mediators of the hypermetabolic response in thermally burned patients. *Ann Surg* 1974; **180**: 280–290.

151. Szabo K. Clinical experiences with beta adrenergic blocking therapy on burned patients. *Scand J Plast Reconstr Surg* 1979; **13**: 211–215.

152. Herndon DN, Barrow RE, Rutan TC, Minifee P, Jahoor F, Wolfe RR. Effect of propranolol administration on hemodynamic and metabolic responses of burned pediatric patients. *Ann Surg* 1988; **208**: 484–492.

153. Minifee PK, Barrow RE, Abston S, Herndon DN. Improved myocardial oxygen utilization following propranolol infusion in adolescents with postburn hypermetabolism. *J Paed Surg* 1989; **24**: 806–811.

154. Baron PW, Barrow RE, Pierre EJ, Herndon DN. Prolonged use of propranolol

safely decreases cardiac work in burned children. *J Burn Care Rehabil* 1997; **18**: 223–227.

155. Honeycutt D, Barrow RE, Herndon DN. Cold stress response in patients with severe burns after beta blockade. *J Burn Care Rehabil* 1992; **13**: 181–186.

156. Aarsland AA, Chinkes DL, Wolfe RR, Barrow RE, Nelson SO, Pierre EJ, Herndon DN. Beta-blockade lowers peripheral lipolysis in burn patients receiving growth hormone. Rate of hepatic very low density lipoprotein triglyceride secretion remains unchanged. *Ann Surg* 1996; **223**: 777–789.

157. Herndon DN, Hart DW, Wolf SE, Wolfe RR. Propranolol decreases muscle catabolism associated with severe burn. *NEJM* 2001, (in press).

158. Chung DH, Evers BM, Townsend CM, *et al*. Burn induced transcriptional regulation of small intestinal ornithine decarboxylase. *Am J Surg* 1992; **163**: 157–63.

159. Huang KF, Chung DH, Herndon DN. Insulin-like growth factor I (IGF-1) reduces gut atrophy and bacterial translocation after severe burn injury. *Arch Surg* 1993; **128**: 54.

160. Chung DH, Evers BM, Townsend CM, Huang KF, Herndon DN, Thompson J. Role of polyamine biosynthesis during gut mucosal adaptation after burn injury. *Am J Surg* 1993; **165**: 144–49.

161. Carter EA, Tompkins RG. Injury-induced inhibition of fat absorption. *J Burn Care Rehabil* 1994; **15**: 154–57.

162. Ryan CM, Yarmush ML, Burke JF, Tompkins RG. Increased gut permeability early after burns correlates with the extent of burn injury. *Crit Care Med* 1992; **20**: 1508–12.

163. LeVoyer T, Cioffi WG, Pratt L, *et al*. Alterations in intestinal permeability after thermal injury. *Arch Surg* 1992; **127**: 26–30.

164. Wolf SE, Ikeda H, Matin S, *et al*. Cutaneous burn increases apoptosis in the gut epithelium of mice. *JACS* 1999; **188**: 10–16.

165. Carter EA, Udall JN, Kirkham SE, Walker WA. Thermal injury and gastrointestinal function. I. Small intestinal nutrient absorption and DNA synthesis. *J Burn Care Rehabil* 1986; **7**: 469–74.

166. Carter EA, Tompkins RG, Schiffrin E, Burke JF. Cutaneous thermal injury alters macromolecular permeability of rat small intestine. *Surgery* 1990; **107**: 335–41.

167. Ryan CM, Bailey SH, Carter EA, Schoenfeld DA, Tompkins RG. Additive effects of thermal injury and infection on gut permeability. *Arch Surg* 1994; **129**: 325–28.

168. Berthiaume F, Ezzell RM, Toner M, Yarmush ML, Tompkins RG. Transport of fluorescent dextrans across the rat ileum after cutaneous thermal injury. *Crit Care Med* 1994; **22**: 455–64.

169. Tokyay R, Zeigler ST, Traber DL, *et al*. Postburn gastrointestinal vasoconstriction increases bacterial and endotorin translocation. *J Appl Physial* 1993; **74**: 1521–27.

170. Horton JW. Bacterial translocation after burn injury: the contribution of ischemia and permeability changes. *Shock* 1994; **1**: 286–90.

171. Gianotti L, Alexander JW, Fukushima R, Childress CP. Translocation of Candida albicans is related to the blood flow of individual intestinal villi. *Circ Shock* 1993; **40**: 250–57.

172. Wolf SE, Jeschke MG, Rose JK, Desai MH, Herndon DN. Enteral feeding intolerance: An indicator of sepsis associated mortality in burned children. *Arch Surg* 1997; **132**: 1310–14.

173. Herndon DN, Barrow RE, Stein M, *et al*. Increased mortality with intravenous supplemental feeding in severely burned patients. *J Burn Care Rehabil* 1989; **10**: 309–13.

174. Hastings PR, Skillman JJ, Bushnell LS, Aarsland AA, Silen W. Antacid titration in the prevention of acute gastrointestinal bleeding. A controlled randomized trial of 100 critically ill patients. *N Eng J Med* 1978; **298**: 1041–45.

175. Moscona R, Kaufman T, Jacobs R, Hirshowitz B. Prevention of gastrointestinal bleeding in burns: the effects of cimetidine or antacids combined with early enteral feeding. *Burns Incl Therm Inj* 1985; **12**: 65–67.

176. Rath T, Walzer LR, Meissl G. Preventive measures for stress ulcers in burn patients. *Burns Incl Therm Inj* 1988; **14**: 504–07.

177. Raff T, Germann G, Hartmann B. The value of early enteral nutrition in the prophylaxis of stress ulceration in the severely burned patient. *Burns* 1997; **23**: 313–18.

178. Lam NP, Le PD, Crawford SY, Patel S. National survey of stress ulcer prophylaxis. *Crit Care Med* 1999; **27**: 98–103.

Chapter 31

Burn nursing
Mary Gordon, Janet Marvin

Acute care

Pulmonary Priorities

Inhalation injury continues to be the most serious and life-threatening complication of burn injury today. Early diagnosis and treatment greatly impact the outcome of care.

Impaired gas exchange is a potential problem for patients who have face and neck burns and/or inhalation injury. Inhalation injury may include carbon monoxide poisoning, upper airway injury (heat injury above the glottis), lower airway injury (chemical injury to lung parenchyma), and restrictive defects (circumferential third-degree burn around the chest). Upper airway edema causes respiratory distress and is the primary concern during the initial 24–48 hours postburn phase. Tracheobronchitis, atelectasis, bronchorrhea, pneumonia, and Adult Respiratory Distress Syndrome (ARDS) may occur during the acute, postburn stage either related or unrelated to inhalation injury.

Nursing care of a patient with inhalation injury begins with a detailed history of the accident. Inhalation injury is suspected when the accident occurred in a closed space. Close observation of the patient and frequent respiratory assessments are made throughout the initial and acute phase postburn. Initially, the patient is observed for hoarseness and stridor, which indicate narrowed airways. Emergency equipment is placed at the bedside to facilitate intubation if necessary. Observing the frequency of cough, carbonaceous sputum, and increased inability to handle secretions may indicate possible inhalation injury and the potential for impaired gas exchange. Other important observations include respiratory rate, breath sounds, use of accessory muscles to aid in respiratory effort, nasal flaring, sternal retractions, increased anxiety, and complaint of shortness of breath. Disorientation, obtundation, and coma may be due to significant exposure to smoke toxins such as carbon monoxide or cyanide. These conditions are managed emergently with 100% oxygen.

Bronchoscopy may be done early to diagnose inhalation injury as well as facilitate airway clearance. Humidified oxygen should be readily available and applied to patients who have evidence of impaired gas exchange (especially pediatric patients). Aggressive nasotracheal suction may be indicated if the patient has difficulty with managing secretions either because of the increased amount of secretions and/or the decreased effectiveness of the cough. In addition, aggressive pulmonary toilet, including turning, coughing, and deep breathing, up and out-of-bed rocking in mother's arms may be done regularly and frequently. Elevation of the head of the bed, unless contraindicated, will also support and possibly improve ventilation. Trends and changes should be correlated with laboratory results and shared with the team.

Another complication is circumferential third-degree burns around the chest and neck, which often cause restrictive defects. The increased amount of edema combined with decreased chest excursion may greatly decrease tidal volume. This condition may progress and can become life-threatening, in which case chest escharotomy may be necessary to release the constricting eschar. The procedure may be done at the bedside or in the operating room. Equipment includes sterile drapes, scalpel, and Bovie (to control bleeding).

Intubation and mechanical ventilation may be required to improve gas exchange. Tube placement should be checked and documented frequently and verified daily by x-ray. Securing the endotracheal tube requires a standard technique for stabilization and prevention of pressure necrosis. Adequate humidity is necessary to prevent secretions from drying and causing mucous plugging. Remember to provide pre/post-suctioning hyperoxygenation. Sterile technique is used when suctioning to prevent infection. Attention to the details of oral hygiene will provide tremendous comfort for the patient.

Criteria for extubation depend on why the tube was inserted initially, but, overall, stable vital signs and hemodynamic parameters will support the plan for extubation. The patient should be awake and alert in order to protect the airway; therefore pain medications may be reduced before extubation. Ventilatory measurements and blood gas analysis should be within normal limits.

Immediately following extubation, the nurse must be alert for signs and symptoms of respiratory distress, administer suction as needed, monitor blood gas measurements, provide optimal positioning for ventilation, as well as provide reassurance and support to decrease anxiety.

Age, burn size, and the presence of inhalation injury and pneumonia have been identified as major contributors to mortality.[5] Thus, vigilant nursing care (frequent nursing assessments, aggressive pulmonary toilet, etc.) combined with anticipating potential problems and being prepared to deal with the problems will add to the team effort and possibly improve the patient outcome.

Burn Wound Care

The primary goal for burn wound management is to close the wound as soon as possible. Prompt surgical excisions of the eschar and skin grafting have contributed to reduced morbidity and mortality in severely burned patients.[6–8]

Wound care in the burn unit has become an art of burn nursing practice. It can be extremely challenging and complicated and, for a new nurse, it can be the most difficult and misunderstood part of burn nursing. The complexity exists because there are many different wounds that require different interventions in relation to time postburn or time postoperative. Wound assessment and care is a learned skill that develops over time. The expert burn nurse must teach these skills to new burn nurses in the bathroom, and operating room, and at the bedside.

Wounds may consist of eschar, pseudoeschar, skin buds, autograft, donor sites, hypermature granulating tissue, blisters, and exposed bone and tendon cavities. Besides the many kinds of possible wounds, there are many topical antibacterial agents available for managing wounds. These choices raise many decisions for the team to address. Topical antimicrobial creams and ointments include mafenide acetate, silver nitrate, silver sulfadiazine, petroleum and mineral oil-based antibacterial products, and Mycostatin powder. Wounds may be treated in the open fashion (topicals without dressings) or closed fashion (topicals with dressings or soaks). Also there are many, many techniques for applying dressings to every area of the body to withstand exercise, ambulation, and moving around in bed. Biological dressings such as homograft or heterograft may be used as temporary wound coverage. Dressings may also be synthetic or biosynthetic or silver impregnated. Selection is based on the present condition of the wound and the expected outcome.

Secondary goals of wound care are to promote healing and to maintain function of the affected body part. These goals are accomplished by preventing wound infection, treating wound infection, preventing graft loss and tissue necrosis, providing personal hygiene, and maintaining correct positioning and splinting throughout hospitalization. To prevent burn wound infection, the burn nurse must use clean technique: cleanse the wound with soap and water; debride the wound of loose necrotic tissue, crusts, dried blood and exudate; and apply topicals and/or dressings and change as often as ordered. The nurse must inspect the wound for evidence of infection: cellulitis, odor, increased wound exudate, and/or change in exudate; change in wound appearance; and increased pain in the wound. The physician should be notified so that changes in wound care can be made. Cultures and biopsies may be ordered to identify the organisms and treat with a specific systemic antibiotic and/or topical dressing and/or soak. The wound is often the source of sepsis in the bloodstream. The five cardinal signs of sepsis are: hyperventilation, thrombocytopenia, hyperglycemia, disorientation, and hypothermia.[10]

Preventing graft loss is another wound care challenge for nursing. Usually the patient returns from the operating room in a position that is maintained for 3 or 4 days. Any interaction with the patient during this time of graft immobilization requires creativity and care in order to prevent shearing of the graft. Postoperative dressings on the thighs and back are protected with polymycin, fine-mesh gauze to prevent soiling by feces and to minimize cleanup. The dressings are continuously monitored for increased drainage and odor, which would indicate possible wound infection. If infection is suspected, then the postoperative dressings may be removed early for a closer inspection of the wound.

Donor sites will also require additional care to prevent infection. Of course, the care postoperatively depends on the coverage of the donor site. If the donor site is covered with fine-mesh gauze, the initial care is to ensure homeostasis and adherence of the gauze to the wound. Therefore the post-op pressure dressing remains intact for 6–12 hours and then removed. The focus of managing the donor site is to keep the wound dry. If grafts/donor sites are on the back or backs of the legs, the patient is placed in a Clinitron bed for 4–5 days to promote drying. If the donor site remains wet, additional drying techniques (hair dryers, external heaters) may be used periodically during the day.[13]

If the donor site is covered with a synthetic or biologic dressing, the same principles apply. Basically, apply a pressure dressing to ensure adherence to the wound for a short period of time postoperative and then expose to the air to support drying of the wound. A bed cradle is used to keep bed linen from contacting the wounds. The location of the graft, donor site, and eschar may all be on the same extremity, which again requires creativity to accomplish all three interventions of care.

Patients are at high risk for pressure necrosis postoperatively, but of course the potential exists at any time. Prevention is the goal and may include frequent turning schedules, rotating splint schedules, or use of air-fluidized or air-loss beds or other special devices to decrease pressure over bony prominences. Prone positioning poses even more of a challenge.

All patients, except those with skin grafts postoperatively, will benefit from a bath or shower. Large acute burns are placed on a shower cart and the wounds are gently showered with warm water. The overhead heater is on and the room temperature is 85°F (29°C) or above. Large acute burns are not immersed in a tub of water, so as to prevent autocontamination and electrolyte imbalance.[9] Time in the bathroom can be used for careful observation of the wound as well as personal hygiene such as shampoo, mouth care, face care, and perineal care.

The bathroom affords an excellent opportunity for teaching the patient and family about wound care and dressing application. As the patient gets closer to discharge, families are required to do more of the care. The trend for earlier release from the hospital poses additional challenges for nursing since it reduces the time available to prepare the patient for discharge. The better the patient and families are educated, the better the outcome will be. Early involvement with patient and family helps identify potential obstacles at discharge and facilitates care coordination in the discharge process.

Metabolic and Nutritional Support

Hypermetabolism, or metabolic stress, is the direct response to a burn injury. The amount of stress increases proportionally to the extent of the injury and strongly influences a patient's nutritional requirements. This response can magnify the normal metabolic rate by 200%. Malnutrition, starvation, and delayed wound healing will result if calories are not provided consistently to meet nutritional requirements. Children require more calorie and protein replacement than adults, because they have additional nutritional demands to support growth and development.

Monitoring output and managing nutritional intake are among nursing's primary responsibilities. An accurate record of intake and output is critical to patient care because potential problems can be detected early and alternate options of care can be individualized to help the patient achieve his/her goals. Accurate weights, daily or as ordered, are also important. Remember to record whether dressings, splints, or linens are included in the weight. Obviously, including additional elements does not reflect an accurate weight, but trends in weight either up or down may be identified and may be helpful in the overall management of the patient.

Typically, when patients cannot consume enough calories by mouth, then enteral feedings are begun. Sometimes enteral feedings are started before the patient is given the option of eating because the amount of calories is so great and/or the condition of the patient is unstable. Parenteral nutrition is used when enteral fails. The goal is to provide adequate nutrients, calories, and protein. A nasogastric tube is inserted initially and used to decompress the stomach until bowel sounds return. Then tube feedings are started at a very low volume per hour to act as a buffer against ulcer formation. The nasogastric tube allows for checking hourly gastric residuals, gastric pH, and guaiac. If the gastric pH falls below 5, or if the guaiac is positive, Maalox and Amphagel given every 2 hours alternately every hour.

Aspiration of stomach contents is a potential complication and always a concern. Gastric residuals are checked before suctioning to prevent the patient from vomiting and possibly causing aspiration. Another precaution is to keep the head of the bed elevated somewhat. A Dobhoff tube is also inserted initially, and feedings are begun as soon as 6 hours postburn. The rate starts slow and is advanced as tolerated to meet the calculated amount of nutritional replacement. Tube feedings continue until the patient can take the required amount of calories by mouth.

Another potential problem with both tubes is dislocation; therefore it is important to check placement periodically throughout the day. When gastric residuals start climbing, it may be because the

Dobhoff tube has slipped into the stomach or the patient is septic. Because tube feedings may become the source of contamination, routine care should include cleaning the blender (if used in tube feeding preparation) in a commercial dishwasher daily and limiting to 4 hours the amount of time that tube feedings can be hung at the bedside. The tubing and container should be changed every 24 hours.

Sometimes when patients are encouraged to begin taking food by mouth, it will help to stop the tube feedings during the day and feed only at night. Not scheduling painful activities around mealtime and providing frequent mouth care will also contribute to improved oral intake.

Regular bowel patterns are expected in the postburn period. Patients are given many medications during hospitalization that may contribute to either diarrhea or constipation. Patients are expected to have at least one bowel movement per day. If not, then a bowel evacuation regimen should be initiated. If diarrhea is the problem and the volume exceeds 1500 ml/day, then bulking agents and/or antidiarrhea medication may be useful to promote routine bowel elimination.

The importance of monitoring and documenting the many parameters of intake and output cannot be overemphasized. Established clinical protocols and guidelines facilitate the implementation and evaluation of the nutritional program.

Other strategies to support the hypermetabolic phenomenon of the burn patient are to keep the room temperature above 85°F (29°C) and to keep the room door closed to prevent drafts across the room. Also frequent rest periods must be provided during the day. Nursing generally makes the schedule of activities for the day, so including frequent rest periods is just as important as anything else that needs to be done during the day. Adequate sleep during the night is also very important: it oftentimes is what makes the difference between a good day and a bad day. A quiet comfortable environment without sensory overload (lights and noise) is essential for the patient to sleep.

Nurses are the grand communicators of progress and/or problems. Nurses work closely with dietitians, physicians, patients, and families to ensure that optimal metabolic and nutritional support is achieved during the postburn period.

Pain and Anxiety Assessment and Management

The expected outcome for pain and anxiety management is for the patient to achieve a balance between successful participation in activities of daily living and therapies and being comfortable enough to rest and sleep as needed. The ultimate goal is for the patient to be satisfied with the pain management plan as it is implemented. Assessment of pain and anxiety provides a baseline for evaluation of pain and anxiety relief measures. Pain and anxiety scales are essential to quantify painful episodes and to evaluate effectiveness of medication. Knowing when and how much to intervene is guided by knowing the baseline pain and anxiety rating for the individual. Patients and families should be given information upon admission on how to use the assessment scales and to identify an acceptable level of pain and anxiety. The assessment scales should be age appropriate. Common pain assessment scales include the visual analog scale, color scale, adjective scales, and faces scale. A pain history may provide valuable insight into how to individualize the pain management plan. A young child may be assessed for pain by crying, irritability, lethargy, depression, facial grimacing and tensing, increased heart rate and blood pressure, abnormal sleep/wake patterns, and withdrawal of a body part when touched.

Intravenous administration of opioids and anxiolytic agents is essential to manage pain and anxiety during the initial stage of injury due to the altered absorption and circulation volume following a major burn injury. A PCA (patient controlled analgesia) pump is useful on children older than 5 years of age and adults. It is important to manage background pain as well as procedural pain for which medication should be given 15–30 minutes prior to a painful procedure. Constipation is frequently a complication of pain management; thus a bowel management program should be instituted at the same time. Relaxation, guided imagery, music therapy, hypnosis, and therapeutic touch are adjunct techniques to complement analgesia and reduce anxiety.[11] Emotional support and patient and family education decrease fear and anxiety, thereby enhancing the pain management plan.[12]

Patient/family education

In order for nurses to be competent teachers, they must be competent practitioners with solid theoretical foundations. Continuing education is key to maintaining competency of a staff as educators of patients and families. Reinforcement of the educational process (assess, plan, implement, evaluate, and document), characteristics of patient population, updates on educational strategies, age-appropriate interventions, and ways to evaluate learning are topics that will sharpen educator competency.

Discharge planning and education begins upon admission. It begins with a thorough assessment of the patient's life prior to the injury. Identifying knowledge deficits and barriers to education, prioritizing strategies for education, projecting supplemental educational handouts and/or classes as well as developing a plan for evaluating the effectiveness of the teaching opportunity are integral parts of the educational process.

Assessment provides essential information for planning an educational program to meet the specific individual needs of each patient and family. It is also done periodically during different stages of the educational process to determine if the plan remains valid or changes need to be made.

The assessment findings become part of the educational plan, in that the plan is tailored to meet the needs and concerns of the patient and family. The plan includes the learning objectives, the strategies for education, and the learning materials. All of these parts of the educational goal are agreed upon by the patient/family and the educator.

Implementation of the plan is the next step, followed by a thorough evaluation of the effectiveness of learning and/or determination of whether the education goal is being accomplished. Alterations in the original plan may be needed any time during the educational process depending on unforeseen situations or changes in conditions that were not anticipated.

The plan and how it was implemented and evaluated are documented on a multidisciplinary education documentation form. All disciplines document the educational encounters on the same form (required by JCAHO).[14] The benefits are many. This process ensures communication of educational topics among the team members, provides a historical account of education, and documents progress and/or changes in the plan. It benefits the patient

and family by making them competent in their role as care provider when discharged from the hospital. Knowledge allays anxiety about the unknown and aids in compliance with recommended care after discharge, improving the long-term outcomes.[15] Patients and families can be empowered to become active participants in the burn care team early in the postburn course through a well-structured educational plan.

Rehabilitation of the burn injured patient

A major burn is one of the most devastating injuries, both physically and emotionally, known to man. After weeks of being an invalid, undergoing repeated surgeries, fighting infection, having the body ravaged by the metabolic consequences of injury, and enduring pain and anxiety, the patient now faces months of continued physical therapy to regain the level of function that they had known before the injury. Most patients who have sustained a major burn will continue to have a higher than normal metabolic rate and find that they do not have the stamina to easily regain their lifestyle.[16] In children, bone metabolism is affected and these children are more prone to fractures.[17] Although these patients must continue to exercise to prevent contractures, they may not have the physical strength to actively participate in such programs. Likewise these patients frequently become depressed, as they face an altered self-image and fear that they will not be able to return to a normal life. For the adult, the concerns of whether they will be able to return to work or have to change their occupation is also a factor. What is the role of the nurse at this phase of treatment? Although nurses have been very involved in the care of the patient in the early phases of care, many nurses do not see how they can continue to be involved. The transition from the hospital to home care is often difficult for both the patient and family. It is important prior to discharge that the patient and family be educated in the care of wounds and healed skin before they leave the hospital. They also need information about the normal depression that occurs post-hospitalization and resources in their home community to which they have access. This is where the nurse case manager becomes an integral part of the patient care team. Nurse case managers that are hospital based can begin to work with the patient and family soon after admission to assess the patient's future needs and coordinate these with outside agencies to ensure that the transition goes smoothly. Often case managers from workman's compensation carriers or HMOs are involved during the early phase as well. Coordination of activities between case managers is important to provide seamless care. With children, it is important for the nurse case manager to begin working with the school nurse or community health nurses to provide for this seamless transition in care.

Although the rehabilitation therapist plays an important role in providing referrals to community therapists and psychologists, and social workers frequently make referrals to community mental health providers, the nurse case manager should be involved in the overall coordination of these and other services to foster a unified approach. The free flow of communication between all providers is necessary for optimal rehabilitation of the patient.

Work Hardening Programs for Adults
Work hardening programs have been shown in adults to more rapidly return the patient to their optimum level of functioning.[18]

These programs may be available through community rehabilitation facilities, Vocational Rehabilitation Agencies, Health Maintenance Organizations, Hospitals or Health Centers with Cardiac Rehabilitation Programs or through Workmen's Compensation Carriers. The major concern for the nurse case manager and the burn team is which patients need these programs and at what point the patient will benefit the most from such intensive programs.

Assessment

Burn patients, like those recovering from coronary heart disease and surgery, find themselves deconditioned. Even 3 weeks at bed rest in a healthy subject can result in a 25% decrease in maximal oxygen consumption. Thus burn patients who are hospitalized for two or more weeks may need to be considered for such programs. Burn patients should be first assessed for risk factors associated with coronary heart disease. Such risk factors include:

- age and sex,
- elevated blood lipids,
- hypertension,
- cigarette smoking,
- physical inactivity,
- obesity,
- diabetes mellitus,
- diet,
- heredity,
- personality and behavior patterns,
- high uric acid levels,
- pulmonary function abnormalities,
- ethnic race,
- electrocardiographic abnormalities during rest and exercise,
- tension and stress.

Cardiac stress testing is usually recommended prior to beginning an exercise program. If the patient has several risk factors, the exercise program can be tailored to fit the patient's needs.[19]

Planning

What is available? Often the major issue is what is available and who will pay for this care. When an adult is injured on the job this is often arranged and paid for by the compensation carrier, since they have a vested interest in returning the patient to work as soon as possible.

Implementation

Once the details are worked out the next hurdle is to get buy-in from the patient and family. Some programs require the patient to be in a facility some distance from their home; this may present issues for both the patient and family. Similarly, if the program is in the local community, daily visits to the rehabilitation facility may pose transportation issues, especially if the patient is unable to transport him or herself. These details can usually be worked out with cooperation of all caregivers and the family involved. Motivation and the determination are often the most difficult factors to overcome. This is especially true if the patient is suffering from depression. The nurse case manager can be very instrumental in rallying the burn team and caregivers in the community to help the patient and family to see this as a way to return the patient to more normal function.

Evaluation

Success in such programs requires that all involved have the same goals and that these goals result in measurable outcomes. The goal of such programs is not only to increase the patients tolerance to exercise, but also to improve their psychological and social functioning and to return the patient to work or to the same level of functioning pre-injury.

Extensive Exercise in Children

Children may suffer from the same deconditioning as adults, especially if they have suffered 40% or greater burns. Cucuzzo et al., have shown that children with greater than 40% burns have bone demineralization.[20] Treatment of these patients with long-term anabolic steroids and intensive exercise programs can return the patients metabolic status and bone re-mineralization to normal much sooner.

Assessment

Children seem to do better if they are at least 4 years old when they begin this exercise program. The best time to start such a program is approximately 6–9 months postburn. With most patients this is after they have had 2–3 months away from the hospital after discharge from their initial injury. Like adults, individualized programs considering their current general state of health is necessary. When children enter these intensive exercise programs it is important for the parent or a responsible adult member of the family to be involved. This may be a significant factor in when the patient is able to start such a program.

Planning

Although, cardiac rehabilitation programs and the like may be readily available in most major towns and cities in this country, often they do not take children. Children's hospitals often have rehabilitation units or outpatient programs for children that can offer similar programs to the adult cardiac programs. Children's hospitals are usually found in major cities; thus these programs may not be as accessible as programs for adults. In some communities, school-age children may be able to obtain help within the school sport programs, especially if they have qualified athletic trainers. Children aged 4 to 6 may have more difficulty finding programs outside of children's hospitals.

Another question is who pays for this care? Unlike the adult with insurance or workman's compensation insurance, children are often without funding for this rehabilitative care. State programs for children with special need (i.e. Title V programs) are one avenue to explore. Other sources of funding may come from private or public charities, school-mandated programs, or vocational rehabilitation programs for the older teenager.

Implementation

Motivating the child and parent can be a major task. Often the parent and child have spent weeks or months during the acute phase of care away from home. If there are other children in the home or if the parent normally works outside the home, the parent may not feel that he/she can be away from home again for 2–3 months. The child may also not want to leave the safety of the home environment. Thus motivating the child and parent is often difficult. Helping the parent see this as a valuable program will require the whole burn team to work together with the patient and family.

Evaluation

The outcome of these programs for the child can be measured in increased exercise tolerance and improved psychological and social adjustment. A major function of these programs is to convince the child and parent that the patient is a normal child and can succeed mentally and physically. The child returns home and can keep up with his/her peers. This alone improves the child's self-esteem.

Reconstructive surgery

Assessment

The role of the nurse in the reconstructive surgery phase is to be an advocate for the patient and family. Education of the patient and family throughout the course of burn care is an important nursing function. Many people have unrealistic expectations for reconstructive surgery. The nurse's role in the outpatient clinic or physicians office is to listen to the patient and family and to understand their hopes and expectations. Often when the surgeon discusses what should or could be done to improve the patient's appearance or function, the patient and family member are reticent to ask questions or to describe what they want. Patient's priorities are often different from the surgeons and this leads to dissatisfaction. Most surgeons prefer to wait until the scar has matured to begin reconstructive surgery. Occasionally, if the scar tissue is interfering with function, correction of the scar will be attempted. This is especially true in children where scar tissue may cause bone deformity if left until it has matured. In children, some reconstructive procedures are best postponed until the child has matured. Usually, surgery is best accepted by the child at the beginning of high school or just prior to starting further education. Although it is difficult to continue to be supportive of the patient and family during the scar maturation process, the nurse's role is one of education, support, and encouraging the patient to continue with exercise, splints and pressure garments, if ordered.

Planning

Once again, the nurse case manager can be instrumental in helping the family find the funding and resources to provide reconstructive surgery for the patient. If the patient is working or in school planning, the procedures should accommodate the patient's school or work schedule as much as possible. For children funding through Services for Children with Special Needs may be available. Working with insurance companies and HMOs can be tricky if the surgery is presented as cosmetic rather than corrective surgery.

Implementation

Preparing the patient for surgery is the responsibility of the nurse and physician. Providing the patient with realistic expectations is often difficult. Many times, immediately after the surgery, the area will look worse and the patient may feel dissatisfied and depressed. Preoperative preparation of the patient and family may allay some of these issues. Surgery, itself, is frightening enough for the patient and family. In children, this can be especially frightening because it may bring up memories of their original burn treatment and the pain associated with this treatment. Postoperatively, the nurse should teach the patient and family how to care for the wound to prevent infection and further scaring.

Evaluation

Whose body is it anyway! A line from a famous play actually sums up the evaluative process for reconstructive surgery. As professionals, we may see great improvement in the patient's condition after surgery. But if the patient is not satisfied with his or her appearance little has been gained by the surgery. This is the reason that the patient and family must have realistic expectations prior to surgery.

References

1. Baxter CR. Fluid volume and electrolyte changes in the early postburn period. *Clin Plast Surg*; 1974; 1(4): 693–703.
2. Demling RH. Fluid replacement in burned patients. *Surg Clin Nort Am* 1987; 67(1): 15–30.
3. Demling RH. *Pathophysiologic changes after cutaneous burns and approaches to initial resuscitation*. In: Martyn JAJ (ed.) Acute Management of the Burn Patient 1990; WB Saunders, Philadelphia.
4. Carleton Sc, Tomassoni AJ, Alexander JK. The cardiovascular effects of environmental trauma *Cardiol Clin*; 1997; 13(2): 257–262.
5. Shirani KZ, Pruitt BA Jr, Mason AD. The Influence of Inhalation Injury and Pneumonia on Burn Mortality. *Ann Surg* 1987; 205: 82–87.
6. Tompkins RG, Burke JF, Schoenfield DA, *et al*. Prompt Eschar Excision: A Treatment System Contributing to Reduced Burn Mortality. *Ann Surg* 1986; 204: 272–281.
7. Herndon DN, Gore D, Cole M, *et al*. Determinants of Mortality in Pediatric Patients with Greater Than 70% Full Thickness Total Body Surface Areas Thermal Injury Treated by Early Total Excision and Grafting. *J of Trauma* 1987; 27: 208–212.
8. Tompkins RG, Remensnyder JP, Burke JF, *et al*. Significant Reductions in Mortality for children with burn injuries through the use of prompt eschar excision. *Ann Surg* 1988; 208: 577–585.
9. Carrougher, Gretchen, 'Burn Wound Assessment and Topical Treatment'. Burn Care & Therapy. Ed. Carrougher. *Mosby, St. Louis, MO*, 1998; 133–165.
10. Ramzy PI. 'Infections in Burns.' Burn Care. Eds Steven E. Wolf & David N. Herndon. *Landes Bioscience, Austin, TX:* 1999; 73–80.
11. Patterson DR. Non-opioid based approaches to burn pain. *J Burn Care Rehabil* 1995; 16: 372–376.
12. Marvin JN. Pain assessment versus measurement. *J Burn Care Rehabil* 1995; 16: 348–357.
13. Dziewulski P, Barret J. 'Assessment, Operative Planning and Surgery for Burn Wound Closure.' Burn Care. (eds) Wolf Steven E & Herndon David N. *Landes Bioscience, Austin, TX.* 1999; 19–51.
14. *Patient and Family Education the Compliance Guide to the JCAHO Standards*. (eds). Iacono & Campbell. Opus Communications, Inc., Marblehead, MA: 2000.
15. Falvo, Donna R. *Effective Patient Education*. Aspen Publishers, Inc., Gaithersburg, MD: 1994.
16. Hart DW, Wolf SE, Klein G, Lee SB, Celis M, Chinkes DL, Herndon, DN. Attenuation of post-traumatic muscle catabolism and osteopenia by long-term growth hormone. 2000; *Ann Surg* Submitted
17. Klein, GL. Bone loss in children following severe burns: Increase risk for fractures in osteoporosis. Osteoporosis Update 1999: Proceedings of the Third International Congress on Osteoporosis, Xian, PR. China, pp. 63–68.
18. Zeller J, Strum G, Cruse C. Patients with burns are successful in work hardening programs. *J Burn Care Rehabil* 1993; 14: 189–196.
19. Adams RB, Tribble GC, Tafel AC, Edlich RF. Cardiovascular rehabilitation of patients with burns. *J Burn Care Rehabil* 1990; 11: 246–255.
20. Cucuzzo N, Ferrando A, Herndon D. A comparison of a progressive resistance exercise program and traditional outpatient therapy for severely burned children. *Journal of Burn Care and Rehabilitation*. Accepted 2000.

Chapter 32

Special considerations of age: the pediatric burned patient

Deb Benjamin, David N Herndon

Introduction

Accidents are the leading cause of childhood deaths in the United States. Each year injuries claim approximately 8000 lives among children 0–14 years. Burns are the third most common injury causing death in children, following motor vehicle and drowning accidents.[1] Burn injuries have the greatest length of stay (average of 7.8 days) for all hospital admissions due to injuries. Approximately 11 000 children are hospitalized each year for burn injuries.[2]

House fires injure or kill over 10 000 people per year, in a place where people usually feel safest, their homes. Home fires are among the leading causes of burn-related deaths in children at a rate of 12%; they are the leading cause of injury-related deaths for black children between the ages of 1 and 9 years. Children between 0 and 5 years of age are at a greater risk as a disproportionate number of fire deaths occur in homes. Deaths among preschool children are at a rate of more that twice the national average (29.6

deaths/million children) or an average of 20% of the total percentage of all home fire deaths.

The greatest cause of home fire deaths (36%) in children 0–5 years is when children 'play with fire'. One-third of this group were classified as having physical and developmental limitations (too young to act). The leading cause of fatal fires for children 6–9 years was heating devices, with the second leading cause being 'playing with fire'. Incendiary or suspicious causes was the lead reason for fire deaths for ages 10–19 years, and heating devices was listed as second. The most common times fires occur for victims in each age group are 6:00AM–3:00PM for ages 0–5 years, 9:00PM– 3.00AM for ages 6–9 years, and 3:00PM–9:00PM for ages 10–19 years.[3]

A child playing with fire is a serious problem. Three out of four cases of children playing with fire involve matches or lighters. Three out of five fatal home fires started by children playing with fire involve initial ignition of bedding, mattress, upholstered furniture or clothing. Over half of these are started in the bedroom. The victims related to fire-play were often younger than the ones who started the fire.[4]

Scalds are another common burn injury in children 2 years and under. Scald injuries may be due to household accidents or deliberate abuse. These may include spilling hot coffee or water, children reaching up to counter tops pulling pot handles or cords attached to cooking appliances and spilling the contents onto themselves, unknowingly putting body parts under a hot water faucet or climbing into a hot tub without realizing the water was too hot, and intentionally or unintentionally being placed into or brought in contact with a hot substance by another individual.

Great strides have been made in the reduction of mortality related to thermal injuries over the past few decades. Current approaches to care have altered the mortality curves such that a child with an uncomplicated burn injury of 95% total body surface area (TBSA) has a 50% chance of survival.[5] The unprecedented survival of these severely injured children can be attributed to the advances in resuscitation, surgical techniques, infection control, pulmonary support, and nutritional support.

The burn injury produces overwhelming physiological and psychological challenges to a pediatric victim. The unique anatomical and physiological attributes of the child require the attention of physicians and nurses who are trained not only in burn care, but also in the specifics of pediatric care. The provision of medical care can induce an additional trauma if developmental needs are not addressed. The most obvious differences between adults and children are in size and body proportion. Shorter lengths, tighter angles, and smaller diameters of various anatomic structures and spaces make certain manipulations more difficult. These differences also require the provision of special equipment and supplies, which reflect the configurations of pediatric anatomy. In addition to anatomical differences there are also many physiological differences between children and adults, which must be considered and will be discussed concerning the treatment of the pediatric burn patient.

Resuscitation

Differences in Children

In a review of 103 children with greater or equal to 80% TBSA burns over a 15-year period, it was found that 69 survived with an overall mortality of 33%. Mortality was greatest in children under 2 years of age and in burns greater than 95% TBSA (**Figures 32.1** and **32.2**). Another major predictor in mortality was the length of time to intravenous access (**Figure 32.3**). Burns that received resus-

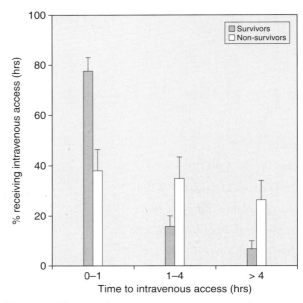

Fig. 32.3 Time to intravenous access in survivors and nonsurvivors. Mortality increases with delays in starting an intravenous line and instituting volume resuscitation.

citation fluids within the first hour had a significantly higher chance of survival.[6] No pediatric patient, no matter how large the burn, how young or with what type of inhalation injury could be accurately predicted whether they would live or die at the time of admission.

Due to their small body weight to body surface area ratio, fluid losses are proportionally greater in children. Normal blood volume in children is approximately 80 ml/kg body weight, compared to the adult whose normal volume is 60 ml/kg. Evaporative water losses in a 20% TBSA burn in a 10 kg child are 475 ml or 60% of the circulating volume, while the same size burn in a 70 kg adult causes the loss of 1100 ml or only 25% of the blood volume. Although fluid losses after a burn injury are directly proportional to the burned surface area, the commonly used 'rule of nines', useful in adults, does not accurately reflect the surface area of children under 15 years of age (**Figure 32.4**). The standard relationships between surface area and weight in adults do not hold true in growing children as infants possess a larger cranial surface area with less area in the extremities than adults. Most routinely used resuscitation formula were developed using adult patients and are almost exclusively weight-based. Since the linear relationship between weight and surface area does not exist in children (surface area varies to weight as a 2/3 function), use of these formulas in children results in under- or over-resuscitation (**Table 32.1**).

Pediatric burned patients should be resuscitated using formulas based on body surface area, which can be calculated from height and weight using standard nomograms (**Figure 32.5**) and which also consider maintenance fluid needs. The most commonly used resuscitation formula in pediatric patients, calls for the administration of 5000 ml/m² body surface area (BSA) burn plus 2000 ml/m² BSA given over the first 24 hours after burn, with half the volume administered during the first 8 hours and the second half given over the following 16 hours.[7] The subsequent 24 hours, and for the rest of the time their burn is open, call for 3750 ml/m² BSA burn (for evaporation from wound) plus 1500 ml/m² BSA (for mainte-

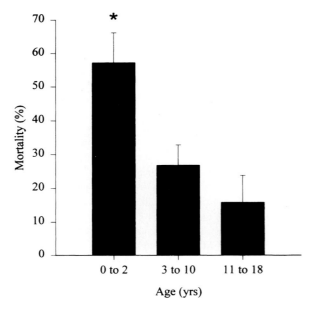

Fig. 32.1 Mortality in burns >80% total body surface area for various ages.

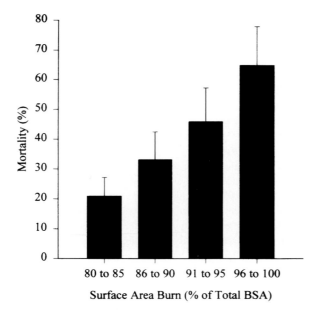

Fig. 32.2 Mortality for increasing burn size.

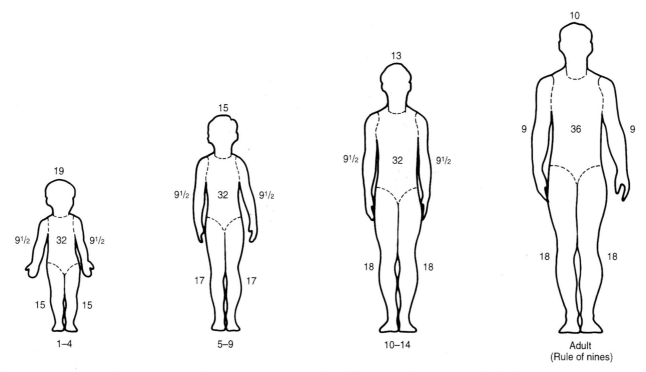

Fig. 32.4 The 'rule of nines' altered for the anthropomorphic differences of infancy and childhood.

nance requirements). As in the adult patient, resuscitation formulas offer *guides* to the amounts necessary for replacing lost volume in children.

Fluid administration should be titrated to achieve a urine output of 1 ml/kg/h. An indwelling urinary catheter is essential for burns greater than 20%. During the early phase of resuscitation urine output should be assessed as frequently as every 15 minutes and titrated appropriately. Initial fluid boluses should be administered in amounts appropriate for the size of the child and should represent no more than 25% of the total circulating volume (10 ml/kg).

Intravenous resuscitation fluid should be isotonic and replace lost electrolytes. Lactated Ringer's is the most suitable solution for the first 24 hours postburn and should be replaced by a 5% dextrose solution during subsequent days. Infants less than 2 years can become hypoglycemic as their glycogen stores are limited, and for them the resuscitation fluid should be LR during the first 24 hours postburn for wound needs but maintenance fluid should be given as D5LR at 1500 ml/m² of total body weight.

Route of administration

It is crucial that venous access be obtained early postburn, even though such access may be extremely difficult to obtain. Due to the small circulating volume, delays in resuscitation for periods as short as 30 minutes can result in profound shock. Small-bore catheters limit the rates at which fluid can be administered; therefore, children with large burn injuries may require two large vessels to be cannulated so that sufficient fluid can be given. The

Table 32.1 Resuscitation by the parkland formula only compared to maintenance fluid requirements alone					
		Calculated needs		Replacement burn loss	
Example	% Burn	Resuscitation*	Maintenance†	ml	ml/kg/%
1-year-old	15	600	800	−200	−1.33
10 kg	30	1200	800	400	1.33
0.48 m² BSA	60	2400	800	1600	2.67
	90	3600	800	2800	3.11
4 years old	15	990	1200	−210	−0.85
16.5 kg	30	1980	1200	780	1.58
0.68 m² BSA	60	3900	1200	2760	2.79
	90	5940	1200	4940	3.33
12 years old	15	2400	2250	1150	1.92
40 kg	30	4800	2550	2550	2.12
1.13 m² BSA	60	9600	2250	7350	3.06
	90	14 400	2250	12 150	3.38

*4 ml/kg/% burn, †2000 ml/m² BSA.

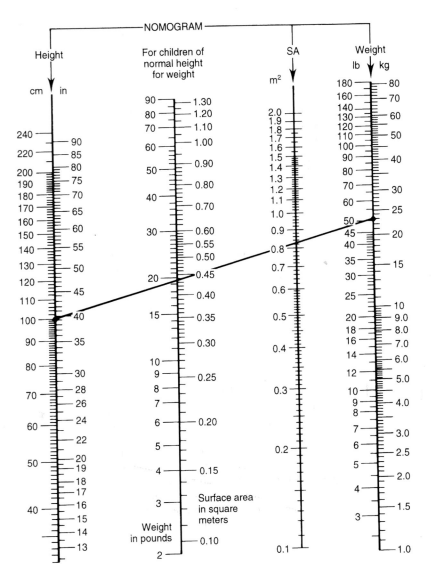

Fig. 32.5 Standard nomogram for the determination of body surface area based on height and weight. The example depicted is for a child of 100 cm in height and 23 kg in weight. (Reprinted with permission from Eichelberger MR, ed. *Pediatric Trauma: Prevention, Acute Care and Rehabilitation.* St Louis: Mosby Year Book, 1993: 572.)

presence of two IVs also provides a safety margin if one infiltrates to allow continued resuscitation while the 'safety' line is reestablished. Intravenous cannulation of the major central vessels is arduous in children. The short thick neck of children makes jugular access difficult. The subclavian vein lies within a protective triangle of shoulder, jaw, and neck; attempted cannulation of this vein when patients are hypovolemic often results in pneumo- and hemothoraces. The femoral or the saphenous veins offer the best temporary alternative for large vein access via surgical cut-down when percutaneous cannulation is unsuccessful.

When venous cannulation cannot be accomplished with dispatch, children can be administered fluid volumes in excess of 100 ml/h directly into the bone marrow.[8] There is a very rare incidence of embolic complications with this procedure. A 16–18 gauge bone marrow aspiration needle can be used to cannulate the bone marrow compartment, although spinal needles and even butterfly needles can be pushed through the soft bone of a child. Although previously advocated only for children younger than 3 years of age, intraosseous fluid administration can be safely performed in children under 8 years of age, if the bone is sufficiently soft to allow needle penetration.[9] The anterior tibial plateau, medial malleolus, anterior iliac crest, and the distal femur are preferred sites for intraosseous infusion. The needle should be introduced into the bone, taking care to avoid the epiphysis, either perpendicular to the bone or at a 60° angle with the bevel facing the greater length of bone (**Figure 32.6**). The needle has been properly inserted when bone marrow can be freely aspirated. Fluid should be allowed to infuse by gravity drip. The use of pumps should be discouraged in case the needle is dislodged from the marrow compartment.

Assessment of resuscitation

Evaluation of the efficacy of resuscitation is difficult. The routine clinical signs of hypovolemia for the adult burn victim, low blood pressure, and decreased urine output, are late manifestations of shock in the pediatric patient and tachycardia is omnipresent. Children have remarkable cardiopulmonary reserve, often not exhibiting clinical signs of hypovolemia until more than 25% of the circulating volume has been lost and complete cardiovascular decompensation is imminent. They frequently develop a reflex

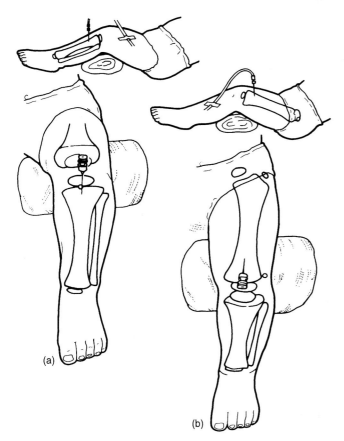

Table 32.3 Modification of the Glasgow Coma Scale for the altered cognition and verbalization skills of the young child

Glasgow Coma Scale		'Pediatric' modifications	
Eye opening			
Spontaneous	4	Spontaneous	4
To speech	3	To speech	3
To pain	2	To pain	2
None	1	None	1
Best verbal response			
Oriented	5	Coos, babbles	5
Confused	4	Irritable cries	4
Inappropriate words	3	Cries to pain	3
Incomprehensible sounds	2	Moans to pain	2
None	1	None	1
Best motor response			
Obeys commands	6	Spontaneous movement	6
Localizes pain	5	Withdraws to touch	5
Withdraws	4	Withdraws to pain	4
Flexion posturing	3	Abnormal flexion	3
Extensor posturing	2	Abnormal extension	2
None	1	None	1

Fig. 32.6 Intraosseous line placement in the proximal tibia (a) and distal femur (b). Reprinted with permission from Fleisher G, Ludwig S, eds. *Textbook of Pediatric Emergency Medicine*, 2nd edn. Baltimore: Williams & Wilkins, 1988: 268.

tachycardia after even the most trivial injury due to an overexuberant catecholamine response to the trauma or anxiety. Systolic blood pressures of less than 100 mmHg are common in children younger than 5 years of age (**Table 32.2**). Young children with immature kidneys have less tubular concentrating ability than adults, and urine production may continue in spite of hypovolemia. Mental clarity, pulse pressures, arterial blood gases, distal extremity color, capillary refill, and body temperature reflect volume status. The Glasgow Coma Scale has been modified to reflect the immature cognition and verbal skills of the infant and young child (**Table 32.3**). A child with normal blood pressure and acceptable heart rate, but with cool clammy extremities, mental obtundation, and a delayed capillary refill, is a child in dire danger. Measurement of arterial blood pH with attention to base deficit is of particular importance in this age group.

Volume overload must be avoided. Although children possess a large cardiopulmonary reserve, the young heart is less compliant, and stroke volumes plateau at relatively low filling pressures, shifting the Starling curve to the left. Cardiac output is almost completely dependent upon heart rate, and the immature heart is more sensitive to volume and pressure overload.

Children are particularly prone to the development of edema from both vasogenic and hydrostatic sources. Vasogenic edema occurs within the early postburn period when vascular integrity is impaired. Of particular concern is the development of cerebral edema. Care should be taken in order to maintain cerebral elevation, particularly during the initial 24–48 hours postburn and avoid hypercarbia. The maintenance of intravascular osmotic pressures decreases the likelihood of edema development. Salt-poor albumin can be expected to remain in the intravascular space if administered after 8 hours postburn in amounts necessary to maintain serum albumin levels at more than 2.5 g/dl. Albumin deficit can be calculated using the formula of:

$$[2.5 \text{ g/dl} - \text{current serum albumin (g/dl)}] \times [\text{wt (kg)} \times 3]$$

The deficit can be administered as 25% albumin and given in three divided doses gradually.

Table 32.2 Normal pediatric vital signs

Age	Minimum heart rate (beats/min)	Systolic BP (mmHg)	Respirations (breaths/min)	Minimal hemoglobin (g/dl)	Minimal hematocrit (%)
<2 years of age	100–160	60	30–40	11.0	33.0
2–5 years of age	80–140	70	20–30	11.0	33.0
6–12 years of age	70–120	80	18–25	11.5	34.5
>12 years of age	60–110	90	16–20	12.0	36.0

Pulmonary edema is more frequently caused by hydrostatic pressures. If identified during the early postburn period without the presence of an inhalation injury, it is usually due to iatrogenic overhydration. Management of volume overload should include restriction of fluid intake and pharmacologic diuresis. A patient who has had a delay in starting adequate resuscitation may also develop permeability pulmonary edema, which is also caused by acute inhalation injury.

Following the first 24 hours postburn, evaporative water loss of 1500 ml/m^2 for maintenance and 3750 ml/m^2 burn area can be expected. Loss of renal medullary concentrating capacity is usual secondary to washout of the medulla during resuscitation and immature kidneys inherent inability to concentrate. Delivery of volume to achieve sufficient calories to support the hypermetabolic response usually exceeds fluid requirements. Hyponatremia is a frequently observed complication in pediatric patients after the first 48 hours post-injury. Frequent monitoring of serum sodium is necessary to guide appropriate salt or water supplementation. Children of less than 1 year of age may require more sodium supplementation due to higher urinary sodium losses. Further, potassium losses should usually be replaced with oral potassium phosphate rather than potassium chloride as hypophosphatemia is frequently observed in this population.[10] Calcium and magnesium losses must also be supplemented.

Evaluation of airways

Inhalation injury, and its sequelae of infection and pulmonary failure, are major determinants of mortality after thermal injury. More than 50% of children ≤9 years of age involved in home fires received smoke inhalation injuries alone.[1] Often children are discovered within the burned shells of their homes, huddled deep within closets where the flames did not touch them, but they are nevertheless dead. Carbon monoxide poisoning coupled with hypoxia is the most frequent cause of death due to 'smoke inhalation'. Any flame-related injury, particularly if it is incurred indoors, should be evaluated for an inhalation component. Children may be spared some of the overt signs of inhalation injury due to their short stature and proximity to the floor-level cool air. Yet, as with adults, the only definitive method to diagnose an inhalation injury is through direct visualization of the airway and early examination of arterial carboxyhemoglobin levels. Signs of potential inhalation injury include facial burns, singed nasal hairs, carbonaceous sputum, abnormal mental status (agitation or stupor), respiratory distress (dyspnea, wheezing, stridor), or elevated carboxyhemoglobin level >10%.[11] (Note CO levels must be calculated from the time drawn, back to the time of the accident with arrest or for O_2 given as described in the chapter on this subject.)

The smaller aperture of the pediatric trachea predisposes it to obstruction. Equal amounts of airway edema in pediatric and adult airway results in significantly disproportionate increases in amounts of resistance and decreases in cross-sectional area. A 1 mm increase in tissue thickness of a 4 mm diameter pediatric trachea results in a 16-fold increase in resistance with a 75% decrease in cross-sectional area. The same edema in an adult airway would increase the airway resistance threefold and reduce airway area by 44%.[12] As edema develops promptly following injury, airway evaluation and management must be given priority in pediatric

patients. During emergent conditions when edema is present, inability to secure the airway with an endotracheal tube is a clear indication of the need for surgical airway control.

Hyperextension of the neck is contraindicated in the pediatric patient. Due to the tight angle between the mouth, pharynx, and trachea, hyperextension will obstruct the airway. Additionally, due to the relatively large tongue and hypertrophied tonsils in young children, hyperextension encourages epiglottal obstruction in the unconscious. The head should be positioned with a slight tilt so that the chin and tip of the nose are level. This should provide optimal alignment of the oropharynx and trachea. Direct laryngoscopy or bronchoscopy is necessary to inspect the larynx and cords for accumulation of soot or the development of erythema or edema. In children under 6 years of age, a straight blade should be inserted below the epiglottis and gently lifted to allow clear visualization of the vocal cords. Care should be taken to avoid the highly vascular adenoidal tissue. In children under 8 years of age, the developing cricoid cartilage creates the narrowest part of the airway just below the glottis, so cuffed endotracheal tubes are rarely needed. The cricoid cartilage is the only circumferential support for the trachea. Open cricothyroidotomy is discouraged in children under the age of 12 years.[13] Formal tracheostomy between cervical ring 2 and 3 is the procedure of choice when required.

Potential hemorrhage and prompt edema formation make emergency intubation difficult. Concurrent placement of an endotracheal tube via bronchoscopy should be considered. A readily available estimate of airway diameter is the width of the patient's little finger. A potential complication of intubation is to intubate the right mainstem bronchus, because of the short distance between the mouth and the bronchial carina.

Following placement of the ET tube, it must be adequately secured. With a squirming child, oozing wounds and moist dressings, this can be a difficult task. One successful approach is to attach the ET tube with tape around the back of the head both above and below the ears. An additional piece of tape over the top of the head, secured to the tape behind the head will prevent accidental extubation in most children.[14] Common treatment modalities for inhalation injury include airway maintenance, clearance, and pharmacologic management (**Table 32.4**). A recent study has shown that a group of children treated with a regimen of heparin and acetylcysteine had a significant decrease

Table 32.4 Airway maintenance, clearance and pharmacologic management	
Turn side to side	q 2 h
Sitting or rocked in chair	as soon as physiologically stable
Ambulation	early
Chest physiotherapy	q 2 h
Suctioning and lavage (nasal/oral tracheal)	q 2 h
Bronchodilators	q 2 h
Aerosolized heparin/ acetylcysteine	q 2 h alternating Heparin 5000–10 000 units with 3 ml NS q 4 h Alternated with acetylcysteine 20% 3 ml q 4 h

in, reintubation rates, atelectasis and mortality when compared to a control group.[15]

Metabolic considerations

Hypermetabolism, fed by protein and lipid catabolism, is a characteristic response to major trauma and infection. No other disease state produces as dramatic an effect on the metabolic rate as burn injury. In the pediatric patient, there are limited glycogen stores to meet the augmented energy demands; therefore, the initiation of protein and lipid catabolism for gluconeogenesis is accelerated. Available stores to support prolonged starvation are critically absent in children. The hypermetabolism that occurs with burn injury is thought to slow wound healing and prolong generalized weakness, weight gain and rehabilitation. This prolonged metabolic dysfunction can lead to loss of lean body mass and increase morbidity.

Thermoregulation

Core body temperature is consistently elevated after a major trauma. A hypothalamic reset induced by various inflammatory cytokines and pain causes this elevation even in the absence of infection. The temperature reset is thought to be an adaptive mechanism to bolster host defense against potential pathogens. Burned patients strive for temperatures of about 38°C. Depressed or 'normal' temperatures are more likely indicative of overwhelming sepsis or exhausted physiological capabilities to maintain temperature and should be viewed as an ominous sign. After major thermal injuries, routine methods of heat conservation are inadequate due to the extensive heat loss through convection and evaporation. Infants and toddlers, with their increased surface area/volume ratios, less insulating fat, and lower muscle mass for shivering are particularly susceptible to hypothermia.

Hypothermia produces numerous consequences. The heart is particularly sensitive to temperature, and ventricular arrhythmias are not uncommon. Hypothermia also increases the susceptibility of the myocardium to changes in electrolyte concentrations. The oxyhemoglobin dissociation curve is shifted to the left by lowered body temperature, impairing peripheral oxygenation. In extreme cases, hypothermia produces central nervous system and respiratory depression, coagulopathies, and loss of peripheral vasomotor tone.

Every effort should be made to reduce the heat loss experienced by pediatric patients. Ambient temperatures and humidity should be maintained at 30–33°C and 80%, respectively, in order to decrease energy demands and evaporative water losses. Wet dressings should be avoided or at least wrapped, and wet bedding promptly changed so as to decrease evaporative or conductive cooling. The patient should be positioned so that drafts are avoided, including the inlets and outlets for air-conditioning and heating ducts. Bathing or showering should be expeditiously completed, avoiding undue environmental exposure.

Nutritional Support

In addition to the increased metabolic demands made by the burn injury itself; essentially all the routine events associated with burn care increase the catecholamine release and metabolic rate through increasing pain and anxiety. Adults rarely are able to voluntarily consume adequate calories needed to meet metabolic demands, despite mature cognitive function. Children will simply refuse, and rational conversation will not sway their adamant refusals.

Those children with small injuries (i.e. less than 30% TBSA) can usually be coaxed to take sufficient calories to support their metabolic response; sometimes their wounds are closed sufficiently quickly so that their endogenous calorie stores are not depleted during their acute postburn period. On the other hand, those children with injuries of greater than 30% TBSA burn will require some form of caloric supplementation.

Calories should be provided through the enteral route via tubes placed in the stomach or duodenum. Most children will tolerate enteral feedings as early as 1–2 hours postburn, if not immediately. Several studies have demonstrated the efficacy of early alimentation and the additional salutary effects.[16,17] Enteral feedings can be given through a flexible silastic duodenal feeding tube, bypassing the stomach, which may be experiencing decreased peristaltic action.

Milk has been demonstrated to be one of the least expensive and best tolerated of all enteral formulas. Additionally, it is palatable and easily recognized by children when they are able to take oral feedings. Because of the low sodium content of milk, sodium supplementation may be needed. Hyperosmolar feedings, commercially available, should be diluted because of the high incidence of subsequent diarrhea if used as sold. Diarrhea is particularly troublesome in children because of their increased sensitivity to volume deficits.

Since caloric demands are related to burn size, caloric support should be given in amounts calculated on body surface area. A series of different formula have been developed at Shriners Burns Hospital – Galveston to meet the differing requirements of the various age groups.[18–20] The Curreri formula has likewise been amended to reflect the differing demands of the pediatric group (**Table 32.5**). Pediatric patients lack the endogenous calorie stores, which permit lengthy fasts in adults. Preoperative NPO orders should consider this unique physiologic aspect of the pediatric patient.

Body Composition

Weight gain in children is extremely rapid during the first 3 years of life, particularly during the first year. Gains in height are not as rapid, rendering an infant chubby. As height growth rates increase, toddlers take a more 'child like' body silhouettes and are said to be '. . . losing their baby fat'. During the remainder of childhood, children 'leapfrog' their growth by first gaining weight and then height. Fat is, therefore, the most variable body tissue component.

Table 32.5 Nutritional requirements for children		
	Galveston	Modified Curreri
Infant	2100 kcal/m² + 1000 kcal/m² burn	BMR + 15 kcal/% burn
Toddler		BMR + 25 kcal/% burn
Child	1800 kcal/m² + 1300 kcal/m² burn	BMR + 40 kcal/% burn
Adolescent	1500 kcal/m² + 1500 kcal/m² burn	

Fat and subcutaneous tissue provides some protection from injury. The accumulation of fat increases rapidly after birth, reaching maximal thickness at about 9 months of age. The thickness of this tissue then begins to slowly decrease until about age 6 years, but it accumulates again during preadolescence, allowing the post-pubertal sex-specific fat deposition. In girls, the percentage of body fat increases gradually up to about 25% in adult women. In contrast, pubescent boys gradually lose fat, eventually reaching about 12% total body weight in adult men. Lean muscle comprises about 25% of birth weight and gradually increases to about 40% in both sexes at puberty; shortly after this time, boys gain an additional 10% in muscle mass.

Growth

Metabolic rates of growing children are significantly higher than those predicted by the Harris–Benedict equation for adults. This elevation is necessary to meet the metabolic demands of growth. Major catastrophic illnesses and traumas have been demonstrated to produce both transient and permanent changes in growth patterns,[21] which may be an adaptive mechanism designed to promote reparative processes. In severely burned patients, nail and hair growth are attenuated during the acute postburn period, and bone growth is slowed.[22-24] Dampened height and weight gain velocities have been documented in children during the first 3 years post-burn, thereby rendering these burned children slighter and shorter than their age-matched peers.[25]

Wound closure

One of the more important advances in the last 20 years has been the development of early excision and early wound closure. Two decades ago third degree burns were treated by removing small amounts of eschar at a time, approximately 10–15%, and then grafting. Today massive excision can be easily managed in children providing results of decreased mortality and decreased length of stay.[26,27] Early excision even in the first 24 hours is safe and effective.[28] Performing early excision within the first 48 hours can significantly reduce blood loss.[29] By using skin substitutes such as cadaver skin, AlloDerm, Integra and TranCyte, the burn wound can be covered and protected for many weeks until enough donor site is available for grafting. Cultured Epidermal Autografts (CEA) is a popular treatment for massive burn injuries. Although it is an effective way to cover large burns with limited donor sites, it may

not be the most cost-effective approach. A group of patients treated with CEA had greater hospital costs, a longer length of stay and more reconstructive admissions than conventional treatment with meshed autografts. CEA did however, provide an advantage of decreased scarring, which is an important factor in long-term outcome.[30]

Scald burns in young children are best managed with delayed treatment. Unless the wound is clearly third degree, the scald injury should be conservatively managed for approximately 2 weeks to allow the wound to heal or determine itself as a third degree wound. This conservative treatment results in less wound excised, less blood loss, and less apparent scarring.[31] Recently, treatment methods for the conservative care of scald burns were analyzed. Scald injuries greater the 20% TBSA (mean 31%) were randomized to treatment with allograft versus topical antimicrobial therapy. Treatment with allograft led to decreased time to healing and decreased pain.[32] In another study, patients greater than 40% TBSA burn (mean 65%) were randomized to homograft or topical antimicrobial. Patients who received treatment with homograft had a significantly decreased length of stay.[33] The current recommended treatment for second burns primarily scalds less than 30% TBSA is immediate application of Biobrane. Biobrane can be safely used in children, even in infants less than 2 years of age. When applied within 48 hours of injury there is no difference in infection between Biobrane and topical antimicrobials. Further, application of Biobrane versus topical antimicrobials leads to decreased pain, decreased length of hospitalization and decreased healing time.[34,35]

Whether or not surgery is required in the treatment of acute burns, there is still the need for many dressing changes. Dressing changes are stressful and painful no matter what type of pain control is used. Proper pain management in children must consider both the child's neurocognitive development for proper psychological support and the child's age and weight for determining proper medication doses.

Pharmacologic support

Pharmacologic management is an important part of total burn care. **Table 32.6** lists pediatric dosages for vitamins, H_2 blockers, diuretics, β-blockers, anabolic agents, and various antibiotics.[36] For more details on the use of some of these agents refer to the chapters on nutrition, metabolism, and infection control.

Table 32.6 Medication Dosage Guidelines

		0–2 Years	2–12 Years	>12 Years
Vitamins and Minerals	Multi Vitamin	Poly Vi Sol 1 ml	Poly Vi Sol 1 ml or Chewable Tab	Vi Deylin 5 ml or Theragran
	Ascorbic acid	250 mg qd	250 mg qd	500 mg qd
	Folic acid	1 mg q MWF	1 mg q MWF	1 mg q MWF
	Vitamin A	2500 U	5000 U	10 000 U
	Zinc sulfate	55 mg	110 mg	220 mg
	Elemental iron	<30 kg dose = 2 mg/kg/dose po TID		
		≥30 kg dose = 65 mg po TID or FeSO$_4$ 325 mg po TID		
H_2 Blockers	Ranitidine	2 mg/kg/dose po or IV q 8 h		
		If gastric pH is less than 4, increase dose by 1 mg/kg up to maximum of 8 mg/kg/dose		

Table 32.6 Medication dosage guidelines (contd)

		0–2 Years	2–12 Years	>12 Years
Diuretics	Furosemide	IV: 0.25 mg/kg/dose q 6 h up to 1 mg/kg/dose po: 0.5 mg/kg/dose q 6 h up to 2 mg/kg/dose		
	Spironolactone	6.25 mg po q 12 h	12.5 mg po q 12 h	25 mg po q 12 h
Beta Adrenergic Blockers	Propranolol	0.25–0.5 mg/kg/dose IV q 6 h, titrate to decrease heart rate by 25%		
	Metoprolol	0.75 mg/kg/dose IV q 12 h, titrate to decrease heart rate by 25%		
Anabolic agents	Growth hormone	0.2 mg/kg/dose sq q day		
	Oxandrolone	0.1 mg/kg/day		
Amebicides and antiprotozoals	Mebendazole	100 mg po BID × 10 days (round, hook or whipworm)		
	Metronidazole	Giardiasis-5 mg/kg/day po TID × 10 days Amebiasis-35–50 mg/kg/day po TID × 10 days		
Aminoglycosides	Amikacin	22.5 mg/kg/day q 8 h IV; 1.5 g max/day		
	Gentamycin	<40 kg = 7.5 mg/kg/day q 8 h IV; >40 kg = 5 mg/kg/day q 8 h IV		
	Tobramycin	<40 kg = 7.5 mg/kg/day q 8 h IV; >40 kg = 5 mg/kg/day q 8 h IV		
Antifungals	Mycostatin	5 ml QID		
	Amphotericin B	Test dose: 0.1 mg/kg × 1 up to 1 mg Initial dose: 0.25 mg/kg/day as tolerated infuse over 6 hours (given q day or qod). Premedicate with acetaminophen and diphenhydramine.		
	Fluconazole	3–6 mg/kg/day IV or po. Immunocompromised: 12 mg/kg/day IV or po		
	Itraconazole	3–10 mg/kg/day q 12–24 h po		
	Miconazole	Children > 1 yr 20–40 mg/kg/day q 8 h IV		
Antivirals	Acyclovir	Mucocutaneous ASV 750 mg/m²/day; 8 mg/kg/24 h q 8 h IV × 7 days Herpes zoster in Immunocompromised Patients: 7.5 mg/kg/dose q 8 h IV; 250–600 mg/m²/dose 4–6 × day po. Varicella-Soster: 1500 mg/m²/day q 6 h or 30 mg/kg/day q 8 h IV; 20 mg/kg/dose (max 800 mg/dose) po 4–5 × day × 6 days. Begin treatment at earliest sign or symptom.		
Cephalosporins	Cefazolin	25–100 mg/kg/day q 8 h IV; 12 g max/day		
	Cefoperazone	25–100 mg/kg/day q 12 h IV; 16 g max/day		
	Cefotaxime	<50 kg = 100–200 mg/kg/day q 6–8 h IV; >50 kg =1–2 g q 6–8 h IV; 12 g max/day		
	Cefotetan	40–60 mg/kg/day q 12 h IV		
	Cefoxitin	80–160 mg/kg/day q 6 h IV; 12 g max/day		
	Ceftazidime	90–150 mg/kg/day q 8 h IV; 6 g max/day		
	Ceftriaxone	50–75 mg/kg/day q 12 h IV; 4 g max/day		
	Cefuroxime	50–100 mg/kg/day q 6 h IV		
Macrolide Anti-infectives	Erythromycin	10–20 mg/kg/day q 8 h IV; 30–50 mg/kg/day q 8 h po		
Penicillins	Amoxicillin	25–40 mg/kg/day q 8 h po; >20 kg = 250–500 mg q 8 h po		
	Ampicillin	50–100 mg/kg/day q 4 h IV (mild to moderate infection); 150–200 mg/kg/day q 4 h IV (severe infection); 50–100 mg/kg/day or if >20 kg = 250–500 mg q 6 h po (mild to moderate infection)		
	Augmentin	<40 kg = 20–40 mg/kg/day q 8 h po		
	Dicloxacillin	12.5–50 mg/k/g/day q 8 h po (up to 2 g/day); >40 kg = 125–250 mg q 8 h po		
	Nafcillin	100–200 mg/kg/day q 4 h IV		
	Penicillin G	25,000–100,000 units/kg/day q 4 h IV		
	Penicillin VK	25–50 mg/kg/day q 6 h po; >12 yr = 125–500 mg q 6–8 h po		
	Piperacillin	200–300 mg/kg/day q 4 h IV		
	Ticarcillin	200–300 mg/kg/day q 4 h IV (24 gm max/day)		
	Zosyn	100 mg/kg/day q 6 h IV		
Misc. Anti-infectives	Aztreonam	200 mg/kg/day q 6 h IV (8 gm max/day)		
	Chloramphenicol	50–100 mg/kg/day q 6 h IV or po		
	Clindamycin	16–40 mg/kg/day q 8 h IV (2.7 gm max/day); 8.58 mg/kg/day q 8 h po (3 gm max/day)		
	Imipenem/Cilastatin	<12 yr = 50 mg/kg/day q 6 h IV >12 yr = 75 mg/kg/day q 6 h IV (4 gm max/day)		
	Vancomycin	40 mg/kg/day q 6 h IV CNS infections 60 mg/kg/day		

Pain Management

A frequent myth in pediatrics is that children do not feel pain as intensely as adults do. What may be more accurate is that children do not always express their pain in the same way as adults.[37] Children may display pain through behaviors of fear, anxiety, agitation, anger, aggression, tantrums, depression, withdrawal and regression.[38,39] How the child's experience of pain from the burn injury and anxiety from the hospitalization are clinically managed will have lasting psychological effects for many months and years to follow. A severe burn injury brings many weeks of surgeries, dressing changes and exercises that can cause intense pain. Pain can also exist as a constant state throughout the hospitalization. This constant or background pain can often be managed with Tylenol alone.[40] Additional medications can be given for more severe pain and procedural pain as described in **Table 32.7**.[36] The first rule for pain control should always be, if a patient says they have pain, then they have pain.

Psychosocial factors

Neurocognitive Development

Delivery of care must be tailored to the specific needs of each patient. The maturing cognitive abilities of the growing child dictate the need for a variety of interactive models for primary care providers. Additionally, knowledge of the neurocognitive stage of the child may indicate the probable method of injury. With recognition of the particular needs of the child within a particular developmental stage, medical care can be safely and effectively delivered with the cooperative participation of the pediatric burned patient.

An infant under 1 year of age is completely dependent; consequently, burn injuries in children of this age are frequently a result of abuse or neglect. Infants are relatively immobile and unable to verbalize needs, so their requirements must be anticipated and met by the health care team. During this period, infants are developing a trusting relationship with their parents or primary care providers. This relationship is essential as it forms the basis for all subsequent social development. A hospitalization during this period is a terrifying experience for which the infant possesses no coping skills. Parental or primary caretaker involvement in care is requisite and should be initiated as soon as possible.

During toddler years, children attempt to separate self from others and the environment and this results in two relevant consequences. Burn injuries to children between 1 and 2 years of age are frequently the result of exploratory behaviors, whereby toddlers differentiate themselves from objects in their environments, including electrical cords and boiling pots. When providing care, it is important to realize that strangers and unfamiliar environments frighten toddlers; this may create difficulties for caregivers. Although verbal skills remain immature, cognitive skills have developed sufficiently that children of this age are receptive to simple verbal explanations and assurances given by the burn care team or parents. These verbalizations must be given in friendly tones and with simple language. Parental or primary caretaker involvement remains critical, for they provide necessary security to the toddler. Comfort may also be sought from special toys, blankets, or other objects brought from home.

Preschool children, aged 2–5 years, can be characterized by their imitative behaviors, which occasionally result in burn injuries due to their immature judgement skills. The propensity of these children for this type of behavior, however, can be used to facilitate their care. Children of this age can assist with their dressing changes and other wound care activities. Additionally, exercise routines can be facilitated with imitative games such as 'Simon says'. Preschool children, although possessing a limited vocabulary, can directly express their fears and anxieties. Regression to toddler-like behavior is to be expected, and parents should be prepared for this occurrence.

Most often, burn injuries to the school-aged child are the results of true accidents or inappropriate judgement. Cognitively, these

Table 32.7 Pain control regimen	
Event	Pain medication guidelines
Background pain	All patients receive acetaminophen 15 mg/kg po q 4 h
	If more background medication is required:
	a. (>3 years) MSO4 0.3 mg/kg po q 4 h
	b. (<3 years) MSO4 0.1 mg/kg po q 4 h or 0.03 mg/kg IV q 4 h
Immediately postoperative (24 h)	1. MSO4 0.3 mg/kg po and Versed 0.5 mg/kg po q 3–4 h or alternate each q 3–4 h
	2. MSO4 0.03 mg/kg IV and Versed 0.03 mg/kg IV q 2–4 h or alternate each q 2–4 h
	3. Patients >5 years, MSO4 PCA pump (patient controlled analgesia)
	a. PCA dose: 0.05 mg/kg MSO4
	b. PCA lockout interval: 6–15 minutes
	c. PCA 4 h limit: 0.2–0.3 mg/kg
Dressing changes and tubings	1. MSO4 0.3 mg/kg po and Versed 0.3 mg/kg po
	2. MSO4 0.03 mg/kg IV and Versed 0.03 mg/kg IV
	3. Ketamine 0.5–2 mg/kg IV
	4. Propofol 0.5–1 mg/kg IV
	5. Nitrous oxide 50% by patient controlled face mask
Rehabilitation therapy	1. MSO4 0.1–0.3 mg/kg po
	2. MSO4 0.03 mg/kg IV
Reconstructive surgery Postoperative period	Hydrocodone 0.1–0.2 mg/kg po q 4–6 h using:
	a. Vicodin (hydrocodone 5 mg/acetaminophen 500 mg)
	b. Lortab elixir (5 ml contains hydrocodone 2.5 mg/acetaminophen 167 mg)

children can understand basic explanations of the procedures to be performed, and such explanation usually elicits the cooperation of a child with the health care provider. The child of 6–10 years is attempting to gain competence in basic interpersonal and social skills and has well-developed gender identification. Modesty should be scrupulously observed; a samesexed individual should perform intimate procedures, such as catheterization or bedpan assistance.

Preadolescent children draw their personal identities from their peer group. They prefer to be grouped with other similarly aged and sexed children or in a private room. Most commonly, injuries in this group are the result of true accidents. Health care providers should interact with these children with the same consideration they would give to adults, observing their rights to privacy and confidentiality. The preadolescent often reacts to hospitalization with withdrawal, particularly if isolated from the peer group. If similarly aged children are unavailable, facilitating their interaction with younger children in an 'older sibling' role can provide social stimulation.

Adolescents are preparing to assume adult roles. Their judgement is limited by their experience, however, and their emotional responses are dramatized. Burn trauma in this group may be the result of homicidal or suicidal attempts in addition to accidents. All interactions with these young people should be conducted as with other adults, and they must feel respected. They will refuse to cooperate with procedures, which they perceive to be forced on them autocratically.

With injury, illness, and hospitalization, children can be expected to exhibit regressive behavior, reverting to behaviors, which brought comfort at an earlier developmental age. Parents and caretakers should understand these behaviors as the child attempts to cope with a very difficult situation. Adult responses to the child should promote comfort and security and should not punish the child. As the child recovers, the behaviors also can be expected to return to preburn maturity.

Family Support

Parents and other family members can provide necessary support, comfort, and guidance for their children. Health care providers can promote family involvement in patient care by encouraging a parent to sleep in the room with a frightened child or by showing the adult how to hold the child safely for cuddling and rocking. Family members can also be invited to feed the patient, participate in dressing changes, or simply to sit and talk or play games. On the other hand, parents and other family members may themselves require psychological support, encouragement, and specific guidance from the health care team in order to interact optimally with the child. Such care of the family is an inseparable aspect of good care of the pediatric patient.

Recovery and long-term outcome

Children with burns of even 100% (99% third degree) TBSA can survive a burn injury.[41] The question that follows is what are their rehabilitative needs and what kind of life can they lead. It may be assumed that these severely burned children will become psychologically impaired, functionally dependent and social outcasts. In a review of patients with burns >80% TBSA, a group of plastic surgeons evaluated their scarring as moderately severe, estimated that at least eight reconstructive surgeries would be required and that their future employability was moderately low.[42] A clinical investigation published in the year 2000 assessed the functional outcomes for 41 burned children with a mean of 88% TBSA and 85% third degree burns. Twenty children were considered massively injured which included amputations of fingers, hands, arms or legs, or brain anoxia. Eighty percent of the 41 children were considered independent in basic ADL skills. Patients with amputations were significantly more dependent in ADL skills than those without amputations.[43] Measures of psychosocial adaptation in children with burns >80% TBSA have shown that pediatric survivors and their parents are within normal limits. Specific measures show behavior problems and social competence at slightly below average and stress to be at the upper limit of normal.[44] These results do not differ significantly to a similar study performed in 1988.[45] Surprisingly, children who have been burned have a positive self regard with a higher self concept and self worth than age-matched peers.[46] Burned children are mostly satisfied with themselves in the areas they consider important. Psychological and functional longitudinal studies provide evidence that children who survive massive burn injuries with the tremendous lifestyle changes it brings, make a positive adaptation and can lead happy successful lives.

Prevention

Prevention remains the single best way to manage pediatric burn injuries. National prevention and education efforts have positively impacted the number of pediatric burns each year. Lowering the temperature set point on hot water heaters and teaching families to check the bath water temperature before placing a child in the bath has decreased hot water scald injuries. Prevention groups have worked with gas hot water heater companies and the Consumer Product Safety Commission (CPSC) to provide education to raise gas water heaters 12 inches off the ground, which significantly reduces the risk of accidental explosions and fires.[47]

Much work still needs to be done in the area of 'child fire play'. Three-fourths of 'child fire play' involves matches or lighters. All matches and other ignition sources must be placed out of reach of children. A positive step toward prevention occurred in 1994 when CPSC placed into effect a child-resistant lighter to protect children under 5 years of age. The importance of placing smoke detectors in multiple areas in a house has received much public education over the last several years. Current prevention education focuses on children, and especially infants that are not able to remove themselves from a fire. Since the CPSC has reduced flammability standards on children's sleepwear in 1997, there has been an increased incidence of sleepwear-related burn injuries in children.[48] One way to protect infants and children is to dress them in fire-resistant sleepwear and clothing to protect them from a burn injury if a fire does occur.

Children have no idea of the dangerous situations they place themselves in. Educating children as early as possible that fire is dangerous is imperative. Providing safe environments for our children and providing appropriate education to them is the responsibility of health care providers, the adults that care for them and the community at large.

References

1. National Vital Statistics System. Deaths: final data for 1997. *Center for Disease Control and Prevention*, 1999; **47(19)**: 1–105.

2. National Center for Health Statistics. Hospitalizations for injury, United States 1996. *Center for Disease Control and Prevention*, **(318)** 1–10.

3. National Fire Protection Association. Patterns of fire casualties in home fires by age and sex. Quincy, MA, April 2000.

4. National Fire Protection Association. Children playing with fire. Quincy, MA, January 2000.

5. Herndon DN, Rutan RL, Alison WE, Cox CS. Management of burn injuries. In: Eichelberger MR, ed. *Pediatric Trauma: Prevention, Acute Care and Rehabilitation*. St Louis: Mosby Year Book, 1993; 568–90.

6. Wolf SE, Rose JK, Desai MH, Mileski JP, Barrow RE, Herndon DN. Mortality determinants in massive pediatric burns: An analysis of 103 children with 80% TBSA burns (70% full thickness). *Ann Surg* 1997; **225(5)**: 554–69.

7. Carvajal HF. A physiologic approach to fluid therapy in severely burned children. *Surg Gynecol Obstet* 1980; **150**: 379–84.

8. Tocantins LM, O'Neill JF. Infusions of blood and other fluids into the general circulation via the bone marrow. *Surg Gynecol Obstet* 1941; **73**: 281–7.

9. Fiser HD. Intraosseous infusion. *N Engl J Med* 1990; **322**: 1579–81.

10. Kruesser W, Ritz E. The phosphate depletion syndrome. *Contrib Nephrol* 1978; **14**: 162–6.

11. Bennett JDC, Milner SM, Gherandini G, Phillips LG, Herndon DN. Burn inhalation injury. *Emergency Med* 1997; **12(17)**: 22–24, 31, 32.

12. Ryan JF, Todres ID, Cotes CJ, *et al*., eds. *A Practice of Anesthesia for Infants and Children*. New York: Grune & Stratton, 1986: 39.

13. Magnason DK, Maier RV. Pathophysiology of injury. In: Eichelberger MR, ed. *Pediatric Trauma: Prevention, Acute Care and Rehabilitation*. St Louis: Mosby Year Book, 1993: 61.

14. Mlcak R, Cortiella J, Desai MH, Herndon DN. Emergency management of pediatric burn victims. *Pediatr Emerg Care* 1998; **14(1)**: 51–4.

15. Desai MH, Mlcak R, Richardson J, Nichols R, Herndon DN. Reduction in mortality in pediatric Patients with inhalation injury with aerosolized heparin/N-acetylcysteine therapy. *J Burn Care Rehabil* 1998; **19(3)**: 210–2.

16. Enzi G, Casadei A, Sergi G, *et al*. Metabolic and hormonal effects of early nutritional supplementation after surgery in burn patients. *Crit Care Med* 1990; **18**: 719–21.

17. McDonald WS, Sharp CW, Deitch EA. Immediate enteral feeding in burn patients is safe and effective. *Ann Surg* 1991; **213**: 177–83.

18. Hildreth MA, Herndon DN, Desai MH, Broemeling DL. Caloric requirements of patients with burns under 1 year of age. *J Burn Care Rehabil* 1993; **14(1)**: 108–12.

19. Hildreth MA, Herndon DN, Desai MH, Duke MA. Caloric needs of adolescent patients with burns. *J Burn Care Rehabil* 1989; **10(6)**: 523–6.

20. Hildreth MA, Herndon DN, Desai MH, Broemeling LD. Current treatment reduces calories required to maintain weight in pediatric patients with burns. *J Burn Care Rehabil* 1990; **11(5)**: 405–9.

21. Prader A. Catchup growth. *Postgrad Med J* 1978; **54(S)**: 133–46.

22. Artz CP, Moncrief JA. *Treatment of Burns*, 3rd edn. Philadelphia, PA: WB Saunders, 1974.

23. Artz LP, Stern PJ, Wurick JD. Skeletal changes after burn injuries in an animal model. *J Burn Care Rehabil* 1988; **9**: 148–51.

24. Klein GL, Herndon DN, Rutan TC, *et al*. Bone disease in burn patients. *J Bone Miner Res* 1993; **8(3)**: 337–45.

25. Rutan RL, Herndon DN. Growth delay in postburn pediatric patients. *Arch Surg* 1990; **125**: 392–5.

26. Herndon DN, Parks DH. Comparison of serial debridement and autografting and early massive excision with cadaver skin overlay in the treatment of large burns in children. *J Trauma* 1986; **26(2)**: 149–52.

27. Thompson P, Herndon DN, Abston S, Rutan T. Effect of early excision on patients with major thermal injury. *J Trauma* 1987; **27(2)**: 205–7.

28. Barret JP, Wolf SE, Desai M, Herndon DN. Total burn wound excision of massive paediatric burns in the first 24 hours post-injury. *Ann Burns Fire Disasters* 1999; **XIII(1)**: 25–7.

29. Herndon DN, Barrow RE, Rutan RL, Rutan TC, Desai MH, Abston S. A comparison of conservative versus early excision therapies in severely burned patients. *Ann Surg* 1989; **209(5)**: 547–53.

30. Herndon DN, Parks DH. Comparison of serial debridement and autografting and early massive excision with cadaver skin overlay in the treatment of large burns in children. *J Trauma* 1986; **26(2)**: 149–52.

31. Desai MH, Rutan RL, Herndon DN. Conservative treatment of scald burns is superior to early excision. *J Burn Care Rehabil* 1991; **12**: 482–4.

32. Rose JK, Desai MH, Mlakar JM, Herndon DN. Allograft is superior to topical antimicrobial therapy in the treatment of partial-thickness scald burns in children. *J Burn Care Rehabil* 1997; **18(4)**: 338–41.

33. Lal SO, Barrow RE, Heggers JP, Hart DW, Herndon DN. Biobrane, a synthetic skin substitute, improves wound healing without increased risk of infection. *Surgical Infection Society*, April 2000 (Abstract 33).

34. Barret JP, Dziewulski P, Ramzy PI, Wolf SE, Desai MH, Herndon DN. Biobrane versus 1% silver sulfadiazine in second-degree pediatric burns. *Plastic Reconstr Surg* 2000; **105(1)**: 62–5.

35. Naoum JJ. The use of homograft compared to topical antimicrobial therapy in the treatment of second-degree burns of more than 40% total body surface area. American College of Surgeons Committee on Trauma, October 2000 (Abstract).

36. Wolf SE, Herndon DN. *Burn Care*. Georgetown, TX: Landes Bioscience, 1999.

37. Schecter N, Allen DA, Hanson K. Status of pediatric pain control: a comparison of hospital analgesic usage in children and adults. *Pediatrics* 1986; **77**: 11–5.

38. Stevens B, Hunsberger M, Browne G. Pain in children: theoretical research and practice dilemmas. *J Pediatr Nurs* 1987; **2**: 154–66.

39. Staddard FJ. Coping with pain: a developmental approach to treatment of burned children. *Am J Psychiatry* 1982; **139**: 736–40.

40. Meyer WJ, Nichols RJ, Cortiella J, *et al*. Acetaminophen in the management of background pain in children post-burn. *J Pain Symptom Manage* 1997; **13(1)**: 50–5.

41. Barret JP, Desai MH, Herndon DN. Survival in paediatric burns involving 100% total body surface area. *Ann Burns Fire Disasters* 1999; **12(3)**: 139–41.

42. Herndon DN, LeMaster J, Beard S, *et al*. The quality of life after major thermal injury in children: An analysis of 12 survivors with greater than or equal to 80% total body, 70% third-degree burns. *J Trauma* 1986; **26(7)**: 609–19.

43. Meyers-Paal R, Blakeney P, Robert R, *et al*. Physical and psychologic rehabilitation outcomes for pediatric patients who suffer 80% or more TBSA, 70% or more third degree burns. *J Burn Care Rehabil* 2000; **21** (pt 1 of 1): 43–9.

44. Blakeney P, Meyer W, Robert R, Desai M, Wolf S, Herndon DN. Long term psychosocial adaptation of children – an 8-year follow-up. *Burns* 1998; **24(3)**: 213–6.

45. Blakeney P, Herndon DN, Desai MH, Beard S, Wales-Seale P. Long-term psychosocial adjustment following burn injury. *J Burn Care Rehabil* 1988; **9(6)**: 661–5.

46. LeDoux JM, Meyer WJ, Blakeney P, Herndon DN. Positive self-regard as a coping mechanism for pediatric burn survivors. *J Burn Care Rehabil* 1996; **17(5)**: 472–6.

47. Benjamin D, Herndon D. Successful prevention programs for gas hot water heater burn injuries. *J Burn Care Rehabil* 2000; **21**(1 part 2): S152.

48. Benjamin DA, Tompkins RG, Warden GD, Greenhalgh DG, Herndon DN. Increasing incidence in sleepwear related burns. *J Burn Care Rehabil* 2001; **21(2)**: S67.

Chapter 33

Care of geriatric patients
Robert H Demling

The geriatric patient, usually defined as over 65 years of age, now comprise about 10% of the major burn population, with an anticipated progressive rise as the geriatric population in the United States continues to increase. The number of elderly people seeking medical attention for minor burns is also increasing, making the recognition of the physiologic and metabolic changes which occur with age even more important for the burn care professional.[1-3]

Epidemiology

Confact with flame is the main (65%) cause of burn injury, while one-third of injuries due to cooking accidents – scalds in 15% and contact with hot objects close to 15%.[1-4] The latter cause is much more prevalent in the elderly, reflecting increasing psychological and physical disability. This fact is also reflected in the statistic that the rate of fire-related deaths in an individual over 75 years of age is four times the national average. The male to female ratio is nearly even compared to the 5 to 1 male to female ratio for the young adult burn victim. This ratio is explained by the fact that 95% of burns in elderly people occur in the home compared to less than half for the younger adult. Prevention therefore must be focused on the home. Prevention should also focus on the fact that

30% of geriatric patients are the victims of self neglect and at least 10% are the victims of elder abuse.[4]

Outcome

As expected, mortality and morbidity is higher for the geriatric patient with a burn.[1-5] Mortality in a young adult with a burn 80% total body surface area (TBSA) is 50%; in a person aged 60–70 years a burn 35% TBSA has a 50% mortality and in a person over 70 years old, a 20% TBSA burn will have a 50% mortality.

In addition, the long-term disability is much greater in the geriatric patient. Approximately 50% of elderly patients with a major burn return to a home environment within the first year[2,3,6] compared to nearly 90% for the younger adult. The increased risk factors present in this population explains these outcome statistics. However, it is important to recognize that despite these risk factors the elderly burn patient has been repeatedly demonstrated to tolerate multiple and early surgical procedures, and early wound closure corresponds to a better outcome.[7-9]

Risk factors

There are a number of well-recognized risk factors, present in elderly people, which will lead to increased morbidity after a burn. Some of the more prominent factors are shown in **Table 33.1**.

Table 33.1 Risk factors in elderly people
- Chronic illness, e.g. adult diabetes
- Cardiovascular disease, e.g. previous infarct
- Pulmonary reserve decreased with age
- Unintentional weight loss
- Decrease in lean body mass
- Impaired nutrition with presence of deficiency states in energy, protein, and macronutrients
- Decreased endogenous anabolic hormones
- Skin aging (thin, decreased synthesis)

Decreased Cardiopulmonary Reserve
Aging is known to decrease pulmonary reserve for both gas exchange and lung mechanics.[10] Elderly people are more prone to pulmonary failure, which is the major cause of death in all burns. The presence of atherosclerosis, coronary artery disease, and previous myocardial infarcts are also common.

Chronic Illness Including Malnutrition
A number of disease states are commonly seen, such as adult onset diabetes and a previous or current cancer. Some degree of protein–energy malnutrition and unintentional weight loss is seen in over one-quarter of the population over 70 years of age.[11-13] Micronutrient deficiency is particularly prevalent. A well

recognized alteration in the gastrointestinal tract is a decrease in the ability to breakdown whole proteins and to tolerate a carbohydrate load, which leads to inadequate calories and protein.[12]

Decreased Lean Body Mass

There is a progressive decrease in lean body mass with aging.[14] The lean mass or body protein compartment is responsible for all the physiologic and metabolic activity needed for survival, and any significant decrease is detrimental since a burn injury characteristically leads to catabolism-induced loss of lean mass. Any pre-existing loss will result in increased morbidity, especially the early onset of immune deficiency, weakness, and impaired healing.[15,16] The cause of the loss is multifactorial. Impaired nutrition, decreased activity, and a decrease in levels of the endogenous anabolic hormones, human growth hormone and testosterone are causative.[10]

Decreased anabolic activity leads to a longer recovery time as well as causing the restoration of muscle to be very slow. Of importance is the fact that elderly people respond to exogenous anabolic stimuli such as testosterone analogs, human growth hormone, and resistant exercise in a similar fashion to the younger population. Therefore, exercise, high protein nutrition, and anabolic agents are essential for recovery.[17–19]

Aging skin and wound healing

There are significant changes in the skin with aging which are responsible for the greater percent of deep burns in the elderly, even after scalds, compared to a younger patient.[20–22] A 50% decrease in the turnover rate of the epidermis is present after age 65, as well as a flattening of the rete pegs and fewer epidermal-lined skin appendages. These properties will significantly decrease the healing rate of a partial-thickness burn.

In addition, there is a progressive thinning of the dermis and a decrease in both collagen content and matrix, especially glycosamino glycan. The latter is responsible for loss of skin turgor. In addition, there is a decrease in vascularity and in the key resident cells, i.e. macrophages and fibroblasts. The thinner dermis with less blood flow explains the greater amount of deep burn, and the decreased cellularity explains a decrease in all phases of healing[20–22] (**Table 33.2**).

Table 33.2 Aging of skin
■ Decreased epidermal turnover
■ Decrease in skin appendages
■ Thinning of dermis
■ Decreased vascularity
■ Decreased collagen and matrix
■ Decreased fibroblasts, macrophages

Treatment

In general, treatment is identical to that for the younger patient except for the fact that massive burns are more commonly managed expectantly.

Initial Resuscitation

In general, more fluid is required to resuscitate the same burn size and avoid hypovolemia.[23] The reason is likely the decreased skin turgor which decreases the resistance to fluid accumulation or edema production. Another possible factor is some improvement in cardiac function. Early ventilatory support is more commonly required due to decreased lung reserve and earlier fatigue.

Wound Management

The same aggressive approach at wound closure used in the younger patient applies to the elderly.[7–9] As older patients tolerate operative procedures, a conservative approach is not warranted. However, thinner skin grafts are necessary due to the thinner skin, and a longer healing time is expected.

Metabolic and Nutritional Support

Although elderly patients do not generate the degree of hypermetabolism seen with younger patients, the catabolic response is comparable, necessitating a 1.5 g/kg/day protein intake.[24,25] Since many patients already have a lean mass deficit evidenced by prior weight loss,[13] the goal of nutritional support must not be 'maintenance' alone, but rather replacement therapy, especially of micronutrients, as preexisting deficiency states are common. Nutrient supplements are invariably required. As supplements are protein hydrolysates, the gut is more capable of absorbing the peptides and amino acids compared to the breakdown of whole proteins.[26,27] Anabolic agents can be valuable adjuncts to optimal nutrition.[28]

Pain and Sedation

There is increasing evidence that the geriatric burn patient is undertreated for pain due to the misconception that there is less pain with age.[30] Both pain and anxiety further increase catecholamine levels which is deleterious. Management using standard drug therapy is affected by the decreased clearance of many of these agents requiring decreased dosages[34] (**Table 33.3**).

Rehabilitation

The elderly patient needs to be aggressively managed to avoid any early loss of function or strength which will be difficult to recover.

Table 33.3 Commonly used drugs requiring decreased doses in elderly patients*	
Drug	**Comments**
Barbiturates (should be avoided in elderly)	Paradoxical pharmacologic response often leading to restlessness, agitation, or psychosis; decreased rate of elimination
Benzodiazepines	Increased sensitivity to pharmacologic effect; some benzodiazepines may be metabolized more slowly
Narcotic analgesics	Increased sensitivity to analgesic effects; possibly impaired clearance
Tricyclic antidepressants	Increased incidence of cardiac and hemodynamic adverse effects; urinary retention and other anticholinergic effects; decreased drug clearance
*Decreased dose in part due to decreased renal function in the elderly	

As previously described, the geriatric patient is capable of restoring muscle strength with resistance exercise and should not be managed conservatively.[32] As with children, providing support and guidance for family or caretakers is an integral part of care. The patient will depend on these individuals for their well-being on discharge.[33,34]

References

1. O'Neill A, Rabbits A, Hamel H, Yurt R. Burns in the elderly; our burn centers' experience with patients over 75 years old. *J Burn Care Rehabil* 2000; **21**: 183.
2. Kravitz M, Elliott S, Weissman M, Saffle JR, Warden GD. Thermal injury in the elderly; incidence and cause. *J Burn Care Rehabil* 1985; **6**: 487–9.
3. Rossignol AM, Locke JA, Boyle CM, Burke JF. Consumer products and hospitalized burn injuries among elderly Massachusetts residents. *J Am Geriatr Soc* 1985; **33**: 768–72.
4. Bird P, Narrington D, Bavillo D, *et al*. Elder abuse: a call to action. *J Burn Care Rehabil* 1998; **19**: 522–7.
5. Fratianni R, Brandt C. Improved survival of adults with extensive burns. *J Burn Care Rehabil* 1997; **18**: 347–51.
6. Larson C, Soffle J, Sullivan J. Lifestyle adjustments in elderly patients after burn injury. *Burn Care Rehabil* 1992; **13**: 48–52.
7. Frye K, Luterman A. Management of the burn wound requiring excision. *Geriatric Patients* 2000; **21**: 200.
8. Kara M, Peters WJ, Douglas LG, Morris SF. An early surgical approach to burns in the elderly. *J Trauma* 1990; **30**(4): 430–2.
9. Burdge JJ, Katz B, Edwards R, Ruberg R. Surgical treatment of burns in elderly patients. *J Trauma* 1988; **28**: 214–17.
10. Goldstein S. The biology of aging. *N Engl J Med* 1977; **285**: 1120–9.
11. Russell R, Sahyoun N. The elderly. In: Parge EM, ed. *Clinical Nutrition*. London: CV, Mosby, 1988: 110.
12. Ausman L, Russell R. Nutrition and the elderly. In: Linden M, ed. *Nutritional Biochemical and Metabolism*. New York: Elsevier, 1991: 120.
13. Wallace J, Schwartz R. Involuntary weight loss in older patients: incidence and clinical significance. *J Am Geriatric Soc* 1975; **43**: 229–37.
14. Forbes G. Body composition: influence of nutrition, disease growth and aging. In: Shils M, ed. *Modern Nutrition in Health and Disease*. Philadelphia: Lea and Febiger, 1994: 781.
15. Kotler P. Magnitude of cell body mass depletion and timing of death from wasting. *Am J Clin Nutr* 1989; **50**: 440–7.
16. Windsor J. Weight loss with physiologic impairment: a basic indication of surgical risk. *Ann Surg* 1988; **207**: 290–6.
17. Demling R, DeSanti L. The rate of restoration of lean mass after burn injury, using the anabolic agent oxandrolone, is not age-dependent. *Burns* 2000 (in press).
18. Rudman P, Fillor A. Effect of growth hormone on body composition in elderly men. *Horm Res* 1991; **36**: 73–81.
19. Fralarone M, O'Neil E. Exercise training and nutritional supplements for physical frailty in very elderly people. *N Eng J Med* 1994; **330**: 1769–75.
20. Goodson W, Hunt T. Wound healing and aging. *J Invest Dermatol* 1979; **73**: 88–91.
21. Jacobsen R, Flowers F. Skin changes with aging and disease. *Wound Rep Reg* 1996; **4**: 311–15.
22. Kurban R, Bharvan T. Histologic changes in skin associated with aging. *J Dermatol Surg Oncol* 1990; **16**: 908–14.
23. Bowser-Wallace BH, Cone JB, Caldwell FT. Hypertonic lactated saline resuscitation of severely burned patients over 60 years of age. *J Trauma* 1985; **25**(1): 22–6.
24. Wolfe R. Relation of metabolic studies to clinical nutrition: the example of burn injury. *Am J Clin Nutr* 1996; **64**: 800–8.
25. Bessy J. Stress response to injury: endocrinologic and metabolic response. In: Greenfield L, ed. *Current Practice of Surgery* New York: Churchill Livingstone, 1995; 1–12.
26. Lupschitz D. Approaches to the nutritional support of the older patient. *Clinic Geriatr Med* 1995; **11**: 715–25.
27. Larsson J, Masson M. Effect of a dietary supplement on nutritional status and clinical outcome: a randomized geriatric study. *Clin Nutr* 1990; **9**: 179–84.
28. Demling R, DeSanti L. Oxandrolone, an anabolic steroid, significantly increases the rate of weight gain in the recovery phase after burn surgery. *Trauma* 1997; **43**: 47–51.
29. Ziegler T. Growth hormone administration during nutritional support: what is to be gained. *New Horizons* 1999; **2**: 249–56.
30. Honari S, Patterson D, Gibbons J, *et al*. Comparison of pain control medication in three age groups of elderly patients. *J Burn Care Rehabil* 1997; **18**: 500–4.
31. Tsujimoto G, Hashimoto K, Hoffman B. Pharmacokinetic and pharmacodynamic principles of drug therapy in old age. *Clin Pharmacol Ther Toxicol* 1989; **27**: 13–26.
32. Franberg W, Meredith C, O'Reilly K, Evans W. Strength conditioning in older men: skeletal muscle hypertrophy and improved function. *J Appl Physiol* 1988; **64**: 1038–44.
33. Manktelow A, Meyer AA, Herzog SR, Peterson HD. Analysis of life expectancy and living status of elderly patients surviving a burn injury. *J Trauma* 1989; **29**: 203–7.
34. Suter-Gut D, Metcalf AM, Donnelly MA, Smith IA. Post-discharge care planning and rehabilitation of the elderly surgical patient. *Clin Geriatr Med* 1990; **6**(3): 69–83.

Chapter 34

Surgical management of complications of burn injury

Dai H Chung, Daniel K Robie, Ambrosio Hernandez
Carlos Angel, David N Herndon

Introduction

Burn injury can produce general surgical problems, which are secondary to both burns and a body's physiological response produced by burn injury. These problems can occur concomitantly with a burn injury, or during a complicated postburn course. Immediate surgical problems associated with burn injury include traumatic injuries sustained from associated blunt or penetrating trauma. At initial evaluation of patients with multiple organ injuries in addition to burns, a physician should follow the Advanced Life Trauma Support protocol to first ensure airway, breathing and circulation. It is often easy to overlook nonthermal injuries when one is assessing a patient with major burn injury, but in fact, these nonthermal injuries can potentially be more life-threatening. Additional surgical complications encountered during the management of major burn patients include a multitude of gastrointestinal tract problems, such as stress-induced gastritis, duodenal ulcers, acalculous cholecystitis, superior mesenteric artery (SMA) syndrome and ischemia-reperfusion injury of the gut. Other surgical complications can result from catheter-related problems and surgical incisions. As a consequence of major burn patients requiring central venous lines for monitoring as well as infusion of fluids and blood products, catheter-related complications are occasionally encountered. Immediate problems include pneumothorax and hemothorax. Potential delayed problems associated with central venous line are infections and thrombosis. A majority of these diagnoses can be difficult to identify, especially in patients with major burns. However, early detection of these conditions and complications is essential if treatment is to be effective. Thus, a surgeon must remain constantly vigilant in order to recognize causes other than burn wound sepsis and 'burn shock' for the clinical deterioration of a burned patient.

Three previously published reports show the significance of general surgical problems in burned patients (**Table 34.1**)[1-3]. Kirksey reported a large series of burned patients with general surgical problems of whom 210 (65%) suffered gastroduodenal ulceration or gastritis.[1] Counce and associates identified the cause of occult sepsis in ten patients to be from intra-abdominal sources (ischemic bowel, acute cholecystitis, abscess formation, and gastric perforation).[2] Marzek and associates reported ten deaths among 45 burned patients resulting from general surgical problems.[3] All three reports emphasized the fact that surgical complications occur in older and more severely burned patients and the delay in diagnosis of surgical complications resulted in poor prognosis of patients. In our own experience at SBI-Galveston, we reviewed 15 general surgical problems occurring in 14 patients in 1994. These patients required a total of 31 operations and exhibited a mortality rate of 50%. Specific problems encountered were enterocolitis, gastrointestinal ulceration, septic thrombophlebitis, mesenteric ischemia, and small bowel obstruction. In addition, 18 patients underwent tracheostomy due to chronic respiratory failures. There were six deaths, with three attributable to sudden tracheal decannulation at home.

Clearly, these secondary and sometimes fatal complications in burn-injured patients deserve attention. Immediate problems seen in burn patients with multiple organ injuries require systematic initial evaluation, and major burn patients need diligent care and attention throughout their hospital course to avoid complications arising from other organ systems. This chapter reviews the frequently encountered general surgical problems in burn patients with respect to diagnosis, management, and prevention.

Table 34.1 Reported series of nonthermal complications in burned patients

	No.	%*	Age (avg)	TBSA (avg)	Complications (n)	Mortality (%)
Kirksey (1968)[1]	322	45	–	–	322	18(–)
Counce (1988)[2]	26	0.02	35	43	32	15(58)[†]
Marzek (1991)[3]	23	7	52	36	45	10(44)[†]
SBI–Galveston (1994)	14	0.01	7	61	15	7(50)[†]

*Percent of total burned patients.
[†]Significant difference vs all burn.

Pathophysiology

Burn wounds of sufficient size (30% in the average size adult) initiate a generalized physiologic response, which affects other organ systems. These pathophysiologic alterations include hypoperfusion due to massive fluid loss and vasoactive hormones, hypermetabolism leading to profound catabolic state and malnutrition, and immunosuppression with a breakdown of normal barriers to bacterial invasion in the gastrointestinal tract. Combinations of these derangements initiate various organ dysfunctions, resulting in nonthermal complications of burn injury.

Massive burn injury results in diffuse capillary leak, hypovolemia, and release of vasoconstrictive hormones, which cause selective decrease in splanchnic blood flow (**Figure 34.1**)[4,5]. The splanchnic hypoperfusion, which has been shown to occur in the early postburn period,[6–8] along with inadequate fluid resuscitation contribute to variable degrees of tissue ischemia. In the gastrointestinal tract, burn injury can result in decreased blood flow to the gut by one-third, despite maintaining adequate cardiac output with fluid resuscitation.[6] A 40% flame-burned pig model showed an early reduction in superior mesenteric blood flow associated with intestinal mucosal hypoxia, acidosis, and increased bacterial translocation despite adequate fluid resuscitation.[9] Sepsis and burn

injuries have additive effects on intestinal integrity.[10] Multiple factors can influence intestinal blood flow and it may be improved by enteral feeding.[8] Furthermore, increased levels of thromboxane, which is a vasoactive inflammatory mediator, have been noted both in the acute stage (3 days postburn) and in association with sepsis.[11] A selective reduction in blood flow to specific abdominal organs (liver, small intestine, kidney) and preservation of blood flow to others (stomach, duodenum, large intestine, spleen, pancreas) have been demonstrated and can lead to specific surgical complications.[6] Hypoperfusion along with ischemia to the gallbladder can contribute to bile stasis, leading to acalculous cholecystitis.[12] Ischemic insults to gastrointestinal mucosa can induce formation of ulcers (Curling's ulcer) and enterocolitis severe enough to cause full-thickness necrosis and even intestinal perforation.[13] Poor renal and hepatic perfusions result in organ dysfunction and failure, which lead to high mortality. In addition to complications involving gastrointestinal tract organs, decreased perfusion to burn wounds results in poor wound healing and increased incidence of wound infection.

The hypermetabolic response to burn injury and alterations in immunological function can also cause nonthermal complications in burn-injured patients. The hypermetabolic response causes a profound catabolic state, which can inhibit wound healing and immunological function. The increase in metabolic rate approaches twice the normal; this can result in excessive weight loss in the absence of adequate caloric intake.[14] This pathophysiological response includes activation of the hypothalmic–pituitary axis, sympathetic outflow, and the acute phase response.[15] The result includes fat and protein breakdown, and increases in gluconeogenesis. Defective fibroblast function occurs with possible delayed wound healing. Leukocyte dysfunction and reduced cellular immunity cause immunological compromise. Various attempts at blunting the hypermetabolic response have been studied;[16–20] however, maintaining a higher ambient temperature, administering systemic steroids, and adrenalectomy have failed in clinical and experimental trials.[14] Intravenous propranolol leads to increased protein catabolism despite decreasing myocardial workload.[16] Excess administration of glucose and insulin improves protein synthesis but increases metabolic rate.[14] Early enteral feeding blunts the response period.[17–19] Growth hormone, monoamine oxidase inhibitors, adrenalectomy, and prostaglandin synthetase inhibitors have all resulted in a decreased hypermetabolic response.[14,20]

The combined effects of splanchnic hypoperfusion and the hypermetabolic response to burn injury can lead to a breakdown of immunological barriers and, specifically, bacterial translocation from the gut, which can initiate systemic inflammatory response and contribute to sepsis. Numerous studies have shown the association of burn injury and bacterial translocation.[21–25] Intervention

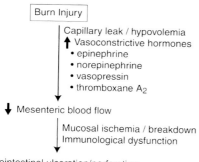

Fig. 34.1 Massive burn injury initiates events, which can cause mesenteric ischemia. The diffuse capillary leak reduces intravascular volume with resultant hypoperfusion. A massive outpouring of vasoconstrictive hormones contributes to hypoperfusion and selective organ ischemia. The reduction in splanchnic circulation can cause mucosal ischemia, intestinal perforation, breakdown of immunological barriers, and bacterial translocation, which then leads to systemic inflammatory response.

aimed at preventing splanchnic perfusion and the hypermetabolic response to burn injury may prevent immunological dysfunction and the occurrence of many nonthermal complications of burn injury.

Burns and multiple trauma

Major burn injury in association with multiple trauma poses an unusual yet complex challenge for the surgeon. As many as 24% of military burn casualties and 5–7% of civilian burn injuries are associated with trauma to other organs.[26,27] Knowing the mechanism of injury helps to predict the type of traumatic injury. For example, 88% of burn patients injured in motorcycle accidents and 36% of those injured in other motor vehicle accidents have additional injuries other than burns. Mortality is directly related to the number and severity of associated injuries in the burn patient (**Table 34.2**). Of 2914 major burn patients admitted over a period of 10 years to Los Angeles County and University of Southern California burn center, combined injuries accounted for approximately 5% of admissions with an overall mortality of 13%, which is double that of burns without associated trauma. Inhalation injury further compromises the prognosis with a mortality of 41% in the group of patients with major burns, multiple trauma and smoke inhalation.[28]

Understanding the mechanism of injury is the key to assess and predict the type of potential traumatic injuries that are associated with burns. Motor vehicle accidents account for the majority of victims followed by attempts to escape housefires and explosions. Patients that are extricated from their vehicles and those that are ejected typically have the most severe injuries. Musculoskeletal injuries are the most frequently encountered associated injuries (59–82%), followed by injuries involving the cardiothoracic (26%), head (24%), abdominal (12%), and genitourinary (9%) systems. Over half of the patients with associated abdominal trauma require operative intervention.[28] Attempts to escape from buildings during a fire commonly result in falls and multiple trauma. The median lethal height for this mechanism of injury is 40 feet (four floors) and spinal injuries can often be overlooked.[29] High-voltage electrical burns can be associated with loss of consciousness, falls, tetanic contractures and massive neurovascular, orthopedic and soft-tissue destruction. Spinal cord lesions are seldom complete and they may not necessarily present with obvious evidence of associated vertebral fractures.[30,31]

A mechanism of injury of particular interest is that of non-accidental trauma, as seen in cases of abuse and assault. Assault-provoked burns carry a 7–16% risk of associated injuries.[28,32] Burn injury is found in 10–20% of documented cases of child abuse.[33] This form of abuse is more common in children younger than 5 years (median age 1.5 years). Inconsistent history involving the burns, delay in seeking help, history of previous trauma, and spe-

cific patterns of the lesions (symmetry, dependent location, tide or splash marks, and marks left by cigarettes, irons, heaters and curling devices) should alert the physician of possible child abuse. A skeletal survey may confirm the presence of old fractures of ribs and long bones and, in those children with altered state of consciousness or developmental delay, a CT scan of the head may reveal the punctate hemorrhages, typical of the 'shaken baby syndrome'.

In many instances, the spectacular nature of the burn injury may shift attention away from the seemingly underwhelming associated injuries, resulting in delay of diagnosis, which can lead to increased morbidity and mortality. Initial management of patients with combined thermal and nonthermal injuries focus on the ATLS protocol, as recommended by the Committee on Trauma of the American College of Surgeons. The most immediate threats to the life of the patient do not come from the burn injury itself, but rather from asphyxia, airway obstruction, impaired breathing from neurologic injury, hypovolemia, exsanguination, tension pneumothorax or cardiac tamponade. Life-threatening thoracic injuries should be managed as in any other thoracic trauma patient. Chest tubes, if possible, are placed away from burned skin to decrease the risk of infective complication such as empyema. Pericardial tamponade can be confirmed by echocardiogram and managed appropriately with needle pericardiocentesis or pericardial window.

Orthopedic injuries comprise the most commonly associated injuries in burn patients. Decisions regarding the optimal management of these patients are made jointly by the burn surgeon and the orthopedist. Therapeutic decisions are based on the following considerations: stability of the wound need for excision and grafting, wound care, and early aggressive physical therapy after the injury. Although fractures away from the burns can be managed with reduction and casting, in cases in which fractures are associated with severe soft-tissue damage, internal or external fixation should be carried out prior to wound colonization (within 24–48 hours) during a period of relative hemodynamic stability. This mode of treatment has resulted in decreased orthopedic complications without additional risks of infection, poor fracture healing, or amputation.[29,32,34–36] Skeletal traction is used infrequently due to resultant patient immobility; however, this can be an option in patients with severe hemodynamic instability. Antibiotic coverage is given appropriately to patients with orthopedic injury. Most dislocations can be managed with closed reduction; however, when open reduction through a burn wound is inevitable, the wound is closed to the level of the fascia without routine drainage.[35,37]

As mentioned above, approximately 5% of combined injury patients have associated intra-abdominal trauma. Diagnostic tools such as diagnostic peritoneal lavage, CT or ultrasonography that are currently used to evaluate any trauma patient with blunt or penetrating injuries should also be considered when evaluating a

Table 34.2 Association between number of organ systems injured and mortality				
Systems injured	Patients	Age (years)	TBSA burned	Mortality (%)
One	29	28.3	35.7	17.2
Two	23	31.7	29.0	21.7
Three or more	13	26.8	28.1	36.4
Totals	65	29.2	31.8	23.1
Reproduced with permission from Purdue and Hunt.[27]				

patient with suspected intra-abdominal injury in addition to major burns. It is imperative to minimize nontherapeutic celiotomies while at the same time avoiding missed injuries that can compromise the overall outcome of the patient. Vascular injuries can be difficult to diagnose due to the appearance of the burned skin, edema, compartment syndrome, or hypotension. Angiography continues to be the gold standard in the diagnosis of these lesions; however, due to the invasive nature of the study, Doppler duplex scan is the preferred initial study to assess any patient with potential vascular injuries. As is standard in all trauma patients, the cervical spine should be considered unstable until a complete work-up has been performed. True unstable cervical spine fractures should be treated with traction via halo or thongs, which can be placed through the burn, along with compulsive site care and early excision. For intracranial pressure (ICP) monitoring, bolts placed through healthy skin are preferred to ventriculostomies.

Gastrointestinal tract complications

Severe burn is associated with transient mesenteric hypoperfusion and impaired gut barrier function, which can subsequently lead to bacterial translocation and systemic sepsis. Early mucosal atrophy that occurs after burn injury has been found to be a major contributing factor for impaired gut barrier function. Recently, Wolf *et al.* has demonstrated that an increase in intestinal epithelial cell turnover in mice is due to increases in both apoptosis and proliferation of gut epithelial cells.[38] Furthermore, this increase in intestinal apoptosis that occurs after cutaneous burn injury has not been found to be the result of mesenteric hypoperfusion alone, and is speculated to be primarily related to proinflammatory mediators produced by the burn wound.[39]

Systemic responses to these severe burn injuries as well as the psychological burden manifest in other organ system, such as gastrointestinal tract and can result in various surgical conditions. They include Curling's ulcer, acalculous cholecystitis, duodenal obstruction secondary to superior mesenteric artery syndrome, and enterocolitis.[40] Goodwin reported a series of 149 intra-abdominal operations in 103 burn patients.[41] The mean total body surface area (TBSA) burn was 43% and the overall mortality was 63%. The most common operative indications were for complications of Curling's ulcer and placement of feeding tubes. The experience at SBI-Galveston with 29 abdominal operations in 13 burned children demonstrates that operative indications were enterocolitis, gastrointestinal ulcer/perforation, and one each for obstruction, possible appendicitis, pneumoperitoneum, and open gastrostomy. Four patients died following the first operation (31%). The overall mortality was 54% and the average TBSA burn was 58%. Various gastrointestinal tract complications can occur in burn patients and they require prompt recognition and treatment to minimize the associated significant morbidity and mortality.

Curling's Ulcer
The changing incidence of gastroduodenal stress ulceration in burn patients reflects both improvement in the treatment of acutely burned patients and success of specific prophylactic measures. The incidence of gastroduodenal ulcer disease was previously reported

as high as 86%, depending on the method of diagnosis (postmortem, gastrointestinal bleeding, routine endoscopic evaluation).[42,43] Since the introduction of aggressive fluid resuscitation, antacid therapy, and early enteral feeding, the incidence of clinically significant gastroduodenal ulcer disease has fallen below 2%.[42,44] They occur more frequently in those patients with larger burns and in the presence of sepsis.[42] Gastric ulcers are usually multifocal and duodenal ulcers are usually solitary; 15% of these patients have both gastric and duodenal ulcerations. Patients present predominantly with hemorrhage, which is often massive, and perforation of ulcer occurs in 12% of the patients.

A significant number of patients with major burn injury can develop mucosal changes within 72 hours and they can progress to ulceration, predominantly in association with subsequent septic episodes and hypoxemia. Multiple factors are implicated as potential causes of stress ulcers in burn patients.[42] They are mucosal ischemia, increased acid production, increased acid back-diffusion, energy depletion, duodenogastric reflux of bile, and direct mucosal injury due to the presence of intraluminal tubes. The state of mucosal perfusion is dependent on a complex interplay of local and systemic factors, and inadequate perfusion can contribute to breakdown of mucosal barrier function to acids.

Preventing stress ulcers requires eliminating or minimizing risk factors, which are important in mucosal injury. Aggressive fluid resuscitation aids in minimizing the reduction in mucosal blood flow. Administration of various medications is also important in reducing gastric acid production. Excellent prospective studies have shown the efficacy of either H_2 blockers or antacids in decreasing the incidence of stress ulceration.[45,46] However, early enteral feeding has been shown to be the most important step in preventing formation of stress ulcers in the gastrointestinal tract after burn injury. In 4107 patients treated at the SBI-Galveston burn center since 1964, only four patients have undergone operations to treat complications arising from ulcer disease. This significantly low incidence emphasizes the important role of early enteral feeding in preventing ulcer complication in addition to providing valuable nutrition in all burn patients.

Proper treatment of established stress ulcers includes those measures currently in use for prevention. More aggressive medical therapy may include combined treatments of intravenous or intra-arterial vasopressin, intravenous somatostatin, and/or interventional endoscopy. The surgical option should be utilized early in order to prevent the profound effects of bleeding and hypotension on a maximally stressed burn patient. Specific surgical indications include ongoing uncontrolled blood loss, massive bleeding (>2.5 liters in adult, >60% blood volume in child), and gastroduodenal perforation. For these hemodynamically unstable patients, a definitive operation with vagotomy and antrectomy has been recommended as the operation of choice.[42] Death occurs in approximately half of patients who undergo surgical correction for ulcers due to the severity of their burn injuries.

Although Curling's ulcers are far less frequent today, they remain a potential hazard to all burn patients. The low incidence of stress ulceration is due to successful aggressive burn injury management and the use of specific preventive measures, especially the early enteral feeding. Surgical therapy is required in a small number of patients; however, when necessary, operative resections are favored.

Acalculous Cholecystitis

Acute cholecystitis is a rare complication of burn injury, and acalculous form predominates in burn patients as it does in ICU or multiple trauma patients. Its incidence is estimated at 0.4–3.5% in burn patients[47,48] and the diagnosis depends on recognizing a combination of signs and symptoms, which are often attributed to other problems in a burn patient. It is associated with high mortality, and the ideal treatment method depends on a patient's overall stability.

Forty cases of acute acalculous cholecystitis have been reported since 1960, and 24 cases have been reported since 1981 (**Table 34.3**)[12,47–52]. In this collective review, the mean TBSA burn was 51%, with a predominance of male patients. Ages ranged from 3 to 65 with an average of 30 years, and disease onset occurred between 17 and 30 days postburn. Interestingly, two cases immediately followed the initiation of enteral feedings after long-term parenteral nutrition. Two other cases occurred in patients who were exclusively fed enterally. Clinical sepsis and positive blood cultures were common.

Proposed etiologies for acalculous cholecystitis include bile stasis, acute decrease in perfusion to gallbladder due to third space fluid loss, and systemic sepsis with the resultant effects of circulating vasoactive mediators on local tissue perfusion.[49–51] These factors can result in local ischemia of the gallbladder wall, leading to inflammation, gangrene, and perforation in unrecognized cases. The common histological finding consists of intense injury to blood vessels within the muscularis and serosa. Additionally, lack of enteral feeding and resultant decreased secretion of cholecystokinin, along with narcotic use, can further contribute to bile stasis. The composition of the bile can also change due to multiple blood transfusions that are frequently required in major burn patients. Sepsis and endotoxemia can also cause decreased perfusion and bacterial invasion of the gallbladder wall.

Acute acalculous cholecystitis commonly presents with fever, right upper quadrant tenderness, leukocytosis, and elevated liver function tests. These findings are also common in any severely burned patient, especially when the overlying abdominal wall is burned. Therefore, a high index of suspicion is necessary in order to avoid a delay in diagnosis. The percentage of gangrenous changes (33–100%) and the rate of gallbladder perforation (12%) noted in recent cases of acalculous cholecystitis in burn patients underlie the continuing difficulty of diagnosing this condition. Ultrasound evaluation is the preferred diagnostic study and findings such as thickened gallbladder wall, pericholecystic fluid, and intraluminal sludge can confirm a clinical suspicion. A positive HIDA scan can also confirm the diagnosis but is often unavailable and difficult to obtain for ICU patients. Once diagnosis is confirmed, cholecystectomy should be performed. A recent report by McClain *et al.* demonstrates that laparoscopic cholecystectomy can be safely performed in burn patients with acalculous cholecystitis with minimal morbidity.[48]

Superior Mesenteric Artery Syndrome

Superior mesenteric artery (SMA) syndrome is usually precipitated by rapid and substantial weight loss. It occurs due to extrinsic compression of the duodenum by the superior mesenteric vascular pedicle. Loss of retroperitoneal fat through malnutrition and weight loss, laxity of abdominal wall muscles, and a recombinant position occurs in burn patients and contributes to the severity of this compression. However, it is a rare complication in burn patients, especially with special emphasis on aggressive early enteral feeding. Typical symptoms are bilious emesis, and intolerance to tube or oral feedings. The diagnosis is established by findings of dilated duodenum and extrinsic compression of the third part of the duodenum on upper gastrointestinal series study. Management is primarily medical via improved nutrition and weight gain with nasojejunal enteral feeding or parenteral nutrition. Surgical procedures are rarely indicated, but when they are necessary, the goal of any procedure is to bypass the point of obstruction created by superior mesenteric vascular pedicle.

Lescher reported a series of 37 patients treated for SMA syndrome at the United States Army Institute of Surgical Research.[53] Eighteen patients were successfully managed medically, mainly with intravenous nutrition and nasogastric decompression. Operative intervention was necessary in 30%, either for failed medical therapy or perforated ulcer. The operation of choice was a side-to-side duodenojejunostomy. There were three postoperative deaths and eight deaths following medical therapy alone for an overall mortality rate of 27%. They recommended intravenous nutrition and nasogastric decompression as the treatment of choice for superior mesenteric artery syndrome in burn patients.

The experience with SMA syndrome in children at both SBI–Cincinnati and SBI–Galveston has shown uniform success with medical management alone without mortality. MacMillan reported a series of 11 patients treated over a 15-year period.[54] The average burn size for these patients was 64% and their weight loss ranged from 10 to 30%. They recommended nasogastric decompression and intravenous nutrition for a period of 3–4 weeks in order to relieve the obstruction. Only one case occurred during the second 5 years of their review. This decrease in incidence of SMA

Table 34.3 Published series of acute acalculous cholecystitis in burn patients							
	No.	Sex (m;f)	Age (avg)	Sepsis	G/P*	Rx (E/O/PM)†	Outcome (S/D)‡
Glenn (1981)[49]	3	2:1	42	3	0/0	1/0/2	0/3
Gately (1983)[47]	1	1:0	19	–	–	1/0/0	1/0
McDermott (1985)[52]	4	4:0	29	2	2/1	2/3/0	4/0
Ross (1987)[50]	3	2:1	39	2	2/0	2/0/1	3/0
Slater (1989)[12]	5	–	26	4	5/0	4/1/0	4/1
Polacek (1991)[51]	1	1:0	3	–	0.1	0/0/1	0/1
McClain (1997)[48]	7	6:1	43	–	3/0	5/0/1	6/1
Total	24	1:2	30	11	12/2	15/3/5	18/6

*G, gangrenous; P, perforation; †E, cholecystectomy; O, cholecystostomy; PM, postmortem diagnosis; ‡S, survival; D, death.

syndrome in recent years was attributed to more aggressive enteral nutritional support, limiting weight loss to under 5% of preburn weight. At SBI–Galveston, only one patient received intravenous nutrition while the other six were managed with nasojejunal feedings and positioning. Nasojejunal tubes were easily placed under fluoroscopic guidance. Positional therapy required placement in either a left-side down or prone position for enteral feeding. The overall incidence of SMA syndrome was low (0.03%), and this was attributed to aggressive early enteral feeding of all burn patients.

A policy of aggressive early enteral feeding as well as ongoing physical rehabilitation results in a very low incidence of SMA syndrome in burn patients. Almost all patients can be managed medically through positioning and nasojejunal feeding, avoiding the potential complications of central venous hyperalimentation or surgical interventions.

Enterocolitis

Splanchnic hypoperfusion may occur as a result of hypovolemia and circulating vasoactive mediators. The degree of intestinal injury is related to the severity and duration of ischemia as well as reperfusion established by fluid resuscitation. Complications of intestinal injury may span from intestinal necrosis with perforations to mucosal barrier breakdown with subsequent bacterial translocation.

Etiology of enterocolitis is multifactorial. Ischemia-reperfusion injury to the gut as well as the presence of virulent bacteria and fungi in the immunocompromised state contribute to intestinal complications. Desai and associates reported a series of both clinically recognized ischemic intestinal complications in burn patients (incidence 1%) and those identified at autopsy (incidence 55%).[13] Seven children and nine adults underwent initial laparotomy for suspected necrotic intestine. Fourteen additional laparotomies were performed in the children, with three survivors. One particular patient underwent seven laparotomies after initial presentation with enterocolitis and eventually survived. Another patient, exhibiting symptoms of sepsis and abdominal distension, underwent five laparotomies for continued clinical deterioration, but subsequently died. The nine adult patients underwent 11 additional laparotomies with two survivors. Additional resection of necrotic bowels was required at each reoperation. All of the children and 89% of the adults were septic and had positive blood cultures during their postburn courses. Sixty-one percent of autopsies performed on children who had succumbed to burn injury showed ischemic intestinal changes. Of these, 66% of patients were septic at the time of death. At autopsy, 53% of adults had ischemic intestinal findings and 86% were septic at the time of death. These results show both the high mortality associated with intestinal ischemic complications in burn patients as well as the high incidence of sepsis in patients with compromised intestines. Other series report additional experience with ischemic intestinal complications in burn patients.[2,3,40]

In a recent review of 2114 patients with burn injury during an 8-year period (1988–1995), Kowal-Vern et al. found that 10 patients experienced ischemic necrotic bowel disease;[40] an additional nine patients suffered other gastrointestinal tract complications. Patients with ischemic bowel disease were found to have dilated bowel loops, intolerance to tube feeding, and high gastric residual volumes. One patient even demonstrated findings consistent with pneumatosis intestinalis. Seven patients required an intestinal resection and one patient had a perforation in the ascending colon. Overall mortality rate was 60% among patients with ischemic necrotic bowel disease. The authors concluded that the severity of thermal injury, the presence of systemic infection and systemic antibiotic therapy resulting in alteration of intestinal flora to make the bowel less 'tolerant' to the enteral feeding contributed to ischemic intestinal complications.[40] A high index of suspicion is essential in these seriously ill patients to diagnose ischemic bowel condition early to intervene and prevent their devastating outcome.

Although the incidence of clinically recognized intestinal ischemic complications is low (1–3%), early recognition and intervention require a high level of suspicion. Signs and symptoms may be falsely attributed to a burn wound and delay identifying intra-abdominal pathology. A high index of suspicion and an aggressive surgical approach must be maintained in order to successfully treat this complication. If bowel rest and broad-spectrum antibiotic coverage do not immediately improve a patient's condition, early surgical approach is desired. At exploration, obviously necrotic intestine should be resected; however, extensively involved segments of compromised bowel may require a predetermined second look operation within 24–48 hours. The primary goal of a surgical approach is to eliminate infarcted bowel with preservation of any viable intestine to avoid short bowel syndrome.

Pseudomembranous colitis is caused by the overgrowth of toxigenic strains of *Clostridium difficile*, which derives its virulence from an alteration of the intestinal bacterial flora. It occurs most commonly as a result of systemic antibiotic therapy; however, oral or topical administration of antibiotics has also been linked to development of pseudomembranous colitis. Topical silver sulfadiazine, used commonly in all burn patients, has recently been reported to cause toxic megacolon, which then can progress to perforation of the colon.[55] Especially in major burn patients, who frequently receive various combinations of systemic antibiotics, physicians must promptly recognize any patient who develops signs of colitis, such as abdominal pain associated with distention and diarrhea. Presence of bloody or guaiac positive stool should immediately alert one to further investigate an overgrowth of *C. difficile* with toxin assay. Elimination of unnecessary systemic antibiotic therapy is the key to prevent this disease process, and when it does occur, oral Flagyl or Vancomycin is the appropriate treatment of choice.

Ileus and Pseudoobstruction

Sepsis, electrolyte imbalance, narcotic use, and renal failure are common conditions in a burn patient that can contribute to generalized ileus. In the presence of ileus, aggressive enteral feeding with continued introduction of significant volume further exacerbates the intestinal complication. Patients will experience abdominal distension and pain. This can then be further complicated by the overuse of narcotics in an attempt to alleviate pain. Therefore, physicians and nursing staff must always be aware of the fact that intestinal ileus is frequently the earliest sign of systemic sepsis in burn patients and have a high index of suspicion to diagnose this condition early and treat properly.

In addition to small intestinal ileus, pseudo-obstruction of the colon (Ogilvie's syndrome) is commonly encountered in burn patients.[56] Presenting symptoms include abdominal distention with constipation or diarrhea. Diagnosis is established by a plain abdominal radiograph, which shows massive colonic distension. Signs and symptoms are usually minimal or attributable to the burns. Optimal therapy should be based on the degree of cecal distension. Distension less than 10 cm is treated conservatively with saline enemas and rectal tubes for decompression, and colonoscopic decompression is the preferred treatment option for persistently dilated cecum lasting more than 3 days or distension greater than 10 cm. However, a special consideration must be used to appropriately adjust the 'acceptable' size of cecal distension based on the patient's size and weight, especially in pediatric patients. An operative intervention is rarely necessary with the creation of a cecostomy or occasionally with resection accompanied by diversion.

Pancreatitis

Acute pancreatitis may affect burn patients.[3] The etiology is usually idiopathic but may be attributable to ischemia, sepsis, and medication use. The diagnosis may be difficult and masked by overwhelming burn injuries. Symptoms of epigastric abdominal pain along with hyperamylasemia confirm the diagnosis. Treatment is similar to pancreatitis in patients without burn injury and consists of supportive care such as bowel rest with NPO, fluid resuscitation, and intravenous nutrition. Abdominal ultrasound examination of the biliary tract should be performed to assess the presence of gallstone. Occasionally, detailed work-up with abdominal CT scan is necessary to identify complications such as pseudocyst formation, pancreatic necrosis, and pancreatic abscess. Operative intervention is rarely indicated unless infective complications occur.

Enteral Feeding Access

The superiority of enteral nutrition over the intravenous route has been well established to specifically avoid complications of central venous lines. Parenteral nutrition has been associated with increased risks for line sepsis, concomitant intestinal atrophy and bacterial overgrowth. However, the excessive caloric intake required in a burn patient, coupled with associated appetite suppression, necessitates alternative means of delivering calories than simple oral route. Nasogastric, nasojejunal, gastrostomy, and jejunostomy tubes can all deliver enteral nutrition but each of these options has its own unique advantages and disadvantages. Selecting the incorrect enteral formula can also cause diarrhea and malabsorption, which complicate wound healing and local wound care, especially in the areas of perineum. The optimal choice would include a method of delivery which impacts least on patient care and a formula which rapidly achieves a positive nitrogen balance without associated diarrhea.

A clear advantage of nasogastric tubes is the avoidance of an abdominal operation and its associated complications. Nasogastric tubes are soft, thin, and pliable, and they avoid the gastric, pulmonary, and nasal complications of large decompression nasogastric tubes. However, these tubes are difficult to maintain, and can inadvertently be displaced or migrate into the pulmonary tree, resulting in potentially serious complications of aspiration. Placement of nasoduodenal or nasojejunal feeding tubes under fluoroscopic guidance has become a standard practice for many burn centers. With its tip placed well beyond the pylorus, risk of aspiration of enteral feeding is negligible. This method is especially useful in major burn patients who frequently experience gastric ileus during immediate postburn period. Immediate enteral feedings can be initiated at the same time the gastric decompression is accomplished with a nasogastric tube. Nasoduodenal or nasojejunal feedings require careful titration to avoid overly aggressive introduction of enteral nutrition.

Surgically placed gastrostomy tubes are maintained for long periods and require minimal experience to manage;[57] however, the surgical site care may be complicated by the presence of a burn wound. Although alternate techniques of placement such as percutaneous endoscopic[58] and laparoscopic-assisted[59] methods are now available to minimize the morbidity associated with surgically placed gastrostomy, it still requires diligent care to avoid complications related to the gastrostomy tube itself. Furthermore, a gastrostomy tube is not adequate for effective gastric decompression in major burn patients. Although jejunostomy feeding can eliminate a risk of gastroesophageal reflex associated with aggressive gastric tube feedings, it also carries the disadvantages of an operative procedure.

Diarrhea in enterally fed burn patients has been extensively reviewed by Gottschlich and associates.[60] They prospectively followed the course of 50 enterally fed postburn patients. Enteral formulas were chosen at the discretion of an attending physician or nutritional specialist. One formula available was a modular tube-feeding recipe specifically prepared for burn patients. It was composed of 85% carbohydrate (nonlactose), 15% fat (50% fish oil, 50% safflower oil), provided 1 kcal/ml, and had a osmolality of 549 mosmol/kg H_2O. Of the patients studied, 50% received this formula. The incidence of diarrhea (defined by >4 bowel movements per day, or large (>200 g) liquid stools) was 32%. Significant variables for the increased occurrence of diarrhea were age (older patients), percent of third-degree burn (average 40%), treatment with antibiotics, high fat intake (>25 g), inadequate vitamin A intake (<10 000 IU), late initiation of tube feedings (>48 hours postburn), and the use of a formula other than the modular tube feeding recipe. Neither osmolality of the formula nor low serum albumin correlated with the occurrence of diarrhea. Given these findings, enteral feeding should be initiated early after burn injury, specifically formulated to avoid diarrhea.

Catheter-related complications

The establishment of vascular access in burn patients is one of the most routinely performed but crucial procedures. It is imperative that patients have adequate vascular access to receive aggressive fluid resuscitation during the critical immediate postburn period. Although peripheral vascular access with large-bore catheters is the preferred route, the placement of a peripheral intravenous line can be extremely difficult in major burn patients with extensive burns over their extremities. The use of central venous lines has become the standard practice in major burn patients to provide secure vascular access for administration of fluid and blood products as well as perioperative monitoring of intravascular volume status. However, central venous line placement can be associated with potentially serious complications. Particular attention should be given to the use of various available cannulation sites depending on the size of the patient, as well as taking into consideration clinical conditions of burn wounds. Arterial monitoring is frequently necessary in critically-ill burn patients. Although placement of arterial cannula in the radial or pedal artery has become routine, the placement of femoral arterial cannula should be considered with extreme caution due to potential ischemic complication to distal limb.

Suppurative Thrombophlebitis

In 1980, Pruitt and associates first reported the significance of suppurative thrombophlebitis in burn patients.[61] Their report included 193 patients treated over an 18-year period, and this represented 4% of all burns seen at the United States Army Institute for Surgical Research. Other centers have, since then, also reported experience with suppurative thrombophlebitis involving peripheral veins in burn patients.[2] More recently, experience with catheter-related septic central venous thrombosis has been reported. Not all of these infections occur in association with venous thrombosis, and specific risk factors for developing suppurative thrombophlebitis include both burn injury and prolonged intravenous catheterization (**Table 34.4**)[62].

The presentation of suppurative thrombophlebitis is often occult with approximately 20% of patients showing no local clinical signs (**Table 34.5**)[62]. In burn patients, occult suppurative thrombophlebitis is most frequent; only 36% of patients reported by Pruitt exhibited local signs.[63] Burn patients frequently display a positive blood culture and clinical sepsis without obvious source. Clinical sepsis is accompanied by hyperpyrexia, hypothermia, change in mental status, hyperglycemia, and hypotension. Diagnosis in these cases requires thorough exploration of all catheter sites. The absence of pus at the site or within the vein does not necessarily rule out suppurative thrombophlebitis.[62,63] Proper exploration of a vein requires surgical cut-down and expression of vein contents. If pus or a clot is found, the involved vein should be completely excised to a normal appearing vein (usually at the first uninvolved tributary). If exploration is negative at one site, then sequential exploration of other sites is absolutely necessary until

Table 34.4 Factors that increase risk of septic thrombophlebitis

Prolonged catheterization (greater than 72 hours)
Concentrated intravenous solutions (K+, antibiotics)
Venous cut-downs
Plastic catheters
Lower extremity access
Poor sterile technique
Emergency catheterization
Frequent intravenous line manipulation
Burns

Reproduced with permission from Golueke and Zinner.[57]

Table 34.5 Local clinical signs of septic phlebitis

Clinical sign	Percentage of patients
Erythema	50.9
Edema	49.0
Local tenderness	45.1
Palpable cord	35.3
Purulent drainage	16.6
Asymptomatic	20.4

Reproduced with permission from Golueke and Zinner.[57]

the source of infection is identified. Besides surgical excision, systemic antibiotics must be administered to eradicate the involved organisms. The most commonly found organisms in infected veins in burn patients reflect those cultured from a burn wound.[63] In nonburn patients, *Staphlococcus, Klebsiella*, and *Candida* are cultured in descending order of frequency.[62] Antibiotics are chosen based on sensitivities and administered until clinical cellulitis resolves.

Catheter-related septic central venous thrombosis has increasingly been recognized in the burn population as it parallels the increased use of central venous catheters in these patients.[63] Kaufman and associates reported five patients diagnosed with septic evidence of thrombosis, catheter infection diagnosed by positive catheter tip and blood culture, and ongoing bacteremia after catheter removal.[64] All of these patients had local evidence of disease manifested by ipsilateral upper extremity swelling. Catheter-related thrombosis can be managed by removal of catheter alone; however, if significant obstruction of flow is present, full systemic heparinization may be required.[64] No surgical intervention was required in these cases; however, surgical therapy may be warranted if medical therapy fails. Three burn patients with septic central venous thrombosis, reported by Pruitt, survived with nonoperative therapy.[63] The prevention of catheter-related suppurative thrombophlebitis requires avoidance of specific risk factors (**Table 34.4**). The incidence of catheter-related infection ranges considerably due to frequent lack of proper documentation of systemic sepsis. When infection occurs without an identifiable source, a sequential exploration of all catheter sites should be performed early in order to avoid the potential catastrophe of death from suppurative thrombophlebitis. The catheter should be removed and its tip cultured for confirmation of diagnosis as well as identification of involved organisms. Appropriate antibiotic coverage should be started immediately. In order to minimize the incidence of these catheter-related complications of thrombosis or infection, the current standard practice for central venous access at SBI–Galveston consists of meticulous aseptic care at the catheter insertion site along with regularly scheduled catheter change. Central venous catheters are changed over a guidewire placed through an existing catheter every 3 days and a new central venous cannula on a fresh site is placed every 6 days.

Thoracic Complications

With the frequent use of central venous lines in major burn patients, the risk for potential thoracic complications associated with placement of central venous lines must be recognized. Although the overall incidence is quite small (1–4%), any thoracic complications can lead to life-threatening conditions. Pneumothorax is caused by lung parenchyma injury during venipuncture of central veins, and can be treated with observation or small chest tube placement. However, if unrecognized, especially in patients receiving positive ventilatory pressure support, it can rapidly progress to tension pneumothorax with hemodynamic compromise. In order to reduce the risk of puncturing the lung parenchyma during attempted central venous line placement, it is crucial to be familiar with the central venous anatomy in the neck and chest areas. Especially in small pediatric patients, percutaneous access to subclavian veins may required more acute cephalad angle of approach under the clavicle due to its venous anatomical differences when compared to adults.[65] Proper shoulder roll should be placed to maximally enhance the space between the first rib and the clavicle for easier access to subclavian veins. The patient should be adequately sedated and given sufficient pain medication to avoid any movement during the procedure. If one fails to access a central vein on one side, immediate chest radiography should be obtained to rule out pneumothorax before proceeding to the other side.

Bleeding related to placement of central venous catheters varies in location and can be subcutaneous, mediastinal, intrathoracic, or pericardial. Subcutaneous hemorrhage occurs typically in patients with a coagulopathy but should be controlled with local pressure. Hemorrhage into the thoracic space can occur at the time of catheter insertion or after the catheter has been in place, from erosion through the vein wall. Blood may accumulate into the mediastinum, pleural space or pericardium. The most common situation leading to venous wall perforation occurs during an insertion of percutaneous introducer sheath over a guidewire. As the sheath is introduced, it can fail to negotiate a path of a vein and traumatize the vein wall. If the injury is small, it can resolve on its own with thrombosis formation; however, in cases of larger venous tear, rapid bleeding into the thoracic cavity can occur and emergent thoracotomy may be necessary. In order to reduce the risk of bleeding complication, many burn centers rely on guidance of fluoroscopy during the insertion of central venous lines. Pericardial tamponade can also occur with high mortality. Bleeding or infusion of fluid into pericardial space can rapidly compromise the cardiac function and results in hemodynamic collapse. Patients typically manifest hypotension, muffled heart sounds and distended neck veins (Beck's triad). However, the classic triad of symptoms is rarely all present and a physician must have a high index of suspicion in order to recognize this condition early. Echocardiogram can confirm the clinical suspicion and pericardiocentesis or pericardial window can return the cardiac function to baseline.

Arterial injury

Arterial monitoring is frequently required in managing patients with major burns, especially during the perioperative period. Although radial and pedal arterial cannulas are routinely placed without significant complications, it can be associated with problems such as hematoma and pain. The larger and more proximal femoral artery can also be considered for access. In pediatric burn patients, the femoral artery can be very small and catheter within the vessel can result in near complete occlusion of blood flow to distal aspect of the limb. If this occurs, the catheter should be immediately removed and the Doppler flow study should be obtained to assess for the presence of intimal flap. Conservative treatment with optimizing the hemodynamics and systemic heparinization are usually adequate to restore blood flow. Surgical intervention is rarely necessary. Mostly importantly, arterial cannulas should be removed as soon as their potential benefit of invasive monitoring is no longer present for the care of major burn patients.

Summary

Surgical problems, which are secondary to burn injury, can cause devastating physiological responses. Physicians must have a high index of suspicion to identify any associated nonthermal injuries when evaluating patients with major burn injury. When presented with patients with multiple organ injuries, the protocols for ATLS should be followed, ensuring the airway, breathing and circulation. Injuries to other organ system should be handled in a systemic fashion with involvement of appropriate consultant surgeons. A multitude of gastrointestinal complications can occur during the course of prolonged hospitalization for major burn patients. Ulcers and other complications must be prevented when possible and detected and treated when present. Finally, medical professionals must be constantly on the alert for problems related to intravenous catheters and tube feedings, as related infections and complications can be fatal.

References

1. Kirksey TD, Moncrief JA, Pruitt BA, O'Neill JA. Gastrointestinal complications in burns. *Am J Surg* 1968; 116: 627–33.
2. Counce JS, Cone JB, McAlister L, Wallace B, Caldwell FT. Surgical complications of thermal injury. *Am J Surg* 1988; 156: 556–7.
3. Marzek PA, Miller FB, Cryer HM, Polk HC. Nonthermal surgical complications in burn patients. *South Med J* 1991; 84: 689–91.
4. Banks RO, Gallavan RH, Zinner MJ, *et al.* Vasoactive agents in control of the mesenteric circulation. *Fedn Proc* 1985; 44: 2743–9.
5. Hilton JG, Marullo DS. Trauma induced increases in plasma vasopressin and angiotensin II. *Life Sci* 1987; 41: 2195–200.
6. Asch MJ, Meseral PM, Mason AD, Pruitt BA. Regional blood flow in the burned unanesthetized dog. *Surg Forum* 1971; 22: 55–6.
7. Jones WG, Minei JP, Barber AE, Fahey TJ, Shires GT III, Shires GT. Splanchnic vasoconstriction and bacterial translocation after thermal injury. *Am J Physiol* 1991; 261: H1190–6.
8. Inoue S, Lukes S, Alexander JW, Trocki O, Silberstein EB. Increased gut blood flow with early enteral feeding in burned guinea pigs. *J Burn Care Rehabil* 1989; 10: 300–8.
9. Tokyay R, Ziegler ST, Traber DL, *et al.* Postburn gastrointestinal vasoconstriction increases bacterial and endotoxin translocation. *J Appl Physiol* 1993; 74: 1521–7.
10. Jones WG, Minei JP, Barber AE, *et al.* Additive effects of thermal injury and infection on the small bowel. *Surgery* 1990; 108: 63–70.
11. Herndon DN, Abston S, Stein MD. Increased thromboxane B₂ levels in the plasma of burned and septic burned patients. *Surg Gynecol Obstet* 1984; 159: 210–3.
12. Slater H, Goldfarb IW. Acute septic cholecystitis in patients with burn injuries. *J Burn Care Rehabil* 1989; 10: 445–7.
13. Desai MH, Herndon DN, Rutan RL, Abston S, Linares HA. Ischemic intestinal complications in patients with burns. *Surg Gynecol Obstet* 1991; 172: 257–61.
14. Herndon DN, Curreri PW, Abston S, Rutan TC, Barrow RE. Treatment of burns. *Curr Prob Surg* 1987; 6: 349–57.
15. Kupper TS, Deitch EA, Baker CC, Wong W. The human burn wound as a primary source of interleukin-1 activity. *Surgery* 1986; 100: 409–41.
16. Herndon DN, Barrow RE, Rutan TC, *et al.* Effect of propranolol administration on hemodynamic and metabolic responses of burned pediatric patients. *Ann Surg* 1988; 208: 484–92.
17. McArdle AH, Palmason C, Brown RA, Brown HC, Williams HB. Early enteral feeding of patients with major burns: prevention of catabolism. *Ann Plastic Surg* 1984; 13(5): 396–401.
18. Mochizuki H, Trocki O, Dominioni L, Brackett KA, Joffe SN, Alexander JW. Mechanism of prevention of postburn hypermetabolism and catabolism by early enteral feeding. *Ann Surg* 1984; 200: 297–310.
19. Sologub VK, Zeats TL, Tarasov AV, Mordkovitch MR, Yashin AY. Enteral hyperalimentation of burned patients: the possibility of correcting metabolic disorders by the early administration of prolonged high calorie evenly distributed tube feeds. *Burns* 1992; 18: 245–9.
20. Fleming YD, Rutan RL, Jahoor F, Barrow RE, Wolfe RR, Herndon DN. Effect of recombinant human growth hormone on catabolic hormones and free fatty acids following thermal injury. *J Trauma* 1992; 32: 698–703.
21. Jones WG, Minei JP, Barber AE, *et al.* Bacterial translocation and intestinal atrophy after thermal injury and burn wound sepsis. *Ann Surg* 1990; 211: 399–405.
22. Carter EA, Tompkins RG, Schiffrin E, Burke JF. Cutaneous thermal injury alters macromolecular permeability of rat small intestine. *Surgery* 1990; 107: 335–41.
23. Levoyer T, Cioffi WG, Pratt L, *et al.* Alterations in intestinal permeability after thermal injury. *Arch Surg* 1992; 127: 26–30.
24. Deitch EA, Winterton J, Berg R. Thermal injury promotes bacterial translocation from the gastrointestinal tract in mice with impaired T-cell mediated immunity. *Arch Surg* 1986; 121: 97–101.

25. Alexander JW, Gianotti L, Pyles T, Carey MA, Babcock GF. Distribution and survival of *Escherichia coli* translocation from the intestine after thermal injury. *Ann Surg* 1990; 213(6): 558–66.

26. Pruitt BA. Management of burns in the multiple injury patient. *Surg Clin N Am* 1970; 50: 1283–300.

27. Purdue GF, Hunt JL. Multiple trauma and the burn patient. *Am J Surg* 1989; 158: 536–9.

28. Dougherty W, Waxman K. The complexities of managing severe burns with associated trauma. *Surg Clin N Am* 1996; 76(4): 923–58.

29. Wong L, Grande CM, Munster AM. Burns and associated nonthermal trauma: An analysis of management, outcome, and relation to the injury severity score. *J Burn Care Rehabil* 1989; 10: 512–6.

30. Briggs D, Kirwin M, Morrison KM. Severe occupational traumatic injuries. *Primary Care* 1994; 21(2): 363–4.

31. Baxter CR. Present concepts in the management of major electrical injury. *Surg Clin North Am* 1970; 50(6): 1913–4.

32. Purdue GF, Hunt JL, Layton TR, Copeland CE, delMundo AG, Baxter CR. Burns in motor vehicle accidents. *J Trauma* 1985; 25: 217–9.

33. Sharp RJ. Burns. In: Ashcraft, Murphy, Sharp, Sigalet, Snyder, eds. *Pediatric Surgery*. Philadelphia: WB Saunders, 2000; 159–60.

34. Dossett AB, Hunt JL, Purdue GF, Schlegel JD. Early orthopedic intervention in burn patients with major fractures. *J Trauma* 1991; 31: 888–93.

35. Saffle JR, Achnelby A, Hofmann O, Warden GD. The management of fractures in thermally injured patients. *J Trauma* 1983; 23: 902–10.

36. Curtis MJ, Clarke JA. Skeletal injury in thermal trauma: a review of management. *Br J Accid Surg* 1989; 20: 333–6.

37. Frye KE, Luterman A. Burns and fractures. *Orthopedic Nursing* 1999; Jan/Feb: 30–5.

38. Wolf SE, Ikeda H, Matin S, *et al.* Cutaneous burn increases apoptosis in the gut epithelium of mice. *J Am Coll Surg* 1999; 188: 10–6.

39. Ramzy RI, Wolf SE, Irtun O, Hart DW, Thompson JC, Herndon DN. Gut epithelial apoptosis after severe burn: Effects of gut hypoperfusion. *J Am Coll Surg* 2000; 190: 281–7.

40. Kowal-Vern A, McGill V, Gamelli RL. Ischemic necrotic bowel disease in thermal injury. *Arch Surg* 1997; 132: 440–3.

41. Goodwin CW, McManus WF, Mason AD, Pruitt BA. Management of abdominal wounds in thermally injured patients. *J Trauma* 1982; 22: 92–7.

42. Pruitt BA, Goodwin CW. Stress ulcer disease in the burned patient. *World J Surg* 1981; 5: 209–22.

43. Czaja AJ, McAlhany JC, Pruitt BA. Acute gastroduodenal disease after thermal injury. *N Engl J Med* 1974; 18: 925–9.

44. Yao-Liang L, Ke-Jian Y. Clinical characteristics and operative treatment of postburn stress ulcers. *Burns* 1983; 10: 30–3.

45. McAlhany JC, Czaja AJ, Pruitt BA. Antacid control of complications from acute gastroduodenal disease after burns. *J Trauma* 1976; 16: 645–8.

46. McElwee HP, Sirinek KR, Levine BA. Cimetidine affords protection equal to antacids in prevention of stress ulceration following thermal injury. *Surgery* 1979; 86: 620–6.

47. Gately JF, Thomas EJ. Acute cholecystitis occurring as a complication of other diseases. *Arch Surg* 1983; 118: 1137–41.

48. McClain T, Gilmore BT, Peetz M. Laparoscopic cholecystectomy in the treatment of acalculus cholecystitis in patients after thermal injury. *J Burn Care Rehabil* 1997; 18: 141–6.

49. Glenn F, Becker CG. Acute acalculous cholecystitis. *Ann Surg* 1981; 195: 131–6.

50. Ross DC, Lee KC, Peters WJ, Douglas LG. Acalculous cholecystitis in association with major burns. *Burns* 1987; 13: 488–91.

51. Polacik V, Broz L, Kripner J, Bouska I, Liska E. Unexpected gastrointestinal complications in severely burned children. *Acta Cir Plast* 1991; 33: 98–109.

52. McDermott MW, Scudamore CH, Boileau LO, Snelling CF, Kramer TA. Analculous cholecystitis: its sole as a complication of major burn injury. *Can J Surg* 1985; 28: 529–33.

53. Lescher TJ, Sirinek KR, Pruitt BA. Superior mesenteric artery syndrome in thermally injured patients. *J Trauma* 1979; 19: 567–71.

54. Ogbuokiri CG, Law EJ, MacMillan BG. Superior mesenteric artery syndrome in burned children. *Am J Surg* 1972; 124: 75–9.

55. Jennings LJ, Hanumadass M. Silver sulfadiazine induced *Clostridium difficile* toxin megacolon in a burn patient: A case report. *Burns* 1998; 24: 676–9.

56. Talamani MA. Ogilvie's syndrome. In: Cameron JL, ed. *Current Surgical Therapy*, 4th edn. St Louis: Mosby-Year Book, 1992; 168–70.

57. Gauderer MW, Stellano TA. Gastrostomy tubes. *Curr Prob Surg* 1986; 9: 658–717.

58. Grant JP. Comparison of percutaneous endoscopic gastrostomy with Stamm gastrostomy. *Ann Surg* 1988; 207: 598–603.

59. Chung DH, Georgeson KE. Fundoplication and gastrostomy. *Semin Pediatr Surg* 1998; 7(4): 213–9.

60. Gottschlich MM, Warden GD, Michel M, *et al.* Diarrhea in tube-fed burn patients: incidence, etiology, nutritional impact, and prevention. *J Parenter Enteral Nutr* 1988; 12: 338–45.

61. Pruitt BA, Stein JM, Foley FD, Moncrief JA, O'Neill JA. Intravenous therapy in burn patients. *Arch Surg* 1970; 100: 399–404.

62. Golueke PJ, Zinner MJ. Management of septic thrombophlebitis. In: Ernst CB, Stanley JC, eds. *Current Therapy in Vascular Surgery*. Philadelphia: BC Decker, 1991; 1014–9.

63. Pruitt BA, McManus WF, Kin SH, Treat RC. Diagnosis and treatment of cannula-related intravenous sepsis in burn patients. *Ann Surg* 1980; 191: 546–54.

64. Kaufman J, Demas C, Stark K, Flancbaum L. Catheter-related septic central venous thrombosis – current therapeutic options. *West J Med* 1986; 145: 200–3.

65. Cobb LM, Vinocur CD, Wagner CW, Weintraub WH. The central venous anatomy in infants. *Surg Gynecol Obstet* 1987; 165: 230–4.

Nonthermal injuries

Chapter 35a

Electrical injuries
Gary F Purdue
John L Hunt

bility. Electrical burns are classified as low and high voltage injuries, with 1000 volts being the dividing line. At high voltages, the cutaneous burn is associated with deep, underlying tissue damage very closely resembling a crush injury.[1] Low voltage injuries have a more localized area of tissue destruction. Nearly all burns occurring indoors except in specialized industrial settings are of the low voltage type. While the victim or witness(es) often know the voltage involved, the amount of current is unknown. Current flow is related to voltage by Ohm's Law where: Current (l) = Voltage (E)/Resistance (R).

Animal experiments have demonstrated that resistance varies continuously with time, initially dropping slowly, then much more rapidly until arcing occurs at the contact sites. Resistance then rises to infinity and current flow ceases.[2] Temperature measurements taken at the same time, showed that the rate of temperature rise paralleled the changes in amperage. Tissue temperature was the critical factor in the magnitude of tissue damage. Interestingly, there was no increase in temperature distal to the contact points.

More than 99% of all electrical burns are caused by 60 cycle-per-second commercial alternating current, which reverses its polarity 120 times per second. Only an occasional industrial low or high frequency injury is encountered. With one-half of the time spent positive with respect to ground and one-half spent negative, the verbiage 'entrance' and 'exit' wound is archaic, as one does not know whether a given point on the body contacted the wire or the ground. These terms should be replaced by the term contact point. A descriptive term such as blow-out type injury describes concentration of current and not its causation (**Figure 35a.1**).

Introduction

Electricity is a ubiquitous part of civilization, which we often take for granted. Unfortunately, electrical burns are the most devastating of all thermal injuries on a size for size basis, usually involving both the skin and deeper tissues. They affect primarily young, working males, often have legal involvement and are the most frequent cause of amputations on the Burn Service. In addition to power company linemen and electricians, crane operators and construction workers are at special risk. Electrical burns have multiple acute and chronic manifestations not seen with other types of thermal injury. Morbidities, lengths of hospital stay and number of operations is much higher than expected, based on burn size alone.

Pathophysiology

Electrical burn severity is determined by voltage, current, type of current (alternating or direct), path of current flow, duration of contact, resistance at the point of contact, and individual suscepti-

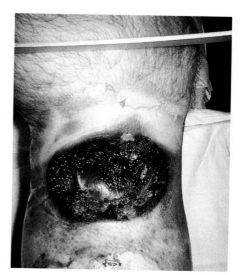

Fig. 35a.1 High voltage contact point. Blowout type injury below knee resulting in an above knee amputation.

The path of current makes a significant difference in fatality rates, but in patients reaching the hospital alive, current path determinations are often less than precise. The patient may have none, one, or many visible contact points and an untold number of invisible contacts. An example of this is the electrocautery where the large grounding pad site is not visible (hopefully). Despite some misconceptions, the term 'electrocution' does not apply to these living patients, as electrocution is defined as 'to kill by electric shock'.[3]

Alternating current causes tetanic muscle contractions, which may either throw the victim away from the contact or draw them into continued contact with the electrical source, creating the potential for continually increasing severity. Altered levels of consciousness, reported in about one-half of high voltage victims,[4] also contribute to prolonged periods of contact. Resistance at the point of contact varies from very low values for sweat-soaked hands or skin in the summer to more than 100 000 ohms for heavily calloused hands or feet during very dry winter weather. Individual susceptibility is a nonquantifiable term to explain why two or more individuals exposed to the same situation have extremely varied injuries.

The burn injury has the potential for three different components; the true electrical injury caused by current flow, an arc injury resulting from the electrical arc generated as the current passes from the source to an object, and a flame injury caused by ignition of clothing and/or surroundings. Electricity arcs at a temperature of up to 4000°C generating a flash type injury,[5] most often seen in electricians working in close proximity to an electric source with metal objects. These injuries, when occurring without actual current flow, are treated and classified the same as any flash burn.

The exact mechanism of injury continues to be the subject of much research, very often appearing clinically to be a multifactorial combination of both thermal and nonthermal causes. Electricity flowing through tissue generates heat, much as it does flowing through the wire of a toaster, with Joule's law defining the amount of power (heat) delivered to an object:

$$\text{Power (J-Joule)} = I^2 \text{ (Current) times R (Resistance)}$$

Tissue resistance from lowest to highest is nerve, blood vessels, muscle, skin, tendon, fat, and bone. Theoretically, current flow would be distributed in proportion to resistance, with tissues having the highest resistance generating the most heat. In the animal model the body acts as a single uniform resistance rather than a collection of different resistances, that is a volume conductor.[2] Deep tissues appear to retain heat and hence more severe injury is seen in the periosseous tissues, especially between two bones (i.e. tibia–fibula, radius–ulna) which usually sustain a more severe injury than superficial tissue. The associated macro- and microscopic vascular injury appears to occur nearly immediately and is not reversible.[6]

Direct and indirect electrical destruction of cells also plays a role in tissue injury. This appears to be especially important for nervous system cells as their injury is not well explained by heating alone. Cells maintaining their integrity with a sodium–potassium–ATPase pump operating at −90 millivolts direct current, certainly have the potential for disruption with high voltage alternating current. Breakdown of cell membranes is one of the mechanisms by which cell damage can occur.[7] This process of electroporation of membranes may explain the injury not apparently caused by heat.[8]

Acute care

Severity of injury is inversely proportional to the cross-sectional area of tissue able to carry current. The most severe injuries are seen at the wrists and ankles, with decreasing severity proximally. Thus, in hand–foot current flow, 30% of the resistance is in the ankle and 25% in the wrist.[9] The extremities are the most frequently injured body parts, with severe injury often occurring in the arm and hand (**Figure 35a.2**). As current follows the path of least resistance it may generate small deep arc injuries in the axilla, groin, popliteal, and antecubital fossae.

Electrocardiographic Monitoring

While ventricular fibrillation is the most common cause of death at the scene of injury, virtually any cardiac arrhythmia can be precipitated by an electrical injury. Arrhythmias are treated using the same indications and modalities as for medical causes. In the author's experience, new onset atrial fibrillation has been the most common arrhythmia seen in patients reaching the hospital alive. All have responded to appropriate medical management.

Direct myocardial injury may also result. This injury behaves more like a traumatic myocardial contusion than a true myocardial infarction, not having the hemodynamic or recurrence consequences of atherosclerotic myocardial infarctions. Housinger et al. have shown that creatine kinase (CK) and MB-creatine kinase (MB-CK) levels are poor indicators of myocardial injury in the absence of ECG finding of myocardial damage, especially in the presence of significant skeletal muscle injury.[10–12] Recent studies have shown that both arrhythmias and muscle damage are manifested very soon after injury.[13] All patients should be monitored during transport and in the emergency room. Rather than a policy of more prolonged cardiac monitoring for all patients, a selective policy makes most efficient use of expensive medical resources.

Indications for cardiac monitoring include:

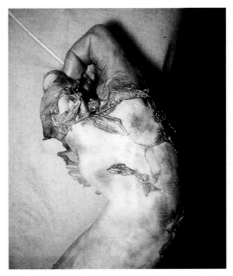

Fig. 35a.2 Characteristic contracted arm and hand following high voltage contact to the hand with extensive myonecrosis to the entire forearm.

- Documented cardiac arrest
- Cardiac arrhythmia on transport or in the Emergency Room
- Abnormal EKG in the Emergency Room (other than sinus brady- or tachycardia)
- Burn size or patient age would require monitoring.

Myoglobinuria

The presence of pigmented (darker than light pink) urine in a patient with an electrical burn usually indicates significant muscle damage. Myoglobin and hemoglobin pigments present risk of acute renal failure and must be cleared promptly. While low levels are of little clinical concern, grossly visible urinary pigmentation requires rapid response to minimize tubular obstruction (**Figure 35a.3**). The urine dispstick is too sensitive for both pigment and hematuria to serve as a guide for treatment. Evaluation of the serum to differentiate myoglobin from hemoglobin depends on the fact that the smaller myoglobin complex is cleared by the kidney at a threshold below visibility, while hemoglobin as a polymer bound to albumen, has a much higher renal threshold. Differentiating between the two is of little clinical significance. Both require prompt clearance and must be treated. Urine color darker than a light pink is promptly treated with two ampules of mannitol (25 grams) given intravenous (IV) push, followed immediately by two ampules of sodium bicarbonate, also given IV push. Ringer's lactate is administered at a rate sufficient to grossly clear the urine of pigment. The rational of this protocol is to create a rapid, osmotic diuresis with initial alkalinization to minimize pigment precipitation in the renal tubules. If adequate organ perfusion is maintained, repeat administration of either mannitol or bicarbonate is not required. Loop diuretics are not as efficient as mannitol. The required urinary output is generally very high for several hours following injury, followed by significant reduction in urine requirements, as the venous return from the injured part to the central circulation is thrombosed. Using this protocol, the authors have had a zero incidence of acute renal failure in 154 consecutive patients with grossly visible urinary pigment.

Resuscitation

The hidden injury associated with an electrical burn makes the use of burn resuscitation formulas based on body surface area burned inaccurate, except to establish a minimum volume required. In the absence of gross myo/hemoglobinuria, the goal of resuscitation is to maintain normal vital signs and a urine output of 30–50 ml/h with Ringer's lactate; the rate is adjusted on an hourly basis to achieve those goals.

Traumatic Injuries

Approximately 15% of electrical burn victims sustain traumatic injuries in addition to their burn, a rate nearly double that of other burn patients. Most of these injuries are caused by falls from a height or being thrown against an object, with some resulting from the tetanic muscle contractions associated with the electrical shock itself; forces strong enough to cause compression fractures.[14] A careful history and physical examination should separate those patients who require a full trauma evaluation.

Compartment Syndrome

Patients with high voltage electrical injuries of the extremities are at risk for development of compartment syndromes during the first 48 hours post-injury. Damaged muscle swelling within the investing fascia of the extremity may increase pressures within the muscle compartment to the point where blood flow to muscle tissue is compromised. Loss of pulses is one of the last signs of a compartment syndrome. A high index of suspicion is paramount for the early diagnosis (either by serial examinations of the affected extremities or measurement of compartment pressures) and prompt treatment of these increased compartment pressures. While a very aggressive approach to fasciotomies has been advocated in the past, significant morbidity attends a fasciotomy and its closure. Mann et al. have made a convincing argument for a conservative course regarding the indications for fasciotomies, that is for the usual clinical signs of compartment syndrome, progressive nerve dysfunction or failure of resuscitation with other patients undergoing exploration and aggressive debridement on the third to fifth postburn day.[15]

Four compartment fasciotomies of the lower leg and anterior/posterior fasciotomies[16] of the upper extremity are performed in the operating room under general anesthesia. Rarely, medial and lateral fasciotomies of the thigh and upper arm are required to complete release. Incisions can be made with either a knife or cautery. Care is taken to assure complete release of all of the affected muscle groups. Coverage of the ensuing wound is with a biologic dressing such as porcine heterograft[17] and the extremity is kept elevated to hasten resolution of edema. At this initial operation, we place a silk suture in the muscle at the proximal limit of gross necrosis. While a great deal of discussion concerns the progressive nature of electrical burns, ultimate division of the muscle is seldom more than 1 cm proximal to that seen at initial evaluation. The initial operation is followed by a second-look operation in 24–48 hours with debridement/amputation and the earliest possible closure. Fasciotomy wound closure is facilitated by use of traction on the affected skin edges by carefully placed sutures, vessel loop tensioning[18] or commercially available tension and device. Skin grafting is minimized if fasciotomy closure is appropriately planned. In order to minimize operating time and blood loss at the initial operation, primary amputations are not generally performed except to remove mummified contracted extremities.

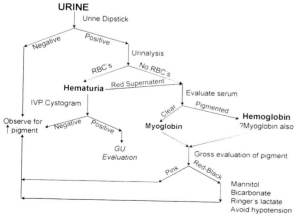

Fig. 35a.3 Work-up and treatment of pigmented urine. Algorithm enclosed.

Wound Care

Local burn care is performed using mafenide acetate (Sulfamylon) on the thick eschar of the contact points, because of its excellent penetration. Silver sulfadiazine is used for microbial control on the deep flash/flame components and a biologic dressing used on more superficial areas. Surgical excision is begun 2–3 days postburn either as a second-look operation following a fasciotomy or as the first procedure in patients not requiring fasciotomies. All obviously necrotic tissue is removed, but tissues of questionable viability are retained and reevaluated every 2–3 days until wound closure can be achieved. A very conservative course of tissue removal and wound closure with a combination of skin grafts and/or flaps for soft-tissue coverage gives the best functional results. An ongoing program of physical therapy and functional splinting is begun the day of admission and continued throughout the hospital stay. Serial neuromuscular examinations are performed to document neurologic status. Regional anesthesia is best avoided to minimize medicolegal complications should late neurologic dysfunction arise.

Diagnosis

Multiple diagnostic modalities have been investigated attempting to speed up the process of identifying the extent of deep tissue necrosis. Radionucleotide scanning with xenon-133[19] and technicium pyrophosphate[20,21] have been shown to be accurate predictors of tissue damage. Hammond showed that scanning did not decrease hospital stay or number of operations required.[21] Magnetic resonance imaging (MRI) provides poor sensitivity for evaluation of muscle damage in nonperfused areas. Gadolinium-enhanced MRI demonstrates potential viability in zones of tissue edema and good correlation with histopathology.[22–24] While very sensitive and specific, diagnostic scans often add little to direct clinical evaluation and create logistical problems of their own. For all practical purposes, the use of the above cited techniques are expensive and unnecessary.

Problem Areas

Contact areas on the scalp, chest, and abdomen provide additional management problems. The scalp must be searched carefully for these lesions as scalp burns are rarely painful and are easily missed on cursory physical examinations (**Figure 35a.4**). Scalp burns that spare the galea are managed by excision and skin grafting directly onto the galea, while wounds that penetrate to the outer table of the skull or deeper require a different approach. Exposure of nonviable calvarium has historically been approached by providing a viable wound bed by removing the dead bone with an osteotome or a dental-type burr. Drilling multiple holes in a close set pattern, deep enough to cause bleeding from viable cancellous bone, is another method to develop granulation tissue that eventually covers the entire area. The latter method is still useful in situations where a patient's advanced age or large burn size precludes more aggressive approaches to wound closure. All of the above methods require weeks to months of wound care before the wound is ready for an autograft. The best and most expedient approach to these deep skull burns is a rotation scalp flap(s) over the burned area. Split-thickness skin grafts cover the resulting adjacent defect. This provides rapid closure and is associated with minimal morbidity (**Figure 35a.5**).[25] Skin expansion of the hair-bearing area can be performed 12–18 months later to obliterate the areas of alopecia.

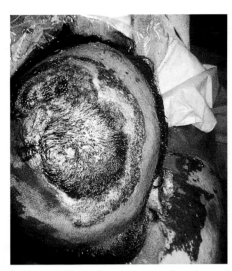

Fig. 35a.4 Deep full-thickness burn of scalp, extending into bone.

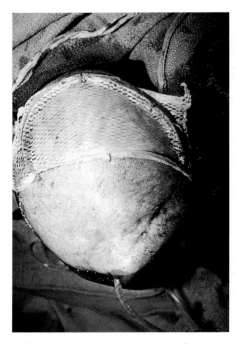

Fig. 35a.5 Postoperative rotation scalp flap used to cover the excised wound with the resulting defect covered with a split-thickness autograft.

Larger scalp defects are closed with free flaps anastomosed to appropriate vessels lying outside the zone of injury.

In addition to the myocardial effects of electricity enumerated above, injury to the deep structures including the phrenic nerve and direct thermal injury to the heart may occur. Chest wall injuries present special closure problems (adjacent or remote soft-tissue flaps) for coverage of exposed bone and cartilage. Costal chondritis is the most frequent complication becoming a source of long-term morbidity, requiring multiple débridements.

Abdominal wounds provide the potential for internal injuries both directly under contact points and remotely as the result of late ischemic necrosis.[26,27] Patients must be evaluated frequently for changes in the abdominal examination and/or feeding tolerance. Deterioration mandates laparotomy. Repair of large abdominal wall wounds requires careful planning and often a multidisciplinary team for optimal results.

Lightning injury

Approximately 100 000 thunderstorms occur in the US each year with lightning killing more people than any other weather phenomena causing about 80 fatalities per year, with Florida and Texas having the most deaths.[28–30] While lightning strikes involve millions of volts of electricity, the spectrum of burn injury is extremely varied, from minimal cutaneous burn to significant burns equal in depth to commercial high voltage electricity. Major cutaneous injury is rare unless a nearby object is turned incandescent, causing a flash/flame type injury, as when a bag of golf clubs on the victims back is struck. The pathognomonic cutaneous sign of a lightning strike is a dendritic arborescent or fern-like branching erythematous pattern on the skin which appears within an hour of injury and fades rapidly, much like a wheal and flare reaction.[31] Full-thickness isolated burns on the tips of the toes has also been reported as being characteristic. Both findings are useful in determining the cause of injury in the patient found down under uncertain circumstances.[32]

Lightning may cause both respiratory and cardiac standstill for which CPR is especially effective when promptly initiated.[33] The ears should be carefully examined as injuries are frequent, ranging from ruptured tympanic membranes (most common) to destruction of the middle and inner ear.[34]

Neurologic complications are relatively common and include unconsciousness, seizures, paraesthesias and paralysis, which may develop over several days after injury. The term keraunoparalysis has been used to describe the latter symptom complex and is associated with vasomotor disorders. Fortunately these are usually transient. Surgically treatable lesions including epidural, subdural and intracerebral hematomas may occur, mandating a high index of suspicion for an altered level of consciousness.[29] The prognosis of many of the neurologic injuries are generally better than for other types of traumatic causes, although subtle neurologic changes may persist, suggesting a very conservative, watchful waiting and supportive approach with serial neurologic examinations after an initial CT scan to rule out correctable causes.

Low voltage burns

Low voltage direct current injuries are most often due to the heating effect of electricity turning a ring, wristwatch, bracelet or necklace incandescent, resulting in a deep circumferential thermal burn. These are treated in the same manner as other thermal burns.[35] Mechanics and persons working on automobiles are at greatest risk for this injury as automotive electrical systems are the most common source of low voltage–high amperage electricity.

Low voltage alternating current injury is usually localized to the points of contact, although with prolonged contact, tissue damage may extend into deep tissues with little lateral extension as seen in high voltage wounds. These wounds are treated by excision to viable tissue and appropriate coverage based on wound depth and location.

Burns of the oral cavity are the most common types of electrical burn in young children. Most of these injuries result from the child chewing on an electrical cord or on the male–female plug interface between two cords. Injuries involving only the oral commissure are initially treated very conservatively, as the extent of injury is difficult to predict. Simple wound care is performed as an outpatient.[36,37] The most serious complication is bleeding from the labial artery, occurring 10–14 days after injury. Families are instructed to digitally compress the labial artery if bleeding occurs and return to the Emergency Room. Following healing, treatment varies by the severity of injury. Gentle stretching and the use of oral splints gives good cosmetic and functional results in most patients, with reconstructive surgery being reserved for the remainder. Severe microstomia is corrected by mucosal advancement flaps. Burns of the mid-portions of mouth heal very poorly and require a much more aggressive surgical approach with carefully planned reconstruction.[38,39]

Complications

The primary early complications of electrical injury include renal, septic, cardiac, neurologic, and ocular. Renal failure and sepsis are preventable by adequate resuscitation and rapid removal of necrotic tissue, while cardiac damage is recognized and treated on admission. Neurologic deficits may be present on admission or develop in the days to weeks after injury.

Cataract formation is the most frequent ocular complication of electrical injury, although ocular manifestations may affect all portions of the eye.[40,41] The exact pathophysiology appears to be unknown, but ocular changes may affect as many as 5–20% of patients with true electrical burns. Saffle reported on seven patients with 13 cataracts, noting a high rate of bilaterality and little association with voltage or location of contact points,[42] although often thought of as being more frequently associated with contact points of the head, neck, and upper trunk. Seventy-seven percent eventually progressed to the point where surgical therapy was necessary, the results of, which were uniformly good. Lag time before appearance may be as short as 4 weeks and as long as 11 years after injury.

Neurologic complications are protean in their diversity and may present either early or late. They can occur up to 2 years after injury. Neuromuscular defects including paresis, paralysis, Guillian–Barré syndrome, transverse myelitis or amyotrophic lateral sclerosis can be caused by electrical injury.[43] A study by Grube puts the incidence into perspective.[4] Of 64 patients with high voltage burns, 67% developed immediate central or peripheral neurologic symptoms. One-third had peripheral neuropathies, with one-third of those persistent. Twelve percent had delayed onset of peripheral neuropathy, with 50% of those resolving. They reported no late onset, central neuropathies. The most common peripheral defect is a peripheral neuropathy, with weakness being the most commonly found clinical finding.[44] In general, resolution of early onset lesions is much better than for late onset, spasticity is more frequent than flaccidity and function is affected more than sensation. Sympathetic over-activity with changes in bowel habits, urinary and sexual function is the primary autonomic complex complication. Although the exact mechanism of nerve injury has not been explained, both direct injury by electrical current and/or a vascular cause receive the most attention. To date imaging studies, including angiography and MRI, have not been helpful in either predicting or evaluating extent of deficit. Very often, neuropsychological status is often abnormal. In a study comparing electrical burn patients with nonburned electricians, Pliskin showed significantly higher cognitive, physical and emotional complaints not related to injury or litigation status.[45] A full neurologic examination must be performed on admission documenting initial presentation. Consistent long-term follow-up with careful neuromuscular examinations becomes an important part of patient care. Electrodiagnostic evaluation may be helpful in delineating the defect. Early involvement of an experienced, interested physiatrist is important in assessing long-term needs and participating in the creation of a therapy plan.

Heterotopic ossification occurring at the cut ends of amputation sites is unique to the electrically burned patient. This occurs in about 80% of patients with long bone amputations, but not in patients with disarticulations or small bone amputations. Ossification was severe enough to require surgical revision of the bone end in 28%.[46] This is easily accomplished by opening the stump incision and using a bone rongeur to remove the soft heterotopic bone and reclosing the stump. Although electrical burns comprise only about 3% of all burn injuries, they consume enormous amounts of resources, requiring a carefully planned team approach for optimal care.

References

1. Artz CP. Electrical injury simulates crush injury. *Surg Gynecol Obstet* 1967; **125**: 1316–17.
2. Hunt JL, Mason AD, Masterson TS, Pruitt BA. The pathophysiology of acute electric burns. *J Trauma* 1976; **16**: 335–40.
3. Webster's third new international dictionary of the English language. Unabridged. Springfield, MA: Merrian-Webster, 1993: 732.
4. Grube BJ, Heimbach DM, Engrav LH, Copass MK. Neurologic consequences of electrical burns. *J Trauma* 1990; **30**: 254–8.
5. Nichter LS, Braynt CA, Kenney JG, *et al.* Injuries due to commercial electric current. *J Burn Care Rehabil* 1984; **5**: 124–37.
6. Hunt JL, McManus WF, Haney WP, Pruitt BA. Vascular lesions in acute electric injuries. *J Trauma* 1974; **14**: 461–73.
7. Lee RC, Kolodney SB. Electrical injury mechanisms: electrical breakdown of cell membranes. *Plas Reconst Surg* 1987; **80**: 672–80.
8. Lee RC, Canaday DJ, Hammer SM. Transient and stable ionic permeabilization of isolated skeletal muscle cells after electrical shock. *J Burn Care Rehab* 1993; **14**: 528–40.
9. Freiberger H. The electrical resistance of the human body to commercial direct and alternating currents. (Der elektrische widerstand des menschilichen Koepers gegen technischen gleich und wechselstrom.) Berlin. *Elertrizitatswirtschaft* 1933; **2**: 442–6.
10. Housinger TA, Green L, Shahangian S, Saffle JR, Warden GD. A prospective study of myocardial damage in electrical injuries. *J Trauma* 1985; **25**: 122–4.
11. McBride JW, Labrosse KR, McCoy HG, Ahrenholz DH, Solem LD, Goldenberg IF. Is serum creatine kinase-MB in electrically injured patients predictive of myocardial injury? *JAMA* 1986; **255**: 764–8.
12. Dilworth D, Hasan D, Alford P, Baker C, Driswold JA. Evaluation of Myocardial Injury in Electrical Burn Patients. *J Burn Care Rehabil* 1998; **19**(1 Pt 2): S239.
13. Purdue GF, Hunt JL. Electrocardiographic monitoring after electrical injury: Necessity or luxury. *J Trauma* 1986; **26**: 166–7.
14. Layton TR, McMurtry JM, McClain EJ, Kraus DR, Reimer BL. Multiple spine fractures from electric injury. *J Burn Care Rehabil* 1984; **5**: 373–5.
15. Mann R, Gibran N, Engrave L, Heimbach D. Is immediate decompression of high voltage electrical injuries to the upper extremity always necessary? *J Trauma* 1996; **40**: 584–9.
16. Fazi B, Raves JJ, Young JC, Diamond DL. Fasciotomy of the upper extremity in the patient with trauma. *Surg Gyn Obstet* 1987; **165**: 447–8.
17. Parshley P, Kilgore J, Pulito J, Smiley P, Miller S. Aggressive approaches to the extremity damaged by electric current. *Am J Surg* 1985; **150**: 78–82.
18. Berman SS, Schilling JD, McIntyre KE, Hunter GC, Bernhard VM. Shoelace technique for delayed primary closure of fasciotomies. *Am J Surg* 1994; **167**: 435–6.
19. Clayton JM, Hayes AC, Hammel J, Boyd WC, Hartford CE, Barnes RW. Xenon-133 determination of muscle blood flow in electrical injury. *J Trauma* 1977; **17**: 293–8.
20. Hunt J, Lewis S, Parkey R, Baxter C. The use of technetium-99 m stannous pyrophosphate scintigraphy to identify muscle damage in acute electric burns. *J Trauma* 1979; **19**: 409–13.
21. Hammond J, Ward CG. The use of technetium-99 pyrophosphate scanning in management of high voltage electrical injuries. *Am Surg* 1994; **68**: 886–8.
22. Fleckenstein JL, Chason DP, Bonte FJ, *et al.* High-voltage electric injury: Assessment of muscle viability with MR imaging and Tc-99 m pyrophosphate scintigraphy. *Radiology* 1993; **195**: 205–10.
23. Ohashi M, Koizumi J, Hosoda Y, Fikosjorp Y, Tuyuki A, Kikuchi K. Correlation between magnetic resonance imaging and histopathology of an amputated forearm after electrical injury. *Burns* 1998; **24**: 362–8.
24. Lee RC. Injury by electrical forces: Pathology, manifestations and therapy. *Curr Prob Surg* 1997; **34**: 738–40.
25. Hunt J, Purdue G, Spicer T. Management of full-thickness burns of the scalp and skull. *Arch Surg* 1983; **118**: 621–5.
26. Newsome TW, Curreri PW, Kurenius K. Visceral injuries- An unusual complication of an electrical burn. *Arch Surg* 1972; **105**: 494–7.
27. Reilley AF, Rees R, Kelton P, Lynch JB. Abdominal aortic occlusion following electric injury. *J Burn Care Rehabil* 1985; **6**: 226–9.
28. Lightning-Associated deaths- United States, 1980–1995. *MMWR* 1998; **19**: 391–4.
29. Hiestand D, Colice GL. Lightning-strike injury. *J Intensive Care* 1988; **3**: 303–14.
30. Tribble CG, Persing JA, Morgan RF, Kenney JG, Edlich RF. Lightning injury. *Curr Concept Trauma Care* 1984; **Spring**: 5–10.
31. ten Duis HJ, Klasen HJ, Nijsten MWN. Superficial lightning injuries – their 'fractal' shape and origin. *Burns* 1987; **13**: 141–6.
32. Fahmy FS, Brinsden MD, Smith J, Frame JD. Lightning: the multisystem group injuries. *J Trauma* 1999; **46**: 937–40.
33. Moran KT, Thupari JN, Munster AM. Electric- and lightning-induced cardiac arrest reversed by prompt cardiopulmonary resuscitation. Letter. *JAMA* 1986; **255**: 2157.
34. Bergstrom L, Neblett LM, Sando I, Hemenway WG, Harrison GD. The lightning-damaged ear. *Arch Otolaryngol* 1974; **100**: 117–21.
35. Manstein CM, Manstein ME, Manstein G. Circumferential electric burns of the ring finger. Letter to the editor. *J Hand Surg* 1987; **12A**: 808.
36. Leake JE, Curtin JW. Electrical burns of the mouth in children. *Clin Plas Surg* 1984; **11**: 669–83.
37. D'Italia JG, Hulnick SJ. Outpatient management of electric burns of the lip. *J Burn Care Rehabil* 1984; **5**: 465–6.
38. Sadove AM, Jones JE, Lynch TR, Sheets PW. Appliance therapy for perioral electrical burns: A conservative approach. *J Burn Care Rehabil* 1988; **9**: 391–5.
39. Pensler JM, Rosenthal A. Reconstruction of the oral commissure after an electrical burn. *J Burn Care Rehabil* 1990; **11**: 50–3.
40. Johnson EV, Klien LB, Skalka HW. Electrical cataracts: A case report and review of the literature. *Opthomal Surg* 1987; **18**: 283–5.
41. Boozalis GT, Purdue GF, Hunt JP, McCulley. Ocular changes from electrical burn injuries: A literature review and report of cases. *J Burn Care Rehabil* 1991; **5**: 458–62.
42. Saffle JR, Crandall A, Warden GD. Cataracts: A long-term complication of electrical injury. *J Trauma* 1985; **25**: 17–21.
43. Petty PG, Parkin G. Electrical injury to the central nervous system. *Neurosurg* 1986; **19**: 282–4.
44. Haberal MMMA, Gureu S, Akman N, Basgoze O. Persistent peripheral nerve pathologies in patients with electric burns. *J Burn Care Rehabil* 1996; **17**: 147–9.
45. Pliskin NH, Capelli-Schellpfeffer M, Law RT, Malina AC, Kelley KM, Lee RC. Neuropsychological symptom presentation after electrical injury. *J Trauma* 1998; **44**: 709–15.
46. Helm PA, Walker SC. New bone formation at amputation in electrically burn-injured patients. *Arch Phys Med Rehabil* 1987; **68**: 284–6.

Suggested reading

Kurtz EB, Shoemaker TM. *The Lineman's and Cableman's Handbook*, 7th Edn. New York: McGraw-Hill, 1985.

Andrews CJ, Cooper MA, Darveniza M, Mackerras D. *Lightning Injuries: Electrical, Medical and Legal Aspects*. Boca Raton: CRC Press, 1992.

Chapter 35b

Electrical injury: reconstructive problems

Thomas Muehlberger, Marcus Spies
Peter M Vogt

Introduction

Severe cases [of electrical injury] coming for reconstruction present a formidable problem of flexion contracture and loss of many tendons and nerves, new pedicled skin and grafted-in tendons and nerves usually being necessary. One encounters inside the limb the same type of destruction and cicatrix as is found after any severe infection.

Sterling Bunnell, 1948

This chapter will focus on the multitude of surgical and reconstructive problems that result from electrical injury. The spectrum of electrical injuries is complex due to various factors determining manifestation, severity, and distribution of the resulting tissue damage. In common with conventional thermal trauma, the consequences of electrical injuries may affect a wide range of physiological functions. However, distinct features warrant a differentiated approach to this unique kind of trauma. The resulting tissue loss and the damage to essential structures of the involved body areas often require extensive plastic-reconstructive procedures.

Although the incidence of low-voltage burns steadily declined over the last decades, electrical injuries still account for 3–5% of all admissions to major burn centers.[1,2] Electrical fatalities are relatively uncommon and most of them occur accidentally. Although earlier reported limb amputation rates of up to 71% decreased over the last decades with the increasing ability to reconstruct anatomic parts and restore function, limb salvage remains a surgical challenge.[3]

Physiological basis of tissue destruction

The traditional pathophysiological understanding of electric injury was based on the assumption that the passage of electric current produces heat and triggers tissue damage.[4] Thus tissue specific susceptibility (and vulnerability) is considered to increase progressively from nerve to blood vessels, muscle, skin, tendon, and fat to bone. As osseous tissue shows the highest electrical resistance it will generate the most heat. It was also assumed that electric current would preferentially take the path of least resistance through the body, in particular along the neurovascular bundles. This theory further postulated that the lesions produced by the current would result in delayed vascular occlusions and progressive tissue necrosis.[5]

In high-voltage injuries the internal milieu acts as a single uniform resistance.[6] Instead of conduction through specific preferential tissues, the body conducts the current with a composite resistance of all tissue components.[7] The crucial factor in determining the resistance and thus the magnitude of tissue damage is the cross-sectional diameter of the affected body part. Devastating injuries to the extremities occur with a significantly higher frequency than tissue damage to the thorax and abdomen[8] (**Figure 35b.1**). As muscle tissue occupies the largest cross-sectional area in the limb it also carries the predominant electric current. In a primate model the heat generated by electric current at energy levels of 40 kJ resulted in increased tissue temperature at specific areas along the upper extremity.[7] The maximal temperatures were found at the elbow, and even higher at the wrist. As joint areas are regions where the cross-sectional tissue composition changes from low resistant muscle to high resistant bone, tendon and skin, a

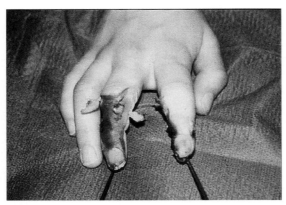

(A)

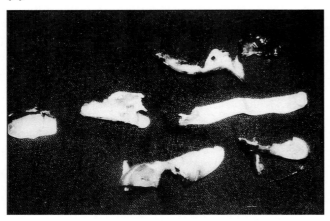

(B)

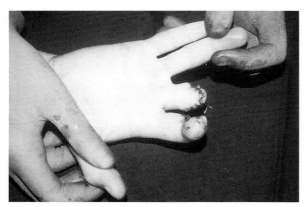

(C)

Fig. 35b.1 Electrical burn from a domestic water heater (220 V). The 13-year-old girl manipulated the device while being immersed in the bathtub. She sustained third and fourth degree burns of the digits (A). Debridement revealed full-thickness injuries involving tendons, nerves, and phalangeal bones (B), which necessitated primary amputation (C).

proportionally higher current and heat are produced in these areas according with Ohm's Law.[9] The resulting large transdermal potential in the extremities, especially around the joints, leads to a breakdown of skin, most commonly seen in the axilla, elbow, and

wrist. These burns occur in specific regions because of the redirection of current flow from underlying muscle tissue to the surface and are often referred to as 'kissing lesions'. Other skin burns occur at the contact points, from igniting clothing or by heat generated by electric arcing. Arcing describes the energy transmission by a hot electrically conducting gas. However, this requires a voltage of more than 20 000 V to bridge even a short distance of 1 cm.[10] The effects on tissue vary from minimal skin wounds to charring and tissue vaporization. In angiographic studies of 28 high-tension electrical injuries with absent peripheral pulses, 82% of arterial occlusions occurred in joint areas.[11] All examined extremities with angiographic signs of damage to large vascular structures also had severe neuromuscular injuries. Electrical damage to a large artery represents a grave prognostic sign for limb survival. The reported risk of amputation is high, between 37 and 65%.[12–14]

With increasing focus on events at the cellular level, further nonthermal mechanisms of cellular injury have been defined. This includes a voltage-induced loss of semipermeability of cell membranes, which can be used experimentally to introduce targeted gene sequences or drugs into cells.[15–17] When the integrity of the cell membrane is lost, however, the impedance is decreased markedly, leading to a simultaneous increase of the area exposed to current flow.[18] Thus cells with larger surface areas, such as muscle and nerve cells, are more susceptible to electrical fields and this may explain in part the pattern of tissue injury found at sites that are distant from contact areas and entry wounds. In addition to breakdown in cellular integrity electrical fields also induce denaturation of membrane proteins by altering their structural conformation and rendering them non-functional.[19] This process which occurs milliseconds after exposure can lead to the dissolution of membrane components. Both mechanisms are responsible for rhabdomyolysis and secondary myoglobin release, which depends directly on the imposed electric current and is not a thermal effect.[20]

In summary, the physiology of electrical injury is complex. Besides enhanced conductivity through nerves and blood vessels, in low-voltage injuries, but not high-voltage injuries, a heat effect on tissue and cellular damage through electroporation are superimposed and cumulative in effect.

Diagnosis and acute treatment

Diagnosis and acute treatment of electrical injury have been described in Chapter 35a. However, several important characteristics need to be emphasized.

Assessment of Tissue Damage

The correct assessment of the extent of tissue damage is difficult. The percentage of burned body surface area grossly underestimates the injury to underlying tissue. Electrical burns may appear as mere pinpoint marks. In contrast, fatal electrocution may even take place without any visible skin burns in case of a large contact area. In a series of 59 patients with high-voltage injuries, the extent of visible burns showed no correlation to any other complications or sequelae.[21] The actual cutaneous resistance depends on contact size, pressure applied during contact, the magnitude and duration of the current, and the moisture status of the skin.

In contrast to thermal burns, deposition of metallic iron and copper is found on the epidermis after electrical injuries as electrolysis occurs in the extracellular fluid of the skin.[22] These metal

Table 35b.1 Dependency of cutaneous resistance on skin moisture.[6]

	Resistance (Ω)
Dry skin	100 000
Wet skin	2 500
Skin immersion	1 500
Rubber soles	70 000

Table 35b.2 Recommendation for cardiac monitoring in the absence of other injuries

Admission and cardiac monitoring	Discharge
Loss of consciousness[36]	Asymptomatic patient[37]
Extensive burns[32]	Normal initial ECG[38]
Current passing through the thorax[34]	Uneventful 4-hour observation[39]
Cardiac dysrhythmias[36]	Voltage less than 240/260 in adults[37,38]
	Voltage less than 120/240 in children[30,39]

condensations produce a black coating of the skin resembling an eschar.

Clinical determination of tissue viability is based on inspection and the demonstration of muscle contractility. As yet, there are no other diagnostic tools available to accurately assess the extent of tissue damage in the early phase following electrical injuries. The value of magnetic resonance imaging (MRI) for the detection of nonperfused nonedematous muscle is debated.[23,24] Serial measurement of skin temperature, muscle perfusion scintigraphy, Xe-133 clearance test, and radionuclide arteriography with labeled microspheres show no significant advantages.[25] Angiography, although not providing information on tissue viability, demonstrates the absence of tissue perfusion, and may lead to an early indication of limb amputation.

Rhabdomyolysis and Myoglobinuria

Rhabdomyolysis leads to hyperkalemia, calcium deposition in damaged muscle cells, release of intracellular phosphate and eventually hypocalcemia. Destroyed muscle cells release myoglobin, resulting in myoglobinemia. However, hemolysis also often occurs with electrical injury, resulting in concurrent hemoglobinemia. Thus urine measurements of hemochromogens cannot be used as a guide to adequate therapy.[26,27] Serum levels of creatinine and creatinine phosphokinase (CPK) are used as indicators of rhabdomyolysis. However, it is important to note that the destruction of 2 g of skeletal muscle can already yield a 10-fold increase of the normal CPK level. After a muscle injury the CPK level will peak by 24 hours and return to baseline within 48–72 hours. This diminishes the diagnostic value of serum and urine chemistry testing.[27,28]

Renal Failure

Myoglobinuria has traditionally been considered a major risk factor for the development of acute renal failure. Recently, patients with electrical injuries have been shown to have a surprisingly low risk for renal failure.[29] In 162 patients, only 14% had myoglobinuria and none developed renal failure. Suggested criteria to evaluate the risk of acute renal failure after electrical injury include: prehospital cardiac arrest, full-thickness burns, compartment syndrome, and high-voltage injury. Presence of at least two criteria should instigate immediate treatment, as the time-frame to prevent the progression to acute renal failure is limited to a few hours postinjury. Renal complications after low-voltage injuries are rare.

Cardiac Monitoring

The need for cardiac monitoring after electrical injuries is highly controversial. The literature review allows the following recommendation. If an initial 12-lead ECG shows no abnormalities, the delayed development of cardiac problems is very unlikely, irrespective whether the patients sustained high- or low-voltage injuries.[30–32] The presence of arrhythmias or conduction abnormalities on initial presentation, electrical injury in children, or if the projected path of the current transversed the thorax, prolonged cardiac monitoring may be warranted.[33,34] However, studies on large series demonstrated no general need for cardiac monitoring in patients with electrical injury.[35,36]

Acute treatment of patients with electrical injuries adheres to guidelines of ABLS, ATLS and current practice of intensive care medicine. This includes the maintenance of a patent airway, effective ventilation, and systemic circulation to provide adequate tissue perfusion and oxygenation. The reduced extent of visible skin burns may lead to underestimation of resuscitation fluid requirements. The patients must be continuously monitored for signs of neurovascular compromise, and deranged tissue perfusion and oxygenation. Pulse oximetry may be useful for this purpose.

Surgical Debridement

Clinical outcome of patients with severe electrical injuries has not changed substantially during the last two decades.[14] Although mortality rates of electrical injury are lower compared to thermal burns, patients have a significantly higher risk of developing complications during hospitalization.[2] Especially amputation rates of affected extremities are still high, at around 50%, despite all attempts at limb preservation.[12,13,40–42]

In the last decades, the concept of progressive tissue necrosis has led to the treatment strategy of early debridement and fasciotomy, followed by serial debridement and delayed wound closure. However, extensive studies have failed to support the notion that electrical injury causes progressive ischemia secondary to electrically induced endothelial damage.[9,40,43,44] In serial arterial angiograms of electrical injured extremities no vascular changes could be found.[45] The observed changes may more likely be explained by vascular changes similar to ischemia–reperfusion injury with immediate cessation of capillary blood flow in response to current passage. This event is followed by vascular spasms lasting for extended time, with subsequent vasodilatation and restoration of flow.[46]

Although still controversial, these findings may shift the acute treatment paradigm. While there is little discussion about the early time point of debridement, several recent studies question the need of extensive and total necrectomy and advocate the approach of delayed soft tissue coverage. 'Conservative debridement' consisting of removal of charred and obviously necrotic tissue has been promoted in a study on 40 patients.[47] In this study partially damaged tendons, muscles, and nerves were preserved, and wound closure was achieved by immediate flap coverage. Patients treated in this manner with immediate soft tissue coverage showed significantly better outcome compared with a control group who had serial

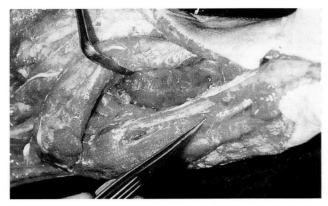

(A)

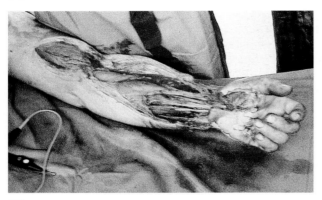

(B)

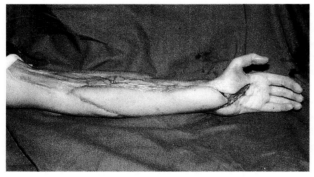

(C)

Fig. 35b.2 High-voltage injury from an overhead power line (30 000 V). The teenager climbed a train and was struck by an arc without touching the power line. The spectrum of injury included third and fourth degree burns and deep tissue necrosis of the forearm (A). After fasciotomy due to impending compartment syndrome (B). Coverage with free latissimus dorsi flap after 'conservative' debridement. Significant functional deficits after 4 years (C).

debridement procedures. Similar results were found in a study using early free-flap coverage for electrical injuries,[41] suggesting that careful limited initial debridement is an adequate measure. According to this study overly extensive and repeated debridement to ensure viability of all remaining tissue appears not only unnecessary but quite likely harmful. It appears safe to abandon these strategies and to perform an early extensive, but selective debridement in order to preserve continuity of functionally important structures (**Figure 35b.2**). Available options for wound closure encompass the total range of plastic reconstructive procedures, from skin grafts and local flaps to free tissue transfer.[48] Pedicled flaps should be considered in cases of suspected arterial compromise.

Despite the encouraging results of the studies recommending early soft tissue reconstruction by all means it should be noted that for the extent of electrical injury no scoring system has been established so far. Therefore, the comparison of different studies using both aggressive debridement alone or selective debridement and early soft tissue coverage is difficult with respect to the severity of tissue damage treated.

The salvage of damaged extremities with functional preservation of vital structures should be attempted and may require revascularization using segmental vein grafts or segmental cable grafting of nerves. Alternative approaches to cases with devastating segmental injury to the upper arm, such as the temporary ectopic implantation of undamaged hands, have been reported, but cannot be considered standard of care.[49] The condition of the individual patient and the level of tissue destruction varies considerably and determines the available therapeutic options.

Compartment Syndrome

Muscle compartment pressure should be monitored clinically and by invasive pressure measurements. In contrast to blunt trauma, pain is not a reliable indicator of increased compartment pressure due to the high incidence of electrical nerve injury. When compartment pressures exceed 30 mmHg surgical decompression by open fasciotomy becomes necessary to prevent ischemic muscle injury. In case of lower compartment pressure, progression may be prevented by administration of nonsteroidal anti-inflammatory drugs and antioxidants, protective splinting, and rest without elevation of the affected extremities. However, general operative decompression in high-voltage injuries of extremities appears not to be warranted. In a cohort study, Mann *et al.* found an increased amputation rate of 45% with immediate operative decompression compared with patients undergoing selective fasciotomy, and they recommend fasciotomy only in case of progressive peripheral nerve dysfunction, manifested compartment syndrome, or other major injuries.[40] With a fixed neurological deficit, however, surgical decompression shows no influence on outcome.[50] If the clinical situation remains doubtful, however, the performance of open fasciotomy with early debridement may be preferred.

Reconstructive challenges

When treating a patient with severe electrical injury, the plastic reconstructive surgeon encounters many surgical challenges. The anatomic regions most often concerned are the head and the extremities, especially the upper extremities. Bearing that in mind, the appropriate reconstruction is of utmost importance for the functional outcome and the resulting quality of life of the injured.

Head: Scalp, Skull and Mouth

The head is a common injury site in electrical burns. The resulting injury usually appears as a circular area with a central full thickness damage of the scalp, often reaching through galea, periosteum, and sometimes bone. Exposure and necrosis of bone may consequently lead to osteomyelitis and even an epidural abscess. Treatment strategies depend on the extent of the injury to the bone. In case of only a partial necrosis of the bone the outer table of the skull can be tangentially removed with a high-speed bone drill and the viable diploic cavity exposed. In case of sufficient vascularization the exposed bone can be grafted immediately or, when blood supply is questionable grafted when suitable granulation tissue has developed.[51] A vacuum sealing system of the wound may be of significant efficiency in growing adequate amounts of granulation tissue. When the initial wound debridement is delayed, necrotic and infected bone might become the source of a full thickness skull defect. However, with grafting of skin on partially debrided viable bone the lack of a subcutaneous or galea layer often causes long-term problems, such as ulceration and scar formation. Full thickness injury of the skull theoretically requires a complete excision of the necrotic bone to prevent infectious complications. However, this poses the patient at risk for a neurosurgical procedure and requires coverage of the excised area by a rotation flap or even a microvascular graft.

Another approach suggested is the partial debridement followed by definitive flap coverage of the exposed bone, which requires early debridement and the prevention of localized bacterial colonization and infection.[52,53] Fortunately, involvement of the dura occurs rarely. This operation usually requires an extensive free-flap procedure.[54] We prefer to use the latissimus flap connected to cervical vessels, and occasionally employ interpositional vein grafts. This reduces the risk of perfusion problems considerably. When these options are not available the use of acellular human dermis to reconstruct the dural defect, followed by split thickness skin grafting after vascularization may be an option.[55]

In children, especially toddlers, common sites of low tension injury include the mouth and occur usually in the area of the oral commissure affecting the commissure, the lips, and the tongue. The injury happens when the child bites into a cord or a light switch, or touches the 'male' end of an improperly connected cord. The injury usually results in a localized partial necrosis of the lips and the commissure; the subsequent contracture results in microstomia. The treatment strategies, conservative versus early surgical intervention, are debated. The more aggressive early approach of excision and reconstruction results in faster healing, shorter length of hospital stay, and fewer surgical procedures.[56,57] However, in this sensitive age group early excision and reconstruction may also result in a tightened lower lip, and consequent inhibition of normal mandible growth.[58,59] The conservative management, which is favored by us, performs the reconstructive procedure after maturation of the burn-wound scar. Thus the extent of the damage is more apparent and the reconstruction can be performed electively.[60] Oral splinting has been advocated during the initial healing period to decrease the need for reconstructive surgery. However, this more likely reduces scar contractures, so the planned reconstructive procedure can be performed after scar maturation.[62–63] The risk of acute hemorrhage by erosion of the oral arteries after sloughing of the necrotic tissue appears low in our patient population. With adequate caution and education of the patient, this does not prohibit the conservative approach.

Thorax and Abdomen

Electrical injury to the trunk is commonly of minor concern. However, high-tension injuries can cause damage to underlying parenchymatous organs such as the lung. Clinically, this may lead to atelectasis and edema, requiring aggressive ventilator support. Intra-abdominal injuries are uncommon, but may require treatment. When exploration during escharectomy and debridement reveals necrotic underlying muscle and fascia, exploratory laparotomy may be indicated. Potential bowel injury may require segmental bowel resection. Reconstructive options for the closure of chest or abdominal wall defects include direct closure or placement of a synthetic mesh covered by local fasciocutaneous or musculocutaneus flaps. However, the potential negative effects of direct closure on intraabdominal pressure with subsequent development of an abdominal compartment syndrome or compromise of respiratory function must be considered.

Extremities

Electrical injuries to the extremities, especially to the arms and hand, are more common in adult members of the workforce. The actual effects and the sequelae depend on the current, the path of the current and the patient's medical condition. Often the electrical source is grasped by the hand, leading to entry wounds at the hands and upper extremities and exit wounds at the lower extremities. As the resistance and thus the local energy production are dependant on the tissue mass and the cross-sectional diameter of the injured body part, high tension injuries often lead to extensive tissue damage and loss of the involved extremity. Despite aggressive treatment strategies with early debridement and decompression of neurovascular structures the likelihood of amputation is high.[12,13,40–42,64] Even if amputation can be avoided the resulting outcome may be a non-functioning extremity. Kissing lesions may incur extensive tissue damage with resulting thermal necrosis of muscle, tendon, nerves, and blood vessels. The superficial injury may appear innocuous, but the operative debridement shows deep tissue destruction often mandating limb amputation. The role of initial debridement cannot be overstated, as remaining non-viable tissue leads to infection and tissue loss. In our view the early debridement of non-viable tissue prevents this fatal development. Imminent or suspected compartment syndrome should always trigger open fasciotomy to prevent further compromise to the involved extremity. With involvement of the hand and the wrist region in the form of an 'arcing phenomenon' release of the Guyon canal and the carpal tunnel, in addition to fasciotomy of the forearm, appears necessary. The reconstruction and coverage at this injury site may require microvascular reconstruction using nerve cable grafts for the median or ulnar nerve and vein grafts for reconstruction of the radial and ulnar artery in combination with coverage by free flaps. However, these options require sufficient soft tissue coverage and absence of any infection. If in doubt, it appears wise to perform a simple skin grafting procedure followed by elective secondary flap coverage and nerve cable grafting. Other regions of selective destruction in the upper extremity are elbow and axilla. The visible amount of tissue damage does not correlate with the destruction found on exploration. The underlying neurovascular structures, such as brachial artery, median and ulnar nerve or the brachial plexus in the axilla, are at risk. Debridement often leaves a vast tissue defect, which may be covered by rotation flaps from anterior or posterior chest wall in the axilla. Microvascular free flaps at the level of the elbow are rarely used. For extensive defects of the hand and forearm, pedicled groin flaps provide good coverage providing independent blood supply (**Figure 35b.3**). The groin flap also avoids a vascular 'steal phenomenon' as it can be seen after microvascular free flaps in such a severely injured extremity.

Despite all surgical options available, when exploration and initial debridement yield vast irreversible destruction of vital structure the decision for amputation is justified and should be made early.

Amputations

Although distressing to the patient, amputation often remains the only option. The main surgical objective is the achievement of a stably covered stump, allowing early fitting and adaptation of prosthetic devices. The optimal level of amputation is determined by the extent of remaining viable tissue and the intention to create sufficient stump length for function and cosmetic appearance of a prosthesis.

In electrical injury involving the lower extremity, this often requires higher amputation than initially anticipated in order to achieve sufficient stability of the stump and thus allow early prosthetic fitting and ambulation. The local situation often is similar to peripheral vascular disease and the amputation techniques should be appropriately chosen. However, open (guillotine) amputation should be avoided wherever possible. Split thickness skin-grafting onto open stumps is an additional but less preferable approach, as breakdown of the skin occurs more often in grafted areas, especially at graft borders or at points where grafts adhere to underlying bone and further surgical interventions will be required. However, if valuable stump length can be maintained by skin-grafting it should be attempted, as secondary plastic surgical correction and specific prosthetic fitting are available.

In the upper extremity, more length should be preserved, as the resulting weight-bearing load to the stump is less compared to the lower extremity. This allows for better control of the prosthesis by the patient and thus enhanced functionality. In the forearm the muscle length of the flexor–extensor system should be preserved to improve function. In long forearm stumps, atraumatic handling of tendons and muscles is necessary to preserve pronation and supination. Upper arm amputations should be made to preserve as much length as possible as this eases subsequent kineplastic procedures for a functional prosthesis. As in the forearm, muscular length of the flexor–extensor system is maintained by joining them over the bone end. Although it is technically feasible to maintain extremity length by coverage with a free flap, this appears only useful in upper extremity amputation where the functional implications warrant such large-scale operation and the load on the stump is reduced.

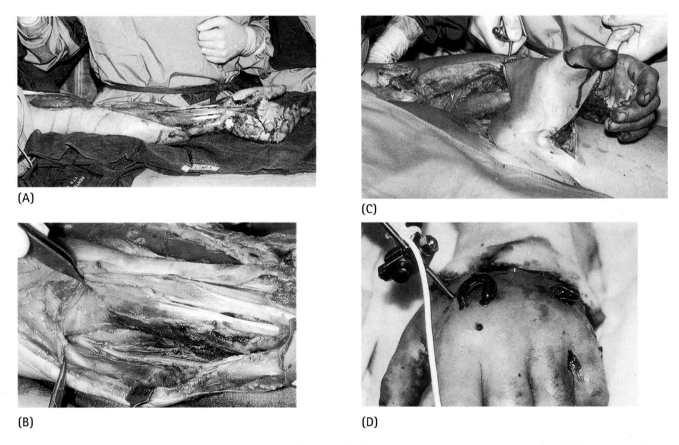

(A)

(B)

(C)

(D)

Fig. 35b.3 High–voltage injury from a power line (50 000 V). Presentation with primary loss of perfusion, loss of function and compartment syndrome. Initial operation with fasciotomy, revascularization of the radial artery and necrectomies. On the following days adequate perfusion with a patent radial artery without coexisting veins. Coverage with groin flap on day 6. Venous congestion and subsequent malperfusion was temporarily treated with leeches. Secondary amputation on day 10 due to late occlusion of the radial artery.

Despite the availability of sophisticated modern myoelectric prostheses the old techniques of surgical rehabilitation should be kept in mind. This includes the Sauerbruch kinematomyoplasty of the biceps humeri muscle and the Krukenberg plasty of the forearm, which provide sensible chopstick-like stumps. Especially for upper-arm amputations, distraction–osteogenesis procedures (Ilizarov technique) provide valuable options to lengthen a short amputation stump.

Peripheral Nerve Injury

Peripheral nerves are very sensitive to electric alterations, and even minor injury may cause transient dysfunction. Clinical findings may be anesthesia, paresthesia, or dysesthesia of usually short-term duration. In rare cases, minor electrical injury may cause temporary autonomic dysfunction and trigger a complex regional pain syndrome (sympathetic reflex dystrophy). Treatment for reflex sympathetic dystrophy should be initiated early and include elevation of the extremity to reduce edema formation, active exercise, non-steroidal anti-inflammatory drugs, and adequate pain relief. The autonomic dysfunction may be influenced by α-adrenergic antagonists, Ca-channel blockers, and low dose diazepam medication, or may require intravenous regional blocks and sympathetic ganglion blockade.[65]

Electrical injury of the upper extremity commonly results in peripheral nerve injury of median and ulnar nerves. The clinical findings may resemble upper extremity compression syndromes or peripheral neuropathy.[66,67] Nerve lesions may be caused by secondary factors such as incorrect positioning and splinting, constricting dressing, or delayed inadequate escharotomy or fasciotomy. Due to accompanying severe muscle loss and scarring, the extent of pure nerve damage is sometimes difficult to determine.

Direct damage to peripheral nerves occurs following the above-mentioned mechanisms of local heat production, depending on cross-sectional resistance or the proximity of peripheral nerves to underlying bone. The local thermal effect produces thrombosis, necrosis or hemorrhage of epineural vessels. Delayed development of fibrosis and therefore a delayed onset of symptoms are not uncommon. Other mechanisms of nerve injury are development of focal axonal degeneration following axonal excitation,[68] or electroporation, which more likely affects myelinated axons.[69,70]

Complications

Central nervous system

Electrical injuries are dramatic events with sometimes devastating consequences. Approximately 60% of all patients with high-voltage injury present with immediate neurological complications, loss of consciousness being the predominant symptom.[71] The involvement of the spinal cord has been described in 2–27% of patients with an entry point of the current located in the head region.[72–74] The incidence of a delayed paralysis progressing to tetraplegia followed by partial remission has been described.[75] However, the cause and mechanism of this phenomenon remain unclear.

The neuropsychological effects of electric injury have been described, mainly in case reports and retrospective studies. Typical consequences and complaints are related to physical, cognitive, and emotional changes.[76,77] The existing problems could not be directly attributed to physical manifestations of injury, and are similar to problems associated with prolonged stress, sleep deprivation, or after blunt head injury. In a study on 481 professional electricians, 97% reported having experienced an electrical shock at some point in their career.[78] The low incidence of neuropsychological dysfunction in this study differed from other findings about the nature and progression of a characteristic neuropsychological syndrome of electrical injury.[77,79] Although the development of transient and progressive neuropsychiatric complications is possible and undisputed, and actual specific effects of electrical injury are difficult to determine. Other confounding factors such as the posttraumatic stress disorder, the grief reaction to disfigurement or extremity loss, and the disposition of the individual, all influence systematic evaluation.

Cataracts

An increased incidence of cataract formation has been described after electrical injury. The incidence in different reports varies from 1% to 8%.[80,81] Patients with head and neck wounds appear to be most at risk. However, the path of the current and the location of the entry point were not related to the development of ocular sequelae.[21] Cataracts may also occur without injury to the head and appear even years after injury. Common initial complaints are blurred vision or diminished visual acuity.[82]

Skeletal Injury

Besides direct tissue destruction through electrical energy, additional trauma can be indirectly inflicted by electric current. Fractures occur due to secondary falls or with forceful tetanic muscle contractions. These are mostly seen in the shoulder,[83] wrists,[84] femurs,[85] and the spine,[86] and may require open reduction and internal fixation. Late sequelae of electrical injury similar to severe thermal burns include major joint contractures and limited function of the extremities.

Another common late complication of electrical burns are heterotopic calcifications in periarticular tissue of large joints, especially elbows. Causative factors include forced passive mobilization, secondary articular bleeding, and calcium precipitation and deposition in damaged or degenerating muscle and connective tissue. Particularly for electrical injury, heterotopic bone formation also occurs in amputation stumps of long bones. This, as well as the common formation of bone cysts in the amputation stump, may lead to secondary skin erosion, inflammation, and difficult adjustment of prosthesis. In both situations surgical excision and wound closure may provide adequate therapy.[87]

Summary

Electrical injuries result in deceptively large tissue loss, often leading to amputation of involved extremities. After initial resuscitation, early debridement, necessary decompression of neurovascular structures, and early wound closure are essential to successful restoration of function. Extensive surgical procedures including free soft-tissue transfer may be necessary to achieve wound closure, and to save and restore limb function. Sometimes, however, early amputation may provide easier and earlier recovery and reintegration into daily life. Long-term complications such as central nervous sequelae, cataracts, and heterotopic ossification must be considered and addressed early in the rehabilitation process.

References

1. Rai J, Jeschke MG, Barrow RE, Herndon DN. Electrical injuries: A 30-year review. *J Trauma* 1999; **46**: 933–936.
2. Tredget EE, Shankowsky HA, Tilley WA. Electrical injuries in Canadian burn care. *Ann N Y Acad Sci* 1999; **888**: 75–87.
3. Rouge RG, Dimick AR. The treatment of electrical injury compared to burn injury: A review of patholphysiology and comparison of patient management protocols. *J Trauma* 1978; **18**: 43.
4. Lewis GK. Trauma resulting from electricity. *J Int Coll Surg* 1957; **28**: 724–727.
5. Artz CP. Electrical injury simulates crush injury. *Surg Gynecol Obstetrics* 1967; **125**: 1316–1317.
6. Wehrmacher WH. The dual challenge of electric injury. *Compr Ther* 1995; **21**: 308–312.
7. Daniel RK, Ballard PA, Heroux P, *et al.* High voltage electrical injury: acute pathophysiology. *J Hand Surg* 1988; **13A**: 44–49.
8. Haberal M, Ucar N, Bayraktar U, *et al.* Visceral injuries, wound infection and sepsis following electrical injuries. *Burns* 1996; **22**: 158–161.
9. Zelt RG, Daniel RK, Ballard PA, *et al.* High-voltage electrical injury: chronic wound evaluation. *Plast Reconstr Surg* 1988; **82**: 1027–1041.
10. Marc B, Baudry F, Douceron H, *et al.* Suicide by electrocution with low-voltage current. *J Forensic Sci* 2000; **45**: 216–222.
11. Vedung S, Arturson G, Wadin K, Hedlund A. Angiographic findings and need for amputation in high tension electrical injuries. *Scand J Plast Reconstr Hand Surg* 1990; **24**: 225–231.
12. Butler ED, Grant TD. Electrical injuries with special reference to the upper extremities. *Am J Surg* 1977; **134**: 95–99.
13. Hunt JL, Mason AD, Masterson TS, *et al.* The pathophysiology of acute electrical injuries. *J Trauma* 1976; **16**: 335–340.
14. Lee RC, Capelli-Schellpfeffer M. Electrical and lightning injuries. In: Cameron JL, ed. *Current Surgical Therapy.* St Louis, MO: Mosby, 1998; 1021–1023.
15. Sugar IP, Foster W, Neumann E. Model of cell electrofusion: membrane electroporation, pore coalescence and percolation. *Biophys Chem* 1987; **26**: 321–335.
16. Tsong TY. Electroporation of cell membranes. *Biophys J* 1991; **60**: 297–306.
17. Coster HG. A quantitative analysis of the voltage–current relationships of fixed charge membranes and the associated property of 'punch-through'. *Biophys J* 1965; **5**: 669–686.
18. Lee RC, Gaylor DC, Bhatt D, Israel DA. Role of cell membrane rupture in the pathogenesis of electrical trauma. *J Surg Res* 1988; **44**: 709–719.
19. DeBono R. A histological analysis of a high-voltage electric current injury to an upper limb. *Burns* 1999; **25**: 541–547.
20. Bhatt DL, Gaylor DC, Lee RC. Rhabdomyolysis due to pulsed electric fields. *Plast Reconstr Surg* 1990; **86**: 1–11.
21. Ferreiro I, Melendez J, Ragalado J, *et al.* Factors influencing the sequelae of high tension electrical injuries. *Burns* 1998; **24**: 649–653.
22. Jacobsen H. Electrically induced deposition of metal on the human skin. *Forensic Sci Int* 1997; **90**: 85–92.
23. Ohashi M, Koizumi J, Hosoda Y, *et al.* Correlation between magnetic resonance imaging and histopathology of an amputated forearm after an electrical injury. *Burns* 1998; **24**: 362–368.
24. Fleckenstein JL, Chason DP, Bonte FJ *et al.* High voltage electric injury: assessment of muscle viability with MR imaging and Tc-99m pyrophosphate scintigraphy. *Radiology* 1995; **195**: 205–210.
25. Sayman HB, Urgancioglu I, Uslu I, Kapicioglu T. Prediction of muscle viability after electrical burn necrosis. *Burns* 1998; **24**: 649–653.
26. Brumback RA, Feedback DL, Leech RW. Rhabdomyolysis following electrical injury. *Sem Neurol* 1995; **15**: 329–334.
27. Feinfeld DA, Cheng JT, Beysolow TD *et al.* A prospective study of urine and serum myoglobin levels in patients with acute rhabdomyolysis. *Clin Nephrol* 1992; **38**: 193–195.
28. Grossmann RA, Hamilton RW, Morse BM, *et al.* Nontraumatic rhabdomyolysis and acute renal failure. *N Eng J Med* 1974; **291**: 807–811.
29. Rosen CL, Adler JN, Rabban JT, *et al.* Early predictors of myoglobinuria and acute renal failure following electrical injury. *J Emerg Med* 1999; **17**: 783–789.
30. Bailey B, Gaudreault P, Thivierge RL, Turgeon JP. Cardiac monitoring of children with household electrical injuries. *Ann Emerg Med* 1995; **25**: 612–617.
31. Arrowsmith J, Usgaocar RP, Dickson WA. Electrical injury and the frequency of cardiac complications. *Burns* 1997; **23**: 576–578.
32. Fish RM. Electric Injury, part III: cardiac monitoring indication, the pregnant patient, and lightning. *J Emerg Med* 2000; **18**: 181–187.
33. Guinard JP, Chiolero R, Buchser E, *et al.* Myocardial injury after electrical burns: short and long term study. *Scand J Plast Reconstr Hand Surg* 1987; **21**: 301–302.
34. Jensen PJ, Thomsen PE, Bagger JP, *et al.* Electrical injury causing ventricular arrhythmias. *Br Heart J* 1987; **57**: 279–283.
35. Wilson CM, Fatovich DM. Do children need to be monitored after electric shocks? *J Paediatr Child Health* 1998; **34**: 474–476.
36. Purdue GF, Hunt JL. Electrocardiographic monitoring after electrical injury: necessity or luxury. *J Trauma* 1986; **26**: 166–167.
37. Cunningham PA. The need for cardiac monitoring after electrical injury. *Med J Aust* 1991; **154**: 765–766.
38. Fatovitch DM, Lee KY. Household electric injury: who should be monitored? *Med J Aust* 1991; **155**: 301–303.
39. Garcia Ct, Smith GA, Cohen DM, Fernandez K. Electrical injuries in a pediatric emergency department. *Ann Emerg Med* 1995; **26**: 604–608.
40. Mann R, Gibran N, Engrav L, Heimbach D. Is immediate decompression of high-voltage electrical injuries to the upper extremities always necessary? *J Trauma* 1996; **40**: 584–587.
41. Chick LR, Lister GD, Sowder L. Early free-flap coverage of electrical and thermal burns. *Plast Recontr Surg* 1992; **89**: 1013–1019.
42. Garcia-Sanchez V, Morell PG. Electric burns: high- and low-tension injuries. *Burns* 1999; **25**: 357–360.
43. Luce EA, Gottlieb SE. 'True' high-tension electrical injuries. *Ann Plast Surg* 1984; **12**: 321–325.
44. Jaffe RH, Willis D, Bachem A. The effect of electric currents on the arteries. *Arch Pathol* 1929; **7**: 244–249.
45. Ponten B, Erikson U, Johansson SH, Olding L. New observations on tissue changes along the pathway of the current in an electrical injury. *Scand J Plast Reconstr Surg* 1970; **4**: 75–82.
46. Hussmann J, Zamboni WA, Russell RC, *et al.* A model for recording the microcirculatory changes associated with standardized electrical injury of skeletal muscle. *J Surg Res* 1995; **59**: 725–732.
47. Zhi-Xiang Z, Yuan-Tie Z, Xu-Yuan L, *et al.* Urgent repair of electrical injuries: analysis of 40 cases. *Acta Chir Plast* 1990; **32**: 142–151.
48. Yang JY, Noordhoff MS. Early adipofascial flap coverage of deep electrical burn wounds of upper extremities. *Plast Reconstr Surg* 1993; **91**: 819–825.
49. Godina M, Bajec J, Baraga A. Salvage of the mutilated upper extremity with temporary ectopic implantation of the undamaged part. *Plast Reconstr Surg* 1986; **78**: 295–299.
50. Engrav LH, Gottlieb JR, Walkinshaw MD, *et al.* Outcome and treatment of electrical injury with immediate median and ulnar nerve palsy at the wrist: a retrospective review and a survey of members of the American Burn Association. *Ann Plast Surg* 1990; **25**: 166–168.
51. Sheridan RL, Choucair RJ, Donclean MB. Management of massive calvarial exposure in young children. *J Burn Care Rehabil* 1998; **19**: 29–32.
52. Luce EA, Hoopes JE. Electrical burns of the scalp and the skull. *Plast Reconstr Surg* 1974; **54**: 359.
53. BizhkoIP, Slesarenko SV. Operative treatment of deep burns of the scalp and skull. *Burns* 1992; **18**: 220–223.
54. Miyamoto Y, Harada K, Kodama Y, *et al.* Cranial coverage involving scalp, bone and dura using free inferior epigastric flap. *Br J Plast Surg* 1986; **39**: 483–490.
55. Barret JP, Dziewulski P, McCauley RL, *et al.* Dural reconstruction of a class IV calvarial burn with decellularized human dermis. *Burns* 1999; **25**: 459–462.
56. Zarem HA, Greer DM. Tongue flap for reconstruction of the lip after electrical burns. *Plast Reconstr Surg* 1974; **53**: 310.
57. DeLaPlaza R, Quetgals A, Rodriguez E. Treatment of electrical burns of the mouth. *Burns* 1983; **10**: 49.
58. Hartford CD, Kealy GP, Lavelle WE, Buckner H. An appliance to prevent and treat microstomia from burns. *J Trauma* 1975; **15**: 356.
59. Ortiz-Monasterio F, Factor R. Early definitive treatment of electric burns of the mouth. *Plast Reconstr Surg* 1980; **65**: 169.
60. Pensler JM, Rosenthal A. Reconstruction of the oral commissure after an electrical burn. *J Burn Care Rehabil* 1990; **11**: 50–53.
61. Leake JE, Curtin JW. Electrical burns of the mouth in children *Clin Plast Surg* 1984; **11**: 669.
62. Dado DV, Polley W, Kernahan DA. Splinting of oral commissure electrical burns in children. *J Pediatr* 1985; **107**: 92.
63. Silverglade D, Ruberg RL. Nonsurgical management of burns to the lips and commissures. *Clin Plast Surg* 1986; **13**: 87.
64. Luce EA, Dowden WL, Su CT, Hoopes JE. High tension electrical injury of the upper extremity. *Surg Gynecol Obstet* 1978; **147**: 38.
65. Gellman H, Nichols D. Reflex Sympathetic Dystrophy in the Upper Extremity. *J Am Acad Orthop Surg* 1997; **5**: 313–322.
66. Still JM, Law EJ, Duncan W, Hughes HF. Long thoracic nerve injury due to an electric burn. *J Burn Care Rehabil* 1996; **17**: 562–564.
67. Haberal MA, Gürer S, Akman N, Basgöze O. Persistent peripheral nerve pathologies in patients with electric burns. *J Burn Care Rehabil* 1996; **17**: 147–149.
68. Agnew WF, McCreery DB, Yuen TG, Bullara LA. Local anaesthetic block protects

against electrically induced damage in peripheral nerve. *J Biomed Eng* 1990; **12:** 301–308.

69. Abramov GS, Bier M, Capelli-Schellpfeffer M, Lee RC. Alteration in sensory nerve function following electrical shock. *Burns* 1996; **22:** 602–606.

70. Gaylor DC, Prakah-Asante K, Lee RC. Significance of cell size and tissue structure in electrical trauma. *J Theoret Biol* 1988; **133:** 223–237.

71. Grube BJ, Heimbach DM, Engrav LH, Copass MK. Neurologic consequences of electrical burns. *J Trauma* 1990; **30:** 254–257.

72. Koller J, Orsagh J. Delayed neurological sequelae of high tension electrical burns. *Burns* 1989; **15:** 175–178.

73. Varghese G, Mani H, Redford SH. Spinal cord injuries following electric accident. *Paraplegia* 1986; **24:** 159–162.

74. Levine NS, Atkins A, McKeel DW *et al.* Spinal cord injury following electrical accidents: case reports. *J Trauma* 1975; **15:** 459–463.

75. Breugem CC, van Hertum W, Groenevelt F. High voltage electrical injury leading to a delayed onset tetraplegia, with recovery. *Ann N Y Acad Sci* 1999; **888:** 131–136.

76. Janus TJ, Barrash J. Neurologic and neurobehavioural effects of electric and lightning injuries. *J Burn Care Rehabil* 1996; **17:** 409–415.

77. Pliskin NH, Capelli-Schellpfeffer M, Law RT, Malina AC, Kelley KM, Lee RC. Neuropsychological symptom presentation after electrical injury. *J Trauma* 1998; **44:** 709–715.

78. Tkachenko TA, Kelley KM, Pliskin NH, Fink JW. Electrical injury through the eyes of professional electricians. *Ann N Y Acad Sci* 1999; **888:** 42–59.

79. Pliskin NH, Fink J, Malina A, Moran S, Kelley KM, Capelli-Schellpfeffer M, Lee R. The neuropsychological effects of electrical injury. *Ann N Y Acad Sci* 1999; **888:** 140–149.

80. Boozalis GT, Purdue GF, Hunt JL, McCulley JP. Ocular changes from electrical burn injuries: a literature review and report of cases. *J Burn Care Rehabil* 1991; **12:** 458–462.

81. Solem L, Fisher R, Strate R. The natural history of electrical injury. *J Trauma* 1977; **17:** 487–492.

82. Saffle JR, Crandall A, Warden GD. Cataracts: A long-term complication of electrical injury. *J Trauma* 1985; **25:** 17.

83. Dumas JL, Walker N. Bilateral scapular fractures secondary to electrical shock. *Arch Orthop Trauma Surg* 1992; **111:** 287–288.

84. Adams AJ, Beckett MW. Bilateral wrist fractures from accidental electric shock. *Injury* 1997; **28:** 227–228.

85. Tompkins GS, Henderson RC, Peterson HD. Bilateral simultaneous fractures of the femoral neck: case report. *J Trauma* 1990; **30:** 1415–1416.

86. van den Brink WA, van Leeuwen O. Lumbar burst fracture due to low voltage shock. A case report. *Acta Orthop Scand* 1995; **66:** 374–375.

87. Helm PA, Walker SC. New bone formation at amputation in electrically burn-injured patients. *Arch Phys Med Rehabil* 1987; **68:** 284–286.

Chapter 36

Cold-induced injury: frostbite

Stephen E Morris

Frostbite is a traumatic injury that is caused by the failure of the normal protective mechanisms against the thermal environment that classically results in localized tissue temperatures falling below freezing, although cold-induced injury can result from nonfreezing environmental insults. Cold-induced injury continues to be a relatively frequent injury in the United States due to increasing interest in out-of-door winter recreational activities as well as the high prevalence of homeless and socioeconomically disadvantaged individuals in large urban centers.[1,2]

One of the earliest cases of frostbite has been found in a preColumbian Chilean mummy from about 3000 BC.[3] Much knowledge about the incidence and circumstances surrounding this injury has been derived from the extensive military experiences of the past.[4] Hannibal lost nearly half of his army of 46 000 soldiers during a 2-week crossing of the Pyrenean Alps due to frostbite injury. During the Revolutionary War, it is recorded in 1778 that Washington lost 10% of his army to cold-related casualties during a single winter.[5]

The first modern published report of cold-induced injury did not occur until 1805,[6] and Baron Larrey produced the first systematic medical observations of frostbite during the Russian campaign of 1812–1813.[7] As Surgeon General of Napoleon's forces in Russia, Dominique Larrey was able to produce classic descriptions of frostbite and trench foot, and to identify the severe effects of refreezing that occurred with bonfire thawing and subsequent marching in frigid conditions. With this information, Larrey made therapeutic recommendations that were adhered to for more than 150 years of military medicine. This included the use of friction massage with snow or ice rather than rapid thawing over an open fire as he had seen more severe injuries subjected to such freeze-thaw-freeze conditions. He also noted that the number of cold-induced injuries were much greater during periods of wet, near-freezing conditions as opposed to similar periods when conditions were dry, but below freezing. He described the loss of all but 360 troops due to cold in a division of 12 000 men. Larrey reported essentially the total loss of one-quarter million troops within a 6-month period due to cold and starvation. Over the past century, military medical experience has only been somewhat better. It is estimated that World Wars I and II and the Korean conflict included one million frostbite injuries. The United States Army reported 90 000 cold injuries during World War II. German troops underwent 15 000 amputations during the winter of 1942,[8] and Greek troops 25 000 amputations due to frostbite alone during the course of the war.[9] High altitude bomber crews suffered from frostbite more than any other injury.[10] Modern military cold-induced injury data continue to accrue.[11–16] Interestingly, the Vietnam War and other military conflicts fought in tropical climates produced substantial nonfreezing cold injuries in soldiers exposed to wet environments in the temperature range of 35–40°F (1.6–4.4°C).[10,17,18] Although there has been little epidemiological data in the civilian population, significant numbers have accumulated in relatively few series.[19,20] This significant body of military and emerging civilian data stimulated first basic laboratory investigations, starting with Merryman[21–23] and, subsequently, clinical research that has taken us from the empiric recommendations of Larrey to the rapid rewarming[24] recommendations of Mills[25,26] and others.[27] Such efforts have paved the way to more systematic investigation and eventually to refinement of patient care practices.

Physiology of temperature regulation

In the human, temperature regulation is achieved through a complex interaction of heat production, loss, and conservation mechanisms that require both autonomic and voluntary functions. Normal body temperature ranges from 36.2 to 37.7°C. Any impairment of autonomic or voluntary behavioral functions may result in dysregulation of thermal homeostasis. Control of thermal homeostasis resides in the central nervous system. Core blood cooling will result in hypothalamic–pituitary axis stimulation of catecholamine release, peripheral vasoconstriction, and inhibition of sweating to conserve heat as well as thyroid hormone release with upregulation of oxidative metabolism and shivering for an increase in heat production. Core temperature, which may be measured by rectal thermometer, is generally expected to be 0.5°C higher than surface temperatures, which may be measured orally or tympanically. Peripheral extremity skin temperature is expected to fluctuate much more widely. In a warm environment, temperature of the distal extremities may substantially exceed core temperature, while the reverse may be true in the heat conservation mode in a cold environment.[28] Acral blood flow may vary from 0.5 to 100 ml/min/100 g of tissue.[29] When blood flow falls below this range, eventual tissue necrosis may occur. With environmental conditioning the maximal blood flow may exceed 100–122 ml/min/100 g of tissue. Such range in peripheral blood flow response affords the core body temperature substantial thermal homeostasis at a relatively cheap metabolic price, but the cost is at the expense of the extremities. The primary function of this response is to maintain core blood temperature. Sir Thomas Lewis described a vasomotor response in cold environments and termed it the 'hunting reaction'.[30–33] In this response, vasoconstriction alternates with vasodilation in 5–10-minute cycles. The cycling is somewhat irregular and results in nonuniform changes in peripheral temperature, but this cycling both conserves core heat and allows extremity viability. The hunting reaction is more pronounced in people indigenous to colder climates. There appears to be maintenance of higher extremity temperature with more rapid cycling and rewarming.[31] Voluntary behaviors may be important in protection of extremities from cold injury and, as such, mental status impairment can constitute a substantial risk for frostbite in the cold environment.[34] Consequently, alcohol and drug intoxication have been roundly implicated among the risk factors for cold-induced injury.[35–39]

Pathophysiology of cold-induced injury

A number of factors have been associated with the development of frostbite. One well-recognized factor is that of ethanol consumption. Valnicek reviewed their 12-year experience in Saskatchewan with patients admitted for frostbite and identified ethanol use in 46%, psychiatric disorders in 17%, vehicular trauma in 19%, vehicular failure in 15%, and drug abuse in 4% of patients.[38] Overt or covert manifestation of psychiatric disease[39] as well as neurovascular factors such as smoking and diabetes mellitus, homelessness, fatigue, improper clothing, previous cold weather injury, high altitude, extremes of age, and male gender[19,40] have all been cited in cold injury. A number of physical factors appear to play a role in the development of frostbite. The duration and efficiency of tissue cooling understandably have a marked effect on the extent of cold injury. Moist or wet skin is substantially more susceptible to frostbite than dry skin.[41] Efficiency of thermal conduction is important as evidenced by the effectiveness of metal contact as opposed to fabric or wood contact. Windchill is a principle of physiologic importance that was demonstrated by Paul Siple who was well-known for his physiologic observations with the Antarctic Byrd Expeditions.[42] He developed formulas, taking into account the effects of temperature and wind speed on tissue cooling, that are a basis for the wind chill charts published by the US Air Force. Thus, exposed skin may suffer similar injuries exposed to air at 0°F in calm conditions or to a 15 mile-per-hour breeze at 25°F.[26] Although high-altitude conditions have been associated with cold injury, there has been no independent risk-factor associated with this environment.[41] The physical state of skin can have an effect on the development of cold injury. Water in the stratum corneum can predispose to water crystallization in the skin and deeper tissue.[43] This may explain recommendations of using oil or ointment on exposed skin at risk for frostbite and the practice of polar explorers to avoid washing during expeditions. The nature of clothing also plays a significant role. Mills[25] documented the association of ill-fitting boots and the development of frostbite. Similarly, some authors have touted the relationship of snug-fitting or damp clothing and cold-induced injury, reporting

the effect of clothing on circulation or the thermal conduction of moisture compared to dry air by a factor of 25.[44] Cigarette smoking is cited as a cause of local circulatory compromise. This has been demonstrated with smoking nude models as well as random skin flaps.[45,46] Chronic smoking does not appear to have an effect on cold-induced injury. Lastly, a history of previous cold injury places the patient at substantial risk for frostbite.[47,48] Not only the incidence of injury, but also the extent may be increased with previous exposure.[44] There is no real evidence of tolerance or indigenous adaptation to the cold environment that is intrinsically protective against frostbite.[16,49]

The injury associated with frostbite is attributed to two broad mechanistic categories: the first is that of direct cellular damage and death due to the cold insult, and the second is the more delayed process mediated by progressive tissue ischemia.[50–56] The immediate effects of frostbite are evidenced by formation of extracellular ice crystals. These crystals cause direct injury to the cell membrane, resulting in cellular dehydration due to a change in the osmotic gradient.[22,57] The rate of cooling is reported to have an effect on the development of extracellular or intracellular ice crystals.[58] Rapid cooling results in intracellular freezing which causes more severe cellular damage and cell death, while a slower rate of cooling produces extracellular ice crystals. This slower process, nevertheless, results in transmembrane osmotic shift that drives water from within the cell and produces intracellular dehydration. This dehydration causes changes in protein[59,60] and lipid conformation, as well as changes in pH and other biochemical processes such as electrolyte concentration that are deleterious to intracellular homeostasis.[61–64] As temperature continues to fall, intracellular crystals develop regardless of cooling rate[20,65] with a loss of the linear relationship of temperature to metabolism,[31,66] decreased DNA synthesis[67] and the vascular response that has been called the 'triple response of Lewis', which is characterized by localized reddening of the wheal and may indicate release of histamine from injured cells.[68]

Microvascular pathophysiology may be even more important in outcome than the direct thermal injury to the cell. This was suggested by studies showing survival of full-thickness skin subjected to freezing and thawing that progressed to necrosis when left in situ but survived when transplanted to a normal, uninjured recipient site.[50] Zacarian identified a number of processes that may play a role in the microcirculatory changes of frostbite. There appears to be a transient vasoconstriction of both arterioles and venules with subsequent resumption of capillary blood flow. Concomitantly there have been microemboli observed.[65] With thawing, the capillaries demonstrate restoration of blood flow, but this diminished within minutes. Complete cessation of blood flow is often seen within 20 minutes after rewarming of frozen tissue. Such similar changes have been seen with random skin flap models after reperfusion which has suggested reactive oxygen species as mediators of injury.[69] Within 72 hours there is a significant de-epithelialization in the capillary bed and deposition of fibrin. Examination of the endothelial ultrastructure has shown swelling, fluid extravasation, vascular endothelial cell dilation and significant projection of the cell into the vascular lumen prior to cell lysis.[70] There is regional variation in the extent of injury with venules being most profoundly affected[71] with the hypothesis that as evidences by lower flow, stasis must play a role in this pathophysiologic process.

Pathobiochemistry of frostbite has been closely compared to the inflammatory response in the burn wound.[27,72] Inflammatory mediators such as eicosanoids in burns,[73–76] in burn blister fluid,[77,78] as well as bradykinin[79] and histamine[80] draw parallels with findings in cold-induced injury. This has prompted investigators to hypothesize a model similar to that of Jackson including zones of necrosis and stasis.[81] Similar to their burn blister analysis, Robson and Heggers examined the fluid in frostbite blisters and found high levels of prostaylandin $F_{2\alpha}$ and thromboxane B_2. These agents or their precursors have been implicated in vasoconstriction and leukocyte adherence.[72] The inhibition of these eicosanoids has had a salubrious effect in animal models.[82,83] Clinical efficacy has been suggested by the use of thromboxane inhibition.[20] It appears that this process is significantly different than the previously proposed mechanism of vasospasm, thrombosis, and fibrin deposition.[2] Much about this mechanism has yet to be elucidated including the nature of microemboli that have been observed.[84]

Signs and symptoms of frostbite injury

Most frequently, the patient is basically unaware that frostbite injury is occurring. The association of hypothermia and the use of substances known to alter mental status may contribute to this problem. Typical distribution in 90% of patients is acral, with others suffering injuries to ears, nose, cheeks and penis.[13,19,38,40] The patient may note insensitivity and clumsiness of the affected part. This complex of symptoms rapidly reverses upon rewarming. Insensitivity is rapidly replaced by severe pain during and immediately after the rewarming process. The pain is often described as throbbing in character sometimes requiring parenteral opioids for relief. Pain symptoms increase for the first few days and gradually abate during the following 3 weeks. Assessment of injury must be deferred until rewarming of the affected part is complete.

A condition often termed 'frostnip' may be present in which there is not true tissue injury; the condition may be manifested by numbness and pallor of exposed skin. This will often affect skiers and others exposed to cold winds for brief periods of time. Rewarming results in near-complete resolution of symptoms and physical findings, with the possible exception of some hyperemia, edema, and tingling in the region. The nonfreezing manifestation of mild cold injury is often termed chilblains, pernio, kibes or cold urticaria. These are often chronic in nature with itching and erythema as more prominent findings. True frostbite, on the other hand, always involves some degree of tissue injury. Classification of severity of cold injury can be helpful in planning medical management. It must be emphasized that clinical appearance will evolve over a period of time after rewarming. Even after rewarming, the initial appearance is often deceptive.[11,19] Most injuries appear hyperemic after rewarming regardless of the degree of involvement. The development of skin blebs is a time-dependent process that often requires many hours to days. Sensation returns during this period, which is often replaced by bothersome tingling and pain. This may develop into severe neuropathic pain that can be aggravated by warm environments and dependent position of the injured member. After 12–24 hours the character of the blebs becomes apparent and an assessment of the degree of involvement may be helpful in planning management of the injury. Traditional classification is similar to that of the burn injury. First degree injury is superficial without formation of vesicles or blebs. There may initially be an area of pallor with surrounding erythema that evolves into general edema and erythema without long-term sequelae. Second degree injury has associated light-colored blisters and subsequent peeling. This often correlates with dermal involvement but has a generally favorable prognosis. Third degree frostbite typically has dark or hemorrhagic blisters that evolve into thick, black eschar over 1–2 weeks. Fourth degree injury involves bone, tendon or muscle and will result in definite tissue loss. Exactness in depth of injury cannot be expected and some favor more general classification of superficial (first and second degree injury) or deep (third and fourth degree) frostbite injury. Poor prognostic findings include hemorrhagic blisters and a woody or nondeforming tissue consistency. Preservation of pin-prick sensation and light-colored and large blebs predict less risk of tissue loss. Long-term symptoms include hypersensitivity to cold, sensory deficits, chronic pain, and hyperhidrosis.[1] Growth abnormalities and heterotopic calcification have also been described as long-term complications of frostbite.[33,85]

Diagnostic methods and management

The time-dependent evolution of the clinical manifestations of frostbite and the inability to assess tissue involvement deep to the skin are significant limitations in the prompt management of this injury. A number of imaging methods have been explored in an attempt to decrease the duration of disability and the length of stay in hospitals. Plain radiographs can demonstrate soft-tissue swelling or, as time progresses, tissue loss, bone demineralization or periosteal inflammation. Arteriography has constituted the traditional method for assessment of distal perfusion, but its usefulness is limited by the same factors as clinical assessment in the early phases of injury.[2] The usefulness of laser Doppler flowmetry in frostbite injury is presently unknown. Radioisotope scintigraphy has emerged as an early diagnostic modality.[86–89] Magnetic resonance imaging is now being proposed as a method to evaluate even individual vessel status and as a means to identify a line of demarcation earlier in the clinical course.[90]

Only a few general principles of frostbite care are generally accepted. Larrey's methods of rubbing the affected area with snow or with vigorous massage have only recently fallen out of usage in the main medical community. Mills and others at the Arctic Aeromedical Laboratory have documented the results of thawing and refreezing with the resultant worsening of outcome.[48] Thus it is recommended that partial or slow rewarming during transport should be avoided. Rapid rewarming means warming at the temperature of 40°C with a protocol such as that based upon the work of McCauley et al.[27]

Frostbite care protocol

- Admit frostbite patient to a specialized treatment unit
- Transfer of acute frostbite patient should be avoided unless necessary for specialized care with great care to protect patient from further cold exposure
- Immediate rapid rewarming should be performed at a temperature of 40–42°C for 15–30 minutes or until rewarming is complete.

After Complete Rewarming:

- White blisters are debrided and topical treatment with Aloe vera (Dermaide aloe) q6h is initiated
- Hemorrhagic blisters are left intact
- Injured parts are elevated and splinted as required
- Tetanus prophylaxis is followed
- Appropriate analgesia is administered
- Ibuprofen 400 mg PO q12h is administered
- Antibiotic prophylaxis is administered as appropriate
- Hydrotherapy or gentle wound care is provided daily
- Photodocumentation is essential upon admission, at 24 hours and at every 2–3 days during hospitalization
- Outpatient care must be tailored to patient situation to maintain adequate wound care and appropriate medical follow-up.

A number of adjunctive therapeutic modalities have been suggested with some experimental rationale, but there is minimal clinical evidence in support of the therapies. Sympathectomy has been examined with mixed results.[91,92] The series by Taylor is of interest with favorable outcomes in a small number of patients. Although suggestive of more rapid resolution of edema and possibly decreased tissue loss, there is no randomized controlled study to answer this question. As is suggested by basic science investigation, the use of anticoagulation does not appear to have any clinical application in frostbite.[49]

Dextran has been thought to have some theoretical utility because of the appearance of microemboli in this disease process. These have been poorly characterized, but basic animal experiments have demonstrated some decrease in tissue loss with the administration of dextrans.[50] Again, this has not been examined in a rigorous fashion clinically.

Vasodilators have been used widely in the past. Intra-arterial reserpine has been used successfully for vasospasm but there are no clinical data to recommend its use for frostbite at the present time. Other efforts to improve tissue oxygenation such as hyperbaric oxygen have likewise been inconclusive and no substantial clinical or laboratory investigation has been produced recently.

In the past decade, the use of thrombolytic agents has been examined in a collected series of patients[93] as well as in an animal model.[94] A multicenter trial will be necessary to measure the effects in a controlled fashion.

Surgical intervention is often required with frostbite injury, but as the adage has been often repeated, 'Frostbite in January, amputate in July',[95] a conservative approach is needed in the present management scheme. Mills described the need for early escharotomy or fasciotomy in certain individuals, but this is indeed rare.[26] He likewise suggested that skin grafting after development of healthy granulation tissue may decrease the amount of post-frostbite pain. Meticulous debridement and gentle but thorough wound care is important in the maintenance of the frostbitten part which is an effort to allow complete demarcation prior to amputation. This is not always possible and surgical intervention may be needed for control of infection as well as wound closure after clinical wound demarcation or as guided by technetium scintigraphy. The need for improved treatment of frostbite has become widespread, with this disease being seen more frequently in the general population over the past few decades. There has been some fascinating progress in the understanding of this injury process, but

clinical investigations are presently lacking in most aspects of care for the frostbite injury. Biochemical intervention and improved imaging methods can help to speed the recovery and enhance the ultimate functionality of these patients.

References

1. Edlich R, Chang D, Birk K, RF M, Tafel J. Cold injuries. *Compr Ther* 1989; **15**: 13–21.
2. Purdue G, Hunt J. Cold injury: a collective review. *J Burn Care Rehabil* 1986; **7**: 331–42.
3. Post PW, Donner DD. Frostbite in a pre-Columbian mummy. *Am J Phys Anthropol* 1972; **37**: 187–91.
4. Schechter D, Sarot L. Historical accounts of injuries due to cold. *Surgery* 1968; **63**: 527–35.
5. Smith D, Robson M, Heggers J. Frostbite and other cold-induced injuries. In: Puerbach P, Geehr E, eds. *Management of Wilderness and Environmental Emergencies*. St Louis: CV Mosby, 1989: 101–18.
6. Zingg W. The management of accidental hypothermia. *Can Med Assoc J* 1967; **96**: 214.
7. Larrey D. *Memoirs of Military Surgery*, Vol. 5. Baltimore: Joseph Cushing, 1814: 156–64.
8. Vaughn P. Local cold injury – menace to military operations. A review. *Military Med* 1980; **145**: 305.
9. Katsas A, Agnantis J, Smyrnis S. Carcinoma on old frostbites. *Am J Surg* 1977; **133**: 377–8.
10. Dembert M, Dean L, Noddin E. Cold weather morbidity among US Navy and Marine Corps personnel. *Military Med* 1981; **146**: 771–5.
11. Orr K, Fainer D. Cold injuries in Korea during the winter of 1950–1951. *Medicine* 1952; **31**: 177–84.
12. Taylor M, Kulungowski M, Hamelink J. Frostbite injuries during winter maneuvers: a long-term disability. *Military Med* 1989; **154**: 411–3.
13. Lehmuskallio E, Lindholm H, Koskenvuo K, Sarna S, Friberg O, Viljanen A. Frostbite of the face and ears: epidemiological study of risk factors in Finnish conscripts. *Br Med J* 1995; **311**: 1661–3.
14. Marsh A. A short but distant war: the Falklands campaign. *J R Soc Med* 1983; **76**: 972–82.
15. Groom A, Coull J. Army amputees from the Falklands: review. *J R Army Med Corps* 1984; **130**: 114–6.
16. Candler WH, Ivey H. Cold weather injuries among US soldier in Alaska: a five-year review. *Military Med* 1997; **162**: 788–91.
17. Allen A. Tropical immersion foot. *Lancet* 1983; **1**: 1185–9.
18. Hanifin J, Cuetter A. In patients with immersion type of cold injury diminished nerve conduction velocity. *Electromyogr Clin Neurophysiol* 1974; **14**: 173–8.
19. Boswick J, Thompson J, Jonas R. The epidemiology of cold injuries. *Surg Gynecol Obstet* 1979; **149**: 326.
20. Heggers J, Robson M, Manavalen K. Experimental and clinical observations on frostbite. *Ann Emerg Med* 1987; **16**: 1056.
21. Kulka J. Histopathologic studies in frostbitten rabbits. In: Ferrer M, ed. *Cold Injury*. New York: Josiah Macy Jr. Foundation, 1956: 94–151.
22. Merryman H. Mechanics of freezing in living cells and tissue. *Science* 1956; **124**: 515–21.
23. Merryman H. Tissue freezing and local cold injury. *Physiol Rev* 1957; **37**: 233–51.
24. Mills W, Whaley R, Fish W. Frostbite: experience with rapid rewarming and ultrasonic therapy. *Alaska Med* 1961; **3**: 28.
25. Mills W. Out in the cold. *Emerg Med* 1976; **18**: 134.
26. Mills W. Summary of treatment of the cold injured patient. Frostbite. *Alaska Med* 1983; **35**: 61–6.
27. McCauley R, Hing D, Robson M. Frostbite: a rational approach based on the pathophysiology. *J Trauma* 1983; **23**.
28. Holm P, Vanggard L. Frostbite. *Plast Reconstr Surg* 1974; **54**: 544–51.
29. Barton A. Physiology of cutaneous circulation, thermoregulatory functions. In: Rothman S, ed. *The Human Integument*. Washington, D.C.: American Association for the Advancement of Science, 1959.
30. Lewis T. Observations upon the reactions of the vessels of the human skin to cold. *Heart* 1930; **15**: 177–208.
31. Dana A, Rex I, Samitz M. The hunting reflex. *Arch Dermatol* 1969; **99**: 441–50.
32. Adams T, Smith R. Effect of chronic local cold exposure on finger temperature responses. *J Appl Physiol* 1962; **17**: 317–22.
33. Britt L, Dascombe W, Rodriguez A. New horizons in management of hypothermia and frostbite injury. *Surg Clin N Am* 1991; **71**: 345–70.
34. Cold Hypersensitivity [editorial]. *Br Med J* 1975; **1**: 643–4.
35. Hashmi M, Rashid M, Haleem A, Bokharie S, Hussain T. Frostbite: epidemiology

at high altitude in the Karakoram mountains. *Ann R Coll Surg Engl* 1998; **80**: 91–5.

36. Kyosola K. Clinical experiences in the management of cold injuries: a study of 110 cases. *J Trauma* 1974; **14**: 32–6.

37. Urschel J. Frostbite. Predisposing factors and predictors of poor outcome. *J Trauma* 1990; **30**: 340–2.

38. Valnicek S, Chasmir L, Clapson J. Frostbite in the prairies: a 12-year review. *Plast Reconstr Surg* 1993; **92**: 633–41.

39. Pinzur M, Weaver F. Is urban frostbite a psychiatric disorder? *Orthopedics* 1997; **20**: 43–5.

40. Hermann G, Schecter D, Owens J. The problem of frostbite in civilian medical practice. *Clin North Am* 1963; **43**: 519–36.

41. Washburn B. Frostbite – what it is – how to prevent it – emergency treatment. *N Engl J Med* 1962; **266**: 974–89.

42. Siple PA, Passel CF. Measurements of dry atmospheric cooling in sub-freezing temperatures. *Proc Am Phil Soc* 1945; **89**: 177–99.

43. Lewis T. Observations on some normal and injurious effects of cold upon the skin and underlying tissues: III. Frostbite. *Br Med J* 1941; **2**: 869.

44. Knize D. Cold injury in reconstructive plastic surgery. In: Conversen J, McCarthy J, Littler J, eds. *General Principles*, Vol. 1. Philadelphia: WB Saunders, 1977: 516–30.

45. Lawrence WT, Murphy RC, Robson MC. The detrimental effect of cigarette smoking on flap survival: an experimental study on the rat. *Br J Plast Surg* 1984; **87**: 216.

46. Reus WF, Robson MC, Zachary L. Acute effects of tobacco smoking on blood flow in the cutaneous micro-circulation. *Br J Plast Surg* 1984; **37**: 213.

47. Whayne TJ, DeBakey MF. Cold injury, ground type. Washington, DC: US Government, 1958.

48. Mills WJ, Whaley R. Frostbite: a method of management. *Proceedings of the Symposium on Arctic Biology and Medicine: IV. Frostbite*, 1964, Fort Wainwright, Alaska. Arctic Aeromedical Laboratory.

49. McCauley RL, Smith DJ, Robson MC, Heggers JP. Frostbite and other cold-induced injuries. In: Auerback PS, ed. *Wilderness Medicine*. St Louis: Mosby, 1995: 129–45.

50. Weatherly-White R, Sjostrom B, Paton B. Experimental studies in cold injury II: the pathogenesis of frostbite. *J Surg Res* 1964; **4**: 17–22.

51. Weatherly-White R, Paton B, Sjostrom B. Experimental studies in cold injury III: observations on the treatment of frostbite. *Plast Reconstr Surg* 1965; **36**: 10–8.

52. Quintanilla R, Krusen F, Essex H. Studies on frostbite with special reference to treatment and effect on minute blood vessels. *Am J Physiol* 1947; **149**: 149–61.

53. Eubanks R. Heat and Cold injuries. *J Arkansas Med Soc* 1974; **71**: 53–8.

54. Furhman F, Crismon J. Studies on gangrene following cold injury, II. General course of events in rabbit feet and ears following untreated cold injury. *J Clin Invest* 1947; **47**: 236–44.

55. Rasmussen D, Zook E. Frostbite: a review of pathophysiology and newest treatments. *J Indiana State Med Assoc* 1972; **65**: 1237–41.

56. Welch G. Frostbite. *Practitioner* 1974; **213**: 801–4.

57. Moran T. Critical temperature of freezing living muscle. *Proc R Soc B* 1929; **105**: 107.

58. Merryman HT. The exceeding of a minimum tolerable cell volume in hypertonic suspension as a cause of freezing injury. In: Walstenholme G, O'Conner M, eds. *The Frozen Cell*. London: Churchill, 1970: 51.

59. Shikama K, Yamazaki I. Denaturation of catalase by freezing and thawing. *Nature* 1961; 190.

60. Marhert C. Lactate dehydrogenase isozymes: dissociation and recombination of subunits. *Science* 1963; **140**: 1629.

61. Lovelock JE. Physical instability in thermal shock in red blood cells. *Nature* 1954; **173**: 659.

62. Lovelock JE. The denaturation of lipid-protein complexes as a cause of damage by freezing. *Proc R Soc Biol* 1957; **147**: 427.

63. Mazur P. Studies in rapidly frozen suspension of yeast cells by differential thermal analysis and conductometry. *Biophys J* 1963; **3**: 323.

64. Mazur P. Causes of injury in frozen and thawed cells. *Fed Proc* 1965; **24**(suppl 14–15): 5.

65. Zacarian SA. Cryogenics: the cryolesion and the pathogenesis of cryonecrosis. In: Stone D, Clater H, eds. *Cryosurgery for Skin and Cutaneous Disorders* Vol. 7. St Louis: CV Mosby, 1985: 27.

66. Vanggaard L. Arteriovenous anastomosies in temperature regulation. *Acta Physiol Scand* 1969; **76**: 13A.

67. Johnson BE, Daniels F Jr. Enzyme studies in experimental cryosurgery of the skin. *Cryobiology* 1974; **11**: 22.

68. Lewis T. *The Blood Vessels of the Human Skin and Their Responses*. London: Shaw and Sons, 1927: 147–50.

69. Bulkley GB. The role of oxygen free radicals in human disease processes. *Surgery* 1983; **94**: 407.

70. Rabb JM, Renaud ML, Brandt PA. Effect of freezing and thawing on the microcirculation and capillary endothelium of the hamster cheek pouch. *Cryobiology* 197; **11**: 508.

71. Zacarian SA, Stone D, Clater H. Effects of cryogenic temperatures in the microcirculation in the holden hamster cheek pouch. *Cryobiology* 1970; **7**: 27.

72. Robson MC, Heggers JP. Evaluation of hand frostbite blister fluid as a clue to pathogenesis. *J Hand Surg [Am]* 1981; **6**: 43–7.

73. Nakae H, Endo S, Inada K. Plasma concentrations of type II phospholipase A_2, cytokines and eicosanoids in patients with burns. *Burns* 1995; **21**: 422–6.

74. Huribal M. Endothelin-1 and prostaglandin E_2 levels increase in patients with burns. *J Am Coll Surg* 1995; **180**: 318–22.

75. Harms BA, Bodai BI, Smith M, Gunther R, Flynn J, Demlings RH. Prostaglandin release and altered microvascular integrity after burn injury. *J Surg Res* 1981; **31**: 274–80.

76. Robson MC, Del Beccaro EJ, Heggers JP. The effect of prostaglandins on the dermal microcirculation after burning, and the inhibition of the effect by specific pharmacological agents. *Plast Reconstr Surg* 1979; **63**: 781–7.

77. Heggers JP, Ko F, Robson MC, Heggers R, Craft KE. Evaluation of burn blister fluid. *Plast Reconstr Surg* 1980; **65**: 798–804.

78. Heggers JP, Loy GL, Robson MC, Del Beccaro EJ. Histological demonstration of prostaglandins and thromboxanes in burned tissue. *J Surg Res* 1980; **28**: 110–7.

79. Back N, Jainchill J, Wilkens HJ, Ambrus JL. Effect of inhibitors of plasmin, kallikrein and kinin on mortality from scalding in mice. *Med Pharmacol Exp Int J Exp Med* 1966; **15**: 597–602.

80. Tanaka H, Wada T, Simazaki S. Effects of cimetidine on fluid requirement during resuscitation of third-degree burns. *J Burn Care Rehabil* 1991; **12**: 425–9.

81. Jackson DM. The diagnosis of the depth of burning. *Br J Surg* 1953; **40**: 588–96.

82. Raine TJ, London MD, Goluch L. Antiprostaglandins and antithromboxanes for treatment of frostbite. *Surg Forum* 1980; **31**: 557.

83. Bourne MH, Piepcorn MW, Clayton F. Analysis of microvascular changes in frostbite injury. *J Surg Res* 1986; **40**: 26.

84. Zook N, Hussmann J, Brown R. Microcirculatory studies of frostbite injury. *Ann Plast Surg* 1998; **40**: 246–53.

85. Reed MH. Growth disturbances in the hands following thermal injuries in children, II. frostbite. *Can Assoc Radiol J* 1988; **39**: 95–9.

86. Cauchy E, Chetaille E, Lefevre M, Kerelou E, Marsigny B. The role of bone scanning in severe frostbite of the extremities: a retrospective study of 88 cases [In Process Citation]. *Eur J Nucl Med* 2000; **27**: 497–502.

87. Greenwald D, Cooper B, Gottlieb L. An algorithm for early aggressive treatment of frostbite with limb salvage directed by triple-phase scanning. *Plast Reconstr Surg* 1998; **102**: 1069–74.

88. Kenney A, III., Vyas P. Frostbite injury: appearance on three-phase bone scan. *Clin Nucl Med* 1998; **23**: 188.

89. Sarikaya I, Aygit AC, Candan L, Sarikaya A, Turkyilmaz M, Berkarda S. Assessment of tissue viability after frostbite injury by technetium-99m-sestamibi scintigraphy in an experimental rabbit model. *Eur J Nucl Med* 2000; **27**: 41–5.

90. Barker JR, Haws MJ, Brown RE, Kucan JO, Moore WD. Magnetic resonance imaging of severe frostbite. *Ann Plast Surg* 1997; **38**: 275–9.

91. Taylor MS. Lumbar epidural sympathectomy for frostbite injuries of the feet. *Mil Med* 1999; **164**: 566–7.

92. Boumand DL, Morrison S, Lucas CE. Early sympathetic blockade for frostbite: is it of value? *J Surg Res* 1980; **20**: 744–7.

93. Salimi Z, Wolverson MK, Herbold DR, Vase W, Salimi A. Treatment of frostbite with streptokinase: an experimental study in rabbits. *Am J Roentgenol* 1987; **149**: 773–6.

94. Skolnick AA. Early data suggest clot-dissolving drugs may help save frostbitten limbs from amputation. *JAMA* 1992; **267**: 2008–10.

95. Erikson U, Ponten B. The possible value of arteriography supplemented by a vasodilator agent in the early assessment of tissue viability in frostbite. *Injury* 1974; **6**: 150–3.

Chapter 37

Chemical burns

Arthur P Sanford

David N Herndon

Introduction

We live in a world increasingly dependent on chemical agents. Our cars are powered by petroleum distillates in the combustion chambers of the engine and chemical reactions in the batteries, our gardens are fertilized by specially enriched products, and our houses are kept clean by powerful agents to dissolve and remove dirt. This makes chemical burns more commonplace in the household, and industrial applications to provide these chemicals are also expanding. Whenever the news of an armed conflict with a country not armed with nuclear weapons is broadcast, the possibility of chemical warfare is included. The variety of chemical exposures is so vast that a short chapter cannot describe all of the agents and their treatments, but this chapter can provide general principles for the treatment of chemical injuries. The importance of understanding these principles is underscored by the fact that while only 3% of all burns are due to chemical exposures, approximately 30% of burn deaths are due to chemical injuries.[1]

Pathophysiology

All burn wounds, whether due to chemical or thermal sources, have the denaturation of proteins in common. The structure of biological proteins involves not only a specific amino acid sequence, but also a three-dimensional structure dependent on weak forces, such as hydrogen bonding or Van der Waals' forces. These three-dimensional structures impart the biological activity on the proteins, and are easily disrupted by outside influences. Heat energy breaks these weak bonds to unfold and denature proteins, just as changes in pH or dissolution of surrounding lipids that may stabilize a protein disrupt its function. Direct chemical effects on a reactive group in a protein will similarly render it ineffective. In addition, chemical agents may act in a systemic fashion as their elements are circulated throughout the victim, with potential toxicity. Severity of a chemical burn injury is determined by several factors: (a) strength (concentration), (b) quantity of burning agent, (c) manner and duration of skin contact (progression), (d) penetration, and (e) mechanism of action. Broadly classified, there are six mechanisms of action for chemical agents in biological systems.[2]

Reduction

Reducing agents act by binding free electrons in tissue proteins. Examples include hydrochloric acid, nitric acid, and alkyl mercuric agents.

Oxidation

Oxidizing agents are oxidized on contact with tissue proteins. The byproducts are also often toxic and continue to react with the surrounding tissue. Examples of oxidizing agents are sodium hypochlorite (Clorox, Dakin's Solution), potassium permanganate, and chromic acid.

Corrosive Agents

Corrosive substances denature tissue proteins on contact. Typically, eschar formation and a shallow ulcer represent their injury. Examples of corrosive agents include phenols and cresols, white phosphorus, dichromate salts sodium metals, and the lyes.

Protoplasmic Poisons

These agents produce their effects by binding or inhibiting calcium or other organic ions necessary for tissue viability and function. Examples of protoplasmic poisons include 'alkaloidal' acids, acetic acid, formic acid, and metabolic competitors/inhibitors such as oxalic and hydrofluoric acid.

Vesicants

Vesicant agents produce ischemia with anoxic necrosis at the site of contact. For example, substances such as cantharides (Spanish Fly), dimethyl sulfoxide (DMSO), mustard gas, and Lewisite.

Desiccants

These substances cause damage by dehydrating tissues and at the same time are involved in exothermic reactions to release heat into the tissue. Examples here include sulfuric and muriatic (concentrated hydrochloric) acid.

Within these groups, there are different categories of compounds, each with their own characteristics. This method of describing burn injuries as acid or alkali is less accurate than describing the classes by how they coagulate proteins. Although the mechanisms of action for individual acids or alkali may differ, the resulting wounds are similar enough to warrant consideration as separate groups.[1] Acids act as proton donors in the biological system, and strong acids have a pH <2. The best predictor of ability of an acid to cause injury, however, is the amount of neutralizing material to correct the pH of the acid to neutral.[3] Alkali, or basic material, capable of producing injury typically has a pH >11.5.[1] In general, alkaline material causes more injury than acidic compounds because acids cause coagulation necrosis with precipitation of protein, while the reaction to alkali is 'liquefaction' necrosis, allowing the alkali to penetrate deeper into the injured tissue.[1] The alkalis dissolve and unite with the proteins of the tissues to form alkaline proteinates, which are soluble and contain OH⁻ ions, causing further reactions deeper into tissue.[4] Organic solutions will tend to dissolve the lipid membrane of cell walls and cause disruption of cellular architecture as their mechanism of action. Inorganic solutions would tend more to remain on the exterior of cells, but may act as vehicles to carry the above-mentioned agents that denature proteins or form salts with proteins themselves.

General principles of management

The most important aspects of first aid for chemical burn victims involve removal of the offending agent from contact with the patient. This requires removal of all potentially contaminated clothing and copious irrigation. Important principles in the irrigation of chemical burn patients involve protection of health care providers to prevent additional injuries. Further, the wounds should not be irrigated by placing the patient into a tub, thereby spreading the injurious material to previously unexposed tissue. Irrigation should be large volume, and 'to the floor' or out an appropriate drain. Lavage of chemical injuries is meant to dilute the agent already in contact with the skin, and prevent additional agent from being exposed to the skin. Early, copious lavage has been shown to reduce the extent and depth of full-thickness injury.[5] No measure of adequacy of lavage has been developed, but monitoring of the pH from the effluent can provide quantifiable information as to adequacy of lavage, but quite often a period of 30 minutes to 2 hours of lavage may be necessary. Clinically, the input of the patient is important to tell that the symptoms of the injury have been reduced and lavage may be stopped. The adage 'Dilution as the solution to the pollution' applies.

Material Safety Data Sheets (MSDS) are mandated to be available for all chemicals present in the workplace. These can be valuable resources for potential systemic toxicity and side-effects of an agent. Plant safety officers should be available at all times to provide this information in cases of industrial accidents. Further assistance is available from regional poison control centers for household chemicals or unidentified agents.

One of the most controversial areas of chemical burn treatment involves the use of neutralizing agents. In theory, they should effectively remove the active chemical from a wound and provide relief from further injury. However, because of the wide range of chemicals potentially involved, their correct use cannot be assured, so they are generally discouraged. The practical problems encountered with their use are exothermic reactions (i.e. when an acid is used to neutralize an alkali solution, the resulting reaction may liberate a large amount of heat) causing further thermal damage on top of the preexisting chemical injury. When the burning agent is known and an appropriate antidote is known there is some benefit demonstrated in its use.[6] Despite this, no agent has been found to be more effective than plain water for irrigation.[5]

General principles of trauma management are followed (The ABCs). Airway patency is assured, followed by adequate air movement, and maintenance of hemodynamics. Despite the increasing awareness of chemical burns, no one burn center has undertaken a study of the resuscitative needs of a chemical burn victim, and hence we rely on the conventional thermal burn formulas for resuscitation. Monitoring of urine output remains paramount to assessment of adequacy of end organ perfusion and hence resuscitation. Systemic disturbances of pH are potential complications and must be monitored until electrolyte trends are stabilized.

The typical large volume lavage required to adequately dilute chemical exposures puts the victim at potential risk for hypothermia, both from evaporative cooling losses and the use of unwarmed lavage fluid. Recognition of this complication can prevent added complications.

Principles of wound care for chemical burns are typically the same as for thermal injuries. Early excision and grafting of obvious nonviable tissue is advocated, particularly in light of the observation that chemical burns tend to heal more slowly than thermal burns. Topical application of antimicrobials can be useful for partial-thickness injury.[7]

Specific agents

Acetic Acid

Table vinegar, a dilute solution of acetic acid, is usually harmless. Glacial, or nearly 100% pure, acetic acid acts as a metabolic poison by forming esters with proteins of metabolic pathways.

Strong Alkali

Lime, sodium hydroxide, and potassium hydroxide are common alkali agents that burn. They are present in many household-cleaning solutions, and have historically been ingested as well as causing cutaneous burns. Dry residues of alkali (e.g. lime) must be brushed away to reduce the total amount of alkali present, then copious irrigation is undertaken. Attempts to neutralize alkali are not recommended. Alkali injury to the eye is particularly devastating. These compounds penetrate the cornea quickly, causing scarring, opacification of the cornea, and perforation.[8]

Assorted Acids

Acids tend to cause hard, dry eschars on contact with skin, sparing deeper tissue. In fact, tannic acid has been described as a treatment for thermal injury,[9] and even Native American people have used unrefined products in the treatment of burns since prehistory. Many of these compounds are absorbed as protoplasmic poisons and are renal and hepatic toxins.

Alkyl Mercuric Compounds

Skin reaction with these substances releases free mercury, which can be found in blister fluid. With time, this mercury is absorbed, which can cause systemic effects. After blisters are debrided, repeat washing to lavage the blister fluid contents away is necessary.

Cantharides

'Spanish Fly' is used as an aphrodisiac that acts as a vesicant upon contact with the skin. This leads to multiple, small blister formation.

Cement

Cement acts both as a desiccant and an alkali. It penetrates clothing and combines with sweat, causing an exothermic reaction. The dry powder is very hygroscopic and will cause desiccation injury if not hydrated or washed away. Cement is calcium oxide, which becomes calcium hydroxide upon exposure to water. Injury results from the action of the hydroxyl ion.[10,13]

Chromic Acid

Contact with chromic acid, a powerful oxidizing agent used to clean other metals, will cause protein coagulation. The lethal dose for ingestion is between 5 and 10 g, and results in gastroenteritis, followed by vertigo, muscle cramps, peripheral vascular collapse, and coma. Water lavage is again the primary treatment for exposure, but in an industrial setting where this acid is used; washing

with a dilute solution of sodium hyposulfite, followed by rinsing in a buffered phosphate solution may be a more specific antidote. Dimercaprol may be used at 4 mg/kg intramuscularly every 4 hours for 2 days, followed by 2–4 mg/kg/day for 7 days total to treat the systemic effects.

Dichromate Salts

A highly corrosive substance with similar symptoms of systemic toxicity as chromic acid. Lethal dose is 50–100 mg/kg. Emergency treatment is by lavage, but more specific treatments include lavage with 2% hyposulfite solution, or a buffer of 7% potassium dihydrogenphosphate and 18% disodium hydrogen phosphate.

Dimethyl Sulfoxide

This is a powerful organic solvent, with the ability to carry non-lipid-soluble compounds quickly across cell membranes. It is used commonly in 'alternative medicine' as a relief for joint pain itself, but commonly is the vehicle for other agents. If implicated in a cutaneous injury, it is likely the dissolved substance, rather than the DMSO itself that will cause injury.

Formic Acid

All patients injured by formic acid should be hospitalized due to multiple systemic effects of this metabolic poisoning agent. These problems include metabolic acidosis, intravascular hemolysis with hemoglobinuria, renal failure, pulmonary complications, and abdominal pain with necrotizing pancreatitis and vomiting.[11]

Hydrocarbons

Prolonged contact with petroleum distillates results in dissolution of lipid cell membranes and cell death.[4] These burns tend to be superficial and heal spontaneously.[12] Systemic toxicity includes respiratory depression, and when lead additives were present, systemic lead poisoning was common. The present epidemic of 'huffing' or inhaling volatile hydrocarbons has produced a syndrome of neurological damage as well.

Hydrochloric Acid/Muriatic Acid

Muriatic acid is the commercial grade of concentrated hydrochloric acid. Once in contact with the skin, it denatures proteins into their chloride salts. Most significantly, hydrochloric acid fumes can cause inhalation injury with a sudden onset pulmonary edema.

Hydrofluoric Acid

Hydrofluoric acid (HF) is a commonly used acid with industrial applications. It is used as a cleaning agent in the petroleum industry and glass etching. It is also one of the strongest inorganic acids known. Hydrofluoric acid is particularly lethal due to its properties both as an acid and as a metabolic poison. The acid component causes coagulation necrosis and cellular death. Fluoride ion then gains a portal of entry that then chelates the positively charged ions like calcium and magnesium.[13] This causes an efflux of intracellular calcium with resultant cell death. The fluoride ion remains active until it is completely neutralized by the bivalent cations, including penetration to bone. This may exceed the body's ability to mobilize calcium and magnesium rapidly enough and muscle contraction and cellular function, dependent on these cations will become dysfunctional. Fluoride ion is also a metabolic poison and inhibits the Na-K ATPase allowing efflux of potassium as well.[14]

These electrolyte shifts at nerve endings are thought to be the cause of the extreme pain associated with HF burns.[15]

HF burns are classified based on the concentration of the exposure according to a system developed by the National Institutes of Health-Division of Industrial Hygiene.[16] Concentrations greater than 50% cause immediate tissue destruction and pain. Concentrations of 20–50% result in a burn becoming apparent within several hours of exposure. Injuries from concentrations less than 20% may take up to 24 hours to become apparent. Studies on the protective properties of skin correlate well with this scheme, as there was noted to be some protection for a period at all acid concentrations, then the still undefined barrier broke down allowing the HF to penetrate.[17] Interestingly, the barrier was disrupted by nicks in the skin and organic solvents, suggesting that some lipid element is lost as the wound turns from superficial to full-thickness.

The systemic symptoms typical of hypocalcemia or hypomagnesemia are generally absent. Serum calcium levels and electrocardiogram are important monitors of patient status.[18] Once cardiac dysrythmias develop, they are hard to restore to a normal rhythm.[19] Compounding the problem of hypocalcemia, the fluoride ion may be acting as a metabolic poison in the myocardium to promote the irritability. The typical electrocardiographic change is Q-T interval prolongation. The fluoride ions can be removed by hemodialysis or cation exchange resins.[19,20]

Treatments of HF exposure are designed to neutralize the fluoride ion and prevent systemic toxicity. Calcium gluconate gel (3.5 g of 2.5% calcium gluconate mixed with 5 oz of water-soluble lubricant is applied to the wound 4–6 times each day for 3–4 days) can be used after the wounds have been copiously irrigated.[7] Calcium gluconate injections into the area of the wound (0.5 ml/cm[2] of 10% calcium gluconate) have also been used with good success.[21] Pain relief with these treatments is often swift, and it is felt that return of symptoms indicate need for repeat treatment. Calcium chloride delivers more milliequivalents per ml of solution, but is contraindicated in subcutaneous injection due to its tissue irritating properties. Burns to the hand with HF are common in workplace accidents, and present special problems; how to deliver large amounts of calcium to limited areas. Palmar fasciotomy may be needed to relieve the pressure after tissue injections.[22] Another option is intra-arterial injections of dilute calcium salts (10 ml of 10% calcium gluconate or calcium chloride in 40 ml of 5% dextrose) into the radial artery that would supply the injured area.[23] Infusion continues until the patient is symptom free of pain in the injured extremity. Injury to eyes by HF is treated with copious irrigation with water or saline, not calcium chloride which is associated with increased corneal ulceration.[24] After the acute period is over, the eye may be irrigated with 1% calcium gluconate every 2–3 hours and recovery usually occurs in 4–5 days. Pulmonary reaction to HF vapor may persist for up to 3 weeks after exposure. Nebulized solutions of calcium gluconate and intermittent positive pressure breathing device support are recommended.[25]

Hypochlorite Solutions

These are potent oxidizers delivered in alkaline solution used as bleaches and household cleaners. Commonly available solutions are 4–6% and are lethal only when a large surface area is involved; however, exposure to 30 ml of 15% solution is potentially fatal. Systemic manifestations of toxicity include vomiting, dyspnea, and edema of the airway, confusion, cardiovascular collapse, cyanosis, and coma.[7]

Nitric Acid

A strong acid that can combine with organic proteins to produce organonitrates which act as metabolic poisons.

Oxalic Acid

This is a potent metabolic poison that combines with calcium to limit its bioavailability. After exposure, serum calcium should be monitored closely, as well as signs of cardiac or respiratory muscle dysfunction. One-half gram oxalic acid exposure or ingestion may be fatal.

Phenol (Carbolic Acid)

This substance was originally used as an antiseptic, but its use declined after serious side-effects were noted. It is bound irreversibly to albumin after exposure and ingestion of as little as 1 g may cause death. Cardiovascular effects include ventricular arrhythmias,[26] and skin necrosis also results from prolonged contact.

Industrial use of this compound and its derivatives (resorcinol or 1,3-dihydroxybenzene) has shown the most common adverse effects to be dermatitis and depigmentation of the skin.[27] Acute poisonings are potentially fatal; so prompt action is necessary with copious irrigation to decontaminate the wound.[28] Polyethylene glycol (PEG molecular weight 300 or 400) has been shown to be of potential benefit,[29,30] but large volume lavage should not be delayed while PEG application is begun. Reports in the literature indicate intravenous sodium bicarbonate may be of use to prevent some of the systemic effects of phenol.[31] The mechanism is not clear, as phenol is not dissociated from albumin by this treatment.

Phosphoric Acid

An industrial acid used in strong concentrations. Lavage followed by electrolyte monitoring (phosphorus is a strong calcium binder) is the treatment of choice.

Phosphorus

Phosphorus has both military and civilian uses. It is an incendiary agent found in hand grenades, artillery shells, fireworks, and fertilizers.[32] White phosphorus ignites in the presence of air and burns until the entire agent is oxidized or the oxygen source is removed (for example, as with immersion in water). The wounds are irrigated with water, the easily identifiable pieces of phosphorus are removed from the wound, and soaked dressings are applied for transport. Ultraviolet light can be used to identify embedded particles through phosphorescence, or a solution of 0.5% copper sulfate can be applied which will impede oxidation and turn the particles black to aid in their identification and removal. Hypocalcemia, hyperphosphatemia, and cardiac arrhythmias have been reported with phosphorus burns.[33]

Potassium Permanganate

This is an oxidizing agent that is highly corrosive in dry, crystalline form. It is poorly absorbed, so systemic effects are rare.

Sulfuric Acid

Sulfuric acid and its precursor, sulphur trioxide, are strong acids and desiccants with many industrial applications. Copious irrigation and early excision are the treatments of choice.[34]

Vesicant Chemical Warfare Agents (Lewisite, Nitrogen Mustard)

These agents were historically used during the trench warfare of World War I. They affect all epithelial tissues, including skin, eyes, and respiratory epithelium. Symptoms described after exposure to mustard gas include burning eyes and a feeling of suffocation associated with a burning throat.[35] This is followed by erythema of the skin in 4 hours, with blisters developing in 12–48 hours. Severe pruritis develops, particularly in the moist areas, such as the axilla and perineum. When the blisters rupture, they leave painful, shallow ulcers. Exposure to larger quantities of these agents produces coagulative necrosis of the skin with either no blistering or 'doughnut blisters' surrounding a central necrotic zone.[36] Secondary respiratory infection and bone marrow suppression often lead to death. Lewisite (2-chlorovinyl-dichloroarsine) is the best known arsine. It is more powerful than the mustards, and the symptoms occur sooner. Phosgene oxime is another common agent in chemical warfare. It is the most widely used halogenated oxime and has the immediate effect of stinging, likened to contact with a stinging needle.[37] Affected areas quickly become swollen with blister formation, and eschars develop over the next week, but wound healing is slow (over 2 months). Eye involvement is extremely painful and can result in permanent blindness. Inhalation leads to hypersecretion and pulmonary edema.

Treatment primarily includes prophylaxis against exposure, and those administering aid to victims should be suitably protected with respirator, butyl rubber gloves, and boots. Clothing is removed from the victims and large volume lavage of the skin is undertaken. Eyes are irrigated with water or 'Balanced Salt Solution'. Symptomatic relief of itch is provided with benzodiazepines, antihistamines, or phenothiazines. Blisters are debrided and dressed with topical antimicrobials (but silver sulfadiazine neutralizes Dimercaprol). Dimercaprol is a chelating agent that is an antidote for Lewisite poisoning, available as an ointment, eyedrops or intramuscular preparation. There is no specific antidote for nitrogen mustard, but sodium thiosulfate and cysteine may be helpful to reduce the effects if administered early.[38] Early excision and grafting has not been shown to be of benefit with nitrogen mustard burns, but the deeper lesions seen with the other agents seem best suited to treatment as if they were full-thickness thermal burns. The blister fluid from nitrogen mustard injuries does not contain active agent and is hence harmless.[39] Symptomatic treatment of ocular and respiratory complications is undertaken. Agranulocytosis or aplastic anemia can result from exposure to these agents, as was seen in Iranian casualties from the Iran–Iraq war.[40] Transfusion of blood products was not helpful, and in the appropriate setting, bone marrow transplantation may be considered. Other marrow stimulators (e.g. granulocyte maturation colony stimulating factor or lithium carbonate) have not been tried.

Oral ingestions

Ingestions of caustic substances are common in young children as they begin to explore their environment and get into the household chemicals, or in adults as a suicide gesture. In a 15-year review of chemical burn injuries at our institution, we identified 154 chemical burn injuries, with 26 patients involved with ingestion injuries (17% incidence), but significantly 14 patients were under age 4 years (unpublished data). Management of these injuries is not necessarily undertaken in a specialized burn unit, but can be handled by a General Surgeon, or Foregut Surgery specialist. Similar principles apply, with neutralization, lavage, and avoidance of vomiting which might reexpose tissue to the offending agent. Early endoscopic evaluation of the oral pharynx, esophagus, and stomach/proximal duodenum with endoscopy will help to define extent of injury before scarring eliminates access to these structures. Particularly vulnerable areas include compromise of the upper airway due to the concentrated exposure in this area and subsequent risk requiring intubation. In general, endoscopic gastrostomy tubes should be considered early in the course of treatment to provide feeding access to the stomach and a guide string should be left in the lumen of the esophagus. The reader is referred to an appropriate General Surgery text for the current management of this problem.

References

1. Luterman A, Curreri P. Chemical burn injury. In: Jurkiewcz M, Krizek T, Mathes S, eds. *Plastic Surgery: Principles and Practice*. St Louis: CV Mosby, 1990: 1355–440.
2. Jelenko C. Chemicals that burn. *J Trauma* 1974; **14**(1): 65–72.
3. Moriarty R. Corrosive chemicals: acids and alkali. *Drug Therapy* 1979; **3**: 89.
4. Mozingo DW, *et al.* Chemical burns. *J Trauma* 1988; **28**(5): 642–7.
5. Leonard LG, Scheulen JJ, Munster AM. Chemical burns: effect of prompt first aid. *J Trauma* 1982; **22**(5): 420–3.
6. Yano K, *et al.* Effects of washing with a neutralizing agent on alkaline skin injuries in an experimental model. *Burns* 1994; **20**(1): 36–9.
7. Milner S, *et al.* Chemical injury. In: Herndon D, ed. *Total Burn Care*. Philadelphia: WB Saunders, 1996: 415–24.
8. Pfister RR. Chemical injuries of the eye. *Ophthalmology* 1983; **90**(10): 1246–53.
9. Cope Z. General treatment of burns. In: *Medical History of the Second World War: Surgery*. London: HMSO, 1953: 288–312.
10. Pike J, Patterson A Jr, Arons MS. Chemistry of cement burns: pathogenesis and treatment. *J Burn Care Rehabil* 1988; **9**(3): 258–60.
11. Naik RB, *et al.* Ingestion of formic acid-containing agents–report of three fatal cases. *Postgrad Med J* 1980; **56**(656): 451–6.
12. Hunter GA. Chemical burns of the skin after contact with petrol. *Br J Plast Surg* 1968; **21**(4): 337–41.
13. Mistry DG, Wainwright DJ. Hydrofluoric acid burns. *Am Fam Physician* 1992; **45**(4): 1748–54.
14. McIvor ME. Delayed fatal hyperkalemia in a patient with acute fluoride intoxication. *Ann Emerg Med* 1987; **16**(10): 1165–7.
15. Klauder J, Shelanski L, Gavriel K. Industrial uses of compounds of Fluride and oxlic acid. *Arch Ind Health* 1955; **12**: 412–9.
16. Division of Industrial Hygiene, National Institutes of Health, Hydrofluoric acid burns. *Int Med* 1943; **12**: 634.
17. Noonan T, *et al.* Epidermal lipids and the natural history of hydrofluoric acid (HF) injury. *Burns* 1994; **20**(3): 202–6.
18. Mayer TG, Gross PL. Fatal systemic fluorosis due to hydrofluoric acid burns. *Ann Emerg Med* 1985; **14**(2): 149–53.
19. McIvor ME, *et al.* Sudden cardiac death from acute fluoride intoxication: the role of potassium. *Ann Emerg Med* 1987; **16**(7): 777–81.
20. Yolken R, Konecny P, McCarthy P. Acute fluoride poisoning. *Pediatrics* 1976; **58**(1): 90–3. .
21. Dibbell DG, *et al.* Hydrofluoric acid burns of the hand. *J Bone Joint Surg [Am]* 1970; **52**(5): 931–6.
22. Anderson WJ, Anderson JR. Hydrofluoric acid burns of the hand: mechanism of injury and treatment. *J Hand Surg [Am]* 1988; **13**(1): 52–7.
23. Vance MV, *et al.* Digital hydrofluoric acid burns: treatment with intraarterial calcium infusion. *Ann Emerg Med* 1986; **15**(8): 890–6.

24. McCulley JP, et al. Hydrofluoric acid burns of the eye. *J Occup Med* 1983; **25(6)**: 447–50.
25. Caravati EM. Acute hydrofluoric acid exposure. *Am J Emerg Med* 1988; **6(2)**: 143–50.
26. Miller F. Poisoning by phenol. *Can Med Assoc J* 1942; **46**: 615.
27. Saunders A, Geddes L, Elliott P. Are phenolic disinfectants toxic to staff members? *Aust Nurses J* 1988; **17(10)**: 25–6.
28. Abbate C, et al. Dermatosis from resorcinal in tyre makers. *Br J Ind Med* 1989; **46(3)**: 212–4.
29. Schutz W. Phenoldermatosen. *Berufsdermatosen* 1959; **7**: 266.
30. Brown VKH, Box VL, Simpson BJ. Decontamination procedures for skin exposed to phenolic substances. *Arch Environ Health* 1975; **30(1)**: 1–6.
31. Bennett I, James D, Golden A. Severe acidosis due to phenol poisoning. Report of two cases. *Ann Intern Med* 1959; **32**: 214.
32. Summerlin WT, Walder AI, Moncrief JA. White phosphorus burns and massive hemolysis. *J Trauma* 1967; **7(3)**: 476–84.
33. Bowen TE, Whelan TJ Jr, Nelson TG. Sudden death after phosphorus burns: experimental observations of hypocalcemia, hyperphosphatemia and

electrocardiographic abnormalities following production of a standard white phosphorus burn. *Ann Surg* 1971; **174(5)**: 779–84.
34. Sawhney CP, Kaushish R. Acid and alkali burns: considerations in management. *Burns* 1989; **15(2)**: 132–4.
35. Willems J. Clinical management of mustard gas casualties. *Ann Med Milit (Belg)* 1989; **3(suppl)**: 1–61.
36. Papirmeister B, et al. The sulfur mustard injury: description of lesions and resulting incapacitation, In: *Medical Defence against Mustard Gas*. Florida: CRC Press Inc: 1990: 13–42.
37. Vesicants. In: *NATO Handbook on the Medical Effects of NBC Defensive Operations: AMedP-6 Part III-Chemical*. Amended final draft. (NATO Unclassified).
38. Parpmeister B, et al. Pretreatments and therapies. In: *Medical Defense Against Mustard Gas*. Florida: CRC Press, 1990.
39. Sultzberger M, Katz J. The absence of skin irritants in the contents of vesicles. *US Navy Med Bull* 1943; **43**: 1258–62.
40. Vedder E. *The Medical Aspects of Chemical Warfare* Baltimore: Williams and Wilkins, 1925.

Chapter 38

Radiation injuries, vesicant burns and mass casualties

Stephen M Milner

David N Herndon

Introduction

Only 4 months after Roentgen reported the discovery of X-rays, Dr John Daniel observed that irradiation of his colleague's skull caused hair loss. Since this finding was reported in 1896, many biomedical effects of radiation have been described.[1] Knowledge of nuclear physics was rapidly amassed in the early part of the twentieth century leading eventually to the Manhattan project and the development of the atomic bomb. The last 50 years have also seen widespread deployment of energy-generating nuclear reactors, and the expanding use of radioactive isotopes in industry, science, and health care.[2] More recently, major industrial accidents of note at Three Mile Island in Pennsylvania, Chernobyl in the Ukraine, and at Goiania, Brazil have resulted in potential or real radiation injuries to hundreds of people. Given the devastating medical consequences that would follow a nuclear detonation or accident, the training of medical personnel in treating radiation injury is a crucial factor in the effective management of such casualities.

Exposure to ionizing radiation can follow one of three patterns: (1) small scale accidents which might occur in a laboratory or from an X-ray device in a hospital setting; (2) large industrial accidents (like those mentioned above) stretching the need for treatment beyond available resources; and (3) detonation of a nuclear device in military conflict where resources are totally overwhelmed or unavailable and associated multiple and combined injuries also exist.

This chapter first describes the terminology used in standard measurement of radiation exposure and discusses the frequency of radiation accidents, injuries, and fatalities. The effects of exposure to ionizing radiation and triage and care protocols are considered according to known and projected prognostic factors. The complications that arise specifically with this injury and the supportive measures that need to be taken will be addressed.

Vesicant agents are characterized by their ability to produce cutaneous blisters resembling 'burns'. Although most physicians are unlikely to encounter casualities of chemical weapons, the proliferation of these agents has increased the risk to both military and civilian populations. They are likely to require expertise found in burn centers and for this reason an account of the management of these injuries is included in this text. Finally, the problem of mass casualties is examined, and recommendations for management are made.

Radiation injuries

Terminology

Damage to biological tissue by ionizing radiation is mediated by energy transference. This can be the result of exposure to electromagnetic radiation (e.g. X-rays and gamma rays) or particulate radiation (e.g. alpha and beta particles or neutrons). The severity of tissue damage is determined by the energy deposited per unit track length, known as linear energy transfer (LET).[3] Electromagnetic radiation passes through tissue almost unimpeded by the skin and is called low-LET since little energy is left behind. In contrast, neutron exposure has high-LET, resulting in significant energy absorption within the first few centimeters of the body. Alpha and low-energy beta particles do not penetrate the skin, and represent a hazard only when internalized by inhalation, ingestion, or absorption through a wound.

Radiation dosing can be expressed in several ways (**Table 38.1**):

1. The Roentgen (R) is the unit of exposure and is related to the ability of X-rays to ionize air. It is defined as the quantity of low energy X-rays or gamma rays required to produce 1.61×10^{15} ion pairs per kilogram of air.
2. The Curie (Ci) or Becquerel (Bq) is the unit of activity (rate of decay) of a radioactive material. One Curie equals 3.7×10^{10} decays per second, a definition originally based on the rate of decay of 1 g of radium.[4] The Becquerel is a smaller but more basic unit and equals one decay per second.
3. The rad is the unit of absorbed dose of radiation and corresponds to an energy absorption of 100 ergs/g. A newer international unit, the gray (Gy), is now in use and is defined as 1 Joule (J) of energy deposited in each kg of absorbing material, and is equal to 100 rads.[5]

Table 38.1 Radiation Units and Conversion Factors

Old Unit	New Unit	Conversion Factor
Rad (rad)	Gray (Gy)	1 Gy = 100 rad
Rem (REM)	Seivert (Sv)	1 Sv = 100 REM
Curie (Ci)	Becquerel (Bq)	1 Bq = 2.7×10^{-11} Ci

Not all radiation is equally effective in causing biological damage, although it may cause the same energy deposition in tissue. For example, 1 Gy of neutron radiation will not have the same effect as 1 Gy of gamma or X-radiation. For this reason, a unit of dose equivalence was derived that allows radiations with different LET values to be compared. One such unit is the REM (acronym of roentgen equivalent human). The Dose in rem is equal to the dose in rads multiplied by a quality factor (QF).[6] The QF takes into account the linear energy transfer and has a different value for different radiations; for X-rays it is 1.0, for neutrons 10. The international unit, now more widely in use, is the sievert (Sv). One sievert equals 100 REM; 1 REM equals 10 mSv. This allows radiations with different LET values to be compared, since 1 Sv of neutron radiation has the same biological effect as 1 Sv of low-LET gamma or X radiation.

Incidence

A significant radiation accident is one in which an individual exceeds at least one of the following criteria:[7]

- Whole body doses equal to or exceeding 25 REM (0.25 Sv).
- Skin doses equal to or exceeding 600 REM (6 Sv).
- Absorbed dose equal to or greater than 75 REM (0.75 Sv) to other tissues or organs from an external source.
- Internal contamination equal to or exceeding one-half the maximum permissible body burden (MPBB) as defined by the International Commission on Radiological Protection (this number is different for each radionuclide).
- Medical misadministrations, provided they result in a dose or burden equal to or greater than the criteria already listed above.

Radiation accidents within the United States should be reported to the federally funded Radiation Emergency Assistance Center/Training Site (REAC/TS). This is operated by Oak Ridge Institute for Science and Education (ORISE) at Oak Ridge, Tennessee, 37831–0117 (Tel. +1 (865) 576–3130). A radiological emergency response team of physicians, nurses, health physicists, and support personnel provides consultative assistance on a 24-hour basis and has the capability of providing medical treatment, whenever a radiation accident occurs. REAC/TS also maintains a Radiation Accident Registry System.

The number of accidents, number of persons involved, as well as the number of fatalities, in the United States and worldwide is shown in **Tables 38.2** and **38.3**. There have been a total of 127 fatalities recorded by the Registry worldwide.[7] The majority of the

Table 38.2 Major radiation accidents: human experience (1944–March 2000)*

Location	No. of Accidents	No. of Persons Involved	Significant Exposures**	Fatalities
US	245	1351	792	30
Non-US	169	132 391	2206	97
Total	414	133 742	2998	127

*Source: DOE/REAC/TS Radiation Accident Registry.
**DOE/NRC dose criteria

Table 38.3 Major radiation accidents worldwide (1944–March 2000)

United States				Other	
New Mexico	3	Algeria	2	Marshall Islands	1
Ohio	10	Argentina	1	Mexico	5
Oklahoma	1	Belarus	1	Morocco	8
Pennsylvania	1	Brazil	4	Norway	1
Rhode Island	1	Bulgaria	1	Russia	5
Texas	9	China (PR)	6	Spain	10
Wisconsin	1	Costa Rica	7	Thailand	3
		El Salvador	1	USSR	29
		Estonia	1	United Kingdom	3
		Israel	1	Yugoslavia	1
		Italy	1		
		Japan	1		

Table 38.4 Major radiation accidents worldwide (1944–March 2000): Classification by Device

Criticalities		22
Critical assemblies	9	
Reactors	7	
Chemical operations	6	
Radiation devices		307
Sealed sources	203	
X-ray devices	79	
Accelerators	24	
Radar generators	1	
Radioisotopes		85
Transuranic tritiums	27	
Fission products	2	
Radium spills	11	
Diagnosis and therapy	38	
Other	6	
Total		414

From REAC/TS (Radiation Accident Registries).

radiation deaths occurred as a result of the Chernobyl accident in the USSR (now Ukraine) in 1986, when 30 people were killed immediately. The classification of radiation accident by device for the period 1944 until March 2000 and their frequency distribution is illustrated in **Table 38.4** and **Figure 38.1**.[7] The majority of radiation accidents are associated with encapsulated, highly radioactive sources used for industrial radiography. Next most frequent accidents are radioisotope accidents that involve radioactive materials, which are unsealed such as tritium, fission products, radium, and free isotopes used for diagnosis and therapy. Uncommon criticality accidents occur when enough fissionable material, such as enriched uranium, is brought together to produce a neutron flux so high that the material undergoes a nuclear reaction (becomes critical).

The most devastating radiation injuries and fatalities yet seen, however, resulted from detonation of nuclear weapons at Hiroshima and Nagasaki during World War II. Since 1945, nuclear weapon technology has developed enormously and current strategic thermonuclear warheads dwarf those weapons used in Japan.[8]

Pathophysiology

The detonation of a nuclear device over a population center will produce an extremely hot, luminous fireball, which emits intense thermal radiation capable of causing burns and starting fires at considerable distance. This is accompanied by a destructive blast wave moving away from the fireball at supersonic speed and the emission of irradiation, mainly gamma rays and neutrons.[9] The result of a combination of thermal and radiation injuries is said to have a synergistic effect on the outcome. Several animal experiments have demonstrated a significant increase in mortality when a standard burn wound model is irradiated, over and above that expected from either injury alone.[10,11]

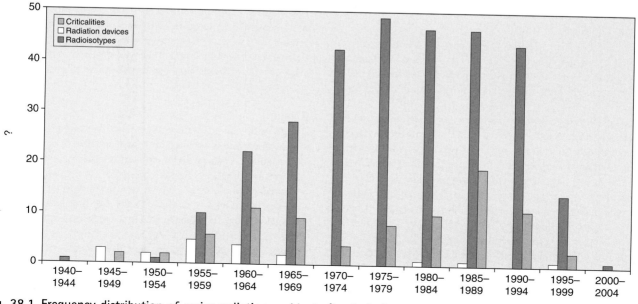

Fig. 38.1 Frequency distribution of major radiation accidents (by device) worldwide: 1940–March 2000.

Thermal Effects

Exact information about the cause of fatalities in a nuclear blast is not available, but from the nuclear attack on Japan, it has been estimated that 50% of deaths were due to burns and some 20–30% were flash burns.[12] The clinical picture may range from an erythema of the exposed areas (most commonly face, hands, arms and legs), to a charring of the superficial layers of the skin. Secondary flame burns may be present following the ignition of the victim's clothing or environment. The physicians at Hiroshima and Nagasaki observed that the 'flame' burn wound seemed to heal at first. However, between 1 and 2 weeks later, a serious relapse occurred. Wound infection set in; there was a disorder in granulation tissue formation; a gray, greasy coating would form on the wounds. Thrombocytopenia resulted in spontaneous bleeding both into the wound and elsewhere. Histologically, the normal collection of leukocytes delineating a necrotic area were found to be absent due to agranulocytosis, and gross bacterial invasion was evident;[13] both these changes obviously affected the prognosis of these otherwise relatively small injuries.

Radiation Effect

Damage to biological tissue by ionizing radiation is mediated by energy transference. The transference of this energy can damage critical parts of the cell directly or indirectly by formation of free radicals (such as the hydroxyl radical). The primary targets are cellular and nuclear membranes and DNA.[14]

The morbidity of radiation is dependent on its dose, the dose rate, and the sensitivity of the cell exposed. Cells are most sensitive when undergoing mitosis so that those that divide rapidly such as bone marrow, skin, and the gastrointestinal tract are more susceptible to radiation damage. Radiation to an organ such as brain or liver, which has parenchymal cells with a slow turnover rate, results in damage to the more sensitive connective tissue and microcirculation.

The overall effect on the organism depends on the extent of the body surface involved, duration of exposure, and homogeneity of the radiation field. It is convenient to consider radiation injuries as localized or whole body (acute radiation syndrome).

Localized Injury

In a localized injury a relatively small part of the body is affected without significant systemic effects.[15] The skin and subcutaneous tissue alone may be involved after exposure to low-energy radiation. Exposure to high-energy radiation may injure deeper structures.

Radiation damage depends on the dose of exposure and several progressive features are observed in skin: erythema is equivalent to a first degree thermal burn and occurs in two stages. Mild erythema appears within minutes or hours following the initial exposure and subsides in 2–3 days. The second onset of erythema occurs 2–3 weeks after exposure and is accompanied by dry desquamation of the epidermal keratinocytes. Epilation (loss of hair) may occur as soon as 7 days post-injury. It is usually temporary with doses less than 5 Gy but may be permanent with higher doses. Moist desquamation is equivalent to a second degree thermal burn and develops after a latent period of about 3 weeks with a dose of 12–20 Gy. The latency period may be shorter with higher doses. Blisters form, and are susceptible to infection if not treated.

Full-thickness skin ulceration and necrosis are caused by doses in excess of about 25 Gy. Onset varies from a few weeks to a few months after exposure. Blood vessels become telangiectatic and deeper vessels occluded. Obliterating endarteritis results in fibrosis atrophy and necrosis. Skin cancers may be evident after months or years.

The Acute Radiation Syndrome

The physiological effects of whole-body radiation are described as the acute radiation syndrome (ARS). The clinical course usually begins within hours of exposure. Prodromal symptoms include nausea, vomiting, diarrhea, fatigue, fever, and headache. There then follows a latent period, the duration of which is related to the dose. Haemopoietic and gastrointestinal complications follow this. The ARS can be subdivided into three overlapping sub-syndromes, which are related to the dose exposure.

Haemopoietic syndrome

This may occur after an exposure of between 1 and 4 Gy. The bone marrow is the most sensitive and pancytopenia develops. Opportunistic infections result from the granulocytopenia and spontaneous bleeding results from thrombocytopenia. Hemorrhage and infection are the usual cause of death.

Gastrointestinal syndrome

This requires a larger dose exposure usually in the range of 8–12 Gy. Severe nausea and vomiting associated with bowel cramps and watery diarrhea occur within hours of irradiation. There is a shorter latent period of 5–7 days, which reflects the turnover time of the gut epithelium (3–5 days). The epithelial damage results in loss of transport capability, bacterial translocation with sepsis, bowel ischemia, and bloody diarrhea. Large fluid imbalances can result in hypovolemia, acute renal failure and anemia from both bleeding and the loss of erythropoiesis. Critical exposure will lead to rapid deterioration with unrelenting bloody diarrhea, fever, refractory hypovolemic shock, sepsis, and death.

Neurovascular syndrome

An exposure to a dose of 15–30 Gy or greater can cause an immediate total collapse of the vascular system superimposed on the aforementioned syndromes. This may be due to the massive release of mediator substances, nitric oxide abnormalities or destruction of endothelium.[10] This syndrome can progress rapidly with variable neurological symptoms, respiratory distress, cardiovascular collapse, and death.

Triage

Triage is the initial classification of casualties into priority groups for treatment and is essential in the management of large numbers of casualties. Those patients unlikely to survive should not be allowed to overwhelm available resources, so that adequate treatment reaches those most likely to survive. In most circumstances, ionizing radiation is not immediately life-threatening and any associated injury should be treated first. Once life-saving measures have been carried out and the patient stabilized, assessment of radiation exposure can proceed. If large-scale casualties are encountered, triage may, of necessity, seem to be Draconian. In conventional warfare with limited medical resources, 50% of soldiers with thermal injuries of up to 70% total body surface area (TBSA) will be expected to survive (**Table 38.5**). This survival

Table 38.5 Survival rates

Burn alone	<70% TBSA	50% survival
Burn alone	>70% TBSA	Probably fatal
Burn plus radiation	<30% TBSA	May survive
Burn plus radiation	>30% TBSA	Probably fatal

TBSA, total body surface area.

rate should be bettered in a smaller civilian major accident. Thus, burns alone over 70% TBSA should receive expectant treatment and those under 20% can have their treatment delayed. If there has been a significant exposure to radiation as well as a thermal injury, individuals with over 30% TBSA burns are unlikely to survive without the use of major resources.[16]

Treatment

The treatment of any burn requires massive support from a dedicated team. This will be available for small accidents. With larger accidents or a nuclear attack, the number of victims could swamp the services; treatment facilities may be destroyed; normal supply channels would be drastically reduced, if present at all; production, distribution and transportation of supplies may be greatly impaired and local care workers may also be the victims.[17]

First Aid

The injured must be evacuated from the source of radiation in order to limit the exposure. Normal resuscitation procedures must be followed (i.e. airway, breathing, circulation etc.). Contaminated clothing must be removed and the skin wounds decontaminated by copious but gentle irrigation with water or saline. The goal of decontamination is to dilute and neutralize particles without spreading them to unexposed areas. Thus, patients should not be immersed in tubs. Irrigation should be continued until a dosimeter such as a Geiger–Muller counter indicates a steady state or minimum radiation count has been reached. Intact skin may also be irrigated with a soft brush or surgical sponge, preferably under a stream of warm water. If this is inadequate, a second scrubbing with mild soap or detergent (pH 7) for 3–4 minutes is recommended. This is followed by application of providone–iodine solution or hexachlorophene soap, which is then rinsed again for 2–3 minutes and dried. If the patient is known to have had less than 100 REM he can be followed as an outpatient. Exposures greater than 100 REM require full evaluation in hospital. Patients with exposures over 200 REM or who have symptoms of ARS should preferably be sent to specialist centers with facilities to treat bone marrow failure.[18]

Assessment

The assessment of thermal injury has been covered in preceding chapters. Exposure to radiation can be estimated clinically, by noting the onset of symptoms of ARS, supported by biological parameters. A complete blood count, including platelets and differential count, should be performed immediately and repeated at 12–24 hours if indicated by a change in the absolute lymphocyte count. If the patient sustains a fall in lymphocyte count of 50% or an absolute count less than 1200/mm³ in a time period of 48 hours post-exposure, a moderate dose of radiation has been encountered.[19] Levels of serum amylase and diamine oxidase (produced by intestinal villi) may be useful biological dosimeters of the future. Amylase levels are only reliable when the salivary glands have been exposed and diamine oxidase has not yet been fully assessed in humans. Lymphocyte chromosomal analysis allows very accurate measurement even at low levels of exposure. However, the need for the test to be performed in cell cultures in laboratories over 48-hour incubation would render this test impractical with large numbers of casualties.[20]

General Care of the Irradiated Patient

Where possible, a history should be obtained from the patient or others. Factors such as age, concurrent medical problems, smoke inhalation, and multiple trauma will affect the prognosis. With this in mind, a full physical examination is carried out to exclude other injuries. Victims of radiation exposure may not appear to differ clinically from the thermally injured and should receive the same care. Those exposed to lethal doses of radiation will exhibit early signs of radiation sickness and should be triaged accordingly.

All patients should be given adequate analgesia. Opiates or opioids are the drugs of choice. They must be titrated to effect and administered by the intravenous route. Early nausea and vomiting will be distressing and must be treated with available antiemetic drugs. Prochlorperazine has to be given by intramuscular injection but the newer agent, ondansetron, may prove successful as it is used against the similar symptoms encountered in radiotherapy and chemotherapy. It can also be used in children.

Patients with thermal burns in excess of 7% TBSA, or with associated inhalation or major trauma, should be treated expectantly in the mass casualty situation. They should be made comfortable and given adequate analgesia and/or sedatives, if available and thought appropriate. Resuscitation should be the same as that for an uncomplicated thermal injury. Any resuscitation formula can be used, but it must be closely monitored and altered as necessary to maintain an adequate urine output. The fluid requirement will be increased as fluid is sequestered into damaged internal organs, especially the gut. Fluid losses from diarrhea and vomiting may also be excessive and need to be replaced. Intravenous fluids may be limited and the victims may be advised to take oral fluids consisting of balanced salt solutions and to maintain a large urine output. A number of oral fluid replacement formulae exist although the best known, Moyer's solution, can be readily formulated by mixing a teaspoon (5 ml) of sodium chloride and a teaspoonful of sodium bicarbonate in a liter of tap water.

Care of the Burn Wound

The patient is bathed gently to remove loose nonviable skin, the remnants of burnt clothing, and any other external debris which may be contaminated with radioactive material. After the patient has been cleaned, decontaminated and debrided, the extent of any thermal burn and its depth can be ascertained more accurately. The major problems that will be experienced with a radiation burn and/or thermal injuries are those associated with sepsis, fluid balance and the nonhealing wound. Mild erythema may require little treatment; however, it is important to avoid further irritation of the skin by exposure to abrasive decontamination, irritating solutions and sunlight. With a slightly higher radiation dose causing dry desquamation, a bland lotion and loose clothing to alleviate itching may be all that is required. Deeper burns with moist desquamation are treated like conventional thermal injuries. Topical chemotherapeutic agents can be used and regularly applied as described elsewhere. In a mass causality situation, dilute safe hypochlorite solution can be easily made (**Table 38.6**). Burns are best treated closed because of the high risk of sepsis in immunosuppressed patients whose wounds are susceptible to dehydration, colonization, and portal entry of organisms. Deep burns may convert to full-thickness wounds because of endarteritis obliterans. Early tangential excision and split skin grafting provides early wound closure, decreased burn wound colonization and sepsis, and shortened hospital stay.[21,22] This technique is recommended by the authors and probably has advantages where the potential to develop septic wounds is great. Information regarding the grafting of radiation burns is not yet available but is probably best delayed. Dubos *et al.*,[23] performing early excision and grafting of burns in irradiated monkeys, have shown that healing occurred fully by the end of the second week, although histologically there was a slight delay in the healing process. The procedure, however, is not without risks. Blood loss in excess of 300 ml/% TBSA excised presents an increased anesthetic hazard. In irradiated tissue that is severely injured, definitive management usually involves resection of damaged tissue and replacement with well-vascularized nonradiated tissue, usually from a distant site.

Hyperbaric oxygen therapy (HBO) may be combined with surgical treatment potentially to enhance wound healing in irradiated tissue. The mechanism of action is not certain but appears to be related to the creation of a high oxygen gradient across the irradiated tissues, which stimulates capillary ingrowth. Hyperbaric oxygen treatments have been devised using an empirical approach.[24] A single treatment or 'dive' consists of 90 minutes in the chamber breathing an oxygen-rich mixture at 2.4 ATA. Soft-tissue defects are usually treated with 30 dives. When combined with surgery a '20/10 protocol' is used in which the operative procedure is 'sandwiched' between 20 preoperative and 10 postoperative dives.

Table 38.6 Ingredients for common mass casualty solutions		
Product	Ingredients/liter of water	
Normal saline	Table salt 9 g = 6.5 ml	
Dextrose 5%	Corn sugar 50 g	
Ringer's lactate	NaCl	102 mEq = 5.96 g
	Na Lactate	28 mEq = 3.14 g
	KCl	4 mEq = 298 mg
	CaCl2	8 mEq = 333 mg
Dakins	Clorox	5 ml
	Sodium Biocarbonate powder 3 gm (baking soda)	2.5 ml
Disinfectant	Grapefruit seed extract (benzochlonium chloride)	5 ml
Water purification	Sodium hypochloride tablets or 2–3 drops of grapefruit seed extract or boil 10 minutes	

Treatment of Complications

Hematological

Blood and platelets are administered to maintain an adequate hemoglobin concentration and a platelet level of 20×10^9 per liter. If surgery is contemplated, this level should be raised to 75×10^9 per liter. All blood products should be irradiated to avoid graft versus host disease.

Bone marrow transplantation is the treatment of choice following total body irradiation. It should be performed between 3 and 5 days post-exposure as the immunosuppression is at its peak. The use of hemopoietic growth factors such as granulocyte colony stimulating factor (G-CSF) and granulocyte-macrophage colony stimulating factor (GM-CSF) have shown increased survival in animals and primates, but their success is not yet proven in humans.[25]

Infection

The immunosuppression associated with irradiation makes the victim susceptible to exogenous and endogenous pathogens. Exogenous infection can be limited by adequate aseptic technique and nursing the patient in a sterile environment. Monitoring the patient adequately will allow the early diagnosis of sepsis and its treatment before it becomes well established. The antibiotic chosen should reflect the current pattern of susceptibility and nosocomial infections in that particular unit at that time. Combination therapy will be required where there is a profound neutropenia. With the large fluid losses and shifts, gentamicin is not recommended unless there is no other choice. Therapeutic levels will be difficult to obtain without risking toxicity and there are now safer broad-spectrum antibiotics (imipenem, ceftazidime and levofloxacin). If Gram-positive infection is suspected, vancomycin or the newer and safer teicoplanin should be administered. If there is an inadequate response, an antifungal agent must be added. Itraconazole with terbenetrine has a synergistic action against most fungi, including aspergillus. The use of fresh frozen plasma, gamma globulin solutions and monoclonal antibodies is at present speculative, but if resources allow and the patient's condition is not stabilizing, these agents should be considered.

Cardiovascular collapse

This complication may occur due to the exposure, sepsis, fluid loss, or hemorrhage. The patient should be given adequate fluid resuscitation, the airway must be protected, and oxygen therapy instituted. Sedation and mechanical ventilation will decrease the oxygen debt that will inevitably occur. Inotropic support may become necessary and should be started as early as possible, accompanied by the relevant cardiovascular monitoring. Invasive monitoring will aid in the treatment of volume replacement, but invasive intravenous lines must be inserted in aseptic conditions, kept meticulously clean, changed regularly, and removed when no longer indicated. Agents that manipulate the release of nitric oxide may become available in the near future and may turn out to be the agents of choice in the treatment of septic shock.

Occupational Exposure

In clinical practice, there are concerns that relatively low levels of radiation delivered over a long period of time might induce cancer and/or exert genetic or teratogenetic effects. The radiation dose can be limited by reducing the duration of exposure, or by increasing the distance from the source of radiation. Since distance and radiation intensity obey the inverse square law, the latter is particularly effective. While the efficacy of shielding devices will be determined by the type and thickness of the material and the energy and type of radiation, **Table 38.7** illustrates the effectiveness of these devices when used at diagnostic X-ray energies. It should be noted that the bodies of others provide very effective shielding. Cumulative doses of radiation can be recorded on radiation badges containing photographic emulsion. The personnel dosimeter is relatively cheap and accurate, but has limitations. The smallest exposure that can be measured is 10 milliREM, film badges can be exposed by heat, giving false readings, and they are analyzed only at monthly intervals.

Table 38.7 The effectiveness of shielding devices	
Device	Transmission
Lead apron	<10%
Thyroid shield	<10%
Leaded glasses	<10%
Unleaded glasses	50%
Human body	1%
Human body wearing lead apron	0.1%
Portable lead shields	<1%

Summary

Treatment of radiation injury, whether or not it is combined with other injuries, requires specialized knowledge and resources. The combination of radiation injury with associated injuries appears to have a synergistic effect on outcome. Significant increases in mortality occur because of immunosuppression secondary to radiation exposure in patients already vulnerable to infections. For localized radiation injury, it is often difficult to assess the level of severity quickly and with accuracy, because of the delay between exposure and appearances of lesions, and because of hidden lesions in underlying tissues. Medical treatment deals with inflammation, moist desquamation, and chronic pain; the most favorable time for surgical intervention is difficult to specify. Full intensive care support is needed for whole-body irradiation causing ARS, and is available only if small numbers are involved. Those that survive and show signs of regeneration of tissues will warrant late surgical intervention. Aplastic anemia, immunosuppression, hemorrhage, and sepsis will be major problems for survivors. The improving therapy of bone marrow transplantation is the treatment of choice. Large numbers of casualties will necessitate expectant treatment only. Evacuation of survivors will take days and a natural selection will take place.

Vesicant burns

Vesicant agents are characterized by their ability to produce cutaneous blisters resembling 'burns'. They have posed a major military threat since the use of sulfur mustard [bis (2-chloroethyl) sulfide] in the trenches of World War I. Since this time, various nations have deployed chemical weapons, and terrorist organizations have used it in public places.[26] The conflict between Iraq and Iran in the 1980s displayed the most open and widespread use of chemical weapons on a battlefield in recent decades. Chemical weapons were believed to have been deployed by Iraq in the 1990

Persian Gulf War, at which time nerve gas and blister agent were detected in the theater of operations.[27,28] Although sulfur and nitrogen mustard are the most important vesicants militarily, the vesicant category includes other agents, such as Lewisite and phosgene oxime. These compounds affect not only skin but all epithelial tissue with which they come into contact, particularly the eyes and respiratory tract.

Mechanisms of Action

The mechanism of action of mustard has eluded identification; however, most of the toxic effects are believed to be related to alkylation of DNA and critical target molecules. The resulting DNA crosslinks prevent replication and repair of DNA, ultimately leading to cell death. The dermal epidermal separation, which causes skin lesions, is believed to be due to release of proteases and other enzymes. Breakage of anchoring filaments connecting the basal cell layer to the basement membrane results in a blister with the basement membrane on its dermal side. There are two main hypotheses to explain the biochemical processes leading to enzyme release.

The first proposes that depurination of the crosslinked DNA results in strand breaks which activate the nuclear DNA repair enzyme poly (ADP-ribose) polymerase. This initiates a cascade of reactions in which cellular stores of nicotinamide adenine dinucleotide (NAD) are depleted, glycolysis is inhibited, and the hexose monophosphate shunt is stimulated. This is thought to lead to induction and secretion of proteases.[29]

The second hypothesis proposes a mechanism based on an interaction between mustard and the intracellular scavenger glutathione (GSH).[30] This is thought to inactivate thiol proteins, including calcium and magnesium adenosine triphosphatases, which regulate calcium levels. Elevation of cytosolic calcium concentration activates production of proteases, phospholipases and endonucleases, which break down membranes, cytoskeleton and DNA, leading to cell death. A separate consequence of depleted GSH could also be lipid peroxidation with the formation of lipid peroxides toxic to cell membranes.[31]

The exact mechanism of action of the other agents is unknown, although Lewisite has been shown to inhibit several important enzyme systems, such as the pyruvate dehydrogenase complex.

Clinical Features

Early symptoms ascribed to mustard gas include an ocular burning sensation and a feeling of suffocation associated with a burning throat.[32] After 4 hours, erythema is seen; in 12–48 hours, blistering appears, accompanied by severe pruritus which has a predilection for moist areas such as the axilla and perineum. The blisters tend to rupture, discharging an amber serious fluid and leaving painful shallow ulcers. Greater exposure produces coagulative necrosis of skin, with either no blistering or 'doughnut blisters' surrounding a central necrotic zone.[33] This will be accompanied by severe conjunctivitis, corneal erosion, and necrotizing bronchitis. A secondary respiratory infection may develop over the next few days which, coupled with associated marrow suppression, could prove fatal. Following absorption of large amounts of mustard, other systems may be affected. Severe stem cell suppression may lead to pancytopenia, and involvement of the gastrointestinal tract can have effects ranging from nausea and vomiting to severe hemorrhagic diarrhea. Excitation of the CNS, resulting in convulsions, has been reported.[34] Mustard may also affect other organs, but rarely do these produce clinical effects.

Lewisite (2-chlorovinyl-dichlorarsine) is the best known arsine. It is more powerful than the mustards, and symptoms occur sooner. Eye irritation is produced immediately, and sneezing, salivation and lacrimation occur thereafter. Nonlethal chronic exposure may lead to arsenical poisoning.

Exposure to phosgene oxime, the commonest halogenated oxime, has the immediate effect of stinging, and is likened to contact with a stinging nettle.[35] Within a minute, the affected area becomes swollen and solid lesions resembling urticaria are seen. An eschar will form after 1 week, but healing is often delayed beyond 2 months. Contamination of the eyes is extremely painful and may result in permanent blindness. Inhalation causes irritation and coughing, hypersecretion, and pulmonary edema.

Treatment for Exposure to a Vesicant Agent

The only prophylaxis against these agents is butyl rubber gloves, boots, and a respirator. The clothing of a victim must either be removed or decontaminated with Fuller's earth powder. Fuller's earth consists of: aluminium, silica, iron oxides, lime, and magnesia. Eyes can be irrigated with water but, if available, 1.26% sodium bicarbonate solution or 0.9% saline should be used. Upon reaching a treatment facility, patients must have all their clothing removed, if this has not already been done, and all the exposed areas must be cleansed with copious water lavage. Attendants should also be suitably protected and contaminated clothing must be placed in special bags.

Itching can be treated with sedatives (benzodiazepines or phenothiazines). Antihistamines may be tried. Blisters should be deroofed and dressed with topical antimicrobials. The mustard blister fluid is harmless.[36] Early excision and grafting of mustard burns has been shown to be of value in the treatment of full-thickness and deep dermal burns in an animal model, although it is not yet of proven value in humans.[37] Dimercaprol (British antilewisite), a chelating agent, is a specific antidote for Lewisite poisoning. It is of note that it is incompatible with silver sulfadiazine. It is available as an ointment for skin lesions, as drops for eye applications (5–10% in oil), and in an intramuscular preparation for systemic toxicity. Other chelating agents such as:

- DMSA-mesodimercaptosuccinic acid;
- DMPS-2,3-dimercapto-1 propanesulfonic acid sodium; and
- DMPA-N-(2,3-dimercaptopropyl) phthalamidic acid

have a higher therapeutic index, are water-soluble, and are effective orally. There is no specific antidote to mustard poisoning and no pretreatments or treatments exist that provide practical or effective protection against mustard toxicity.[38]

Affected eyes should be irrigated, treated with antibiotics, and inspected at the earliest time by an ophthalmologist. Respiratory injury requires symptomatic treatment according to its severity. Inhalation of high-dose steroids is controversial at present. Severe exposure will lead to agranulocytosis or aplastic anemia.[39] The pancytopenia seen after 7 days in Iranian casualties did not appear to be helped by transfusion of relevant blood products. Bone marrow transplantation may prove useful, although of little practical value with large numbers of casualties. The effect of bone marrow stimulants such as oxymetholone and lithium carbonate is

unknown but may be considered. Fluid replacement may be carried out dynamically with adequate cardiovascular monitoring. The maximum fluid loss occurs during blister formation and not necessarily in the first 24 hours.

Long-term Effects of Acute Exposure

Individuals who sustain mustard injury may experience difficulties even after the initial effects of the injury have subsided. Destruction of melanocytes leaves hypopigmented areas, otherwise hyperpigmentation tends to predominate. Acute and severe exposure can also lead to chronic skin ulceration, scar formation, and the development of skin cancer. Recurrent or persistent corneal ulceration can occur after latent periods of 10–25 years. Chronic conjunctivitis and corneal clouding may accompany this delayed keratopathy.[40]

Clinical follow-ups on 200 Iranian soldiers who suffered injuries from mustard during the Iran–Iraq War indicate that about one-third had experienced varied respiratory ailments, such as chronic bronchitis, asthma, recurrent pneumonia, bronchiectasis and even tracheobronchial stenosis, more than 2 years after exposure. Some 12% of all British soldiers exposed to mustard in World War I were awarded disability compensation for respiratory disorders believed to have been due to mustard exposures during combat.[41]

Summary

The vesicant agents are perhaps poorly named since they have the ability to affect all epithelial surfaces, particularly the eyes and respiratory surfaces, and not just the skin. The most important vesicant is sulfur mustard, which acts as an alkylating agent, causing a series of clinical reactions ranging from vesicles to severe skin necrosis. Systemic effects are seen with high doses and the combination of depressed bone marrow activity and respiratory involvement often proves fatal. There is no effective antidote, and treatment depends on prevention of contact and local therapy to achieve wound healing, which tends to be slow. There is no risk to the caregiver and no active agent in the blister fluid.

Mass burn casualties

Burn injured patients should ideally be managed individually with treatment tailored to their personal needs. However, with mass casualties, following monumental disasters, whether natural or otherwise, lack of experienced staff, paucity of equipment, and insufficient time to perform all relevant tasks may make this an impossible goal. Nevertheless, every medical facility should be prepared at a moment's notice to cope with such situations. The handling of mass casualties is not confined to hospitals and the success of medical support will depend on adequate planning. It is informative to consider past disasters where mass casualties have involved large numbers of burned patients.[42] These have fared badly over the last 30 years and have included the circus fires in Nitroi, Brazil[43] in 1961, and at Bangalore[44] in 1981, and the camping ground explosion in 1978 at Los Alfaques[45] where more than 400, 100 and 200 victims died, respectively. European disasters have been smaller but have included the Bradford Football Stand Fire[46] in 1985, and the Ramstein Air Show disaster[47] in 1988.

Principles of Triage

Triage is the process by which casualties are sorted on the basis of treatment priorities. It must first facilitate the application of maneuvers that are life-saving.[48] The ABCs of trauma management are carefully followed so that a patient with an airway or breathing problem takes priority over a patient with a circulatory disability. Remember, the overall severity of the injury is determined by the combined effect of different injuries. For instance, the priority of a 40% burn will be increased if there is an associated fracture which may contribute to overall fluid loss. In a mass casualty situation, the patient with the most severe injury or greatest threat to life is not necessarily the patient that receives first priority. Consideration must be given to likelihood of survival, to optimize available resources. Furthermore, if patients' needs exceed available resources (equipment and personnel) they may be given a lower priority for triage until the necessary resources are secured. It is important to note that the triage should be performed by the person with the greatest experience of the types of injuries expected.

Management

Clinical management must continue throughout the chain of evacuation and can be divided for descriptive purposes into that occurring at the site of injury, the receiving (trauma or accident and emergency) center, and the specialist burns unit. At each site the overall management of large-scale burn disasters revolves around the three principles of triage, treatment and transport.

On Site

Triage

Casualties at the site of the accident are triaged according to:

- The general condition of each patient, the extent and depth of the burn injuries and a patient's ambulatory status.
- Availability of facilities and personnel in the adjacent hospitals.

All patients undergoing triage must be adequately labeled. This will enable them to be identified according to their group. Large colored labels that are waterproof should be attached to each victim. The label will denote the triage group, treatment, drugs administered, and time given. Cases can be graded as follows:[49]

A. Ambulant patients with less then 10% burns – wounds are dressed and treatment is continued as an outpatient unless there is a reason for admission, i.e. extremes of age, deep burns requiring surgery, areas requiring special nursing.
B. 10–30% burns – after first aid these patients can be moved to distant hospitals initially, so as not to overload burn centers.
C. Serious burns involving 30–50% TBSA – these patients may be saved by energetic measures and should be transferred immediately to specialist centers for optimum treatment of shock and respiratory problems.
D. More than 50% TBSA burns, especially those with respiratory burns and the elderly, are unlikely to survive. These patients should be transferred to the nearest hospital but admitted to a separate ward.

In any disaster it is advisable to group similar injured casualties in the same installations. Certain hospitals near the disaster should be designated as 'burn centers' and all cases requiring immediate and intensive care should be sent to these institutions.

Treatment

At this level, treatment of casualties may be limited to maintenance of airway, management of respiratory problems, commencement of intravenous infusions, protection of the burn wound, and analgesia. Escharotomy should be carried out for full-thickness circumferential burns, and antitetanus prophylaxis given.

Transport

The transportation of the burned patient between the site of injury and the receiving hospital is known as *primary transport*. The initial call will reveal the location; the number of injuries; the approximate time of the incident. This information will aid in decisions regarding the personnel, vehicles, equipment, and protective clothing that must be sent. On arrival at the scene, vehicles must be parked where they are out of danger and not blocking essential access or exits.

Most burn patients can be safely transported provided that they are properly stabilized and accompanied by competent medical personnel. The patient's physiology should be monitored throughout the journey.[50] Treatment including additional analgesia must be continued en route as necessary. Transfer itself can exacerbate the existing deleterious physiological changes. The parameters that should be monitored continually during transfer are listed in **Table 38.8**.

Accepting Hospital

Triage

Cases greater than 70% TBSA probably will not survive in the mass casualty situation. They should be made comfortable with adequate analgesia and sedation if thought necessary. They should be treated after patients in the more salvageable groups (see above).

Treatment

Mass nuclear casualties have been dealt with previously. When supplies and facilities are overloaded, compromises will be necessary. These are:

- Plasma and blood products are reserved for cases with associated trauma. Electrolyte solutions are effective in uncomplicated burns for the first 24 hours.
- Local wound care. Exposure method may be useful in this situation.

Table 38.8 Parameters to be Monitored Continually During Patient Transfer
Respiratory rate and pattern
Heart rhythm and rate
Capillary refill time
Blood pressure
Level of consciousness
Blood and fluid loss
Oxygen saturation
Drugs and fluids administered

▪ Grafting. Lack of operating space may be a problem. Patients whose wounds can be covered by a single grafting procedure take priority to allow early discharge.

With larger burns temporary biological cover may be necessary until space becomes available.

Away from the site of the disaster, opportunity is taken to carry out the 'secondary survey', a full examination from head to foot. A full history is recorded and an assessment of the extent of the burn and associated injuries is included. A respiratory evaluation based clinically, together with arterial blood gases and fiberoptic bronchoscopy (if practical), enables an early decision on whether patients require intubation and ventilation. This decision can be made by analysis of frequent arterial Po_2 measurements on a constant Fio_2 to detect early shunting. A pulse oximeter may provide a more practical substitute for arterial catheterization.

If the casualty is unconscious, attention must be paid to the possibility of associated head and neck injury, pneumothorax and carbon monoxide poisoning.[51] The burn wounds are then cleaned with a mild antiseptic solution and debrided. The extent and depth of burns are then estimated which, together with the weight of the patient, can be used to guide intravenous fluid resuscitation along well-established formulae. Success is measured by careful cardiovascular monitoring, aiming to produce a urine output in the range of 0.5 ml/kg/h in adults and 1.0 ml/kg/h in children.

Ideally each patient should have their fluid requirements calculated on an individual basis. However, when large numbers of casualties are involved, problems can occur in applying the standard formulas.[52] To obviate this problem the Burns Calculator has been developed[53] to assist nonexperienced personnel to prescribe fluid to adults and children over the first 8 hours.

Transport

Transfer from the receiving hospital to the Burns Unit is known as *secondary transport*; it is established that full assessment and resuscitation before moving the patient is invaluable in preventing cardiovascular and respiratory disasters.[54,55] A full examination may reveal other injuries, e.g. ruptured spleen that could prove fatal if not diagnosed. Biochemical and hematological parameters are optimized. For example, abnormal potassium predisposes to arrhythmias. Equally, transferring a hypoxic patient increases the morbidity and mortality. Airway problems need managing definitively before transport. Any suggestion of airway involvement must alert the need for intubation. There is no place for intubated patients breathing spontaneously during transfer. Adequate analgesia, sedation, and muscle relaxation should be given so that pain, anxiety, or restlessness does not interfere with the clinical picture. Attention must be paid to the wound, the immobilization of fractures and need for escharotomy before transport is commenced. All the necessary drugs and equipment needed during transfer must be available. It is wise to assume that the journey time will be twice that normally encountered so that enough drugs and oxygen are available in case of delays. All documents, including drugs and fluids administered, must be taken with the patient. A contemporaneous record of events during the journey must be kept.

Tertiary Referral Center

At the burn center, the patient is reassessed. Physiological stabilization is obtained and those with lesser injuries may be transferred to peripheral hospitals with their treatment plan so as to reduce the strain on the facilities of the burn center. Similarly, cases found to require grafting at a later date can be sent back to the unit so that a two-way traffic is established. It is important that only those needing the tertiary center remain there. Transportation between tertiary referral centers is very similar to that already mentioned.[56]

Summary

In mass casualty situations involving burns, local resources may not be able to cope with the large and unexpected number of victims. The system is therefore so stressed that treatment must be prioritized. Patients with the most urgent needs are given the earliest care. This may differ from nonmass casualty situations in that the most critically injured may be placed in an expectant category, to allow resources to be distributed to as many victims as possible. The objective is to provide a protocol for assessment of injured patients, and transportation to appropriate hospital facilities.

Conclusion

Planning for mass casualties is important. Well-trained personnel, preset protocols, specialized transport, and adequate supplies of documents, drugs and equipment will ensure minimal mortality and proper use of facilities. Paradoxically, the threat of chemical and thermonuclear injury is heightened by the breakup of the Soviet Union, producing a glut of weapons specialists on the world employment market. Also small chemical industries can produce dangerous chemicals with ease and minimal cost. Health care workers serving a civilian population or military force have the obligation to learn the basics of management of radiation and chemical injury to achieve the greatest good for the greatest number of injured.

References

1. Daniel J. The X-rays. *Science* 1896; 3: 562–3.
2. Hirsch EF, Bowers GJ. Irradiated trauma victims: the impact of ionizing radiation on surgical consideration following a surgical mishap. *World J Surg* 1992; 16: 918.
3. Rubin P, Casarett GW. *Clinical Radiation Pathology*, Philadelphia: Saunders, 1968.
4. Luckett LW, Vesper BE. Radiological considerations in medical operations. In: Walker RI, Cerveny TJ, eds. *Textbook of Military Medicine–Medical Consequences of Nuclear Warfare*, Virginia: TMM Publications, Office of The Surgeon General, 1989: 227–44.
5. Hall EJ. *Radiobiology for the Radiologist*, Maryland: Harper & Rowe, 1994: 2–13.
6. Mettler FA, Kelsey CA. Fundamentals of radiation accidents. In: Mettler FA, Kelsey CA, Ricks RC, eds. *Medical Management of Radiation Accidents*, Boca Raton: CRC Press, 1990: 2.
7. DOE/REAC/TS Radiation Accident Registries, personal communication and unpublished data, June 2000.
8. Eisman B, Bond V. Surgical care of nuclear casualties. *Surg Gynecol Obstet* 1978; 146: 877–83.
9. Lewis KN. The prompt and delayed effect of nuclear war. *Sci Am* 1979; 241(1): 35–47.
10. Kelleher D. Acute effects of ionizing radiation. In: *United States Navy, Royal Navy Workshop on Nuclear Warfare Combat Casualty Care*, 1983: 71–80.
11. Brooks JW, Evans EI, Han WT, *et al*. The influence of external body radiation on mortality from thermal burns. *Ann Surg* 1953; 136(3): 533–4.
12. Glasstone S, Dolan PJ. The effects of nuclear weapons, United States Department of Defense and the United States Department Of Energy, 1977: 541–628.
13. Oughterson AW, Warren S. Medical effects of the atomic bomb in Japan. New York: McGraw-Hill Book Co, 1956.
14. Need JV. Update on the genetic effects of ionizing radiation. *JAMA* 1991; 32: 698.
15. Nenot JC. Medical and surgical management for localized radiation injuries. *Int J Radiat Biol* 1990; 57: 784.
16. Becker WK, Buescher TM, Cioffi WG, McManus WF, Pruitt BA. Combined

radiation and thermal injury after nuclear attack. In: Browne D, Weiss JF, MacVittie, Madhavan VP eds. *Treatment of radiation injuries*, New York: Plenum Press, 1990: 145–51.

17. Hirsch EF, Bowers GJ. Irradiated trauma victims: The impact of ionizing radiation on surgical considerations following a nuclear mishap. *World J Surg* 1992; **16**: 918.

18. Radiation Injury. American Burn Association Advanced Burn Life Support Course Provider's Manual. Appendix 1, 1999: 66.

19. Browne D, Weiss JF, MaVittie TJ, Madhavan VP (eds). Consensus summary. In *Treatment of Radiation Injuries*, New York: Plenum Press, 1990: 10.

20. Walden TL, Farzaneh MS. Biological assessment of radiation damage. In: Walker RI, Cerveny TJ eds. *Textbook of Military Medicine – Medical Consequences Of Nuclear Warfare*. Virginia: TMM Publications, Office of the Surgeon General, 1989: 85–104.

21. Burke JF, Bondoc CC, Quinby WC. Primary burn excision and immediate grafting: A method shortening illness. *J Trauma* 1974; **14**: 389–95.

22. Gray D, Pine R, Harnar T, Marvin J, Engrav L, Heimbach D. Early surgical excision versus conventional therapy in patients with 20 to 40 percent burns. *Am J Surg* 1982; **189**: 147–51.

23. Dubos M, Neveux Y, Monpeyssin M, Drouet J. Impact of ionizing radiation on response to thermal and surgical trauma. In: Walker RI, Gruber DF, MacVittie TJ, Conklin JJ eds. *The pathophysiology of combined injury and trauma*. Baltimore, 1985: 19–25.

24. Kindwall EP. Hyperbaric oxygen's effect on radiation necrosis. *Clin Plast Surg* 1993; **20**: 473–83.

25. Antin JH. Use of rhGM-CSF in bone marrow failure. In: Browne D, Weiss JF, MacVittie, Madhavan VP eds. *Treatment of radiation injuries*, New York: Plenum Press, 1990: 11–18.

26. Sidell FR, Urbanetti JS, Smith WJ, Hurst CG. Vesicants. In: Zajtchuk R, Bellamy RF eds. *Textbook of Military Medicine – Medical aspects of Chemical and Biological Warfare*. Office of the Surgeon General, Department of the Army, Washington DC, 1997: 197–228.

27. New York Times News service, 20,000 troops may have faced gas. The Sun. 23 Oct 1996: A–1.

28. Eddington PG. Gassed in the Gulf, xiii. Washington: Insignia Inc, 1997: 72–82.

29. Papirmeister B, Feister AJ, Robinson SI, Ford RD. Molecular mechanisms of cytotoxity. In: *Medical Defense against Mustard gas: Toxic mechanisms and pharmacological Implications*. Boca Raton: CRC Press Inc, 1990: 155–97.

30. Orrenius S, McConkey DJ, Nicotera P. Biochemical mechanisms of cytotoxicity. *Trends Pharmacol Sci Fest Suppl* 1985; **15**: 18–20.

31. Somani SM. Toxicokinetics and toxicodynamics of mustard. In: Somani SM ed. *Chemical Warfare*, San Diego: Academic Press, Inc., 1992: 13–45.

32. Willems JL. Clinical management of mustard gas casualties. *Ann Med Milit (Belg)* 1989; 3 (suppl): 1–61.

33. Papirmeister B, Feister AJ, Robinson SI, Ford RD. The sulfur mustard injury: description of lesions and resulting incapacitation. In *Medical Defense against Mustard gas: Toxic mechanisms and pharmacological Implications*. Boca Raton: CRC Press Inc., 1990: 13–34.

34. Vesicants (blister agents), Mustard and nitrogen mustards. In: *NATO Handbook on the Medical Aspects of NBC Defensive Operations*. Washington DC: U.S. Army, U.S. Navy, U.S. Air Force, 1984; **3**: 12–15.

35. Blister agents (vesicants) In *Treatment of Chemical Agent Casualties and Conventional Military Chemical Injuries*. Virginia: U.S. Army Technical Manual No.

8–285, U.S. navy NAVMED Publication No. P-5041, U.S. Air Force Manual No. 160–11, 1990; **4**: 14.

36. Sultzberger MB, Katz JH. The absence of skin irritants in the contents of vesicles. *US Nav Med Bull* 1943; **43**: 1258–62.

37. Graham JS, Braue EH, Schomacker KT. Laser debridement and autologous split-thickness skin grafting promotes improved healing of deep cutaneous sulfur mustard burns. *Biosicience 2000 Medical Defense Review*, Hunt Valley.

38. Papirmeister B, Feister AJ, Robinson SI, Ford RD. Pretreatments and therapies. In *Medical Defense against Mustard gas: Toxic mechanisms and pharmacological Implications*. Boca Raton: CRC Press Inc., 1990: 243–87.

39. Anslow WP, Houck CR. Systemic pharmacology and pathology of sulfur and nitrogen mustards. In *Chemical Warfare Agents and Related Chemical Problems*. DTIC No AD-234-249, Summary Technical Report of Division 9, National Defense Research Committee of the Office of Scientific research and Development, Washington DC, 1946: Pts 3–4.

40. Blodi FC. Mustard gas keratopathy. *Int Ophtalmol Clin* 1971; **2**: 1.

41. Gilchrist HL (1928) A comparative study of world war casualties from gas and other weapons. Washington DC: Government Printing office.

42. Barclay TL. Planning for mass burns casualties. Royal Society of Medicine Services. Round Table Series No 3. In: Wood C (ed). *Accident and Emergency Burns: Lessons from the Bradford Disaster*. Oxford: Alden Press, 1986: 81–8.

43. Pitanguy I. Treatment of victims from the great catastrophe of the Gran Circus at Niteroi (Brazil). In Wallace AB, Wilkinson AW (eds) *Research in Burns*. Edinburgh: E & S Livingstone, 1966: 216–21.

44. Das RAP. Circus fire at Bangalore. *Burns* 1983; **10**: 17–29.

45. Arturson G. The Los Alfaques disaster: a boiling liquid expanding vapour explosion. *Burns* 1981; **7**: 233–51.

46. Sharpe DT, Roberts AHN, Barclay TL, Dickson WA, Settle JAD, Crockett DJ et al. Treatment of burns casualties after fire at Bradford City Football Club ground. *Br Med J* 1985; **291**: 945–9.

47. Seletz JM. Flugstag-88 (Ramstein Air Show Disaster): An Army response to a MASCAL. *Military Med* 1990; **155**: 153–5.

48. Advanced Trauma Life Support for Doctors. Student Course Manual 6th edn. Chicago, American College of Surgeons, 1997.

49. Low Chee Ann W. Mass casualty organisation in burn disasters. *Med J Malaysia* 1977; **31**: 349–52.

50. Edbrooke DL, John RE, Murray RJ. Transportation. In: Rylah LTA (ed). *Critical Care of the Burned Patient*. Cambridge: Cambridge University Press, 1992.

51. Safar P, Pretto EA, Bircher NG. Resuscitation medicine involving the management of severe trauma. In: Baskett P, Weller R (eds). *Medicine for Disasters*. London John Wright, 1988: 36–87.

52. Milner SM, Rylah LTA. Burn casualties in war: a simplified resuscitation protocol. *Br J Hosp Med* 1993; **50**: 163–7.

53. Milner SM, Hodgetts TJ, Rylah LTA. The burns calculator: a simple proposed guide for fluid resuscitation. *Lancet* 1993; **341**: 1089–91.

54. Bion JF, Edlin SA, Ramsey G, McCabe S, Ledingham IM. Validation of a prognostic score in critically ill patients undergoing transport. *Br Med J* 1985; **291(6493)**: 432–4.

55. Ehrenworth J, Sorbo S, Hackel A. Transport of critically ill adults. *Crit Care Med* 1986; **14**: 534–7.

56. Ellis A, Rylah LTA. Transfer of the thermally injured patient. *Br J Hosp Med* 1990; **44**: 206–8.

Chapter 39

Exfoliative and necrotizing diseases of the skin

Marcus Spies, Maureen Hollyoak, Michael J Muller
Cleon W Goodwin, David N Herndon

Introduction

Acute, severe exfoliative, and necrotizing diseases of skin and underlying structures may cause significant morbidity in the afflicted patient. The problems associated with these diseases, such as wound infection, sepsis, adequate nutrition, and pain are similar to those seen in patients with major burns. Burn centers provide expertise in the treatment and management of critically ill patients with skin loss from all causes, not solely from thermal injury. This chapter describes the pathophysiologic processes of severe exfoliative skin disorders, their diagnosis, and the specialized treatment offered by burn units.

Severe exfoliative disorders

Erythema multiforme minor (EM), Stevens–Johnson syndrome (SJS), and toxic epidermal necrolysis (TEN) are severe exfoliative diseases of skin and mucous membranes. There is great controversy on the classification of these exfoliative skin disorders and the terminology is confusing. Most authors consider SJS and TEN to be the same disease entity, differing only by the area of involved skin. In this classification, SJS is considered to affect less than 10% total body surface area (TBSA), whereas TEN covers greater than 30% TBSA, leaving a zone of overlap between 10 and 30% TBSA, which is referred to as SJS/TEN.[1,2] The most common characteristics of these disease entities are defined in **Table 39.1**.[3,4] The incidence of TEN is estimated at 0.4–1.2 cases per million persons per year. The incidence of SJS has been reported to be 1–7 cases per million persons per year.[5–9] These exfoliative disorders occur in all age groups; however, the incidence is increased in the elderly and females.[3,10–13] In addition, TEN is seen more often in patients with HIV infection[14] and in bone marrow transplant recipients.[15] Mortality of TEN ranges from 25 to 80%. However, reports are variable and usually based only on small patient populations.[16–18] Death may occur early in the course of the disease, with sepsis being the most frequent cause. *Pseudomonas aeruginosa* and *Staphylococcus aureus* are the predominant organisms involved.[16] Pulmonary embolism and gastrointestinal hemorrhage are other causes of death.[10,16] The prognosis of SJS/TEN is worse than that of a burn victim with the same extent of skin loss.[16] Mortality is increased significantly in those patients at the extremes of age, and in relation to the percentage of denuded skin and serum urea nitrogen levels.[16,19] SJS is associated with a mortality rate of 0–38%.[11,20] Erythema multiforme rarely causes death.[20]

Etiology

TEN and SJS both appear to be caused by immunologic reactions to foreign antigens. TEN, as the more severe entity, has a much higher percentage associated with antecedent drug therapy. Drugs are implicated in 77–94% of cases of TEN.[21,6] Antibacterials and antifungals (36%), anticonvulsants (24%), analgesics and nonsteroidal anti-inflammatory agents (38%), and even corticosteroids (14%) have been implicated.[21,22] Attempts to identify drugs suspected of having caused exfoliative necrolysis by skin test and laboratory tests seldom have been rewarding.[16] Upper respiratory tract infections, pharyngitis, otitis media, or viral illness are frequently reported.[10–12,23–25] *Mycoplasma pneumoniae* and herpes viruses (cytomegalovirus, Epstein–Barr virus, herpes simplex, and varicella zoster) have been implicated in the cause of EM and SJS, but not TEN.[11,26,27] It can be difficult to differentiate some prodomal symptoms as due to viral or other infectious agents, or due to the primary disease process. Recently, the incidence of HIV infection in patients with toxic epidermal necrolysis has risen.[14,28] Whether this increase is due to their immunocompromised state or to the increased prescription of high risk drugs, particularly sulfonamides, is debated. No history of drug ingestion or preceeding illness may be noted in these patients. Many of these cases may

Table 39.1 Characteristics of Erythema multiforme, SJS and TEN

	Erythema multiforme	Stevens–Johnson syndrome	Toxic epidermal necrolysis
Prodrome	Absent	High fever, malaise	High fever, malaise
Acute phase	4–8 days	4–8 days Sensation of skin burning or tenderness	Sudden onset, 1–2 days Sensation of skin burning or tenderness
Skin lesions	Symmetrical, primarily located on the extremities, some target lesions without blisters	Variable distribution, individual vesicles on an erythematous base <10% TBSA Nikolsky's positive	Diffuse generalized epidermal detachment, absence of target lesions, large confluent plaques >30% TBSA Nikolsky's positive
Mucosal involvement	Absent or limited to one surface, usually oral	Severe, two or more surfaces involved	Severe, two or more surfaces involved
Histopathology	Dermoepidermal separation, mononuclear perivascular cell infiltrate, small areas of epidermal detachment associated with target lesions	Dermoepidermal separation, more intense dermal infiltrate, areas of epidermal detachment	Epidermal necrosis, dermoepidermal separation, minimal dermal inflammatory infiltrate, large areas of epidermal detachment
Recovery	1–4 weeks	1–6 weeks	1–6 weeks
Mortality	0%	0–38%	25–80%

actually suffer from lack of patient recall of current medication because of the severity of the underlying disease or the patient's age. Idiopathic cases, not related to drugs, accounted for only 3–4% of TEN.[6,7]

Morphology/Histopathology

An early skin biopsy is essential for diagnosis. Skin manifestations vary from patient to patient and with the age of the lesion (**Figure 39.1**). Skin lesions may evolve to different stages of development with recurrent attacks of EM in a single patient.[29] Advancing edges of the target lesions show scattered necrotic keratinocytes in the epidermis and only mild dermal inflammation. In older lesions and central zones of target lesions, the dusky appearance corresponds to areas of extensive keratinocyte necrosis, often with the formation of subepidermal bullae and dermoepidermal separation. The surrounding erythematous zone shows papillary dermal edema, vascular dilation with endothelial cell swelling, and perivascular

mononuclear cell infiltrate.[13] Extravasated erythrocytes may be seen in the surrounding papillary dermis. The reticular dermis is normal.

Epidermal and dermoepidermal suppressor/cytotoxic T lymphocytes in addition to dermal infiltrates of helper T lymphocytes have been demonstrated.[30–32] Hertl has confirmed that these epidermal cells are cytotoxic T-cells.[33] Langerhans cells appear to be reduced in the epidermis, although numerous dermal macrophages are observed.[34] A more intense dermal cell infiltrate is present in SJS, especially in postherpetic cases.[26,30] Dendritic lymphoid cells are observed, opposed to damaged dermal macrophages and necrotic keratinocytes. Further, at the point where the cytoplasmic processes contact the keratinocyte, the plasma membrane of the keratinocyte is absent.[34] Aberrant expression of HLA-DR on keratinocytes has been observed, a phenomenon which has been observed in many other inflammatory skin disorders.[31,35]

Immunofluorescence microscopy has demonstrated IgM and C3 along the dermoepidermal junction and dermal vessels in cases of postherpetic SJS and EM.[26,30] There have been only two reports of basal cell immunofluroscence in TEN.[34,36] The pathogenesis of TEN is not completely understood. Type IV delayed hypersensitivity reaction, type II cytotoxic reaction, keratinocyte cytotoxicity mediated by lymphocytes, drug-related nonimmunologic mechanisms, and keratinocyte apoptosis mediated by receptors of the TNF superfamily are possible mechanisms which amplify predisposing factors of infection and genetic susceptibility.[14,37–39] Positive patch tests in patients with TEN have been used to support the delayed hypersensitivity hypothesis.[32] This view is somewhat at odds with the fact that HIV patients display increased frequency of TEN.[14,40]

Suppression/cytotoxic T-cell infiltrates are observed in the epidermis in TEN[32,34] and graft versus host disease.[41] It is hypothesized that cytotoxic T-cells recognize drug metabolites which are complexed with the MHC-I molecule on the surface of keratinocytes, migrate into the epidermis, react with keratinocytes, and cause epidermal necrosis. The occurrence of sicca syndromes in patients

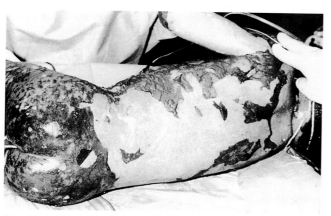

Fig. 39.1 Topical epidermal necrolysis (TEN) is characterized by massive sloughing of the epidermal tissue.

with TEN and graft versus host disease further supports the autoimmune theory.[42] The observation of blebbing of the keratinocyte plasma membrane in TEN is considered a reliable morphologic finding of cytotoxic T-lymphocyte cytolysis.[34] Further, the observation that cyclophosphamide aids TEN patients supports this theory, as cyclophosphamide is known to inhibit cytotoxic T-lymphocyte activity.[34] Type II cytotoxic reactions involve the binding of either IgG or IgM antibodies to a cell-bound antigen. The antigen–antibody complex then activates the complement cascade and results in the cell destruction. This mechanism is not generally supported since nuclear fragmentation, common to keratinocytes of toxic epidermal necrolysis patients, is not a consequence of complement-mediated cytolysis.[34,36,43] Keratinocyte apoptosis as the primary mechanism in the pathogenesis of TEN has been favored recently.[38] This event is thought to be mediated by ligand/receptor interaction of the tumor necrosis factor (TNF)-superfamily (as TNFα/TNFreceptor or FasL/Fas interaction).[38,44] In SJS, keratinocyte DNA fragmentation has been found in about 90% of cases associated with dermal perforin-positive lymphocytes.[39] Nonimmunological mechanisms include keratinocyte injury by either drug, drug metabolite, or toxic products derived from a drug in the epidermis.[14,28,45]

Clinical Features

A prodromal phase of TEN/SJS is identified frequently and usually consists of low-grade fever, malaise, and cough, all of which may suggest a respiratory tract infection. These symptoms may precede any cutaneous manifestation by 1–21 days, but usually last for 2–3 days.[2,11] Additionally, patients may present with conjunctivitis, sore throat, and generalized, tender erythema. This may evolve from morbilliform eruptions or discrete erythematous or purpuric macules.[37] Later, vesicles and large bullae emerge from areas of erythema. Patients may exhibit diffuse red erythema immediately followed by epidermolysis.[16] On light digital pressure, the epidermis desquamates in sheets: Nikolsky's sign is positive. Generally, a lag period of 1–3 weeks is observed from initiation of drug until skin eruption, which may be shorter on reexposure of a previously sensitized individual.[1,2]

Two or more areas of mucosa involvement are typical of SJS or TEN. Mucosal involvement precedes skin lesions by 1–3 days in one-third of cases.[13,46] Several sites are usually affected, in the following order of frequency: oropharynx, ocular, genitalia, and anus. Most TEN patients have multiple mucosal lesions, and they generally persist longer than cutaneous lesions.[16]

Complications

Toxic epidermal necrolysis is frequently associated with serious complications. The skin reepithelializes from the dermal elements without scarring. Some patients experience hemodynamic instabilty and shock, and secondary full-thickness necrosis of the skin may develop; however, abnormal pigmentation is common (**Figure 39.2**). Nail plates are frequently lost and nail regrowth may be abnormal or absent.[13] Mucosal membrane erosions may result in cicatricial lesions causing phimosis in men and vaginal synechiae in women. Oropharyngeal involvement is common and often results in severe dysphagia.[47] Although mucocutaneous erosions are the most common features of TEN/SJS, the disease may present with multisystem involvement. The onset of intestinal symptoms generally occurs concurrently with the cutaneous lesions.[48] Epidermal and epithelial sloughing may extend into the

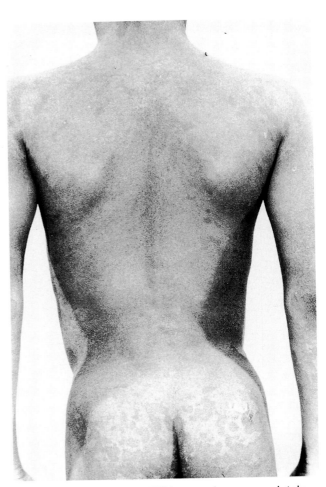

Fig. 39.2 One year post-TEN, wounds are completely closed with minimum of residual scarring but with abnormal pigmentation.

gastrointestinal mucosa, and may induce esophagitis with frequent subsequent stricture formation.[45] Gastrointestinal erosions macroscopically resemble ulcerative or pseudomembranous colitis and massive hemorrhage requiring resection has been reported.[10,16,23] Intestinal involvement worsens the prognosis.[16,48] Respiratory tract involvement occurs and is associated with increased mortality.[47,49] These complications include diffuse erythema to extensive confluent tracheal and bronchial erosion covered by fibrinous exudate.[37,47] Epiglottal swelling, necessitating intubation, has been reported.[47] Desquamation of alveolar lining cells also has been reported and these patients require frequent tracheobronchial toilet.[48] Subclinical interstitial edema is often noticed and 30% of cases progress to frank pulmonary edema and respiratory decompensation.[13,50] Bronchopneumonia was found to be the most frequent complication, occurring in 50% of patients.[20,23,49] Pulmonary embolism is an important cause of death in patients with TEN.[16] Renal manifestations like glomerulonephritis and acute tubular necrosis,[51] as well as hepatitis and hepatocellular necrosis, have been described.[13,37] Hypoalbuminemia, increased erythrocyte sedimentation rate, leukocytosis, thrombocytopenia, and normochromic and normocytic anemia are common.[20,47] Leukopenia is a frequent and poor prognostic sign.[12,13,16,23] This is due, in part, to depletion of the T-helper/inducer lymphocyte population (CD4+).[52] Ocular sequelae are the most severe long-term complications and occur in half of the survivors. Pseudomembranous or membranous conjunctivitis resulting from coalesced fibrin and necrotic debris can lead to opacification, secondary infection, and blindness.[4] Conjunctival scarring may result in lacrimal duct destruction leading to reduced tear production and keratoconjunctivitis siccal, a Sjögren-like syndrome. Ectropion, entropion, trichiasis, and symblepharon can also occur.[11,42]

Management

Toxic epidermal necrolysis is a life-threatening disease and such a patient is best managed in an intensive care burn unit where vigorous fluid resuscitation, nutritional support, wound care, physical therapy, and social services are provided routinely in a multidisciplinary team approach.[10,12,17,18,23,24,37]

Surgical Approach

Debridement of necrotic epidermis and coverage of the large wound surface with biological or synthetic dressings are essential.[10,53–55] Sloughed epidermis should be removed in order to reduce bacterial growth and the risk for infection. The exposed and tender dermis should be covered. Debridement is best undertaken under general anesthesia as soon as diagnosis by histology is established. Blood loss associated with debridement is minimal, so over-resuscitation must be avoided. Synthetic dressings, such as Biobrane™, and biological dressings, such as homograft (cadaver allograft) and porcine xenograft skin, greatly reduce the pain, decrease fluid loss, promote healing, and reduce the risk of wound infection and sepsis (**Figure 39.3**).[10,53–56] Biobrane™ is readily available as a commercial shelf product; however, in our own experience it is associated with increased local infection when covering greater than 40% TBSA wound areas. Porcine xenograft adheres well to the skin and is commercially available in large quantities.[54,55] Homograft is more likely to become vascularized and therefore reduces the number of graft changes.[10,57] All biological or synthetic dressings must be secured in place. Grafted areas must be immobilized and protected from shear forces. In children, Steinmann pins to suspend extremities may be useful.[54] In both adults and children, continuous rotation or air fluidized (Clinitron) beds frequently are used.

Topical Therapy

As separation occurs at the dermal–epidermal junction, varying depths of viable dermis remain. If this dermis can be protected from toxic detergents, desiccation, mechanical trauma, and wound infection, then rapid reepithelialization by proliferation of basal keratinocytes from the skin appendages will occur.[53] However, bacterial proliferation on the unprotected wound surface with invasive infection leads to full-thickness skin necrosis. Hydrotherapy and topical antimicrobials provide debridement and infection control which should be initiated early in the course of the disease.[11,25] Effective topical antimicrobial agents include silver sulfadiazine cream,[29] silver nitrate solution,[13,23,25] chlorhexidine gluconate solution,[13] and polymyxin-bacitracin ointment.[11] Silver sulfadiazine is widely used but may exacerbate the disease process due to its sulfonamide component. Additionally, an inhibitory effect on epithelialization and leukopenia requiring discontinuation has been observed. Silver nitrate solution does not contribute to the ongoing drug reaction, and epithelialization is not inhibited. However, frequent and painful dressing changes are required and serum electrolytes and osmolarity must be carefully monitored. For patients with contaminated wounds due to delayed initiation of treatment, silver nitrate soaks can reduce contamination and prepare the wound for eventual biological dressing. Chlorhexidine gluconate and polymyxin ointment are effectively against Gram-negative organisms, including *P. aeruginosa*, with low incidence of sensitivity. Moreover, chlorhexidine gluconate also show bactericidal effects against Gram-positive organisms.

Corticosteroid Therapy

Corticosteroid treatment of toxic epidermal necrolysis has promoted much controversy. In regard to the delayed hypersensitivity reaction or antibody-dependent cytotoxicity theories of pathogenesis corticosteroids would seem to be an appropriate form of medical therapy.[37,58] However, the practice of administering continuous high-dose corticosteroid in an attempt to stop the progression of the disease is widely rejected.[11–13,37,41,45,59,60] Rational assessment of the benefit of corticosteroids administration is not possible due to the lack of randomized, controlled, prospective trials. Many authors feel that steroids enhance the risk of sepsis,[23,54] increase protein catabolism, delay wound healing,[16] cause severe gastrointestinal bleeding,[16,23] prolong hospitalization,[60] and increase mortality.[12,23,61] Lyell states that the indication for the use of steroids in the treatment of toxic epidermal necrolysis is vague.[45]

One study found no decrease in the progression of SJS with steroids, but instead found significant morbidity.[61] In a prospective, although not randomized, study increased survival (66%) was seen in matched patients who did not receive steroids compared to only 33% survival in those who did receive steroids.[23] Pediatric SJS patients treated with steroids had a longer hospital stay and a complication rate of 74% compared to 28% in those without steroids.[60] Another study demonstrated 80% mortality associated with steroid therapy which was reduced to 20% when steroids were withheld.[12] In several studies, patients with antecedent glucocorticoid therapy before the onset of TEN showed no significant survival benefit,[62,63] and corticosteroid use itself has been linked to an increased risk for developing TEN.[22] Corticosteroids may have a place in the

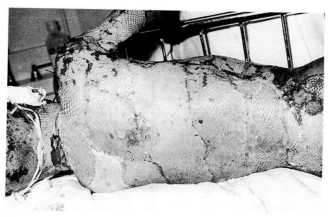

Fig. 39.3 As with many partial-thickness wounds, biological dressings do much to encourage reepithelialization and reduce the pain associated with these wounds.

treatment of TEN during the very early erythrodermic stages of the disease, before major skin loss has occurred, but it needs to be emphasized that steroid therapy is detrimental and thus contraindicated with skin loss of more than 20% TBSA.[59]

General Management

Drugs suspected of having initiated the disease should be discontinued immediately. Administration of pain medication is of high priority and antipyretic agents may be required. The empirical use of broad-spectrum antibiotics may be necessary if neutropenia exists, as these patients are prone to septic complications. The white blood cell count generally returns to normal levels after 2–5 days. The cause of this immunosuppression is unclear; it may be part of the primary disease or a secondary event.[58] Neutropenia is the only complication in which 'prophylactic' antibiotics are indicated. Otherwise, systemic antibiotics only should be used for documented infections or suspected sepsis. Oral nystatin prevents intestinal overgrowth of *Candida* and decreases the risk of *Candida* sepsis.[23,58] Frequent monitoring of urinary tract, respiratory tract, skin, and catheters allows early detection of systemic infection and identification of organisms.

Intravenous replacement of fluid losses through the exposed body surface is required. However, as patients do not develop the massive edema and fluid losses evident in burn patients, fluid resuscitation formulas commonly employed in the management of thermal injuries overestimate the actual need.[13,37,53–55] Ringer's lactate solution is given at a rate determined by close monitoring of the patient's condition and urine output. Once wound coverage is accomplished, fluid requirements usually decrease. Colloid is administered if serum albumin is less than 2.5 g/dl. Central line placement should be avoided, if possible, to reduce the risk of infection and sepsis. To further minimize this risk, lines should be placed, in areas of uninvolved skin. Invasive devices are removed as soon as possible, and oral and nasogastric routes are utilized at earliest convenience. Environmental temperature should be raised to 30–32°C to reduce metabolic energy expenditure. Heat shield and infrared lamps are beneficial in patients' rooms, bathrooms, and operating rooms.

Stress ulceration prophylaxis is advisable. Mouth erosion, resulting in severe dysphagia, can be alleviated by the use of viscous lidocaine or cocaine rinses, and thus ease oral administration of nutrients and fluids. Oral debris should be removed and the mouth sprayed with antiseptic several times a day.[59] Pulmonary involvement requires close supervision, with careful toileting including bronchoscopy, incentive spirometry, mobilization, and coughing to prevent infections and complications. If mechanical ventilatory support is necessary, the prevention of bronchopulmonary infection gains even more importance. Daily monitoring by blood assessment, including blood gas analysis, chest X-ray, and bacteriological culture, are required to initiate timely antibiotic therapy or ventilatory support. Measures to prevent thromboembolism, such as low-dose or low-molecular-weight administration of heparin, should be instituted on admission.

Ocular involvement should be assessed daily by an ophthalmologist. Conjunctival crusting can be minimized by the application of saline eye drops every hour. Any adhesions should be broken using a blunt instrument, and bland eye drops or ointment applied frequently.[11,53] Documented ocular infections are treated with antibiotics instilled frequently (10–24 times daily). After recovery, special ophthalmologic follow-up is needed to prevent and address ocular long-term sequelae. Lacrimal duct obstruction may be detected early by performing Schirmer's test.[11,59]

During hospitalization, patients with TEN and SJS may demonstrate limitations in mobility, decreased strength, postural and gait deviation, contractures, and impaired coordination. Therefore, patients should be treated and closely followed throughout the course of the disease by a physiotherapist.[64]

Nutritional Support

Enteral nutrition should be started on admission. Due to the frequent presence of oral mucosal ulcerations, patients may be reluctant to take nutrition orally, and thus require a nasogastric tube placement. Unlike burned patients who have significantly elevated metabolic rate, these patients appear to have metabolic rates only slightly above basal requirements.[53,58] Weight stabilization and a positive nitrogen balance have been achieved in adults with 2500 kcal/day.[53] If gastrointestinal function becomes impaired or sepsis intervenes, requirements may increase. Total parenteral nutrition should be avoided.

Adjunctive Treatment Strategies

In the search of better treatment modalities, the use of immunomodulating approaches may prove useful. Recent trials include the use of drugs, such as cyclosporin A,[65,66] cyclophosphamide,[67] thalidomide,[68] the administration of intravenous immunoglobulins,[69,70] and plasmapheresis.[71,72] In a recent study, cyclosporin A showed superior beneficial effects when compared to cyclophosphamide treatment.[66] The use of thalidomide, a potent inhibitor of TNFα action, to counteract TNF effects and potential TNF-induced apoptosis of keratinocytes, yielded excess mortality resulting in termination of the study.[68] A similar approach uses intravenous immunoglobulins to block Fas ligand (FasL)-mediated keratinocyte cell death, as TEN patients have been shown to express lytically active FasL. Uncontrolled trials in TEN patients showed promising results; however, data from controlled prospective studies are still missing.[69,70] In several uncontrolled trials, plasmapheresis showed beneficial effects.[71,72] The implied underlying mechanisms are the removal of the initiating drug, its metabolites, and the mediators of inflammation.

Until these treatment modalities have proven their efficacy in controlled trials, the gold standard of treatment for TEN patients consists of a multidisciplinary approach, such as used in severe burns, focusing on wound care, infection control, and prevention of complications. The specific requirements of these patients are best met in an intensive burn care unit, so early referral to a burn center is strongly recommended. Guidelines for the transfer decision may rely on the referral criteria for severe burn injury established by the American Burn Association (see also algorithm in **Figure 39.4**). The multidisciplinary burn team for specialized treatment of patients with extensive skin loss with trained critical care physicians, surgeons, critical care nursing specialists, respiratory therapists, physical and occupational therapists is able to provide the best acute care as well as early and adequate rehabilitation.

Skin and soft-tissue infections

Staphylococcal scalded skin syndrome, necrotizing fasciitis, and purpura fulminans are examples of a group of conditions

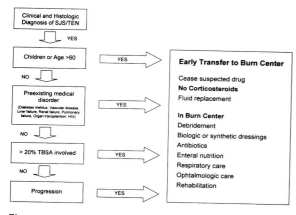

Fig. 39.4 Algorithm for management of SJS/TEN.

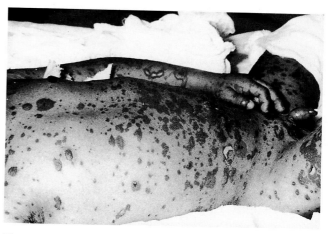

Fig. 39.5 Staphylococcal scalded skin syndrome is characterized by diffuse, erythematous lesions with bullae formation (see left forearm). Epidermis is shed in sheets with minimal abrasion. The wounds are partial-thickness and heal without surgical intervention.

characterized by extensive soft-tissue loss, rapid onset of critical illness, and death. Early, accurate diagnosis is essential to initiate appropriate action, such as extensive surgical excision in the case of necrotizing fasciitis or crepitant soft-tissue infections. Burn care centers with their acute and reconstructive capacities have much to offer these patients with extensive skin loss.

Staphylococcal Scalded Skin Syndrome

Staphylococcal scalded skin syndrome is the severe condition caused by exfoliative staphylococcal toxins and is characterized by systemic signs and symptoms and generalized involvement of the skin (**Figure 39.5**). It is important to make a diagnosis early, particularly to differentiate it from TEN, which has a different management and much greater mortality. Staphylococcal scalded skin syndrome is predominantly a disease of infancy (Ritter's disease) and early childhood, with most cases occurring before the age of 5 years.[73] Newborn nurseries are often the sites of outbreaks. Attendant staff may be infected or colonized with *Staphylococcus aureus* strains producing epidermolytic toxin, thus emphasizing the importance of standard hygienic measures. Adult staphylococcal scalded skin syndrome syndrome is rare and usually associated with compromised renal function. Mortality is generally only 4%, but can be much higher in adults (40%) depending on underlying diseases.[73,74]

Two distinct epidermolytic toxins (ETA and ETB), are responsible for the blistering in staphylococcal scalded skin syndrome.[45] ETA is heat-stable, whereas ETB is heat-labile and encoded by a bacterial plasmid. Most toxigenic strains of *S. aureus* are identified as group 2 phage.[75] The exfoliative toxin is metabolized and excreted by the kidneys, leading to a predisposition of patients with renal immaturity (children) or renal compromise. The exfoliative toxins produce blistering by disrupting the epidermal granular cell layers through interdesmosomal splittings but without epidermal necrosis and with very few inflammatory cells. The exact mechanism of action of the toxins has not been determined, although it is felt that the toxins directly affect desmosomes. One might be proteolytic disruption of desmosomes with the toxin or part of its sequence acting as a serine protease.[73,76,77]

Diagnosis of staphylococcal scalded skin syndrome can be made rapidly with a skin biopsy. The characteristic intraepidermal level of splitting is seen, with the split occurring at the granular layer level (stratum granulosum) with no epidermal necrosis or inflammatory cells in the corium.[73] Immunofluorescent studies of the skin are negative.[75] A Tzanck preparation from a scraping of the base of a freshly denuded area will reveal the affected cell population, i.e. acanthocytic keratinocytes.[75] Bullae, denuded skin and blood are usually sterile, however, and staphylococci can usually be cultured from nares, conjunctiva, or pharynx.[78]

Management

Onset may be marked by fever, malaise, and irritability. Scarlatiniform erythema is often accentuated in flexural and periorificial areas.[73] The skin is generally tender to touch, and sheets of skin may peel away in response to minor trauma (Nikolsky's sign). Blisters appear within 24–48 hours of rupture, leaving a characteristic moist erythematous epidermal base. Severe mucosal involvement is not a typical feature. With diagnosis antibiotics should be started, and semisynthetic penicillinase-resistant penicillin analogs are indicated (e.g. methicillin or oxacillin), since the majority of group 2 staphylococci show resistance to penicillin. Administration of steroids to these patients is contraindicated.[75] After screening for colonization, decontamination of colonized areas, especially the nasopharyngeal region in patients and nursing staff, may be advisable to prevent further spread. Fluid resuscitation is usually required at a lesser volume compared to a burn patient with a similar involved body surface area. Fluid substitution should be guided by urine output, hemodynamic parameters, electrolyte, and colloid status.

Until skin barrier function is restored, patients should receive appropriate wound dressings to prevent secondary wound infection. Topical agents are soothing and bacteriostatic. It needs to be pointed out that the wound initially is not colonized or infected, so alternatively, large areas can be more effectively managed with biological or synthetic dressings. They have the advantage of eliminating the need for frequent dressing changes which can be particularly traumatic for young children. Mortality usually is low, but may occur in very young and adult patients, usually from sepsis or electrolyte imbalance on the basis of underlying disease.[75] Complete wound healing is usually observed within 7 days, and scarring and altered pigmentation are not common.

Necrotizing Fasciitis and Bacterial Myonecrosis

Necrotizing fasciitis is a soft-tissue infection which is characterized by widespread necrosis of fascia and subcutaneous tissue which may progress to muscle and skin necrosis. Overall mortality may still be as high as 50%.[74,79] Most cases of necrotizing fasciitis are due to polymicrobial infections including both anaerobic Gram-positive cocci and Gram-negative bacilli.[79] *Streptococcus*, *Staphylococcus*, *Enterococcus*, and *Bacteroides* are commonly found. Infection with many bacterial species may result in bacterial myonecrosis. However, gas gangrene by *Clostridia* spp. results in severe systemic toxicity and higher mortality than necrotizing fascitis. A deep contaminated wound frequently preceeds the severe soft-tissue infection. Streptococcal myositis has a mortality rate of between 80 and 100%.[80] Risk factors for both necrotizing fasciitis and bacterial myonecrositis have been identified as diabetes mellitus, intravenous drug use, age greater than 50 years, hypertension, and malnutrition/obesity. The presence of three or more of these risk factors was found to give a predictive mortality rate of 50%[81] (See **Figure 39.6**).

Diagnosis

Early diagnosis is of extreme importance and consequence. Initial presentation is deceptive as the findings may be localized pain and edema without discoloration of the skin. Later, induration and erythema may be evident. Paresthesia of overlying skin and eventual dusky discoloration and local blistering may occur in the later course. Severe toxemia may develop, usually out of proportion to the local signs. Severe systemic alterations are characteristic of myonecrosis. Gas inclusion may be evident in subcutaneous tissues on X-ray. CT and MRI may help in the diagnosis and provide information on the nature and extent of the infection.[82] Frozen section biopsies may provide early histologic evidence of infection.[83] Gram stains and microbiological testing are very important diagnostic tools and guide antibiotic treatment. However, a definite distinction between necrotizing fasciitis, myonecrosis, and other soft-tissue infections often can only be established during surgery.

Management

The key to successful management of necrotizing infections is early diagnosis and radical surgical intervention. Surgical exploration involves complete excision of all necrotic tissues. If more than one operation for debridement of infected necrotic tissue is needed, mortality increases from 43 to 71%; this outcome drastically highlights the importance of adequate initial necrosectomy.[84] In patients with many risk factors, early amputation of the extremity, especially in cases of myonecrosis, should be considered. Broad-spectrum antibiotics are started preoperatively, although high-dose penicillin is appropriate for clostridial infections. However, antibiotic treatment is no substitution for surgical intervention. Adequate fluid resuscitation and nutritional support are also required. Wounds are packed open with antiseptic soaked dressings, which need to be changed frequently. Kaiser and Cerra have reported unsatisfactory results with either early application of porcine xenografts or burn wound topical antimicrobials.[85] Complete control of local and systemic infection is required before wound closure is addressed.

As in burns, secondary infections must be prevented by proper wound management, Biological or synthetic dressings offer the advantages of decreased pain, decreased fluid loss, and prevention of secondary infection. Frequently, large areas of skin and soft-tissue loss result from this disease and will eventually require extensive surgery to achieve adequate closure. Some authors advocate the use of hyperbaric oxygen and claim that it results in decreased mortality and reduced need for debridement; however, most of these reports are case reports or uncontrolled trials and adequate prospective controlled trials in patients are still lacking.[86,87] In animals, hyperbaric oxygen therapy alone did not improve survival or bacterial colonization, but did show adjuvant effects to antibiotic treatment.[88] In summary, hyperbaric oxygen therapy, if available, should not delay radical surgical debridment and should be used as an adjunct to radical surgery and antibiotic therapy.[87,89]

Purpura Fulminans

Purpura fulminans is a term that describes an acute syndrome of rapidly progressive hemorrhagic necrosis of the skin due to dermal vascular thrombosis associated with vascular collapse and disseminated intravascular coagulation (DIC).[90] It may occur in individuals with dysfunction of the protein C anticoagulant system, with acute severe infection, or idiopathically without any coagulation dysfunction or infection.

It has been associated with systemic infection by *Meningococcus*, Gram-negative bacilli, *Staphylococcus*, *Streptococcus*, and *Rickettsia* organisms. Skin necrosis begins in a region of dermal discomfort, which rapidly progresses to evanescent flush, followed by petechiae. Hemorrhagic bullae progress to frank skin necrosis. The process generally involves the skin and subcutaneous tissues, without involvement of muscle. Skin involvement is frequently an early manifestation of the disease process. Skin biopsy will, therefore, allow an earlier diagnosis.[90] Mortality in the acute phase is 18–40%.[91]

Management is directed at halting progression of the underlying infectious disease, preventing secondary infections, and removing nonviable tissue. Early heparin administration and replacement of clotting factors have proven useful to stop intravascular clotting.[91] Shock from blood extravasation and sepsis require extensive volume replacement. Limb vascular and compartmental pressure should be monitored closely to enable early escharotomy and/or fasciotomy, when needed. Skin lesions resulting only in blisters should

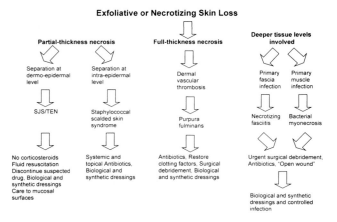

Fig. 39.6 Flowchart of management of exfoliative and necrotizing conditions of the integument.

be treated with topical antimicrobials (e.g. silver sulfadiazine) to prevent secondary infection. Nonviable tissue should be removed as soon as the patient's condition allows. Small areas can be covered with autografts but as large areas are frequently involved, allograft or xenograft skin coverage may be required. Limb amputations may be frequently required due to vascular compromise, as well as revisions for progression of disease.[92] Isolation of the affected patient, as well as monitoring and prophylactic treatment of patients and staff, may be necessary to prevent further spread and outbreaks of the disease, especially in case of meningococcal infection.

Conclusion

Inflammatory and infectious conditions of the skin and underlying tissues represent a major diagnostic and therapeutic challenge. The team approach to their care is essential, and wound management is paramount. Burn units are ideally suited to deal with patients with these conditions and should be considered as the appropriate site of referral for these critically ill patients.

References

1. Rasmussen JE. Erythema multiforme. Should anyone care about the standards of care? *Arch Dermatol* 1995; **131**: 726–9.
2. Becker DS. Toxic epidermal necrolysis. *Lancet* 1998; **351**: 1417–20.
3. Patterson R, Dykewicz MS, Gonzales A, *et al.* Erythema multiforme and Stevens–Johnson syndrome: descriptive and therapeutic controversy. *Chest* 1990; **98**: 331–6.
4. Wilkins J, Morrison L, White CR. Oculocutaneous manifestations of the Erythema multiforme/Stevens–Johnson syndrome/toxic epidermal necrolysis spectrum. *Dermatol Clin* 1992; **10**: 571–82.
5. Chan HC, Stern RS, Arndt KA, *et al.* The incidence of erythema multiforme, Stevens–Johnson syndrome and toxic epidermal necrolysis. *Arch Dermatol* 1990; **126**: 43–7.
6. Roujeau JC, Guillaume JC, Fabre JP, *et al.* Toxic epidermal necrolysis (Lyell syndrome): incidence and drug etiology in France, 1981–1985. *Arch Dermatol* 1990; **126**: 37–42.
7. Schoepf E, Stuehmer A, Rzany B, *et al.* Toxic epidermal necrolysis and Stevens–Johnson syndrome: an epidemiologic study from West Germany. *Arch Dermatol* 1991; **127**: 839–42.
8. Naldi L, Locasti F, Marchesi, Cainelli T. Incidence of toxic epidermal necrolysis in Italy. *Arch Dermatol* 1990; **126**: 1103–4.
9. Strom BL, Carson JL, Halpern AC, *et al.* A population-based study of Stevens–Johnson syndrome: incidence and antecedent drug exposures. *Arch Dermatol* 1991; **127**: 831–8.
10. Halebian P, Corder V, Herndon D, Shires GT. A burn center experience with toxic epidermal necrolysis. *J Burn Care Rehabil* 1983; **4**: 176–83.
11. Prendiville JS, Hebert AA, Greenwald MJ, Esterly NB. Management of Stevens–Johnson syndrome and toxic epidermal necrolysis in children. *J Pediatr* 1987; **115**: 881–7.
12. Kim PS, Goldfarb IW, Gaisford JC, Slater H. Stevens–Johnson syndrome and toxic epidermal necrolysis: a pathophysiologic review with recommendations for a treatment protocol. *J Burn Care Rehabil* 1983; **4**: 91–100.
13. Roujeau JC, Chosidow O, Saiag P, Guillaume JC. Toxic epidermal necrolysis (Lyell syndrome). *J Am Acad Dermatol* 1990; **23**: 1039–58.
14. Saiag P, Caumes E, Chosidow O, *et al.* Drug-induced toxic epidermal necrolysis (Lyell syndrome) in patients infected with the human immunodeficiency virus. *J Am Acad Dermatol* 1990; **26**: 567–74.
15. Villada G, Roujeau J, Cordonnier C, *et al.* Toxic epidermal necrolysis after bone marrow transplantation: study of nine cases. *J Am Acad Dermatol* 1990; **23**: 870–5.
16. Revuz J, Penson D, Roujeau JC, *et al.* Toxic epidermal necrolysis: clinical findings and prognostic factors in 87 patients. *Arch Dermatol* 1987; **123**: 1160–6.
17. Murphy JT, Purdue GF, Hunt JL. Toxic epidermal necrolysis. *J Burn Care Rehabil* 1997; **18**: 417–20.
18. McGee T, Munster A. Toxic epidermal necrolysis syndrome: mortality rate reduced with early referral to regional burn center. *Plast Recon Surg* 1998; **102**: 1018–22.
19. Scully MC, Frieden IJ. Toxic epidermal necrolysis in early infancy. *J Am Acad Dermatol* 1992; **27**: 340–4.
20. Ruiz-Maldonado R. Acute disseminated epidermal necrosis type 1, 2 and 3: study of sixty cases. *J Am Acad Dermatol* 1985; **13**: 623–35.
21. Guillaume JC, Roujeau JC, Revuz J, *et al.* The culprit drugs in 87 cases of toxic epidermal necrolysis (Lyell syndrome). *Arch Dermatol* 1987; **123**: 1166–70.
22. Roujeau JC, Kelly JP, Naldi L, *et al.* Medication use and the risk of Stevens–Johnson syndrome or toxic epidermal necrolysis. *N Engl J Med* 1995; **333**: 1600–7.
23. Halebian PH, Madden MR, Finkestein JL, *et al.* Improved burn center survival of patients with toxic epidermal necrolysis managed without corticosteroids. *Ann Surg* 1986; **204**: 503–11.
24. Adzick NS, Kim SH, Bondoc CC, *et al.* Management of toxic epidermal necrolysis in a pediatric burn center. *Am J Dis Child* 1985; **139**: 499–502.
25. Yetin J, Bianchini JR, Owens JA. Etiological factors in Stevens–Johnson syndrome. *South Med J* 1980; **73**: 599–602.
26. Howland WW, Golitz LE, Weston WL, Huff JC. Erythema multiforme: clinical histopathologic, and immunologic study. *J Am Acad Dermatol* 1984; **10**: 438–46.
27. Avakian R, Flowers FP, Araulo OE, *et al.* Toxic epidermal necrolysis: a review. *J Am Acad Dermatol* 1991; **25**: 69–79.
28. Goldstein SM, Wintroub BW, Elias PM, Wuepper KD. Toxic epidermal necrolysis: unmuddying the waters. *Arch Dermatol* 1987; **123**: 1153–5.
29. Huff JC, Weston WL, Tonnesen MG. Erythema multiforme: a critical review of characteristics, diagnostic criteria and causes. *J Am Acad Dermatol* 1983; **8**: 763–75.
30. Merot Y, Gravallese E, Guillen FJ, Murphy GF. Lymphocyte subsets and Langerhans' cells in toxic epidermal necrolysis. *Arch Dermatol* 1986; **122**: 455–8.
31. Villada G, Roujeau JC, Clerici T, *et al.* Immunopathology of toxic epidermal necrolysis. Keratinocytes, HLA-DR expression, Langerhans cells and mononuclear cells: an immunopathologic study of five cases. *Arch Dermatol* 1992; **128**: 50–3.
32. Miyauchi H, Hosokawa H, Akaeda T, *et al.* T-cell subsets in drug-induced toxic epidermal necrolysis. *Arch Dermatol* 1991; **127**: 851–5.
33. Hertl M, Merk HF, Bohlen H. T-cell subsets in drug-induced toxic epidermal necrolysis. *Arch Dermatol* 1992; **128**: 272.
34. Heng MC, Allen SG. Efficiency of cyclophosphamides in toxic epidermal necrolysis: clinical and pathophysiologic aspects. *J Am Acad Dermatol* 1991; **25**: 778–86.
35. Roujeau JC, Huynh TN, Bracq C, *et al.* Genetic susceptibility to toxic epidermal necrolysis. *Arch Dermatol* 1987; **123**: 1171–3.
36. Stein KM, Schlappner OL, Heaton CL, Decherd JW. Demonstration of basal cell immunofluorescence in drug-induced toxic epidermal necrolysis. *Br J Dermatol* 1972; **86**: 246–52.
37. Parson JM. Toxic epidermal necrolysis. *Int J Dermatol* 1992; **31**: 749–68.
38. Paul C, Wolkenstein P, Adle H, *et al.* Apoptosis as a mechanism of keratinocyte death in toxic epidermal necrolysis and Stevens–Johnson syndrome. *Br J Dermatol* 1996; **134**: 710–4.
39. Inachi S, Muizutani H, Shimuzu M. Epidermal apoptotic cell death in erythema multiforme and Stevens–Johnson syndrome. Contribution of perforin positive cell infiltration. *Arch Dermatol* 1997; **133**: 845–9.
40. Correia O, Chosidow O, Saiag P, *et al.* Evolving pattern of drug-induced toxic epidermal necrolysis. *Dermatology* 1993; **186**: 32–7.
41. Paller AS, Nelson A, Steffen L, *et al.* T-lymphocyte subset in the lesional skin of allogenic and autologous bone marrow transplant patients. *Arch Demartol* 1988; **124**: 1795–801.
42. Roujeau JC, Philippoteau C, Koso M, *et al.* Sjögren-like syndrome following toxic epidermal necrolysis. *Lancet* 1985; **1**: 609–11.
43. Hensen EJ, Claas FHJ, Vermeer BJ. Drug-dependent binding of circulating antibodies in drug-induced toxic epidermal necrolysis. *Lancet* 1981; **2**: 151–2.
44. Haake AR, Polaskowska RR. Cell death by apoptosis and epidermal biology. *J Invest Dermatol* 1993; **101**: 107–12.
45. Lyell A. Toxic epidermal necrolysis (the scalded skin syndrome): A reappraisal. *Br J Dermatol* 1979; **100**: 69–86.
46. Rasmussen J. Toxic epidermal necrolysis. *Med Clin N Am* 1980; **64**: 901–20.
47. Wahle D, Beste D, Conley SF. Laryngeal involvement in toxic epidermal necrolysis. *Otolaryngol Head Neck Surg* 1992; **6**: 796–9.
48. Chosidow O, Delchier JC, Chaumette MT. Intestinal involvement in drug-induced toxic epidermal necrolysis. *Lancet* 1991; **337**: 928.
49. Lebargy F, Wolkenstein P, Gisselbrecht M, *et al.* Pulmonary complications in toxic epidermal necrolysis: A prospective clinical study. *Intensive Care Med* 1997; **23**: 1237–44.
50. McIvor R, Zaidi J, Peters W, Hyland R. Acute and chronic respiratory complications of toxic epidermal necrolysis. *J Burn Care Rehabil* 1996; **17**: 237–40.
51. Krumlovsky F, Del Greco F, Herdson P, Lazat P. Renal disease associated with toxic epidermal necrolysis (Lyell's disease). 1975; **57**: 817–25.

52. Roujeau JC, Moritz S, Guillaume JC, et al. Lymphopenia and abnormal balance of T-lymphocyte subpopulation in toxic epidermal necrolysis. *Arch Dermatol Res* 1985; **277**: 24–7.

53. Heimbach DM, Engrav LH, Marvin JA, et al. Toxic epidermal necrolysis: A step forward in treatment. *JAMA* 1987; **257**: 2171–5.

54. Marvin JA, Heimbach DM, Engrav LH, Harner TJ. Improved treatment of the Stevens–Johnson syndrome. *Arch Surg* 1984; **119**: 601–5.

55. Taylor JA, Grube B, Heimbach DM, Bergman AB. Toxic epidermal necrolysis: a comprehensive approach. *Clin Pediatr* 1989; **28**: 404–7.

56. Sowder LL. Biobrane wound dressing used in the treatment of toxic epidermal necrolysis: a case report. *J Burn Care Rehabil* 1990; **11**: 237–9.

57. Birchall N, Langdon R, Cuono C, et al. Toxic epidermal necrolysis: an approach to management using cryopreserved allograft skin. *J Am Acad Dermatol* 1987; **16**: 368–72.

58. Halebian PH, Shires GT. Burn unit treatment of acute, severe exfoliating disorders. *Ann Rev Med* 1989; **40**: 137–47.

59. Revuz J, Roujeau JC, Guillaume JC, et al. Treatment of toxic epidermal necrolysis: Creteil's experience. *Arch Dermatol* 1987; **123**: 1156–8.

60. Ginsburg CM. Stevens-Johnson syndrome in children. *Pediatr Infect Dis* 1982; **1**: 155–8.

61. Rasmussen JE. Cause, prognosis and management of toxic epidermal necrolysis. *Compr Ther* 1990; **16**: 3–6.

62. Rzany B, Schmitt H, Schoepf E. Toxic epidermal necrolysis in patients receiving glucocorticosteroids. *Acta Derm Venereol* 1991; **71**: 171–2.

63. Guibal F, Bastuji-Garin S, Chosidow O, et al. Characteristics of toxic epidermal necrolysis in patients undergoing long-term glucocorticoid therapy. *Arch Dermatol* 1995; **131**: 669–72.

64. McDonald K, Johnson B, Prasad JK, Thomson PD. Rehabilitative considerations for patients with severe Stevens-Johnson syndrome and toxic epidermal necrolysis: a case report. *J Burn Care Rehabil* 1989; **10**: 167–71.

65. Wilkel CS, McDonald CJ. Cyclosporine therapy for bullous erythema multiforme. *Arch Dermatol* 1990; **126**: 397–8.

66. Arevalo JM, Lorente JA, Gonzalez-Herrada C, Jimenez-Reyes J. Treatment of toxic epidermal necrolysis with cyclosporin A. *J Trauma* 2000; **48**: 473–8.

67. Heng MCY, Allen SG. Efficacy of cyclophosphamide in toxic epidermal necrolysis: clinical and pathophysiological aspects. *J Am Acad Dermatol* 1991; **25**: 778–86.

68. Wolkenstein P, Latarjet J, Roujeau JC, et al. Randomized comparison of thalidomide versus placebo in toxic epidermal necrolysis. *Lancet* 1998; **352**: 1586–9.

69. Sanwo M, Nwadiuko R, Beall G. Use of intravenous immunoglobulin in the treatment of severe cutaneous drug reactions in patients with AIDS. *J Allergy Clin Immunol* 1996; **98**: 1112–5.

70. Viard I, Wehrli P, Bullani R, et al. Inhibition of toxic epidermal necrolysis by blockade of CD95 with human intravenous immunoglobulins. *Science* 1998; **282**: 490–3.

71. Yamada H, Takamori K, Yaguchi H, Ogawa H. A study of the efficacy of plasmapheresis for the treatment of drug induced toxic epidermal necrolysis. *Therapeutic Apheresis* 1998; **2**: 153–6.

72. Egan CA, Grant WJ, Morris SE, et al. Plasmapheresis as an adjunct treatment to toxic epidermal necrolysis. *J Am Acad Dermatol* 1999; **40**: 458–61.

73. Resnick SD. Staphylococcal toxin-mediated syndromes in childhood. *Semin Dermatol* 1992; **11**: 11–8.

74. Canoso JJ, Barza M. Soft tissue infections. *Rheum Dis Clin North Am* 1993; **15**: 235–9.

75. Elias PM, Fritsch P, Epstein EH. Staphylococcal scalded skin syndrome: clinical features, pathogenesis, and recent microbiological and biochemical developments. *Arch Dermatol* 1977; **113**: 207–19.

76. Dancer SJ, Garratt R, Sanhanha J, et al. The epidermolytic toxins are serine proteases. *FEBS Letts* 1990; **268**: 129–32.

77. Vath GM, Earhart CA, Rago JV, et al. The structure of the superantigen exfoliative toxin A suggests a novel regulation as a serine protease. *Biochemistry* 1997; **36**: 1559–66.

78. Itani O, Crump R, Minouni F, et al. Ritter's disease (neonatal staphylococcal scalded skin syndrome). *Am J Dis Child* 1992; **146**: 425–6.

79. Patino JF, Castro D. Necrotizing lesions of soft tissue: a review. *World J Surg* 1991; **15**: 235–9.

80. Steven DL. Invasive group A streptococcal infections. *Clin Infect Dis* 1992; **14**: 2–13.

81. Francis KR, Lamaute HR, Davis JM, Pizzi WF. Implications of risk factors in necrotizing fasciitis. *Am J Surg* 1993; **59**: 304–8.

82. Sharif HS, Clark DC, Aabed MY, et al. MR Imaging of thoracic and abdominal wall infections: comparison with other imaging procedures. *Am J Roentgenol* 1990; **154**: 989–95.

83. Stamenkovic I, Lew PD. Early recognition of potentially fatal necrotizing fasciitis: the use of frozen-section biopsy. *N Engl J Med* 1984; **310**: 1689–93.

84. Freischlag JA, Ajalat G, Busuttil RW. Treatment of necrotizing soft tissue infection: the need for a new approach. *Am J Surg* 1985; **149**: 751–7.

85. Kaiser RE, Cerra FB. Progressive necrotizing surgical infections: A unified approach. *J Trauma* 1981; **24**: 349–52.

86. Risemann JA, Zamboni WA, Curtis A, et al. Hyperbaric oxygen therapy for necrotizing fasciitis reduces mortality and the need for debridement. *Surgery* 1990; **108**: 847–50.

87. Green RJ, Dafoe DC, Raffin TA. Necrotizing fasciitis. *Chest* 1996; **110**: 219–29.

88. Zamboni WA, Mazolewski PJ, Erdmann D, et al. Evaluation of penicillin and hyperbaric oxygen in the treatment of streptococcal myositis. *Ann Plast Surg* 1997; **39**: 131–6.

89. McHenry CR, Piotrowski JJ, Petrinic D, et al. Determinants of mortality for necrotizing soft-tissue infections. *Ann Surg* 1995; **221**: 558–65.

90. Adcock DM, Hicks MJ. Dermatopathology of skin necrosis associated with purpura fulminans. *Semin Thromb Hemost* 1990; **16**: 283–92.

91. Chasan PE, Hansbrough JF, Cooper ML. Management of cutaneous manifestations of extensive purpura fulminans in a burn unit. *J Burn Care Rehabil* 1992; **13**: 410–3.

92. Genoff MC, Hoffer MM, Achauer B, et al. Extremity amputation in meningococcemia induced purpura fulminans. *Plast Reconstr Surg* 1992; **89**: 878–81.

Pathophysiology

Chapter 40

The burn problem: a pathologist's perspective

Hal K Hawkins

Hugo A Linares

Introduction

'Burns are not a simple injury, but a very complicated disease.' This statement, published by J. Long in 1840 and cited by Dr Linares in the first edition of this book, holds true even more in 2001.[1] Massive destruction of viable tissue which occurs in burn injury, and injury to the airways by inhalation of toxic products of combustion, stimulate complex reactions which are only beginning to be understood. Certainly, burn injury is frequently complicated by malfunction of every organ system. The nature of this malfunction is often clarified by examination of the body after death. Postmortem examination also has the potential to reveal adverse effects of therapy, which might not be clear during life. An important example of this is that the treatment of burned skin with tannic acid was popular until degeneration of the liver was

described in autopsies of burned patients treated with tannic acid. The causative link was later confirmed experimentally.[2] In addition, every death after burn injury has medicolegal implications. Postmortem examination often contributes substantial evidence in this regard. The process of analysis of an entire case from the point of view of pathogenesis often clarifies the nature of the patient's most significant problems. This chapter systematically reviews the observations made at autopsy in patients who have died after burn injury. Where possible, hypothetical interpretations of the mechanisms of disease are suggested, often on the basis of comparison of autopsy findings with results of animal experiments. To quote Dr Linares on this method, 'Pathology combines anatomy, physiology, and theories of disease, and it is a point of convergence for medicine and the biological disciplines.' The observations reviewed here include our experience of 269 autopsies performed on burned children at the Shriners Burns Hospital in Galveston from 1966 to the present.

To introduce the sections that follow, the major medical problems that complicate burn injury are summarized here. The degree of disruption of normal physiologic processes after burn injury is extreme. Immediately after burn injury, massive loss of intravascular fluid into the burned tissue begins to occur.[3,4] Unless this fluid loss is replaced by the physician very promptly and carefully, serious *hypovolemia* develops.[5-7] The consequences of hypovolemia often include the death of neurons in the brain, focal necrosis of the intestinal epithelium, and necrosis of the proximal tubules of the kidneys. The neural and endocrine responses to the traumatic injury may lead to recognizable lesions in the stomach and in the heart. Thermal injury to skeletal muscle, or lack of perfusion of muscle, may lead to local exudation of fluid and development of such high pressure in muscle compartments that arterial perfusion is prevented. This 'compartment syndrome', unless relieved by prompt surgical intervention, leads to necrosis of muscle throughout the entire compartment.[8] The consequences of massive necrosis of muscle often include secondary injury to the lungs, due to release of reactive oxygen species, and myoglobinuria with secondary renal damage.[9] At the time of injury, patients frequently inhale sufficient carbon monoxide to seriously impair the oxygen carrying capacity of the blood. The resultant tissue *hypoxia* can cause death at the scene, and if the patient survives, it can be sufficient to lead to irreversible neuronal injury and brain death. Hypoxia, sometimes related to carbon monoxide intoxication, also contributes to cardiac and renal injury. In addition, when fires occur in closed spaces, the 'flashover' process consumes all available oxygen, so that the patient's environment may contain too little oxygen to sustain life. Occasionally, a burn victim is found without pulse or respiratory effort, probably as a consequence of hypoxia, and is revived by cardiopulmonary resuscitation. In such cases, ischemic and hypoxic injury may be profound in multiple organs, and there may be significant 'ischemia/reperfusion injury' to the lungs after resuscitation. Patients injured in house fires often suffer injury to the respiratory tract caused by inhalation of toxic products of combustion.[10] This *smoke inhalation* injury stimulates an intense inflammatory reaction, which can lead to obstruction of airways and further tissue injury. This problem is discussed below in the section on the respiratory system. *Infection* is the next major risk experienced by patients after burn injury. Necrotic skin provides an excellent environment for proliferation of bacteria and fungi, and as long as necrotic tissue remains, the risk of infection remains high. Injury to the intestinal epithelium by hypoxia or ischemia leads to translocation of intestinal bacteria into the portal circulation. In addition, patients all experience substantial immunosuppression, probably as a result of excessive secretion of endogenous glucocorticoids, and release of cytokines into the circulation which lead to ineffective host defense. *Coagulopathy* may be a very serious complication of burn injury. It may lead directly to tissue ischemia, or the resultant hemorrhage may lead to secondary hypovolemia. Patients often require transfusion of very large quantities of blood products during their treatment.

Disease processes involving multiple organ systems

Hypoxia and Ischemia

All cells require a constant supply of oxygen and metabolic substrates, such as glucose, to remain viable. This is largely because animal cells exist in a state of dynamic equilibrium which requires membrane transport to maintain integrity. In hypoxia, when the supply of oxygen is insufficient, cells generate a limited amount of metabolic energy by anaerobic glycolysis, releasing lactic acid. With ischemia, when the flow of blood is insufficient, this metabolic perturbation is complicated by a lack of supply of glucose and other fuels, and the extracellular fluid composition may change dramatically. Tissues vary greatly in their sensitivity to injury by hypoxia or ischemia. In general, tissues with the greatest metabolic activity are the first to lose viability under conditions of hypoxia and ischemia. These tissues include the neurons of the central nervous system, the myocytes of the heart, the epithelial cells of the small intestine, and the proximal tubular cells of the kidney. The location and extent of necrosis in these organs depends on the severity and duration of the ischemic or hypoxic injury.

After ischemia and hypoxia have led to irreversible injury and death of selected cell types or whole segments of organs (infarcts), responses are generated which may lead to further injury of remote organs. Cellular necrosis stimulates an intense acute inflammatory reaction, probably by means of activation of the complement cascade, degranulation of mast cells, and other processes. This reaction surrounds an infarct, or proceeds throughout a region of tissue injury if the local circulation is sufficient. Monocytes recruited to the regions of injury secrete cytokines in large quantities, and polymorphonuclear neutrophils activate their antibacterial mechanisms. Both of these have effects throughout the body, the most important probably being tumor necrosis factor alpha (TNFα) and superoxide. In addition, in endothelial cells injured by hypoxia, the enzyme xanthine dehydrogenase is converted to xanthine oxidase, which releases superoxide during degradation of adenosine, which in turn is released by necrotic cells. Superoxide, released into the circulation by this metabolic process and by neutrophils, can injure the lung by damaging both endothelial and epithelial cells and allowing protein-rich fluid to exude into alveoli. The inflammatory

reaction to thermal tissue injury also stimulates an intense influx of neutrophils, which undoubtedly contribute to this injury by releasing superoxide. In experimental models of burn injury, as well as in models of ischemia-reperfusion injury, the lungs have been shown to be injured by these processes.[11] Endogenous antioxidants such as glutathione are depleted, and conjugated dienes appear, indicating that cell membrane injury due to lipid peroxidation has occurred in the lung.[12]

Infection and Sepsis

The skin normally provides a highly effective barrier against invasion of tissues by infectious agents. Necrotic tissue, in the skin as elsewhere, provides an excellent culture medium, and the body surface is inevitably exposed to multiple potential pathogens. Patients who are treated for deep burn injury with traditional debridement and washing for several days generally arrive at this institution with large quantities of multiple microorganisms growing in the necrotic skin. The bacteria appear to proliferate initially in areas with insufficient circulation to develop a significant inflammatory response. As large numbers of bacteria accumulate, those with high pathogenic capacity invade the adjacent viable tissue, produce further necrosis, and gain access to the circulation. This is the condition of burn wound sepsis, which historically has been the leading cause of death in burn patients. In Dr Linares' series of 100 autopsies, sepsis was present in 73%, as documented by positive blood culture and demonstration of invasive infection of viable tissue.[13] In 80% of these fatal cases of sepsis, the burn wound was the source of the infection. The pathogens which were most important were *Pseudomonas aeruginosa*, *Staphylococcus aureus*, *Klebsiella pneumoniae*, *Escherichia coli*, *Enterobacter*, and *Candida* species.

Burn wound sepsis is suspected clinically when a burn wound is the site of proliferating microorganisms exceeding 10^5/g of tissue, and there is histologic evidence of active invasion of subjacent unburned tissue.[14] In our institution, the wounds of burn patients, especially the open areas, are routinely sampled for quantitative culture and for histologic study when excision and grafting procedures are done, and whenever clinical examination suggests the possibility of tissue infection. The histologic classification used and its rationale are discussed below under the integumentary system. Once septicemia occurs, there is a generalized reaction which often includes hypotension, tachycardia, increased hyperthermia or hypothermia, and poor perfusion of the intestines and other viscera.[15] In the case of Gram-negative bacteria, the endotoxin stimulates monocytes via their CD14 receptors to become activated and set up a cascade of release of proinflammatory and anti-inflammatory mediators which affect all organs and tissues in the body.[16-18] Coagulopathy is also an important complication of sepsis.[19] In addition, once bacteria have gained entrance to the general circulation, it becomes possible for foci of tissue infection to develop at distant sites. This is most likely to occur in sites of tissue necrosis or on cardiac valves. Abscesses in distant organs can allow the infection to resist eradication by specific antibiotics, and thus allow sepsis to develop again after initially effective therapy. The risk of infection is proportional to the severity of the burn, the time before the initiation of fluid therapy, the presence of metabolic alterations, the development of immunologic deficiency, the concurrence of trauma, the local evolution of wounds, and the age of a patient. An infection may begin in a burn wound, the respiratory system, the gastrointestinal tract, the urinary tract, the blood vessels, and from localized infection in any area of the body. Although most serious infections in burn patients appear to be due to endogenous flora, and many derive from wound infections present at the time of admission, nosocomial infection is a constant hazard.

The problem of burn wound sepsis is amenable to therapy. The strategy of excision of the potentially infected burn wound as early as possible, together with judicious administration of effective antibiotics, has greatly reduced the number of deaths due to infection. Coincident with the institution of early excision and grafting of burn patients in our institution, the incidence of burn wound sepsis as a cause of death has declined dramatically.[20] In one recent year, no patient death was related to infection. The problem of sepsis has not disappeared, however. Certain organisms can evade the best current efforts at management, and have caused death in recent cases, including bacteria resistant to nearly all available antibiotics, and invasive fungi. Those patients who are referred for therapy more than 1 week after burn injury often have extensive invasive wound infection and sepsis, which may be difficult or impossible to eradicate.

Coagulopathy

The burn wound has procoagulant effects, and may induce coagulation throughout the circulation (DIC, disseminated intravascular coagulation).[21,22] Tissue necrosis, particularly lethal injury to endothelial cells, with exposure of subendothelial collagen, and release of tissue thromboplastin, can activate coagulation and lead to coagulopathy. Systemic release of active thrombin not only leads to generation of fibrin peptides but also stimulates acute inflammatory reactions, including increased vascular permeability and upregulation of adhesion molecules on neutrophils and endothelial cells.[23] Generation of fibrin degradation products may be sufficient to interfere with normal thrombosis, and thrombocytopenia can develop in response to abnormal intravascular fibrin generation.[24] Activation of the kinin system can stimulate further abnormal vascular permeability and hypotension.[18] Consumption of coagulation factors can lead to abnormal bleeding, which can cause extensive tissue injury secondarily. It is important to note that the acute phase response to burn injury includes increased synthesis of fibrinogen and factor VIII. During the first 3–10 days after burn injury, patients often have supranormal clotting activity. This may increase their susceptibility to development of DIC, especially if sepsis supervenes. It also implies that laboratory testing of levels of fibrinogen and factor VIII may yield normal values even in the presence of abnormal consumption of these factors. When DIC occurs in the patient's terminal course, as was the case in a majority of the autopsies reviewed by Dr Linares, microscopic fibrin thrombi are seen in many organs at the time of autopsy. These microthrombi are seen most commonly in the lungs, the skin, the kidneys, and the gastrointestinal tract.[25,13]

Integumentary System

The skin is the site of initial injury in burn patients, and many of the events that lead to dysfunction or failure of other organs begin in the skin. Thermal injury rapidly produces irreversible injury and cell death in epidermal keratinocytes, in the epidermal appendages including hair follicles and their attached sebaceous glands and sweat glands, and in the connective tissue cells of the dermis. In many cases, the burn wound excised within 48 hours of injury

shows that the entire dermis and all of the hair follicles are necrotic, but that much of the subcutaneous adipose tissue remains viable. It appears that the greater insulating capacity of adipose tissue protects it to some extent. In some cases, of course, the necrosis of the initial thermal injury may extend deep into the subcutaneous tissue. In extreme cases, the underlying skeletal muscle may become necrotic as a result of thermal injury. Necrosis of skeletal muscle is especially prominent in the case of electrical injury, in which more heat may be generated adjacent to bone than near the body surface. An interesting observation (**Figure 40.1a**) is that there is often a band-like infiltrate of degenerating polymorphonuclear neutrophils in the midst of a totally necrotic dermis. This suggests that the boundary between necrotic and viable tissue may have extended deeper after the initial burn injury and its inflammatory response. There is experimental evidence that burn wounds often evolve from an initial level of necrosis to a deeper level of necrosis, even from second to third degree, as a result of poor perfusion of the tissue immediately deep to the initial burn injury. This process of vascular stasis deep to the burn is undoubtedly due in part to the rapid loss of intravascular fluid from the damaged capillaries and venules just below the necrotic burn wound. In addition, there is evidence that neutrophils contribute to this process of burn wound extension, most likely by adhering to endothelium and to each other, with resulting obstruction of the microvasculature.[26]

It is important to assess the presence and extent of infection within the burn wound, both in the excised wound during therapeutic procedures, and by biopsy of suspicious areas in open foci after grafting procedures. A high index of suspicion serves the burn patient well. All biopsy and excision specimens in our institution are sampled and studied histologically with stains for bacteria (Brown and Hopps) and fungi (methenamine silver). Within large excision specimens, samples are taken from sites of especially deep tissue injury and sites which show abnormal discoloration of dermal or subcutaneous tissue. When infectious microorganisms are found, it is important to determine their location with respect to the boundary between living and necrotic tissue. This boundary may be irregular. It is generally distinct and marked by inflammation in wounds several days old, but may be somewhat indistinct in very fresh specimens, as karyolysis takes some time to develop in burn wounds. As noted above, wound infections generally begin with colonization of the skin surface and proliferation of organisms on the surface, often with extension into hair follicles, followed by growth within the necrotic tissue. Both the coagulum on the surface and the necrotic epidermis and dermis are considered part of the burn eschar. Growth within necrotic tissue is considered evidence of tissue infection, however, and potentially more dangerous than growth on the surface of necrotic skin, under a layer of fibrin and debris. Even when quantitative cultures show more than 10^5 bacteria per gram of tissue, when careful histologic study shows that the organisms are limited to the skin surface or the superficial necrotic tissue, the risk of sepsis appears to be quite low. Such growth on or in necrotic tissue, however, does set the stage for invasion of viable tissue. The finding of clusters of bacteria or fungi within viable tissue does imply a serious risk of sepsis and further tissue invasion. As a rule, bacterial invasion of viable tissue is quite apparent by histologic study of appropriate tissue samples, and often includes a zone of tissue necrosis surrounded by intact tissue. Invasive fungal infection presents a somewhat different pattern, in that there is often a

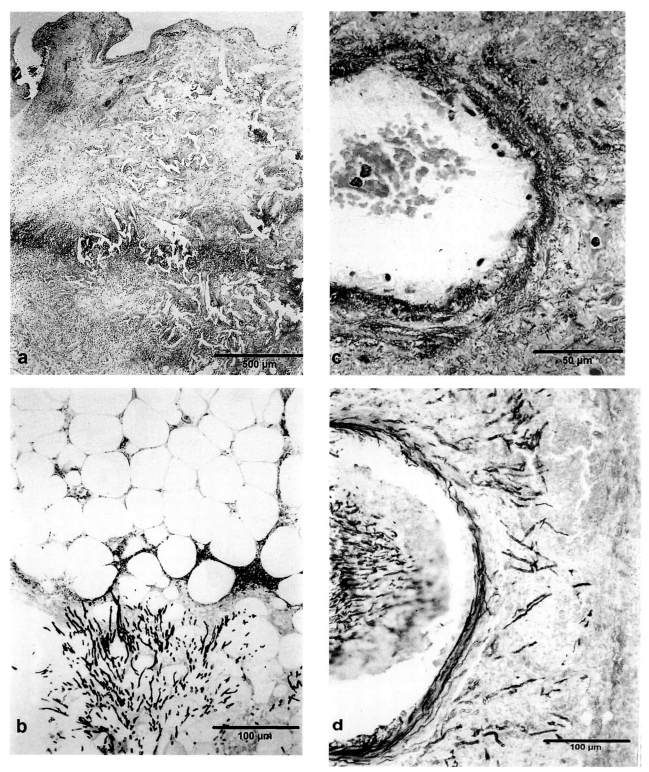

Fig. 40.1 (a) This low-magnification view of a freshly excised burn wound shows degenerative remnants of a band-like acute inflammatory infiltrate in the midst of the necrotic dermis. Hematolylin and eosin (H&E), bar = 500 μm.
(b) Filamentous fungal hyphae extend to the boundary between necrotic and viable tissue. This is considered evidence of invasion of viable tissue. Grocott methenamine silver stain, bar = 100 μm. (c) Lung tissue from a patient who had sepsis due to *Pseudomonas* which originated in the skin. This pulmonary artery is necrotic, and innumerable bacilli are present in its wall. Brown–Hopps tissue Gram stain, bar = 50 μm. (d) A filamentous fungus (*Fusarium*) penetrates the wall of a pulmonary artery in another patient with burn wound sepsis. Methenamine silver stain, bar = 100 μm.

wavefront of necrosis that accompanies fungal invasion (**Figure 40.1b**). Thus fungal infection which extends to a boundary between necrotic and viable tissue is considered evidence of fungal invasion of viable tissue. On this basis, infections identified within burn wounds are reported as surface colonization, invasion of necrotic tissue, which may be superficial or deep, and invasion of viable tissue. The responsible surgeon is called immediately when invasion of viable tissue is found. If the level of clinical suspicion is especially high, frozen sections have been found useful for this determination, using a tape transfer device to facilitate handling of these difficult specimens, and confirming the results with routine sections on the following day.

Respiratory System

In recent years respiratory failure, defined as inability to maintain adequate oxygen saturation while administering 100% oxygen by ventilator, has been the most common immediate cause of death in patients at the Shriners Burns Hospital in Galveston. The causes and mechanisms of respiratory failure are multiple, and will be addressed separately, although more than one mechanism operates in many cases. Direct thermal injury to the airways probably does not occur, except in cases of burn injury due to exposure to large quantities of steam. In addition to these processes which are specifically related to burn injury, patients may also develop problems related to the airways such as pneumothorax or interstitial emphysema, aspiration of gastric contents, pulmonary embolism, and nonspecific pulmonary edema due related to increased venous pressure. In Dr Linares' series of 100 burn autopsies, every patient had severe lung lesions of various kinds.[27]

Infection

In most patients who die with respiratory failure, postmortem cultures of lung tissue are sterile. However, in those patients who have sepsis at the time of death, extensive infection of the lungs is commonly present, and it may represent a terminal event. As is true of sepsis in general, fatal pneumonia is most often seen as a consequence of infection with a highly resistant bacterial strain, an invasive fungal infection, or in a compromised host with renal failure or some other cause of severe immunodeficiency. Virulent and antibiotic-resistant strains of *Pseudomonas* may produce an angioinvasive infection in the lung, with massive proliferation of bacteria within the walls of pulmonary arteries and consequent ischemic necrosis of segments of lung tissue (**Figure 40.1c**).[28] A similar angioinvasive pattern of pulmonary infection can be seen with generalized infection due to *Aspergillus* or similar filamentous fungi (**Figure 40.1d**).

Diffuse alveolar damage

This process affects the pulmonary parenchyma in all lobes and segments, and begins with exudation of protein-rich fluid into alveolar spaces. This proteinaceous exudate, representing the vascular phase of the acute inflammatory reaction, is a consequence of damage or increased permeability of both capillary endothelial cells and the epithelial type I cells of the alveolar lining. Within hours, the exudates form the hyaline membranes which are one histologic hallmark of this disease process. Within a few days, the exudate begins to undergo organization by spindle-shaped fibroblasts, and collagenous fibrosis develops, which obliterates alveoli and greatly thickens the septa between alveoli. Macrophages accumulate within alveoli, and alveolar epithelial type II cells multiply. In the late stages, there is severe interstitial fibrosis.

There are multiple pathogenetic mechanisms that may be responsible for this process, but it is not clear which of these are most significant in patients with burn injury.[29,30] The burn injury itself stimulates activation of complement, liberating peptides including C5a and C3a, which could, in spite of their short half-lives, directly stimulate vascular leakage in the pulmonary bed. More likely, these and many other peptides activate circulating neutrophils, which produce secondary injury to the vascular and epithelial membranes in the lung.[31,32] Conversion of xanthine dehydrogenase to xanthine oxidase in the burn wound can cause release of superoxide into the venous circulation, stimulating endothelial injury and oxidative stress in the lung. The neutrophils reacting to the burn wound also undergo an oxidative burst, contributing to the release of superoxide into the circulation. This process is greatly enhanced if the patient's course is complicated by ischemic injury of muscle compartments, limbs or other organs.

Lipid peroxidation is a recognized consequence of burn injury. Superoxide can also react with nitric oxide, produced in the lung, to form peroxynitrite, a highly toxic substance.[33] Thrombin peptides, released during thrombosis of blood vessels in the wound, can also activate neutrophils.[34] The kinin system can be activated during thermal injury, with its systemic consequences. When patients develop sepsis, additional pulmonary damage can be produced by release of proinflammatory cytokines and augmentation of the processes that lead to inflammatory injury of the lung.[13,35] Finally, the presence of oxygen in high concentration within the lung can itself lead to injury, and this injury can be manifest in the form of diffuse alveolar damage.[36–38] Despite this plethora of mechanisms which can lead to pulmonary injury in burn patients, many patients with massive burn injury do not develop clinically apparent respiratory difficulty. The conditions which seem to be most strongly associated with this form of pulmonary injury are delayed fluid resuscitation, limb ischemia, and, of course, sepsis.

Smoke inhalation injury

Patients often inhale products of combustion in house fires, and the toxic effects of these gases and fumes directly injure tissues within the lung. These patients are recognized clinically by observing prominent hyperemia of the tracheobronchial mucosa, and small particles of carbonaceous soot within the airways, during bronchoscopy. Associated findings include facial burns and singed nasal hairs. These patients usually do not require ventilator therapy for several days, but are at high risk of developing respiratory failure, which responds poorly to ventilator therapy and may prove fatal even when the burn injury is small. Experimental studies in sheep and dogs have partially clarified the mechanisms of smoke inhalation injury.[39] The immediate reactions to inhalation of toxic smoke, in animals, include detachment of numerous ciliated columnar cells from the tracheobronchial epithelium, secretion of all stored mucus by secretory cells, and a dramatic increase (10-fold or greater) in tracheobronchial blood flow. Within a few hours, an intense acute inflammatory reaction develops, with exudation of numerous neutrophils into the airways, and release of protein-rich fluid which may coagulate within airways, forming occlusive 'casts' containing mucus and desquamated cells. After 48 hours, the exudate of neutrophils, which is most intense in the trachea at earlier times, fills many terminal bronchioles, and begins to extend into the lung parenchyma. This inflammatory reaction resolves in the experimental animal, and the epithelium slowly regenerates. However, autopsy evidence suggests that the exudation of neutrophils and protein into the airways does not resolve in humans, but may persist for weeks. The loss of airway epithelium, which may be complete, does not regenerate for long periods of time. Perhaps because of failure of the mucociliary escalator, mucus can be seen to accumulate around terminal bronchioles focally. These lesions are illustrated in **Figure 40.2a–d**.

Multiple mechanisms may be responsible for the respiratory disease evoked by inhalation of toxic smoke. As in the case of diffuse alveolar damage, the available evidence indicates that neutrophils may be responsible for much of the injury, but the locus of injury appears to be different, centered on the airways rather than the pulmonary parenchyma. Factors which may be likely to lead to selective damage to the airways include local release of neuropeptides by afferent C-fibers in the airways, and activation of proinflammatory processes in reaction to injury to the airway mucosa, particularly local production of interleukin-8.[40–43] These concepts are hypothetical, not yet confirmed experimentally. Local activation of thrombin during the formation of fibrin clots, and local production of endothelin-1 may further enhance the inflammatory reaction in the airways. Secretory cells appear to be especially sensitive to smoke inhalation injury. Obstruction of small bronchi and bronchioles is thought to lead to failure of ventilation of multiple small segments of lung tissue, and inappropriate vasodilation in these poorly ventilated segments may well contribute to the failure of adequate oxygenation. Segmental atelectasis and prominent vasodilation in focal areas are features of smoke inhalation injury seen in experimental animals, and also in patients examined at autopsy after burn injury and smoke inhalation injury. As is the case with diffuse alveolar damage, the toxic effects of high concentrations of oxygen may complicate the reaction to injury.

Cardiovascular System

Despite the tachycardia and increased output common to patients with burn injury, structural lesions of the heart have been uncommon in our autopsies done on a pediatric population of patients. Cardiac dilation and clinical evidence of poor myocardial contractility do develop in some patients after burn injury. Bacterial endocarditis occurs in occasional patients with sepsis complicating burn injury. Nonbacterial thrombotic endocarditis (marantic endocarditis) has also been seen, and may also give rise to embolic complications (**Figure 40.3a**). When the endocardial region of the left ventricle is examined at autopsy, small foci of necrosis associated with local hemorrhage are often observed. (**Figure 40.3b**) Contraction band necrosis is sometimes the only evidence of myocardial injury. These lesions may represent poor perfusion of a tissue with high metabolic demands during terminal episodes of hypotension. In some cases, they may represent the effects of endogenous or exogenous adrenergic stimulation. Rona and his associates have demonstrated that β-adrenergic agents, at high doses, stimulate development of small foci of myocyte necrosis and hemorrhage in the subendocardial region of the heart.[44,45]

Urinary System

Patients with extensive burn injury, if resuscitated adequately during the first few hours after injury, may have normal renal func-

tion throughout their hospital course. It is not uncommon, however, especially when the initial fluid resuscitation was not optimal, or when patients develop episodes of sepsis, for acute renal failure to develop. In such cases, the autopsy frequently reveals evidence of acute tubular necrosis, the morphologic expression of which depends upon the timing of the injury.[46] In Dr Linares' autopsy series, evidence of acute tubular necrosis was present in 86% of the cases, and all of these patients had clinical evidence of renal failure.[27] The morphologic features of acute tubular necrosis include edema of the entire kidney with substantial increase in weight, necrosis of proximal tubular cells with karyolysis, karyorrhexis, and sloughing of the injured cells from the tubular basal lamina (**Figure 40.3c**). Within 48 hours, these events are followed by evidence of regeneration of surviving cells of the renal tubule, which flatten, become basophilic, and undergo mitosis as they migrate to reconstitute the epithelial lining. Vasodilation and accumulation of erythroblasts in small blood vessels often accompany this lesion. Clinical renal failure was an independent factor associated with increased mortality in the analysis of prognostic factors in patients with greater than 80% TBSA burns in our institution.[47] Patients with renal failure seem to be at especially high risk for the infectious complications of burn injury.

Digestive System and Hepatobiliary Tract

The association of duodenal ulcers with burn injury, described by Curling, is a classical lesion which may occur in patients with burn injury.[48] In a pediatric population treated prophylactically with inhibitors of gastric acid secretion, these lesions are distinctly uncommon. Local mucosal necrosis and hemorrhage, an early manifestation of this process, is seen with some frequency (**Figure 40.3d**). Such defects in the mucosa are often multiple, typically small and round, and can be associated with significant hemorrhage from the exposed blood vessels deep to the lesion. They heal rapidly and rarely lead to serious complications.

The intestinal tract is especially susceptible to ischemic and hypoxic injury, and lesions related to poor perfusion are often found at the time of autopsy. Decreased blood flow in the splanchnic circulation is a well-established physiologic consequence of endotoxemia.[14,49] Thus sepsis is associated with an increased risk of intestinal injury. Hypoxic or ischemic injury of the intestinal epithelium, which may be very limited, can lead to translocation of intestinal flora into the mesenteric lymphatic circulation and into the portal venous circulation.[50–53] Additional factors favoring the escape of bacteria from the intestine include alterations in the bacterial ecology of the gut.[54] Thus, hypotension and hypoxia can also be causes of sepsis. In our autopsy experience, formation of abscesses or foci of tissue infection in the intestinal tract was uncommon, except when many organs including the skin were heavily infected in patients with generalized sepsis. The intestinal lesion most commonly seen at autopsy is the presence of transverse streaks of hemorrhage in the small intestine in a 'ladder' pattern, associated with focal necrosis of folds of mucosa. This lesion is called superficial hemorrhagic necrosis.[55] Perhaps surprisingly, perforation of the intestinal tract is an uncommon occurrence in patients with burn injury.

The liver is enlarged in most autopsies of children who succumb to burn injury, often to double or triple its normal weight. Occasionally such hepatomegaly is thought to compromise ventilation. The lesions often seen at autopsy include steatosis, with

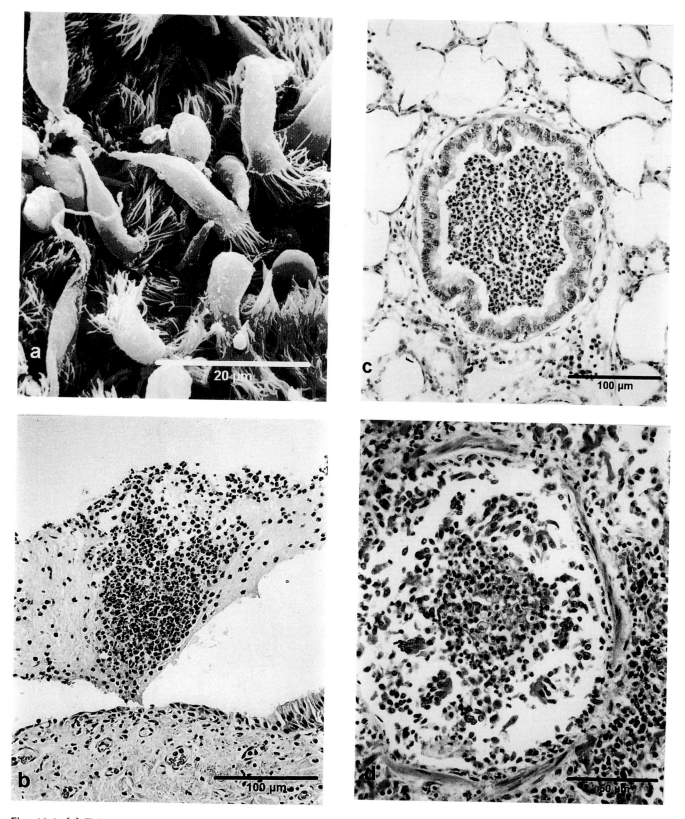

Fig. 40.2 (a) This scanning electron micrograph demonstrates desquamation of intact ciliated cells from the tracheal mucosa in a sheep, 15 minutes after insufflation of cotton smoke. Bar = 20 μm. (b) Extensive exudation of polymorphonuclear neutrophils into the trachea is seen 3 hours after insufflation of cotton smoke in the sheep model. H&E, bar = 100 μm. (c) A small bronchiole is filled with polymorphonuclear neutrophils in a sheep 72 hours after insufflation of cotton smoke and 40% TBSA burn injury. H&E, bar = 100 μm. (d) In a human autopsy, similar occlusion of a small bronchiole by polymorphonuclear neutrophils is seen, 24 days after burn injury. H&E, bar = 50 μm.

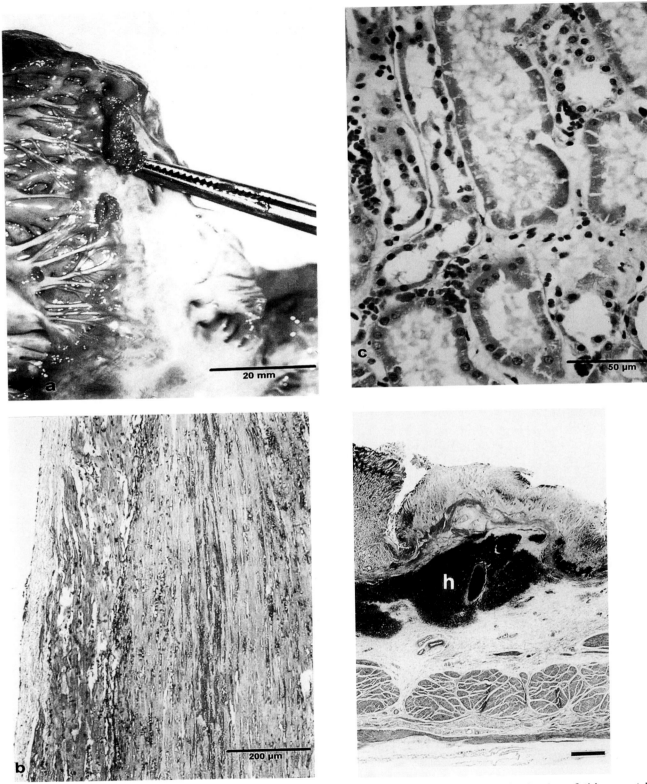

Fig. 40.3 (a) A nodular lesion of nonbacterial thrombotic endocarditis is present on the mitral valve of this recent burn patient; there is no destruction of the valve. Bar = 20 mm. (b) A small focus of necrosis of cardiac muscle cells in a left ventricular papillary muscle in a patient who had burn wound sepsis. H&E, bar = 200 μm. (c) Changes of acute tubular necrosis are seen in this micrograph of the kidney of a child who developed acute renal failure after inadequate fluid resuscitation after burn injury. The proximal tubular cells show karyolysis. H&E, bar = 50 μm. (d) A gastric lesion in a burn patient. There is focal necrosis of the mucosa and submucosal hemorrhage. H&E, bar = 200 μm.

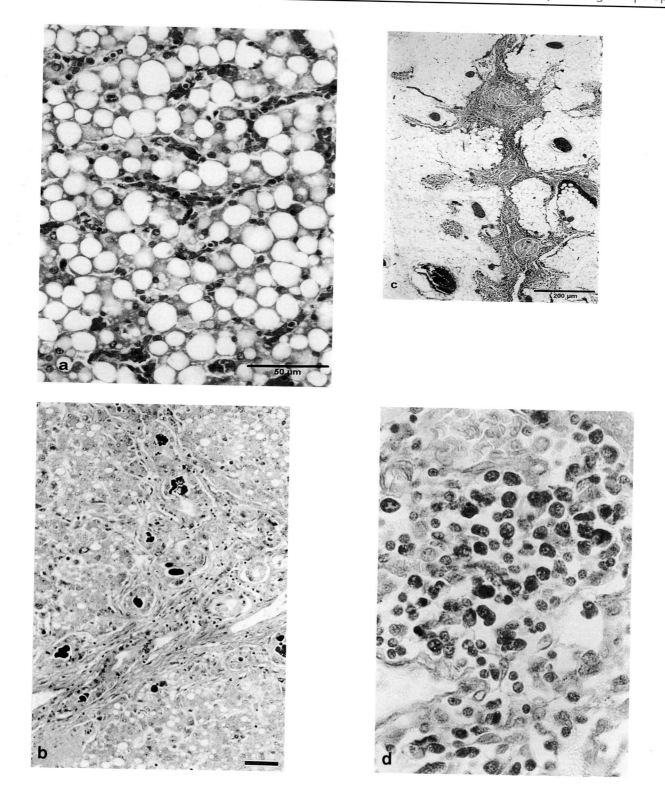

Fig. 40.4 (a) Steatosis in liver cells in a burn patient. Large round lipid droplets distend hepatocytes in this micrograph at high magnification. H&E, bar = 50 μm. (b) Intrahepatic cholestasis complicating burn injury. H&E bar = 100 μm. (c) Striking atrophy of the thymus is seen in this 13-year-old patient who died 8 days after burn injury. H&E, bar = 200 μm. (d) A lymph node at high magnification showing a medullary cord filled with pyroninophilic cells. Methyl-green-pyronine stain, bar = 50 μm.

deposition of large and small lipid droplets in hepatocytes (**Figure 40.4a**), and congestion, often with centrilobular necrosis. This pattern of central necrosis may be a consequence of reduced splanchnic blood flow in patients with sepsis. Cholestasis is commonly observed in patients with burn injury (**Figure 40.4b**) The basis for this abnormality is not clear, although multiple physiologic derangements could be expected to lead to cholestasis.[56,57]

Lymphoid System

Depletion of lymphocytes from lymphoid tissues throughout the body is a consistent feature seen at autopsy in patients with burn injury. The abnormalities were well described by Dr Linares in 1978.[58] The thymus is consistently very small, even in young children (**Figure 40.4c**). The lymph nodes often lack germinal centers, and may be strikingly depleted of lymphocytes. Sinus histiocytosis is often present, and pyroninophilic cells resembling plasma cells are often prominent, in the portions of the node normally occupied by B cells (**Figure 40.4d**). The splenic white pulp is deficient, sometimes strikingly so. The gastrointestinal lymphoid tissue of the terminal ileum is generally atrophic, in spite of its normal prominence in children, the appendix often shows a striking lack of normal lymphoid tissue in its wall. These abnormalities of lymphoid tissue correlate with the deficient immune responsiveness typical of patients with extensive burn injury. To some extent they may represent the effects of high levels of endogenous glucocorticoids in burn patients.

Musculoskeletal System

Lesions of skeletal muscle are uncommon in burn patients, but are ominous when they occur. Occasionally, direct thermal injury extends into deep muscle, and at times this injury can be so severe that adequate debridement is not practical. Electrical injury, not uncommonly, is associated with extensive necrosis of muscle. When invasive bacterial or fungal infection extends into muscle, it may not be feasible to treat adequately by excision of the infected tissue, and the infection may be resistant to antibiotic therapy and likely to disseminate. Atrophy of skeletal muscle occurs as part of the catabolic state of burn patients, and represents a challenge for those involved in rehabilitative efforts.

Central Nervous System

When the brain and spinal cord are examined carefully at autopsy, abnormalities can be found in the great majority of patients who die after burn injury. The commonest lesion is degeneration or loss of neurons in the portions of the cortex most susceptible to hypoxic and ischemic injury. These lesions can be a result of hypovolemia during resuscitation, shock developing as part of the syndrome of sepsis, or as a consequence of respiratory failure. Of course, extensive hypoxic brain injury may occur in patients who are asphyxiated during the initial burn injury. Some patients who require cardiopulmonary resuscitation at the scene of injury develop massive cerebral edema and brain death several days after the initial injury, reflecting the response to extensive hypoxic/ischemic injury in the brain. Severe hypoxic brain injury also can occur in burn patients who are deprived of oxygen during the progress of a house fire, or who are poisoned by carbon monoxide at the scene of

the burn. Another special case is the patient who has direct thermal injury to the brain. Such lesions, which occur occasionally in young children, can be detected by radiologic imaging studies, and are represented at autopsy by small foci of tissue necrosis on the cortical surface, surrounded by a hyperemic reaction.

The burn autopsy

As long as patients continue to develop complications of burn injury which are difficult to manage, and as long as the pathogenesis of these complications remains uncertain, careful postmortem examination of patients who do not survive will continue to contribute to patient care. There is a paradox here. Tissue injury occurs due to elevated temperature, a very simple physical alteration. However, there is no disease with more complex clinical and physiopathologic derangements than an extensive burn. Observations made at the time of autopsy often clarify the nature of the problems that have led to the patient's demise. Sometimes the findings lead to suggestions for changes in procedure that may lead to improved patient safety. Often a causal sequence of events can be reconstructed by including the clinical evidence and the autopsy findings. Infectious processes, for example, often can be traced from their sites of origin, in the skin or elsewhere, to the fatal conclusion. The emergence of unusually resistant bacterial strains can be traced. The autopsy should always be approached from the point of view of using both clinical and autopsy evidence to better understand the reactions of the patient to the burn injury and to the treatments provided. In other words, the burn autopsy can provide not only an appropriate morphologic analysis, but also a dynamic interpretation of the pathogenesis of the disease processes of importance in an individual patient. When approached in this way, investigation of patient deaths becomes a valuable learning experience for all those who participate in it. Not infrequently, unexpected lesions are found which were likely to have been significant in the patient's course. Of course, the circumstances of burn injury may have legal implications, and documentation of the patient's injuries and careful interpretation of the hospital course can have the beneficial effect of providing factual evidence where only supposition would be available otherwise. We advocate a policy of carrying out complete autopsies on all patients who die after burn injury, whenever possible, including microscopic study and consultation with specialists, in collaboration with the local medical examiner or coroner.

References

1. Long J. Post-mortem appearances found after burns. *Lond Med Gaz* 1840; **25**: 743–50.
2. McClure RD, Lam CR, Romence H. Tannic acid and the treatment of burns: an obsequy. *Ann Surg* 1944; **120**: 387–98.
3. Harkins HN. Experimental burns. I. The rate of fluid shift and its relation to the onset of shock in severe burns. *Arch Surg* 1935; **31**: 71–85.
4. Underhill FP, Kapsinow R, Fisk M. Studies on the mechanism of water exchange in the animal organism. *Am J Physiol* 1930; **95**: 302–14.
5. Cope O, Moore FD. The redistribution of body water and the fluid therapy of the burned patient. *Ann Surg* 1947; **126**: 1010–45.
6. Evans EI, Purnell OJ, Robinett PW, Batchelor A, Martin M. Fluid and electrolyte requirements in severe burns. *Ann Surg* 1952; **135**: 804–17.
7. Demling RH. Fluid replacement in burned patients. *Surg Clin N Am* 1987; **67**: 15–30.
8. Justis DL, Law EJ, MacMillan BG. Tibial compartment syndromes in burn patients. A report of four cases. *Arch Surg* 1976; **111**: 1004–8.

9. Rosen CL, Adler JN, Rabban JT, *et al*. Early predictors of myoglobinuria and acute renal failure following electrical injury. *J Emerg Med* 1999; **17**: 783–9.

10. Aub JC, Beecher HK, Cannon B, *et al*. *Management of the Cocoanut Grove Burns at the Massachusetts General Hospital*. Philadelphia: JB Lippincott Co., 1943.

11. Sakano T, Okerberg CV, Shippee RL, Sanchez J, Mason AD, Pruitt BA. A rabbit model of inhalation injury. *J Trauma* 1993; **34**: 411–6.

12. Clements NC, Jr, Habib MP. The early pattern of conjugated dienes in liver and lung after endotoxin exposure. *Am J Respir Crit Care Med* 1995; **151**: 780–4.

13. Linares HA. Sepsis, disseminated intravascular coagulation and multiorgan failure: catastrophic events in severe burns. In: Schlag G, Redl H, Siegel JH, Traber DL, eds., *Shock, Sepsis, and Organ Failure*. Berlin: Springer-Verlag 1991; 370–98.

14. Teplitz C. The pathology of burns and the fundamentals of burn wound sepsis. In: Atrz CL, Moncrief JA, Pruitt BA, eds., *Burns. A Team Approach*. Philadelphia: Saunders, 1979: 45–94.

15. Bone RC, Sibbald WJ, Sprung CL. The ACCP-SCCM consensus conference on sepsis and organ failure. *Chest* 1992; **101**: 1481–2.

16. Fredholm B, Hagermark O. Studies on histamine release from skin and from peritoneal mast cells of the rat induced by heat. *Acta Derm Venereol* 1970; **50**: 273–7.

17. Horakova Z, Beaven MA. Time course of histamine release and edema formation in the rat paw after thermal injury. *Eur J Pharmacol* 1974; **27**: 305–12.

18. Olsson P. Clinical views on the kinin system. *Scand J Clin Lab Invest* 1969; **24**: 123–4.

19. Effeney DJ, Blaisdell FW, McIntyre KE, Graziano CJ. The relationship between sepsis and disseminated intravascular coagulation. *J Trauma* 1978; **18**: 689–95.

20. Hawkins HK, Linares H, Desai MH, Herndon DN. Declining incidence of burn wound sepsis at autopsy. *J Burn Care Rehabil* 1999; **20**: 211.

21. Curreri PW, Kak AF, Dotin LN, Pruitt BA. Coagulation abnormalities in the thermally injured patient. In: Skinner DB, Ebert PA, eds. *Current Topics in Surgical Research*. New York: Academic Press, 1970: 401.

22. McManus WF, Eurenius K, Pruitt BA. Disseminated intravascular coagulation in burned patients. *J Trauma* 1973; **13**: 416–22.

23. Alkjaersig N, Fletcher AP, Peden JC, Monafo WW. Fibrinogen catabolism in burned patients. *J Trauma* 1980; **20**: 154–9.

24. Bick R. Disseminated intravascular coagulation and related syndromes: a clinical review. *Semin Thromb Hemost* 1988; **14**: 299–337.

25. Watanabe T, Imamura T, Nakagaki K, Tanaka K. Disseminated intravascular coagulation in autopsy cases: its incidence and clinico-pathologic significance. *Pathol Res Pract* 1979; **165**: 311–22.

26. Mileski WJ, Borgstrom D, Lightfoot E, Rothlein R, Faanes R, Lipsky P, Baxter C. Inhibition of leukocyte-endothelial adherence following thermal injury. *J Surg Res* 1992; **52**: 334–9.

27. Linares HA. Autopsy findings in burned children. In: Carvajal HF, Parks DH, eds. *Burns in Children*. Chicago: Year Book, 1988.

28. Teplitz C, Davis D, Mason AD, Moncrief JA. Pseudomonas burn wound sepsis. 1. Pathogenesis of experimental pseudomonas burn wound sepsis. *J Surg Res* 1964; **4**: 200–22.

29. Demling RH, Wong C, Jin LJ, Hechtman H, LaLonde C, West K. Early lung dysfunction after major burns: role of edema and vasoactive mediators. *J Trauma* 1985; **25**: 959–66.

30. Clowes GHA, Zuschneid W, Dragacevic S, Turner M. The nonspecific pulmonary inflammatory reactions leading to respiratory failure after shock, gangrene and sepsis. *J Trauma* 1968; **8**: 899–914.

31. Swank DW, Moore SB. Roles of the neutrophil and other mediators in adult respiratory distress syndrome. *Mayo Clin Proc* 1989; **64**: 1118–32.

32. Mulligan MS, Smith CW, Anderson DC, *et al*. Role of leukocyte adhesion molecules in complement-induced lung injury. *J Immunol* 1993; **150**: 2401–6.

33. Huie RE, Padmaja S. The reaction of NO with superoxide. *Free Rad R* 1993; **18**: 195–9.

34. Cooper JA, Solano SJ, Bizios R, Kaplan JE, Malik AB. Pulmonary neutrophil kinetics after thrombin-induced intravascular coagulation. *J Appl Physiol: Respir Environ Exercise Physiol* 1984; **57**: 826–32.

35. Lentz LA, Ziegler ST, Cox CS, Traber LD, Herndon DN, Traber DL. Cytokine response to thermal injury, shock sepsis and organ failure. The second Wiggers Bernard Conference. 1993; 245–64.

36. Fukushima M, King LS, Kang KH, Banerjee M, Newman JH. Lung mechanics and airway reactivity in sheep during development of oxygen toxicity. *J Appl Physiol* 1990; **69**: 1779–85.

37. Moran JF, Robinson LA, Lowe JE, Wolfe WG. Effects of oxygen toxicity on regional ventilation and perfusion in the primate lung. *Surgery* 1981; **89**: 575–81.

38. Barazzone C, Horowitz S, Donati YR, Rodriguez I, Piguet PF. Oxygen toxicity in mouse lung: pathways to cell death. *Am J Respir Cell Mol Biol* 1998; **19**: 573–81.

39. Linares HA, Herndon DN, Traber DL. Sequence of morphologic events in experimental smoke inhalation. *J Burn Care Rehabil* 1989; **10**: 27–37.

40. Veronesi B, Carter JD, Devlin RB, Simon SA, Oortgiesen M. Neuropeptides and capsaicin stimulate the release of inflammatory cytokines in a human bronchial epithelial cell line. *Neuropeptides* 1999; **33**: 447–56.

41. Zimmerman BJ, Anderson DC, Granger DN. Neuropeptides promote neutrophil adherence to endothelial cell monolayers. *Am J Physiol* 1992; **263**: G678–82.

42. Lentz CW, Abdi S, Traber LD. The role of sensory neuropeptides in inhalation injury. *Proc Am Burn Assoc* 1992; **10**: 27–37.

43. Kunkel SL, Standiford TJ, Kasahara K, Strieter RM. Interleukin-8 (IL-8): The major neutrophil chemotactic factor in the lung. *Exp Lung Res* 1991; **17**: 17–23.

44. Rona G, Boutet M, Huttner I, Peters H. Pathogenesis of isoproterenol-induced myocardial alterations: functional and morphological correlates. *Recent Advances in Studies of Cardiac Structure and Metabolism* 1973; **3**: 507–25.

45. Kahn DS, Rona G, Chappel CI. Isoproterenol-induced cardiac necrosis. *Ann N Y Acad Sci* 1-31-1969; **156**: 285–93.

46. Martineau PP, Hartman FW. The renal lesions in extensive cutaneous burns. *JAMA* 1947; **134**: 429–36.

47. Wolf SE, Rose JK, Desai MH, Mileski JP, Barrow RE, Herndon DN. Mortality determinants in massive pediatric burns. An analysis of 103 children with > or = 80% TBSA burns (> or = 70% full-thickness). *Ann Surg* 1997; **225**: 554–65.

48. Curling TB. On acute ulceration of duodenum in cases of burn. *Trans R Med Chir Soc Lond* 1842; **25**: 260–81.

49. Fronek K, Zweifach BW. Changes of splanchnic hemodynamics in hemorrhagic hypotension and endotoxemia. *J Surg Res* 1971; **11**: 232–7.

50. Berg RD, Garlington AW. Translocation of certain indigenous bacteria from the gastrointestinal tract to the mesenteric lymph nodes and other organs in a gnotobiotic mouse model. *Infect Immun* 1979; **23**: 403–11.

51. Deitch EA, Berg R. Bacterial translocation from the gut: a mechanism of infection. *J Burn Care Rehabil* 1987; **8**: 475–82.

52. Wells CL, Maddaus MA, Simmons RL. Proposed mechanisms for the translocation of intestinal bacteria. *Rev Infect Dis* 1988; **10**: 958–79.

53. Baker JW, Deitch EA, Berg RD, Specian RD. Hemorrhagic shock induces bacterial translocation from the gut. *J Trauma* 1988; **28**: 896–906.

54. Berg RD, Wommack E, Deitch EA. Immunosuppression and intestinal bacterial overgrowth synergistically promote bacterial translocation. *Arch Surg* 1988; **123**: 1359–64.

55. Ahren C, Haglund V. Mucosal lesions in the small intestine of the cat during low flow. *Acta Physiol Scand* 1973; **88**: 541–50.

56. Hurd T, Lysz T, Dikdan G, McGee J, Rush BF, Machiedo GW. Hepatic cellular dysfunction in sepsis: an ischemic phenomenon? *Curr Surg* 1988; **45**: 114–9.

57. Cano N, Gerolami A. Intrahepatic cholestasis during total parenteral nutrition. *Lancet* 1983; **1**: 985.

58. Linares HA, Beathard GA, Larson DL. Morphological changes of lymph nodes of children following acute thermal burns. *Burns* 1978; **4**: 165–70.

Chapter 41

Pathophysiology of the burn wound

W Geoff Williams

The burn wound is the source of virtually all ill-effects, local and systemic, seen in a burn patient. Removal of the burn wound (excision) results in a much improved patient and, when done early, yields improvements in survival as well as a decline in morbidity. It could be said that a burn wound and all of the subsequent events observed in the patient represent a continuum, without any clear points of separation. While recognizing this, the focus of this chapter concerns the events occurring in and surrounding the burned skin and subcutaneous tissues during the acute and subacute period. Only brief references are made to remote systemic effects and to healing and scarring, all of which are covered in other chapters.

Anatomy and physiology of normal skin (Figure 41.1)

The surface of the skin ranges from 0.2 to 0.3 m² in an average newborn and 1.5 to 2.0 m² in an adult. The skin consists of two layers: the epidermis, ranging from 0.05 mm thick (in areas such as the eyelids) to over 1 mm thick on the soles; and the dermis, usually at least 10 times thicker than the associated epidermis. An average total skin depth is 1–2 mm. Males generally have thicker skin than females. Skin is very thin in infants, increasing in thickness until age 30 or 40, and then progressively thinning with age. The epidermis, originating from ectoderm, is composed primarily of epithelial cells, specifically keratinocytes, as well as other cell types including: melanocytes, which function to produce pigment for the purpose of ultraviolet radiation protection; Langerhans cells which serve an immune function; and Merkel cells which serve as mechanoreceptors. The basal layer of keratinocytes is called the stratum germinativum and contains young cells, which are mitotically active, providing generation of outwardly migrating epidermal cell layers. From this layer, cells migrate outward and mature along the way to become the stratum spinosum, a layer where mitosis no longer occurs but protein synthesis is prominent. The next outward layer of maturation is the stratum granulosum where specialization into keratin production predominates. The next stage of migration is the stratum lucidum, where cells lose their nuclei and flatten, evolving into a dead layer called the stratum corneum. This layer, composed of keratin, along with cellular debris, is a compact, relatively impervious layer, which eventually desquamates. The entire process of epidermal maturation and turnover from the basal layer to desquamation takes approximately 2–4 weeks. Epidermal appendages (i.e. hair follicles, sebaceous glands, and sweat glands) are comprised of special cell types but are also lined with epidermal cells. These structures extend from the epidermis downward, residing mostly in the dermis.

The dermis, derived from mesoderm, is a relatively thick layer comprised of fibrous connective tissue. The primary cell type is the fibroblast, a spindle-shaped cell which does not frequently replicate but is very active in producing extracellular protein, primarily collagen and elastin. Collagen is secreted into the intercellular matrix, where it undergoes maturation (crosslinking and coiling) into strong fibers oriented so as to allow stretchability while providing tensile strength. Elastin is processed to form elastic fibers, imparting a degree of resting tension to the skin. Constant turnover (i.e. degradation, remodeling, and production of collagen) occurs at a low rate in unstressed skin and at higher rates when chronic mechanical stress is applied or when healing is occurring. This, along with plasticity in the arrangement of cells, grants the skin a great capacity to comply, over time, with two- and three-dimensional stresses. The ground substance of the skin is a nonfibrous bulk of glycosaminoglycans, proteoglycans, and similar macromolecules. Hyaluronic acid is an example of a well-known and important glycosaminoglycan. The ground substance provides a semifluid matrix that lubricates the cellular and fibrillar components. It is through this ground substance that inflammatory and other cells may migrate and nutrients diffuse.

The dermis is subdivided into a thin, superficial layer known as the papillary dermis and a thicker, deep portion called the reticular dermis. A large plexus of vessels beneath the dermis, known as the

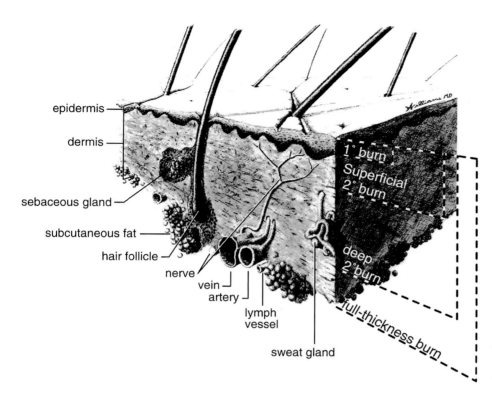

epidermis

dermis

sebaceous gland

subcutaneous fat

hair follicle

nerve

vein

artery

lymph vessel

sweat gland

1° burn
Superficial 2° burn
deep 2° burn
full-thickness burn

Fig. 41.1 Diagram of the skin including description of the various depths of burn injury. (Reproduced with permission from William G. Williams MD.)

subdermal plexus, sends vessels upward to again form a plexus between the reticular and papillary dermis. More superficial yet, exist a network of smaller vessels, the papillary plexus. Other structures found in the dermis include lymphatics and nerve fibers, which are bare-ended as well as receptor-associated. At the dermoepidermal junction exists a basement membrane, a layer composed of mucopolysaccharides but also rich in fibronectin. Cells of the basal epidermal layer are joined to the basement membrane by hemidesmosomes. The basement membrane, in turn, is anchored to the dermis with the aid of specialized fibrils.

Although the skin is often not thought of as an organ, its specific and vital functions clearly define it as such. These include:

- Protective – guards the body from harmful environmental entities, including radiation, weather, etc.
- Immunological – assists in the presentation of antigens to immune cells. Sebum possesses antibacterial properties owing to its high levels of long-chain fatty acids, particularly oleic acid.[1] Skin prevents entry of microorganisms and actually disposes of invasive bacteria through the desquamation process.
- Fluid, protein, and electrolyte homeostasis – prevents the excessive loss of these substances and participates in the control of fluid and electrolyte excretion.
- Thermoregulation – along with its appendages, prevents heat loss but also allows for rapid cooling during times of exercise through evaporation of sweat as well as vasodilation of dermal vessels.
- Neurosensory – possesses nerve endings and receptors which enable the nervous system to process and interpret information (pain, touch, hot and cold) from the environment.

- Social-interactive – when intact, aids in certain social, interpersonal reactions (sexual identity and attraction, body image, etc.).
- Metabolism – vitamin D production.

Thermal energy and its early molecular, cellular, and tissue effects

Thermal energy or heat is a manifestation of random molecular kinetic energy. This energy is easily transferred from high-energy molecules to those of lower energy during contact, via a process referred to as *conduction* of heat. An example of this process is a hot stove coil transferring heat to a pot. Conduction is greatly enhanced when the molecules that are giving up heat to a body or, alternatively, removing heat from a body are rapidly whisked away and replaced. This occurs when currents of air or liquid are involved, a process referred to as *convection*. An example would be the cooling of a hot object in a cool wind. *Radiation* describes a process whereby a molecule may give up kinetic energy through conversion to electromagnetic energy. The electromagnetic energy then travels through space to where it may be absorbed by another molecule, imparting kinetic energy (i.e. heat), again to a receiving molecule. An example would be the electric coil of a light bulb emitting infrared electromagnetic radiation, which travels through space to heat an observer's hand several inches away. All of these mechanisms affecting heat transfer may deliver heat to, or away from, living tissues. Radiation is a relatively inefficient method of heat transfer; and, for significant tissue injury to occur, it must involve either a very hot temperature source such as an electric arc flash, or a long duration of exposure such as lying under a heat lamp. Conduction is more efficient, as is the case of burning a hand with a hot iron or by immersion in scalding water. In many burn injuries, more than one of these mechanisms may be a factor as is the case when ignition of clothing is involved. Intense infrared radiation is emitted from a source of ignition (the clothing), heat is conducted from the hot fabric to the skin, and hot gases liberated from the flame heat the skin through convection.

When contemplating the effect of heat on a cell, one must consider the temperature to which the cell is heated as well as the time period for which the temperature is sustained. These two factors together determine the degree of damage incurred by a cell. Moritz and Henriquez[2] were among the first to work out the time–temperature relationship in thermal injury to skin (**Figure 41.2**). At sustained temperatures between 40 and 44°C,[2] various enzyme systems begin to malfunction, and early denaturation of protein occurs. Cellular functions are impaired, one of which is the membrane Na^+ pump; and the result is a high intracellular Na^+ concentration and concomitant swelling. As the temperature reaches 44°C and higher, damage accumulation outruns the cell's inherent repair mechanisms, assuming exposure time is long enough, and leads to eventual necrosis. Plasma membrane modifications that are significant enough to cause necrosis have been observed in cells exposed

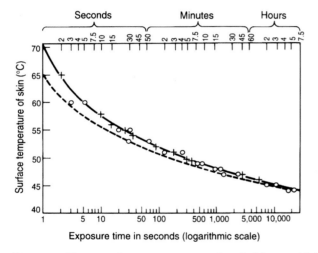

Fig. 41.2 Time–surface temperature thresholds at which cutaneous burning occurs. The broken line indicates the threshold at which irreversible epidermal injury of porcine skin is first sustained. The solid line indicates the threshold at which epidermal necrosis of porcine skin occurs. Critical exposures of porcine skin are represented by crosses. Each cross denotes the shortest exposure time at the temperature indicated which resulted in transepidermal necrosis. The results of critical experimental exposures of human skin are indicated by circles. The open circles represent the longest exposure at the temperature indicated that failed to destroy the epidermis, and the solid circles represent the shortest exposure at the temperature indicated that resulted in transepidermal necrosis. (Reproduced with permission from Moritz AR and Henriques FC. Studies of thermal injury II. The relative importance of time and surface temperature in the causation of cutaneous burns. Am J Pathol 1947; 23: 695–720.)

to 45°C for 1 hour.[3] Also occurring as part of the damage process is the production of oxygen free radicals, a class of oxygen species exhibiting an unpaired electron. These highly reactive molecules are capable of promoting further cell membrane abnormalities, leading to death. If the heat source is suddenly withdrawn, damage accumulation will continue until the cooling process brings cells back down to a tolerable temperature range. If, therefore, the cell is rapidly cooled, a significant amount of damage is obviated, which may determine whether a cell survives or dies.

As temperatures increase, protein destruction increases in severity. The early denaturation described above gives way to severe alteration of protein, a process referred to as coagulation. This phenomenon involves destruction of all levels of protein architecture. New aberrant bonds are formed, creating macromolecules not resemblant of original structures. This condition may be reached immediately in cases where skin is exposed to high temperatures or, alternatively, where lower temperature is applied for longer duration. In either case, cell necrosis is universal and complete, usually beginning at the skin surface where the heat energy was most directly received, and extending downward. This zone is called the *zone of coagulation* and is the first of three zones of burn injury (**Figure 41.3**) described by Jackson.[4] This zone comprises the initial burn eschar. Lying deep and peripheral to the zone of coagulation is a zone of lesser injury where most cells are initially viable. Here, however, circulation becomes progressively impaired leading to cessation of blood flow, hence the term *zone of stasis*. The development of ischemia within this zone is devastating to already compromised cells. Necrosis follows and in some cases may convert the entire zone of stasis to essentially dead eschar. Impairment of blood flow begins with events occurring in the microvasculature, including platelet microthrombus formation, neutrophil adherence to vessel walls, fibrin deposition endothelial swelling, and vasoconstriction.[5] Heat-injured erythrocytes lose the ability to deform,[6] impeding their passage through microvessels. Impairment of blood flow ensues within a couple of hours in more severe areas of a burn and is delayed for up to 16–24 hours[7] in less severe regions. Slowed blood flow progressing to cessation in this region proceeds for up to 48 hours postburn. This should not be confused with the coagulation of blood vessels seen immediately in severe injuries. Given optimal conditions, stasis may be reversed with cell recovery occurring within 1 week.[8] Even if recovery does occur, epithelial cell loss is high throughout this zone. During the recovery period, the tissues are very tenuous and susceptible to additional insult. Dehydration, pressure, hypovolemia, over-resuscitation, infection and even hypernatremia[9] may lead to further necrosis. The burn physician, therefore, should take extra care to address these concerns. Zawacki,[8] accordingly, has demonstrated that, through rigorous but careful wound care, progressive burn wound ischemia may be reversed and necrosis prevented. Nondesiccating dressings, topical antimicrobial agents, and adequate fluid resuscitation, along with frequent monitoring of the wound all are essential. Robson *et al.*[10] have explored extensively the pathophysiology of progressive burn wound ischemia, looking for more specific treatments. This work was preceded by the knowledge that various vasoactive inflammatory mediators are formed in burned tissues, most notably thromboxane A_2 and prostaglandin $F_{2\alpha}$.[11] In using specific thromboxane inhibitors, Robson[10] and others[12] have been able to demonstrate significant improvement in dermal perfusion as well as reduced necrosis

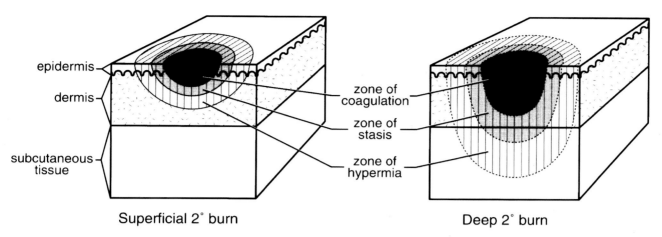

epidermis
dermis
subcutaneous tissue

zone of coagulation
zone of stasis
zone of hypermia

Superficial 2° burn

Deep 2° burn

Fig. 41.3 Diagrammatic rendition of Jackson's three zones of burn injury. Superficial 2° injury on left, deeper 2° injury on right. (In deep 2° burn note potential for conversion to full-thickness tissue loss if zone of stasis progresses to necrosis.)

within the wound. Platelet adherence and vasoconstriction, known effects of thromboxane,[13] were all ameliorated. More generalized inhibitors of prostanoids including steroidal and nonsteroidal anti-inflammatory agents,[13] have been tried, with some success, but are problematic because of the blockage of some related beneficial events. Peripheral to the zone of stasis lies the *zone of hyperemia*, characterized by minimal cellular injury but also prominent vasodilation with increased blood flow due to vasoactive mediators produced as part of the inflammatory response. Complete cellular recovery usually prevails in this zone, barring complications such as infection or trauma. The concept of the three zones of the burn wound is important because it underscores the three-dimensional aspect of this injury as well as providing a framework for understanding its progressive nature.

Burn wound edema

Burn wound edema is a concept of paramount importance owing to its deleterious effect on oxygen and nutrient delivery as well as its role in systemic hypovolemia. Edema formation is a process, which in many nonburn injuries may serve a useful purpose by delivering bacteria-fighting substances into the interstitium[14] and providing a mechanism (with the aid of lymphatics) for bacteria and debris removal. These beneficial effects are heavily outweighed by negative ones in a burn wound, where edema, most dramatic in the zone of ischemia, further compromises oxygen delivery to already ischemic tissues.[15]

Burn wound edema formation has been clearly documented[16,17] using a model wherein lymph flow from scalded dog and cat paws was measured and found to be elevated soon after burning. Furthermore, large amounts of protein in the draining lymph were noted, suggesting that the microvasculature in burned tissue had become much more permeable so as to allow leakage of plasma proteins into the interstitium. This was further documented in studies using radiolabeled albumin.[18] The causes of increased vessel permeability are poorly elucidated but are vital to understand if this process is to be modulated. One cause may be heat-mediated damage to capillary and venular endothelial cells. This results in

cell swelling, which disrupts intercellular connections and creates avenues for fluid loss (**Figure 41.4**).[19] Chemical mediators liberated within a burn wound have also received attention as causes of increased vessel permeability, primarily in postcapillary venules. These include histamine,[20] bradykinins,[21] oxygen free radicals,[22] and sensory neuropeptides.[23]

Casting doubt on vessel permeability as the sole cause of burn edema formation is evidence that larger protein molecules are retained within the vasculature to a greater degree than are smaller ones,[24] despite the knowledge that capillary pore sizes are much larger[25,26] than the largest protein molecule (**Figure 41.4**). Specifically, analysis of burn edema fluid revealed a disproportionately low ratio of large molecules, such as globulins and fibrinogens, compared to small molecules such as albumin. These facts suggest that despite large vessel pore sizes, there remains an apparent degree of selective permeability against larger molecules and a tendency to retain them within the vessel. Possible explanations lie within the interstitium. For instance, the capillary basement membrane that often appears to remain intact after heat injury may function as a back-up permeability barrier, retaining molecules, which were allowed initial passage by damaged endothelium. Further evidence for an interstitial role is the observation that edema can arise in special settings where the endothelium remains intact but the interstitium is selectively injured as occurs in oxygen free radical damage of hyaluronic acid and collagen.[27] Creating a need for further explanations of edema formation were Arturson's calculations which suggest that in order to develop the massive amounts of edema seen in burn wounds, fluid-driving pressures in the ranges of 200–300 mmHg would be needed.[28] Attention was soon turned to elevated capillary hydrostatic pressure as a possible additional cause. Indeed, Pitt[29] found that capillary pressures are nearly doubled early after burn injury. One of the first proposed mechanisms for this process was the involvement of chemical mediators such as histamine, known for its ability to dilate arterioles[30] and also known to be released from mast cells upon injury.[31] Accordingly, histamine receptor antagonists have been studied in burn edema models. Several reports of success, especially with H_2 blockers,

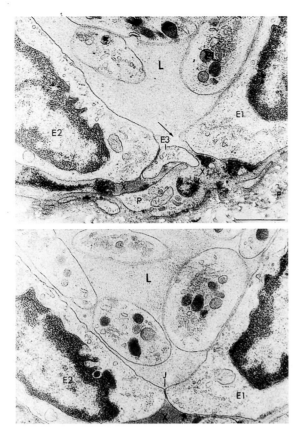

Fig. 41.4 Electron micrograph showing burn–induced endothelial cell gap. (Reproduced with permission from Cotran RS. The delayed and prolonged vascular leakage in inflammation. II. An electron microscope study of the vascular response after thermal injury. Am J Pathol 1965; 46: 589–620.)

have come forth.[32,33] Adding more knowledge regarding histamine is the recent finding that its vasodilatory effect is mediated through nitric oxide release.[34] Yet another mechanism for histamine's role in the production of burn edema may occur through its stimulation of oxygen free radical formation[35–37] (to be discussed later in this chapter).

Various prostanoids (**Figure 41.5**), found in burn fluid[38–40] may also have roles in edema production. This line of thinking is supported by several studies using inhibitors of prostaglandin production, including indomethacin,[17] nicotinic acid,[41] and ibuprofen.[42] Results show that edema formation within a burn is reduced but without a significant change in lymph protein content. This suggests that the size of capillary pores is unchanged by the drug, pointing to increased capillary pressure through vasodilation, rather than increased permeability, as the prostaglandins primary mechanism of action in causing edema.[39] Capillary filtration pressures may also be raised by impairment of venular outflow caused by erythrocyte sludging and agglutination[43] in postcapillary venules. This sludging could be a result of fluid loss from a more proximal capillary, as well as heat-damaged erythrocytes having lost some of their ability to bend and deform for passage through small vessels.[6] Adherence of platelets and neutrophils to capillary

and venular endothelial surfaces probably also contributes. Yet another cause of elevated capillary filtration pressure may be venular constriction, caused by mediators such as serotonin. Systemic conditions that may increase capillary filtration pressure include hypertension and fluid overload.

Remaining explanations for burn edema formation deal with events and conditions existing in the interstitium. Perhaps the most relevant recent discovery in this area is by Lund and co-workers,[44] and confirmed by Kramer and co-workers,[45] who found that interstitial hydrostatic pressures are dramatically reduced in the early postburn period, depending on the severity of the burn. Intravascular sources were eliminated as possible causes of this phenomenon when Lund's group further demonstrated similar dramatic tissue pressure drops in human skin, which had been excised and then burned.[46] The explanation given is that collagen fibers and their ties to cells are damaged, and this is followed by an unleashing phenomena causing a mechanical expansion of the interstitial space creating a vacuum effect. These negative pressures measured by micropipette to be as much as 120 mmHg in severe burns may explain the rapid achievement of significant edema levels seen in burn wounds by 2–3 hours. Additionally, these high negative pressures, when added to other forces present, are severe enough to account for Arturson's calculated pressure requirements for the formation of burn edema. In addition to hydrostatic pressure changes, interstitial osmotic pressure increases significantly through several mechanisms. The breakdown of collagen and other interstitial proteins into smaller more osmotically active particles,[47] the sequestration of sodium by damaged collagen,[48] and the flux of plasma proteins through enlarged vessel pores into the interstitium, may be involved. The causes of burn wound edema may be summarized as follows:

- increased capillary and venular permeability resulting from direct effects of heat on endothelium as well as from the action of mediators produced in a burn wound;
- increased hydrostatic pressure within microvessels as a result of chemical mediators causing proximal vasodilation or distal vasoconstriction, as well as impedance of flow distally by endothelial damage and related events;
- dramatic decreases in interstitial hydrostatic pressure resulting from heat-related disturbances of collagen architecture; and
- relative increases in interstitial oncotic pressure due to creation of greater osmotic loan in the interstitium.

It is important to summarize the time course of burn edema since the ability of the tissues to receive oxygen[15] and nutrients is reduced during this period, while susceptibility to infection is increased.[49] Edema formation is rapid, achieving significance within 2–3 hours. This process is generally biphasic, with an immediate, transient phase lasting 10–15 minutes followed by a sustained phase. The rapidity and extent of edema formation is dependent upon the severity of burn injury. Lymphatic resorption begins immediately (although evidence suggests that it may be impeded early on due to blockage from fibrinous debris)[50] and continues as long as the edema is present. The amount of edema in a wound is maximal by 12–24 hours after injury, and persists at a high level for 48–72 hours. Subsequently, a slow resolution of edema occurs, depending on the physiological condition of the wound and the patient.

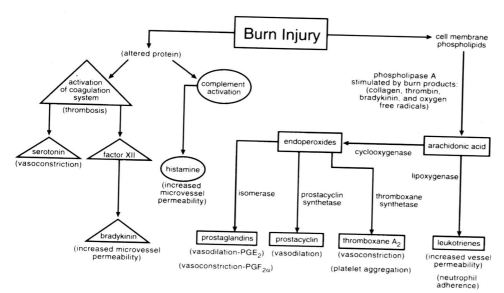

Fig. 41.5 Flow diagram showing several of the major molecular pathways activated and resultant mediators produced by thermal injury. (End responses listed in parentheses.)

Burn inflammation

Many of the above processes are either part of, or a result of, the inflammation process. For example, mediators responsible for the increased vessel permeability and hydrostatic pressure leading to burn edema, arise from inflammation within a wound. Inflammation begins via several mechanisms, most notably when cell membrane phospholipids are destroyed or altered by thermal insult. Phospholipase A, stimulated by a number of burn injury by-products,[51] then acts to convert the phospholipids to arachidonic acid which then feeds into the arachidonic acid cascade (**Figure 41.5**). The various prostanoids and leukotrienes that are produced go on to mediate vasodilation, or in some cases vasoconstriction, increased capillary permeability, neutrophil chemotaxis, and dia-pedesis, as well as chemoattraction of other inflammatory cells. Several of these phenomena, in particular neutrophil activity, are stimulated by another set of key reactions, which comprise the complement cascade (**Figure 41.5**), which is activated in heat-damaged tissues.[52] Thirdly, burn injury activates the coagulation system (**Figure 41.5**) yielding products responsible for vasocon-striction, such as bradykinin[53] and serotonin, as well as mediators of neutrophil activation and increased vessel permeability. Cellular infiltration,[54] initiated by inflammatory mediators from a burn wound, begins with the arrival of neutrophils at 4–5 days postburn, followed by macrophages. The neutrophil, long known to be an important component of burn inflammation, has continued to be the center of much interest. Recent work has shown that post-burn administration of antibodies which block neutrophil adher-ence to endothelial walls significantly reduces local edema and necrosis.[55] Further antibody studies, however, indicate that block-ing neutrophil function rather than adherence and aggregation may be more important when treating the progressive aspect of necro-sis.[56] A means by which neutrophils mediate damage is through their release of oxygen free radicals,[57] which in turn react with and damage cell components, primarily membrane lipids, to create detectable lipid peroxidation products. Superoxide dismutase, an enzyme that inactivates the hydroxyl radical, has been found to reduce lipid peroxidation in burn settings,[58] suggesting a role for oxygen radical antagonists in ameliorating damage to cell mem-branes. Oxygen free radicals not only inflict damage directly on cell membranes, but also stimulate the activity of phospholipase A, which triggers the arachidonic acid cascade and thus furthers inflammation. In addition to being produced by neutrophil-specific mechanisms, oxygen radicals are produced in microvascular endothelial cells as by-products when hypoxanthine is converted to xanthine via the enzyme xanthine oxidase. This fact was linked to burn wound pathophysiology by Ward's group of investigators[35] who discovered that oxidative damage was reduced by the drug, allopurinol, a xanthine oxidase inhibitor. They further identified histamine as a promoter of xanthine oxidase activity and, thus, established a link between histamine and oxygen free radical pro-duction.[35] This was verified by observing a decreased production of lipid peroxidation products when H_2 receptor antagonists as well as cromolyn, a mast cell stabilizer, were administered.[31] Reestablish-ment of blood flow in the zone of stasis is yet another setting wherein oxygen free radicals are produced.[27] This phenomena occurs as oxygen, a driving force in oxygen free radical produc-tion, is restored to the tissues. Part of this process involves ischemia-related alterations in purine metabolism, which results in increased xanthine oxidase activity.[59] The renewed oxygen free radical production and subsequent damage in this and other post-ischemic settings is known as ischemia-reperfusion injury and may account for some of the late necrosis occurring in a burn wound.

After the arrival of inflammatory cells and the propagation of the above events within a burn wound, inflammation becomes prominent at 7–10 days. Consequently, blood flow is maximal at this stage, creating a troublesome and hazardous setting for surgi-cal excision of the eschar. Accordingly, many surgeons plan surgery much earlier in order to avoid high operative blood loss.

Burn wound depth

First Degree Burns

First degree injury involves damage to the epidermis only and is rarely clinically significant other than being painful. The involved area is initially erythematous due to vasodilation. Eventually, desquamation ensues but is followed by complete scarless healing within 7 days.

Second Degree Burns

Second degree burns are partial-thickness by definition but are further categorized into superficial and deep. In superficial injuries, all of the epidermis is destroyed as well as varying superficial portions of the dermis. These lesions are usually very painful due to survival of nerve endings in the mid and superficial dermis. Blistering is often present. Healing will generally occur rapidly and completely through migration to the surface by epithelial cells, which survive in deeper portions of hair follicles, as well as sweat and sebaceous glands.[60] Relatively little scarring occurs in a superficial injury, owing to the contracted inflammatory phase, which is cut short by wound closure (reepithelialization) occurring within 2 weeks. It is, however, this type of injury, that may have a significant zone of stasis underlying the superficial necrosis and thus, be, predisposed to further necrosis and possible conversion to a much deeper wound. Unless complications occur, the treatment for superficial wounds consists of supportive dressing changes. Deep partial-thickness wounds are a very different story and, for all intents and purposes, are treated like full-thickness injuries. Most of the dermis is destroyed, and what few epithelial cells remain are located in the deepest recesses of the epidermal appendages. Heat kills the nerve endings, rendering a wound relatively insensate. Pressure sensation may remain, owing to survival of deeply-situated pressure receptors. Blistering is usually absent due to the thicker adherent overlying eschar, which prevents the lifting effect of edema. Due to the depth from which migrating epithelial cells must travel, reepithelialization is greatly retarded in these wounds. When healing does occur, often weeks down the road, the epidermis is very thin, tenuous and sometimes nonfunctional. Due to the prolonged period before wound closure, the inflammatory phase is protracted, allowing extensive deposition of collagen, which is manifested as copious scarring.

Third Degree Burns

Third degree, or full-thickness, burns involve necrosis of the entire thickness of skin, leaving no chance for healing except for small wounds which may heal by contraction and epithelialization from the wound edges, but will likely incur profuse scarring. Third degree wounds routinely are treated with excision and grafting.

Fourth Degree Burns

Fourth degree injury refers to situations where heat damage extends to deep structures, such as muscle, tendon, bone, etc. Treatment may require elaborate debridement and reconstruction, or even amputation.

The burn eschar

There are several issues involving a burn eschar itself, which must be addressed. Essentially the eschar represents an open wound. Nearly all of the properties of, and benefits provided by, normal skin are lost. The eschar no longer provides a barrier – mechanical, immunological, or otherwise – to infection. In fact, it provides a medium for bacterial growth.[61] This problem may be enhanced as the eschar takes up water from surrounding tissues or from topically applied drug vehicles. The ability of skin to prevent loss of fluids, electrolytes, and plasma components likewise is absent in the eschar due to its high degree of permeability.[62] It has been shown that ongoing protein loss occurs at a high rate through the eschar even after capillary permeability decreases.[63] The loss of complement components[64] and immunoglobulins[65] aggravates burn-induced immune suppression, while loss of protein, in general, impairs nitrogen balance and wound healing. The eschar may at times play a role in impairment of hemostasis as it promotes consumption of clotting and related factors, i.e. platelets, fibrinogen, etc.[66] This process may, in turn, give rise to some of the burn wound mediators discussed earlier, namely bradykinins and serotonin (**Figure 41.5**). The thermoregulatory function provided by normal skin is absent in eschar. Although the tissue within the eschar is metabolically dead, it contains heat-derived products and toxins, which may diffuse into the circulation causing distant organ dysfunction and other problems. Excision of the eschar and grafting of autogenous or nonautogenous skin greatly ameliorates many of these problems. Subeschar tissue fluid has in fact been shown to invoke a systemic inflammatory response as well as multisystem organ dysfunction when administered to nonburned animals.[67] Excision of the eschar may additionally contribute to regional morbidity (i.e. cause compression syndromes), requiring escharotomy. Even breathing may be mechanically impaired by a tight thoracic eschar.

The blister

The blister arises usually in the setting of superficial partial-thickness injury; an exception is in infants and elderly people because of their thinner skin. Here, a relatively deep second degree burn may have a thin eschar, which may allow for blister accumulation. A blister is formed by leakage of fluid from heat-injured vessels deep to the zone of coagulation. The fluid enters and collects, usually in the area of the damaged dermoepidermal junction, lifting the epidermis away from the underlying dermis. Release of plasma proteins and skin degradation products into the blister osmotically draws yet more fluid, causing enlargement of the blister over time. Many of the mediators located in the blister are harmful, while only a few are beneficial.[68] Furthermore, wound healing growth factors exist in lower than normal quantities.[68] Therefore, there appears to be evidence supporting the concept that blisters should generally be debrided and the bed carefully dressed, although this topic is often debated. Like the eschar, the blister does not generally provide the function of intact skin and therefore should not be considered a closed wound.

Systemic effects

As alluded to previously, many of the systemic phenomena observed in burn patients are direct results of either toxins produced by heat damage, or of mediators produced by inflammation and related processes within the burn wound. These systemic effects, summarized in (**Figure 41.6**), will be dealt with in detail in other chapters.

Conclusion

The burn wound is a serious injury, progressive in nature, causing a myriad of effects far beyond its bounds. Much knowledge has

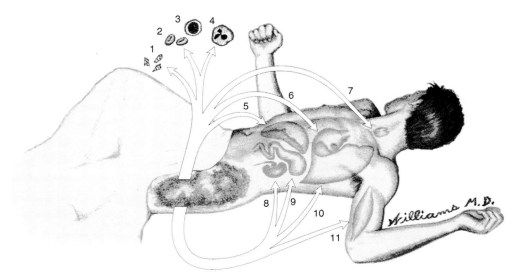

Fig. 41.6 Summarization of some of the major systemic effects of the burn wound. (1) platelets and other clotting factors are consumed in the burned tissue leading to systemic clotting derangements; (2) red cells are heat damaged leading to their early destruction as well as decreased flexibility; (3) suppression of cellular immunity by various burn-related by-products and mediators; (4) impairment of neutrophil function by burn mediators; (5) peroxidation of hepatocytes; (6) myocardial depression mediated by unknown factors produced in the burn wound; (7) multiple endocrine aberrations including hypermetabolism, produced in part by inflammatory mediators from the burn wound; (8) renal tubule damage from various burn wound products; (9) decreased blood flow to gut caused by burn mediators; (10) pulmonary hypertension and edema caused by burn inflammatory products; (11) fat and skeletal muscle catabolism caused by events initiated in the burn wound. (Reproduced with permission from William G. Williams MD.)

been gleaned regarding its pathophysiology, yet more remains to be uncovered. As more information comes forth, much morbidity and mortality surrounding this dreadful injury can be circumvented.

References

1. Ricketts CR, Squire JR, Topley E. Human skin lipids with particular reference to the self-sterilizing power of the skin. *Clin Sci Mol Med* 1951; **10**: 89–111.
2. Moritz AR, Henriquez FC. Studies of thermal injury II. The relative importance of time and surface temperature in the causation of cutaneous burns. *Am J Pathol* 1947; **23**: 695–720.
3. Bass H, Moore JL, Conkley WT. Lethality in mammalian cells due to hyperthermia under oxic and hypoxic conditions. *Int J Radiat Biol* 1978; **33**: 57–67.
4. Jackson DM. The diagnosis of the depth of burning. *Br J Surg* 1953; **40**: 588–96.
5. Boykin JV, Eriksson E, Pittman RN. Microcirculation of scald burn: an *in vivo* experimental study of the hairless mouse ear. *Burns* 1980; **7**: 335–8.
6. Johnson GS, Lineberger T, Hothem AL, Adams K, Hinson T, Winkenwerder W. Erythrocyte flexibility in the burned patient. *Burns* 1979; **6**: 91–5.
7. Zawacki BE. The local effects of burn injury. In: Boswick JA, ed. *The Art and Science of Burn Care*. Rockville, MD: Aspen, 1987: 29.
8. Zawacki BE. Reversal of capillary stasis and prevention of necrosis in burns. *Ann Surg* 1974; **180**: 98–102.
9. Harada T, Izaki S, Tsutsumi H, Kobayashi M, Kitamura K. Apoptosis of hair follicle cells in the second-degree burn wound under hypernatremic conditions. *Burns* 1998; **24**: 464–9.
10. Robson MC, Del Becarro EJ, Heggers JP, *et al*. Increasing dermal perfusion after burning by decreasing thromboxane production. *J Trauma* 1980; **20**: 722–5.
11. Johnson CE, Granström E, Hamburg M. Prostaglandins and thromboxane in burn injury in man. *Scand J Plast Reconstr Surg* 1979; **13**: 45.
12. Del Becarro EJ, Robson MC, Heggers JP, *et al*. The use of specific thromboxane inhibitors to preserve the dermal microcirculation after burning *Surgery* 1980; **87**: 137–41.
13. Robson MC, Del Becarro EJ, Heggers JP. The effect of prostaglandins on the dermal microcirculation after burning and the inhibition of the effect by specific pharmacological agents. *Plast Reconstr Surg* 1979; **63**: 781–7.
14. Warden G. Immunological response to burn injury. In: Boswick JA, ed. *The Art and Science of Burn Care*. Rockville, MD: Aspen, 1987: 113.
15. Remensnyder JP. Topography of tissue oxygen tension changes in acute burn edema. *Arch Surg* 1972; **105**: 477–82.
16. Arturson G. The change in transcapillary leakage during healing of experimental burns. *Acta Chir Scand* 1967; **133**: 609–14.
17. Arturson G. Microvascular permeability to macromolecules in thermal injury. *Acta Physiol Scand Suppl* 1979; 111–22.
18. Brouhard BH, Carvajal HF, Linares HA. Burn edema and protein leakage in the rat. I. Relationship of time to injury. *Microvasc Res* 1978; **15**: 221–8.
19. Cotran RS. The delayed and prolonged vascular leakage in inflammation II. An electron microscope study of the vascular response after thermal injury. *Am J Pathol* 1965; **46**: 589–620.
20. Robson MC, Smith DJ, Heggers JP. Innovations in burn wound management. In: Habal MB, ed. *Advances in Plastic and Reconstructive Surgery*, Vol. 4 Chicago, IL: Year Book, 1987: 149.
21. Demling RH. Pathophysiology of burn injury. In: Richardson JD, ed. *Trauma, Clinical Care and Pathophysiology*. Chicago, IL: Yearbook, 1987: 128.
22. Hatherill JR, Till GO, Bruner LH, Ward PA. Thermal injury, intravascular hemolysis and toxic oxygen products. *J Clin Invest* 1986; **78**: 629–36.
23. Siney L, Brian SD. Involvement of sensory neuropeptides in the development of plasma extravasation in rat dorsal skin following thermal injury. *Br J Pharmacol* 1996; **117**: 1065–70.
24. Davies JWL. Capillary permeability, oedema and lymph PG1. In: *Physiological Responses to Burn Injury*. London: Academic Press, 1982: 61.
25. Demling RH, Kramer GC, Gunther R, *et al*. Effect of nonprotein colloid on postburn edema formation in soft tissues and lung. *Surgery* 1984; **95**: 593–602.
26. Honeycutt D, Traber L, Toole D, Herndon DN, Traber DL. Colloid resuscitation of ovine burn shock. *Circ Shock* 1990; **31**: 72.
27. Kaufman T, Neuman RA, Weinberg A. Is postburn dermal ischemia enhanced by oxygen free radicals? *Burns* 1989; **15**: 291–4.
28. Arturson G, Mellander S. Acute changes in capillary filtration and diffusion in experimental burn injury. *Acta Physiol Scand* 1964; **62**: 457–63.

29. Pitt RM, Parker JC, Jurkovich GJ, Taylor AE, Curreri PW. Analysis of altered capillary pressure and permeability after thermal injury. *J Surg Res* 1987; **42**: 693–702.

30. Douglas WW. Histamine and 5-hydroxytryptamine (serotonin) and their antagonists. In: Gilman AG, Goodman LS, Rall TW, Murad F, eds. *The Pharmacological Basis of Therapeutics*. New York, NY: Macmillan, 1985: 605.

31. Friedl HP, Till GO, Trentz O, Ward PA. Roles of histamine, complement and xanthine oxidase in thermal injury of the skin. *Am J Pathol* 1989; **135**: 203–17.

32. Brimblecombe RW, Farrington HW. Histamine H_2 receptor antagonists and thermal injury in rats. *Burns* 1976; **3**: 8–13.

33. Till GO, Guilds LS, Mahrougui M, Friedl HP, Trentz O, Ward PA. Role of xanthine oxidase in thermal injury of skin. *Am J Pathol* 1989; **135**: 195–202.

34. Leurs R, Brozius MM, Jansen W, Bast A, Timmerman H. Histamine H-1 receptor-mediated cyclic GMP production in guinea pig lung tissue is an L-arginine-dependent process. *Biochem Pharmacol* 1991; **42**: 271–7.

35. Friedl HP, Till GO, Ryan VS, Ward PA. Mediator-induced activation of xanthine oxidase in endothelial cells. *FASEB J* 1989; **3**: 2512–8.

36. Granger DN, McCord JM, Parks DA, Hollwarth ME. Xanthine oxidase inhibitors attenuate ischemia-induced vascular permeability changes in the cat intestine. *Gastroenterology* 1986; **90**: 80–4.

37. Granger D, Rutili G, McCord J. Superoxide radicals in feline intestinal ischemia. *Gastroenterology* 1981; **81**: 22–9.

38. Änggard E, Arturson G, Jonsson CE. Efflux of prostaglandins in Lymph from scalded tissues. *Acta Physiol Scand* 1970; **80**: 46A–7A.

39. Arturson G, Hamberg M, Jonsson CE. Prostaglandins in human burn blister fluid. *Acta Physiol Scand* 1973; **87**: 270–6.

40. Heggers JP, Loy GL, Robson MC, Del Beccaro EJ. Histological demonstration of prostaglandins and thromboxanes in burned tissue. *J Surg Res* 1980; **28**: 110–7.

41. Hilton JG, Wells CH. Nicotinic acid reduction of plasma volume loss after thermal trauma. *Science* 1976; **191**: 861–2.

42. Demling RH, LaLonde C. Topical ibuprofen decreases early postburn edema. *Surgery* 1987; **102**: 857–61.

43. Robb HJ. Dynamics of the microcirculation during a burn. *Arch Surg* 1967; **94**: 776–80.

44. Lund T, Wiig H, Reed RK. Acute postburn edema: role of strongly negative interstitial fluid pressure. *Am J Physiol* 1988; **255**: H1069–74.

45. Kinsky MP, Guha SC, Button BM, Kramer GC. *J Burn Care Rehabil* 1998; **19**: 1–9.

46. Lund T. The 1999 Everett Idris Evans memorial Lecture; Edema Generation Following Thermal Injury: An Update. *J Burn Care Rehabil* 1999; **20**: 445–52.

47. Lund T, Onarheim H, Wiig H, Reed RH. Mechanisms behind increased dermal inhibition pressure in acute burn edema. *Am J Physiol* 1989; **256**: H940–8.

48. Leape L. Tissue changes in burned and unburned rhesus monkeys. *J Trauma* 1970; **10**: 488–92.

49. Knighton D, Halliday B, Hunt TK. Oxygen as an antibiotic. *Arch Surg* 1984; **119**: 199–204.

50. Glenn WWL, Gilbert HH, Drinker CK. The flow of lymph from burned tissue with particular reference to the effects of fibrin formation upon lymph drainage and composition. *Surgery* 1942; **12**: 685–95.

51. Arturson G. The pathophysiology of severe thermal injury. *J Burn Care Rehabil* 1985; **6**: 129–46.

52. Fjellstrom KE, Arturson G. Changes in the human complement system following burn trauma. *Acta Pathol Microbiol Scand* 1963; **59**: 257–70.

53. Nwariaku FE, Sikes PJ, Lighfoot E, Mileski WJ, Baxter C. Effect of Bradykinin antagonist on the local W.J. inflammatory response following thermal injury. *Burns* 1996; **22(4)**: 324–27.

54. Shilling JA. Wound Healing. *Physiol Rev* 1968; **48**: 374–423.

55. Bucky LP, Vedder NB, Hong CHZ, May JW, Ehrlich HP. A monoclonal antibody which blocks neutrophil adhesion prevents second degree burn becoming third degree burns. *Proc Am Burn Assn* 1991; **23**: 133.

56. Gasser H, Paul E, Redl H, Schlag G, Traber D, Herndon DN. Loss of plasma antioxidants after burn injury. *Circ Shock* 1991; **34**: 13.

57. Nwariaku FE, Sikes PJ, Lightfoot E, Mileski WJ. Inhibition of selectin- and integrin-mediated inflammatory response after burn injury. *J Surg Res* 1996; **63**: 355–8.

58. Thomson PD, Till GO, Woolliscroft JO, Smith DJ, Prasad JK. Superoxide dismutase prevents lipid peroxidation in burned patients. *Burns* 1990; **16**: 406–8.

59. Fantone JC, Ward PA. Oxygen-derived Radicals and Their Metabolites: Relationship to Tissue Injury. Kalamazoo, MI: Upjohn 1985: 32.

60. Zawacki BE. The natural history of reversible burn injury. *Surg Gynecol Obstet* 1974; **139**: 867–72.

61. Pruitt BA, Moncrief JA. Current trends in burn research. *J Surg Res* 1967; **7**: 280–93.

62. Jelenko C III, Ginsburg JM. Water holding lipid and water transmission through homeothermic and poikilothermic skins. *Proc Soc Exp Biol Med* 1971; **139**: 1059–62.

63. Waymau K. Protein loss across burn wounds. *J Trauma* 1987; **27**: 136–40.

64. Heggers JP, Ko F, Robson MC, Heggers R, Craft KE. Evaluation of burn blister fluid. *Plast Reconstr Surg* 1980; **65**: 798–804.

65. Heggers JP, Heggers R, Robson MC. The immunological deficit encountered in thermal injury. *J Am Med Technol* 1982; **44**: 99–102.

66. Simon TL, Curreri PW, Harker LA. Kinetic characterization of hemostasis in thermal injury. *J Lab Clin Med* 1977; **89**: 702–11.

67. Jing Chen, Yi-Ping Zhou, Xin-Zhou Rong. An experimental study on systemic Inflammatory response syndrome induced by subeschar tissue fluid. *Burns* 2000; **26**: 149–55.

68. Wilson Y, Goberdhan N, Dawson RA, *et al.* Investigation of the presence and role of calmodulin and other mitogens in human burn blister fluid. *J Burn Care Rehabil* 1994; **July/Aug**: 303–14.

Chapter 42

Wound healing
David G Greenhalgh

Introduction

The ultimate goal of all burn team members is to heal the patient's wounds with the least scarring and to maximize the functional and cosmetic outcome. The management of the burn wound depends on the depth and extent of the injury. Those wounds that are superficial need to reepithelialize. Smaller, but deep, wounds heal by scar formation and contraction. These processes are beneficial at times, but detrimental at other times. Understanding how these wounds heal will help with choosing an appropriate treatment. Larger wounds require grafting. By understanding how a graft heals, one can optimize the outcome. It is clear that all patients with burns greater than 20–25% total body surface area (TBSA) develop systemic changes that influence their survival. The burn wound is a major source of inflammatory

mediators that lead to hypermetabolism, muscle wasting and, potentially, dysfunction of multiple organ systems. The best way to treat these systemic problems is to eliminate the source of the inflammatory mediators by expeditiously removing the source of the mediators and covering the wound. The strategies for covering these massive wounds will be discussed in the chapter. The factors that influence wound healing will also be described. Finally, much of our time is devoted to the management of scars. While relatively little is known about reducing scar formation, more options are available to us compared to the past. Hopefully, we will gain further insights into the control of scar formation in the future.

There are several basic principals the burn team must remember when treating a wound.

1. The goal is to maximize the functional and cosmetic outcome of the burn.
2. Optimizing initial wound care will minimize the need for scar management and reconstructive surgery. (Do it right from the start.)
3. If a burn heals within 2 weeks, then scarring is minimal. If the wound has not healed within 2 weeks, then grafting is probably indicated.
4. Topical agents reduce infection risks but do not eliminate bacteria. Target the topical agent for the wound type and the likely bacterial flora.
5. Make treatment simple (especially in the outpatient setting).

  A. Sterile techniques are unnecessary. Use clean techniques.
  B. The patient may get into the shower or bath.
  C. Caregivers should wash their hands and use clean barriers (gowns, gloves) in the inpatient setting.
  D. At home, barrier techniques are probably not indicated.
  E. Try to minimize pain.

The goal of this chapter will be to describe the types of wound healing in order to promote better principals of wound management that will lead to the best possible outcome for burn patients.

Types of burns

In order to optimally treat burn wounds, one must first know the types of burn injuries that exist. The type of healing that is involved in each type of wound changes, depending on wound depth.

Skin can be simply considered to consist of two major components: the epidermis and dermis (**Figure 42.1**). The major function

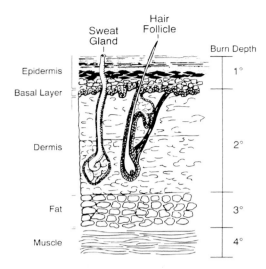

Fig. 42.1 A schematic drawing that demonstrates the major layers of the skin. The type of healing that occurs after a burn depends on which layers of the skin are damaged. A first degree burn does not extend deeper than the basal layer of the epidermis. A second degree burn involves the dermis and a third degree burn extends beneath the dermis and into the fat. A fourth degree burn involves tissue beneath the fat.

of the epidermis is to keep invading organisms 'out' and keep water 'in'. At the base of the epidermis are the basal cells, which are the only keratinocytes of the epidermis that can proliferate and migrate. These cells are attached to a basement membrane that separates the epidermis from the dermis. The basal cells differentiate as they leave the basement membrane and eventually die and slough in the more superficial layers of the epithelium. The detachment, migration away from the basement membrane, differentiation, and sloughing is the normal life cycle of the keratinocytes. The dermis adds the strength to the skin, since it is made of collagen and other extracellular matrix (ECM) proteins. The dermis also contains a vascular and neural plexus. The vascular plexus is vital for temperature control, and the neural plexus gives the skin the ability to sense the environment. The neural network also produces the sharp pain that results from superficial burns. The dermis also contains the skin adnexa (hair follicles, oil glands, sweat glands) which are lined by epithelial cells. These adnexa are essential for the healing of superficial burns.

The depth of burn has traditionally been divided into first, second, third, and fourth degree (**Figure 42.1**). A first degree burn does not extend below the basal cell layer of the epidermis. These burns are dry, red, and painful. The second degree burn extends into the dermis and is characterized by being moist, painful and red with blanching. The wound is moist because of the loss of the barrier function of the epidermis. The pain and blanching redness exist because the dermal nerves and blood supply persist. A third degree burn extends completely through the dermis and into the subdermal fat. These burns are dry, less painful, and do not blanch because the dermal nerves and blood supply are destroyed. These burns can be almost any color (white, tan, black, brown, and red) and tend to be leathery as a result of the 'eschar' produced from the

coagulated proteins that result from the burn. The eschar should not be confused with the 'scab' that develops over time on a second degree burn. This scab is the result of fibrin and cellular deposition from the exuding wound fluid. Finally, a fourth degree burn is one that extends to fascia, bone, tendon, muscle, or other tissue beneath the subcutaneous fat.

Types of tissue repair

Reepithelialization

Since first and second degree burns leave behind remnants of epithelium, the major form of healing for these types of wounds is reepithelialization. For first degree burns, such as sunburns, the basal cell layer of keratinocytes persists. The basal cell layer simply differentiates to recreate the multiple layers of the epidermis. This process is usually complete within 3–4 days. Little treatment is needed to manage these wounds other than possibly a moisturizer.

Once the burn extends into the dermis (second degree), then the entire epidermis has to be reconstructed from the skin adnexa. Fortunately, the skin adnexa (hair follicles, sweat glands, oil glands, and others) are lined with epithelial cells. There are several stimuli for the basal keratinocytes at the wound edge and the adnexal epithelial cells to migrate on to the surface of the wound.[1] First, the loss of basal cell–cell contact leads to signals for the keratinocytes to migrate. In addition, growth factors that target epithelial cell growth and migration are released from the wound to stimulate migration. Growth factors that specifically target epithelial cells include epidermal growth factor (EGF), transforming growth factor-α (TGF-α), and keratinocyte growth factors-1 and -2 (KGF-1 and KGF-2).[2-6] Other growth factors stimulate keratinocyte growth and migration either directly or indirectly in addition to having other wound healing activities (TGF-β and interleukin-1 [IL-1]).[6,7] Finally, if keratinocytes come in contact with specific proteins, then they are stimulated to migrate. For instance, basal cells are content to stay put if they are in contact with proteins that are in the basement membrane (such as laminin or collagen type IV). When they come in contact with proteins found in the wound, such as fibrin, fibronectin, or collagen type 1, then they are stimulated to migrate.[8] All of these stimuli are produced in a second degree burn or split-thickness skin graft (STSG) donor site.

The keratinocytes then migrate from the original wound edge and from the skin adnexa, and travel over the viable wound bed (**Figure 42.2**). If there is a moist and viable surface, then the cells can migrate most rapidly. As the epithelial cells march up from the adnexa, whitish dots (epithelial buds) appear on the reddish background of the wound (**Figure 42.3**). When the cells regain contact with other migrating keratinocytes (cover the wound), they differentiate and form all of the layers of the epidermis. The wounds with the highest concentration of skin adnexa heal the fastest. This is why the scalp heals within 4–5 days, while areas lacking hair, such as the lower leg in older people, tend to take a longer time to reepithelialize. If the wound dries and forms a 'scab' (composed of fibrin, dead neutrophils, and other debris), then the keratinocytes have to 'cut' their way along the viable surface by releasing proteases and other enzymes. If a thick scab does develop, then light debridement will assist with healing. One must be careful, however, to avoid pulling off the new epithelium. It has been shown

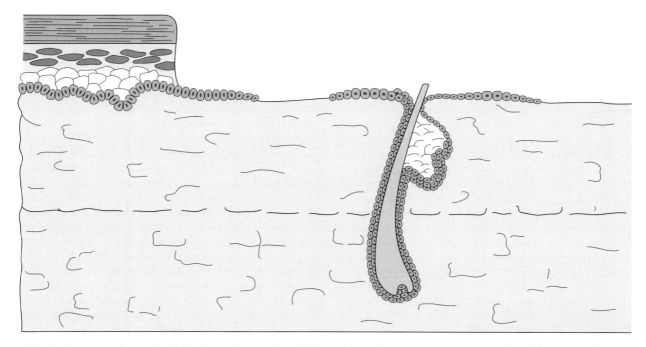

Fig. 42.2 A diagram of reepithelialization. Basal cells of the epidermal edge migrate across the viable wound bed. In addition, skin adnexa, such as hair follicles also contain epithelial cells that migrate onto the surface and participate in the resurfacing. If the surface is moist and free of fibrinous exudate, then reepithelialization proceeds the fastest.

that by maintaining the moist environment, reepithelialization occurs more rapidly than if the wound is allowed to dry. Many ointments and dressings have been designed to assist with optimizing healing of these superficial wounds. For instance, an ointment such as bacitracin prevents drying while at the same time decreasing Gram-positive organisms. Dressings have also been designed to maintain the moist environment. These 'biologic dressings' are designed to cover the wound and maintain the optimal environment until reepithelialization is completed. Transparent polyurethane dressings were designed with this in mind. Other dressings are designed to stick to the wound and allow for healing. Biobrane™, which has a layer of collagen type I sticks to the wound until reepithelialization is complete. Trancyte™ uses

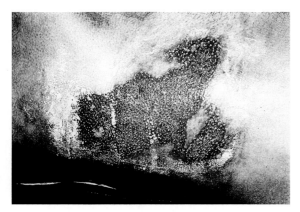

Fig. 42.3 Epithelial buds are the white dots in the middle of the red wound in this burn that is reepithelializing.

the same principal but has fibroblasts in the dressings that release a variety of growth factors. Some of the older biologic dressings are pigskin and human allograft. All of these biologic dressings have many advantages as well as disadvantages. These agents stick to the wound and allow for protected reepithelialization under the dressing. The biologic dressings that contain live cells also have the advantage of releasing growth factors and other agents that may accelerate healing. One problem is cost; some of the viable biologics can cost thousands of dollars just to cover a relatively small area. These costs must be balanced with the advantages of each dressing. A jar of bacitracin may reduce costs by a factor approaching hundreds to a thousand times.

Another approach to accelerating healing of superficial burn wounds and STSG donor sites has been to apply exogenous growth factors. At one time, there was a great deal of interest in applying these cytokines to a wound to accelerate reepithelialization. Many animal studies have demonstrated accelerated healing of superficial wounds.[2-6] Several controlled, randomized, prospective and double-blinded clinical trials have been performed using different growth factors.[9-11] Most of the trials were performed using small donor sites on opposite sides of the body and revealed that a statistically significant improvement in tissue repair was found. Unfortunately, what proved to be statistically significant was not clinically relevant. Wounds would heal a day or two faster compared to the control. Since the healing of small donor sites does not impact length of stay, the benefit did not justify the cost. It is difficult to accelerate greatly the healing of small donor sites. The healing of donor sites in massive burns, however, often appears to be slower than that of small wounds. Herndon's group has treated children with relatively large burns (>40%) with systemic human recombinant growth hormone and found that the time to reharvest donor sites was significantly shortened.[12] With the requirement for multiple reharvests, the length of stay per percent burn was also significantly shortened. The decrease in length of stay more than counteracts the increased cost of the recombinant protein.

Scar Formation

A second form of healing involves recreating the 'tough' component of the tissue. For skin, the body attempts to form a 'new dermis'. During this process, new connective tissue consisting of the extracellular matrix (ECM), which gives tissue its strength, is created. In simpler forms of life, and in the fetus, skin and other tissues can be regenerated. In mammals (at least after birth), wounds are closed by creating a less than perfect scar. No one knows why scars form instead of regeneration, but one can guess that in our contaminated world, more expeditious closure at the expense of regeneration may have been an evolutionary compromise for controlling bacterial invasion. Scar formation is both essential (to prevent dehiscence) and a hindrance, in that excessive fibrosis is an ultimate complication of many disease processes (contractures, hypertrophic scars, keloids, pulmonary fibrosis, cirrhosis, arthritis, etc.). Investigators are trying to understand the controls of these processes. Much more is known about the factors that turn on the process than is known about what turns off the process. These factors will be discussed in this section.

Scar formation is usually divided into three phases. The three phases were originally determined by measuring the tensile strength of incisions over time (**Figure 42.4**). During the first 4–5 days after closing an incision, little change in wound strength is noted. During this time, inflammatory cells invade the incision, so it is called the *inflammatory* or *lag phase*. After this period, there is a rapid increase in collagen content in the incision that is associated with a rapid increase in tensile strength. This phase is called the *proliferative* or *collagen phase*. Two key events occur during this phase, the deposition of the ECM and the ingrowth of new vessels. Finally, there is a prolonged phase where the incision

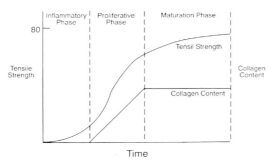

Fig. 42.4 The phases of scar formation are based on the changes of tensile strength and collagen deposition in an incision. For the first 4–5 days after closing an incision, there is little increase in strength. During this inflammatory phase, inflammatory cells prepare the wound for the arrival of fibroblasts. Once the fibroblasts arrive in the proliferative phase, there is a rapid increase in tensile strength as collagen content increases. After 2–3 weeks, there is no more increase in collagen content but the incision strength continues to increase in the maturation phase.

continues to gain strength (up to approximately 80% of the original skin) but there is no increase in collagen content. Also during this *maturation phase*, the wound tends to become less cellular and vascular until a quiescent, white scar is formed.

The inflammatory phase prepares the wound for the subsequent repair process. The main role of this phase is to eliminate invading organisms and remove foreign tissue. The inflammatory phase is divided into vascular and cellular components. All of the components of healing are controlled by the release of local and systemic mediators. In the *vascular response*, there is a release of local catecholamines that induce vasoconstriction in an attempt to control bleeding. In addition, when platelets and coagulation factors are exposed to the proteins outside the vessels (collagen type I, thrombin, tissue factor, Hageman factor), hemostasis is initiated. After bleeding is controlled, different mediators (histamine, serotonin, kinins, nitric oxide, prostaglandins and leukotrienes) induce vasodilation and increased permeability. The increase in permeability allows for the leakage of serum proteins and water into the local wound area. When the wound is large enough, such as after a burn that is greater than 20% TBSA, then the mediators 'spill over' into the systemic circulation and cause the total body edema that we are familiar with in major burns.

In the *cellular response*, multiple signals are released to attract inflammatory cells to the wound. Platelets contain multiple growth factors in their alpha granules that attract the cells. Other factors such as complement (C3a and C5a) and clotting factors (thrombin and fibrin) are chemotactic for inflammatory cells. The first cells to arrive in the wound are neutrophils. These cells are mainly responsible for killing invading organisms. They release many mediators, such as proteases and oxygen radicals, which can be destructive to tissues if produced in excessive amounts. Several investigators also implicate an excessive neutrophil response that is responsible for the 'systemic inflammatory response syndrome' (SIRS). Studies performed in the 1970s, however, suggest that neutrophils are not essential for the healing process.[13]

Macrophages (and monocytes) have been found to be the major regulators of the healing process.[14-17] When these cells were eliminated from a wound, very little tissue repair took place. Macrophages release multiple cytokines and growth factors that stimulate the migration and proliferation of fibroblasts, keratinocytes, endothelial cells, and other cells involved in tissue repair. The list of growth factors released by these cells has become quite large and is best reviewed in other publications.[17] Macrophages are found in the wound in relatively high numbers after 3–4 days. In the incision, fibroblasts follow very soon after the arrival of macrophages. The role of lymphocytes in the healing process is less clear. Lymphocytes release multiple cytokines that influence macrophages.[18,19] Tissue repair is not greatly affected, however, in mice with severe-combined immunodeficiency (lacking lymphocytes).[20] As discussed below, lymphocytes do release interferons (IFNs), which appear to have antifibrotic tendencies.

Once fibroblasts arrive in the wound, the proliferative phase begins. Two events occur in the proliferative phase: the *synthesis of the extracellular matrix* (ECM: collagens and other matrices) and *re-creation of a blood supply* (angiogenesis, vasculogenesis, and arteriogenesis). Fibroblasts are the cells that produce the majority of the ECM. Since collagen is the major strength of tissues, its biosynthesis has been well studied and will only be briefly mentioned here. Excellent reviews describe the details of collagen production.[21,22] There are at least 19 types of collagen. All collagens can be divided into fibril-forming and nonfibrillar collagens. All collagens have at least some component of amino acid triplet repeats of 'glycine-X-Y', with the 'X' often being proline and the 'Y' frequently being hydroxyproline or hydroxylysine. The peptide chains then form into a triple helix that give collagen its strength. One of the most important biochemical reactions in the biosynthesis of collagen is the hydroxylation of proline or lysine. The enzyme 'protocollagen hydroxylase' required for this reaction requires oxygen, iron (Fe^{++}), α-ketoglutarate and, most importantly, vitamin C. In vitamin C deficiency (scurvy), the hydroxylation does not occur and the triple helix fails to form. The malformed collagen collects within the fibroblasts and healing is markedly impaired. There are many other steps in the biosynthesis of collagen where abnormalities can occur. Another key stage is during the creation of intercollagenous bonds that help bind fibrils of collagen together. Lysyl oxidase, the enzyme required for this process can be blocked by such agents as penicillamine and β-aminopropionitrile (BAPN). The role of these agents and the other steps in collagen synthesis are reviewed elsewhere.[23–25] The deposition of the other ECM components also is essential for normal healing. The role of these other proteins includes glycosaminoglycans (GAGs) and elastins. Their synthesis will not be covered here.

In order to create the ECM, fibroblasts require oxygen and nutrients. In order for healing to continue, a new blood supply must be created. A great deal has been learned about the creation of a new blood supply, and the process has become quite complex. Three processes occur in the creation of a new blood supply: vasculogenesis, angiogenesis, and arteriogenesis. In addition, vascular myogenesis (recruiting the smooth muscle cells to surround the vessels) must also occur. Excellent reviews give more detail.[26,27] Most new vessel development involves angiogenesis and arteriogenesis. With *vasculogenesis*, undifferentiated precursor stem cells to endothelial cells (angioblasts) arrive in the site of injury and differentiate to form new vessels. This type of vessel development is important in embryogenesis, but does not appear to be as involved after birth. The stem cells do persist into adulthood and thus there is a potential for vasculogenesis to occur.

Angiogenesis involves sprouting of endothelial cells from postcapillary venules (**Figure 42.5**). Several stimuli can activate the process. Low oxygen levels and lactic acid are two stimuli that can induce the process.[22,28] In addition, there are multiple angiogenic factors (such as fibroblast growth factor-2 [FGF-2] and vascular endothelial growth factor [VEGF]) that stimulate endothelial migration and proliferation.[30–33] After an injury, hypoxia and lactic acid are commonly present. In addition, macrophages release angiogenic growth factors in response to the hypoxic environment. The endothelial cells lining the postcapillary venules release proteases that digest the basement membrane. The endothelial cells then migrate towards the chemotactic signals (the concentration gradient of growth factors). As the endothelial cells migrate, endothelial cells in the original venule proliferate to replace those that have migrated away. As the sprout migrates towards the stimulus a lumen is formed to create a new vascular pathway. Recent data also suggest that angiogenesis involves other methods to modify the primitive vascular complex by causing the sprout to divide by intussusception or creating transendothelial cell bridges.[26]

For larger vessels, *arteriogenesis* completes the process by adding the smooth muscle wall of the vessel. The process of *vascular myogenesis* involves the migration of smooth muscle cells along the perimeter of the endothelial sprout. Growth factors, such as platelet-derived growth factor-BB (PDGF-BB), are involved in this process. The smooth muscle cells stabilize the new vessel and at the same time limit its growth.

The process of neovascularization is important to other fields besides wound healing. Many tumors produce increased angio-

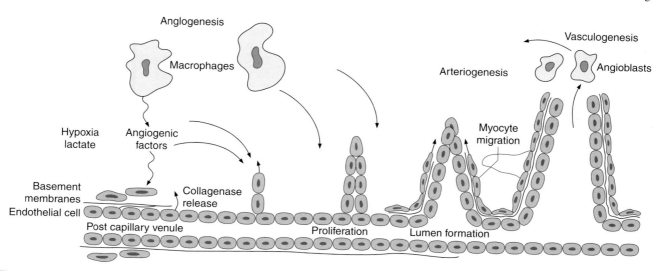

Fig. 42.5 Neovascularization of a wound involves three components. Angiogenesis involves the release of angiogenic factors from cells (macrophages) in a hypoxic environment. These angiogenic factors stimulate endothelial cells to release collagenases and proteases that digest the basement membrane. Endothelial cells then migrate towards the angiogenic stimuli. The migrating endothelial cells eventually form a lumen at the original vessel. During arteriogenesis, smooth muscle cells migrate along the newly formed vessel to recreate the muscle layer. A third type of process is called vasculogenesis. This process of angioblasts migrating into a tissue to initiate new blood vessel formation dominates embryonic development but appears to play a lesser role in adults.

genic factors or have mutated angiogenic receptors. A great deal of research is being performed to understand this process. Investigators have also found inhibitors of the angiogenic process (such as angiostatin)[34,35] that may be useful for cancer chemotherapy and possibly scar control.

The final phase of scar formation is maturation. During this phase, in an incision, there is no net increase in collagen content, despite an increase in tensile strength. When studying these wounds, collagen synthesis is occurring, but there is an equal rate of collagen breakdown by collagenases. Collagen tends to be broken down where it is not needed and it is increased along lines of stress. In essence, fibroblasts are attempting to reorganize the scar to the most efficient configuration possible. In addition, intermolecular bonds are formed between collagen fibrils which tend to increase the strength of the protein (especially collagen type I, the most common collagen in the scar). Lysyl oxidase is the key enzyme required for this process. Any inhibition of the enzyme will lead to a weaker scar. If there is an imbalance between collagen synthesis and breakdown, then pathologic healing occurs. If there is too little synthesis or excessive collagenase activity, then chronic wounds develop. Studies have demonstrated that there is both a decrease in growth factor synthesis and increased collagenase activity in chronic, nonhealing ulcers.[36–39] On the opposite extreme, if the balance is shifted to excessive collagen deposition, then hypertrophic scarring or keloids may form. Unfortunately, the controls of the collagen synthesis/breakdown balance are not well understood and are the topics of many investigations.

During the maturation process, the wound goes from being highly cellular and vascular to one that is relatively acellular and avascular. For burn patients, we know that the burn wound tends to get redder and more raised before it matures. The duration of the maturation process can vary depending on how long the wound remains open. Wounds that heal rapidly, such as sunburn, tend to remain red for a very short time. Those that are open for weeks tend to require 1–2 years to fade out and flatten. The controls of the maturation process are just starting to become known and are discussed below.

The wounds that the burn team deals with do not follow the simplified healing of an incision. With large wounds, all three phases tend to blend together (**Figure 42.6**). If one examines the histology of a 10-day open wound, the center is full of inflammatory cells. The original wound edge tends to be less cellular and has a great deal of collagen deposition. At the edge of the migrating epithelium, there appears to be a transition between inflammation and wound maturation. In essence, all of the three phases of healing are blended together, with the edge of the migrating epithelium being the center of transition. In the center, where the wound is exposed to chronic bacterial invasion, there is a persistent stimulus for inflammation (thus the presence of the inflammatory phase). This tissue is full of inflammatory cells, immature vessels, and collagen. When the inflammatory response is not eliminated, the tissue becomes the moist, red and raised 'granulation tissue' we are familiar with. Once the epithelium marches across the wound, then the inflammatory stimuli are eliminated and fibroblasts tend to predominate. In addition, there appears to be signal from the epithelial cells that induces apoptosis in the nearby inflammatory cells.[40,41] As one follows the wound farther behind the migrating epithelium, there appear to have fewer and fewer fibroblasts. In

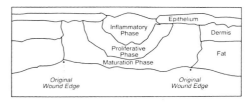

Fig. 42.6 In large open wounds, the phases of scar formation blend together. In the middle of the open wound there is a continuous inflammatory stimulus. Inflammatory cells persist in this area. When the epithelium covers the wound, the inflammatory cells undergo apoptosis and disappear. Fibroblasts dominate this part of the wound which resembles the proliferative phase in an incision. Farthest from the center and nearest to the original wound edge, maturation of the wound is evident with a less cellular and more organized collagen pattern being found.

essence, the wound covered with an epithelium appears to be going through a maturation phase.

The relationship between wound coverage and maturation has been known for some time. Deitch *et al.* noted that wounds that healed within 2–3 weeks tended not to scar.[42] If exposure persisted for longer periods, then the wounds tended to develop hypertrophic scarring. Other investigators have demonstrated that the apoptosis was induced in fibroblasts after epithelial closure[40,41,43] or coverage of a wound with a flap.[44] Apparently, the epithelium has signals that regulate the amount of scar formation. If the wound is left open for too long, then the usual controls that prevent an excessive scar are lost. Several investigators have demonstrated that TGFβ is a likely candidate for a factor that is involved in excessive scar formation.[45–48] Tredgett's group has demonstrated that patients with hypertrophic scars tend to have increased serum levels of TGFβ.[1,47,48] He and others have demonstrated that different isoforms of interferon (IFN) may reverse the effects of TGFβ1.[49–51] Others have found that elimination of TGFβ1 (by knockout technology) leads to the eventual death of the animal from overwhelming inflammation.[52,53] The lymphocytes are involved in the regulation since elimination of both TGFβ1 and lymphocytes leads to the elimination of the inflammatory response.[20] One hypothesis is that, in its attempt to control inflammation and at the same time wall off the inflammatory source by inducing fibrosis, TGFβ1 regulation may be lost.[40] Interestingly, Ferguson's group has shown that only the TGFβ1 and TGFβ2 isoforms appear to induce scarring, while TGFβ3 has antiscarring effects.[54] Eventually, we will be able to understand the controls of collagen deposition enough to greatly reduce excessive scar formation.

Contraction

The final type of healing is contraction. This process must be differentiated from contracture, which is the pathologic result of the long-term shrinkage of a scar. Contraction is the relatively rapid, mechanical reduction in size of a wound.[55,56] The classical example of contraction occurs in open wounds in rodents. If one creates a sizable open wound in a mouse, the wound edges 'pull' together to heal the wound within 10–14 days. An open wound will actually contract to 80–90% of the original wound size. The rest of the wound closure occurs by creation of a new scar and reepithelialization. Most likely, the process of contraction evolved as a rapid and efficient way to close an open wound. It certainly makes more sense for a wound to shrink rapidly than to regenerate over a much longer period.

Contraction also occurs on wounds in people. The wounds that contract the most are those that tend to be surrounded by loose skin. Small, open wounds on the buttocks (as for the small but deep electric burns) are amenable to contraction. The elderly, with their much looser skin, also can have wounds that can be left to contract. In areas where the skin is tight, such as over the dorsal fingers or ankles, wounds tend to resist contraction. These wounds tend to take much longer to heal and lead to scar problems.

There are three phases of contraction, just as there are for scar formation. Initially, there is a 'lag period' while waiting for new fibroblasts to enter the wound. Then there is a phase of rapid contraction, which is followed by a slower and more drawn-out contraction phase. The contraction of the wound is the result of specialized fibroblasts that contract to shrink the wound. These fibroblasts express α-actin, one of the key components of muscle, so they are called 'myofibroblasts'. There is considerable debate as to whether these cells are just a different phenotype of fibroblasts or whether they are a different type of cell. That debate is not essential for this chapter. As fibroblasts synthesize their collagen, they maintain contact so that millions of cells are intertwined with the new matrix. As the cells contract through a actin/myosin interaction process, the ECM, which is attached to the wound edge, also contracts.

Scar contracture is a more gradual process that may partially involve the same process. Contracture occurs over months as opposed to weeks for contraction. Scar maturation involves the continual remodeling of collagen. During the synthesis of the new collagen along lines of stress, fibroblasts probably contract in an attempt to continually shrink the wound. If there is little resistance, as for those patients who do not participate in a therapy program, then the scar contractures can be profound. Lips can be pulled to the chest and fingers extended to the forearm. Fortunately, the forces of contracture can be counteracted with stretching and massage. Compliant patients may end up with little functional abnormality. The ability of something to splint the contraction also applies to thicker grafts. Thin grafts have little resistance to shrinkage, while thicker grafts shrink less. The splinting ability also applies to the surrounding tissue. Areas where the skin is tight, such as over the forehead, tend not to shrink. When a graft is placed on looser skin, then the contraction process is more noticeable. While there is a great interest in the control of the contracture process, relatively little is known at this time. Hopefully, the future will bring better preventative treatments.

Types of Wound Coverage

Different strategies are required for closing different sized wounds. The goal should always be to obtain the most cosmetic and functional wound closure the first time. Small and clean wounds may be treated by *primary closure*. A small burn wound or scar can be excised and reapproximated with sutures or staples. This closure tends to lead to relatively narrow scars. The limitation on this type of closure is the tension of the wound and whether it is relatively free of contamination. If there is a concern about the bacterial load, a *delayed primary closure* can be performed. These wounds are left open and treated with dressing changes for 4–5 days and then closed. Since this period is during the inflammatory (lag) phase, then little inhibition in wound strength occurs. For larger wounds, the tension of a closure can lead to a scar that widens over time. Placement of tissue expanders beneath nearby healthy skin may be used as a strategy for 'stretching' the healthy skin to accommodate a larger wound. The best example of this technique is for the removal of burn alopecia (baldness) from the scalp. Surgeons can cover the scalp with as little as one-third of the hair-bearing skin. If a wound is too large or dirty to be closed, then a *secondary closure* is an option. This term is a euphemism for leaving the trunk or thigh wound to heal on its own. This strategy is useful for relatively large burns in older patients (with loose skin) and who could not tolerate an operative treatment. Sizable areas heal amazingly well in these high-risk patients.

There are many other strategies for covering larger areas of skin loss. Burn caregivers routinely deal with these types of wounds. Open wounds that need to be closed can be closed with a skin graft. Areas that are functionally important (such as fingers and hands), or cosmetically important, are best treated with a sheet graft. If possible, the thickest graft (full-thickness skin graft [FTSG]) should be used if the skin is readily available.[57] As stated before, the thicker the graft, the less the contraction. One must balance the need for a thick graft with the potential scar that a donor site may make. One strategy is to use the thickest skin possible for split-thickness skin grafts (STSG). The back has very thick skin and tends to scar less than other areas.[58] Another strategy is to use the scalp for a donor site. The scalp matches the color of the face nicely and, if not taken too thickly, will not transfer hair. The scalp heals extremely rapidly and the hair hides the donor site.

There are three phases of skin graft healing.[59] Initially, the graft survives by diffusion of nutrients from the wound bed. Since the skin 'imbibes' nutrients from the wound bed, the phase is called the *phase of imbibition*. If any barrier forms between the wound bed and the graft (such as a hematoma, a seroma, pus, or nonviable tissue from inadequate excision), then the graft dies. Since the graft is only held in place by the natural fibrin, there is little resistance to shear so staples or sutures are required. After 2–3 days, blood vessels invade the graft in the *phase of neovascularization*. New blood vessels invade through angiogenesis (as described above) by a process of 'inosculation', where old capillaries in the wound bed are said to 'hook up' with those in the graft. Any shear at this time leads to hematoma formation and loss of the graft. Gradually, new collagen bridges form between the wound bed and the graft in the final *phase of maturation*. This process takes months as the graft tends to get thicker and more vascular for 3–4 months before finally fading out over the ensuing months (**Figure 42.7**). This maturation process parallels the maturation phase described earlier and can take 1–2 years for completion.

Since grafts require a viable wound bed, flap techniques have been developed to cover difficult wound beds where exposed bone or tendons exist. A flap contains its own blood supply and thus does not depend on the 'imbibition' from the wound bed. Flaps also have the benefit of being thicker than skin grafts and thus tend to prevent contraction. One must remember that a flap leaves a defect that must be closed. A local flap involves transfer of a nearby tissue by rotation, advancement or transposition. Part of the skin must stay attached to the original donor site until a new blood supply develops from the recipient site. A 'random' flap has its

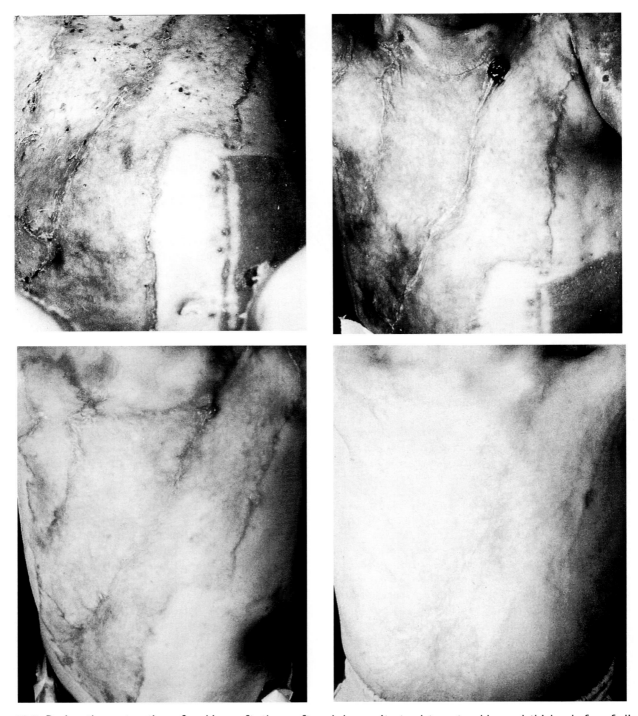

Fig. 42.7 During the maturation of a skin graft, the graft and donor site tend to get redder and thicker before fading into the more supple and naturally colored mature wound. At 5 days after grafting (upper left), both the graft and donor site are pink and dry. At 4 months (upper right), the wound has become thicker, tighter and redder. If the patient continues therapy and massage, the wounds begin to smooth out and become less red at 8 months (lower left). The mature wound becomes flat, supple, and loses its redness (lower right).

blood supply maintained by the dermal plexus. Other flaps, such as a groin flap, have an axial vessel that travels with the tissue. Myocutaneous flaps utilize the underlying muscle in transfer since the skin derives its blood from that muscle. Finally, free flaps are myocutaneous flaps that have their main vessels separated and reattached to distant vessels. For a more detailed review of flaps, check plastic surgery textbooks.

Cosmetically and functionally, sheet grafts are the best type of skin graft for covering large areas of the body.[60] By reharvesting donor sites, relatively large areas can be covered with sheets of skin without significant donor site morbidity. The author has covered as much as 55% TBSA of a patient with sheet grafts. Unfortunately, as wounds cover more of the body surface area, different strategies are required for wound coverage. *Meshing* skin grafts has become the standard method for covering large areas. The size of the mesh can be increased to cover larger and larger areas. Healing of the mesh graft requires not only skin graft 'take' but also the interstices must undergo scar formation, contraction and reepithelialization. These grafts lead to a permanent mesh pattern, because of this required interstice healing.

Once massive wounds are encountered, then new strategies are required. It is clear that the large burn wound leads to a massive and continuous SIRS that is a major contributor to patient mortality. Most burn surgeons believe that the source of the inflammatory stimulus should be expeditiously excised and covered with some type of permanent or temporary material that functions as skin. Some feel that the wound should be closed within hours, while others feel that the wound should be closed within days. Most cover the wound with as much autograft as possible; then they use some other form of coverage. The 'gold standard' has been to use allograft (cadaver skin) as a temporary wound cover. If fresh skin is available, then the skin will 'take' as a viable skin transplant until the body rejects. Patients with massive burns, however, are significantly immunosuppressed, so rejection may take several weeks to months. During that time, the donor sites can be recropped as they heal to gradually replace the allograft.

Other strategies have been developed. Cultured epithelial autografts can be grown from the patient's skin and massively expanded to cover the entire body.[61] Unfortunately, the lack of a dermis leads to prolonged fragility and significant scarring, so most believe that a 'dermis' is required along with an epithelium.[62] One strategy has been to place allograft and then, when the cultured epithelium has been prepared, apply it to the dermal allograft. Since it has been found that the epithelium is the major source of the immune reaction, and not the dermis, this technique is possible.

Others have developed dermal substitutes that can be used with very thin autografts.[64–66] One of the most commonly used dermal substitutes is Integra™, which is a dermis that is created from collagen type I and chondroitin-6-sulphate. The dermis is covered with a silicone 'epithelium' that reduces water loss and bacterial invasion. The dermal substitute is applied to the excised wound and allowed to vascularize. After 2–4 weeks, the silicone can be removed and a thin, meshed autograft applied over the surface. Other dermal substitutes exist. Alloderm™ is a freeze-dried human dermis that can be applied beneath a thin autograft. Transcyte™ is silicone/nylon membrane that has allogeneic neonatal fibroblasts cultured in its ECM. This material is sold as both a dermis and a temporary dressing that releases growth factors and thus can accelerate healing of superficial burns.

Several others have described developing composite skins that are composed of a viable dermis (often containing fibroblasts) and cultured keratinocytes.[67–69] These 'skins' are available on the market as allogeneic products (Apligraf™), while investigators are using biopsies from patients to grow a new composite skin. Recent reports suggest that there is excellent graft take with some types of composite skin. All of these 'skin substitutes' do have the problem of being expensive and having lower resistance to infection than autografts. Great progress has occurred and, someday, autografting may be a procedure of the past.

Factors affecting wound healing

Age

The basic components of tissue repair do not change throughout the life of an individual. There are some relatively minor differences that are dependent upon age but, for the most part, healing occurs efficiently throughout life. The most profound differences of tissue repair occur before birth. In the 1980s, surgeons began to experiment with trying to operate on fetuses to treat congenital abnormalities such as diaphragmatic hernias. They discovered that incisions produced in the fetuses healed without a noticeable scar. Soon, many investigators were studying fetal healing in an attempt to determine the factors that were involved in 'scarless' tissue repair.[70,71] It became clear that there was a period when healing transformed from scarless to 'scar forming', and that gestational time was consistent for each species and occurred before birth. Prior to that period, an incision would regenerate to the normal 'scarless' architecture of the surrounding tissue. It was discovered that TGFβ was not present during scarless healing but it was present later during the creation of a scar. In addition, there appeared to be a paucity of inflammatory cells with scarless healing, but increased inflammation during the creation of a scar. Another finding in the early fetal wound was a higher concentration of hyaluronic acid than that which was found in the more mature animals. Teleologically, these findings make sense. During the period of fetal organ growth and differentiation, the animal exists in an environment of minimal risk from outside invasion. The fetus can afford to 'take the time' to regenerate that tissue. If a wound developed later in life, then that organism needs to be ready for fighting outside invaders. The development of an inflammatory response is essential to survival. Unfortunately, in order to close a wound rapidly and fight invasion, the body sacrifices regeneration for a more expeditious but less than perfect scar. There is a great deal of research on fetal wound healing that cannot be covered here but many reviews exist for those interested.[70,71]

There is feeling among many burn team members that the very young child heals differently than the adult. It has been stated that younger children tend to take longer to mature their wounds than adults. To examine the question of whether scar maturation was different in younger children versus teenagers, the time to maturation was followed for different ages in children.[72] It was found that there was no difference in scar maturation in the very young when compared with teenagers. It has also been put forward that therapy is of no assistance in the prevention of scar contractures in children. While different strategies are necessary for children, their scars can be modified by occupational and physical therapists. Wounds in children can mature very nicely. One problem with children is that their bones tend to grow faster than their scars do. They must be followed as they grow as they may develop contractures that may need reconstructive surgery later in their teen years.

One difference does exist, however – the skin is thinner in the very young child. Strategies to utilize thicker skin, such as from the back, do help with avoiding donor site scarring.[58]

At the other extreme, the very elderly patient tends to have looser and thinner skin. Any experienced burn caregiver will know that a burn that appears to be superficial in an elderly person will often tend to 'convert' to third degree. The burn does not 'convert' but, instead, the skin is much thinner and thus the wound is deeper from the start. Another problem with the geriatric patient is that the blood supplies to some areas of the skin decrease. Along with the decrease in vascularity, the same area will often have decreased hair and other skin adnexa. The classic signs of vascular insufficiency to extremity are decreased hair density, and thinner, more fragile skin. These changes, along with relative hypoxia, lead to delayed healing. The thinner skin in an elderly person must be kept in mind when planning grafting procedures. It is not uncommon for the recipient site to have excellent graft take but to have the donor site fail to heal. Donor sites should be harvested as thinly as possible. In addition, using dermal substitutes that allow for the use of ultrathin donor sites should be of benefit. It is covered elsewhere in this text, but one must also be aware that the elderly patient has much less ability to survive larger burns when compared with younger patients. Relatively small burns often lead to multiple organ failure and critical illness that impairs tissue repair. Many elderly burn patients are treated nonoperatively since their operative risks are prohibitive.

Not all healing is impaired in the elderly. The older patient does have looser skin that allows for contraction of larger wounds. Larger wounds can be allowed to contract with less disfigurement. For example, I have treated a 90-year-old woman with a tea spill to the thigh without grafting. A large open area on the anterior thigh healed over months without range of motion problems. Her family was taught care and she was discharged in their care within days of admission. The ultimate treatment of any elderly patient does require different strategies when compared to the younger patient.

Nutrition

The importance of adequate nutrition for the healing of wounds has been known for over a century. Studies at the beginning of the last century proved that healing was impaired with either total protein-calorie or just isolated protein malnutrition.[73,74] These studies have been repeated hundreds of times.[75,76] The aggressive nutritional support of burn patients has contributed not only to improved healing but also improved survival. While growth factors potentially may improve healing during malnutrition, there is no substitute for aggressive nutritional support. One should assess the nutritional state of the patient prior to injury. Those patients who were malnourished prior to their burn will be at higher risk for complications and death.

There have been many investigations to determine whether the addition of specific nutrients may improve healing. Certain amino acids have been given in excess to animals to determine whether healing could be augmented. Several amino acids (methionine, cysteine, arginine) have provided statistically significant improvements in tissue repair, but whether their addition leads to clinical improvement is not clear.[77,78] Arginine has been shown to improve collagen deposition and tensile strength.[79] In addition, it stimulates the immune system and thus may benefit the patient. Several 'immune-stimulating' tube-feeding formulas include arginine. Glutamine is another nutrient that has been found to protect the enterocytes of the gut. The amino acid has not been proven to improve tissue repair.[80]

Other nutrients, such as vitamins and trace elements, are essential for wound healing. The importance of vitamin C has already been discussed. Without vitamin C, collagen synthesis is impaired at the same time as collagen breakdown continues.[81] Since the balance between collagen synthesis and breakdown is lost, old incisions may break down. The other important vitamin for tissue repair is vitamin A. Vitamin A has been found to accelerate tissue repair and even may reverse the healing deficit after radiation or steroid treatment.[82,83] The vitamin is proinflammatory and stimulates fibroblast function. Some of the B vitamins may also improve some aspects of wound healing.[84] The one vitamin that is commonly felt to improve healing but has no studies to support that contention is vitamin E. At least one study has demonstrated that vitamin E fails to accelerate tissue repair.[85] While it may not have profound effects on healing, vitamin E is essential for other aspects of burn treatment.

Trace elements are also known to improve healing. Zinc is the most notable mineral that has been found to reverse healing defects.[86] The mineral is essential for many enzymes that are involved in tissue repair. The commonly used Unna boot contains zinc oxide. Zinc deficiency also leads to impaired tissue repair. Copper is essential for lysyl oxidase, the enzyme that is required for crosslinks between collagen molecules.[87] Other trace elements may play a lesser role in tissue repair. Most burn centers supplement patients with extra vitamins and minerals. Whether the extra supplements help burn patients has not been proven. It does appear that extra vitamin C may be helpful for reducing fluid requirements during resuscitation.[88]

Infection

It is well known that infection has profound effects on tissue repair. Surprisingly, infection does not always lead to impaired healing. Some studies have demonstrated that contaminating a wound with bacteria led to impaired tissue repair.[89–91] Others attempted similar experiments but found that tissue repair was improved.[92–94] It appears that, if minor contamination occurs, then inflammation is augmented and the result is improved healing. If, on the other hand, large amounts of virulent bacteria are present then the host is overwhelmed and the infection is destructive. The same may be true for skin graft take. Robson has stated that if a wound bed has greater than 10^5 bacteria, then a graft will not take.[95] Lesser numbers tend not to have an effect.

The systemic effects of infection also affect tissue repair. An abscess distant from the wound has been found to impair tensile strength.[96] At least a portion of the decrease was attributed to impaired nutritional intake. It is most likely that sepsis does lead to alter tissue repair. Experience suggests that donor sites heal poorly and graft take is decreased in profound sepsis. Just the burden of a large burn wound appears to decrease the rate of donor site closure.

Associated Illnesses

There are several systemic problems that have adverse affects on tissue repair. The most recognized disease affecting healing is *diabetes mellitus*.[97,98] Diabetes can affect healing by several causes. First, the disease leads to both macrovascular and microvascular disease. The altered perfusion may lead to impaired nutrient and oxygen delivery. Second, the peripheral neuropathy of diabetes mellitus contributes to the tendency to develop ulcers. Insensate feet will not feel minor injury so that a minor irritation may turn into a more serious wound. Loss of the normal reflexes of the muscles that maintain the arch of the foot may lead to increased pressure areas, especially over the second metatarsal. Finally, the wounds in diabetic patients tend to have a higher propensity to become infected. A minor wound frequently becomes infected and more extensive. Diabetic patients tend to have a higher risk for amputation when compared to patients without the problem. Fortunately, a growth factor (Regranex™ [PDGF-BB] is available to treat these wounds. The growth factor does appear to help healing in these problem wounds.[99]

Other diseases do affect healing. Obviously, any vascular abnormality that leads to tissue hypoxia has adverse effects.[28,29,100] In addition, uremia[101] and liver failure[102] have adverse affects on tissue repair. Malignancy has been known for a long time to have adverse affects on wound healing.[103,104] It is likely that the body shunts nutrients away from the wound and to the cancer. In addition, cancer patients tend to have anorexia and weight loss, both of which contribute to impaired wound closure. Any other disease that impairs nutrition will predispose the patient to altered healing.

Cytotoxic Treatments (Steroids, Chemotherapy, Radiation)

Any agent that impairs cellular proliferation will lead to some impairment in tissue repair. Steroids are the most notable class of drug that leads to alteration of healing.[105,106] Steroids decrease the inflammatory response and decrease collagen production. The inhibition of collagen production is occasionally used as a strategy to decrease scar formation in those patients with a tendency towards hypertrophic scarring. Its efficacy varies from patient to patient. Growth factors have been found to reverse some of the adverse affects of steroids.[107–109]

Most chemotherapy agents lead to altered healing.[110,111] These agents are designed to kill rapidly proliferating cells. Unfortunately, the cells required for tissue repair must also grow rapidly. The agents affect healing if given systemically and lead to chronic nonhealing ulcers if they extravasate into the subcutaneous tissues. Growth factors have had some beneficial effects in animal studies.[112] Finally, radiation leads to similar problems as for chemotherapy agents.[113,114] The effects can also be improved with topical growth factors.[115] Other drugs may have effects on healing but are not of major clinical importance.

Scar control

A great deal of knowledge has been gained about the factors that accelerate healing. Growth factors and other agents have been developed to reverse healing abnormalities of all kinds. The factors that 'turn off' the healing process have not been elucidated. Failure to control healing leads to excessive scarring that affects other organs beside the skin (hypertrophic scars and fibrosis). The same processes lead to impaired cardiac function after a myocardial infarction, pulmonary fibrosis, cirrhosis, arthritis, and many other fibrotic diseases. If one were able to control scar formation, then a great deal of diseases would have a better outcome.

In order to stop healing, inflammation must stop. It appears clear that covering a wound with an epithelium is required to begin stopping the inflammatory response. As long as there is exposure to foreign antigens and organisms the body will continue to 'try to protect' the organism with an inflammatory response. Studies have demonstrated that the epithelium induces apoptosis (programmed cell death) in inflammatory cells as it marches across a wound.[40,41] In addition, as a wound is covered with a graft or flap, apoptosis is induced in fibroblasts and other inflammatory cells.[44] The signal produced by the covering epithelium has not yet been elucidated, but studies suggest that factors that affect apoptosis are produced in the migrating keratinocytes.[116] More studies are needed to understand how the epithelium influences the ultimate scar.

We do know that if a wound is left open for too long, then it has a tendency to develop hypertrophic scarring.[42] Several investigators have demonstrated that TGFβ plays a role.[45–48] Those patients with a greater tendency to scar have higher serum levels of TGFβ1.[47,48] One study has revealed that antibodies to TGFβ1 can reduce the amount of scarring that is present in a rat wound.[54] In addition, TGFβ3 may have antiscarring effects.[54] In addition, interferons may reverse the tendency towards hypertrophic scarring. Both IFN-γ and IFN-α2b have been found to reverse some of the scarring tendencies in patients.[49–51] In addition, tension that is produced in a scar contracture increases TGFβ1 production and increases collagen production. Releasing the tension in a scar band by performing a release will decrease TGFβ1 expression.[117] Hopefully, more therapeutic agents will be available in the future.

Finally, there are a few clinical modalities used for scar control in patients. Scar massage and stretching (therapy) appear to be very efficacious. Patients who are compliant with a therapy program do much better than those who do not. Silicone is another product that is available for the treatment of scarring. The exact mechanisms of how silicone works is not clear.[118,119] Finally, pressure through hard materials or stretchy cloth (garments) have been used for decades to reduce hypertrophic scarring. There are some studies being published that suggest pressure garments are not effective, but there are also many years of experience that suggest they are very helpful. Hopefully, third party support for garments is not lost before well-controlled studies are completed to answer the question of their efficacy.

Understanding the principals of wound healing is essential to the adequate treatment of burn patients. The skin is the first barrier to the outside world. If enough of the skin is lost, then any other defense will be overwhelmed. In addition, it is now known that the wound is not an isolated event that affects only the local tissues. An open wound leads to a profound systemic response that, if large enough, will lead to major systemic changes and potentially the ultimate failure of the organism (through multiple organ failure). Our job as caregivers of the burn patient is to heal the wound as expeditiously as possible, while at the same time maintaining the best cosmetic and functional outcomes as possible. The best way to succeed in completing that goal is to have as good a knowledge of tissue repair as possible.

References

1. Woodley DT, O'Keefe EJ, Prunieras M. Cutaneous wound healing: a model for cell-matrix interactions. *J Am Acad Dermatol* 1985; 12: 420–33.
2. Barrandon Y, Green H. Cell migration is essential for sustained growth of keratinocyte colonies: The roles of transforming growth factor-α and epidermal growth factor. *Cell* 1987; 50: 1131–7.
3. Cooper ML, Hansbrough JF, Foreman TJ, et al. The effects of epidermal growth factor and basic fibroblast growth factor on epithelialization of meshed skin graft interstices. *Prog Clin Biol Res* 1991; 365: 429–42.
4. Staiano-Coico L, Kreuger JG, Rubin JS, et al. Human keratinocyte growth factor effects in a porcine model of epidermal wound healing. *J Exp Med* 1993; 178: 865–78.
5. Jimenez PA, Rampy MA. Keratinocyte growth factor-2 accelerates wound healing in incisional wounds. *J Surg Res* 1999; 81: 238–42.
6. Hebda PA. Stimulatory effects of transforming growth factor-beta and epidermal growth factor on epidermal growth factor from porcine skin explant cultures. *J Invest Dermatol* 1988; 91: 440–5.
7. Chen JD, Lapierre J-C, Suder D, Peavey C, Woodley DT. Interleukin-1 alpha

stimulates keratinocyte migration through an EGF/TGF-alpha independent pathway. *J Invest Dermatol* 1995; **104**: 729–33.

8. Woodley DT, Wynn KC, O'Keefe EJ. Type IV collagen and fibronectin enhance human keratinocyte thymidine incorporation and spreading in the absence of soluble growth factors. *J Invest Dermatol* 1990; **94**: 139–43.

9. Falanga V, Eaglstein WH, Bucalo B, *et al.* Topical use of human recombinant epidermal growth factor (h-EGF) in venous ulcers. *J Dermatol Surg Oncol* 1992; **18**: 604–10.

10. Brown GL, Nanney LB, Griffin J, *et al.* Enhancement of wound healing by topical treatment with epidermal growth factor. *N Engl J Med* 1989; **321**: 76–83.

11. Greenhalgh DG, Rieman M. Effects of basic fibroblast growth factor on the healing of partial-thickness donor sites: A prospective, randomized, double-blinded trial. *Wound Rep Reg* 1994; **2**: 113–21.

12. Herndon DN, Barrow RE, Kunkel KR, *et al.* Effects of human growth hormone on donor-site healing in severely burned children. *Ann Surg* 1990; **212**: 424–32.

13. Simpson DM, Ross R. The neutrophilic leukocyte in wound repair: A study with antineutrophil serum. *J Clin Invest* 1972; **51**: 2009–23.

14. Leibovich SJ, Ross R. The role of the macrophage in wound repair. A study with hydrocortisone and antimacrophage serum. *Am J Pathol* 1975; **78**: 71–100.

15. Korn JH, Halushka PV, LeRoy EC. Mononuclear cell modulation of connective tissue function. *J Clin Invest* 1980; **65**: 543–54.

16. Diegelmann RF, Cohen IK, Kaplan AM. The role of macrophages in wound repair: A review. *Plast Reconstr Surg* 1981; **68**: 107–13.

17. Riches DWH. Macrophage involvement in wound repair, remodeling, and fibrosis. In: Clark RAF, ed. *The Molecular and Cellular Biology of Wound Repair* 2nd edn. New York: Plenum Press, 1996; 95–141.

18. Wahl SM, Wahl LM, McCarthy JB. Lymphocyte-mediated activation of fibroblast proliferation and collagen production. *J Immunol* 1978; **121**: 942–6.

19. Barbul A. Role of T cell-dependent immune system in wound healing. *Prog Clin Biol Res* 1988; **266**: 161–75.

20. Crowe MJ, Doetschman TC, Greenhalgh DG. Expression of TGF-β isoform mRNAs during wound healing in immunodeficient TGF-β1 knockout mice. *J Invest Dermatol* 2000; **115**: 3–11.

21. Prockop DJ, *et al.* The biosynthesis of collagen and its disorders. Part I. *New Engl J Med* 1979; **301**: 13–23.

22. Prockop DJ, *et al.* The biosynthesis of collagen and its disorders. Part II. *New Engl J Med* 1979; **301**: 77–85.

23. Fuller GC, Cutroneo KR. Pharmacological interventions. In: Cohen IK, Diegelmann RF, Lindblad WJ, eds. *Wound Healing. Biochemical and Clinical Aspects*. Philadelphia: WB Saunders, 1992; 311–13.

24. Bamert W, Stojan B, Wiedman V. D-penicillamine and wound healing in patients with rheumatoid arthritis. *Z Rheumatol* 1980; **39**: 9–13.

25. Arem AJ, Misiorowski R, Chvapil M. Effects of low-dose BAPN on wound healing. *J Surg Res* 1979; **27**: 228–32.

26. Carmeliet P. Mechanisms of angiogenesis and arteriogenesis. *Nature Med* 2000; **6**: 389–95.

27. Folkman J. Towards an understanding of angiogenesis: search and discovery. *Perspect Biol Med* 1985; **29**: 10–36.

28. Hunt TK, Pai MP. The effect of varying ambient oxygen tensions on wound metabolism and collagen synthesis. *Surg Gynecol Obstet* 1972; **135**: 561–7.

29. LaVan FB, Hunt TK. Oxygen and wound healing. *Clin Plast Surg* 1990; **17**: 463–72.

30. Roesel JF, Nanney LB. Assessment of differential cytokine effects on angiogenesis using an *in vivo* model of cutaneous wound repair. *J Surg Res* 1995; **58**: 449–59.

31. Roberts AB, Sporn MB, Assoian RK, *et al.* Transforming growth factor type beta: Rapid induction of fibrosis and angiogenesis *in vivo* and stimulation of collagen formation *in vitro*. *Proc Natl Acad Sci USA* 1986; **83**: 4167–71.

32. Davidson JM, Benn SI. Regulation of angiogenesis and wound repair. Interactive role of the matrix and growth factors. In: Sirica AE, ed. *Cellular and Molecular Pathogenesis*. Philadelphia: Lippincott-Raven, 1996; 79–106.

33. Folkman J, Klagsbrun M. Angiogenic factors. *Science* 1987; **235**: 442–7.

34. Crum R, Szabo S, Folkman J. A new class of steroids inhibits angiogenesis in the presence of heparin or a heparin fragment. *Science* 1985; **230**: 1375–8.

35. Brem H, Gresser I, Grosfeld J, Folkman J. The combination of antiangiogenic agents to inhibit primary tumor growth and metastasis. *J Pediatr Surg* 1993; **28**: 1253–7.

36. Werner S, Breeden M, Greenhalgh DG, Hofschneider PH, Longaker MT. Induction of keratinocyte growth factor is reduced and delayed during wound healing in the genetically diabetic mouse. *J Invest Dermatol* 1994; **103**: 469–72.

37. Frank S, Hubner G, Breier G, Longaker MT, Greenhalgh DG, and Werner S. Regulation of vascular endothelial growth factor expression in cultured keratinocytes. *J Biol Chem* 1995; **270**: 12607–13.

38. Brown DL, Kane CD, Chernausek SD, Greenhalgh DG. Differential expression and localization of IGF-I and IGF-II in cutaneous wounds of diabetic versus nondiabetic mice. *Am J Pathol* 1997; **151**: 715–24.

39. Trengove NJ, Stacey MC, MacAuley S, *et al.* Analysis of the acute and chronic wound environments: The role of proteases and their inhibitors. *Wound Rep Reg* 1999; **7**: 442–52.

40. Greenhalgh DG. The role of apoptosis in wound healing. *Internat J Biochem Cell Biol* 1998; **30**: 1019–30.

41. Brown DL, Kao WW-Y, Greenhalgh DG. Apoptosis down-regulates inflammation under the advancing epithelial wound edge: Delayed patterns in diabetes and improvement with topical growth factors. *Surgery* 1997; **121**: 372–80.

42. Deitch EA, Wheelahan TM, Rose MP, Clothier J, Cotter J. Hypertrophic scars: Analysis of variables. *J Trauma* 1983; **23**: 895–8.

43. Desmouliere A, Redard M, Darby I, Gabbiani G: Apoptosis mediates the decrease in cellularity during the transition between granulation tissue and scar. *Am J Pathol* 1995; **146**: 56–66.

44. Garbin S, Pittet B, Montandon D, Gabbiani G, Desmouliere A. Covering by a flap induces apoptosis of granulation tissue myofibroblasts and vascular cells. *Wound Rep Reg* 1996; **4**: 244–51.

45. Bettinger DA, Yager DR, Diegelmann RF, Cohen IK. The effect of TGF-β on keloid fibroblast proliferation and collagen synthesis. *Plast Reconstr Surg* 1995; **98**: 827–33.

46. Lin RY, Sullivan KM, Argenta PA, Meuli M, Lorenz HP, Adzick NS. Exogenous transforming growth factor-beta amplifies its own expression and induces scar formation in a model of human fetal skin repair. *Ann Surg* 1995; **222**: 146–54.

47. Ghahary A, Shen YJ, Scott PG, Gong Y, Tredget EE. Enhanced expression of mRNA for transforming growth factor-beta, type I and type III procollagen in human post-burn hypertrophic scar tissues. *J Lab Clin Med* 1993; **122**: 465–73.

48. Wang R, Ghahary A, Shen Q, Scott PG, Roy K, Tredget EE. Hypertrophic scar tissues and fibroblasts produce more transforming growth factor-β1 mRNA and protein than normal skin and cells. *Wound Rep Reg* 2000; **8**: 128–37.

49. Harrop AR, Ghahary A, Scott PG, *et al.* Regulation of collagen synthesis and mRNA expression in normal and hypertrophic scar fibroblasts *in vitro* by interferon-γ. *J Surg Res* 1995; **58**: 471–7.

50. Granstein RD, Rook A, Flotte TJ, *et al.* A controlled trial of intralesional recombinant interferon-gamma in the treatment of keloidal scarring. *Arch Dermatol* 1990; **126**: 1295–301.

51. Tredget EE, Shen YJ, Liu G, *et al.* Regulation of collagen synthesis and messenger RNA levels in normal and hypertrophic scar fibroblasts *in vitro* by interferon alfa-2b. *Wound Rep Reg* 1993; **1**: 156–65.

52. Shull MM, Ormsby I, Kier AB, *et al.* Targeted disruption of the mouse transforming growth factor-β1 gene results in multi focal inflammatory disease. *Nature* 1992; **35**: 693–9.

53. Brown RL, Ormsby I, Doetschman TC, Greenhalgh DG. Wound healing in the transforming growth factor-β1-deficient mouse. *Wound Rep Reg* 1995; **3**: 25–36.

54. Shah M, Foreman DM, Ferguson WJ. Neutralization of TGF-β1 and TGF-β2 or exogenous addition of TGF-β3 to cutaneous rat wounds reduces scarring. *J Cell Sci* 1995; **108**: 985–1002.

55. Montandon D, D'Andiran G, Gabbiani G. The mechanism of wound contraction and epithelialization. *Clin Plast Surg* 1977; **4**: 325–46.

56. Tranquillo RT, Murray JD. Mechanistic model of wound contraction. *J Surg Res* 1993; **55**: 233–47.

57. Schwanholt C, Greenhalgh DG, Warden GD. A comparison of full-thickness versus partial-thickness autografts for the coverage of deep palm burns in the very young pediatric patient. *J Burn Care Rehabil* 1993; **14**: 29–33.

58. Greenhalgh DG, Barthel PP, Warden GD. Comparison of back versus thigh donor sites in pediatric burn patients. *J Burn Care Rehabil* 1993; **14**: 21–5.

59. Greenhalgh DG and Staley MJ. Burn Wound Healing. In: Richard RL, Staley MJ, eds. *Burn Care and Rehabilitation: Principles and Practice*. Philadelphia: FA Davis, 1994; 70–102.

60. Archer SB, Henke A, Greenhalgh DG and Warden GD. The use of sheet autografts to cover patients with extensive burns. *J Burn Care Rehabil* 1998; **19**: 33–8.

61. Gallico GG, O'Connner NE, Compton CC, Kehinde O and Green H. Permanent coverage of large burn wounds with autologous cultured human epithelium. *N Engl J Med* 1984; **311**: 448–511.

62. Rue LW, Cioffi WG, McManus WF and Pruitt BA. Wound closure and outcome in extensively burned patients with cultured autologous keratinocytes. *J Trauma* 1993; **34**: 662–8.

63. Cuono C, Langdon R, McGuire J. Use of cultured epidermal autografts and dermal allografts as skin replacement after burn injury. *Lancet* 1986; **1**: 1123–4.

64. Heimbach D, Luterman A, Burke J, *et al.* Artificial dermis for major burns. A multi-center randomized clinical trial. *Ann Surg* 1988; **208**: 313–20.

65. Hansbrough JF, Dore C and Hansbrough WB. Clinical trials of a dermal tissue replacement placed beneath meshed, split-thickness skin grafts on excised burn wounds. *J Burn Care Rehabil* 1992; **13**: 519–29.

66. Wainwright DJ. Use of an acellular allograft dermal matrix (Alloderm) in the management of full-thickness burns. *Burns* 1995; **21**: 243–8.

67. Hansbrough JF, Boyce ST, Cooper ML, Foreman TJ. Burn wound closure with cultured autologous keratinocytes and fibroblasts attached to collagen-glycosaminoglycan substrate. *J Am Med Assoc* 1989; **262**: 2125–30.

68. Boyce ST, Goretsky MJ, Greenhalgh DG, Kagan RJ, Rieman MT, Warden GD. Comparative assessment of cultured skin substitutes and native skin autograft for the treatment of full-thickness burns. *Ann Surg* 1995; **222**: 743–52.

69. Hansbrough JF, Morgan JL, Greenleaf GE, Bartel R. Composite grafts of human keratinocytes grown on a polyglactin mesh-cultured fibroblast dermal substitute as a bilayer skin replacement in full-thickness wounds in thymic mice. *J Burn Care Rehabil* 1993; **14**: 485–94.

70. McCallion RL and Ferguson MWJ. Fetal wound healing and the development of antiscarring therapies for adult wound healing. In: Clark RAF, ed. *The Molecular and Cellular Biology of Wound Repair*, 2nd edn. New York: Plenum Press, 1996; 561–99.

71. Mast BA, Nelson JM and Krummel TM. Tissue repair in the mammalian fetus. In: Cohen IK, Diegelmann RF, Lindblad WJ, eds. *Wound Healing. Biochemical and Clinical Aspects*. Philadelphia: WB Saunders, 1992; 326–43.

72. Schwanholt CA, Ridgway CA, Greenhalgh DG, *et al.* A prospective study of burn scar maturation in pediatrics: does age matter? *J Burn Care Rehabil* 1994; **15**: 416–20.

73. Howes EL, Briggs H, Shea R, *et al.* Effect of complete and partial starvation on the rate of fibroplasia in the healing wound. *Arch Surg* 1993; **26**: 846–58.

74. Rhoads JE, Fliegelman MT, Panzer LM. The mechanism of delayed wound healing in the presence of hypoproteinemia. *J Am Med Assoc* 1942; **118**: 21–5.

75. Daly JM, Vars HM, Dudvich SJ. Effects of protein depletion on strength of colonic anastomoses. *Surg Gynecol Obstet* 1972; **134**: 15–21.

76. Irvin TT. Effects of malnutrition and hyperalimentation on wound healing. *Surg Gynecol Obstet* 1978; **146**: 33–7.

77. Localio SA, Morgan ME, Hinton JW. The biological chemistry of wound healing. The effect of methionine on the healing of wounds in protein-depleted animals. *Surg Gynecol Obstet* 1948; **86**: 582–9.

78. Williamson MB, Fromm HJ. The incorporation of sulphur amino acids into proteins of regenerating wound tissue. *J Biol Chem* 1955; **212**: 705–12.

79. Seifter E, Rettura G, Barbul A, *et al.* Arginine: an essential amino acid for injured rats. *Surgery* 1978; **84**: 224–30.

80. McCauley R, Platell MB, Hall J, McCulloch R. Effects of glutamine on colonic anastomotic strength in the rat. *J P E N* 1991; **15**: 437–9.

81. Bartlett MK, Jones CM, Ryan AE. Vitamin C and wound healing. I. Experimental wounds in guinea pigs. *N Engl J Med* 1942; **226**: 469–73.

82. Ehrlich HP, Hunt TK. Effects of cortisone and vitamin A on wound healing. *Ann Surg* 1968; **167**: 324–8.

83. Levenson SM, Gruber CA, Rettura G, *et al.* Supplemental vitamin A prevents the acute radiation-induced defect in wound healing. *Ann Surg* 1984; **200**: 494–512.

84. Alvarez OM, Gilbreath RL. Thiamine influence on collagen during the granulation of skin wounds. *J Surg Res* 1982; **32**: 24–31.

85. Ehrlich HP, Tarver H, Hunt TK. Inhibitory effects of vitamin E on collagen synthesis and wound repair. *Ann Surg* 1972; **175**: 235–40.

86. Pories WJ, *et al.* Acceleration of healing with zinc oxide. *Ann Surg* 1967; **165**: 432–6.

87. Pinnell SR, Martin GR. The cross linking of collagen and elastin. *Proc Natl Acad Sci USA* 1968; **61**: 708–14.

88. Tanaka H, Hanumadass M, Matsuda H, Shimazaki S, Walter RJ, Matsuda T. Hemodynamic effects of delayed initiation of antioxidant therapy (beginning two hours after burn) in extensive third-degree burns. *J Burn Care Rehabil* 1995; **16**: 610–5.

89. Smith M, Enquist IF. A quantitative study of impaired healing resulting from infection. *Surg Gynecol Obstet* 1967; **125**: 965–73.

90. Irvin TT. Collagen metabolism in infected colonic anastomoses. *Surg Gynecol Obstet* 1976; **143**: 220–4.

91. Bucknall TE. The effect of local infection upon wound healing. *Br J Surg* 1980; **67**: 851–5.

92. Tenorio A, *et al.* Accelerated healing in infected wounds. *Surg Gynecol Obstet* 1976; **142**: 537–43.

93. Raju DR, *et al.* A study of the critical inoculum to cause a stimulus to wound healing. *Surg Gynecol Obstet* 1977; **144**: 347–50.

94. Levenson SM, *et al.* Wound healing accelerated by *Staphylococcus aureus*. *Arch Surg* 1983; **118**: 310–20.

95. Krizek TJ, Robson MC, Kho E. Bacterial growth and skin graft survival. *Surg Forum* 1967; **18**: 518–9.

96. Greenhalgh DG, Gamelli RL. Is impaired wound healing caused by infection or nutritional depletion? *Surgery* 1987; **102**: 306–12.

97. McMurry JF, Jr. Wound healing with diabetes mellitus. *Surg Clin N Am* 1984; **64**: 769–78.

98. Goodson WH, III, Hunt TK. Wound healing and the diabetic patient. *Surg Gynecol Obstet* 1979; **149**: 600–8.

99. Steed DL, the diabetic study group. Clinical evaluation of recombinant human platelet-derived growth factor for the treatment of lower extremity diabetic ulcers. *J Vasc Surg* 1995; **21**: 71–7.

100. Wu L, Mustoe TA. Effect of ischemia on growth factor enhancement of incisional wound healing. *Surgery* 1995; **117**: 570–6.

101. Yue DK, McLennan S, Marsh M, *et al.* Effects of experimental diabetes, uremia, and malnutrition on wound healing. *Diabetes* 1987; **36**: 295–9.

102. Bayer I, Ellis HL. Effect of obstructive jaundice on wound healing. *Br J Surg* 1976; **63**: 392–6.

103. Devereux DF, Thistlewaite PA, Thibault LF, *et al.* Effects of tumor bearing and protein depletion on wound breaking strengths in the rat. *J Surg Res* 1979; **27**: 233–8.

104. Weinzweig J, *et al.* Supplemental vitamin A prevents the tumor-induced defect in wound healing. *Ann Surg* 1990; **211**: 269–76.

105. Howes EL, Plotz CM, Blunt JW, *et al.* Retardation of wound healing by cortisone. *Surgery* 1950; **28**: 177–81.

106. Sandberg N. Time relationship between administration of cortisone and wound healing in rats. *Acta Chir Scand* 1964; **127**: 446–55.

107. Laato M, Heino J, Kahari VM, *et al.* Epidermal growth factor (EGF) prevents methylprednisolone-induced inhibition of wound healing. *J Surg Res* 1989; **47**: 354–9.

108. Pierce GF, Mustoe TA, Lingelbach J, *et al.* Transforming growth factor β reverses the glucocorticoid-induced wound healing deficit in rats: Possible regulation in macrophages by platelet-derived growth factor. *Proc Natl Acad Sci USA* 1989; **86**: 2229–33.

109. Beck LS, DeGuzman L, Lee WP, *et al.* TGF-β1 accelerates wound healing: Reversal of steroid-impaired healing in rats and rabbits. *Growth Factors* 1991; **5**: 295–300.

110. Ferguson MK. The effects of antineoplastic agents on wound healing. *Surg Gynecol Obstet* 1982; **154**: 421–9.

111. Falcone RE, Napp JF. Chemotherapy and wound healing. *Surg Clin N Am* 1984; **64**: 779–5.

112. Lawrence WT, Sporn MB, Gorschboth C, *et al.* The reversal of an Adriamycin induced healing impairment with chemoattractants and growth factors. *Ann Surg* 1986; **203**: 142–7.

113. Reinisch JF, Puckett CL. Management of radiation wounds. *Surg Clin N Amer* 1984; **64**: 795–802.

114. Luce EA. The irradiated wound. *Surg Clin N Am* 1984; **64**: 821–9.

115. Mustoe TA, Purdy J, Gramates P, *et al.* Reversal of impaired wound healing in irradiated rats by platelet-derived growth factor-BB. *Am J Surg* 1989; **158**: 345–50.

116. Kane CD and Greenhalgh DG. Expression and localization of p53 and bcl-2 in healing wounds in diabetic and nondiabetic mice. *Wound Rep Reg* 2000; **8**: 45–58.

117. Grinnell F, Zhu M, Carlson MA, Abrams JM. Release of mechanical tension triggers apoptosis of human fibroblasts in a model of regressing granulation tissue. *Exp Med Res* 1999; **248**: 608–19.

118. Perkins K, Davey R, Wallis KA. Silicone gel: a new treatment for burn scars and contractures. *Burns* 1982; **9**: 201–4.

119. Ahn ST, Monafo WW, Mustoe TA. Topical silicone gel for the prevention and the treatment of hypertrophic scar. *Arch Surg* 1991; **126**: 499–504.

Chapter 43

Molecular and cellular basis of hypertrophic scarring

Paul G Scott, Aziz Ghahary

Edward E Tredget

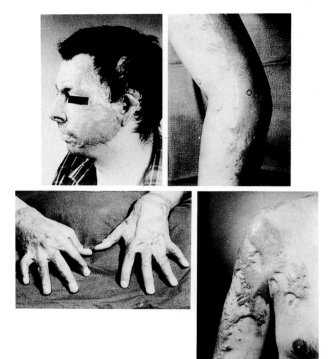

Fig. 43.1 Hypertrophic scarring in a 34-year-old white man, 8 months following a 60% total body surface area burn involving the face, upper extremities and hands. (From reference 36, with permission.)

Introduction

The postburn hypertrophic scar presents as a raised, erythematous, pruritic, and inelastic mass of tissue. If left untreated it may undergo a reorganization of the collagen within its dermal matrix, leading to the development of contractures and thus adding functional impairment to the discomfort and cosmetic problems already suffered by the recovering burn patient (**Figure 43.1**). The undesirable physical properties of hypertrophic scar tissue can be attributed to the presence of a large amount of extracellular matrix that is of altered composition and organization, compared to normal dermis or mature scar. This matrix is the product of a dense population of fibroblasts (and other cell types) maintained in a hyperactive state by inflammatory cytokines such as transforming

growth factor β (TGF-β) and other factors, some of which may be physical in origin. Eventually, most hypertrophic scars undergo at least some degree of spontaneous resolution: a process that may have led to some of the conflicting descriptions of the histology, cell biology or chemistry of hypertrophic scar that have appeared in the literature from time to time. This chapter will review what is known about the molecular and cellular characteristics of the postburn hypertrophic scar and how these help to explain its development, drawing comparisons with normal wound healing and mature scars. While it would be misleading to suggest that the etiology of this debilitating condition is completely understood, it is nevertheless our hope that the better understanding of its pathogenesis now emerging will lead eventually to more rational and successful, non-surgical treatments.

Chemical composition and organization of the extracellular matrix

Collagen

Collagen is the predominant extracellular matrix protein in both normal dermis and hypertrophic scar, where it is responsible for the tensile strength of the tissue. However, collagen constitutes a smaller proportion (about 30% less of the dry weight) of the latter because there are greater increases in other components such as the proteoglycans and glycoproteins[1] (see below). The major genetic form of collagen in skin and scars is type I, which characteristically assembles into thick fibrils, fibers, and fiber bundles. In normal dermis there are smaller amounts of type III (10–15% of the total) and very small amounts of type V and type VI collagens. Pure types III and V collagens assemble *in vitro* into thin fibrils[2–4] but are found in tissues mainly in heterotypic fibrils mixed with larger amounts of type I collagen.[5–7] Both types III and V collagens are considered to reduce the diameters of the collagen fibrils of which they form part. Hypertrophic scars generally contain thinner collagen fibrils than normal dermis (averaging around 60 nm in diameter compared to 100 nm).[8] This difference may possibly be explained by the higher proportions of types III and V collagens, reported to be about 33%[9,10] and 10%[11], respectively. Type III collagen appears in healing wounds within a few days after injury,[12] and its persistence at high levels in hypertrophic scars is probably a reflection of their biological immaturity. Type VI collagen does not assemble into fibrils, but rather into thin beaded filaments, 5–20 nm wide, that are seen to run perpendicular to the fibrils and possibly to link them together.[13] These may constitute the interfibrillar elements that have been described in hypertrophic scar.[14]

In the light microscope, much of the collagen in hypertrophic scars is seen to be arranged in 'whorls' or 'nodules', rather than the thick fibers or fiber bundles that are characteristically oriented parallel to the surface in normal dermis.[8] In some specimens (e.g. **Figure 43.2**) there are extensive regions of almost hyaline appearance where little organization of the fine-fibered collagen is apparent. In the electron microscope the narrow collagen fibrils in these regions are seen to be more widely spaced than in normal dermis or mature scar and to be ovoid or irregular in cross-section.[14] The interfibrillar space in fibrous connective tissues is occupied mainly by two other classes of matrix macromolecules: the proteoglycans and glycoproteins.

Proteoglycans and Glycoproteins

Proteoglycans influence physical properties of connective tissues such as turgor, resilience and resistance to compression, while glycoproteins such as fibronectin and tenascin are involved in cell–matrix adhesion and have effects on cell behavior mainly through this mechanism. Proteoglycans also influence cellular activity, but through a variety of mechanisms including both positive and negative modulation of growth factor activity. The morphology of collagen fibrils and their organization are profoundly affected by the nature and amounts of proteoglycans present in the connective tissue. Consequently, there are good reasons to study these noncollagen matrix macromolecules in postburn hypertrophic scar.

Proteoglycans consist of one or more glycosaminoglycan chains, which are themselves linear polymers of anionic disaccha-

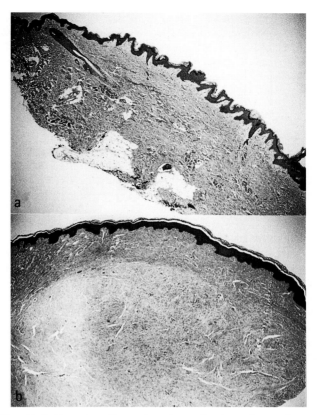

Fig. 43.2 Hemotoxylin and eosin–stained sections of normal skin (a) and a hypertrophic scar containing a nodule (b) (original magnification × 10). (From Scott PG, Ghahary A, Tredget EE, Molecular and cellular aspects of fibrosis following thermal injury. Hand Clinics 2000; 16: 271–87, with permission.)

rides, covalently attached to a protein core. In the most common glycosaminoglycans (dermatan sulfate, chondroitin sulfate, heparan sulfate and hyaluronic acid), one unit of the repeating disaccharide is a uronic acid. Early chemical analyses of hypertrophic scars revealed elevated concentrations of uronic acid (and hence glycosaminoglycans).[15] Since it is the anionic polysaccharide glycosaminoglycan chains that are mainly responsible for the water-holding capacity of connective tissues,[16] it is not surprising that hypertrophic scars are hyper-hydrated relative to normal dermis or mature scars. However the 2.4-fold increase in glycosaminoglycan content (and presumably osmotic pressure) is disproportionately high relative to the 12% increase in water content.[1] Since the collagen fibers normally restrict swelling of connective tissues, it may be proposed that the high concentration of glycosaminoglycans in hypertrophic scars is responsible for their enhanced turgor.

Following the initial analyses of total glycosaminoglycan content in hypertrophic scars, it was reported that the nodular areas were virtually devoid of dermatan sulfate (the major glycosaminoglycan in normal dermis) and contained instead chondroitin sulfate which is usually only a minor component.[17] The corresponding changes in the proteoglycans were defined more recently, when it was reported that hypertrophic scars contain on average only 25% of the amount of the small dermatan sulfate proteoglycan decorin (the major proteoglycan found in normal dermis) and six-fold higher concentrations of a large proteoglycan resembling versican.[1] This latter proteoglycan, which carries 12–30 chondroitin sulfate chains, is normally present only in the proliferating zone of the epidermis and in association with elastin in the dermis.[18] Decorin and versican, as detected by immunohistochemistry, show a strikingly inverse distribution in the nodules,[19] thus explaining the earlier observations on the distribution of dermatan and chondroitin sulfates.

Decorin is implicated in the regulation of collagen fibril formation and in the organization of fibrils into fibers and fiber bundles.[20,21] In the decorin-null mouse recently described, collagen fibrils were found to be variable in diameter and irregular in outline.[22] This latter characteristic was described earlier for the collagen fibrils in the nodules of hypertrophic scar[8] and may be explained by the virtual absence of the decorin that normally serves to define and delimit the fibril surface. A second small proteoglycan, biglycan, present in lesser amounts than decorin in normal dermis, is found at elevated levels in postburn hypertrophic scars.[1,19] In most connective tissues, biglycan is found close to the cell surface[23] but in hypertrophic scars it is associated with the collagen in the extracellular matrix;[19] possibly because there is little decorin to compete for the restricted number of proteoglycan core protein binding sites on the collagen fibrils.[24]

The differences in proteoglycan proportions and distributions between normal dermis and hypertrophic scars could in principle result either from altered biosynthesis or altered degradation. There is evidence for the former mechanism, since fibroblasts cultured from postburn hypertrophic scar contain less decorin mRNA and synthesize less of the protein than do normal fibroblasts.[25] It was recently shown by *in situ* hybridization that there are relatively few cells expressing mRNA for decorin in healing burn scars until about 12 months after injury.[26] Surprisingly, in fibroblasts cultured from hypertrophic scars, there were no differences in contents of mRNAs for versican or biglycan, suggesting that other factors such as TGF-β (see below) were influencing fibroblast behavior and responsible for the elevated amounts of these two proteoglycans in the scars.[25]

As hypertrophic scars mature, the collagen fibrils become coarser and better organized and there is an increase in immunohistochemically detectable decorin (**Figure 43.3**). At about 12 months after injury, a time when many scars start to resolve spontaneously,[27] there is a large increase in numbers of cells expressing decorin (**Figure 43.4**), suggesting that this proteoglycan may play an active role in the resolution. Mature scars show contents of collagen, proteoglycans, and water that are indistinguishable from those in normal dermis.[1]

The results of early chemical analyses of hexose and sialic acid contents[15] showed that hypertrophic scars contained elevated concentrations of glycoproteins, at least part of which is fibronectin.[28] This extracellular matrix macromolecule has effects on cell attachment and activity (reviewed in reference 29) that could be important in the development and organization of hypertrophic scar, but its role does not appear to have been investigated directly.

The hypertrophic scar fibroblast phenotype

Many laboratory investigations have been based on the premise that the fibroblasts that can be grown from tissue explants retain

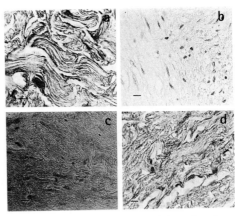

Fig. 43.3 Immunohistochemical staining for decorin in normal skin from the abdomen of a 39-year-old female (a), postburn hypertrophic scar from the neck of a 4-year-old male, 5 months (b) and 12 months (c) after burn injury and postburn mature scar from the neck of a 22-year-old female, 216 months after burn injury (d). Bars = 10 μm. (From reference 26, with permission.)

the hypertrophic scar phenotype in culture. This is at least partly justified since these cells show characteristics that would be predicted from what is known about the tissue. Some strains of hypertrophic scar fibroblasts synthesize more collagen[30] and fibronectin[31] than normal dermal fibroblasts and all strains investigated make less decorin,[25] collagenase[32,33] and nitric oxide.[34] Rather less consistent are the reports of altered cell replication rates *in vitro*. Since hypertrophic scar has a greater density of fibroblast-like cells than normal dermis or mature scar,[26] it might be predicted that these cells would divide more rapidly in culture but the consensus is that population doubling times are unchanged or slightly longer.[31,35,36] Possible explanations for this apparent anomaly are the absence *in vitro* of stimulatory cytokines, such as TGF-β (see below), that are present in the tissue,[19,37] or that the cells that grow out of the explants are approaching the end of their replicative life-span. There have been reports of enhanced incorporation of bromodeoxyuridine into hypertrophic scar fibroblasts *in vitro*,[38] but labeling with tritiated thymidine led Oku and colleagues to conclude that most fibroblasts in hypertrophic scar are dormant, although there may be a small population of more rapidly proliferating cells.[39]

Myofibroblasts and Delayed Apoptosis in Hypertrophic Scars

The presence of myofibroblasts, cells characterized by an indented nuclear envelope and well-developed stress-fibers, has been considered pathognomonic for fibrous tissue that is prone to undergo contracture.[40] Hypertrophic scar tissue contains elevated numbers of cells identified as myofibroblasts on morphological criteria.[41] Myofibroblasts are now usually identified by their positive staining for α-smooth muscle actin;[42] such cells are especially prominent in palmar fascia in Dupuytren's disease[43] and in hypertrophic scar but not in keloid.[44] All fibroblasts probably have some contractile ability, as seen in experimental model systems such as the fibroblast-populated collagen lattice where myofibroblasts do not appear until contraction is complete.[45]

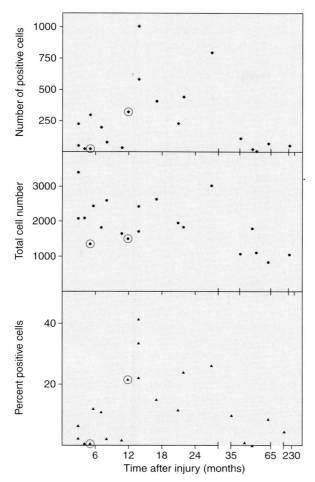

Fig. 43.4 Expression of mRNA for decorin, as assessed by *in situ* hybridization, in healing burn wounds as a function of time after injury. Note the large increase in numbers and percentages of positive cells between 12 and 36 months. Also note the decrease in total cell number after 36 months. The circled data points were obtained for tissue from the same patient sampled twice. (From reference 26, with permission.)

Moreover, cells with the morphological characteristics of myofibroblasts can be induced in skin by the application of tension in the absence of wounding.[46] Nevertheless, electroinjected antibodies against α-smooth muscle actin block the contraction of the fibroblast-populated collagen lattice,[47] indicating that this minor actin isoform (normally accounting for about 14% of the total actin in fibroblasts) is an integral component of the contractile apparatus.

The reduction in cellularity that accompanies the conversion of granulation tissue into scar tissue or of hypertrophic scar into mature scar, is associated with induction of apoptosis (programmed cell death).[48] (See reference 49 for a brief review of this complex process.) The myofibroblast has been suggested to be a terminally differentiated pre-apoptotic cell.[40] However, this suggestion appears inconsistent with the reports that organization of α-smooth muscle actin into stress fibers protects fibroblasts

against the induction of apoptosis,[50] and with the different distributions of α-smooth muscle actin staining and apoptotic cells in skin wounds in guinea pigs treated with IFN-α2b.[51] The prevalence of myofibroblasts in hypertrophic scar may actually be a sign of a delay in the normal onset of apoptosis in the healing wound and this delay may be responsible at least in part for the hypercellularity.

Influence of Extracellular Matrix on Fibroblast Survival

The extent and strength of interactions between attachment-dependent cells such as fibroblasts and epithelial cells and the underlying extracellular matrix are important factors determining cell survival. Detachment of such cells often leads to apoptosis, a phenomenon for which the term 'anoikis' (Greek for hopelessness) was coined.[52] In this context, the high concentration of fibronectin in hypertrophic scars might be important, since binding of the α5β1 integrin to this adhesive glycoprotein has been shown to inhibit Chinese hamster ovary (CHO) cells from undergoing apoptosis.[53] Results obtained with the fibroblast-populated collagen lattice also support the paradigm that the extracellular matrix regulates fibroblast behavior in healing wounds ('outside-in signaling'). In the anchored lattice, which resists deformation in all but the short vertical dimension, the cells continue to proliferate, while in floating or stress-relaxed collagen lattices that are rapidly reorganized, they are triggered to undergo apoptosis.[54,55] In the nodules of the postburn hypertrophic scar, the abundant glycosaminoglycans might inhibit reorganization of the collagen matrix by the fibroblasts, thereby maintaining their proliferative phenotype and delaying the onset of apoptosis.[55] Treatment of hypertrophic scars with pressure therapy has been used for many years and is generally considered beneficial. Recently it was shown that such treatment promotes the reorganization of postburn scar tissue and the disappearance of α-smooth muscle actin staining myofibroblasts, probably by accelerating the onset of apoptosis.[56]

Modulation of fibroblast behavior by fibrogenic and anti-fibrogenic cytokines

Two general mechanisms might be suggested to account for the altered phenotype of fibroblasts in hypertrophic scars. The first, and simplest idea is that the thermal injury selectively destroys certain cells, for example those in the superficial dermis, while the second, and more extensively investigated possibility, is that the proliferation and/or activities of certain subsets of fibroblasts are affected by fibrogenic cytokines present in the wounds. These two mechanisms are not mutually exclusive. Some of the activities of the cytokines in healing wounds are shown in **Figure 43.5**.

Transforming Growth Factor-β

The best-characterized fibrogenic cytokine is TGF-β actually a family of (in mammals) three closely-related proteins (for review see reference 57). Cellular sources of this cytokine include degranulating platelets, macrophages, T-lymphocytes, endothelial cells, smooth muscle cells, epithelial cells, and fibroblasts, i.e. all the major cell types participating in wound healing.[57] Transforming growth factor-β1 is a potent chemoattractant for monocytes[58] and fibroblasts.[59] It stimulates fibroblasts to synthesize collagen,

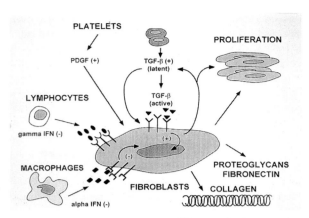

Fig. 43.5 The fibrogenic and antifibrogenic factors that modulate fibroblast function during wound healing. (From Tredget EE, Nedelec B, Scott PG, Ghahary A, Hypertrophic scars, keloids and molecular basis for therapy. *Surgical Clinics of North America* 1997; 77: 701–30, with permission.)

fibronectin, and glycosaminoglycans,[60–62] downregulates decorin synthesis while upregulating production of versican and biglycan,[63] enhances neovascularization,[64] and modulates production of a variety of proteinases and their inhibitors.[65,66] Subcutaneous injection of TGF-β1 into newborn mice stimulates formation of granulation tissue[64] and accelerates healing of incisional wounds in rats.[67] Many of the effects of TGF-β1 on mesenchymal cells may actually be mediated by connective tissue growth factor. This protein, which stimulates the proliferation of fibroblasts and synthesis of extracellular matrix proteins,[68] is coordinately expressed with TGF-β in several fibrotic conditions.[69]

Transforming growth factor β stimulates the expression of α-smooth muscle actin in fibroblasts and may delay the onset of apoptosis by this pathway.[50] Fibroblasts cultured from hypertrophic scar synthesize more TGF-β1 than do normal dermal fibroblasts[70] and the protein has been detected in the scar by immunohistochemistry.[19,37] The serum of recovering burn patients contains levels of TGF-β1 about twice those in control patients.[71] All these observations, and evidence implicating it in other fibrotic conditions (reviewed in reference 72), point to the probable involvement of TGF-β in the pathogenesis of postburn hypertrophic scarring.

The activity of TGF-β in connective tissue may be modified by interaction with components of the extracellular matrix, such as the proteoglycans. Decorin has been shown to bind and neutralize at least some of the activities of TGF-β,[73,74] and mature postburn scars stain intensely for TGF-β which appears to be codistributed with the decorin.[19] Consequently it could be suggested that decorin, which is massively reexpressed in healing burn wounds starting around 12 months after injury,[26] plays a role in the downregulation of TGF-β activity and hence in the natural resolution of hypertrophic scarring.

Insulin–Like Growth Factor-1

Other cytokines that may play a role in hypertrophic scarring include insulin-like growth factor-1 (IGF-1). Like TGF-β1, IGF-1 is expressed locally in response to tissue injury,[75,76] including post-burn hypertrophic scar tissue.[77] Insulin-like growth factor-1 is mitogenic for fibroblasts and endothelial cells, stimulates collagen production by osteoblasts,[78] lung[79] and dermal[80] fibroblasts, and in growth plate chondrocytes,[81] and reduces expression of collagenase by dermal fibroblasts.[33] The remarkable similarity in activities of IGF-1 and TGF-β1 can now be explained by the observation that IGF-1 induces transcription of the gene for TGF-β1, so that at least some of its actions on fibroblasts might be mediated through this indirect mechanism.[82] Expression of IGF-1 in uninjured skin seems to be restricted to epidermis, sweat and sebaceous glands[83] but in a healing burn wound these elements are disrupted and epithelial cells migrating towards the wound surface could possibly secrete IGF-1 in proximity to fibroblasts and affect their activity.

Interferons

The interferons (IFNs) are naturally occurring cytokines that were originally detected as proteins expressed in response to viral infection[84] but which may have therapeutic application in the treatment of hypertrophic scars and keloids. There are two main classes of interferon: type I, comprising IFNs-α and -β (produced by leukocytes and fibroblasts, respectively), and type II (IFN-γ, produced by activated T-lymphocytes). They are distinguished by the degree of their amino acid sequence similarity and by their receptors and intracellular signaling pathways.[84] Treatment of fibroblasts *in vitro* with either type of interferon inhibits cell proliferation and reduces expression of type I and III collagens,[85,86] fibronectin,[87] and TGF-β.[71] Interferon-α2b, but not IFN-γ, also induces the expression of collagenase, suggesting that it may possibly be of greater benefit than the latter in the treatment of fibroproliferative disorders where an excessive amount of collagen is present.[88] Treatment of fibroblasts in the collagen lattice with IFNs reduces the rate of lattice contraction,[89,90] probably by downregulating the expression of the genes for the major β and γ isoforms of actin.[91] Administration of IFN-α2b through an osmotic mini-pump reduces the rate of wound closure and the frequency of α-smooth muscle actin positive cells, and increases the frequency of apoptotic cells at late stages in healing.[51] Although keloids in patients treated with IFN-α2b showed only limited improvement,[92,93] early (phase II) trials in postburn hypertrophic scar patients have shown promising results, associated with a reduction in scar height, increase in scar suppleness and reduced levels of circulating methylhistamine and TGF-β.[71] In these same patients, there was an increased frequency of apoptotic cells following treatment with IFN-α2b.[94] Induction or augmentation of apoptosis by IFNs has been demonstrated in activated T-cells, squamous cell carcinoma cells, and non-myeloma skin cancer cells.[95–97] It does not appear to have been previously shown in fibroblasts but is consistent with the report that IFN-γ downregulates α-smooth muscle actin.[98]

Given the evidence, reviewed above, that interferons can modify fibroblast behavior both *in vivo* and *in vitro*, the question naturally arises of whether depressed intrinsic levels of these cytokines might play a role in the pathogenesis of aberrant scarring. This question has been investigated indirectly. McCauley and colleagues isolated peripheral blood mononuclear cells (PBMC) from black keloid patients and from a control group of patients who had suffered equivalent trauma but did not develop keloids.[99] After appropriate stimulation, PBMC from the keloid patients secreted less IFN-α and IFN-γ, but more IFN-β. Cytokine production by T-cell clones that could be grown from active hypertrophic scar tissue and scars undergoing remission were compared by Bernabei and colleagues.[100] In both cases, clones producing IFN-γ predominated but the amounts released were 4–6 times lower in clones from scars undergoing remission. It was suggested that the IFN-γ, a potent proinflammatory cytokine, was responsible for the prolonged inflammation in active hypertrophic scars.

Possible Role of T-lymphocytes

It has long been recognized that hypertrophic scars are heavily infiltrated with lymphocytes, often forming perivascular cuffs.[8] These lymphocytes are surrounded by a proteoglycan-rich matrix that they may have secreted themselves.[101] The largest population of lymphocytes in hypertrophic scars is activated (CD4+) T-helper cells, found especially in the subpapillary dermis but also in the epidermis and reticular dermis.[102] There are also increased numbers of macrophages and Langerhan's cells but B-lymphocytes are not seen. Two subsets of T-helper cells (Th1 and Th2) can be differentiated by the cytokines that they synthesize.[103] Th1 cells secrete IFN-γ, interleukin-2 (IL-2) and tumor necrosis factor β (TNFβ) and are principally involved in cell-mediated immunity, whereas Th2 cells secrete IL-4, IL-5 and IL-10 and induce antibody production. The activation of naïve mouse CD4+ T-lymphocytes to secrete TGF-β is promoted by the Th-2 cytokine IL-10, and the amounts of TGF-β secreted are greater in T-cell populations from IFN-γ null mice and lower in IL-4 null mice.[104] In burned mice there is a depletion of splenocytes synthesizing IFN-γ and IL-2 (Th1 cytokines) and an increase in synthesis of IL-5 (a Th2 cytokine).[105] There is also evidence for a similar 'Th2 response' in human burn victims. Stimulated PBMC from patients with 25–90% surface area burns showed diminished production of IL-2.[106] Increased production of IL-4 accompanied by decreased IFN-γ was subsequently reported in a group of burn and major trauma patients.[107] Although the stimulus for most investigations of T-lymphocytes in burn victims was presumably to understand the basis of the reduced resistance to infection in these patients, these results also suggest that a systemic (immune) response to injury may modulate the localized (fibroproliferative) response. A link between the type of Th response to injury and the severity of fibrosis has been demonstrated in mice. Hepatic fibrosis is much more severe in BALB/c mice, which show a Th2 response to chemically-induced liver injury, than in C57BL/6 mice which respond with a Th1 cytokine profile.[108] Moreover, shifting the Th2 response toward a Th1 response by treatment with a neutralizing antibody to IL-4 or with IFN-γ itself, ameliorated the fibrosis in BALB/c mice. It is possible that the systemic administration of IFN-α2b to recovering burn patients has a similar effect on the T-helper cell phenotype and that its beneficial effects are mediated in part through this mechanism.[71]

Summary

The postburn hypertrophic scar consists of a mass of hypercellular and disorganized connective tissue overlain with a thickened epidermis. Within the connective tissue, much of the collagen is arranged in whorls and nodules, rather than the thick fibers and fiber bundles running parallel to the surface that are characteristic of normal dermis. This abnormal arrangement of collagen,

together with the very high content of glycosaminoglycans, accounts for the inelasticity and turgor of the tissue. Abnormalities in the extracellular matrix may result from the selection and stimulation of subpopulations of fibroblasts, synthesizing increased amounts and altered proportions of specific types of collagens and proteoglycans, and reduced amounts of proteolytic enzymes such as collagenase, that are normally responsible for the remodeling phase of wound healing. Increased levels of circulating and local fibrogenic cytokines, such as TGF-β and IGF-1, and decreased antifibrogenic cytokines such as the interferons, are believed to mediate these shifts in phenotype. The hypercellularity of hypertrophic scar may result in part from a blockade in the induction of the programmed cell death (apoptosis) that normally accompanies scar maturation, consequent upon altered cytokine profiles and signals from the altered extracellular matrix.

References

1. Scott PG, Dodd CM, Tredget EE, Ghahary A, Rahemtulla F. Chemical characterization and quantification of proteoglycans in human post-burn hypertrophic and mature scars. *Clin Sci* 1996; 90: 417–25.
2. Adachi E, Hayashi T. *In vitro* formation of hybrid fibrils of type V collagen and type I collagen. Limited growth of type I collagen into thick fibrils by type V collagen. *Connect Tissue Res* 1986; 14: 257–66.
3. Lapiere CM, Nusgens B, Pierard GE. Interaction between collagen type I and type III in conditioning bundles organization. *Connect Tissue Res* 1977; 5: 21–9.
4. Birk DE, Fitch JM, Babiarz JP, Doane KJ, Linsenmayer TF. Collagen fibrillogenesis *in vitro*: interaction of types I and V collagen regulates fibril diameter. *J Cell Sci* 1990; 95: 649–57.
5. Henkel W, Glanville RW. Covalent crosslinking between molecules of type I and type III collagen. The involvement of the N-terminal, nonhelical regions of the α 1 (I) and α 1 (III) chains in the formation of intermolecular crosslinks. *Eur J Biochem* 1982; 122: 205–13.
6. Keene DR, Sakai LY, Bachinger HP, Burgeson RE. Type III collagen can be present on banded collagen fibrils regardless of fibril diameter. *J Cell Biol* 1987; 105: 2393–402.
7. Birk DE, Fitch JM, Babiarz JP, Linsenmayer TF. Collagen type I and type V are present in the same fibril in the avian corneal stroma. *J Cell Biol* 1988; 106: 999–1008.
8. Linares HA, Kischer CW, Dobrkovsky M, Larson DL. The histiotypic organization of the hypertrophic scar in humans. *J Invest Dermatol* 1972; 59: 323–31.
9. Bailey AJ, Bazin S, Sims TJ, LeLous M, Nicoletis C, Delaunay A. Characterization of the collagen of human hypertrophic and normal scars. *Biochim Biophys Acta* 1975; 405: 412–21.
10. Hayakawa T, Hashimoto Y, Myokei Y, Aoyama H, Izawa Y. Changes in type of collagen during the development of human post-burn hypertrophic scars. *Clin Chim Acta* 1979; 93: 119–25.
11. Ehrlich HP, White BS. The identification of αA and αB collagen chains in hypertrophic scar. *Exp Mol Path* 1981; 34: 1–8.
12. Gay S, Viljanto J, Raekallio J, Penttinen R. Collagen types in early phases of wound healing in children. *Acta Chir Scand* 1978; 144: 205–11.
13. Engel J, Furthmayr H, Odermatt E, *et al.* Structure and macromolecular organization of type VI collagen. *Ann N Y Acad Sci* 1985; 460: 25–37.
14. Kischer CW. Collagen and dermal patterns in the hypertrophic scar. *Anat Rec* 1974; 179: 137–45.
15. Shetlar MR, Dobrkovsky M, Linares L, Villarante R, Shetlar CL, Larson DL. The hypertrophic scar. Glycoprotein and collagen components of burn scars. *Proc Soc Exp Biol Med* 1971; 138: 298–300.
16. Ogston AG. In: Balazs EA, ed. *Chemistry and Molecular Biology of the Intercellular Matrix*. New York: Academic Press, 1970; 1231–40.
17. Shetlar MR, Shetlar CL, Linares HA. The hypertrophic scar: location of glycosaminoglycans within scars. *Burns* 1977; 4: 14–9.
18. Zimmerman DR, Dours-Zimmerman NT, Schubert M, Bruckner-Tuderman L. Versican is expressed in the proliferating zone in the epidermis and in association with the elastic network of the dermis. *J Cell Biol* 1994; 124: 817–25.
19. Scott PG, Dodd CM, Tredget EE, Ghahary A, Rahemtulla FR. Immunohistochemical localization of the proteoglycans decorin, biglycan and versican and transforming growth factor-β in human post-burn hypertrophic and mature scars. *Histopathology* 1995; 26: 423–31.

20. Scott JE, Orford CR, Hughes EW. Proteoglycan-collagen arrangements in developing rat tail tendon. *Biochem J* 1981; **195**: 573–81.

21. Scott JE. Proteoglycan-fibrillar collagen interactions in tissues: dermatan sulphate proteoglycan as a tissue organizer. In: Scott JE, ed. *Dermatan Sulphate Proteoglycans: Chemistry, Biology, Chemical Pathology.* London: Portland Press, 1993; 165–82.

22. Danielson KG, Baribault H, Holmes DF, Graham H, Kadler KE, Iozzo RV. Targeted disruption of decorin leads to abnormal collagen fibril morphology and skin fragility. *J Cell Biol* 1997; **136**: 729–43.

23. Bianco P, Fisher LW, Young MF, Termine JD, Robey PG. Expression and localization of the two small proteoglycans biglycan and decorin in developing human skeletal and non-skeletal tissues. *J Histochem Cytochem* 1990; **38**: 1549–63.

24. Brown DC, Vogel KG. Characteristics of the *in vitro* interaction of a small proteoglycan (PGII) of bovine tendon with type I collagen. *Matrix* 1989; **9**: 468–78.

25. Scott PG, Dodd CM, Ghahary A, Shen YJ, Tredget EE. Fibroblasts from post-burn hypertrophic scar tissue synthesize less decorin than normal dermal fibroblasts. *Clin Sci* 1998; **94**: 541–7.

26. Sayani K, Dodd CM, Nedelec B, *et al.* Delayed appearance of decorin in healing burn scars. *Histopathology* 2000; **36**: 262–72.

27. Reid WH, Evans JH, Naismith RS, Tully AE, Sherwin S. Hypertrophic scarring and pressure therapy. *Burns* 1987; **13**: S29–S32.

28. Kischer CW, Hendrix MJC. Fibronectin (FN) in hypertrophic scars and keloids. *Cell Tissue Res* 1983; **231**: 29–37.

29. Hynes RO. *Fibronectins*, New York: Springer-Verlag, 1990.

30. Ghahary A, Scott PG, Malhotra SK, *et al.* Differential expression of type I and type III procollagen mRNA in human hypertrophic burn fibroblasts. *Biomed Letts* 1992; **47**: 169–184.

31. Kischer CW, Wagner HN, Pindur J, *et al.* Increased fibronectin production by cell lines from hypertrophic scar and keloid. *Connect Tissue Res* 1989; **23**: 279–88.

32. Arakawa M, Hatamochi A, Mori Y, Mori K, Ueki H, Moriguchi T. Reduced collagenase gene expression in fibroblasts from hypertrophic scar tissue. *Br J Dermatol* 1996; **134**: 863–8.

33. Ghahary A, Shen YJ, Nedelec B, Wang R, Scott PG, Tredget EE. Collagenase production is lower in post-burn hypertrophic scar fibroblasts than normal fibroblasts and is down-regulated by insulin-like growth factor-1. *J Invest Dermatol* 1996; **106**: 476–81.

34. Wang R, Ghahary A, Shen YJ, Scott PG, Tredget EE. Nitric oxide synthase expression and nitric oxide production are reduced in hypertrophic scar tissue and fibroblasts. *J Invest Dermatol* 1997; **108**: 438–44.

35. Savage K, Swann DA. A comparison of glycosaminoglycan synthesis by human fibroblasts from normal skin, normal scar, and hypertrophic scar. *J Invest Dermatol* 1985; **84**: 521–6.

36. Scott PG, Ghahary A, Chambers MM, Tredget EE. Biological basis of hypertrophic scarring. In: Malhotra SK, ed. *Advances in Structural Biology*, Vol. 3. Greenwich, Connecticut: JAI Press, 1994; 157–202.

37. Ghahary A, Shen YJ, Scott PG, Tredget EE. Immunolocalization of transforming growth factor-β1 in human hypertrophic and normal dermal tissue. *Cytokine* 1995; **7**: 184–90.

38. Zhou L-J, Ono I, Kaneko F. Role of transforming growth factor-β 1 in fibroblasts derived from normal and hypertrophic scarred skin. *Archs Dermatol Res* 1997; **289**: 646–52.

39. Oku T, Takigawa M, Fukamizu H, Inoue K, Yamada M. Growth kinetics of fibroblasts derived from normal skin and hypertrophic scar. *Acta Dermato-Venereol* 1987; **67**: 526–8.

40. Desmouliere A, Gabbiani G. The role of the myofibroblast in wound healing and fibrocontractive diseases. In: Clark RAF, ed. *The Molecular and Cell Biology of Wound Repair*, 2nd edn. New York: Plenum Press, 1996; 391–423.

41. Baur PS, Larson DL, Stacey TR. The observation of myofibroblasts in hypertrophic scars. *Surg Gynecol Obstet* 1975; **141**: 22–6.

42. Skalli O, Ropraz P, Trzeciak A, Benzonana G, Gillessen D, Gabbiani G. A monoclonal antibody against α-smooth muscle actin: a new probe for smooth muscle differentiation. *J Cell Biol* 1986; **103**: 2787–96.

43. Skalli O, Schurch W, Seemayer T, *et al.* Myofibroblasts from diverse pathological settings are heterogeneous in their content of actin isoforms and intermediate filament proteins. *Lab Invest* 1989; **60**: 275–85.

44. Ehrlich HP, Desmouliere A, Diegelmann RF, *et al.* Morphological and immunochemical differences between keloid and hypertrophic scar. *Am J Pathol* 1994; **145**: 105–13.

45. Ehrlich HP, Rajaratnam JB. Cell locomotion forces versus cell contraction forces for collagen lattice contraction: an *in vitro* model of wound contraction. *Tissue Cell* 1990; **22**: 407–17.

46. Squier CA. The effect of stretching on formation of myofibroblasts in mouse skin. *Cell Tiss Res* 1981; **220**: 325–35.

47. Arora PD, McCulloch CAG. Dependence of collagen remodelling on α-smooth muscle actin expression by fibroblasts. *J Cell Physiol* 1994; **159**: 161–75.

48. Desmouliere A, Redard M, Darby I, Gabbiani G. Apoptosis mediates the decrease in cellularity during the transition between granulation tissue and scar. *Am J Pathol* 1995; **146**: 56–66.

49. Orrenius S. Apoptosis: molecular mechanisms and implications for human disease. *J Intern Med* 1995; **237**: 529–36.

50. Arora PD, McCulloch CAG. The deletion of transforming growth factor-β-induced myofibroblasts depends on growth conditions and actin organization. *Am J Pathol* 1999; **155**: 2087–99.

51. Nedelec B, Dodd CM, Scott PG, Ghahary A, Tredget EE. Effect of interferon-α2b on guinea pig wound closure and the expression of cytoskeletal proteins *in vivo*. *Wound Rep Reg* 1998; **6**: 202–12.

52. Frisch SM, Francis H. Disruption of epithelial cell-matrix interactions induces apoptosis. *J Cell Biol* 1994; **124**: 619–26.

53. Zhang Z, Vuori K, Reed JC, Ruoslahti E. The α5β1 integrin supports survival of cells on fibronectin and up-regulates Bcl-2 expression. *Proc Natl Acad Sci USA* 1995; **92**: 6161–5.

54. Varedi M. The effects of reorganization of cytoskeleton and matrix on gene expression, growth and apoptosis of dermal fibroblasts. *Ph.D. Thesis*, University of Alberta, 1997.

55. Varedi M, Tredget EE, Ghahary A, Scott PG. Stress-relaxation and contraction of a collagen matrix induces expression of TGF-β and triggers apoptosis in dermal fibroblasts. *Biochem Cell Biol* 2000; **78**: 427–36.

56. Costa AM, Peyrol S, Porto LC, Comparin JP, Foyatier JL, Desmouliere A. Mechanical forces induce scar remodeling. Study in non-pressure-treated versus pressure-treated hypertrophic scars. *Am J Pathol* 1999; **155**: 1671–9.

57. Roberts A, Sporn MB. Transforming growth factor-β. In: Clark RAF, ed. *The Molecular and Cell Biology of Wound Repair*, 2nd edn. New York: Plenum Press, 1996; 275–308.

58. Wakefield LM, Smith DM, Masui T, Harris CC, Sporn MB. Distribution and modulation of the cellular receptor for transforming growth factor-β. *J Cell Biol* 1987; **105**: 965–75.

59. Postlethwaite AE, Keski-Oja J, Moses HL, Kang AH. Stimulation of the chemotactic migration of human fibroblasts by transforming growth factor-β. *J Exp Med* 1987; **165**: 251–6.

60. Ignotz RA, Massague J. Transforming growth factor-β stimulates the expression of fibronectin and collagen and their incorporation into the extracellular matrix. *J Biol Chem* 1986; **261**: 4337–45.

61. Sporn MB, Roberts AB, Wakefield LM, de Crombrugghe B. Some recent advances in the chemistry and biology of transforming growth factor-β. *J Cell Biol* 1987; **105**: 1039–45.

62. Varga J, Rosenbloom J, Jimenez SA. Transforming growth factor β causes a persistent increase in steady state amounts of type I and type III collagen and fibronectin mRNAs in normal human dermal fibroblasts. *Biochem J* 1987; **247**: 597–604.

63. Kahari V-M, Larjava H, Uitto J. Differential regulation of extracellular matrix proteoglycan (PG) gene expression. *J Biol Chem* 1991; **266**: 10608–15.

64. Roberts AB, Sporn MB. In: Sporn MB, Roberts AB, eds. *Peptide growth factors and their receptors.* New York: Springer-Verlag, 1990; 421.

65. Edwards DR, Murphy G, Reynolds JJ, *et al.* Transforming growth factor-β stimulates the expression of collagenase and metalloproteinase inhibitor. *EMBO J* 1987; **6**: 1899–1904.

66. Overall C, Wrana, JL, Sodek J. Independent regulation of collagenase, 72 kDa progelatinase, and metalloendoproteinase inhibitor expression in human fibroblasts by transforming growth factor-β. *J Biol Chem* 1989; **264**: 1860–9.

67. Mustoe TA, Pierce GF, Thomason A, Gramates P, Sporn MB, Deuel TF. Accelerated healing of incisional wounds in rats induced by transforming growth factor-β. *Science* 1987; **237**: 1333–6.

68. Grotendorst GR. Connective tissue growth factor: a mediator of TGF-β action on fibroblasts. *Cytokine Growth Factor Rev* 1997; **8**: 171–9.

69. Igarashi A, Nashiro K, Kikuchi K, *et al.* Connective tissue growth factor gene expression in tissue sections from localized scleroderma, keloid and other fibrotic skin disorders. *J Invest Dermatol* 1996; **106**: 729–33.

70. Wang R, Ghahary A, Shen Q, Scott PG, Roy K, Tredget EE. Hypertrophic scar tissue and fibroblasts produce more TGF-β1 mRNA and protein than normal skin and cells. *Wound Rep Reg* 2000; **8**: 128–37.

71. Tredget EE, Shankowsky HA, Pannu R, *et al.* Transforming growth factor-β in thermally injured patients with hypertrophic scars: effects of interferon-α2b. *Plast Reconstr Surg* 1998; **102**: 1317–28.

72. Ghahary A, Pannu R, Tredget EE. Fibrogenic and anti-fibrogenic factors in wound repair. In: Malhotra SK, ed. *Advances in Structural Biology*, vol. 4. London, JAI Press, 1996; 197–232.

73. Yamaguchi Y, Mann DM, Ruoslahti E. Negative regulation of transforming growth factor-β by the proteoglycan decorin. *Nature* 1990; **346**: 282–4.

74. Hausser H, Groning A, Hasilik A, Schonherr E, Kresse H. Selective inactivity of TGF-β/decorin complexes. *FEBS Letts* 1994; **353**: 243–5.

75. Blatti SP, Foster DN, Ranganathan G, Moses HI, Getz MJ. Induction of fibronectin gene transcription and mRNA is a primary response to growth-factor stimulation of AKR-2B cells. *Proc Natl Acad Sci USA* 1988; **85**: 1119–23.

76. Edwall D, Schalling M, Jennische E, Norstedt G. Induction of insulin-like growth factor-1 messenger ribonucleic acid during regeneration of rat skeletal muscle. *Endocrinology* 1989; **124**: 820–5.

77. Ghahary A, Shen YJ, Nedelec B, Scott PG, Tredget EE. Enhanced expression of mRNA for insulin-like growth factor-1 in post burn hypertrophic scar tissue and its fibrogenic role by dermal fibroblasts. *Mol Cell Biochem* 1995; **148**: 25–32.

78. McCarthy TL, Centrella M, Canalis E. Regulatory effects of insulin-like growth factor I and II on bone collagen synthesis in rat calvarial cultures. *Endocrinology* 1989; **124**: 301–9.

79. Goldstein RH, Poliks CF, Pilch PF, Smith BD, Fine A. Stimulation of collagen formation by insulin and insulin-like growth factor I in cultures of human lung fibroblasts. *Endocrinology* 1989; **124**: 964–70.

80. Bird JL, Tyler JA. Dexamethasone potentiates the stimulatory effect of insulin-like growth factor-1 on collagen production in cultured human fibroblasts. *J Endocrinol* 1994; **142**: 571–9.

81. Hill DJ, Logan A, McGarry M, De Sousa D. Control of protein and matrix-molecule synthesis in isolated bovine fetal growth-plate chondrocytes by the interactions of basic fibroblast growth factor, insulin-like growth factor-I and II, insulin and transforming growth factor-β1. *J Endocrinol* 1992; **133**: 363–73.

82. Ghahary A, Shen Q, Shen YJ, Scott PG, Tredget EE. Induction of transforming growth factor-β1 by insulin-like growth factor-1 in dermal fibroblasts. *J Cell Physiol* 1998; **174**: 301–9.

83. Ghahary A, Shen YJ, Wang R, Scott PG, Tredget EE. Expression and localization of insulin-like growth factor-1 in normal and post-burn hypertrophic scar tissue in human. *Mol Cell Biochem* 1998; **183**: 1–9.

84. Sen GC, Lengyel P. The interferon system. A bird's eye view of its biochemistry. *J Biol Chem* 1992; **267**: 5017–20.

85. Harrop AR, Ghahary A, Scott PG, Forsyth N, Uji-Friedland A, Tredget EE. Effect of γ-interferon on cell proliferation, collagen production and procollagen mRNA expression in hypertrophic scar fibroblasts *in vitro*. *J Surg Res* 1995; **58**: 471–7.

86. Tredget EE, Shen YJ, Liu G, *et al.* Regulation of collagen synthesis and mRNA levels in normal and hypertrophic scar fibroblasts *in vitro* by interferon-α2b. *Wound Rep Reg* 1993; **1**: 156–65.

87. Ghahary A, Shen YJ, Scott PG, Tredget EE. Expression of fibronectin messenger RNA in hypertrophic and normal dermis tissues and *in vitro* regulation by interferon-α2b. *Wound Rep Reg* 1993; **1**: 166–74.

88. Ghahary A, Shen YJ, Nedelec B, Scott PG, Tredget EE. Interferons γ and α2b differentially regulate the expression of collagenase and tissue inhibitor of metalloproteinase-1 messenger RNA in human hypertrophic and normal dermal fibroblasts. *Wound Rep Reg* 1995; **3**: 176–84.

89. Sahara K, Kucukcelebi A, Ko F, Phillips L, Robson M. Suppression of *in vitro* proliferative scar fibroblast contraction by interferon-α2b. *Wound Rep Reg* 1993; **1**: 22–7.

90. Dans MJ, Isseroff R. Inhibition of collagen lattice contraction by pentoxifylline and interferon-α, -β and -γ. *J Invest Dermatol* 1994; **102**: 118–21.

91. Nedelec B, Shen YJ, Ghahary A, Scott PG, Tredget EE. The effect of interferon-α2b on the expression of cytoskeletal proteins in an *in vitro* model of wound contraction. *J Lab Clin Med* 1995; **126**: 474–84.

92. Al-Khawajah MM. Failure of interferon-α2b in the treatment of mature keloids. *Internat J Dermatol* 1996; **35**: 515–7.

93. Wong TW, Chiu HC, Yip KM. Intralesional interferon-α2b has no effect in the treatment of keloids [letter]. *Br J Derm* 1994; **130**: 683.

94. Nedelec B. The effect of interferon-α2b on wound contraction and scar contractures. *PhD Thesis*, University of Alberta, 1997.

95. Dao T, Ariyasu T, Holan V, Minowada J. Natural human interferon-α augments apoptosis in activated T cell line. *Cell Immunol* 1994; **155**: 304–11.

96. Egle A, Villunger A, Kos M, *et al.* Modulation of Apo-1/Fas (CD95)-induced programmed cell death in myeloma cells by interferon-α2. *Eur J Immunol* 1996; **26**: 3119–26.

97. Rodriguez-Villanueva J, McDonnell TJ. Induction of apoptotic cell death in non-melanoma skin cancer by interferon-α. *Int J Cancer* 1995; **61**: 110–4.

98. Desmouliere A, Rubbia-Brandt L, Abdiu A, Walz T, Macieira-Coelho A, Gabbiani G. α-smooth muscle actin is expressed in a subpopulation of cultured and cloned fibroblasts and is modulated by γ-interferon. *Exp Cell Res* 1992; **201**: 64–73.

99. McCauley RL, Chopra V, Li Y-Y, Herndon DN, Robson MC. Altered cytokine production in black patients with keloids. *J Clin Immunol* 1992; **12**: 300–8.

100. Bernabei P, Rigamonti L, Ariotti S, Stella M, Castagnoli C, Novelli F. Functional analysis of T lymphocytes infiltrating the dermis and epidermis of post-burn hypertrophic scar tissues. *Burns* 1999; **25**: 43–8.

101. Linares HA. Proteoglycan-lymphocyte association in the development of hypertrophic scars. *Burns* 1990; **16**: 21–4.

102. Castagnoli C, Trombotto C, Ondei S, *et al.* Characterization of T-cell subsets infiltrating post-burn hypertrophic scar tissues. *Burns* 1997; **23**: 565–72.

103. Mosmann TR, Coffman RL. Th1 and Th2 cells: different patterns of lymphokine secretion lead to different functional properties. *Annu Rev Immunol* 1989; **7**: 145–73.

104. Seder RA, Marth T, Sieve MC, *et al.* Factors involved in the differentiation of TGF-β-producing cells from naïve CD4+ T cells: Il-4 and IFN-γ have opposing effects while TGF-β positively regulates its own production. *J Immunol* 1998; **160**: 5719–28.

105. Hunt JP, Hunter CT, Brownstein MR, *et al.* The effector component of the cytotoxic T-lymphocyte response has a biphasic pattern after burn injury. *J Surg Res* 1998; **80**: 243–51.

106. Horgan AF, Mendez MV, O'Riordain DS, Holzheimer RG, Mannick JA, Rodrick ML. Altered gene transcription after burn injury results in depressed T-lymphocyte activation. *Annals Surg* 1994; **220**: 342–51.

107. O'Sullivan ST, Lederer JA, Horgan AF, Chin DH, Mannick JA, Rodrick ML. Major injury leads to predominance of the T helper-2 lymphocyte phenotype and diminished interleukin-12 production associated with decreased resistance to infection. *Annals Surg* 1995; **222**: 482–90.

108. Shi Z, Wakil AE, Rockey DC. Strain-specific differences in mouse hepatic wound healing are mediated by divergent T helper cytokine responses. *Proc Natl Acad Sci USA* 1997; **94**: 10663–8.

Chapter 44

Pathophysiology of the burn scar

Hugo A Linares

Introduction

Cutaneous wound repair is a complex, multistep physiologic, biochemical, cellular, and molecular process of restoring the anatomical and biological integrity of damaged skin. Skin, the largest organ of the body, is multistructural and multifunctional and exhibits substantial regional variations. It is composed of two distinct layers of different embryonic origins, the ectodermal vascular epidermis and the vascularized mesodermal dermis, lying over a fibroadipose connective tissue which, in turn, attaches the skin to the underlying musculoskeletal system. Separating, but at the same time binding, the epidermis and dermis is a zone of attachment called the basement membrane, or epidermal–dermal junction. This biological complex zone (basal membrane zone) is composed of both ectodermal and mesodermal elements. It forms a specialized bridge which integrates epidermis and dermis, and it contains at least three major matrix molecules (laminin, type IV collagen, and bullous pemphigoid antigen) and provides a functional supporting structure for cellular and extracellular activities.[1] Restoration of skin continuity requires ectodermal and mesodermal repair with epithelial resurfacing, synthesis of connective tissue, and active centripetal movements aimed at diminishing a defect. The ability to replace destroyed tissue with identical anatomical and functional structures has been lost during the evolutionary process for most mammalian tissues. Only certain tissues with expanding cell population (i.e. liver) or with cell renewal systems (i.e. epithelium) are capable of a certain degree of regeneration. In general, mesodermal injuries will be repaired through a fibroplastic mechanism (scar formation). Clearly, acceptable wound repair will depend not only on the ability of cells to proliferate, but also on the degree of preservation and reconstruction of the stromal architecture.

Wounds and loss of tissue

Vertical cutaneous injuries, such as surgical incisions which have a minimal loss of tissue, will essentially heal through the formation of a blood clot (fibronectin, plasma glycoprotein), rapid epithelialization, and fibroblast proliferation. Progressive collagenization and increased strength, which reach normal levels within weeks, will complete the healing process and leave imperceptible scarring, in most cases. On the other hand, cutaneous wounds with a predominant horizontal loss of tissue (ulcerations, lacerations, burns) exhibit a healing which proceeds through a variety of mechanisms according to the extent and level of the involved structures. Superficial epidermal damage, with intact basal membrane, requires only the replacement of epithelial cells. Stimulation of physiologic epimorphic mechanisms of epithelial renewal leads to rapid repair. Lesions involving epidermis and superficial dermis (i.e. deep donor site, superficial partial-thickness burns) which leave intact hair follicles or sweat glands, heal by migration of epithelial cells from the edge of the wound and from epithelial appendages together with a prompt and fairly uncomplicated mesenchymal activity. Burn injuries delay epithelial migration, proliferation, and intercellular adhesions (integrins) by 1–2 weeks; and infection further retards this process. Burn injury may also interfere with the normal sequence of growth factors involved in this form of repair.[2] The combined epidermal and dermal healing may leave minimal or no scarring, especially in areas where skin appendages are numerous (i.e. scalp). In full-thickness skin loss where all epithelial sources are destroyed, the reepithelialization occurs only from the edges.

There is a critical level of damage (deep partial-thickness burns) in which mesodermal healing takes between 2 and 6 weeks, and frequently results in abnormal scarring. Most mesenchymal wounds, which are caused by horizontal damage, heal through the formation of granulation tissue. Granulation tissue is a specialized young connective tissue, so called because of its bright red granular surface created by multiple, raised capillary loops which form a structural axis surrounded by cells and extracellular matrix. It is basically a highly cellular, vascular, and fairly organized anatomical, physiologic, and functional structure directed primarily 'to clean' damaged areas (via macrophages), 'to fill' existent gaps (via collagen) and 'to feed' growing active new mesenchymal tissue (via neovessels). It is a very dynamic cellular and extracellular matrix which, in time, will progressively be replaced by a permanent, distinct, mature connective tissue called a scar.[3]

The burn wound

Cutaneous repair after burning is accomplished through a series of complex, biological mechanisms. Burns are very peculiar injuries because they force an organism into a tremendous biological task of equilibrating its deranged internal homeostasis and, at the same time, reconstituting its destroyed protective barrier against the external environment. Paradoxically, the same systemic and potentially damaging inflammatory response triggered by extensive thermal destruction of the cutaneous envelope will provide the basic stimulus for the reconstitution of the skin barrier. A burn wound becomes ischemic, hypoxic, and highly edematous; so healing follows a slow course in comparison with other types of wounds.

The immediate first response is to control the damage produced to the vascular system. A hemorrhage is always sensed by the body as a threat. The first reaction is prompt vasoconstriction, platelet aggregation, and activation of the coagulation system. The ensuing response starts a wide spectrum of structural physiologic actions and reactions guided by molecular signals within the frame of a nonspecific inflammatory response. The initial neurohormonal and immune response is followed by release of mediators (cytokines), by macrophages, and by lymphocytes within a wound. With this active intervention of the host environment, cellular and extracellular elements will converge in order to achieve epidermal and mesenchymal closure of the defect followed by a lengthy period of remodeling (maturation) which may last several months or years. Permanent scarring will result.

The mesenchymal response

Platelets, in contact with thrombin and subendothelial collagen surrounding a vascular gap, not only contribute to hemostasis but

trigger the healing process by releasing a variety of local and circulating growth factors, fibrinopeptides, von Willebrands factor VIII, glycoproteins, vasoactive substances, adenosine diphosphate, chemoattractants, and other inflammatory mediators.[4,5] A classic inflammatory response involving intravascular and extravascular processes is then evoked. Proteases not only attack the damaged tissue but, as a product of their activity, promote the formation of important peptides which locally and systemically elicit the activity of different systems of defense. Liberated peptides provide the signals for chemotactic attraction of leukocytes, monocytes, and mast cells; they also provide the amino acid essentials for the protein synthesis which is required for the reparative process.

Polymorphonuclear leukocytes, in a rapid response to the messages sent by platelets and also through factors produced by the activation of the complement system, form the first line of defense against local bacterial contamination. Usually within 24–72 hours, the polymorphonuclear cells will gradually be superseded by monocytes which acquire the characteristics of tissue macrophages and become a central mediator of the process. The macrophages not only help to clean a wounded area of undesirable debris and bacteria (including effete neutrophils) but, through the release of biologically active mediators (growth factors, enzymes, reactive oxygen intermediates, prostaglandins, etc.), stimulate the attraction of the fibroblasts to the area.[6]

It has been demonstrated that activated T lymphocytes, following the influx of neutrophils and macrophages, enter a wound area by day 4 or 5 and become an important part of the modulation of the healing process.[7,8] The polymorphonuclear leukocyte has been claimed to be nonessential to the wound healing process in the absence of bacterial contamination. On the contrary, activated macrophages and T lymphocytes are a consistent part of the repair mechanisms. Macrophages are essential for fibroblast function; the presence of an intact T-cell immune system is essential, at least indirectly, for a normal healing outcome.[9] An adequate balance of monokines and cytokines, which have both stimulatory and inhibitory activity, will lead to a regulated normal repair.[7]

Granulation tissue

Granulation tissue is the framework for the repair processes and provides provisional support for the resurfacing epithelium.[4–6,10] Fibroblasts, macrophages, and new blood vessels form a structural trinity embedded in a loose, gel-like, extracellular matrix of collagen, hyaluronic acid, fibronectin, and other glycosaminoglycans which move into a wound space as a unit under the direction and regulation of orchestrated biomolecular messages.[10] Fibronectin, a glycoprotein found in serum, precedes the appearance of collagen which later is deposited in a fibronectin-bearing matrix. Fibronectin gives direction to migrating processes and disappears as soon as mature collagen bundles are formed.[11] Through a variety of still not well understood mechanisms, an ambivalent activity will promote the growth of this reparative tissue. The same cellular and molecular structures aimed at destroying and eliminating wounded tissue will now change functions and will proceed to a very opposite task, which is the build up of a new connective tissue (cells and extracellular matrix), first as a provisory assurance of tissue continuity and later as a permanent fibrous bridge between the edges of the wound (scarring).

There is increasing evidence that the complex processes involving the formation and activity of granulation tissue, as well as other aspects of wound healing, are highly influenced by a group of multifunctional polypeptides (growth factors, cytokines). These substances may influence *angiogenesis* by transforming growth factor alpha and beta (TGFα, TGFβ), fibroblast growth factor (FGF), tumor necrosis factor alpha (TNFα), or platelet-derived endothelial cell growth factor (PDECGF). They also affect *collagenogenesis* by TGFβ, platelet-derived growth factor (PDGF), or insulin-like like growth factor (IGF). Further, they influence *fibroblast proliferation* and *activation* via PDGF and macrophage-derived proliferation factor (MDPF). *Epithelial cell proliferation* is altered via epidermal growth factor (EGF), TGFα and basic fibroblast growth factor (bFGF). These polypeptides can also regulate *chemotaxis* by influencing interleukin-1 (IL-1) and IL-6, or *contraction* via endothelin-1.[12–14] TGF seems to be essential in attracting the right cells to a wound area and promoting the stimulation of angiogenesis as well as a variety of cells involved in wound healing, including epithelial cells and fibroblasts.[15] The TGF family of five different peptides seems to have a unique and specific intervention in the building regulation of the extracellular matrix and in control over cell–matrix and cell–cell interaction mediated by integrin receptors.[16] Multifunctional activities of most of these polypeptides are unclear. At different times or concentrations, they may be stimulators or inhibitors to one another and to other wound healing processes.[17–19]

The 'Feeding' Network

One of the main developing features of granulation tissue is the formation of a capillary network. Capillaries originating as sprouts of proliferating endothelial cells from the vascular net of viable connective tissue, which surrounds the hyperlactated, acidotic, and hypoxic wounded area, form the axis of each of the 'red granules' of the wound bed. The anoxic environment of the wound not only stimulates fibroblasts but induces macrophages to secrete angiogenic factors.[20] The newly formed vessels run predominantly parallel to each other and perpendicular to the open surface of the wound; to some extent, they send off lateral sprouts to their neighbors' capillaries, thereby producing an arced plexus. The development of new capillaries follows a sequence of structural and biochemical steps, beginning with the vasodilation of a preexisting vessel (usually another capillary or a venule). This facilitates the arrival of messages sent through angiogenic factors to stimulate the migration of endothelial cells from the donor vessel. The stimulated endothelial cell produces plasminogen activator and collagenase, which degrade the basement membrane of the vessel wall. The endothelial cells then migrate, proliferate, and mature. In as little as 24–36 hours, it is possible histologically to detect the formation of capillary sprouts and the progressive formation of a capillary tube which includes a new basement membrane and pericytes.[21] The leakiness of the new interendothelial junctions frequently results in edema.[22]

Fibroblasts

Fibroblasts are of the juvenile type, with a large and hyperchromatic nucleus, one or more prominent nucleoli, intense cytoplasmic basophilia, and a plump fusiform or stellate appearance. They demonstrate an increased amount of ribonucleoproteins and an active synthesis of proteoglycans and collagen. In the beginning, the fibroblasts are loosely and irregularly arranged and lay down collagen fibers which first run in a predominantly parallel orientation with respect to the neovessels. As the granulation tissue matures and gets older, the new formed collagen fibers tend to be oriented parallel to the surface, at right angles to the direction of the growing neovessels and usually parallel also to the lines of tension. This pattern of orientation is lost on hypertrophic scars, as will be described later[23] (**Figure 44.1**). Because of the sequenced growing of the granulation tissue, it is possible to distinguish in the same histological section the younger, superficial, unorganized layer from the progressively dense fibroplastic organized, older, and deeper layer. Fibroblasts synthetize many of the components of the extracellular matrix, including glycosaminoglycans (proteoglycans), fibronectin, laminin, and elastic fibers.

Collagen

Collagen, the most common mammalian protein and an essential product of fibroblasts, will undergo structural modifications so as to provide adequate tensile strength. At least 17 types of collagen have been already described. Of those, the most known in skin are the types I, III, IV, V, VI, and VII. The fibrillar types I, III and V, and the beaded filaments type VI, are normal components of dermal collagen. The sheet forming collagen IV, fibrillar type V, anchoring forming collagen VII, and collagen XVII are found at the dermoepidermal interface.[24,25] Fibrillar collagens I and III are the primary fibroplastic molecules associated with granulation tissue and the development of scars. Type III forms within 24 hours after injury, while type I and its precursor molecules can be seen between 4 and 7 days.[26,27] Type III fibrillar collagen is produced first and is the most abundant.[28] The high lactate and low oxygen concentration in the wound alters the normal skin I:III collagen ratio and regulates collagen synthesis and deposition.[29] This is gradually reversed, and as healing progresses, type I collagen becomes predominant. Mature dermal tissue has a normal I:III collagen ratio of 4:1;[30] however, this normal proportion is never achieved by scar tissue.

Proteoglycans

Fibroblasts produce and secrete several complex carbohydrates, and many of them are associated with proteins (glycosaminoglycans/proteoglycans). Proteoglycans are very versatile and striking molecules with essential functions. They interact with other substances and cells, and they bind to several extracellular matrix molecules, cell–cell adhesion molecules, and growth factors.[31] Proteoglycans have one or more attached glycosaminoglycan chains covalently bound to a core protein. The core protein molecular structure has been recommended as the base for the classification of proteoglycans.[32] It is possible to differentiate at least five groups according to their molecular sizes and site of activity:[33]

- large extracellular proteoglycans with multiple glycosaminoglycan chains (aggrecan, versican, perlecan);
- small connective tissue proteoglycans with no more than two chains (decorin, biblycan, fibromodulin);
- basement membrane heparan sulfate proteoglycans;
- cell surface proteoglycans (syndecan, betaglycan, thrombomodulin); and
- intracellular proteoglycans (serglycin).

The role of proteoglycans in the wound healing process (i.e. regulation of collagen fibrillogenesis) is currently a subject of great

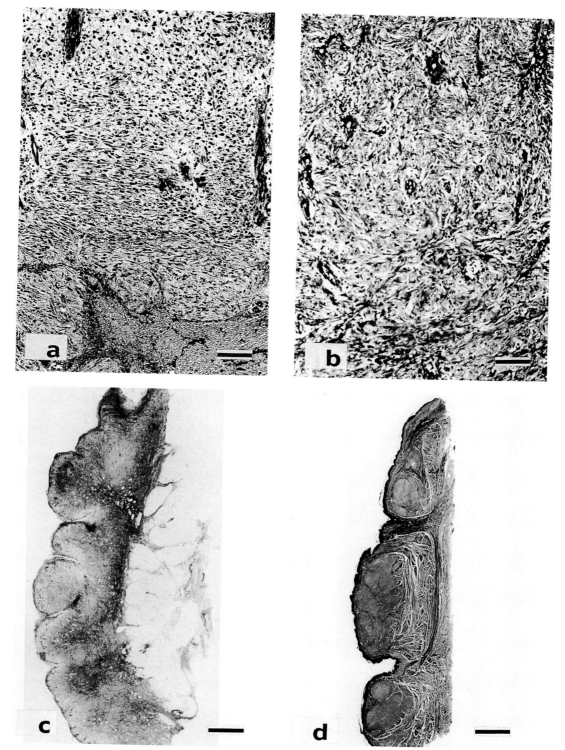

Fig. 44.1 Granulation tissue. (a) Normal healing with a predominant parallel orientation of collagen fibers. Masson stain. Bar 100 m. (b) Granulation tissue leading to a hypertrophic healing showing the collagen fibers in a predominant whorl-like pattern. Masson stain. Bar 100 μm. (c) and (d) Hypertrophic granulation tissue matching the developed hypertrophic scar depicted in (d). Masson stain c: Bar 1 mm; (d) Bar 2.5 mm.

interest.[34,35] Early in granulation tissue, fibroblasts deposit a matrix of fibronectin and hyaluronic acid which promotes cell migration and proliferation. Later, fibroblasts produce collagen and proteo-

glycan matrix, which increase tissue tensile strength and resilience.[6,36] It has been suggested that fibronectin may be essential in the organization of the granulation tissue matrix and may form the scaffold in which collagen is organized, in addition to sending chemotactic signals for neutrophils and macrophages.[37]

Hyaluronic acid is the most abundant glycosaminoglycan present during the first week of healing and has its highest concentration at about 5 days after injury. It is required for fibroblast mitosis.[38] Gradually, the concentration of hyaluronic acid diminishes in favor of dermatan sulfate and chondroitin sulfate (decorin, versican, aggrecan) which peak at about 2 weeks after wounding so as to progressively decline in the following weeks.[39] These macromolecules are an integral part of the healing process and are the proteoglycans which actively participate in the differentiation and stabilization of the connective tissue extracellular matrix.

Contraction

About 1 week post-injury, when fibrillar collagen type I starts to build up the strength of the fibrous tissue, another mechanism commences. Along with efforts to epithelialize a denuded area, an organism tries also to achieve a spatial reduction of a wounded area by means of centripetal movements of the surrounding skin and shrinkage of the wound contents. This active process of contraction is in contrast to the deforming contracture which is a late end result. The contractile forces, it is suggested, are produced by fibroblasts and their functional and structural phenotypic modulated versions, the myofibroblast.[40,41] A specialized interconnection of intracellular actin-like microfilaments and extracellular fibronectin across the cellular membrane of the myofibroblast form a cohesive complex of cell–cell and cell–matrix links, called a 'fibronexus'.[42] Contraction should cease when its force is exceeded by the opposite force of the surrounding skin[43] (**Figure 44.2**).

The process of reepithelialization

Within hours after injury, epithelial cells from wound margins or adnexal structures, if a wound is superficial, will initiate a series of specific mechanisms, directed to cover a new surface. In burns, this epithelial response may be delayed up to several days. The early phases of the reepithelialization process are marked by the centripetal and epibolic migration of epithelial cells from the margins of the wound. This is followed within 24–48 hours by the proliferation of new cells behind the migrating front to provide an additional population of cells to cover the gap.[44] The rate of movement varies from 0.1 to 1 mm per day according to local conditions. The initial stimulus is largely unknown, but several possible mechanisms have been suggested. The migration may be induced by loss of attachment to neighboring damaged cells ('free edge effect'), active contact guidance, or the presence of soluble mediators such as fibronectin, chalones, epibolin, or PDGF. Cellular proliferation may be assisted by EGF.[45,46] Through phenotype modulation (cellular metamorphosis), the epidermal basal cells lose their desmosomes and hemidesmosomes; and the intracellular tonofilaments are retracted, form peripheral actin filaments (pseudopodia), and express fibronectin receptors.[46] This change in phenotype, similar to the one observed in cultured epidermal cells, has been called regenerative maturation.[47,48] The cells, without hemidesmosomal links, start their lamellipodial crawling over a provisional matrix of fibrin, fibrinogen, fibronectin, and tenascin while secreting plasminogen activators and collagenases in order

to open a way through desiccated tissues. The cells migrate on fibronectin using integrin receptors.[49] Fibronectin and thrombospondin promote keratinocyte mobility while laminin, an adhesion factor in intact epidermis, is lost after wounding.[1] The mechanisms involved in the epithelial movement are controversial and include the 'leapfrog model' (pulling and sliding), whereby cells above and behind the leading cell stream over the latter to attach to the wound bed,[50] or the model of the formation of a chain of cells which advances while individual cells maintain their original position in the chain.[46] It seems that in the skin the epithelial cells migrate in clusters or sheets of cells rather than in a single dissociated cell migration as seen in the monolayer epithelia of the cornea.[44] These cellular activities need a new supporting structure to replace the damaged original basement membrane and facilitate movement. Epithelial cells traverse the surface of granulation tissue by gliding over a new provisional matrix synthesized by themselves.[51] It seems that a fibronectin substrate, a critical component, appears first and is gradually supplemented by collagen IV, heparin sulfate and, finally, laminin.[52]

Epithelial reparation and granulation tissue formation take place simultaneously. Both of these processes advance through devitalized tissue to cover a wound. This is accomplished by the release from the advancing epithelium of several proteases, including collagenase to denature collagen and plasminogen to dissolve blood clots. Epithelial cells advance more rapidly if the wound bed has adequate humidity.[53,54] For this reason, if enough devitalized tissue still covers the area, the leading cellular front seeks a more favorable environment by gliding underneath the eschar, crust, or scab. The epithelial migration ceases when the advancing epithelium meets its counterpart growing from the opposite direction. The microvillous processes of the encountering cells contact one another and form attachments which could result in contact inhibitions. The cells which were migrating in a lateral motion across the wound surface then regain the normal vertical direction of differentiation toward the surface so as to become cornified cells. Probably laminin is the 'stop signal' to cease the horizontal motion and start ascending vertically.[55] The same migrating epidermal cells, from the wound margins inwards, will reconstitute the basal membrane which is discernible by day 5 and exhibits complete development 2 weeks post-injury.[26]

The beginning of a permanent scar

When the migrating epithelium has completed resurfacing the new connective tissue matrix, the building up of granulation tissue stops. The mechanisms involved in the termination of the healing processes are largely unknown, although the intervention of angiogenic inhibitor factors may be an important feature. The former granulation tissue becomes true scar tissue, and is inelastic and somewhat brittle. The tensile strength, which initially is very low, increases in subsequent weeks as the scar matures, although it never regains the strength of the original tissue.[56]

The remodeling of the collagen meshwork includes increased crosslinking, breakdown activity of collagenases, decrease in glycosaminoglycans, regression of the capillary neovascularity, maintenance of an adequate I:III collagen ratio, and reorientation of collagen fibers in response to mechanical stress. The latter is a very characteristic feature of normal scarring in which collagen bundles of the dermis run in a distinct parallel orientation with

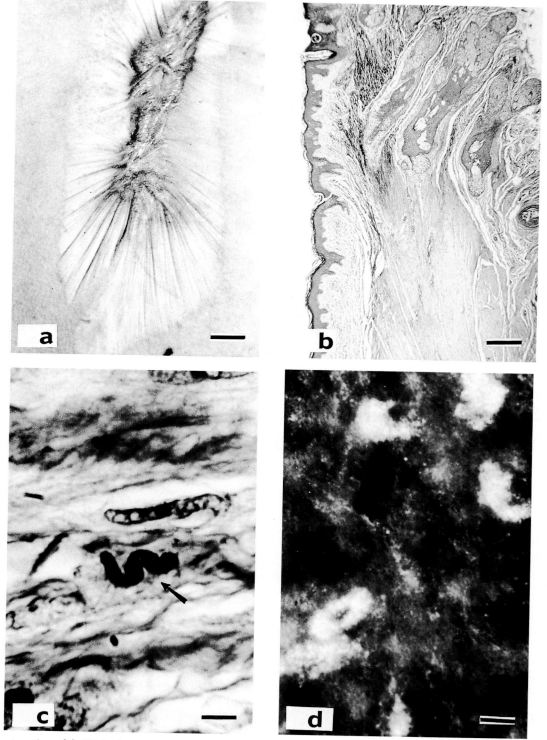

Fig. 44.2 Contraction. (a) Clinical appearance of a scar with clear contraction marks. Bar 1 cm. (b) Histological appearance showing the stretched morphology of the dermal tissue due to contraction. Movat stain. Bar 100 μm. (c) Contracted myofibroblast (arrow) Masson stain. Bar 10 μm. (d) Immunocytoplasmic labeling of myofibroblasts with human antismooth muscle serum followed by antihuman IgG. Immunofluorescence. Bar 10 μm.

respect to the surface of the skin. Clinically, the original redness, elevation, and firm consistency of the new scar tissue gradually evolves into a pale, flat, soft scar tissue which is level with the adjacent skin surface. This phase of 'maturation' includes a gradual replacement of the original scar tissue over a period of at least 6 months.

Wound healing interferences

It is obvious that any factor capable of disturbing the complex mechanisms of tissue repair will interfere with adequate wound healing. The more common problems are associated with:

- local factors (impaired circulation, denervation, infection, mechanical stress, foreign bodies, dehiscence, trauma);
- systemic factors (age, nutritional deficits, illness, metabolic disturbances); or
- iatrogenia (surgical technique and material, medications, physicochemical treatments).

These adverse wound conditions will increase the possibility of abnormal healing, either hypotrophic or hypertrophic.

Abnormal healing

The healing of a wound is a very complex nonspecific process which requires a delicate equilibrium of opposing actions. Cell proliferation must be balanced by cell necrosis, and collagenosis must be paired with collagenolysis, and angiogenesis with capillary obliteration. A resulting scar may be depressed with respect to the surrounding normal skin level, show hypotrophic or even atrophic tissue features, be darker or lighter than the surrounding skin, or become hypertrophic.

The distinction between keloids and hypertrophic scars

The differentiation between true, genuine, spontaneous, or idiopathic keloid, and false, spurious, traumatic, or cicatricial keloid was introduced by Alibert almost 200 years ago, leading to a controversy which still continues.[57]

According to Alibert, true keloids have a lancinating, pungent, and burning pruritus with a painful sensation, while false keloids result only from inflammation of a scar after burns or ulcerations. Although this division was generally accepted in the beginning, the false keloid started to be designated as a cicatrix, warty tumor of the cicatrix, or vegetations of the cicatrix. By the end of the nineteenth century, 'hypertrophic scar' became a differentiating term. It is in Kaposi's chapter on keloids, in 1874,[58] that the differentiation among 'true keloid, cicatricial keloid, and hypertrophied scar' was first made. He stated that scars 'which remain within the limits of the loss of substance of the skin represent so-called hypertroid scars, looking, however, exactly like keloids. Does this kind of scar belong also to the class of false, or cicatricial keloids? Where does keloid cease; and where does hypertrophied scar commence? Or is it probable that the so-called spontaneous keloid is only hypertrophied scar?' Since then, repeated efforts have been made to solve such a controversial issue. Perhaps two of the most currently used criteria of differentiation are that keloids exceed the limits of the initial injury as defined by Kaposi in 1874[58] and that keloids have conspicuous thick, glassy, faintly retractile collagen bundles, as described by Blackburn and Cosman in 1966.[59] Histologic studies show that the growing of scars over the limits of a wound is related not only to the activity of the scar itself but also to the structure and opposing forces of the surrounding normal tissue. This 'trespass' of boundaries may be seen in clinically diagnosed hypertrophic scars as well as in scars clinically classified as keloids. Also, thick, glassy, faintly retractile collagen bundles may be seen in the same histologic section of a scar sharing large areas with collagen bundles of opposite characteristics[60] (**Figure 44.3**). Several biochemical profiles of skin and scar samples have shown that hypertrophic scar and keloid are not distinct pathologic entities, but are similar aberrations with quantitative differences, and keloids show greater deviation from normal healing.[61–63] We support the concept that the differences are essentially quantitative and that keloids are extreme variants of hypertrophic scars. Therefore, no distinction will be made, and thus hypertrophic scars as well as keloids will be termed either as hypertrophic healing or as hypertrophic scars, unless the term keloid is used to maintain a specific reference.

Toward a hypertrophic healing

The development of a new mesenchymal matrix in granulation tissue follows a fairly predictable pattern, as was previously described for normal wound healing. At the surface of normal granulation tissue, fibroblasts and collagen fibers have a predominant parallel orientation with respect to the vertical proliferating neovessels. In the lower layer, however, collagen fibers and fibroblasts adopt a transverse orientation with respect to the neovessels and a parallel orientation with respect to the surface of the skin (see **Figure 44.1a**). By the time a wound is completely reepithelialized and the granulation phase is complete, all the collagen fibers of the dermis will present the predominant parallel orientation which is characteristic of normotrophic scars (see **Figure 44.4b**).

In previous works, it has been shown that the events differentiating normal healing from hypertrophic healing actually start during the development of granulation tissue and become fairly evident 3–5 weeks after injury.[64,65] One of the most notable differences is the orientation of collagen fibers. If the healing process will result in hypertrophic healing, it is possible to see, in the granulation tissue, a tendency for collagen fibers to run in a haphazard direction with a tendency toward a whorl-like pattern which is characteristic of hypertrophic scars (see **Figure 44.1b**).

Although the cell population of granulation tissue, as seen with light microscopy, does not show qualitative differences between normal and hypertrophic development, they show a marked difference in their cyclic evolution. The structural characteristic of immature connective tissue, which normally disappears within several weeks, will persist for several months if hypertrophic healing develops. In many cases, a chronic inflammatory reaction of variable degree may persist. The collagen pattern, persistent cellularity, abundance and composition of proteoglycans, and the prolonged chronic inflammatory reaction are the most common morphologic features which distinguish hypertrophic healing from normal healing.[66–68]

Clinical appearance and histiotypic organization

Hypertrophic scars are depicted as tumor-like lesions raised above the level of the skin with a wide spectrum of variations in shape, size, color, and consistency. These characteristics usually correspond to the site and extent of an injury, time of evolution, and individual susceptibility. In certain areas (chest, shoulders, lobules of the ears) the hypertrophic healing tends to be prominent, nodular, pedunculated or semipedunculated, round or oval, smooth and

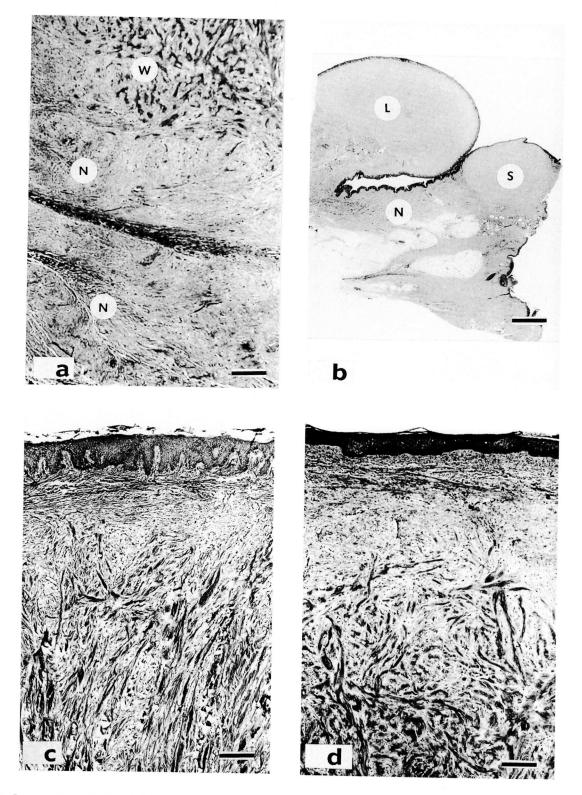

Fig. 44.3 Scars differentiation. (a) Hypertrophic healing showing two different collagen patterns in the same section: whorls (W) and nodules (N). Masson stain. Bar 100 μm. (b) Two hypertrophic scars (S and L) bridged by a section of normal skin (N). The hypertrophic scar (S) shows a moderate expansion above the level of the normal skin (N) while the hypertrophic scar (L) shows the excessive tumor-like growth producing the 'trespass' of the original limits of the wound. HE stain. Bar 3 mm. (c and d) Hypertrophic healing with rete ridges (c) compared to a hypertrophic healing without rete ridges as depicted in (d) Masson stain. Bar 100 μm.

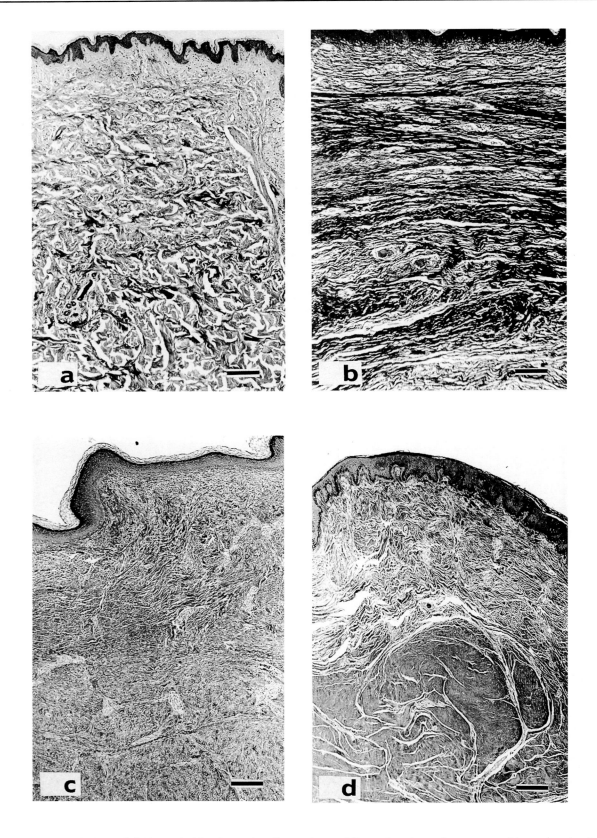

Fig. 44.4 Histomorphology. (a) Normal skin. Dermal collagen in a tridimensional regular pattern. Masson stain. Bar 200 μm. (b) Normotrophic healing. Dermal collagen in a parallel orientation. Masson stain. Bar 100 μm.
(c) Hypertrophic healing. Dermal collagen in a predominant whorl-like pattern. Masson stain. Bar 100 μm.
(d) Hypertrophic healing. Dermal collagen in a predominant nodular pattern. Masson stain. Bar 100 μm.

shiny, hard, and somewhat elastic. In other areas, it usually has an irregular surface and is rarely elevated more than 15–20 mm above the level of the surrounding skin. The edges are usually prominent and end abruptly, sometimes with finger-like or chain-like prolongations. Initially, a scar is red or pink (so-called immature); but after a period of time, months or even years, the scar flattens, softens, and blanches (maturation). In immature scars, redness and turgidity are due to increased active vascularity. Immature scars sometimes display a minute pinkish, bluish, or purplish superficial net of small blood vessels. The scar does not adhere to the subcutaneous tissue and appears to grossly exceed the limits of the original injury[60] (see **Figure 44.3b**).

Histologically, the appearance of a scar depends on the evolutionary state during which a sample is taken. Also, scars from different anatomical sites display histologic differences. Those located on ears or shoulders show very broad, thick collagen fibers more frequently than scars from other sites. It is also possible to observe that there is no 'invasion' of surrounding normal tissues but that the overgrown healing really pushes apart the surrounding normal tissue without invading it. The gross anatomy appearance of lesions which exceed the limits of the original injury appears to be produced by tumor-like growth pushing the epithelium upward. This suggests that the clinical appearance will depend, in part, on the forces generated by the opposing superficial layers of the skin in the area and on the skin's resistance to deformation.

The histologic appearance of the epidermis is also variable. It may appear hyperplastic, with visible rete ridges, or thin and smooth. The typical histologic features of the hypertrophic healing reside in the reticularis layer of the dermis. In early stages, there is hypercellularity (fibroblasts, myofibroblasts) and hypervascularity. The collagen fibers run in curvilinear, whorl-like arrangements which, in most cases, progress to distinct nodular forms. Whorls and nodules may be seen in the same histologic section[66] (**Figure 44.4**). These structures never involve the subcutaneous tissue, from which they are often separated by somewhat compact parallel bands of connective tissue with nearly normal characteristics. The increased cellular population is composed of young, active fibroblasts and myofibroblasts. Mast cells appear increased over the number observed in normal skin. Plasma cells and lymphocytes are usually present at the beginning of the formation of a scar and form a perivascular cuff, which may persist for a long time as scattered foci or chronic inflammation. The vascular structure is prominent and the capillary network appears to follow the arrangement of the collagen fibers. Skin appendages are atrophic, destroyed, or displaced by the scar. At times they do not slough, but elicit a foreign-body reaction. Usually, no elastic tissue can be found except in the papillary areas of the dermis and in the normal dermal areas surrounding the scar. The interstitium shows a significant amount of ground substance (glycosaminoglycans), which has been shown to contain an elevated amount of chondroitin-4-sulfate.[68]

With time, the thickened hyaline fibers of nodules and whorls become elongated and elastic fibers reappear. This is indicative of a regression pattern, which proceeds toward 'mature' scar. The reorientation of the collagen fibers in a parallel arrangement, as found with nonhypertrophic healing, is accompanied by a progressively reduced number of fibroblasts and myofibroblasts, and a pronounced decrease in vascularization, which corresponds to the flattening, blanching, and softening of a mature scar described above. Tissue structure never recovers its original appearance.

Scanning electron microscopy

Under a scanning electron microscope (SEM), nodules appear as fused masses of tissue in stark contrast to the adjacent collagen filaments and fibers. The individual collagen filaments present in normal skin are rarely seen. The dermal matrix appears as an adhesive mass of material, as though the filaments were 'glued' together. Fiber diameter is about one-half to three-quarters that of normal skin, and cross-stranding is frequent. The large bands of collagen appear also to be oriented in every direction except directly across the wound.[69,70]

Transmission electron microscopy

The modules of active hypertrophic scars consist of tightly packed collagen with a reduced amount of total interstitial space. The collagen filaments have a predominant diameter of 600 Å (60 nm). The lumen of the vessels is often partially or completely occluded, and the basal lamina in most of the vessels is greatly thickened. In early stages, the number of fibroblasts and myofibroblasts is significant. Fibroblasts have an active appearance, with vast arrays of rough endoplasmic reticulum and Golgi membranes. Myofibroblasts appear with folded or grooved nuclei containing fine contractile filaments, and with a variable number of free ribosomes, mitochondria, glycogen, vacuoles, and pinocytotic vesicles. The structural appearance of hypertrophic scars under electron microscopy parallels that under light microscopy at any stage of hypertrophic healing.[70]

In search of etiopathogenic explanations

The biological mechanisms responsible for the deviation of the normal healing process toward an excessive reparative response are still elusive. The lack of a reproducible laboratory animal models adds a very frustrating circumstance. On the other hand, increasing technology and firm interest from many researchers are providing, piece by piece, the elements which hopefully will solve the hypertrophic healing puzzle.

The Collagen/Fibroblast Factor

Evidently, the most visible feature of a hypertrophic scar is the excess of collagen deposition, suggesting that the essential balance between collagen synthesis and degradation is missing. An increased proline hydroxylase activity and an increased collagenase activity insufficient to counteract the exuberant collagen synthesis have been described by many authors.[71–73] Despite equal or increased levels of activity of lysyl oxidase, it seems that hypertrophic scars have a decreased content of highly crosslinked collagen and also an increased amount of soluble collagen.[63,74,75] A proper degradation of collagen may be inhibited by the action of α_1-antitrypsin and α_2-macroglobulin which were found in the extracellular matrix of hypertrophic scars.[71,76] Some researchers report a significant increase in the I:III collagen ratio,[77] while others describe just the opposite.[78,79] Since the report from Conway et al.,[80] which describes the characteristics of cultured fibroblasts in keloids and hypertrophic scars, an increased number of workers have followed this line of research. Diegelmann[81] shows that cultured keloid fibroblasts synthesize two to three times more collagen than normal skin fibroblasts, without significant differences in collagen degradation rate. An intriguing observation was made by Abergel et al.[77] that the increase in collagen synthesis was not a constant characteristic of keloids. It was speculated that the heterogeneous population of normal skin fibroblasts which can strongly differ in the amount of collagen synthesized among them may be also reflected in keloid fibroblast cultures. Thus, it may be that keloids have a normal or a very high production of collagen.[82,83] Although the growth of keloid fibroblasts is normal, the cells seem to be modulated to some specific function, such as the production of more collagen.[81] Cultures with an excessive production of collagen may also have high levels of type 1 collagen-specific mRNA which suggest a loss of regulatory control at the transcriptional level.[77,82]

Two conflicting reports of similar studies raise some speculation about the possibility of racial factors and also reflect the concept that production of collagen is not the sole problem in hypertrophic healing. Procollagen synthesis was found to be increased in five of nine keloid fibroblast cultures from black patients,[77] while, despite increased levels of intracellular prolyl-4-hydroxylase and glucosyltransferase, a normal synthesis was found in eight of nine keloid fibroblast cultures from white patients.[83] The initial rate of collagen synthesis in hypertrophic scars is about twice that in normotrophic scars and fell to the same level as in normal scars about 2–3 years after injury.[84]

The Glycosaminoglycan/Proteoglycan Factor

Proteoglycans affect the ultimate physical characteristic of the mature collagen within a scar because of their intervention in the extracellular formation of collagen fibrils. They influence the aggregation of collagen monomers.[85] There is evidence from a variety of studies that the composition of glycosaminoglycans and proteoglycans in wound healing and in hypertrophic healing differs from normal skin. While, in normal skin, human dermis shows a much greater amount of decorin than chondroitin sulfate proteoglycans, the reverse occurs in granulation tissues and scars.[86] In particular, chondroitin-4-sulfate has been identified as the main contributor to the striking increase of proteoglycan levels in hypertrophic scars.[68,87] It has also been demonstrated that the strong association between collagen and proteoglycans in hypertrophic scars may prevent collagenase from breaking down collagen. The excessive presence of chondroitin-4-sulfate may contribute to the overabundance of collagen deposition which is characteristic of hypertrophic scars.[67,88] Furthermore, it has been observed that, in hypertrophic scars, there is a persistent presence of a perivascular cuff of variable density, mainly composed of lymphocytes[60,66] and that the proteoglycan associated with this perivascular T-cell infiltration is mainly chondroitin-4-sulfate.[89] Fibroblasts derived from hypertrophic scars incorporated proportionally more radiolabeled precursors into chondroitin sulfate and hyaluronic acid in vitro than did normal skin fibroblasts.[90]

Other Factors

The immunological explanation has been explored by several researchers. Chytilova et al. were able to produce hypertrophic healing in rabbits, during the course of autoimmune disease, by the repeated injection of lyophilized autologous skin.[91] People who carry HLA-B14 or HLA-Bw16 antigens have been shown to have a greater risk of developing hypertrophic healing;[92,93] but it was also found that there were no significant differences in the incidence of HLA-A and B antigens in keloid and nonkeloid formers.[94] Abdalla-Osman et al. developed a sebum autoimmune theory.[95] Other researchers found antinuclear antibodies directed against fibroblasts in those who form keloids and increased levels of IgA, IgG, and IgM.[96] Immunoperoxidase techniques performed on hypertrophic scar sections showed an anomalous expression of HLA class II molecules on keratinocytes and fibroblasts and dense infiltrates of IL-2R positive cells and Langerhans (CD1) cells.[97,98] Fibroblasts from hypertrophic healing were shown as having an increased fibronectin production, suggesting the presence of specific mechanisms controlling fibronectin expression.[99] A heavy fibronectin deposition was found to be predominantly located in the nodular structures of hypertrophic healing sections.[100] A recent study showed an increased production of IL-6, TNF and IFN in hypertrophic healing, suggesting that the altered levels of immunoregulatory cytokines may play a significant role in the overproduction of collagen.[101] It has been also suggested that the excessive and inappropriate action of TGF may promote abnormal healing.[102–105]

The search for solutions

Therapeutic solutions to hypertrophic scars have been met with the same degree of confusion and controversy as their morphologic and etiopathogenic descriptions. Proposed solutions have been innumerable, but in most instances frustration has been the net result. Unfortunately, the present state of knowledge of the etiopathogenic mechanisms responsible for hypertrophic healing is still inadequate to formulate a sound biological basis for a routinely effective treatment. It is possible to achieve, if not ideal, at least satisfactory results with several different approaches using surgical, pharmacologic, and physical methods. Surgery, corticoids, and pressure, alone or in combination, are currently the most universally used methods of treatment. Because of the altered disposition of collagen fibers in dermal hypertrophic healing and the possibility of modifying it by mechanical methods, a special consideration concerning the use of pressure may be worthwhile. (**Figure 44.5**). The influence of mechanical forces on the clinical course of hypertrophic scarring has been known for centuries, although it was not until recent years that its use was particularly stressed. As early as in the sixteenth century, Ambroise Paré advised: 'if the scar be too big, or high, it shall be plained by making convenient ligation and straight binding to the part a Plate of Lead rubbed over with Quick Silver'.[106] It was not until the early 1970s that the use of pressure for the treatment of hypertrophic scars and contractures after burns became a standard treatment in every burn facility. This universal use of pressure originated and was promoted by the Shriners Burns Institute at Galveston.[106] As was described in the preceding pages, a granulation tissue showing collagen fibers in a disorganized, whorl-like arrangement will develop into hypertrophic scarring. If pressure is applied for a variable period of time, however, the collagen fibers will modify their disorganized orientation and will adopt a definite parallel arrangement which is characteristic of the pattern of the granulation tissue which leads to normotrophic healing. Likewise, under constant pressure, the whorl-like arrangement of collagen fibers and nodular formation seen in immature hypertrophic scars assumes a progressive predominantly parallel arrangement similar to that found in normotrophic scars (**Figure 44.6**). Constant pressure will decrease the vascularity, decrease the

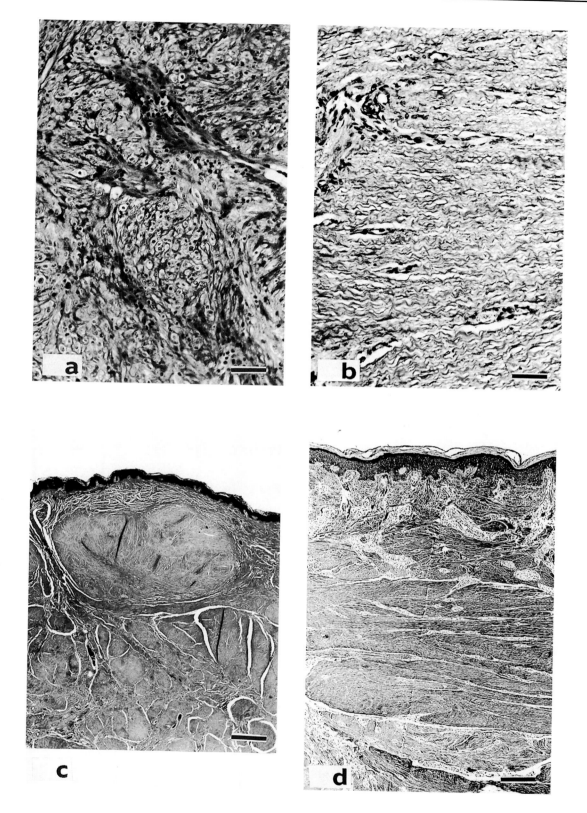

Fig. 44.5 Influence of pressure. (a) Granulation tissue with collagen fibers in a whorl-like pattern. Masson stain. Bar 100 μm. (b) Granulation tissue after 25 days of pressure showing the 'parallelization' of the collagen fibers. Masson stain. Bar 100 μm. (c) Hypertrophic healing with collagen fibers in a nodular pattern. Masson stain. Bar 250 μm. (d) Hypertrophic healing after several months of pressure showing the 'parallelization' of the collagen fibers. Masson stain. Bar 150 μm.

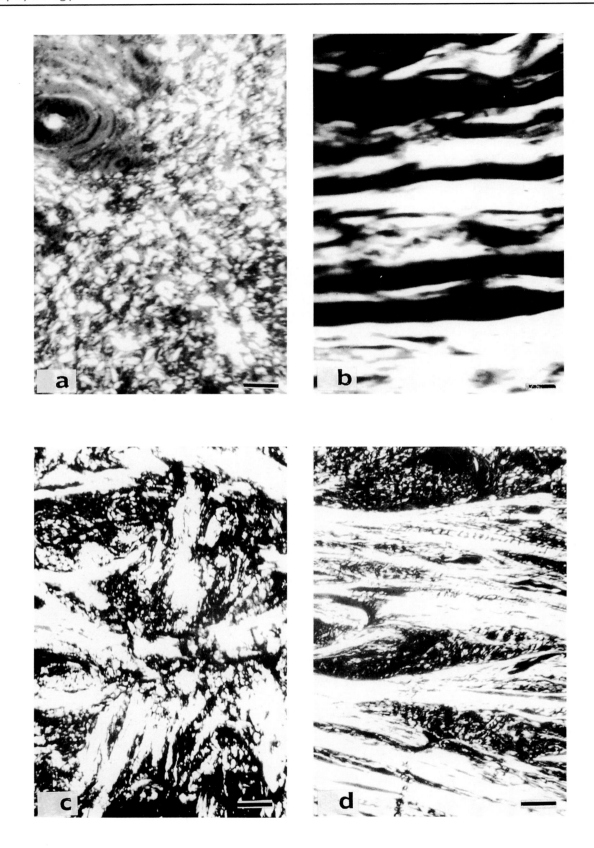

Fig. 44.6 Polarized light pictures of collagen fibers depicting (a) the tridimensional pattern of collagen in normal skin, (b) the parallel orientation in normotrophic scars, (c) the whorl-like arrangement in hypertrophic scars, and (d) the 'parallelization' of collagen fibers after pressure. (a–d) Bar 200 μm.

tissue partial pressure of oxygen, decrease the amount of proteo-glycans, and decrease the cellular response as well as the collagen deposition (**Figure 44.7**).[107–110]

Toward the future

Recent progress in molecular biology has shown that many cell functions are brought about by an interaction among macromole-cules. The binding between macromolecules, therefore, has far-reaching physiologic implications. The study of proteoglycans in hypertrophic scars can be of great interest because the organiza-tion of collagen fibrils in tissues may be related to amounts and kinds of proteoglycans, and because the binding of proteoglycans to collagen can influence fibril formation. Research should include the study of factors which influence the structure, migration, func-tion, and modulation of the cells which control the synthesis and degradation of the intercellular matrix. In essesnce, the leading cells are ten: neutrophils, eosinophils, basophils, monocytes, T-lymphocytes, B-lymphocytes, natural killer cells, platelets, endothelial cells, and fibroblasts. All of these or their precursors are circulating within the blood vessels, including fibroblasts pre-cursors.[111] This is important to note because it means that all the elements including those capable of producing collagen such as

endothelial cells and fibroblasts are ready to act in the healing area. Through mediators, each cell is submitted to a myriad of variable and sometime contradictory messages. How it chooses the appropriate response, is still unknown to researchers. During the inflammatory war aimed to conquer the healing of a wound, the cells may read these correctly, but the messages may be false. It is not known how much and how long a 'false' message may be transmitted among cells, and how long wound healing abnormali-ties may be maintained. It is not known very well how to read and how to interpret those messages correctly, and how to correct them if they are wrong. Thus, to learn the cell's wound healing language should be the focus of future research.[112] The immuno-logic and genetic interference should be thoroughly explored. Biochemical analysis and structural events could be important in determining the role of the sulfate glycosaminoglycans in the development and aggregation of collagen fibers. Several possible mechanisms might be involved in producing the excessive amount of collagen deposition which is characteristic of these scars including: an actual increase in the rate of collagen synthesis; the presence of inhibitors for the enzymatic breakdown of collagen and/or glycosaminoglycans; the absence or defective production of the specific enzymes; the presence of physical barriers oppos-ing a proper enzymatic attack; growth activity promoted by sul-fated proteoglycans; or other causes, yet unknown.

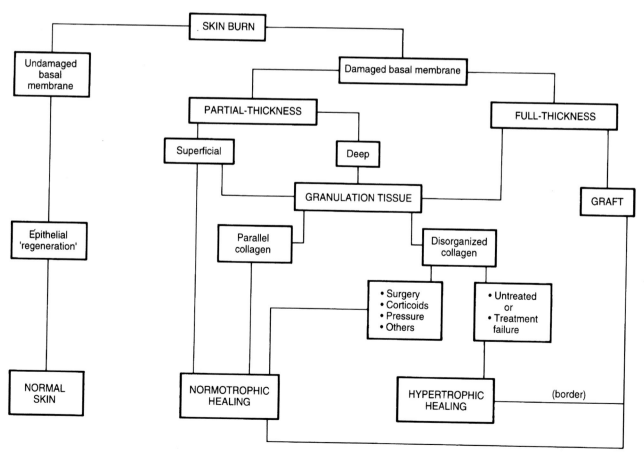

Fig. 44.7 The healing of skin after a burn injury.

References

1. Gamelli RL. Wound healing. In: Gamelli RL, Dries DJ, eds. *Trauma 2000*. Austin: RG Landes, 1992; 139–45.

2. Dover R, Wright NA. The cell proliferation kinetics of the epidermis. In: Goldsmith LA, ed. *Physiology, Biochemistry, and Molecular Biology of the Skin*. New York: Oxford University Press, 1991; 239–65.

3. Larson DL, Abston S, Dobrkovsky M, *et al. The Prevention and Correction of Burn Scar Contracture and Hypertrophy*. Galveston: Shriners Burns Institute, 1973; 1–21.

4. Kloth LC, Miller KH. The inflammatory response to wounding. In: Kloth LC, McCulloch JM, Feedar JA, eds. *Wound Healing: Alternatives in Management*. Philadelphia: FA Davis, 1990; 3–13.

5. Knighton DR, Fiegel VD. Regulation of cutaneous wound healing by growth factors and the microenvironment. *Invest Radiol* 1991; **26**: 604–11.

6. Clark RAF. Cutaneous wound repair. In: Goldsmith LA, ed. *Physiology, Biochemistry, and Molecular Biology of the Skin*. New York: Oxford University Press, 1991; 576–601.

7. Barbul A. Immune aspects of wound repair. *Clin Plast Surg* 1990; **17**: 433–42.

8. Efron JE, Frankel HL, Lazarou SA, Wasserkrug HL, Barbul A. Wound healing and T-lymphocytes. *J Surg Res* 1990; **48**: 460–3.

9. Regan MC, Barbul A. Immune control of wound healing. In: Gamelli RL, Dries DJ, eds. *Trauma 2000*. Austin: RG Landes, 1992; 146–50.

10. Hunt TK. Physiology of wound healing. In: Clowes GHA, ed. *Trauma, Sepsis and Shock*. New York: Marcel Dekker, 1988; 443–71.

11. Lambert WC, Cohen PJ, Klein KM, Lambert MW. Cellular and molecular mechanisms in wound healing: selected concepts. *Clin Dermatol* 1984; **2**: 7–23.

12. Appleton I, Tomlinson A, Chander CL, Willoughby DA. Effects of endothelin-1 on croton oil-induced granulation tissue in rat: a pharmacological and immunohistochemical study. *Lab Invest* 1992; **67**: 703–10.

13. Kingsnorth AN, Slavin J. Peptide growth factors and wound healing. *Br J Surg* 1991; **78**: 1286–90.

14. Dijke PT, Iwata KK. Growth factors for wound healing. *Biotechnology* 1989; **7**: 793–8.

15. Schultz G, Bennett N, Rotatori S, Macaully S, Moser M. EGF and TGF-in wound healing: analysis of wound fluids and effects of exogenous factors on wound healing. *J Cell Biol* 1993; **S17E**: 109.

16. Roberts AB, Flanders KC, Heine UI. Transforming growth factor- multifunctional regulator of differentiation and development. *Phil Trans R Soc Lond B* 1990; **327**: 145–54.

17. Sporn MB, Roberts AB. Peptide growth factors are multifunctional. *Nature* 1988; **332**: 217–8.

18. Hunt TK, La Van FB. Enhancement of wound healing by growth factors. *N Engl J Med* 1989; **321**: 111–2.

19. Hunt TK. Wound fluid: the growth environment. In: Barbul A, Caldwell MD, Eaglstein WH, *et al.*, eds. *Clinical and Experimental Approaches to Dermal and Epidermal Repair: Normal and Chronic Wounds*. New York: Wiley-Liss, Inc, 1991; 223–30.

20. Anderson GR, Stoler DL. Anoxia, wound healing, VL30 elements, and the molecular basis of malignant conversion. *Bioessays* 1993; **15**: 265–72.

21. Folkman J, Brem H. Angiogenesis and inflammation. In: Gallin JI, Goldstein IM, Snyderman R, eds. *Inflammation: Basic Principles and Clinical Correlates*. New York: Raven Press, 1992; 821–39.

22. Schoefl GI. Studies of inflammation. III. Growing capillaries: their structure and permeability. *Virchows Arch Pathol Anat* 1963; **337**: 97–104.

23. Linares HA, Kischer CW, Dobrkovsky M, Larson DL. The histiotypic organization of the hypertrophic scar in humans. *J Invest Dermatol* 1972; **59**: 323–31.

24. Claudy AL. Les Collagenes. *Ann Dermatol Venereol* 1988; **115**: 767–71.

25. Uitto J, Christiano AM, Chung-Honet LC, Greenspan DS, Li K, Tamai K. Molecular complexity of the cutaneous basement membrane zone: perspectives on wound healing. *J Cell Biol* 1993; **S17E**: 109.

26. Eisenmenger W, Nerlich A, Gluck G. Die Bedeutung des Kollagens bei der Wundaltersbestimmung. *Z Rechtsmed* 1988; **100**: 79–100.

27. Hopkinson I. The extracellular matrix in wound healing: collagen in wound healing. *Wounds* 1992; **4**: 124–32.

28. Gay S, Viljanto J, Raekallio J, Penttinen R. Collagen types in early phases of wound healing in children. *Acta Chir Scand* 1978; **144**: 205–11.

29. Hunt TK. The physiology of wound healing. *Ann Emerg Med* 1988; **17**: 1265–73.

30. Peacock EE, Cohen IK. Wound healing. In: McCarthy L, ed. *Plastic Surgery*. Philadelphia: WB Saunders, 1990; 161–85.

31. Ruoslahti E. Proteoglycans in cell regulation. *J Biol Chem* 1989; **264**: 13369–72.

32. Kjellen L, Lindahl U. Proteoglycans: structures and interactions. *Annu Rev Biochem* 1991; **60**: 443–75.

33. Templeton DM. Proteoglycans in cell regulation. *Crit Rev Clin Lab Sci* 1992; **29**: 141–84.

34. McPherson JM, Piez KA. Collagen in dermal wound repair. In: Clark RAF, Henson PM, eds. *The Molecular and Cellular Biology of Wound Repair*. New York: Plenum Press, 1988; 471–96.

35. Sugumaran G, Baldwin CT. The diversity of proteoglycans. *Wounds* 1992; **4**: 248–55.

36. Hascall VC, Hascall GK. Proteoglycans. In: Hay ED, ed. *Cell Biology of Extracellular Matrix*. New York: Plenum Press, 1981; 39–63.

37. Grinnell F. Fibronectin and wound healing. *J Cell Biochem* 1984; **26**: 107–16.

38. Turley EA, Torrance J. Localization of hyaluronate-binding protein on motile and non-motile fibroblasts. *Exp Cell Res* 1984; **16**: 17–28.

39. Bently JP. Rate of chondroitin sulfate formation in wound healing. *Ann Surg* 1967; **165**: 186–91.

40. Gabbiani G, Ryan GD, Majno G. Presence of modified fibroblasts in granulation tissue and their possible role in wound contraction. *Experientia* 1971; **27**: 549–53.

41. Ehrlich HP. Wound closure: evidence of cooperation between fibroblasts and collagen matrix. *Eye* 1988; **2**: 149–57.

42. Singer II. The fibronexus: a transmembrane association of fibronectin-containing fibers and bundles of 5 nm filaments in hamster and human fibroblasts. *Cell* 1979; **16**: 675–85.

43. Pollack SV. The wound healing process. *Clin Dermatol* 1984; **2**: 8–16.

44. Stenn KS, Malhotra R. Epithelialization. In: Cohen IK, Diegelmann RF, Lindblad WJ, eds. *Wound Healing*. Philadelphia: WB Saunders, 1992; 115–27.

45. Goslen JB. Wound healing for the dermatologic surgeon. *J Dermatol Surg Oncol* 1988; **14**: 959–72.

46. Daly TJ. The repair phase of wound healing – re-epithelialization and contraction. In: Kloth LC, McCulloch JM, Feedar JA, eds. *Wound Healing: Alternatives in Management*. Philadelphia: FA Davis Company, 1990; 14–30.

47. Hennings H, Michael D, Cheng D, Steinert P, Holbrook K, Yuspa SA. Calcium regulation of growth and differentiation of mouse epidermal cells in culture. *Cell* 1980; **19**: 245–54.

48. Mansbridge JN, Knapp AM. Changes in keratinocyte maturation during wound healing. *J Invest Dermatol* 1987; **89**: 253–63.

49. Grinnell F. Fibronectin and wound healing. *Am J Dermatopathol* 1982; **4**: 185–8.

50. Krawczyk WS. The pattern of epidermal cell migration during wound healing. *J Cell Biol* 1971; **49**: 247–63.

51. Stenn KS, Madri JA, Roll FJ. Migrating epidermis produces AB2 collagen and requires continued collagen synthesis for movement. *Nature* 1979; **277**: 229–32.

52. Davidson JM. Wound repair. In: Gallin JI, Goldstein IM, Snyderman R, eds. *Inflammation: Basic Principles and Clinical Correlates*. New York: Raven Press, 1992; 809–19.

53. Winter GD. Formation of the scar and the rate of epithelialization of superficial wounds in the skin of the young domestic pig. *Nature* 1962; **193**: 293–4.

54. Hinman CD, Maibach H. Effect of air exposure and occlusion on experimental human skin wounds. *Nature* 1963; **200**: 377–8.

55. Woodley DT, Bachmann PM, O'Keefe ED. The role of matrix components in human keratinocyte re-epithelialization. In: Barbul A, Caldwell MD, Eaglstein WH, *et al.*, eds. *Clinical and Experimental Approaches to Dermal and Epidermal Repair*. New York: Wiley-Liss, 1991; 129–40.

56. Forrest L. Current concepts in soft connective tissue wound healing. *Br J Surg* 1983; **70**: 133–40.

57. Alibert JLM. *Description des Maladies de la Peau Observées à l'Hôspital Saint-Louis et Exposition des Meilleurs Methodes Suivés pour leur Traitement*. Paris: Barrois l'Aîné et Fils, 1806; 113.

58. Hebra F, Kaposi M. *On Diseases of the Skin Including the Exanthemata*. London: The New Sydenham Society, 1874; 272.

59. Blackburn WR, Cosman B. Histologic basis of keloid and hypertrophic scar differentiation. *Arch Pathol* 1966; **82**: 65–71.

60. Linares HA. Hypertrophic healing: controversies and ethiopathogenic review. In: Carvajal HF, Parks DH, eds. *Burns in Children*. Chicago: Year Book Medical Publishers, 1988; 305–19.

61. Murray JC, Pinnell SR. Keloids and excessive dermal scarring. In: Cohen IK, Diegelmann RF, Lindblad WJ, eds. *Wound Healing, Biochemical and Clinical Aspects*. Philadelphia: WB Saunders Co, 1992; 500–22.

62. Craig P. Collagenase activity in cutaneous scars. *Hand* 1973; **5**: 239–43.

63. Knapp TR, Daniels JR, Kaplan EN. Pathologic scar formation. *Am J Pathol* 1977; **86**: 47–67.

64. Linares HA, Kischer CW, Dobrkovsky M, *et al.* On the origin of the hypertrophic scar. *J Trauma* 1973; **13**: 70–5.

65. Linares HA, Larson DL. Early differential diagnosis between hypertrophic and nonhypertrophic healing. *J Invest Dermatol* 1974; **62**: 514–6.

66. Linares HA, Kischer CW, Dobrkovsky M, *et al.* The histiotypic organization of the hypertrophic scar in humans. *J Invest Dermatol* 1972; **59**: 323–31.

67. Linares HA, Larson DL. Proteoglycans and collagenase in hypertrophic scar formation. *J Plast Reconstr Surg* 1978; **62**: 589–93.

68. Shetlar MR, Shetlar CL, Linares HA. The hypertrophic scar: location of glycosaminoglycans within scars. Burns 1977; 4: 14–9.

69. Hunter JAA, Finlay JB. Scanning electron microscopy of normal human scar tissues and keloids. Br J Surg 1976; 63: 826–30.

70. Kischer CW, Linares HA, Dobrkovsky M, Larson DL. Electron microscopy of the hypertrophic scar. In: Arceneaux CJ ed. 29th Ann Proc Electron Microscopy Soc Amer. Boston, MA 1971; 302–3.

71. Cohen IK, Keiser HR, Sjoerdsma A. Collagen synthesis in human keloid and hypertrophic scar. Surg Forum 1971; 22: 488–9.

72. Craig RDP, Schofield JD, Jackson SS. Collagen biosynthesis in normal human skin, normal and hypertrophic scar and keloid. Eur J Clin Invest 1975; 5: 69–74.

73. McCoy BJ, Cohen IK. Collagenase in keloid biopsies and fibroblasts. Connect Tissue Res 1982; 9: 181–92.

74. Harris ED Jr, Sjoerdsma A. Collagen profile in various clinical conditions. Lancet 1966; 2: 707–19.

75. Di Cesare PE, Cheung DT, Perelman N, Libaw E, Peng L, Nimni ME. Alteration of collagen composition and cross-linking in keloid tissues. Matrix 1990; 10: 172–8.

76. Cohen IK, Beaven MA, Horakova Z, Keiser HR. Histamine and collagen synthesis in keloid and hypertrophic scar. Surg Forum 1972; 23: 509.

77. Abergel RP, Pizzurro D, Meeker CA, et al. Biochemical composition of the connective tissue in keloids and analysis of collagen metabolism in keloid fibroblast cultures. J Invest Dermatol 1985; 84: 384–90.

78. Bailey AJ, Bazin S, Sims TJ, LeLous M, Nicoletis C, Delaunay A. Characterization of the collagen of human hypertrophic and normal scars. Biochim Biophys Acta 1975; 405: 412–21.

79. Weber L, Meigel WN, Spier W. Collagen polymorphism in pathologic human scars. Arch Dermatol Res 1978; 261: 63–71.

80. Conway H, Gillette R, Smith JW, Findley A. Differential diagnosis of keloids and hypertrophic scars by tissue culture technique with notes on therapy of keloids by surgical excision and decadron. Plast Reconstr Surg 1960; 25: 117–32.

81. Diegelmann RF, Cohen IK, McCoy BJ. Growth kinetics and collagen synthesis of normal skin, normal scar and keloid fibroblasts in vitro. J Cell Physiol 1979; 98: 341–6.

82. Abergel RP, Chu ML, Bauer EA, Uitto J. Regulation of collagen gene expression in cutaneous diseases with dermal fibrosis: evidence for pretranslational control. J Invest Dermatol 1987; 88: 727–31.

83. Ala-Kokko L, Rintala A, Savolainen ER. Collagen gene expression in keloids: analysis of collagen metabolism and type I, III, IV, and V procollagen mRNAs in keloid tissue and keloid fibroblast cultures. J Invest Dermatol 1987; 89: 238–44.

84. Craig RDP, Schofield JD, Jackson DS. Collagen biosynthesis in normal and hypertrophic scars and keloid as a function of the duration of the scar. Br J Surg 1975; 62: 741–4.

85. Hardingham TE, Fosang AJ. Proteoglycans: many forms and many functions. FASEB J 1992; 6: 861–70.

86. Yeo TK, Brown L, Dvorak HF. Alterations in proteoglycan synthesis common to healing wounds and tumors. Am J Pathol 1991; 138: 1437–50.

87. Shetlar MR, Larson DL, Shetlar CL, et al. The hypertrophic scar, glycoprotein and collagen components of burn scars. Proc Soc Exp Biol Med 1971; 138: 298–300.

88. Linares HA. Measurement of collagen-proteoglycans interaction in hypertrophic scars. Plast Reconstr Surg 1983; 71: 818–9.

89. Linares HA. Proteoglycan-lymphocyte association in the development of hypertrophic scars. Burns 1990; 16: 21–4.

90. Savage K, Swann DA. A comparison of glycosaminoglycan synthesis by human fibroblasts from normal skin, normal scar, and hypertrophic scar. J Invest Dermatol 1985; 84: 521–6.

91. Chytilova M, Kulhankek V, Horn V. Experimental production of keloids after immunization with autologous skin. Acta Chir Plast 1959; 1: 72–9.

92. Laurentaci G, Dioguardi D. HLA antigens in keloids and HS. Arch Dermatol 1977; 113: 1726.

93. Castagnoli C, Peruccio D, Stella M, et al. The HLA-DR 16 allogenotype constitutes a risk factor for hypertrophic scarring. Human Immunol 1990; 29: 229–32.

94. Cohen IK, McCoy BJ, Mohanakumar T, Diegelmann RF. Immunoglobulin, complement, and histocompatibility antigen studies in keloid patients. Plast Reconstr Surg 1979; 63: 689–92.

95. Abdalla-Osman AA, Gumma KA, Satir AA. Highlights on the etiology of keloid. Int Surg 1978; 63: 33–7.

96. Kischer CW, Shetlar MR, Shetlar CL, Chavapil M. Immunoglobulins in hypertrophic scars and keloids. Plast Reconstr Surg 1983; 71: 821–5.

97. Castagnoli C, Stella M, Magliacani G, Alasia ST, Richiard P. Anomalous expression of HLA class II molecules on keratinocytes and fibroblasts in hypertrophic scar consequence to thermal injury. Clin Exp Immunol 1990; 82: 350–4.

98. Cracco C, Stella M, Alasia ST, Filogamo G. Comparative study of Langerhans cells in normal and pathological human scars. II. Hypertrophic scars. Eur J Histochem 1992; 36: 53–65.

99. Babu M, Diegelmann R, Oliver N. Fibronectin is overproduced by keloid fibroblasts during abnormal wound healing. Mol Cell Biol 1989; 9: 1642–50.

100. Kischer CW, Hendrix MJC. Fibronectin (FN) in hypertrophic scars and keloids. Cell Tissue Res 1983; 231: 29–37.

101. McCauley RL, Chopra V, Li YY, Herndon DN, Robson MC. Altered cytokine production in black patients with keloids. J Clin Immunol 1992; 12: 300–8.

102. Davidson JM, Broadley KN, Benn SI. Cytokine influences on ECM metabolism during wound healing. J Cell Biol 1993; S17E: 109.

103. Sporn MB, Roberts AB. Introduction: what is TGF-β. In: Clinical Applications of TGF-Beta. Ciba Foundation Symposium 157. Wiley, Chichester, 1991; 1–6.

104. Babu M, Diegelmann R, Oliver N. Keloid fibroblasts exhibit an altered response to TGF-β. J Invest Dermatol 1992; 99: 650–5.

105. Martin P, Hopkinson-Woolley J, McCluskey J. Growth factors and cutaneous wound repair. Prog Growth Factor Res 1992; 4: 25–44.

106. Linares HA, Larson DL, Willis-Galstaun BA. Historical notes on the use of pressure in the treatment of hypertrophic scars or keloids. Burns 1993; 19: 17–21.

107. Larson DL, Evans EB, Abston S, Dobrkovsky M, Linares HA. Techniques for decreasing scar formation and scar contractures in the burn patient. J Trauma 1971; 11: 807–23.

108. Linares HA, Larson DL, Baur PS. Influence of mechanical forces on burn scar contracture and hypertrophic. In: Krizek Th J, Hoopes JE, eds. Symposium on Basic Science in Plastic Surgery. St Louis: CV Mosby, 1976; 101–27.

109. Larson DL, Willis B, Linares HA, Shetlar MR, Kischer CW. Burn scar changes associated with pressure. In: Longacre JJ, ed. The Ultrastructure of Collagen. Springfield: CC Thomas, 1976; 269–74.

110. Larson DL, Huang TT, Linares HA, Dobrkovsky M, Baur PS, Parks DH. Prevention and treatment of scar contractures. In: Artz CP, Moncrief JA, Pruitt B, eds. Burns, A Team Approach. Philadelphia: WB Saunders, 1979; 466–91.

111. Bucala R, Spiegel LA, Chesney J, et al. Circulating fibrocytes define a new leukocyte subpopulation that mediates tissue repair. Mol Med 1994; 1: 71–81.

112. Linares HA. Solving the hypertrophic healing problem: are we searching in the right direction? In: Magliacani G, Teich Alasia S, eds. La Cicatrice Patologica. Napoli: Giuseppe de Nicola Editore da Pronto Stampa, 1998; 7–12.

Rehabilitation

Chapter 45

Comprehensive rehabilitation of the burned patient

Michael A Serghiou, E Burke Evans, Sheila Ott
Jason H Calhoun, Dan Morgan, Les Hannon

With burns, as perhaps with any other order of trauma, there is urgent need for immediate and aggressive initiation of patient specific rehabilitation programs. Distribution and depth of burn so clearly define and predict the patterns of deformity from wound to scar contracture that it is possible on burn day 1 to design a program and establish short- and long-term goals. The more extensive the burn, the greater the rehabilitation challenge. A seriously burned extremity in an otherwise modestly burned patient is much easier to restore to function than an extremity similarly burned in a patient with full-thickness burns involving trunk, neck, head, and other extremities. Among seriously burned patients, the immediate and primary treatment goals will always be preservation of life and wound coverage. These basic treatment priorities, however, do not preclude the development and implementation of an aggressive rehabilitation program.

The short-term rehabilitation goal is to preserve the patient's range of motion and functional ability. Long-term rehabilitation goals include the return of the patient to independent living and training on how to compensate for any functional loss suffered as a result of the burn injury in order to be as productive as possible in their physical environment reintegration.

This chapter begins with addressing positioning, splinting, serial casting, skeletal suspension, traction, prosthetics and orthotics utilized in burn rehabilitation during the emergent, acute, and rehabilitative phases of recovery. Scar management, which includes pressure therapy, inserts, massage, and heat modalities utilized during the rehabilitative phase of recovery, is then discussed. The latter portion of this chapter discusses exercise ambulation and activities of daily living which are vital in the patient's functional recovery. The burn team should involve the patient and/or their caregivers in their care, as this is critical in bringing about the most desirable outcome in burn rehabilitation. This chapter concludes with addressing the importance of patient/caregiver education in burn rehabilitation.

Positioning and splinting of the burned patient for the prevention of contractures and deformities

Appropriate positioning of the burned patient is vital in bringing about the best functional outcomes in burn rehabilitation. It should begin immediately upon admission to the burn center and continue throughout the rehabilitation process when the scars from the last operative procedure (including reconstructive surgery) are matured. The role of the burn therapist is invaluable in designing a positioning program, which counteracts all contractive forces without compromising positive functional outcomes. In planning and implementing an effective patient-specific positioning program the therapist should be aware of the patient's total body surface area (TBSA) of burns, the depth of all injuries, respiratory status, and associated injuries such as exposed tendons/joints or fractures. All positioning programs are individualized and are monitored closely for any necessary adjustments depending on the patient's medical status. The frequently stated quote that 'the position of comfort is the position of deformity' applies to every burned patient who sustained a serious injury.

Antideformity positioning is achieved through splinting, mechanical traction, cutout foam troughs and mattresses, pillows, strapping mechanisms, serial casting and, in some cases, through surgical application of pins. The burn therapist needs to be aware of physician-specific protocols and to work closely with the entire burn team in designing the most effective positioning program. Orthotics and splinting devices are vital in burn rehabilitation as they are utilized throughout the burn recovery in obtaining appropriate positioning of the entire body and counteract the contractile forces, which lead to deformity. No matter how the burn therapist approaches splinting (material choice, design, application schedules) the goal is to bring about the best functional outcome at the completion of rehabilitation. When fabricating a splint or orthosis the burn therapist must be aware of the anatomy and kinesiology of the body surface to be splinted. Also, the therapist should be well aware of all mechanical principles of splinting and how they relate to pressure, mechanical advantage, torque, rotational forces, first class levels, friction, reciprocal parallel forces and material strength.[1]

Positioning/splinting must be designed in a way that:

- allows for edema reduction;
- maintains joint alignment;
- supports, protects and immobilizes joints;
- maintains and/or increases range of motion;
- maintains tissues elongated;
- remodels joint and tendon adhesions;
- promotes wound healing;
- relieves pressure points;
- protects newly operated on sites (grafts/flaps);
- stabilizes and/or positions one or more joints enabling other joints to function correctly;
- assists weak muscles to counteract the effects of gravity and assist in functional activity; and
- strengthens weak muscles by exercising against springs or rubber bands.[1]

All devices should:

- not cause pain;
- be designed with function in mind;
- be cosmetically appealing;
- be easy to apply and remove;
- be lightweight and low profile;
- be constructed out of appropriate materials; and
- allow for ventilation in preventing skin/wound maceration.[1]

Head

In aiding with facial edema reduction, the head may be positioned by elevating the head of the bed at 30–45° if the patient's hips are not involved. In cases where the hips are burned, the entire bed may be elevated at the head of the bed with the use of shock blocks (wood blocks 8–12 inches high with recessed slots for bed legs). This will avoid positioning the hips in a flexion contracture prone position. In the cases where the ears are burned, they may be protected from wrapping on pillows with ear cups made of thermoplastic materials or foam.[2] Serial splinting to maintain open nostrils may be required and is accomplished with the fabrication of nasal obturators. These are serially adjusted as the circumference of the nostril increases. In cases of severe ear burns, a splint may be fabricated to prevent the rim of the ear from contracting toward the head. Internal ear canal splints may also be fabricated and adjusted serially as the circumference of the canal increases. Mouth splints are utilized for the prevention of microstomia. These devices are custom-made by the therapist or they may be obtained commercially. Mouth splints may be static or dynamic for the horizontal or vertical opening of the mouth.[3–6] In cases of severe microstomia where compliance is an issue, an orthodontic commissure appliance may be custom-fabricated by an orthodontist.[7] The use of stacked tongue blades is an acceptable technique to aid in reversing microstomia. The number of tongue blades stacked in the patient's mouth are increased daily with rewards to the patient. Ongoing work looks at the development of a microstomia device that circumferentially opens the mouth according to its anatomy. Facial scar hypertrophy may require fabricating a high thermoplastic transparent mask such as the Uvex™ and W-clear masks or a silicone elastomer face mask.[8–10] A semi-rigid low thermoplastic opaque mask may also be fabricated depending on the state of scar maturation.

Neck

The neck is positioned in neutral or in slight extension of approximately 15° without any rotation. The amount of neck extension must not be so great that traction on the chin causes the mouth to open. Positioning may be achieved with a short mattress supine, a rolled towel or foam cushion placed behind the upper back on the scapular line. Pillows should be avoided in the cases of anterior neck burns as they may lead to flexion contractures. In the case of anterior neck burns, a conforming custom thermoplastic collar may be fabricated (**Figure 45.1**).[11] A soft neck collar or a Watusi type collar may also be fabricated.[10,12,13] It has been observed that, in some cases, acute patients rotate their neck or laterally flex it on one side, which may lead to a lateral neck contracture (torticollis). If the patient is to remain in bed for a while, a dynamic head strap mechanism may be fabricated to counteract the lateral neck contractile forces and bring the neck in the neutral position (**Figure 45.2**). For the prevention of torticollis, the therapist may fabricate a lateral neck splint which conforms to the head of the patient, the lateral neck, and anterior/posterior shoulder (**Figure 45.3**)

Spine

Contracture resulting from unilateral or asymmetric burns of the neck, axilla, trunk, and groin will cause lateral curvature of the spine (scoliosis). The level and amplitude of curvature will vary with the site and severity of the contracture. In addition, pelvic obliquity accompanying asymmetric hip or knee flexion contracture will impose a lateral lumbar curve. With none of the scoliotic curves associated with burns is there an intrinsic spinal deformity, and permanent spinal deformity will never result if the extrinsic

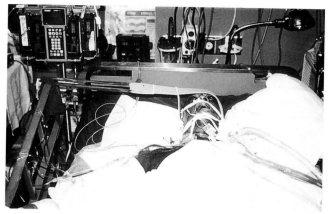

Fig. 45.2 A dynamic head strap mechanism aids in positioning the neck in a neutral position during a prolong ICU bed confinement.

cause, i.e. scar contracture, is eliminated. On the other hand, if the contracture is allowed to persist through several years of growth, the vertebral deformity will become structural and permanent.

As long as the patient is recumbent, lateral curvature can be prevented by maintaining straight alignment of the trunk and neck.

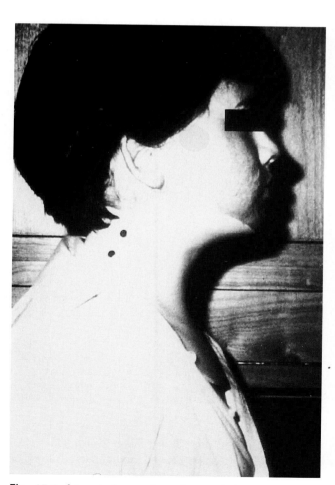

Fig. 45.1 An anterior neck conformer helps prevent neck flexion contractures.

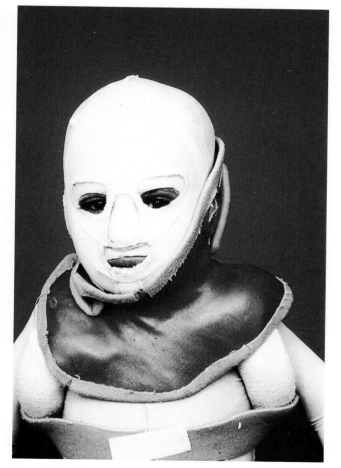

Fig. 45.3 A lateral neck splint is utilized to prevent lateral neck flexion contractures (torticollis).

However, the curve is often insidious in onset and will not be recognized until the patient begins to walk. Trunk list observed early in the ambulation period can be simply a transient accommodation to pain and wound tightness, but a persistent list may herald the development of scoliosis. Other subtle signs of spinal curvature are asymmetry of shoulder levels, scapular asymmetry, asymmetry of dependent upper extremity alignment to the trunk, and asymmetry of pelvic rim levels (**Figure 45.4a,b,c**). Once there is an established asymmetric contracture it is difficult by therapeutic means to stretch it out, so it is probably better to deal surgically with a deforming scar early than to permit even minor scoliosis to persist.

Exaggerated thoracic kyphosis secondary to anterior chest and neck burn is difficult to prevent because the recumbent position cradles the back and encourages protraction of the scapulae. The two-plane contracture extending from chin and neck to thorax and from shoulder to shoulder anteriorly pulls the chin down, flexes the neck and pulls the scapulae forward. Protraction of the scapulae alone may cause a normal thoracic kyphosis to appear to be exaggerated. However, if the protraction posture is not corrected, it tends to become habitual, and the final result features a prominent and rounded thoracic spine (**Figure 45.5a,b**). As this spinal deformity in its genesis is linked to neck and shoulder contractures, the measures for its prevention and correction are discussed in the section dealing with neck and shoulders.

Exaggeration of spinal lumbar lordosis is rarely related to overlying burn of the back. On the other hand, full-thickness burns of the abdomen are occasionally deep enough to compromise or even eliminate abdominal muscle function. In this circumstance the pelvis, for lack of support of anterior motors, will roll forward and lumbar lordosis will increase (**Figure 45.6**). The hamstring and gluteus maximus muscles, though strong posterior stabilizers of the pelvis, cannot compensate for loss of abdominal muscle power. If all abdominal muscles are lost, viscera will protrude, shifting the center of gravity forward. To compensate and achieve balance the patient must lean backwards, further increasing the lumbar lordosis. There is no way to prevent this sequence if abdominal muscle function is lost and since surgical correction often is not practical, the only treatment recourse may be sturdy external abdominal support to relieve the burden of protruding viscera.

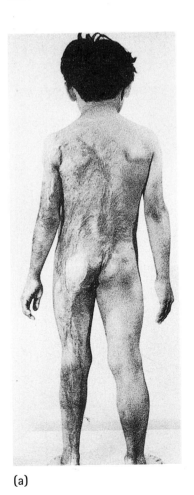

(a)

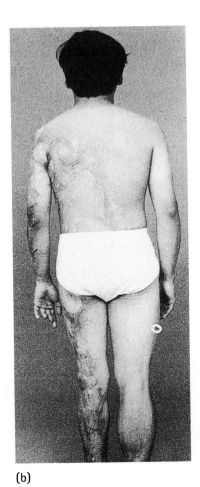

(b)

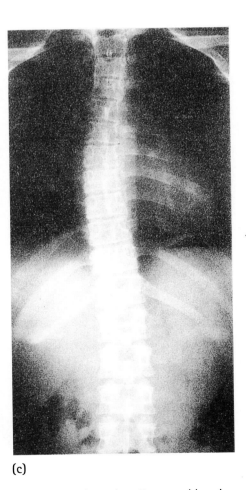

(c)

Fig. 45.4 (a) Six years after 45% TBSA burn involving mainly the left side of the chest and trunk, a 7-year-old male stands with a trunk list to the right which compensates for a scar-imposed unbalanced thoracic spinal curve convex to the right. (b,c) At age 17 spinal alignment has improved. Thoracic asymmetry and shift of the trunk toward the left are due to fixed structural thoracic scoliosis extending from the third thoracic vertebra through the first lumbar vertebra.

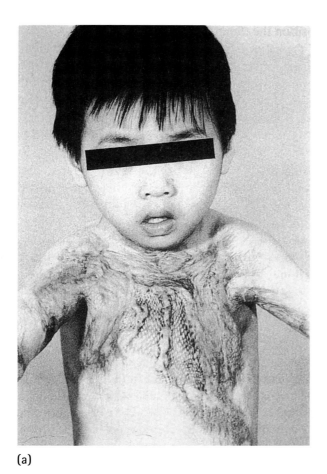

(a)

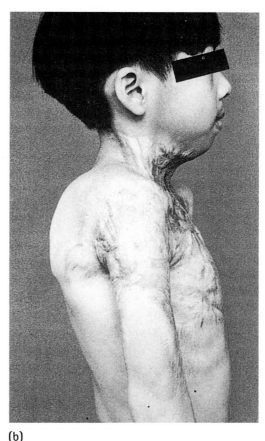

(b)

Fig. 45.5 (a) A 3-year-old boy as he appeared 14 months after a full-thickness anterior burn of neck, chest, and shoulders. Scar contracture has flexed the neck and protracted the scapulae. (b) Three years later, after several release and graft procedures, the shoulders remain protracted, the scapulae are winged, and the thoracic kyphosis is exaggerated.

Shoulder Girdle/Axilla

Elevation of the arms should be in the corono-sagital plane with the glenoid at approximately 15–20° of horizontal flexion. Abduction in the coronal plane places the glenohumeral joint in relative extension and uncovers the head of the humorous, rendering it more prone to anterior subluxation if the position is chronically maintained. Also, abduction in the coronal plane may cause excessive tension to the brachial plexus over time, resulting in a neuropathy such as radial nerve palsy. Positioning may be achieved with splints, pillows, bedside tables, foam arm troughs, and thermoplastic slings suspended from an overhead trapeze mechanism (**Figure 45.7**). Airplane splints are custom-fabricated or obtained commercially for the prevention of axillary contractures. To accommodate wound dressings and promote healing, a three-piece airplane splint may be fabricated (**Figure 45.8**). This splint connects the patient's arm thermoplastic piece to the one on the lateral trunk with a thermoplastic custom-made rod. Commercially available airplane splints come equipped with a mechanism that allows for adjustments, depending on available shoulder abduction ranges.[10,11,13] A figure-of-eight axillary wrap may be fabricated to provide pressure and stretch the axillary skin surfaces (**Figure 45.9**).

Elbow/Forearm

With severe burns involving the upper extremity, the elbow will be held in flexion. This position favors flexion contracture and threatens posterior exposure of the joint if there is dorsal full-thickness burn. Full extension is the protecting position for the elbow. If the joint remains exposed posteriorly, extension may need to be rigidly maintained for several weeks. If the joint is not exposed, mobilization into increasing flexion range can begin very soon after the burn. The elbow is integral to the so-called delivery system for the hand, and elbow range to full or near-full flexion is more important for overall function than range to full or near-full extension. Flexion is required for grooming, eating and toileting; extension, for reach and stabilization.

Radial head rotation for pronation and supination is less often affected by burn than flexion and extension. The pronators and supinators are frequently injured in electrical accidents where bone being a poor conductor heats destroying the muscles closest to it. Forearm rotation is essential for accurate hand placement and the rehabilitative program must seriously address that function. Depending on the location and severity of the injury, the forearm may be positioned in neutral or in slight supination. Static elbow splints may be soft or custom-fabricated of thermoplastic

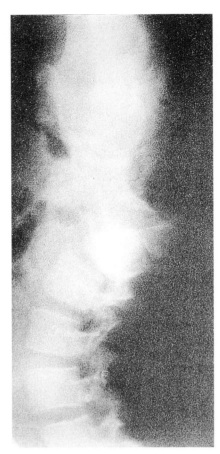

Fig. 45.6 In this 17-year-old male, 3 years after a 90% TBSA burn, total loss of abdominal musculature has resulted in pronounced forward pelvic tilt, an almost horizontal sacrum, and an exaggerated lumbar lordosis.

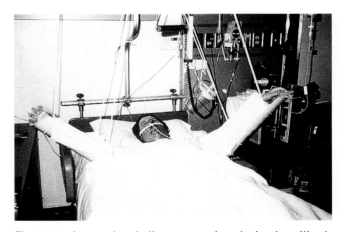

Fig. 45.7 An overhead sling suspension device is utilized for positioning the shoulders in bed.

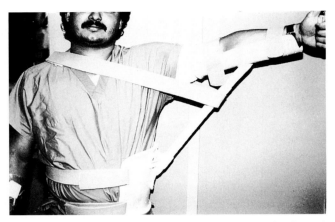

Fig. 45.8 A three-piece airplane splint may be fabricated to accommodate wound dressings and promote healing while maintaining the shoulder abducted.

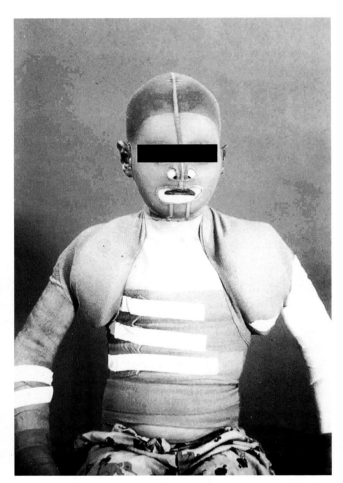

Fig. 45.9 A figure-of-eight axillary wrap provides a constant stretch of the axillary skin surfaces.

materials. An anterior elbow conformer may be fabricated over the burn dressing, or a three-point elbow extension splint can be made avoiding sheering of fresh grafts/flaps by not making contact with the operated on sites. Dynamic elbow extension or flexion splints may be utilized in providing prolonged gentle sustained stretch aiding in the correction of contractures.[14] Forearm dynamic pronation/supination splints may be custom fabricated or obtained commercially for the correction of contractures.[10,11,13]

Wrist/Hand

The usual posture of the unsupported burned hand is wrist flexion, metacarpophalangeal extension, interphalangeal flexion, and first metacarpal extension and adduction. Metacarpophalangeal extension·is imposed to some degree by dorsal swelling of the hand and the overall posture may be the position of greatest comfort. If the hand rests unsupported on the bed, all features of the deformity may be positionally reinforced with the first metacarpal being pushed farther into extension and adduction. The overall appearance is that of an intrinsic minus or claw deformity (**Figure 45.10a,b**).

If, in the acute burn phase, the wrist is securely supported in extension, the metacarpophalangeal joints of digits 2–5 will tend to fall into flexion because of gravity if the forearm be pronated or the hand elevated and because of the reciprocal tendering action between digital flexors and extensors. The first metacarpal will likewise fall forward into flexion. Wrist extension is, thus, basic to control of hand and digit position and to prevention of hand and wrist deformity.

Among the digits, the second and fifth most easily drift into metacarpophalangeal extension because each has a proper extensor and has relative functional freedom from the third and fourth digits. The fifth is occasionally pulled into extreme abduction and extension by scar contracture. The thumb may become similarly displaced, and to a lesser degree the index finger. The severe displacement of these digits gives a grotesque, but characteristic, deformity (**Figure 45.11ai, aii, b, ci, cii**).

For adults, adolescents and older children, preventive static positioning with a custom thermoplastic splint can be relatively efficient. There are, however, two common faults in custom splints that are designed to gain metacarpophalangeal flexion and to position the thumb in flexion and abduction. If the transverse fold of the splint is not proximal to the metacarpophalangeal joints of digits 2–5, the splint will impede rather than favor metacarpophalangeal flexion. If the thumb component of the splint applies

volar rather than medial pressure the metacarpophalangeal joint will extend and the metacarpal will become correspondingly more adducted. The first metacarpophalangeal joint should be maintained in slight flexion and pressure from the splint should be applied just to the medial surface of the digit. Any degree of first metacarpal adduction contracture increases the likelihood that the proximal phalanx will be pushed into hyperextension and eventually into subluxation by the splint. The optimal position for the burned hand and wrist includes 15–40° wrist extension, 70–90° metacarpophalangeal (MCP) joint flexion and neutral interphalangeal (IP) joint position. The thumb should be positioned in a combination of palmar and radial abduction with the first MCP joint slightly flexed as mentioned above. This positioning which resembles the intrinsic plus position of the hand is achieved through a burn hand splint fabricated by the therapist (**Figure 45.12**). Superficial hand burns should not be splinted in order to allow for frequent movement and the freedom to function independently. In the case of circumferential hand burns, a hand extension splint may also be fabricated to prevent flexion contractures and cupping of the palm. The flexion and extension splints are alternated depending on the burn center's protocols. A 'sandwich' hand splint may be fabricated which includes the volar burn hand splint with a dorsal platform over the interphalangeal joints in order to prevent flexion of the digits. The splint may be secured with an elastic bandage or with velcro strapping (**Figure 45.13**).[15] Individual static finger splints may include a digital gutter splint for the prevention of flexion contractures or a Boutonniere deformity, a thumb c-bar for the prevention of syndactyly in the first web space, and figure-of-eight digital splint for the prevention/correction of swan neck deformity and a distal interphalangeal joint extension splint for the prevention of mallet finger deformity. Dynamic splinting of the hand may include MCP extension or flexion splints, PIP/DIP flexion or extension splints, thumb outriggers, digital knuckle benders, or flexion/extension spring-loaded splints. The therapist must moni-

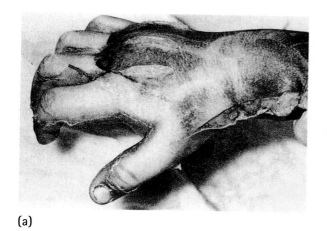

(a)

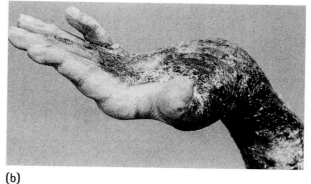

(b)

Fig. 45.10 (a) Edema following a full-thickness burn of the dorsum of the right hand of a 4-year-old boy – imposed metacarpophalangeal extension and digital flexion just 1 day after a 73% TBSA burn. (b) Two months after burn, the hand shows the common progression of the deformity with wrist flexion and fixed hyperextension of all metacarpophalangeal joints.

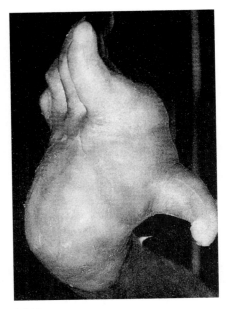

(a)(i)

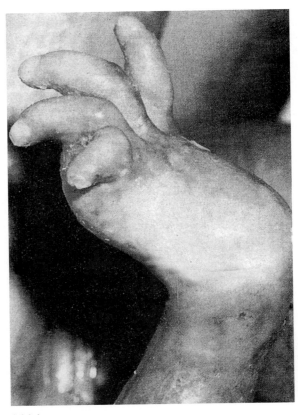

(a)(ii)

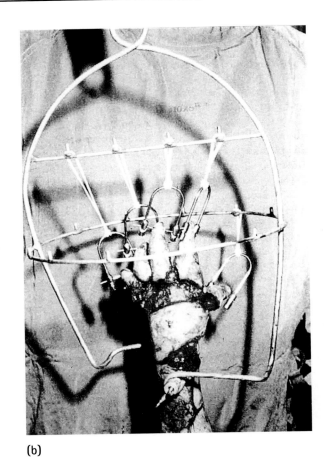

(b)

Fig. 45.11 (a) Severe wrist flexion and digital extension deformities of the left upper extremity of a 6-year-old boy 7 months after 40% TBSA burn. (b) After surgical release of wrist and digits and split-thickness autogenous skin grafting, the corrected position was maintained with digital pin traction in a halo splint proximally fixed at the wrist.

tor dynamic splinting closely and make frequent adjustments to the outriggers in maintaining a 90° angle of pull at all times. Wrist splints may be fabricated dorsally, volarly, or in the cases of a deviation contracture they may be constructed on the medial or lateral aspect of the joint. The therapist should design these splints having in mind the importance of the wrist joint in the performance of activities of daily living. A dynamic wrist splint may be utilized which provides a prolonged stretch in counteracting any contractile forces. In treating the edematous hand, it is important to position the hand above the heart level at all times, to aid edema

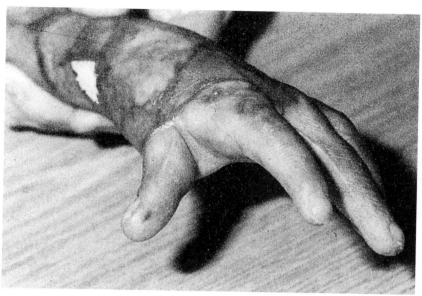

(c)(i)

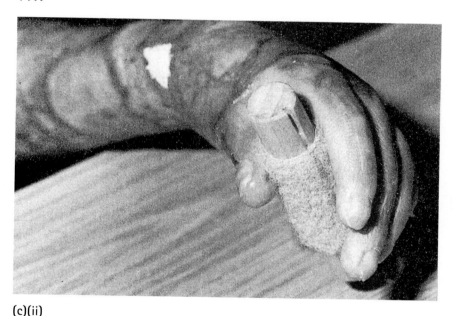

(c)(ii)

Fig. 45.11 (c)(i, ii) Six months after surgical release, there is active wrist extension to neutral, and digital grasp and release have been restored. The skeletal traction splint was removed 2 weeks after its application when an exercise program was begun. Position was maintained at rest with an orthoplast splint.

reduction. Elevation should not compromise the vascular supply to the hand.[10,11,13]

Once wrist and digital contractures are established, their severity and maturity of the scar determine if the deformities can be best managed by splinting, serial casting, skeletal traction or will require surgical release followed by splinting or traction (**Figure 45.11 b, ci, cii**).

Hip

When anterior burns extend from abdomen to thigh, hip flexion is the position of comfort. If the hip is fixed in any degree of flexion, posture will be modified. Bilateral symmetric contractures impose increased lumbar lordosis or knee flexion or both. Asymmetric contracture will cause pelvic obliquity and scoliosis. In adults and older children, thighs are more likely to be held in adduction than in abduction, whereas in preambulatory infants the secondary component of the contracture is abduction. Thus, for the hips the preventive position is full extension, 0° rotation and symmetric abduction of 15–20°. If elevation of the upper body is needed for edema reduction then the entire frame of the bed is elevated with the use of shock blocks placed at the head of the bed. Soft mattresses should be avoided as they may promote hip flexion. Hip positioning is accomplished with the use of abduction pillows and other strapping mechanisms eliminating hip rotation. If the patient wears bilateral foot splints then connector bars may be utilized on the splints to bring about the desired bilateral hip positioning stated above. Hip flexion contractures may be serially corrected with an anterior hip spica (**Figure 45.14**) or with a 3-point hip extension

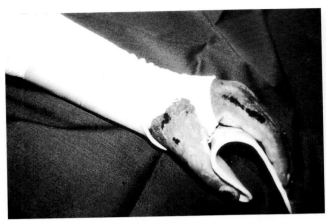

Fig. 45.12 The intrinsic plus position hand splint positions the hand appropriately in preventing contractures and preserving function.

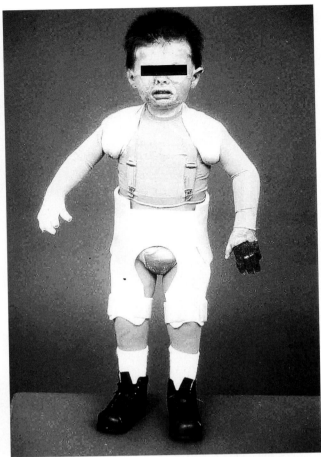

Fig. 45.14 An anterior hip spica splint is utilized to prevent anterior hip flexion contractures.

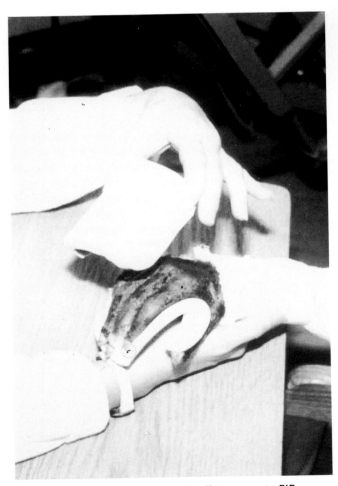

Fig. 45.13 The 'sandwich' hand splint prevents PIP flexion contractures.

splint.[10,11,13] Subtle hip flexion contractures can easily be overlooked when the patient stands, there being only a slight increase in lumbar lordosis or forward or lateral shift of the trunk. If established hip flexion contractures are not surgically corrected, body posture is likely to be permanently altered with scoliosis or exaggerated lordosis.

Knee

Whether a deep burn injury crossing the knee is mainly anterior or posterior, the patient will more often than not flex the knee. Deep anterior burns may expose the joint, occasionally destroying the patellar tendon. Deep posterior burns result in bridging scar formation. The appropriate position for the knee is full extension to be maintained by splint or skeletal traction until there is efficient quadriceps function and the patient is ambulatory. Thereafter, night splints must be used until scar contracture is no longer a threat. Knee splints may include a posterior custom-made thermoplastic knee conformer or a soft knee immobilizer.

Persisting bilateral knee flexion contractures will impose hip flexion. Persisting unilateral contractures may impose pelvic obliquity and scoliosis. As with the hip, posture alteration may be so subtle as to be overlooked. Correction of even a slight contracture should be a surgical priority, as should elimination of a soft bridging scar band that does not prevent complete willful knee extension but causes the patient habitually to hold the knee in slight flexion.

Foot/Ankle

Ankle equinus is the most frequently occurring deformity involving the foot. Initially it is related more to gravity and failure to support the foot at neutral (90°) at the talotibial joint than to the early effect of the burn. Loss of deep and superficial peroneal nerve function will compound the problem by encouraging the foot to drift into inversion as well as equinus because of loss of dorsiflexion and eversion motors. In the end, the total deformity for the unsupported foot may be ankle equinus, hind-foot inversion, and forefoot varus and equinus. Ankle equinus quickly becomes a resistant deformity so that within a few days or even hours the foot can no longer be positioned at 90° of dorsiflexion. Eventually the contractures of scar, muscle, and capsular structures combine to fix the deformity.

Equinus deformity and the attending inversion and forefoot varus can be prevented by accurate and unyielding support of the foot in neutral alignment at 90° or greater of dorsiflexion. If the patient must be nursed prone, the feet must be allowed to fall free from the mattress. Static splinting, if not performed correctly by an experienced therapist, is often unsuccessful because of the patient's desire and tendency to plantarflex strongly, displacing the splint and leading to ulcers of the heel, malleoli, toes, and where the splint edges touch the skin. A stable footboard may be effective if the feet are kept securely and totally against it. For large burns, and particularly for circumferential burns of the lower extremities, skeletal suspension incorporating calcaneal traction will support the foot at neutral if the traction pin is placed in the calcaneus well behind the axis of ankle motion. A balanced traction system demands that the knees be supported in flexion with tibial pins at the level of the tibial tubercle. Calcaneal pins will not prevent forefoot equinus. If traction must be employed for several weeks, proximal pull dorsal pins in the first or first and second metatarsals may be required for support of the forefoot. Transmetatarsal pins are also useful when calcaneal traction alone is not sufficient to correct equinus.

Minor established equinus deformity will yield with a standing and walking program. At the outset, graduated heel lifts may be used to accommodate to the deformity. If the patient must be confined to bed, skeletal traction through the calcaneus may be the quickest and most efficient way to correct the deformity. Traction is effective even if scar contracture contributes to the deformity. Serial corrective casts or posterior splints alone are useful mainly for minor contractures. For the treatment of circumferential foot/ankle burns, anterior foot splints are also fabricated and their application is alternated with the posterior foot splints in preventing plantar or dorsal foot contractures.[10,11,13] The Multi Podus® System foot splints are frequently utilized for the positioning of the burn foot/ankle as they relieve heel pressure in preventing pressure ulcers (**Figure 45.15**). For fixed, unyielding deformity, scar release combined with tendoachillis lengthening with or without posterior capsulotomy is a standard surgical procedure that yields inconsistent results. The correction achieved is often just to neutral or slightly more. The Ilizarov system has been used with generally satisfactory immediate results in severe cases. However correction

is achieved, if there are no dorsiflexion motors and if the range of ankle motion is only a few degrees, ankle fusion may in the end yield the best functional result.

The most common intrinsic deformity of the foot is extreme extension of the toes due to dorsal scar contracture. This deformity is insidious in onset and is difficult to prevent as there is no type of nonskeletal splinting that will hold the toes flexed. In its extreme, the deformity includes dorsal metatarsophalangeal subluxation which may involve one or all toes, depending on the location of the scar. The metatarsal heads become prominent on the plantar surface and walking may be painful. Correction of the deformity requires dorsal surgical release of the contracture, manual correction of the deformity and, in severe cases, intrinsic or extrinsic pinning of the digit or digits in an overcorrected position, i.e. metatarsophalangeal and interphalangeal flexion. The deformity will commonly, if not inevitably, recur to some degree unless the patient is able to achieve active metatarsophalangeal flexion in all digits after the operation.

Dorsal scar contractures extending from leg to foot to toes may pull the foot into marked inversion if the scar is medial or into eversion if the scar is lateral. The fifth and first toes may be separately displaced by the same scar bands. These contractures must always be surgically corrected. Their persistence will lead to bone deformity in a growing child and will permanently adversely affect foot and ankle function. Even slight inversion, whether imposed by scar contracture or motor weakness, will increase pressure on the lateral border of the foot, leading to callous formation and a painful inefficient gait. Occasionally, the base of the fifth metatarsal is so offensive as to require partial surgical ostectomy.

When there is both anterior and posterior scar contracture, the talus will remain aligned with the calcaneus in a relatively plantar flexed position as the midfoot and forefoot are pulled into dorsiflexion. The result is so-called 'rocker bottom foot' with the head of the talus prominently the principal weight-bearing feature. This deformity, once established, defies correction by usual surgical means because of the shortage of soft tissue and because vessels and nerves cannot be stretched to accommodate to the corrected

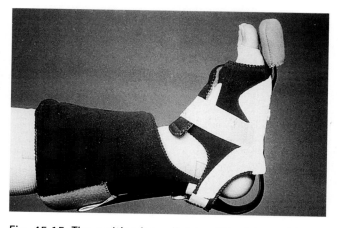

Fig. 45.15 The multipodus splint is utilized to position the burned feet appropriately and prevent heal and malleoli skin breakdown.

position. The Ilizarov system may offer partial solution to the problem (see Ilizarov External Fixator discussion below). Removal of the head of the talus may give a reasonable weight-bearing surface. With chronic painful ulceration, amputation is the best treatment (**Figure 45.16a,b**).

An Unna's boot may be applied at time of skin grafting to the lower extremity and contribute to early patient ambulation. Unna's boot is a bandage impregnated with calamine lotion and zinc oxide which, when applied over the grafted lower extremity (6 layers), hardens to a semirigid dressing resembling a plaster cast. This cast-like total contact dressing provides uniform support to the fresh skin graft and, when reinforced with a thermoplastic or plaster splint, facilitates early ambulation. Unna's boot may be applied for up to 7 days post-grafting, although it could be removed earlier for the inspection of the skin graft. Once removed, a new Unna's boot needs to be fabricated, depending on the burn center's lower extremity postoperative immobilization protocol.[16]

Serial Casting

Serial casting is frequently utilized in burn rehabilitation for the correction of significant contractures. Joints with over 30° of contracture respond well to casting. The applied cast provides total contact with circumferential and evenly distributed pressure. The prolonged gentle sustained stretch provided by the cast aids in tissue elongation without causing microtrauma to the surfaces targeted for the correction of contractures (**Figure 45.17**). Casting is a relatively simple, fast and painless intervention and provides an alternative to dynamic splinting when patient compliance is an issue (i.e. pediatrics).

Plaster casting bandages come in different widths and may also be cut in strips by the therapist prior to casting a patient. Plaster casts are inexpensive, easy to fabricate, are light-weight, and allow for ventilation down to the skin surface thus avoiding skin/wound maceration. Plaster is fast-setting when reacting with warm water.

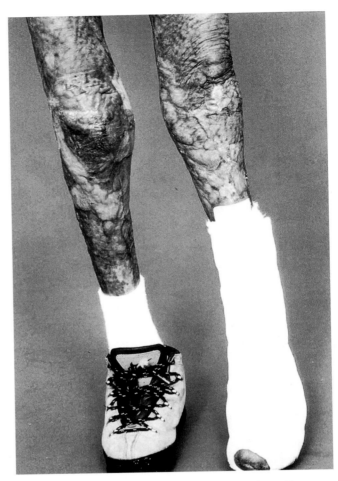

Fig. 45.17 Serial casting provides prolonged gentle sustained stretch and aids in tissue elongation and correction of contractures without pain.

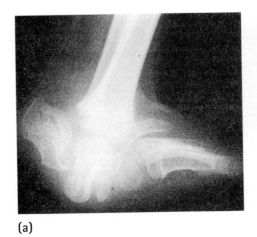

(a)

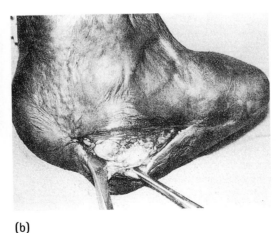

(b)

Fig. 45.16a,b Extreme rocker–bottom deformity of the left foot of a 7-year-old boy 6 years after a 35% TBSA burn. The deformity is too far advanced for surgical reconstruction. (b) The head of the talus was removed to relieve painful weight-bearing pressure.

Disadvantages of this technique include the decreased water resistance of plaster and breakage if not constructed strongly enough to withstand the patient's own muscle strength.

Fiberglass casts are an alternative technique to plaster casts. Fiberglass bandages are fast-setting when reacting with water, they are lightweight and the casts are stronger (mostly preferred for lower extremity walking casts). Fiberglass is more expensive than plaster; because of its abrasive properties, therapists must wear gloves prior to handling it.

A light dressing and padding on the bony prominences should be applied prior to either casting technique. Prior to casting, the therapist should consider therapeutic heat, massage and stretching of the joints about to be casted. When casting is completed, the patient should feel a gentle, but not painful, stretch. The first cast should be removed at approximately 24 hours and thereafter, depending on the patient's tolerance, it could be applied up to a week at a time. In cases of casting over wounds, the cast should be removed at 1–2 days in order to avoid complications in wound healing.[17,18]

Skeletal suspension, traction and stabilization systems in burn management

Skeletal suspension and traction systems have been used to a limited extent in burn management for a number of years. The early reports of Larson[19] and Evans[20-22] described the use of skeletal suspension for positioning and for extremity elevation for open wound management and of skeletal traction for prevention and correction of contractures. The later reports of Harnar[23] and Youel[24] deal mainly with the management of hand burns with the skeletally anchored digital traction splints bearing the names banjo, halo, and hay rake. Evans[25] has reported using a rigid external fixator for treatment of an exposed unstable knee. Calhoun[26] has reported his experience with the use of the Ilizarov system in the correction of severe burn contractures and deformities.

Skeletal Suspension and Traction

The adaption of skeletal suspension and traction systems to burn management grew out of earlier experience with traction to correct the elbow and knee contractures of patients with rheumatoid disease, and of traction and suspension as definitive means for treating certain extremity fractures. In its earliest application to burn management, skeletal suspension was used for extremity elevation only to facilitate wound care. From this experience, evolved better defined traction systems, including those expressly designed for hands and feet.

Upper Extremity

For suspension or traction of upper extremity, pins may be directed through distal radius or through the second and third metacarpals. The radial pin is directed from dorsal to ventral, 1–2 cm proximal to the radioulnar joint, exiting the bone between the median nerve and the radial artery alongside the flexor carpi radialis. The traction bow must extend beyond the hand. Hand support can be supplied with a thermoplastic splint or padded grab bar attached to the bow. The transmetacarpal pin is introduced anterolaterally in the second metacarpal just proximal to the head and is directed so as to exit the posteromedial surface of the third metacarpal, at the same level. Transfixation of the two functionally fixed units does not inhibit digital or palmar motion. If the hand is burned, suspension of the extremity can be achieved with one of the skeletally anchored traction splints which position wrist and digits through pins in the distal phalanges or hooks attached to the nails (**Figure 45.18a,b**)

Lower Extremity

For lower extremity suspension or traction, pins are introduced through the distal femur, proximal tibia, distal tibia, calcaneus and the first and second metatarsals (**Figure 45.18a**). The femoral pin is inserted from lateral to medial, at or just above the condylar flair. The tibial pin is inserted at the level of the tibial tubercle, sufficiently posterior to that structure to traverse securely two cortices. The distal tibial pin is introduced laterally, proximal to the growth plate in children and 1–1.5 cm proximal to the talotibial joint in adults.

Placement of the calcaneal pin depends upon the reason for insertion. If the pin is only for elevation of the extremity, it is placed transversely in the calcaneus, from lateral to medial, in line with the axis of motion of the talotibial joint, to allow free active motion of that joint. If the pin is being used to gain or maintain dorsiflexion of the talotibial joint it is placed well posterior to the axis of motion (**Figure 45.18c,d**). The transmetatarsal pin is inserted inferomedially into the shaft of the first metatarsal, just proximal to the head. It is directed to exit the dorsolateral surface of the second metatarsal at the same level. This pin is used when calcaneal traction is insufficient to maintain ankle dorsiflexion, when there is threat of development of forefoot equinus, or simply to control rotation of the leg. Skeletally anchored traction splints can be used for hands to control or position digits.

In the suspension mode for both upper and lower extremities, distal weight is such as to maintain desired position of the extremity when the patient is asleep or inactive, but is not so great as to prevent active motion or functional exercise. In the traction mode, weight must be sufficient for constant uniform pull to correct a contracture or to maintain surgically gained positioning. With lower extremity suspension or traction, a proximal tibial pin is always required to control rotation of the extremity and to prevent hyperextension of the knee. In the management of a patient with extensive burns, lower extremity weights for the proximal tibia and calcaneus can be alternately increased or decreased to favor flexion or extension of the knee. In the upper extremity, elbow flexion can be gained just by decreasing the distal weight. Occasionally when there is an elbow extension contracture, it is necessary to insert an olecranon pin for traction to gain elbow flexion.

Technique

Threaded Steinmann pins are preferred for major bones, non-threaded pins being used solely for digital traction. Pin size depends on patient size and anticipated weight load. The pin must be strong enough not to bend when traction is applied. When a pin bends with traction it becomes less efficient and erodes the cortical bone more quickly. For only one of the usual pin sites is there hazard in insertion: the distal radial pin, whether inserted on volar or dorsal surface, must deal with radial artery and median nerve. With insertion from dorsal to volar, the pin enters the bone just radial to the extensor bundle so as to emerge between the nerve and artery. Just as the pin penetrates the volar cortex, the speed of the

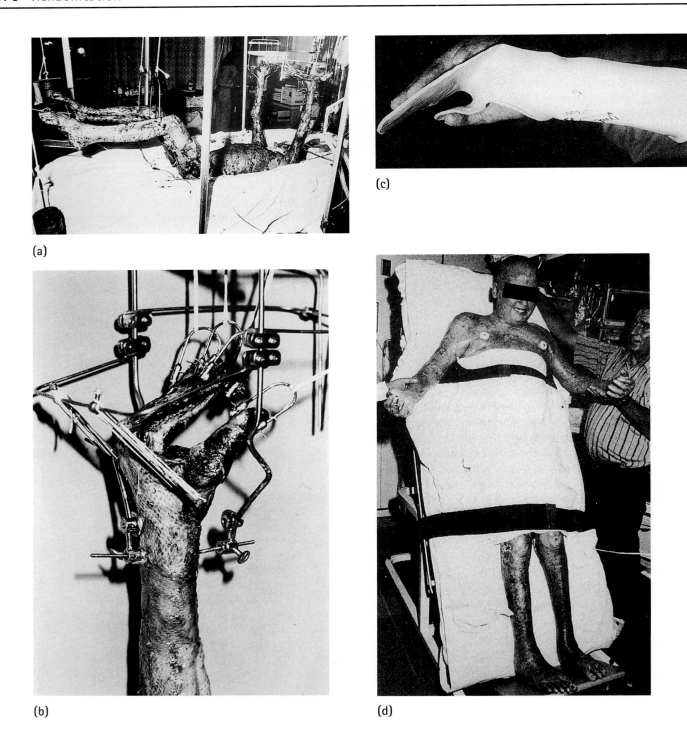

(a)

(c)

(b)

(d)

Fig. 45.18a,b This 16-year-old male with 94% mainly full-thickness total body surface burn and comatose from anoxic brain injury was placed in skeletal suspension and traction after an initial excision and grafting procedure. Pins were inserted in wrist, hands, tibiae, and calcanei. Forefoot equinus was controlled with foam slings (not shown) rather than transmetatarsal pins. Traction was discontinued on the 63rd postburn day. (b) On postburn day 14, the hand is shown as positioned in hay rake splint with pins through distal radius, second and third metacarpals, and distal phalanges of all digits. The wrist is in approximately 20° of extension, metacarpophalangeal joints in 90° of flexion and digits 2–5 in interphalangeal extension. The thumb is in metacarpal abduction and flexion and in metacarpophalangeal extension. When grafts were secure, traction was released twice daily for exercise. (c) When traction was removed, hand position was maintained with a thermoplast splint. (d) In a standing table, 4 months after burn, feet, ankles, hands and wrists remain in good position. Patient has emerged from a coma.

drill should be slowed a great deal to avoid ensnarement of the artery or nerves which would be lifted from the bone with the dorsal approach. There is no record of acute injury with pin insertion of either the radial artery or the median nerve.

Complication

Complications recorded by Youel among 1128 extremities in 626 patients treated with skeletal suspension and traction included 30 pin track infections and 14 bone infections.[24] The overall infection rate was 4.0%. This is a low incidence considering the population treated. In fact it is likely that all pin sites become infected to some extent regardless of the quality of pin site care. If traction for any condition is continued for several weeks there will be trabecular concentration along the pin tracks. If this denser bone becomes nonviable because of infection along the track, it will separate from the surrounding bone to from a so-called cigarette sequestrum. This kind of bone infection is usually benign and, like simple pin track infection, will resolve after the pin is removed. A diagnosis of osteomyelitis requires positive culture of curetted bone in addition to radiographic changes. The organisms in all infections of pin site origin are those found on the surface wounds. *Staphylococcus* and *Pseudomonas* are the most common. Only one of Youel's[24] cases of osteomyelitis required surgical debridement. All others responded favorably to an average of 2 weeks of antibiotic therapy. Infection related to skeletal pins will always be more common in patients with acute burns than in those whose burn wounds have healed. Youel's study confirms this expected difference. Pin site infection can be kept to a minimum if pins are observed closely for loosening and the pin sites are kept clean and open. Loose pins should be replaced with a larger one at the same site or a new site chosen.

With prolonged transmetacarpal pin traction, a synostosis may develop along the pin track between the second and third metacarpals. This phenomenon is more likely to be observed in patients who develop heterotopic bone at other sites. There is no reason to remove the bridging bone as the two affected metacarpals make up the fixed part of the hand.

Rigid External Fixators

In acute burn states, rigid external fixators are useful in the management of fractures and for the stabilization of exposed and unstable major joints. The advantage of rigid external fixation for fractures as compared to balanced free skeletal traction is that the patient can be moved about easily for wound management. The disadvantage is that the four or more transosseous pins are required to align and immobilize the fracture and can complicate management of wounds of the affected extremity.

For exposed and/or unstable major joints, there is no more secure or accurate way to gain and maintain alignment than with an external fixator (**Figure 45.19a–c**). In children it is not necessary to use a commercial fixator; as one fabricated of methyl methacrylate-filled plastic tubing and threaded pins will work very well. The advantage of a commercial product is its being readily adjustable. For elbow or knee stabilization, there must be at least four pins traversing eight cortices, two above and two below the joint. For the knees of larger patients it is better to have six pins through 12 cortices. Commercial unicortical screw systems for fracture stabilization may be as useful in burn treatment for unstable joints as for fractures if need for fixation is relatively short-

term. There is the concern that, in the rapidly demineralizing bone of seriously burned patients, pin purchase in only one cortex might not give continuing stability. In a fixed system, just as with free traction pin, loosening and untidy pin sites are the prime causes of pin site and pin track infection.

In chronic burn states, a rigid pin system is occasionally useful for maintaining skeletal position after contracture release and grafting. The best example of this application is with reestablishment of the first intermetacarpal space after first metacarpal extension–adduction contracture (**Figure 45.20a–c**). Multiple pin fixation is distinctly better than transmetacarpal pinning because it permits fine adjustment and is secure enough for free movement of the metacarpophalangeal and interphalangeal joints of the first and second digits. There are commercial external fixation systems for small bones; however, the most practical system combines commercial threaded pins with methyl methacrylate-filled plastic tubing.

Ilizarov External Fixator

The Ilizarov system seems to be ideally suited for the correction of chronic skeletal deformities in burns in which there is extreme fixed malposition, tight and unyielding soft tissue contracture, diminishing articular cartilage space, shortened blood vessels and nerves, and loss of skeletal length. Surgical correction is often out of the question because of inadequate soft tissue and because shortened nerves and vessels cannot tolerate abrupt major stretch. However, these same structures seem to tolerate well the spaced micro-incremental stretch imposed by the Ilizarov external fixator. In his report, Calhoun lists four major foot and ankle deformities (equinus, cavus, rocker bottom, and toe dislocation) as indications for use of the Ilizarov system in burn contracture management[26] (**Figure 45.21a–d**). Of the 48 patients treated with the Ilizarov fixator since 1988 at the Shriners Burns Hospitals in Galveston, Texas only two involved the upper extremity.

An advantage of the Ilizarov system is that the fixation is stable enough to permit the patient to bear weight on an affected lower extremity. In that respect, thus, it is a functional device. On the other hand, to gain correction of deformity requires that the device be in place for a long time. Among the 48 patients cited above, the average fixator time was 2.5 months. As with other means of skeletal fixation, infection about the pins is a common complication that is readily controlled with antibiotics or with pin removal.

In general, results of correction of burn deformity with the Ilizarov fixator are satisfactory; however, the final attained position cannot be considered to be stable. After removal of the fixator maintenance of position may require casts, expressly fabricated splints or braces and aggressive physical therapy. Motor weakness or absence further complicates rehabilitation. In children, the deformities may gradually recur with growth, necessitating reapplication of the device. If after correction there is minimum or no motion in a major joint, fusion is the best way to prevent deformity and to gain maximum stable function.

Prosthetic and orthotic intervention

The Prosthetist's Role

To date, little has been published regarding prosthetics relating to thermal injury, yet patients with burn injuries can present interest-

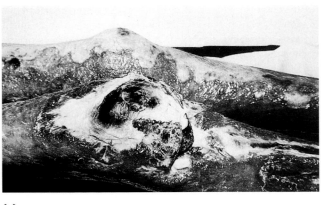

(a)

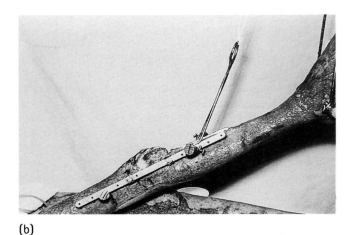

(b)

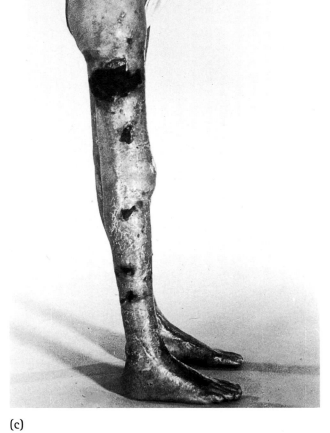

(c)

Fig. 45.19 (a) Widely exposed right knee joint and anterior tibia in an 8-year-old girl, 30 days after a 41% TBSA burn. (b) For repeated wound debridement and to facilitate eventual wound closure, the knee was stabilized in extension with four pins through medial and lateral external splints fabricated of stock strap aluminum. (c) Four months after burn, the right knee joint and tibia were completely covered with autogenous skin grafts. The knee was completely extensible and could be flexed 30°. The external fixator was removed 2 months after application.

ing problems which are simultaneously the same as with other patients and yet unique. Patients who have suffered severe burns have complex, long-term problems and considerable self-care to provide. The challenge to the orthotist and prosthetist is to design a device which is maximally useful to a patient who may have multiple limitations. To be useful, a device must be as easy to use as possible. Simplicity often determines whether the device is successful or discarded by a patient.

Planning for Function

Prosthetic rehabilitation begins with surgery and progresses to splinting, exercise therapy, preparatory, and then definitive prosthetics. Surgeons performing amputations must be familiar with optimal levels for function and growth. Consultation with rehabilitation team members prior to surgery regarding the planned surgi-

cal level, weight-bearing areas and alternatives can provide useful information in providing a patient with optimum function while using a prosthesis.

Additional Multiple Involvement

Many burned patients have severe limitations in the function of intact extremities which affect their ability to utilize a prosthesis. Their limitations and strengths are important considerations when planning treatment. For example, functional status has been improved in patients with considerable knee instability secondary to burn trauma by performing below-knee rather than above-knee amputation, stabilizing the knee with prosthetic components, and allowing knee stability to improve over time with the formation of scar tissue. Salvaging part of the forearm where there is an active elbow flexor and no extensor, or even extremely limited range of

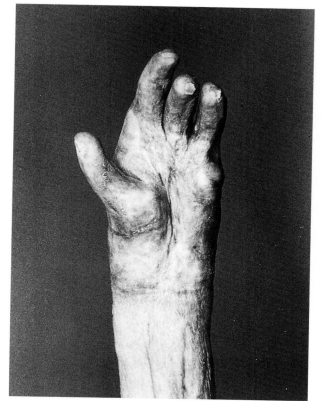

(a)

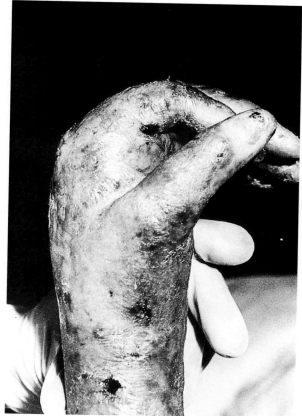

(c)(i)

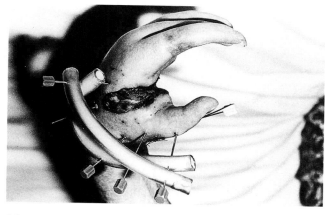

(b)

Fig. 45.20 (a) Left hand of a 15-year-old female, 1 year after a 53% TBSA burn. The fifth digit has been amputated at the metacarpophalangeal joint. The first metacarpal has become fixed in flexion and adduction. The first metacarpophalangeal joint is subluxated in extension. (b) The first metacarpal has been freed from the palm and the first metacarpophalangeal and subluxation has been reduced. The thumb ray is held in metacarpal abduction and flexion and in metacarpophalangeal flexion by terminally threaded pins stabilized by two methyl methacrylate filled plastic tubing splints. (c)(i,ii) Two months after corrective surgery, grasp and pinch have been restored. External fixators were removed six weeks after application. Position is maintained with splint and through active and passive exercise.

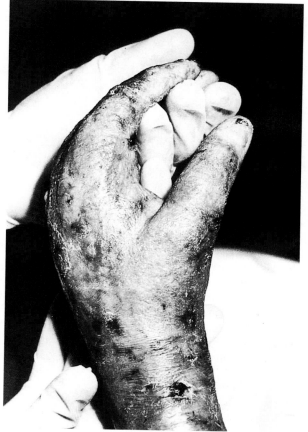

(c)(ii)

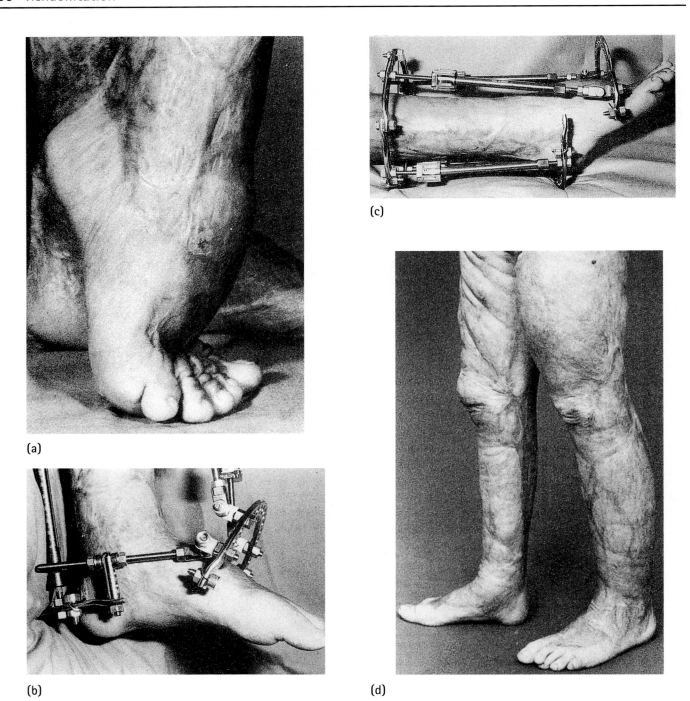

(a)

(b)

(c)

(d)

Fig. 45.21 (a) Extreme equinus deformity of the right foot and ankle of an 11-year-old male, 8 years after a 92% TBSA burn. The deformity was due to scar and triceps surae contracture. (b) To correct an equinus deformity, Ilizarov components were applied so as to gain anterior shortening through a distal transmetatarsal pin and posterior lengthening through a distal calcaneal pin. (c) Correction to 5–10° above neutral was attained in 6 weeks. Walking on the affected extremity was permitted throughout correction period. No soft-tissue release was required. The Ilizarov components were removed 13 weeks after application. (d) Four years after removal of the Ilizarov fixator, correction has been maintained and there is active dorsiflexion of 10° from neutral.

motion, can provide increased function both with and without a prosthesis compared to a higher amputation level with better skin coverage. Limited function of the contralateral extremity, especially the hand, will affect decisions regarding amputation, ampu-tation level, and reconstructive surgery. Severely burned patients may need to use their remaining functioning extremities differently than patients without total body involvement. Prosthetic rehabilitation should enhance adaptations.

Prosthetic Components

Standard prosthetic texts are useful in providing broad basic information and explanation of the many components available and their use.[27,28] Components for various regions are described below.

Hand

Improved techniques of plastic surgery of the partial hand have greatly reduced the need for partial hand prosthesis other than those for cosmesis. On the other hand, opposition posts can be useful for patients awaiting further surgical improvement.

Below elbow

- Wrist flexion units, especially when there is contralateral upper extremity involvement.
- Distal cushions in below-elbow sockets.
- Padding – which can be attached to a harness ring so as to distribute pressure from straps.
- Rapid adjust buckles for donning and doffing for patients with limited range of motion at the glenohumeral joint.
- Cross-chest straps for patients with protracted scapulae and/or scarring and poor definition in the deltopectoral area.
- Utilization of 'preflexion' of the forearm relative to the socket to compensate for limited range of motion.

Above elbow and shoulder level

- A flexible thermoplastic inner socket provides reduction in shear stress at trim lines and enhanced adjustability and socket replacement.
- For extremely short above-elbow and shoulder level cases, chest expansion is rarely useful for activating the elbow lock. Other means, such as attaching the elbow lock cable to a waistband may be necessary.
- Electronics have been used rarely due to physiological and environmental factors.

Lower extremity

Choice of prosthetic components for the lower extremity is based on a patient's functional ability and physiology pertaining to the maintenance of skin integrity. When these criteria are satisfied, cosmesis is addressed. Severely burned patients may exhibit muscle weakness not usually seen at the same amputation levels in the non-burn patient. These should be noted and compensation such as increasing stability of a prosthetic knee through alignment or components should be provided.

Below knee

Proximal weight-bearing components, such as knee joints/thigh lacer or ischialgluteal weight-bearing brims can be helpful with patients who have problems tolerating full weight bearing on the amputation stump or who have the sagittal plane leverage which a below-knee residual limb can provide but lack the frontal plane stability at the knee. They also assist a patient with diminished thing strength. For partial feet, several types of prostheses have been utilized. Pressure, especially for dorsal foot burns, should be incorporated into the prosthesis or the shoe so as to inhibit hypertrophic burn scar formation. Where bony overgrowth and bone spurs occur, the use of extra socket depth with replaceable distal

cushions is helpful. Use of suspension sleeves with and without suction valves has been rewarding.

Above the knee

Neoprene-type suspension belts are well tolerated. Suction, especially suction using 'hypobaric sheaths', can work if no excessively deep scarring is present. Where scarring is present, the sockets are contoured to the shape presented. Ischial containment with utilization of large surface areas, increased stump to socket stability, and flexible inner sockets are routinely prescribed.

Socket Fitting

With early fitting, some skin problems will be encountered, but these have not been of major significance. Silicone gel or urethane socket inserts have been used successfully, but they create extra bulk, weight, and replacement expense (especially with still growing pediatric patients). They are used when other methods are unsuccessful. Distal cushions made from the usual prosthetic materials such as silicone foam are used. On occasion, patients have removed the distal cushions on their own, and no distal edema problems have been noted.

Initial Prosthetics

Initial and early prosthetic treatment of an upper extremity amputee includes splinting for the prevention of contracture. A splint may be extended past the distal end of a residual limb to match the length of the whole limb, thus assisting a patient in retaining the concept of length. This is especially useful for patients whose active participation in a rehabilitation program is delayed. A preparatory prosthesis is provided when early definitive fitting is not prudent, e.g. when reduction of stump volume is anticipated or when fitting over a bulky dressing is necessary. For young children, a socket with harness/cable and PVC tube extension has been used.[29] The distal tube is filled with plastic resin, drilled, and tapped to accept a prosthetic device. Friction is provided through a set screw on the side of the distal tube. Wrist flexion units can be added, but they add weight and require maintenance, as well as careful training by an occupational therapist. Unless this component significantly increases a patient's function, it may be more of an irritant than an aid. Standard figure-of-eight harnessing can be used to attach a prosthesis. To distribute pressure, pads are placed under the harness from C7 to the distal scapular area and extend laterally the width of the back.

Preparatory weight-bearing treatment is provided through an air bag system, utilizing air bags designed for stabilization of a lower extremity. Containers have been fabricated from laminated plastics or polypropylene, using neoprene on the distal end or a solid ankle cushion heal foot with adapters built into the containers (**Figure 45.22**). Treatment usually begins on a tilt table, progressing to standing and then ambulation in the parallel bars. Most below-knee prosthetic devices are self-suspending. A belt with straps attached to the containers (when fabricated) has been used for above-knee cases. When a patient experiences hypersensitivity at the amputated sites and the skin at those sites is very fragile, a hybridized prosthesis/orthosis (prosthesis) may be fabricated. This allows for early ambulation by having patients shift their weight from side to side (**Figure 45.23a,b**). In the cases where bilateral amputations occur above the knee, an Ilizarov external fixator may be applied to lengthen the femoral bones bilaterally and prevent

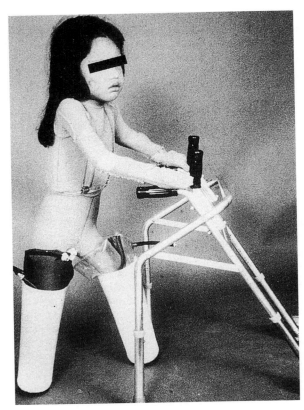

Fig. 45.22 This girl is walking on a set of temporary prostheses which employ air bags surrounding the partially healed stumps. These air bag prostheses allow the patient to begin weight bearing and practice walking before full healing has occurred.

hip contractures. A 2–3-inch gain bilaterally will eventually make the fitting of prosthesis much easier. Pillions may be attached to the orthotic fixators in order to allow for some weight bearing before the lengthening and healing of the bones is completed (**Figure 45.24**).

Definitive Prosthetics

Knowledge about a patient's prosthetic ability, work, and recreational activities will have been accrued by the time of definitive fitting. Most patients welcome the opportunity to provide feedback regarding changes in components or changes for function and fit with the definitive prosthesis. Information is provided to a patient regarding available options. Some patients will sacrifice cosmesis for hi-tech, maximum function such as a thermoplastic socket with a frame for a hydraulic knee and energy return foot with no cosmetic covering. Others will part with some function in order to achieve a desired level of cosmesis. The current array of the available prosthetic socket/weight-bearing and suspension combination, as well as application and use of the many component combinations, is beyond the scope of this chapter. In general, the simplest system which provides the most functional-cosmetic level is accepted by the amputee as the best choice.

Some patients will continue to use their preparatory prosthesis for extended periods of time while other areas of the body are treated. Prior to definitive fitting, body weight, residual limb volume, wear and use patterns should be stable in order to optimize the long-term result with the definitive prosthesis. Return clinic visits should include prosthetic evaluation. Children may require length adjustments even prior to definitive fitting. Other patients may leave the hospital with the prosthetic knee locked and may need additional therapy and prosthetic alignment for improved ambulation with swing phase knee flexion. The overall process of prosthetic evaluation and fitting is illustrated in **Figure 45.25**.

The Orthotist's Role

The role of the orthotist in treating the burn patient is similar to treating any other patient with orthopedic deficits. Soft-tissue deformities involving structural and mechanical properties are addressed by the same forces which are harnessed and applied to any orthotic user. Treating the burn patient for his orthotic needs may, however, pose a significant challenge of the orthotist in the cases where fitting of an orthosis may be completed by poor skin integrity, fragile and/or sensitive skin, and fluctuation in the volume of the extremity to be treated. Additional factors which may have an influence on the type of the orthosis used may include the patient's neurological status, pressure points due to pressure garment presence, projected duration of the orthotic utilization, geographic location or a patient's proximity to a clinic for follow-up visits and orthotic modifications, and language/cultural barriers which may affect the compliance with an orthosis.

Orthotic treatment of the lower extremity

The approach of the orthotist in treating the injured foot depends on the extent of the burn injury. Orthotic shoes, which are the fundamental component of most lower extremity orthotics, may be utilized with some modifications in correcting deformities of the burned foot. Modifications of these shoes may include arch pads, molded foot thermoplastics, tongue pads, and metatarsal bars. The orthotic shoes should distribute all forces to the foot appropriately and should reduce pressure on sensitive or deformed structures. Inserts for plantar foot support such as the University of California Biomechanical Laboratory Type (UCBL) may be utilized as indicated.

Occasionally, during the preambulation stage a patient may be fitted with orthotic shoes and a modified Dennis Brown Bar. This device, if properly utilized, may position the ankle joint appropriately, thus preventing or correcting plantar/dorsal contractures and inversion/eversion of the foot. If hip abduction is required, the specific length of the bar can be established prior to fitting the Dennis Brown Bar.

Leg length discrepancies are seen frequently in the cases of severe lower extremity burn injuries and they should be addressed with a shoe lift. The ankle/foot complex is difficult to address, especially in the case of a severe thermal injury. In most cases, the resultant deformity is the equinovarus foot. Both conventional and thermoplastic systems may be designed to treat the equinovarus or equinovalgus foot. Such systems may include a metal ankle foot orthosis (AFO) with a plastic shoe insert, polypropylene plastic posterior AFO (solid or with a posterior leaf spring), an AFO with stirrup attachment, an AFO with stirrups and patellar tendon support. A dorsiflexion spring assist may be incorporated in the stirrups of an AFO to aid weak ankle motion. Different straps such as

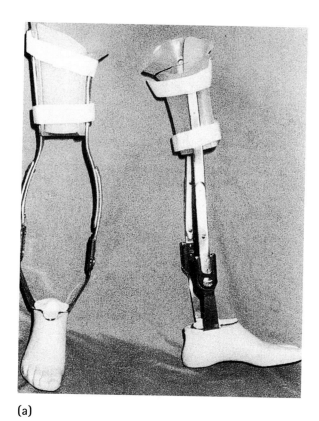

(a)

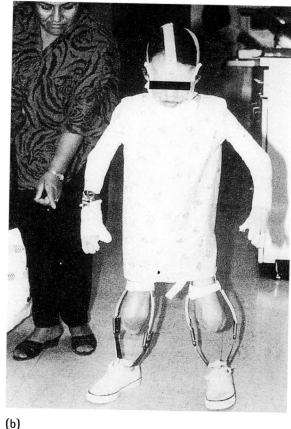

(b)

Fig. 45.23 (a) When the skin at the stump is too fragile to permit weight bearing, a hybridized prosthetic/orthotic device such as this can allow a patient to begin walking (b) by shifting the weight to a proximal site (in this case the ischium) when it cannot be borne distally.

a valgus correction strap may be attached to the AFO for the correction of specific problems. During more complicated cases, and depending on the anatomy and function of the lower extremities, a knee ankle foot orthosis, hip knee ankle foot orthosis or a trunk knee ankle foot orthosis may also be designed for the best functional outcome.[30]

Burn scar management

History

The burn wound, like any other wound, heals by the formation of scar at the injured site in order to replace the destroyed tissues. Scar is defined as the fibrous tissue replacing normal tissues destroyed by injury or disease.[31] In the case of a burn injury the scars, if not managed appropriately, have the potential of becoming thick and raised, resulting in scar hypertrophy. Hypertrophic scars are not cosmetically appealing and if they cross any joints they may restrict function. Pressure therapy for scar management is a very old and established component of a recovering burn patient's continuing rehabilitation program. Extensive historical notes on the earliest references to scarring are provided by Linares and colleagues who attribute the first full medical

description of scars to Petz in 1790.[32] They also state that the first medical reference to the use of pressure for treatment was written by Johnson in 1678 referring to the work of Ambroise Paré in the sixteenth century.[32] Other historical events noted by Linares *et al.* are: first known accounts of the use of pressure for treatment of children in 1859, use of elastic bandages in 1860, adhesive plaster for pressure in 1881, and use of traction to treat scars in 1902. Linares' review includes descriptions of Nason's work in 1942 in which he noted that ischemia produced by pressure arrests the overproduction of scar tissue, 'where the imprint of the elastic of an undergarment or a belt may be seen – no keloid is present.'[32] Another historical review, by Ward,[33] reveals that Blair in 1924 reported the positive influence of pressure on healing wounds. Nason's application of the 'constant pressure' principle included developing a type of neck splint made of a piece of dental impression compound or a piece of heavy felt strapped tightly over the scar for 6–8 weeks and possibly longer. Later, various splints were developed utilizing pressure and immobilization.[32] In the 1960s, Drs Silverstein and Larson observed the influence of pressure on healing burns. Their observations led to the manufacture of customized pressure garments that revolutionized scar management in the 1970s, which continues to date with some modifications.[32,33]

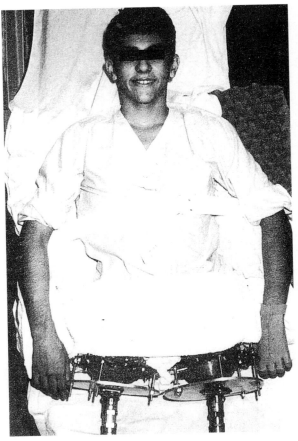

Fig. 45.24 When a bilateral amputation occurs high above the knee, a prosthesis cannot readily be fitted. An orthotic external fixator can be used to lengthen the bones and reduce contractures. In this case, the 2–3 inch bones were stretched to about 6 inches, while prosthetic pillions were attached to the orthotic fixators in order to allow some weight bearing before the lengthening and healing process were complete.

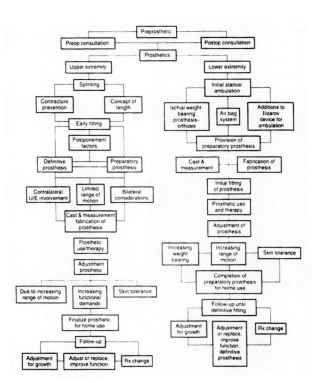

Fig. 45.25 Algorithm showing the process of prosthetic evaluation and fitting.

The Scar

As the burn wound progresses toward healing or after skin grafting operations take place, scars begin to form. Generally, the deeper the burns are the higher the risk is for the development of hypertrophic scars. Also, the longer a wound remains open the higher the chances for hypertrophic scar formation.[34,35] As the wound begins the healing process, collagen fibers develop to bridge the wound, forming an immature (active) scar which appears as a red, raised and rigid mass.[36–39] Abston reported that pressure therapy during maturation lead to a flatter, softer, and more devascularized scar.[40] Burn scars may take up to 2 years to mature. Factors contributing to the formation of hypertrophic scars may include: wound infection, genetics, immunologic factors, repeated harvesting of donor sites, altered ground substance, age, chronic inflammatory process, location of the injury, and tension.[41] Scar hypertrophy may be evident at 8–12 weeks after wound closure.[42]

Assessment

In order to better study the process of scar maturation, ongoing research is looking at alternative techniques in assessing the state of scars. Hambleton and colleagues studied the thickness of scars with ultrasonic scanning. This method, which is completely noninvasive, allows for a comparison of the thickness of dermal tissue in the traumatized area with that in the normal skin at regular intervals following initial healing.[43] Darvey et al. described a technique for the objective assessment of scars utilizing a video camera image on a computer and quantitatively analyzing the color of the scars using a custom written computer program.[44] Esposito used a modified tonometer to measure skin tone which correlates to skin pliability and tension.[45] Bartell and co-workers used the elastometer properties of normal versus injured skin. In his study, Bartell showed that scars, if left untreated, will show improvement overtime.[46] The Vancouver Burn Scar Assessment developed by Sullivan and colleagues is a subjective way of rating the burn scar pigmentation, vascularity, pliability, and height.[47] Hosoda utilized laser flowmetry to determine the perfusion of hypertrophic scars versus nonhypertrophic scars.[48] Other studies suggest that laser Doppler flowmetry and monitoring of transcutaneous oxygen tension may become ways of determining scar maturation.[49]

Treatment of Hypertrophic Scars

To date, hypertrophic scars remain very problematic and difficult to manage. Even though the mechanism of scar maturation is not well understood, clinically the accepted protocol to treat hypertrophic scars includes the use of pressure therapy which should be instituted early on in the maturation process of the burn scar. Means of pressure therapy include pressure garments, inserts, and conforming orthotics. Once the skin has healed enough to withstand sheering, massage and heat modalities may be utilized as an adjunct in scar management. The use of pressure in effectively depressing scars was well documented by Drs Silverstein and Larson in the 1970s, their observation and studies sparked the near universal use of pressure garments. When an active scar is compressed it blanches, which indicates decreased blood flow in the area.[50] Less blood leads to decreased oxygen in the tissues, which in turns leads into decreased collagen production, causing a balance between collagen synthesis and collagen breakdown (lysis). When a balance in the production and breakdown of collagen is established, the resultant scar appears flatter.[51] The efficacy of custom pressure garments in treating hypertrophic scars was first questioned by Kealey *et al.* in 1990.[52] In a prospective study, they compared prefabricated cotton tubular elastic Tubigrip™ garments to custom-made Jobst pressure garments. Their study showed that Tubigrip™ and Jobst pressure garments are equally efficacious in the treatment of hypertrophic scars.[52] The results of this study raised the question of how much pressure is really needed in effectively treating scar hypertrophy. At the Shriners Hospital for Children in Galveston, Texas, Groce *et al.* are studying the effects of high versus low pressure in treating hypertrophic scars. Preliminary results of the study show no significant difference in scar pigmentation, vascularity, and pliability in the patients receiving high versus low pressure therapy.[53] Another study at the Shriners Hospital for Children in Galveston, Texas by Groce, *et al.* is examining the effects of pressure versus no pressure in treating hypertrophic scars in children with small burns. Preliminary results show significant differences in scar height in the extremities of children with small burns receiving pressure therapy. No significant differences, however, are noted in the vascularity, pigmentation and pliability of the scars in the pressure receiving versus the nonpressure receiving groups.[54] Moore, *et al.* in a prospective study at the University of Washington, Harborview have looked at the effectiveness of custom pressure garments in wound management. In this study, one-half of a grafted wound was covered with a custom garment of verified pressure and compared to the other half without pressure. The results of this study suggest that custom pressure garments do not alter the ultimate appearance of burn wounds which have been excised and grafted.[55] In a prospective randomized study in 1995, Change *et al.* showed that pressure garment therapy does not affect the rate of burn scar maturation.[56]

Pressure Therapy

As long as the scars are active they may be influenced by pressure therapy. However, not all burn scars require pressure. Patients with burn wounds which heal within 7–14 days do not need pressure therapy. Those patients whose wounds heal within 14–21 days are closely monitored for pressure therapy needs and may be generally advised to use pressure garments prophylactically. A wound that heals after 21 days will require the use of pressure garments.[51] The correct amount of pressure in suppressing the hypertrophic scar has not yet been determined. Pressure of as little as 10 mmHg may be effective in remodeling the scar tissue over time; pressures over 40 mmHg may be destructive to tissues and cause paresthesias.[42] Early forms of pressure therapy include the use of elastic ace bandages directly applied on the newly healed skin or on top of the

burn dressings. The use of conforming thermoplastics along with elastic bandages may also be utilized as means of early pressure therapy.[57] Once the wounds are almost or completely closed, tubular elastic bandages such as Tubigrip™ may be utilized. These tubular bandages are offered in different sizes and accommodate all anatomical circumferences. Care should be taken in applying these tubular bandages so that fragile skin or freshly applied skin grafts do not sheer, or the minimal dressing underneath is not disturbed. The burn therapist should be aware that these tubular bandages are materials made of a single elastic thread spiraling through the weave of the fabric, disturbance of the continuous elastic by cutting holes into it will alter the pressure gradient provided by these materials. The tubular elastic bandages should be doubled over the skin surface area treated in order to provide adequate pressure.[58] Early pressure application over the hand and digits can be accomplished by the use of thin, elastic, and self-adherent wraps such as Coban™ (**Figure 45.26**). This form of pressure is excellent for adult and pediatric patients for controlling edema and aid in the early scar management of hands when the shearing forces of a glove cannot be tolerated. Small children are excellent candidates for Coban gloves versus a garment glove because of compliance issues, comprehension of instructions in

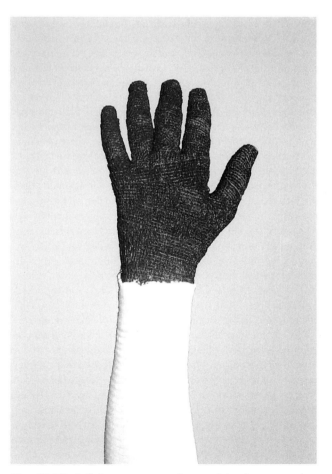

Fig. 45.26 A Coban wrap can be used to decrease edema and aid in the effective management of hand scar hypertrophy.

assisting with the application of the glove, and difficulties in obtaining accurate measurements for a garment glove. Coban may be applied over the burn dressings or directly onto the healed digits. The burn therapist needs to be aware that, if coban is wrapped too tight, it may deform the interosseous structures of the healing hand. However, if Coban is wrapped too loosely, it may encourage swelling of the hands when used in combination with arm elastic garments. Coban strips are pre-cut approximately twice the length of the digits to be wrapped. Each strip is wrapped in a spiral fashion beginning at the nail bed of each digit, overlapping half of the Coban width and ending in the adjacent web space. Each fingertip needs to be exposed so that blood circulation can be monitored at all times. The Coban is stretched from 0 to 25% of the entire elasticity of each strip. Once all web spaces are covered, the rest of the hand is wrapped with Coban extending approximately 1 inch past the wrist joint. No skin areas should be visible once the Coban glove is completed. If small hand areas remain uncovered, a small piece of Coban is stretched over the area and adheres to the rest of the Coban. When the glove is completed the therapist should very superficially lubricate the entire glove with lotion in order to eliminate the adherent effect of the Coban and to allow for the functional use of the hand. Coban should be removed on a daily basis by the therapist or the caregiver. Removal of coban should be done carefully by cutting off or unwrapping each digit strip individually to avoid disturbing any small wound healing. The use of prefabricated interim pressure garments is widely accepted and utilized in burn rehabilitation. These garments provided commercially by different companies include pieces for the entire body and are offered in different sizes. Interim garments made of softer materials introduce the burn patient to circumferential pressure and protect the newly healed skin. Another reason for using these garments prior to ordering custom-made garments is to allow for the patient's weight to stabilize (post-acute hospitalization) and any remaining edema to subside. In some cases, where obtaining custom-made garments at regular intervals (approximately 12 weeks) is not an option, the recommendation should be that interim garments should be the choice for long-term pressure therapy. Once the patient's weight has stabilized, edema has subsided and the skin is able to withstand some shearing (approximately 3–4 weeks post wound closure), measurements are taken for the fabrication of custom-made pressure garments (**Figure 45.27**). Today, several companies specialize in the fabrication of these garments. Clinically, custom therapeutic pressure for the prevention, control and correction of scar hypertrophy averages 24–28 mmHg, which is equal and opposing to the capillary pressure (25 mmHg). At this pressure level many researchers believe that scars may be altered.[59] In order for pressure therapy to be effective, pressure garments need to be worn at all times, day and night. They should only be removed for bathing and on occasion during exercises, if they interfere with movements. Each order is duplicated so one set of garments can be worn while the other is being washed. Today, pressure garment companies offer multiple colors of materials and, for the pediatric population, Disney characters may be sewed on the garments to make them cosmetically appealing and improve the patients' compliance.[60] The burn therapist should choose a reputable company, which provides excellent service and support for the patient and the therapist. The company's willingness and flexibility to manufacture nonstandard garments, availability of special options, cost and turnaround time should be taken into con-

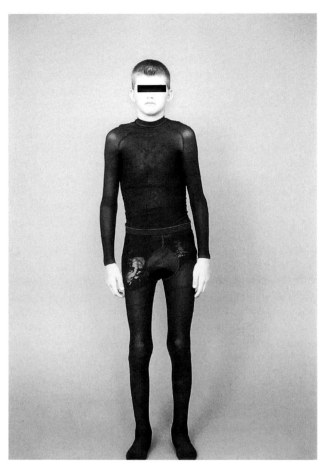

Fig. 45.27 Custom-made pressure garments may be fabricated for the entire body.

sideration when selecting the burn center's pressure garment provider.[61]

Inserts

Inserts are widely utilized in burn rehabilitation as an adjunct in achieving effective pressure over certain anatomical locations where pressure garments do not provide adequate pressure. These locations include concave body areas such as the face, neck, antecubital fossae, sternum, palm of the hands, web spaces, upper back, and arches of the feet. These materials come commercially prefabricated or may be custom-made by the burn therapist or the medical sculpture technician. Inserts come in different forms such as silicone gels, elastomers, putties mixed with silicone catalyst, skin care silastic pads, foam, and even in the form of hard thermoplastic materials contouring to different anatomical locations. The experienced burn therapist chooses the appropriate insert material best suited to the patient according to their stage of scar maturation and skin sensitivity. Generally, pressure therapy begins with a soft, thin and elastic insert and progresses to a more rigid insert in depressing the more unyielding burn scar. Inserts need to be worn underneath pressure garments starting with a few hours of application and progressing as tolerated, toward a 24-hour application. They should be removed frequently for cleaning (warm water and soap), drying and application of cornstarch in avoiding scar maceration and skin breakdown. Patients may be allergic to certain insert materials so the burn therapist should try different inserts until one is found to be best tolerated by the patient's skin. In cases of scar maceration, blisters, skin breakdown, contact dermatitis and a rash or an allergic reaction, inserts should be removed until healing occurs. Silicone, a polymer based on the element silicon, appears to be the trend in the treatment of hypertrophic scars. To this date the mechanism of how silicone affects the burn scar is not known. Clinically, silicone has been observed to depress the height of hypertrophic scars, prevent shrinking of fresh skin grafts (hard elastomer silicone pads versus silicone gel pads), and increase the pliability of a scar thus allowing for increase in the range of motion of affected joints. Patients report that silicone is soothing to the skin and aids in decreasing pain. Silicone being occlusive may cause the collection of excessive moisture and cause skin maceration if not removed frequently for cleaning and drying. Its disadvantages are that it is very expensive and short-lived.[62-64] The therapist should look for silicone gel pads with a nonshearing protective medium on the nonskin surface in order for the gel to last longer. Also, buying larger size gel pads and cutting them to fit the patient's need may be a cost-effective method for today's shrinking clinic budgets.

Other insert materials include liquid silicone elastomer which when mixed with a catalyst forms a solid but elastic insert. The experienced therapist could create custom inserts for difficult anatomic locations such as the face and web spaces using this technique. Prosthetic Foam™ is a liquid-based silicone elastomer which when mixed with a catalyst solidifies in the form of a very pliable foam insert, it works best for the palm of the hands where function needs to be preserved while pressure is applied. These foam inserts also work best for applying pressure to contour surfaces on the face (around eyes, mouth, nose) while protecting these sensitive areas from excess and rigid pressure. Elastomer putties such as Otoform K™ (**Figure 45.28**) or Rolyan Ezemix® form semirigid but still elastic inserts for different areas of the body where the scar can tolerate more pressure, such as in the web spaces to prevent syndactyly.[63] Early on in scar management a soft foam such as Plastizote™, Velfoam™ or Betapile™ may be utilized to apply gentle pressure to the very fragile and sensitive scar.

High thermoplastic transparent masks were developed in 1968 by Padewski to be applied directly to the face to prevent, control, and reverse scar hypertrophy. These masks require the moulaging of the patient in creating a negative facial mold. A positive mold of the face is fabricated with the use of plaster. The patient's positive facial mold is then 'sculptured' in an attempt to recreate the patient's nonburned face. A high thermoplastic material such as Uvex™ (**Figure 45.29**) or W-Clear™ is then pulled over the positive mold in order to create the hard plastic mask. Holes for the eyes, nose, and mouth are cut. The mask is worn under pressure garments or with a head strapping mechanism. In cases of significant scar hypertrophy on the face, the positive mold is 'sculptured' sequentially over a period of time in order to avoid excessive pressure over facial scar leading to skin breakdown. A silicone elastomer face mask (**Figure 45.30**) may be created utilizing the existing positive facial mold and is worn under facial pressure garments. The use of the clear and silastic masks is preferred over the use of just a facial garment as they provide conforming pressure around facial openings (eyes, nose, and mouth). Frequently, the

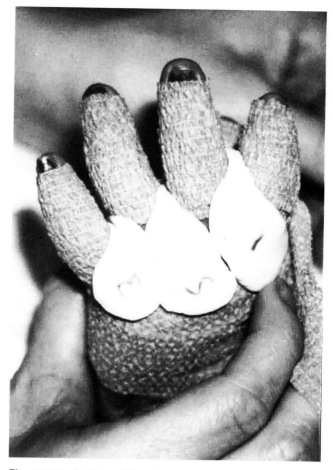

Fig. 45.28 Otoform K™ web space inserts are utilized for the prevention of syndactyly in the hand.

burn therapist manufactures the clear mask to be worn during the day and the silastic mask along with the facial mask to be worn at night.[32,65-67]

Burn Scar Massage

Once the burn scars have matured enough to tolerate sheering forces, massage may be incorporated into the scar management regimen. Scar massage is an effective modality for maintaining joint mobility in the case of contractures. It aids in softening or remodeling of the scar tissues by freeing adhering fibrous bands, allowing the scars to become more elastic and stretchy, thus improving joint mobility. Initially, the therapist may utilize a nonfrictional massage, applying mostly stationary pressure to skin blanching and mobilizing the skin surface without friction. Utilization of lubricants during this massage technique should be avoided. As the skin begins to tolerate frictional massage, the scar tissue is manipulated in rotary, parallel and perpendicular motions, using a lubricant and pressing the skin to blanche. Clinically, massage is found to alleviate itching. It is also used for desensitization purposes. An electrical massager with a heat attachment may be used along with lubrication as heat and massage in combination may increase scar pliability. Massage should be performed at least twice daily (× 3–5 preferred) for 5–10 minutes on each treated body surface. The burn therapist should frequently assess the skin

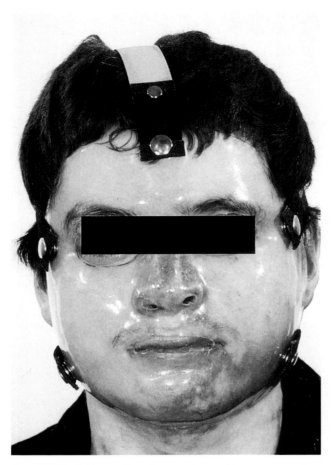

Fig. 45.29 A Uvex clear facemask provides pressure to the face so as to prevent scar hypertrophy and to preserve facial features.

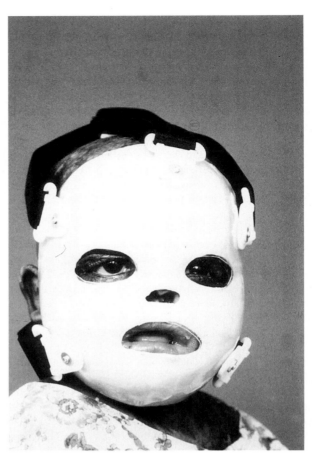

Fig. 45.30 A silicone elastomer facemask provides pressure to the face in preventing facial scar hypertrophy and preserve facial features.

condition in avoiding further injuries. The patient and/or family are instructed on home massage techniques and electrical massagers may be issued for home use. Other therapeutic modalities for scar management may include the use of heat. Heat relaxes tissues and makes them pliable in preparation for mobilization. Heat modalities may include hot packs, paraffin wax, fluidotherapy, and ultrasound. Even though the use of therapeutic heat as an adjunct to rehabilitation is well documented, therapeutic heat modalities are infrequently being utilized in burn rehabilitation.[68,69]

Burn scar management is a complicated and lengthy process and for it to be successfully completed the patient and caregivers should be committed to follow the therapist's recommendations. Extensive training should take place addressing the use and care of pressure garments, inserts, lubrication, and other therapeutic scar management procedures to be performed by the patients and their caregivers. Lubricants which do not contain perfume and other skin irritants should be selected and applied frequently (5–6 times daily) to the healing skin. Lubricants with sun protection factor (SPF) of at least 15 are recommended.[70] Written instructions with pictures and diagrams along with videos addressing scar management should accompany the patient home upon discharge from the hospital. Follow-up visits to the burn or rehabilitation clinic for the assessment of overall recovery to include garments, inserts and

other home therapeutic interventions are needed for the patient to successfully complete his burn rehabilitation. The therapists' knowledge, creativity and continuing research in improving the currently existing scar management techniques may be the key to positive outcomes in pressure therapy.

Exercise and Ambulation of the Burn Patient

Exercise

An underlying principle of physical recovery is that the promotion of purposeful activity in patients with dysfunction requires the application of professional hands directed by minds abundant with relevant information.[71] Therapeutic exercise is motion of the body or its parts to relieve symptoms or to improve function.[72] The need for exercise to enhance mobility of the burn patient begins acutely and continues throughout the months of healing. Even though painful and extensive therapy is required during the long rehabilitation process, the results are for the most part dependent upon the patients' and families understanding, involvement, and dedication to the treatment.[68] The therapist is challenged to be creative and insightful enough to enlist the patient's cooperation and participation in tedious, painful and purposeful activity over a long period of time.

The goals of exercise in burn rehabilitation are to:

- reduce the effects of edema and immobilization;
- maintain functional joint motion and muscle strength;
- stretch the scar tissue; and
- return the patient to optimal level of function.

Scar bands crossing a joint may lead to contractures limiting the range of motion of the affected joint and burn scars which cross joints, if left untreated, will prevent motion. Muscle and fibrous contracture of the joint structure can cause the deformity to become irreversible. The therapist should educate both the burn patient and their support group as to how to maintain the patient's functional mobility. For maximum benefit, all instructions should be simple, concise, and pertinent to the individual being treated. Both verbal and written instructions, as well as detailed demonstrations, are necessary. The patient and their caregivers should be given time to practice in the presence of the therapist. Early education reduces apprehension and provides a message that therapy is an ongoing evolutionary process.[73]

Exercise sessions depend upon the patient's physical, psychological, and medical status. In the conservative treatment of burn wounds, a vigorous physical therapy program is instituted immediately so as to maintain function.[74] Postoperatively exercises involving autografted joints are discontinued for 4–5 days. Escharotomies, fasciotomies, heterografts, and synthetic dressings are not contraindications for exercise.[75] Early mobilization to prevent edema, proper exercise techniques, and accurate documentation of function are more important than the type of wound closure.[74]

Scar contracture and joint mobility limitations are the result of the shortening of immature connective tissue. Therapy aims to prevent deformity and the subsequent limitation of movement. In circumferential burns, both the flexor and extensor surfaces are at risk of contracture. Exercise in conjunction with splinting should promote antagonistic movements around those joints in order to bring about the most mobile results.[73] Treatments are tailored to each individual patient with independent living being the ultimate goal throughout the rehabilitation continuum.

To achieve optimal results the goals of burn rehabilitation should include:

- stretching of the healing skin;
- maintaining or regaining normal joint range of motion;
- preserving motor skill coordination;
- maintaining or regaining strength and endurance to minimize muscular atrophy; and
- promoting functional independence.[75]

There are a variety of exercise techniques which can be incorporated into a therapy session to accomplish these objectives. Exercise techniques can be described in four categories: stretching, strengthening, cardiovascular, and functional activity exercises.

'Stretching' exercises are performed with a slow, prolonged force. Gentle, sustained stretch is more effective than multiple repetitive movements in gaining length of burned tissues. An indication of effective stretching is that the scar tissue will blanche. If scars extend across more than one joint, each joint should be stretched individually, and then the skin stretched as a whole unit across the involved joints. 'Passive' exercise is a form of stretching exercise which is performed without voluntary muscle contribution. It is a slow, gentle stretch provided by an outside force with the prime result being the stretching of tissue. There is no muscular action, and thus, there are no gains in muscle strength. The use of a continuous passive motion (CPM) device has been documented to be an effective modality for improving joint range of motion.[75] Advances have shown CPM treatment to be a viable option because of its benefits to soft-tissue remodeling, joint nutrition, wound healing, and venous dynamics.[76,77] Active and active-assistive exercises should become the focus of the session in lieu of passive stretch once the patient has achieved full range of motion. All passive exercise should be performed cautiously when there is evidence of bone or tendon exposure.

'Strengthening' exercise improves the muscles' ability to perform work. Strengthening exercises utilize muscular power thus promoting an increase in muscle strength. 'Active' exercise is performed independently by a patient. This is the form of exercise most recommended because it stretches healing skin and provides a strengthening component. Frequent exercise performed actively by a patient promotes the greatest increase in movement. 'Active-assistive' exercise utilizes the same principles; however, a patient is 'assisted' by an outside force (therapist or assistive device) to achieve the full range of motion. A patient will achieve improvements in strength and range of motion, but not equal to those provided by active exercise. Active-assistive exercise is suggested for those patients who are too weak to perform a full range of motion exercise independently. In 'resistive' exercises, manual or mechanical resistance is applied to a movement. A variety of modalities offer resistance, ranging from traditional weights to innovative combinations of rubber bands. Resistive exercises can begin in an 'assistive' fashion with minimal resistance and assistance provided to complete the range of motion.

'Cardiovascular' exercises are designed to improve a patient's endurance level. These activities are performed for prolonged periods of time with minimum resistance and can be designed to involve activities which are enjoyable for the patient.

'Functional' exercise includes those activities which incorporate all types of the above-mentioned exercises. They are designed to improve the coordination and performance of patients in tasks which are relevant to activities of daily living. For example, feeding requires both coordination and strength as well as stretching to take the hand to the mouth. Performing functional activities is generally rewarding to patients. The goal(s) and purpose of these activities are clearly defined and understood. Completion of these tasks requires concentration and appears to distract a patient from the pain of movement. Functional tasks also seem to provide a feeling of accomplishment and encouragement to a patient who wants to regain independence.

Some basic physiology principles should be kept in mind when a patient is exercising. The average pulse rate should not exceed 60–75% of the predicted maximum heart rate. In adults, the systolic blood pressure should not exceed 225–230 mmHg. The diastolic blood pressure should be monitored and exercise stopped if the values suddenly and rapidly increase 20 mmHg or more or exceed 130 mmHg. A patient should not become dyspneic or exhibit labored breathing. The nonburned skin of a patient should be closely watched; and it should not become increasingly pale, cool or moist. An increase in body temperature, malaise, fatigue, and heat prostration should be avoided.[73]

Exercise begins immediately postburn. For a patient being treated conservatively, movement helps maintain strength and range of motion, and aids in circulation and healing. For a patient who has been grafted, isometric exercises can be performed during the immobilization period. The benefit of isometrics is that a patient does not 'forget' how to contract the muscle, a common phenomenon with periods of prolonged immobilization. Isometric exercise also helps in maintaining muscle strength, though not as profoundly as active strengthening exercise. When skin grafts have become stable, active exercise may begin. Active exercise is initially performed by allowing a patient to limit the intensity by pain. It is followed by passive stretching exercise and strengthening to maintain mobility.

Exercise can be performed with dressing and wraps in place. Care should be taken when dressings are applied so that joint range of motion is not restricted. Dressings which have been correctly applied will minimize discomfort and promote movement, while dressings applied too tightly will limit mobility, increase pain, and may create pressure-induced neuropathies. Exercise can also be performed while the patient is in the bath where the buoyancy of the water and the absence of confining dressings can make exercise less painful. Exercise is initially painful and the very first repetition is often the most difficult. Discomfort is due to stretching skin which has lost its natural lubricating mechanism and has become dry and tight. Movement itself decreases pain. Each subsequent repetition will be easier as the skin stretches, and the muscle pumping action of active movement helps resolve edema, thus significantly reducing pain.

Specific movements can be targeted to prevent burn scar contracture. In burn rehabilitation, we find that the patients tend to position themselves in a comfortable position, which most frequently is the position of contracture. Based on knowledge about typical contractures, the following movements are encouraged: neck extension and lateral flexion, shoulder abduction and flexion, elbow extension and supination, metacarpophalangeal flexion, interphalangeal extension, wrist extension, knee extension, ankle dorsiflexion, and metatarsophalangeal flexion. Exercise sessions may be indicated three to four times daily for more involved areas. Patients should be encouraged to exercise between therapy sessions.

Ambulation

To walk again following a burn injury is an important goal shared by patients of all ages. The benefits of ambulation are to:

- help maintain range of motion;
- maintain strength in the lower extremities;
- prevent thromboemboli;
- maintain bone density via weight-bearing; and
- promote independence in functional activities.[73]

Ambulation exercises may also help prevent decubiti, provide mild, cardiovascular conditioning, and increase appetite. Ambulatory patients have fewer problems with lower extremity contractures and endurance.[75]

Opinions differ as to when ambulation can begin. The patient's medical status, including the stability of skin grafts, is usually the prime indicator for the commencement of ambulation. As with other exercise, proper positioning facilitates proper gait.[73] The patient who has been allowed to assume a position of comfort will have difficulty extending the hips and knees during ambulation. The ankle may be tight, limiting plantigrade position when in the

upright position. If the joints are in the normal alignment, the amount of pain and energy are greatly reduced.

All wounds must have the proper dressings prior to ambulation. Lower extremity burn wounds should be wrapped with elastic bandages in order to facilitate capillary support. Wrapping will decrease edema and therefore decrease pain and promote healing. The extremities should be wrapped distal to proximal from the toes to the groin crease. The foot should always be included to avoid excess edema. Those extremities which have had skin grafting generally have less graft loss when there is a second elastic wrap to provide further support. Lower extremity donor sites are less painful when wrapped with elastic bandages. Wrapping which incorporates the 'figure of eight' pattern has been reported to provide better pressure than the spiral wrap[39] perhaps due to increased vascular support.

The use of a tilt table (**Figure 45.31**) can assist in beginning ambulation for those patients who may have difficulty assuming the upright position. There are a variety of reasons why erect positioning may prove difficult: for example, extended periods of bed rest which influence blood pressure or ankle tightness may inhibit plantigrade position. The tilt table can be used to overcome these obstacles and assist a patient with early ambulation.

Patients tend to perform much better when given an achievable

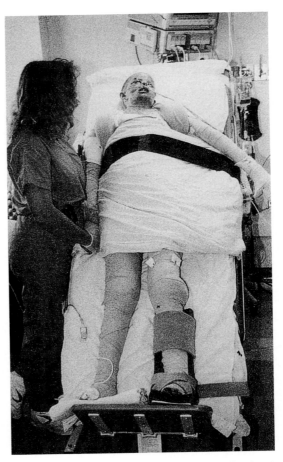

Fig. 45.31 The tilt table may be utilized prior to ambulation for those patients who may have difficulty assuming the upright position.

goal such as walking a specific distance or to a certain place. Children do well when provided with a desired incentive such as a toy or a game. Frequent rest periods may be necessary secondary to decreased endurance levels or increased pain. Patients should be encouraged to ambulate further distances each day. Care should be taken to avoid prolonged periods of standing so that hypotension does not develop. The lower extremities, even when properly wrapped for support, will show signs of vascular insufficiency when dependent for too long a period of time. The use of assistive devices, i.e. crutches or walkers, is discouraged because the legs need the muscle pumping action to prevent edema.[73] Exercise and ambulation are integral parts in the rehabilitation of burn patients. Both allow a patient to resume a lifestyle as active and independent as possible.

Patient and/or Caregiver Education

When the patient is being discharged from the acute hospital stay, it is vital that they leave with an individualized home exercise instruction program. Splinting and positioning, exercises, activity of daily living performance, scar control measures, and psychosocial issues are addressed. This program can then be updated and upgraded to allow for progression during the ever-changing phases that the burn patient goes through, in what may be in excess of a 2-year recovery period. During follow-up visits, screening and monitoring of the patient's progress regarding the above categories is performed and the necessary changes are completed. This detailed knowledge of the patient's status will allow the burn team to coordinate the care for the patient so that recommendations can be followed through. Providing the patients with a checklist is a valuable tool to enable the patient to assume some control of their rehabilitation process, enable them to track their progress and encourage their continuation of the program. Many patients and their caregivers are often overwhelmed by the rehabilitation program. It takes an extraordinary amount of time and energy to plan and participate in the home exercise/instruction program. Continuous communication among the patient, caregiver and the burn team will ease the patient's transition into recovery.

References

1. Fess EE, Philips CA. *Hand Splinting – Principles and Methods*, 2nd edn. Part II: Principles. St Louis: CV Mosby, 1987; 125–254.
2. Harries CA, Pegg SP. Foam ear protectors for burned ears. *J Burn Care Rehabil* 1989; 10: 183–4.
3. Ridgway CL, Warden GD. Evaluation of a vertical mouth stretching orthosis: two case reports. *J Burn Care Rehabil* 1995; 16(1): 74–8.
4. Taylor LB, Walker J. A review of selected microstomia prevention appliances. *J Pediatric Dent* 1997; 19: 413–8.
5. Heinle JA, et al. The microstomia prevention appliance: 14 years of clinical experience. *J Burn Care Rehabil* 1988; 9(1): 90–1.
6. Maragakis GM, Tempone MG. Microstomia following facial burns. *J Pediatr Dent* 1999; 23: 69–73.
7. Sykes L. Scar traction appliance for a patient with microstomia: a clinical report. *J Prosthet Dent* 1996; 76(1): 464–5.
8. Rivers, et al. The transparent face mask. *Am J Occup Ther* 1979; 33: 108–13.
9. Linares HA, Larson DL, Willis-Galstraun B. Historical notes on the use of pressure in the treatment of hypertrophic scar and keloids. *Burns* 1993; 19(1): 17–21.
10. Malick MH, Carr JA. Manual on management of the burned patient, including splinting, mold and pressure techniques. Pittsburgh: Harmarville Rehabilitation Center, 1982.
11. Leman CJ. Splints and accessories following burn reconstruction. *Clini Plast Surg* 1992; 19(3): 721–31.
12. Walters CJ. Splinting the Burn Patient. Maryland: RAMSCO Publishing Company, Laurel, 1987.
13. Richard R, Stalay M. Burn care and rehabilitation principles and practice. Philadelphia: F.A. Davis Company, 1994; Chapter 11 242–323.
14. Richard RL. Use of the dynasplint to correct elbow flexion contracture: A case report. *J Burn Care Rehabil* 1986; 7: 151–2.
15. Ward RS, et al. Have you tried the sandwich splint? A method of preventing hand deformities in children. *J Burn Care Rehabil* 1989; 10: 83–5.
16. Harnar T, Engrav L, Marvin J. et al. Dr. Paul Unna's boot and early ambulation after skin grafting of the leg. *Plast Reconstr Surg* 1982; 69: 359–60.
17. Bennett GB. Serial casting: a method of treating burn contractures. *J Burn Care Rehabil* 1989; 10(6): 543–5.
18. Ridgway CL, et al. Serial casting as a technique to correct burn scar contractures: a case report. *J Burn Care Rehabil* 1991; 12: 67.
19. Larson DL, Evans EB, Abston S, Lewis SR. Skeletal suspension in traction in the treatment of burns. *Ann Surg* 19868; 168(6): 981–5.
20. Evans EB. Orthopedic measures in the treatment of severe burns. *J Bone Joint Surg (Am)* 1966; 48: 643–69.
21. Evans EB, Larson DL, Abston S, Willis B. Prevention and correction of deformity after severe burns. *Surg Clin North Am* 1979; 50(6): 136–75.
22. Evans EB, Larson DL, Yates S. Preservation and restoration of joint function in patients with severe burns. *JAMA* 1968; 204: 843–8.
23. Harnar T, Engrav L, Heimbach D, Marvin J. Experience with skeletal immobilization after excision and grafting of the severely burned hands. *J Trauma* 1985; 25: 299–302.
24. Youel L, Evans EB, Heare TC, Herndon DN, Larson DL, Abston S. Skeletal suspension in the management of severe burns in children. *J Bone Joint Surg (Am)* 1986; 68: 1375–9.
25. Evans EB. Musculoskeletal changes complicating burns. In: Epps CH Jr, ed. Complications in Orthopaedic Surgery. Vol 2. Philadelphia: JB Lippincott Co, 1978; 113–58.
26. Calhoun JH, Evans EB, Herndon DN. Techniques for the management of burn contractures with the Ilizarov fixator. *Clin Orthop Rel Res* 1993; 280: 117–24.
27. Bowker JH, In: Michael JWM, ed. Atlas of Limb Prosthetics: Surgical Prosthetic and Rehabilitation Principles. St Louis, MO: CV Mosby, 1992.
28. Pritham CH. Cumulative volume of clinical orthotics and prosthetics. Alexandria, VA: The American Academy of Orthotists and Prosthetists 1988: 8(3)–12(3).
29. Fletchall S, Tran T, Ungarao V, Hickerson W. Updating upper extremity temporary prosthetics. Thermoplastics. *J Burn Care Rehabil* 1992; 13: 584–6.
30. O'Sullivan SB, Schmitz TJ. Physical rehabilitation assessment and treatment, edn 3. Chapter 30, Orthotic Assessment and Management, 655–84. Philadelphia: F.A. Davis Company, 1994.
31. Stedman's Medical Dictionary. 23rd edn, Baltimore: Williams and Wilkins, 1976.
32. Linares HA, Larson DL, Willis-Galstraun B. Historical notes on the use of pressure in the treatment of hypertrophic scars and keloids. *Burns* 1993; 19(2): 17–21.
33. Ward RS. Pressure therapy for the control of hypertrophic scar formation after burn injury, a history and review. *J Burn Care Rehabil* 1991; 12(3): 257–62.
34. Linares HA. Hypertrophic healing: Controversies and etiopathogenic review. In: Carvajal HF, Parks DH eds. Burns in children: Pediatric Burn Management. Chicago: Yearbook Medical Publishers, 1988, 305–323.
35. Shakespeare PG, Renterghem L. Some observations on the surface structure of collagen in hypertrophic scars. *Burns* 1985; 11: 175–80.
36. Hayakawa T, Hino M, Fuyamada H, et al. Lysyl oxidase activity in human normal skins and post-burn scars. *Clin Chim Acta* 1976; 7: 245–50.
37. Hayakawa T, Hino M, Fuyamada H, et al. Prolyl hydroxylase activity in human normal skins and post-burn scars. *Clin Chim Acta* 1977; 75: 137–42.
38. Hayakawa T, Hashimoto Y, Myokei Y, et al. Changes in type of collagen during the development of human post-burn hypertrophic scars. *Clin Chim Acta* 1979; 93: 119–25.
39. Hayakawa T, Hashimoto Y, Myokei Y, et al. The effects of skin grafts on the ratio of collagen types in human post-burn wound tissues. *Connect Tissue Res* 1982; 9: 249–52.
40. Abston S. Scar reaction after thermal injury and prevention of scars and contractures. In: Boswick JA, ed. The Art and Science of Burn Care. Rockville: Aspen Publishers, 1987; 360–1.
41. Staley M, Richard R. Burn Care and Rehabilitation Principles and Practice. Philadelphia: F.A. Davis Company, 1994; Chapter 14 380–418.
42. Reid WH, Evans JH, Naismith RS, et al. Hypertrophic scarring and pressure therapy. *Burns* 1987; 13 (suppl): S29.
43. Hambleton J, Shakespeare PG, Pratt BJ. The progress of hypertrophic scars monitored by ultrasound measurements of thickness. *Burns* 1992; 18(4), 301–7.
44. Davey RB, Sprod RT and Neild TO. Computerized colour: a technique for the assessment of burn scar hypertrophy. A preliminary report. *Burns* 1999; 25(3): 207–13.
45. Esposito G, et al. The use of a modified tonometer in burn scar therapy. *J Burn Care Rehabil* 1990; 11: 86–90.
46. Bartell TH, Monafo WW and Mustoe TA. A new instrument for serial

measurement of elasticity in hypertrophic scar. *J Burn Care Rehabil* 1988; **9**: 657–60.

47. Sullivan T, *et al*. Rating the burn scar. *J Burn Care Rehabil* 1990; **11**: 256–60.

48. Hosoda G, Holloway GA, Heimback DM. Laser Doppler flowmetry for the early detection of hypertrophic burn scars. *J Burn Care Rehabil* 1986; **7**: 490–7.

49. Berry RB, *et al*. Transcutaneous oxygen tension as an index of maturity in hypertrophic scars treated by compression. *Br Plast Surg* 1985; **38**: 163–73.

50. Reid WH, Evans JH, Naismith RS, *et al*. Hypertrophic scarring and pressure therapy. *Burns* 1987; **13 (suppl)**: S29.

51. McDonald WS, Deitch EA. Hypertrophic skin grafts in burn patients: a prospective analysis of variables. *J Trauma* 1987; **27**: 147–50.

52. Kealey GP, Jensen KL, Laubenthal KN, Lewis RW. Prospective randomized comparison of two types of pressure therapy garments. *J Burn Care Rehabil* 1990; **11**: 334–6.

53. Groce A, McCauley R, Herndon D, Serghiou M, Chinkes D. The effects of high pressure vs. low pressure garments in the control of hypertrophic scarring in the burned child: a preliminary 6-month report. Abstract presented at American Burn Association Annual Meeting, March 14–17, 2000.

54. Groce A, Herndon D, McCauley R, Serghiou M, Chinkes D. The effects of pressure garments vs. no pressure for the control of hypertrophic scarring in children with small burns: a preliminary 6-month report. Abstract presented at American Burn Association Annual Meeting, March 14–17, 2000.

55. Moore M, Engrav LH, Calderon J, *et al*. Effectiveness of custom pressure garments in wound management: a prospective trial within wounds and with verified pressure. Abstract presented at American Burn Association Annual Meeting, March 14–17, 2000.

56. Chang P, Laubenthal KN, Lewis RW, Rosenquist MD, Lindley-Smith P, Kealey GP. Prospective randomized study of the efficacy of pressure garment therapy in patients with burns. *J Burn Care Rehabil*. 1995; **16**: 473–5.

57. Engrav LH, *et al*. Do splinting and pressure devices damage new grafts? *J Burn Care Rehabil* 1983; **4**: 107–8.

58. Rose MP, Deitch GA. The effective use of a tubular compression bandage, Tubigrip, for burn scar therapy in the growing child. *J Burn Care Rehabil* 1983; **4**: 197–201.

59. Cheng JCY, *et al*. Pressure therapy in the treatment of post-burn hypertrophic scar – A critical look into its usefulness and fallacies by pressure monitoring. *Burns* 1984; **10**: 154–63.

60. Thompson R, Summers S, Rampey-Dobbs R, Wheeler T. Color pressure garments vs traditional beige pressure garments: perceptions from the public. *J Burn Care Rehabil* 1992; **13**: 590–6.

61. Ward RS. Reasons for the selection of burn-scar-support suppliers by burn centers in the United States: a survey. *J Burn Care Rehabil* 1993; **14**(3): 360–7.

62. Van den Kerchove E, Boechx W, Kochreyt A. Silicone patches as a supplement for pressure therapy to control hypertrophic scarring. *J Burn Care Rehabil* 1991; **12**(4): 361–9.

63. McNee S. The use of silicone gel in the control of hypertrophic scarring. *Physiotherapy* 1990; **76**: 194–7.

64. Quinn KJ. Silicone gel in scar treatment. *Burns* 1987; **13**: 533–40.

65. Derwin-Baruch L. UVA therapists meet the challenge of scar management. OT Week 1993; April 15: 15–17.

66. Rivers, EA, Strate RG, Solem LD: The transparent facemask. *Am J Occup Ther* 1979; **33**: 108–13.

67. Gallagher J, Goldfarb W, Slater H, Rososky-Grassi M. Survey of treatment modalities for the prevention and treatment of hypertrophic burn scars. *J Burn Care Rehabil* 1990; **11**(2): 118–20.

68. Miles WK, Grigsby, de Linde L. Remodeling of scar tissue in the burned hand. In: Hunter JM, *et al*. eds. Rehabilitation of the hand, edn 4, Vol II. St. Luis: CV Mosby, 1995; 1267–94.

69. Wood, EC: Beard's massage: Principles and techniques, edn 2. Philadelphia: WB Saunders, 1974; 48–59.

70. Huruitz S. The sun and sunscreen protection: recommendations for children. *J Dermatol Surg Oncol* 1988; **14**(6): 657–60.

71. Wolf SL. Morphological functional considerations for therapeutic exercise. In: Basmajian JV, ed. Therapeutic Exercise. 4th edn. Baltimore, MD: Williams & Wilkins, 1984: Chapter 2.

72. Licht S. History. In: Basmajian JV, ed. Therapeutic Exercise. 4th edn. Baltimore, MD: Williams & Wilkins, 1984: Chapter 1.

73. Johnson CL. The role of physical therapy. In: Boswick JA, ed. The Art and Science of Burn Care. Rockville: Aspen, 1987: Chapter 34, 304.

74. Robson MC, Smith DJ, VanderZee AJ, Roberts L. Making the burned hand functional. *Clin Plast Surg* 1992; **19**(3): 663–71.

75. Fisher SV, Helm PA. Rehabilitation of the patient with burns. In: DeLisa, Gans, Currie, *et al*. eds. Rehabilitation Medicine Principles and Practice. 2nd edn. Philadelphia: JB Lippincott Company 1993: Chapter 53.

76. Salter RB, Hamilton HW, Wedge JH, *et al*. Clinical application of basic research on continuous passive motion for disorders and injuries of synovial joints: a preliminary report. *J Orthop Res* 1983; **1**(3): 325–42.

77. Lynch JA. Continuous passive motion: a prophylaxis for deep vein thrombosis following total knee replacement. *Orthop Trans* 1984; **8**(3): 400.

Chapter 46   Musculoskeletal changes secondary to thermal burns

E Burke Evans

metabolism.[10,14] In this section only what is clinically apparent will be discussed.

The more extensive the burn and the greater the number of complications, the longer the patient will be bed confined and relatively immobile. It is easy to understand that the onset of osteoporosis might be accelerated and its intensity more marked in the burn illness which features a hypermetabolic state. If a single extremity of an otherwise normal person is immobilized for a long period of time because of local trauma, as with a fracture, the bones of that extremity will lose mineral to a degree that loss of density can easily be seen in a plain radiograph. So with burns isolated to the extremities, the bones of the affected extremities become osteoporotic; and, in persons with generalized burns, the bones of deeply burned extremities may show more profound mineral loss than is observed in nonburned extremities or in the axial

Table 46.1 Classification of musculoskeletal changes secondary to burns

Alterations limited to bone
  Osteoporosis
  Periosteal new bone formation[1]
  Irregular ossification[1]
  Diaphyseal exostosis[1]
  Acromutilation of fingers[2]
  Pathologic fracture
  Osteomyelitis
  Necrosis and tangential sequestration
Alterations involving pericapsular structures
  Pericapsular calcification
  Heterotopic para-articular ossification
  Osteophyte formation
Alterations involving the joint proper
  Dislocation
  Chondrolysis[3]
  Septic arthritis
  Spontaneous dissolution[4-6]
  Ankylosis
Alterations involving muscles and tendons
  Desiccation of tendons[7]
  Fibrosis of muscles[8]
Alterations secondary to soft tissue
  Muscle and joint contractures
  Malposition of joints
  Scoliosis
Soft tissue injury
  Compartment syndrome
  Nerve injury
Abnormalities of growth
  Acceleration and retardation
  Destruction of growth plate

Among trauma states, the burn is alone in the ability and tendency of its wound, even as it heals, to create major musculoskeletal deformity. In addition, the protracted burn illness which accompanies severe burns may result in other skeletal change. **Table 46.1** presents a classification of musculoskeletal changes secondary to burns; from that, the most commonly occurring and clinically significant alterations have been selected for discussion in detail.

Changes confined to bone

Osteoporosis

Osteoporosis is the most frequently occurring postburn change involving the bone. In Shiele's radiographic study of patients with burns confined to the upper extremities, osteoporosis was found in 24 of 70 patients.[9] Klein's ongoing studies suggest that, among persons with serious burns, reduction of bone mass density is pervasive.[10] Stated causes of osteoporosis in thermal burns are bed confinement, immobilization, hyperemia,[11] reflex vasomotor phenomena,[12] and adrenocortical hyperactivity.[13] In Chapter 22 of this book, Klein thoroughly reviews the effects of burn injury on bone skeleton (**Figure 46.1**). Van Der Wiel *et al.*[15] found, in an X-ray absorptiometry study of 16 adults with fractures of one tibia, that there was eventual loss of bone mineral density in the contralateral femur and in the lumbar spine, but to a lesser degree than in the ipsilateral femur. These findings, though not strictly analogous to those observed in burns, nevertheless point to the occurrence of generalized osteoporosis in other trauma states and the difference in loss of bone density relative to local factors. In fractures or in burns, impaired mobility and local hyperemia could account for this difference.

Another characteristic of the osteoporosis of burns that seems to set it apart is its persistence, not just until restoration of the anabolic state, but for months and years after the burn has healed (**Figure 46.2**). This phenomenon may be most clearly observed in patients who have survived 90% burns, but Klein records less than normal bone among even moderately burned children as long as 17 months after injury.[10] It seems obvious that muscle atrophy and/or the failure or inability of the person to return to the preburn level of physical activity surely account in part for this protracted state of reduced bone mineralization.

There is probably no way to prevent osteoporosis in any patient whose burn is of such severity as to require an extended period of bed confinement. On the other hand, the advance of bone atrophy can at least be modified favorably even among patients with large burns if mobilization and active exercise are initiated soon after the burn. The bones of the axial skeleton, pelvis, and lower extremities are most efficiently stressed by weight bearing. Thus, standing is a priority measure. Muscle contraction alone may help to forestall bone atrophy and bone is better stressed if the contraction is resisted. Incrementally increasing resistance during motion or at the termination of an arc of motion or to muscle contraction in an extremity which may not be moved can be supplied by anyone who attends the patient. Isometric muscle contraction can be exacted from even seriously burned patients and is important for bone stress, for maintaining muscle tone and bulk, and for the patient's continuing ready identification of the affected extremity. Passive motion has little or no effect on bone and thus does not figure in the prevention of osteoporosis. Other preventive measures. e.g. closure of the wound and maintenance of nutrition, are routine in critical burn care. Treatment of established osteoporosis involves the more aggressive employment of measures for prevention. There are no long-term studies, however, which measure the effectiveness of exercise, diet, medication, or modality in the treatment of osteoporosis in any state.

Osteomyelitis

In burns, bones can become infected by exposure of bone by the burn; by an open fracture accompanying the burn; by extension of infection from a septic joint, introduction of organisms along traction pins, internal fracture fixation devices; or by blood-borne organisms of bacteremia. Considering the apparent great liability of seriously burned patients for developing osteomyelitis, it is

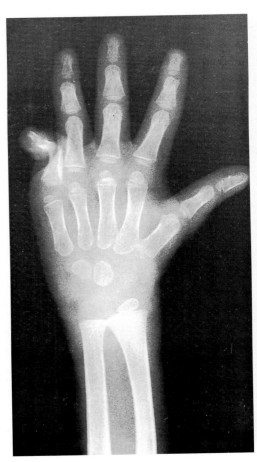

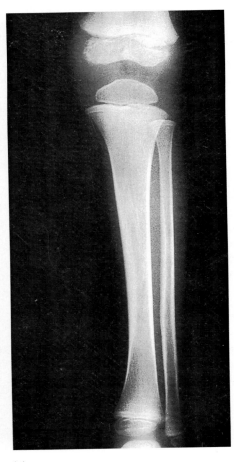

(a) (b)

Fig. 46.1 (a) Six months after injury there is the coarsened trabeculation of marked osteoporosis of bones of left hand and forearm of a 4-year-old male whose 70% full-thickness burn involved head, chest, and both upper extremities. (b) A roentgenogram of the left tibia and fibula obtained the same date as that of the hand shows minimal atrophy.

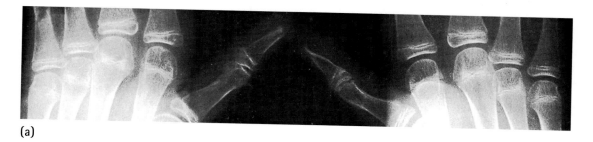

(a)

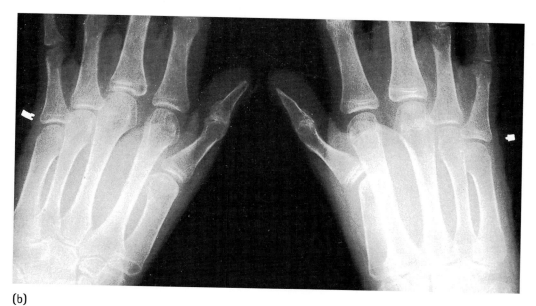

(b)

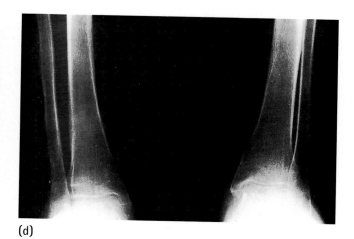

(c)

(d)

Fig. 46.2 (a) Advanced osteoporosis in the hands of a 14-year-old male 9 months after 100% TBSA burn. All growth plates are open. (b) Twenty-four months after injury, osteoporosis persists and there is irregular closure of metacarpal and phalangeal growth plates. (c) Eight months after injury, growth plates of distal tibiae and fibulae remain open. (d) Twenty-four months after injury, distal growth plates of tibiae and fibulae are closed. Other major growth plates remain open. Osteoporosis is unchanged.

surprising that it does not regularly occur. As it turns out, clinically significant osteomyelitis in burned patients is rare. Antibiotics given for the general state may prevent seeding of the bone or may repress any small focus of bone infection.

The cortex of long bones is a good barrier to surface organisms.

Even exposure of cortex will have little adverse effect if the blood supply of the bone remains intact. Prolonged exposure will kill the outer layer of the cortex which will in time sequestrate, separating at a well defined cleft between dead and living bone. With minor or moderate exposure, the bone will usually survive long enough for bordering granulation tissue to cover it. For larger defects, it is common practice to drill closely spaced holes through the exposed cortex so as to encourage buds of granulation tissue to emerge from the still vascular medullary canal. With this practice, there seems to be little risk of infecting the bone, no matter how contaminated the rest of the limb. It may be that there is sufficient centripetal pressure to discourage the invasion of organisms when the holes are fresh and that the holes are rapidly sealed by blood clot and advancing tissue. There are no reports of deep bone infection related to cortex drilling.

With open fractures which remain at the base of part of a major soft tissue burn wound, bone infection is probaby inevitable. Even so, the infection tends to remain at the fracture site and not to involve the rest of the bone, so that local debridement and stabilization of the soft-tissue wound are all that are required for treatment. Dowling reported osteomyelitis of the tibia related to an open bimalleolar fracture in an extensively burned extremity.[16] On the other hand, osteomyelitis developed in neither of the two open fractures reported separately by Choctaw[17] and Wang.[18] Three patients have been treated in whom open fractures of the femur complicated thigh burns. Each case required aggressive and repeated debridement. One fracture was treated in traction, while the other two were treated with external fixators. In one of the patients who was admitted 8 months after acute burn, there was established osteomyelitis of the femur in relation to the exposed fracture. Osteomyelitis did not develop in either of the other patients; in the end, all three had sound femurs.

When traction pins are directed through burned skin for the treatment of fractures or for suspension of a burned extremity, the factors favoring development of infection along the pin track and the formation of cigarette sequestra are:

- the introduction or migration of organisms from the burn wound;
- linear pressure of the traction pin;
- prolonged traction;
- excessive movement of the extremity leading to loosening of the pin; and
- sealing of the pin sites.

For traction or suspension, pins may be inserted through acutely burned skin, through eschar, through granulation tissue, or later through ischemic burn scar which may be colonized with uncommon and antibiotic-resistant organisms. No amount of local cleaning is likely to sterilize the surface through which the pin must pass, yet it seems that organisms in sufficient numbers to colonize are rarely introduced in this manner.

Local low-grade infections usually resolve when pins are removed if the pin sites are vigorously curetted of granulation tissue. In one case in which a four-pin custom external fixator was used in the treatment of an open infection of the elbow, there resulted diffuse osteomyelitis of humerus and radius. The infection was controlled with antibiotics and without surgery after the pins were removed. In experience with the use of the Ilizarov system for correction of skeletal deformity in burns, one patient developed a pin track infection of such severity as to require removal of the pin, curettage, and intravenous antibiotics for control of methicillin-resistant staphylococcus.[19]

Hematogenous osteomyelitis and that due to spread from an infected joint are rare. The literature entertains no report of the occurrence of either entity in association with burns. Were bone infection of this sort to be recognized, effective treatment would depend upon the identification of the offending organisms for organism-specific antibiotic regimen.

Fractures

Pathologic fractures were at one time common in burn management because of the practices of delayed excision of eschar and of keeping patients in bed until wounds were completely covered. During that time, fractures occurred because of bone collapse when patients first stood or walked after a prolonged period of bed confinement or when stiff joints were manipulated[20] (**Figure 46.3**). The bones most commonly affected were the femur at its distal metaphysis and the tibia at its proximal one. The only treatment required was support of the extremity until the fracture consolidated, usually in 4–6 weeks. Children were more often affected than adults and the fractures usually compressed one cortex, producing an angular deformity which rapidly corrected with growth. More currently, Klein's study strongly suggests that fractures occur more frequently in burned children than in a matched normal population even months after the acute burn. Now, however, in acute burn management, the most frequently seen fractures are those occurring at the time of, or in association with, the burn

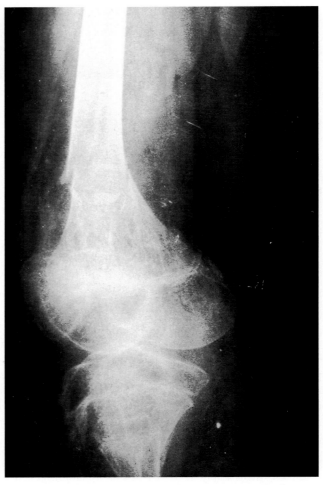

Fig. 46.3 Pathologic fracture of the osteoporotic femur of a 9-year-old girl sustained on the first day she stood after 5 weeks of confinement for 40% TBSA burn.

injury. Falls or violent trauma account for many of the fractures, and the sites are those common to the causes, bearing no relation to the burn itself. Reports indicate that fractures associated with burns occur in all bones of the axial and appendicular skeleton.

Although fractures complicate burn treatment and occasionally delay mobilization of patients, their management need not be complex. Fractures in extremities not burned can be treated in a routine manner by manipulative reduction and plaster immobilization, by open reduction and internal fixation, with an external fixator, or with skeletal traction (**Figure 46.4**). Fractures in extremities with

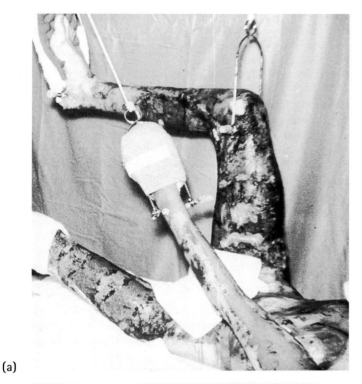

(a)

Fig. 46.4 (a) This 15-year-old male sustained closed fractures of the right femur, left tibia and left humerus at the time of a 46% TBSA burn involving mainly trunk and right lower extremity. The femur and humerus fractures were treated in skeletal traction. Suspension of the right lower extremity aided management of circumferential deep burns of that extremity. Lesser burns of the left leg made it possible to treat the minimally displaced fracture of the left tibia in a circular cast. All fractures consolidated in 6 weeks in satisfactory alignment. (b) Fractures of the left humerus as it appeared at the time of admission to the hospital. (c) Five weeks after injury, the fracture showed maturing callus. Traction was discontinued at 6 weeks.

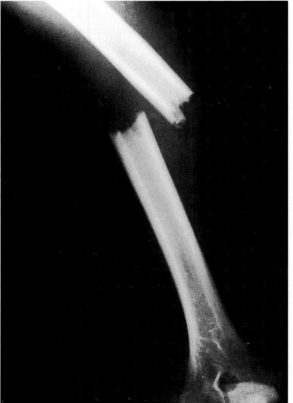

(b)

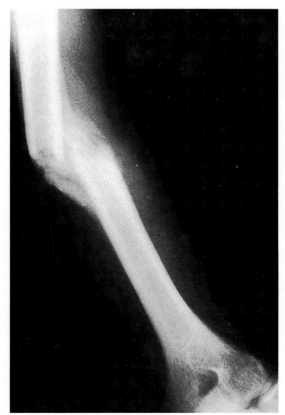

(c)

first degree or superficial second degree burns can be managed in the same way. Deep second degree and third degree burns present a different problem only with respect to the early bacterial colonization of third degree burns and the degradation of deep second degree burns to full-thickness burns which will, in turn, become colonized. There is, thus, a precious window of time when fractures requiring open reduction and internal fixation can be definitively treated without increased risk of infecting the bone however, fracture reduction and stabilization are so important in the functional management of a severely burned patient that the risk of bone infection should be acknowledged and shouldered at any postburn stage. Skeletal traction can often be the management choice, particularly in children and adolescents, even if the treatment protocol requires that the patient be moved from bed for tubbing, dressing change, or additional surgery. The disadvantages of skeletal traction are the confinement to bed and the imposed relatively fixed position of the affected extremity. External fixators, now in common use, have made it possible to align and stabilize fractures in burned extremities without open operation. In fact, external fixation may be the treatment of choice for open fractures in burns, as it often is for open fractures not associated with burns. There is the added functional advantage of patient mobility. Brooker's extensive favorable experience supports this concept.[21] With both skeletal traction and external fixation, there is an added risk of bone infection because of the path from surface to bone provided by the pins. This is a risk worth taking, and it is minimized by scrupulous pin site care and by removal and replacement of any loosening pin. Frye recognized and discussed the specific and continuous difficulties encountered in the management of fractures and burns.[54]

When casts are used for stabilization of fractures in burned extremities, the wound is made inaccessible and there is an abiding fear that the unattended wound will seriously degrade or at best not improve. Those fears may be well founded, however, Wang[18] showed that a bivalved circular cast could be used effectively for an open comminuted fracture of a proximal tibia with overlying deep burns, and Choctaw[17] reported successful use of a cast for immobilization of an open comminuted fracture after immediate postburn grafting of the affected extremity. Common sense should dictate which fractures can be treated with circular or bivalved casts or with splints. If a reduced or moderately displaced but aligned fracture is so stable as to require external support only for maintenance of alignment, then cast or splint immobilization should be all that is needed. On the other hand, if a fracture, because of instability, requires, for maintenance of reduction, three-point pressure or molding of the cast material, then it will be better treated by other means.

Dowling[16] reported osteomyelitis resulting from open bimalleolar fracture in an extremity with extensive deep burns. In neither of the cases reported by Wang and Choctaw did the bone become infected. There were also no infections among Saffle's 42 fractures, nine of which were treated by open reduction and internal fixation.[22] With two fractures of the femur, each of which was exposed at the base of a deep chronic burn, aggressive debridement of the wounds and the fracture ends was followed by treatment with skeletal traction in one and by external fixation with the Ilizarov system in the other. Both fractures healed without further complication.

Fractures in burned patients heal quickly. There is no recorded experience which suggests that healing is delayed by the burn. Neither is there any record of failure of union. Callus formation may be abundant.

Among severely burned patients, nondisplaced or minimally displaced fractures may not be detected until unusual local pain in an affected extremity prompts roentgenographic examination or when a roentgenogram obtained for other reason reveals the fracture as an incidental finding. These fractures are usually of no functional significance. Modest angular deformity near a joint may be a problem in adults, though not in children. On the other hand, undetected transphyseal fractures in children can be a major functional threat.

Changes involving pericapsular structures

Heterotopic Bone

Heterotopic bone formation is a rare, but functionally important, complication of thermal burns. The incidence in a general burn population is reported to be somewhere between 1 and 3%.[1,23-26] In select populations, the incidence may be higher as it will be if patients with periarticular calcification are included in the statistics. For example, Tepperman et al. reported a 35.3% incidence among patients referred to a tertiary care center for rehabilitation.[27] Jackson made the observation that the incidence of heterotopic bone could be expected to be less in institutions which admit patients with minor burns.[28] Munster's[29] roentgenographic survey of 88 adult and teenage patients with 160 burned upper extremities yielded a 16% incidence of pericapsular calcification; and the 23% incidence reported by Schiele et al.[9] included both heterotopic ossification and calcification. In the early routine roentgenographic study reported by Evans,[20] periarticular calcification which did not progress to heterotopic bone was excluded from the final calculation of an incidence of 2%. The 3.3% incidence recorded by Kolar and Vrabec[30] included patients with pericapsular calcification. Even if heterotopic bone occurs infrequently in thermal burns, it remains that once it develops, it often compromises joint motion and is difficult to treat. In addition, its pathogenesis is still incompletely understood; and, thus, protocols for prevention may in fact miss the mark.

Pathogenesis

The metabolic changes occurring after thermal burn are increased metabolic rate; protein catabolism; ureagenesis; fat mobilization; glucogenolysis; gluconeogenesis; elevated glucose flow; and eventual total body weight loss.[31,32] There is an accompanying suppression of the immune system which favors wound infection, but, at the same time, favors survival of skin allografts. Infection, failure of skin graft take, or anything which delays closure of a burn wound, will extend the altered metabolic state. Though it might be assumed that there occurs, along with the metabolic upheaval, an adverse change in connective tissue milieu, the exact nature of such a change is not known. It is also not known what the metabolic changes have to do with the development of heterotopic bone, but it is clear that the burn disease is necessary to its formation. Other factors to be considered in the genesis of heterotopic bone are percentage of burn, location of burn, period of confinement, osteoporosis, superimposed trauma and genetic predisposition. These factors, though identifiable, are not easy to implicate.

Percentage of burn

Most reported cases of heterotopic bone have had a 20% or greater total body surface area (TBSA) burn; however, heterotopic bone has been found in patients with as little as 10% third degree burn.[20] Peterson et al.,[5] Munster et al.,[29] and Elledge et al.[25] have reported affected patients with TBSA burns of 8, 14, and 12% respectively. In addition, with the now extensive experience in salvage of patients with 80% or greater burns, it is clear that heterotopic bone occurs no more frequently among these patients at the other end of the percentage spectrum than in the general burn population. It cannot be said, thus, that the percentage of burn is a determining factor.

Location of burn

A high percentage, but by no means all, of the reported heterotopic bone has occurred in joints with overlying deep burn. In their initial report, Evans and Smith described heterotopic bone occurring a distance from any third degree burn involvement.[1] Johnson, in his early report, noted that in one of his three patients, the skin overlying one affected joint was not even superficially burned.[33] If it be assumed that degradation of connective tissue milieu in burns is a total body phenomenon, it follows that heterotopic bone formation need not be burn site-dependent. Thus, the location of the burn cannot alone be a determining factor.

Period of confinement

Evans and Smith expressed the belief that length of bed confinement was perhaps the most important factor in the development of heterotopic bone.[1] At the time of that report, patients with even moderate burns might be kept in bed for several weeks. The consequences of prolonged confinement were loss of active range of joint motion and bone demineralization; it was thought that each of these adverse changes might contribute to the formation of heterotopic bone. Thus, any maloccurrence which necessitated longer confinement could be a factor in the pathogenesis. Kolar implicated wound sepsis as such an independent factor along with the length of confinement.[30] Other investigators have not addressed the period of confinement as specifically as Kolar, and there have been no studies of comparative groups of confined and nonconfined patients. Thus, it may never be determined whether or not current aggressive practice of early mobilization of patients will have an effect on the incidence of heterotopic bone.

Osteoporosis

Only Schiele et al. have reported a relationship between heterotopic bone formation and osteoporosis.[9] We have noted previously that, among their group of 70 adults with burns confined to the upper extremities, 11 of the 16 who developed heterotopic bone had roentenographically identifiable osteoporosis. In their series of patients, there were 24 who had osteoporosis. Thus, fewer than one-half of these developed heterotopic bone and there were two in the group that developed heterotopic bone who did not have osteoporosis. If the findings in that study are not altogether persuasive, the matter is further confused by the knowledge that the survivors of extensive TBSA burns who may develop profound osteoporosis seem to have no greater liability to the formation of heterotopic bone than the general burn population.

Superimposed trauma

In one of the patients reported by Evans and Smith, the elbow of the more often used and minimally burned right upper extremity developed heterotopic bone, whereas the elbow of the less used but more seriously burned left upper extremity did not.[1] In the same patient, the right hip spontaneously dislocated. After reduction, that hip developed extensive heterotopic bone in the planes of the rectus femoris and iliopsoas, the muscles stressed by the posterior displacement. The opposite hip developed only a small spicule of heterotopic bone anteriorly at the joint line. Experience with this one patient reinforced the authors' belief that there occurred with burns a general compromise of connective tissue which rendered it particularly susceptible to superimposed trauma and that it was this liability to injury which accounted for the appearance of heterotopic bone at sites of repeated stretching of soft tissue, as at the minimally burned elbow or at sites of recognized abrupt excessive stretching as at the dislocated hip. According to all reports, the elbow is the most common site of heterotopic bone formation in adults and children.[25,26,30,34] Perhaps it is the regular use of this joint which accounts for that orientation. Jackson has pointed out that the elbows are subjected to pressure posteriorly and medially when they are used for leverage or are simply in contact with the bed.[28] He suggests with this observation that external pressure is a factor in the orientation of heterotopic bone to the elbow. There may be other factors as well that favor the elbow. Commonly, the elbow is splinted in extension to prevent flexion contracture. If flexion range is lost, passive stretch and encouragement of active flexion are part of the rehabilitation effort. The posterior structures most affected by this effort are those attached to the olecranon. Thus, it is not surprising that heterotopic bone develops medially in line with and deep to the medial fibers of the triceps. If a flexion contracture develops, the heterotopic bone is commonly in the line of brachialis or biceps attachments to coronoid process and biceps tubercle. And if there is loss of pronation and supination range, stretching may cause heterotopic bone to form in line with the proximal radioulnar ligaments and interosseous membrane. There is an implication here that both the quality and timing of postburn exercise may be important. Gentle passive and active motion should cause less tissue disruption than abrupt passive or active or even chronically repeated motion, and the effect of any mobilization effort must vary with the relative stiffness of the joint and the intrinsic resistance of soft tissue. Thus, the longer a joint is limited in its motion, the stiffer it will become and the greater will be the soft-tissue damage with any forced manipulation.

The concept of superimposed trauma as a cause of heterotopic bone is supported by the experimental work of Evans[35] and of Michelsson and Rauschning.[36] Evans found that all burned and nonburned rabbits given a single necrotizing injection of alcohol in one quadriceps muscle readily healed the lesions, whereas rabbits, burned or nonburned, which were given a second same-site injection 7 days after the first, uniformly developed well defined and histologically identifiable ossicles of heterotopic bone. In this experiment, it was clear that, in susceptible animals, it was not the burn which made the difference, but the chronicity of the wound. Michelsson and Rauschning determined that forceful or regular active remobilization of rabbit knees, which had been immobilized for 1–5 weeks, resulted in the development of heterotopic calcification and ossification in the muscles which were stretched. The response was more consistent in the quadriceps of the knees immobilized in extension than in the hamstrings of those immobilized in flexion. The longer the period of immobilization and the more vigorous the remobilization, the greater the response. Muscle necrosis was a prominent histologic finding.

Superimposed trauma is implicated in the development of

heterotopic bone in head-injured patients or those with post-traumatic or infectious transverse myelitis.[37–39] In these patients, it is assumed that tissue media are altered by injury to the central nervous system. The secondary injury, as in burns, is periarticular. In post-traumatic myositis ossificans, the development of heterotopic bone depends upon persistence of the muscle lesion and local necrosis and, thus, at least by inference, upon repeated insults to the affected muscle.

The development of heterotopic bone in burns has been associated with the agitation of patients and their resistance to physical therapy.[1,40] Two affected adults and one affected child in a 10-year study resisted physical therapy programming.[35] One adult refused to move and the other was extremely apprehensive. The child was likewise apprehensive and refused to cooperate with the therapist. The development in all three of posterior heterotopic bone in both elbows could have been ascribed both to the difficulty encountered in mobilizing the elbows and to the continual pressure on the elbows in bed.

Genetic predisposition

It is difficult to explain the low incidence of heterotopic bone among great numbers of patients similarly burned except on the basis of some, as yet unidentified, inherited factor. It is known that persons with proliferative noninflammatory arthritis of the hip are more likely to develop heterotopic bone after total hip replacement than persons who have hips replaced for other reasons. In this instance, the predisposing inherited abnormality is identifiable. Though heterotopic bone formation may occur more regularly among spinal cord-injured and head-injured patients than among burned ones, by no means do all persons with head and spinal cord injuries develop heterotopic bone. The total burn experience at the University of Texas Medical Branch has yielded only two similarly affected siblings. Twin brothers who had 19 and 20% TBSA burns, and who were mobile throughout much of their treatment and recovery period, developed near identical heterotopic bone of both elbows.[41] There is, however, no scientific proof that genetic predisposition has anything to do with the formation of heterotopic bone in burns. Nor is there any literature to support the idea that a person who develops heterotopic bone when burned will be liable to develop it if they sustain head or spinal cord injury.

Characteristics and Behavior

Heterotopic bone associated with burns has been reported to occur about all major joints. The joints most commonly affected are elbow, shoulder, and hip, in that order of frequency. The early manifestations are joint swelling and tenderness not unlike any acute inflammatory process. The patient may call attention to the process by a reluctance to move the affected joint. Onset may be as early as 1 month and as late as 3 months or more after the burn, but it is more likely to be associated with the acute recovery phase of treatment than later. Crawford et al. reported that the clinical diagnosis was made in advance of roentgenographic changes in nine of his 12 patients.[34] Tepperman et al.[27] and Peterson et al.[26] found that bone scans could help to make a diagnosis before there were roentgenographic changes. The earliest roentgenographic alteration is local periarticular increase in soft tissue density. There follows diffuse stippled calcification in the same distribution in or about the capsule of the joint. It is at this point that the process may reverse itself, perhaps due to the improved state of the patient.

Because of this change in course, there may be many patients whose periarticular calcification is never detected. If the calcification persists, it may be assumed that bone will develop by either the intramembranous or the enchondral route or both as it does in animal models.

The flecks of calcification appear roentgenographically to lie within the capsule, whereas heterotopic bone may involve not only capsular structures but may extend as well into the planes of muscles and tendons. At each major joint there is a more or less characteristic distribution of heterotopic bone which is similar to that associated with patients with head and spinal cord injury. At the elbow, posteriorly disposed bone extends from the olecranon to the medial epicondylar ridge of the humerus in line with the medial border of the triceps muscle (**Figure 46.5a,b**). At the joint, it may extend medially to bridge the ulnar groove.[3,42] The medial, rather than lateral, orientation of the heterotopic bone may be related to the medial position of the olecranon and the greater tension on soft tissue on that side. As Jackson points out, the contact area of the elbow is medial, and continual pressure in this area may have something to do with the orientation.[28] Heterotopic bone on the anterior surface of the elbow develops in the planes of the brachialis and biceps muscles extending from humerus to coronoid process or biceps tubercle. Occasionally, a bridge of heterotopic bone develops between the radius and ulna just distal to the joint. More rarely, bone has been found to fill the olecranon fossa and even to ensheath the entire joint. At the shoulder, bone has been found to extend from the acromion to the humerus in the line of the rotator muscles or deep to the deltoid (**Figure 46.5c**), to lie anteriorly in the plane of the pectoralis major, and, more deeply, to parallel the subscapularis. Hoffer et al.[43] reported that heterotopic bone at the shoulder lay anteriorly in the plane of the capsule. At the hip, heterotopic bone may extend from pelvis to femur in the planes of rectus or iliopsoas anteriorly or in the plane of the gluteal muscles laterally. Jackson has reported heterotopic bone in the plane of the quadratus femoris.[28] Like the shoulder, the hip may be ensheathed anteriorly with heterotopic bone which appears to originate in the capsule.

When heterotopic bone bridges a joint, it becomes part of the skeleton and may, if loaded, increase in dimension as fully developed ossicles with mature cortex and medullary cavity. If the bone does not bridge a joint, it will, in children, gradually disappear when the burn wound has healed and the child is healthy. In recovering adults, nonbridging bone will, in time, diminish in size, but it may never completely disappear. The same tendency for heterotopic bone to regress after resolution of disease was noted by Lorber, who reported on two patients with paraplegia secondary to tuberculosis in whom deposits of heterotopic bone diminished in size, after return of motor function.[37] Bottu and Van Noyen[44] reported a similar experience with a patient who had transient viral meningoencephalitis, and Jacobs reported almost complete resorption of large bilateral deposits of heterotopic bone in a patient who recovered from paralytic measles encephalomyelitis.[38]

Serum levels of calcium, phosphorus, and alkaline phosphatase have been reported by most authors to be normal or, at best, insignificantly higher in burned patients who have developed heterotopic bone.[1,23,29,45,46] In addition, there is no convincing evidence that calcium intake affects heterotopic bone formation one way or the other. Evans' and Smith's limited routine studies of affected and unaffected patients led the authors to believe that the values of

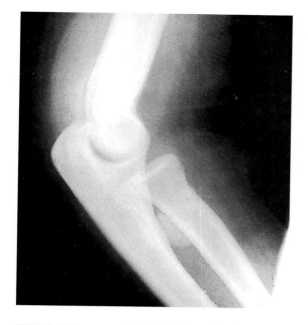

(a)(i)

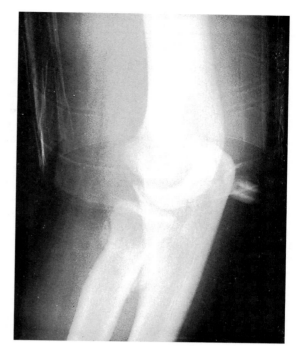

(a)(ii)

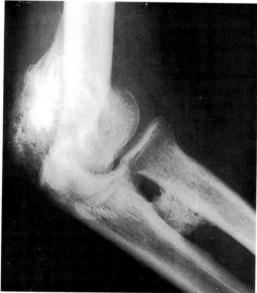

(b)(i)

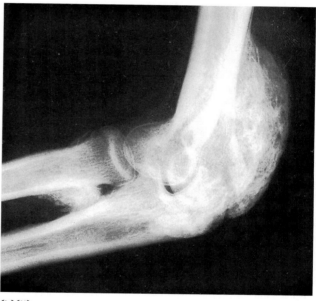

(b)(ii)

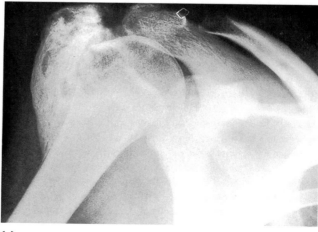

(c)

Fig. 46.5 (a) Three months after 94% TBSA burn of a 16-year-old male, resistance to motion, local swelling, and pain of both elbows prompted obtaining roentgenograms, each of which showed spotty linear soft-tissue calcification and ossification along the distal humerus and between the radius and ulna at the level of the biceps tubercle. (b) Six months after burn, elbow flexion and extension were reduced to 10° on the left and to less than 5° on the right. Bridges of immature heterotopic bone extended from the medial epicondylar ridges to the olecranons. Forearm rotation was 0% due to interosseous bridges of heterotopic bone at the level of the bicipital tuberosities. Prognosis for restoring functional range of motion in the elbows is poor. (c) At 6 months postburn, glenohumeral motion on the right was limited to a few degrees by heterotopic bone underlying the deltoid. At the same time, a lesser deposit of heterotopic at the left hip did not limit motion.

serum calcium, phosphorus, and alkaline phosphatase were so consistently normal as to make further investigation unnecessary.[1] One interesting observation was that of Koepke, whose early, but incomplete, studies suggested that those patients who were susceptible had elevation of serum alkaline phosphatase before development of heterotopic bone, but not afterwards.[24]

Prevention and Treatment

The incidence of heterotopic bone in burns is so low as to make it impractical to administer aspirin or indomethacin or other nonsteroidal anti-inflammatory drugs which are currently used for patients at risk for development of heterotopic bone after major hip surgery. Rather, the thrust in prevention should be toward reducing the period of bed confinement and the duration of the postburn hypermetabolic state. The now prevailing practice of early wound excision and grafting may, in fact, address both of these problems as nearly as it is possible to do so. Even patients with extensive TBSA burns may be out of bed and walking within the first postburn week. Extremity motion is begun as soon as graft and wound stability permit. With this programming, the incidence and intensity of osteoporosis should be reduced as well.

If certain patients are predisposed to the development of heterotopic bone, then the quality and timing of joint mobilization for those patients may be critical. Stretching edematous pericapsular structures in the early postburn period may very well be hazardous if additional tissue damage is the result; however, maintenance of joint motion and muscle function is part of the early excision and grafting program, and it is certain that, the longer joint motion is restricted, the more likely it is that pericapsular structures will be damaged by stretching. We should like to think that any secondary injury to soft tissue could be avoided by controlled and assisted active motion, gentle terminal stretch, and terminal resistance.

When a patient is reluctant to move a joint previously moved with relative ease, and certainly when there is evidence of unusual swelling about the joint, roentgenograms should be obtained to determine if there is pericapsular calcification or ossification. Once heterotopic bone or calcification is recognized, joint exercise should be restricted to gentle passive and assisted active motion only. Crawford et al.[34] observed that ossification progressed to complete ankylosis in all patients who persisted in moving an affected joint beyond the pain-free range. They concluded that active range of motion exercises and stretching were contraindicated if heterotopic bone or calcification was suspected, but that active range of motion could safely be resumed within pain-free range once the diagnosis had been confirmed. In the series of Peterson et al.,[26] 18 patients suspected of having heterotopic bone had active range of motion exercises only; ten regained functional range of motion and eight developed ankylosis.

Surgical excision of heterotopic bone is indicated when joint motion is lost or significantly compromised by bridging bone or exostoses. Evans has suggested that surgery be postponed until the burn wound has healed, scars are soft and associated with no inflammatory response, the patient is healthy, and the offensive bone is roentgenographically mature, i.e. well defined and not increasing in dimension[20] (**Figure 46.6**). This position makes sense considering the behavior of heterotopic bone, i.e. proliferation while there are open burn wounds or active scars and regression with wound healing and scar softening. For removal of heterotopic bone, surgical exposures should be planned with extensible incisions so as to facilitate total excision. When there is a bridge of bone, each end of the bridge should be excavated slightly. When there is attachment at only one end, the cartilaginous or fibrous extension should be removed along with the bone. Capsular sheets of bone should be removed completely. If bridging heterotopic bone is incompletely excised, the bridge is likely to recur. When a joint is bridged by bone in only one plane, removal of the offending bone will usually restore functional motion and the likelihood of recurrence of the bridge is small. When a joint is bridged in more than one plane, recurrence is more likely and the chance for restoration of functional range of motion is correspondingly diminished. When the local inflammatory process has caused intra-articular synovial proliferation and cartilage destruction, the joint is most likely destined for ankylosis. Removal of the heterotopic bone about a joint so affected may allow more functional positioning of the joint, but it is not likely to arrest the process. On the other hand, extra-articular arthrodesis by a bridge of heterotopic bone may preserve the joint. This is particularly the case at the elbow when there is only one posterior bridge of bone from olecranon to medial epicondylar ridge of the humerus. In this situation, the olecranon is fixed in the trochlea, but the radiocapitellar and radioulnar joints remain functional. In Evans' experience with removal of single bridges at the elbow, joint cartilage was found to be healthy as long as 5 years after ankylosis. Preservation of pronation and supination was credited with maintaining the synovial bath to provide nutrition for the humeroulnar cartilage. Indeed, when pronation and supination additionally are blocked by bridging bone, cartilage degradation is certain. Evans' further experience with long-term survival of glenohumeral cartilage after ankylosis by bridging bone from acromion to humerus is not as easily explained.

Reported experience with excision of heterotopic bone in burns has not been uniformly favorable. Dias,[46] Hoffer et al.,[43] and Peterson et al.[26] reported restoration of functional range of motion in most of their patients with timely excision of heterotopic bone. Other surgeons have reported less satisfactory results. In our own experience, results have varied, as anticipated, with severity of affection. We have learned that, if heterotopic bone recurs after excision, it is worthwhile to excise again if the joint affected remains structurally identifiable. For the most part, however, attempts to improve joint function with second operations have failed. We believe that ultimate failure can be predicted at the time of initial surgery; we are convinced that the single most important factor in successful initial excision is in timing surgery to coincide with the patient's return to good health.

Changes involving the joint

Dislocation

Luxations and subluxations of joints in burned patients may occur as a result of direct destruction by the burn of ligaments and capsules, loss of articular cartilage due to infection, faulty positioning, and eventually scar contracture. In all phases of management, but particularly in the acute phase, positioning is of prime importance in the prevention of joint deformity. The preferred positions, listed in **Table 46.2**, serve as a guide for the prevention of dislocation of joints and of malposition secondary to scar contracture.

The joints most liable to structural compromise due to exposure by the burn and loss of soft tissue support are knee, elbow,

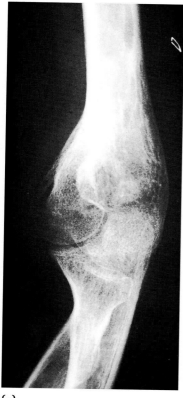

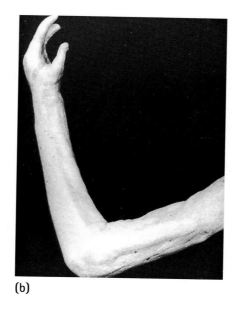

(b)

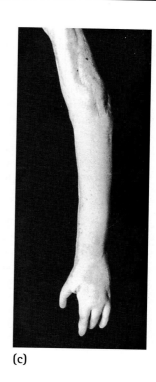

(c)

(a)

Fig. 46.6 (a) A mature sheet of heterotopic bone extends from humerus to olecranon, obliterating the olecranon fossa 11 months after 53% TBSA burn in a 13-year-old female. Elbow flexion and extension range was less than 10%. Pronation and supination were near normal range. (b), (c) Three months after excision of heterotopic bone, the patient had attained 90° of elbow motion and a continuing increase to functional (hand to mouth) range was predicted. Now the patient can extend the elbow and can flex it to 90°.

proximal interphalangeal joints of the hand, and metacarpophalangeal joints. These hinge joints have in common a subcutaneous dorsal surface, accounting for their ready exposure.

The elbow, for its trochlear architecture, is more intrinsically stable than the other joints in this group. It requires loss of collateral support to render it easily displaceable. The knee, on the other hand, is immediately in danger of subluxation if there is loss of continuity of its central slip, the patellar tendon, even if the

Table 46.2 Preferred positions for major joints	
Joint	Preferred position
Neck	Midline in neutral or slight extension
Shoulders	Scapulothoracic retraction and depression 85° of glenohumeral elevation with 20–25° of horizontal flexion
Elbows	Extension
Wrists	Slight extension
Metacarpophalangeal joints 2–5	80–90° of flexion
Fingers	Proximal and distal interphalangeal extension
Thumbs	Carpometacarpal flexion and abduction, metacarpophalangeal flexion 5–10°, interphalangeal extension
Spine	Extension with no lateral deviation
Hips	Extension and slight external rotation in 15° of symmetric abduction
Knees	Extension
Ankles	Neutral
Feet	Neutral

retinacula remain intact. In this circumstance, gravity alone will displace the tibia posteriorly in relation to the femur if the patient is recumbent. The hamstring muscles contribute to the displacement force regardless of the position of the extremity. Loss of collateral ligaments compounds the problem, but loss of collateral ligament stability in the presence of an intact patellar tendon and functioning quadriceps constitutes far less a threat than loss of patellar tendon. For the lower extremity, persistent posterior translation of the tibia beneath the femur with inefficient quadriceps pull is potentially a functional disaster.

For both the elbow and the knee, the protecting position is extension. These two joints are rarely at risk for articular displacement from contracture alone and, if there is no ligament or tendon loss, extension resting splints will give adequate positional support. When there is soft-tissue disruption, splinting may not adequately protect either joint. An external fixator with two-pin, four-cortex fixation above and below the joint will provide stability and will permit access to the wound. For the elbow, it allows fine adjustment to the normal carrying angle as well. If the knee is accurately reducible at the time of application of the fixator, there is a good possibility that the reduction can be maintained. If the tibia cannot be brought forward completely by manual manipulation, it may be necessary to suspend the tibia through a transverse pin at the level of the tibial tubercle. For static vertical traction, the extremity must be elevated from the bed. For dynamic traction, enough weight must be used to accomplish the same elevation. If the tibia can be brought forward by this means, an external fixator will likely hold the reduction. For the knee to remain stable with the tibia forward, the patellar tendon must be reattached and quadriceps integrity reestablished; otherwise, when the fixator is removed, the tibia will once again begin an incremental posterior shift toward its own point of stability. No amount of external splinting or bracing is likely to prevent that shift.

The proximal interphalangeal joints of the hands are more frequently exposed by burn than any others. If the central extensor slip remains intact, there is less risk of subluxation of the joint. Even if there is loss of continuity of the central slip, but preservation of the lateral bands, subluxation is easily prevented if the joint is maintained in extension while soft-tissue cover is being achieved. It is with loss of the support of lateral bands and collateral ligaments that the joints become liable to dislocation. With the metacarpophalangeal joints, the tendency to displacement or subluxation may be greater because these joints are functionally multiplaner, while the interphalangeal joints are uniplaner. Happily, the metacarpophalangeal joints are less often exposed than the interphalangeal ones.

The protecting position for the proximal interphalangeal joints is full extension. If only the central slip is lost, the position may be held with an external splint. In states of greater instability it may be necessary to use intramedullary transarticular Kirschner wires to hold the position. The wires, though reasonably efficient, do not control rotation, and they carry with them a risk of post-treatment joint stiffness. Pin traction through the distal phalanges in a skeletally stabilized metal splint is another method for maintaining extension of threatened digital joints.[47,48] It has the advantages of patient comfort and mobility, secure positioning of hand and upper extremity, easy maintenance of elevation, and easy access for dressings, for additional surgery, and for exercise of lesser affected joints. The system likewise makes it possible to keep digits sepa-

rated, thus facilitating local care. Traction should not be used if collateral ligaments are not intact. By whatever means attained, the corrected position must be maintained until the joint is covered with graft. Protection should continue with a standard splint or brace until the joint is sound.

The two joints most likely to dislocate because of faulty positioning are the shoulder and the hip. These two ball and socket multiplaner joints sacrifice stability in favor of mobility. This is particularly true of the shoulder, where the shallow glenoid contains at any one time only one-third of the head of the humerus. In burns, the head of the humerus may begin to subluxate forward if, during prone positioning for management of back and buttock wounds, the arms are maintained in full abduction in the coronal plane. In this position the arms are in at least 15–20° of extension from the more secure neutral position in line with the scapulae, and the humeral heads are forced forward against the anterior capsule. Even when the patient is supine, full abduction and extension of the arms should be avoided. For short-term management, particularly when the patient gets out of bed every day, this position probably does not threaten the joint. But if the patient is to be bed confined and the position unrelieved for days or weeks, the head of the humerus may begin to subluxate forward. In the extreme situation, the head of the humerus will dislocate to a medial subcoracoid position. In patients with deep burns extending from chin to axillae to chest, the common posture of elevation and protraction of the scapulae may be associated with upward subluxation of the humeral heads. With one patient in whom the right clavicle was sacrificed distally because of the depth of the burn, the head of the right humerus moved forward and then upward because of loss of anterior stabilizers.

The head of the humerus is most secure in the glenoid fossa when the arm is adducted to neutral and internally rotated a position which is incompatible with wound management of burns of the trunk, neck, and upper extremities. The protecting position, which accommodates the need for abduction for axillary burns, is elevation of the arms in line with the scapulae. The arm is then approximately 20° forward of the coronal plane or in 20° of horizontal flexion. When the patient is prone, the protecting position can be gained only if the chest is supported on a chest width mattress or foam rubber pad, either of which will allow the arms to drop forward. When the patient is positioned this way, whether supine or prone, the forearms will be pronated and the arms will be in sufficient internal rotation to favor seating of the head of the humerus in the glenoid.

The hip will tend to subluxate posteriorly if the thigh is persistently allowed to remain flexed, adducted, and internally rotated during the acute burn phase. For the most part, however, the protecting position of extension to neutral or 180° and 15–20° of symmetric abduction is easy to attain and maintain and is, in fact, the most desirable position for wound management.

If dislocation of the head of humerus or femur is undetected, or if reduction is delayed for other reasons, open reduction will likely be required. Reduction of a chronically displaced head of humerus in one seriously burned patient using the Ilizarov technique was hampered by the fragility of the bone. Another head of humerus that had been dislocated anteriorly for several weeks was found at the time of open reduction to have extensive erosion of the articular cartilage.

Infection of a joint may result in its subluxation or dislocation.

Hip displacement because of apparent spontaneous dissolution has been described by Evans and Smith.[1] Eszter and Istvan[6] and Cristallo and Dell'Orto[4] reported similar cases. In none of these cases, however, could it be determined that the joint destruction was due to infection.

Septic Arthritis

A joint exposed by a burn or by removal of burn eschar is presumed to be infected. The joints most frequently exposed are the knee, the elbow, the proximal interphalangeal joints of the hand, and the metacarpophalangeal joints, all on the subcutaneous dorsal surfaces. Wrist and ankle are less often affected and other joints rarely. Treatment requires stable positioning of the joint for maximum reduction of wound size so as to facilitate soft tissue closure or grafting and to allow aggressive daily lavage. The position for all of the joints listed except the ankle is extension. The ankle is positioned in neutral. External fixation, intramedullary pinning, or skeletal traction may be required in order to secure the position. To maintain ankle position it is sometimes appropriate to insert a large vertical Steinmann pin through calcaneus and talus into the tibia. The position should be maintained until the exposed joint is covered with epithelialized granulation tissue or skin graft. Exposed adjacent bone can be shaved or drilled so as to encourage surface granulation. Drilling is particularly useful at the elbow where the olecranon is regularly exposed. Often, however, granulation tissue will quickly extend the wound margins and effectively close the wound so as to allow split-thickness skin grafting. If the burn is isolated to the joint, or if the extremity is not otherwise seriously burned, a local muscle, skin or compound flap may be used to close the joint. Free vascularized flaps are useful and should always be considered if it is anticipated that nerve graft or tendon graft or transfer at the site will be required in the future. Incremental remobilization of the joint may proceed when wound closure is sound. Culture of material from an exposed joint will likely yield a variety of organisms consistent with those of the general burn wound requiring, thus, broad-spectrum antibiotic management.

The incidence of hematogenous septic arthritis is obscured by its frequent association with severe burns and because there are rarely separable clinical signs such as local heat and swelling, elevation of temperature, and elevation of sedimentation rate. Local tenderness and greater than usual pain with motion may focus attention on the affected joint. Aspiration of the joint will confirm a diagnosis. A roentgenogram is helpful, but in the early phases of infection will show only local cellulitis as increased periarticular soft-tissue density. If a patient has been receiving broad-spectrum antibiotics, material aspirated from the affected joint may not grow an organism in culture. Clearly, without organism identification and sensitivity determinations, specific antibiotic therapy cannot be initiated.

We have been of the opinion that debridement and exteriorization of the joint and regular vigorous lavage are as important as antibiotics in the treatment of closed infected joints. We believe now that arthroscopic debridement and closed irrigation should be considered as an alternative method of management whether or not skin over the affected joint is burned. Rarely in burns, a joint may become infected from adjacent metaphyseal osteomyelitis. In this situation, joint preservation is the treatment priority, and measures are the same as for septic arthritis of strictly hematogenous origin.[41] In children, most infected joints can be salvaged. Adult joints are less resilient. Persistent joint infection will destroy cartilage and lead to ankylosis.[5,49] All chronically infected joints are liable to dislocation because of surface destruction and capsular laxity.

Amputations

In burns, major amputations are most often performed because of nonviability of the extremity or because a surviving extremity is rendered useless by scar, deformity or insensitivity. Occasionally, in an extensive burn, a severely burned extremity which might be salvaged in part is sacrificed to reduce the extent of the burn or as a lifesaving measure.

In thermal burns, the level of extremity amputation is determined by the viability of muscles and tendons. The more distal the site the better, and it is important to retain joints even if motion will be restricted. For example, if a forearm or leg must be sacrificed, the elbow or knee should be spared if the more proximal muscles controlling that joint are intact, if the bone bleeds, and if there is the possibility that the remaining tissue of the stump has sufficient blood supply to produce granulations for grafting. Aside from affording a better functional prospect, sparing the joint will provide the surgeon opportunity at a later time to choose an appropriate revision level if the joint does not function. The patient will at that time be healthier and stump closure will be routine. Jackson suggests that it may be technically feasible to cover even nonviable bone with a free flap in order to maintain extremity length.[28]

Prostheses can be fitted easily over stumps covered with split-thickness grafts. Ridges of hypertrophic scar will break down if there is friction within the socket of the prosthesis. A scar often softens and flattens because of the constant, even pressure of a well fitted socket; prostheses fitted early over grafted stumps may prevent scar thickening. Breakdown may occur at points where the graft is adherent to bone. This problem may necessitate surgical freeing of the adherent graft and reshaping of the bone. Minor hip and knee flexion contractures complicate the fitting and function of a prosthesis; thus, every effort should be made to maintain full extension of these joints. Late revisions of amputations in children are required when the bone overgrows in length and when offensive terminal exostoses develop. The overgrowing bone can be shortened and the exostoses removed.

It is important, in the early management of upper extremity amputations in infants and young children, to supply temporary prosthetic extensions. This provides functional orientation to a prosthesis, maintains muscle bulk and tone, and encourages continuing bimanual activity at normal extremity length until a prosthesis with appropriate terminal device can be applied. Children quickly acquire prehension and transfer skills if they have an opposable stump and they may reject prostheses if they are not applied early. It is equally important to restore bipedal function as soon as possible. If delay of healing or ulceration of a lower extremity stump prevents early prosthetic fitting, an ischial weight-bearing device which suspends the stump will permit the child to walk in advance of prosthetic fitting. Inflatable plastic air bags provide both even pressure and accurate fit for weight bearing in container sockets. Early prosthetic fitting is desirable in teenagers and adults as well, but is not as critical as it is in children. As in nonburned persons, an upper extremity prosthesis may be rejected at any age if the opposite extremity is fully functional.[50]

Alterations in growth

In 1959, Evans and Smith reported that a patient who was 24 years of age when burned had a subsequent 1.5 inch increase in height.[1] It was suggested that one explanation for this growth spurt might be local change in hemodynamics with stasis, passive hyperemia, and chronic inflammation. We have not documented height changes in burned adults, but we have observed children whose growth after burn has seemed to be retarded. A study by Klein *et al.*[10] confirms growth delay in seriously burned children, particularly in the first postburn year. If growth plates remain open, it is difficult to explain overall growth retardation except on an endocrine or humoral basis. It is easy, however, to explain extremity length differences on the basis of premature closure of growth plates due to direct involvement of the bone or to severity of overlying burn. Frantz reported lower limb length discrepancy in four patients with foot and ankle burns.[51] Growth plates closed prematurely in only two of the cases. Jackson described two patients with digital and lower extremity deformity respectively due to partial closure of growth plates.[28] In Ritsila's case, contracture alone was apparently the cause of growth retardation in an upper extremity.[52] It seems reasonable, though hard to prove, that growth in a severely burned extremity would be retarded because of functional impairment. One patient, a 3-year-old boy with 80% TBSA burn and sufficiently deep burns of the right upper extremity to require mid-humerus amputation, demonstrated, 4 years after the burn, failure of development of the right shoulder girdle. The factors operant in this case could be premature closure of growth plates of scapula and clavicle, restrictive scar, and disuse atrophy.

There is yet another confusing aspect of premature closure of growth plates in that, within an extremity with total full-thickness burn, only a few of the growth plates will close prematurely. The explanation for this capricious selectivity is at best obscure. Evans and Calhoun recorded an example of spotty closure of growth plates in a 14-year-old male with 90% TBSA burn.[19] There was complete closure of distal tibial and fibular epiphyses 1 year after burn, together with closure of all digital epiphyses in the feet and of several digital epiphyses in the hands. Other major epiphyses were spared (**Figure 46.2**).

In early experience, abnormal growth plate closure was observed in a 6-year-old girl with 50% third degree burn which did not involve legs or ankles.[53] Rapidly destructive septic arthritis of one ankle resulted in closure of the adjacent tibial growth plate.

Only occasionally can growth changes be anticipated because of obvious affection of the bone. More often the changes are subtle. It seems clear, thus, that among seriously burned children, regular height and extremity length measurements must be part of ongoing postburn assessment until it is determined that the extremities and trunk are developing on schedule. Extremity and trunk alignment must likewise be part of the assessment as subtle angular deformity can occur because of partial closure of a growth plate. Jackson's report addresses this problem.[28]

So-called growth arrest lines seen in the roentgenograms of nonburned children, who have serious illness or major trauma other than burns, are commonly observed in burned children. In burns, as in other conditions, these transverse markers of relatively increased mineralization represent normal recovery from an insult to enchondral bone formation due to serious stress. They are of no clinical or functional significance. They are more related to total burn than to involvement of select burned extremities as all major long bones are affected. There is no evidence that growth arrest lines *per se* have any effect on growth.

References

1. Evans EB, Smith JR. Bone and joint changes following burn. *J Bone Joint Surg (Am)* 1959; 41: 785.
2. Rabinov D. Acromutilation of the fingers following severe burns. *Radiology* 1961; 77: 968–73.
3. Peters WJ. Heterotopic ossification: can early surgery be performed, with a positive bone scan? *J Burn Care Rehabil* 1978; 11(4): 318.
4. Cristallo V, Dell'Orto R. Pathological dislocation of the hip. *Arch Ortop* 1966; 79: 57–61.
5. Evans EB, Larson DL, Abston S, Willis B. Prevention and correction of deformity after severe burns. *Surg Clin N Am* 1970; 50: 1361–75.
6. Eszter V, Istvan S. Atipusos septicus arthritisek spontan luxatiok egesi serulteken. *Orv Hetil* 1972; 113: 48.
7. Jozsa L, Reffy A, Menesi L. Thermal injuries of human tendons. *Acta Chir Hung* 1985; 26: 113–8.
8. Salisbury RE, McKeel DW, Mason AD. Ischemic necrosis of the intrinsic muscles of the hand after thermal injuries. *J Bone Joint Surg (Am)* 1974; 56: 1701–7.
9. Schiele HP, Hubbard RB, Bruck HM. Radiographic changes in burns of the upper extremity. *Diagn Radiol* 1972; 104: 13–7.
10. Klein G, Herndon H, Rutan T, *et al*. Long term reduction in bone mass after severe burn injury in children. *J Pediatr* 1995; 126(2): 252–6.
11. Owens N. Osteoporosis following burns. *Br J Plast Surg* 1949; 1: 245–56.
12. Colson P, Stagnara P, Houot H. L-osteoporose chez les brules des membres. *Lyon Chir* 1953; 48: 950–6.
13. Artz CP, Reiss E. *The Treatment of Burns*, 1st edn. Philadelphia: WB Saunders, 1957.
14. Klein G, Herndon D, Rutan T, *et al*. Bone disease in burn patients. *J Bone Miner Res* 1993; 8(3): 337–45.
15. Van Der Wiel H, Lips P, Naura J, Patka C, Harma J, Teule G. Loss of bone in the proximal part of the femur following unstable fractures of the leg. *J Bone Joint Surg (Am)* 1994; 76: 230–6.
16. Dowling JA, Omer E, Moncrief JA. Treatment of fractures in burn patients. *J Trauma* 1968; 8: 465–74.
17. Choctaw WT, Zawacki BE, Dorr L. Primary excision and grafting of burns located over an open fracture. *Arch Surg* 1979; 114: 1141–2.
18. Wang Xue-wei, Zhang Zhong-ning. The successful treatment of a patient with extensive deep burns and an open comminuted fracture of a lower extremity. *Burns* 1984; 10: 339–43.
19. Evans EB, Calhoun JH. Musculoskeletal changes complicating burns. In: Epps CH Jr, ed. *Complications in Orthopaedic Surgery*, Vol. 2. Philadelphia: JB Lippincott, 1994; 1239–78.
20. Evans EB. Orthopaedic measures in the treatment of severe burns. *J Bone Joint Surg (Am)* 1966; 48: 643.
21. Brooker AF. The use of external fixation in the treatment of burn patients with fractures. In: Brooker AF, Edwards CC, eds. *Fracture Fixation: The Current State of the Art J Pediatr* 1995; 126, 2: 252–6.
22. Saffle JR, Schnelby A, Hoffmann A, Warden G: The management of fracture in thermally injured patients. *J Trauma* 1983; 23: 902–10.
23. Boyd BM, Robers WM, Miller GR. Periarticular ossification following burns. *South Med J* 1959; 52: 1048.
24. Koepke GD. Personal communication, 1964.
25. Elledge ES, Smith AA, McManus WF, Pruitt BA. Heterotopic bone formation in burned patients. *J Trauma* 1988; 28: 684–7.
26. Peterson SI, Mani MM, Crawford CM, Neff JR, Hiebert JM. Postburn heterotopic ossification: insights for management decision making. *J Trauma* 1989; 29: 365.
27. Tepperman PS, Hilbert L, Peters WJ, Pritzker KPH. Heterotopic ossification in burns. *J Burn Care Rehabil* 1984; 5: 283.
28. Jackson D MacG. Destructive burns: some orthopaedic complications. *Burns* 1979; 7: 105–22.
29. Munster AM, Bruck HM, John LA, Von Prince K, Kirkman EJ, Remig RL. Heterotopic calcification following burns: a prospective study. *J Trauma* 1972; 12: 1071–4.
30. Kolar J, Vrabec R. Periarticular soft-tissue changes as a late consequence of burns. *J Bone Joint Surg (Am)* 1959; 41: 103–11.
31. Heggers JP, Heggers R, Robson MC. Biochemical abnormalities in the thermally injured. *J Am Med Technol* 1981; 43: 333.
32. Herndon D. Mediators of metabolism. *J Trauma* 1981; 12: 701.
33. Johnson JTH. Atypical myositis ossificans. *J Bone Joint Surg (Am)* 1957; 39: 189–94.

34. Crawford CM, Varghese G, Mani MM, Neff JR. Heterotopic ossification: are range of motion exercises contraindicated. *J Burn Care Rehail* 1986; **7**: 323.
35. Evans EB. Heterotopic bone formation in thermal burns. *Clin Orthop* 1991; **263**: 94–101.
36. Michelsson JE, Rauschning W. Pathogenesis of experimental heterotopic bone formation following temporary forcible exercising of immobilized limbs. *Clin Orthop Rel Res* 1983; **176**: 265–72.
37. Lorber J. Ectopic ossification in tuberculous meningitis. *Arch Dis Child* 1953; **28**: 98.
38. Jacobs P. Reversible ectopic soft tissue ossification following measles encephalomyelitis. *Arch Dis Child* 1962; **37**: 90.
39. Garland DE, Blum CE, Waters RL. Periarticular heterotopic ossification in head-injured adults. *J Bone Joint Surg (Am)* 1985; **62**: 1261.
40. VanLaeken N, Snelling CT, Meek RN, Warren RJ, Foley B. Heterotopic bone formation in the patient with burn injuries. A retrospective assessment of contributing factors and methods of investigation. *J Burn Care Rehabil* 1989; **10**: 331.
41. Evans EB. Musculoskeletal changes complicating burns. In: Epps CH Jr, ed. *Complications in Orthopaedic Surgery*, Vol 2. Philadelphia: JB Lippincott, 1978: 1133–58.
42. Cope R. Heterotopic ossification. *South Med J* 1990; **83**(9): 1058.
43. Hoffer M, Brody G, Ferlic F. Excision of heterotopic ossification about elbows in patients with thermal injury. *J Trauma* 1978; **18**: 667–70.
44. Bottu Y, VanNoyen G. Un cas d'ossification reversible des tissus mous chez une petite patiente paraplegique. *Acta Paediatr Belg* 1963; **17**: 223.
45. Proulz R, Dupuis M. Ossifications et calcifications para-articulaires à la suite de brulures: revue de la literature et présentation de 3 cas. *Union Med Can* 1972; **101**: 282–93.
46. Dias D. Heterotopic para-articular ossification of the elbow with soft tissue contracture in burns. *Burns* 1982; **9**: 128–34.
47. Harnar T, Engrav L, Heimbach D, Marvin J. Experience with skeletal immobilization after excision and grafting of the severely burned hands. *J Trauma* 1985; **25**: 299–302.
48. Youel L, Evans E, Heare TC, Herndon DN, Larson DL, Abston S. Skeletal suspension in the management of severe burns in children. *J Bone Joint Surg (Am)* 1986; **68**: 1375–9.
49. Jackson D MacG. Burns into joints. *Burns* 1976; **2**: 90–106.
50. Malone JM, Fleming LL, Roberson J, *et al.* Immediate, early and late postsurgicial management of upper-limb amputation. *J Rehabil Res Dev* 1984; **21**: 33–41.
51. Frantz CH, Delgado S. Limb-length discrepancy after third-degree burns about the foot and ankle. *J Bone Joint Surg (Am)* 1966; **48**: 443–50.
52. Ritsila V, Sundell B, Alhopura S. Severe growth retardation of the upper extremity resulting from burn contracture and its full recovery after release of the contracture. *Br J Plast Surg* 1976; **29**: 53–5.
53. Evans EB, Larson L, Yates S. Preservation and restoration of joint function in patients with severe burns. *JAMA* 1968; **204**: 843–8.
54. Frye KE, Luterman A. When burn injury and skeletal trauma are two components of the multiple trauma. *Orthop Nurs* 1999; **18**(1): 30–5.
55. Nassabi H, Raff T, Germann G. Manifestation of multifocal heterotopic ossifications with unusual locations as a complication after severe burn injury. *Burns* 1996; **22**: 500–3.
56. Holguin PH, Rico AA, Garcia JP, Del Rio JL. Elbow anchylosis due to postburn hetertopic ossifcation. *J Burn Care Rehabil* 1996; **17**(2): 150–4.
57. Djurickovic S, Meek RN, Snelling CF, *et al.* Range of motion and complications after postburn heterotopic bone excision about the elbow. *J Trauma* 1996; **41**(5): 825–30.

Reconstruction

Chapter 47   Prolonged hypermetabolic response over time, the use of anabolic agents and exercise, and longitudinal evaluation of the burned child

Patricia E Blakeney, Robert L McCauley, David N Herndon

vivors, to assist them to achieve the best possible outcomes, physically and psychologically and socially. Without such effort to always learn from our patients, we would produce a growing population of children with severe burns who must contend with disabilities, disfigurements, and social prejudices that are everyday obstacles to success in school and play, as well as to their potential achievements and contributions to society as adults.

Treatment of pediatric burns is similar in many ways to that for adults; however, pediatric injuries present unique challenges, both at the time of acute treatment and throughout rehabilitation. The adult body is mature and relatively static, whereas the body and brain of a child are constantly evolving. Skin grafts in children must be placed with a consideration for the changes that occur during growth and development. Scar contractures limiting movement are more common. The child's self concept and cognitive schema of the world are rudimentary. There is little known of how severe burns and intrusive treatments may impact children cognitively and emotionally; even less is understood about the varying impact at different developmental stages. Although the goals of rehabilitation are similar for children and adults, the techniques useful for motivating children to participate in uncomfortable exercises are quite different. This chapter focuses on children with very large and very severe burns because of the special challenges. We describe what is known currently about their outcomes; and we report methods, procedures, and technologies that are currently being explored to maximize the full potential of these children to become self-sufficient adults who are integrated and contributing members of society.

Introduction

Burns in children remain major challenges to medical science, not only in terms of mortality, but in discovering ways to improve their recoveries; the ultimate goal is for young burn survivors to grow into active, self supporting, happy adults, i.e. to achieve an optimal quality of life. As advances in burn care have reduced the high mortality associated with even massive burns to children, burn team scientists and clinicians have barely begun to know what the long-term quality of life for these survivors can be.[1-5] Rehabilitative challenges with such children are numerous, and the best methods of achieving good outcomes for children with big burns are still being developed.[6] Following the survivors, longitudinally and systematically collecting information from them in several domains of their lives, we can use these data not only to guide our treatments of current patients but also of future sur-

Long-term outcomes of children with massive burn injuries

For the past decade, doctors at Shriners Burns Hospital in Galveston have followed, longitudinally, children who survived massive injuries, assessing physical and psychosocial adaptation on an annual basis with standardized measures when available. In 1986, assessments of 12 survivors of such massive injuries were reported.[4] Of the 12, eight (66%) were found to be well adjusted; four were described as regressed with excessive fear, neurotic symptoms, and somatic complaints. A later follow-up report of eight of the children found satisfactory adjustment in six (75%) and two who were not doing well.[7] Four years later, we reported the results of psychosocial assessments of 25 children with total body surface area (TBSA) 80% burned in which the burned children appeared, as a group, to have no more behavioral problems than their age-matched cohorts in a normative reference group.[8] The burned children also had positive self-esteem, equal to and sometimes surpassing, that of the nonburned reference group. Examining the impact of physical impairment upon the psychosocial competence of 19 survivors of massive burns, we found the competence scores of the burned children, as reported by both the parents of the children and the children themselves, to be equal to those of the normal, age-matched reference group.[9] Physical impairment was related to competence only in the area of activity, and not in academic or social competence. Perhaps most surprising to us was that two of the 19 children had ratings of 'no physical impairment' based upon range of motion measurements according to AMA guidelines. We concluded that severe childhood burn injury does not necessarily induce onerous physical impairment, and even severe impairment does not necessarily lead to poor psychosocial adjustment.

In a more recent examination of the psychological and behavioral adjustment of 74 of our survivors of massive injury (TBSA ≥80%, ≥70% full-thickness), we found that 70% of the children and young adults had no significant difficulty; most were doing well and described themselves as being 'happy'. Most were still in school. Three young adults had married or were living with a committed partner and had become parents.[10]

Of 41 who were also assessed for physical functioning, 32 patients were independent with completion of age-appropriate activities of daily living skills. Only the amputation of fingers seemed to impede the self-sufficiency of these individuals.[11] Although some, like those with finger amputations, required adaptive devices and compensations such as extra time to achieve successful performance, most of these survivors of massive injury had managed the skills required to meet developmental milestones, to develop appropriate autonomy, and to achieve psychological and social well-being.

In a study conducted at our sister institution, the Shriners Hospital in Boston, 80 survivors of burns involving >70% TBSA were evaluated almost 15 years following their injuries.[12] The investigators used a quality of life assessment tool to measure achievement in several domains, including general health, psychological health, family function, physical function, and physical role. The scores of these young people were similar to those of the normal population with the exception of physical functioning and physical role. In these areas, the scores were more than 2 standard deviations below the age- and gender-matched norms, indicating that some had continuing serious physical disabilities. Thus, while some children surviving severe burns had, as young adults, lingering physical disabilities, most reported having accomplished a satisfying quality of life.

Difficulties associated with large burn injuries

The generally positive outcomes reported above present an even more optimistic view when one considers that the majority of children and young adults described in these studies were treated initially many years ago. With experience and increased data, gathered in large part from these courageous young people, burn team clinicians and scientists have identified many long-term problems associated with large burns. Problems have been identified with overall growth and development of the soft tissues, muscle, and bone. Difficulties related to the scarring process, contractures limiting mobility, disfigurement, and the consequent psychosocial problems are all problems the burn survivors must face

and conquer in some way. Large burns, i.e. >40% TBSA, are complex injuries, affecting every body system.

Managing the hypermetabolic response to burn injury

The hypermetabolic response (discussed in detail in Chapters 20–28 of this book) appears to play an early and central role in many of the long-lasting difficulties children with severe burn injury have encountered; thus, it will be reviewed here. In response to a severe burn injury, afferent stimuli are activated causing a hypothalamic thermoregulatory re-setting to occur. This results in increased heat production, increased heart rate and cardiac output; resting energy expenditure increases to about 150% of normal.[13] The stress response to burn injury is characterized by a cascade of hormones with increased circulating levels of catecholamines, cortisol and glucagon that result in a hypercatabolic state.[14] The effects of this hypermetabolic, hypercatabolic state are rapid muscle breakdown[15] and reduced bone formation, resulting in severe osteopenia or osteoporosis.[16] Some of the deleterious effects of this early disruption, e.g. linear growth retardation and weakness of the bones, appear to contribute to life-long disabilities, remaining problems even years after the body's metabolism has returned to normal.[17-19] One can think of this state as the body running at almost twice its normal rate even though the individual is lying at rest. The patient requires enormous amounts of nutrient calories to keep up with the energy expenditure. Even with adequate calories, individuals in this state lose muscle mass and bone density. Conventional thinking has been that this state should dissipate with full healing of the burn wound. However, in our clinical work, we observed that the children fail to develop muscle, to grow, and to gain weight for a period of time extending far beyond wound healing. Recently, we were able to follow systematically 25 severely burned children for 1 year to ascertain the duration of the hypermetabolic-hypercatabolic state. Stable isotope metabolic and body composition studies were performed during acute hospitalization, at initial hospital discharge, and at 6, 9, and 12 months postburn. The resting energy expenditure of these children peaked at 1-week post-injury, with a metabolic rate of 180% of normal and progressively declined with time. At the time of exit from the study, i.e. 12 months, their resting energy expenditure was still 15% above basal metabolic rate. Catabolism persisted for at least 9 months, which was 7 months after complete wound healing. This is the first scientific documentation that the physiologic derangement incited by acute burn injury continues for many months after full healing of all wounds.[20,21]

During these long months, the children's linear growth is arrested. They fatigue easily. They often have difficulty concentrating and may be irritable and emotionally labile, compounding problems for themselves and for their friends and families. At the time immediately following discharge from the hospital and when they are facing the most difficult challenges of resuming 'normal' life, the children are literally exhausted and physically weak. The first months following the injury are especially arduous, for during those early months the child and family are still grieving the loss of the pre-burn child; they often are grieving other losses as well – loss of loved ones, loss of home and possessions, loss of dreams. Developing methods for facilitating participation in rehabilitation while the children and families are simultaneously struggling to cope with life's sadness, and while the child is so weak and easily fatigued, is a major challenge for burn care specialists.

Recognition that many of the difficulties of the first year post-burn are part of the illness of severe burns should remove some of the strife from the process of rehabilitation. In the past, burn care professionals and patients and their families, all feeling frustrated, have alternated between blaming themselves and blaming each other for their failures during this first terrible year post-injury. With the evidence that this extraordinary physical disruption continues for most of that first year, the informed team can teach the family about this part of the illness and assist them in planning to manage this phase just as they have managed the acute phase.

However, knowledge of the duration and extensive harm resulting from the catabolic effects of the trauma has also led to efforts to better delineate mechanisms of catabolism[22,23] and to a vigilant pursuit of early interventions that could attenuate the effects of the hypermetabolic response. As will be seen through the remainder of this discussion, administration of an anabolic agent such as growth hormone (GH) during the acute treatment of severely burned children has been demonstrated to be extremely beneficial in promoting healing and health.[14] Studies of GH demonstrate that it can be given safely to severely burned children,[24] and that it accelerates wound healing[25] and reduces tissue wasting commonly seen in the hypercatabolic patient.[26] Knowledge gained from such studies suggests improved treatment approaches that can be evaluated. For most of the issues evolving from massive burn injury, we are still in the early stages of this process – still learning about problems and devising methods of improving our treatments.

Growth Delay and Anabolic Agents

In 1990, Rutan and Herndon demonstrated a dampened growth curve for both height and weight in male and female patients who had sustained major thermal injury.[17] The growth velocities were delayed up to 3 years after burn injury. Even after the return to normal growth velocities, the burned patients lagged behind age- and sex-matched peers.

Normal linear growth and weight gain in children are dependent upon a number of factors. The prenatal environment, adequate nutritional intake, and an emotionally nurturing household environment are crucial. Long hospitalizations alone have been known to produce profound arrests in growth and development in children. The management of massively burned children includes multiple operations and prolonged hospitalization. In cases of fascial excision, subcutaneous fat layers in the injured area are also removed. Fat stores are further depleted in providing energy for the process of gluconeogenesis from existing protein stores for dietary supply. All the reasons for the growth delay following severe burns are not currently known. However, plasma growth hormone levels have been shown to decrease in severely burned adults,[27] and it is likely that children experience a similar decrease. Using recombinant human growth hormone (rhGH) in the acute treatment of children with severe thermal injuries has been shown to improve net muscle protein synthesis[26] as well as to accelerate wound healing and reduce length of hospital stay.[25,28] Improvement in each of these areas could contribute to improved growth and weight gain; therefore, administration of GH was perceived as a probable advantageous tool in the management of pediatric burn patients toward normal growth.

Low et al.[29–31] tested the hypothesis that rhGH would ameliorate the growth delay by following, for 3 years, 49 children in a prospective, randomized, masked study. Twenty-six children received 0.2 mg/kg rhGH during their acute hospitalizations; 23 children received 0.9% saline as placebo during the same time periods of acute hospitalization. They found that the children who were treated with rhGH during their acute care maintained their stature (height for age percentile and height-velocity), whereas untreated children who were not in a growth spurt at the time of burn remained delayed in linear growth at the end of the study 3 years post-injury. Continuing with this study, Low et al. found that the differences in height percentiles had nearly resolved at 5 years postburn.[32] Short-term (average of 6 weeks) administration of rhGH did not attenuate the hypermetabolic state; resting energy expenditures remained elevated for both groups of children during the time they were being treated acutely. However, the administration of rhGH apparently made up for a deficit that commonly occurs following severe burn injury. Children burned during a growth spurt are thought to have the advantage of higher levels of growth hormone available and thus can maintain normal growth without exogenous hormone.

Currently, we are administering GH over a period of 1 year post-injury to a randomized sample of severely burned children to attempt to improve prolonged muscle protein metabolism. A difficulty confronted in this study is that GH is administered via daily injections. Although these injections are virtually painless (the investigators have first given them to themselves to be sure of this), they are a daily source of irritation and tension to parent and child. Therefore, we are seeking a less intrusive means of accomplishing this end. Oxandrolone is an anabolic steroid that has been used in cachectic hepatitis and AIDS patients and can be administered orally. We have now begun a series of studies to determine whether oxandrolone is as efficacious as growth hormone in impeding the chronic muscle protein catabolism in burned children. The first of these studies demonstrates that oxandrolone, given for only 1 week to 14 children, significantly increased protein synthesis. This study suggests that this orally administered anabolic agent is a promising alternative to growth hormone in mitigating the catabolic effects of the hypermetabolism of severely burned children.[33,34]

Loss of strength and endurance mitigated by exercise

Resistance exercise also has an established influence on muscle strengthening and muscle protein synthesis. The beneficial effects have been well documented adults, adolescents, and older children.[35–40] Ferrando et al. demonstrated that moderate resistance exercise is capable of ameliorating the decreases in skeletal muscle protein synthesis and strength that accompany inactivity.[41] The acute stimulatory effects of resistance exercise may last up to 48 hours.[42] An intensive, rehabilitation program that includes resistance exercise, then, would be expected to improve the heightened protein synthesis initiated during acute hospitalization by the administration of rhGH. The combination of GH and exercise should therefore provide for a synergistic effect on skeletal muscle protein synthesis by addressing separate stimulatory mechanisms for an extended period of time. Each intervention is a compliment of the other, and the combination should provide for a synergistic effect on protein synthesis. Additionally, aerobic and resistance exercise should strengthen the cardiovascular system which has also been shown to be diminished over time with large burns, especially for those individuals who also suffered inhalation injuries (see Chapters 17–19).[43–45] However, the degree to which a rehabilitation program for severely burned children could safely incorporate progressive resistance and aerobic exercises has been a question.

In 1998, our team in Galveston began a study to do just that. The study is currently on-going so data presented here should be considered preliminary. The purpose of the study is, first, to test whether the program can be safely completed by severely burned children 6 months post injury and, second, to test whether such children can develop greater muscular strength and greater endurance with this addition to the more traditional outpatient therapy program.[46–48] Whereas traditional rehabilitation therapy programs emphasize the relief of scar contractures, this program incorporates an exercise prescription to increase musculoskeletal and cardiovascular strength and function. Patients included in this program have burns ≥ 40% TBSA, are 6 years or older, and are designated by a random selection process to be compared to a similar control group who receive traditional outpatient therapy in their home communities. They participate in this program from the 6th through the 8th month after their burn injury. During these 3 months, the children receive moderate intensity, progressive resistance training using free weights as well as aerobic and general conditioning exercises, supervised by an exercise physiologist, for 1 hour three times each week. They also receive 1 hour of occupational and physical therapy twice daily for 5 days a week, 2 hours of school daily for 5 days a week, play therapy daily, and psychological counseling for at least 3 hours a week.

When Cucuzzo et al.[46–48] reported their results, they had 11 patients who had participated in the intensive in-house exercise program and 10 in the control group. On testing at 6 months, there were no differences between the groups. However, testing at 9 months, after the 3-month trial, revealed that, although muscular strength had increased for both groups, the improvement in the group who had intensive training was over twice that of the group who had outpatient therapy at home. The program had succeeded in increasing the strength for those 11 children and had done so safely; there were no injuries or contraindications to exercise during 479 exercise and testing sessions.

As of this writing, 22 individuals have completed the 9-month (post-3-month training or at home rehabilitation program) assessments. Those in the intensive program continue to demonstrate significantly improved muscle strength (100% over their 6-month ability) compared to the group who receive outpatient therapy at home (39% improvement over their 6-month ability). In addition, cardiovascular fitness (walking on a treadmill) improved by 30% for the in-house group while the at-home group actually lost 3% fitness. Data analyses have not yet looked for effects of an anabolic agent in conjunction with the exercise program; however, the results of these preliminary analyses are very exciting in their promise of enhanced overall well-being for survivors of very large severe burn injuries.

Bone loss and other skeletal changes

Skeletal changes (see Chapters 24–26, 44) are associated with severe burn injury as a result of damage to the epiphyseal plate,[49] as a result of joint contractures and joint dislocations,[50] and consequently to bone atrophy or osteoporosis.[51,52] In some situations it is unclear whether a failure in normal bone maturation is a result of the burn injury itself or is secondary to the compression therapy applied to assist in the maturation of burn scars or skin grafted areas. McCauley et al. documented significant delay in the development of the mandible in children who had been burned in the head/neck region; however, all of the children had also required compression therapy that may have restricted normal growth.[53]

Osteoporosis in burned children was noted as a significant concern in 1966 by Evans.[51] Recent work indicates that a critical event that immediately contributes to this burn-associated bone loss is decreased bone formation (discussed in detail in Chapter 23). Within 48 hours of burn injury of ≥ 40% TBSA burns, children experience a decrease in serum osteocalcin, a biochemical marker of bone formation.[54,55] At 3.5 weeks postburn, iliac crest bone biopsies revealed reduced bone formation in children and in adults.[51,53] How long bone formation is reduced is not known; however, in a cross-sectional study of children comparably burned a mean of 5 years previously, bone formation was still reduced in approximately half the patients studied.[55,57] Preliminary data obtained from longitudinal studies of severely burned patients, with measures taken at 6 weeks through 9–14 months following injury, show no significant improvement in bone density, and this phenomenon appears to be due to absolute loss of bone mineral content.[58] Thus, data to date indicate that severely burned children lose bone relative to age-matched unburned children and fail to regain the quantity of bone mass sufficient to approximate normal. This failure leaves them with weakened bones, susceptible to bone fractures[55] and puts them at increased risk for the development of adult onset osteoporosis.[59]

Likely contributors to reduced bone formation are the endocrine change related to the hypermetabolic response and immobilization.[59] The short-term administration (6 weeks) of an anabolic agent, rhGH, was not effective in preserving bone density.[60] Interventional trials of long-term administration of anabolic agents are now underway in Galveston. However, the strength-building and endurance training in the exercise program described above does seem to contribute positively to bone re-mineralization.[48]

Joint Contractures

Joint contractures are a frequent muscular skeletal complication, particularly in children. Bhattachara[50] noted a 10% incidence in a group of 50% patients; 64% of these contractures were in patients younger than 10 years of age. The rapid rate of children's limb growth relative to the rate of growth of burn scar or grafted areas probably contributes significantly to this major problem. One study suggests that the type of graft bed can make a difference in contracture development; Jones et al. reported that patients with tangential excision down to fat had better joint mobility at 1 year post-injury than did those with excisions to fascia.[61] It is apparent that children requiring fascial excision experience a number of problems including the development of contour deformities secondary to hypertrophy of the remaining fat cells and marked differences in muscular development.

Heterotopic Bone Formation

Decrease in joint mobility can develop from heterotopic bone formed late in acute hospitalization or during recovery. Although the etiology of heterotopic bone formation is unknown, it is known that it does not necessarily occur over burned tissue. The incidence of heterotopic bone formation varies between 1% in a retrospective study to 23% in a prospective study.[62,63] Heterotopic bone remains a mystery at this writing. Not only are factors influencing the development of heterotopic bone unclear, but also the techniques that contribute to the successful surgical management and postoperative care of these patients. Consequently, surgical outcome tends to be less than optimal, and recurrence rates remain high.

Integument

Hypertrophic scar formation is a sequela of burn wound healing that we have found no way to avoid; we continue to look for techniques for better management of the scarring process in order to obtain improved functional and cosmetic results. The medical and surgical management of hypertrophic scar formation has been detailed in Chapters 37 and 43–45 of this text, and will be discussed only briefly here as a reminder that management of hypertrophic scars is an extremely important component in the care and long-term outcomes of severely burned individuals. Compression therapy to minimize scarring and contractures, which was popularized in the late 1960s and early 1970s, continues to be the mainstay for the nonsurgical management of hypertrophic scar formation.[65–68] However, its effectiveness has never been scientifically proven and is currently a subject of debate.[69] In 1999, a study at Shriners Burns Hospital in Galveston revealed no significant differences in burn scars at 6 months postburn in patients receiving high pressure versus low pressure.[70] An ongoing study at Harborview Medical Center applies pressure to one-half, and no pressure to the other half, of the same wound. Their findings are that, at 6 and 9 months postburn, the halves treated with pressure were softer than the halves without, and the scars without pressure were higher; however, the difference was undetectable at 12 months post burn. The assessments were made using highly objective, technical assessments using ultrasound, color chromometer, and durometer.[71] Although less technically sophisticated, another ongoing study in Galveston compares patients with ≤ 30% TBSA who do and do not receive pressure garments according to a random design. At 6 months, the only significant difference between the two groups was the height of the burn scars. There were no differences in mobility or in other characteristics of scar, i.e. pigmentation, vascularity, or pliability. A panel of blinded observers, 10 plastic surgeons and seven rehabilitation therapists, could not distinguish significant differences between the groups when evaluating pigmentation, color or overall aesthetics from photographs.[72]

Thus, the studies and debates continue, and, at least until more evidence is gathered, pressure therapy with the familiar elastic garments is still prescribed. Patients vary in their ratings of comfort of the garments once applied, but all agree they are difficult to put on and that they are very hot in warm temperatures. Their application is the fuel for daily tensions in the homes of some burned children whose parents want to adhere to the prescribed wearing of the garments for 23 hours per day. Such children and their families would no doubt feel relieved if the data eventually show that pressure does not make a significant difference in long-term outcomes. However, it should be noted that the studies thus far include neither the examination of burns over joints nor do they include burns of the hands, neck and face. In addition, none of the studies to date question the use of pressure in the form of splints, another source of discomfort and tension for burned children and their families.

None of the known studies yet have broached the face with an attempt to determine the efficacy of pressure versus no pressure. The elastic hood and underlying silicone face pad present special problems for patients, and some extreme challenges for the adults trying to assist a burned child or adolescent. The elastic mask and hood, covering head, face, and hair, effectively hides the identity of the person wearing it. It is perceived by children as sinister, associated with 'bad men' or Hallowe'en monsters, and most children who have worn this garment can relay stories of being ridiculed by strangers who did not know the purpose of the garment. Emotional expressiveness, usually apparent in facial movements, is hidden by the hood. More than one child has explained nonadherence with the prescribed wearing of the elastic mask with a statement similar to 'I want my friends to see me laugh'. A study by Groce *et al.* compared the elastic mask and hood with silicone pad to the transparent silicone face mask and found no significant differences between the amount of pressure applied by each to the forehead, cheeks, and chin.[73] Many children have expressed a preference for, and seem to wear more readily, the transparent mask. This study should make it easier for them to be granted their choice – an important event during a time when so much is happening to them outside of their control.

Longitudinal planning for reconstructive surgery

The complex reconstructive needs of patients with large and deep burns, small areas of good donor sites and large areas of burn scar and grafted tissue, dictate the development of a mechanism by which reconstruction can proceed in a rational and orderly fashion. The team in Galveston modified a form devised by the American Burn Association Rehabilitation Committee which it uses to record potential reconstructive needs and to allow systematic planning for future operations. This form is intended to cover all body regions with subdivisions into anatomical units (**Figure 47.1**). Brou *et al.* demonstrated the usefulness of this inventory of potential reconstructive needs in 25 patients with a mean TBSA burn of 71%. The total number of potential reconstructive needs was 512, of which 235 were in the head/neck region. The average number of problems per patient was 21.[74] Obviously, relying on plastic surgery to correct all potential problem areas presents very real risks. Rather, the coordination of efforts by plastic surgeons, general surgeons, orthopedic surgeons, respiratory therapists, physical therapists, and occupational therapists has been proven to be of significant importance in the long-term maximal recovery and rehabilitation of these patients.

Sexual Maturation

Although we have used the Tanner scale to assess our prepubertal and adolescent patients on an annual basis for many years postburn, we have found no evidence that sexual maturation is significantly affected by severe burn injury. It is important to note that questions about breast development, ability to have children, and future sexual abilities are not infrequent worries posed even by young children. Certainly as adolescents, children with disfiguring burn scars have thoughts, feelings *and* behaviors similar to those of nonburned adolescents.[75]

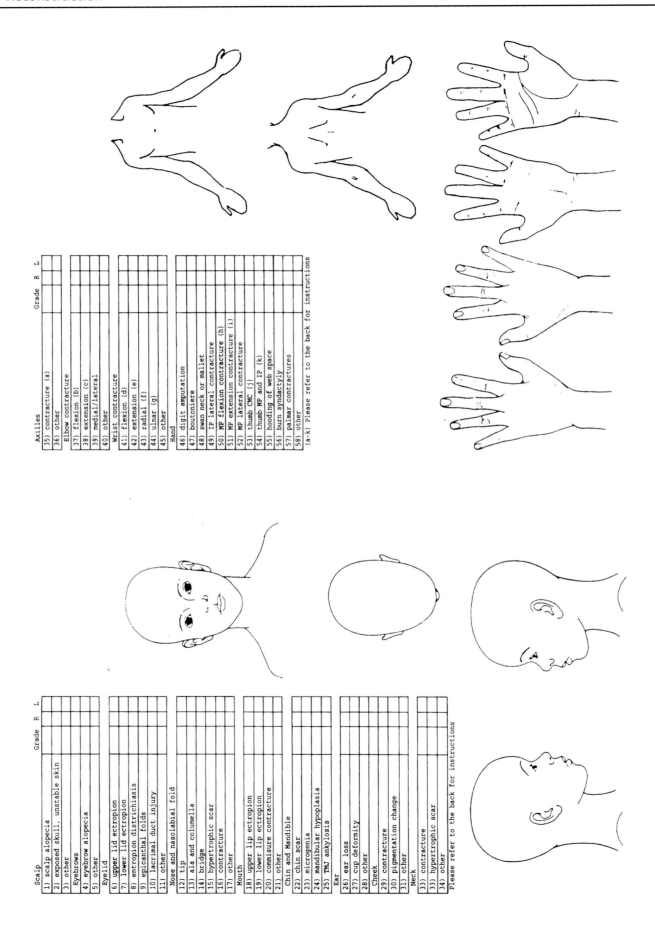

Axilles	Grade	R	L
35) contracture (a)			
36) other			
Elbow contracture			
37) flexion (b)			
38) extension (c)			
39) medial/lateral			
40) other			
Wrist contracture			
41) flexion (d)			
42) extension (e)			
43) radial (f)			
44) ulnar (g)			
45) other			
Hand			
46) digit amputation			
47) boutoniere			
48) swan neck or mallet			
49) IP lateral contracture			
50) MP flexion contracture (h)			
51) MP extension contracture (i)			
52) MP lateral contracture			
53) thumb CMC (j)			
54) thumb MP and IP (k)			
55) hooding of web space			
56) burn syndactyly			
57) palmar contractures			
58) other			

(a–k) Please refer to the back for instructions

Scalp	Grade	R	L
1) scalp alopecia			
2) exposed skull, unstable skin			
3) other			
Eyebrows			
4) eyebrow alopecia			
5) other			
Eyelid			
6) upper lid ectropion			
7) lower lid ectropion			
8) entropion districhiasis			
9) epicanthal folds			
10) lacrimal duct injury			
11) other			
Nose and nasolabial fold			
12) tip			
13) ala and columella			
14) bridge			
15) hypertrophic scar			
16) contracture			
17) other			
Mouth			
18) upper lip ectropion			
19) lower lip ectropion			
20) commisure contracture			
21) other			
Chin and Mandible			
22) chin scar			
23) microgenia			
24) mandibular hypoplasia			
25) TMJ ankylosis			
Ear			
26) ear loss			
27) cup deformity			
28) other			
Cheek			
29) contracture			
30) pigmentation change			
31) other			
Neck			
33) contracture			
33) hypertrophic scar			
34) other			

Please refer to the back for instructions

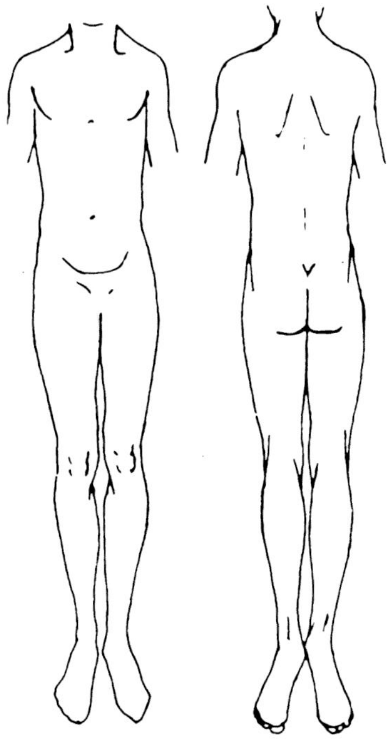

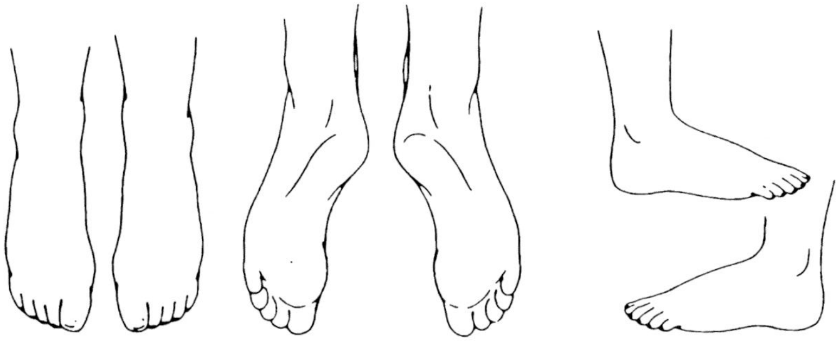

INSTRUCTIONS

I) Identify the patient's abnormality and check the appropriate box (R) for right and (L) for left or both for single or midline structures. Use the empty space in each line to write additional information.

II) Use the diagram to draw the observed abnormality when needed for more detailed information.

III) Signal each abnormality in the diagram by writing the corresponding number.

IV) Grade each observed abnormality as (S) for severe, (Mo) for moderate, and (Mi) for mild.

V) Some items have specific grading criteria such as:

  (a) Shoulder abduction (normal ROM 0 to 180 degrees)
    Severe: 0 to 60 degrees
    Moderate: 0 to 120 degrees
    Mild: 0 to 180 degrees

  (b) Elbow flexion (normal ROM 0 to 150 degrees)
    Severe: 100 to 150 degrees
    Moderate: 50 to 100 degrees
    Mild: 0 to 50 degrees

  (c) Elbow extension (normal ROM 150 to 0 degrees)
    Severe: 0 to 50 degrees
    Moderate: 0 to 100 degrees
    Mild: 0 to 150 degrees

  (d) Wrist flexion (normal ROM 0 to 70 degrees)
    Severe: 60 degrees or more
    Moderate: 60 to 20 degrees
    Mild: 20 to -20 degrees

  (e) Wrist extension (normal ROM 0 to -60 degrees)
    Severe: -60 degrees or more
    Moderate: -60 to -40 degrees
    Mild: -40 to -20 degrees

  (f) Wrist ulnar deviation (normal ROM 0 to 30 degrees)
    Severe: 30 degrees or more

  (g) Wrist radial deviation (normal ROM 0 to 20 degrees)
    Severe: 20 degrees or more

  (h) MP flexion (normal ROM 0 to 90 degrees)
    Severe: 90 degrees or more
    Moderate: 90 to 45 degrees
    Mild: 45 to 0 degrees

  (i) MP extension (normal ROM 90 to 0 degrees)
    Severe: less than 0 degrees

  (j) Thumb CMC
    Severe: no opposition or pinch possible
    Moderate: lateral pinch only
    Mild: opposition present

  (k) Thumb MP and IP
    Severe: no opposition or pinch possible
    Moderate: laters. pinch only
    Mild: opposition present

  (l) Hip
    Severe: affects gait and posture
    Moderate: affects sporting activities
    Mild: no functional impairment

  (m) Knee
    Severe: affects gait and posture
    Moderate: affects sporting activity
    Mild: no functional impairment

	Grade	R	L
Trunk			
59) kyphosis			
60) scoliosis			
61) lordosis			
62) breast, nipple, areola			
63) abdominal scar			
64) other			
Perineum			
65) penile scars/deformities			
66) vulvar scars/deformities			
67) perineal contractures			
68) anal stenosis			
69) anal incompetence/prolapse			
70) other			
Hip and Thigh			
71) contractures (l)			
72) amputation/stump			
73) other			
Knee and Leg			
74) contractures (m)			
75) unstable skin			
76) osteomyelitis			
77) amputation/stump			
78) other			
Ankle and Foot			
79) equinus			
80) varus			
81) valgus			
82) cavus			
83) calcaneus			
84) unstable heel pad			
85) toe hyperextension			
86) toe hyperflexion			
87) toe/foot amputation			
88) other			

(l–m) Please refer to the back for instructions

Fig. 47.1 Inventory form for potential reconstructive needs.

McCauley *et al.* documented the growth and development of 28 female patients with significant burn injury to the anterior chest wall involving the nipple-areola complex.[76] The mean age at the time of the burn injury was 5.9 years with a mean follow-up of nearly 9 years. At this time, patients were treated with either epluchage or delayed tangential excision. This study provided the first longitudinal assessment of breast development in adolescents with burns; it also documents that, with conservative management of tissue during the acute phase of injury, chances of breast development are optimized. Second, even with loss of the nipple – areola complex, the underlying breast bud is rarely injured. Such studies bring to light the impact of acute management on subsequent growth and development of children and clearly demonstrate the need for acute burn surgeons to preserve tissue in critical areas. McCauley *et al.* also documented the absence of prenatal complications associated with mature circumferential truncal burns. In seven patients with 14 pregnancies, the mean time of follow-up from burn injury to the first pregnancy was more than 12 years.[77]

Summary: longitudinal evaluation

The long-term outcomes reported in the beginning of this chapter are impressive even without the information just discussed. Reviewing the difficulties those very survivors taught us about and that they had to deal with makes their positive accomplishments very impressive. Psychologically, they have struggled to adapt, and we have learned from those struggles and developed interventions to ease the burden of being a child burn survivor living in a world where burn scars and pressure garments are largely unknown and misunderstood. Those concerns and interventions are discussed in the chapter on Psychosocial Recovery and Reintegration in this book. We are grateful that these young people have shared their time and experiences with us so that we could learn and try to improve.

Because children's bodies, brains, and social experiences are in a constant state of flux, the need to follow them longitudinally is quite apparent. Just as we assess the children with massive injuries on at least an annual basis, so do we assess children with lesser burn injuries regularly, systematically, and with standardized instruments to the extent possible so that we can compare our patients to the normative unburned samples reported. And, just as the coordination of many disciplines is necessary during the emergency and acute phases of injury, so must many disciplines be involved, working in coordination, in the long-term assessment and treatment of burned children. The focus of our treatment must always be on the ultimate endpoint which is the burn survivor, injured as a child and developed into an autonomous adult with maximum functioning, physically and psychologically. The focus of longitudinal studies such as those reported in this chapter must always be on identifying problems and looking for ways to improve our care to reduce the difficulties of the future.

References

1. Herndon DN, Parks DH. Comparison of serial debridement and autografting and early massive excision with cadaveric skin overlay in the treatment of large burns in children. *J Trauma* 1986; **26**: 149–52.
2. Herndon DN, Barrow RE, Rutan RL, Rutan TC, Desai MH, Abston S. A comparison of conservative versus early excisional therapies in severely burned patients. *Ann Surg* 1989; **209**: 547–53.
3. Wolf S, Rose JK, Desai M, Mileski J, Barrow R, Herndon D. Mortality determinants in massive pediatric burns: an analysis of 103 children with ≥80% TBSA burns (≥70% full-thickness). *Ann Surg* 1997; **225**(5): 554–69.
4. Herndon D, LeMaster J, Beard S, et al. The quality of life after major thermal injury in children: an analysis of 12 survivors with ≥80% TBSA, 70% third degree burns. *J Trauma* 1986; **26**: 609–18.
5. Herndon DN, Rutan R, Desai M, Blakeney P, Womack J. What size burns should be resuscitated? *Proc Am Burn Assoc* 1993; **25**: 106.
6. Constable JD. The state of burn care: past, present, and future. *Burns* 1994; **20**: 316–24.
7. Beard S, Desai M, Herndon D. Adaptation of self-image in burn disfigured children. *Proc Am Burn Assoc* 1989; **21**: 154.
8. Blakeney P, Meyer W, Moore P, et al. Psychosocial sequelae of pediatric burns involving 80% or greater Total Body Surface Area. *J Burn Care Rehabil* 1993; **14**: 684–9.
9. Moore P, Moore M, Blakeney P, Meyer W, Murphy L, Herndon D. Competence and physical impairment of pediatric survivors of burns of more than 80% total body surface area. *J Burn Care Rehabil* 1996; **17**: 547–51.
10. Blakeney P, Meyer W, Robert R, Herndon DN. Long-term psychosocial adaptation of children who survive burns involving 80% or greater Total Body Surface Area. *J Trauma* 1998; **44**: 625–34.
11. Meyers-Paal R, Blakeney P, Murphy L, et al. Physical and psychological rehabilitation outcomes for pediatric patients who suffer > 80% total body surface area burn and >70% 3rd degree burns. *J Burn Care Rehabil* 2000; **21**: 43–9.
12. Sheridan R, Hinson M, Liang M, et al. Long-term outcome of children surviving massive burns. *JAMA* 2000; **283**: 69–73.
13. Wolfe RR, Herndon DN, Jahoor F, Miyoshi H, Wolfe M. Effects of severe burn injury on substrate cycling by glucose and fatty acids. *N Engl J Med* 1987; **317**(7): 403–8.
14. Ramirez RJ, Wolf SE, Herndon DN. Is there a role for growth hormone in the clinical management of burn injuries? *Growth Hormone IGF Res* 1998; **8**: 99–105.
15. Sakurai Y, Aarsland A, Herndon DN, et al. Stimulation of muscle protein synthesis by long-term insulin infusion in severely burned patients. *Ann Surg* 1995; **222**: 283–97.
16. Klein GL, Herndon DN, Goodman WG, et al. Histomorphometric and biochemical characterization of bone following acute severe burns in children. *Bone* 1995; **17**: 455–60.
17. Rutan RL, Herndon DN. Growth delay in post-burn pediatric patients. *Arch Surg* 1990; **125**: 392–5.
18. Klein GL, Herndon DN, Rutan TC, Sherrard DJ, Coburn JW, Langman CB. Bone disease in burn patients. *J Bone Miner Res* 1993; **8**: 337–45.
19. Klein GL, Herndon DN, Langman CB, Rutan TC, Young WE, Pembleton G. Long term reduction in bone mass following severe burn injury in children. *J Pediatr* 1995; **126**: 252–6.
20. Hart DW, Wolf SE, Mlcak R, et al. Persistence of muscle catabolism after severe burn. Presented at the *Society of University Surgeons* 2000, Toronto.
21. Hart DW, Wolf SE, Mlcak R, et al. Persistence of muscle catabolism after severe burn. *Surgery* 2000, (in press).
22. Hart DW, Wolf SE, Chinkes DL, et al. Determinants of catabolism after severe burn. Presented at the *Am Surg Assoc* 2000; Philadelphia.
23. Hart DW, Wolf SE, Chinkes DL, et al. Determinants of catabolism after severe burn. *Ann Surg* 2000, (in Press).
24. Ramirez RJ, Wolf SE, Barrow RE, Herndon DN. Growth hormone treatment in pediatric burns: A safe therapeutic approach. *Ann Surg* 1998; **228**(4): 439–48.
25. Gilpin DA, Barrow RE, Rutan RL, Broemeling L, Herndon DN. Recombinant human growth hormone accelerates wound healing in children with large cutaneous burns. *Ann Surg* 1994; **220**: 19–24.
26. Gore DC, Honeycutt D, Jahoor F, Wolfe RR, Herndon DN. Effect of exogenous growth hormone on whole-body and isolated-limb protein kinetics in burned patients. *Arch Surg* 1991; **126**: 38–43.
27. Jeffries MK, Vance ML. Growth hormone and cortisol secretion in patients with burn injury. *J Burn Care Rehabil* 1992; **13**(4): 391–5.
28. Herndon DN, Barrow RE, Kunkel KR, Broemeling L, Rutan RL. Effects of recombinant human growth hormone on donor-site healing in severely burned children. *Ann Surg* 1990; **212**(4): 424–31.
29. Low JFA, Herndon DN, Barrow RE. Effect of growth hormone on growth delay in burned children: a 3-year follow-up study. *Lancet* 1999; **354**: 1789.
30. Low JA. Growth hormone prevents delay in height development in burned children. Abstract of the 59th Ann Meeting of the Amer Assoc for the Surg of Trauma. 1999 Boston.
31. Low A, Jeschke M, Barrow R, Herndon D. Attenuating growth delay with growth hormone in severely burned children. Abstract of the Seventh Vienna Shock Forum 1999 Vienna.

32. Low JFA, Barrow RE, Mittendorfer B, Jeschke MG, Chinkes DL, Herndon DN. The effect of short-term growth hormone treatment on growth and energy expenditure in burned children. *Pediatrics* 2000; (pending).

33. Hart DW, Wolf SE, Ramzy PI, *et al.* Anabolic effects of oxandrolone following severe burn. Presented at the Society of Critical Care Medicine 2000, Orlando.

34. Hart DW, Wolf SE, Ramzy PI, *et al.* Anabolic effects of oxandrolone following severe burn. *Lancet* 2000; (pending).

35. Biolo G, Maggi SP, Williams BD, Tipton KD, Wolfe RR. Increased rates of muscle protein turnover and amino acid transport following resistance exercise in humans. *Am J Physiol (Endocrinol Metab)* 1995; **268**: E514–20.

36. Chesley A, MacDougall JD, Tarnopolsky MA, Atkinson SA, Smith K. Changes in human muscle protein synthesis after resistance exercise. *J Appl Physiol* 1992; **73**: 1383–8.

37. MacDougall JD, Gibala MJ, Tarnopolsky MA, MacDonald JR, Interisano SA, Yarasheski KE. The time course for elevated muscle protein synthesis following heavy resistance exercise. *Can J Appl Physiol* 1995; **20**: 480–6.

38. Blimkie CJR. Resistance training during preadolescence. *Sports Med* 1993; **15**(6): 389–407.

39. Blimkie CJR. Resistance training during pre-early puberty: efficacy, trainability, mechanisms, and persistence. *Can J Spt Sci* 1992; **17**(4): 264–79.

40. Ramsay JA, Blimkie CJR, Smith K, Garner S, MacDougall JD, Sale DG. Strength training effects in prepubescent boys. *Med Sci Sport Exerc* 1990; **22**: 605–14.

41. Ferrando AA, Tipton KD, Bamman MM, Wolfe RR. Resistance exercise maintains skeletal muscle protein synthesis during bed rest. *J Appl Physiol* 1997; **82**: 807–10.

42. Phillips SM, Tipton KD, Aarsland A, Wolf SE, Wolfe RR. Mixed muscle protein synthesis and breakdown following resistance exercise in humans. *Am J Physiol (Endocrinol Metab)* 1997.

43. Mlcak RP, Desai MH, Carp SS, *et al.* Increased physiological dead space/tidal volume ratio during exercise in burned children. *Proc Am Burn Assoc* 1991; **23**: 24.

44. Desai MH, Mlcak RP, Robinson G, *et al.* Does inhalation injury limit exercise endurance in children convalescing from thermal injury. *J Burn Care Rehabil* 1993; **14**: 16–20.

45. Mlcak RP, Desai MH, Robinson E, *et al.* Cardiopulmonary stress testing in children convalescing from thermal injury. *Proc Am Burn Assoc* 1991; **23**: 161.

46. Cucuzzo N, Herndon DN. The effects of aerobic exercise in the rehabilitation of severely burned children. *Proc Am Burn Assoc*, 2000; Las Vegas **21**: 203.

47. Cucuzzo N, Farmer S, Sesostris I, Herndon DN. Three repetition maximum strength testing in burned children.

48. Cucuzzo NA, Ferrando AA, Herndon DN. A comparison of a progressive resistance exercise program and traditional outpatient therapy for severely burned children. *Med Sci Sport Exerc* 2000 (submitted).

49. Jackson DM. Destructive burns some orthopedic complications. *Burns* 1981; **7**: 105–22.

50. Bhattachara V, Singh J, Sinha F, *et al.* Macroradiographic study of post-burn contracture of limbs. *Burns* 1984; **10**: 379–87.

51. Evans EB. Orthopedic measures in the treatment of severe burns. *J Bone Joint Surg (Am)* 1966; **48**: 643–9.

52. Klein GL, Herndon DN, Rutan TC, *et al.* Long-term reduction in bone mass and increased fracture risk in children following severe burns. *J Bone Miner Res*, S232: 1993.

53. McCauley RL, Fairleigh JF, Robson MC, Herndon DN. Effects of facial burns on facial growth in children: preliminary report. *Proc Am Burn Assoc* 1991; **23**: 137.

54. Klein GL, Herndon DN, Goodman WG, *et al.* Histomorphometric and biochemical characterization of bone following acute severe burns in children. *Bone* 1995; **17**: 455–60.

55. Klein G, Herndon DN, Langman CB, *et al.* Long-term reduction in bone mass following severe burn injury in children. *J Pediatr* 1995; **126**: 252–6.

56. Klein GL, Herndon DN, Rutan TC, *et al.* Bone disease in burn patients. *J Bone Mine Res* 1993; **8**: 337–45.

57. Klein GL, Wolf SE, Goodman WG, Phillips WA, Herndon DN. The management of acute bone loss in severe catabolism due to burn injury. *Hormone Res* 1997; **48**(Suppl. 5): 83–7.

58. Klein GL, Nusynowitz ML, Herndon DN. Reduction in bone mineral density following burn injury is due to fall in bone mineral content. Abstract of the Bone and Tooth Society, 2000.

59. Klein GL, Herndon DN. The role of bone densitometry in the diagnosis and management of the severely burned patient with bone loss. *J Clin Densitometry* 1998; **2**(1): 11–5.

60. Klein GL, Wolf SE, Langman CB, *et al.* Effect of therapy with recombinant human growth hormone on insulin-like growth factor system components and serum levels of biochemical markers of bone formation in children after severe burn injury. *J Clin Endocrinol Metab* 1998; **83**: 21–4.

61. Jones T, McDonald S, Deitch E. Effect of graft bed on long term functional results of extremity skin grafts. *J Burn Care Rehabil* 1988; **9**: 72–4.

62. Jackson DM. Destructive burns some orthopedic complications. *Burns* 1981; **7**: 105–22.

63. Heslop J. Heterotopic periarticular ossification in burns. *Burns* 1982; **8**: 436–8.

64. Schiele H. Radiographic changes in burns of the upper extremity. *Diagn Radiol* 1972; **104**: 13–7.

65. Larson DL, Abston S, Evans EB, Dobrkosky M, Linares HA. Techniques for decreasing scar formation and contractures in the burned patient. *J Trauma* 1971; **11**: 807–23.

66. Kloti J, Pochon JP. Long-term therapy of second and third degree burns in children using Jobst compression suits. *Scand J Plast Recon Surg* 1979; **13**: 163–8.

67. Robertson JC, Drett JE, Hodgson B, Druett J. Pressure therapy for hypertrophic scarring: preliminary communication. *J R Soc Med* 1980; **73**: 348–54.

68. Ward R. Pressure therapy for the control of hypertrophic scar formation after burn injury a history and review. *J Burn Care Rehabil* 1991; **12**: 257–62.

69. Chang P, Laubenthal KN, Lewis RW II, Rosenquist MD, Lindley-Smith P, Kealey GP. Prospective randomized study of the efficacy of pressure garment therapy in patients with burns. *J Burn Care Rehabil* 1995; **16**: 473–5.

70. Groce A, McCauley R, Herndon DN, Serghiou M, Chinkes D. The effects of high pressure vs. low pressure garments in the control of hypertrophic scarring in the burned child: a preliminary 6-month report. *J Burn Care Rehabil* 2000: (submitted).

71. Moore M, Engrav LJ, Calderon J, *et al.* Effectiveness of custom pressure garments in wound management: A prospective trial within wounds and with verified pressure. Abstract of the Am Burn Assoc Annual Meeting, 2000; Las Vegas.

72. Groce A, Herndon DN, McCauley R, Serghiou M, Chinkes D. The effects of pressure garments vs. no pressure for the control of hypertrophic scarring in children with small burns: A preliminary 6-month report. *J Burn Care Rehabil* 2000 (submitted).

73. Groce A, Meyers-Paal R, Herndon DN, McCauley RL. Are your thoughts of facial pressure transparent? *J Burn Care Rehabil* 1999; **20**: 478–81.

74. Brou JA, Robson MC, McCauley RL, *et al.* Inventory of potential reconstructive needs in the patient with burns. *J Burn Care Rehabil* 1989; **10**: 550–60.

75. Robert RS, Blakeney PE, Meyer WJ III. Impact of disfiguring burn scars on adolescent sexual development. *J Burn Care Rehabil* 1998; **19**: 430–5.

76. McCauley RL, Beraja V, Rutan RL *et al.* Longitudinal assessment of breast development in adolescent female patients with burns involving the nipple areola complex. *Plast Recon Surg* 1989; **83**: 676–80.

77. McCauley RL, Stenberg BA, Phillips LG, Blackwell SJ, Robson MC. Long-term assessment of the effects of circumferential truncal burns in pediatric patients on subsequent pregnancies. *J Burn Care Rehabil* 1991; **12**: 51–3.

Chapter 48

Overview of burn reconstruction
Martin C Robson

Introduction

'Beauty is only skin deep.' The very denial in this statement emphasizes the importance of appearance in society today.[1] Body image is a basic part of personal identity. It incorporates physical characteristics with an individual's attitude toward these characteristics. It emanates from both conscious and subconscious sources.[2] These sources are established by perceived standards of how people look and what is normal. Thus, the final outcome is determined separately by a patient and by society as a whole.[2] In the integumentary system involved in burn injury, even though the processes of wound healing have apparently progressed normally, proliferative scar formation may result. This can occur even though a physician understands normal wound healing and performs all therapeutic maneuvers correctly. Still, too much collagen is laid down with the end result of proliferative scar formation.

Wound healing

What causes normal wound contraction to result in contracture and hypertrophic scars so frequently seen after burns? It appears that the normal wound healing process begins and seems to continue. It does not shut off, so normal wound contraction becomes contracture and ends with a hypertrophic scar. It is important to remember that contraction is a normal part of the physiology of wound healing; therefore, it is neither possible nor desirous to prevent wound contraction.[3] On the other hand, one may be able to prevent the abnormal continuation of wound contraction which leads to a contracture and deformity. One way to reduce contracture and hypertrophic scar formation is to minimize the time in which normal wound contraction takes place. We can reduce the amount and the intensity of the inflammation. In the burn wound, we can excise and close the wound very early so as to decrease the inflammatory phase.[3] It is desirable to reduce this time because it has been demonstrated that hypertrophic scars are related to the amount of time a wound is allowed to remain in the inflammatory phase before it moves into the proliferative phase.[4] Recent data suggest that excess inflammation increases the amount of the fibrogenic cytokines transforming growth factor (TGF)-β1 and TGF-β2 and decreases normal fibroblast apoptosis.[5–7] The inflammatory phase should be reduced not only in wounds healing by secondary or tertiary intention but also in those healing by primary intention. This emphasizes the need for successful skin graft 'take' at the time of initial excision and grafting during the acute care of the burn wound.[3] Another technique for decreasing hypertrophic scar is to minimize or eliminate a deficiency of tissue. In closing burn wounds initially, it is important to make sure that an adequate amount of tissue is placed. Whenever possible, this means using sheet grafts instead of meshed grafts or postage stamp grafts.[3] Despite aggressive and improved acute care, healing of burns too frequently leaves residual deformities. Wound contraction, a normal and necessary part of healing, promotes distortions which produce visual disfigurement and functional limitation. A wound continues to contract until it achieves a comfortable position or an equal opposing force.[8]

Reconstruction

All members of a burn team should participate in the overall reconstruction planning; otherwise, reconstruction degenerates into a goal.[2,9] Psychological support, splinting, exercises, and pressure garments all affect the surgical result. A patient must also be included in this planning and understand the surgical objectives.[10] Dreams of miracles too often overshadow realistic goals and expectations. Along with other members of a burn team, a physician encourages a patient through the difficult acute period. This can lead to a false optimism on patients' part because they assume that once this initial period is conquered, everything will return to 'normal'. Even the most honest physician implicitly encourages a patient through this period while privately thinking that the final result will be far from satisfactory. Thus, a patient often will wonder, 'When does the plastic surgery begin?'[11] Preoperative discussion minimizes postsurgical depression by improving patient acceptance. This ultimately helps integrate a patient back into society.

Timing of Reconstruction

If possible, reconstruction is postponed until wounds have matured.[3] Frequently, postponement is not possible if the deformity is progressive or causing a functional deficit. In these cases, reconstruction is initiated early. An example of this might be a severe ectropion of the eyelid. This early reconstruction is usually undertaken to correct significant tissue deficiency. In planning, appreciation of this deficiency is important. In fact, the diagnosis of a true tissue deficiency may be the most important step in reconstruction.[2] The surgical plan involves recreating the initial tissue loss and then adding appropriate tissue.

Priorities for reconstruction

Reconstruction proceeds stepwise, with priorities given to certain anatomical areas. The first priority must always remain the prevention of deformity.[2,3] Obviously, this receives great emphasis in acute therapy, but the importance of postoperative splinting or pressure garments must be remembered after each reconstructive procedure.[4] Lack of attention to these details jeopardizes optimal functional and aesthetic results. The next priority is reconstruction of active function.[2,3] The final priority is restoration of passive function.

Although functional reconstruction is afforded the first operative priority, resurfacing procedures of lesser priority may be combined with these functional reconstructions.[2,3] What should be reconstructed becomes clear when one considers a patient as a whole.[12] Confusion occurs when an inexperienced surgeon views a contracture amenable to flap reconstruction as an isolated event unrelated to age, lifestyle, occupation, and physical demands.[3] The complications of a major burn often require multiple procedures and can take several years to reconstruct. A surgeon should document every deformity with possible surgical alternatives and then assign priorities. Brou *et al.* designed a very useful inventory (illustrated in Chapter 47) for potential reconstructive needs to allow a more systematic evaluation guided by body regions, divided into anatomical units.[13] All the somatic abnormalities caused by burns are included, as well as a system for grading severity of the defect. Additionally, a donor tissue surveillance form has been reported to further coordinate a systematic method of management.[14] A priority rating for the use of the available tissue ranges from function salvage, through improvement of function, to cosmetic. Restoring function, obviously, is a higher priority than improving cosmetic appearance; however, cosmetic reconstruction will also help patients improve their activities of daily living, improve function, or return to a job.

After the reconstructive needs are prioritized according to anatomical body region and functional severity in order to compile a priority list of reconstructive needs, the list is matched with the available donor tissue sites and a preliminary operative strategy is formulated.[14] Then a patient, parent, surgeon priority survey is consulted to match desires with feasibilities.[10] Once the priorities of reconstruction have been determined, multiple diverse techniques are available. Simplicity is often a virtue.[3]

Closures

Whenever possible, closure of wounds by direct approximation and primary healing is desirable, whether dealing with a primary injury or a reconstructive procedure. Often, however, defects exist which cannot be directly sutured. In such situations, grafts or flaps are required. Traditionally, closure by grafts is considered first; then the possibilities of local flaps and distant flaps are evaluated, choosing the simplest method which will produce the desired result. In burn reconstruction, the z-plasty, which is in reality two random flaps, often is considered before a skin graft.[3] With better understanding of the blood supply to the skin through axial, musculocutaneous, and fasciocutaneous vessels, flaps and free tissue transfer using microvascular anastomoses have assumed a more prominent place in the hierarchy of techniques. Skin expansion techniques have also proven their utility. It is clear that direct closure, grafts, flaps, free tissue transfer, and tissue expansion comprise the armamentarium of the reconstructive burn surgeon; each must be understood to be properly utilized.

Direct closure

Direct closure in burn reconstruction is the simplest form of scar revision following excision of the scar.[3] Scar formation is the fundamental phenomenon of wound healing in most human tissues, including the dermis. An understanding of normal wound healing and insight into the factors which make a scar less than optimal are both essential to planning scar revisions.[3] All scars proceed through the inflammatory, proliferative, and maturation phases of wound healing, and will therefore require time to reach their final appearance. A normal scar which appears hypertrophic at 6 weeks may be quite satisfactory after 6–12 months. If the mature scar is not satisfactory, application of the basic principles of reconstruction can then be expected to result in an improved scar.

The most common mechanical reasons for unacceptable scars are an unfavorable direction of the original wound in regard to the normal lines of skin tension, failure of proper dermal approximation, and a pathologic extension of normal wound contraction which results in a contracture.[3,15] Molecularly, there appears to be an overexpression or dysregulated function of inflammatory cytokines, particularly the isoforms of TGFβ.[5,6] If the excessive scarring was due to an improper direction of the original wound, the wound direction should be realigned so that the new scar will fall in the lines of minimum resting tension.[3] These lines, in general, will run perpendicular to the fibers of the underlying muscle. Realigning a scar to the minimum resting skin tension lines will often allow it to become almost invisible. When a wound is reapproximated, the dermis is carefully approximated with an inverted suture. This supports the tissues until the tensile strength of the new collagen is sufficient to prevent spreading of the scar. Although a degree of wound contraction is a normal part of wound healing, contracture is preventable. Placing the direction along the lines of minimum resting tension will greatly help.

The z-plasty technique

The line of contracture can be lengthened either by excising the old scar as an ellipse, thus elongating each side of the wound slightly, or by adding tissue by introducing a z-plasty, skin graft, or a flap. This is a technique by which two triangular skin flaps are interchanged in position to gain length along a scar or skin fold at the expense of the adjacent tissues.[3] It is used in burn reconstruction so frequently that it almost can be viewed as a extension of the direct closure technique. Understanding the geometry and principles of the z-plasty allows reconstructive surgeons to lengthen a contracted scar, obliterate a web contracture, add to an area of deficient tissue and change the direction of the scar, thus giving them an important technique of scar revision.[16] The incisions are designed with three lines of equal length: a central member, and two limbs extending from its ends to resemble the letter Z or its mirror image (**Figure 48.1**). The angles formed by the limbs with the central member can vary depending on the desired final result; angles of 60° can be shown mathematically to give the maximum practical increase in length. When the flaps are mobilized and

transposed, the flap bases lie along the line formerly occupied by the central member, resulting in a gain in length. This gain in length is approximately 25% for 30° angles, 50% for 45° angles and 75% for 60° angles.

Skin Grafting

When reconstructive needs are such that excision and direct closure are insufficient, skin grafting is the next most common technique.[3] When a scar contracture is incised or excised, the wound edges will retract widely and the tissue deficiency will become apparent. A split-thickness or full-thickness skin graft will replace the deficiency and improve the scar. Skin grafts are also useful for scar revision in areas where previous scars or skin grafts are of poor quality or have a poor color match.[3] Following excision, a carefully tailored full-thickness skin graft will improve quality and color match. Skin grafts remain the mainstay of burn reconstruction. These grafts may be of the split-thickness, full-thickness, or composite variety depending on the specific needs of a patient. A split-thickness or partial-thickness skin graft includes epidermis and part of the dermis. A full-thickness skin graft includes epidermis and full thickness of the dermis. A composite graft, although not strictly a skin graft, includes the full thickness of the skin and a portion of the underlying tissue such as subcutaneous tissue, muscle, cartilage, or bone.[15]

Split-thickness skin grafts

These can vary in thickness depending on the amount of dermis included. Thin split-thickness grafts contain little dermis and are cut only to the level of the subpapillary vascular plexus. Medium split-thickness grafts contain most of the dermis, approximately three-quarters thickness. The thickness of the graft is relative, depending on the age and sex of a patient and the region of the body of the donor site.[15] Clinically, the translucency of the graft and the pattern of bleeding from the donor site help determine the thickness. The thicker the graft, the more opaque it becomes. A thinner translucent graft will come from a bed with many closely spaced, fine, bleeding points of the subpapillary plexus.[15] For thicker grafts a deeper layer is cut, leaving a bed with fewer larger vessels from the dermal plexus. Split-thickness skin grafts are best used to cover large denuded surfaces occurring after contracture release or excision of unacceptable burn scar (**Figure 48.2**). They are also used when recurrent wound contraction is of lesser consequence. A great advantage of these grafts is that their donor sites heal themselves from the remaining skin appendages, such as hair follicles and sweat glands.[15] This allows harvesting of the grafts of almost any size needed to close a defect. They can also be harvested from previously healed partial-thickness burn wounds or donor sites.

The thickness of a graft is a matter of preference of the surgeon, but several guidelines are helpful. The thinner the graft, the higher is the chance of survival on the recipient site. Thinner grafts have fewer cells to be nourished prior to establishment of the blood supply. Also, since the undersurface of the graft has a higher density of vessels, vascular ingrowth can proceed more rapidly. Further, the donor site of a thin split-thickness graft will epithelialize more rapidly. Thin grafts have disadvantages which must be considered by the reconstructive surgeon. The thinner the graft, the more the interface of the fibrous tissue between the graft and the recipient site will contract during the maturation phase. Therefore,

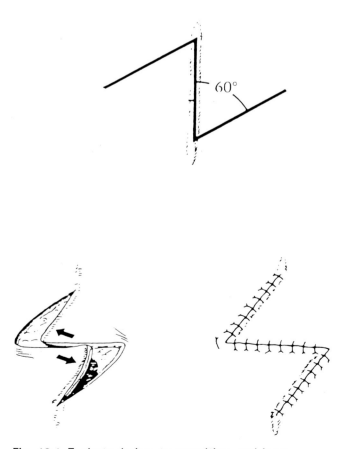

Fig. 48.1 Z-plasty design, transposition, and inset.

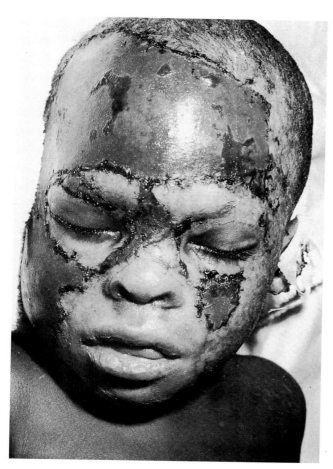

Fig. 48.2 Split-thickness graft to resurface areas of unacceptable scar.

the wound beneath a thicker split-thickness graft will contract minimally, if at all. Thicker grafts will more closely resemble their donor site in color, texture, and hair distribution.

Full-thickness skin grafts

These tend to resemble normal skin better than split-thickness grafts. They provide more padding, a better color match, a more nearly normal hair pattern, and inhibit wound contraction in the recipient site. Because they require near ideal conditions for survival, they must be placed in a vascular recipient site. Their thickness requires more nourishment prior to the establishment of vascular integrity. The major disadvantage of full-thickness grafts is that their donor sites cannot heal spontaneously since no skin appendages are left behind. Therefore, the size of the graft is limited to dimensions which will allow primary closure of the donor site. If this practice is not followed, the donor site from a large full-thickness graft must be closed by a split-thickness graft.[15] Only rarely is this approach used for burn reconstruction, since donor sites are often limited in a burn patient.

Composite graft

Occasionally, a defect requires underlying supportive tissue as well as skin. Most frequently this is reconstructed with a flap, which will be discussed later. If the area is small enough, a skin graft containing underlying tissue (a composite graft) can be used. The risk of nonvascularization of this type of graft severely limits its usefulness. If no portion of the graft is more than 0.5 cm from the wound edge, the survival rate is good.[15] The blood supply to a composite graft comes through its margin instead of its base, which accounts for the strict size limitation. Despite these limitations, the composite graft may be the first choice in reconstruction of areas of the face such as the nasal alae.

Choice of donor site

When skin grafts of any variety are chosen for reconstruction, choosing a donor site requires some thought. The color, texture, vascularity, thickness, and hair-bearing nature to the skin varies from one area of the body to another.[3] The nearer the donor site is to the recipient site, the more closely the skin will match. Skin grafts to the face taken from above the clavicle tend to retain their natural blush state, whereas those from below the clavicle tend to take on a yellowish or brownish hue.[3,15] The donor site of a split-thickness skin graft is like a partial-thickness burn or deep abrasion. It must be protected from trauma and bacteria in order to epithelialize satisfactorily.

Postoperative care

Finally, postoperative care of a skin graft is as important as the grafting operative technique. The graft should be inspected by 48–72 hours after placement, using an aseptic technique. Any fluid found beneath the graft should be aspirated or evacuated by making a small nick in the graft to express it.[15] If fluid is not removed by 96 hours, evidence has been presented that the graft epithelializes on the undersurface, preventing satisfactory vascularization.[17] The graft must be immobilized and protected for at least 5–7 days. Edema should be prevented in the recipient bed for 4–6 months. This becomes of great practical importance in grafts applied to the lower extremity. In this situation, support such as an elastic stocking is required to overcome the hydrostatic pressure until the collagen of the graft is totally incorporated into the extremity.

Reconstruction Using Flaps

Burn deformities and defects are best corrected by excision, primary approximation, or z-plasty whenever possible. Skin grafting is usually thought of as a second choice. Cases do exist, however, where skin grafting is either not possible or not desirable. The area in need of reconstruction, such as bare bone or tendon, may lack the vascularity necessary to support a skin graft. Tissue to reconstruct these defects must carry its own blood supply. When two surfaces must be reconstructed, an inherent blood supply is obviously necessary.[3] An example of this is the full-thickness loss of an eyelid or lip. There are also situations where a skin graft could theoretically close a defect but would not serve the final purpose as well as vascularized composite tissue.[3] This occurs when deeper tissue is desired for contouring but the defect is too large for a composite graft or when padding is required over a bony prominence. Occasionally a skin graft can correct a deformity or close a defect but is not the most desirable type of reconstruction. If future surgery will be necessary beneath a reconstructed area, if near-normal sensation is required of a reconstructed tissue, or if a hoped-for esthetic result cannot be achieved by a skin graft, then a skin graft is not the best choice. In all of these circumstances, reconstruction can be better effected by a flap.

A skin flap by definition is a segment of skin and subcutaneous tissue which is transferred from its original position on the body to another site while maintaining its own inherent vasculature for nourishment.[15] In some cases of burn reconstruction, deeper tissue such as muscle or bone is carried with the skin flap. All flaps have a 'pedicle', which is their vascular base of attachment.

In order to understand skin flaps, a thorough knowledge of their blood supply is necessary. There are two main anatomical patterns of blood supply to the skin. The first of these depends upon vessels from the aorta or its major branches which lie deep to the muscles.[15] Perforating branches through the muscles along fascial planes become the musculocutaneous and fasciocutaneous arteries and terminate by supplying the dermal–subdermal plexus of the skin. This vascular pattern forms the predominant blood supply to the skin. In the other anatomical pattern, vessels from the aorta or its major branches form direct cutaneous arteries which lie superficial to the muscles and parallel to the skin for long distances and supply the dermal–subdermal plexus directly.[15]

Cutaneous or random pattern flap

This is a flap based on a blood supply from musculocutaneous arteries penetrating perpendicularly into its base, supplying the length of the flap through the longitudinal dermal–subdermal plexus[15] (**Figure 48.3**). The surviving length of this flap is limited by the perfusion pressure in the vessels. Since these flaps lack an anatomically recognized arteriovenous system, they have strict length limitations. The length cannot survive beyond the blood supply of the dermal–subdermal anastomotic plexus perfused by the perforating musculocutaneous arteries without special conditioning of the flap.[15]

Cutaneous pattern flaps can be subclassified as local flaps or flaps from a distance. The z-plasty and its modifications are literally two or more interpolated cutaneous flaps; however, beyond the z-plasty, they have lost their great utility for burn reconstruction except for the face. Local flaps in the face are still excellent if there is an adjacent unscarred area to serve as donor tissue. Although great amounts of tissue were once moved from far distant sites on the body by the ingenious use of tubed pedicles and delay procedures, those methods have been supplanted by free flaps and skin expansion.

Axial or arterial pattern flap

This receives its blood supply from a direct cutaneous artery which enters its base and runs longitudinally within the flaps[15] (**Figure 48.3**). The length of the flap is determined by the length of the direct cutaneous artery supplying it, plus an additional random portion at the termination of the artery supplied by the dermal–subdermal plexus. Since axial or arterial pattern flaps are supplied by a specific longitudinal arteriovenous network, traditional length: base width ratios play no role in the designing of the flap. In fact, no skin is necessary at the base of these flaps, and the artery and vein alone can serve as the base of pedicle.[15] This type of axial flap is called an island flap. Often, the nerve is preserved with the vessels in the pedicle, making it a neurovascular island flap.

Axial flaps can be very useful in reconstructive surgery for burns. The key to their use is an exact knowledge of the anatomy of the direct cutaneous arteries. Since the skin is unimportant in the flap's base, the pivot point becomes the artery itself and the arc of the flap can be 360° within the reach of the artery.[15] This type of

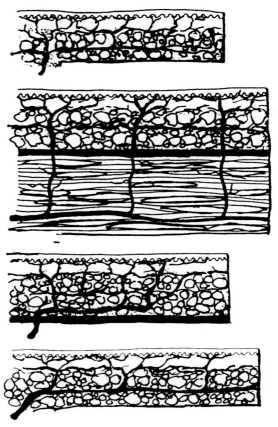

Fig. 48.3 A random flap (top) has a muscular perforator artery, cut from the underlying muscle. If the muscle is included (second from top), the flap is musculocutaneous and brings its own blood supply. The length of an arterial flap (bottom two figures) is dictated by the length of the artery.

flap is particularly useful for reconstruction of facial parts such as the ears and eyebrows, and for the upper extremity. The radial forearm flap is a classic example of the island neurovascular island pedicle flap that has proven very useful for reconstruction of the upper extremity.

Musculocutaneous or myocutaneous flap

If a muscle is adequately supplied with blood flow through a single dominant vascular pedicle, the muscle with its overlying skin and subcutaneous tissue can be raised as a flap and transferred as a unit on the segmental vascular pedicle[15] (**Figure 48.3**). In this case, a large area of skin can be transferred on multiple muscle perforators which are fed by the pedicle without the limitations imposed on cutaneous or random flaps. Likewise, a fasciocutaneous flap may be raised by including the vascularized fascia in the same way. This type of flap can be quite helpful to reconstruct patients with massive burns where most of the body surface consists of healed skin grafts over fascially excised muscles. Raising the muscle as the blood supply to the previously applied skin graft obviates the lack of cutaneous or axial vessels in the skin.

Free flap

Any of the types of flaps can be transferred by dividing its vascular pedicle and reanastomosing it in a recipient site.[15] When this technique is used, the flap is classified as a free flap. A free flap is not considered a graft since vascularization and nourishment is immediately reestablished through the pedicle. It is feasible to anastomose arteries and veins of less than 1 mm diameter.[3,18]

Microsurgical technique, understanding of flap physiology, and the definition of skin territories have rapidly improved over the past 20 years. This has allowed the almost routine successful free transfer of composite tissue from distant areas.[3] Free flaps have great utility in cases involving a burned patient in which local tissue is not available because it is included in the area of injury. In addition, although most acute wound closures and late reconstructions can be effected by split-thickness skin grafts, there are occasionally cases in need of reconstruction in which the underlying bed following contracture release will not support a graft or which would benefit from subcutaneous padding so as to achieve a more esthetic result.[18] Similarly, subcutaneous tissue is desirable if future tendon or bone reconstruction will be necessary beneath the reconstructed integument.[3] The methodology is being applied more frequently to severely burned patients and especially in cases of electrical injury. When used judiciously, it helps to solve many of the problems which previously resulted in limb amputation. As free flaps are used more frequently in the acute postburn period, reconstruction will be affected at the time of the initial operation.

Expanded skin

Expansion of skin can now be performed to yield tissue for reconstruction. Expanded tissue can be considered another type of flap. Based on the observations that tissue expands in biological conditions of pregnancy, obesity, and pathologic conditions such as tissue overlying neoplasms, Neumann used a subcutaneous balloon to artificially expand an area of the skin to reconstruct an ear.[19] After more frequent reports of tissue expansion, animal experiments by Cherry and his associates reviewed the biology of the phenomenon.[20] It appears that gradual stretching of the skin can usually occur with minimal risk of cell necrosis and dermal rupture. Epidermal cells appear to be essentially unaltered, and the thickness of the epidermis remains unchanged. The dermis thins, and there is an increase in the number of fibroblasts and myofibroblasts. There is marked thinning of the subcutaneous tissue and atrophy of muscle both above and below the expander. None of these changes would seem to be detrimental in using expanded skin for reconstruction.[3,18]

In a situation of insufficient unburned skin, any chance of damaging the skin to be used for reconstruction must be viewed from a perspective of proper risk: benefit ratio.[18] Despite this worry, there are areas in which burn scars cannot be adequately reconstructed with conventional means.[3] These include areas of alopecia on the scalp and the male face, where expanded hair-bearing adjacent skin would seem ideal. Other burn deformities of the head and neck call for reconstruction with skin of similar color, tone, texture, thickness, and composition.[3] In these cases, results with tissue expansion are frequently far superior to those possible with available alternative techniques.[3,18,21] Once the methods available for burn reconstruction are understood and technically mastered, they can be applied to all parts of the body as needed; however, the principles remain the same: perform a careful evaluation and inventory of deformities, prepare a detailed prioritized plan, and proceed using the principles enumerated here.

Postoperative Principles for Reconstruction

Regardless of what type of operative reconstruction is required on what specific anatomical body part, there are some postoperative principles. Pressure is an effective adjunct in the control of scar maturation. Kischer has shown that in hypertrophic scars treated with pressure, the collagen nodules common in untreated hypertrophic scars disappear and the collagen bundles become oriented parallel to the skin.[22] Pressure garments customized to an individual should be applied as soon as possible after wound healing is completed so as to prevent further shortening of the collagen. Measurements should be taken before healing is complete, as it takes time to receive custom-made garments. The pressure gradient garments may last 1–3 months, depending on activity and weight change; however, they should be replaced before they are completely worn out and lose their effectiveness. Pressure is continued from 6 to 24 months or until it is clinically apparent that the scars have matured and redevelopment of deformity is unlikely. In addition to the pressure garments, the use of flexible elastomer in such concave areas as the axilla, clavicle, neck, hand, and inferior chest has been extremely helpful in producing smooth, nonerythematous healed wounds.[12] The silicone is spread directly on the body part and covered with a compression garment. This technique is also very useful if tried early on fresh scars. Increased skin pliability and range of motion have been noted with its use.

Reconstruction of a burned patient can restore more function, as well as result in a subjective and objective sense of greater worth for the patient. It is well known that there may be little correlation between the severity of the physical defect estimated by the physician and the functional limitation perceived by a patient. This is equally true of aesthetic appearance. Because of this, many patients become depressed and ultimately resort to social isolation. Therefore, it is no longer enough to be technically able to perform the reconstructive procedures described or have the judgement to choose the appropriate type and timing of the reconstruction. A surgeon must also be a sympathetic physician who not only reconstructs a patient anatomically and functionally, but also considers the cosmetic or esthetic result and how it will aid the patient in total rehabilitation.[2]

Summary

Postburn reconstruction is complicated by the frequent occurrence of multiple reconstructive needs in a single patient. This chapter presents a simple, comprehensive approach to burn scar reconstruction. The primary aim of the surgeon is to prevent burn scar deformity by rapid wound closure, correction of tissue deficiencies, and assiduous attention to postoperative splinting and compression therapy. The initial step in managing secondary deformities is to identify and prioritize reconstructive needs. Reconstruction is then performed in a stepwise fashion aiming to restore active function first, followed by passive function, and finally addressing esthetic reconstruction. Reconstructive techniques are applied in a hierarchy from simplest to most complex (**Figure 48.4**). Primary excision and closure of scars by reorienting the scar to the lines of relaxed skin tension can significantly

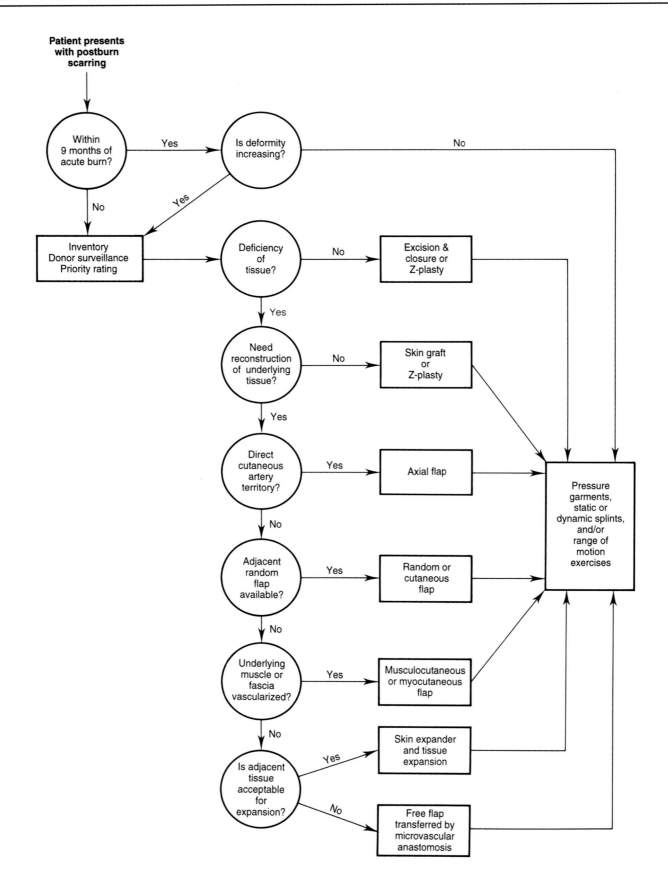

Fig. 48.4 Algorithm outlining series of decisions required on patient presenting with postburn scarring.

improve appearance. The use of z-plasty, flap repair, and tissue expansion are also reviewed. Skin expansion, in particular, has become the standard management of postburn alopecia and, although associated with a relatively high complication rate, has significantly improved the aesthetic appearance of patients. The reconstruction of a burned patient is often a long process which requires multiple procedures. The approach presented here advocates a stepwise, prioritized approach aiming at both maximum function as well as optimal appearance.

References

1. Bernstein NR. *Emotional Care of the Facially Burned and Disfigured*. Boston: Little, Brown, 1976.
2. Robson MC, Smith DJ. Reconstruction of the burned face, neck and scalp. In: Boswick JA, ed. *The Art and Science of Burn Care*. Rockville: Aspen Publishers, 1987.
3. Robson MC, Barnett RA, Leitch IOW, Hayward PG. Prevention and treatment of postburn scars and contracture. *World J Surg* 1992; **16**: 87–96.
4. Robson MC. Disturbances of wound healing. *Ann Emerg Med* 1988; **17**: 1274–8.
5. O'Kane S, Ferguson MWJ. Transforming growth factor-βs and wound healing. *Int J Biochem Cell Biol* 1997; **29**: 63–78.
6. Polo M, Smith PD, Kim Y-J, *et al.* Effect of TGF$_{\beta2}$ on proliferative scar fibroblast cell kinetics. *Ann Plast Surg* 1999; **43**: 185–90.
7. Wassermann RJ, Polo M, Smith P, *et al.* Differential production of apoptosis-modulating proteins in patients with hypertrophic burn scar. *J Surg Res* 1998; **75**: 74–80.
8. Larson DL, Abston S, Evans EB, *et al.* Techniques for decreasing scar formation and contractures in the burn patient. *J Trauma* 1971; **11**: 807–23.
9. Bernstein NR, Robson MC. *Comprehensive Approaches to the Burned Person*. New Hyde Park, NY: Medical Examination Publishing, 1983.
10. Bjaranson D, Phillips LG, McCoy B, *et al.* Reconstruction goals in burn children: are our goals the same? *J Burn Care Rehabil* 1992; **13**: 389–90.
11. Constable JD. The limitations of esthetic reconstruction. In: Bernstein NR, Robson, MC, eds. *Comprehensive Approaches to the Burned Person*. New Hyde Park, NY: Medical Examination Publishing, 1983.
12. Salisbury RE, Petro JA, Winski, FV. Reconstruction of the burn patient. In: Boswick, JA, ed. The Art and Science of Burn Care, Rockville: Aspen, 1987.
13. Brou J, Robson MC, McCauley RL, *et al.* Inventory of potential reconstructive needs in the patient with burns. *J Burn Care Rehabil.* 1989; **10**: 555–60.
14. Burns BF, McCauley RL, Murphy FL, *et al.* Reconstructive management of patients with greater than 80 percent TBSA burns. *Burns* 1993; **19**: 429–33.
15. Robson MC, Parsons RW. Reconstructive and plastic surgery. In: Cushieri A, Giles GR, Moosa AR, eds. Essential Surgical Practice. Bristol, England: John Wright and Sons, Ltd, 1982: Chapter 22.
16. Koss N. The mathematics of flap design. In: Krizek TJ, Hoopes JE, eds. Symposium on Basic Science in Plastic Surgery. St Louis: CV Mosby, 1976: 274.
17. Littlewood, AHM. Seroma: an unrecognized cause of failure of split-thickness skin grafts. *Br J Plast Surg* 1960; **13**: 42–6.
18. Robson MC, Smith DJ, Heggers JP. Innovations in burn wound management. In: Habal MB, Morain WD, Lewin ML, Parson RW, Woods JE, eds. Advances in Plastic Surgery. Chicago: Yearbook Medical, 1987: 149.
19. Neumann CG. The expansion of an area of skin by progressive distention of a subcutaneous balloon. *Plast Reconstr Surg* 1957; **19**: 124–30.
20. Cherry GW, Austad E, Pasyk K, *et al.* Increased survival and vascularity of random pattern skin flaps elevated in controlled, expanded skin. *Plast Reconstr Surg* 1983; **72**: 680–5.
21. Gottlieb LJ, Parsons RW, Krizek TJ. The use of tissue expansion techniques in burn reconstruction. *J Burn Care Rehabil* 1986; **7**: 234–7.
22. Kischer CS. Collagen and mucopolysaccharides in the hypertrophic scar. *Connect Tissue Res* 1974; **2**: 205–13.

Chapter 49 Reconstruction of the burned hand

Joseph M Mlakar
William R Dougherty

Little solace can be garnered from survival if due diligence were not given to the importance of rehabilitation of the patient as a fully functional person.

Luce[1]

Introduction

Although the hand accounts for only 3% of the total body surface area (TBSA),[2,3] it is involved in more than 70% of treated burn injuries.[4] The hand is commonly burned as an isolated injury, and is rarely spared in burns greater than 60% TBSA.[5,6] Burns of the hand may account for up to 8% of emergency room visits for hand injuries[7] and are often an indication for referral to a regional burn center.[8]

Typically, hand burns are an injury of the working class.[9] Most hand burn injuries occur to employed males.[10,11] Injuries that occur on the work site are more likely to be flame burns or electrical burns.[12] Injuries that occur at home are more likely to be a scald, explosions or open flames.[12] However, contact burns to the hand intend to involve more small children.[13,14]

In a review of their experience with 1705 burn injuries over 10 years, Tredget et al.[15,16] reported an incidence of 54% with hand and upper extremity injuries. Hand burn patients were 80% male. One-third were children. Half of the patients were employed at the time of injury, and one-third of injuries occurred at work. Mean burn size was approximately 15% TBSA. Three-quarters of all hand and extremity burn injuries occurred with less than 20% TBSA burned. Flame burns accounted for 60% of injuries, scald burns for 19%, and electrical burns for 7%. Other hand burns accounted for the remaining 14%, and included burns from tar, grease, steam, friction and chemicals. Tredget stressed that burn injuries are a frequent form of upper extremity trauma.

Unlike the foot, which may still function as a cold, stiff lifeless stump, the function of the hand depends upon stability, sensibility, mobility, dexterity, and controllable power. This requires stable skin coverage, an adaptable skeletal framework, and gliding balance of multiple tendon/muscular forces. The function of an individual is very dependent on the use of their hands. Our hands are organs of *both* function and beauty, interacting with our environment and with others. As an organ of social interaction, the hand needs to look and feel normal to others to prevent social embarrassment. One of the most difficult social barriers for burn patients is shaking hands in greeting other people, especially if the hand has partial amputation or loss. Because of hand deformity, many burn patients spend years with their hands in their pockets attempting to hide their deformity.[17]

The hand is a delicate balance of light touch and power grip, sensitivity versus strength. Loss of hand function negatively impacts on occupation, activities of living, and self-worth.[18,19] Loss of hand use results in impairment rating of 95% for the involved extremity, and 57% loss of the function of the whole person.[20,21] Thumb loss accounts for approximately 50% of the function of the whole hand.[21] Our opposable thumb helps differentiate us (humans) from other primates.

Much has been written on the management of the burned hand and its subsequent reconstruction.[22-28] In fact, in the last 34 years, over 500 articles related to hand burn injuries have been written in the English language alone. Many are case reports or small series. A few are large retrospective reviews of outcomes with a given protocol. Prospective randomized trials are rare. Among those reporting the best outcomes, common treatment priorities include: optimize function early, minimize deformity, and prevent disability.[28]

Sheridan et al.[29,30] examined their recent 10-year experience in managing 1645 burned hands (495 children and 659 adults). Many of the patients had bilateral injuries. Their approach to the burned hand emphasizes: (1) ranging and splinting through hospitalization; (2) prompt sheet autograft wound closure as soon as practical; and (3) the selective use of axial pin fixation and flaps. Using this approach, hand function was subsequently judged to be normal in 97% of partial-thickness (second degree) burns in both adults and children, and 81–85% of deep partial-thickness burns or full-thickness (third degree) injuries requiring grafting.[29,30]

In contrast, the patients with so-called 'fourth degree' hand burns – those involving underlying extensor tendons, joint capsules or bone – faired much worse in their functional recovery.[29,30] Only 20% of children and 8% of adults achieve normal function

following fourth degree burns. However, 70% of these same children, and 90% of these adults, were able to independently perform activities of daily living (**Figure 49.1**). In this series, 65% of children with fourth degree burns required secondary late postburn reconstruction, compared to 32% of third degree burns, and 4.4% of second degree burns. Together, these reviews comprise the largest series of hand burn patients reported in the English literature, and are the current benchmark for comparisons of other treatment strategies.

Decision-making with acute injuries

The best means to return function to a burned hand is to prevent the need for reconstruction and rehabilitation.[11] The first surgeon addressing the needs of the burn-injured patient has the best opportunity to correct subsequent problems and deformity.[31]

Acute hand treatment principles are similar to that for other injuries. First and foremost, do no harm. In the treatment of the burned hand, that means specifically preventing desiccation of the burn wounds. Desiccation destroys tissue and increases the zone of stasis and depth of injury.[32] Wound care also should prevent

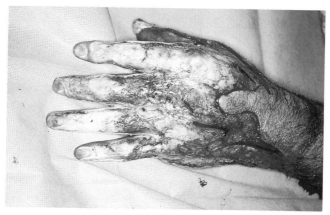

(a)

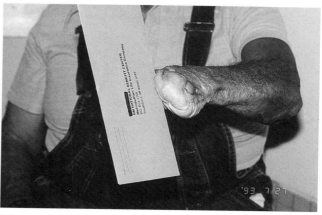

(b)

Fig. 49.1 Fourth-degree burns of the hand (a) usually result in a loss of normal hand function, but the majority of treated patients can perform independent activities of daily living (b).

infection.[33] The second principle is to maintain circulation. Keep edema in check and watch for evidence of decreased hand circulation. Intrinsic musculature is extremely sensitive to the effects of soft-tissue ischemia.[34] Loss of function of the intrinsic muscles creates a tendon imbalance and clawing, which is very difficult to correct in the burn-injured hand.[35]

In prioritization of needs, survival of the acute burn patient takes precedence over function.[36] Therefore, initial grafting is generally performed to maximize surface wound coverage.[36,37] This expedites wound closure and increases probability of survival. The goal of treatment of the whole burned person includes wound closure by 14 days, as delay in healing results in hypertrophic scars, contracture formation, limitations in motion, decreased strength and endurance, and poor overall outcome.[38–40] In general, deeper burns are managed by surgical intervention as soon as practical, to minimize immobility and to decrease duration of both illness and discomfort.[41] Traditionally, maximization of function is the second priority. Therefore, hands take high priority.[42,43] With the advent of synthetic dermal and skin substitutes, e.g. Integra™, hands can be afforded greater priority in grafting without compromise of survival.

The hand is specifically prone to thermal injury. The hand is the only appendage that operates outside of a 2-foot circle from our central axis. The dorsal hand has non-glabellar skin, which is thin and mobile, allowing for individual joint motions. A thin areolar tissue layer overlies the tendons and the surface of the joints. The separation between dorsal skin and extensor tendons gets extremely thin, especially over the joints, making extensor tendon and dorsal hood involvement more likely. In contrast, the palmar aspect has a glabrous, thick, hairless skin-bearing surface. There is minimal skin mobility, allowing for extreme grip stability and a higher concentration of sensory receptors. Palmar skin is heavily anchored to underlying fascia by fibrous septae. Flexor tendon burn injuries are less likely to occur than in their extensor counterparts. Burn-related changes in palmar skin integrity or hypertrophic scarring may result in loss of long-term instability of overlying skin coverage and contractures.

Initial evaluation of the burned hand

> Management of the acutely burned hand begins with a careful evaluation of the patient to whom the hands are attached.
>
> Sheridan[29]

In large burns, life-threatening injuries may supersede the treatment of the burned hand. It is important that the hand not be overlooked.[44] If the patient does survive, neglect of the hand during acute treatment results in increased morbidity and decreased total functioning.[42]

Evaluation of the burned hand begins with a careful history of the injured person, if possible. Character of the burning agent should be identified, along with the mechanism of hand injury. The temperature and time of contact with the noxious agent should be carefully noted. Hand dominance and occupation become extremely important for rehabilitation and possible occupational retraining, as does a history of prior hand problems. A history of habits and past medical history can also delineate problems that may arise during the acute or reconstructive period, including factors such as smoking, diabetes, or vascular disease.

On physical examination, it is important to make an estimation of the extent and depth of the burn injury. Areas of circumferential involvement are documented. Assessment of associated injuries should include radiographs when appropriate. Verification of perfusion should include attention to color, warmth, softness, sensation, and Doppler flow. Maintenance of circulation is vital (**Figure 49.2**).

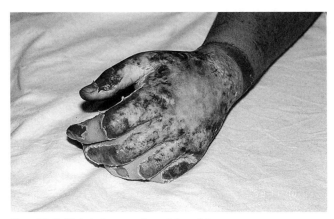

Fig. 49.2 Third degree dorsal hand burn.

Assessing Depth

Assessment of burn depth is an inexact science at best.[45,46] Evaluation accuracy by experienced burn surgeons has been identified to be approximately 64%.[47] There is some evidence that laser Doppler flowmetry may be of some assistance.[48] Other modalities for assessing depth have included ultrasound, intravenous (IV) fluoroscein, and fluorescence of IV indocyanine green dye.[49–52] However, none has been proven to be more accurate than an expert observer.[46]

Burns at the extremes are usually easy to classify in terms of depth,[46,53] but burn depth progresses over the first 48 hours post-injury, making early assessment inaccurate and difficult.[54] Deep second degree (which will heal) are most difficult to call at a single observation.

Superficial partial burn injuries typically appear erythematous with some blistering and pain. If the blisters have ruptured, the exposed, moist dermal bed appears pink and moist. Pain from these injuries is significant. Deep partial-thickness burns, sometimes referred to as indeterminate burns, have a moist mottled and/or petechial dermal surface and may either be pale or erythematous depending on the mechanism of injury. Typically, these still blanch with pressure and are painful, but variable, in their sensation. Full-thickness burn injuries appear leathery with a pale to brown eschar surface. Coagulated vessels are sometimes visible and the wound is anesthetic. However, depth classification rarely falls into such clear categories. Depth determination often proceeds by serial observation of progression of healing.

Outpatient Versus Inpatient Treatment

The first decision when assessing a hand burn is location of subsequent treatment. Patients with small superficial burns can be treated as outpatients if there is adequate home support and no other injuries. Outpatient management assumes the patient can maintain good follow-up and can follow prescribed treatment/ regiments reasonably. In light of possible suboptimal outpatient management, the risks of the initial burn treatment of the burned hand are high.[42] Burned hands can develop infection and contraction quickly, delaying return to work and impairing subsequent hand function. Therefore, if the depth of burn or home environment is in question, it may be cost-effective to provide inpatient treatment for 24–48 hours, until wound progression is clearer.

Management of burn blisters in the hands remains somewhat controversial. Some advocate leaving the blisters intact to provide sterile wound coverage and reduce discomfort. However, blister fluid in burns is rich in prostaglandin, especially thromboxane, which may in turn increase burn wound depth by increasing zone of stasis and further accentuating burn injury.[55,56] Therefore, it seems prudent to remove blisters of the dorsum of the hand or digits, given the close proximity of skin to tendon in these locations. In palmar blisters, or blisters less than 2 cm,[2] fluid can be aspirated and the keratin shell left in place to provide for temporary biologic coverage to reduce discomfort.

Typically, patients with smaller burns of the hands are allowed to go home. Treatment is begun on an outpatient basis. The family is recruited to help do the dressings. The wounds should be seen again at least daily in the first 48 hours to verify the initial presentation and assessment. At home, wounds are typically washed with warm water and mild soap. The use of sterile technique is both unrealistic and unnecessary.[57] There is no evidence that oral antibiotics have a positive impact on outcome or subsequent infection.[58] Wound care is kept simple, and may include either topical agents or biologic dressings. The goal is to minimize pain, prevent infection, prevent discomfort, and optimize motion.

If burn wounds are thought to be full-thickness, but not requiring admission, antimicrobial dressings such as Bactroban™ or silver-sulfadiazine can be utilized until grafting can be appropriately arranged. During outpatient treatment, range of motion exercises for the hand, especially active range of motion, is encouraged. Hand elevation is maintained to reduce edema.

For the inpatient treatment of burns, it is necessary to document the severity of the burn injury, including percent of TBSA involvement, depths of burns of the hands and elsewhere, and whether or not there is evidence of circumferential injury. Larger burns result in increased edema, increasing the risk of capillary stasis and digital compartment syndromes.

Escharotomies

Compartment syndrome of the hand can occur in large hand burns that are not always completely circumferential.[59] Loss of pulse is a typically late finding in compartment syndromes.[34] Early signs would include coolness of the fingertips, delayed capillary refill, subjective numbness, complaint by the patient, and altered sensation in the fingertips. One of the strongest indicators of ischemia is pain upon passive stretch of the intrinsic musculature.[34] Intrinsic musculature is stretched when metacarpal–phalangeal joints are held in extension and digits are stretched at the PIP joints in flexion (**Figure 49.3**). Clinically, if there is question about need for escharotomy, subeschar and intramuscular compartment pressures can easily be measured. A needle can be inserted into the muscular compartment and attached to an arterial pressure line to monitor intra-compartmental pressures if needed. Indications for escharotomy include subeschar pressures greater than 30 mmHg, diminishing perfusion despite resuscitation, diminishing temperature, increase firmness of

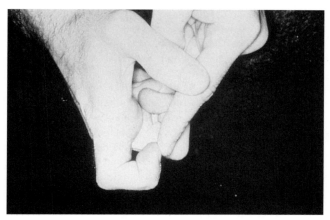

(a)

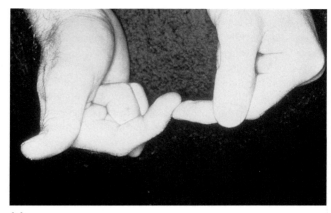

(b)

Fig. 49.3 Intrinsic tightness (IT) test (right hand tested). In the absence of intrinsic tightness, PIP joint flexion is greater when the MCP joint is extended (a) than when the MCP joint is flexed (b). This demonstrates a negative (normal) IT test.

upper arm, forearm or hand muscular compartments, decreasing capillary refill, and increase numbness.[35] Nurses can also be trained to monitor pulsatile perfusion of superficial palmar arch vessels or digital vessels using a bedside Doppler.[42]

If there is any doubt about need for the procedure, escharotomies are generally completed. Moreover, evidence of escharotomy is usually removed at the time of excision and grafting of the burn.[57] Escharotomies should be checked for completeness by re-measuring the subeschar pressures. Fasciotomy may be required if the escharotomy does not reduce the pressures or restore circulation. Escharotomies are completed in axial-oriented incisions along the medial and lateral arm and forearm, through the eschar extending into normal fat. At the elbow, the incision is completed anterior to the ulnar styloid process to avoid injury to the ulnar nerve. At the wrist, the cut is taken along the radial dorsal aspect to avoid the superficial sensory branch of the radial nerve. Incisions are extended into the burned hand to the metacarpal–phalangeal joints. If needed, dorsal escharotomies can be completed in the web spaces of the hand to provide for decompression of the intrinsic muscular compartments.

Escharotomies of the digits are not generally required if release of hand, forearm, and upper arm are adequate. Often, perfusion is reestablished in the fingertips and hands following escharotomies of the rest of the upper extremity burns.[60] If escharotomies are required, they may be completed along the radial aspect of the thumb, the ulnar aspect of the index, middle and ring fingers, and the radial aspect of the small finger to diminish the possibility of inadvertent damage to the neurovascular bundles of selected digits. Escharotomy is recommended on the radial side of the little finger to preserve ulnar sensation along this border digit.

Previously, chemical escharotomies using Travase™ ointment had been well described, obviating the need for surgical escharotomies of the digits.[61] Subsequently, similar chemical escharotomy has been completed using collagenase ointment. Ointment is placed over the digit, which is wrapped loosely circumferentially using a moist gauze; circulation of the digit is reassessed in 1 hour. This maneuver can be repeated if the initial chemical escharotomy is incomplete.

The utility of escharotomies in digits in children continues to be debated.[29,35,38] However, in adults, digital escharotomies improve survival of the digits.[29,35,38] The incidence of necrosis with escharotomy has been reported at 7.1% compared with 20% necrosis when digital escharotomies are not performed. Use of chemical escharotomy, however, eliminates the risk of inadvertent nerve disruption with escharotomy, justifying its recommended use in any severely burned digit.

If intrinsic muscle tightness with pain is present, recommendation is dorsal hand fasciotomies, in addition to escharotomy. Fasciotomy is completed through 2–4 dorsal hand incisions. Interosseous muscular fascia is divided using blunt hemostat dissection. Fasciotomies are indicated if intra-compartmental pressures are greater than 30 mmHg several minutes following escharotomy. Fasciotomies are most commonly indicated in electrical burns and combined crush/burn injuries (**Figure 49.4**).

Special consideration in hand burns

Hand Burns in Children
In children, contact burns of the hands are much more likely[60] (**Figure 49.5**). Due to small cross-sectional diameters, children are more prone to compartmental syndromes and digital tip necrosis.[59] Dorsal hand skin is thinner, resulting in much deeper injuries.

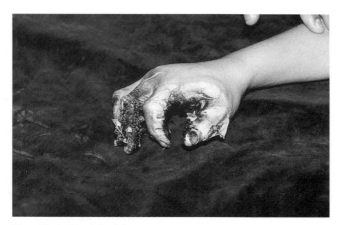

Fig. 49.4 Electrical burn.

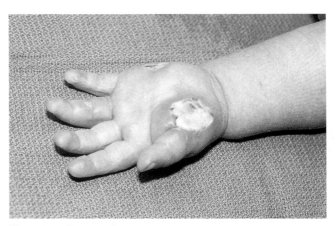

Fig. 49.5 Contact burn.

Splinting and rehabilitation therapy is much more difficult in the small hand.[62] However, children rarely have a problem with the development of chronic joint stiffness and can be kept immobilized without sequellae much longer than their adult counterparts.[63] In children, however, growing scars often do not keep up with the growth of the child. Therefore, secondary reconstruction of the burned pediatric hand is much more likely.[64]

Chemical Burns
About 60% of all chemical burns involving the hand are work-related injuries.[65] Initial management consists of copious and continues water irrigation immediately following chemical exposure, which is critical to limiting injury[66] (**Figure 49.6**). However, water irrigation is contraindicated in chemical burns from elemental sodium, potassium or lithium, which react to water with actual thermic reaction. In these, the particles are covered with mineral oil prior to their surgical removal.

If nail beds are burned, nails may need partial removal to allow for adequate irrigation treatment of the subungual inflammation and contamination.[65]

Hydrofluoric acid deserves special mention, as one of the most painful of chemical burns. Hydrofluoric acid is prevalent in photography lab products in industrial processes such as glass etching, and household products such as rust removers. Hydrofluoric acid is also used in petrochemical refining. The fluoride ion rapidly extends through the epithelium into subcutaneous tissues and binds with calcium, producing extreme pain.[67] If greater than 2.5% TBSA is involved, the patient can develop systemic hypocalcemia and shock.[68]

Specialized treatment of a hydrofluoric acid burn consists of neutralization using topical calcium gluconate 10% prepared as a slurry by crushing calcium gluconate tablets into an aqueous gel.[69] Typically, this is applied with gloves until pain is gone. If this is ineffective, subcutaneous injection is possible using calcium gluconate or magnesium sulfate in concentrations of 0.5 ml/cm.[2,69] However, in fingertip injuries, fingertip pulp[21] is tightly confined, and injection creates increased discomfort. As an alternative, hydrofluoric acid burns can be neutralized by giving 10 ml of 10% calcium gluconate mixed with 40 ml of 0.9% normal saline solution delivered intravenously by regional Bier block over 20–30 minutes, or intra-arterially over 4 hours.[70]

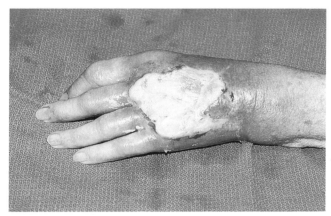

(a)

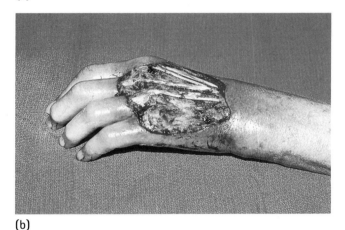

(b)

Fig. 49.6 Chemical burn (a) before debridement and (b) after debridement.

Combined Thermal and Crush Injuries

Combined thermal and crush injuries such as injuries from hot presses, are far more common in industry than in a domestic setting.[71] This injury is more severe than the additive effect of either injury alone.[72] Initial management includes fasciotomy, which is generally required to reduce intercompartmental pressure within the deep spaces of the hand. In spite of appearances at early debridement, these injuries are usually deceptively deeper. The full extent of burn is manifested only with time, usually as a failure of the initial grafting procedure. Many protocols propose a 'second look' at deep tissues after 48 hours, as the extent of injury can be misjudged easily initially.[72] It is recommended to avoid temptation to graft during the first operative intervention, which usually occurs within the first 48 hours postburn. Typically, patients have an accumative effect from both injuries. Recovery and return to work is quite drawn out.[72]

Fourth Degree Hand Burns

Fourth degree hand burns are defined by burns that involve or lead to exposure of a tendon, bone, joint, or nerve, obviating the presence of a graftable wound bed.[73] Coverage requires either a flap for presentation of exposed vital structure, or Kirshner wire (K-wire) fixation of the involved joint or segment. The 'K-wire' fixation

promotes adequate wound stability for healing by secondary intention with granulation formation, and then subsequent skin grafting. Fourth degree injuries commonly result in stiff joints, and many require amputations for adequate functional treatment.[42]

Electrical injuries account for approximately 30–65% of fourth degree hand burns, depending on the country.[13] Most high-voltage injuries occur at work.[74] Twenty percent of fourth-degree injuries occur from hot rollers producing burn-plus-crush effects. Contact burns account for 14% of fourth degree hand burns, and most often occur at a time of loss of consciousness, as seen with epileptics, diabetic comas or explosion-type injuries.

Nonsurgical treatment strategies

Wound care of the burned hand has the same requirements as all burn wounds: (1) dressing should allow healing while providing for unimpeded range of motion; (2) progressive range of motion therapy; and (3) early excision of burn eschar and coverage (if appropriate) to facilitate wound closure and healing.[75]

Wound Care Dressings

A variety of products and materials are currently available for dressing of both partial-thickness and full-thickness hand burns. The goal of the dressings is to protect the wound from infection and desiccation, either prior to healing as for partial-thickness burns, or prior to grafting as for deep-partial- and full-thickness burns. Ideally, a dressing should be easy to change, semi-permeable, and prevent maceration from exudate.[75] In the hand, it should also be thin to allow movement. Last, but not least, a dressing should be comfortable.

For superficial second degree burns, as long as desiccation and infection are prevented, healing occurs quickly without long-term sequelae. Almost any wound care dressings are successful. If second degree burns are deeper, however, wounds become more problematic and wound dressings more selective. During wound care, it is essential that the patient be cooperative and able to follow instructions. It is not harmful to wait up to 2 weeks to determine whether wounds of questionable depth will heal. If healing does not occur, then grafting can be performed with excellent results.[57] Wounds that heal in less than 2 weeks will produce minimal scarring, but if wounds take longer than 2 weeks to heal, the risk of scarring increases. Deitch documented a 21% incidence of hypertrophic scarring in wounds that healed in 14–21 days, but 78% incidence of hypertrophic scarring in wounds that took longer than 21 days to heal.[40]

Options for dressings are varied. Successful wound care treatment protocols have been reported with 0.5% silver-nitrate solution, mafenide acetate, Bactroban™ ointment, polysporin ointment, and silver sulfadiazine cream, which remains the most popular.[75] Newer dressings include a silver-coated barrier dressing called Acticoat.™ Acticoat™ is applied and left in position for several days. Fewer dressings are required, and it negates the need for daily hydrotherapy.[76]

Biobrane™ is a bilaminate semi-permeable silicone membrane bonded to a thin layer of nylon fabric. Modified porcine dermal collagen is bound to the nylon, which helps hold the dressing in place until the partial-thickness wound heals. Biobrane™ is available as a glove, and allows for active range of motion during the healing process. However, Biobrane™ cannot be used for deeper or full-thickness injuries.[77]

Procel Gore-Tex™ gloves have an expanded outer layer bonded to an inner layer of polymetric non-woven fabric. These reusable, water vapor-permeable polytetrafluoroethylene bags, popularized in Great Britain, are applied with silver sulfadiazine and changed daily.[78–80] Bags can be washed and reused. Range of motion is well maintained with decreased pain. With use of the Gore-Tex™ gloves or bags, it was noted that patients had a decreased exudate, skin maceration, and pain, and increased mobility and independence.[81] The bags result in a high patient-satisfaction rate, with 92% having good mobility during use.

Superficial partial-thickness burns, regardless of topical treatment, usually will heal well. Burns that heal within 14 days will recover aesthetically and functionally better than grafted burns.[38,39] Therefore, it is important to avoid unnecessary operations on wounds that will heal in this time frame in the non-critical burn patient.

Hand therapy for the acute burn injury

For acute injuries, edema management consists of a simple program of elevation to decrease both edema and pain. Active and passive range of motion exercises are begun as soon as possible. Protective splinting is required to maintain joint and hand posture.

In a hospital setting, different methodologies have been used to elevate the hand.[82] A towel can be used as a sling to suspend the arms to about 45 degrees.[10,15] Alternately the hand is suspended straight up, with the elbows bent, resting the elbows to provide maximal stable elevation of the hands in supine patients.[83]

One message is clear from the volume of burn literature: prevention of hand deformities is more successful than the subsequent treatment. Edema of the hand causes a loss of joint and dorsal skin laxity and impairs flexions at the metacarpal–phalangeal (MCP) joints. Some state that the keystone to positioning the hand properly is maintenance of dorsal flexion of the wrist at approximately 15–20°.[10,15] The flexor tendons remain in tension, pulling the hand into a more flexed hand posture, if the wrist is kept at slight extension.

However, we believe that the key to the positioning maintenance of the burned hand is control of the MCP joint.[84] The MCP joint is a cam-lever, eccentric joint. When the joint is in extension, the collateral ligaments are loose. When the joint is in full flexion, the collateral ligaments are tight (**Figure 49.7**). In extension, loose collateral ligaments allow the joints to move back and forth, and the fingers can move from side to side. In full flexion, such as in the full fist, the fingers are stable.

During the edematous phase of hand burn injuries, tissue swelling occurs within the hand and the joints. Because the joint has more laxity in an extended position, edema naturally drives the MCP joint into an extended posture. However, if the hand remains in this posture for too long, the collateral ligaments shorten and tighten. Once the hand gets stiff with a MCP extended posture, the contractual forces of the shortened collateral ligaments can be tough to overcome. In addition, with the MCP joints in extension, increased tension on the balance of the extrinsic and intrinsic tendons drives the IP (interphalangeal) joints of the digits into acute flexion. The hand is naturally moved to a posture of MCP-extension/IP flexion during the course of scar contracture and healing. If unchecked, end-stage contracture disease of the burned hand results, called the claw-hand deformity.[85] This deformity is defined by wrist flexion, MCP joint hyperextension, PIP flexion, boutonniere deformities of the digits (PIP flexion and slight DIP extension), and a thumb adduction contracture. The postburn claw-hand is a useful image to consider when splinting, positioning, and ranging the hand. It is the forces that produce the claw hand deformity that the surgeon and hand therapists hope to overcome (**Figure 49.8**).

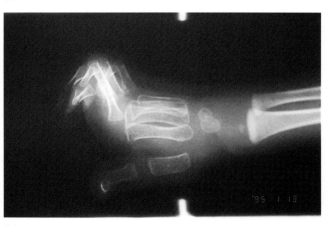

(a)

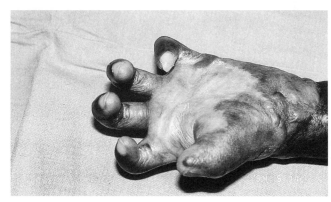

(b)

Fig. 49.8 (a) Claw hand deformity: a therapist's nightmare. Notice the severe MCP hyperextension in the X-ray (b).

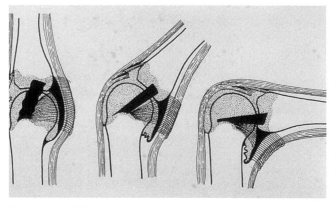

Fig. 49.7 MCP collateral ligaments are loose in extension, and tight in flexion.

Splinting

During the splinting process, the hand should remain elevated at least to 45°. Depending on the status of the rest of the extremity, if the elbow region is not burned, it is possible to keep the patient in the flexed elbow posture and elevate the hands even to 90°. Stockinet™ (osborne sling) placed around the arm and suspended to an IV pole, sometimes is helpful in this maneuver.

Much has been written on the proper splinting position of the hand. It has erroneously called the position of function.[86-88] The position of function is like the hand reaching to catch a ball. Splinting should be done in the position of protection, which places the hand in the best position to help overcome imbalance of tendon forces working on the hand during the edema phase. The position of protection keeps the collateral ligaments of the MCP joint in a flexed position, at 70–90° (**Figure 49.9**). Wrist extension is maintained at 20–30°, IP joints are held in full extension, and the thumb is kept adducted and slightly opposed. The proper position of the thumb during the splinting process is argued between a position of full adduction versus in a position of full extension.[89]

The ideal posture of the thumb is to separate the first metacarpal and second metacarpal heads at a maximum distance. This occurs when the first metacarpal is about 45° from both the plane of the palm and 45° from a line drawn along the first ray extending into the radius. In a severely burned hand, the position of the thumb is very difficult to maintain.

A temporary pre-manufactured splint can be placed on the patient with the initial dressing and first assessment. A customized manufactured splint can then be made over the first 1–2 days. Pre-manufactured splints sometimes create pressure points in the hand. Most therapy programs recommend removal of the splints for range of motion activities at least twice a day.[90] However, one program recommends applying the initial dressing, splint and bandage on, and keeping the hand maximally elevated without range of motion for 5 days.[1] There has not been demonstrated to be either an advantage or disadvantage to this approach.

All splinting and ranging programs are designed to maximize active use of the hand, maintaining function and protecting posture. Patients should be encouraged to use the hands for self-care activities, as this speeds return to functional activities.[91] Static splinting is used mainly to hold position between therapy sessions, or if active participation with the range of motion program is not possible. Vigorous stretching programs that emphasize passive range of motion are associated with tearing of tendons, scar tissue, vessels and joint capsules. A passive stretching should not be overused.[92-94]

Some protocols provide for passive range of motion activities primarily by the use of continuous-passive motion (CPM) devices.[44] One such protocol was used for 43 patients from a mass casualty accident with an average burn size of 19.4% TBSA burns including hands. In this program, if the patient was actively able to obtain a full fist, or the MCPs could be actively brought into greater than 70° flexion, the patient was started on a program of active movement with activities of daily living, along with progressive resistance exercises. If the patient could only obtain a half-fist, or MCP flexion was less than 70°, the patient was started on a program of alternating intervals of CPM machines. Static splinting was used at night and active movement with activities of daily living during the day, alternating every 4 hours with CPM use. If the patients could obtain no active movement due to severe injury or coma, then the CPM was used on 4-hour intervals with static splinting maintained in between. If hand motion failed to improve over 72 hours, then the patients were started on a program of dynamic splinting for 5 days. If this program failed, then position of the hand was maintained by use of K-wires. K-wires were also used for treatment of open joints. Use of this CPM-based program in these patients resulted in good to excellent function for all hands. They recommend use of this or similar protocols so that hand injuries are not overlooked or ignored in seriously injured patients.[44]

However, the use of CPMs in hand burns remain somewhat controversial. The use of CPMs was prospectively tested on nine patients with symmetric hand burns.[15] One hand was maintained in a CPM for an average of 5 days, for up to 18 hours a day. CPMs were started after skin grafting in these patients along with standard motion exercises. This study demonstrated no improved range-of-motion at the point where the CPM discontinued. There was no significant improvement in edema or pain with the hand treated with CPM. Interestingly, the total act of range of motion was less in the hand treated with the CPM versus the nontreated hand. Most of the total active motion improvements occurred with active range motion and activities of daily living. It appears that stressing the active movement of the burned hand improves outcomes, and not necessarily use of CPMs.[15]

Alternatives to Early Motion

At the University of Louisville, a different approach is used for hand burns. Patients are immobilized immediately using Xeroform™ (bacteriostatic petroleum gauze), splinted in an intrinsic-plus splint, and elevated to 90°.[1] The splint and dressings are maintained for 5 days and the blood flow and circulation of the hands are monitored. In this program, digital escharotomies are rarely necessary if the strict program of hand elevation is maintained. Hands are reassessed at 5 days; if burns are felt to be full-thickness, then the patient undergoes skin grafting. If the hand burn is felt to be indeterminate and the patient is cooperative, then a program of twice-daily Silvadene dressings are started along with twice daily therapy. If the range of motion decreases during the time of observation, then the program is halted and the patients are taken for surgical grafting. Success of this program depends upon the vigilant observations of the therapist and surgeon to

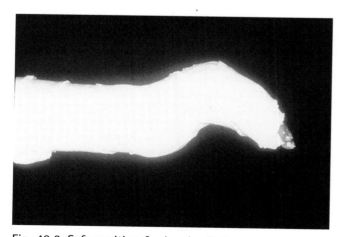

Fig. 49.9 Safe position for hand splinting.

assure that active range of motion of the healing burned hands is maintained.

Surgical treatment of acute hand burns

Surgical Principles

In patients with large burns, the priority of the burn places survival over function. Therefore, the priority is placed in the first operative procedures on maximizing initial surface coverage. Available donor sites are used to obtain large area coverage of trunk and upper portions of upper and lower extremities. Hands are often excised, covered with allograft or protective dressings, and grafted at a later time once survival is assured.

Majority opinion currently in the surgical literature suggests that the earlier surgery is achieved for the burned hand, the better functional results and the less need for reconstructive surgery.[89,95–102] However, in controlled clinical trials, this has not yet been proven as true. However, if a more deliberate waiting period is followed prior to grafting of the burn wound hand position and range of motion of the hand must be strictly maintained.[103] If motion and position are maintained, then a burned hand can be grafted later (i.e. during the second or even third week postburn) and still have excellent results. Prolonged immobilization in adults, however, is felt to be detrimental.[104,105]

When is Surgery Needed

Modern principles of burn management have led to excellent results for treatment of second and third degree hand burns.[10] Second degree burns are treated nonsurgically with expected return to full function and healing. Deep second and third degree burns are excised and grafted early, thereby decreasing hospital length of stay (LOS) hospital costs and time to return to work.[89,95–102]

Debate remains on the optimal treatment of indeterminate depth hand burns. Although most advocate early excision of these indeterminate burns, several prospective studies have failed to show that early excision and grafting of indeterminate burns failed to improve hand function compared with conservative dressing treatments.[10,96,97,106] Early excision and grafting of these burns, however, may be justified to shorten LOS decrease pain, reduce complications from prolonged immobilization and allow earlier self-feeding.[89,95–102]

Early Versus Late Surgery

Although early excision of localized deep hand burns were proposed as early as the 1940s, the standard treatment remained topical antimicrobials which allowed for primary eschar separation, then skin grafting.[107,108] In the 1970s, emphasis shifted to early excision of deep hand burns with reported improved functional results and reduced subsequent need for reconstructive procedures.[109] Burke's[23] classic paper in the mid 1970s showed good to excellent results in 99% of patients with partial-thickness burns treated nonsurgically and in 93% of patients with deep partial-thickness or full-thickness burns treated with excision and grafting. These were classified as Class 1- and Class II-type burn injuries respectively. However, in Burke's report of fourth degree burns (or Class III hand burns) only one of six patients showed an outcome better than poor results.

Surgery within 2 weeks trends to a better functional results and fewer reconstructive procedures than delayed surgeries.[10,89,95–102,106]

Early excision and grafting also produces shorter, less costly hospital stays.[24,84] In a 10-year follow-up of hand burns taking longer than 21 days to heal, 100% of patients required reconstructive surgeries.[24,84] By contrast, in a similar group operated on within 5–10 days, there was only a 26% incidence of reconstruction required.[24,84] Still, some surgeons assert that if an intensive dedicated hand therapy program is available, 1-year functional results for both early and late excisional treatment remains the same.[25,96,110] Tangential excision versus conservative early management failed to detect any difference in function in late follow-up care.[96,97,111] The singe preeminent caveat of conservative treatment is the careful monitoring of the patient's functional status so that one can switch treatment and graft if indicated.[1]

Hand Burn Treatment Algorithms

A number of algorithms exist for the treatment of acute hands,[44,112,113] all of which follow a similar pattern. Partial-thickness injuries or second degree burns are typically treated with topical agents. There are a number of dressings available. Patients tend to do well and heal without any difficulties. Full-thickness burns or third degree burns are typically excised and grafted. No one has shown any adverse effect waiting for 2 weeks to determine whether or not the burn is full-thickness.[30,57] Following excision and grafting, patients' hands tend to do well. In fourth degree burns, choices for treatment includes flap coverage, amputation or stabilization of the area prior to granulation and skin grafting. In patients with significant neurovascular injury or significant injuries to tendon, bone or joint, amputation is often recommended or required.[42]

In Sheridan's series of adult patients, 5% of the patients were classed third or fourth degree burn injuries.[30] Of these, 89% had K-wires and stabilization of one or more joints; 69% required amputation of one or more digital stumps, either partial or complete. Thirteen percent of patients had reconstruction using a pedicle flap, either a groin or an abdominal flap with the groin flap preferred.

Wound Closure Options

In full-thickness and deep full-thickness burn injuries, wound closure options are standard as for any surgical wound, and include: skin grafts, skin substitutes, local flaps, pedicle flaps, and microvascular free tissue transfers. Skin grafts remain the standard and acceptable coverage of full-thickness graftable burn wounds of the hand.[114,115] Does the type of skin graft for hand burns matter? Many authors argue that sheet grafts and mesh grafts are functionally equivalent in the hand burn.[15,101] Studies support that sheet grafts and 1.5:1 mesh grafts have the same functional outcome.[84] However, most authors report that the aesthetic outcome is better with sheet grafts.[29,42] As an aesthetic organ, hand appearance should not be ignored (**Figure 49.10**). But in a controlled trial of sheet grafts versus mesh grafts, the color, shape and texture of both hands was judged as similar by a three-person panel.[15] Furthermore, a study of thick versus thin split-thickness grafts utilized as sheet grafts for the burned hands coverage reported no differences in range of motion, appearance or patient satisfaction at 1 year.[116]

Skin substitutes are being used with more frequency in the coverage of hands. Integra™, which is a completely synthetic dermal-analog, has been used in a number of patients, long-term data are

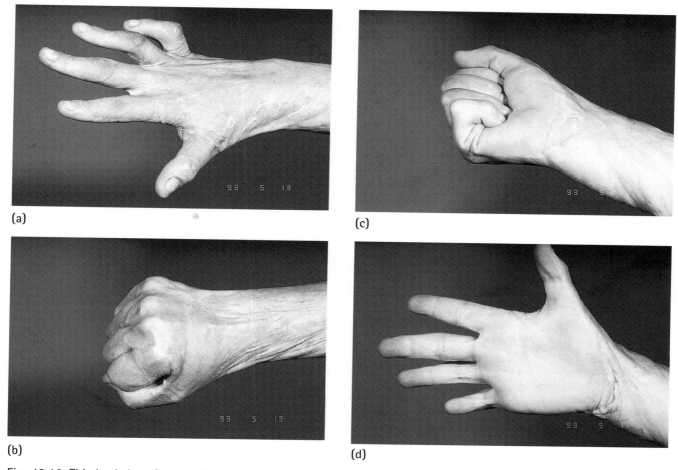

(a)

(b)

(c)

(d)

Fig. 49.10 This healed grafted hand shows normal hand function and motion, despite mild postburn postural deformities and scarring.

still forth coming (W. Dougherty, personal communication). Alloderm™, an immunologically inert dermis derived from human cadaver, has also been used in burned hands with accepted healing.[114,117] However, no one had documented superiority of these new materials over conventional skin grafts for reconstruction of the burned hand.

In patients with small areas of exposed bone, joint or tendons, local flap surgery will provide acceptable coverage.[118] In larger exposed areas, skin resurfacing can be completed with pedicle groin flaps, pedicle radial forearm flaps, random abdominal flaps or free-tissue transfers. (This is discussed in further detail in the discussion of the fourth degree burn.)

For nonexpanded mesh grafts or sheet grafts to be successful, perfect homeostasis of the excised burn wound is imperative. To achieve this, most surgeons recommend use of a tourniquet with exsanguination of the hand, prior to tangential excision. Tangential excision is typically performed with the knife of choice, down to pearly white, moist dermis or bright yellow subcutaneous fat.[119] Excision should continue until any evidence of thrombosed small vessels or extravascular hemosiderin staining is completely removed from tissues. Loupe magnification and adequate time for excision both allow for a more controlled tangential excision.

Other strategies for providing hemostasis include: the use of temporary topical epinephrine soaked dressings, 1:10 000, use of a

soaked nonadherent dressing such as Telfa pads, use of topical thrombin, and in some cases, insufflation of wounds with 1–400 000 to 1–1 000 000 epinephrine solution.[120] Hemostasis is finalized with judicious use of electrocautery, being careful to avoid injury to neurovascular structures. Bipolar electrocautery in digits and palmar surfaces can be extremely helpful.

Some burn centers recommend use of fibrin glue underneath the sheet grafts to improve graft 'take' and to provide for improved hemostasis.[118,121] Fibrin glue is prepared by mixing of cryoprecipitate, calcium, and thrombin. This has been demonstrated to decrease the subgraft hematoma rate and increase wound healing.[122] It was also shown to improve two-point discrimination neurologic testing of the grafted hand during follow-up.[122]

Skin Grafting Techniques

Many programs currently use exclusively sheet grafts for coverage of the burned hand, while others still prefer covering debrided wounds with 1:1 or 1.5:1 mesh unexpanded. Sheet grafts typically are preferred in women, in unilateral injuries, or by request of the patient.[15] Tourniquet typically should be deflated prior to skin graft placement to assure adequate homeostasis of the wound. Some surgeons, when using mesh grafts, do not deflate the tourniquet, reducing blood loss and operative time.[97]

Following graft placement, grafts are either covered with a

gentle compressive dressing or left open to allow direct observation of the mesh grafts. Grafts are secured in place with combinations of staples, absorbable sutures or surgical tape. For sheet grafts, they are typically examined at least within the first 24 hours to remove blood and hematomas. Hands are positioned either with splints or K-wires. Many surgeons prefer the use of fingernail hoods, hooks with elastic band to provide for slight distraction of the digit into a ukulele or hayrake or Banjo type splint (W. Dougherty, personal communication). This allows for stabilization without penetrating directly into the joint with a K-wire.

Hands are kept elevated following application of the grafts. After about a week, programs of active and passive range of motion are resumed. Some recommend use of a Coban or Unna boot wrap to secure bandages.[111] As in many aspects of surgical treatment, techniques of grafting and dressing hands remain more art form than science, with acceptable results reported by all authors.

Hand Position with Grafting

The majority of grafted hands have dorsal burns.[6] Debate exists on the best position for the hand during initial healing of skin graft coverage. Most authors tend to favor the safe position (intrinsic-plus) of the hand following the application of the grafts.[123] This is especially true if there is risk of PIP extensor hood exposure. However, grafting of the dorsal hands with the patient in intrinsic-plus posturing may fail to add an adequate volume of skin overlying the dorsum of the hand, especially at the level of the PIP joints.[124,125] Patients may be best stabilized in a full-flex hand posture post-grafting with flexion at the DIP, PIP, and MP joints. No adverse consequences have been shown with this method, and it may reduce stiffness in the digits following grafting.[84,126] This fist position increases the length of the hand 20–32 mm in index to little fingers and 9 mm in the thumb.[125] The fist position increases the dorsal skin length on the hand 11–20%, and along each finger approximately 12–17%. Assuming that the average hand width is approximately 10 cm, the difference in dorsal skin is more than 21 cm^2,[125] when placing the hand in the safe position versus the fist position. In the safe position, the dorsal hand may be covered with too little skin, especially if the split in the split graft contracts to 30–50% of its original size with healing.[127,128]

Management of Exposed Tendons or Joints

The most common area of exposed extensor tendon is at the PIP joint on the digits.[85] This is due to the thin skin and adipose tissue overlying this area. Commonly, most authors recommend stabilization of the joint using an axial K-wire and maintaining the area through a regular program of dressings.[30] Once granulation has formed over the area of the joint, skin graft coverage is completed. However, if there is little risk of a boutonniere deformity, the splinting of the area can be used rather than K-wires. If there are extensive areas of exposed tendons or joints, early debridement is completed, and acute coverage is provided by groin flaps, abdominal flaps or other local flaps[73] (**Figure 49.11**). Typically, isolated, unstable open joints are treated with K-wire fixation, allowed to granulate, and are subsequently grafted.[30] If the joint remains unstable, the patient could go onto a program of joint fusion.[42] Amputations typically are delayed to maintain maximal length. Exposed tendons must be kept moist and not stretched with passive range of motion activities.[90]

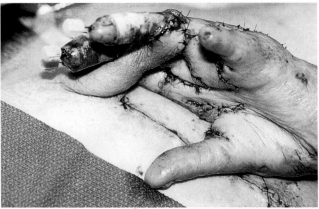

(a)

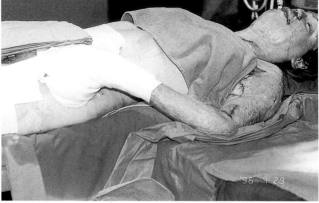

(b)

Fig. 49.11 (a) Groin flap–volar digital reconstruction (b) The hand is secured to avoid inadvertent pulling for 10–21 days.

Special Management of Children

In treatment of the burned hand in children, most surgeons recommend using the thickest donor sites available, such as the back or scalp, with less of a tendency to scar.[64] A two-stage procedure has been preferred by many that have managed children[128] but has never been shown to be more effective. Sheet grafts are felt to be more cosmetically and functionally acceptable. It has been reported that up to 55% TBSA of burns can be covered in sheet grafts including the hand.[130] In children, hand stiffness is usually not a problem and dressing and passive splints can remain in place longer without a fear of functional delay.[131]

Treatment of Palmar Burns

Typically, palmar burns are managed more conservatively compared to dorsal burns. The palms tend to be protected during massive burn injuries as a clenched fist posturing is a protective reflex during severe burn injuries. Most surgeons allow palmar burns up to 3 weeks to heal since typically they do not require grafting.[132] Glabella skin of the palm is extremely thick and tends to recover from burn injuries. In Sheridan's series, 58% of the hands had palmar burns, but only 18% required grafting.[29] His experience is limited with isolated palmar burns, accounting for only 1% of his patients. During the early healing period of palmar burns, the hands are splinted in extension alternating with flexion if a combination of dorsal and volar burns is present.

Barret *et al.*[132] reported a 10-year experience of isolated palmar burns in 120 children; of these, 110 (92%) were partial-thickness and healed without surgery. Only 8% (10 patients) were felt to be full-thickness injuries, but only 4 (3%) of these required excision and grafting. All of the hands that required excision and grafting subsequently developed postburn contractures. Grafting was typically treated with a split-thickness graft, harvested from the sole of the foot. Ten percent of the partial Class I burns developed postburn sequellae, and 50% of the full-thickness burns developed postburn sequellae. Thirteen percent of the total population developed contractures and 56% required subsequent reconstruction. In this series, contact burns accounted for 84% of palmar burns; the most common sources include a hot iron, an oven door, a heater or hot coals. If healing of the burn took longer than 3 weeks, the patients developed scarring functional and sequelae.

Treatment of Fourth Degree Hand Burns

As previously identified, a fourth degree hand burn is a burn with an exposed area of vessels, nerves, tendons, joints or bones. By definition, skin grafts cannot be used to cover these exposed areas primarily. Options include either K-wire or coverage with flaps. Cross-finger flaps,[133] can be useful for either dorsal or volar cover, with little functional deficit in the donor digit. Cross-finger flaps require a two-stage approach with formation of the flap and then secondary flap division (**Figure 49.12**). For limited defects in the area at the base of the digit or at the lower aspect of the PIP, small defects can be covered with homodigital flaps.[134] These are designed on the nonopposing side of the digit, if unburned, and are longitudinal and proximally based. The base of the flap should be distal to the proximal digital crease for more proximal flaps or distal to the neck of the proximal phalanx for flaps commencing around the PIP joint, so as to preserve the dorsal digital artery necessary to nourish the flaps. The lateral digital donor defect is covered immediately with a full-thickness skin graft. These are transferred expeditiously in a single stage and do not require sacrifice of a digital vessel. Dorsal metacarpal flaps (distally based) are also available for coverage of small defects at the base of the digits. However, all of the local flaps are very limited in their coverage area.

For more severe or larger burn injuries, distal flaps, vascular pedicle flaps, or free flaps are needed to provide immediate soft-tissue coverage, and hand resurfacing. Abdominal or groin flaps remain the workhorse flaps for coverage of acutely burned fourth degree hand injuries[135] (**Figure 49.13**). They provide for adequate protection in a complicated hand wound with minimal morbidity to the donor areas. However, they require immobilization for 1–2 weeks in a multistaged pedicle procedure. They are insensate and sometimes bulky.

Vascularized pedicle flaps are much thinner and do not require the same degree of immobilization. These include the radial forearm flap,[136] the Chinese flap (ulnar artery forearm flap),[137] and the reverse posterior interosseous flap.[138] The first two require sacrifice of a major artery in a traumatized extremity. Flaps are hirsute and insensate when based distally and do have some limitation of reaching distal defects in the hand. The use of microvascular free tissue transfers or free flaps has greatly expanded the volume of options available for acute reconstruction of the burned hand; however, it

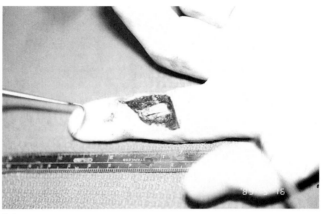

(a)

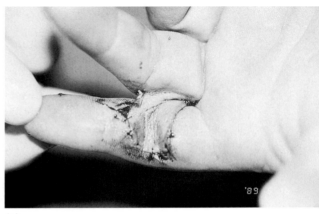

(b)

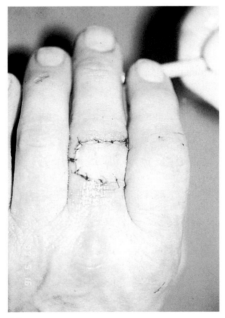

(c)

Fig. 49.12 Cross-finger flap reconstruction: (a) wound, (b) flap, (c) full-thickness skin graft coverage.

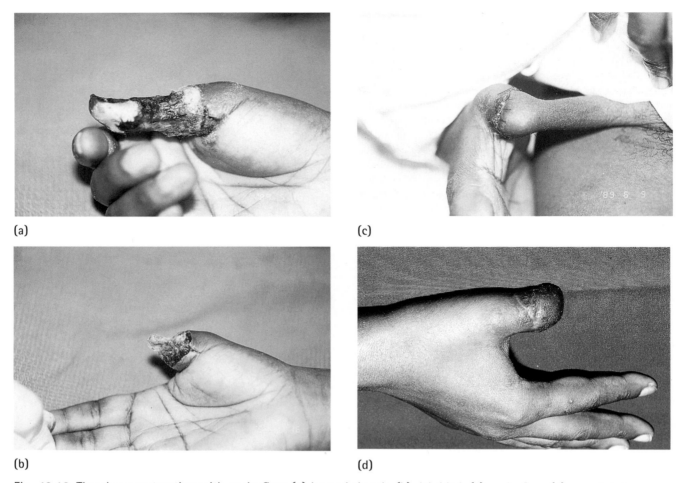

Fig. 49.13 Thumb reconstruction with groin flap: (a) burned thumb, (b) debrided, (c) groin flap, (d) completed.

requires a stable patient and an experienced microvascular surgery team. Free flaps can be used safely in acute electrical injuries.[139]

Engrav and associates[73] reported on their treatment of fourth degree hand burns. This included 35 hands in 25 patients (22 male and three female predominantly working men). Average burn size was 24% with flame and high voltage injuries accounting for 65% of injuries shared equally. Most flame burns occurred outside of the work place, while electrical injuries in their series typically occurred while working. Neurovascular injury to the hand or digits was noted in 100% of the amputated parts and 7% of nonamputated parts. On average, each patient had 4.5 operations. Use of flaps resulted in a shorter healing time by 36%, one less procedure and a better functional outcome than use of K-wire stabilization. They noted, however, that in their series, patients treated with K-wire, granulation and grafting were much larger burns compared to patients treated with flaps. Average burn size was approximately 61% in those treated with K-wires versus 15% of those treated with flaps.[73]

Fourth degree burns represented 5% of hand injuries reported in the Alberta series, which consisted of seven hands in five patients, two of which were bilateral.[15] All were treated with groin flaps, left in place 14–27 days, and later divided, thinned, and subsequently grafted. They reported a 97% success rate with 89% successful coverage in one try and 11% requiring a second flap. Total active motion only obtained 30–38% of normal long-term difficulties.

However, most of these patients had no long-term difficulties with activities of daily living or work activities.

Use of the Crane Principle for Fourth Degree Burns

The crane principle was first described by Millard in 1969 to provide a platform for complex soft-tissue reconstructions.[140] A flap is transposed to cover a defect. The flap is then split into two lamina, with the skin and outer lamina being returned to the original site and the soft-tissue now adherent to the wound providing for a stable platform for skin grafting. Engrav reported their results of 11 patients, six underwent hand reconstruction using the crane principle and five had abdominal flaps.[141] In their series, the crane patients had better cosmetic outcomes, better TAMs, required no secondary debulking procedures, and had similar hand function as the abdominal skin flap group. Engrav and colleagues recommended use of a distal flap with crane principle reconstruction and subsequent grafting instead of relying on cumbersome distal flaps or complex thin free tissue transfers. The patients' systemic condition and depth of burn prior to treatment must be considered (**Figure 49.14**).

Microvascular Reconstruction of Acute Hand Burn

Microvascular reconstruction is feasible for acute hand burn injuries.[142,143] Although, many seriously injured patients are unable

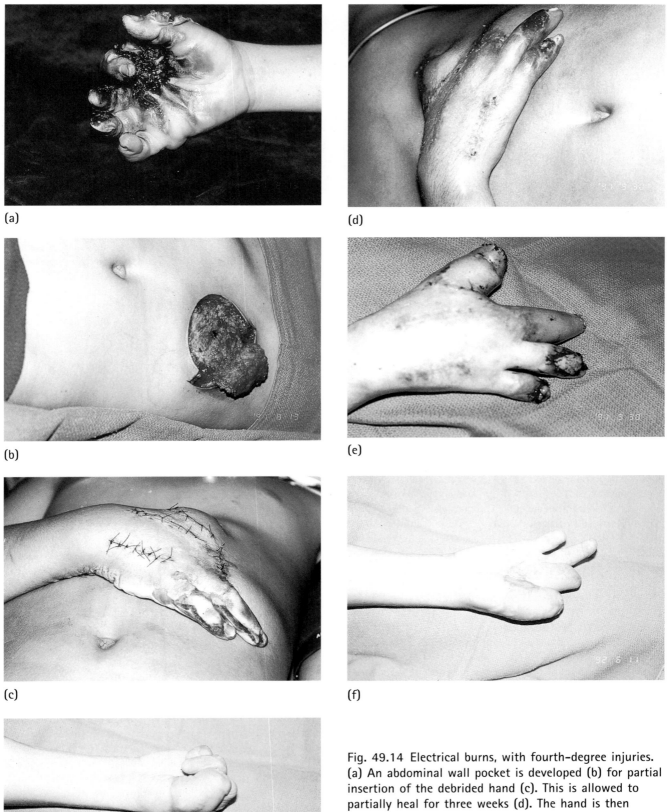

(a)

(b)

(c)

(d)

(e)

(f)

(g)

Fig. 49.14 Electrical burns, with fourth-degree injuries. (a) An abdominal wall pocket is developed (b) for partial insertion of the debrided hand (c). This is allowed to partially heal for three weeks (d). The hand is then removed, and rebuilt with a combination of flaps and skin grafts (e). Following healing, good hand function is preserved in opening (f) and closing (g), allowing activities of daily living (h).

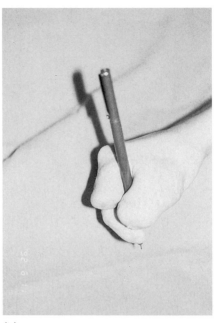

(h)

Fig. 49.14b Final outcome, electrical burn from previous page.

to undergo the prolonged operative time and exposure required for these delicate but complex procedures, microvascular reconstruction remains a useful option for selected patients with deep fourth degree hand burns. They are best for patients who have localized wounds, very deep wounds, limited wounds elsewhere outside of the body and a low risk of mortality.[143] These include electrical injuries, frostbite, some contact burns, and abrasion/friction burns. In all, microvascular free-tissue transfers are more commonly used in late reconstruction of the burned hand.[143]

Principles of rehabilitation hand therapy

Role of the Hand Therapist

No treatment of hand injuries or hand reconstruction is complete without some mention of the hand therapist. Outcomes in hand surgery can be made or broken by the participation and skill of these trained professionals.[144] The hand therapist is a critical member of the burn team,[142,145] providing education to the patient, the family, and the medical staff. The hand therapist is a primary player in edema management, which reduces inflammation and to allow for early mobilization. Therapists assist with range of motion exercises, with active range preferred over passive movement. This is especially true at the elbow where risk of heterotopic ossification is highest.[10] Hand therapists are responsible for: (1) splint maintenance; (2) patient positioning; (3) functional activity support; (4) strength development in both fine pinch and power grip; (5) psychosocial support for the recovering patient and their family; and (6) assistance in pain management techniques.

Record-keeping in Hand Therapy

In order to provide useful comparative data, and objectively to evaluate patients during the recovery phase of acute burn hand injuries, record keeping is key to documentation for an accurate accountability of the patient's rehabilitation and progress. A hand record should contain information on six different parameters.[146–149] These include some record of pain rating, strength, goniometry, sensation, volumetry, and dexterity. Pain is recorded as a subjective rating by the patient. This serves as a good backdrop to determine the progress of rehabilitation therapy. Strength ratings include a grip dynamometer and a pinch strength gauge. Goniometry is completed under the guidelines established by the American Society of Hand Therapists. Sensation is documented by the use of monofilaments and the two-point discrimination test. Volumetry is measured by water displacement. Dexterity is typically measured by a sequential occupational dexterity assessment (SODA). In the future, many of our assessments may be computerized, which would speed the process to 20 minutes compared to an hour manually.[149]

Challenges of the Burned Hand

The most common challenges after an acute burn hand injury include the thumb web contractures, PIP joint contractures of the digits, and fifth-finger boutonniere deformities.[4,150,151] In spite of early splinting, adequate therapy, and vigilant treatment, these deformities continue to develop.[152]

Common treatment obstacles in acute hand therapy include: (1) inappropriate positioning of poorly fitting splints, (2) prolonged immobilization, (3) delays initiation of acute range of motion and participation of functional activities, and (4) problems with lack of communication and support.[145]

Common treatment obstacles during the rehabilitation phase include: (1) non-compliance in the application of garments and splints, by either patients or staff; (2) delayed rehabilitation progression with delay in implementation of either range of motion, casting or dynamic splinting; (3) and delayed referral to outpatient therapy after hospitalization.[145]

There are a number of current factors that continue to jeopardize patient recovery following acute hand injury: (1) sensitivity to the needs of the burned hand may often be overlooked in the face of other, more overwhelming burn injuries; (2) confused jumbles of treatment priorities during rehabilitation that refer the patient back and forth between multiple specialists; (3) fragmented care which treats the patient as a series of parts instead of a whole; and (4) fiscal pressures or restraints from the insurer have become a distasteful part of any treatment program.[152]

Returning the Patient to Work

In the burned hand, timing of return to work is a very useful indication of early hand care outcome. Hand burns may or may not have a significant influence on the ultimate return to work of acutely injured patients.[153–157] Of patients with severe burn injuries, 80–86% will return to work despite face and hand burns.[156] Typically, patients with burns involving less than 5% TBSA including the hands were returned to work in less than a month. If TBSA burns are approximately 10%, return to work is variable. However, in this group, if the patient has not returned to work within 6 months, they are unlikely to ever return. In patients with burns greater than 30% TBSA, approximately one-third do not ever return to work. Studies looking at return to work and independent living have identified hand injuries as significant in delaying return to full function.[154,158,159] In England, about 80% of those who return to work return to their same jobs. If hospitalization was less than 10 days during the entire course of treatment, the patients typically were able to return to work in less than 2 months.

Complications in Burn Hand Rehabilitation

All patients with significant hand burns will have some setbacks and delays in the course of their rehabilitation and retraining. Commonly, despite excellent care and state of the art wound dressings, wound excision and skin resurfacing patients will continue to be plagued with a number of postburn sequellae and less than optimal outcomes related to the depth of their original injury.[152] These include problems with wound healing and development of deformities of the thumb or small finger. Boutonniere deformities remain common, as do contracted burned palms, especially in pediatric patients. Furthermore, patients who suffer from burns of the hand also can develop significant bouts of depression and post-traumatic stress disorders, which impair the burned survivors ability to participate fully with the rehabilitation progress. Peripheral neuropathies are reported resulting in weakness and altered sensations in the hands. Some patients also develop problems of reflex sympathetic dystrophy as with other hand injuries. Heterotopic ossification is reported much less commonly now, probably due to a heightened awareness of its development.

Postburn reconstruction

There is no 'cookbook' for reconstructing the burned hand. Multiple issues can color the chances for a successful outcome. What is the endpoint of surgical effort? Is it when the patient tires, becomes discouraged, or ceases to return? These questions are not rhetorical. Whereas an appendectomy cures appendicitis, no single procedure or series of procedures cures burns … A thoughtful surgical plan set up in conjunction with the burn team and with timed goals gives the patient the best chance for success.

Salisbury, 2000[152]

Developing a Reconstructive Plan (Figure 14.15)

Half of the reconstructive demands for patients with severe burns involve the upper extremity, and half again of these involve the hand.[160] However, the presence of an anatomic abnormality is not an automatic indication for surgical treatment[152] (**Figure 49.16**). Timing of a surgical plan revolves around therapy and vocational rehabilitation. Patients may place a higher value on a facial reconstruction, even if purely aesthetic, than they do with many of the postburn deformities.[152] Many patients simply adapt to their boutonniere fingers or slight contractures, and tire of the surgical process following recovery from their acute injury. Other patients are not compliant with their hand therapy and therefore, will not be good candidates for completing complex reconstructive maneuvers.

The key to the plan is an ability to communicate between surgeon and patient.[164] Patients need to understand from the surgeon what is possible and what is realistic. Surgeons need to listen to the patients to determine exactly what they need and what they desire. For some patients, the loss of self-image associated with the burn

of the hand or with other burns, is so devastating that they may not want additional deformity, but opt for another treatment regardless of advantages or expected gains. For example, a young woman who has lost multiple fingers may opt for a metacarpal stacking as opposed to a toe-to-hand transfer simply because her feet are still normal.

In formulating the plan for the reconstruction of the burned hand, it is important to take into account the rest of the extremity[25] (**Figure 49.17**). In the upper extremity, function of the elbow is critical to adequate positioning of the hand, given deformity at all three major joint levels. It is often appropriate to do releases of wrist, elbow and axilla, and complete large motion reconstructions prior to attempting finer motion reconstruction of the hand. However, it is also possible to complete all of the releases at a single setting. The most common contracture of the upper extremity is the axilla.[41] The most common reconstruction need of the post-burn hand is a web space release.[160] Timing of initiation of burn reconstruction is patient-dependent. Early releases can be performed during early active scar maturation.[64]

Common Sequellae of Hand Burns

Postburn deformities are still common despite improvements in acute care.[152] These include:

- first webspace thumb adduction contractures;
- other webspace contractures;
- dorsal skin contractures;
- fifth-finger abduction deformity;
- metacarpal phalange joint extension deformities;
- extensor tendon adhesions;
- Boutonniere deformities;
- PIP flexion deformities;
- median and ulnar nerve compression eropathies;
- amputation effect secondary to ischemic gangrene;
- elbow and axillary contractures; and
- heterotopic ossification of elbow or wrist.[152]

Obviously, most of hand contractures do not occur in isolation, but as combinations of the above. Also, hand problems commonly exist with other body part deformities.[162] Reconstruction of other areas often takes priority and precedence over reconstruction of the hand, especially if the patient is able to adapt to the deformity. Subsequent reconstructive surgery is needed in only 0.65% of Class I hand burn injuries. In Class II injuries, 6.5% of the patients require reconstruction. In Class III injuries, approximately 66% of the patients require one or more post-reconstructive procedures. In spite of this, only about 9% of these Class III patients cannot perform activities of daily living with their reconstructed hands.

Surgical Treatment of Burn Scar Contractures

Principles for reconstruction of burn scar contractures include:

1. incisional release of scars at each joint level to allow for maximum restoration of movement;
2. excisional removal of hypertrophic scars when feasible;
3. restoration of transverse and longitudinal hand arches;
4. release or lengthening of deep tissue contractures including but not limited to extensor tendons, lateral bands and/or accessory collateral ligaments;
5. stabilization of bones and joints in positions of function

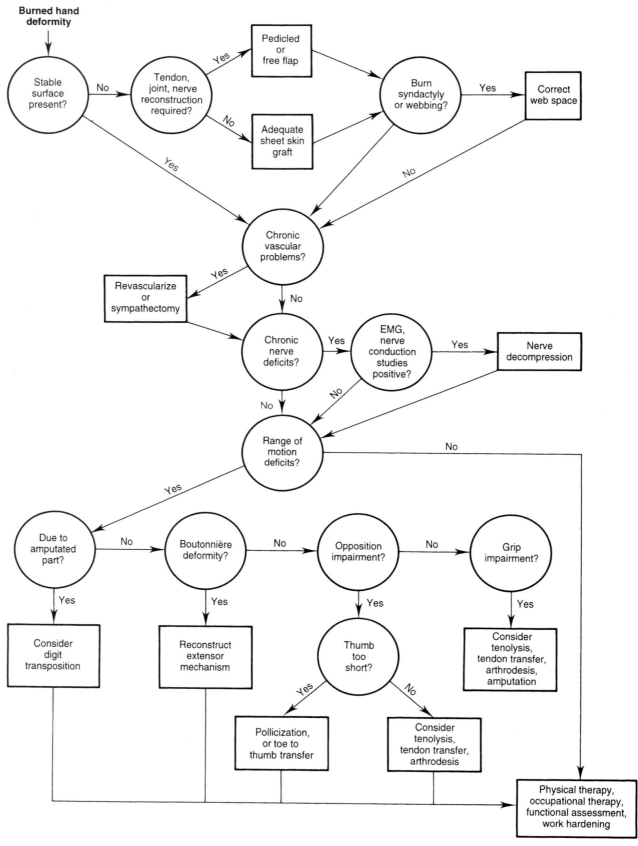

Fig. 49.15 Algorithm for reconstruction of the burned hand deformity. (Courtesy of Louis Strock, Robert McCauley *et al.* in *Total Burn Care* 1st Edition.)

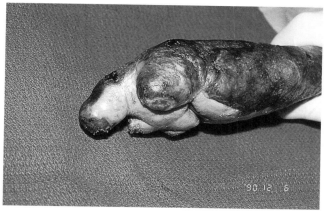

(a)

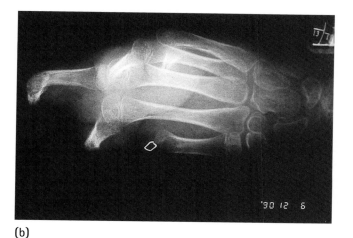

(b)

Fig. 49.16 (a) Mitten hand and (b) Mitten hand X-ray.

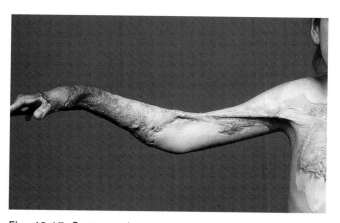

Fig. 49.17 Contracted upper arm.

with either internal K-wires, external splints or external skeletal fixation;

6. resurfacing of hand and digits with thin pliable acceptable tissues, skin grafts if tendons are protected – flaps if joints or tendons are apparent; and

7. use of flaps whenever feasible for reconstruction of web spaces.

McCauley and Barret[163] documented that the surgical correction of Grade IV contractures of the hand could produce excellent functional results in children. They recommended using skin graft coverage whenever possible for children due to ease and thinness and reserved flaps for teens. McCauley and co-workers stress long-term K-wire fixation of the MCP joints and IP joints to achieve maximal function, keeping pins in place for 4–6 weeks. The fingers are fixed using axial K-wires with MCPs at 80–90° and IPs at 180° for most pediatric hand contractures. In spite of long periods of internal fixation stabilization, reported hand results were excellent (**Figure 49.18**).

Thicker the Graft the Less the Contracture

It has been argued for some time whether split-thickness grafts or full-thickness grafts are better in the release of hand contractures. The general thinking is still thicker is better, especially for burns of toddlers.[24,64,127,164–166] In a study done by Pensler et al.,[167] however, there was no difference in treatment of contractures using split-thickness versus full-thickness grafts.

In a study of 129 patients comparing full-thickness and split-thickness grafts, 63% of patients underwent full-thickness

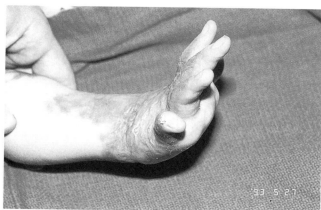

(a)

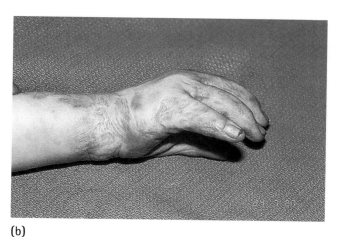

(b)

Fig. 49.18 Extensor contracture; (a) contracted hand; (b) released hand.

grafting.[168] The most common areas of grafting included axilla, hand and wrist, and head and neck. Greater patient satisfaction was reported with the full-thickness grafts. Children tended to require re-release of grafted areas during growth spurts. Split-thickness grafts required more re-releases than full-thickness grafts and recurred earlier.[168]

The largest problem with the use of full-thickness graft for postburn reconstruction is its lack of ability for coverage. It also requires more time to apply. One way to overcome this shortcoming is through the use of expanded full-thickness grafts, which have been shown to behave identically to a regular full-thickness graft.[169]

There have been anecdotal reports of use of Integra™ for release of contractures. FDA approval for Integra™ reconstruction is expected at the time of this writing. Currently, long-term data are not available for effectiveness in its long-term use.

Skin grafting can also be extremely useful for treatment of hypopigmentation of the hand. Hypopigmentation areas can be treated by dermabrasion and epithelial sheet graft application.[170,171]

Flaps for Hand Resurfacing

A number of flaps have been reported in the literature as being extremely useful for resurfacing the postburn hand. Although it is beyond the scope of this chapter to present all flaps, they include:

- reverse proper digital artery flap;
- reverse dorsal digital flap;
- reverse first and second metacarpal flaps;
- reverse forearm flaps including ulnar, radial, posterior interosseous;
- pedicle distal flaps; and
- free tissue free flap transfer.[136,172-174]

The reverse forearm flaps have shown extreme versatility and usefulness in closure and coverage of the postburn hand following contracture, and scar release. They are thin, pliable, close to the site of coverage and extremely versatile in their use. Flaps can be harvested as fascial only flaps and covered with skin grafts to provide some of the advantages of flap coverage, but donor site morbidity is limited. Each, however, does sacrifice a major vessel to the hand. The dorsal ulnar artery flap, which is based on a small segment of the ulnar artery, does not require sacrifice of the entire vessel.[175-177]

Pedicle distal flaps, such as the groin flap or abdominal flap, remain a workhorse of hand reconstruction.[135,178] Generally, they involve a multistaged procedure for attachment, separation and subsequent debulkings.

Free flaps have become the new standard for reconstruction of a multitude of soft-tissue defects, including burned and postburned hands. Use of free flaps requires presence of satisfactory recipient vessels, which must be documented in postburn hand injuries. The presence of the vessels can be determined by Doppler flowmetry, color flow duplex ultrasound, or angiographic flow. A segment of vessel is chosen for an anastomosis, which is close to the reconstruction but outside the zone of injury. Adequacy of flow and patency is determined by intraoperative inspection under the microscope. The vessel is deemed suitable for anastomosis if there is a good spurt test.[179] In the burned hand, flaps can usually be connected into the radial artery and the cephalic vein in the anatomic snuffbox. Due to the three-dimensional curved surface of the dorsum of the hand, skin surface coverage required is often larger than expected with free tissue transfers.[143]

Free-flap Selection for the Hand Reconstruction

A number of flaps are available for thin free flap surfacing of the hand. Some of the old workhorse flaps for free tissue transfer, including the latissimus, muscle, scapular flap, the periscapular flap and the rectus abdominal flap, although useable, typically are not suitable due to their thickness and bulk. Streamline flaps offer a better alternative for free flap and resurfacing during reconstruction.[143] The five most commonly used flaps are the free radial forearm flap, the dorsalis pedis free flap, the temporoparietal fascial flap, the lateral arm flap or the arterialized venous free flap.[143]

The free radial forearm flap is often harvested from the opposite arm to provide a large surface area. Flap dimensions can easily cover the entire dorsum of the hand and digits. The flap is thin and supple and can be harvested as an innervated flap by including the lateral and medial antebrachial cutaneous nerves. However, the flap does require a sacrifice of a major vessel of the opposite arm. It also produces a large donor site deformity on the opposite arm, which typically is skin grafted.

The dorsalis pedis free flap may be harvested as a sensate flap by including the superficial peroneal cutaneous nerve. It is not large enough to cover the entire hand, but it does provide good coverage for the dorsum and proximal digits. It can be harvested with extensor tendons of the foot, allowing for composite reconstruction of the dorsal hand and tendons if needed. The dorsalis pedis flap can also be harvested with portions of the second metatarsal for bony reconstruction or MCP joint reconstruction. However, it does produce a significant donor deformity for the donor defect is generally skin grafted.

The temporoparietal fascial flap is harvested from the scalp as a fascial free flap, then covered with the skin graft. As a vascular fascia, it is extremely thin and pliable. Donor site morbidity is minimal as the scalp can be closed without evidence of harvest (**Figure 49.19**). The flap easily can resurface the entire dorsum of the hand. The flap can be harvested as a sensory flap if needed by including a portion of the auricular temporal nerve, but this is generally not indicated. The temporoparietal flap also has variable venous outflow making this somewhat more tenuous of a flap than the other two mentioned.

The lateral arm flap offers many of the advantages of the radial free forearm flap with greatly reduced donor site morbidity. This fasciocutaneous flap is harvested from the upper lateral arm. It is a thin flap with consistent vessels, easy to harvest. Donor defects less than 6 cm wide can be closed primarily. The flap can be made sensate by including a portion of the posterior brachial cutaneous nerve. However, the flap size is still smaller than that available with either the radial forearm or temporoparietal free flaps.

Arterial venous free flaps offer the advantages that they preserve major arteries and can be elevated easily without deep dissection. They are thin, nonbulky tissues with flap sizes up to 14×9 cm. In experienced hands, harvest has been reported to take no longer than 25 minutes, with subsequent anastamosis of an artery to a vein and at least two vein to veins to improve venous outflow.[180,181] These can provide for a large vascular pedicle, are quick and easy to harvest, and do not require sacrifice of a major vessel. However, they undergo a prolonged phase of congestion and ecchymosis and may be more problematic in early healing.

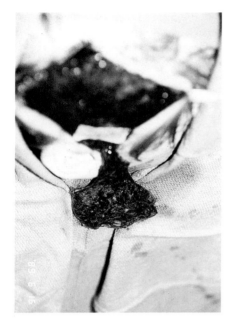

(a)

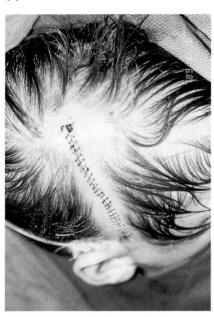

(b)

Fig. 49.19 (a) Temporoparietal flap, (b) donor site.

Surgical treatment of specified deformities

Chronic Postburn Joint Problems

In many patients, the involvement of contractures is not limited to the skin and soft tissues alone. The joints and associated supporting structures including ligaments and capsules are also involved.[182] At the time of scar release, MCP and proximal IP capsulotomies can be very helpful in improving motion, power, and dexterity to the hand if combined with an appropriate post-operative hand therapy program.[151] Without appropriate postoperative therapy, capsulotomies will increase scars and can result in poor

postoperative function. A program of capsulotomies should be discussed preoperatively with the designated therapist to assure adequate follow-up and treatment.[183]

If joints are severely damaged and painful, arthrodesis remains the procedure of choice.[42] Artheoplasties are fraught with hazard in the light of severe overlying scar and poor soft-tissue mobility. Attempted arthroplasties can result in chronic pain and eventual extrusion.[42] Arthrodesis typically eradicates pain and provides stability to the joint to allow for function. Arthrodesis may be the best alternative in significant boutonniere deformities, especially in the absence of a stable skin coverage or if the joints are already dislocated.

Volar Contractures

Since volar contractures generally involve the fingers, they are often included in management of release of the postburn contracted hand. The advantage over dorsal contractures is that tendons typically do not come into play with release of volar contractures. Adequate peritenon is present over the flexor sheaths to allow for direct application of skin grafts. On occasion, release is better achieved with the application of small, localized flaps to prevent subsequent graft contracture and recurrence of the contractures. Finger volar contractures can be released using a series of z-plasty flaps, which also provide better long-term stability than a skin graft.[184]

With release of volar contractures, nerve vascular bundles can easily be cut. Nerve vascular bundles become displaced volarly by getting encased in the scar. Furthermore, release of the contracture can produce vascular ischemia of the digits.[185] Once the nerve vascular structures become foreshortened in a long-standing contracture, attempting over-aggressive release can produce irreversible spasm within the vessel with phalangeal loss. Release the tourniquet and evaluate digits prior to completion of volar contracture release. These digits need to be monitored carefully during the postoperative period.

Web Contractures

Web contractures remain the bane of existence of many reconstructive burn and hand surgeries. Despite release, they often recur.[186] Web contractures, most commonly, merely consist of a dorsal hooding. On occasion, they could represent true interdigital contractures with burns syndactyly. Web contractures remain the most common sequelae of the burn hand injury despite newer and better methods for protection of the webs. Unless the web contractures involved the first web, they rarely cause significant functional deficits. Dorsal hooding can be released with multiple z-plasties, five-flap z-plasties or a series of release and grafting. For significant burn syndactyly, formation of a dorsal pedicle flap from the remaining soft tissues on the digits can be elevated to interpose within the base of the web. Reconstruction on either side of the central flap is completed using skin grafting (**Figure 49.20**).

Thumb Adduction Contraction

As previously noted, the thumb is responsible for 50% of the hand function. Thumb contractures remain a very difficult problem in the postburn reconstructed hand (**Figure 49.21**). In long-standing contracture there is shortening of the adductor musculature, changes in the balance of tendons, and contractures of the joint capsules. In less severe contractures, release can be completed

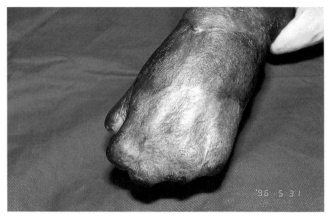

(a)

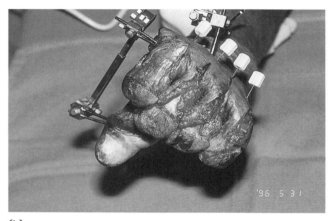

(b)

Fig. 49.20 Release of mitten hand (a) before and (b) after.

using a five-flap or jumping man z-plasty. A four-flap z-plasty can also be used. Typically, a simple z-plasty is not used because it produces too deep of a web space. Following a release, if there is significant carpal/metacarpal joint exposure, flap reconstruction is needed.

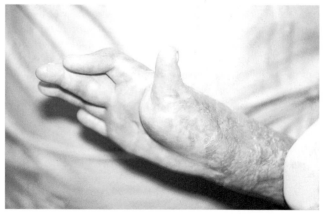

Fig. 49.21 Thumb adduction contracture and boutonniere deformity of the index finger.

Another option for first web release and reconstruction is to do a release with the aid of an external skeletal distracter[186,187] (**Figure 49.22**). The scar is released as soon as possible and the web reconstructed using full-thickness graft. An external skeletal fixation distracter is placed at the time of surgery and distracted maximally. Tourniquet is released and if there is a problem with blood flow or capillary blushing, the distracter is relaxed. The distracter is left in position and gradually expanded 1–2 mm a day until optimal positioning between first and second metacarpal heads is achieved. The external distracter can either remain in place or be replaced using a methacrylate bar. The hand function can continue with active and passive therapy during the healing phase. The external fixator can be removed 2–4 weeks after release following adequate healing.

Boutonniere Deformity

Boutonniere deformity involving the PIP joint digit in the postburn hand is the most common bone and joint defect[188] (**Figure 49.21**). It results from destruction of the central slip of the extensor tendon. The lateral bands on the extensor hood then slips past the volar axis of the PIP joint. The bands, therefore, become flexors at the PIP joint but remain extensors at the DIP joint.

Much has been written in the hand literature on the reconstruction of boutonniere deformities in general. Typically, reconstruction is performed by reconstruction of the central slip, either by taking portions from the distal central slip and rotating it backwards or taking portions of the lateral bands and interweaving them to reconstruct a stable central segment. However, repair in the burn patient often fails due to poor coverage over the PIP joint. Furthermore, with long-standing, boutonniere deformities, capsular contractures can occur along with bony changes within the joint itself. Therefore, in complicated boutonniere injuries, PIP fusion at 25–50° increasing towards ulnar digits may be the best surgical treatment.[150]

Complex Thumb Reconstruction

Options for thumb reconstruction include metacarpal stacking, distraction osteogenesis and pedicle flaps, pollicization, or toe-to-hand transfers. The goal in all of these is to provide for pinch or key grip. All are useful and feasible, but need to be adapted by the patient's desires and the state of the postburn hand at the time of reconstruction.

Partial thumb reconstruction can be completed using island pedicle flaps taken from other digits to provide for a sensate stable pad. This is done, however, with loss of sensation to the donor digit. Free tissue transfer options for simple soft-tissue reconstruction of the thumb include wrap-around flaps, first web space flaps taken from the foot for base reconstruction and toe pulp flaps to rebuild a sensate digital tip. All of these are useful for coverage of finger defects as neurosensory flaps and are based upon the first dorsal metatarsal artery and plantar digital nerves.

Metacarpal stacking has shown great utility in reconstruction of the first burned hand by providing a viable pinch-grip even in some of the most devastated multiple amputation hands (**Figure 49.23**). This procedure was first used by Littler in multiple digital reconstruction, and repeated in burn patients.[189] Metacarpal stacking provides for a stable vascularized osteocutaneous transfer with concomitant deepening of a first web.

Distraction osteogenesis and pedicled flaps do provide for a stable post with coverage. However, their usefulness is limited due

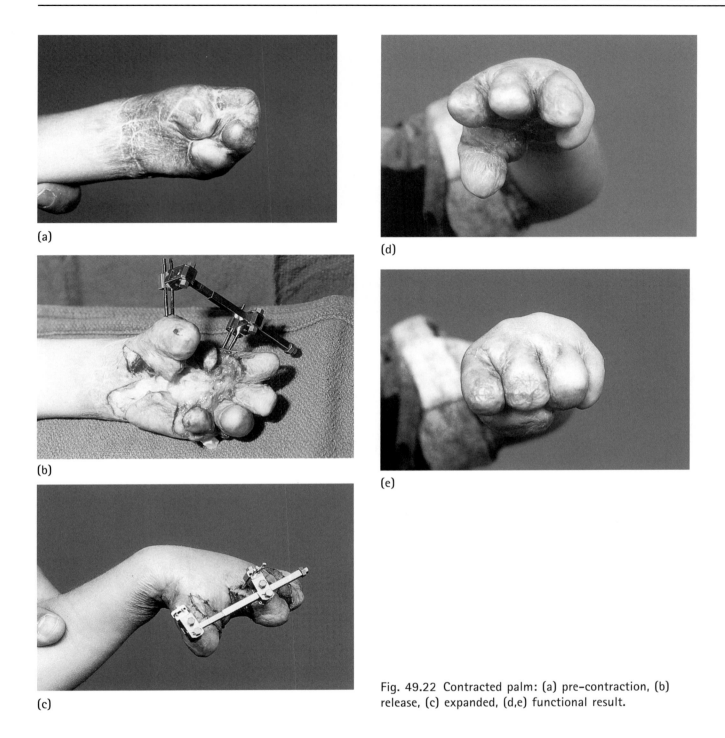

(a)

(b)

(c)

(d)

(e)

Fig. 49.22 Contracted palm: (a) pre–contraction, (b) release, (c) expanded, (d,e) functional result.

to poor sensation and less mobility than with either pollicization or toe-to-hand transfers. Pollicization is most commonly done for congenital deficiencies of the hand where forearm musculature is deficient and nerve and functional retraining occurs at a younger age.[190] Although useful in the burn hand, its popularity has been transplanted by toe-to-hand transfers.

Digital transfers in the hand allows for reestablishment of a functioning sensate thumb and provides opportunity for maximum recovery of thumb function (**Figure 49.24**). It requires, however, an intelligent cooperative patient for retraining and the availability of an experienced microvascular team.

Summary

Reconstruction of the burned hand begins with acute care. Early therapy, edema control, and adequate positioning are integral to the successful outcome of the burned hand. In the acute setting, the positioning of the MCP joint helps determine the position of

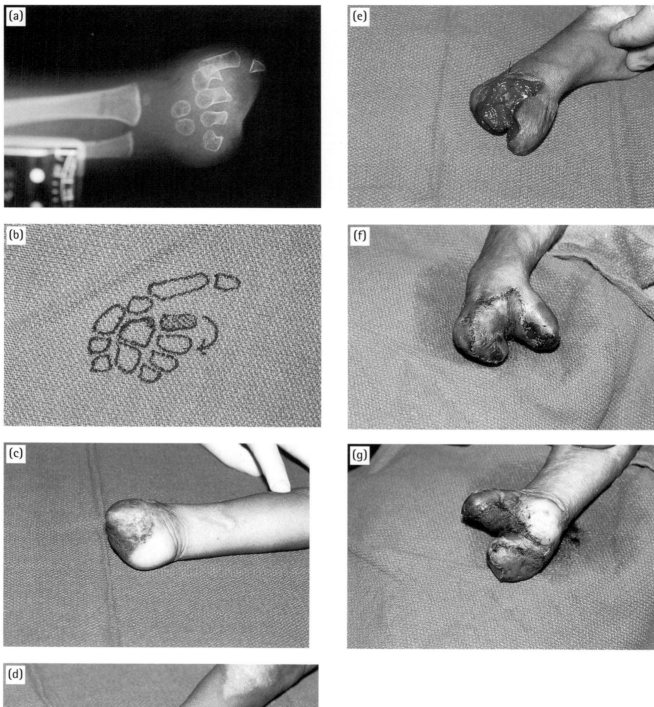

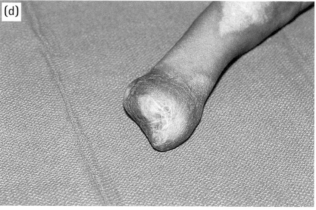

Fig. 49.23 In cases of an amputated mitten hand (a), metacarpal stacking may be helpful in restoring some function (b). Pre-op volar (c) and dorsal surfaces (d) are shown. The hand is split (e), and the residual second metacarpel and its overlying soft tissue is transferred on its vascular pedicle to the end of the residual third metacarpal. The residual soft tissue defect is skin grafted (f). Metacarpal stacking is used to deepen the first web space and lengthen either opposing hand pillars (g).

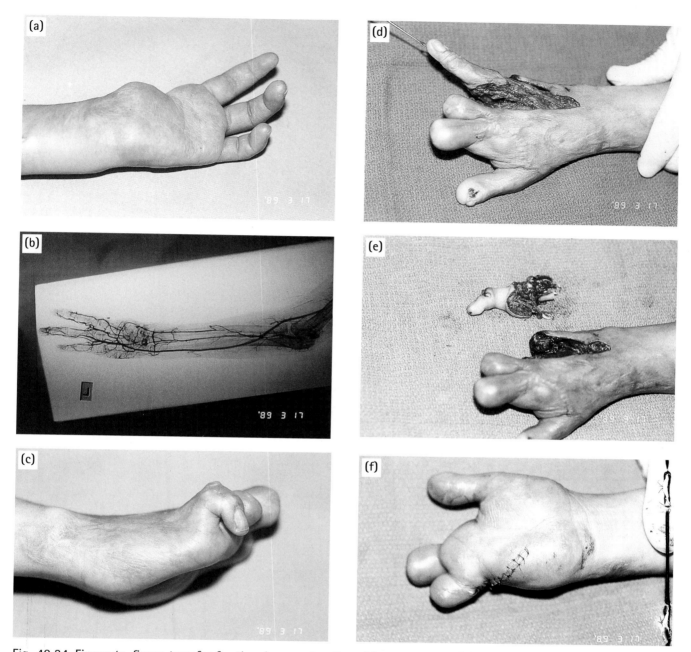

Fig. 49.24 Finger–to–finger transfer for thumb reconstruction: (a) pre-receptor. (b) Angiogram of the recipient hand. (c) A useless contracted opposite fifth digit is chosen for transfer. It is harvested (d), separated (e), and its defect closed (f).

the hand. Acute soft-tissue coverage is chosen based on limitations versus needs. Successful outcomes require cooperation of patient, surgeon and therapist in formulating an acceptable plan for maximum rehabilitation and recovery of the burned person. Despite adequate care in the initial period, a number of postburn sequellae and contractures still occur. Digital and hand recon-

struction require formulation of a well thought out plan. Microvascular transfer of thin, soft-tissue substitutes, provides further options for postburn reconstruction. Outcome of burned hand treatment is related to function and appearance as determined by return to work, quality of daily living and patient self-acceptance.

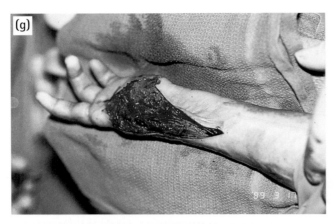

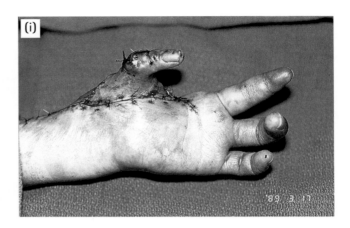

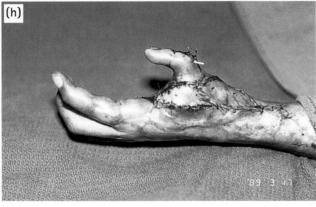

Fig. 49.24 (contd) Finger-to-finger transfer for thumb reconstruction: (g) The recipient hand is prepared for microvascular reanastomoses. A vascularized, sensate, but immobile thumb post is recreated with the transferred digit (h & i).

References

1 Luce MD, Edward The Acute and Subacute Management of the Burned Hand. *Clinics in Plastic Surgery* 2000; **27**: 49–63.

2 Rossiter ND, Chapman P, Haywood IA. How big is a hand? *Burns* 1996; **22**: 230–1.

3 Lund CC, Browder NC. The estimation of areas of burns. *Surg Gynecol Obstet* 1944; **79**: 352–8.

4 Helm PA. Burn rehabilitation: dimensions of the problem. *Clinic Plast Surg* 1992; **19**: 551–60.

5 Belliappa PP, McCabe SJ. The burned hand. *Hand Clin* 1993; **9**(2).

6 Pruitt BA. Epidemiology and general considerations. In: Salisbury RE, Pruitt BA, eds. Burns of the upper extremity. Philadelphia, PA: WB Saunders, 1976.

7 Bhende MS, Dandrea LA, Davis HW. Hand injuries in children presenting to a pediatric emergency department *Ann Emerg Med* 1993; **22**(10): 1512–3.

8 Gultespie et al, ABA Criteria for referral to a regional burn center, in Advanced Burn Life Support Course, 2000.

9 Griffin P, Leitch I. Burns to the Hand. Australian Family Physician Vol. 24, No. 2, February 1995; 166–72.

10 Salisbury RE, Dingeldein GP. The burned hand and upper extremity. In: Green, ed. Operative hand surgery. Churchill Livingstone, 1993, Chap 55, 2007–31.

11 Robson MC, Smith DJ. Burned Hand. In: MJ Jurkiewicz Ed., *Plastic Surgery: Principles and Practices*. St. Louis: CV Mosby, 1990.

12 Vidal-Trecan G, et al. 'Differences between burns in rural and in urban areas' *Burns* 2000; **26**(4): 351–8.

13 Bucek S. The primary treatment of severe burn hand by flap plastic. *ACTA Chirurgiae Plasticae* 1995: **37**(3): 83–8.

14 Salisbury RE, Pruitt BA. Burns of the Upper Extremity. Philadelphia: WB Saunders, 1976.

15 Tredget E. 'Management of the acutely burned upper extremity' Hand Clinics Vol. 16 No. 2 May 2000; 187–202.

16 Tredget EE, Shankowsky HA, Taerum TV, *et al.* The role of inhalation injury in burn trauma: A Canadian experience. *Ann Surg* 212: 720, 1991.

17 Quayle B. 'Tools For Burn Survivors' Presented at the Phoenix Society World Burn Congress, Atlanta Sept 1999.

18 Bostwick JA. Early management of burns of the hand. In: Bostwick JA, ed. *The art & science of burn care*. Rockville: Aspen Publ, 1987: 347.

19 Sheriff MM, Sato RM. Severe thermal hand burns – Factors affecting prognosis *JBCR* 1989; **15**: 42–6.

20 Engrav LH, Dutcher KA, Nakamura DY. Rating burn impairment. *Clin Plast Surg* 1992; **19**: 569–98.

21 American Medical Association. Guides to the evaluation of permanent impairment. 4th edn. Chicago: American Medical Association, 1994.

22 Magliacani G, Bormioli M, Cerutti V. Late results following treatment of deep burns of the hand. *Scand J Plast Reconstr Surg* 1979; **13**: 137.

23 Burke JF, Bondoc CC, Quinby WC. Primary surgical management of the deeply burned hand. *J Trauma* 1976; **16**: 593.

24 Bondoc CC, Quinby WC, Burke JF. Primary surgical management of the deeply burned hand in children. *J Pediatr Surg* 1976; **11**: 355.

25 Robson MC, Smith DJ, Vanderzee Roberts L. AJ. Making the burned hand functional. *Clin Plast Surg* 1992; **19**(3): 663–71.

26 Salisbury RE, Bevin AG. Atlas of Reconstructive Burn Surgery. Philadelphia: WB Saunders, 1981.

27 Howell JW. Management of the burned hand. In: Richard RL, Staley MJ, eds. Burn care and rehabilitation: principles and practice. Philadelphia: FA Davis Co, 1994: 531.

28 Pruitt BA: The burned patient: I. Initial care. *Curr Probl Surg* 1979; **16**: 13–27.

29 Sheridan RL, Baryza MJ, Pessina MA, *et al.* Acute hand burns in children: management and long-term outcome based on a ten-year experience with 698 injured hands. *Ann Surg* 1999; **229**: 558–64.

30 Sheridan RL, Hurley J, Smith MA, *et al.* The acutely burned hand: management and outcome based on a ten-year experience with 1047 acute hand burns. *J Trauma* 1995; **38**: 406–11.

31 Robson MC. Reconstruction and rehabilitation from admission. In: Bernstein NR, Robson MC, eds: Comprehensive approaches to the burned person. New Hyde Park, NY: Medical Exam Publishing 1983; 35–48.

32 Zawacki BE. Reversal of capillary stasis and prevention of necrosis in burns. *Ann Surg* 1974; **180**: 98–102.

33 Robson MD. Burn Sepsis. *Crit Care Clin North AM* 1988; **4**: 281–98.

34 Salisbury RE, McKeel DW, Mason AD. Ischemic necrosis of the intrinsic muscles of the hand after thermal injuries. *J Bone Joint Surg* 1974; **56A**: 1701.

35 Salisbury RE, Levine NS. The early management of upper extremity thermal injury. In: Salisbury RD, eds. *Burns of the Upper Extremity*. Philadelphia: WB Saunders, 1976: 36–46.

36 Muller MJ, Nicolai M, *et al*. Modern treatment of a burn wound. In: Herndon, ed. *Total Burn Care*. Philadelphia: WB Saunders, 1996, 136–47.

37 Tompkins RG, Remensnyder JP, Burke JF, *et al*. Significant reductions in mortality for children with burn injuries through the use of prompt eschar excision. *Ann Surg* 1988; **208**: 577–85.

38 Deitch EA, Wheelahan TM, Rose MP: Hypertrophic burn scars: Analysis of variables. *J Trauma* 1983; **3**: 895.

39 Fraulin FOG, Illmayer SJ, Tredget EE: Assessment of cosmetic and functional results of conservative versus surgical management of facial burns. *J Burn Care Rehabil* 1996; **17**: 19.

40 Tredget EE, Nedelec B, Scott PG, *et al*. Hypertrophic scars, keloids, and contractures: The cellular and molecular basis for therapy. *Surg Clin North Am* 1997; **77**: 701.

41 Frist W, Ackroyd R, Burke JF, *et al*. Long-term functional results of selective treatment of hand burns. *Am J Surg* 1985; **149**: 516.

42 Smith MA, Munster AM, Spence RJ. Burns of the hand and upper limb-a review. *Burns* 1998; **24**: 493–505.

43 Covey MH, Dutcher K, Heimbach DM, Marvin JA, Engrav LH, DeLateur B. Return of hand function following major burns. *J Burn Car Rehabil* 1987; **8**: 224–6.

44 Barillo DJ, Harvey KD, Hobbs CL, Mozingo DW, Cioffi WG, Pruitt BA. Prospective outcome analysis of a protocol for the surgical and rehabilitative management of burns to the hands. *Plast Reconstr Surg* 1997; **100**: 1442–51.

45 Heimbach D, Mann R, Engrav L. Evaluation of the Burn Wound. Management Decisions' In: Herndon, ed. Total Burn Care, 1996: 81–8.

46 Heimbach D, Engrav L, Grube B, *et al*. Burn depth: a review. *World J Surg* 1992; **16**: 10.

47 Heimbach DM, Afromowitz MA, Engrav LH, Marvin JA, Perry B. Burn depth estimation-man or machine. *J Trauma* 1984; **24**: 373–7.

48 Schiller WR, Garren RL, Bay RC, *et al*. Laser Doppler evaluation of burned hands predicts need for surgical grafting. *J Trauma* 1997; **43**: 35–40.

49 Stern MD. In vivo evaluation of microcirculation by coherent light scattering. *Nature* 1975; **254**: 56–8.

50 Holloway GA Jr, Watkins DW. Laser Doppler measurement of cutaneous blood flow. *J Invest Dermatol* 1977; **69**: 306–9.

51 Waxman K, Lefcourt N, Achauer B. Heated laser Doppler flow measurements to determine depth of burn injury. *Am J Surg* 1989; **157**: 541–3.

52 Green M, Holloway GA, Heimbach DM. Laser Doppler monitoring of microcirculatory changed in acute burn wounds. *J Burn Care Rehabil* 1988; **9**: 57–62.

53 Jackson DM. The diagnosis of the depth of burning. *Br J Surg* 1953; **40**: 588–96.

54 Robson MC, Del Becarro ET, Heggers JP *et al*. Increasing dermal perfusion after burning. *J Trauma* 1980; **20**: 722–5.

55 Heggers JP, Ko F, Robson MC, *et al*. Evaluation of burn blister fluid. *Plast Reconstr Surg* 1980; **65**: 798.

56 Robson MC, Del Beccaro EJ, Heggers JP. The effect of prostaglandins on the dermal microcirculation after burning, and the inhibition of the effect by specific pharmacological agents. *Plast Reconstr Surg* 1979; **63**: 781–7.

57 Greenhalgh, D. Management of acute burn injuries of the upper extremity in the pediatric population. *Hand Clinics*: 2000; Volume 16; No 2: 175–186.

58 Heggers J, Linares HA, *et al*. Treatment of infections in burns in Herndon: *Total Burn Care* 1996: 98–136.

59 Brown RL, Greenhalgh DG, Kagan RJ, *et al*. The adequacy of limy escharotomites/fasciotomies after referral to a major burn center. *J Trauma* 1994; **37**: 916.

60 Greenhalgh DG, Barthel PP, Warden GD. Comparison of back versus thigh donor sites in pediatric burn patients. *J Burn Care Rehabil* 1993; **14**: 21.

61 Gant TD. The early enzymatic debridement and grafting of deep dermal burns to the hand. *Plast Reconst Surg* 1980; **66**: 185.

62 Schwanholt CA, Daugherty MB, Gaboury T, *et al*. Splinting the pediatric palmar burn. *J Burn Care Rehabil* 1992; **13**: 460.

63 McCauley, R. Reconstruction of the pediatric burned hand. *Hand Clin* May 2000; **16**(2): 249–59.

64 Schwanholt C, Greenhalgh DG, Warden GD. A comparison of full-thickness versus partial-thickness autografts for the coverage of deep palm burns in the very young pediatric patient. *J Burn Care Rehabil* 1993; **14**: 29.

65 Reilly D, Garner W. Management of Chemical Injuries to the Upper Extremity. *Hand Clin*, May 2000; **16**(2): 215–23.

66 Gruber RP, Laub DR, Vistnes LM. The effect of hydrotherapy on the clinical course and pH of experimental cutaneous chemical burns. *Plast Reconst Surg* 1975; **55**: 200–4.

67 Kirkpatrick JJ, Enion DS, Burd DA. Hydrofluoric acid burns: A review. *Burns* 1995; **21**: 483–93.

68 Anderson WJ, Anderson JR. Hydrofluoric acid burns of the hand: Mechanism of injury and treatment. *J Hand Surg (Am)* 1988; **13**: 52–7.

69 Kirkpatrick JJ, Burd DA. An algorithmic approach to the treatment of hydrofluoric acid burns. *Burns* 1995; **21**: 495–99.

70 Aaron CK, Fudem GM, Hartigan CF. Treatment of extremity hydrofluoric acid burns: An in vivo histopathologic comparions of topical, locally infiltrated, intra-arterial, and regional IV calcium gluconate [abstract]. *Acad Emerg Med* 1996; **5**: 419.

71 Tajima T. Treatment of open crushing type industrial injuries of the hand and forearm. *J Trauma* 1974; **14**: 995–1011.

72 Sagi A, Amir A, Fliss DM, Van Straten O, Ofer G, Rosenberg L. Combined thermal and crush injury to the hand and fingers. *Burns* 1997; **23**: 176–81.

73 Nuchtern JG, Engrav LH, Nakamura DY, Dutcher KA, Heimbach DM, Vedder NB. Treatment of Fourth-Degree Hand Burns. *J Burn Care Rehabil* Jan/Feb 1995: 36–41.

74 Saffle JR, Davis B, Williams P. The American Burn Association Registry Participant Group. Recent outcomes in the treatment of burn injury in the United States: a report from the American Burn Association patient registry. *J Burn Care Rehabil* 1995; **16**: 219–232.

75 Logsetty S, Heimbach DM. Modern techniques for wound coverage of the thermally injured upper extremity. *Hand Clin* 2000; **16**: 205–214.

76 Tredget EE, Shankowsky HA, Groeneveld A, *et al*. A matched-pair, randomized study evaluating the efficacy and safety of Acticoat silver-coated dressing for the treatment of burn wounds. *J Burn Care Rehabil* 1998; **19**: 531.

77 McHugh TP, Robson MC, Heggers JP, *et al*. Theraputic efficacy of Biobrane in partial thickness and full thickness thermal injury. *Surgery* 1986; **100**: 661–4.

78 Terril PJ, Kedwards SM, Lawrence JC. The use of Gore-Tex bags for hand burns. *Burns* 1991; **17**: 161–5.

79 Bache J. Clinical evaluation of the use of Op-Site gloves for the treatment of partial thickness burns of the hand. *Burns* 1998; **14**: 413–6.

80 Hall M. Minor burns and hand burns: comparing treatment methods. *Professional Nurse* April 1997, Vol 12, No 7; pp 489–91.

81 Jostkleigrewe F, Brandt KA, Flechsig G, Bruck JC, Henckel von Donnersmarck G, Muhlbauer W. Treatment of partial thickness burns of the hand with the preshaped, semipermeable Procel Burn Cover: results of a multicentre study in the burn centres of Berlin, Duisburg and Munich. *Burns* 1995; **21**: 297–300.

82 Tilley W, McMahon S, Shukalck B, Rehabilitation of the Burned Upper Extremity. *Hand Clin* May 2000; **16**(2): 303–17.

83 Settle J. Hand burns. In Simon KL ed. Principles and Practice of Burns Management. New York: Churchill Livingston, 1996: 385–93.

84 Salisbury RE. Acute Care of the Burned Hand. In JW May Jr, JW Littler eds, Plastic Surgery, Vol. 8. Philadelphia: Saunders, 1990: 5399–417.

85 Donelan MB. Reconstruction of the burned hand and upper extremity. In: McCarthy, ed. Plastic Surgery. Philadelphia, PA: WB Saunders, 1990: 5452–482.

86 Newton N, Bubenicova M. Rehabilitation of the autografted hand in children with burns. *Physical Therapy* 1977; **57**: 1383.

87 Strickland JW. Biological basis for hand splinting. In: Fess EE, Philips CA, eds. Hand splinting: principles and methods. 2nd edn, St. Louis: Mosby, 1987: 43.

88 Littler JW. The finger extensor mechanism. *Surg Clin North Am* 1967; **47**: 415–432.

89 Moncrief JA, Switzer E, Rose LR. Primary excision and grafting in the treatment of third-degree burns of dorsum of the hand. *Plast Reconstr Surg* 1964; **33**: 305–16.

90 Boswick JA Jr. Management of the burned hand. *Hand Clin* 1990; **6**: 297–303.

91 Levine NS, Buchanan RT. The care of burned upper extremities. *Clin Plast Surg* 1986; **13**: 107.

92 Edstrom LE, Robson MC, Headley BJ. Evaluation of exercise techniques in the burn patient. *Burns* 1977; **4**: 113.

93 Covey M. Occupational Therapy. In: Boswick JA Jr. ed., *The Art and Science of Burn Care*. Rockville, Md.: Aspen Publishers, 1987.

94 Boswick JA Jr. Rehabilitation and Reconstruction of the Burned Hand. In: Boswick JA Jr. ed.. *The Art and Science of Burn Care*. Rockville, Md.: Aspen Publishers, 1987.

95 Tompkins RG, Burke JF, Schoenfeld DA, *et al*. Prompt eschar excision: A treatment system contributing to reduced burn mortality. A statistical evaluation of burn care of the Massachusetts General Hospital. *Ann Surg* 1986; **204**: 272–81.

96 Edstrom L, Robson M, Machioverna JR, *et al*. Management of deep partial thickness dorsal hand burns: Study of operative vs. non-operative therapy. *Orthop Rev* 1979; **8**: 27.

97 Goodwin CW, Maguire MS, McManus WF, Pruitt BA Jr. Prospective study of burn wound excision of the hands. *J Trauma* 1983; **23**: 510–517.

98 Salisbury RE, Wright P. Evaluation of early excision of dorsal burns of the hand. *Plast Reconstr Surg* 1982; **69**: 670–5.

99 Hunt JL, Sato RM. Early excision of full thickness hand and digit burns: Factors affecting morbidity. *J Trauma* 1982; **22**: 414–9.

100 Harden NG, Luster SH. Rehabilitation considerations in the care of the acute burn patient. *Crit Care Nurs Clin* 1991; **3**: 245.

101 Hunt JL, Sato R, Baxter CR. Early tangential excision and immediate mesh autografting of deep dermal hand burns. *Ann Surg* 1979; **189**: 147, 151.

102 Burke JF, Bondoc CC, Quinby WC. Primary burn excision and immediate grafting: A method of shortening illness. *J Trauma* 1974; **14**: 389.

103 Levine BA, Sirenik K, Peterson H, *et al.* Efficacy of tangential excision and immediate autografting of deep second degree burns of the hand. *J Trauma* 1979; **19**: 670.

104 Peacock EE Jr, Madden JW, Trier WC. Some studies on the treatment of burned hands. *Ann Surg* 1970; **171**: 903.

105 Bondoc CC, Quinby WC Jr, Siebert J, *et al.* Management of acute thermal hand injuries. In: Tubiana R ed. *The Hand*. Philadelphia: WB Saunders, 1988: 766–74.

106 Kalaja E. Acute excision or exposure treatment? *Scand J Plast Reconstr Surg* 1984; **18**: 95.

107 Cope O, Langohr JL, Moore FD, *et al.* Expeditious care of full-thickness burn wound by surgical excision and grafting *Ann Surg* 1947; **125**: 1.

108 McCorkle HJ, Silvani H. Selection of the time for grafting of skin to extensive defects resulting from deep thermal burns. *Ann Surg* 1945; **121**: 285.

109 Moncrief JA. Third degree burns of the dorsum of the hands. *Am J Surg* 1958; **96**: 535.

110 Labandter H, Kaplan I, Shavitt C. Burns of the dorsum of the hand: Conservative treatment with intensive physiotherapy versus tangential excision and grafting. *Br J Plast Surg* 1976; **29**: 352.

111 Sanford S, Gore D. Unna's Boot dressings facilitate outpatient skin grafting of hands. *J Burn Care Rehabil* 1996; **17**: 323–6.

112 Falcone PA, Edstrom LE. Decision making in the acute thermal hand burn: An algorithm for treatment. *Hand Clin* 1990; **6**: 233.

113 Sykes PJ. Severe burns of the hand: a practical guide to their management. *J Hand Surg (Br)* 1991; **16**: 6–12.

114 Lorenz C, Petriac A, Hohl HP, Wessel L, Waag KL. Early wound closure and reconstruction. Experience with a dermal substitute in a child with 60 percent surface area burn. *Burns* 1997; **23**(6): 505–8.

115 Griffin PA, Leitch IO. Burns to the hand. Australian Family Physician 1995; **24**(2).

116 Mann R, Honari S, Meyer NA, *et al.* Prospective randomized trial of thick versus medium-thickness grafts for dorsal hand burns. In: American Burn Association Annual Meeting. Chicago, IL: Mosby, 1998.

117 Janzekovic Z. A new concept in the early excision and grafting of burns. *J Trauma* 1970; **10**: 1103–8.

118 Hallock GG. Distal Based Flaps for Reconstruction of Hand Burns. *J Burn Care Rehabil* 1997; **18**: 332–7.

119 Janzekovic Z. A new concept: Early excision and immediate grafting of burns. *J Trauma* 1970; **10**: 1103.

120 Fraulin FOG, Tredget EE: Subcutaneous instillation of donor sites in burn patients. *Br J Plast Surg* 1993; **46**: 324.

121 Vedung S, Hedlung A: Fibrin glue: Its used for skin grafting of contaminated burn wounds in areas difficult to immobilize. *J Burn Care Rehabil* 1993; **14**: 356–8.

122 Boeckx W, Vandevoort M, Blondeel P, *et al.* Fibrin glue in the treatment of dorsal hand burns. *Burns* 1992; **18**: 395–400.

123 Strock LL, McCauley RL, Smith DS, *et al.* Reconstruction of the burned hand. In: Herndon DN, *Total Burn Care*. Philadelphia: WB Saunders, 1996: 506.

124 Burm MD, Jin Sik and Oh MD, Suk Joon. Fist Position for Skin Grafting on the Dorsal Hand: II. Clinical Use in Deep Burns and Burn Scar Contractures. *Plast Reconstr Surg* 2000; **105**: 581.

125 Burm JS, Chung CH, Oh SJ. Fist position for skin grafting on the dorsal hand: I. Analysis of length of the dorsal hand surface in hand positions. *Plast Reconstr Surg* 1999; **104**: 1350.

126 Brody GS. Management of Stiff Metacarpophalangeal and Interphalangeal Joints. In: May JW Jr, and JW Littler eds, Plastic Surgery, Vol. 7. Philadelphia: Saunders, 1990.

127 Fifer TD, Pieper D, Hawtof D. Contraction rates of meshed, nonexpanded split-thickness skin grafts versus split-thickness sheet grafts. *Ann Plast Surg* 1993; **31**: 162.

128 Vande Berg JS, Rudolph R. Immunohistochemistry of fibronectin and actin in ungrafted wounds and wounds covered with full- and split-thickness skin grafts. *Plast Reconstr Surg* 1993; **91**: 684.

129 Warden GD, Saffle JR, Kravitz H. A two-stage technique for excision and grafting of burn wounds. *J Trauma* 1982; **22**: 98.

130 Archer SB, Henke A, Greenhalgh DG, *et al.* The use of sheet autografts to cover patients with extensive burns. *J Burn Care Rehabil* 1998; **19**: 33.

131 Schwanholt C, Daugherty MB, Gaboury T, Warden GD. Splinting the pediatric palmar burn. *J Burn Care Rehabil* 1992; **13**: 460.

132 Barret JP, Desai MH, Herndon DN. The isolated burned palm in children: epidemiology and long-term sequelae. *Plast Reconstr Surg* 2000; **105**: 949–52.

133 Hallock GG. The simple cross-finger flap: technique and vascularanatomy. *Orthop Rev* 1984; **13**: 91–6.

134 Hallock GG. Homodigital flaps: Especially for treatment of the burned hand. *J Burn Care Rehabil* 1995; **16**: 503–7.

135 Hanumadass M, Kagan R, Matsuda T. Early coverage of deep hand burns with groin flaps. *J Trauma* 1987; **27**: 109.

136 Hallock GG. Distal-based flaps for reconstruction of hand burns. *J Burn Care Rehabil* 1997; **18**: 332.

137 Grobbelaar AO, Harrison DH. The Distally Based Ulnar Artery Island Flap in Hand Reconstruction. *The Journal of Hand Surgery*. Vol22 B No. 2 April 1997: 204–211.

138 Zancolli EA, Angrigiani C. Posterior interosseous island forearm flap. *J Hand Surg (Br)* 1988; **13**: 130.

139 Chick LR, Lister GD, Sowder L. Early free-flap coverage of electrical and thermal burns. *Plast Reconstr Surg* 1992; **89**: 1013.

140 Millard RD. The crane principle for the transport of subcutaneous tissue. *Plast Reconstr Surg* 1969; **43**: 451–67.

141 Matsumura H, Engrav LH, Nakamura DY, Vedder NB. The use of the Millard 'Crane' Flap for deep hand burns with exposed tendons and joints. *J Burn Care Rehabil* 1999; **20**: 316–9.

142 Asko-Seljavaara S, Pitkanen J, Sundell B. Microvascular free flaps in early reconstruction of burns in the hand and forearm. Case reports. *Scand J Plast Reconstr Surg* 1984; **18**: 139–44.

143 Takeuchi M, Nozaki M, Sasaki K, Nakazawa H, Sakurai H. Microsurgical reconstruction of the thermally injured upper extremity. *Hand Clinics*; Vol 16; No 2; May 2000: 261–268.

144 Habel MB. The burned hand: A planned treatment program. *J Trauma* 1978; **18**: 587.

145 Torres-Gray, Johnson J, Mlakar J. 'Rehabilitation of the Burned Hand'. *Journal of Care and Rehabilitation*, 1996; **17**(2): 161–4.

146 Rice S, Fish J, Gomez M. The role of digital imaging in the treatment of the burn patient. In Proceedings of the Canadian Burn Special Interest Group, American Burn Association Meeting, Orlando, FL, 1999.

147 Brandsma JW. Development of a uniform record for patients with burns of the hand. *J Hand Therapy* 1999; **12**: 333–6.

148 American Society of Hand Therapists. Clinical Assessment Recommendations. 2nd edn. Chicago, Ill: ASHT, 1992.

149 Harvey KD, Barillo DJ, Hobbs CL, *et al.* Computer-assisted evaluation of hand and arm function after thermal injury. *J Burn Care Rehabil* 1996; **17**: 176–80.

150 Beasley RW. Secondary repair of burned hands. *Hand Clin* 1990; **6**: 319–41.

151 Parry SW. Reconstruction of the burned hand. *Clin Plast Surg* 1989; **16**: 577–86.

152 Salisbury, RE. Reconstruction of the burned hand. *Clin Plast Surg* 2000; **27**: 65–9.

153 Helm PA, Walker SC, Peyton SA. Return to work following hand burns. *Arch Phys Med Rehabil* 1986; **67**: 297–8.

154 Tanttula K, Vuola J, Asko-Seljavaara S. Return to employment after burn. *Burns* 1997; **23**: 341–4.

155 Engrav LH, Covey MH, Dutcher KD, Heimbach DM, Walkinshaw MD, Marvin JA. Impairment, time out of school, and time off from work after burns. *Plast Reconstr Surg* 1987; **79**: 927–34.

156 Saffle JR, Tuohig GM, Sullivan JJ, Shelby J, Morris SE, Mone M. Return to work as a measure of outcome in adults hospitalized for acute burn treatment. *J Burn Care Rehabil* 1996; **17**: 353–61.

157 Helm PA, Walker SC. Return to work after burn injury. *J Burn Care Rehabil* 1992; **13**: 53–7.

158 Hu X, Wesson DE, Logsetty S, *et al.* Functional limitations and recovery in children with severe trauma. A one-year follow-up. *J Trauma* 1994; **37**: 209–13.

159 Baker RA, Jones S, Sanders C, *et al.* Degree of burn, location of burn, and length of hospital stay as predictors of psychosocial status and physical functioning. *J Burn Care Rehabil* 1996; **17**: 327–33.

160 Brou JA, Robson MC, McCauley RL, *et al.* Inventory of potential reconstructive needs in the patient with burns. *J Burn Care Rehabil* 1989; **10**: 555–60.

161 Mlakar J 'The reconstructive process: On the Road to Recovery' Presented at World Burn Congress, San Francisco, July 2000.

162 Achauer BM. Burns of the upper extremity in burn reconstruction. New York: Thieme Medical Publishers, 1991: 100–33.

163 McCauley RL, Barrett JP. Management of extreme burn hand deformities in children. *Proc Am Burn Assoc* 1999; **20**: S214.

164 Sloan DF, Huang TT, Larson DL, Lewis SR. Reconstruction of eyelids and eyebrows in burned patients. *Plast Reconstr Surg* 1976; **58**: 340.

165 Merrell SW, Saffle JR, Schnebly A, Kravitz M, Warden GD. Full-thickness skin grafting for contact burns of the palm in children. *J Burn Care Rehabil* 1986; **7**: 501.

166 Blair VP, Brown JB. The use and uses of large split skin grafts of intermediate thickness. *Surg Gynecol Obstet* 1929; **49**: 82.

167 Pensler JM, Steward R, Lewis SR, Herndon DN. Reconstruction of the burned palm: full thickness versus split-thickness skin grafts long term follow up. *Plast Reconstr Surg* 1988; **81**: 46.

168 Iwuagwu FC, Wilson D, Bailie F. The use of skin grafts in postburn contracture release: a ten-year review. *Plast Reconstr Surg* 1999; **103**: 1198–1204.

169 Bauer BS, Vicari F, Richard ME, *et al*. Expanded full-thickness skin grafts in children: case selection, planning, and management. *Plast Reconstr Surg* 1993; **92**: 59.

170 Kahn AM, Cohen MJ, Kaplan L. Treatment for depigmentation resulting from burn injuries. *J Burn Care Rehabil* 1991; **5**: 468–73.

171 Kahn A, Cohen M. Vitiligo: Treatment by dermabrasion and epithelial sheet grafting. *Journal of the American Academy of Dermatology*; Oct 1995: 646–8.

172 Martin D, Bakhach J, Casoli V, *et al*. Reconstruction of the hand with forearm island flaps. *Clin Plast Surg* 1997; **24**: 33–48.

173 Chang SM. The distally based radical forearm fascia flap. *Plast Reconstr Surg* 1990; **85**: 150–1.

174 Foucher G, Khouri RK. Digital reconstruction with island flaps. *Clin Plast Surg* 1997; **24**: 1–32.

175 Hallock GG. Distal-based flaps for hand coverage. *Contemp Orthop* 1995; **31**: 83–9.

176 Song RY, Gao YZ, Song YG, *et al*. The forearm flap. *Clin Plast Surg* 1982; **9**: 21.

177 el-Khatib H, Zeidan M. Island adipofascial flap based on distal perforators of the radial artery: An anatomic and clinical investigation. *Plast Reconstr Surg* 1997; **100**: 1762–6.

178 Rose EH. Small flap coverage of hand and digit defects. *Clin Plast Surg* 1989; **16**: 427–42.

179 Wei FC, Chen HC, Chuang DCC, *et al*. Second toe wrap-around flap. *Plast Reconstr Surg* 1991; **88**: 837.

180 Nakayama Y, Soeda S, Kasai Y. Flaps nourished by arterial inflow through the venous system: an experimental investigation. *Plast Reconstr Surg*, **67**: 328–334.

181 Woo SH, Jeong JH, Seul JH. Resurfacing Relatively Large Skin Defects of the Hand Using Arterialized Venous Flaps. *J Hand Surgery* April 1996; **21B**(2): 222–9.

182 Stern PJ, Neale Mw, Graham JJ, *et al*. Classification and treatment of postburn proximal interphalangeal joint flexion contractures in children. *J Hand Surg* 1987; **12A**: 450–7.

183 Salisbury FR. Hand management. In: Fisher SV, Helm PA, eds. Comprehensive rehabilitation of burns. Baltimore: Williams and Wilkins, 1984: 218.

184 Ebbehoj J. Y to V instead of Z to N. *Burns Incl Therm Inj* 1983; **10**: 121.

185 Roberts L, Meyers R, Pierre E, *et al*. Sensory analysis of nerve grafting in children with electrical burns of the upper extremity. *Proc Am Burn Assoc* 1996; **27**: 123.

186 Mancoll JS, Mlakar JM, McCauley RL, *et al*. Burn web space contractures – are they just a bad penny? *Proc Am Burn Assoc* 1996; **28**: 111.

187 Hirshowitz B, Karev A, Rousso. Combined double Z-plasty and V-Y advancement for thumb web contracture. *Hand* 1975; **7**(3): 291–3.

186 Mlakar JM, Rose K, Evans EB. 'Treatment of Pediatric First Web Contractures with External Skeletal Distraction', *Proc Am Burn Assoc (abstract)*, 1996.

188 Simpson RL, Flaherty ME. The burned small finger. *Clin Plast Surg* 1992; **19**: 673–82.

189 Littler JW: The neurovascular pedicle method of digital transposition for reconstruction of the thumb. *Plast Reconstr Surg* 1953; **12**: 303.

190 Ward JW, Penler JM, Parry SW: Pollicization for thumb reconstruction in severe pediatric hand burns. *Plast Reconstr Surg* 1985; **76**: 927.

Chapter 50

Reconstruction of the head and neck

John P Remensnyder

Matthias B Donelan

Introduction

Reconstruction of the severe deformities and scars of the face, head, and neck following healing from burns confronts the surgeon with some of the most challenging problems in reconstructive surgery. Two of the major issues requiring facial reconstruction of burn deformities are: (1) psychological problems due to facial abnormalities in patients of all ages and (2) potential inhibition of various forms of facial growth in children with severe facial scars. Facial deformities caused by the way facial burns heal and create scars of various varieties pose problems of the necessity of various approaches to burn facial reconstruction. Through knowledge of available reconstructive techniques, accurate diagnosis of tissue deficiency and secondary distortion, imaginative planning and definitive, careful execution of one's surgical plan are the bare minimum items for achieving improvements in a burn deformed face. The following are general considerations of various techniques needed for planning burn scar reconstruction of the face, head, and neck.

Nonoperative techniques

There are a number of nonoperative techniques available which may either produce a definitive improvement of facial burn scarring or make it possible to carry out subsequent surgery to greater advantage. Frequent elastic compression to recently healed facial burns offsets the tendency of the burned face to develop hypertrophic scars which can become aesthetically unattractive and devastating in producing facial distortions by scar contractures. Elastic facemasks that can be custom-designed and fitted are available. When used on recently healed burns of the face, elastic facemasks can avoid the development of heavy scars and also can help reduce hypertrophic scars that develop in a nontreated postburn face. In addition to elastic face masks, there are a variety of thermoplastic materials that are used to create rigid, custom-molded face masks retained by means of elastic straps around the head. Such rigid facemasks can press on healing areas or hypertrophic scars. The materials of rigid facemasks can be either transparent or opaque; there is an advantage to having a transparent facemask because alterations of the areas under pressure can be directly inspected through the facemask and timing of alterations or new procedures can be made accurately. Experience and technical finesse provide essentials in the fabrication and use of rigid face masks, which may require remodeling one or more times in order to control facial scar formation.

Other useful nonoperative techniques for partially restricting major facial scar formation is the topical use of certain pharmacological agents. The use of topical vitamin E (alphatocopherol) and the topical or intralesional injection of fluoridated steroids can be very useful. If the scarring is not extensive and treatment begun early, many patients will benefit from twice-daily application of concentrated vitamin E oil. Unfortunately, not all respond by scar softening and some patients have skin hypersensitivity to the carrier oil. Triamcinolone 0.025% can be used in the same way. One of the regular benefits of the topical use of triamcinolone is the relief of itching frequently caused by hypertrophic scars. If the topical use is not effective in reducing scar hypertrophy, 0.1% triamcinolone solution can be injected into multiple sites of the scar being careful not to exceed the proper dose. Improvement may not be seen for a few weeks or a month.

Scar Revision

A wide variety of local scar revisions are useful in burn face reconstruction but are often overlooked when preoccupied with more extensive procedures. Direct excision of limited burn scars with primary closure can be gratifying, particularly with careful attention to postoperative wound care. This is also applicable to excessively prominent scars of the edges of previously placed skin grafts and flaps. Z-plasties are one of the most reliable and dependable of techniques for revision of limited facial scars. These techniques break up scar lines, redirect tension forces and can reset misplaced features. Z-plasties are particularly useful in correcting specific forms of scar in the nasolabial area, the oral commissures, the para-alar nasal regions, the medial and lateral periorbital canthi, and the ear lobe. Occasionally, burn scars produce relatively limited but complicated areas of scarring, particularly in the cheek and mandibular areas. Often, scars of this type in these areas are susceptible to correction by excision and single or multiple local flap rotation – the exact configuration of which is determined by the nature of the scar.

Split-thickness Skin Grafts

One must be cautious in using split-thickness skin grafts for major facial reconstruction because they do not, by their nature, offset subsequent wound contraction. If such skin grafts are to be used at all, they should be used as medium-thickness skin grafts so that subsequent contractures will be lessened. Post-graft contracture is particularly noticeable in soft, pliant areas such as the cheek, where there is no underlying firm support to offset the contracting tendency. Areas that lend themselves to reconstruction utilizing split-thickness skin grafts are the chin complex, forehead, and the total aesthetic unit of the nose. Excision of hypertrophic or contracting scars of these areas with subsequent resurfacing by a split-thickness skin graft yield satisfactory results as the tendency to contraction is well offset by the underlying rigidity of the bony structures. Certainly one of the commonest applications of split-thickness skin grafting of the head and neck reconstruction is its use in correcting cervical contractures. Surgical releases of neck contractures often produce very large tissue defects which are most expeditiously resurfaced with a medium-thickness split-thickness skin graft which when healed must be maintained by a rigid neck collar for several weeks postoperatively.

Full-thickness Skin Grafts

The full-thickness skin graft is clearly the preferred skin graft for reconstruction of facial areas and structures. Because it includes the entire dermis and satisfies the full thickness requirement of a wound, there is little, if any, postoperative wound contraction. Color match is more critical using full-thickness skin grafts as opposed to split-thickness grafts as the ultimate skin graft color is more predictable. For this reason, it is important to use full-thickness skin grafts, when possible, from areas close to the face which will provide grafts that will match the special characteristics of facial skin better than such grafts from more distant sites. The appropriate regional donor sites for providing full-thickness skin grafts for facial reconstruction are the neck, upper chest, upper lateral chest and the retroauricular area (if not unduly ruddy). The temptation to excise small areas of hypertrophic scars, particularly about the upper and lower lips and the nose, and replacing with small full-thickness skin grafts must be avoided as small full-thickness skin grafts have the tendency to heap up due to minor graft edge contracture and produce unattractive results in the postoperative months. Full-thickness skin grafts are best used in the face to replace full aesthetic units of the face after complete scar excision. This concept extends to the use of full-thickness skin grafts from appropriate donor sites to replace scarred aesthetic facial units such as the cheek, chin and lower lip, upper lip, nose, and lower eyelids. Large aesthetic unit full-thickness skin grafts are usually removed from the upper anterior of lateral chest and the large donor sites must be resurfaced with split-thickness skin grafts. Full-thickness skin grafts applied to the face heal well, but require optimal postoperative compression and care to achieve best results; even then, later edge scar revision is occasionally necessary to give blending and smoothing to the final results.

Composite Grafts

Composite grafts are defined as free grafts of two or more kinds of tissue. Great care must be exercised for their use in order to achieve best results: a well vascularized bed to receive composite grafts is absolutely essential for their successful use as is careful postoperative compression to prevent early venous engorgement and loss. In addition, careful diagnosis of the exact extent of the anticipated defect ensures that a composite graft suffices for repair. Donor site considerations are paramount since one does not wish to inflict secondary deformity due to the donor site in otherwise normal structures. The ear is a common donor site of composite grafts and, in some burned patients, the ear also has scars. Composite skin–cartilage grafts from the ear for nasal alar reconstruction work best when the alar defect is modest and symmetry can be achieved. Hair-bearing full-thickness skin grafts from the scalp for eyebrow reconstruction, while technically not a composite graft (since hair follicles are epidermal derivatives), are practically thought of and treated as composite grafts.

Pedicle Flaps

The use of pedicle flap tissue, when available from nonburn scarred donor sites, provides some of the finest results seen in burn reconstruction of the face. On the other hand, the inappropriate application of pedicle flaps result in grotesque reconstructive deformities due to excessive flap thickness, and generally require extensive secondary surgery to correct. Pedicle flaps for facial reconstruction, because they must be constructed in a very thin fashion, entail multiple preliminary surgical delays to create safe vascular supply for their eventual transfer. The certain special pedicle flap for major nasal reconstruction includes forehead flaps, scalping flaps and Tagliocozzi (upper arm) flaps. Pedicle flaps used for covering the releases of neck contractures often do not create appropriate results because the flaps are too bulky and do not match the active neck motion.

Hard-Tissue Replacement

Since most of the facial deformities imposed by thermal injury are fairly superficial, although some burns create very deep injuries, there are relatively few requirements for hard-tissue replacement in postburn reconstruction of the face and head. One of the most specific and frequent hard tissues is the use of rib cartilage superficially carved to replace missing ear cartilage framework as a result of burn injury. Bone grafts are needed for replacement of skull defects following electrical injuries, and split ribs are most useful for such reconstruction, although occasionally plates of synthetic material can be used for skull reconstruction. Rib grafts are also useful in replacing destroyed nasal bones and are most frequently used by a cantilever technique. Synthetic (such as silicone) implants properly placed against the bone can be useful in bulking out the deficient deep soft tissue of the chin pad lost due to burn injury.

General principles of head and neck reconstruction

The clinical activity of reconstruction of head and neck deformities due to burns has several general principles as described below. Each general principle provides a basis for approach to plan reconstruction with appropriate specific goals and techniques. Each of the important general principles is listed below with explanation of the principle and including specific example or requirements.

Gain Healing As Rapidly As Possible in Acute Facial Burns

By avoiding the storms of prolonged eschar separation, granulation tissue formation and secondary healing, one should be able to minimize scar formation and, hence, subsequent contracture and distortion of facial features. To avoid severe scar formation, one must not hesitate to excise early obvious full-thickness or deep partial-thickness burns and provide immediate autogenous grafts. Particularly in patients who have suffered extensive burns, burns of the face should be treated with topical antiseptic agents for 7–10 days in order to determine the burn depth and, at that point, deep facial burns should be tangentially excised and grafted with sheet grafts. There is virtually no indication for using meshed grafts in facial resurfacing because the mechanical appearance of healed meshed grafts create additional facial deformity.

Figure 50.1a shows the deeply burned face of a 5-year-old Native American girl 3 days after sustaining a 20% total body surface area (TBSA) flame burn involving her face, hands, and lower abdomen. On the 10th postburn day, the burn wound of her face was carefully excised tangentially using a free-hand skin graft knife leaving a well-vascularized wound bed and normal facial contour. **Figure 50.1b** shows the sheet autografts 4 days after application with the graft edges placed in esthetically acceptable locations. **Figure 50.1c** demonstrates her condition 5 years later, after a subsequent nasal reconstruction but no further surgery on her face or forehead, with a reasonable facial contour, soft and gratifying lack scar contracture. A few minor scar revisions were performed in the succeeding years.

Use Time, Physical Means and Pharmacologic Agents to Hasten Scar Maturation

Orderly scar maturation is essential in order to obtain good surgical and esthetic result, especially in the burned face. (**Table 50.1**) lists the familiar nonoperative adjuncts that are clinically useful in helping to control burn scar formation and hasten its maturation.

In selected instances, time alone will allow normal bodily processes to improve facial scars with softening and return to normal coloration, texture, and contour. Unfortunately, it is not always possible to identify a burn scarred patient who will undergo long-term satisfactory healing without active intervention. Massage of facial scars, using skin softeners to reduce friction, results in scar improvement but must be done regularly over a period of weeks or months. Occasionally, massage using steroid ointments or vitamin E will hasten the scar maturation and improvement process. Injection of steroid suspensions in multiple locations in a developing hypertrophic scar can occasionally prevent the development of unsightly scars. One of the keys to insuring good scar formation following burn healing or surgical procedures is the relief of excessive motion or tension by the use of facial splints and/or neck splints to relieve tension facial tissues. Prolonged elastic pressure plus the use of rigid facial conformers represents one of the most reliable methods of preventing hypertrophic scar formation following excision and grafting of the acutely burned face (see **Figure 50.2**). **Figure 50.2a** is an intraoperative photograph showing the wound bed following tangential excision of a deep facial burn in a 15-year-old boy who sustained a 51% TBSA flame burn. His deep facial burn was excised on the 7th postburn day and grafted with sheets of autografts. After good initial healing, he was fitted with an opaque plastic facial conformer which was held in place by an elastic facemask (**Figure 50.2b**) which he wore for several months after healing. **Figure 50.2c** shows his condition 5 years later, demonstrating absence of distorting contractures, softly texture grafts, and a well-maintained facial contour.

Do Not Wait for Scar Maturation in Areas of High Functional Priority

Contracture and hypertrophic scar formation in certain facial areas of high priority must be relieved early, even during the acute coverage phase, if necessary in order to prevent severe functional disability. Areas of such high priority include upper and lower eyelids, upper and lower lips, and the neck. Prolonged contracture of eyelids creates chronic conjunctivitis and exposes the cornea to irritation, which may lead to corneal ulceration. Failure to relieve lip contractures makes eating and fluid retention difficult. If allowed to persist too long, lip contractures destroy the normal tongue–lip balance, and the teeth of growing children will begin to incline labially and impair the normal bite.

This principle is further illustrated in **Figure 50.3**. This 11-year-old girl rapidly developed a profound cervical contracture only 2 months after healing of a 76% TBSA burn (**Figure 50.3a**). Mouth closure was difficult, her head position was extremely uncomfortable, and motion was markedly limited. At this point, she was treated with a wide cervical release and scar excision, and resurfacing of the area with split-thickness skin graft (**Figure 50.3b**). This achieved a good neck–chin relation and relieved the contracting forces affecting her lower lip and face. Eighteen years later (**Figure 50.3c**), with only one further minor lower neck graft, her condition shows that she maintained a good release, had reasonably flat scars, and a pleasing normal contour of her lower face and neck was preserved.

Conserve Best Donor Areas in Extensive Burns when Possible for Facial Reconstruction

In extensively burned patients whose faces will need future reconstruction, the best remaining donor area, if such exists, should be saved for facial reconstruction. Obviously, in an extensively burned individual all the limited donor sites have to be used in order to preserve life and gain initial healing. If the face will clearly need reconstruction at a later date, extra careful attention must be paid to avoiding infection and other complications in the limited donor sites. In this way, the donor sites will be available for later facial reconstruction.

A good example of this situation is shown in **Figure 50.4**. This 5-year-old boy suffered 86% TBSA flame burn from a gasoline explosion and it was anticipated that he would need complex facial reconstruction following healing. His initial treatment involved early excision with allografting, followed by

Table 50.1 Physical and pharmacological agents
Time
Massage
Steroids
Vitamin E
Skin softeners
Splints and collars
Elastic pressure
Rigid conformers

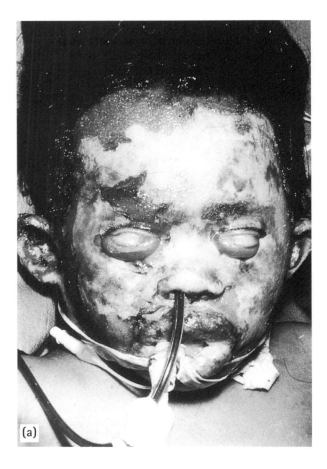

(a)

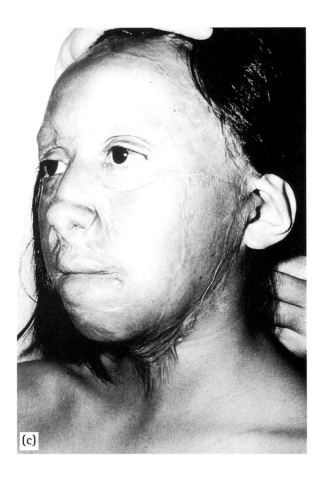

(c)

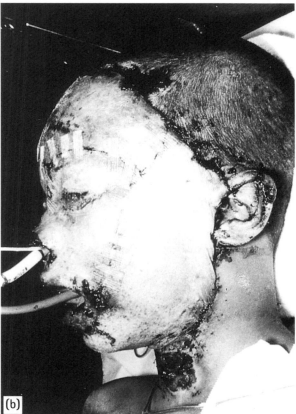

(b)

autografting and part of his wounds covered with laboratory-grown cultured epidermal cells. This shows the unburned buttock area which was the source of countless autografts – with especial attention paid to getting good healing of the donor site after each harvesting. As a result, when he was finally covered and healed, his buttock skin was able to serve as a future reconstructive donor site.

Correct The Contractures In One Facial Area That Produce Deformities In Other Areas

Not infrequently, burns will produce scar contractures such as those shown in **Figure 50.5a**, in which an intrinsic contracture in one area will produce an extrinsic contracture in another area. This 5-year-old girl had an intrinsic contracture in the cheek and para-commissural area, which produced extrinsic contractures in other regions, in this instance the orbital area, nose, lips and neck. In such a complex situation, she required scar releases and grafting of

---

Fig. 50.1 (a) A 5-year old Native American girl 3 days after sustaining 20% TBSA flame burn with deep burns of her face. (b) Sheet autografts applied to her face after tangential excision of her deep facial burns on the 10th postburn day. (c) Condition 5 years after facial excision and grafting having had only a subsequent nasal reconstruction.

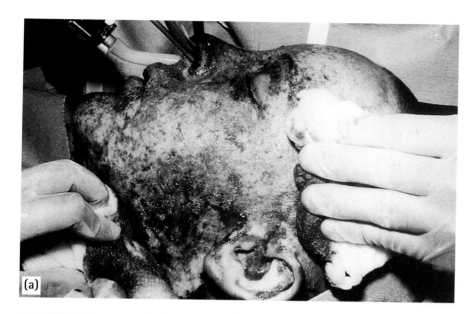

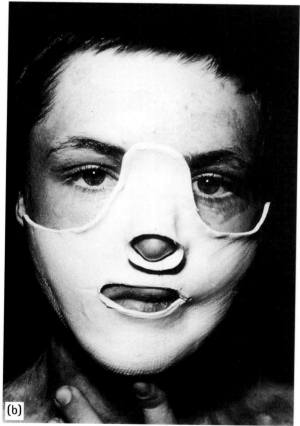

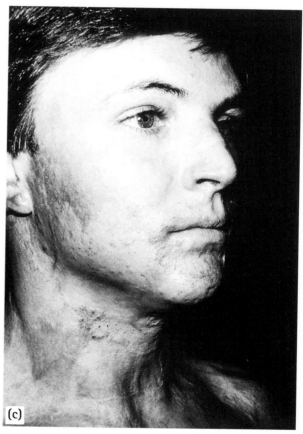

Fig. 50.2 (a) Tangentially excised facial burn wound of a 15-year-old boy 7 days after sustaining a 51% TBSA flame burn. (b) Opaque plastic facial mask which was held in place with an elastic mask which he wore for several months after excision and grafting. (c) Condition 5 years after facial burn excision and immediate grafting.

a whole series of her intrinsic contractures in order to gain an acceptable result. She required, in sequence, releases and grafting of her lower lid and cheek area, neck, upper lip, paracommissural area and lateral nasal area. Six years later (**Figure 50.5b**), she was finally free of both intrinsic and extrinsic contractures of her face and neck, leaving her with a fairly normal, well-balanced appearance but still with a little more work to do in the nasal and lateral cervical areas.

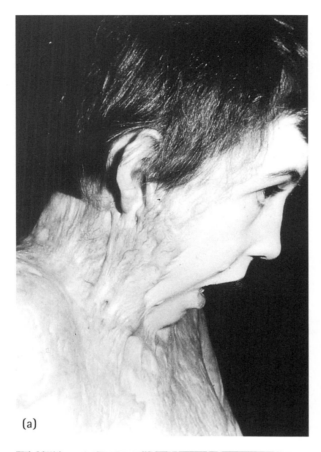

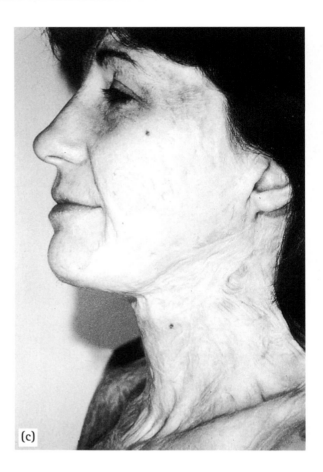

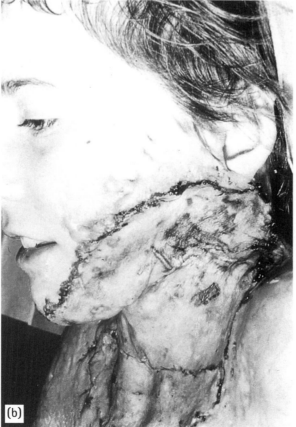

Plan As Comprehensively As Possible for Facial Reconstruction

With the wide variety of techniques available today to burn reconstructive surgeons, it becomes imperative to work out as detailed and complete a plan as possible when beginning the reconstructive sequence of restoring a burn-distorted face. The plan should be developed with specific desires of the patient combined with reconstructive possibilities as outlined by the surgeon. An example of this form of planning and reconstructive sequence is represented by the 11-year-old girl shown in **Figure 50.6**. She had suffered severe facial and hand burns, which healed with the result shown, following a considerable amount of delayed healing and some late grafting. She was particularly disturbed by the appearance of her eyelids and was also concerned about the condition of her cheeks and nose. Therefore, a comprehensive plan involving numerous reconstructive procedures was created based on her request and her family's concerns.

Fig. 50.3 (a) An 11-year-old girl with profound cervical contracture 2 months after healing from a 76% TBSA flame burn. (b) Split-thickness skin grafts in place after extensive release and excision of mento-cervical burn scar contracture. (c) Condition 18 years later with well maintained mento-cervical relation and lower face and cervical contours.

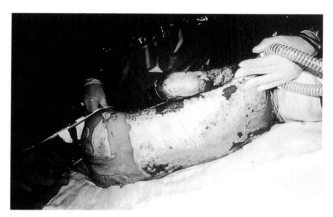

Fig. 50.4 Back and unburned buttocks of a 5-year-old boy who suffered an 86% TBSA burn. Buttock skin served as a donor site for repeated grafts during the acute phase and was carefully maintained to serve as a donor site for late facial reconstruction.

Work for Fullness of Features and a Three-Dimensional Result Whenever Possible

One of the most difficult problems in reconstructing the burned face is the avoidance of a two-dimensional, flat appearance that burns and surgical scars tend to impose. Achieving the third-dimensional aspect is essential in restoring a normal appearance to such detailed and complex area as the nose, lips, inner canthus, philtral dimple, the infralabial hollow, and a projecting chin.

A complex example of the necessity to reconstruct facial features with important three-dimensional qualities is shown in **Figure 50.7a**. The lips and lower one third of the nose of this female burn patient were destroyed by a contact burn from the hot exhaust pipe in a motorcycle accident. Not only was she missing the lower part of her nose, but the upper lip was contracted by scar, and her missing lower lip exposed her teeth and made holding liquids in her mouth impossible. Her lower lip was restored by means of a transverse cervical flap (**Figure 50.7b**) migrated in stages. This provided the basic lower lip tissue, which was surgically thinned three times. Since she refused a forehead flap, a Tagliacozzi flap from her left upper arm (**Figure 50.7c**) was used to rebuild the lower part of her nose, initially leaving it long and tailoring it into place secondarily. **Figure 50.7d** shows her profile 4 years later, with still a little more work to be done on her upper lip, but with a good three-dimensional restoration of her lower lip and lower nose.

Use Local Tissue When Available for Good Tissue Character Match

This aphorism is well known to reconstructive surgeons, but is sometimes difficult or impossible to achieve in burned patients

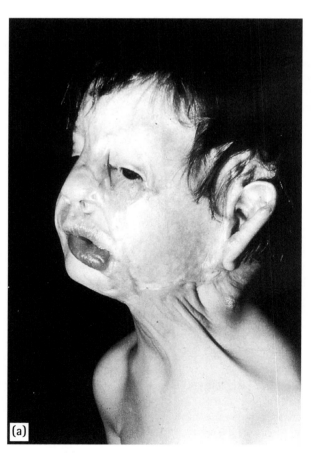

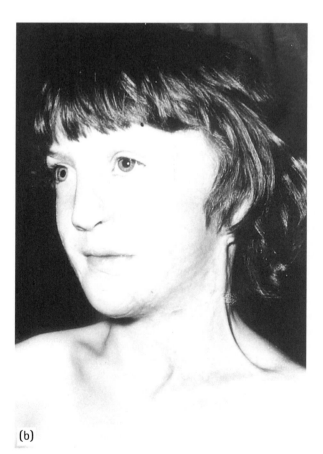

Fig. 50.5 (a) A 5-year-old girl with multiple scars of her face producing intrinsic and extrinsic facial and cervical contractures. (b) Condition 6 years later after several reconstructive procedures to release the intrinsic contractures which also resulted in release of extrinsic contractures.

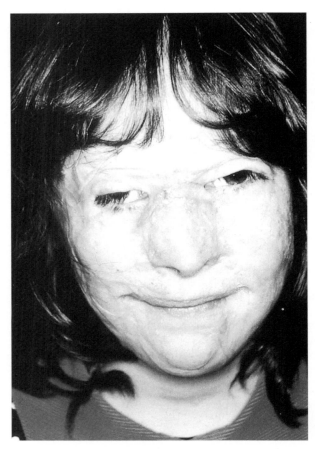

Fig. 50.6 An 11-year-old girl with multiple facial scars and contractures several months after facial burns from a burning car blanket.

Avoid Mosaicism or a Patchwork Appearance by Resurfacing Single or Transfacial Units with Large Grafts or Flaps

This final principle is the critically important idea that one of the most valuable goals in extensive facial reconstruction should be to provide repair tissue that covers entire major esthetic areas, or even a combination of esthetic units, with no interposing scar junction lines and placing edge scars in inconspicuous locations. When this is possible, one can achieve an uniformity in appearance which is difficult, if not impossible, to accomplish any other way. To this end, one should use large transunit, full-thickness skin grafts or radically thinned adjacent cervico-pectoral flaps. Such flaps can only be used if there are nonburned areas of the cervico-pectoral region.

Figure 50.9 shows a patient who illustrates the use of this principle in reconstructing an extensively burn-scarred face. This 13-year-old boy was first seen 4 months after healing from a 30% TBSA upper body and facial burn. His entire middle and lower face had diffuse hypertrophic scars which produced local distortions of his facial features (**Figure 50.9a**). To provide the basic resurfacing of his face, an upper chest flap was designed encompassing the remaining normal chest skin which required three surgical delays before elevation for reconstruction. **Figure 50.9b** shows his condition after the scars of the left side of his face were excised, the flap transferred, and the chest donor site closed with split-thickness skin grafts. Subsequently, he had the right facial scars excised and the remaining flap divided from its pectoral origin and inset into the right facial esthetic unit. **Figure 50.9c** shows his condition 9 years after beginning his reconstructive surgery, having had some scar revisions, a full-thickness skin graft to resurface his entire nose, followed by a cosmetic rhinoplasty and, finally, a scalp flap to create a mustache. The chest flap provided a good tissue character base for his extensive facial reconstruction.

Developmental aspects of burned face deformities in children and their correction

Serious burns of a child's face which produce substantial scarring may create not only externally visible deformities, but also may influence or alter certain physical and psychological growth and developmental aspects of the child. Fortunately, though, such impairments generally are only temporary and can be restored to normal either spontaneously or corrected by surgical, psychological or rehabilitative actions. Rarely, though, such growth and developmental problems associated with burn facial deformities may create long-term problems that may require future correction.

There have been many clinical studies of both physical and psychological changes and impairments of children's certain processes of growth and development caused by facial and other burn deformities. Such studies discuss the nature of the problems, methods of management and correction, and the results and outcomes. Most studies indicate that such developmental problems are correctable either with time or direct professional treatment. The following items are some of the most important physical and psychological developmental and growth problems caused by major facial burn scars and deformities.

because of the distribution of their scars. For facial reconstruction, adjacent local tissue generally gives the best result – retroauricular, neck, upper chest, and upper arm skin are areas which give the best color match to facial skin, as well as providing tissue of the same thin, supple character as facial skin.

An example illustrative of using local skin for facial reconstruction is shown in **Figure 50.8a**. This 8-year-old girl had extensive partial thickness burns of her face when her sweater caught on fire. She healed spontaneously with nonoperative therapy, but unfortunately developed large, unsightly hypertrophic scars in the mandibular and lower facial areas of both sides of her face despite continuous pressure therapy, night splints, and steroid massage. Her condition 9 months after her initial burn is shown in **Figure 50.8a**. Her scars were serially excised utilizing the redundancy and elasticity of her neck skin after removing the scars. She had three procedures on each side of her face, each time undermining the skin of her neck at the supraplatysmal level down to her clavicles and advancing the neck skin to replace the amount of scar excised. This ultimately left only a single narrow linear scar. **Figure 50.8b** shows her result 5 years after her procedures were begun with a good tissue character match and the normal contours of her neck maintained.

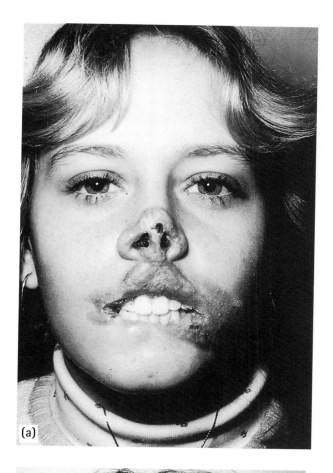

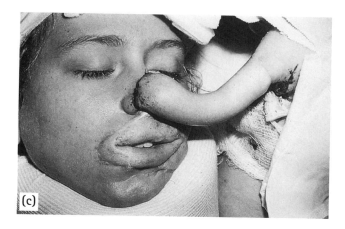

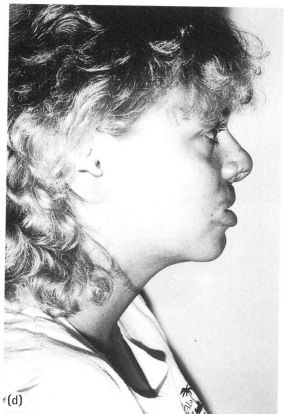

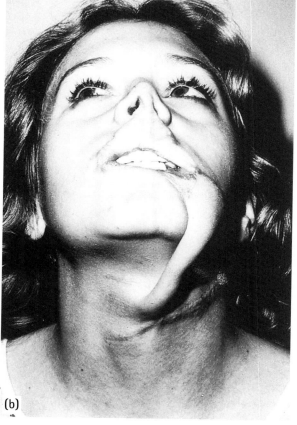

Fig. 50.7 (a) A 15-year-old girl with destroyed lips and lower nose due to a contact burn from motorcycle exhaust pipe. (b) First stage of transfer of cervical flap for reconstruction of upper and lower lips. (c) Tagliacozzi from left arm applied to nose for reconstruction of lower one-third of her nose. (d) Profile view 4 years later showing restoration of three-dimensional aspects of her nose and lips.

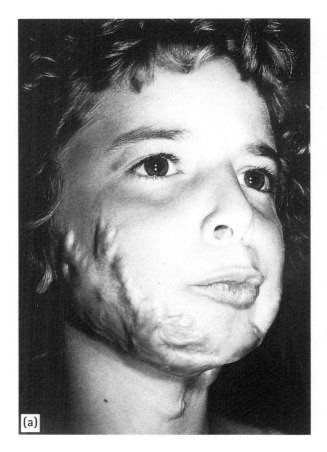
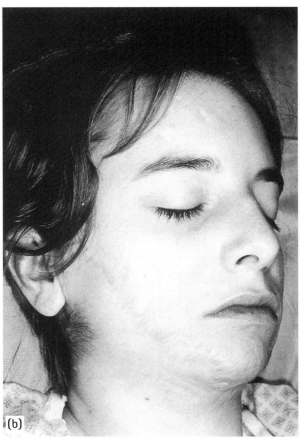

Fig. 50.8 (a) Right side of face of an 11-year-old girl with heavy hypertrophic scars 9 months after partial thickness burn to her lower face. (b) Condition and remaining scar 5 years after three operative procedures of partial excision and cervical skin advancement.

Physical

- Impaired nasal growth by hypertrophic nasal scars;
- Dental displacement due to scar contracture of the lower lip;
- Impaired mandibular growth by heavy hypertrophic scars of the lower anterior face and also by excessive facial scar pressure therapy;
- Danger of cortical blindness or occlusion amblyopia due to prolonged eyelid closure by surgical tarsorrhaphy.

Psychological

- Alteration of the child's body-image and general psychological growth due to facial deformities;
- Retardation – temporary or permanent – of intellectual and cognitive development;
- Alteration social confidence and development of social abilities and concerns which may cause more social, antisocial and/or self-isolated behavior;
- In teenaged children, psycho-sexual behavior confidence and development of sexual maturity, abilities, activities and concerns may be influenced by facial deformities. Such changes would tend to limit normal psycho-sexual

development and therefore as such a teenagers enter adulthood, they may lack normal sexual interests and activities.

Physical Problems

Impaired nasal growth

Burn scars of the face which cover the nose, as occurred in a 7-year-old boy who had just recovered from 65% TBSA burn (**Figure 50.10a**), may cause excess pressure and growth limitation to a burned child's nose. In the normal growth of the nose and face, in general, there are two forms of growth of cartilage and facial bones. The process of cartilage enlargement involves two separate, basic growth mechanisms; appositional and interstitial.[1] Appositional growth of cartilage occurs as a result of accumulation of entirely new cell layers and intercellular matrix on the outer surfaces of cartilage due to perichondrial activities. Interstitial growth and enlargement of cartilage occurs due to three processes:

1. division and multiplication of existing chondrocytes within the cartilage mass;
2. increase in the size of each individual chondrocytes; and
3. formation and continued accumulation of cartilaginous matrix due to chondrocytes activity.

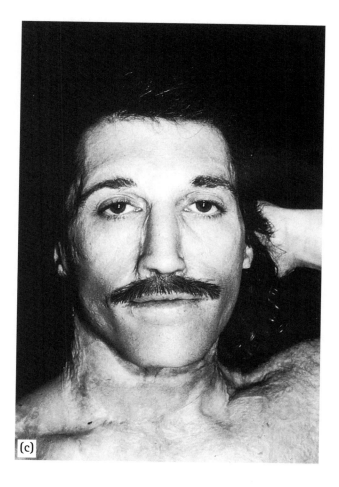

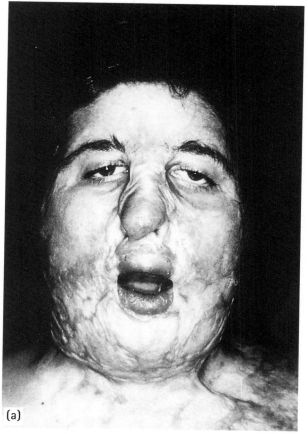

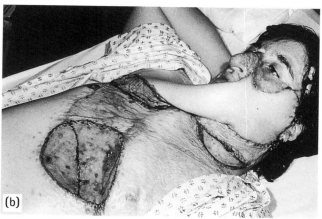

Fig. 50.9 (a) A 13-year-old boy 4 months after healing from a 30% TBSA flame burn with middle and lower face replaced by hypertrophic scar causing multiple contractures of his facial features. (b) Condition following excision of left facial scar and application of an upper chest flap as the first stage of complete facial resurfacing. (c) Condition 9 years after beginning reconstructive sequences with chest flap resurfacing his entire middle and lower face, with additional subsequent nasal resurfacing, rhinoplasty and scalp flap to create a mustache.

Interestingly, facial bone growth also involves osteal forms of appositional and interstitial bone growth. Facial bones are related to each other by bone sutures where bone growth continues to keep the facial bones in contact with each other. Nasal growth both in vertical length and horizontal projection in children is primarily influenced by the cartilaginous growth of the nasal septum, which has a very active anterior growth center. The nasal and anterior maxillary bones get moved out into a projected position by the actively growing nasal septum, and the facial bones are moved away from the cranial base. In this process, additional bone growth at the various facial bone sutures maintains the position of the facial bones with each other and help them enlarge in both vertical and horizontal directions.[2] Scars on the nose such as this little boy

had, and also more hypertrophic nasal scars, cause pressure and limitation of the nasal cartilage growth and resultant nasal bone growth. In order to maintain normal nasal growth as much as possible, it is critical to remove the nasal scars and resurface the nose with a skin graft, or in more destructive cases with a flap. **Figure 50.10b** shows his appearance 2 weeks after scar removal and skin grafting. In general, it is best to excise and graft the full esthetic unit of the nose in order to achieve both acceptable functional and esthetic results in the future. **Figure 50.10c** shows the result of his nasal scar release and graft 2 years later. While the nose is still a little flat and limited in projection, it is evident that there is some active nasal growth due to release of restriction on the active growth of the nasal septum. **Figure 50.10d** shows his condition

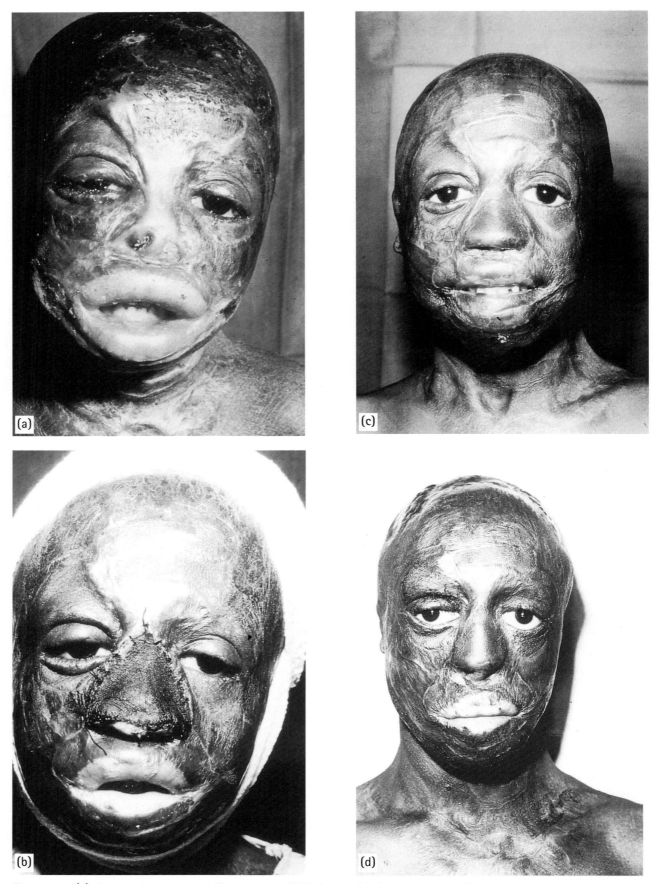

Fig. 50.10 (a) A boy who recovered from a 65% TBSA burn with heavy scars on his nose that could cause growth limitation. (b) Appearance two weeks after excising nasal esthetic unit containing heavy scars and covered with a skin graft. (c) Result 2 years postoperatively showing slow nasal growth. (d) Result 12 years post-operatively showing relatively normal nasal growth and projection.

12 years later, at the age of 19 years. Even though he still has some facial scarring that needs correction, it is evident that his nose has grown more normally and has an almost normal adult appearance and projection as a result of the scar resection and grafting 12 years before.

Dental displacement

Another physical developmental problem in children with burned facial scars is the displacement of growing teeth of the anterior mandible due to contracture of the lower lip such as the little girl shown in **Figure 50.11a** had. In terms of normal dental positioning, one of the main reasons that teeth remain in the upright position and maintain normal bite is the normal muscular balances between tongue and lip musculature. In a child with inhibited tongue function, the teeth lean inward in a lingual direction due to the pressure of lip musculature. In a child like this, with her lower lip pulled out and down by burn scar, the teeth begin to lean out in a labial direction, as is evident in this picture. Another growth aspect of normal dental positioning is the fact that young children have permanent teeth in an early stage of development, with each tooth having its own rate of development. If a burned child has excessive and contracting lip scars or excessive scar pressure on the mandible, severe permanent damage can occur either to the crown or root of the potentially permanent teeth, depending on the

stage of development at the time of abnormal pressures from burn scars. In very young children, the teeth have more developmental time and such burn scars could cause very harmful damage to the child's permanent teeth development. In a child such as this, with her lip contracted and her teeth tilting our labially, it is critical to have orthodontic treatment in addition to surgical correction. Prior to lip contracture correction, it is very useful to have a dental brace placed to begin to pull the teeth back to a more normal upright position. Following the application of the dental braces to help correct the teeth positions, the chin and lip scar should be excised and replaced with either a free skin graft of local flap. **Figure 50.11b** shows this little girl's condition 2 years after lower lip and chin scar excision and grafting with split-thickness and full-thickness skin grafts. Six weeks after her surgical correction, she no longer needed her dental brace. Once the lip has been restructured and the perioral muscles are acting more normally, the dental muscle balance is restored and teeth remain upright and the dental brace is no longer needed.

Reduction of mandibular growth

As stated in the discussion of nasal deformities due to scars, mandibular growth can be impeded, and possibly permanently altered, by pressure due to facial scaring, especially in the lower face and also by treatment of facial scarring by use of pressure

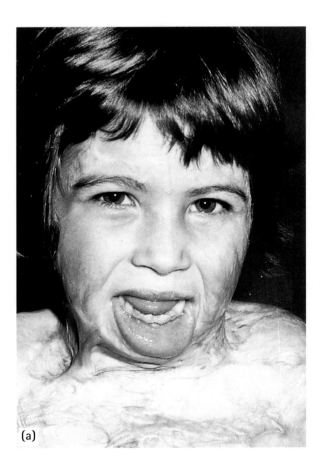

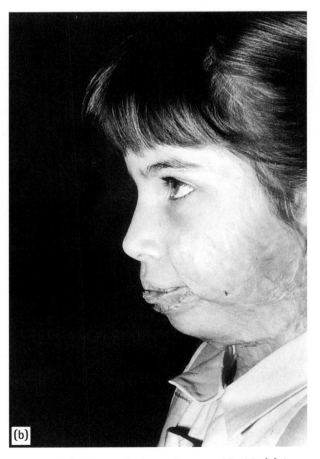

Fig. 50.11 (a) Labial displacement of lower teeth due to contracture of the lower lip in an 8-year-old girl. (b) Lower lip condition 2 years after contracture release and grafting of the lower lip and chin after which she recovered normal position of her teeth.

devices and garments. The boy shown in **Figure 50.12** had this picture taken 9 years after he had suffered an 89% TBSA burn which included a large amount of facial scarring that was treated temporarily with a pressure garment attempting to reduce the scarring. As a result of the facial scarring and pressure garment treatment, he had diminished mandibular growth, causing a recession of his chin, as is obvious in his profile. Since the chin is composed mostly of mandibular bone, the pressure exerted on the chin by burn scars and/or pressure garment can be very high. It creates a backward force through the rami of the mandible to the mandibular condyle which is the major source of mandibular growth-and the excess pressure prevents forward growth of the mandible.

A long-term study from the Burn Center at the University of Washington, in Seattle, Washington concerning mandibular growth in children with burn scars of the face who were treated with pressure devices and garments has been reported in 1996 and 1999 with very critical and important results.[3,4] Their 11-year studies indicate that both facial scarring and use of pressure garments contribute to, or are responsible for, deviations from the normal directions of facial growth, especially the mandible. Initially, they studied patients who wore pressure garments for several months or more than a year. **Figure 50.13** shows the kind of pressure garment and device that are used to help control facial scarring. This boy

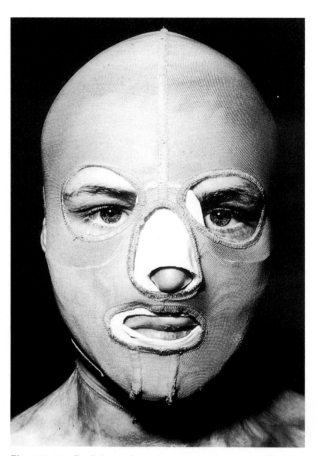

Fig. 50.13 Facial mask and pressure garment that may cause reduction of mandibular growth while treating facial scars.

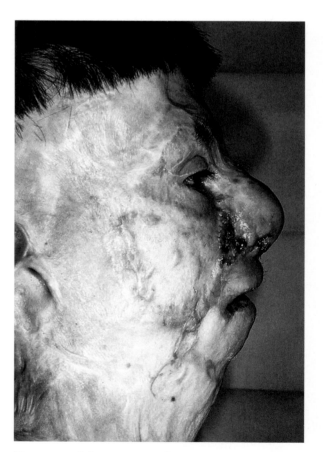

Fig. 50.12 A boy 9 years after recovering from an 89% TBSA burn who had diminished mandibular growth and mandibular recession due to heavy lower face scars and treatment with pressure garments.

had an Isoprene plastic mask molded to his lower face and then an elastic garment placed over it to create pressure through the plastic device on the lower face and by means of the elastic garment on the upper face and forehead. Because the clinical investigators at the University of Washington found results of limited mandibular growth in patients using pressure garments for long periods of time, they recommended that pressure garments be used for shorter times and that patients be followed and treated by orthodontic consults to help correct mandibular, malocclusion, and dental deformities. In their follow-up study in which they did sequential lateral cephalograms and panmandibular X-rays to define the nature of facial growth in their patients, they found that some of their patients with severe scarring and pressure garment use showed a directional change of mandibular growth from a normal anterior–inferior direction to exclusively inferior direction. Because of this directional change, some of the children as they matured had somewhat longer than normal faces. More importantly, they found that many of the children who had directional changes in the growth of the maxilla and mandible improved towards normal growth and appearance after discontinuing the pressure garments. In a few of the children, although the direction of their facial growth returned to normal in the years after their burn and use of pressure garments, the changes in the appearance and development of their faces persisted. The general explanation of inhibition of mandibular growth due to facial scarring and pressure garment use is that the mandibular endochondral growth center was inhibited by the effect of pressure on the bones as described in Wolff's law,[5] which was devised in the later part of the nineteenth century. Wolff's law points out that the orientation and architecture of the medullary trabeculae of growing bones are very sensitive and responsive to external stresses, pressures, and tensions. As a result, the bone growth is inhibited, and bone shape and growth direction are altered. Just to reiterate as a summary concerning limitation of mandibular growth in facially burn-scarred children, prevention and treatment of children with heavy facial scarring who are being treated with pressure garments should include the following points:

1. limited time in using pressure garments;
2. early surgical removal of heavy facial scars and replacement with skin grafts or flaps; and
3. use of orthodontic consults to follow the children's mandibular and dental growth and correct any detected problems with orthodontic braces or ultimately with orthodontic surgery.

Occlusion amblyopia

The fourth physical developmental growth process that may affect children with burn-scarred faces is a variable loss of sight due to excessive length of time of eyelid closure, which is technically referred as 'occlusion amblyopia' and some refer to as 'cortical blindness'. One example of occlusion amblyopia is a young girl who had facial burns and scars from a fire inside her parent's automobile. She was referred to us 18 months later for treatment of her remaining facial scars and deformed nose. When we examined her, it was evident that she was blind in her right eye. Her mother told us that she had been blind ever since her right upper and lower eyelids were closed over her right eye for 6 or 8 weeks. Tarsorrhaphy had been used to repair her upper lid contracture with a skin graft. Occlusion amblyopia persisted in her right eye for a total of 2.5 years, at which point she gradually regained vision, although it was not totally normal for a long period of time. After a few years, this patient regained normal vision and ocular refraction. Occlusion amblyopia occurs mostly in children, aged 6 months to 9 years, when their lids are forced to cover the eye, excluding the pupil from vision. Several factors can cause this problem, including: severe congenital ptosis, lid tumors, hemangiomas of the orbital region, prolonged eye patches, and tarsorrhaphies.[6] Very young children are more susceptible to occlusion amblyopia than older children. Studies of eye-patching duration have indicated that, for infants, the duration should not exceed 3 days; for 1–3-year-old children, no more than 2 weeks; and for 3–9-year-old children no more than 3 months. If these durations are exceeded, the child will very likely get occlusion amblyopia, which produces either decreased vision or total blindness. Most children are not permanently blind, but, as they recover, they have limited visual acuity and may have unequal refractive power in their eyes. There is no known ophthalmological treatment for children who get occlusion amblyopia. The best active form of aid is to remove or correct the various factors that cause long-term eyelid closure. In children with burn contractures of their eyelids, prolonged tarsorrhaphies should not be used in maintaining the correction of the contracture because of the danger of causing occlusion amblyopia in a growing child with developing optic functions.

Psychological Problems

In addition to pure physical growth problems, children with extensive facial scarring from burns may have alterations in their processes of psychological growth and development. The face of a child is not only a critical element of interpersonal and social relations, it represents one of the largest elements of a child's concept of their body image. Therefore, facial deformities create not only physical problems for growing children but may create changes or limitations in their psychological growth and development. Not all children with facial deformities have severe psychological changes and growth limitations. There have been a number of studies concerning this indicating that, in general, no more than 50% of children with this type of disfigurement had significant emotional and psychological disturbances. Pless and Pinkerton, two very experienced American child psychiatrists, have described the sequence of the adjustment to a childhood disorder such as facial disfigurement.[7] They indicate that a child's personality components are influenced by their family and social environment, which can create the child's emotional reactions to severe disabilities or defects such as burn facial deformities. When children react psychologically to a disability of deformity, they are also influenced externally by reactions from both family and other social contacts; these reactions then influence the children's body image and how they will deal with their problem. The child's changes in body image and psychological management then create an altered personal psychological functioning, with either normal adjustment or maladjustment, all of which ultimately influences the child's reaction to their facial disfigurement.

A study by Adullah et al.,[8] addresses specific psychological reactions of children to burn facial deformities but also provides generalizations concerning the children's reactions. Their data demonstrated generalized emotional reactions on the part of burn-scar disfigured children and indicated that the greater number of head and neck scars the children had, the less happiness and self-satisfaction they felt. All their data indicated that among the facially burn-disfigured children they studied, there were many psychological and emotional changes and problems. The authors stated two important conclusions related to psychological reactions of children with facial burn deformities:

- facial disfigurement has a more deleterious effect on a childs psychosocial adjustment than severe burn deformities of other parts of their bodies; and
- children with facial burn scarring may seem to be superficially adjusting satisfactorily to their problems, but in fact may harbor more deeply very severe and grave self-deprecating feelings.

Summaries of these studies clearly indicate that children with facial burn deformities may have moderate to severe changes in their psychological reactions which may significantly influence their emotional and psychological growth and development either temporarily or permanently.[9]

Alteration of body image and general psychological growth

The first major psychological reaction that children with burn-scarred disfigured faces may have is an alteration in their body image, and in some cases a limitation of their general psychological growth. Bernstein[10] pointed out that awareness of body image, which in children begins about the age of 3 or 4 years, consists of at least the following factors:

- the practical image of how a child feels they look and how it affects people;
- the image the child thinks that other people would like; and
- the conceptual image, i.e. what the child thinks he or she would or should look like.

Bernstein also described that the organization and development of the body image in children is a complex psychophysiological process that depends on several factors, such as

- immediate contact with other children;
- self-touching sensation;
- spatial organization;
- resolution of inner tension;
- the openness for exploration of parts of the body; and
- cultural and parental taboos.

Many other psychiatrists agree that the face and its condition is both the most socially critical instrument of interpersonal communication and the most complex area of a child body image. It is generally agreed that a burned child's emotional reactions to facial disfigurement involves severe internal changes in their body image concept which may cause emotional reactions such as: depression, feelings of self-guilt, loss of self-confidence, and other elements having to do with general psychological growth and development.

Many children with burned facial deformities have problems that cause diminution of general psychological growth. Psychiatrists agree that severe burned facial deformity can damage the developing personality apparatus, as well as damaging the social role of a growing child and can distort general psychological life course.[11] In addition, some facially disfigured children are bothered by feelings of guilt, self-blame, badness and being unlovable – all of which can potentially slow down the child's general psychological growth. Adolescent children who have grown up with burn facial deformities have difficulty beginning to mature. One normal psychological step of adolescents is progressively moving away from their parents towards independence. It has been observed that adolescents with facial deformities are less able to move towards independence because they tend to need more parental help, support and guidance. As a result, many facially deformed adolescents do not emotionally mature normally and grow up looking and acting more childlike.[12]

Intellectual and cognitive impairment

Unreconstructed burn deformities of the face can cause problems which result in impairment of a child's intellectual and cognitive functioning and which might diminish their ability to function well in school. Bernstein[13] studied children with persistent facial deformities and demonstrated that the emotional effects of a child's facial deformities negatively influenced other ego functions, which harmed peer relationships and diminished school performance. Poor school performance was attributed to the consequences of the child's psychological withdrawal from confidence and maladaptation to academic requirements. The disfigured child's altered self-perception of being, which includes a feeling of diminished worth

and an injured body image, is also considered likely to contribute to underachievement in school performance.

Social confidence alteration

Another specific psychological difficulty of children with burn-scarred facial deformities is the progressive lack of social confidence and social emotional abilities, causing them to become socially isolated. These reactions, which may persist for months and years, are expressed in several ways.

Bernstein[10] pointed out that many facially disfigured children tend to be very shy and sensitive, and comparison with their normal peers, appear to be less socially involved and tend to have less social experience as a result of their more limited social contacts. Also, children with burned facial deformities tend to find it very difficult to obtain social acceptance from their peers; they feel that they have social disapproval and do not feel they are included in the social activities of their peer groups. More specifically, many of these facially deformed children feel that they encounter social barriers in their relations and feel that they are being left out of multipersonal social activities, peer relationships, and dating and intimate relationships. One other devastating social issue involving a child with facial burn scar deformities has to do with the fact that it is difficult for the child to physically cover up the face. Therefore, people of all ages living nearby will see their deformities and the child may be constantly questioned about what happened. Because this does happen, the child must learn to deal with such questions, which may have a very profound negative psychological and social effect.

Psycho-sexual behavior growth changes

Psycho-sexual development and growth may be retarded or changed in burn-scarred adolescents as they approach adulthood. Late teenagers who have burn scars in their faces for more than a year or two may have no interest, or confidence, in achieving normal affections or sexual relations, both of which are psychological areas of interest in normal late teenagers as they approach adulthood. Bernstein[10] also indicated that the normal middle adolescent must play out his sexual fantasies with the body of a child, in effect, at least compared with the larger, complete body of an adult. In late adolescence the normal individual is biologically, and in some cases socially, on a par with adults, if not in a superior position. The achievement of the late adolescent's stable body image is the result of unimpaired psychological development over previous years. Many adolescents with burned facial deformities have limited body image growth and wind up with an unstable body image and lack of confidence that causes a reduction in sexual progression and interest. In some such adolescents, they have had persistent self-anger as a result of their facial deformities, which may then inhibit their psycho-sexual growth and development. It is understood that psychological development, in general, can be damaged or impaired by such critical events as burns and subsequent facial deformities due to burn scars. When such an event occurs and persists at the particular age at which adolescents are initiating or continuing their psycho-sexual development, then clear sexual identity and confidence do not occur at that time in the teenage child's development; these children will tend not to reach full normal psycho-sexual development as they approach adulthood.

Clearly, as described in many psychiatric studies, a certain percentage of growing adolescents with persistent facial deformities due to burn scarring experience inhibition of their normal psychological patterning of potential sexual roles which diminishes the psychological route to normal sexual maturation and fulfillment.

Summary

There are several methods of trying to correct the growth and development problems of children with burn deformed faces who have both physical and psychological difficulties. Correction of children with only physical facial deformities but no psychological problems requires only surgical treatments as described. Facial reconstructive surgery in children with burn scar facial deformities, but who have no obvious psychological alterations, may help improve the body image that was altered by the presence their facial deformities. Surgically improving the appearance of their faces is capable of creating a parallel improvement in the child's deformed body image. On the other hand, children with psychological problems created by burn scar facial deformities require help from various professionals using several methods, both surgical and psychological. Psychological treatment of burn-facially-deformed children would follow surgical correction and include individual psychotherapy, possible group psychotherapy, and play therapy. In addition, it is critical for facially and psychologically deformed children to learn new psychological coping mechanisms to enable them to maintain a sense of growth continuity and confidence in their identity and body image. Psychotherapy to improve their self-esteem, even though they may have acquired surgically improved faces, is necessary to assure a recurrence of normal psychological growth and development and advancement to normal maturity.

Specific facial and head areas of reconstruction

Reconstructive surgery of the face and neck following burn injuries can be divided into acute and late reconstructive phases. As a general principle, reconstructive surgery is best carried out when the scars are mature and the patient has recovered from the trauma of the acute burn injury. Acute reconstructive intervention is indicated in the eyelid, perioral, and cervical areas when acute deformities severely compromise function and patient care.

Acute Phase Reconstruction

Eyelids

Upper and lower eyelid ectropion can occur from burn injuries to the periorbital region (intrinsic contracture) or may arise secondarily as a result of the contracture of open wounds and skin grafts at more distant sites (extrinsic contracture). With severe ectropion such as shown in **Figure 50.14a**, early intervention is mandatory in order to prevent irreversible injury to the cornea. Conservative measures to protect the cornea, such as temporary sutures or contact lenses, are often ineffective. Tarsorrhaphy can cause irreversible iatrogenic injury and should not be used. The best treatment is early intervention with release of contracture and resurfacing with split-thickness skin grafts (**Figure 50.14b**). Release of even extreme contractures with grafting can be done in the presence of open wounds and effectively restores protective eyelid function.

Perioral deformities

Microstomia occurs from circumferential scarring at the junction between lips and cheek. Perioral scarring from either open wounds or contraction of skin graft suture lines can act as a pursestring resulting in diminished oral opening (**Figure 50.15**). This can compromise alimentation and airway access. Microstomia is best addressed by the acute release of the oral commissures taking care to avoid extensive transverse releasing incisions in the aesthetic units of the cheek. Overcorrection can easily result in macrostomia. As soon as adequate oral opening is achieved for feeding and airway access, definitive reconstruction is best left for the post-acute period.

Macrostomia results from rapid contraction of open wounds or grafts in the cheek and perioral region, resulting in eversion of the upper and lower lips and lateral movement of the oral commissures (**Figure 50.16**). The loss of an effective oral sphincter results in drooling desiccation of the oral mucosa and can result in irreversible damage to the dentition. Early intervention with release and grafting of the lower and/or upper lips can be carried out as soon as possible. Definitive reconstruction is best carried out at a later period.

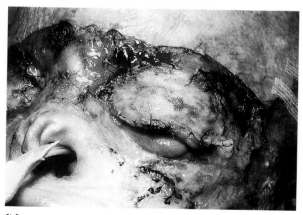

(a)   (b)

Fig. 50.14 (a) Extreme eyelid ectropion during early acute phase. (b) Successful correction of ectropion with release and graft despite operative wounds.

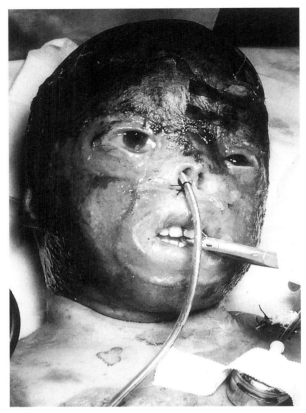

Fig. 50.15 Microstomia during acute phase as a result of circum-oral contracture.

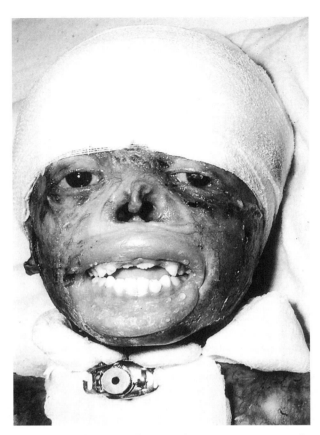

Fig. 50.16 Macrostomia secondary to contracture of open wounds and grafts with lip eversion and loss of oral competence.

Cervical deformities

Anterior neck contractures in the acute period are best prevented by aggressive splinting and early excision and grafting when indicated. When severe anterior neck flexion contractures occur, early release and grafting is necessary to allow for adequate airway access and to minimize hypertrophic scarring as a result of excessive and persistent tension.

Late Phase Reconstruction

Most facial burns result in focal scarring without excessive distortion of facial features. Early surgical intervention is rarely indicated and scar maturation over a period of several years can often give remarkable improvement. Scars may heal better than grafts or flaps, and the gradual transition from uninjured to burned skin is often less conspicuous than junctional scars. When scars are not maturing favorably, early conservative intervention such as massage, pressure, topical steroids, steroid injection, or treatment with pulse dye laser may be efficacious. If scars remain hypertrophic and do not respond to conservative measures, tension is often the culprit. Judicious intervention with release and graft or appropriate revision with z-plasties can favorably influence scar maturation. In patients with focal scarring, one must avoid the temptation to excise all scars if such aggressive excision is likely to result in iatrogenic secondary deformities.

A separate and distinct group of facial burn patients are those with pan-facial deformities. This group of patients is marked by distortion of facial features with displacement of mobile structures

and compression of soft-tissue contours. In addition, there may be loss or amputation of body parts such as eyebrows or ears. Patients with pan-facial burn deformities require careful strategic planning in which reconstructive options are analyzed and areas requiring reconstructive surgery are carefully prioritized. Each patient presents a unique challenge and must be approached individually in close consultation with the patient and family.

Eyebrows

Eyebrow reconstruction following complete loss is an unsolved surgical problem. Composite grafts of hair-bearing scalp from carefully selected sites in the retroauricular area can satisfactorily transfer hair.[14-16] Unfortunately, the hair is scalp hair which grows rapidly and is more projecting than the tangential delicate hair of the normal eyebrow. For complete eyebrow replacement, the technique of composite grafting as described by Brent[14] is most useful. For partial eyebrow loss, micro- and mini-grafting of scalp hair can be efficacious. Occasionally, borrowing composite grafts from a contralateral unburned eyebrow is appropriate. Temporal artery island flaps for eyelid or eyebrow reconstruction have been used for many years.[15,17,18] When used for eyebrow reconstruction, they can be bushy and conspicuous and should be used with caution, particularly when carrying out unilateral eyebrow reconstruction.

Eyelids

Correction of upper and lower eyelid contractures in the late reconstructive period can be a daunting and humbling challenge. The periorbital region is made up of the complex three-dimensional anatomy and requires abundant skin to appropriately drape the complex contours of both the upper and lower eyelids. The slightest amount of excessive tension from either the eyelid skin itself or contractures in adjacent regions such as the forehead or cheek can profoundly and adversely effect eyelid function and appearance. Reconstructive goals should be restoration of a normally shaped palpebral fissure with appropriate orientation of upper and lower eyelashes at rest and in the open position whenever possible. This often requires extensive releasing incisions extending medial to the medial canthus and lateral to the lateral canthus in order adequately to release all the contracted tissues. When ectropion is the result of a distant contracture, the normal eyelid skin should always be returned to it normal location. Incisions should not be made at the eyelid margin thereby separating the normal eyelid skin from the ciliary line and replacing it with a graft. When overlying scar is released, care must be taken to prevent injury to the underlying orbicularis oculi muscle. This is often rolled up and contracted and is rarely completely lost. It must be unfolded to its normal flat broad shape and the resulting defect resurfaced with abundant skin graft. Upper eyelid resurfacing is best carried out with split-thickness skin grafts from the best available donor site.[15] Lower eyelid resurfacing may be done with either split-thickness skin grafts or appropriate full-thickness grafts when indicated. Full-thickness skin grafts in the upper eyelid usually transfer thick dermal component which compromises the delicate folding of the normal supratarsal fold. For minor contractures of either upper or lower eyelids, the perfect reconstructive material can be obtained from an unburned contralateral upper eyelid. Medial canthal folds are best corrected with z-plasties where there is not a significant tissue deficiency.[19]

Lower lip and chin

Deformities of the lower lip and chin usually occur in combination. Contracting forces result in inferior dislocation and eversion of the lower lip. In addition, there is compression of the soft-tissue contours of the chin prominence. Release should be carried out at the vermillion scar junction and the lower lip carefully unfurled taking care to prevent iatrogenic injury to the underlying orbicularis oris muscle.[20] The resulting defect is then resurfaced with split-thickness skin grafts or full-thickness grafts when indicated. Restoration of chin contour can be improved with chin implants.

Upper lip deformity

The upper lip is usually shortened and retruded by severe facial burn injuries. Releasing and grafting should be carried out taking care not to over correct the deformity and create a long upper lip.[20] Reconstruction of the philtrum when indicated is best performed by the technique of Schmidt[21] using a composite graft from the triangular fossa of the ear.

Ears

Improved care in the acute phase of burn injury has greatly decreased the incidence of helical chondritis and the resulting associated deformities of crumpled or lost cartilage. Minor ear

deformities are often seen in patients with little or no hair loss and can easily be camouflaged. Larger defects can be treated by myriad local reconstructive techniques.[22–25] Subtotal ear amputation (**Figure 50.17a,b**) often lends itself to reconstruction with a conchal transposition flap and skin graft.[26] Complete ear loss can be masked by the use of a prosthesis. Fixation has been improved by the use of osteo-integrated implants but cost and color changes remain problematic. Selected patients can be appropriate candidates for total ear reconstruction using autologous cartilage and soft-tissue coverage from either temporalis fascia flaps or expanded local tissue.[27] Alloplastic materials should not be used in the reconstruction of postburn ear deformities due to an acceptably high extrusion rate.[28]

Nasal and perinasal areas

Burns of patients' faces involve many structures creating scar deformities, but because the nose is prominent and projecting in the central part of the face it is one of the most commonly burn-injured facial structures with ultimate nasal deformities due to burn scars. Serious burns of faces involving the nose result in either partial or total loss of the nose or produce scar deformities of the nasal area. Since the nose is in the center of the critical esthetic facial triangle, the most visible portion of the face in the triangle from both

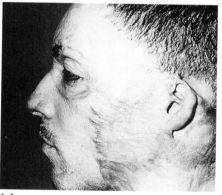

(a)

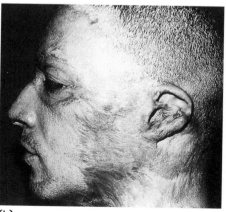

(b)

Fig. 50.17 (a) Typical postburn pattern of peripheral helical loss. (b) Reconstructed ear following expansion with conchal transposition flap and skin grafts.

outer ocular canthi down to the point of the chin, restoration of normal nasal appearance in a burned patient's face has both physical and psychological importance. In adults and children there are several methods of reconstruction of partial and total nasal losses and deformities caused by burns. Good nasal reconstructive results in the child will remain when they reach maturity and any applied flaps will grow with the child and these are important reasons for not delaying to restore as much as possible normal nasal appearances and structures in burn deformed children.

The following nasal problems are among the commonest formal of burn nasal deformities that need either simply direct or complex reconstructive procedures:

1. mild or hypertrophic scarring of the nasal skin;
2. various forms of partial nasal loss such as nasal ectropion, nostril stenosis and columellar loss; and
3. extensive or total nasal loss.

There are both physical reasons and psychological and emotional needs for burned nasal reconstruction. Patients of any age with burn facial deformities including scarred and distorted noses may have impaired self-images and fear of what people think about their appearance. The aesthetic facial triangle is the area of the face most easily seen, therefore, any deformities of the nose in the center of the aesthetic triangle are always easily seen by both the burned patient in a mirror and by the other people nearby. Because of the prominence of nasal deformities in this region, they can be strongly emotionally disturbing to the patient, which would be a major indication for surgical repair.

There are also important physical indications for correcting burn nasal deformities in patients of various ages. Heavy scarring of the nose can produce abnormal pressure on the growing bones and cartilages of the nose and, unless corrected, will impair nasal growth. The most important nasal growth center is in the anterior portion of the nasal septum and pressure from excessive nasal scarring will not only distort the septum and nasal shape, but also will prevent effective nose growth from the septal growth center. Heavy burn scarring with contractures in noses already grown also create structural deformities because of the flexibility of the cartilaginous nasal structures. Another physical indication for nasal deformity correction has to do with abnormal or absent valving of the nasal airways. If they are too wide in patients with extensive nasal loss, symptoms of nasal crusting of the mucosa occur including nasal bleeding and they also will have a very uncomfortable sensation of getting too much air. If the nostrils are too narrow, the deformed patient will have difficulty breathing through the nose and will be obliged to continuously breathe through the mouth. Extensive mouth-breathing can have serious problems such as aspiration of food and liquids when eating.

One diagnostic mode of determining the distortions and losses of a patient's burn-scarred nose can best be determined by using a close-up photograph of the burn-deformed nose with an overlay drawing of what its normal shape should be. The difference between the two graphic representations will show what the exact losses are and their locations.

Methods of Nasal Reconstruction

The following list includes the various useful methods of repair and reconstruction of the various forms of burn nose deformities and losses.

- *Nasal hypertrophic scarring*
  1. split thickness skin graft;
  2. full thickness skin graft.
- *Partial nasal loss*
  1. nasal ectropion – local flaps from scarred tissue, ear composite cartilage grafts, rim turn-down with split-thickness or full-thickness skin grafts;
  2. nostril stenosis – circular full thickness skin grafts, z-plasties, paranasal flaps;
  3. columellar loss – nasolabial flaps, upper lip flaps, composite ear cartilage, forehead flap.
- *Extensive or total loss*
  1. forehead flaps;
  2. scalping flaps;
  3. Tagliacozzi flap;
  4. chest flap.

Nasal Hypertrophic Scarring and Skin Graft Replacement

The following points are major considerations in skin graft replacement of nasal scarring:

1. Both split-thickness and full-thickness skin grafts are used to replace scarred nasal tissue, but the results from using full-thickness skin grafts are in general better than the results of using a split-thickness skin graft
2. Burn scarring tends to create a very flattened appearance to the nasal area and appears to destroy the dorsal nasal support; therefore, when the tense and heavy scar is removed in an appropriate design then the appearance of dorsal nasal projection is usually restored.
3. In general, hypertrophic scars covering the nose should be removed and the complete esthetic unit of the nose should be uniformly grafted with a single sheet of normal skin.
4. Proper color match is important to achieve with a proper colored graft and the best unscarred donor sites for good color match are the supraclavicular area, the retroauricular area and the inner aspect of the upper arm, but unfortunately, however, the postauricular area does not have enough skin to replace the complete aesthetic unit of the nose and it is also important to recognize that using grafts from the lower parts of the body results in dark or yellowish-brown grafts to the nose.

Figure 50.18 a shows a small boy who sustained facial burns in a house fire. The thick hypertrophic scar across his nose needed removal to allow normal growth and improve his appearance and his feelings about himself. **Figure 50.18b** shows that the entire nasal esthetic unit was surgically removed and replaced with a full-thickness skin graft taken from his nonscarred upper inner arm. All the stitches were tied over the graft's stent which stayed in place for 2 weeks to assure that the graft took well. **Figure 50.18c** shows his nasal appearance 18 months later with a smooth skinned, relatively normal looking nasal surface. He had also had full-thickness skin grafts to replace the scars of his upper lip and chin and, just a month before this picture, a full-thickness skin graft was used to replace scar in his upper neck.

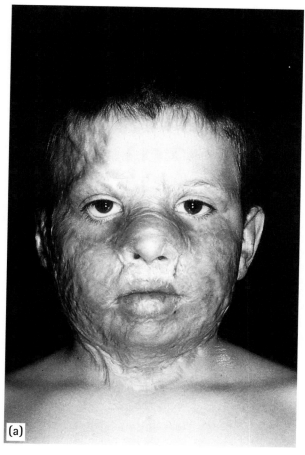

(a)

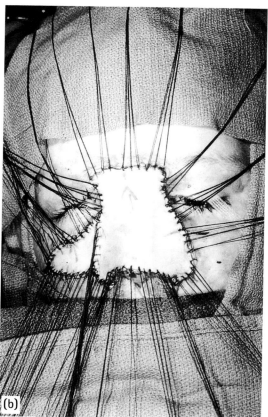

(b)

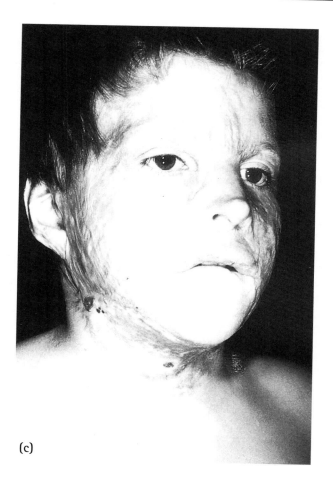

(c)

Nasal Ectropion Reconstruction

Burn scar contractures of the nose tend to pull the tissue of the lower and alae up to abnormal positions and creating nasal ectropion and lower deformities. There are at least four technical considerations that may be involved in the correction of burned nasal ectropion.

Full release of alar contraction

The alar margin in most cases is release with a curved incision in the region of the alar crease that extends medially into the nasal tip as far as needed. If this does not drop the alar margin far enough, then the incision can be deepened between the lateral crus of the alar cartilage and the caudal border of the upper lateral cartilage leaving the underlying mucous membrane intact.

Local flaps from scarred tissue

Local flaps of normal or scarred tissue can be designed and raised to replace the missing alar tissue and correct the nasal ectropion.

Fig. 50.18 (a) Thick nasal scar preoperatively prior to excision and full thickness skin grafting. (b) Full-thickness skin graft from upper inner arm sewn into the full nasal esthetic unit after nasal scar excision. (c) Result 18 months following nasal scar excision and full-thickness skin grafting.

Flaps of tissue are elevated from the naso-labial area and if the tissue is scarred then one must include some underlying subcutaneous fat with the flap in order to preserve the flap's blood supply. Occasionally, it is helpful to do a surgical delay of scarred flaps a week or two before transposition. Once the flaps are ready they are then rotated into the releasing incisions in the alar margins.

Use of ear composite cartilage grafts

Composite cartilage grafts from the ear are very useful to replace the alar tissue after releasing the alar margins to a normal level. The composite grafts of skin and cartilage are generally taken from the posterior conchal area of the ear. If the alar margin is missing, the composite graft may have to be taken from the helical margin to provide a normal appearing edge.

Turning down supra alar tissue

Nasal ectropion involving the whole nasal tip as well as the alar margins can be repaired by excising the scar across the entire lower nose, turning down some of the tissue to create a more normal tip and then grafting the defect with either a split-thickness or full-thickness skin graft.

Nostril Stenosis Correction

Nostril stenosis of varying degrees is a common burn deformity of the nose and needs correction to permit normal and more comfortable breathing and the following are three common methods of correcting burn nostril stenosis.

Circular full-thickness grafts

After excising the scarred area of a nostril and enlarging it to normal again a full-thickness skin graft can be stitched into the defect and a nostril stent kept in place for 2 or 3 weeks until full healing occurs. It is best to use a full-thickness skin graft in this situation rather than split-thickness skin graft because the full-thickness skin graft will have very little postoperative contracture, whereas a split-thickness skin graft always contracts to a varying degree postoperatively.

Z-plasties

For relatively minor nostril stenosis, local z-plasties generally can provide a release and correction to more normal nostril size again.

Paranasal flaps

The use of paranasal flaps is perhaps one of the most reliable techniques for nostril stenosis repair. Paranasal flaps of the tissue lateral to the ala with an inferior base can be elevated and transferred to the lower nostril defect created by the nostril release. With satisfactory blood supply, the paranasal flaps survive well and keep the nostril open and hence this technique has a great advantage for the repair of burned nostril stenosis.

Columellar Loss Reconstruction

Columellar loss does not always occur due to a burn unless virtually the entire nose including the columella is lost. Perhaps the commonest cause for columellar loss in a burned patient is due to a prolonged nasotracheal intubation during which the nasotracheal tube creates pressure necrosis on the columella and even occasionally on the alar. Four methods of reconstruction of columellar loss in burned patients is listed as following.

Nasolabial flaps based superiorly are elevated and placed in the columella position by elevating the alar base temporarily. If the nasolabial area is basically unscarred, this technique generally creates a good new columella. If there is much scar it does not work as well because of loss of flexibility and possibly lack of good blood supply.

Upper lip flaps are useful for only minimal columellar loss because the lip does not provide as much tissue for a rotation flap as the nasolabial area of the face.

Composite cartilage grafts from the ear likewise, for minimal loss of the columella, can replace the straight portion of the columella both from the functional and appearance standpoint. Again, however, the healing is a problem of the composite graft in a position like the columella where it is not easy to provide post-operative pressure to keep the graft in place and assure proper healing. Flaps are more reliable for healing in a location such as this.

Relatively small-sized forehead flaps can also be used to reconstruct a destroyed columella. A properly designed forehead flap based on the supra-trochlear artery and vein can be turned down to replace the columella by raising up the alar area of the nose until the flap is healed in place.

Extensive or Total Nasal Loss Reconstruction

In patients with extensive facial burns and major or total loss of their noses, reconstruction of the nose requires the use of a major pedicle flap of tissue of various kinds. Such flaps are valuable in total nasal reconstruction of burned nasal losses in both adults and children. In the past, it has been felt that reconstructing the nose of a child with flap was not indicated because the flap would not grow with the child. Our experience has indicated that this is not so because we have done total nasal reconstructions in children under the age of 10 and have followed them into adulthood when they had the nasal flap grown to proper size. The following paragraphs list the four types of nasal reconstruction flaps that are used and, generally, one wants to use a flap that has no scar on it in order to get the best result. However, it is possible to replace burn scars of the forehead with a uniformly smooth skin graft and then after complete healing use the grafted forehead provide a forehead flap to create a reasonably attractive new nose.

Forehead flaps

Forehead flaps are flaps using forehead tissue down to and including the frontalis muscle and grafted skin. Such flaps are based either on the supratrochlear or supraorbital vascular supply depending on the location of the flap design.[29] Prior to transfer of the flap to the nasal region, it is generally necessary to create a surgical delay of the flap in order to assure excellent vascular supply to the flap as it is transferred. The shaping of the nasal tip when using a forehead flap or a scalping flap is created by the design of the flap on the forehead but also in shaping the end of the flap when it is placed in the nasal position at which time the columella and the nostril edges are formed by appropriate suturing. Occasionally one may need forehead tissue expansion in order to provide enough tissue for reconstruction of the nose and be able to close the forehead defect primarily. When this is necessary the tissue expander is placed beneath the frontalis muscle in order to assure safe tissue expansion. The use of a tissue expander for this purpose is only rarely needed because the forehead most often provides enough tissue for creating a new nose and the defect can often be closed satisfactorily by using a skin graft. **Figure 50.19a** shows that extensive loss

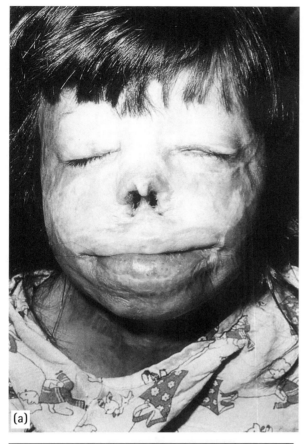

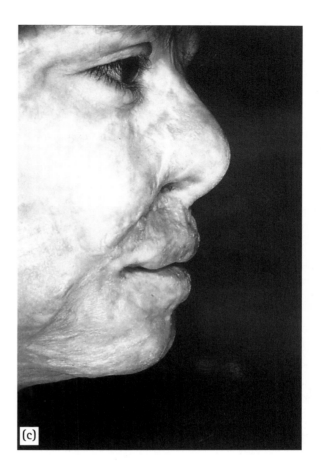

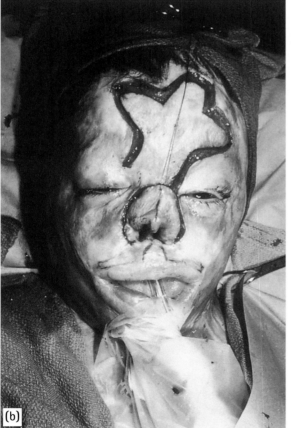

of the nose of a 10-year-old girl who had recovered from an 80% total body surface area (TBSA) burn several months before this picture was taken. Most of the tip, the alae and the columella had been destroyed requiring a major nasal reconstruction. Because her forehead was not too badly scarred, it was decided to reconstruct her nose by using a forehead flap. **Figure 50.19b** shows the outline of the forehead flap which had just been surgically delayed and was based on the right supratrochlear blood supply. Also the area of the scar of the nose was incised and a portion of the scarred remaining nasal skin was turned down to provide part of the new nasal lining. At the end of the operation the forehead flap was sewn into place as well as creating new nostrils and the forehead donor site was covered with a sheet of split-thickness skin graft. **Figure 50.19c** shows her result 16 months later with a relatively normal appearing nose and adequate sized nostrils.

Scalping flaps

Scalping flaps are a variety of forehead flaps where the blood supply is based on a large area of the scalp and not on the supratrochlear or supra-orbital vessels.[30] In creating a scalping flap the

Fig. 50.19 (a) Major loss of nose in a 10-year-old girl after recovery from an 80% TBSA burn. (b) Surgical elevation of forehead flap to reconstruct her nose after removal of the residual scarred nasal skin. (c) Result of forehead flap nasal reconstruction 16 months postoperatively.

portion to create the new nose is designed on the forehead using either normal or grafted skin and the frontalis muscle. From the upper portion of the design, an incision is made curving well back into the scalp which then allows the forehead portion of the whole flap to be dropped down to the nasal region. The open area of the scalp can either be temporarily grafted or dressed until the nasal portion is headed and the scalp portion is returned to its normal location in the scalp. **Figure 50.20a** shows an 11-year-old boy who had suffered an 86% TBSA burn, and after complete healing and recovery he had only a portion of his nose left that had been grafted

and had gross distortion of the remaining alae and nostrils. To replace his nose a portion of the forehead that had been regrafted one month previously and then was outlined in design and underwent a surgical delay. **Figure 50.20b** shows that 1-month later the forehead portion was elevated and the superior line of the flap was incised in a curving manner back to just above his right ear. The scarred tissue of the upper portion of the nose was outlined for removal and the lower portion designed to be turned down to be included in the nostrils as shown here. Following the excision of the nasal scar and turn-down of the nostril flaps, the forehead tissue

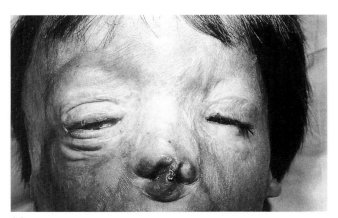

(a)

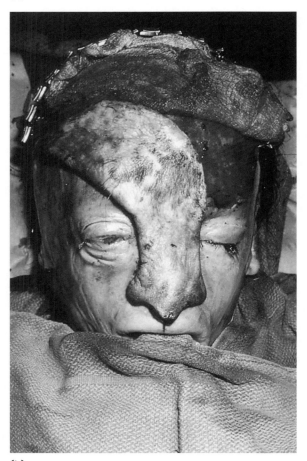

(b)

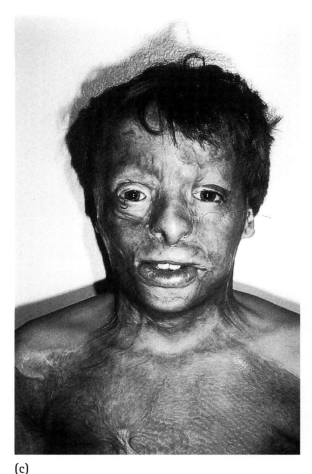

(c)

Fig. 50.20 (a) Major loss of nose of 11-year-old boy after recovery from an 86% TBSA burn. (b) Scalping flap with forehead-designed tissue brought down to reconstruct his nose. (c) Result of scalping flap reconstruction of nose 2.5 years postoperatively.

with its scalp base was brought down and sewn into place. The large raw area of the scalp was closed with a temporary skin graft which was removed when the scalp portion of the flap was divided and replaced in the normal cephalic location. **Figure 50.20c** shows his result 2.5 years later with a reasonably attractive nose on a still somewhat scarred face. His hair grew relatively normally on the portion of the scalp that had been part of the scalping flap. He was also able to breathe normally through his reconstructed nostrils.

Chest flaps

When the forehead is not available for use as a flap to reconstruct the nose, in some cases it is necessary to use a surgically delayed tube flap from an unscarred portion of the anterior chest or clavicular area to replace extensive loss of the burned nose. Such flaps must be carefully designed and surgically delayed in order to insure that the flap's random blood supply would be sufficient to support the flap when it is transferred. One of the major problems with such flaps is the fact that flaps from the chest area bring too much fat to the new nose and create an unattractive enlarged new nose. Such unattractive reconstructions require one or more surgical procedures later to defat the flap and improve its appearance.

Tagliacozzi flap

The technique of using an upper inner arm flap with good color match and minimal subcutaneous fat for nasal reconstruction was created by Gaspar Tagliacozzi who lived from 1545 to 1599 in Italy and published a book in 1597 describing how to do an upper arm flap to replace a missing nose.[31] This flap has, since that time, been referred to as a Tagliacozzi flap and continues to be used for this purpose 4 centuries later. In burned patients, many of them have unburned skin in the upper inner arm region suitable for a Tagliacozzi flap, if they require reconstruction of extensive loss of their nose due to a major burn. Tagliacozzi flaps are very useful in children because attachment of the flap to the nose requires that the arm be held up on the head for a minimum of 2–4 weeks and children do not suffer any joint disorders in the shoulder to the prolonged abnormal position. In adults over the age of 40, placing their arm up on their head for several weeks in order to transfer a Tagliacozzi flap may create major shoulder joint problems or restriction due to capsular fibrosis. There is a variation from the standard Tagliacozzi flap that was designed and recommended by Dr Fermando Monasterio, a plastic and reconstructive surgeon in Mexico. He recommended attaching the flap to the forehead first and then dividing if from the arm so there would be less scarring in the nasal tip region which would allow creating a better shape. **Figure 50.21a** shows a little 9-year-old boy who had extensive burns of his face and upper body. He had a considerable amount of his nasal structure lost and a skin graft placed on the upper part of his nose. To recreate his nose it was decided to use a Tagliacozzi flap based on the inner aspect of his left arm which had no burn scars. **Figure 50.21b** shows the delay of the flap which was surgically created into a tube and the arm defect repaired with a skin graft. **Figure 50.21c** shows that 2 weeks later, the proximal end of the Tagliacozzi tubed flap was attached to the surgically debrided nose and his arm was attached to his head similar to Tagliacozzi's attachment method for 3 weeks while the flap got solidly healed. After 3 weeks, the distal end of the flap was divided and the excess amount of tissue was left hanging with a proper dressing for 2 weeks to ensure a good blood supply to the nasal tip tissue. After

the 2 weeks of the excess tissue hanging it was surgically fashioned to create the new nasal tip nostrils. **Figure 50.21d** shows that 5 months after the nose was moderately well constructed but had a bit of excess tissue which was later revised and corrected.

Burn neck contractures and their influence on facial deformities

One of the most difficult problems in reconstructing the major deformities of patients who were burned is that of the various forms of neck contractures caused by burn scarring which may limit both neck and jaw mobility and also may influence and increase facial deformities. Patients who suffer both limited and extensive facial burns often sustain significant burns to the cervical region which may produce neck contractures after initial healing. In order to achieve optimal correction of burned facial deformities of patients who have scarring of both the face and neck, it is necessary to correct the neck contracture first in order to attain the best possible results of successive facial reconstruction. Burn scar contracture in the cervical region can cause at least four significant deformities in the face:

1. pulling down the lower lip, which in some cases makes it difficult to close the mouth;
2. pulling down lower eyelids by tension through either normal or scarred cheek skin;
3. increased tension in facial scars caused by burn contractures of the neck can create increases in the size, thickness and contracture of hypertrophic scars of the face; and
4. complex combinations of the three problems noted above caused by neck scar contractures.

The critical procedures for the surgical correction of the various deforming neck scar conditions are the wide release and deep removal of all the contracting scar and replacement with healthy new tissue to maintain the release. The various aspects and problems of burned neck deformities and their correction will be delineated in the following portion of this section:

- classification of types of burn neck contractures;
- prevention methods;
- problems of various types faced by patients;
- surgical treatment; and
- the use of grafts and flaps for correction and coverage.

Classification

In reviewing all the patients with cervical burn contractures there are three main groups of neck contractures defined by the degree of involvement and functional deformity and described by the abnormal joining up of various anatomical areas by the contractures.

1. Severe neck contractures
   a. Labio-sternal
   b. Mento-sternal
2. Moderate neck contractures
   a. Cervico-sternal
   b. Heavy multiple bands
   c. Upper neck involvement exclusively
3. Mild neck contractures
   a. Discrete linear bands
   b. Isolated cervical scars.

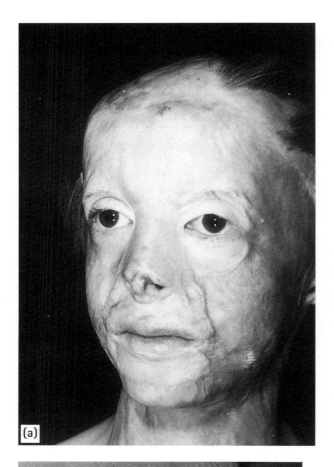

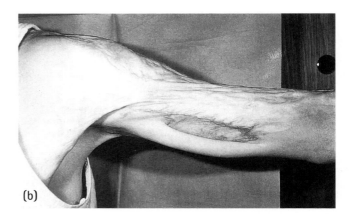

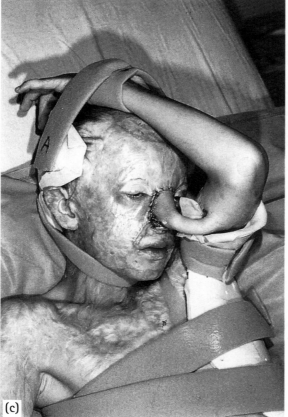

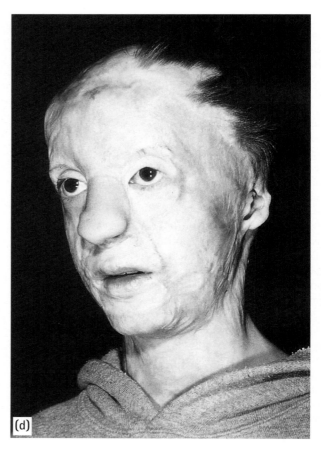

Fig. 50.21 (a) A 9-year-old boy who suffered extensive burns and loss of nose that was grafted during acute burn phase. (b) Delayed tubed Tagliacozzi flap on left upper inner arm. (c) Tagliacozzi flap sutured in place to replace his nose. (d) Result 5 months after Tagliacozzi flap to reconstruct his burn destroyed nose with some excess tissue that was later revised.

There are several pictures of patients with the various kinds of burn neck contractures mentioned in the list above. **Figure 50.22** represents a patient who had a labio-sternal contracture which is a very distressing problem with the burn scar extending directly from the lower lip down to the sternum and chest, which stoutly tethers the head down on the chest. **Figure 50.23** demonstrates a mento-sternal contracture which is slightly less severe than the labio-sternal variety because the lip is not pulled down, but the boy's chin is uncomfortably fused to the chest as shown in the profile view. In both of these two severe contracture groups, the mandible is involved and patients with such contractures are unable to look up without opening their mouths, and such patients tend to walk around constantly with their mouths open to reduce the tension of the contracture. **Figure 50.24** has a patient with a cervico-sternal contracture with burn scars that mainly connect the neck down to the upper chest which also tends to limit head motion to a limited degree. The girl in this picture has considerable neck scarring some of which also extends up to the face without pulling facial structures down to the chest which labio-sternal and mento-sternal contractures. **Figure 50.25** shows a girl with heavy multiple bands that do not limit the emotion of the neck but do cause discomfort. **Figure 50.26** shows a young boy with the mildest of

burn neck deformities, namely discrete linear bands, and he has only a single band extending up his neck which to a minor degree can create tension on various of the lower facial features.

Prevention of Burn Neck Contractures

Several neck contractures prevention methods can be employed during the treatment of an acutely burned patient and some of the methods listed will tend to prevent burn neck contractures or reduce the severity of a subsequent contracture:

- early grafting;
- physical therapy;
- short mattress use;
- TV placement;
- use of neck collar; and
- possible use of a mandibular wire.

Early excision and grafting of a recently healed burn scar of the neck can be useful in preventing the development of a later severe neck contracture. Also, since the neck is an area of high priority, an acutely burned patient should have the burn eschar excised and grafted early in the course of acute treatment which is another way to prevent later contracture.

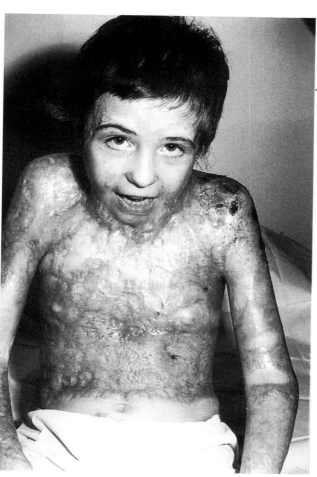

Fig. 50.22 Labio-sternal burn neck contracture in a girl who sustained a 65% BSA burn with her lip pulled down to her chest.

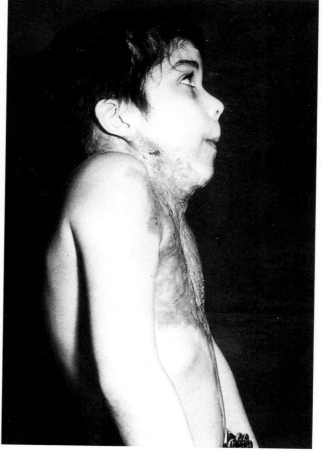

Fig. 50.23 Mento-sternal burn neck contracture with chin pulled down to chest.

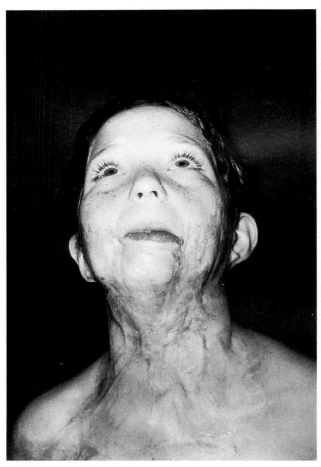

Fig. 50.24 Cervico–sterna burn neck contracture with burn scar from the neck to the chest.

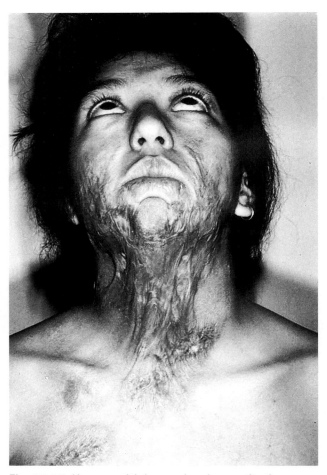

Fig. 50.25 Heavy multiple scar bands constituting a moderate neck contracture.

Physical therapists caring for acutely burned patients can perform several procedures to help prevent neck contractures. Such important activities include:

- making sure the patient is positioned correctly, with mild flexion of the neck, hyperextension of the anterior neck and rotating the neck towards the unburned side if possible;
- beginning neck exercises immediately after entry to the burn area of the hospital and continue such activities up to the time that excision and grafting is done; then appropriate exercises should be resumed about 7–10 days after grafting;
- the use of exercises when sitting or standing also can be done, particularly using a mirror to assure that the patient sees her or his position, the range of available motion and helping maintain proper posture; and
- during important careful exercises, other parts of the body should be maintained in proper alignment, e.g. to prevent shoulder elevation or forward contraction, and also to prevent dropping of the jaw or lower lip.

A short mattress can be very helpful for certain burned patients. When a burned patient with neck involvement is placed in bed, a short mattress can be placed on top of a regular one so that the patient's head and neck tend to fall off the end of the short mattress into hyperextension and tends to help resist the contracting force of the healing burn scar.

In addition, if there is a television above the acutely burned patient's bed, the overhead TV could be mounted in a correct position in combination with a short mattress so that the patient's head will be maintained in a hyperextended position while they are watching a television program.

Neck collars used appropriately for acutely burned patients as they heal can also be helpful in preventing burn neck contractures. A neck supporting collar or brace used early in the treatment of a burned patient or just after initial healing can be very useful in preventing a neck contracture. Such collars placed in a sterile fashion can be either commercially made collars of a custom-made, well fitting isoprene plastic collar made by a burn physio-occupational therapist.

Mandibular wires are not always possible to use to keep an acutely burned neck in a hyperextended position because the wire placed through the mandibular bone and applied with weighted traction frequently causes severe unnecessary pain for the burned patient. However, the use of a mandibular wire to keep the neck extended may work comfortably in a limited number of burn patients.

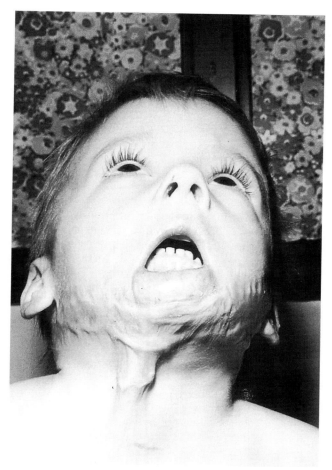

Fig. 50.26 A discrete scar band in the anterior neck which is one of the mildest burn neck contractures.

Problems due to Neck Contractures

Patients with burn neck contractures have several kinds of problems which are caused by the various physical characteristics of the neck contractures.

Discomfort

A patient who has a significant burn contracture of the neck has the head solidly encased in scar and is unable to move the head in a normal fashion. In addition, the miseries of a thoroughly uncomfortable position accumulate and cause continual aching of the muscle and vertebral joints. Patients with such severe neck contractures are very limited in normal and comfortable flexion, extension and rotation of the head.

Sense of deformity

Patients of all ages who are afflicted with neck contractures of various degrees not only experience different forms of discomfort, but also may have deep negative feelings of their appearance which may create a substantial distortion of the patient's self-image. In addition, they may also feel that they look like a freak or a monster.

Drooling

Severe forms of neck contractures, such as labio-sternal type, cause constant drooling of saliva which leads to discomfort and is due to the fact that the patient is unable to keep their lower lip in a normal closed position. Also, because of the inability to keep normal lip closure, some patients will find it impossible to retain flood and ingested liquids in their mouths and in the most severe cases, this can lead to nutritional problems.

Airway problems

Neck contractures can cause mild to severe airway distortions which may complicate the ability of anesthetists to place intraoral airways. In addition, children with marked neck contractures and enlarged tonsils may commonly develop severe respiratory distress with intermittent hypoxia and cyanosis. The probable mechanism of this form of upper airway obstruction is that the chin is drawn down to the chest which forces the laryngo-hyoid complex up to a position which further narrows the already constricted part of the airway because of the enlarged tonsils and creates interference with normal laryngeal function.

Abnormal position problems

A patient with almost any degree of neck contracture will tend to develop a compensatory kyphosis posture in order to be able to look directly ahead. The kyphosis position does not become permanent if a proper neck release is done early. An even more distressing problem caused by an unrelieved lateral neck contracture is the production of a torticollis-like uncomfortable condition. In adults and children this can be very uncomfortable. However, in young children if the neck contracture creating a torticollis position remains untreated for an abnormally long time, the growing skeletal areas may have permanent changes created by the torticollis deformity on the bones.

Dental imbalance

One of the most unusual, but important, problems caused by neck contracture which also causes significant lower lip contractures is the tendency for the lower anterior teeth to lean outward from their normal position. Teeth are held in their normal vertical position by the balance supported by the combination of tongue and labial musculature. When the lower lip pulled down by the scar of neck contractures for a significant period of time, the lower teeth will be inclined to a flattened position in the labial direction.

Surgical Treatment

The definitive surgical treatment of burn neck contractures is ideally done at the proper time and responding to the correct desires and reasoning of the patient. In performing the effective surgical correction of neck contractures, each of the following items must be properly done.

Incision depth

In order to correct a neck contracture of any type, it is necessary to incise the correct depth where normal tissue is by sequentially incising through the contracture scar and occasionally necessary through the normal skin at the scar edge. On occasion in extreme cases, incision must be carried on through the platysma down to the anterior cervical musculature thus allowing the wound to gape as much as possible which will then make it easier to do scar excision of proper size and breadth. In addition, special attention must be paid to removing all deep scars such as collagen tension bands and plates of scar which will create an optimal bed for the skin graft or flap and also release the tensions in the face.

Excision width

It is imperative not only to cut deeply enough, but also to excise widely enough and in the proper functional zones so as to remove both the heavy superficial and deep scars in order to permit a full release of the contracture. Occasionally, it is necessary to cut into the normal tissue at the scar edge in order to make the edge design correct so that a scar band is not formed after healing. In certain cases, in order to get a proper release, a very wide excision of all the scar must be carried out either back to the lower areas of the infra-mastoid regions or to the region of the sterno-cleido mastoid muscle, which is the neutral active portion of the lateral neck. By carrying out appropriate width of excisions, the scar edges in those regions will not hypertrophy post-operatively because of lack of excess motion on the healing edge scar.

Edge design

Proper edge design of neck contracture release by wide and/or complete scar excision will prevent linear scar contractures from developing in the late postoperative period. In general, a single or several V-shaped designs of the excision edges will prevent hypertrophic edge scar contractures from developing.

Thickness of skin graft

When skin grafts are placed on neck contracture releases, they must be proper thickness in order to achieve satisfactory results. A major problem following neck scar releases and excisions is a recurrence of the neck contracture due to initial application of too thin a skin graft. Depending on the age and skin type of the patient receiving neck contracture correction, a maximal thickness split-thickness skin graft should be taken with the dermatome at between 18 and 20/1000th of an inch thick and provide extremely careful postoperative care of the donor site.

Immediate postoperative care

There are several special procedures in carrying out successful early and later postoperative care. The stent tied over the skin graft must be stabilized with a soft dressing covered by a well designed solid neck splint and left in place until the graft is well healed. In particular, with large grafts of virtually the entire anterior portion of the neck, it is critical to keep the patient on a full-liquid diet postoperatively until the stent is removed in order to minimize swallowing action. When swallowing solid foods, the laryngeal cartilage ('Adam's apple') is moved very actively during the swallowing action. Such motion of the laryngeal cartilage tends to rub against the under side of the skin graft held stably by the tend and neck splint, and the constant laryngeal motion frequently will cause a loss of the central portion of the graft. Later, when the stent is taken down and the graft is solidly healed, a carefully fitted neck splint with soft conformer should be applied for several weeks or months to help continue late healing and modeling of the graft.

Coverage Choices – Use of Skin Grafts or Pedicle Flaps

The two major choices of coverage for excised neck scar contractures are free split-thickness skin grafts and various forms of pedicle flaps. Rarely, full-thickness skin grafts and free flaps may be used. The following are some of the advantages and disadvantages of the use of free skin grafts and pedicle flaps for the repair of burn neck contractures.

Split-thickness skin grafts

The *advantages* of the use of free split-thickness skin grafts include:

- a single operative procedure is used with a free graft;
- the hospital time is usually much shorter when using free grafts comparing it using complex pedicle flaps;
- donor site deformities for both split- and full-thickness skin grafts are generally not very substantial;
- if further releases are necessary, it is relatively simple to use free grafts in successive stages.

The *disadvantages* of using free split-thickness skin grafts can occur in the following situations:

- split-thickness skin grafts are not always esthetically satisfactory because they can become a little stiff and wrinkled and, if taken from the very lower part of the body, will appear darker than the surrounding cervical and upper chest skin;
- free skin grafts, both split-thickness and full-thickness, need prolonged immobilization and pressure – for several months in some cases – in order to get a good result;
- split-thickness skin grafts can become lost due to action of the laryngeal cartilage moving during swallowing or lost due to subgraft hematoma formation and recurrent contractures can occur if there is some graft loss or too thin a graft was used.

Pedicle flap

The *advantages* of the use of pedicle flaps in correcting neck contractures include:

- pedicle flaps bring full-thickness skin plus determined subcutaneous tissue to the defect;
- pedicle flaps can be easily remodeled later by thinning the flap which has protective vasculature – the pedicle edge scars tend to look more attractive than graft edge scars;
- pedicle flaps tend to bring normal tissue fullness to areas of the neck which have lost tissue fullness due to acute burns and deep scarring.

The *disadvantages* of the use of pedicle flaps can occur due to the following instances:

- the use of preparing pedicle flaps occasionally need several operative stages which makes a longer hospital stay;
- the donor site of a good-sized pedicle flap usually needs skin grafting which tends to create nonesthetic scarring in the previously normal skin areas;
- occasionally, pedicle flaps moved to the repaired area get fat if the patient gets obese later in life and, also usually, the use of free flaps brings too much bulk to areas like the neck;

- unfortunately, if the flap gets ischemic necrosis due vascular problem, then the patient will get additional scarring.

Figure 50.27 and 50.28 illustrate successful examples of correcting burn neck contractures by using split-thickness skin grafts and pedicle flaps.

Figure 50.27 illustrates a child with correction of her neck contracture using a split-thickness skin graft that has several of the important points of surgical correction of burn neck contractures:

1. **Figure 50.27a** shows her preoperative condition with a moderately severe cervico-sternal contracture;

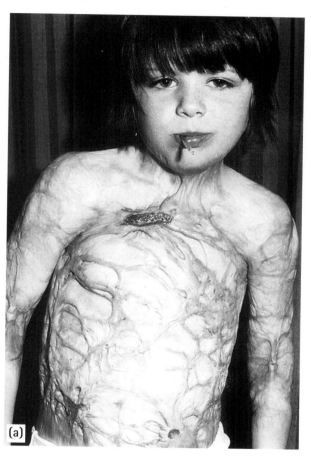

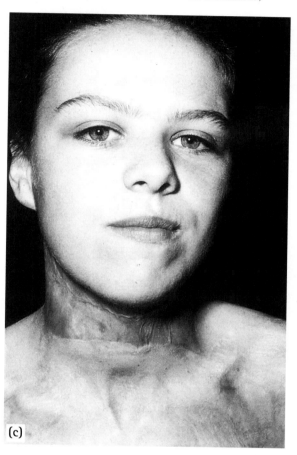

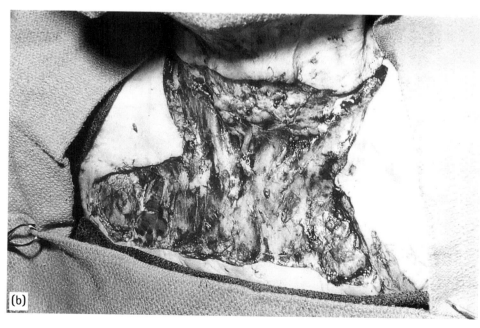

Fig. 50.27 (a) Preoperative condition of girl with severe cervico–sterna burn neck contracture. (b) Neck defect after excision of neck scar with V-shaped edge design at both sides. (c) Result of neck contracture scar excision and skin graft with V-shaped edge designs 8 years postoperatively.

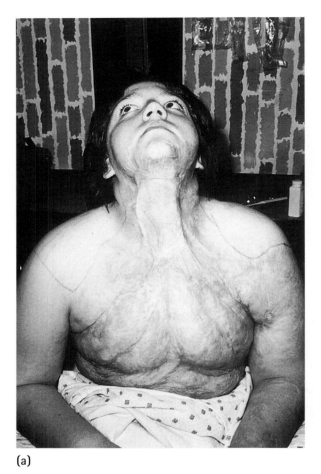

(a)

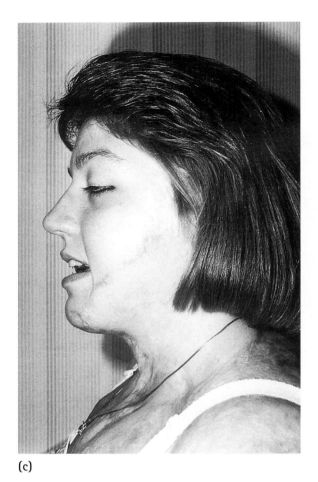

(c)

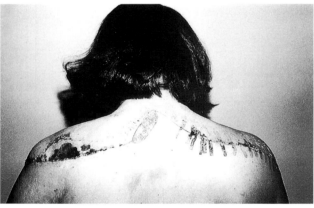

(b)

Fig. 50.28 (a) Preoperative status of a teenaged girl with recurrent burn neck contracture with anterior designs of epaulette shoulder flaps. (b) Surgical design and delay of epaulette shoulder flaps to replace the recurrent burn neck contracture. (c) Result 6 years postoperatively after epaulette shoulder flaps to correct recurrent burn neck contracture.

2. **Figure 50.27b** shows the neck defect after excision of the scar contracture with the depth down to the surface of the anterior cervical musculature with the width of excision back to the sternocleido mastoid region and the edge created with a large V-shaped design on each side;
3. **Figure 50.27c** shows her result 8 years postoperatively.

Figure 50.28 illustrates a young woman who had a labio-sternal neck contracture corrected when she was young, but then

partially recurred later in her life requiring re-correction using pedicle flaps:

1. **Figure 50.28a** shows her neck contracture recurrence, which seriously impaired her neck motion, her self-image and self-confidence and also shows the anterior portions of the epaulette flaps to be used in correction;
2. **Figure 50.28b** shows the posterior portion of the design of

the epaulette flaps which had been incised and elevated during initial surgical delays of the flaps; and

3. **Figure 50.28c** shows the good result that she had 6 years later which improved her neck mobility and helped her return to more normal self-image and greater self-confidence.

References

1. Enlow D. *The Human Face. An Account of the Postnatal Growth and Development of the Craniofacial Skeleton.* New York: Harper and Row, 1968; **8**, 39.

2. Enlow D. *The Human Face. An Account of the Postnatal Growth and Development of the Craniofacial Skeleton.* New York: Harper and Row, 1968: 236.

3. Fricke NB, Omnell L, Dutcher KD, *et al.* Skeletal and dental disturbances after facial burns and pressure garment use: a 4-year follow-up. *J Burn Care Rehabil* 1999; **20**: 239–49.

4. Fricke NB, Omnell L, Dutcher KD, *et al.* Skeletal and dental disturbances after facial burns and pressure garments. *J Burn Care Rehabil* 1996; **17**: 338–45.

5. Enlow D. *The Human Face. An Account of the Postnatal Growth and Development of the Craniofacial Skeleton.* New York: Harper and Row, 1968; 79.

6. Harley RD. *Pediatric Ophthalmology*, 2nd edn, Vol. 1. Philadelphia: WB Saunders, 1983; **294**, 327–30.

7. Pless IB, Pinkerton P. *Chronic Childhood Disorders: Promoting Patterns of Adjustment.* Chicago: Year Book Medical, 1975.

8. Adullah A, Blakeney P, Hunt R, *et al.* Visible scars and self-esteem in pediatric patients with burns. *J Burn Care Rehabil* 1994; **15**: 164–8.

9. Bernstien NR In: Noshpitz J, ed. *Basic Handbook of Child Psychiatry*, Vol 1. New York: Basic Books, 1979: 432–6.

10. Bernstein NR, Robson MC. *Comprehensive Approaches to the Burned Person.* New Hyde Park, NY: Medical Examination, 1983; 49–77.

11. Bernstein NR, Robson MC. *Comprehensive Approaches to the Burned Person.* New Hyde Park, NY: Medical Examination, 1983; 57.

12. Bernstein NR, Robson MC. *Comprehensive Approaches to the Burned Person.* New Hyde Park, NY: Medical Examination, 1983: 63–5.

13. Bernstein NR. *Emotional Problems of the Facially Burned and Disfigured.* Boston: Little Brown, 1976.

14. Brent B. Reconstruction of ear, eyebrow and sideburn in the burned patient. *Plastic Reconstr Surg* 1975; **55**: 312–7.

15. Sloan DF, Huang TT, Larson DL, Lewis SR. Reconstruction of the eyelids and eyebrows in burned patients. *Plastic Reconstr Surg* 1976; **58**: 240–346.

16. Pensler JM, Dillan B, Parry SW. Reconstruction of the eyebrow in the pediatric burned patient. *Plastic Reconstr Surg J* 1985; **76**: 434–9.

17. Monks GH. The restoration of a lower eyelid by a new method. *Boston Med Surg J* 1898; **139**: 385–7.

18. Conway H, Stark RB, Kavanaugh JD. Variations of the temporal flap. *Plastic Reconstr Surg* 1952; **9**: 410–23.

19. Converse JM, McCarthy JG, Dobhovsky M, *et al.* Facial burns. In: Converse JM, ed. *Plastic Reconstr Surg.* Philadelphia, PA: WB Saunders, 1977; 1628–31.

20. Engrav LH, Donelan MB. Face burns: acute care reconstruction. In: *Operative Techniques in Plastic and Reconstructive Surgery*, No. 2. Philadelphia, PA: WB Saunders, 1997; 4.

21. Schmid E. The use of auricular cartilage and composite grafts in reconstruction of the upper lip, with special reference to reconstruction of the philtrum. In: Broadbent TR ed. *Transactions of the Third International Congress of Plastic Surgery, Amsterdam.* The Netherlands: Ecerpta Medica, 1964; 306.

22. Antia NH, Buch VJ. Chondrocutaneous advancement flap for the marginal defect of the ear. *Plastic Reconstr Surg* 1967; **39**: 472.

23. Brent B. Reconstruction of the auricle. In: McCarthy JG, ed. *Plastic Surgery*, Vol. 3. Philadelphia, PA: WB Saunders, 1990; 2094–152.

24. Feldman J. Facial burns. In: McCarthy JG, ed. *Plastic Surgery*, Vol 3. Philadelphia, PA: WB Saunders, 1990; 2153–236.

25. Davis J. *Aesthetic and Reconstructive Otoplasty.* New York: Springer-Verlag, 1987.

26. Donelan MB. Conchal transposition flap for post-burn ear deformities. *Plastic Reconstr Surg* 1989; **83**: 641–52.

27. Lynch JB, Pousti A, Doyle J, Lewis S. Our experiences with silastic ear implants. *Plastic Reconstr Surg* 1972; **49**: 283–5.

28. Brent B, Byrd HS. Secondary ear reconstruction with cartilage grafts covered by axial, random and free flaps of temporoparietal fascia. *Plastic Reconstr Surg* 1983; **72**: 141–51.

29. Strauch B, Vasconez LO, Hall-Findlay EJ, eds *Grabb's Encyclopedia of Flaps.* Vol 1. 181–94. Boston: Little Brown & Co.

30. Strauch B, Vasconez LO, Hall-Findlay EJ, eds Vol 1. Ibid. 195–203.

31. Tagliacozzi G. *De Curtorum Chirurgia per Insitionem (Icones).* Venice: Bindoni, 1597.

Chapter 51

Correction of burn alopecia
Robert L McCauley

Introduction

Burns to the head and neck represent some of the more challenging problems in acute wound care, subsequent rehabilitation, and reconstruction. The defects are not easily hidden. Initial reports documented a 25% incidence of burn injuries involving the head and neck region.[1] In 1989, Brou *et al.* noted that defects in the head and neck region constituted 235 of 517 (45%) problems in 25 pediatric patients with a 71% mean TBSA burn.[2] In a more recent study of 194 pediatric burned patients, alopecia was noted in 32% of the patient population.[3] Although this study documented a 61% incidence of burn alopecia occurred because of the burn itself or because of the harvesting to scalp skin grafts. Later data documented a 2.2% incidence of complications, including scar alopecia, secondary to the use of the scalp doner site in burn patients.[4] Regardless of the etiology, alopecia in burned patients continues to pose a significant problem for the reconstructive surgeon.

Approaches to correction of burn alopecia

Reconstruction of scalp defects with the use of excision and primary closure has proven to be applicable in regions with small defects.[5,6] Indeed, several excisions have been reported to be successful in the correction of burn alopecia which is less than 15% of the hair-bearing scalp. In 1977, Huang *et al.* reported that the use of primary excision and/or rotation flaps was useful in the correction of defects covering 15–20% of the hair-bearing scalp.[1]

Although these methods remain useful in the correction of small scalp defects, larger defects require more involved surgical techniques.

In 1968, Ortichochea introduced the four-flap technique for reconstruction of scalp defects.[7] This was subsequently modified to the three-flap scalp reconstruction in 1971.[8] Although it is difficult to gauge the extent of alopecia covered using these techniques, these methods have been quite useful in the correction of moderate size alopecia defects. The primary disadvantage associated with the use of these techniques relates to the use of blood transfusions, the extensive scarring which results from mobilization of the multiple scalp flaps and their inability to close very large defects.[9] Also taking advantage of the profuse vascular supply of the scalp, Juri *et al.* used a variety of monopedicled scalp flaps to cover segmental areas of alopecia, especially in the frontal region.[10-12] The use of this pedicled flap was limited in that size of the alopecia segment to be corrected was small. However, Feldman showed coverage of patients with significant burn alopecia when horizontal scalp reduction was used in combination with the Juni flap.[13] More recently, Barrera has shown that the use of micrografts and minigrafts can be very successful in the correction of large alopecia segments in 32 burn patients.[14] Because of the size of micrografts (1–2 hair follicles) and minigrafts (3–4 hair follicles), the metabolic rate is quite low, allowing them to survive in scar tissue. However, the clinical application of tissue expansion to the closure of large scalp defects without excessive scarring revolutionized the approach to this problem.

Tissue expansion

Skin expansion is based on the dynamic fashion in which living tissue responds to a constant mechanical stress load. The growth of the gravid uterus and our ability to gain or lose massive amounts of weight demonstrates the ability of the skin to develop independently. Tissue expansion represents a medical application of the normal physiologic process for the correction of significant traumatic defects using adjacent, identical tissue.

As part of the exotic esthetics of various cultures, tissue expansion has achieved significant social implications in a variety of societies throughout the world. The enlarged lips of the Acaridan women were primarily developed to accentuate their own sense of beauty. The elongated necks that were subsequently produced in the Padugung women of Burma also attest to the exotic aesthetics associated with tissue expansion.[15]

Clinical uses of soft-tissue expansion did not gain significance until 1905 when bone-lengthening by distraction resulted in expansion of soft tissue.[16] These experiments were initially conducted by Codivilla, with subsequent follow-up by Putti in 1921.[17] The first reported clinical case of pure soft-tissue expansion was reported in 1956 by Neumann for the reconstruction of a traumatic ear defect by expansion of postauricular skin using a subcutaneous balloon.[18] In 1975, Radavan and Austed, working independently, developed the concept of soft-tissue expansion using a silicone implant.[19–21] Although Radavan became the first surgeon to gain extensive experience in the use of silicone expanders, Austed first reported the laboratory and clinical experience with tissue expanders prior to subsequent clinical use.

Biology of tissue expansion

Histologic Studies of Skin

Experimental data on the biology of tissue expanders have resulted from animal experimentation.[21–23] Subsequent human studies were noted to be similar to the animal data.[24] Initial studies by Paysk *et al.* showed that, although cellular retraction was normal, the epidermis appeared thicker and was associated with the loss of rete ridges. Histologic examination of the dermis revealed a thinner dermis. It is clear that the most significant changes occur with thinning of the reticular dermis. Although the papillary dermis also thins out, its response to tissue expansion is less dramatic when compared to the reticular dermis.[25] Also noted was an increase in dermal collagen content with breakage of elastic fibers; however, no significant changes in skin appendages were seen. Electron microscopy also documented the absence of significant physiologic changes of skin associated with soft tissue expansion. In 1998, Takei *et al.* investigated the molecular basis for tissue expansion. This group suggested that the protein kinase, a transductive pathway, is involved in the increased mitotic activity observed in the epidermis after skin expansion[26] (**Figure 51.1**).

Vascular Supply of Expanded Skin

Several investigators have observed a significant increase in vascularity associated with soft-tissue expansion both histologically

and clinically. Cherry *et al.* noted an increase in the surviving length of expanded skin flaps when compared to delayed skin flaps.[27] Sasaki *et al.*, using labeled microspheres, confirmed these earlier studies while also documenting an increase in blood flow associated with expanded skin flaps.[28] More recently, Lantieri *et al.* suggested that vascular endothelial growth factor (VEGF) may play a role in the development of the increased vascularity noted in expanded flaps. A comparison of immunolocalization of VEGF in expanded versus unexpanded skin demonstrated VEGF was only expressed in expanded tissue.[29] The ability of soft tissue to expand is based on several physiological properties. The skin has a constant ability to adapt, although this depends primarily on the amount and distribution of structural proteins and tissue fluids. Collagen fibers become parallel with the stretching of the tissue. Although elastin fibers are important for recoil after stretching, collagen fibers lengthen permanently.

Clinical Application in Burn Alopecia

The role of tissue expansion in the correction of pediatric burn alopecia has slowly become recognized as the gold standard with which other reconstructive methods must be compared. With the increased survival of children suffering massive total body surface area burns, reconstruction of significant defects have become quite a challenge.

In 1978, Huang *et al.* classified the extent of burn alopecia as it related to the correction of this problem.[1] At this time, the authors used primary excision and rotation flaps as a means to either eliminate or camouflage burn alopecia. These investigators felt that alopecia greater than 15% of the hair-bearing scalp was not amenable to correction with serial primary excision. A major thrust in the clinical application of tissue expansion for the correction of burn alopecia developed with the 1984 report of Manders *et al.*[30] This group of investigators demonstrated the efficacy and safety of soft-tissue expansion in the correction of scalp defects in pediatric patients.[30] Later reports confirmed the feasibility of tissue expansion in the correction of burn alopecia despite moderately high complication rates.[30–33] Subsequently, McCauley *et al.* further classified burn alopecia based on not only the pattern of the alopecia but also the extent of the alopecia.[34] This classification was designed as a means by which reconstructive efforts could be designed so as to correct specific problems of burn alopecia (**Table 51.1**). In this report, patients with types IA and IB burn alopecia were corrected via a single expansion, although overinflation of the scalp expander may be required (**Figure 51.2**). Patients with type IC and ID burn alopecia required sequential expansion in order to obtain complete coverage (**Figure 51.3**). Patients who

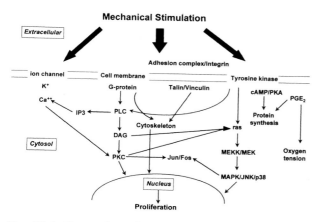

Fig. 51.1 Illustration of possible signal transduction pathways induced by mechanical strain to increase flap length. EGF, epidermal growth factor; TGFα and β, transforming growth factor α and β; PDGF platelet-derived growth factor; CTGF, connective tissue growth factor; IGF, insulin–like growth factor; phospholipase C; IP3, inositolphosphate 3; PKC, protein kinase C; DAG, diacylglycerol; MAPK, mitogen-activated kinases; MEKK, MAPK kinase; MEK, MAPK kinase; JNK, c–jun amino terminal kinase.

Table 51.1 Classification of burn alopecia	
Type I	Single alopecia segment
	A Less than 25% of the hair-bearing scalp
	B 25–50% of the hair-bearing scalp
	C 50–75% of the hair-bearing scalp
	D 75% of the hair-bearing scalp
Type II	Multiple alopecia segments amenable to tissue expansion placement
Type III	Patchy burn alopecia not amenable to tissue expansion
Type IV	Total alopecia

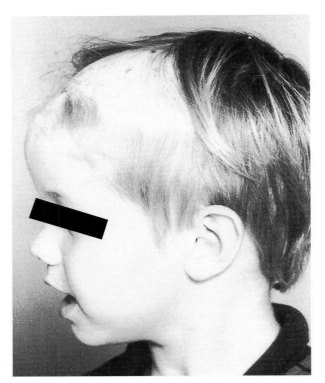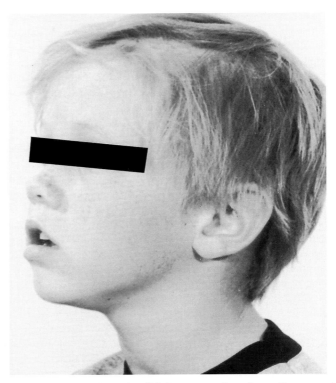

Fig. 51.2 (a) Preoperative view of 6-year-old white male with type 1A burn alopecia. (b) Postoperative view after correction of alopecia with a single expansion.

presented with type II burn alopecia were corrected with a single expanded scalp flap; however, patients with type IIB, C or D required multiple expanders if the adjacent alopecia segment could accommodate an expander. Alternatively, if the hair-bearing segments could not accommodate an expander, this tissue was incorporated around the larger expanded flap. Once the wound matured, the anterior portion of the uniform hair-bearing scalp was lifted and advanced as a single flap. Obviously patients with type III and type IV burn alopecia were not candidates for tissue expansion.

Complications

Complications associated with tissue expanders can be subdivided into those that are major, and those, that are minor. Major complications have been reported to be as low as 3% and as high as 49%.[30–32,34,35] It appears that the incidence of complications associated with tissue expanders continues to remain around 15–20%. The major complications are usually defined as those requiring removal of the expander. Such complications may be secondary to infection, exposure of the expander from traumatic extrusion, wound dehiscence, or erosion of an envelope fold or reservoir through the skin.[33] Implant failure, which requires removal of the implant, also is considered a major complication as would be ischemia of the expanded scalp flap, resulting in necrosis. Manders *et al.* reported a major complication rate of 24%.[9] Several investi-

gators have reported similar complications ranging from 17 to 24%.[31,34] Neale *et al.* have shown that, with proper protocols and patient selection, the major complication rate (those requiring additional surgery for expander replacement of additional procedures) has decreased from 22 to 12%.[25] Minor complications have been documented with these patients and have been defined as poor compliance, intolerance of the injection to fill the expanders, and alterations in the early preoperative plans secondary to incomplete coverage following expansion. Rates of such minor complications have been reported to be between 17 and 40%, with a mean still in the range of 20%.[9,31]

Conclusion

It is clear that tissue expansion has become a permanent member in the armamentarium of the reconstructive surgeon for the correction of soft-tissue defects. This role in the correction of burn alopecia has been one with tremendous impact. Numerous reports detailing the success of tissue expansion in the reconstruction of scalp defects are available. With so many burn injuries occurring to the head and neck, reconstructive surgeries, such as those designed to correct alopecia, are becoming more common and are experiencing new improvements in technique.

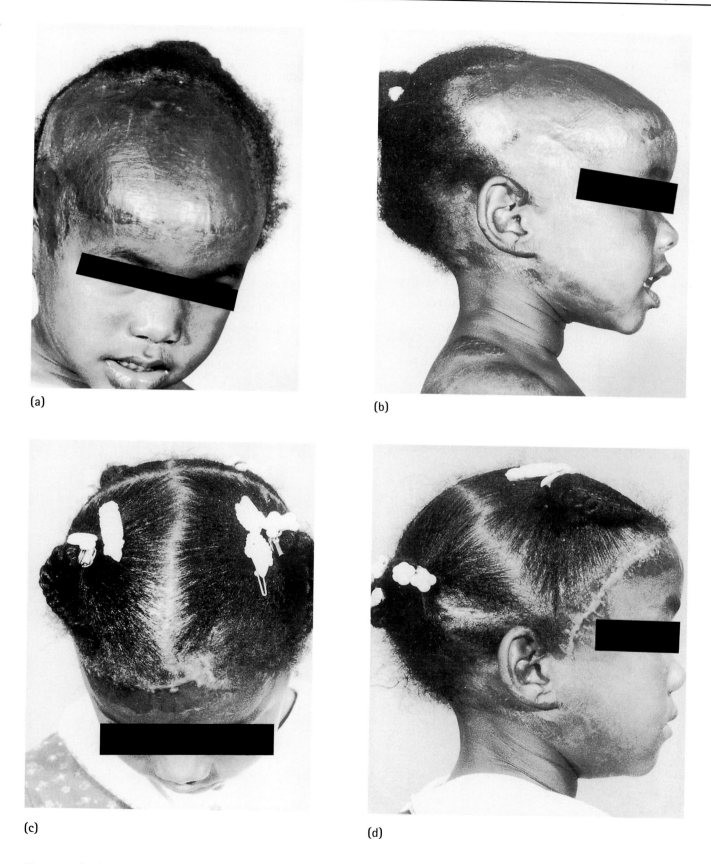

Fig. 51.3 (a,b) Preoperative views of a 6-year-old black female patient with type IC burn alopecia. (c,d) Postoperative views after correction using sequential expansion.

References

1. Huang TT, Larson DL, Lewis SR. Burn alopecia. *Plast Reconstr Surg* 1977; **60**: 762.
2. Brou JA, Robson MC, McCauley RL, *et al.* Inventory of potential reconstructive needs in the burn patient. *J Burn Care* 1989; **10**: 555.
3. Brou JA, Vu T, McCauley RL, *et al.* The scalp as a donor site: revisited. *J Trauma* 1990; **30**: 579.
4. Barret JP, Dziewulski P, Wolf SE, Desai MH, Herndon DN. Outcome of scalp donor sites in 450 consecutive pediatric burn patients. *Plast Reconstr Surg* 1999; **103**: 1139–42.
5. Paletta C. Surgical management of the burned scalp. *Clin Plast Surg* 1982; **9**: 167.
6. Vallis CP. Surgical management of cicatricial alopecia of the scalp. *Clin Plast Surg* 1982; **9**: 179.
7. Ortichochea M. Four flap scalp reconstruction technique. *Br J Plast Surg* 1967; **20**: 159–71.
8. Ortichochea M. New three flap scalp reconstruction technique. *Br J Plast Surg* 1971; **24**: 184–8.
9. Manders EK, Schendon MJ, Fussey JA, *et al.* Soft tissue expansion: concepts and complications. *Plast Reconstr Surg* 1984; **74**: 493–504.
10. Juri J. Use of parieto-occipital flaps in the surgical treatment of baldness. *Plast Reconstr Surg* 1975; **55**: 456.
11. Juri J, Juri C, Arufe HN. Use of rotation scalp flaps for the treatment of occipital baldness. *Br J Plast Surg* 1978; **61**: 23.
12. Juri J, Juri C. Aesthetic aspects of reconstructive scalp surgery. *Clin Plast Surg* 1981; **8**: 243–54.
13. Feldman G. Post-thermal burn alopecia and its treatment using extensive horizontal reduction in combination with a Juni flap. *Plast Reconstr Surg* 1994; **93**: 1268–73.
14. Barrera A. The use of micrografts and minigrafts for the treatment of burn alopecia. *Plast Reconstr Surg* 1999; **103**: 581–9.
15. Saszki G. Tissue expansion. In: Jurkiewicz MJ, Krizek TJ, Mathes S, Ariyan S, Saszki G, eds. *Plastic Surgery: Principles and Practice*. St Louis: CV Mosby, 1990; 1608.
16. Codiville A. On the means of lengthening the muscle and tissues in the lower limbs which are shorted and high deformity. *Am J Orthop Surg* 1905; **2**: 353.
17. Putti, V. Operative lengthening of the femur. *JAMA* 1921; **77**: 937.
18. Neumann CG. The expansion of an area of skin by progressive distention of a subcutaneous balloon. *Plast Reconstr Surg* 1957; **19**: 124.
19. Austed ED, Thomas SV, Pasyk K. Tissue expansion: dividend or loan? *Plast Reconstr Surg* 1986; **78**: 63.
20. Radavan C. Tissue expansion in soft tissue reconstruction. *Plast Reconstr Surg* 1984; **74**: 491.
21. Austed ED, Pasyk KA, McClatchey KD, Cherry GW. Histomorphometric evaluation of guinea pig skin and soft tissue after controlled tissue expansion. *Plast Reconst Surg* 1982; **70**: 704–10.
22. Pasyk KA, Austed ED, McClatchey KD, Cherry GW. Electron microscopic evaluation of guinea pig skin and soft tissues expanded with a self-inflating silicone implant. *Plast Reconstr Surg* 1982; **70**: 37.
23. Pasyk KA, Argenta LC, Hasseh C. Quantitative analysis of the thickness of human skin and subcutaneous tissue following controlled expansion with a silicone implant. *Plast Reconstr Surg* 1988; **81**: 516.
24. Pasyk KA, Argenta LC, Austed ED. Histopathology of human expanded tissue. *Clin Plast Surg* 1987; **14**: 435–45.
25. MacLennan SE, Corcoran JF, Neale HW. Tissue expansion in head and neck burn reconstruction. *Clin Plast Surg* 2000; **27**: 121–132.
26. Takei T, Mills I, Arai K, Sumpio BE. Molecular basis for tissue expansion: clinical implications for surgeons. *Plast Reconstr Surg* 1998; **102**: 247–58.
27. Cherry GW, Austed ED, Pasyk KA, McClatchey KD, Romich RJ. Increased survival and vascularity of random pattern skin flaps elevated in controlled, expanded skin. *Plast Reconstr Surg* 1983; **72**: 680–5.
28. Sasaki GH, Pang CY. Pathophysiology of skin flaps raised on expanded skin. *Plast Reconstr Surg* 1984; **79**: 59–65.
29. Lantieri LA, Martin-Garcia N, Wechsler J, Mitrofanoff M, Raulo Y, Bauch. Vascular endothelial growth factor expression in expanded tissue: A possible mechanism of angiogenesis in tissue expansion. *Plast Reconstr Surg* 1998; **101**: 392–8.
30. Manders EK, Graham WP, Schendon MT, Davis TS. Skin expansion to eliminate large scalp defects. *Ann Plast Surg* 1984; **12**: 305–12.
31. Neale HW, High RM, Billmon DA, *et al.* Complications of controlled tissue expansion in the pediatric burn patient. *Plast Recontr Surg* 1988; **82**: 840–5.
32. Buhrer DP, Huang TT, Yee HD. Treatment of burn alopecia with tissue expanding in children. *Plast Reconstr Surg* 1988; **82**: 840–5.
33. Ortega MT, McCauley RL, Robson MC. Salvage of an avulsed expanded scalp flap to correct burn alopecia. *South Med J* 1988; **23**: 220–3.
34. McCauley RL, Oliphant JR, Robson MC. Tissue expansion in the correction of burn alopecia: classification and methods of correction. *Ann Plast Surg* 1990; **25**: 103–15.
35. Sasaki GH. Intraoperative sustained limited expansion (ISLE) as an intermediate reconstructive technique. *Clin Plast Surg* 1987; **14**: 563–71.

Chapter 52

Management of contractural deformities involving the shoulder (axilla), elbow, hip, and knee joints in burned patients

Ted Huang

Contractural deformities

The Factors Leading to Contractural Deformities

Folding bodily joints in flexion, so called a posture of 'comfort' is a characteristic body posture seen commonly in a distressed individual. Although the exact reasons are not entirely clear, contraction of muscle fibers at rest, and contractile force difference between the flexor muscle and the extensor muscle may play an important role in the genesis of this body posture. The magnitude of joint flexion, furthermore, increases as an individual loses voluntary control of muscle movement as frequently occurs in a burn victim (**Figure 52.1**), Prolong period of physical inactivity associated with burn treatment and scar tissue contraction around the joint structures as the recovery ensues further impede the joint mobility.

Incidence of Burn Contracture

The burn treatment that requires a long period of bed confinement and physical inactivity as well as restriction of joint movement will lead to joint dysfunction. Consequently, every bodily joint; i.e. the vertebral, mandibular, shoulder, elbow, finger, hip, knee and toe joints, is susceptible to the change. Of various bodily joints involved, the contractural deformities of the shoulder (axilla), elbow, hip, and the knee are relatively common. Factors such as a wide range of joint movement and an asynchronous muscular control characteristic features of these joints, when combined with a high vulnerability to burn injuries are the probable reasons accounting for the high incidence encountered. Recent review of the records of 1005 patients treated at the Shriners Burns Hospital in Galveston, Texas over the past 25 years indicated that the elbow was the joint

Burn injuries, regardless of the etiology, rarely involve a joint. However, the joint function is often impaired because of burns. The joint problems and joint deformities noted in burn patients are mostly due to physical inactivity combined with limitation of joint movement because of scar contracture. The regimen of burn management, especially during the period immediately following the injury, seldom includes plans to care for the joint. Instead, the treatment is focused upon resuscitative efforts to restore fluid balance and to maintain functional integrity of the circulatory and the pulmonary systems. The consequence of joint dysfunction is usually left for later reconstruction.

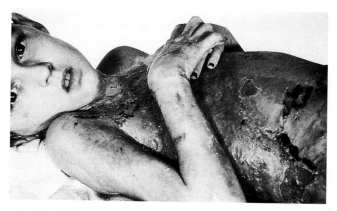

Fig. 52.1 The posture of 'comfort' characterized by flexion of shoulder (axilla) and elbow joints, plus hip and knee joints is assumed by patients under distress, as in burn patients.

most commonly affected. There were 397 patients with elbow joint deformity followed by 283 knee contractures. There were 248 axillay deformities. The hip joint contracture was the deformity least encountered and was noted in only 77 patients (**Table 52.1**).

The Efficacy of Splinting in Controlling Burn Contractures

Although Cronin in 1955 demonstrated that the neck splint was effective in preventing recurrence of neck contracture following surgical release,[1] the routine use of splinting for burn patients did not become a part of the regimen of burn wound care in Galveston until 1968 when Larson, the former Surgeon-in-Chief and Willis, the former Chief Occupational Therapist at the Shriners Burns Institute began to fabricate splints with thermoplastic materials to brace the neck and extremities.[2-5]

For more than three decades, a neck brace, a three-point extension splint, and a molded brace fabricated from thermoplastic materials, the prototypes of devices used to splint the neck, elbow, and the knee joints were used in the management of burn patients at the Shriners Burns Hospital and the University of Texas Medical Branch Hospitals in Galveston, Texas. An 'airplane splint' similarly made of thermoplastic materials was also used to splint the axilla during the period where the use of other splinting and bracing techniques, such as a 'figure-of-eight' bandage is not feasible.

A study was conducted in 1977 to determine the efficacy of splinting across large joint structures such as the elbow, axilla, and knee joints by reviewing the records of 625 patients. There were 961 burns over these joints in this group of patients. Of these, 356 had involved the axillae, while 357 and 248, respectively, involved the elbow and the knee joint. The incidence of contractural deformities encountered in these joints was, as expected, low with the use of splints. The incidence of contractures in these joints was 7.3%, provided that patients had worn the splints for 6 months. The effectiveness of splinting was diminished to 55% if splinting was discontinued within 6 months. For comparison, the incidence of contractural deformity ascertained in 219 patients who had never worn the splint was 62%, (**Table 52.2**).

Table 52.1 The distribution of joint deformities

Joint involved	No.
Shoulder (Axilla)	248
Elbow	397
Hip	77
Knee	283
Total	1005

Table 52.2 The incidence of contractures across the shoulder (Axilla), elbow and knee joints

	Without splint	With splint	
		<6 months	>6 months
Shoulder			
Severe/Moderate	137	24	23
Mild/None	37	6	129
Elbow			
Severe/Moderate	75	17	10
Mild/None	61	33	161
Knee			
Severe/Moderate	26	4	2
Mild/None	45	16	155

Although splinting and bracing were shown to be effective in minimizing joint contracture, it was not entirely clear if restriction of joint movement would affect the quality of scar tissues formed across the joint surface. The effects were assessed by determining the frequency of secondary surgery performed in this group of patients. Over 90% of 219 individuals who did not use the splint/bracing required reconstructive surgery. In contrast, the need for surgical reconstruction in individuals who wore splints was 25%.[6]

Management

The Acute Phase of Recovery

It is believed that inadequate physical exercise and lack of joint splinting and bracing, while allowing a patient to assume the posture of 'comfort', are the main factors responsible for the genesis of contractural deformities seen in burn patients during the *acute phase* of recovery from burn injuries. The deformities, furthermore, are made worse because of skin involvement and burn scar contracture. In order to minimize this undesirable consequence of burn injuries, proper body positioning, and splinting of the joint structures must be incorporated in the regimen of burn treatment. The treatment should be implemented as soon as the patient's condition becomes stable.

Body positioning and joint splinting

Bodily position

Although a supine position is preferred, the patient may be placed in a lateral decubitus position while confined in bed. The head should be placed in a neutral position with the neck slightly extended. For a patient placed in a supine position, neck extension is achieved by placing a small pad between the scapulae to facilitate the scapular traction. A neck brace may be used if a patient is placed in other body positions.

Shoulder (axillary) joint

The shoulder joint is kept at 90–120° of abduction and 15–20° of flexion. This generally results in 60–80° of arm elevation. The position is not only useful in protecting the brachial plexus from traction injury but also effective in maintaining the stability of the glenohumeral joint. The position is best kept with the use of foam wedge, trough, and/or airplane splint. A 'figure-of-eight' wrapping over a pad around the axilla, more frequently used for patients during the intermediate phase of recovery from the injury, is effective in maintaining shoulder abduction. It is also useful in preventing excess shoulder flexion.

Elbow joint

Elbow flexion is commonly seen in a distressed patient. Rigid flexion contracture of the elbow is a common sequela if the elbow is left unattended. With burns of the skin around the olecranon, exposure of the elbow joint is a common sequela if the elbow is allowed to contract freely. Maintaining the elbow in full extension is, therefore, essential. An extension brace (**Figure 52.2**) or a three-point extension splint across the elbow joint is effective for this purpose, (**Figure 52.3**).

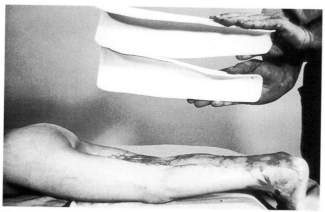

Fig. 52.2 A splint made of thermoplastic material is used to limit joint flexion.

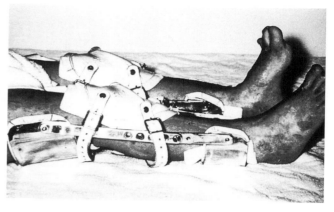

Fig. 52.4 A 'three–point' extension splint can be also used to manage the flexion contractures of a knee joint.

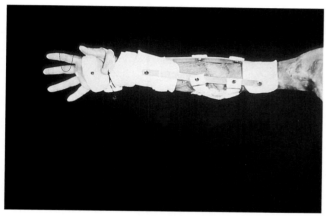

Fig. 52.3 A 'three–point' extension splint manufactured similar to an orthotic device is used either to extend a contracted elbow joint or to immobilize the joint in full extension.

Hip joint

A contractural deformity of the hip is relatively uncommon unless the hip joint is allowed to remained flexed for a long period of time. Hip extension can be achieved by placing the patient in a prone position. In a supine position, 15–20° of abduction is maintained with the use of brace or anklet.

Knee joint

Flexion of the knee is another posture commonly assumed by a burned victim. Similar to the elbow, uncontrolled flexion of the knee joint will lead to exposure of the joint structure especially in instances where the injuries involved the patella surface. Maintenance of knee in full extension is, in this sense, an essential component of therapeutic regimen. This is accomplished by means of a knee brace or a three-point extension splint to assure a full extension of the knee joint, (**Figure 52.4**).

Exercise

Although exercising a burned victim is an integral part of burn therapy, it is seldom implemented until the resuscitative measures are completed and the condition of patient is considered stable.

The primary goal of exercise is to maintain functional integrity of the joint structures and the muscle strength. This is attained by, in most instances, moving the joint manually and muscles passively. Frequency and intensity of an exercise regimen, however, may vary depending upon the magnitude of injury and the extent of joint involvement. The treatment, if possible, should be intensive and is rendered as frequent as possible.

The Intermediate Phase of Recovery

A period starting from the second month following the injury through the fourth month is considered the intermediate phase of recovery from burn injuries. The burn victims typically will have full recovery of physiologic functions with integumental integrity restored. The cicatricial processes around the injured sites, on the other hand, are physiologically active though healing of the burned wound is considered satisfactory. That is, the process is characterized by, in addition to a maximal rate of collagen synthesis, a steady increase in the myofibroblast fraction of the fibroblast population in the wound,[7] the cellular change believed to account for contraction of the scar tissues. Continuous use of splinting and pressure to support the joints and burned sites, in this sense, is essential in order to control changes caused by ensuing scar tissue formation and scar contracture.

Bodily positioning and joint splinting

Joint splinting and bodily positioning are similar to the regimen used during the acute phase of burn recovery. That is, the shoulder is kept at 15–20° flexion and 80–120° of abduction. A 'figure-of-eight' wrapping over an axillary pad is used to maintain this shoulder joint position (**Figure 52.5**). The elbow and knee joints are maintained in full extension by means of a three-point extension splint or brace. A pressure dressing or garment is incorporated in the splint. In instances where the use of 'figure-of-eight' bandage, pressure dressing and/or garment, is not feasible because of recent surgery, devices such as an 'airplane splint' device (**Figure 52.6**) or a three-point extension splint may be used to splint the axilla, elbow and the knee joints.

Pressure dressing

A compression dressing, originally incorporated in the treatment of burned wounds of the upper and lower extremities at the

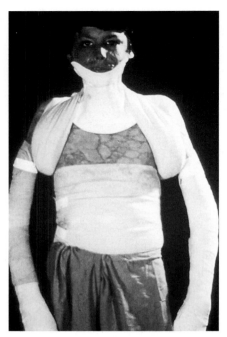

Fig. 52.5 An elasticized bandage is used to wrap around the shoulder (axilla) joints in a 'figure-of-eight' fashion to extend and to abduct the shoulder joints. An axillary pad is included in the wrapping to increase the pressure upon the axillary fold.

Shriners Burns Hospital in 1968 as a means to provide mechanical support to healing wounds, is effective in reducing tissue swelling and in promoting softening of a burned scar. Compression of a

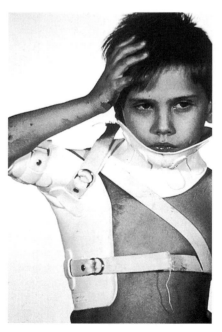

Fig. 52.6 An 'airplane' splint made of thermoplastic materials is used to maintain the shoulder abduction. The angle of separation may be increased, as the joint becomes more mobile.

burned wound even though healing is still in progress, is most easily achieved by means of wrapping the extremity with an elasticized bandage. Wrapping of the extremity should begin at the hand or foot. The bandage is moved cephalad in a crisscross fashion. The splint is reapplied over the bandage. It is important to rewrap the extremity three to four times daily. Wrapping extremity with an elasticized bandage can produce a pressure ingredient of 10–25 mm Hg.[5,8] The use of pressure dressing should be continued for 12–18 months.

Surgical management of established contractural deformities

Contraction of the shoulder, elbow, hip and knee joints can occur despite proper splinting and intensive physical therapy. Surgical reconstruction of contractural deformities, in this sense, remains an essential component of patient care and patient rehabilitation. The task of deciding the timing of surgical intervention, however, can be difficult and requires detailed evaluation of the patient and the deformity. The following are ascertained before surgery:

- the causes of joint immobility;
- the extent and the availability of uninjured skin that could be used for reconstruction; and
- the extent of maturation of scar tissues that surround the joint.

Patient Evaluation

Numerous factors will affect joint movements in burn patients. Although hypertrophy and contraction of scar tissues and/or contracted skin graft around a joint are the most common causes of joint impairment, changes in the ligamentous structures or the joint itself due to burn injuries could also limit the joint mobility. Detailed examination that includes radiographic assessment of the joint structures is essential in order to formulate a definitive treatment plan.

Nonoperative or Minimally Invasive Approach to Correct a Contracted and/or Stiff Joint

Restoration of movements in a contracted and/or stiff joint could be attained by minimally invasive or non-surgical means.[2–6] 'Pushing' and 'pulling' of an extremity that in turn, 'stretches' contracted scars and tissues around an affected joint is the principle behind this modality of managing a contracted and/or stiff joint. The treatment is found to be especially effective in mobilizing a contracted joint caused by a long period of physical inactivity or in some instances, of scar contracture. Although the morbidities associated with this modality of treatment are minimal, break down of the skin due to pressure and/or friction resulting from 'pushing' and 'pulling' of a limb can occur.

Shoulder (axillary) contracture

Tight scars formed across the shoulder joint, usually in the area along the axillary folds, often limit the joint movement. The joint stiffness caused by scar contracture may be further aggravated by physical inactivity, especially if the patient is allowed to remain in the posture of 'comfort'.

There are two nonsurgical methods commonly used to mobilize a contracted shoulder (axilla) joint. One is 'figure-of-eight' compression dressing technique and the other an 'airplane' splinting technique:

A 'figure-of-eight' compression dressing

An elasticized bandage is used to wrap over a pad placed in the axillary fold around the shoulder joint in a 'figure-of-eight' fashion to extend and abduct the shoulder. The dressing must be worn continuously and it is removed only for cleansing. Continuous wear of the dressing for a period of 3–6 months is necessary to obtain the release. The mobility of the joint increases as the scar tissues across the axilla softens. The extent of relief may be limited if the scar is thick and unyielding to the pressure. (**Figure 52.7a–d**).

An airplane splint

The splint is fabricated with a thermoplastic material. The spreading angle of the splint is conformed to the extent of the shoulder (axilla) joint held at maximum abduction plus 10–15° of extension. Abduction and extension of the arm, will be maintained by 'pushing' the arm away from the upper thorax. Care is needed to protect the skin over the inner aspect of the arm and the side of the chest. The splint is changed regularly as the angle of joint abduction increases. One to 3 months of continuous use of this device is usually necessary to achieve needed release in most instances (**Figure 52.6**).

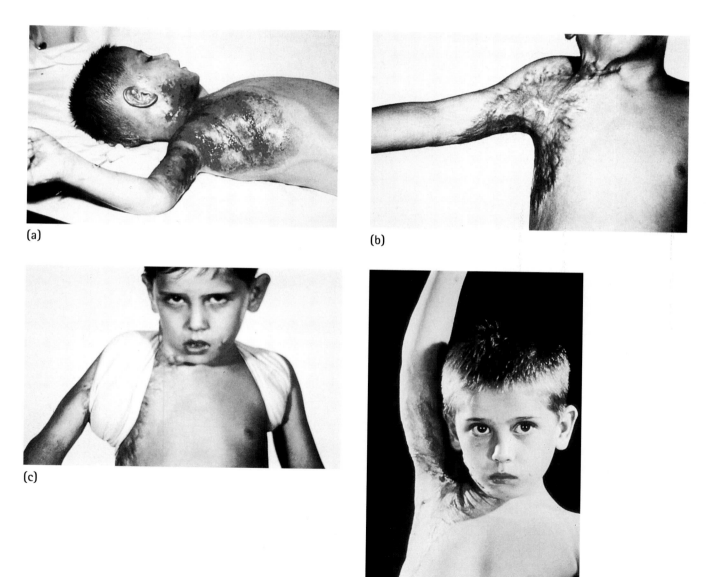

(a)

(b)

(c)

(d)

Fig. 52.7 (a) A 6-year-old body sustained burns of the right side of his body extending from the lower neck to the upper thorax that included the axillary crease. (b) He experienced difficulty in extending both the neck and the right arm because of ensuing contraction of scar tissues around the neck and the axilla. (c) A 'figure-of-eight' dressing was used to maintain the shoulder extension and abduction. The dressing was used for 12 months. (d) He regained the shoulder extension and mobility with the use of pressure dressing.

Elbow and knee contracture

Flexion contracture is the most common deformity encountered in these two joints. The scar formed across the antecubital and the popliteal fossae frequently aggravates the magnitude of contractural problems in these joints. The following techniques are frequently utilized before surgery to obtain joint movement and joint extension.

A three-point extension splint

The splint is assembled similar to a prosthetic/orthotic device. Two sidebars hinged at the middle are connected with a bracing trough at the end. A cap pad is attached at the mid-section of the sidebar to fit over the elbow or the kneecap. The splint is placed across the antecubital fossa or the popliteal fossa. Fitting of the splint is adjusted with the Velcro straps, (**Figures 52.2** and **52.3**). Extending movement of the joint is determined by the extent of preexisting joint stiffness. The angle of extension is initially determined by the angle of joint contracture. The magnitude of extension is controlled by tightening the olecranon or patella pad. It is increased gradually as the joint gains its mobility. The problems encountered with the use of a 'three-point extension splint' are uncommon. However, break down of the skin can occur. Leverage attainable from three-point pressure application may be limited in a young individual because of inadequate leverage due to short limb length. The skeletal traction technique, in such instances, may be used.

A skeletal traction technique

Utilizing a skeletal traction technique to restore movements in a contracted joint typically requires percutaneous insertion of a Steinman pin through the radius for the elbow joint and the tibia for the knee joint. The pin is inserted through both cortices at the junction of proximal two-third and the distal third of the radius or the tibia. A contracted joint can be mobilized by continuous and constant 'pull' of the long bone utilizing gravitational force generated with 10–15 pounds weight placed through a pulley device.

For a flexion deformity of the elbow, the patient is placed in a supine position. The pulley traction device will provide a horizontal and then a vertically downward pull (**Figure 52.8a–d**). A

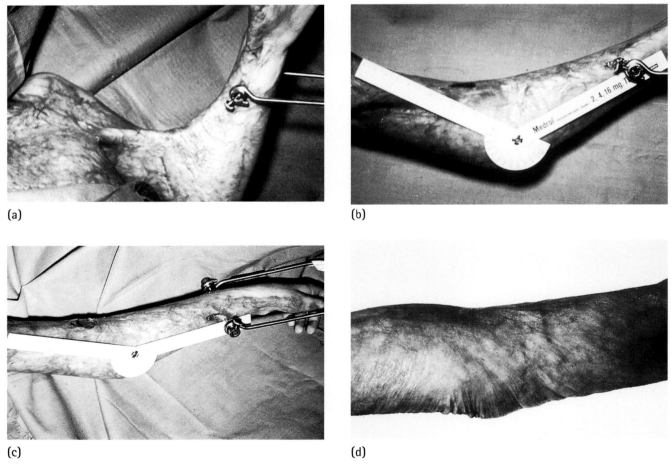

(a)

(b)

(c)

(d)

Fig. 52.8 (a) A skeletal traction technique may be used to extend a contracted joint as in this 8-year-old girl. A Steinman pin was inserted percutaneously through the distal one-third of the radius. The direction of pull was horizontal using 10–15 pound weights. (b) The elbow joint was mobilized in 30–36 hours of constant pull. (c) A near full extension of the elbow joint was achieved in 6 days. (d) This was the appearance of the elbow 2 years after the traction extension treatment for elbow contracture. A minor procedure was, however, needed to release a tight band across the elbow surface.

weight placed around the ankle with the patient being placed in a prone position, instead of a skeletal traction device, may be used to pull the foreleg to loosen a contracted knee. This technique is especially useful in treating individuals with a limited knee flexion contracture. Traction is continued for a period of time and is repeated several times a day (**Figure 52.9a, b**).

Although the morbidities due to infection are uncommon, continuous and constant force of pull can cause break down of the skin typically located in the area across the joint surface. The wound can be temporarily covered with surgical dressing or biological dressing. Closure of the wound is contemplated once the joint contracture is fully corrected.

Surgical Treatment of a Contracted Joint

Surgical treatment of a contracted joint is contemplated in individuals where the use of nonsurgical treatment is ineffective and where functional integrity of a joint is at jeopardy. Surgical intervention, in this regard, is relatively unusual during the acute phase of recovery. Instead, the reconstruction is delayed until the scar tissue becomes fully 'matured', i.e. flattening and softening of the scar tissue.

Presurgical evaluation

The patient is seen and the involved joint is examined before surgery. The following features are assessed:

- The extent of joint contracture is determined and the passive and active range of joint motion is assessed. Radiographic evaluation may be obtained to delineate structural integrity of the joint.
- The magnitude of scarring and scar thickness is assessed. The scar is usually the thickest across the joint surface.
- The location and the size of uninjured skin are delineated. The availability of uninjured skin frequently determines the technique of reconstruction. Skin graft and skin flap donor site is also ascertained.
- The point and the axis of joint rotation are located. The line

of incisional release is in alignment of the axis of joint movement.

Techniques of joint contracture release

Despite detailed examination before surgery, exact cause of joint stiffness can only be delineated with surgery. In practice, contraction of the scar tissues across the joint structure is the most common cause of contractural joint deformities.

Release of joint contracture by incising the scarred tissue

A contracted joint is freed by making an incision in the scar across the joint surface. The incision is placed in line with the axis of joint rotation. The incision is confined within the width of the scar initially and is lengthened as necessary to achieve the intended release. Prior infiltration of the area with lidocaine containing epinephrine in 1:400 000 concentration is useful in obtaining hemostasis and later pain control. The incision, however, must be made with caution to avoid injuring major vessels and nerves. This is achieved by 'pushing' instead of 'slicing' motion of a surgical blade to free the scarred tissues. The extent of release is assessed by the improvement of joint motion gained as the scarred tissue is severed. In rare instances, cicatricial changes could involve the joint capsule. Reconstruction of the capsular structure will be necessary.

The use of z-plasty technique9

A contracted area can be lengthened by use of the z-plasty technique. The technique utilizes the principle that a contracted wound is lengthened by interposing two triangular skin flaps mobilized from an unburned area immediately adjacent to the area of release. The lengthening of the wound is maximally attained by interposing two triangular flaps of 60° angle. While the z-plasty technique is an excellent means to ameliorate the problem of wound contracture; it is not possible if the amount of uninjured skin adjacent to the wound is limited.

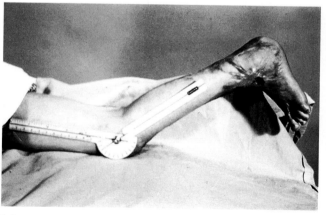

(a)

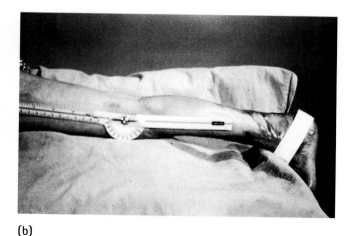

(b)

Fig. 52.9 (a) A knee contracture developed in an 8-year-old male youth due to improper positioning and immobilization of the knee joint. There was no direct injuries involving the knee area. With the patient being placed in a prone position, the ankle was strapped with 10–15 pound weights. (b) The flexion contracture was relieved in 3 days.

Wound coverage

There are six basic techniques of wound coverage. Namely,

1. Primary closure of the wound;
2. A full-thickness or partial-thickness skin graft;
3. An interposition skin flap mobilized from the area adjacent;
4. Combination of an interposition skin flap and skin grafting;
5. A muscle or skin-muscle flap mobilized from the adjacent area; and
6. A free skin or skin-muscle flap harvested from a distant site and is transferred via a microsurgical technique.

Primary closure of the wound

Wound closure *per primum* following burn scar excision is difficult if not entirely impossible. Inelasticity of the skin surrounding the wound and inadequate amount of uninjured skin available for mobilization and closure preclude the use of this method of wound closure. Closure of a resultant wound following release, in practice, would defeat the original objective of contractural reconstruction.

Skin grafting technique

The use of a piece of skin graft, full- or partial-thickness, to cover a wound is the most fundamental technique of wound coverage that is technically simple with minimal morbidities.

Operative technique: A *partial-thickness skin graft* of 15/1000th to 20/1000th in thickness is harvested from an unburned area using a dermatome. The scalp, lower abdomen, and the anterior surface of the upper thigh are the common donor sites. A piece of *full-thickness skin graft* can be harvested from the lower abdomen, above the suprapubic or inguinal area without leaving unsightly donor site defects. The subdermal fatty tissues are removed but attempts should be made to preserve the subdermal capillary plexus (**Figure 52.10a–c**). The donor defect is usually closed primarily. The graft is cut to fit the defect and the edges are anchored with 3–0 silk sutures. The ends are left sufficiently long to tie over a bolster to immobilize the graft. Several anchoring 'mattress' stitches using 4–0 or 5–0 chromic catgut sutures may be placed in the center of the graft to immobilize the skin graft against the base. Hemostasis around the recipient site is essential. Hematoma formed underneath the graft will hinder the 'take' of the graft.

After care: The bolster is usually removed in 4–5 days after the procedure. Bodily fluid or blood elements accumulated underneath the graft; i.e. seroma and/or hematoma are evacuated. This is achieved by making a small 'nick' in the graft with a pair of surgical scissors. The fluid is 'rolled' out with a cotton tip applicator. The joint is immobilized immediately and pressure dressing is used to minimize the consequence of contracture. Physical exercise is resumed in 3 weeks after the surgery.

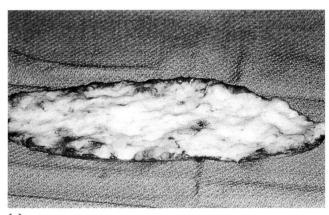

(a)

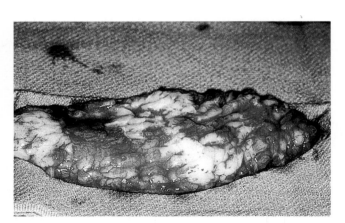

(b)

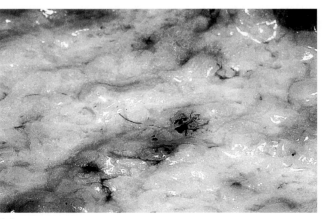

(c)

Fig. 52.10 (a) A piece of skin with subcutaneous tissues is removed from the abdomen that will be used as a full-thickness skin graft. (b) The subcutaneous fatty tissues were sharply removed with a pair of fine scissors. The capillaries were left undisturbed. (c) A close up view to show the capillaries that are left in the graft.

An interposition flap technique

This technique, known by various names such as 'three-quarter z-plasty' technique, a 'banner' flap interposition technique, etc. is the most useful method of wound coverage following a releasing procedure for a contracted joint. The technique is based upon a principle that an open wound consequential to surgical release may be covered with a skin flap mobilized from an adjacent area. While designing of a flap is technically simple, it requires an area of unburned skin adjacent to the released wound.

Operative technique: A triangular skin flap is designed in an unburned area adjacent to the wound following release. A vertical limb of the flap begun at the end of released wound edge, is set at a 90° angle with the end of the wound. The limb length is equal to the wound length. A triangular flap is formed but making the width of flap at mid-section the same as the wound width. The flap can be based either proximally or distally depending upon the direction of the triangular flap designed (**Figure 52.11a**). The flap is dissected out and is rotated 90° to cover the defect (**Figure 52.11b,c**). The

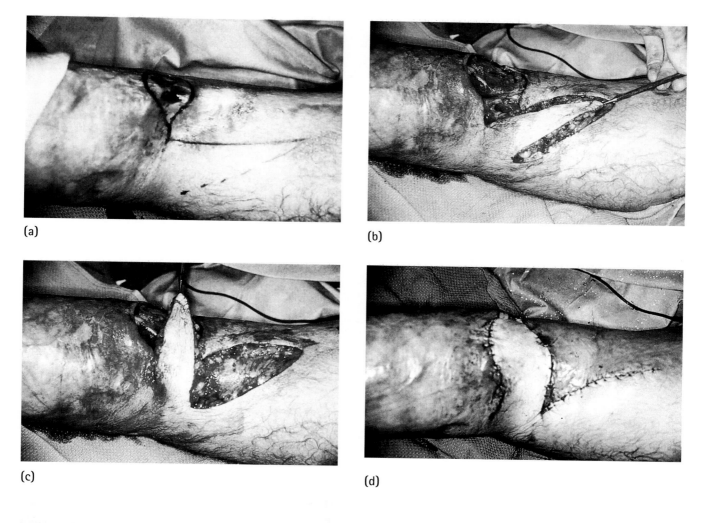

(a)

(b)

(c)

(d)

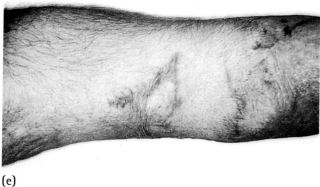

(e)

Fig. 52.11 (a) An interpositional skin flap technique; i.e. a modified z-plasty technique is useful in reconstructing a flexion deformity around the joint, as seen in this 42-year-old individual who had sustained burn injuries around the upper extremity. A triangular flap based distally on the lateral side of the elbow was designed in an uninjured area adjacent to the scarred joint surface. The length of the flap was equal to the length of scar release. (b) The triangle flap was faricated. (c) The skin flap was rotated 90° to make up tissue defect. (d) The donor site was closed primarily. (e) The appearance of the wound a year following the reconstruction.

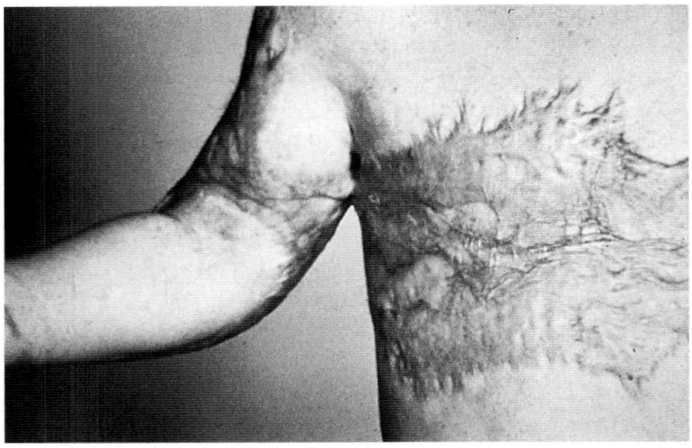

Fig. 52.12 (a) An interpositional skin flap technique of wound closure may be modified as in this 5–year-old girl who had sustained burns around the right axilla that caused contraction of the axillary joint. (b) The skin defect was so extensive that could not be covered completely with a single flap. (c) The uninjured skin raised as a flap was transferred to the middle of the wound leaving the areas proximal and distal to the flap to be covered with skin grafts. (d) The appearance of the wound 10 days following the surgery. (e) The appearance of the wound ten years after the surgery. The flap placed in the middle of the wound had increased in size because of body growth and stretching of the scar tissues.

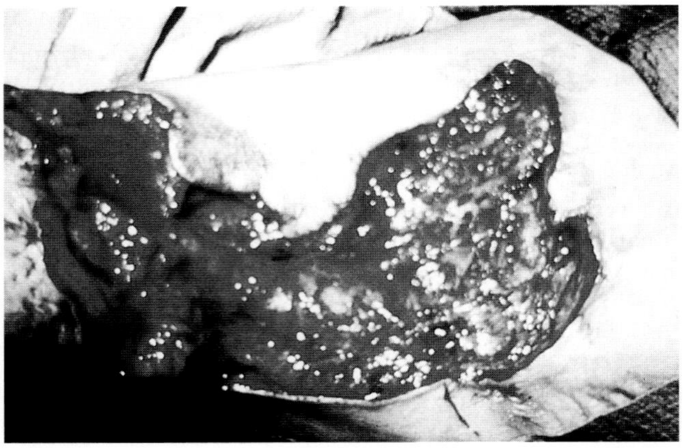

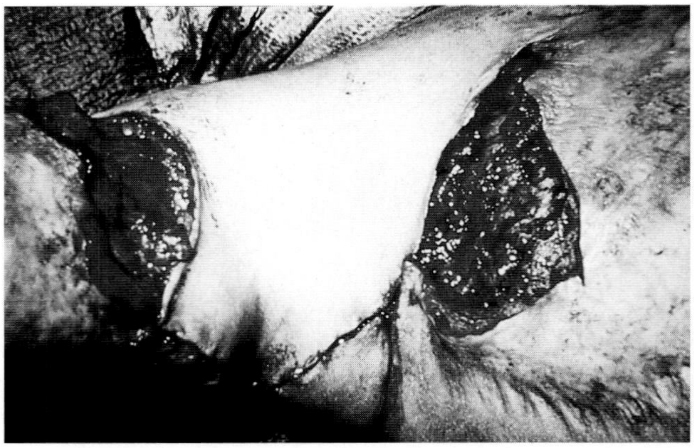

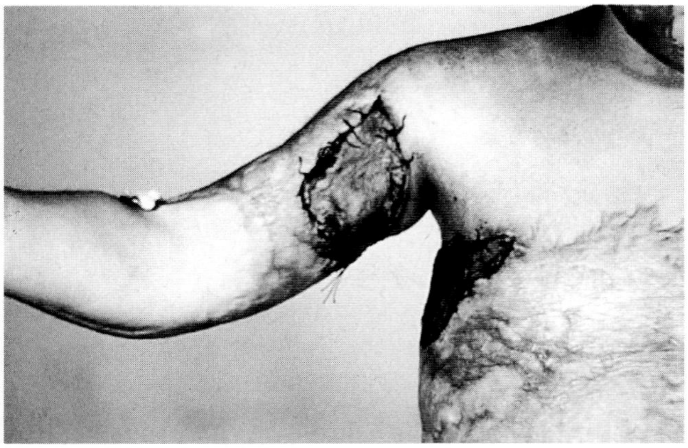

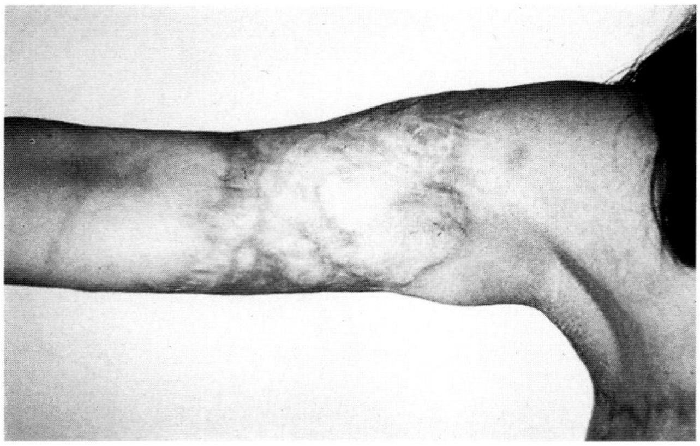

flap donor defect is closed primarily (**Figure 52.11d, e**). The width of flap may be narrow in instances where the size of unburned skin is not enough to fabricate a triangular skin flap sufficiently to cover the wound. The flap, in such an instance, is anchored in the middle of the wound. The two sides not covered by the flap are closed with a piece of skin graft (**Figure 52.12a–e**).

After care: The wound edges are kept clean with antibiotic ointment. Sutures may be removed in 10 days. Splinting of the joint is resumed within 4–5 days and joint exercise in 10–14 days.

A muscle flap or skin-muscle flap technique

The technique is utilized in instances when the resultant defect following release is so extensive that coverage of the wound with a skin flap or a skin graft are not feasible. The latissimus dorsi muscle harvested either as a muscle flap or as a musculocutaneous flap may be used to cover the axilla. The soleus muscle flap or the gastrocnemius muscle-skin flap may be used to cover the wound around the knee joint coverage (**Figure 52.13a–d**).

Muscle or muscle-skin flap, in practice, is seldom used to reconstruct burn deformities unless vital structures such as the brachial or popliteal neurovasculatures became exposed consequential to releasing procedures. Similarly, the indication of microsurgical composite tissue transfer technique is limited in burn scar release. Donor site limitation and technical difficulty encountered in pediatric patients probably account for the infrequent use of this method.

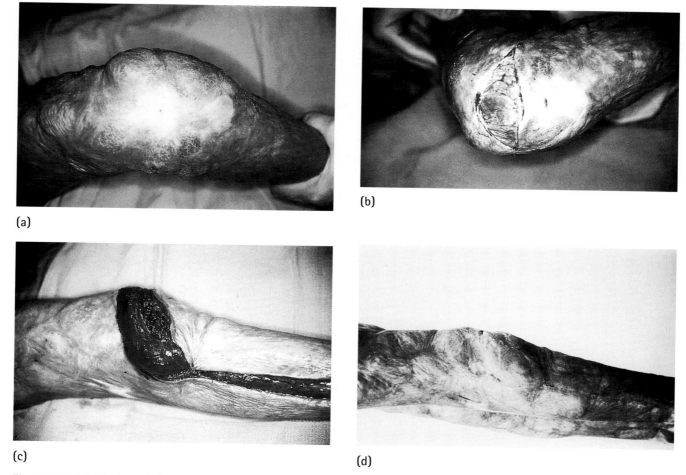

(a)

(b)

(c)

(d)

Fig. 52.13 (a) Flexion of the knee was limited because of tight scars around the patella. (b) An incisional release of the tight area across the patella provided the relief of knee contracture. However, it resulted in an open wound of 4–5 cm in size. (c) A medial segment of the soleus muscle was used to cover the defect. (d) The appearance of the knee area 3 months following the procedure.

Summary

Contractural deformities of the shoulder (axilla), elbow, hip, and knee joint are not uncommon sequelae of burn injuries. Although the injury involving the limbs and the joint structures could account for the deformities encountered, lack of proper positioning and inadequate physical exercise while recovering from the injuries could further contribute to genesis of the problems. The use of brace, splint and pressure dressing is important in minimizing such an undesirable consequence of burn injuries. The treatment for an established joint deformity, on the other hand, requires surgical release of the contracted skin and scars. Various methods of reconstruction have been described to manage the problems encountered. Attempts have been made to outline the approach of managing contractural deformities involving the shoulder (axilla), elbow, hip, and the knee joints.

References

1. Cronin TD. Successful corrections of extensive scar contractures of the neck. Using split-thickness skin grafts. In: *Transactions of the First International Congress on Plastic Surgery*. Baltimore: Williams & Wilkins, 1957: 123.
2. Willis B. The use of orthoplast isoprene in the treatment of the acutely burned child. A follow-up. *Am J Occup Ther* 1970; **24**: 187.
3. Larson DL, Evans EB, Abston S, *et al*. Techniques for decreasing scar formation and scar contractures in the burn patient. *J Trauma* 1971; **11**: 807–23.
4. Larson DL, Abston S, Evans EB, *et al*. Contractures and scar formation in the burn patient. *Clin Plast Surg* 1974; **1**: 653–66.
5. Larson D, Huang T, Linaris H, *et al*. Prevention and treatment of scar contracture. In: Artz CP, Moncrief JA, Pruitt BA, eds. *Burns. A team approach*. Philadelphia: WB Saunders, 1979: 466.
6. Huang TT, Blackwell SJ, Lewis SR. Ten years of experience in managing patients with burn contractures of axilla, elbow, wrist, and knee joints. *Plast Reconst Surg* 1978; **61**: 70–6.
7. Bauer PS, Larson DL, Stacy TR. The observation of myofibroblasts in hypertrophic scar. *Surg Gynecol Obstet* 1975; **141**: 22–6.
8. Linares HA, Larson DL, Willis-Galstaum BA. Historical notes on the use of pressure in the treatment of hypertrophic scars or keloids. *Burns* 1993; **19**: 17–21.
9. McCarthy JG. Introduction to plastic surgery. In: McCarthy JG, ed. *Plastic Surgery*. Philadelphia: WB Saunders, 1990; 55.

Chapter 53

Reconstruction of the trunk and genitalia

Robert L McCauley

Introduction

Recent studies, used to develop an inventory of reconstructive needs in burned children, have documented that burns of the torso and lower extremities eventually result in a significant number of problems. Brou *et al.*, in an evaluation of 25 patients with a mean body surface area burn of 71%, documented 70 problems associated with the trunk and perineum.[1] In 1993, Burns *et al.* analyzed the reconstructive management of patients with greater than 80% total body surface area (TBSA) burns. In the 28 patients analyzed, there were 564 needs identified.[2] This correlated well with previous studies documenting approximately 20 reconstructive needs per patient when the TBSA burn was at least 70%. The trunk was noted to be the most frequently identified area of injury in the torso/lower extremity region. Indeed, this region was only second to the hand as the most frequently injured anatomical unit. Further examination of truncal injuries clearly identified the breast, as the most frequently identified area of reconstruction needs. Subsequent analyses of the donor tissue surveillance form revealed that the necessary donor sites for reconstruction were often not available or were of poor quality when at all feasible. Consequently, it became quite clear that a stepwise plan of action for reconstruction could not be followed. Indeed, patient and family desires must be combined with a projected realistic outcome in order to determine the most judicious and efficacious use of available donor sites.

Historical issues

Evaluation of the management of burns to the truncal region requires longitudinal analysis of parameters of growth and development in order to assess the efficacy of variations in acute burn wound management. Over recent years, an increase in the survival of burned patients has been associated with better resuscitation, improved antimicrobial therapy, and early excisional therapy. Such data are well documented in the burn literature and remain the standard of care today.[3–7] Longitudinal assessment of earlier methods of burn care, which included delayed excision and épluchage, exhibited an increase in hospital morbidity and mortality of burned patients. The conservative management of tissue over the torso however proved to be quite beneficial in female patients who survived this type of management. In 1989, McCauley *et al.* documented that with conservative management of burn tissue over the anterior chest wall, involving the nipple–areola complex it is possible for normal breast development to occur even with nipple loss[8] (**Figure 53.1a, b**). This retrospective study, which ana-

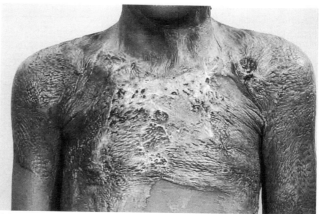

(a)

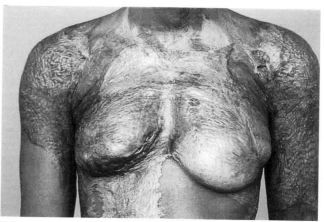

(b)

Fig. 53.1 (a) A 7-year-old female, 1-year s/p 25% TBSA burn with immature hypertrophic scars over the anterior chest wall. Note absence of nipple–areolar complex. (b) Ten-year follow-up at age 17 after burn injury. Reconstruction only required to assist right-sided breast development.

lyzed burn therapy nearly 20 years earlier, revealed that, indeed, conservative management of the nipple–areola complex in these patients was uniformly beneficial. On the other hand, 71% of these patients required incisional releases of the anterior chest wall to assist in breast development. The importance of this study lies in the observation that, even with loss of the nipple–areola complex, the breast bud itself is rarely injured. Although burn management prior to 1970 was quite conservative, the longitudinal effects of blunt eschar separation resulted in maximum tissue preservation, which produced flexible, mature burn scars.

Often it is difficult to evaluate the development of young females who have lost their nipple–areola complex as they proceed to develop in their adolescent years. Many of these patients require frequent follow-up in order to document the early stages of breast development and to plan surgical correction should entrapment of the developing breast in burn scar become a problem. During this period of time, pressure garments are often worn in order to assist the maturity of burn scars to accommodate the developing breast. Many of these patients will require an incisional release to allow the breasts to develop without distortion (**Figures 53.2a–c and 53.3a,b**). Subsequent maturation of skin grafts not only results in blending in with injured tissue but also allows the tissue over the breast to immediately become more relaxed.

In-patients who require global fascial excision of the anterior chest wall, breast development will not occur. In such patients,

maturity of the tissue over the anterior chest wall is of paramount importance if reconstructive methods are to be successful at a later date. Many of these patients will require tissue expansion and subsequent placement of a muscular prosthesis to give the appearance of developed breasts.

The unilateral chest wall burn presents a significant problem. In children, the uninjured side will proceed with uninhibited breast development, whereas the burned side may require surgical procedures in order to assist a developing breast. The development of breast asymmetry and contour deformities are quite common. The burned breast tends to be fuller and does not have the natural ptosis associated with a matured female breast. Mastopexy of the uninjured breast may be performed in order to relieve the grade II or greater ptosis, to realign the nipple–areolar complex, and to give the uninjured breast a fuller appearance. Mudge and McCauley documented significant improvement in breast symmetry and aesthetics using this approach.[9]

Multiple breast releases, conducted to assist development, may result in multiple contour deformities. The lack of fullness and accentuated asymmetry of the infraclavicular area may require reconstruction using pedicled fasciocutaneous flaps or a latissimus dorsi musculocutaneous flap. Even if the level of the nipple–areola complexes are similar, medial or lateral displacement of the nipple may be of significant concern to the patient. If breast contracture is a problem, medial or lateral incisional releases and coverage with

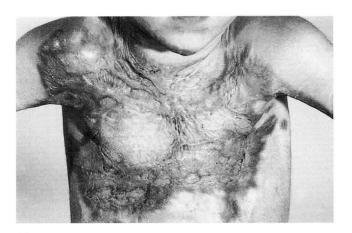

(a)

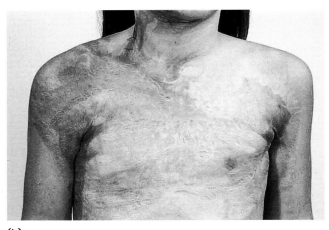

(b)

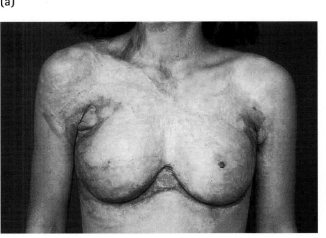

(c)

Fig. 53.2 (a) A 4-year-old female 6 months s/p 20% TBSA burn with immature hypertrophic scars and apparent loss of the nipple–areolar complex. (b) Four-year follow-up of patient at 8 years with maturity of the burn scars over the anterior chest wall. (c) Fourteen-year follow-up of patient at 18 years of age after recreation of the inframammary fold with split-thickness skin grafts.

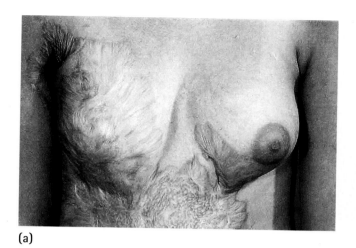

(a)

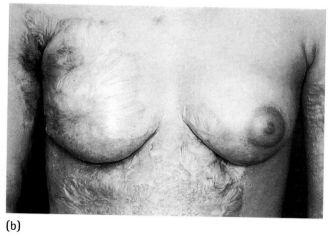

(b)

Fig. 53.3 (a) A 16-year-old female 8 years s/p 38% TBSA burn with neglected burn scar contractures over the anterior chest wall with entrapment of both breast. (b) Two-year follow-up after incisional releases and resurfacing with thick split-thickness skin grafts.

skin grafts will allow better nipple positioning. On the other hand, if breast contracture is not a problem, isolated repositioning of the nipple–areola complex is indicated. Clearly in patients with macromastia and breast deformities correction of the breast contracture prior to reduction mammaplasty assures optimal results.[10]

Reconstruction of the nipple–areola complex is a significant problem and represents the second stage of breast reconstruction. Although many techniques are available, most have been fraught with loss of nipple projection within 6 months. Evaluation of various techniques in the burned breast are still lacking. Recent studies by McCauley *et al.* have documented the safety of using the 'skate' flap as described by Littler. Longitudinal assessment of this procedure has shown that nipple projection is maintained although contraction does occur.[11]

Perineal burn management

The acute management of perineal burns is well documented at the Shriners Burns Institute–Galveston, and protocols for the management of out-patients are well publicized.[12,13] Rutan *et al.*, in a 20-year review of more than 5500 pediatric patients hospitalized at the Shriners Burns Institute in Galveston, showed only 1% of these patients sustained burns to the perineum or genitalia. Boys tend to outnumber girls 3:1, with a majority of these patients having greater than or equal to a 40% TBSA burn. Other investigations have documented the efficacy of conservative management of genital and perineal burns.[14–16] These wounds are treated with topical antimicrobial agents in an open manner. Sharp debridement, particularly over the penis, is discouraged. Urinary catheters are frequently used during the resuscitative periods for the first 48–96 hours, when concomitant injury to the urethra has been ruled out. When required, urinary diversion has been accomplished through suprapubic catheterization. Long-term urethra catheterization has been associated with ureterostenosis, which contributes to urinary tract infections.

Burn scar contractures of the perineum and genitalia are the most frequent long-term sequelae of burn injuries. Perineal webbing can present significant problems with limitation in hip range

of motion as well as hooding of the external genitalia. More extensive burns involving the buttock region can also result in perianal stenosis or hooding, which may impede fecal evacuation. Alghanem *et al.*, in a retrospective review, documented the 5% incidence of rectal prolapse which was related to malnutrition, diarrhea, and constipation.[12] Manual reduction and correction of the instigating factors led to correction of this problem in all patients. Reconstruction of the perineal burn scar bands can usually be accomplished with multiple z-plasties in order to correct banding genitalia hooding (**Figure 53.4a,b**). Patients who present with perianal stenosis may have entrapped unburned tissue in this region.[14] Reconstruction can be accomplished with an incisional release of burn tissue from the perineum body to the coccyx through the stenotic orifice and the eversion of the unburned tissue from the anus. Lateral excision of burn scar tissue will allow recreation of the gluteal folds and access to a normal uninjured anus.

Reconstruction of the male external genitalia represents one of the most challenging problems for reconstructive surgeons. Problems may be minor, as in those which can be corrected using z-plasties or skin grafts to restore function. Major problems in patients are secondary to partial or total loss of the penis. Fortunately, problems associated with full-thickness injuries to the penis in burn patients are relatively few. Consequently, except in electrical injuries, conservative management of burned tissue in this region is the rule.[16–19] The subsequent contractures over the penis are small; however, reconstruction of the penis may be required in the acute phase if a patient complains of significant pain during erection. Here, the immature scar is treated by an incisional release and, if possible, full-thickness skin grafts to alleviate this problem. Complete loss of the penis is a devastating problem and challenges every reconstructive surgeon. Documentation of urinary excretory function is essential in evaluating such patients for further reconstruction. The use of rectus abdominus myocutaneous flap for penal reconstruction is well published.[17,18] However, significant problems have been associated with the development of urethral stenosis. In addition, erotic sensation appears to be limited, although with subsequent placement of a penal implant, intromission is accomplished. A more recently developed technique

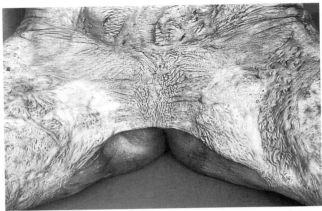

(a)

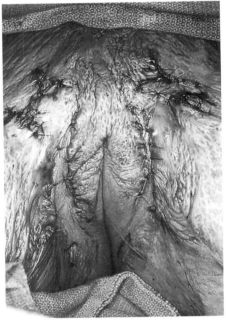

(b)

Fig. 53.4 (a) A 10-year-old female s/p 30% TBSA burn with mature burn scars and hooding of perineal burn scars over the vagina. (b) Correction of the deformity using bilateral local skin flaps.

using the radial artery forearm flap with coaptation of sensory branches of the cutaneous nerves from the forearm to the pudendal nerve has been associated with much improved erotic sensation.[18,19] Stenosis of the urethra continues to be a problem. The use of full-thickness strips of bladder to line the neourethra may improve or eliminate problems associated with urethra stenosis.

Summary

Problems associated with reconstruction of burns to be truncal region continue to represent a challenge. Entrapment of breast tissue in burn scars in female patients can be eliminated with skin grafts. Contour problems which are associated with developing breasts may be corrected with the use of skin grafts and/or fasciocutaneous flaps. Improved symmetry of the breast is of significant importance for patients who have unilateral burns of the breast.

Reconstructive techniques, including mastopexy and reduction mammaplasty, may be required in order to obtain symmetry. In patients requiring fascial excision of full-thickness burns over the anterior chest wall, tissue expansion and subsequent placement of submuscular saline implants have been quite successful for breast reconstruction.

Management of wounds to the perineum and genitalia during the acute phase should be conservative. Perineal burn scar bands remain the most frequent complication associated with burns in these areas. Contractures are corrected with the use of multiple z-plasties. Total effacement of the gluteal folds and perianal stenosis can be addressed with lateral excision of the burned tissue and eversion of the normal tissue. Penile reconstruction continues to remain a significant challenge. Staged pedicle flap reconstruction has been replaced with the use of musculocutaneous flaps and free tissue transfer with subsequent placement of penile implants. Indeed, as we continue to scrutinize the severity and frequency of problems associated with burns in the truncal regions of pediatric patients, the complexity and numbers of reconstructive procedures necessary for complete rehabilitation will undoubtedly continue to grow.

References

1. Brou JA, Robson MC, McCauley RL, et al. Inventory of potential reconstructive needs in the patient with burns. J Burn Care Rehabil 1989; 10: 555–60.
2. Burns BF, McCauley RL, Murphy FL, Robson MC. Reconstructive management of patients with greater than 80% TBSA burns. Burns 1993; 19: 429–33.
3. Burke JF, Bandoc CC, Quinby WC. Primary excision and immediate grafting. A method for shortening illness. J Trauma 1974; 14: 389–95.
4. Herndon DN, Parks DH. Comparison of serial debridement and autografting and early massive excision with cadaveric skin overlay in the treatment of large burns in children. J Trauma 1986; 26: 149–52.
5. Herndon DN, Gore DC, Cole M, et al. Determinants of mortality in pediatric patients with greater than 70% full thickness total body surface area thermal injury treated by early total excision and grafting. J Trauma 1987; 27: 208–12.
6. Herndon DN, Barrow RC, Rutan RL, Rutan TC, Desai MH, Abston S. A comparison of conservative versus early excisional therapies in severely burned patients. Ann Surg 1989; 209: 547–53.
7. Desai MH, Herndon DN, Broemeling L, Barrow RE, Nichols RJ, Rutan RL. Early burn wound excision significantly reduces blood loss. Ann Surg 1990; 211: 753–62.
8. McCauley RL, Beraja V, Rutan RL, Huang TT, Abston S, Rutan TC, Robson MC. Longitudinal assessment of breast development in adolescent female patients with burns involving the nipple-areolar complex. Plast Reconstr Surg 1989; 83: 676–80.
9. Mudge B, McCauley R. Correction of asymmetry in the unilaterally burned breast. Proc Am Burn Assoc 2000; 21(1) Part 2: S221.
10. Thai K, Mertens D, Warden GD, Neale HW. Reduction mammaplasty in post-burn breasts. Proc Am Burn Assoc 1999; 20(1) Part 2: S131.
11. McCauley RL, Robson MC. Reconstruction of the nipple areola complex in the burned breast using the 'skate' flap. Proc Am Burn Assoc 1994; 26: 14.
12. Algahanem AA, McCauley RL, Robson MC, Rutan RL, Herndon DN. Management of pediatric perineal and genital burns: twenty year review. J Burn Care Rehabil 1990; 11: 308–11.
13. Rutan RL. Management of perineal and genital burns. JET Nurs 1993; 20: 169–76.
14. Alghanem AA, McCauley RL, Robson MC. Gluteal pouching: a complication of perineal burn scar contracture. A case report. J Burn Care Rehabil 1990; 11: 137–9.
15. Culp D. Genital injuries: etiology and management. Urol Clin 1977; 4: 143–6.
16. Michielsen D, Van Htee R, Neetens C, La Faire C, Peeters R. Burns to the genitalia and the perineum. J Urol 1998; 159(2): 418–9.
17. Edelman CG, Sweet ME, Messing EM, Helgerson RB. Treatment of severe electrical burns of the genitalia and perineum by early excision and grafting. Burns 1991; 17: 506–9.
18. Garner WL, Smith DJ. Reconstruction of burns of the trunk and breasts. Clin Plast Surg 1992; 19: 683–91.
19. Kao XS, Kao CL, Yang ZN, Shi HR. One-stage reconstruction of the penis with free skin flap: report of three cases. J Reconstr Microsurg 1984; 1: 149–53.

Chapter 54

Management of burn injuries of the perineum

Ted Huang

Burns of the perineal area is quite uncommon even though the lower trunk and the lower extremities are vulnerable to the burn injury. According to Alghanem *et al.*, the incidence of perineal burns was about 12 per 1000 admissions.[1] The incidence was reassessed recently by reviewing the records of 5651 patients admitted to the Shriners Burns Hospital between 1976 and 1998. There were only 91 patients identified to have burn injuries of the perineal area. While overall incidence of the perineal burns has remained unchanged, boys were found to sustain the injury four times more often than girls in this group of patients. Among 44 boys with genital burns, there were 35 penile burns and nine with scrotal injuries. In contrast, there were only four patients who had burns of the labial structures. Burns of the vaginal vault were not encountered in this group of patients.

Management of burns of the perineum during acute phase of injury

A conservative approach is used to manage perineal burns.[1,2] That is, the perineal area is cleansed daily and the wound is covered with antibiotic dressing. The urethral tract is stented with an indwelling Foley catheter as it is also used to decompress the urinary bladder. The perineal area is neither splinted nor braced. The thighs are maintained at 15° of abduction using a wedge splint to minimize contracture of the hip joint. The extent of burns is allowed to demarcate in time and the wound is often left to heal spontaneously. A nonhealing wound is managed with the use of a partial-thickness or a full-thickness skin graft. In rare occasions, a skin flap may be mobilized from the area adjacent to reconstruct defects consequential to full-thickness skin loss of the penis and the scrotum.

Other possible problems seen with burns of the perineum during the acute phase of injury would include necrosis of the penile shaft, testicular necrosis, urethral stricture, and rectal prolapse. Although the Shriners Burns Hospital in Galveston, Texas, has adopted a relatively conservative regimen to manage perineal burns, the approach of wound care in practice, is quite variable and the exact regimen is often modified depending upon the structures involved:

Burns of the Penis

Burn injuries limited to the penis, though possible, is quite rare, (**Figure 54.1**). Concomitant involvement of the penis with burn

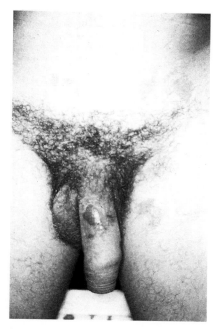

Fig. 54.1 An isolated burn injury of the penis is relatively uncommon. This 27-year-old man sustained scalding burns of penis from accidental spilling hot coffee on the lap.

injuries of the lower trunk and the perineal area, on the other hand, is quite common. The initial regimen of patient management, in addition to resuscitative measures, consists of wound care and urethral stenting (**Figure 54.2a**). An indwelling Foley catheter of appropriate size is inserted into the urinary bladder to stent the urethral tract and at the same time to monitor the urinary output. The catheter is removed once the swelling around the penile shaft is subsided and status of the wound becomes delineated. No attempt is made to debride the burned wound early. Instead, it is allowed to demarcate and is often allowed to heal spontaneously.

Loss of Skin over the Penile Shaft and the Scrotum

Spontaneous healing is expected in most instances with burn injuries of the penis and scrotum since full-thickness injury of the penile and scrotal skin is relatively uncommon. Skin grafting, partial-thickness or a full-thickness, could be used to cover the wound if healing is delayed (**Figure 54.2a,b,c,d**). In rare instances, a skin flap may be needed to reconstruct structures such as urethral tract and/or scrotal sac because of loss of the skin coverage. An inguinopudendal skin flap mobilized from the inguinal crease area may be used if the use of skin graft is judged to be not feasible[3]. The use of muscle-skin flap such as a gracilis MC flap is not

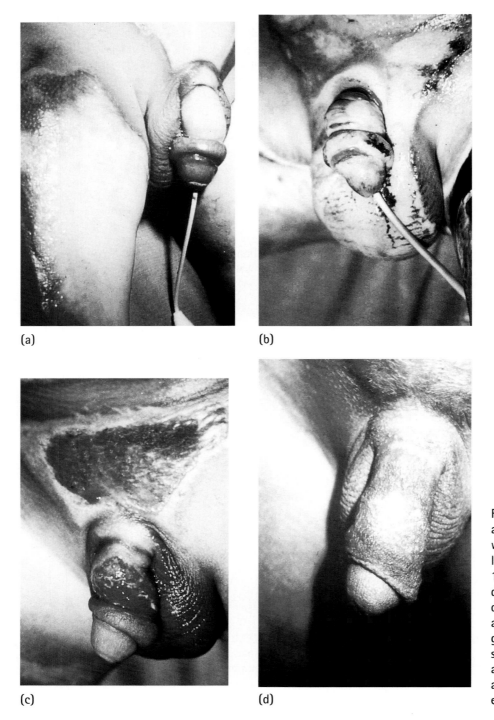

(a)

(b)

(c)

(d)

Fig. 54.2 (a) Burns of the penis are more commonly associated with injuries of the lower trunk-lower extremities, as seen in this 14-year old male youth. (b) The depth of injury became better defined in 4 days. (c) A small area in the shaft of penis was grafted with a partial-thickness skin graft later. (d) The appearance of genitalia 2 years after the accident. The patient experienced no difficulty.

recommended because of high tissue temperature that may interfere with spermatogenesis.

Burn Wound of Labia Majora

Isolated burns of the labial structures are rare. Instead, labial burns are often associated with injuries of surrounding areas such as abdomen and inguinal folds. As in the management of burns of male genitalia, the injured areas are allowed to heal spontaneously. (**Figure 54.3a,b**). Distortion of the labial structures mostly due to contraction of the scar tissues in the pubic and inguinal areas is left for later reconstruction.

Perineal Wound Coverage

An isolated burn injury of the perineal area is extremely rare. On the other hand, the area will become involved if the lower trunk/buttock is injured. The extent of scar contracture varies depending upon the depth of burns. While it may heal spontaneously with minimal scarring, contracture of the perineal area is a common sequela regardless of methods used to care for the wound (**Figure 54.4a–c**). The natural inclination to keep the thigh

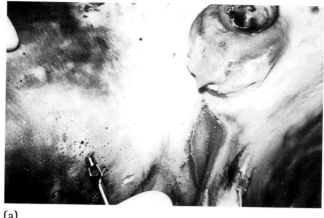

(a)

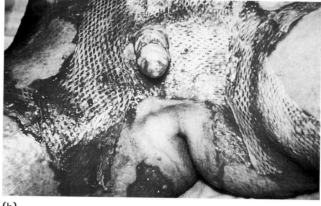

(b)

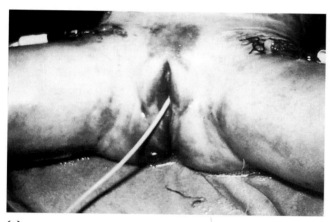

(a)

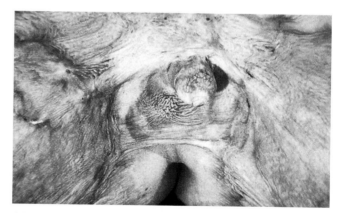

(c)

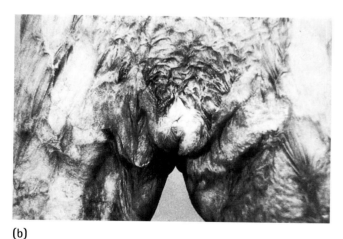

(b)

Fig. 54.3 (a) Burn injuries involved the lower trunk and the thighs that included the labia. While the lower abdomen and the thighs required skin grafting, the labial injury was left to heal spontaneously. (b) The appearance of genitalia 5 years after the injury.

Fig. 54.4 (a) The patient was an 8-year-old who sustained third degree burn injuries of the trunk and the lower extremities that had involved also the penis and the scrotum. (b) The wound including the scrotum was debrided and was grafted with a meshed partial-thickness skin graft. (c) The changes ensued in the genitoperineal area were characterized with scar hypertrophy and burn scar contracture. Tight scars formed across the perineum interfered with thigh movement.

together and hip adducted during the recovery phase of acute burn injuries seems to aggravate scar contraction.

Anal Burns

Burns of the anus is rare, though it could become involved because of extensive burns of the perineum. If the skin injury around the anal opening is full-thickness, the use of a skin flap may be necessary to minimize the consequence of stricture. A piece of skin flap mobilized from the area adjacent will be necessary to graft the perianal area. Wound coverage with a piece of skin graft is technically difficult and it will lead to anal stricture because of graft contracture.

Rectal Prolapse

Rectal prolapse occurs occasionally in young children with extensive burn injuries with or without perineal involvement. The exact reasons for rectal prolapse occurring in burned infants remain unclear. Redundant rectal mucosa, structural relationship of the rectum to other pelvic organs such as sacrum and coccyx, urinary bladder and uterus, and lack of muscular support provided by the pelvic musculatures, the anatomical features uniquely special to infants of 1–3 years of age could account for the incident. Sudden increase in intra-abdominal pressure and malnutrition due to burn injuries could conceivably aggravate the magnitude of descend of the rectal mucosa through the anal opening.[4]

Clinically, in addition to eversion of rectal mucosa, the finding of edematous swelling around the buttocks and perianal area is quite common, even though the area could be spared of burns. The onset can be quite sudden without obvious precipitating event. However, grunting or Valsalva maneuver can precipitate an eversion of the rectal canal through the anal opening.

The regimen of treatment consists of rectal padding, daily cleansing of the perineal and perianal area. Stool softener is added to the dietary regimen to facilitate bowel movement. Spontaneous regression of the prolapse is likely as the nutrition improves and tissue swelling subsides, (**Figure 54.5a–c**). Surgical intervention, though in most instances is unnecessary, is indicated if the prolapse is not readily reducible due to anal sphincteric dysfunction and/or intussusception.[4,5]

Reconstruction of established deformities of the perineum and the perineal structures

Cicatricial contracture around the perineum is the most common sequelae of perineal burns.[1,6] In our group of 91 patients, over one-half suffered contractural deformity in the perineal area. The magnitude of contracture is, furthermore, exaggerated because of contraction of burn scars in the inguinal crease and inferomedial gluteal folds. Other problems, though relatively uncommon, included complete loss of penis, anal stenosis and intractable rectal

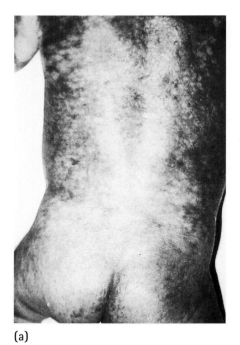

(a)

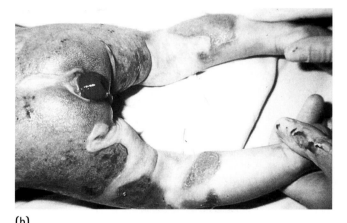

(b)

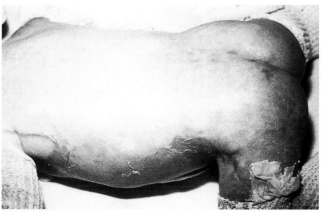

(c)

Fig. 54.5 (a) The patient was a 2-year-old girl who had sustained 65–70% total body surface burns. (b) Prolapse of the rectum appeared 12 days after the accident. The problem was managed nonsurgically. (c) The prolapse receded spontaneously 2 months later as she recovered from the burn injury.

prolapse. There are numerous methods such as the z-plasty technique, an interpositional skin flap technique, incisional release of scarred tissues closed with local skin flap or skin graft available to reconstruct the deformities. In practice, the technique used to reconstruct perineal and genital deformities varies depending upon the magnitude of scarring, scarred deformity around the perineum and the extent of functional impediment encountered.

Reconstruction of Penile Deformity

The task of assessing the exact extent of penile deformities can be difficult. Distortion of the penile configuration attributable to scar contracture could be due to loss of the skin or combination of the skin and the Buck's fascia. In addition, the scarring in the pubic area and/or the inguinal fold could further exaggerate the extent of penile deformity. Engorging the penile shaft is necessary to assess precisely the extent of penile deformity, as the gross appearance of a flaccid penis can be misleading. It is necessary to make the penile shaft engorged; i.e. creating artificial penile erection, in order to determine the extent and the location of scar involvement. Artificial penile erection is created under anesthesia by first placing a tourniquet at the base of the penis. A tourniquet using a piece of one-quarter inch Penrose drain is placed at the base of the penile shaft. Physiologic saline solution is injected into the corpus cavernosum in sufficient amount to induce congestion. The shaft deformity attributable to the skin loss and/or fascial loss will be delineated once the corpus becomes engorged (**Figure 54.6a,b**).

The skin defect resulting from incisional release of the scar is covered with a full-thickness skin graft if the Buck's fascia is spared of scarred injury. In a rare instance with injury that involved the Buck's fascia, surgical release of facial deformity was necessary. A dermal graft harvested from the lower abdomen may be used to reconstruct the fascial defect. A skin flap mobilized from the area along the groin crease, as an island skin pedicle flap will be needed to cover the skin defect.

Complete loss of penis, though devastating, is extremely rare (**Figure 54.7a,b**). Reconstruction of the penis is delayed until puberty. The delay is often necessary due to limited use of soft tissue that can be harvested for genital reconstruction soon after the accident. There are several methods currently available to reconstruct a neophallus. A segment of rectus abdominis MC flap, for instance, may be mobilized from the lower abdomen to form a neophallus. In recent years, a forearm osteocutaneous flap transferred to the pubic area via microsurgical technique has been found to be useful in reconstructing a phallus. A urethral tract could be reconstructed with a piece of full-thickness skin graft or utilizing a tube-within-a-tube technique at the time of phallus reconstruction if a forearm osteocutaneous flap technique is used[7] (**Figure 54.8a,b,c**).

Reconstruction of Scrotal Deformities

Full-thickness burn injuries of the scrotum would result in scar encasement of testicular structures. Reconstruction would, therefore, require surgical release of the scarred areas. A thin skin flap such as the inguinopudendal flap or a flap mobilized from the area adjacent, however, is needed to cover the resultant defect. A musculocutaneous flap such as a gracilis MC flap is not suitable for scrotal reconstruction because of the thickness of the flap and possible impeding spermatogenesis due to high tissue temperature exerted from the flap. Even though contractural deformity is likely to recur, skin grafts may be used to cover the defect.

Reconstruction of Labial Deformity

An isolated contour deformity of the labia majora is relatively uncommon. On the other hand, scar contracture occurring in the

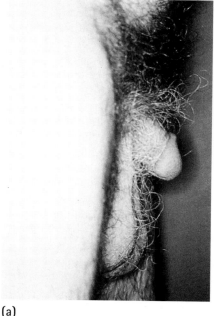

(a)

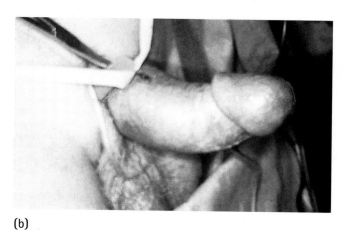

(b)

Fig. 54.6 (a) The technique of eliciting an artificial penile erection requires placement of a rubber tourniquet using a piece of one-quarter inch Penrose drain around the proximal penile shaft. A #22 gauge butterfly intravenous infusion set is used to inject physiologic saline solution into the corpus cavernosum to artificially engorge the penis. (b) The area with Buck's fascia defect is delineated as the corpus cavernosum is filled with saline solution.

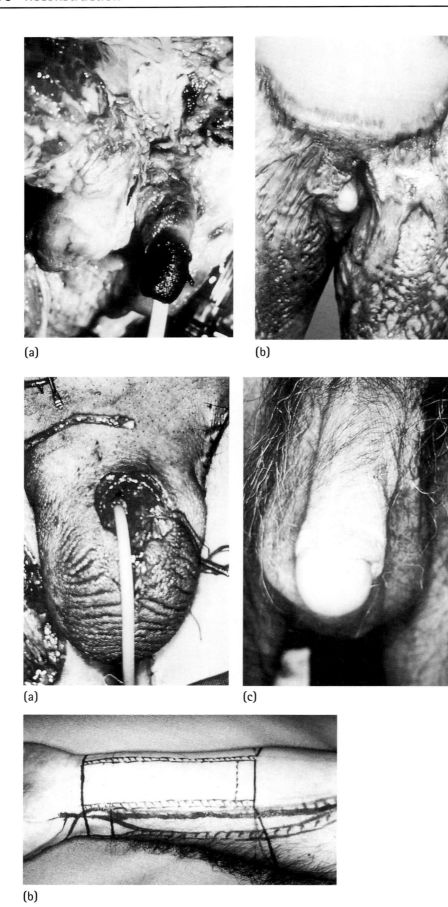

Fig. 54.7 (a) A full-thickness burn of the penis, though uncommon, can occur and the outcome is devastating, as seen in this 12-year-old boy. No attempt was made to remove the penile tissue. Instead, the wound was allowed to demarcate itself. An indwelling Foley catheter was used to stent the urethra. (b) The patient was able to urinate through a short remnant of the penis. Reconstruction of the penile shaft is being planned.

Fig. 54.8 (a) There are various techniques available to reconstruct a penile shaft. A forearm osteocutaneous flap, one of the methods currently in use, was chosen for this 51-year-old man who has lost the penis because of cancer. (Courtesy of Dr Kenji Sasaki. Reprinted with permission from *Plast Reconstr Surg* 1998; **104**: 1054–8.) (b) A section of the skin with a segment of the radius attached is harvested from the volar surface of the forearm and is transferred to the pubic area via microsurgical technique. A tube-inside-the-tube technique was used to reconstruct the urethral tract. In addition, the pulp from the big toe was also used to reconstruct the glans penis. (Courtesy of Dr Kenji Sasaki. Reprinted with permission from *Plast Reconstr Surg* 1998; **104**: 1054–58.) (c) The appearance of reconstructed penis in a 50-year-old man who had lost the penis because of cancer. (Courtesy of Dr Kenji Sasaki. Reprinted with permission from *Plast Reconstr Surg* 1998; **104**: 1054–58.)

suprapubic and pubic area, as well as the inguinal fold could distort the normal configuration of the labia. Prior surgical release of the contracted scar tissues around the pubic and inguinal fold areas is an essential step in order to determine the extent of labial deformity and the method to reconstruct the deformed labia. To restore a contour deformity caused by skin and subcutaneous tissue loss, a skin flap may have to be mobilized from the area adjacent. To reconstruct a contour deformity due to parenchymal tissue loss, injection of free fat cells; i.e. lipoinjection could be useful. To inject free fat cells to augment the labial contour, the cells are aspirated from the lower abdomen using the inner cannula of #14 Intracath® needle attached to a 3 ml syringe. The syringe is moved in a 'back-and-forth' piston-like manner. The fat cells are injected into the labia using the same syringe but connected with a 19 gauge blunt needle.

Reconstruction of Band Deformity Around the Perineum

Scarring and scar contracture of the perineum is a common sequela of perineal burns, especially if it is allowed to heal spontaneously. Although it seldom causes any difficulty at young age, the scars around the perineum could eventually interfere with sitting because of tightness or contraction developed around the buttock. In addition, the patient may encounter difficulty with bowel movement because of gluteal contracture and cicatricial changes involving the anal opening. The deformity resulted in the perineal area is usually consisted of a tight band developed in the suprapubic area (**Figure 54.9a,b**), or between the ischial tuberosities. Inelastic scars causes inadequate spreading of the buttock and is responsible for discomfort with sitting, (**Figure 54.10a,b**).

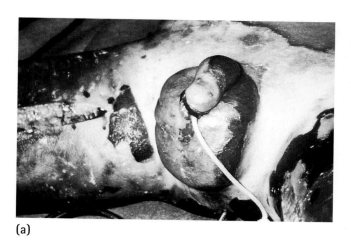

(a)

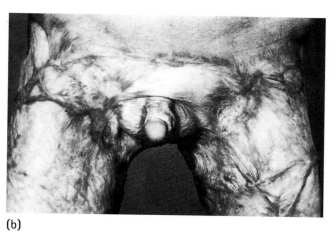

(b)

Fig. 54.9 (a) The patient an 11-year-old boy, sustained burns mostly in the lower trunk and the thigh areas that included lateral scrotal skin and the proximal penile shaft. (b) Debridement and grafting of the burned wound resulted in tight scar bands across the suprapubic and inter-ischial areas.

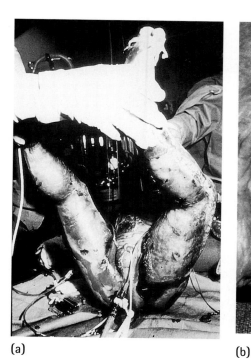

(a)

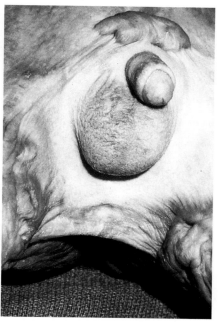

(b)

Fig. 54.10 (a) A 9-year-old sustained deep burns of the lower trunk and the lower extremities. Burns of the genitalia was less severe and the area was allowed to heal spontaneously. (b) A tight band developed across the perineal area as the healing of the perineal wound ensued.

Although a contracted perineal band may be incised to gain release, the task of closing the resultant wound can be difficult. Recurrence of contracture is a common sequela with the use of skin graft. Instead, a multiple z-plasty technique is a preferred method of reconstruction to release scar bands around the perineum.

The technique of multiple z-plasty

The patient is placed in a lithotomy position. Tightness and scar band can be delineated with abduction of the hip joint (**Figure 54.11a**). A line is drawn in the scar band along the horizontal direction of the band. The length of the horizontal line may extend from one side of the scarred area to the other. A triangular flap with its apex at the end of horizontal line is marked. The angle may vary between 30 and 60°, depending upon the uninjured tissues available at both ends of the horizontal line. The length of the limb of each triangle will be the same as the incision made perpendicular to the horizontal line to release the tight band (**Figure 54. 11b**). Two z-plasties; i.e. two triangular flaps with 30–60° and 90° angle, respectively, are formed as the flaps are raised along the skin markings made. Release of a contracted scar

band is achieved by rotating these two flaps at each end (**Figure 54. 11c**). Although the extent of perineal release may be limited because of scarred tissues surrounding the triangular flaps fashioned, the z-plasty technique is useful in changing the pulling direction of scar tissue, thus diminishing tightness around the perineum.

Reconstruction of Anal Stricture

While burn injuries rarely involve the entire anorectal canal, it is not unusual to involve the perianal skin and the external sphincter ani muscle. Stricture of the anal opening due to scar contracture and the cicatricial involvement of the external sphincter ani muscle are common sequelae. Cicatricial changes around the anal opening can and will interfere with bowel movement. The treatment requires surgical release of constricted scar bands around the anal opening. An interpositional skin flap fashioned as an island flap or a modified z-plasty with skin flaps mobilized from the area adjacent, is used to make up the tissue defect (**Figure 54.12a–d**). The method of using a piece of skin graft to reconstruct the defect is not useful. Application of the graft is difficult and recurrence of stricture is common because of scar contracture.

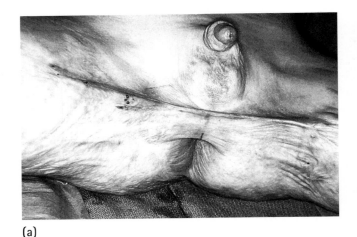

(a)

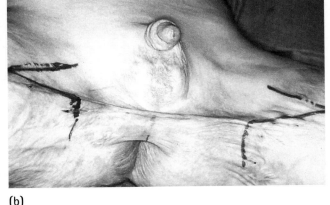

(b)

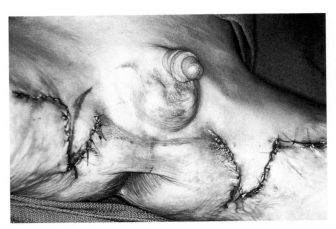

(c)

Fig. 54.11 (a) A tight scar band developed in the perineal area consequential to burn injuries involving the perineum and the lower extremities. (b) Releasing incisions were placed in the areas away from the anal opening to avoid injuring the anal sphincter. A triangular flap was designed in the uninjured area at each end of the scar band. A releasing incision was set perpendicularly to the direction of the scar band. (c) Each triangular flap was rotated 90° to close the open wound resulted from incisional release.

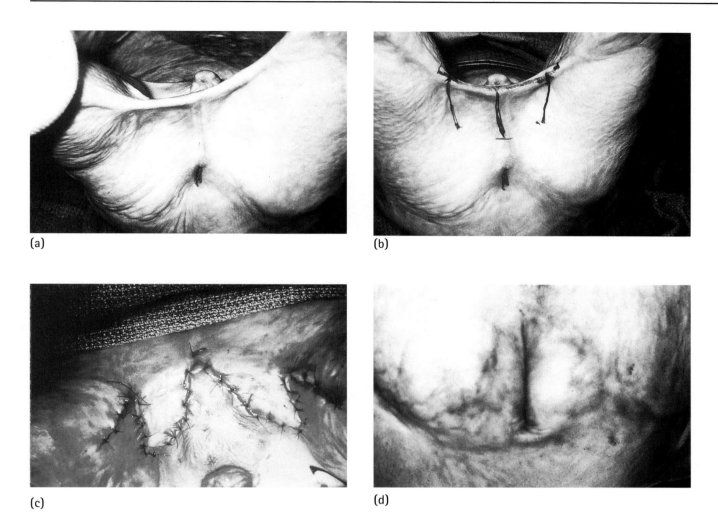

(a)

(b)

(c)

(d)

Fig. 54.12 (a) A 7-year-old boy developed, in addition to a tight scar band across the perineum, anal incontinence because of cicatricial changes that had involved the entire perineal area. (b) A modified multiple z-plasty technique was utilized to reconstruct perineal contracture and anal stenosis. (c) Skin flaps were rotated into the areas to reconstruct the deformity following the surgical release. (d) The appearance of the anal area 8 months after the surgery. Release of the anal stricture restored the anal incontinence.

Reconstruction of Rectal Prolapse

Although the problem, in most instances, is self-limiting and the prolapse will recede spontaneously as nutritional status of the patient and healing of the burned perineum improve, surgical intervention will be necessary if the rectal prolapse becomes intractable[4,5] (**Figure 54.13a–d**).

Summary

Burn injuries of the perineum is relatively uncommon. The regimen of treatment during the acute phase of recovery is conservative. The urethral tract is stented with an indwelling Foley catheter and the wound is cleaned daily. Neither a splint nor a brace is used to immobilize the perineal area. The wound is usually left to heal spontaneously. The resultant deformity, with rare exception of total loss of the penis, is limited. Instead, disfigurement of the scrota/labial contour and/or scar bands around the genitalia is the common complaint presented by the patients. The approach in reconstructing scarred deformities is centered upon release of tight scar bands around the perineal structures as it interferes with sitting and/or bowel movement. Incisional release and reconstruction utilizing a z-plasty technique or an interpositional skin flap technique is effective in correcting the deformities.

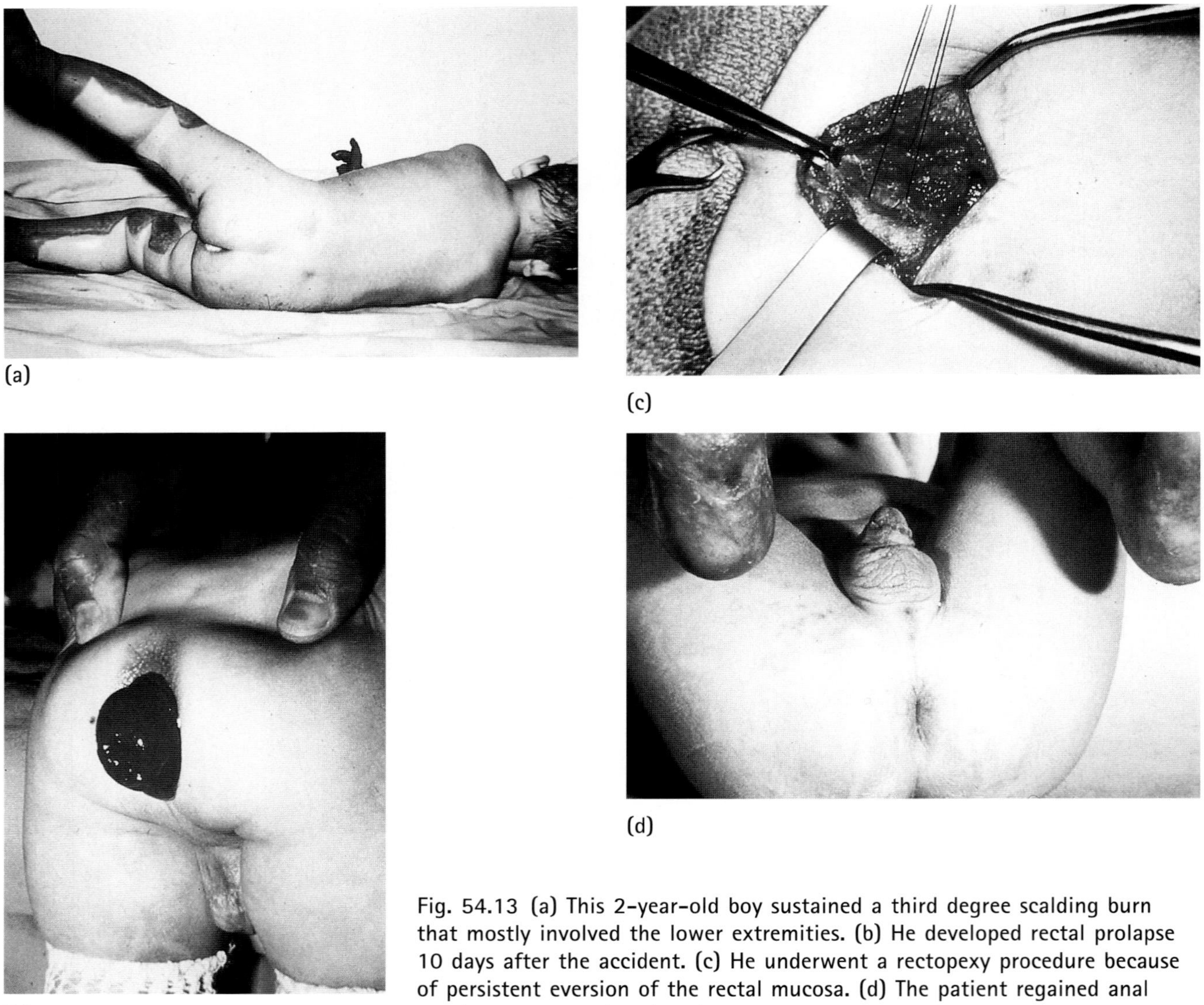

(a)

(b)

(c)

(d)

Fig. 54.13 (a) This 2-year-old boy sustained a third degree scalding burn that mostly involved the lower extremities. (b) He developed rectal prolapse 10 days after the accident. (c) He underwent a rectopexy procedure because of persistent eversion of the rectal mucosa. (d) The patient regained anal continence 6 months after the surgery.

References

1. Alghanem AA, McCauley RL, Robson RC, Rutan AL, Herndon DN. Management of pediatric perineal and genital burns: twenty-year review. *J Burn Care Rehabil* 1990; **11**: 308–11.

2. Rutan RL. Management of perineal and genital burns. *JET Nurs* 1993; **20**: 169–76.

3. Huang T. Twenty years of experience in managing gender dysphoric patients: I. Surgical management of male transsexuals. *Plast Reconst Surg* 1995; **96**: 921–30.

4. Stafford PW. Other disorders of the anus and rectum, anorectal function. In: O'Neill JA, Rowe MI, Grosfeld JL, Fonkalsrud EW, Coran AG, eds. *Pediatric Surgery*, 5th edn. St Louis: Mosby, 1998.

5. Aschcraft KW, Garred JL, Holder TM, Amoury RA, Sharp RJ, Murphy JP. *J Ped. Surg* 1990; **9**: 992–5.

6. Pisarski GP, Greenhalgh DG, Warden GD. The management of perineal contractures in children with burns. *J Burn Care Rehabil* 1994; **15**: 256–9.

7. Sasaki K, Nozaki M, Morioka K, Huang TT. Penile reconstruction: combined use of an innervated forearm osteocutaneous flap and big toe pulp. *Plast Reconstr Surg* 1998; **104**: 1054–8.

Chapter 55   # Foot burns and their complications
Roger E Salisbury

Introduction

Characterized as a major burn by the American Burn Association,[1] burns of the feet present unique and difficult management problems, often causing significant long-term morbidity. Treatment of acute lower extremity burns is initially complicated by a high incidence of cellulitis, poor graft survival, chronic pain, and a prolonged period of immature scar requiring lengthy immobilization and hospitalization. Long-term rehabilitation of foot burns may be complicated by poor patient compliance, chronic edema formation, and complex reconstructive needs resulting from extensive contractures, ligament and tendon injuries, peripheral neuropathies, and bony abnormalities. Thus, isolated foot burns should be given top priority and treated with early, aggressive therapy.

Epidemiology

Annually, approximately 1% of the population of the United States reportedly experiences a thermal injury. Of these 2 million injuries, roughly 100 000 require acute hospitalization.[2] Burns of the feet, either as part of a larger total body surface injury or as isolated injuries, compromise 5–10% of these hospital admissions. Isolated foot burns are most commonly contacted in nature from scald, grease, chemical or electrical injury. Flame injuries are the commonest cause when foot burns are part of a larger total body injury.[3] Age of the injured patient parallels demographics for other burns, the average age of the patient with foot burn being 25 years old.[4] Scald injuries are particularly common in the pediatric age groups and the examining physician must always consider child abuse or neglect.[5] The frequency of the site of the burn depends on the reference source quoted but dorsal foot burns appear more common than plantar surface injuries.[3] A complete assessment of the burn should include mechanisms of injury, location, extent and depth of injury, and age of the patient. Complicating factors such as past medical history and the ability of the patient to care for the injury are also important. These factors provide information, which can significantly affect optimal treatment modalities and eventual outcomes.

General principles – assessment of burn injury

Foot burns are the most common burn injury treated initially on an outpatient basis, but subsequently requiring hospital admission and in-patient care. Nearly 30% of delayed admission foot burns re-present with burn wound cellulitis.[4] Several factors are responsible, the most significant being early local edema. In injured tissue, local edema and positions of dependency increase serum production, which inactivates sebum.[6] Sebum contains high levels of fatty acids, particularly oleic acid, which destroys streptococcal, and to a lesser extent staphylococcal, bacteria.[7] These Gram-positive bacteria are the principle agents in early burn wound cellulitis. Lower extremity cellulitis is associated with increased length of hospitalization, increased need for grafting, and increased hypertrophic scarring.[4] Since simple therapeutic measures to prevent edema, such as strict bed rest, elevation, and wound care are less likely to be performed in the outpatient setting, hospitalization for even simple foot burns is indicated. Short-term admissions of 24–48 hours will improve wound care, decrease the significant period of early edema formation, and allow the physician time to establish adequate arrangements for home care.[5] Limited hospital stay also affords the wound time 'to declare itself', allowing the surgeon further opportunity to determine depth of injury and formulate accurate decisions regarding operative treatments.

Initial assessment of depth of injury is based upon physical appearance, the presence of pain, skin texture, location, and mechanism of injury.[8] Clinical assessment is paramount, as noninvasive diagnostic techniques are not completely accurate. Superficial (first degree) burns of the foot involve only the thinner outer epidermis. Pain and erythema with intact skin are clinical features. These burns heal in 5–10 days with no residual scarring.

Second degree, partial-thickness burns of the foot, are classified as either superficial or deep, depending on extent of dermis injury. Superficial partial-thickness burns involve the epidermis and papillary dermis and are characterized by pain, erythema, and blister formation as plasma leaks under devitalized epidermis. These burns heal within 1–2 weeks (without surgery), generally with minimal scarring. In contrast, deep partial-thickness foot burns extend well into the reticular dermis with minimal viability of epidermal appendages. These wounds are typically erythematous to white in color, without blisters, less painful and less moist than superficial partial-thickness burns, and often indistinguishable from full-thickness (third degree) injury. Mechanism and location influences the depth of injury. Scald burns are associated with more superficial burns. Oil and flame burns typically cause deeper injuries despite initial presenting appearance. Dorsal foot burns, because of minimal subcutaneous tissue and paucity of excess skin tends to be deeper in nature than plantar surface injuries. Spontaneous healing is possible within 3 weeks if optimal conditions persist for the remaining epidermal appendages to regenerate an epithelium. However, these wounds can change in appearance as ischemic injury extends into the zone of stasis. The burns heal initially with a thin epidermis and subsequently develop a dense hypertrophic scar. Because the foot is a highly functional area, predisposed to contracture, deep dorsal partial-thickness burns require surgical intervention with debridement and grafting early. This treatment will decrease the inflammatory period and reduce contracture formation. Deep partial-thickness burns of the plantar surface often can be managed nonoperatively. A thick dermis and epidermis generally protects the area from full-thickness injury typically seen on the dorsal foot. However, if an eschar persists over 3 weeks time, debridement and grafting are necessary. Occasionally, debrided wounds will reepithelialize spontaneously, without the need for grafting.

Full-thickness (third degree) burns involve destruction of the entire dermis and epidermis with no elements remaining for spontaneous healing. These burns are anesthetic and have a characteristic white, dry, waxy appearance. Coagulated capillaries may impart a dark discoloration to the wound. This wound can heal only by contraction and ingrowth of epitheliums from skin margins. Burns of this type require debridement and grafting, and may require extensive reconstructive procedures to reestablish the structural integrity of the foot.

Hospitalization

Acute Care

Once the decision to hospitalize the patient has been made, the wound should be sterilely debrided of any devitalized skin at the bedside. Adequate analgesia is obtained with oral or parenteral narcotics. Early assessment of the wound depth is made at this time. Superficial partial-thickness burns are treated with Xeroform™ fine mesh gauze or a synthetic skin substitute (Biobrane™). Deeper burns are placed in Silvadene™. If cellulitis is present, Sulfamylon™ is used for increased eschar penetration. Either an open or closed dressing method may be utilized. Complete bed rest with extremity elevation above the heart is mandatory. Parenteral antibiotics are not routinely administered unless cellulitis is present. In this instance, wound cultures are obtained and a first-generation cephalosporin antibiotic will provide adequate coverage. Alternative agents, such as ampicillin/sulbactam or vancomycin are employed for more invasive cellulitis or if the patient's medical condition warrants increased coverage. Consideration as to possible need for escharotomies is entertained if circumferential burns involve a more proximal portion of the leg.

Aggressive wound care is essential to prevent cellulitis and burn wound conversion which requires twice daily sterile foot washings and dressing changes with re-application of a topical antimicrobial cream. If burns are to be treated nonoperatively, early passive and active range of motion exercises help to minimize contraction and preserve function.[9] If cellulitis is present, however, range of motion should be delayed, as excessive movement can facilitate the spread of local infection.[9]

Early splinting of foot burns is essential. Unsupported ankles are prone to plantar flexion and there is a pronounced tendency to develop shortening of the Achilles' tendon. This complication is seen too frequently in patients with large total burns on ventilators who are uncooperative and unable to be ambulated. Medical and nursing staff should check the foot daily for evidence of foot drop or ulcer formation. Positioning of the ankles in 90° of dorsiflexion with a footboard or splint will maintain proper tendon positioning for eventual ambulation.[10] While utilizing splints, added heel support with the use of wool boots will help prevent heel breakdown. A pressure of 70 mmHg for as little as 2 hours results in irreversible necrosis. Consideration must also be given to prevention of deep venous thrombosis and its associated morbidity.[11] Subcutaneous administration of mini-dose heparin twice daily is utilized at our institution.

Following healing, ambulation is resumed. Patients are wrapped from the toes to the groins with Ace™ bandages in a figure-of-eight or spiral fashion, reducing venostasis and improving blood flow.[9] Silastic boots formed from a positive plaster mold of the patient's foot have been shown to prevent plantar pressure changes on healing epithelium in other burn centers.[12]

Surgical Care

If surgical wound management is indicated, early excision and grafting of the burn wound should be performed, within 5 days post injury. Early excision and grafting has been shown to decrease hospitalization time.[13] Since foot burns require prolonged bed rest, early surgical debridement decreases the risk of prolonged immobilization and allows for early ambulation.

The depth of burn injury and the position of the burn on the foot dictate the type of surgical modality chosen. The preferred procedure is tangential excision with application of split thickness skin grafts.[5] For both dorsal and plantar injuries, excision to fascia should be avoided since this operation increases complications. Poor distal blood flow makes the clinical end-point of excision difficult to establish. In other areas of the body during excision, punctuate bleeding of a well-vascularized wound bed is noted. However, in the foot, viable deep dermis and subcutaneous tissue may be present with a white, shiny appearance. Deep distal phalangeal burns of the toes are particularly difficult to excise and graft. Thus topical chemotherapy, debridement, and grafting of granulation tissue are a preferred method of treating these burns.

When harvesting skin, thicker skin grafts (more stable) are

preferred, from 16/1000th to 20/1000th of an inch. The grafts are meshed one and a half times the original size and are placed without fully expanding the meshed spaces. Thinner or wider mesh grafts can increase tissue desiccation.[5] Full-thickness skin grafts offer no advantage over split-thickness grafts when adequate subcutaneous tissue is present.

Postoperative Care

Following application of grafts, postoperative care is performed with many of the same principles outlined for nonsurgical management. First, steps must be taken to prevent the complications associated with graft loss, including hematoma, shear injury, and infection. Meticulous intraoperative techniques, including adequate hemostasis and proper placement of the graft, prevent perioperative graft loss secondary to hematoma formation. Complete bed rest and immobilization utilizing splints can best prevent shear injury. Previous methods of skeletal suspension with Steinmann pins placed into the tibia and calcaneus have shown no significant improvement in outcome.[3] Graft maceration and desquamation are prevented by use of a semipermeable, nonocclusive dressing. For large grafts, irrigation with a 0.1% dilute Silvadene™ solution is used several times a day to prevent desiccation and to facilitate graft adherence.

Infection prophylaxis is essential. Strict intraoperative and perioperative sterile techniques must be followed. Topical antibiotic irrigants help provide a bacteriostatic environment for graft growth. Perioperative parenteral antibiotics are routinely administered. Grafts are inspected 2 days postoperatively and daily thereafter to ensure proper adherence and healing. If infection is suspected, cultures are obtained and topical and parenteral antibiotics are changed according to organism sensitivity. Normally, with one and a half-meshing, the graft interstices are completely coalesced by the fifth to seventh postoperative day. Range of motion exercises are re-started just prior to this period. Ambulation is resumed as early as 1 week postoperatively for most dorsal and lateral grafted burns. Plantar grafts are immobilized until 10 days postoperatively. Ace™ bandages are applied in a figure-of-eight or spiral fashion, and are essential to prevent shear injury once ambulation is started. Discharge planning is initiated once graft healing is confirmed and ambulation is tolerated. Discharge plans must include instructions regarding foot care (with special emphasis on proper protection and bathing of the grafted areas) and splints or orthotic devices.

Scar contracture and postoperative complications

While split-thickness skin grafts are optimum for early wound coverage in most foot burns, they are not without complications. Because of the biomechanics of ambulation and the demands placed on the skin of the dorsal and plantar surface of the foot, ulceration, fissure formation, hypertrophic scarring, keloids, chronic pain, gait abnormalities, and scar contracture may occur. These complications can rapidly produce progressive functional impairments and contour deformities, which can increase local tissue destruction. These problems are common over the dorsal aspect of the foot. Scar contracture entraps local tissue and tendons, producing hyperextension of the metatarsal phalangeal joints with flexion of the interphalangeal joints, resulting in a typical hammertoe deformity. This process may progress to the classical

rocker bottom foot. The deformity is accentuated with ambulation and is associated with repeated ulceration secondary to improper shoe fit. Initial treatment involves splinting and range of motion exercises. If these conservative modalities fail, surgical treatment is necessary. Complete excision of the scar tissue including underlying involved structures such as shortened tendons may be necessary, followed by placement of a sheet graft and appropriate postoperative immobilization. Immobilization is facilitated by placement of Kirschner wires through the distal phalanges. These deformities can reoccur if the contracture is inadequately excised.[14]

Web space deformities are also common in distal foot burns and are treated in a similar fashion to web space contractures of the hands. Simple z-plasty is usually effective and further skin grafting will not be necessary.[15]

Plantar surface contractures include phalangeal flexion contractures of the toes. Early treatment involves splinting and range of motion exercises. If this treatment fails, incisional release and skin grafting is utilized. Since there is little resistance in this area to prevent recontracture scar formation, thick sheet grafts are preferred over thin grafts, which are more likely to contract. Postoperative immobilization is essential, and K-wires or splints are utilized for this purpose. Persistent recurrent contracture problems are best managed with local flaps. These are generally obtained from the lateral toes and rotated to cover the tissue defects. Care must be taken to avoid the neurovascular bundles of the toe, which are located on the volar lateral toe margins. For larger contracture deformities complicated by necrosis and/or infection of the underlying metatarsal bone, sacrifice of the distal toe with resection of the distal metatarsal and creation of a toe pedicle flap is required.[14,16,17] Larger injuries involving the metatarsal heads suggest specific plantar surface pressure points and will likely require distant tissue coverage.

Deep posterior heel burns may result in significant contractures. The classical example is Achilles' tendon shortening leading to an equinus type deformity.[15] Splints are essential in the early management of these injuries to prevent this crippling deformity. Early grafting is the treatment of choice. For deeper injuries or for severe contractures, tendon release or lengthening procedures is required. Coverage is then obtained by utilizing a graft or local flap.

Foot reconstruction

If functional anatomy of the hand is glossed over in medical school, the foot is treated as a nonentity. In reality, the foot is easily as complex as the hand but has elicited far less research in reconstruction. Perhaps the fact that general, plastic, and orthopedic surgeons perform upper extremity reconstruction accounts for the disparity. Certainly the anatomy of the foot has presented anatomical challenges to reconstruction that still defy answers. For instance, the fibrous septa binding skin to deep tissues simply has not been duplicated by flap coverage, and shear forces result in frequent ulceration. The gait cycle has been thoroughly analyzed[18] but too few surgeons have used it to evaluate their postoperative results, which the author finds astonishing. Function is truly the test of excellence in reconstruction and must be measured to evaluate the validity of the surgery.

While skin grafts are sufficient for most foot burns, electrical and deep flame burns often present more difficult reconstructive problems to the surgeon. Following a major injury, the remaining soft-tissue coverage may be insufficient to support a graft as tendons and bones may be exposed. Although tendons can be resected and bone decorticated to allow for the ingrowth of granulation tissue prior to grafting, such surgical repair may not adequately address the needs of a functional ambulating individual. Following reconstruction, the foot should be able to withstand the forces of unrestricted motion and weight-bearing during ambulation. The repair must also restore normal anatomic contour to the specific sub-units of the foot and provide adequate sensation and proprioception.

The foot can be divided into the dorsal and the plantar surfaces. The specific sub-units of the plantar foot include the distal plantar surface, the mid plantar surface, and the proximal plantar surface (hind foot) which includes the distal Achilles' tendon and malleolar regions. Reconstruction may require local skin flaps, muscle flaps, fasciocutaneous flaps, free flaps, or even composite tissue transplantation. In some instances a cross leg flap may serve as an adequate alternative.

The dorsal foot

The dorsum of the foot is composed of a thin layer of epidermis, dermis, and subcutaneous tissue allowing for adequate extensor tendon motion. Repair of complex soft-tissue wounds of this area must provide thin, pliable tissue which is durable enough to withstand the pressure of foot wear while protecting the underlying mobile tendons.[18] Small proximal dorsal foot wounds may be adequately closed with the use of a local muscle flap. Myocutaneous flaps such as the abductor hallucis, the abductor digiti minimi, or the extensor digiti brevis muscle are adequate local transpositional flaps for this purpose.[19–21] Historically, larger dorsal foot defects required the use of a cross leg flap.[22] However, the advent of microsurgery with shortened immobilization time and decreased hospitalization has largely outdated these flaps. Fascial and skin free flaps are currently the procedures of choice.[23–26] The radial forearm flap and the temporalis fascia flap have been used successfully to close these defects.[27–29] The specific operative details on the use of flap reconstruction are beyond the scope of this chapter.

The plantar foot

Distal and Mid-distal Plantar Defects

Complex soft-tissue defects of the plantar foot surface are true reconstructive challenges. The plantar skin surface is composed of a glabrous epidermis and dermis (up to 3.5 mm thick) a dense subcutaneous tissue layer, and a vertical fibrous septa.[30]

These components move in unison to absorb and resist the shearing forces of ambulation. Up to 50% of previously placed plantar split-thickness skin grafts may be lost with ambulation due to these sheering forces.[31] Adequate reconstruction of the plantar foot surface must provide a sensate covering that will protect the tissue from further damage while ambulating. Reconstruction of the plantar distal forefoot can be performed utilizing several different procedures. For small defects, the V-Y-advancement flaps or simple toe flaps are effective surgical choices.[9,17,32,33] Neurovascular island flaps provide adequate coverage for larger defects.[34,35] Extensive soft-tissue loss will require the use of a fascial or muscle-based free flap.[36] The mid-plantar foot is usually a nonweight-bearing surface. Injuries to this sub-unit are best managed with a skin graft.[32] Larger defects will require a medial or lateral based fascial or muscle plantar transportation flap.[37,38] Free flaps provide an alternative option for larger defects.[25,26]

Proximal Plantar (Hind foot) Defects

The plantar hind foot presents a unique reconstructive challenge to the surgeon. A durable, thick heel pad cushion is required over the weight-bearing surface of the calcaneus to ensure normal ambulation.[18] Proximally, the nonweight-bearing hind foot is covered with a thin, pliable, fibrous sheet extending from the Achilles' tendon and malleolar area.[39] Tissue utilized in repair of this sub-unit must approximate the strength of the native tissues. Transposition flaps incorporating the proximal plantar subcutaneous plexus can provide adequate coverage for defects of both the weight-bearing and nonweight-bearing portions of the heel.[40,41] For more complex defects of the weight-bearing heel, numerous local muscle or myocutaneous flaps are utilized. The intrinsic muscles, including the abductor hallucis, flexor digitoris brevis and abductor digiti minimi muscles, provide adequate rotational flaps in a single staged repair.[42–44] Fascio-cutaneous flaps generally cover only a limited area and may require a delayed procedure.[37] Reverse pedicled posterior leg fasciocutaneous flaps require division of a major trifurcating artery, usually the posterior tibial artery, and therefore are secondary reconstructive options.[45]

The nonweight-bearing heel and the distal Achilles' tendon region are probably best reconstructed utilizing a lateral calcaneal artery flap.[46] This island pedicle flap will cover 3–5 cm tissue defects.

Subfascial arterialized flaps can be used alternatively.[47,48] Suprafascial flaps, either medial or laterally based are employed for small defects.[49,50] Reconstruction of significant malleolar injuries are best repaired utilizing local muscle transpositional flaps. The extensor digitorum brevis myocutaneous flap is an acceptable choice.[51,52] In addition, the previously described intrinsic muscle flaps, including the abductor hallucis, abductor digiti minimi, flexor digitorum brevis flaps, provide alternative options.[42–44] Excellent sensate coverage for the ankle is also obtained using a dorsalis pedis flap or peroneal artery island pedicle flap, although there is a potential for healing problems over the donor site.[53–55]

Local flaps are not without complications. The majority of local flaps are perfused through the medial and lateral plantar arteries. Therefore an occluded posterior tibial artery will compromise significantly the perfusion of most local flaps, resulting in flap loss. In instances of local flap failure or where significant soft-tissue loss is present, free flaps are necessary.[23,25,26] Adequate donor sites for free flaps include the deltoid, the lateral arm, and the radial forearm.[56,57] Although free flaps are generally durable and provide excellent coverage, they are not without complications. Meticulous microsurgical technique coupled with long operative time is necessary to achieve acceptable results. Complications, including thrombus formation, may lead to failure of these flaps during the first 5 postoperative days. Furthermore, transplanted tissue may provide poor adherence to native foot structures, leading to persistent skin ulceration, and eventual flap loss. These problems may be compounded by poor patient compliance. Although free flaps are associated with certain morbidity, studies show that they cause less postoperative pain and fewer gait changes than local flaps.[58]

Local flaps, because of limited amounts of transposable tissue, may lead to chronic pain with ambulation. Such pain causes patients to avoid weight-bearing over the areas of reconstruction and instead redistribute weight over other areas of the foot.[59] This activity leads to significant changes in gait, which persist with time and are minimally influenced by supportive footwear.[59]

In contrast, patients with sensory free flaps do not demonstrate significant gait changes.[58] Free flaps offer the advantage of abundant transposable tissue which acts as padding over bony prominences. Extra padding helps to minimize the amount of pain and patients are less likely to avoid weight-bearing over reconstructed areas, preventing the gait changes noted in patients with local flaps. The major gait change experienced by patients with sensory free flaps is an increase in the average cycle time of each step.[58] With a slower gait cycle time, fewer vertical and horizontal sheer forces are applied to reconstructed areas and flap survival is improved.

In some instances, free flaps may not be feasible for coverage of large foot tissue defects. The classical cross leg fasciocutaneous muscle or myocutaneous flap offers a viable alternative.[60,61] Cross leg flaps do require prolonged cross leg fixation and are associated with extended hospitalization.[62]

Conclusion

Burns of the feet present complex healing and reconstructive problems to the surgeon. Because of the small surface area involved, the complexity of small foot burns may be underappreciated, resulting in a high rate of complication from early wound cellulitis to late scar contractures. Reconstructive efforts to deal with these problems and provide coverage for open wounds must also incorporate full functional ambulation and weight-bearing as mandatory goals. Surgical procedures performed without regard to this dictum may be technically successful but produce a functionally debilitated patient, potentially creating a further care burden for society. For instance, several articles have appeared in recent years showing a more pleasing aesthetic result due to technical improvements in the surgery. While one cannot deny the importance of appearance, it is most disturbing that significant functional problems still remain to be solved. For instance, free flaps are a technical advance but because they lack the fibrous elements binding skin to underlying tissue, there is minimal resistance to shear forces and ulceration frequently results. May's clinical and gait analysis study[58] following free microvascular muscle flaps with skin graft is an excellent attempt to analyze results and one hopes that other thoughtful studies will follow. To date, nothing has been totally satisfactory to insure painless weight-bearing and further research is warranted. Sommerlad's paper,[59] although published in 1978, still should provoke thoughtful humility in those doing this work. He found that, irrespective of treatment, the average time loss from work was 17 months. More than half of the patients had pain 5 years post-injury. Significantly, patients avoided weight-bearing when possible, regardless of the surgical technique employed for reconstruction, and simply altered their gait. More long-term analyses, such as this paper, are certainly needed.

References

1. Artz CP, Moncrief PA, Pruitt BA, eds. *Burn Care: A Team Approach*. Philadelphia: WB Saunders, 1979.

2. Department of Health, Education, & Welfare. *Reports of the Epidemiology and Surveillance of Injuries*. Atlanta: Center for Disease Control, 1982.

3. Gore D, Desai M, Herndon D, et al. Comparison of complications during rehabilitation between conservative and early stage management in thermal burns involving the feet of children and adolescents. *J Burn Care Rehabil* 1987; 9: 92.

4. Zachary LS, Heggers JP, Robson MC, et al. Burns of the feet. *J Burn Care Rehabil* 1987; 8: 192.

5. Demling R, Lalonde C, eds. *Burn Trauma*. New York: Thieme, 1989.

6. Robson MC, Krizek T, Wray RC. Care of the thermally injured patient. In: Zuidema GD, Rutherford RB, Ballinger WA, eds. *Management of Trauma*. Philadelphia: WB Saunders, 1979.

7. Ricketts LR, et al. Human skin lipids with particular reference to the self-sterilization power of the skin. *Clin Sci Mol Med* 1951; 10: 89.

8. Robson MC, Smith DT. Thermal injuries. In: Jurkiewicz MT, Krizek TS, Mathes SJ, Ariyan S, eds. *Plastic Surgery, Principles and Practice*. St Louis: CV Mosby, 1990.

9. Malick MH, Carr JA, eds. *Manual on Management of the Burn Patient*. Philadelphia: Harmarville Rehabilitation Center, 1982.

10. Robson MC. Reconstruction and rehabilitation from admission: a surgeon's role at each phase. In: Bernstein NR, Robson MC, eds. *Comprehensive Approaches to the Burned Patient*. New York: Medical Examination Publishing, 1983.

11. Kakkar VV, Spindler J, Flute PT, et al. Efficacy of low doses of Heparin in prevention of deep vein thrombosis after major surgery. *Lancet* 1972; 2: 101.

12. Feldman AE, Thompson TT, MacMillan BG. The molded silicone shoe in the prevention of contractures involving the burn injured foot. *Burns* 1974; 1: 5.

13. Burke JF, Bondoc CC, Quinby WC. Primary excision and immediate grafting, a method of shortening illness. *J Trauma* 1974; 14: 389.

14. Salisbury RE, Bevin AG. Atlas of reconstructive burn surgery. Philadelphia: W.B. Saunders, 1981: 249.

15. Witt PD, Achauer BM, eds. *Burn reconstruction*. New York: Thieme, 1991: 134.

16. Snyder GB, Edgerton MT. The principle of the island neurovascular flap in the management of the ulcerated anesthetic weight-bearing areas of the lower extremity. *Plast Reconstr Surg* 1965; 36: 518.

17. Emmertt AJ. The toe flap. *Br J Plast Surg* 1976; 29: 19.

18. Lamont JG. Functional anatomy of the lower limb. *Clin Plast Surg* 1986; 13: 571.

19. Ger R. The management of chronic ulcers of the dorsum of the foot by muscle transposition and free skin grafting. *Br J Plast Surg* 1976; 29: 199.

20. Mathes SJ, Nahai F, eds. Clinical applications for muscle and musculocutaneous flaps. St. Louis: Mosby, 1982.

21. Ishidawa K, Isghiki N, Suywki S, Shimamaura S. Distally based dorsalis pedis island flap for coverage of the distal portion of the foot. *Br J Plast Surg* 1987; 40: 521.

22. Uhm K, Skin KS, Lew J. Crane Principle of the cross-leg fasciocutaneous flap: aesthetically pleasing technique for damaged dorsum of the foot. *Ann Plast Surg* 1985; 15: 257.

23. Daniel RK, Taylor GT. Distant transfers of an island flap by microvascular anastomosis. *Plast Reconstr Surg* 1973; 52: 11.

24. Masquelet MD, Rinaldi S, Mauchet A. The posterior arm free flap. *Plast Reconstr Surg* 1985; 76: 908.

25. Raine TJ, Nahai F. Free tissue transfers to the foot. *Plast Surg Forum* 1984; 7: 112.

26. Swartz WW, Jones NF. Soft tissue coverage of the lower extremity. *Curr Prob Surg* 1985.

27. Chicarilli ZN, Ariyan S, Cuono CB. Free radial forearm flaps versatility for the hand and neck and lower extremity. *J Reconstr Microsurg* 1986; 2: 221.

28. Hallock GG. Simultaneous bilateral foot reconstruction using a single radial forearm flap. *Plast Reconstr Surg* 1987; 80: 836.

29. Hallock GG. The radial forearm flap in burn reconstruction. *J Burn Care Rehabil* 1986; 7: 318.

30. Sarrafian SK. Anatomy of the foot and ankle. Philadelphia: J.B. Lippincott, 1983.

31. Dahl TD, LeMaster JE, Cram AE. Effectiveness of split thickness autografts of plantar aspects of the feet. *J Burn Care Rehabil* 1984; 5: 463.

32. Rooks MD. Coverage problems of the foot and ankle. *Ortho Clin N Am* 1989; 20: 723.

33. Colen LB, Rplogle SL, Mathes SJ. The V-Y plantar flap for reconstruction of the forefoot. *Plast Reconstr Surg* 1988; 81: 220.

34. Snyder GB, Edgerton MT. The principle of the island neurovascular flap in the management of the ulcerated anesthetic weight-bearing areas of the lower extremity. *Plast Reconstr Surg* 1965; 36: 518.

35. Buncke HT, Colen LB. An island flap from the first web space of the foot to cover plantar ulcers. *Br J Plast Surg* 1980; 33: 242.

36. May TW, Gallico GG, Lukash FN. Microvascular transfers of free tissue for closure of burn wounds of the distal lower extremity. *N Engl J Med* 1982; 306: 253.

37. Freeman BS. Plantar flaps used for sole and heel lesions. *Texas J Med* 1968; 64: 64.

38. Colen LB, Buncke HJ. Neurovascular island flaps from plantar vessels and nerves for foot reconstruction. *Ann Plast Surg* 1984; **12**: 327.

39. Scheflan M, Nahai F, Hartrampf C. Surgical management of heel ulcers – a comprehensive approach. *Ann Plast Surg* 1981; **7**: 385.

40. Hidalgo DA, Shaw WW. Anatomic basis of plantar flap design. 1986; **78**: 627.

41. Shaw WW, Hidalgo DA. Anatomic basis of plantar flap design: *Clin Appl* 1986; **78**: 637.

42. Ger R. The surgical management of ulcers of the heel. *Surg Gynecol Obstet* 1975; **140**: 909.

43. Ikuta Y, Murakami T, Yoshioka K, *et al.* Reconstruction of the heel pad by flexor digitorum brevis musculocutaneous flap transfer. *Plast Reconstr Surg* 1980; **66**: 264.

44. Hartrampf CR. Scheflan M, Bostwick J. The flexor digitorum brevis muscle island pedicle flap: a new dimension in heel reconstruction. *Plast Reconstr Surg* 1980; **66**: 264.

45. Hong G, Steffens K, Wang FB. Reconstruction of the lower leg and foot with the reverse pedicled posterior tibial fasciocutaneous flap. *Br J Plast Surg* 1989; **42**: 512.

46. Holmes J. Rayner CR. Lateral calcaneal artery island flaps. *Br J Plast Surg* 1984; **37**: 402.

47. Reiffel RS, McCarthy JG. Coverage of the heel and sole defects: a new subfascial arterialized flap. *Plast Reconstr Surg* 1981; **66**: 250.

48. Shanahan RE, Gingrass RP. Medial plantar sensory flap for coverage of heel defects. *Plast Reconstr Surg* 1979; **64**: 295.

49. Elsahy NI. The use of the bipedicle flap for the repair of ulcers in the non-weight bearing areas of the heel. *Acta Chir Plast* 1978; **20**: 34.

50. Curtin JW. Functional surgery for intractable conditions of the sole of the foot. *Plast Reconstr Surg* 1977; **59**: 806.

51. Land A, Soragni O, Monteleone M. The extensor digitorum brevis muscle island flap for soft tissue loss around the ankle. *Plast Reconstr Surg* 1985; **75**: 892.

52. Leitner DW, Gordon L, Buncke HJ. The extensor digitorum brevis as a muscle island flap. *Plast Reconstr Surg* 1985; **76**: 777.

53. Gould JS. The dorsalis pedis island pedicle flap for small defects of the foot and ankle. *Ortho* 1986; **9**: 867.

54. Yoshimura M, Shimada T, Imura S, *et al.* Peroneal island flap for skin defects in the lower extremity. *J Bone Joint Surg* 1985; **67**: 935.

55. McGraw JB, Furlow LT. The dorsalis pedis arterialized flap. *Plast Reconstr Surg* 1975; **55**: 177.

56. Russell RC, Guy RJ, Zook EG, *et al.* Extremity reconstruction using the free deltoid flap. *Plast Reconstr Surg* 1985; **76**: 586.

57. Scheker LR, Lister GD, Wolff TW. The lateral arm free flap in releasing severe contracture of the first web space. *J Hand Surg* 1988; **13**: 146.

58. May JW, Halls MJ, Simon SR. Free microvascular muscle flaps with skin graft reconstruction of extensive defects of the feet: a clinical and gait analysis study. *Plast Reconstr Surg* 1985; **5**: 627.

59. Sommerland BC, McGrowther DS. Resurfacing the sole: long-term follow-up and comparison of techniques. *Br J Plast Surg* 1978; **31**: 107.

60. Barclay TL, Sharp DT, Chisolm EM. Cross-leg fasciocutaneous flaps. *Plast Reconstr Surg* 1983; **72**: 843.

61. Cervino AL, Thottam JJ. Cross-foot flap for ankle coverage. *Ann Plast Surg* 1979; **2**: 72.

62. Taylor GA, Hopson WL. The cross-foot flap. *Plast Reconstr Surg* 1975; **55**: 677.

Psychological and social issues

Chapter 56   The ethical dimension of burn care

Bruce E Zawacki, Arthur P Sanford

Introduction

In seeking optimum health for each patient, 'total burn care' aspires to integrated excellence in multiple dimensions. It is a 'bio-psycho-social-economic-legal-and-ethical' enterprise, and the many hyphens indicate that all the dimensions of care are connected. Too often, the bio-psycho-social-etc. dimensions are assumed to be interconnected like railway cars, with the biological dimension in front, and the ethical hooked on only if necessary at the end, like an optional caboose. This is a misleading assumption. In our experience, 'total burn care' is most frequently achieved when it is assumed that *all* the dimensions of burn care are *always* present and in need of regular attention. Moreover, highly integrated, team-oriented, interdisciplinary[1] burn centers practice as if *all* the dimensions of care are *always* interpenetrating, like the length, width, and height of a solid object. In their daily work they assume that no one dimension may be changed without affecting all the others, and they depend on frequent detailed rounds, interdisciplinary staff meetings, and ongoing interviews with patients and families to keep all the dimensions of care ever coordinated and up-to-date.

In part because the multiple dimensions of burn care are so intimately interrelated, decisions involving the ethical dimension of burn care are extremely common. They are so common, in fact, that care-providers are usually unaware of them. Ethics, after all, is critical thinking about right and wrong, what should or should not be done, etc.[2] The words 'should', 'should not' and so forth indicate that ethical matters are being addressed. For example, whenever we decide which of several therapeutic alternatives *should* be recommended, we are making an ethical decision.[3] Should we spend more time with patient A than with patient B? Should we catch up on our journal reading as opposed to getting more sleep? Should we spend more time with our families and less at work? All are ethical decisions. Ethical decision making is therefore like breathing:[4] ever necessary and ongoing, but regularly automatic unless the problem is serious enough to be singled out for explicit attention.

What is 'an ethical problem?' When is it serious?

Often significant ethical problems are trivialized by mislabeling them as 'merely problems in communication'.[a] A formal yet practical definition is therefore necessary: an ethical problem is present when it involves a conflict of two or more of the following: rights or rights-claims, obligations, goods and/or values.[b] For example, disputes about writing a 'comfort-measures-only' order for a patient without decision-making capacity and with a very low probability of survival commonly involve a conflict between an obligation and a good: the obligation not to abandon aggressive therapy prematurely, and the good of a maximally pain-free and unprotracted death. In such a case, *the burn team and the patient/surrogate* are ordinarily the major stakeholders and appropriate decision-makers, and we say they are addressing 'a problem in *clinical* ethics'. On the other hand, consider the burn center's or health care organization's (HCO's) responsibility to ICU patients when a safe nurse:patient ratio cannot be consistently met despite the burn center's best efforts? If discerning 'what should be done' in such circumstances requires decision-making at the *managerial level* of the burn center or HCO, a 'problem in *organizational ethics*'[5] is the correct term to use.

As indicated, conflicts among rights, obligations etc, are *very*

---

[a] As we shall explain in detail, 'ethical problems' shared by stakeholders *are*, in fact, optimally resolved by communication . . . but by a very challenging, particular, uncommon, and decidedly untrivial species of communication called ethical dialogue.

[b] Modified slightly from May WW. *Discerning What's Right in Health Care at the Clinical Level*. Lecture at U.S.C. Keck School of Medicine, Los Angeles CA, May 8, 2000. As used here and elsewhere in this chapter, the term 'values' refers to considerations (e.g. principles, laws, rules, roles, assumptions, preferences, goals, etc.) giving direction and/or impetus to decision making.

common and vary greatly in difficulty. When should they be taken seriously? An ethical problem is serious when there are stakeholders involved who stand to be affected seriously by the problem or its outcome. Stakeholders working collaboratively without outside help can successfully manage the vast majority of such problems. When are such problems so serious that assistance should be sought from a health care ethics committee/consultant (HEC) or its equivalent? There are two answers: the first short and crude, the second longer and more precise. An ethical problem is serious enough to refer to a HEC:

- when you suspect the 'New York Times sniff-test' would be positive,[c] i.e. you think a hypothetical newspaper reporter might be interested in making the problem or its solution public;
- when there is persistent disagreement among the major stakeholders; and codes, rules, laws and more discussions fail to lead to a resolution within generally acceptable ethical boundaries.

How should 'clinical ethics' problems be managed?

In the United States, the 'informed consent process' was developed by the American judiciary to safeguard the legal rights and welfare of all the stakeholders participating in 'bedside' or 'clinical' decision-making. Throughout the USA, this legal process has become the foundation of the health care provider's approach to avoiding and managing serious ethical problems at the bedside. Its application in the burn center was explained and diagramed in detail in the first edition of this book,[6] and what follows should be considered an update and development of what is stated there.

On the vast majority of occasions, there is little or no difficulty achieving agreement and patient consent about a proposed course of burn management. Occasionally, however, the process of obtaining informed consent leads to problems involving disagreements, anxieties and/or controversies about 'what should be done'. At this point, the participants must give careful attention to the quality of the discussion or 'ethical discourse' being used in attempting to resolve the problem. Ethical discourse is a skill requiring practice, like playing a musical instrument. No one becomes good at playing the violin or participating in ethical discourse simply by reading books about the subject, or by letting a consultant take over when things get difficult. Avoidance of, or reluctance to participate in, discourse with stakeholders about ethical problems is like a violin player who avoids practice, or won't go near the concert hall: both will perform suboptimally when at last forced by circumstances to act.

Contrary to very common practice, ethical discourse at its best is not merely filling your 'opponent's' heads with what you want them to know so they will say what you want hear. Nor is it simply getting your discourse partners to effectively 'get things off their chests' so they will feel better and then say what you want to hear. Least of all is it engaging in verbal warfare in an effort to 'be victorious over your opponents'. At its best, ethical discourse begins by building a 'safe place for ethical dialogue', i.e. establishing an interpersonal 'relationship' made safe for transparent and self-crit-

ical honesty by making active listening and openness-to-learning the norm.[7]

The Role of the Care-provider in Ethical Dialogue

The care-provider should *develop the trust* necessary to establish the 'safe place for ethical dialogue' described above. To do this, the care-provider should learn the bio-psycho-social-economic- and cultural/religious information required to approach the patient and their family and/or surrogate with empathy for their lives and values. Some religious backgrounds teach us that we have certain limitations to this life and look to the future beyond. Others teach us that within our lives we'll come back and reflect on what our previous lives have been and also place extreme respect on the departed spirit. Finally, there are people who do not have a religious background that live for different goals and different aspirations. All of these must be considered early on when determining what the caregiver's relationship and position will be with the patients and their families. Many patients will decide against extremes of treatment and continuing care with the hope of not burdening their family with large hospital bills. Often these issues must be explored with patients before one can feel comfortable with the decision and its justification.

The care-provider must *discover if the patient has 'decision-making capacity'* sufficient to participate meaningfully in deliberation. To have decision-making capacity, the patient's (or if necessary, the patient's/surrogate's) consent to or refusal of the care-provider's recommendations must be: *informed* (i.e. comprehending and appreciating relevant information); *free* (substantially free of distorting nonrational/emotional influences); *deliberate* (decided after weighing pros versus cons in the light of his or her value system); *voluntary* (reflecting his or her own intentions); and *expressed* (communicated verbally or non-verbally).[8] Decision-making capacity is enhanced by optimizing the patient's physiological stability, consciousness, and pain control as much as possible. It is typically verified by ascertaining orientation, and by asking patients to rephrase the information provided to them in their own words and to say why they have made the decision they have. Determination of decision-making capacity by judicial process (i.e. determination of 'legal competency') is rarely necessary. If despite all efforts, the patient is found to be without decision-making capacity, an appropriate surrogate is commonly available among the patient's family or friends.

The care-provider should *provide appropriate information* about the patient's diagnosis and the therapy proposed, its nature, prognosis, pros and cons, and similar information about plausible alternatives including forgoing the therapy proposed. Prior investigation of the *patient's and/or surrogate's bio-psycho-social-economic-cultural-etc. background* is particularly helpful in the effort to assure clear communication and a common understanding among dialogue partners.

The Role of the Patient or Surrogate

The initial task of the patient is to assimilate the information given by the caregivers. One cannot expect a patient in burn shock to understand or have complete background to understand what medical information is being given to them. There are limitations in their understanding and assimilation of information that must be taken into account. Also, the patients have the right within their own value system to make a decision with their own best interest

---

[c] Comment made at the 5th Annual Conference of the Los Angeles County Bioethics Network, Marina del Rey, CA: 18 April, 1998.

at heart. This includes their aforementioned religious or nonreligious background, their family and what the needs and wants of their family are. It becomes an obligation of the patient or their surrogate to become a member of the team responsible for the individual. This obligation includes the necessity to reveal information completely and honestly, to become actively involved in their care, and participate constructively and sincerely in ethical dialogue about the issues at hand.

We must also consider previous life experiences. For example, the patient may have had family members or relatives with severe or terminal illnesses, themselves. Such experiences may influence their decision making. Religious belief may also be a large factor in people's decisions. A clergyman might be involved at any step of the way to involve the patient's religious resources or spiritual support background in order to try to make the decisions about care and continuing treatments. Finally, there is the perception of what it would be like to survive a significant burn. Many people feel that this is not something that one would wish on anyone, let alone suffer through oneself. Patients may feel that they are not going to be a functional member of society, or that they will lose out on many of the things that they had been previously involved in or hope to achieve. Shriners Burns Hospital–Galveston has performed investigations in this area, looking at children as an example of this outcome; the essence is that children who survive large burn injuries end up at least as well off as their peers.[9] Boys, when they reach maturity, perform better scholastically and have a better self-image than their peers; girls perform at least on an average level with their peers. So, what we are finding is that these people do not become shutins but they do survive and thrive. The philosophy is that if you help the person get through the crisis, their own internal tools dictate whether they are going to fail or succeed. If the patient was going to succeed, they will succeed. If the patient fails, they were going to fail regardless of the burn injury. This can be employed and recognized by these data.

How Should Persistent Ethical Conflict Be Managed?

Even when participants make a sincere effort to establish a 'safe place', 'put relationship before decision-making', and perform their roles well, disagreements about conscientiously held positions occasionally persist. At this point, patience and setting aside adequate time to walk through carefully considered steps in ethical decision-making are necessary. Often, to build up their own skills and enhance chances of success, the patient/surrogate or care-providers will ask a HEC to coach them in pursuing a consensus collaboratively arrived at.

In any serious ethical inquiry, three questions must be answered: What seems to be the problem? What can be done? What should be done?[3] A seven-step decision-making model (illustrated in **Table 56.1**) has been found helpful in answering these questions.

In arranging a conference designed to achieve a consensus resolving ethical conflict at the clinical level, every effort should be made to have all the major stakeholders present to work collaboratively. To discover their current perceptions and level of understanding, to help equalize power, and to model civil discourse, the patient/surrogate and their significant others are asked to speak first as the care-providers listen carefully and respectfully. As indicated by step 1 (see **Table 56.1**), patients are asked to introduce themselves, explain the conflict as they see it, and indicate what

they hope to achieve by the discussion. Thereafter, the care-providers do the same. This step typically takes the most time, but is the most important of all the seven. It 'lets off steam', makes the patient/surrogate and allies feel 'listened to', and optimally leads them to ask for the corrective and supplementary information they need from the care-providers, which (in step 2) they usually can provide or obtain[d]. If successfully carried out, steps 1 and 2 transform a potential or actual power struggle into a collaborative search for the answers to the next and then the final question listed on **Table 56.1**.

Table 56.1 Three questions to be addressed when a clinical ethics problem is serious and persistent, and the steps appropriate for answering each question	
Question to be answered	Steps for answering each question
A. What seems to be the problem?	Step 1: Disclose/discover conflicting values of stakeholders
	Step 2: Disclose/discover the relevant information
A. What can be done?	Step 3: Identify principles, laws, other values relevant to the decision
	Step 4: Identify alternative courses of action
B. What should be done?	Step 5: Compare alternatives and values: is decision clear?
	Step 6: If not, assess consequences
	Step 7: Make decision, collaboratively if possible

Modified with permission from May WW. *Ethics in the Accounting Curriculum: Cases and Readings.* Sarasota, FL: American Accounting Association, 1990: 1.

The conversation of step 3 may address principles (like respect for persons, beneficence, etc.) but more typically cites relevant laws and rules of the community and or institution, and/or other values ('no unnecessary pain', 'what the patient would want if able to speak', etc.). Step 4 is usually best carried out using a blackboard or equivalent to brainstorm and record all the plausible alternative courses of action. In step 5, the group collaboratively may find a principle, rule, value etc., or some combination thereof so compelling that the proper alternative is clear; e.g. because it is considered unlawful homicide in most locations, large doses of narcotic primarily intended to stop breathing rather than control pain will be found unacceptable. If the decision is still not clear, steps 6 and 7 will usually lead to a mutually acceptable decision within boundaries acceptable institutionally, legally, and ethically.

Rarely, consensus will elude the most sincere adherence to the 7-step process. If 'time to sleep on the problem', further discussion, efforts to transfer care of the patient, etc. fail, appeal to the courts, or (in at least one US State[10]) appeal to relevant legislation for relief from responsibility for care of the patient, may be necessary.

---

[d] Note the similarity of these early steps to those of the 'S-P-I-K-E-S' protocol for delivering 'bad news' described by Buckman as quoted by Foley, K. A 44-year-old woman with severe pain at end-of-life. JAMA 1999, 281: 1937–1945.

The patient without decision-making capacity, surrogate or advance directive

In such cases, care-providers typically have no way of knowing or deducing with confidence what the patient's wishes might be in a given set of circumstances. In general, the decision must seek the 'best interest of the patient', but the process required may vary. In some jurisdictions, consultation with another physician, the health care institution's administration, and/or HEC, is mandatory. In others, a court-appointed conservator might be required. In all such cases:

- the search for a surrogate should be diligent;
- all relevant medical information must be obtained and reviewed;
- real or apparent conflicts of interest must be disclosed;
- the opinions of the health care team, and of one or more physicians in addition to the responsible attending, should be reviewed;
- burden versus benefit must be weighed from the patient's point of view; and
- steps should be taken to ensure the benefit of continued life to a disabled patient is not devalued or underestimated.[11]

Some institutions also require that consideration of economic impact on health care providers and the health care institution be excluded from consideration in such cases. Eventually, a surrogate decision-maker is identified and, hopefully, this is a person who has previously known the patient and their values prior to the accident, who has possibly had discussions about extreme end-of-life issues and can speak on the patient's behalf. The surrogate decision-maker must not make the decision based on what they would want for the patient. However, the surrogate decision-maker must know what that patient would prefer and act as an advocate in this situation since the patient is not able to participate in the decision.

How should 'organizational ethics' problems be managed?

Currently, health care decision-making affecting burn care occurs at three levels: in the clinic, in the organization, and in society.[5] The disciplines designed to improve ethical decision-making at the first and last levels are called 'clinical' and 'societal' ethics, respectively. They discern facts and values for guiding *clinical* or *societal* decisions that affect patient care and have received wide attention in both the media and scholarly journals for years. Recently, attention has been called to the need for discernment of facts and values for guiding *managerial* decisions that affect patient care.[5,12] For example, at times problems present as difficulties in clinical decision-making, but have their 'root causes' in areas that require decision-making at the managerial level. With dwindling numbers of nurses entering training, fewer and fewer nurses will be available to provide intensive care, and managerial decisions will be required to produce or recruit more nurses and to judge just when it is no longer safe to admit new patients to beds without adequate staffing. Perhaps rehabilitation services in a given geographical area have not kept up with the ever increasing numbers of patients with large burns who survive but require more, longer, and more expert rehabilitation. Managerial decisions

about the distribution of scarce resources will have to be made if adequate rehabilitation is to be available.

Such decisions are ethical: they involve conflicts of rights, obligations, goods, and/or other values. They tend to be less dramatically immediate and more deferrable, but they usually affect more persons and require more resources and follow-up than clinical ethics decisions.[12] They sometimes appear to be made 'in the front office', apparently without satisfactory input from care-providers, patients or other stakeholders, and without availability of extensive literature or assistance from a committee or consultant skilled in ethical analysis and critique applied at the organizational level.

The development of the discipline of 'organizational ethics' is just beginning, and is overdue in the judgement of JACHO[13] and other authorities.[14] We believe the obligation to be ethical at every level of health care decision-making will become increasingly obvious and pressing with continuing changes in the ways health care is delivered. We hope that future editions of this book will report significantly increasing awareness of, and progress in, this level of health care ethics. Without such progress, the ability of health care ethics to make a difference in practice even at the clinical level will be significantly limited.

Specific problems

Human Research

Many of the modern improvements in health care, particularly burns, have come through active research protocols. Many advances, including fluid resuscitation, excision and grafting, temperature and nutritional control, and modulation of hypermetabolic response are all based on active research in a clinical setting on human patients. It must be remembered that these are volunteers first and patients must not be coerced into the treatment. Institutions involved in human research must have Institutional Review Boards in place to monitor approved protocols and follow-up on patients and complaints with their research driven care-givers. Childhood research is an even more scrutinized area because it is the parent, as a surrogate, who is giving consent for the research. It is a difficult area to approach, however, with the thorough monitoring of Institutional Review Boards and the realization children have a great deal to benefit from advances in health care. Children should be included in research so that they can get the benefits of progress in medicine and science at the earliest possible opportunity. However, this should not be at the expense of their own rights. Many patients feel that, when asked to participate in research protocols they have a duty to those who proceeded them and who helped the physicians reach their current level of care. Patients often feel they should try to give something back to the science of medicine. Patients realize that they cannot fully repay their care-givers and may feel they must participate in research in order to help future victims.

Futility

The concept of futility and hopelessness in the care of a patient has changed drastically over the recent past. At one point any burn over a significant size offered no hope for survival.[15] Through efforts in resuscitation, physicians have pushed this survivability to current levels where even in the youngest of age groups extremely large burn victims can function and survive. At the same time, we are finding that there is no simple definition of futility,[16] making simple pronouncements of futility impossible.

Do Not Resuscitate (DNR) Versus Comfort–Measure–Only Versus Active Withdrawal of Treatment

Once the goals of treatment have been agreed upon, decisions about the end-of-life care of an individual patient are to be made. End-of-life care should be a mutual and agreeable choice from the patient with the understanding by the health care team that treatment has become inappropriate to the goals agreed upon. Even if these conditions are met, it is important to realize that there is a duty to care for the patient. A do not resuscitate order (DNR) is not equivalent to a do not care (DNC) order.

An Allocation of Scarce Resources

In its simplest terms, this becomes a question of who should survive and what is the price of life in an area where health care dollars are less and less available to all people. There is progressive improvement in survival given the concerted efforts of all members of the health care team. However, the reality is that society is providing limited funds for the care of burned patients. It becomes a very difficult personal decision of whether the burn unit should focus on saving money and decline treatment of one burn victim to prepare for the next burn or should resources be expended on a patient who perhaps has a poorer possibility of survival. The only problem with holding back on resources is that this next big burn may never come, and one has not provided the full open access of health care to the first patient. It can always be said that saving for the future in this situation does not benefit either, and one must advocate the use of the resource; once resources are exhausted, the patient should be redirected. Arguments can be made for both sides; however, if there is no other alternative for the patient, clearly they must be cared for in their current setting.

A final note: 'ethical preposterism[17] in burn care'

As conceived in ancient Athens and during most of its history, Western ethics has been an effort to (1) achieve 'the ethical life', i.e. life in all its important dimensions lived at its most flourishing; and (2) solve any problems about 'what should or should not be done' during that quest. The sustained pursuit of excellence in 'total burn care' first achieved momentum in the USA in the mid-twentieth century. It has always drawn its most primal motivation from the fact that burn patients are arguably the most severely injured and utterly vulnerable of human beings, and therefore deserving of the most tender, skillful, and comprehensive care. Commitment to the safety, healing, rehabilitation, and growth of patients during their return to as flourishing a life as possible, has been the spearhead of the quest since its beginning, and both the fire in its belly and the steel in its resolve ever since. Clearly, burn care is an ethical endeavor through and through, not just when and where 'difficult patients' or 'ethical problems' become evident.

In our introduction we observed that the bio-psycho-social-economic-legal-and-ethical dimensions of 'total burn care' are often seen as interconnected like railway cars, with 'bio-' (i.e. the biological dimension) in front, and 'ethical' hooked on only if necessary at the end, like an optional caboose. We believe this to be not only misleading, but also an example of 'preposterism'.[17] Taken from the Latin *pre-* (before) and *posterus* (following), that is 'preposterous' which puts the first last, and what should follow first.[18] We believe the ethical dimension of burn care should be habitually seen not as a sometimes-tacked-on caboose, but as a leading and driving locomotive which extends its influence back through all dimensions of the enterprise like a steel backbone. Were that image actually lived out as dreamed by the early founders of the effort, the providers and receivers of burn care could confidently expect to experience a continually improving 'ethical climate' and fewer 'ethical problems', no matter where history might take the train.

References

1. Fulginiti VA. The right issue at the right time. In: Holmes DE, Osterweis M, eds. *Catalysts in Interdisciplinary Education.* Washington DC: Association of Academic Health Centers, 1999: 7–24.
2. Gillon R. *Philosophical Medical Ethics.* Chichester: John Wiley, 1985: 2.
3. Pellegrino E, Thomasma DC. *A Philosophical Basis of Medical Practice.* New York. Oxford University Press, 1981: 119–52.
4. Maguire DC. *The Moral Choice.* Garden City, New York: Doubleday, 1978: 113.
5. Potter RL. On our way to integrated bioethics: clinical/organizational/communal. *J Clin Ethics* 1999; **10**: 171–7.
6. Zawacki BE. Ethically valid decision-making. In: Herndon DN, ed. *Total Burn Care,* 1st edn. London: WB Saunders, 1996: 575–82.
7. Zawacki BE, Imbus S. Enhancing trust and subjective individual dialogue in the burn center. In: Orlowski JP, ed. *Ethics in Critical Care Medicine.* Haggerstown MD: University Publishing Group, 1999: 489–512.
8. Faden RR, Beauchamp TL. *A History and Theory of Informed Consent.* New York: Oxford University Press, 1986: 235–381.
9. Blakeney P, Herndon D, Desai M, Beard S, Wales-Sears P. Long-term psychological adjustment following burn injury. *J Burn Care Rehabil* 1988; **9**(6): 661–5.
10. Alquist. Health care decisions. (California) Assembly Bill No. 891, Chapter 4, sections 4730–4736; operative July 1, 2000.
11. Ad hoc drafting committee. Guidelines for Forgoing Life-Sustaining Treatment for Adult Patients at the LAC+USC Medical Center. LAC+USC Medical Center, Los Angeles CA, May 5, 1993.
12. Hirsch NJ. All in the family – siblings but not twins: the relationship of clinical and organizational ethics analysis. *J Clin Ethics* 1999; **10**: 210–5.
13. Joint Commission on Accreditation of Healthcare Organizations. *Ethical Issues and Patient Rights.* Oakbrook Terrace ILL: Joint Commission on Accreditation of Healthcare Organizations, 1998: 67–90.
14. Society for Health and Human Values-Society for Bioethics Consultation Task Force on Standards for Bioethics Consultation. *Core Competencies for Health Care Ethics Consultation.* Glenview, IL: American Society for Bioethics and Humanities, 1998; 24–6.
15. Herndon D, *et al.* Teamwork for Total Burn Care: Achievements, Directions and Hopes. In: Herndon DN, ed. *Total Burn Care,* 1st edn. London: WB Saunders, 1996; 1–4.
16. Emmanuel L, *et al.* Medical futility in end of life care: Report of the council on ethical and judicial affairs. *JAMA* 1999; **281**(10): 937–41.
17. Haack S. *Manifesto of a Passionate Moderate.* Chicago: University of Chicago Press, 1998; 180–208.
18. Modified from: Barzun J. *The American University.* New York, Harper and Row, 1968: 221.

Chapter 57a

Functional sequelae and disability assessment
Glenn D Warden, Petra M Warner

really the measure of productivity for our specialty? The real product or measurements of customer service is a patient who can successfully return to society and, even more importantly, be a useful, productive individual who can successfully interact socially within a community. Yes, patients with larger and more severe burns are surviving, but this has created new problems for patients' quality of life. Although the problems are magnified in massively burned patients, they exist even in smaller burns. These problems are best demonstrated in a pediatric burn patient with a 95% TBSA burn (**Figure 57a.1**). Cultured keratinocytes were utilized to achieve wound coverage. The child survived; however, when we examined the patient's current and future reconstructive needs, they totaled 33 potential reconstructive procedures. Thus, the reconstructive problems are monumental in a child with very few donor sites.[3]

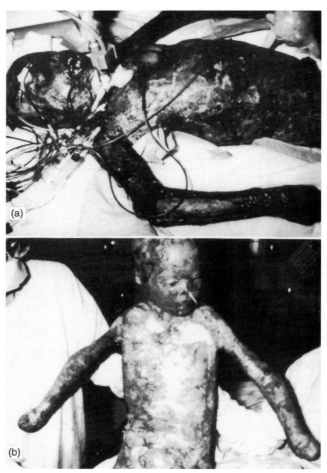

Fig. 57a.1 Pediatric burn patient with 95% total body surface area burn (a) at the time of admission and (b) at discharge. Reproduced from ref. 3 with permission.

Introduction

Advances in acute burn care during the past 25 years. in terms of decreased mortality and decreased length of hospital stay, have been truly outstanding and amazing. In 1971, survival statistics at the Institute of Surgical Research in San Antonio demonstrated an LD_{50} (lethal dose resulting in a 50% survival rate) with approximately 40% TBSA (total body surface area) burn. Thus 50% of the patients with burns of only 40% died. Now, the LD_{50} approaches 80% TBSA, and, if no inhalation injury is involved, patients with burn injuries greater than 80–90% of their TBSA routinely survive. In almost every burn unit in the United States, the length of stay has decreased from nearly 3 days/percent burn to less than 1 day/percent burn. The success can be stated simply: patients with larger, more severe burns are surviving; however, are these patients returning to society to become productive citizens? What is the real outcome of massively burned patients? Do pediatric burned patients become functional adults? How do they function socially later in life? What is the long-term effect on the patient's families and society? Are survival and decreased length of stay

With regard to survival, the results of this patient are impressive; however, we must ask the question: 'Has the medical expertise in terms of survival progressed past the ability to reconstruct and rehabilitate patients?' Unfortunately, the answer is clearly 'yes'. Are we returning our patients to a society which is not ready financially, psychologically, or socially, to accept them? Again, unfortunately, the answer is clearly 'yes'.

Although the American Burn Association has made rehabilitation a major emphasis, quality work still remains to be done. It is important and imperative that burn centers evaluate the functional outcome of a thermally injured patient. This is important, not only for disability assessment, but also for evaluation of our medical management. Outcome studies in the twentieth century will not only emphasize survival and hospital stay, but also patient satisfaction and ability to return to work. The purpose of this chapter is to review the functional sequelae and disability assessment following thermal injury.

Basic considerations – Impairment – Disability – Handicap

The various terms such as 'impairment', 'disability', and 'handicap' appear in laws, regulations, and policies of diverse origin without proper coordination of the ways in which they are used. 'Impairment' refers to an alteration of an individual's physiological, psychological, and anatomical structure or function that interferes with activities of daily living.

'Disability', which is assessed by nonmedical means, means an alteration in an individual's capacity to meet personal, social, or occupational demands or to meet statutory or regulatory requirements. Simply stated, impairment is what is wrong with the health of an individual; disability is a gap between what the individual can do and what the individual needs or wants to do. An individual who is impaired is not necessarily disabled. Impairment gives rise to disability only when the medical condition limits the individual's capacity to meet the demands which pertain to nonmedical fields and activities. On the other hand, if an individual is able to meet a particular set of demands, the individual is not disabled with respect to those demands, even though a medical evaluation may reveal impairment.

The concept of 'handicap' is independent of both impairment and disability, although it is sometimes used interchangeably with either of those terms. Under the provision of federal laws, an individual who is defined as handicapped has an impairment that substantially limits one or more life activities including work, has a record of such impairment, or is regarded as having such an impairment. As a matter of practicality, however, a handicap may be operationally understood as being manifest in association with a barrier obstacle to functional activity. An individual of limited functional capacity is handicapped if there are barriers to accomplishment of tasks or life activities, which can be overcome only by compensating in some ways for the effect of an impairment. If an individual is not able to accomplish a task or activity despite accommodation, or if there is no accommodation that will enable the accomplishment, then in addition to being handicapped, the individual is also disabled. On the other hand, an impaired individual who is able to accomplish a task or activity without accommodation is, with respect to the task or activity, neither handicapped nor disabled. The concept of 'employability' deserves special attention, for, in an occupational setting, if an individual within the boundaries of medical condition has the capacity, with and without accommodation, to meet a job's demands and conditions of employment as designed by the employer, the individual is employable and consequently not disabled. On the other hand, an individual who does not have the capacity or who is unwilling to travel to and from work, to be at work, and to perform assigned tasks and duties, is not employable.

The first critical task in carrying out a medical determination related to employability is to learn about a job, specifically the expectations of the incumbent, with respect to performance, physical activity reliability, availability, productivity, expected duration of useful service life, and any other criteria associated with qualifications and suitability. Sufficient detailed information from a job analysis will provide a basis upon which a physician determines exactly what kinds of medical information are needed and to what degree of detail to assess an individual's health with respect to demand criteria.

Impairment Assessment

Before discussing the medical aspects of evaluating thermally injured individuals, it must be pointed out that no Social Security and Worker's Compensation disability program medical listing exists for burns. Instead, burns must be evaluated under the appropriate body system. Often, more than one system is involved, in other words, musculoskeletal, respiratory, and skin all must be considered in the final decision. Claims must be aimed primarily at resolving the question of onset, whether the impairment can be expected to last 12 months or end in death. The medical evidence needed to document the existence and severity of a medically determinable impairment due to burns must include a history of the impairment, which describes the origin and course of the condition, dates of confinement, nature of treatment, and the claimant's response; current objective findings such as results of examinations, laboratory tests such as blood pressure, electrocardiogram, X-rays, blood tests, range of motion, medical factual data upon which diagnoses are based; and a description of the objective findings of the claimant's limitations and remaining capacities. In other words, how far can the patient walk, which activities cause breath or chest pain, what extent of motion is there in affected parts of the body. Regional specialized burn centers treat many serious burns annually. These centers are excellent sources of medical evidence as they maintain complete detailed records regarding the nature of an injury, treatment, complications, and prognosis. Advances in burn care have improved the survival rate in major burns. Efforts to rehabilitate these survivors and improve their quality of life represent a significant challenge for those involved in their care. The rehabilitation of these survivors is unique and multifaceted, and rarely limited to one system. Many individuals will experience some type of long-term physical impairment or mental limitation, and the rehabilitation process may take years to complete. It must be emphasized that impairments resulting from a burn are not restricted to the skin. Complications may affect any body system; thus, the examiner who is assessing individuals for disability must be attentive to the systemic sequelae of burn injury. The evaluation of a burn victim has some unique features. The necessity to consider such subjective factors as heat and cold intolerance, sensitivity to sunlight, pain, chemical sensitivity, and changes in sweating pattern, as well as the more objective considerations of decreased coordination, sensation, strength, and contracture, lends itself to a unique evaluation.

Disfigurement from scarring, a frequent sequelae of burns, may not affect performance and thereby, in and of itself, causes no impairment. Scarring represents a special type of disfigurement. Again, no percentage of impairment is assigned for the existence of a scar *per se*; however, scars affect sweat glands, hair growth, and nail growth, and cause pigment changes or contractures and may affect loss of performance and cause impairment. Sensory deficit, pain or discomfort from scars needs to be evaluated, as well as the loss of motion of a scar area. An impairment due to disfigurement from scarring may also create behavioral or psychological impairments which subsequently may be rated. The need for intermittent or continuous treatment of the skin with topical agents and pressure garments can impair a person's function and needs to be considered. There is a surprising lack of published literature which relates to the impairment evaluation of a burned patient. The following are concepts which must be kept in mind when evaluating a postburn patient for impairment and resulting deformities.

Skin

Scars and cutaneous abnormalities which result from the healing of burned tissue may represent a special type of disfigurement. Scars should be described by giving their dimensions in centimeters, and by describing their shape, color, anatomical location, and evidence of ulceration; their depression or elevation, which relates to whether they are soft and pliable or hard and indurated, thin or thick and smooth or rough; and their attachment, if any, to underlying bone, joints, muscle and other tissues. Good color photography with multiple views of a defect enhances the description of scars.

The tendency of a scar to disfigure should be considered in evaluating whether impairment is permanent or whether the scar can be changed, made less visible, or concealed. Function may be restored without improving appearance and appearance may be improved without altering anatomical or physiologic function. If a scar involves loss of sweat gland function, hair growth, nail growth, or pigment formation, the effect of such loss on performance of an activity of daily living should be evaluated. Furthermore, any loss of function due to sensory pain, any sensory defect, pain or discomfort in a scar should be evaluated.

Burn scar contracture is probably the most frequently seen cause of impairment in a postburn individual. Every burn, regardless of the depth of injury, heals with some element of contracture. Contractile forces continue long after a wound is healed and can result in severe skin shortage. Inadequate skin prohibits movement to a joint's normal arc of motion and will influence not only the joint underlying the contracture, but also those adjacent to the scar. In the early stages of development, burn scar contractures may often be corrected through the use of splints and pressure garments designed to force developing scar tissue into more normal configurations. In spite of the benefits derived from these modalities, they may also function as a type of impairment, both physically and cosmetically. Understanding the splints which individuals must wear and their limitations are important factors in the assessment of disability. Often, surgical means must be employed in order to restore function. When a surgical release of a contracture is performed, the resultant defect can be of considerable size and will require closure by means of a skin graft or flap of tissue. Burn

scar contracture frequently requires a series of staged surgical procedures before optimal function and cosmesis are achieved. Recovery from surgical intervention must be followed by an extensive rehabilitation program. If an individual does not participate in a rehabilitation program, contractures will reoccur.

The definition of functional impairment should not be limited to an individual's ability or inability to perform joint range of motion. An extremity can exhibit full active range of motion and still be considered impaired due to poor skin quality. Although much can be done to restore function, the skin is never restored to normal. Scar tissue is less tolerant of the everyday stress imposed on it than normal skin. Scar epithelium is thin, fragile, and prone to chronic ulceration. Regardless of the location, these chronic open areas will not heal and eventually require skin grafting. This type of lesion can occur at any time, even years after the initial hospitalization. Skin grafts have the same abnormalities as burn scars in that they all involve contracture formation, have loss of sweat gland function, hair growth, and altered pigment formation. Although frequently cosmetically more acceptable, skin grafts are still not normal skin. Physical limitations such as cold and heat intolerance, difficulty with sun exposure, altered sensation, or painful scars may prohibit individuals from performing their past work or other work.

Musculoskeletal

Functional limitation secondary to burn injury usually results from an anatomical alteration about a major joint. The degree to which the function of a joint is affected is greatly influenced by the amount of soft-tissue loss and the degree of pain associated with movement. Full-thickness burns, those involving all layers of skin, may also result in secondary damage to muscle, bone, tendon, and ligaments. In the acute phase of treatment of such injuries, a joint may be exposed, making it vulnerable, and susceptible to a chronic infection (osteomyelitis), instability, and arthritic changes. Ectopic calcification, the abnormal deposition of calcium around the joints, is usually seen in the elbow, but it can occur in any joint. Symptoms include pain with a significant decrease in motion. These changes in joint structure can be verified by X-ray and will require surgery at a later date for correction. Extensive soft-tissue destruction involving the loss of muscle mass as seen in electrical injuries, will require numerous staged procedures in order to restore function. An individual may never be restored to full function and may be excluded from performing certain types of work which exist in the national economy.

Restriction of normal movement by contracture is not limited to the extremities. When a scar occurs over the trunk or anterior chest, severe and chronic postural changes can result which may cause secondary spinal deformity or altered respiratory functions. Amputations are another leading contributor to postburn impairment. Unlike amputations which are performed for other medical conditions such as peripheral vascular disease, amputation following an extensive thermal injury will often require several staged surgical procedures in order to produce a stump capable of accommodating a prosthesis. It is also important to realize that amputations are not confined to the extremities alone but may also involve skin appendages such as the ears and nose. Complicated stage procedures using local or distant full-thickness skin or muscle-skin flaps are required in order to restore function and cosmesis in these areas. An understanding of how long it will take for an individual's function to be restored is an important factor in deciding about the issue of disability.

Special senses and speech

Impairment to the senses of hearing or vision can occur as a result of a thermal insult, secondary to life-sustaining treatments or as a complication of a healing burn. The loss of central or peripheral vision may begin at the time of contact with a burning agent and can cause the destruction of the eyelids and damage to the cornea. A series of surgical procedures must be performed in order to create a functional eyelid. Contracture of the eyelids, more commonly the lower, may develop quickly resulting in incomplete closure of the eyelid; and potential damage to the cornea can result in conjunctivitis or corneal ulceration. In spite of adequate surgical correction, it is common for such injured individuals to have repetitive episodes of recontracture for up to 2 years post-healing, due to ongoing scar contracture process. Perioral burns that result in lip eversion and microstomia, or contracture of the mouth, may eventually impair mastication and result in drooling as well as inhibiting an individual from producing speech which can be heard or understood. Hearing impairment due to the acute burn is rare, but there may be a loss of the external ear, or deafness secondary to the treatment of life-threatening infections with antibiotics.

Respiratory system

Burns that occur in an enclosed space, such as a building structure, often result in some form of inhalation injury to the respiratory system. Impairment may be limited to a temporary need for ventilatory support or extend to permanent respiratory disease. Chronic and recurrent respiratory infections and pulmonary insufficiency may limit an individual's ability to perform their past work or other work in the national economy, especially when toxic chemicals or dust are present in the workplace. Exposure to irritating gases can also worsen pre-existing asthma or result in irritant-induced asthma. Although this form of reactive airway disease usually resolves with time, some individuals may have persistent respiratory impairment that also may require a change in vocation in order to avoid continued exposure to irritants and exacerbation of symptoms.

Furthermore, patients with severe inhalation injuries may require a tracheostomy long after the burn has healed. Closure of the stoma is often delayed for the purpose of intubation and anesthesia in future reconstructive surgeries. Pulmonary function tests are essential in determining respiratory impairment.

Cardiovascular system

A cardiovascular evaluation should include a good history and electrocardiogram. Patients complaining of chest discomfort thought to be of cardiac origin should have a more extensive workup. There is some evidence of increased incidence of cardiovascular disease in the long-term follow-up of survivors of large thermal injuries.

Neurological system

Neurological impairment caused by a burn may be obvious at the time of admission to a burn center or become clinically apparent up to 2 years following the injury. Patients who are considered at risk include those who have sustained an electrical injury, are predisposed to stroke, or who exhibit signs of peripheral neuropathies secondary to thermal damage. Such patients should be closely monitored for signs of progressive neurological deficit. Electromyography studies will chart the development of degenerative peripheral nerve or spinal cord dysfunction. Dysfunction may be demonstrated in the form of paresis, paralysis, tremor, involuntary movement, or ataxia. Individuals who have suffered an electrical injury may develop a condition characterized by progressive degeneration of fine and gross motor coordination. Resultant complications can range from inability to perform work-related tasks safely to an inability to perform the routine activities of daily living. It is a disease process which takes place over a significant period of time, and may worsen after an individual has returned to work. In addition to the motor deficits caused by electrical injury, those individuals in whom a current passed above the level of the clavicle have a high incidence of cataract formation with the first 3 years post-injury.

Aside from electrical injury, peripheral nerve injury can also result from deep to full-thickness burns. Symptoms of sensory deficits and pain from nerve injury include anesthesia, dysesthesia, paresthesia, hyperesthesia, cold intolerance, and an intense, burning pain. However, behavioral and psychological issues can make it difficult to assess a patient's true impairment and disability due to peripheral nerve injury. To minimize the subjectiveness of pain-related impairment, only persistent pain that leads to permanent loss of function, in spite of maximum effort toward medical rehabilitation and physiological adjustment, can be classified as permanent impairment.[1]

Heme and lymphatic

Full-thickness or deeper burns, particularly of the lower extremities, will also cause damage to the lymphatic system. Such injured individuals often demonstrate a lack of normal lymphatic drainage, resulting in chronic edema and the development of stasis ulcers. There can be little or no improvement expected post-healing. External support in the form of elastic garments is necessary to help replace the normal activity of the lymphatic system in reabsorption of fluid. These individuals frequently have difficulty in standing for long periods of time or working in a hot and humid environment.

Digestive system

The digestive system is not usually a problem except in those individuals who have had superior mesenteric artery syndrome, cholecystitis, or peptic ulcer disease during the acute admission. The post-discharge clinical course of these individuals is never predictable; if affected individuals become symptomatic, they should be followed up by a specialist.

Genitourinary system

The genitourinary system may be a problem if deep perineal or buttock burns occurred. Aside from the obvious psychological problems, partial loss of the penis or scarring of the external genitalia may result in difficulty voiding. A badly scarred perineum or buttocks may make sitting in one position for prolonged periods painful and difficult.

Psychological

The advances of surgical techniques involving early excision and grafting as well as the increased ability to prevent infection allow many patients who would otherwise perish to face life shattered by psychological problems as a result of disfigurement. The onset of a thermal injury is a sudden and frightening experience not only to a patient, but also to his family members. Because of the unexpected nature of onset, all phases of the patient's lifestyle are abruptly changed. Often, the full emotional impact is not felt until the time a patient is discharged from the protected environment of a hospital. At this time, the reality of the emotional, physical, and financial burden of a thermal injury are apparent and must be faced. The extent to which a person can psychologically deal with his injuries varies, as do individual personalities. Each case is unique and must be evaluated as such. Studies on the psychological adjustment of survivors of burns generally reflect a biased adjustment to moderate injuries. Few quantifiable data are available concerning the psychological well-being of long-term survivors of severe injuries. Although most authors conclude that victims of burns make satisfactory adjustments, others report symptoms of the psychopathologic sort which contradict this optimism.[6] Public acceptance is an important problem facing a burn patient. Goffman, in 1963, stated that the way that burn disfigured patients have dealt with the world has generally been shown to be affected by society showing negative responses to visible scars. The burn-disfigured person has to contend with their body image as well as the attitudes of the people and the culture around them. TV and radio have altered not only family standards, but standards of self-perception as well. The young and the beautiful are emphasized. Everyone must be a 'ten'. Patients with burns, like paraplegic or quadriplegic persons, have injuries which can be seen and understood by the public; however, there is also marked ambivalence about a patient with burns as emphasized by the movie industry which has frequently characterized the evil person as being deformed. The 'Phantom of the Opera' is a burn victim, while 'A Nightmare on Elm Street' depicts Freddie Krueger as evil, deformed, and scarred. The burned patient must deal not only with his burn injury, but also with society's built-in impressions which are fostered early in life through cartoons, advertising, television, and movies. This is especially important in the pediatric burned patient for whom returning to school can be difficult, to say the least. Recent studies from the Shriners Burns Institutes in Boston and Galveston emphasize that, in pediatric patients with large thermal injuries, most children appear to be satisfied with their quality of life.[5,7,8] This finding was especially true in children with supportive families who had consistent clinical follow-up and early reintegration into society. However, outcome studies on psychosocial impairment are difficult to assess. It is encouraging to see that the Galveston study reported psychosocial adjustment scores within normal limits, with only diminished social competency skills as issues of concerns among their patient group. Unfortunately, in-depth feelings regarding disfigurement and social integration may not surface with the use of present medical evaluation and further refining and modification, in addition to our current techniques, may be needed to bring out the latent fears and detrimental feelings in these patients.

Impairment Evaluation

The physical examination of a burn victim is much the same as the disability evaluation for any patient. With the information gathered from the history and physical examination, and using the tables in the American Medical Association's *Guide to the Evaluation of Permanent Impairment*,[1] the physician can arrive at an impairment rating. In addition to the usual range of motion form, a questionnaire regarding the special problems related to burns is useful (**Table 57a.1**). The American Medical Association's Guide to the Evaluation of Permanent Impairment is difficult, complex, and time-consuming. It is helpful to have members of a rehabilitation department, namely physical therapy and/or occupational therapy, be familiar with this evaluation. A combined approach with either an occupational therapist or a physical therapist to evaluate actual objective determination such as range of motion, and a burn surgeon performing the subjective rating for the skin or psychological status, is useful. The objective measurements due to restriction of active motion and amputations are well outlined in the *Guide to the Evaluation of Permanent Impairment*. The techniques of measurement are simple, practical, and scientifically sound. For the examination of upper and lower extremities, a large and small portable goniometer are used. The upper extremity, lower extremity, the spine, and the pelvis are considered a unit of the whole person; and Tables are available in the manual to determine impairment ratings of the whole person. The subjective rating for skin or psychological determination is not precise. The criteria for evaluating permanent impairment of the skin is divided into five classes:

■ *Class I impairment of the whole person is 0–9%*. A patient belongs in class I when (a) signs or symptoms of skin disorder are present, and (b) with treatment, there is no limitation or minimal limitation in the performance of the activity of daily living, although exposure to certain physical and chemical agents might increase limitation temporarily.

■ *Class II impairment of the whole person is 10–24%*. A patient belongs in class II when (a) signs and symptoms of skin disorder are present, and (b) intermittent skin treatment is required, and (c) there is limitation in the performance of some of the activities of daily living.

■ *Class III impairment of the whole person is 25–54%*. A patient belongs in class III when (a) signs and symptoms of skin disorder are present, and (b) continuous treatment is required, and (c) there is limitation in performance of many of the activities of daily living.

■ *Class IV impairment of the whole person is 55–84%*. A patient belongs in class IV when (a) signs and symptoms of skin disorder are constantly present, and (b) continuous treatment is required which may include periodic confinement to the home or other domicile, and (c) there is limitation of performance of many of the activities of daily living.

■ *Class V impairment of the whole person is 85–95%*. A patient belongs in class V when (a) signs and symptoms of skin disorder are constantly present, and (b) continuous treatment is required which may include constant confinement to the home or other domicile, and (c) there is limitation of performance of most activities of daily living.

The impairment evaluation is somewhat subjective; however, individual patients can be placed into various categories. The final impairment rating is a combination of the actual objective determinations and the subjective rating for skin and psychological impairment.

Table 57a.1 Patient questionnaire related to burn sequelae

Decreased sensation	Yes ___	No ___	Areas involved _____
Heat intolerance	Yes ___	No ___	Areas involved _____
Cold intolerance	Yes ___	No ___	Areas involved _____
Sensitivity to sunlight	Yes ___	No ___	Areas involved _____
Sensitivity to chemicals	Yes ___	No ___	Areas involved _____
Area of increased perspiration	_____		
Area of decreased perspiration	_____		
Restricted chest motion	Yes ___	No ___	
Restricted abdominal motion	Yes ___	No ___	
Loss of hair	Yes ___	No ___	
Loss of nails or malformed nails	Yes ___	No ___	
Dysesthesias	Yes ___	No ___	Where_____
Hypopigmentation	Yes ___	No ___	Where_____
Hyperpigmentation	Yes ___	No ___	Where_____
Drug use	Yes ___	No ___	
Increased alcohol use	Yes ___	No ___	Amount _____
Donor site scarring	None ___	Minor ___	Moderate ___ Severe ___
Approximate body surface area of donor _____ %			
Gastric pain	Yes ___	No ___	
Joint pain	Yes ___	No ___	Where _____
Tearing, photophobia	Yes ___	No ___	
Decreased vision	Yes ___	No ___	
Shortness of breath	Yes ___	No ___	
Lack of endurance	Yes ___	No ___	
Hoarseness or other vocal cord problem	Yes ___	No ___	Describe _____

Functional outcome

Outcome from thermal injury depends upon many factors other than severity of illness; this may include social status, family support, and patient motivation. A determination of impairment combined with disability is an excellent modality to determine outcome. Presently, we perform formal impairment ratings only when asked by insurance companies, social security, worker's compensation, or the legal system. With emphasis on continuous quality improvement and insurance companies evaluating care by outcome determinations, it is important for burn surgeons to document their outcome. Impairment ratings are time consuming; however, they are an excellent way to evaluate outcomes of care. A systematic approach to evaluating outcomes in this manner should be initiated.

Summary

Disability determination is a difficult and by no means objective procedure. It is not within the scope of this chapter to present all the possible complications and resulting impairments secondary to burn injury.[2,4,7] There are certain concepts which must be kept in mind when evaluating a postburn patient for impairment and resulting deformity. Most burn injuries which are significant enough to require admission to a specialized burn care facility will likely result in some type of temporary or permanent disability. Concepts unique to burn patients include:

- the most common complications arise from burn scar contracture and cosmetic deformity, and will require staged surgical procedures for correction;
- rehabilitation may take several years to return a patient to an acceptable level of functioning;
- postburn cosmetic deformity needs to be confined to areas which are socially visible;
- resulting disabilities are not proportional to the extent of cutaneous injury; and
- certain complications, such as neurological degeneration, may not arise until a few years following an injury and are fairly unpredictable.

Many burned patients will have limitations which, individually, fall short of the criteria needed for evaluating disability. It is important to evaluate the comprehensive result of all limiting factors in order to accurately assess the level of disability.

Chapter 57b

Cost-containment and outcome measures

Juan P Barret

Introduction

Several developments in medicine and burn care have occurred during the last six decades. Patient care, clinical observation, and research have produced important advances in the understanding of the pathophysiology of burns and in the treatment of burn injuries and their complications. As described in the first chapter of this book, the nature of burn injury seemed to require the participation of many different specialities, thus leading to the development of 'burn teams' and 'burn centers'. The result of such collegial effort is state of the art burn care that gathers well-trained personnel with ultimate technology. The drawback of such evolution, though, is complex treatment and a climb in hospital costs. The complexity of burn care in the context of the current health economic era has made outcome measurement, quality assurance, and cost-containment in the burn unit extremely important components of burn care.

The present chapter gives an insight into the relevance of outcome measurement as an objective reflection of the quality of care that is provided in burn centers. The development of quality assurance programs is necessary to maintain excellent outcomes while improving cost-containment. How programs of quality assurance function and how costs are contained with overall improvement of the quality of care are explained below.

Socioeconomic impact of burns

Burn injuries continue to plague the economic systems of both developed and underdeveloped countries. In developed countries, severe disabilities secondary to burns produce significant financial losses; in the developing world, loss of life from burns is extremely high. In the United States, there are 1.2 million burns each year resulting in 60 000 hospitalizations and approximately 6000 deaths. The death toll is highest at the extremes of age; young adults more frequently survive with disabilities that truncate their production in society.[1] Minor burns represent economic loss in the form of sick leaves, and their sequelae sometimes interfere with the productivity of the survivor. Survivors of massive burns are more prone to develop long-term sequelae, and consequences to their families and to society can be devastating.[2,3]

The overall incidence of burns in developed countries is still relatively high, while the numbers of persons who die from burns is remarkably low. It is reported that 820 per 100 000 persons/year are burned, with 30 per 100 000 persons/year requiring specialized treatment. Admissions to burn centers account for 6.5 per 100 000 persons/year. The gross burn mortality in developed countries (people who die at the scene of the accident plus people who die in specialized units) is only 0.6 per 100 000 persons/year. LD50 (the body surface area burned that kills 50% of people) in the pediatric population[4,5] and in young adults[6] is over 90% total body surface area (TBSA) full-thickness burns, and over 40% TBSA full-thickness burns in the elderly.[6] Burn mortality indices under 4% are common among inpatient populations.

The social cost of minor burns in developed countries is significant. In Western Europe, these costs, including the loss of production at work of the individual, social security cost, and the cost of the entire treatment is around 7000 Euro. For severe burns, social costs are much higher and are to be estimated over 40 000 Euro per patient.[8] These are underestimates because the true social costs of long-term disabilities resulting from burn injuries are not yet well determined.

The impact of even the low burn mortality in developed countries is relevant. Beyond the cost of the acute treatment of these severe injuries are the costs of the permanent loss of the individual's productivity at work, social security costs, and insurance costs. When these costs are added, the estimated cost to society upon losing one middle class worker in Western Europe is around 1.1 million Euro.[8]

The world view is more dismal. World statistics put burn injuries to the level of major health problem. Burns described as 'minor' in developed countries produce severe disabilities and even death in developing countries. There are more than 150 000 fire deaths every year in the world, and approximately 30 000 000 people in the world require admission to specialized units. In developing countries, survival of patients with burns over 40% TBSA burned is minimal.[7]

Outcome measures

For a long time, burn mortality has been considered a major outcome measure of the quality of burn care. With the improved survival rates over the last three decades, virtually all pediatric and young adult burn patients should be considered candidates for survival.[5,9] Improvement in burn mortality has produced a change in the expectations of burn care providers. No longer is survival *per se* a sufficient outcome measure, but psychosocial adaptation and physical rehabilitation are of prime importance. Rehabilitation, psychology services, and social support departments are now important members of the burn team. Their care, like that of physicians and nurses, begins with the admission of the patient to the burn center and extends for a long period of time after the patient is discharged. The need for some supportive services may extend throughout the patient's lifetime.

Paralleling the development of modern societies, outcome measurements in health care systems focus more on rehabilitation and quality of life than on raw incidence, prevalence and survival rates. When this principle is applied to trauma and burn care systems, there are three main outcome measurements that are to be considered:

1. Burn mortality (raw and relative mortality);
2. Grade of disability; and
3. Quality of life.

Burn Mortality

As previously mentioned, burn mortality is still one of the major outcome measures in burn centers. Although every burn center has its own particular limitations, it is clear that there exists a minimum standard of burn survival (i.e. LD50 of 90% TBSA burned in children and young adults) that should be met given the social and economic situations are provided. In order to achieve the minimal standards of care, it is important to analyze the comparability of results of every burn center. Since local geographic and social parameters vary, the generation of models of probability of death or probit analysis[10,11] with statistical logistic regression[12] has proven useful for surveying the outcome of burn victims (**Figure 57b.1**). It has the benefit of comparability,[10] but it presents also the benefit of internal control of the burn center, since the logistic model represents the standard of care for that given center. The probability for survival that the model assigns to patients represents the minimum standard. Patients admitted to the burn center with a determined burn injury are plotted in the graphic of probit analysis, and are assigned a probability of death. Afterwards, the real outcome of the patient is compared to the probability for that outcome, and disparities are analyzed on a case per case basis. Relevant data for every new patient are introduced into the logistic regression model, so the probability of survival for the following patient is

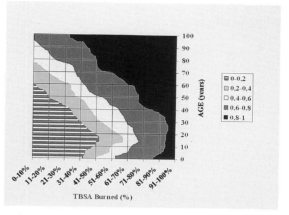

Fig. 57b.1 The generation of computer models of death probabilities helps in decision–making and in quality assurance programs. Mortality, though, should not be used alone as outcome measure, but together with rehabilitation parameters and quality of life.

more accurate. Ideally, the probability of survival should increase with time, reflecting the continuous improvement of the quality of care. The responsibility of the burn team is to continuously improve those results and generate new revised models of probit analysis. The advantage of this analysis is that it includes all the particular social and economic situations of the local geographic area, and on the other hand it is comparable with the results of other centers. One of the main disadvantages is that the prediction is based only on age and TBSA burned.

Other indeces such as the abbreviated burn severity index (ABSI),[13] includes the patient's sex, depth of the injury, and inhalation injury as risk factors that determine the severity of the burn, achieving a more accurate predictive factor. If additional factors are considered, such as preexisting diseases or the abuse of toxic substances, the specificity and sensitivity of the predictors improve.[14] However, even though survival after burn trauma is one of the primary objectives of burn centers, raw mortality and relative mortality (mortality index corrected per age and sex groups in the general population) are no longer the only outcome measures in burn health systems.

Grade of Disability

Currently, the grade of disability and the quality of life achieved by burn survivors are also main outcome measures. In modern society, it is not only survival that is important, but also the quality of life achieved. Survival at any price may lead to subtotal or total disability, which may be not acceptable for all persons. The latest reports of psychosocial adaptation of patients surviving severe or massive injuries show an optimal response and adaptation in society.[2,3] Moreover, most burn survivors achieve social adjustment that is within normal limits. It is not unusual for people surviving these catastrophic injuries to develop and attain goals such that the resultant quality of life is better than the pre-morbid condition. In other words, some people would never have carried out important and relevant projects in society had the injury not happened. Physical disabilities are certainly common. In particular, patients whose injuries and sequelae are located in important functional areas, such as hands, elbows and feet, present with important restrictions in day to day activities. Nevertheless, social adaptation is also good, and some patients develop lives that are very close to 'normal' living. This is particularly true in pediatric patients, whose capacity for adaptation is great. Rehabilitation services, social services, and psychology departments play an important role in the preparation of patients for day to day activities and for coping with society in general. These services are involved early on, during the acute phase, and in the overall treatment plan of patients, so that they can help patients through the acute phase and to make a smooth transition to the reintegration into society (**Table 57b.1**). (For more information see 'Organization of Burn Care' in *A Colour Atlas of Burn Care*.)

The physical examination of a burn victim is much the same as the disability evaluation for any patient. With history and physical examination, and using the tables of the American Medical Association's Guide to the Evaluation of Permanent Impairment, a rating of impairment can be made.[15] The techniques of measuring, although complex and time-consuming, are practical and scientifically sound. A combined approach, with an occupational or physical therapist who makes the objective determination of physical impairment and a burn surgeon who makes the subjective determinations, is advisable. A systematic approach should be followed, including skin assessment, musculoskeletal system, special senses and speech, respiratory system, cardiovascular system, neurological system, hemic and lymphatic systems, digestive system, genitourinary system, and psychological system. After a thorough assessment has been performed, the patient will be placed in one of the categories for permanent impairment and disability (**Table 57b.2**). This evaluation is very important to determine the outcome of burn patients. Impairment and disability assessments are most relevant for insurance companies, social security, worker's compensation, and the legal system. Since the burn team is not only responsible for the acute care, but also for continuous quality improvement and the evaluation of outcome characteristics, disability determination is an integral part of

Table 57b.1 Members of the burn team
Burn surgeons (plastic surgeons and general surgeons)
Nurses (ICU, acute and reconstructive wards, scrub nurses, anesthesia nurses)
Case managers (acute and reconstructive)
Anesthesiologists (experienced in burn anesthesia)
Respiratory therapists
Rehabilitation therapists
Nutritionists
Psychosocial experts
Social workers
Volunteers
Microbiologists
Research nurses
Support services (secretaries, environmental services, medical records, material management, informatics, technicians, etc.)
Adapted from Barret JP, Herndon DN, A Colour Atlas of Burn Care London: WB Saunders.

Table 57b.2 Categories of burn impairment and disabilities
■ Class I: Impairment of 0–10%. No limitation or minimal limitation in the performance of the activity of daily living. Exposure to certain physical and chemical agents might increase limitation temporarily. Skin disorders are present, but no treatment is necessary
■ Class II: Impairment of 10–25%. There is limitation in the performance of some of the activities of daily living. Skin disorders are present and intermittent skin treatment is required
■ Class III: Impairment of 25–50%. There is limitation in performance of many of the activities of daily living. Skin disorders are present, and continuous treatment is required
■ Class IV: Impairment of 55–80%. There is limitation in performance of many of the activities of daily living. Skin disorders are present, and continuous treatment is required, which include periodic confinement to home or health care institution
■ Total impairment

modern burn care. Only with such evaluation can the quality of outcomes be improved.

Quality of Life

Although disability and impairment assessment is one of the main outcome measures, it alone does not describe the quality of life that patients achieve after burns are healed and all formal treatment is finished. One of the measures that adapts to health care systems is the Quality Adjusted Life Years (QALY) introduced by Torrance in 1986.[16] One QALY is a measure of all benefits of health treatment that include increase in life expectancy and enhanced quality of life. The increase in life expectancy is measured in number of years, while quality of life is measured in a scale with a maximum of 1 (perfect health). In this scale, 0 corresponds to death. There are negative numbers, since there are health situations that are considered by patients to be worse than death. The QALY are, therefore, the number of years with perfect health which are also compared to the number of years lived in a specified state of health. For example, if a person lived for 70 years in perfect health and died, they would accomplish 70 QALY. Conversely, if a person lived 45 years in perfect health, and then acquired chronic renal failure, with a quality of life of 0.4 and died at age 70, they would accomplish 55 QALY [45 QALY + 25(0.4)]. There are two sorts of methods to calculate QALY, the 'standard gamble'[17] and the 'time trade-off'.[18] The second method is the simplest and the most used. Patients are confronted with two situations: the situation of disease and/or sequelae for t years and the situation of perfect health for x years followed by death. The utility of any treatment of a chronic condition is represented by x/t. Life expectancy under a certain chronic condition is compiled from medical literature. This time is converted to QALY under perfect health, and the risks of the medical treatment are then evaluated in terms of the effectiveness in producing QALY.

When QALY are applied to burn patients, it is easy to assume that the treatment of severe injuries, which will result in death without treatment, will produce an important number of QALY. Nevertheless, many burn injuries heal with sequelae, so that the quality of life achieved is not that of perfect health, but sometimes quite less than that. Patients that survive life-threatening injuries acquire a high number of years in terms of life expectancy, whereas the total number of QALY is often less than the optimal number. This is confusing since the overall assessment of quality of life that burn patients express in the long run is usually higher than expected.[2,3] As an example, at the Vall d'Hebron Burn Center in Barcelona, Spain, the overall QALY acquired by all patients (minor and major burns) during 1996, based on an estimation of time trade-off, was 3 QALY per patients.[8] QALY acquired by burn patients were less than expected especially in severely burned patients. One of the main problems of QALY assessment as a measure of cost-efficacy and cost-utility is that patients tend to make a short-term estimation of life expectancy and quality of life.[19] Burn sequelae are more dramatic in the first months and years after the injury, resulting in a low estimation of QALY.

Quality assurance

Quality assurance (QA) means a critical appraisal of data collected in the specific system to give assurance to users and to health care providers that quality is achieved. Such appraisal should also result in better management, lower complication rates, and better outcomes. The essence of QA is the idea that real quality improvements involve the continuous search for opportunities for all processes to get better.[20] Quality assurance is essential in the modern health care system where cost-containment and cost-efficacy are primary end-points. QA programs provide data to support requests for funding of burn patient care at an appropriate level. They are primordial to suffice the minimal requirements that are to be met by burn centers in order to be endorsed by national societies and state agencies.

The standard QA program is depicted in **Figure 57b.2** All members of the multidisciplinary burn team (**Table 57b.1**) join together to satisfy common goals and to target all possible problems encountered in day to day work. Should problems arise, an assessment is made; and committees are organized to respond if such a formal response is needed. Actions are carried out in order to solve the problem, and the results of such actions measured. When responses are shown to be effective, the actions and changes in protocols are sustained. Otherwise any new problem that was

encountered with the process is targeted for improvement, and actions carried out to address those problems.

Developing a functional QA program requires that the burn team develop clinical protocols and critical care pathways. Although time-consuming at first, this planning saves much time in the long-term. Members of the burn team are well acquainted with clinical protocols that begin at the exact time point during patient care. Time points, red flags, and self-stopping parameters are necessary. Protocols are essential for a QA program, since deviations from protocols are easily detected, facilitating evaluation and assessment of the deviations.

Clinical indicators of the overall performance of the unit must be established. It is the responsibility of every member and every department involved in the burn care system to provide the burn team and the QA program with indicators of the well-functioning unit, essentially defining what the unit would be if everything goes very well. Deviation from these performance goals are detected and included in the evaluation system. Outcome measures are main clinical indicators of the performance of the burn unit as a whole and should be evaluated periodically. Changes in outcomes must be evaluated carefully to detect any malfunction or deviation and develop an appropriate action. Mortality, probit analysis, disability, and quality of life are outcome measures that need to be surveyed constantly. Every specialty involved in burn care must develop their own specific outcome measures that contribute to overall outcome in order to assess, maintain, and constantly improve their contribution to care. Examples of these secondary outcome measures are graft take, pain control, or infection control.

At the Shriners Burns Hospital in Galveston, Texas, QA staff are active and indispensable members of the burn team. Their constant surveillance helps burn patients and burn team members by assisting to develop protocols and by monitoring achievements according to protocols. They promptly detect deviations so that adequate action can be immediately taken. Their effort assures that no variables will be left to flow without control, so the expected outcome will result. The author finds QA staff to be important back-up aids helping to prevent unwanted surprises.

Finally, QA programs help to maintain cost-efficacy in the burn center. By maintaining outcomes, the investment that society and insurance companies make in the expensive treatment of burn patients is rewarded by provision of state of the art treatment and excellent outcomes. Documentation of such standard of care should result in reimbursement and funding that are maintained if not increased.

Cost-containment in the burn unit

Over the last two decades there has been a continuous change and evolution in health economy. The continuous increase in world population has been joined with an increase in life expectancy, which, along with the decrease in births has led to an increase in the mean age of population. This is particularly true in developed countries where the population pyramids have reversed their shape. The increasing population of 'elders', along with the economic crisis and the expected increase in costs of health care technology and specialists, have provoked an exponential increase in health costs. Economical analysis and cost-containment with an emphasis on cost-efficacy and cost-utility are principle pillars of health economy.

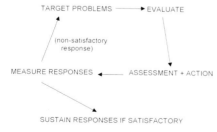

Fig. 57b.2 The cycle of quality assurance. The performance of the unit is continuously assessed. When problems are detected, an action is taken after complete evaluation of the situation. The responses and the new performance of the unit are measured again. If the response is deemed adequate, the action is sustained. Should the response not be appropriate, a new cycle begins.

Assessing the maintenance of good outcomes assures that all economic efforts invested in burn centers produce the expected benefits with a positive cost-efficacy effect. Our resources in contemporary society have become limited, so the best outcomes with good cost-efficacy and cost-utility ratios are essential. It is clear that insurance companies and society, in general, seek health care systems where less investment still results in the best outcome. It is particularly true in burn centers; reimbursement will peak in centers that provide the best functional outcome in a standard period of time. Contracts flow when good return to productive life is achieved.

Burn treatment presents some particularly relevant differences that make it unique in health economy. In contrast with general costs of tertiary hospital treatments, whose costs peak in human resources, burn treatment costs peak in technology and material costs. These can be as high as 70% of all costs in burn centers, leaving the remaining 30% for wages and salaries of personnel. Materials used in the day to day care of burn patients are extremely expensive. However, with cost-containment measures, QA programs and continuous outcome measures, burn centers can benefit the hospital budget via reimbursement from third party providers.

In order to maintain a dynamic and viable center, a cost-containment program must be instituted. These programs are defined as all measures directed to produce the best cost-efficacy and -utility ratios; i.e. to maintain costs within expected margins and optimize burn care providing the best outcomes. The main steps of cost-containment programs are:

1. Data acquisition and outcome measurement;
2. Treatment protocols; and
3. Optimization of resources.

Data Acquisition and Outcome Measurement

The first step to control costs in burn centers is the development of a QA program, as previously described, to include data acquisition and outcome measurement. The flow of economic efforts is then bi-directional, from society to patient care and from burn centers to society. All investments made in the burn center are returned to society in the form of excellent outcomes and social reintegration. On the other hand, the knowledge of the most recent outcome figures for the burn unit alert the burn team to know the point of futility of treatment. Expensive efforts to save patients whose burn injuries are fatal increase costs exponentially, decreasing the resources available for other burn patients. It is particularly true in developing countries, where all efforts need to be concentrated only in those patients who will survive.

However, the equal responsibility of the burn team to improve the outcome of burn patients mandates that they push ahead to achieve better survival and better quality of life for their patients. The line that separates futility from constant improvement is vague. The only way to define it and to improve outcomes without increasing futile efforts is with burn research. Experimental and clinical burn research produces new data, which, after critical evaluation of results, will impact and change clinical protocols and pathways.

Treatment Protocols and Rationalization of Pharmaceutical Costs

Burn care treatment is expensive. State of the art technology, pharmacological treatments, and skin substitutes are at the top of the price ladder in health treatment. A judicious and clear use of these technologies is clearly indicated for such costs to provide benefit. Clinical protocols and critical care pathways are essential elements to control costs. Protocols and pathways are tools developed after consensus conferences over treatments and diagnostic tests. Experts review the quality and effectiveness of these treatments and techniques, and a consensus is generated about the rationale for the use of old, current, and new technology. Consensus declarations are included in clinical pathways. In this way, well thought-out methodology with predicted costs are used to generate outcomes. If no deviations are made and new techniques are not tried without thoughtful consideration, the overall costs of the burn center are contained – provided the annual number of admissions are maintained.

The introduction and testing of new techniques need to be carried out within well-controlled research protocols, and all results need to be critically reviewed. New treatments must be tested versus the standard of care at any given time, and results compared. When better outcomes are achieved with good cost-efficacy results, the new treatment protocol can be general and become standard. As an example, advances that were possible thanks to research supported by the Shriners of North America are prompt eschar excision and immediate wound closure, pressure garments, fluid resuscitation, bacterial translocation control, early enteral nutrition, and improvements in inhalation injury treatment among others. This research was conducted as a comprehensive program of experimental research followed by clinical application in clinical research protocols. Positive results were then applied to routine clinical protocols improving standard patient care.

Cost-containment, besides QA programs and clinical protocols, is based in rationalization of pharmaceutical costs and optimization of resources. Since more than 60% of all costs in burn centers result from the use of topical and systemic treatments, it is of paramount importance that tight control on the use of such treatments exist. In order to reduce and control costs, it is necessary to use generics in place of trademarks when feasible with the same drug activity. The least expensive trademark should be used when no generic suffices. However, an expensive treatment should be used if such practice reduces the length of hospital stay. For instance, when the treatment of superficial second degree burns in children is done with Biobrane™, a more expensive treatment alternative than the traditional treatment with 1% silver sulfadiazine, a significant reduction in pain and hospital stay is achieved. Thus, the overall cost of treatment is reduced, and yet there is a significant improvement in outcome.[21] In this situation, the initial treatment with a much more expensive alternative method results in a better outcome, providing a better cost-efficacy ratio.

Optimization of Resources

The optimization of resources begins with the organization and calculation of burn unit requirements. In order to calculate the number of personnel required to treat all burns in a determined area, the *method of necessity* is very helpful. To determine the desired number of personnel (RT), one must obtain the catchment population (P), the incidence of burns (I) in persons/year, the number of hours of treatment per day (A), the mean hospital stay in days (L), and the mean number of hours that personnel work in the burn unit (W).[22] The basic formula is as follows:

$$RT = \frac{P \times I \times A \times L}{W}$$

For example, in a geographic area with a population of 5 million people, a raw burn incidence (patients admitted to the burn center) of 6.5 per 100 000 persons/year, and 1 admission per patient per year, a mean hospital stay per patient of 16.5 days with full time (40 hours/week) personnel working a total of 1960 hours per year to provide continuous care of a patient per 24 hours, the total number of personnel required for the complete treatment of burn patients is 65.6, calculated as follows:

$$RT = \frac{5\,000\,000 \text{ people} \times 6.5/100\,000 \text{ persons/year} \times 24 \text{ hours} \times 16.5 \text{ days}}{1960 \text{ hours}} = 65.6$$

The number of beds (NB) dedicated to burn treatment is based on the incidence of burn injuries (I), the mean hospital stay (L), and the ideal index of admissions (IO) estimated as 0.85 (85% of beds used for burn treatment, 15% of beds unoccupied).[23] The formula is as follows:

$$NB = \frac{I \times L}{365 \times IO}$$

When this formula is applied to the same example, the number of beds required are 17.3 beds for a geographic area with 5 000 000 population and a burn incidence (admissions to burn center) of 6.5 per 100 000 persons/year:

$$NB = \frac{5\,000\,000 \text{ people} \times 6.5/100\,000 \text{ persons/year} \times 16.5 \text{ days}}{365 \times 0.85} = 17.3$$

Although all parameters are well known for all countries and the theoretical burn care needs can be calculated with them, it is common knowledge that burn incidence and the index of admissions suffer important oscillations throughout the year. The calculation of an optimal burn center occupation at 0.85, which is the index for optimal outcome and cost-efficacy, means that the index of admissions may decrease fewer than 40% in certain periods of the year. Even though it does not affect the actual function of the burn center (it does affect if the index is calculated at 1, with periods of bed occupation over 100%), it makes an important impact in cost-containment, since the maintenance of a full functioning burn center with minimal admissions reduces all benefits, and may produce an important financial loss.

In order to optimize the index of occupation of the burn center, and maintain it at 0.85, it is possible to admit patients at the burn center who present with a spectrum of injuries suitable for treatment at the burn center. Given the nature of burn injuries, the burn team is capable of managing patients with a spectrum of trauma and extensive cutaneous or soft-tissue losses. **Table 57b.3** compiles all patients suitable to be treated at the burn center. Patients that can be successfully treated and benefit from the technology and expertise of the burn team are trauma patients (general multi-trauma and neurological trauma, facial trauma), TEN and dermatoses, plastic surgery patients including free flap reconstruction, and chronic wounds. It must be borne in mind, however, that the burn center is a super-specialized unit created for the care of burns, and that, as such, it may be the only facility for such injuries in that particular area. It is imperative to reach a balance between optimal function and cost-containment with optimal treatment of burn injuries. To achieve that, a set of priorities have to be created for

admission to the burn center so the treatment of other injuries and patients do not challenge the admission of severe burn injuries. In **Table 57b.4**, all patients suitable for treatment in the burn unit are divided into three types of priorities. Priority 1 patients include all burn patients whose injuries are categorized as major injuries by ABA standards. These patients have priority over all other patients. Patients included in priority 2 are patients who may be treated in other specialized units of the hospital, but also can be treated with the same standard of care in the burn unit and will benefit from care by the burn team. These patients are admitted on a bed availability basis, with the main idea of maintaining an optimal IO. Patients included in priority 3 are patients who do not present with acute injuries but who may benefit from treatment in the burn center. These patients are admitted as elective cases.

Table 57b.3 Patients suitable for treatment in a burn center
Acute burns
Rehabilitation and reconstructive burn patients
Toxic epidermal necrolysis and other life-threatening dermatosis
Blunt and penetrating trauma patients
Brain trauma
Maxillofacial injuries
Upper and lower limb reconstruction
Craniofacial surgery
Free flap reconstruction
Traumatic soft-tissue avulsions
Pressure sores
Chronic wounds
Diabetic and vascular ulcers
Adapted from Barret JP, Herndon DN, A Colour Atlas of Burn Care London: WB Saunders.

Table 57b.4 Priority of admissions to the burn center
■ *Priority 1*
1. Severe burns
2. Electrical injuries
3. Burns with inhalation injury
4. Burns in infants
5. Burns in the elderly
6. Burns in patients with chronic or debilitating diseases
7. Toxic epidermal necrolysis
■ *Priority 2*
1. Multiple blunt or penetrating trauma
2. Brain trauma
3. Maxillofacial injuries
4. Upper and lower limb reconstruction following trauma
■ *Priority 3*
1. Free flap surgery
2. Craniofacial surgery
3. Other plastic surgery procedures
Adapted from Barret JP, Herndon DN. 'A Colour Atlas of Burn Care', London: WB Saunders.

When a conflict arises, i.e. there is a shortage of beds and patients included in priority 1 need to be admitted to the burn center, the priority 1 patients have priority over all other patients. Patients included in priority 3 should be moved to another ward in the hospital, followed by patients included in priority 2 if the need for beds is very acute. (Generally, this occurs in response to a major disaster, and the disaster plan will be activated.) It must be borne in mind that all flow of patients must maintain the required standards of care for all patients. The program of optimization should not be carried out until the required standards of care as demonstrated via QA programs can be provided.

Other programs of cost-containment that are very effective in maintaining low costs and improving the quality of care are programs to optimize human resources and programs of day care. Human resources in the burn center can be optimized by planning nurses' shifts. Morning shifts are usually the busiest, and 8-hour shifts are the most effective. Therefore, morning shifts can be scheduled with the largest number of nurses, while afternoon and night shifts can be staffed by fewer. On the other hand, nurses' shifts with flow capabilities increase the overall performance of personnel in the burn center. Personnel that can staff the nursing wards, outpatient clinics, and social services provide more freedom in the organization and optimization of resources, diminishing costs in the burn center.

Another important change in modern health care is the development of day care programs, i.e. major wound care on an outpatient basis and day surgery. Both types of programs diminish the need of admission to the burn center, thereby decreasing costs and increasing performance. This also allows the treatment of other injuries in the burn center which increases reimbursement via third party payors and via the budgets of other departments. Patients who present with burn wounds, even large wounds, that do not need admission for other causes and whose injuries at not at risk of infection at home may be treated as outpatients with daily or periodic dressing changes in the day care unit of the burn center. On the other hand, minor burns, with the advent of new and safer techniques of anesthesia, can be successfully treated surgically in day surgery. These two programs require a strict standardization of protocols so only patients who fit the program are included in the day care unit protocol. Patients must be able to reach the burn center at any time, and all risk factors and warning signs need to be explained verbally and provided in writing to the patient and/or to the person who will take responsibility for the care of the patient. Every effort should be made by the burn team to start a program of day care, since the benefits in patient care, quality of life, and cost-containment are spectacular when the program is fully functioning.

Summary

The relevant socioeconomic impact of burns and the particular characteristics of burn injuries made necessary the development of teams to provide dedicated and specialized treatment of burn injuries. The achievement of total burn care and the current excellent outcomes in burn patients have paralleled a continuous increase in the complexity of treatment of burn victims and concomitant increase in costs of treatment. To contain costs and to prevent decline in standard of treatment, it is necessary to develop clinical protocols providing strict guidelines to health care providers. Thus, quality assurance programs are developed. Outcome measurement is also a part of quality improvement, since it is the main indicator of the quality of care that is performed at the burn center. Outcome data are part of the data acquisition of QA programs, and outcomes are also improved by the actions of such programs. The climb in costs must be contained with specific measures following an overall plan. QA programs provide the tools to assure that measures to control expenses are applied while maintaining the quality of care so excellent cost-efficacy can be obtained. In the modern era of health care management, programs of day care, admission of patients without burn injuries to the center, and optimization of resources (technical and human) are of paramount importance to maintain the gold standard of burn care while containing costs.

References

1. Ramzy PI, Barret JP, Herndon DN. Thermal Injury. *Crit Care Clin* 1999; 15: 333–52.
2. Blakeney P, Meyer W III, Robert R, Desai M, Wolf S, Herndon D. Long-term psychosocial adaptation of children who survive burns involving 80% or greater total body surface area. *J Trauma* 1998; 44: 625–32.
3. Haddadin KJ, Kurdy KA, Haddad AI. Long-term psychological effects of burn unit admission among paediatric patients with minor burns. *Ann Burn Fire Dis* 1999; 12: 168–73.
4. Barret JP, Desai MH, Herndon DN. Survival in paediatric burns involving 100% total body surface area. *Ann Burn Fire Dis* 1999; 12: 139–41.
5. Barret JP, Wolf SE, Desai MH, Herndon DN. Cost-efficacy of cultured epidermal autografts in massive pediatric burns. *Ann Surg* 2000; 231: 869–76.
6. Barret JP, Gomez P, Solano I, Gonzalez-Dorrego M, Crisol FJ. Epidemiology and mortality of adult burns in Catalonia. *Burns* 1999; 25: 325–30.
7. Munster AM. The 1996 presidential address. Burns of the world. *J Burn Care Rehabil* 1996; 17: 477–84.
8. Barret JP, Solan I. Socio-economic impact of adult burns in Catalonia. *Proceedings of the 2nd meeting of the Spanish Burns Association*, Barcelona, 1996.
9. Wolf SE, Rose JK, Desai MH, Mileski JP, Barrow RE, Herndon DN. Mortality determinants in massive pediatric burns. *Ann Surg* 1997; 225: 554–9.
10. Gomez-Cia T, Mallen J, Marquez T, Portela C, Lopez I. Mortality according to age and burned body surface in the Virgen del Rocio University Hospital. *Burns* 1999; 25: 317–23.
11. Finney DJ. *Probit Analysis*, 3rd edn. Cambridge: Cambridge University Press, 1971.
12. Hosmer DW, Lemeshow S. Applied Logistic Regression. New York: John Wiley & Sons, 1989.
13. Tobiasen J, Hiebert J, Edlich RF. The abbreviated burn severity index. *Ann Emerg Med* 1982; 11: 260–2.
14. Germann G, Barthold U, Lefering R, Raff T, Hartmann B. The impact of risk factors and pre-existing conditions on the mortality of burn patients and the precision of predictive admission-scoring systems. *Burns* 1997; 23: 195–203.
15. American Medical Association Committee on rating of Mental and Physical Impairment. Guide to the evaluation of permanent impairment. Chicago: American Medical Association, 1988.
16. Torrance GW. Measurement of health state utilities for economic appraisal: a review. *J Health Econ* 1986; 5: 1–30.
17. Von Neumann J, Morgenstern D. Theory of games and economic behavior. Princeton: Princeton University Press, 1947.
18. Torrance GW, Thomas WH, Sackett DL. A utility maximation model for evaluation of health care programmes. *Health Serv Res* 1972; 7: 118.
19. Ortun-Rubio V. La economia en sanidad y medicina: Instrumentos y limitaciones. Euge, Barcelona, 1991.
20. Wood FM. Quality assurance in burn patient care: the James Laing Memorial Essay, 1994. *Burns* 1995; 21: 563–68.
21. Barret JP, Dziewulski P, Ramzy PI, Wolf SE, Desai MH, Herndon DN. Biobrane versus 1% silver sulfadiazine in second degree pediatric burns. *Plast Reconstr Surg* 2000; 105: 62–5.
22. Hornby R, Ray K. Guidelines for Health Manpower. Geneve: WHO, 1980.
23. Cuervo JL, Varela J, Belenes R. *Gestion de Hospitales*. Barcelona: Vicens Vives, 1994.

Chapter 58

Management of pain and other discomforts in burned patients

Walter J Meyer III, Janet A Marvin, David R Patterson
Christorpher Thomas, Patricia E Blakeney

Introduction

The words 'burn injury' trigger, for almost any adult in the world, immediate and vivid images of excruciating pain and suffering. An early lesson of childhood is that 'hot' 'burns' and hurts. There can be no doubt that complaints of pain are ubiquitous in a burn unit. Burn care professionals should be especially conscious of the management of the pain and suffering endured by their patients. Working to make an acute burn patient comfortable is never ending and fraught with frustration. The experience of pain is complex and dependent upon an interaction of dynamic physical and psychological variables. Beecher[1] observed that soldiers burned in battle could perform heroic feats without apparent pain; yet as soon as they were in a safe place their pain was significant. As noted by Choinière, the pain

expressed by a burned patient varies from day to day and from hour to hour (see **Figure 58.1**).[2] This great variability makes it difficult to give enough medication to relieve a patient's pain without giving too much and causing potentially significant untoward reactions.

Pain is not directly observable. The burn care professional must interpret reports from the patient and other observers to ascertain when, where, and to what level the patient experiences discomfort. More interpretation is required to tease out how much of the discomfort is due to pain and how much is a reflection of fear or anxiety. Adding to this confusion is the fear often expressed – by family members, by patients themselves, and even by well-trained medical professionals – that patients will become addicted to the drugs if they are given 'too much'. Then, just when the professionals seem to have found a good management plan to facilitate

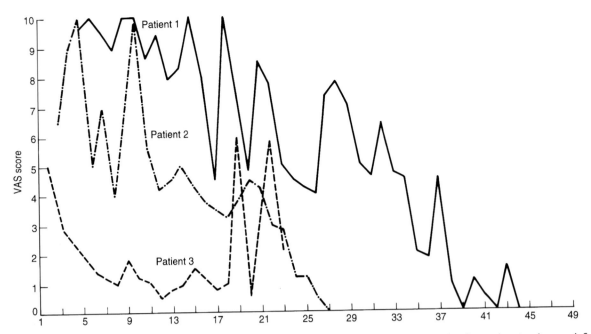

Fig. 58.1 VAS scores for different patients show how variable expressions of pain can be from day to day and from one patient to the next. Reproduced with permission from Choinière et al.[2]

comfort for a particular patient, something changes to upset the balance of factors, and the patient reports suffering again. Thus, frustrated caregivers understandably might concede defeat to the issue of pain and focus on working to heal the patient with the certain knowledge that, as the patient heals, the pain and other discomforts will also diminish.

Pathology of a burn injury as it relates to pain

All burn injuries are painful. First degree or very superficial partial-thickness burns may damage only the outer layers of the skin, the epidermis; but they do produce mild pain and discomfort, especially when something such as clothing rubs against the burned area. Second degree or moderate to deep partial-thickness burns result in variable amounts of pain depending on the amount of destruction to the dermis. Superficial dermal burns are the most painful initially. Even the slightest change in air currents moving past the exposed superficial dermis causes a patient to experience excruciating pain. Without the protective covering of the epidermis, nerve endings are sensitized and exposed to stimulation. In addition, as the inflammatory response progresses with the increase in swelling and the release of vasoactive substances, pain is increased.[3,4]

Areas of deeper partial-thickness burns may display a confusing pattern of pain over the first few days. These areas may show little or no response to sharp stimuli such as a pinprick; yet a patient may complain of deep achy pain related to the inflammatory response. These wounds are more similar to full-thickness burns in their pain response. In a full-thickness burn, the dermis, with its rich network of nerve endings is completely destroyed. This leads to an initial response of a completely anesthetic wound when a sharp stimulus is present. Yet, patients often complain of a dull or pressure type of pain in these areas. Once the devitalized tissue i.e.

eschar, sloughs and is replaced by granulation tissue a patient again experiences the sensation of sharp pain to noxious stimuli.

Pain-generating Mechanisms during an Initial Injury

Although no one would question the fact that burn injuries are painful, there are many reports of burn victims accomplishing extraordinary feats after injury. The dearth of information on the mechanism of pain perception leaves many unanswered questions. Meyer and Campbell[3] attempted to study the mechanism of pain after thermal injury. These studies were accomplished in monkeys and humans exposed to a series of thermal stimuli before and after a 53°C 30-second burn to the glabrous skin of the hand. In monkeys, the response of C and A nociceptive afferents were studied and compared to subjective responses by humans. The burn resulted in increased sensitivity of the A fibers, decreased sensitivity of the C fibers, and increased pain sensitivity (hyperalgesia) in human subjects. This study would suggest that A fibers rather than C fibers are chiefly responsible for the hyperalgesia related to burn injury. To test this hypothesis, Meyer and Campbell[3] used a sphygmomanometer cuff inflated to 250 mmHg 20 minutes after the burn injury. Motor functions and sensitivity to light touch disappeared after 40 minutes. Hyperalgesia at the site was likewise demonstrated, yet pain evoked by the test stimuli applied 5 cm from the injury to uninjured skin was not decreased. It would appear from these experiments that C-nociceptive afferents code for pain intensity of thermal pain near the threshold (43–48°C) of the glabrous skin of the uninjured hand; A fibers code for pain above the threshold during a prolonged, intense heat stimulus and for hyperalgesia which occurs minutes after the injury. Preliminary work by the same investigators in other areas of the body did not produce similar results, which could be related to the difference in intensity of A and C fibers in the skin of different areas of the body. Later studies by Campbell et al.[4] and Coderre and Melzack[5] confirm that burn injuries not only make an injured area and surrounding tissue more painful but also cause hyperalgesia.

Pain-generating Mechanisms Following an Initial Injury

Even less is known about pain-generating mechanisms after an initial injury than during. As a wound remains unhealed for days or weeks, and as various surgical and nonsurgical therapies are applied to a wound during the healing phase, a patient's pain complaints vary considerably. In an attempt to describe the pain experience by burned patients after an initial injury, Charlton and associates[6] used a series of pain measurement tools and standardized psychological tests to measure anxiety and depression. Visual analog pain ratings for overall pain in a group of burned patients were skewed towards the low end of the scale, with a median of 1.75 on a 10-point scale in the study by Charlton et al. Patients in Charlton et al.'s study also completed the McGill Pain Questionnaire. As a group, these patients were comparable to a group of post-herpetic neuralgia patients on the Present Pain Intensity Scale and the Number of Words Chosen Scale, but resembled a group of arthritic patients on the pain rating index.

Choinière et al.[2] utilized the visual analog scale (VAS) on a daily basis and asked patients to rate their worst pain for each day. Patients' scores varied widely from patient to patient. For the same patient, overall pain scores varied widely from day to day, but gradually declined towards the end of hospitalization. In an effort to elucidate the predictor of pain in these patients, Choinière et al. compared pain scores with patient's age, socioeconomic status, and educational level and found no significant correlation. Likewise no significant correlation was found between the pain scores and burn size. These findings are similar to the results in studies by Klein and Charlton[7] and Perry et al.[8] Choinière and associates suggest that perhaps these results are related to two issues:

- assessment of the size of the burn wound is usually made only once at the time of injury; thus the measure does not necessarily reflect the current clinical condition of the patient at the time of pain measurement; and
- calculation of the burn size does not usually include the superficial first-degree burns, which are known to be painful.

Further analysis of the Choinière et al. data to include the first degree areas in total extent of burn and limiting the pain measurements to those obtained during the first week postburn showed a positive correlation of pain with burn size ($p < 0.02$). In addition, they found that pain scores at rest were significantly correlated with extent of first degree burns ($p < 0.04$) and pain at time of treatments was significantly correlated with extent of second degree burns in < 0.02. No correlation was found with the extent of third degree burns.

Atchison et al.[9] measured pain scores in children and found a significant correlation between pain scores during the procedure and both the extent of total burn injury and the extent of third degree burn. However, several issues raise major concerns about the validity of these data:

1. pain scores spanned the time post-injury from 2 to 117 days in burns from 4% to 93% TBSA;

2. pain management was constant for the individual child across the entire period of treatment; and
3. pain medications were not adjusted to a child's weight.

Another source of confusion concerning the amount of pain expressed by burn patients is the role played by psychological problems such as anxiety and depression. Charlton et al.[6] used the State/Trait Anxiety Inventory to measure anxiety and reported that the study sample of adult burned patients was not particularly anxious. Other studies have suggested that burned patients have increased levels of anxiety, especially related to treatment and outcome and that these levels may increase over time.[10–12] Anticipation of pain related to treatments that occur at least daily can increase a patient's perception of pain. Anticipatory anxiety related to treatments leads to perception of increased pain, and the increased pain leads to further increases in anxiety. This reaction may explain some findings which suggest that pain increases over time in burned patients.[13–15]

Using the Zung Depression Scale to measure depression, Charlton et al.[6] found that most patients experienced only mild to moderate depression, with few showing moderate to severe depression. Similar results were found by Choinière et al.[2] who noted that pain at rest was significantly and positively related to levels of anxiety or depression; i.e. with elevated anxiety or depression, pain scores at rest increased. Interestingly, all patients hospitalized more than 3 weeks showed an increase in the depression scores. Although these studies demonstrate the great variability in pain expression in burned patients, they do not identify pain-generating mechanisms, either physiologically or psychologically, in a burn-injured patient. Further work in these areas is needed to better understand the great variability of burn pain.

Pain as a Function of the Healing Process

As a deep dermal or full-thickness burn wound heals, either by primary intention from excision and grafting or by secondary intention through granulation tissue and scar formation, the injured neural tissue is reorganized.[16] Reflex neural function returns to grafted burn skin approximately 5–6 weeks after the burn has been covered by autografted skin.[17] Active vasodilatation, vasoconstriction, and pain sensation all return at this time. These functions also return to the burn wound which heals through scar formation but may take up to 6 months for complete neural reorganization.

Although rare, causalgia, dysesthesia, and phantom pain syndrome can sometimes develop in healing skin. The incidence of these chronic pain syndromes seems to be related to the healing process. Burns that have been excised and grafted on a clean and uniform vascular bed rarely develop one of these chronic pain syndromes. Wounds that heal by granulation and scar formation seem to be more apt to develop a chronic pain problem. Skin biopsies of granulation tissue have clearly shown neuronal tissue entrapment.[17] Pain, in scar tissue, often subsides over time as the scar tissue matures.

Types of Pain in Burned Patients During the Acute Phase of Treatment

As already noted, the pain expressed by a burned patient is extremely variable. In many studies, burned patients have been asked to rate overall pain, pain at rest, overall procedural pain, and worst pain during the procedure. Such perplexing instructions may account for some of the variability in pain reports. For example, if asked to rate one's overall pain for the day, one would expect this rating to include resting pain, pain during normal activity, and pain during painful procedures. A more reasonable approach may be to ask a patient to rate pain as procedural and nonprocedural pain, giving each type of pain an operational definition. Procedural pain would be pain related to wound care and active or passive stretching of the patient's scar tissue, activities that seem to cause the worst pain for burned patients. Nonprocedural pain would be the discomfort experienced at rest and while performing activities of daily living. This nomenclature of procedural and nonprocedural pain allows for planning therapies for pain relief, based on the intensity of pain experienced throughout the day. As therapies for pain management are discussed later in this chapter, the importance of differentiating procedural and nonprocedural pain will become increasingly clear.

Measurement of pain in burned patients

Although pain cannot be measured directly, it can be quantified by using one of the standardized tools described below. Using standardized tools allows us to gauge the effectiveness of our treatment for any one patient. Assessing pain on a scheduled basis, just as vital signs are assessed, and using the same tool for each assessment gives us information about how pain is experienced by a single patient throughout a day; we can note patterns that emerge and schedule medications accordingly. And, of course, using a standardized tool allows us to compare our patients to each other and to patients from other burn units in order to judge, for example, the effectiveness of a new protocol for pain management. A final and very important reason for assessing pain regularly and in standard fashion is that this procedure communicates to patients that we believe they have pain, that pain with this kind of injury is universal and so common that we have tools developed especially for this phenomenon, that we care about our patients' comfort, and, implicitly, we will try to diminish discomfort. This communication reassures the patient, thereby reducing the likelihood that the patient will escalate pain behaviors (e.g. screaming and moaning) in an effort to convince the staff that the pain is severe and requires medication instantaneously.

Pain Measurement Techniques for an Adult Burned Patient

What is the gold standard for the measurement of pain? Gracely,[18] in a recent article on pain measurement, reviewed a number of objective modalities for the measurement of experimental pain. He noted that 'pain arises from and is modulated by, a number of mechanisms'. These mechanisms are not static but change over time and involve all levels of the central nervous system. In an attempt to understand these mechanisms, several experimental tools have been employed to further elucidate the exact pathways involved in pain transmission and to better understand the therapies used to relieve pain.

Some of these tools are: cortical evoked potentials; functional brain imaging (PET or positive emission tomography); functional magnetic resonance imaging (fMRI); source analysis of evoked activity; and electrophysiological recording from the human brain. As noted by Gracely, comparing them with verbal judgements of pain magnitude validates these physiologic measures. 'This

implicitly elevates subjective judgement to the level of a validational standard.'[18] Clinical measurements of pain must continue to rely on standard subjective measures.

A variety of pain measurement techniques have been used with adult burned patients. The more common measures include adjective scales (**Table 58.1**), numeric scales (i.e. rating pain on a scale of 0–5, 0–10 or 0–100), and visual analog scales (**Figure 58.2**). Each of these scales measures the sensory component of a patient's pain. Adjective scales and numeric scales are quick and easy to administer because they do not require a visual representation of the scale. The visual analog scale requires a visual representation of the scale to be presented to a patient. Patients must mark or point to the place on the scale that represents their level of pain. This presents a problem for a burned patient whose hands are burned, so some investigators have used a technique of sliding a line or color strip along the scale with instructions to a patient to direct the movement of the slide, stopping at the point representative of the patient's pain. The visual analog scale has been used in a number of studies with a variety of patient samples and has been shown to be a valid method of measuring the sensory component of a patient's pain. The demonstrated validity of the scale allows for comparisons of visual analog pain assessments between studies with different patient samples.

Motivational-affective and cognitive-evaluative components of pain are most frequently measured using the McGill Pain Questionnaire (MPQ).[19] The MPQ consists of 20 sets of adjectives which describe all three components of pain: sensory, affective, and evaluative. Qualitative profiles and quantitative scores for each dimension as well as a total pain score can be derived from the selected adjectives. The MPQ has been translated into several languages and has been shown to be a reliable and valid measurement tool. The major problem with the tool is that it takes 10–20 minutes to administer and may not be as useful for frequent, repeated measurements. Many studies have employed this measurement on a daily basis to measure either overall or resting pain. Gordon et al.,[20] in a prospective multicenter study, asked 40 adult burned patients to rate their pain on four scales. These scales were: a visual analog scale, a analog chromatic scale,[21] an adjective scale, and a faces scale.[22] At the end of the study, patients were asked to choose their preferred scale. Patients preferred the faces and analog chromatic scales. Although further research is needed to validate these findings, the preference of patients is another variable to be considered.

A major concern in the clinical setting is to use a consistent tool

Table 58.1 Adjective scales in English and Spanish			
0	No pain	0	Nada de color
1	Slight Pain	1	Dolor leve (ligero)
2	Moderate Pain	2	Dolor moderado
3	Severe Pain	3	Dolor severo

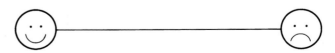

Fig. 58.2 Visual analog scale (VAS) for children to rate their levels of pain from the Varni Thompson Pediatric Pain Questionnaire.[50]

to measure pain and to use it before and 1–2 hours after the administration of a medication for pain relief. For procedural pain management, the same tool should be used to measure pain at the beginning of a procedure (post-premedication), during it, and post-procedure in order to measure the effectiveness of pain management regimens for procedural pain.

Pain Measurement Techniques for Pediatric Patients

The measurement of children's pain is much more complex than it is for adults, especially for preverbal children. For many years it was thought that infants did not feel pain because of incomplete myelinization of the sensory nerves. Anand and colleagues published data in 1987[23] and 1988[24] to suggest that infants do experience pain as evidenced by a variety of physiologic and metabolic responses. Anand and Hickey[25] hypothesize that, although A fibers are not completely myelinated and may not be efficient in transmission of pain, unmyelinated C fibers take over the transmission of noxious stimuli. This research has demonstrated the need for pain assessment and management in infants and preverbal children as well as older children.

The assessment of pain in children has included physiologic measurements, behavioral assessment, and patient reports of pain. The physiologic indicators that have been evaluated are heart rate,[26] respiratory rate,[26] blood pressure,[26] endocrine changes,[26,27] and changes in P_{O_2}.[28] None of these shows promise as an indicator for measuring pain in sick children, since all are affected by a variety of stressors in addition to pain.

A number of behavior scales have been devised to measure pain by providing standardized instructions and guidelines for observing behaviors thought to be specific to pain. A number of investigators[29–34] has looked at infants' cries as measurable behaviors that can be observed in order to evaluate pain. Although these studies demonstrate that length of cry, pitch, intensity, and other characteristics of crying may be used to evaluate pain in infants, the analyses of cry are very time consuming and require elaborate audio equipment. Izard et al.,[35] Craig et al.,[36] and Granau and Craig[33] have attempted to code facial expressions as measures of pain in infants. Their system characterizes nine facial actions involved in the expression of pain, but its use requires videotaping and detailed analyses of an infant's facial movements. Although this method offers excellent research applications, it, like the detailed analyses of crying, is not appropriate for the clinical setting. On the other hand, the studies do provide clinicians with information about various facial actions, as categorized by Granau and Craig, which may be helpful in the clinical identification of pain in infants. Other investigators have devised multidimensional scales that include length of cry, facial expressions, and behavioral

states in order to measure pain in infants.[37–39] These scales are easier to use and allow an observer to assess pain as either present or absent without further quantification.

Examples of observational scales which allow for quantification and may be used with toddlers and preverbal children are the CHEOPS (Children's Hospital of Eastern Ontario Pain Scale)[40] and The Observer Scale.[41] The CHEOPS is a scale of six behaviors, each scored on a numeric range, which yields a total numeric score for pain. This scale has been shown to be valid and to have good interrator reliability. The Observer Scale is another standardized instrument that categorizes overall pain or comfort behaviors on a scale of 1–5. The five categories are: laughing, euphoric; happy, contented, playful; calm or asleep; mild-moderate pain (crying, grimacing, restlessness, but can be distracted with toy, food, or parent); and severe pain (crying, screaming, inconsolable).

A burn-specific observational tool was recently developed by Barone et al. at Shriners Hospitals for Children–Cincinnati.[42] The OPAS (Observational Pain Assessment Scale; see **Table 58.2**) is useful in children 0–3 years of age.

Research suggests that simple self-report scales can be used with preschool children. Examples of such scales include the Oucher Scale (photographs of children with various facial expressions).[43–45] Drawings of faces[22,46] have also been used with preschool age children[47] and school age children (8 years).[48] Preschool children have also used the Poker Chip Tool,[49] color scales,[50,51] and a thermometer[51] to report the degree of pain or hurt. These simple tools allow a preschooler to report pain and are easy to use. One caution with the face scales is that a practitioner must help a child differentiate between physical pain and sadness unrelated to pain. Since there is no evidence that any one of these is more valid than another, it is recommended to pick one and use it consistently. When self-report scales are used in conjunction with observational scales, a practitioner gets a better picture of a child's response to pain and pain therapies.

A school-aged child's cognitive development allows more abstract thinking. In addition to the Faces Pain Rating Scales, which they enjoy,[22] they can use simple numeric scales 0–5 in the early school years (ages 7–8)[53] and more complex scales 0–10 or 0–100 in the later years (age 9–12). Visual analog scales anchored with happy and sad faces[51] and simple adjective scales[51,54] also can be used with this age group. In addition to self-reports of pain, observational scales such as the CHEOPS,[40] or the Procedure Behavior Check List[55] can be used with a school-aged child. Again, the important issue is to use one selected scale consistently since no one has been shown to be more valid than others.

Adolescents can think abstractly and can quantify and qualify phenomena and so can use the same scales as adults. One concern

Table 58.2 Observational Pain Assessment Scale (OPAS)

Assess each of the areas identified in the 'Observed Behavior' column rating each behavior using the 0, 1 or 2 rating. Add the ratings together for each observed behavior. Document your total score.

Observed Behavior	0	1	2
Restlessness	Calm, cooperative	Slightly restless, consolable	Very restless agitated, inconsolable
Muscle, Tension	Relaxed	Slight tenseness	Extreme tenseness
Facial Expression	No frowning or grimacing, composed	Slight frowning or grimacing	Constant frowning or grimacing
Vocalization	Normal tone, no sound	Groans, moans, cries out in pain	Cries out, sobs
Wound Guarding	No negative response to wound	Reaching/gently touching wound	Grabbing vigorously at wound

Reproduced with permission of the publisher from Crome et al.[136]

with adolescents is that, when they are ill, they tend to regress and thus may require the use of a simpler scale during such times.[56] In summary, there are many measurements tools for pain assessment across the life span which can be useful to the researcher and the clinician. **Table 58.3** presents a list of clinically useful tools according to patient age.

Table 58.3 Recommended pain measurement tools for burned patients
Infants and Toddlers
CHEOPS 40
The Observed Pain Scale
Preschooler
Faces Pain Rating Scale[43,44]
Oucher[38–40]
Pediatric Pain Questionnaire[47]
CHEOPS[36]
School age child
Faces Pain Rating Scale[43,44]
Visual analog
Numeric scale
Pediatric Pain Questionnaire[47]
Procedure Behavior Checklist[51]
Adolescents and adults
Visual analog
Numeric scales
Adjective scales
McGill Questionnare[18]

Anxiety Measurement Scale

Anxiety is measured in a variety of ways. Robert *et al.* recently surveyed 64 burn treatment centers to determine how they evaluated and treated anxiety, especially in children.[57] They found that most centers did not use standardized measures of anxiety. Based on that survey and other information, the Shriners Burns Hospital in Galveston has begun using the Fear Thermometer adapted by Silverman and Kurtines[58] from the Walk's Fear Thermometer.[59] That instrument is illustrated in **Figure 58.3**.

Itch Measurement Scale

The severe itching of burn scars and wounds has not been much discussed in the literature, but clinicians can testify that this phenomenon is a very serious problem. Patients who experience such itching often excoriate new grafts or recently healed skin, thus enhancing their susceptibility to infections. When the pruritis is severe, patients can focus on nothing else. Until every recently there have been no tools for measuring itch. Now, Field *et al.*[60] have reported using a visual analog scale of 1–10 to assess itching. Pat Blakeney and Janet Marvin at the Shriners Burns Hospital in Galveston have recently developed a new instrument to measure itch called 'itch man' (**Figure 58.4**). This instrument was based on a patient's drawing of his experience in the hospital.[61] Children seem to be able to relate to 'itch man', but validation studies are still in progress.

Treatment considerations

Once pain has been assessed and quantified, treatment can be considered. Three modalities of treatment are effective with pain secondary to burn injury. They are surgical treatment, pharmacological treatment, and behavioral treatment.

Surgical Treatment of Pain

The pain is predominately related to the open wound. Once the wound is closed, the pain subsidies. The use of resection and grafting of open burn wounds significantly reduces the burn pain. Open wounds should be grafted as soon as they are clean enough to do so. Even temporary coverage with cadaver skin or pigskin reduces pain in the area of the burn. In the case of second degree wounds, the use of Biobrane™, Opsite™, Tegaderm™ or other wound-covering dressings almost immediately eliminates pain in the burn wound site. Duinslaeger *et al.*[62] compared methods of treatment of open donor sites. Cultured allogeneic keratinocyte sheets accelerated healing and thereby reduced pain and suffering compared to Opsite™ treatment. The cultured keratinocyte sheets cut healing time in half. Pain assessment as early as day 3 revealed lower pain scores in those sites treated with keratinocyte sheets.

Pharmacologic Management of Pain

Pharmacologic management of burn pain is the mainstay of therapy. General rules or tenets are helpful in governing the use of pain medication. The first tenet is that if patients say they are having

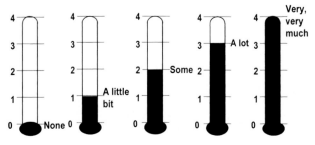

Fig. 58.3 Fear thermometer to rate anxiety level from Silverman and Kurtines.[58]

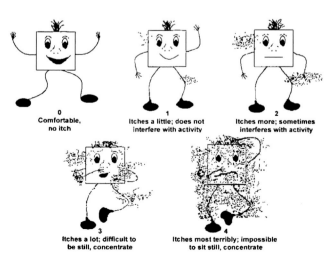

Fig. 58.4 Itch man scale to rate itching intensity in children designed by Blackeney and Marvin.[61]

pain, they are having pain. The second tenet is that analgesics are most effective when given on a regular scheduled basis (not 'as needed' or PRN). Thirdly, pain medication should not be given as an injection since injections themselves cause pain and anxiety. Lastly, dose and type of medication should be reevaluated frequently to make sure pain is continuously controlled and that the patient is experiencing no serious side-effects. The dosing of medication should be adjusted for the general clinical condition of the patients, considering factors of nutritional state, shock, sepsis, age extremes, and concurrent illnesses such as hepatitis etc. Review articles[53-74] recommend a variety of therapeutic modalities for background and procedural pain during the stages of burn treatment. The three stages are:

- the emergency or resuscitative phase (0–72 hours after injury);
- the acute phase (72 hours to 3 or 5 weeks, until the wounds are closed); and
- the rehabilitative phase (from the time of wound closure to scar maturity); this phase may last months to years.

Table 58.4 provides a matrix summary of therapies that are recommended for procedural and background pain over the three phases of burn care. A variety of routes or methods of administration are also suggested. The routes or methods recommended include the intravenous bolus (IVB), intravenous continuous infusion (IVCI), patient-controlled analgesia (PCA), and orally administered agents on a nonpain contingent (NPC) basis. Many patients

also require anxiolytic medication along with the analgesic medication. Therefore, included in **Table 58.4** are the anxiolytic agents suggested for use by several authors.

Emergency phase

For pain management therapy, the emergency or resuscitative phase applies only to patients with burns greater than 10% total body surface area (TBSA). During the emergency phase, the preferred route for most medications is the intravenous route because of potential problems with absorption from the muscles and stomach related to decreased perfusion. Of the agents recommended for the relief of procedural pain, morphine is the most widely used. For procedures, IVB and IVCI are the most common methods of administration used. For extremely painful procedures in both the emergency and acute phase, fentanyl has a major advantage in that it is shorter-acting and avoids oversedation following a procedure as might occur with repeated doses of morphine. In addition to the opiates, analgesic doses of anesthetic agents such as ketamine and nitrous oxide may be used for procedural pain. These two agents, along with anxiolytic agents to be used as adjuncts to pain management, will be discussed later in this chapter.

Acute phase

During the acute phase, the choice of pharmacological agents used to manage procedural pain encompasses a number of orally administered opiates. To control background pain during the acute phase, the use of PCA of NPC (nonpain-contingent) medication regimens

Table 58.4 Pharmacologic therapies for burn pain relief

Procedural Analgesics	Background Analgesics	Anxiolytics
Emergent phase		
Morphine (IVB, IVCI)	Morphine (IVCI, PCA)	Diazepam (IV) (Valium)
Meperidine (IVB)	Meperidine (PCA)	Lorazepam (IV) (Ativan)
Fentanyl (IVB, IVCI)	Methadone (PO, NPC)	Midazolam (IV, IVCI) (Versed)
Hydromorphone (IVB, PO) (Dilaudid)		
Nalbuphine (IVB) (Nubain)		
Ketamine (IV) (Ketalar)		
Nitrous oxide (IH)		
Acute Phase		
Morphine (IVB, IVCI, PCA) Roxanol (oral morphine)	Morphine (IVCI, PCA)	Diazepam (PO) (Valium)
Meperidine (IVB, IM)	Meperidine (IVCI, PCA)	Lorazepam (PO) (Ativan)
Fentanyl (IVB, IM)	Methadone (PO, NPC)	Alprazolam (PO) (Xanax)
Hydromorphine (PO) (Dilaudid)	Sustained release morphine (PO, NPC) (MS Contin)	
Nalbuphine (IVB) (Nubain)	Acetaminophen (PO, NPC)	
Ketamine (IV, IM) (Ketalar)	NSAIDs (PO, NPC)	
Oxycodone (PO) (Percocet)	Choline magnesium trisalicylate	
Rehabilitative Phase		
For severe pain:	**For mild to moderate pain:**	**Anxiolytics**
Hydromorphone (PO) (Dilaudid)	Oxycodone (PO) (Percocet)	Diazepam (PO) (Valium)
	Nonsteroidal anti-inflammatory drugs (NSAIDs) with or without narcotics	Lorazepam (PO) (Ativan)
	Usually not necessary: Acetaminophen NSAIDs	Alprazolam (PO) (Xanax)

are far superior to the PRN (as requested) method. PRN regimens often result in undermedication by one nurse and overmedication by the next nurse. A patient may become angry and confused about what to expect regarding pain control and may feel realistically helpless in an environment where others decide whether relief is necessary. Allowing a patient to medicate himself as needed usually results in better and smoother pain control as well as better staff and patient relationships. An alternative to PCA, which seems to work equally well for background pain, is the use of NPC medication regimens. Such regimens may use methadone in a pain cocktail, slow release morphine (MS Contin™), or other oral agents given on a fixed dosing schedule, the frequency of which will depend on the pharmacologic agent.

For background pain, PCA and IVCI are being used with greater frequency. Both of these methods allow for greater flexibility in dose titration and should avoid over- and undermedication. Since even the more severely burned patients are usually alert and coherent, the PCA method is the ideal method for titration. PCA can be used with or without a background IVCI. For a burned patient with extensive hand burns, the control cord can be fitted with a padded pedal-type apparatus that can be positioned so that the patient can press it with a foot, elbow, etc. Occasional patients will use the highest dose allowed in order to withdraw from the entire treatment setting. If this occurs, confrontation and negotiation are important to get the patient back to the task at hand.

Ventilator patient

Special consideration should be given to managing the pain of a patient on the respirator. If the patient is fighting the respirator and needs to be sedated to provide adequate function of the respirator, then frequent and high doses of intravenous morphine can be given such as 0.03–0.06 mg/kg every hour in order to ensure pain control with adequate sedation. The use of other forms of sedation without opiates may provide sedation without adequate control of pain.

Rehabilitative phase

During the rehabilitative phase, most patients complain more of an aching type of pain, similar to arthritic pain. In this case, mild narcotics, acetaminophen, or nonsteroidal anti-inflammatory drugs (NSAIDs) may be used for either procedural (exercise) or background pain. Ibuprofen has been used at 10 mg/kg with some positive effect, but many individuals have gastrointestinal upset with this type of medication. If a procedure will cause severe pain, morphine, hydromorphone, or one of the other oral opiates should be used.

Age of Patient and Pain Management

Since the pharmacologic management of burn pain not only spans the phases of burn care, but also must be tailored to meet the needs of all age groups, it is important to comment on pain management in both the very young and the elderly. There is a tendency to give less medication to young children because 'they don't complain of pain'. This opinion is supported by the fact that some children become very withdrawn rather than screaming when they are receiving painful stimuli (e.g. abused children). It is unlikely that a burn is any less painful in a 3-month-old than in a 30-year-old; thus, the same therapeutic modalities adjusted for age and size are appropriate for burned children. A major issue of treating pain in young children is the safety risk of using opiates. One example is a

1998 report of the Seattle group concerning respiratory depression in three children treated with standard doses per kilogram of opiates given to other age groups.[75] There has been a similar experience at the Shriners Burns Hospital in Galveston. In all cases the respiratory depression responded well to an opiate antagonist such as naloxone. Young children may have an increased sensitivity to the respiratory depressive effects of opiates.[76]

Many times with children it is very difficult to separate out pain complaints from anxiety complaints, post-traumatic stress complaints or even itch complaints. In this case, the first step is to make sure that the pain medication is adequate and that it is being given. After ensuring that the pain medication is adequate, then one can begin to examine carefully for the other disease problems, all of which can mimic pain.

At the other extreme of age is the elderly patient. Again, the tendency is to give less medication, either because these patients do not complain as much or because they are thought to be 'more sensitive' to pain medications. A realistic and important concern with the elderly is oversedation. Studies in nonburned elderly people have shown that, with increased age, the efficiency of the clearance mechanism for certain drugs is decreased, and repeated doses may lead to drug accumulation. This would suggest that, when managing pain in an elderly burned patient, it is not that the dose *per se* should be decreased, but that the interval between dosing should be lengthened so as to prevent accumulation and oversedation.

Neuropathic or Phantom Pain

Some severely burned patients have partial loss of digits or limbs associated with their burns. This adds a different dimension to the management of their pain since these individuals often have sensations of the existence of these digits or limbs for many years after their loss. This type of pain usually does not respond to traditional pain management with nonsteroidal acetaminophen or opiates. This neuropathic pain often does respond to the use of tricyclics or anticonvulsants. Doses of imipramine or amitriptyline of 1 mg/kg body weight often are effective. In a recent review, Thomas *et al.* reviewed 29 patients who had amputations for either burn or electrical injury.[77] Of the 33% who experienced phantom limb pain, all but one patient's pain responded to amitriptyline, if the pain does not respond to this, then carbinazopine might be utilized in doses which are therapeutic for seizures. Over time, this neuropathic pain seems to become more tolerable and slowly dissipate.

Pharmacologic Agents Used in Management of Pain

The preceding discussion has focused on the reviews and reports of 'how we do it' or the 'bias' of health care professionals in treating burn pain. The following focuses on specific pharmacologic modalities in burn pain management.

Lidocaine and related agents

Beausang *et al.*, recommended adding bupivacaine to the adrenaline solution used in preparing the burn wound eschar site and the grafting site.[78] Their clinical impression was a reduction of pain. Sympathetic nerve blocks with the same medication are effective for blocking thermal pain.[79] Other similar medications such as lignocaine (1 mg/kg) given intravenously has been reported to cause significant relief of pain for up to 3 days.[80] More recently Pedersen *et al.*[81] reported the use of EMLA cream, a prilocaine and lignocaine mixture, to burn wounds in a double blind randomized manner for 8 hours; however, this procedure did not reduce late hyperalgesia. Seizures have been reported following topical lidocaine.[82]

Opioids

Of these agents, morphine has continued to be the mainstay for both background and procedural pain management. Other opiates such as hydromorphone (Dilaudid); levorphanol (Levodromoran), fentanyl, and methadone are all excellent oral agents for the relief of moderate to severe pain when given in equianalgesic doses to morphine. Fentanyl comes in a convenient sucker, especially attractive for use with children. Of concern with hydromorphone is that the period of peak effect varies widely from 45 to 90 minutes; for this reason, the combination of lorazepam given 1 hour before a procedure and hydromorphone given 45–60 minutes before a procedure results in excellent pain control for the majority of adult patients. As with other opiates, tolerance may develop rapidly, so the dose of hydromorphone may need to be adjusted frequently. Methadone has a longer half-life than morphine and therefore can provide coverage for a longer time between doses. In addition, we have seen some patients who did not respond to morphine but did respond to methadone. We do not know if this represents a difference in absorption or a difference in specificity. Also, methadone has been noted to give smoother pain relief for children postoperatively than morphine.[83]

Perry and Inturris[84] reported that the pharmacokinetics of morphine in burned patients were not significantly altered in comparison to normals. They found that the $t_{1/2a}$ (apparent distribution half-life in minutes) was 4.3 ± 3.4 (SD) in burned patients versus $t_{1/2a}$ 1.7 ± 1.2 in normal subjects and that the $t_{1/2b}$ (apparent elimination half-life in minutes) was 98.8 ± 20.8 (SD) in burned patients versus 176.8 ± 70.3 in normal subjects. Likewise, the apparent volume of central compartment, clearance, hepatic extraction, and plasma binding were similar for burned patients and normals. Osgood[66] found in a group of acutely burned children that the distribution and elimination half-life of morphine markedly shortened $[t_{1/2a} = 1.2 \pm 0.39$ (SEM) for burned children vs. 2.2 ± 0.49 minutes in normals; $t_{1/2b} = 36.9 \pm 6.40$ for burned children vs. 126 ± 38.18 minutes in normals (p < 0.05)] and that the rate of clearance was increased for acutely burned children.

Bloedow et al.[85] reported on the pharmacokinetics of meperidine in 11 acute burns (1 week post-injury) and in five convalescent patients (about 6 weeks postburn). The meperidine steady state distribution volume (l/kg) during both the acute and convalescent phases was about half the distribution volume reported in the literature for meperidine in healthy subjects. The meperidine clearance in burned patients (acute, 420 ml/min; convalescent, 600 ml/min) was slower than would be anticipated in the presence of known marked increases in hepatic blood flow in burned patients.

Novoa[86] reported, in 1980, that burned patients could tolerate, for procedural pain, higher doses than the usual 10–15 mg intravenous dose of morphine. She reviewed a 2-year experience in which adults were given from 20 to 35 mg (occasionally as much as 50 mg) of morphine intravenously in incremental doses during debridement. Although the total number of patients treated was not given, she reported only two incidents over the 2 years in which naloxone hydrochloride was needed to correct respiratory depression.

From the published literature concerning the use of opioids in patients with burn injury, one would have difficulty making decisions about the best drug, the best dosage range, or the best route or method (i.e. PCA, PRM, or continuous infusion) of administration of these drugs.[84–92] Morphine or other opioids are considered mainstays of pain relief for burned patients, but many reviewers report less than adequate pain relief for burned patients with the use of opioids. The line between enough opioid to provide pain relief and too much, causing respiratory depression, is difficult to find. Personal experience has shown that even a PCA regimen must be individualized and frequently adjusted. Important caveats for the use of PCA should include:

- an initial bolus in adults of 5–10 mg of morphine or equivalent dose of other drugs;
- increasing the patient-controlled dose as needed to achieve pain relief (recognizing that tolerance develops at varying rates in individual patients);
- planning for a change in dosing regimens at night to include: (a) giving a bolus dose at bedtime; (b) doubling the patient-controlled dose and lengthening the time interval between doses so that when patients awaken in pain, they do not have to lie awake to push a button several times in order to get adequate medication; and (c) if the increased intermittent dosing is not adequate, being lenient with bolus doses or to start a patient on a continuous morphine drip at night.

Fentanyl probably deserves a little special notice. It is becoming more popular since it is now available in a lollipop. Fentanyl is preferred by many because it acts rapidly, has short duration, and involves no histamine release. It does cause some emesis, however, even with the fentanyl lozenges.[93] In nonburned patients the pharmacokinetic data show great variability, especially with the parent compound fentanyl.[94] Thus, further pharmacokinetic studies, in nonburned as well as burned patients, need to be completed in order to better understand the efficacy and safety of this class of drugs.

Transmucosal fentanyl citrate in the form of lollipops provide a new user-friendly form of treating pain in children who have suffered burn injury. In 1998, Sharar et al. carried out a double blind study comparing their use at a fentanyl dose of 10 µg/kg with the more classic oral hydromorphone (60 µg/kg).[95] They found in a double blind crossover design study that the fentanyl lollipops provided safe and effective control of pain. In fact, the pain scores were improved before wound care and anxiolysis was improved during wound care; at other times the two treatments were identical.

Clonidine

Clonidine has been reported to be extremely useful in pain management postburn. It has the advantage of not causing pruritus or respiratory depression. Lyons et al.,[96] noted that the pain of an 11-year-old boy was much better controlled by low dose morphine when he received intravenous clonidine (350 µg/4 hours).

Nonsteroidal anti-inflammatory drugs

Two reports[97,98] were found concerning the use of NSAIDs in burned patients. Neither of these studies reported on the use of NSAIDs for pain management, but one study by Wallace[97] reported a significant reduction in body temperature [0.67°C (p < 0.01)] and a decrease in metabolic rate (11.4%; p < 0.01) with the administration of ibuprofen, suggesting that this drug may attenuate the metabolic response to thermal injury by blunting the temperature elevation associated with burn injuries. The second study of the pharmacokinetics of ibuprofen when given enterally to burned patients reports the half-life to vary from 1.4 to 5.1 hours, depending on whether the drug was given by enteral tube with tube feeding (t_m = 1 hour) or orally with a regular diet (t_m = 5.1 hours).[98] Although ibuprofen was not given for pain control in either study, the results might lead one to ask, concerning the first study, was the decrease in metabolic rate solely related to a decrease in body temperature or was some of the effect a result of better pain control? The second study is important if one is going to use ibuprofen as part of pain management regimen. The results would suggest that different dosing schedules might be necessary if a patient is receiving tube feedings or a regular diet. Nonsteroidals, such as ibuprofen, have, in addition to analgesic effects, anti-inflammatory activity which, in some instances, may be advantageous due to the ability to inhibit prostaglandin biosynthesis. This activity is, however, directly associated with some of the side-effects of these drugs which include gastrointestinal bleeding, hypertension, and congestive heart failure.

Acetaminophen

Because of the significant side-effect profile of nonsteroidal and anti-inflammatory drugs such as ibuprofen, acetaminophen has been considered for the management of chronic pain. In 1991, Bradley *et al.* reported that acetaminophen at a dose of 10–15 mg/kg of body weight given every 4 hours (up to a maximum of 4000 mg/day) was equal in efficacy to ibuprofen at a dose of 10 mg/kg of body weight given every 4 hours (up to a maximum of 2400 mg/day).[99] In addition, acetaminophen is well tolerated and causes almost no side-effects, most particularly gastrointestinal side-effects as with ibuprofen. There is some concern about long-term liver problems with this medication when used in high doses such that blood levels reach 50 µg/ml.[100]

Meyer *et al.*[101] at the Shriners Burns Hospital in Galveston reported an analysis of 395 consecutive acutely burned pediatric patients who were treated in 1993 and 1994 with a pain management protocol that utilized acetaminophen scheduled at 15 mg/kg every 4 hours as background management with morphine added for breakthrough pain and procedures such as tubbing. Background pain for 50.6% of the children was managed with acetaminophen alone, whereas the pain of 44.8% was managed with morphine. Best response to acetaminophen was in the younger age groups where 68% of the children under 3 years had their pain well managed by acetaminophen. The size of the burn also had a significant influence on the effectiveness of using acetaminophen alone. The smaller the burn, the more likely the positive response. For example, 66.4% of those with burns of less than 10% responded to acetaminophen alone, whereas only 9.1% of those with burns greater than 60% could be managed with acetaminophen alone. The study did not include an analysis of the depth of the burns, but there was a mixture of severe second degree and third degree injuries. Acetaminophen can be monitored easily in the blood and, in the authors' experience, 15 mg/kg every 4 hours did not cause blood levels to exceed 10 µg/ml except in very young children or extremely ill children receiving multiple type of other medications that are metabolized by the liver. No child had

levels over 40 µg/ml. Thus, acetaminophen should be safe over a long period of time. It may be given in conjunction with morphine with probably no significant additional side-effects. Acetaminophen is rapidly absorbed from the stomach and small bowel and achieves peak analgesic efficacy more rapidly than even aspirin. It is available in elixir and oral drops. One should be aware that, because acetaminophen is packaged in conjunction with hydrocodone in the form of Vicodin™ and Loratab™, one should be careful *not* to give acetaminophen in addition to either one of these combination medications. This survey has recently been repeated using 225 patients admitted in 1998.[102] Very similar results were found except that acetaminophen alone is used less often. In recent years, more children are now receiving morphine with the acetaminophen, probably because our staff have become more comfortable with giving morphine to even very young children.

Antianxiety drugs

As mentioned above, anxiety medication should be considered *only* after the patient's pain has been aggressively treated. The medical staff often inappropriately attribute the patient's complaint to anxiety ('just anxious' is a frequently used phrase) when, in fact, the patient is really experiencing pain. The three main antianxiety drugs used in the treatment of burn related anxiety are lorazepam, diazepam, and midazolam.

Martyn *et al.*[103] studied the pharmacokinetics of lorazepam in burned patients. The study compared burned patients to controls matched for age and weight. The burned patients were studied at a mean of 22 ± 4.6 (SE) days post-injury. The data showed that with burn injury there is an increased volume of distribution (2.66 ± 0.55 vs. 1.39 ± 0.1 l/kg, p<0.02), an increased clearance (4.28 ± 1.20 vs. 1.16 ± 0.1 ml/min/kg, p<0.01), and a significantly reduced half-life, (9.6 ± 1.3 vs. 13.9 ± 0.9 hours, p < 0.025). Therefore burn patients often need higher than expected doses. Patterson *et al.*[104] reported that, in a double-blind placebo-controlled study of 79 patients, 1 mg lorazepam did significantly reduce procedural pain ratings in those patients with high baseline pain, but did not reduce baseline trait anxiety.

Martyn *et al.*[105] also studied diazepam in burned patients. After a single dose, there was a rapid decline in concentration due to the high lipid solubility and rapid tissue uptake, leading to a shorter hypnotic effect of the drug. Interestingly, the elimination half-life was significantly prolonged for burned patients (72 hours vs. 36 hours for control subjects). Thus, with repeated administration, the tissue could become saturated and then the termination of the effect would depend more on biotransformation by hepatic enzymes. Hepatic enzyme activity has been shown to be quite depressed in burned patients.

Based on Martyn's work, we would conclude that lorazepam would be superior to diazepam in treating anxiety in burned patients.[105] Martyn suggests that, in addition to the fact that the clearance of lorazepam is faster than diazepam in burned patients, two other features of lorazepam make it a more acceptable drug for burned patients. First, it is metabolized by conjugation (a cytochrome P450 independent pathway) to a pharmacologically inactive glucuronide metabolite; and, second, the unbound volume of distribution is much less than for diazepam that causes clinically effective blood concentrations to persist for many hours, resulting in longer lasting sedation. Additionally, unlike diazepam, lorazepam is not affected by the concomitant administration of cimetidine. In a recent survey of the use of antianxiety drugs in burned children, 59% received lorazepam at a dose of 0.03 mg/kg or higher every 4 hours for much of their initial hospitalization; an additional 19% of patients received it for procedures only.[102] Lorazepam provided aid in anxiety control with essentially no side-effects. Fewer than 1% of the children had hallucinations or delirium associated with rapid changes in dose. The authors report that an occasional child responded with increased agitation rather than sedation, an occurrence we have also noticed infrequently.[106]

Although the pharmacokinetics of midazolam have not been reported in burned patients, it has characteristics in nonburned patients that would seem to make it an attractive anxiolytic agent for burned patients. Midazolam has a more rapid onset than either diazepam or lorazepam; thus, it allows for more rapid titration for effect in an individual patient. The elimination half-life of 2.5 hours is considerably shorter than that of lorazepam (13 hours) or diazepam (36 hours) and should result in a shorter recovery time after a procedure.[107] It is better tolerated when given intravenously. The anesthetic effect of midazolam is greater than diazepam.[108,109] Elderly patients have a more consistent response to a given dose.[110] Of the three benzodiazepines reviewed, either lorazepam or midazolam would seem to be more appropriate than diazepam for repeated use in burned patients. However, in our experience, we have found diazepam to be very useful in providing background anxiety control when muscle relaxation is desired (for example, to facilitate rehabilitative exercise) in addition to attenuating anxiety.

Anesthetic Agents Used in Analgesic Doses for Procedural Pain Nitrous oxide

Baskett[111,112] reported the use of nitrous oxide in addition to a neuroleptanalgesic (a combination of dehydrobenzperidol and phenoperidine) during burn dressing changes in children. The addition of 50% nitrous oxide was noted to diminish the respiratory depression associated with neuroleptanalgesia alone and provided a safe, short-acting analgesia. In these studies, patients were fasted for 6 hours before the procedure, but resumed normal oral intake within 2 hours.

Filkin et al.[113] reported results from both a retrospective study and a prospective study on the use of 50% nitrous oxide and 50% oxygen for debridement pain. In the retrospective study, the charts of 52 male patients were reviewed for the number of treatments, the effectiveness of pain relief, and the frequency of side-effects. The average burn size was 19% TBSA (range 2–85%), and the mean age was 28 years (range 16–64 years). The number of treatments varied from 1 to 52 per patient, with a mean of 12 treatments per patient. Of the 52 patients, only one patient reported no pain relief and requested to discontinue the use of the nitrous oxide. Side-effects noted were dizziness, giddiness, increased verbalizations, euphoria, dream-like state, nausea, and nonspecific tremors. Only in two patients were the side-effects considered to be significant enough to withdraw the treatment; these occurred in one patient with nausea and in one patient who developed nonspecific tremors. In the prospective study, all patients were given a standard dose of morphine (0.2 mg/kg) pre-procedure. Patients were then randomized to receive either a 50% nitrous oxide–50% oxygen mixture or compressed air for a given study treatment. Patient and patient care staff were blinded as to the treatment condition. Pain scores were taken at 10, 20, and 30 minutes using a four-point adjective scale, and at 3 hours post-procedure using a

VAS scale. All patients were allowed to use the nitrous oxide mixture in addition to morphine for debridement when they were not being studied. The study was aborted when 80% of the planned 30 patients requested to withdraw from the study because they did not feel that they were getting consistent pain relief on study days, preferring to use nitrous oxide for all treatments.

In addition to both of the above studies, a retrospective study by Marvin,[114] in which charts from 130 patients (65 who received nitrous oxide and 65 patients matched for % TBSA burned who did not), were reviewed, also found excellent patient acceptance and few side-effects. In the study by Marvin, the frequency of specific side-effects related to peripheral neuropathy, changes in liver function, and anemia were noted; no patient in either group showed changes in liver function tests while receiving the nitrous oxide mixture. Anemia as a direct side-effect of nitrous oxide could not be studied in this patient sample because of the frequent surgical procedures requiring blood transfusions in both groups. The only significant finding was that four patients in the group treated with nitrous oxide had a discharge finding of a neurological disorder which included one carpal tunnel injury, an exposed Achilles' tendon, a brachial plexus injury, and 'decreased function related to disuse'. The carpal tunnel injury and the exposed Achilles' tendon were directly related to the initial injury. The brachial plexus injury, noted within 24 hours of an operative procedure, was thought to be due to positioning and was resolving at the time of discharge. The fourth patient had been a very uncooperative patient who had decreased hand function attributed to lack of exercise to maintain function. None of these neurological disorders were similar to the polyneuropathies previously reported in relation to chronic nitrous oxide exposure.[115–117]

Hayden et al.[118] reported one case of progressive myeloneuropathy in burns related to the use of nitrous oxide. In this case, a 23-year-old male with a 46% TBSA burn including the legs, trunk, buttocks, and patchy areas on both arms, used a mixture to 50% nitrous oxide and 50% oxygen PRN (as necessary) for a period of 3 months. During these 3 months, he used 40 000 liters of Entonox™. During treatment, the patient developed bilateral foot drop and weakness of grip in both hands. He also complained of electrical shock sensations radiating from the lumbar spine to both feet with sudden neck flexion. He went on to develop diarrhea (four to five bowel movements/day) and was unable to walk without assistance. Post-discharge, he complained of impotency. At 6 months post-discharge, he had experienced gradual return of all function except power and sensation in his lower extremities. The PRN use reported here varies from the once or twice daily use reported by Basket,[111,112] Filkin,[113] and Marvin;[114] it would seem from the report that the patient consumed vastly larger doses. This may well explain the neurological problems seen in this case, which were similar to those described with chronic abuse of nitrous oxide.[115–118]

Ketamine

Ketamine is used often with children to manage their pain, particularly for protracted wound debridement. The route of administration can be oral, intravenous on intramuscular. In adults, it causes considerable dysphoria with unpleasant hallucinations and flashbacks even after complete recovery. However, it is very safe because it preserves airway reflexes. In children, these side-effects occur much less often.

Slogoff et al.[119] reported their clinical experience with the use of subanesthetic doses of ketamine for 150 debridement and dressing change procedures in 40 burned patients. Fourteen patients had only one exposure and the remainder had 2–13 exposures. The initial dose was 1.6 mg/kg of ketamine given intravenously. The results showed that patients with one or two exposures had coherent conversation or no vocalization 60% of the time; screaming or vocalization unrelated to stimulation occurred 34% of the time; and vocalizations in response to stimulation, 5%. In the group that received two or more exposures, coherent vocalizations dropped to 40%, while screaming or vocalization unrelated to stimulation increased to 49%; and vocalizations related to stimulation increased to 11%. Involuntary movement was rare in either group: 7% in <2 exposures and 8% in ≥2 exposures. One patient developed upper airway obstruction, which responded to manipulation of the mandible, and one patient experienced unpleasant emergence reactions after each of four procedures but did not refuse further treatment with ketamine. Significant findings in this study were:

- all patients who had more than two procedures required higher doses (p < 0.001);
- the duration of analgesia per dose, min/mg/kg was less with subsequent doses (p < 0.001); and
- the time to complete orientation was less with subsequent doses (p < 0.01).

With the increase in dosage after the second exposure, the actual time of analgesia remained constant at about 15 minutes. All patients had complete amnesia for all procedures.

Martinez et al.[120] described a dream state of burned patients treated with ketamine for dressing changes. A randomly selected sample of 15 patients (ten males, and five females, age range from 20 to 85 years) were asked to describe their dreams while under the influence of ketamine. All subjects were prepared by either a nurse or a physician in an unstructured interview to discuss the procedure and 'the likelihood that positive thoughts would result in pleasant experiences'. Twelve of 15 subjects stated that they experienced dreams while under the effects of ketamine. Eight of the 12 described their dreams as pleasant. Subjects were also asked to rate their ketamine experience according to a list of descriptions: seven chose 'frightening', 11 chose 'floating', two chose 'beautiful', eight chose 'helpless', two chose 'powerful', and 11 chose 'confusing'.

Two protocols for the use of ketamine in burned patients were published in the *Journal of Burn Care and Rehabilitation* (March/April, 1987).[121,122] One protocol, from San Francisco General Hospital, allowed a nurse to administer ketamine 2–3 mg/kg body weight intramuscularly for dressing changes under the order and immediate supervision of a physician.[120] The second protocol presented was from the Shriners Burns Hospital in Galveston.[121] This protocol actually described the use of ketamine as an anesthetic, not an analgesic agent. The doses used were 1–2 mg/kg body weight, intravenously, or 8–10 mg/kg body weight given intramuscularly. The procedures required administration by an anesthesiologist. A review by Marlyn[123] of the use of ketamine in burned patients as an analgesic agent was also presented with the above-mentioned protocols. One salient point from the review is that, in low doses (1–3 mg/kg body weight rectally), ketamine can produce short periods of analgesia (5–30 minutes) for dressing changes. Second, with repeated use, tolerance can develop, so increased doses are required over time. Third, despite the maintenance of laryngeal and pharyngeal reflexes, patients should have nothing by mouth for 4–6 hours prior to administration. The side-effects of ketamine include the production of copious upper airway secretions (necessitating the use of drying agents: atropine or glycopyrrolate), hypertension, pulmonary and systemic arterial hypertension, tachycardia, and postoperative emergency reactions. Ketamine is contraindicated for patients with systemic or pulmonary arterial hypertension, myocardial infarction, ventricular failure, history of cerebral injuries, or psychiatric disorders.

More recently, Dimick et al.[124] reported on the use of anesthesia assisted procedures in burned patients. They reported on 109 procedures in 46 patients for staple removal from grafts (34 procedures), massive dressing changes or vigorous debridement (74 procedures), or facial moulage (one procedure). Anesthesia time ranged from 40 to 180 minutes. A variety of different combinations of inhalation and intravenous agents were administered. Ventilation was assisted at the discretion of the anesthesiologist in attendance. Ninety-eight procedures (90%) were uneventful. In the other 11 patients, two lost their intravenous access and had to be recannulated; seven patients had systolic blood pressure and/or pulse rate vary more than 20% from baseline and required treatment; two patients required unplanned intubations, but both were extubated at the end of the procedure. Within 2 hours after the procedure, 72% of patients were able to cooperate fully; and within 4 hours, all were able to cooperate fully. They concluded that anesthesia-assisted procedures in a burn intensive care unit could be performed safely with appropriate professional care and monitoring.

Propofol (diprivan)

At the Shriners Burns Hospital in Galveston propofol, a new sedative hypnotic agent is often used for prolonged pain procedures such as line placement or staple removal. Its onset of action is extremely rapid even with a dose as low as 1.5 mg/kg intravenously.[125] The airway must be closely observed while using the medication. Use over 5 days is associated with renal toxicity.

Itch Medications

Several classes of medications can be used to treat itch. The approaches to treatment are as varied as the presumed causes of the itching.[126] Pruritus associated with burns is poorly understood, so blocking histamine, kinins, proteases, prostaglandins, substance P and 5-HT release and receptors have all been tried. The first line of defense is a series of moisturizing body shampoos and lotions to alleviate itching due to dry scaly skin. Then, failing that, Preparation H™ has been advocated. Topical steroids are not used because of the infection risk. Antihistamine creams such as Benadryl (diphenylhydramine) cream are available. Usually the antihistamines are given orally. Using only one antihistamine results in complete relief for only 10% of the patients.[127] Diphenhydramine orally 1.25 mg/kg every 6 hours is often the first oral medicine used because of its sedative effect as well as helping to control the itch. If itch is not well controlled using only one, then another class of antihistamines can be added, such as hydroxyzine 0.5/kg given orally every 6 hours. Lastly, if the itch is still not well controlled, an antiseritonic agent, such as cyproheptadine 0.1 mg/kg every 6 hours, can be added, scheduled so that one of the medications is given every 2 hours. This is targeted against the 5-HT$_3$ receptors. Care must be made to not use the cyproheptadine with patients who are on serotonergic antidepressants.

Development of Protocols for Comfort

Interest in pain management of burned patients has been a high priority in the treatment of burns only in the last 10–15 years. Several institutions have developed pain and anxiety management protocols. In 1995, the *Journal of Burn Care and Rehabilitation* published a special issue devoted to then current practices of systematic treatment of burn pain. In the first edition of this book, also in 1995, we reported the initial use of a burn pain protocol used at the Shriners Burns Hospital in Galveston.[128] In 1997 the Boston group, headed by Tompkins, published a 3-year history with a similar protocol.[70] They incorporated a distinction in treating ventilated acute patients differently from nonventilated acute patients. Most recently, a national consensus on pain management has been reached. Ulmer[129] brought these to the attention of the burn community in a 1998 article. An updated protocol currently used in the Shriners Burns Hospital in Galveston is in **Table 58.5** and includes management of the most common discomforts of burned patients.

Nonpharmacologic therapies in burned patients

As has been discussed, there is a strong interaction between psychological and physiological factors contributing to the pain experience. Anxiety in particular is prevalent among burn patients and is known to exacerbate acute pain. Nonpharmacologic therapies play an important role in addressing the psychological factors that exacerbate pain as well as having a direct impact on the pain itself.[129]

In understanding how nonpharmacologic approaches can be used with burn pain, it is important to discuss how behavioral principles contribute to the patient's experience.[131] In terms of classical (stimulus–response) conditioning, patients (particularly children) often will develop a conditioned anxiety response to stimuli associated with painful burn procedures. One study demonstrated that the simple appearance of scrubs was enough to elicit a fearful response in burn children.[132] In terms of operant (reinforcement) conditioning, patients can be thought to gain reinforcement by avoiding or escaping painful procedures, perhaps by screaming enough to terminate treatment or to obtain some sort of reinforcement from the staff by showing pain behaviors. Between the stimulus that precedes pain and the pain response that follows, there is the cognitive processing of pain. Such cognition can be modified as can behavior and influence how much pain a patient experiences. Classical and operant conditioning principles, and modifying internal cognitions have bearing on how nonpharmacologic approaches are applied to burn pain. A recent series of articles by Thurber and Martin and colleagues[133,134] provides an extensive discussion of the theory and application of such principles to pediatric wound care pain.

Classical Conditioning

If the stimuli associated with a painful procedure can be conditioned to evoke anxiety or pain, then a logical goal is to reduce the impact that pre-tubbing stimuli have on the fear/pain response. An obvious environmental intervention is to make the wound care

Table 58.5 Shriners Burns Hospital (Galveston) comfort protocol for children
Background Pain
NOTE: Begin bowel prep program simultaneously with beginning opioids
Pre-tub
First choice
PO midazolam 0.3 mg/kg and PO acetaminophen 15 mg/kg
If inadequate,
add PO morphine sulfate solution 0.3–0.6 mg/kg (if > 15 kg) or fentanyl lollipop 10 ug/kg
If NPO,
IV midazolam 0.03 mg/kg and IV morphine 0.05–0.1 mg/kg (if > 15 kg)
Pre-Rehab Therapy
On request of therapist,
PO morphine sulfate solution 0.1–0.3 mg/kg or IV morphine 0.01–0.03 mg/kg
If child is very anxious add 0.1 mg/kg diazepam or 0.03 mg/kg lorazepam
Postoperative Pain
Option A
IV morphine infusion via PCA pump (if > 5 years), total dose 10–20 mg/kg/4 hr
Option B
Attendant administered bolus, slow IV push morphine 0.02–0.05 mg/dose q 2 h (hold if level of responsiveness is decreased)
Background Pain
Oral acetaminophen 15 mg/kg q 4 h
If inadequate,
add oral morphine solution 0.1–0.3 mg/kg q 4 h or MS Contin 0.5 mg/kg PO q 8–12 h
Anxiety
lorazepam PO 0.03 mg/kg q 4–6 h
or if muscle relaxation is also desired, diazepam 0.1 mg/kg
NOTE: Taper benzodiazepines slowly by reducing dose by 50% every 2 days
Acute Stress Disorder or Post Traumatic Stress Disorder Symptoms
Imipramine 1 mg/kg or
Prozac 5 mg if under 6 years of age; for older person begin with 5 mg and increase slowly to 20 mg as needed
Itch
Use skin moistening shampoos & lotions, topical ointments (not hydrocortisone creams)
Begin with diphenhydramine PO 1.25 mg/kg q 6 h; if itch not well controlled add hydroxyzine PO 0.5/kg q 6 h; if itch still not well controlled add cyproheptadine 0.1 mg/kg q 6 hr so that one of the medications is given every 2 hrs.

procedure setting as minimally threatening as possible. For children this might involve making the hydrotherapy tank a 'bath tub play area' with age-appropriate floating toys, etc. Our understanding is that some clever children's hospital staffs have turned their

MRI scan into a 'cave in a jungle'; obviously such a setting will be less threatening to a child than will be the typical location of such radiologic procedures. Similar principles can certainly be applied to burn care.[133,134]

There are other implications of classical conditioning. The best way to prevent a conditioned pain response is to optimize pain control in the first place. By aggressively and proactively treating pain, the contributions of conditioned anxiety will be minimized. Conversely, once a patient undergoes a procedure with inadequate analgesia, concomitant anxiety can be extremely difficult to treat.

Psychological preparation plays an important role in minimizing anticipatory anxiety. Patients can be provided with procedural or sensory preparatory information.[135] With procedural-based preparatory information, patients are explained the mechanics of their procedure (e.g. 'we will unwrap your bandages, wash your wounds and debride necrotic skin and then will apply silver sulfa-diazine cream and rewrap your dressings'). With sensory informa-tion patients are prepared as to what they might feel during a procedure ('You will likely feel a pulling sensation as we remove your dressings and a stinging sensation when we wash your wounds with an antiseptic'). Such information is usually helpful to patients, but we should stress that some patients prefer to have as little information as possible, given their particular coping styles.[131]

Another approach based on classical conditioning is relaxation training. Patients can be taught deep relaxation and imagery prior to undergoing painful procedures. The rationale is to counteract the anxiety stimulated by pre-procedural stimuli with the relax-ation response. If anticipatory anxiety is minimized with deep relaxation, the potential for a cyclical interaction between anxiety and acute pain is reduced. A number of studies have applied relax-ation training and stress inoculation techniques, as well as some of the behavioral techniques discussed below to reduce burn pain.[136–140]

Operant Conditioning

The consequences that patients receive for showing pain can have implications for pain control. Since burn procedures are extremely aversive, it will be the natural tendency of patients, particularly children, to be motivated to escape such events. Staff members who allow patients to terminate procedures might be reinforcing, and potentially exacerbating, such escape behaviors. When left unchecked this process can lead to a hysterical patient that becomes combative rather than tolerating procedures. While such avoidance behavior should alert the staff that analgesia is inade-quate, it can also occasionally suggest a need for further limit set-ting. Rewarding a patient with rest once a stage of wound care is completed rather than based on pain behavior can be a useful means to minimize such escalating behavior. Again, however, the goal of a burn team should be to provide enough preparation and analgesia in a pre-emptive fashion that such problems with escape behavior do not develop in the first place.

Operant conditioning also has implications for the manner in which patients receive pain medication. When patients are med-icated in response to pain behaviors they are potentially receiving social reinforcement in terms of attention from the staff as well as the euphoric effects that the drugs might cause. This is one reason that, as mentioned earlier, it is far preferable that patients are med-icated at regular time intervals rather than on a pain basis in response to their pain complaints, which encourages them to com-plain more often in order to get the reward.[141] A similar application of operant principles is for the patient who excessively complains about pain out of emotional dependency needs, attention seeking, or euphorigenic properties of the pain medications. In such patients, provided that adequate levels of pharmacologic analgesia have indeed been established, it may be important to extinguish pain behavior by distracting the patient from pain and ignoring pain behavior. This is a model more consistent with that used for chronic pain.[142]

A final application of operant principles has to do with token economies for children. It can be extremely useful to reward chil-dren for successful completion of procedures by using star charts or reinforcement schedules of this nature. Thus, a child, upon com-pleting a procedure, may receive a star in a grid that covers a week of burn care. Older children can use an accumulation of points to purchase a desired reward. It is important that children are rewarded for completing procedures rather than for 'not scream-ing' as the latter can serve as a subtle form of punishment to chil-dren.[133,134]

Cognitive Interventions

How patients think about their pain can be regarded as a behavior that can be modified and, in turn, can influence the degree of suf-fering they experience. As such, an important nonpharmacologic approach can be to draw out the thoughts patients have about their pain and modify them accordingly. A particularly salient example is catastrophizing about pain. Catastrophizing thoughts include those such as 'I cannot stand this pain', 'I will never get better', or 'The pain means I will die'. Such catastrophizing thoughts have been associated with greater amounts of pain and less favorable health outcomes in a variety of studies. Patients can be taught to challenge and reinterpret such thoughts. Along the same lines, it can be useful to teach patients to reinterpret the meaning of their pain sensations. For example, the appearance of skin buds and enhanced pain sensation may indicate that a wound is healing and skin grafts may not be necessary.[131]

Under the rubric of cognitive interventions patients may be taught techniques to enhance their ability to cope with pain. Positive self-talk and imagery designed to facilitate coping during periods of pain are examples of this. Thurber and colleagues have described the Two-Process Model of Control as it relates to con-trolling pediatric burn pain.[134] In terms of primary control, the patient attempts to modify the objective conditions of the painful procedure, such as negotiating how and when a dressing change will take place. In secondary control, patients make adjustments so that they can better tolerate the difficult procedures (e.g. positive self-talk, catastrophizing). Thurber et al.[133] and Martin-Herz et al.[134] have recently published a two-part series on a conceptualiza-tion of psychological approaches to burn pain, as well as specific examples for treatment.

Another example of enhancing coping is to give the patient more control during painful procedures. Kavanaugh has described how giving children more control during procedures can reduce the effects of learned helplessness and enhance pain tolerance.[143] Kavanaugh reported that children who were provided with the opportunity to participate in and make decisions about their wound care showed lower depression, anxiety, hostility, and stress scores than did controls. Such findings fit well into the paradigm described by Thurber et al.[134]

Distraction is another cognitively based approach to pain control. Processing pain requires a certain amount of conscious attention and distracting such patients' attention can enable patients to tolerate pain better. Movies, music therapy and games have all been used with some success as distraction techniques for burn pain.[144,145] Music has the additional benefit of inducing a relaxation response. More recently, Hoffman and colleagues have reported on the use of virtual reality (VR) as a powerful analgesic.[145–147] Virtual reality can immerse patients' attention in a computer-generated world, and engage them in interaction with that world. These investigators indicate that VR can significantly reduce pain during wound care and physical therapy,[146,147] even relative to computer game distraction.[148]

Hypnosis

Hypnosis involves a blend of relaxation, imagery and cognitive-based approach. The technique deserves special attention because there are a number of reports on its use with burn pain and, when it is effective, its impact on burn pain can be quite dramatic. There are over a dozen anecdotal reports in the literature that indicate that hypnosis can dramatically reduce pain; such studies, however, lack control groups, standard measures of pain or information about pain medications.[149] More recently, tightly controlled studies with reliable measures of pain have supported hypnosis as an effective nonpharmacologic approach to burn pain.[150,151]

Burn patients are ideal candidates for hypnosis for a number of reasons. In a review of such factors, Patterson *et al.* listed motivation, regression, dissociation, and hypnotizability as factors that promote hypnotic analgesia on the burn unit.[148] Specifically, patients who are faced with the excruciating nature of burn pain are motivated to engage in techniques such as hypnosis. The nature of a burn and its resulting care can cause a patient to become emotionally regressed (i.e. more dependent on the burn staff) and dissociated (i.e. removed from their emotions), and both of these factors seem to be associated with hypnotizability. Such factors likely account for the frequent dramatic effects that are seen with hypnosis and burn care. On the other hand, hypnosis clearly will not benefit some burn patients, and the degree to which patients are inherently hypnotizable almost certainly has some bearing on this issue.[152]

Ewin[153,154] has strongly argued for providing hypnosis within 2–4 hours after a patient sustains a burn injury. He maintains that this approach can serve to impede the progression of the burn as well as facilitate pain control. Unfortunately it is difficult to have a clinician available during this stage of burn care, and Ewin's findings have yet to be tested in other settings. The protocol used by Patterson and colleagues[150–155] is to provide hypnosis prior to wound care and have nurses provide standard post-hypnotic suggestions during wound care. This approach is efficient for both the hypnotist and the nurses. Patterson *et al.* have recommended that hypnosis used in this fashion be an adjunct to, rather than replacement for, pain medication.[150]

Other Approaches

There is some evidence that transelectrical stimulation (TENS) can be effective with burn pain,[156] but we are aware of only one study of this nature. Massage therapy has been reported to be useful in reducing burn pain.[157] We are unaware of any studies on the efficacy of acupuncture on burn pain, although this modality has been useful with pain from a variety of different etiologies. The acute nature and variable distribution of burn pain may make acupuncture a challenging modality to apply to this problem.

For patients in the post-hospital, long-term rehabilitation phase, nonpharmacologic approaches from physical and occupational therapists become critical. Stretching, strengthening, increasing activity, and hot/cold therapy may all become instrumental in enhancing pain control during the rehabilitative stage.

Summary

The state of the art in burn pain management would seem to be based more on personal bias and tradition than on a systematic, scientific approach. As noted above, we have few studies of the pharmacokinetics of opioids and antianxiety drugs in burned patients. Martyn[64] in a review of pharmacologic studies in burned patients, describes a variety of pathophysiologic changes accompanying burn injury which can alter drug deposition. These changes include cardiovascular changes, alteration in renal and hepatic function, and fluctuations in plasma protein concentration which may render pharmacokinetic studies of nonburned patients not applicable to burned patients. In addition, the number of pharmacokinetic studies of pain-relieving drugs of any kind in young children is virtually nil. Since approximately 35% of all burn injuries occur in children under 16 years, with a great majority of these occurring in children under 2 years, we have almost no information on which to base the use of pain-relieving drugs in burned children. It is no wonder that Perry and Heidrick[158] found great disparity in what burn care staff would order or administer to a young child as compared to an adult with burns of similar size and area of distribution on the body. More pharmacokinetic studies in both adults and children with burn injuries must be initiated.

Similar to the lack of conclusive data about the use of the various opioids or anxiolytic agents, is the scarcity of scientific data to recommend any of the nonpharmacologic techniques. However, significant progress has been made just since the last edition of this book 5 years ago. Most burn centers recognize anxiety as contributing to patient discomfort and are beginning to treat both anxiety and pain. Nonpharmacologic techniques are more frequently included in a center's repertoire of tools for managing anxiety, recognized as a definite adjunct to pharmacotherapy. The major problem currently with these techniques is that they are personnel intensive and therefore are often not offered or reimbursed in the current managed care environment in the US.

How, then, can we provide the 'best' pain management for a burned patient? Probably the first answer to that question is vigilance in assessment and flexibility in treatment. Patients show great individual variation in their responses to the variety of agents and modalities presented. A successful approach with a burned patient requires that health care personnel understand the pain associated with the different depths of wounds, the phase of the healing process, and the components of the pain response. For the burned patient during the initial 3–7 days, the more superficial areas give rise to moderate or severe pain, while the full-thickness areas contribute less to the overall pain response.[2] Although moderate to severe pain is usually related to procedures or physical therapy, background pain (or pain at rest) is usually described as mild, or very mild, but may be exacerbated by emotional concerns and anxiety. By the second week postburn, the moderately deep partial-thickness burn with its multitude of skin buds accounts for the majority of the moderate to severe pain. In many burn centers, deep dermal and full-thickness burns are excised and grafted between the third and tenth days postburn. Although this often eliminates the severe pain associated with wound debridement during the second and third week, donor sites are often as painful as the areas of more superficial burns were initially. Dressing changes 3–5 days post-grafting also may be accompanied by the removal of sutures or staples which is usually described by patients as an excruciatingly painful procedure. By the third or fourth week, if the wounds are not mostly healed, anxiety and depression may cause a patient to perceive increased levels of pain. And, within a single phase of recovery and within a single patient, pain frequency and intensity will vary from day to day. A fixed and inflexible approach to treatment is likely to overmedicate on one day and undermedicate the next.

To avoid over- and undermedication in adults, regimens which allow patients to control their own therapy seem most appropriate. This is very important for adults and teenagers, but children also can benefit from having this control. PCA can be used safely by many children and should not be disregarded as a tool on the basis of age alone. For procedural pain, patient control regimens may include self-administered nitrous oxide, PCA, hypnosis, a variety of behavioral approaches, or a combination of these approaches. For background pain, the best control seems to be the use of slow-release opioids or other pain cocktails given on a nonpain contingent basis (i.e. scheduled every 4–6 hours) with the flexibility to supplement this with PRN or 'as desired' medication. Another approach would be to use PCA with or without a continuous low-dose infusion of narcotics. A variety of nonpharmacologic therapies may also help relieve background pain. The most important aspect to remember with all of these regimens, as mentioned before, is flexibility. The other obvious aspect is to remember that a patient is not only the best person to assess their pain, but is also the best to evaluate the success of the therapies provided.

Pain management for children with burns is confusing and difficult. The regimens presented in **Table 58.4**[159] may assist one to manage a burned child's pain. It is important to remember that the regimens presented are only guidelines and must be individualized according to patient response. Certain groups of children are excluded from this protocol because they require a very individualized approach. The exclusions are:

- patients with burns greater than 60% TBSA;
- children less than 12 months of age with weight less than 12 kg;
- children with respiratory difficulty for any reason;
- septic patients; and
- children of any age who are below the tenth percentile in weight for age.

Likewise, all patients are started on a bowel regimen at the time that opioids are initiated.

As challenging as managing comfort is for the health care provider, it is equally important to the burned patients. Recent studies suggest both physiologic and psychological reasons to successfully manage pain. Kavanagh et al.[160] demonstrated that pain in a burned patient adds significantly to the physiologic demands caused by stress. Schreiber and Galai-Gat[161] as well as Ptacek et al.[162] have shown that successful pain management can significantly reduce the occurrence of psychological disorders such as post-traumatic stress syndrome.

Burn care professionals who desire to keep their patients as comfortable as possible can perhaps best prepare themselves by learning to:

- watch and listen to their patients with vigilance;
- use a standardized assessment tool for measuring discomfort on a scheduled basis as well as during moments when the patient is complaining, either verbally or behaviorally, pre- and postadministration of treatment;
- know how discomforts are likely to change as the patient recovers;
- include a variety of pharmacologic and nonpharmacologic methods for managing discomforts and be prepared to change as the patients' needs change; and
- feel comfortable with a process that never ends, but which can bring many moments of relief for the patient and satisfaction for the care givers.

References

1. Beecher HK. Relationships of significance of wound to pain experience. *JAMA* 1958; **161**: 1609–12.
2. Choiniere M, Melzack R, Rondeau J, Girard N, Paquin MJ. The pain of burns: characteristics and correlates. *J Trauma* 1989; **29**: 1531–9.
3. Meyer RA, Campbell JN. Myelinated nociceptive afferent account for hyperalgesia that follows a burn to the hand. *Science* 1981; **213**: 1527–9.
4. Campbell JN, Meyer RA, Roya SN. Hyperalgesia: new insights. *Pain* 1984; **Suppl 2**: Abstract 3.
5. Coderre T, Melzack R. Increase pain sensitivity following heat injury involves a central mechanism. *Behav Brain Res* 1985; **15**: 259–62.
6. Charlton JE, Klein R, Gagliardi G. Factors affecting pain in burned patients: a preliminary report. *Postgrad Med* 1983; **59**: 604–7.
7. Klein RM, Charlton JE. Behavioral observation and analysis of pain behavior in critically burned patients. *Pain* 1980; **9**: 27–40.
8. Perry S, Heidrich G, Ramos E. Assessment of pain by burn patients. *J Burn Care Rehabil* 1981; **2**: 322–6.
9. Atchison NE, Osgood PE, Carr DB, Szyfelbein SK. Pain during burn dressing change in children: relationship to burn area, depth and analgesia regimens. *Pain* 1991; **47**: 41–5.
10. Andreasen NJC, Noyes R, Hartford CE, Bordland G, Proctor S. Management of the emotional reactions in seriously burned adults. *N Engl J Med* 1972; **286**: 65–9.
11. West DA, Shuck JM. Emotional problems of the severely burned patient. *Surg Clin N Am* 1978; **58**: 1189–204.
12. Goodstein RK. Burns: an overview of the clinical consequences afflicting patient, staff and family. *Compr Psychiatry* 1985; **26**: 43–57.
13. Savedra M. Coping with pain: strategies of severely burned children. *Canadian Nurse* 1977; **73**: 28–9.
14. Beales JG. Factors influencing the expectation of pain among patients in a children's burn unit. *Burns* 1983; **9(3)**: 187–92.
15. Mannon JM. *Caring for the Burned: Life and Death in a Hospital Burn Center.* Springfield, IL: CC Thomas, 1985.
16. Ponten B. Grafted skin: observations on innervation and other qualities. *Acta Clin Scan (Suppl)* 1960; **257**: 1–5.
17. Freund PR, Brengelmann, GL, Rowell LB, *et al.* Vasomotor control in healed grafted skin in humans. *J Appl Physiol* 1981; **51**: 168–71.
18. Gracley RH. Pain measurement. *Acta Anaesthesi Scand* 1999; **43(9)**: 897–908.
19. Melzack R. The McGill Pain Questionnaire: major properties and scoring methods. *Pain* 1975; **1**: 277–99.
20. Gordon M, Greenfield E, Marvin J, Hester C, Lauterbach S. Use of pain assessment Tools: Is there a preference? *J Burn Care Rehabil* 19(5): 451–4.
21. Grossi E, Broghi C, Cerchiari EL. Analogic Chromatic Continuous Scale (ACCS): a new method for pain assessment. *Clin Rheumatol* 1983; **1**: 337–40.
22. Wong D, Baker C. Pain in children: comparison of assessment scales. *Pediatr Nurs* 1988; **14**: 9–17.
23. Anand KJS, Sippel WG, Aynsley-Green A. Randomized trial of fentanyl anesthesia in preterm neonates undergoing surgery: effects on the stress response. *Lancet* 1987; **1**: 243–8.

24. Anand KJS, Aynsley-Green A. Does the newborn infant require potent anesthesia during surgery? Answers from a randomized trial of halothane anesthesia. In: Dubner R, Gebhart G, Bond M, eds. *Pain Research and Clinical Management* Vol. 3: Amsterdam: Elsevier, 1988: 329–35.

25. Anand KJS, Hickey PR. Pain and its effects in the human neonate and fetus. *N Engl J Med* 1987; **317**: 1321–9.

26. Attia J, Amiel-Tison C, Mayer N-N, *et al.* Measurement of postoperative pain and narcotics administration in infants using a new clinical scoring system. *Anesthesiology* 1987; **67**: A532.

27. Szyfelbein SK, Osgood PF, Carr DB. The assessment of pain and plasma B-endorphin immunoactivity in burned children. *Pain* 1985; **22**: 173–82.

28. Williamson PS, Williamson ML. Physiologic stress reduction by a local anesthetic during newborn circumcision. *Pediatrics* 1983; **71**: 36–40.

29. Fuller B. FM signals in infant vocalizations. *Cry* 1985; **6**: 5–10.

30. Fuller B, Horii Y. Differences in fundamental frequency, jitter and shimmer among four types of infant vocalizations. *J Commun Dis* 1986; **18**: 111–8.

31. Fuller B, Horii Y. Spectral energy distribution in four types of infant vocalizations. *J Commun Dis* 1988; **20**: 111–21.

32. Franck LS. A new method to quantitatively describe pain behavior in infants. *Nurse Res* 1986; **35**: 28–31.

33. Granau RVE, Craig KD. Pain expression in neonates: facial action and cry. *Pain* 1987; **28**: 395–410.

34. Johnston C, O'Shaughnessy D. Acoustical attributes of infant pain cries: discriminating features. In: Dubner R, Gebhart G, Bond M, eds. *Pain Research and Clinical Management*, Vol. 3. Amsterdam: Elsevier, 1988: 341–7.

35. Izard CE, Heubner RR, Risser D, *et al.* The young infant's ability to produce discrete emotional expressions. *Dcu Psychol* 1980; **19**: 132–40.

36. Craig KD, McMahon RJ, Morison JD, Zaskow C. Developmental changes in infant pain expression during immunization injections. *Soc Sci Med* 1984; **19**: 1331–7.

37. Johnston CC, Strada ME. Acute pain response in infants: a multidimensional description. *Pain* 1986; **24**: 373–82.

38. Katz ER, Kellerman J, Siegel SE. Behavioral distress in children with cancer undergoing medical procedures: developmental considerations. *J Consult Clin Psychol* 1980; **48**: 356–65.

39. Mills N, Preston A. Acute pain behaviors in infants/toddlers. In: Funk S, Tomquist E, Champagne M, *et al.* eds. *Key Aspects of Comfort: Management of Pain, Fatigue and Nausea.* New York: Springer, 1989; 52–9.

40. McGrath PJ, Johnson G, Goodman JT, Schillinger J, Dunn J, Chapman JA. CHEOPS: a behavioral scale for rating postoperative pain in children. In: Fields HL, Dubner R, Cerrera F, eds. *Advances in Pain Research and Therapy.* New York: Raven Press, 1985: 395–402.

41. Tyler DC, Tu A, Douthit J, Chapman CR. Toward validation of pain measurement tools for children: a pilot study. *Pain* 1993; **52**: 301–9.

42. Barone M, McCall J, Jenkins M, Warden G. The Development of a Observational Pain Scale (OPAS) for Pediatric Burns. Abst 230. Presented at the 32nd Annual Meeting of the American Burn Assoc, Las Vegas, Nevada, March 14–17, 2000.

43. Beyer J, Aradine C. Content validity of an instrument to measure young children's perceptions of the intensity of their pain. *Pediatr Nurs* 1986; **1**: 386–95.

44. Beyer J, Aradine C. Patterns of pediatric pain intensity: a methodological investigation of self-report scale. *Clin J Pain* 1987; **3**: 130–41.

45. Beyer J, Aradine C. The convergent and discriminant validity of a self report measure of pain intensity for children. *Children's Health Care* 1981; **16**: 274–82.

46. McGrath PA, de Veber L, Hearn M. Multidimensional pain assessment in children. In: Fields H, Dubner R, Cerrera F, eds. *Advances in Pain Research and Therapy*, New York: Raven Press, 1985: 387–93.

47. Maunuksela EL, Ollskola KT, Korpela R. Measurement of pain in children with self-reporting and behavioral assessment. *Clin Pharma Ther* 1987; **42**: 137–41.

48. Bieri D, Reeve RA, Champion GD, Addicoat L, Zeigler JB. The face pain scale for the self-assessment of the severity of pain experienced by children: development, initial validation, and preliminary investigation of ratio scale properties. *Pain* 1980; **41**: 139–60.

49. Hester NO. The pre-operational child's reaction to immunization. *Nurse Res* 1979; **28**: 250–4.

50. Varni JW, Thompson KL, Hanson V. The Varni/Thompson Pediatric Pain Questionnaire. In Chronic musculoskeletal pain in juvenile arthritis. *Pain* 1987; **28**: 23–38.

51. Eland J. Minimizing pain associated with pre-kindergartner intra muscular injections. *Issues Compr Pediatr Nurs* 1981; **5**: 361–72.

52. Szyfelbein SK, Osgood PF, Murphy JL, Atchison NE. Comparison of fentanyl plasma levels and pain scores in burn children. Abst 107. Presented at the 17th Annual Meeting of the American Burn Association, March 27–30, 1985, Orlando, Florida.

53. McGrath PJ, Unruh AM. *Pain in Children and Adolescents.* Amsterdam: Elsevier, 1987: 351.

54. Sevedra M, Gibbons P, Tesler M, *et al.* How do children describe pain? A tentative assessment. *Pain* 1982; **14**: 95–104.

55. LeBaron S, Zettzer L. Assessment of acute pain and anxiety in children and adolescents by self-report, observer reports, and behavior checklist. *J Consult Clin Psychol* 1984; **52**: 729–38.

56. Beyer J, Wells N. The assessment of pain in children. *Pediatr Clin N Am* 1987; **36**: 837–54.

57. Robert R, Blakeney P, Villarreal C, Meyer WJ. Anxiety: current practices in assessment and treatment of anxiety of burn patients. *Burns* 2000 (in press).

58. Siverman W, Kurtines W. *Anxiety and Phobic Disorders: A Pragmatic Approach.* New York: Plenum Press: 1996.

59. Walk RD. Self-ratings of fear in a fear invoking situation. *J Abnorm Social Psychol* 1956; **52**: 171–8.

60. Field T, Peck M, Hernandez-Reif M, Krugman S, Burman I, Ozment-Schenck L. Postburn itching, pain, and psychological symptoms are reduced with massage therapy. *J Burn Care Rehabil* 2000; **21**: 189–93.

61. Blakeney P, Marvin J. Itch Man Scale. Shriners Hospitals for Children, 2000.

62. Duinslaeger LAY, Verbeken G, Vanhalle S, Vanderkelen A. Cultured allogeneic keratinocyte sheets accelerate healing compared to op site treatment of donor sites in burns. *J Burn Care Rehabil* 1997; **18**: 545–51.

63. Marvin JA, Heimbach DM. Pain management. In: Fisher SV, Helm PA, eds. *Comprehensive Rehabilitation of Burns.* Baltimore: Williams and Wilkins, 1984: 311–28.

64. Martyn JAS. Clinical pharmacology and drug therapy in the burn patient. *Anesthesiology* 1986; **65**: 67–75.

65. Mackersie RC, Karaglanes TG. Pain management following trauma and burns. *Anesthesiol Clin N Am* 1989; **7**: 211–19.

66. Osgood PF, Szyfelbein SK. Management of burn pain in children. *Pediatr Clin N Am* 1989; **36**: 1001–13.

67. Ahremolz DH, Solem LD. Management of pain after thermal injury. *Adv Clin Rehabil* 1987; **1**: 215–29.

68. Judkin KD. Pain control in burns. *Clin Anaesth* 1987; **1**: 635–48.

69. Ross DM, Ross SA. *Childhood Pain: Current Issues, Research and Management.* Baltimore: Urban & Schwarzenberg, 1988; 259–73.

70. Sheridan RL, Hinson M, Nackel A, *et al.* Development of a pediatric burn pain and anxiety management program. *J Burn Care Rehabil* 1997; **18**: 455–9.

71. MacLennan N, Heimbach DM, Cullen BF. Anesthesia for major thermal injury. *Anesthesiology* 1998; **89**: 749–70

72. Beushausen T, Mucke K. Anesthesia and pain management in pediatric burn patients. *Pediatr Surg Int* 1997; **12**: 327–33.

73. Wilson GR, Tomlinson P. Pain relief in burns – how we do it. *Burns* 1988; **14**: 331–2.

74. Hedderich R, Ness TJ. Analgesia for trauma and burns. *Crit Care Clin* 1999; **15**: 167–84.

75. Gibbons J, Honari SR, Sharar SR, Patterson DR, Dimick PL, Heimbach DM. Opiate-induced respiratory depression in young pediatric burn patients. *J Burn Care Rehabil* 1998; **19**: 225–9.

76. Lynn AM, Slattery JT. Morphine pharmacokinetics in early infancy. *Anesthesiology* 1987; **66**: 136–9.

77. Thomas C, Brazeal B, Behrends L, *et al. Phantom Limb Sensation and Pain in Youth Burn Survivors,* 9th Congress of the European Burn Association, 2001 Lyon, France.

78. Beausan E, Orr D, Shah M, Dunn KW, Davenport PJ. Subcutaneous adrenalin infiltration in pediatric burn surgery. *Br J Plastic Surg* 1999; **52**: 480–1.

79. Pedersen JL, Rung GW, Kehlet H. Effect of sympathetic nerve block on acute inflammatory pain and hyperalgesia. *Anesthesiology* 1197; **86**: 293–301.

80. Jonsson A, Cassuto J, Hanson B. Inhibition of burn pain by intravenous lidocaine infusion. *Lancet* 1991; **338**: 151.

81. Pedersen JL, Callesen T, Moiniche S, Kehlet H. Analgesic and anti-inflammatory effects of lignocaine-prilocaine (EMLA) cream in human burn injury. *Br J Anaesthesiol* 1996; **76**: 806–10.

82. Wehner D, Hamilton GC. Seizures following application of local anesthetics to burn patients. *Ann Emerg Med* 1984; **13**: 456–8.

83. Berde CB, Beyer JE, Bournaki MC, Levin CR, Sethna NF. Comparison of morphine and methadone for prevention of postoperative pain in 3 to 7 year old children. *J Pediatr* 1994; **119**: 136–41.

84. Perry SW, Inturrisi LE. Analgesia and morphine deposition in burn patients. *J Burn Care Rehabil* 1983; **4**: 276–9.

85. Bloedow DC, Goodfellow LA, Marvin J, Heimbach D. Meperidine disposition in burn patients. *Res Commun Chem Pathol Pharmacol* 1986; **54**: 87–9.

86. Novoa J. Large dose morphine for pain control. Presented at the 12th Annual Meeting of the American Burn Association, San Antonio, Texas, March 27–29, 1980.

87. Sandidge CH, Marvin JA. Methadone therapy in treating non-procedural pain in burn patients. Presented at the 18th Annual Meeting of the American Burn Association, Chicago. Illinois, April 9–12, 1986.

88. Concilius R, Denson DD, Knarr D, Warden G, Raj PP. Continuous intravenous infusion of methadone for control of burn pain. *J Burn Care Rehabil* 1989; **10**(5): 406–9.

89. Lee JJ, Marvin JA, Heimbach DM. Effectiveness of nalbuphine for relief of burn debridement pain. *J Burn Care Rehabil* 1989; **10**(3): 241–6.

90. Sandidge CH, Marvin JA, Heimbach DM. Patient controlled analgesia (PCA) in treating pain in burn patients. Presented at the 19th Annual Meeting of the American Burn Association, Washington, DC, April 29-May 2, 1987.

91. Wolman RL, Lasecki MH, Alexander LA, Lutemlan A. Clinical trial of patient controlled analgesia in burn patients. Presented at the 19th Annual Meeting of the American Burn Association, Washington, DC, April 29-May 2, 1987.

92. Kinsella J, Galvin R, Reid WH. Patient-controlled analgesia for burn patients: a preliminary report. *Burns Incl Therm Inj* 1988; **14**(6): 500–3.

93. Krauss B, Green SM. Sedation and analgesia for procedures in children. *N Engl J Med* 2000; **13**: 938–56.

94. Mather LE, Phillips GD. Opioids and adjuvants: principles of use. *Clin Crit Care Med* 1986; **8**: 77–103.

95. Sharar SR, Bratton SL, Carrougher GJ, et al. A comparison of oral transmucosal fentanyl citrate and oral hydomorphone for inpatient pediatric burn wound care analgesia. *J Burn Care Rehabil* 1998; **19**: 516–21.

96. Lyons B, Casey W, Doherty P, McHugh M, Moore KP. Pain relief with low dose intravenous clonidine in a child with severe burns. *Intensive Care Med* 1996; **22**: 249–51.

97. Wallace BH, Caldwell FT, Cone JB. Ibuprofen lowers body temperature and metabolic rate of humans with burn injury. *J Trauma* 1992; **32**: 154–7.

98. Cone JB, Wallace BH, Olsen KM, Caldwell FT, Gurley BJ, Bond PJ. The pharmacokinetics of ibuprofen after burn injury. *J Burn Care Rehabil* 1993; **14**: 666–9.

99. Bradly JA, Brandt KD, Katz BP, Kalasinski LA, Ryan SI. Comparison of an inflammatory dose of ibuprofen, an analgesic dose of ibuprofen, and acetaminophen in the treatment of patients with osteoarthritis of the knee. *N Engl J Med* 1191; **325**: 87–91.

100. Temple AR. Pediatric dosing of acetaminophen. *Pediatr Pharmacol* 1983; **3**: 321–7.

101. Meyer WJ, Nichols RJ, Cortiella J, et al. Acetaminophen in the management of background pain in children post-burn. *J Pain Symptom Management* 1997; **13**: 50–5.

102. Meyer WJ, Brown A, Villarreal C et al. *Evolution of a Pain Protocol over a six year period.* 33rd Annual Meeting-American Burn Association, 2001 Boston, MA.

103. Martyn JAJ, Greenblatt DJ. Lorazepam conjugation unimpaired in burn patients. (Abst) *Anesthesiology* 1985; **63**: A 113.

104. Patterson DR, Ptacek JT, Carrougher GJ, Sharar SR. Lorazepam as an adjunct to opioid analgesics in the treatment of burn pain. *Pain* 1997; **72**: 367–74.

105. Martyn JAJ, Greenblatt DS, Quinby WC. Diazepam kinetics following burns. *Anesth Analg* 1983; **62**: 293–7.

106. Stanford GK. Postbum delirium associated with use of intravenous lorazepam. *J Burn Care Rehabil* 1988; **9**(2): 160–1.

107. Greenblatt DJ, Locniskar A, Ochs HR, Lauren PM. Automated gas chromatography for studies of midazolam pharmacokinetics. *Anesthesiology* 1981; **55**: 176–9.

108. McClure JH, Brown DT, Wildsmith JAW. Comparison of the IV administration of midazolam and diazepam as sedation during spinal anaesthesia. *Br J Anaesth* 1983; **55**: 1089–93.

109. Driessen JJ, Booij LH, Vree TB, Crul JE. Midazolam as a sedative on regional anesthesia. *Arzneim Forscl V Drug Res* 1981; **31**: 2245–7.

110. Brophy T, Dundee JW, Heazelwood V, Kawar P, Varghese A, Ward M. Midazolam, a water-soluble benzodiazepine for gastroscopy. *Anaesth Intensive Care* 1982; **10**: 334–47.

111. Baskett PJE, Hyland J, Deane M, et al. Analgesia for patient dressing in children. *Br J Anaesth* 1969; **41**: 684–8.

112. Baskett PJE. Analgesia for the dressing of burns in children: a method using neuroleptanalgesia and Entonox. *Postgrad Med J* 1972; **48**: 138–42.

113. Filkin SA, Cosgrav P, Marvin JA, et al. Self-administered anesthesia: a method of pain control. *J Burn Care Rehabil* 1981; **2**: 33–4.

114. Marvin JA, Engrav LH, Heimbach DM. Self-administered nitrous oxide analgesia for debridement: a five year experience. Presented at the 16th Annual Meeting of the American Burn Association, San Francisco, California, April 11–14, 1984.

115. Layzer RH. Myeloneuropathy after prolonged exposure to nitrous oxide. *Lancet* 1978; **2**: 1227–30.

116. Layzer RB, Fishman RA, Schafer JA. Neuropathy following abuse of nitrous oxide. *Neurology* 1978; **28**: 504–6.

117. Paulson GW. Recreational misuse of nitrous oxide. *J Am Dent Assoc* 1979; **98**: 410–11.

118. Hayden PJ, Hartemink RJ, Nicholson GA. Myeloneuropathy due to nitrous oxide. *Burns* 1983; **9**(4): 267–70.

119. Slogoff S, Allen GW, Wessels JV, Cheney DH. Clinical experience with subanesthetic ketamine. *Anesth Analg Curr Res* 1974; **53**(3): 354–8.

120. Martinez S, Achauer B, Dobkin de Rios M. Ketamine use in a burn center: hallucinogen or debridement facilitator? *J Psychoactive Drugs* 1985; **17**(1): 45–9.

121. Handrop M, Spinella J. Ketamine: featured protocol. *J Burn Care Rehabil* 1987; **8**(2): 148–9.

122. Parker J. Ketamine: review of featured protocol. *J Burn Care Rehabil* 1987; **8**(2): 149.

123. Martyn JAJ. Ketamine pharmacology and therapeutics. *J Burn Care Rehabil* 1987; **8**(2): 146–48.

124. Dimick P, Helvig E, Heimbach D, Marvin JA, Coda B, Edward WT. Anesthesia assisted procedures in a burn intensive care unit procedure room: benefits and complications. *J Burn Care Rehabil* 1993; **14**: 446–9.

125. Cravero JP, Manzi DJ, Rice LJ. The management of procedure-related pain in the child. In: Ashburn MA, Rice LJ, eds. *The Management of Pain*. New York: Churchill Livingstone, 1998.

126. Odom RB, James WD, Berger TG. Pruritus and neurocutaneous dermatoses. In: *Andrews' Diseases of the Skin* New York: WB, Saunders, 2000.

127. Vitale M, Fields-Blache C, Luterman A. Severe itching in the patient with burns. *J Burn Care Rehabil* 1991; **12**: 330–3.

128. Marvin JA, Muller MJ, Blakeney PE, Meyer WJ. Pain response and pain control In: Herndon DN, ed. *Total Burn Care*. Philadelphia: Saunders, 1996.

129. Ulmer JF. Burn Pain Management: A Guideline-bases approach. *J Burn Care Rehabil* 1998; **19**: 151–9.

130. Patterson, D, Sharar S. Burn pain. In: Loeser J. ed. *Bonica's Management of Pain*, 3rd edn. Philadelphia: Lippincot, Williams & Wilkins, 2001: 776–83.

131. Patterson DR. Nonopioid based approaches to burn pain. *J Burn Care Rehabil* 1995; **16**(3): 372–6.

132. Meyer D. Children's responses to nursing attire. *Pediatr Nurs* 1992; **18**: 157–60.

133. Martin-Herz SP, Thurber CA, Patterson DR. Psychological principles of burn wound pain in children: Part II: Treatment applications. *J Burn Care Rehabil* (In Press).

134. Thurber CA, Martin-Herz SP, Patterson DR. Psychological principles of burn wound pain in children: Part I: Theoretical framework. *J Burn Care Rehabil* (in press).

135. Everett JJ, Patterson DR, Chen AC. Cognitive and behavioral treatments for burn pain. *The Pain Clin* 1990; **3**(3): 133–45.

136. Cromes GF, McDonald M, Robinson C. The effects of relaxation training on anxiety and pain during burn wound debridement. Presented at the 12th Annual Meeting of the American Burn Association, San Antonio, Texas, 1980.

137. Fagerhaugh SY. Pain expression and control on a burn care unit. *Nurs Outlook* 1974; **22**(10): 645–50.

138. Knudson-Cooper MS. Relaxation and biofeedback training in the treatment of severely burned children. *J Burn Care Rehabil* 1981; **2**(2).

139. Kueffner M. Passage through hospitalization of severely burned, isolated school-age children. *Commun Nurs Res* 1976; **7**: 181–97.

140. Wernick RL, Jaremko ME, Taylor PW. Pain management in severely burned adults: a test of stress inoculation. *J Behav Med* 1981; **4**(1): 103–9.

141. Melzack R. The tragedy of needless pain. *Sci Am* 1990; **262**(2): 27–33.

142. Fordyce WE. *Behavioral Methods for Chronic Pain and Illness*. St Louis: Mosby Year Book, 1976.

143. Kavanagh CK, Lasoff E, Eide Y, et al. Learned helplessness and the pediatric burn patient: dressing change behavior and serum cortisol and B-endorphin. *Adv Pediatr* 1991; **38**: 335–63.

144. Elliott CH, Olson RA. The management of children's distress in response to painful medical treatment for burn injuries. *Behav Res Therapy* 1983; **21**(6): 675–683.

145. Kelley ML, Jarvie GJ, Middlebrook JL, McNeer MF, Drabman RS. Decreasing burned children's pain behavior: impacting the trauma of hydrotherapy. *J Appl Behav Anal* 1984; **17**(2): 147–58.

146. Hoffman H, Patterson D, Nakamora D, et al. Use of virtual reality for adjunctive treatment of adult burn pain during physical therapy: A case study. *Int J Human-Computer Interaction* (in press-a).

147. Hoffman HG, Patterson DR, Carrougher GJ. Use of virtual reality for adjunctive treatment of adult burn pain during physical therapy: A controlled study. *Clin J Pain* (in press-b).

148. Hoffman HG, Doctor JN, Patterson DR, Carrougher GJ, Furness TA III. Use of virtual reality for adjunctive treatment of adolescent burn pain during wound care: A case report. *Pain* 2000; **85**: 305–9.

149. Patterson DR, Questad KA, Boltwood MD. Hypnotherapy as a treatment for pain in patients with burns: Research and clinical considerations. *J Burn Care Rehabil* 1987; **8**(3): 263–8.

150. Patterson DR, Everett JJ, Burns GL, Marvin JA. Hypnosis for the treatment of burn pain. *J Consul Clin Psychol* 1992; **60(5)**: 713–7.

151. Patterson DR, Ptacek JT. Baseline pain as a moderator of hypnotic analgesia for burn injury treatment. *J Consul Clin Psychol* 1997; **65(1)**: 60–7.

152. Patterson DR, Adcock RJ, Bombardier CH. Factors predicting hypnotic analgesia in clinical burn pain. *Int J Clin Exper Hypn* 1997; **45(4)**: 377–95.

153. Ewin DM. (1983). Emergency room hypnosis for the burned patient. *Am J Clin Hypn* 1983; **26(1)**: 5–8.

154. Ewin DM. Hypnosis in surgery and anesthesia. In: Wester WC, II Smith AH Jr, eds. *Clinical Hypnosis: A Multidisciplinary Approach.* Philadelphia: JB Lippincot, 1984.

155. Patterson DR, Questad KA, DeLateur BJ. Hypnotherapy as an adjunct to narcotic analgesia for the treatment of pain for burn debridement. *Am J Clin Hypn* 1989; **31(3)**: 156–63.

156. Kimball KL, Drews JE, Walker S, Dimick AR. (1987). Use of TENS for pain reduction in burn patients. *J Burn Care Rehabil* 1987; **8(1)**: 28–31.

157. Field T, Peck M, Krugman S, *et al.* Burn injuries benefit from massage therapy. *J Burn Care Rehabil* 1998; **19(3)**: 241–4.

158. Perry S, Heidrick G. Management of pain during debridement: a survey of US burn units. *Pain* 1982; **13**: 267–80.

159. Meyer WJ, Marvin JA, Villereal C, Blakeney PE, Roberts R, Thomas C. Protocol for pain management. Personal communication.

160. Kavanaugh CK, Lasoft E, Eide Y, *et al.* Learned helplessness and the pediatric burn patient: dressing change behavior and serum cortisol and beta endorphins. *Adv Pediatr* 1991; **38**: 335–63.

161. Schneiber S, Galai-Gat T. Uncontrolled pain following physical injury as the core trauma in post traumatic stress disorder. *Pain* 1993; **54**: 107–10.

162. Ptacek JT, Panerson DR, Montgomery B, Ordonez NA, Heimbach DM. The relationship between pain during hospitalization and disability at one month post burn. Abst 46. Presented at the 26th Annual Meeting of the American Burn Association, Orlando, Florida, April 20–29, 1994.

Chapter 59

Psychiatric disorders associated with burn injury

Christopher R Thomas, Walter J Meyer III

Patricia E Blakeney

Introduction

The knowledge and skills of a psychiatrist are often needed in the pharmacologic management of psychiatric symptoms which commonly occur in conjunction with burn injuries.[1] Psychiatric expertise is also an asset to a burn team in addressing multitudes of psychological issues concomitant to burn injuries. Although a psychiatrist is usually sought as a consultant, a psychiatrist is most helpful to patients and to burn teams as an integrated member of the medical staff.

Preexisting psychiatric disorders are relatively common in the histories of burned patients, and frequently appear to have contributed significantly to the etiology of the injury itself.[2-6] Substance abuse,[7] organic brain dysfunction, attention deficit hyperactivity disorder, conduct disorder, and personality disorders have been reported as frequently occurring premorbid conditions. One study found alcohol use disorder in 11% of hospitalized burn patients with almost all of those injuries considered preventable.[8] Patients intoxicated at the time of burn injury also suffer a higher rate of complications in their treatment.[9] Those abusing flammable inhalants are at particular risk for burn injury.[10-12] A small, but important, number of patients are admitted with serious burn injuries resulting from purposeful self-immolation.[13-16] In one study of 67 patients with self-inflicted burns, 75% had a prior psychiatric illness and 20% had a previous suicide attempt.[17] A separate study of 11 patients with self-inflicted burns reported that 10 had a prior psychiatric illness, with two attempting suicide and two motivated by hallucinations.[18] Of patients with self-inflicted burns, those attempting suicide are more likely to have larger burns and longer hospitalizations than those with the intent of self-mutilation.[19] As described by Stoddard and Cabners[15] and by Raskind,[20] burn patients with suicidal intent present emotional, as well as physical, challenges to a treatment team. A suspected suicide attempt will almost invariably elicit requests for psychiatric involvement in management and treatment of a patient. Less dramatic indicators of premorbid psychiatric disorders are also identifiable early in a patient's admission and signal the need for psychiatric consultation. Burn patients with a history of any premorbid psychiatric disorders are more likely to have preventable injuries,[21] require longer hospitalization,[22] and have problems with adjustment early in their recovery.[23,24] The risk of psychiatric complications following burn injury is greater in those patients with a previous history of affective, alcohol or substance use disorders.[25] It is therefore important to screen for any preexisting psychiatric disturbance in burn patients.

In addition to premorbid psychiatric illness, other psychological factors have been found to be associated with an increased risk for psychiatric symptoms following burn injury. Taal and Faber[26] reported that dissociation and anxiety experienced during the burn injury predicted later psychopathology. Tedstone and colleagues[27] found that certain coping styles were predictive of later psychological difficulties. Patients with coping patterns of helplessness, emotion-focused, problem-focused, focusing on the positive, and seeking social support were all at increased risk for subsequent emotional distress. A coping style of acceptance appears to be a protective factor against later anxiety and post-traumatic distress symptoms. While it is understandable to expect patients with major burns to be at risk, even minor burns can result in significant psychological distress and psychiatric symptoms.[28] At the present time, there is no profile that can reliably predict which patients will suffer psychiatric symptoms following burn injury. All patients should be carefully assessed as part of their care.

This chapter will focus on the psychiatric treatment of common mental disturbances that can be expected to occur as part of a symptom complex experienced by any patient who is suffering a serious burn injury. Although preexisting psychopathology alters the expression of a patient's distress and complicates medical management of the patient, the common symptoms described in this chapter are not necessarily indicative of premorbid psychopathology. These symptoms can be very distressing to patient, family, and staff if not well managed by both psychological and pharmacological interventions. The most commonly occurring psychiatric symptoms discussed in this chapter are delirium, organic psychoses, burn encephalopathy, post-traumatic symptoms, sleep disturbances, pain, and depression, which occur during the critical care phase of burn treatment. Psychiatric problems are often noted as part of the long-term process of recovery from burn injury, i.e. phobias and other anxiety disorders, acute stress disorder, post-traumatic stress disorder, major depression, and dysthymia.

Common psychiatric symptoms

Critical Care Phase

Delirium, organic psychoses, and burn encephalopathy

Organic factors and premorbid conditions contribute to symptoms during the initial part of treatment. Disorientation, confusion, sleep disturbance, transient psychosis, and delirium are commonly observed among adolescent and adult patients.[3,29–32] Causes of these symptoms are usually unclear and multifactorial. Hypertension, hypoglycemia, electrolyte imbalance, sepsis, and/or a variety of organic problems can contribute to delirium. The unusual physical surroundings of an intensive care unit heighten the probability of psychoses. The altered state of consciousness may be transitory, wax and wane over several days, or, with large burns, persist for weeks. The picture may be confused further by a suspected occurrence of anoxia. Delirium has been found to occur more often in males who have a history of substance abuse and with burn injuries over 30% total body surface area (TBSA).[30] A past history of substance abuse is often suspected as contributing to delirium, particularly with adolescent and adult patients. Inhalant abuse or intoxication at the time of a fire are factors to be considered. Another potential cause of disorientation, hallucinations, and agitation may be medications used in the treatment of the acute burn patient. Morton and colleagues[33] reported severe psychotic symptoms in a patient following treatment with anabolic steroids.

In an altered state of consciousness, patients may misinterpret their surroundings, resulting in potentially frightening illusions of reality. Patients may misperceive lines and hoses as snakes. A patient may shout about the fire or the accident, describe symbols of death, monsters, or the devil. A patient may misidentify the people in the room, seeing instead absent friends or dead people, or may identify a treatment team as prison guards. The content of the illusions or hallucinations may be so bizarre and morbid as to suggest a schizophrenia, a brief reactive psychosis, or a psychotic depression (e.g. dead bodies, dead people, or angels). Sometimes patients are so frightened by these visions that they try to escape or become combative. Such psychotic symptoms are understandably frightening to the family of the patient and disconcerting to even experienced staff. Hallucinations are uncommon in children, but when they do occur, the most likely cause is stress, followed by pain and medications.[34] While less frequent, sepsis and metabolic condition have also resulted in hallucinations in young burn patients.

In our experience, symptoms of delirium and transient psychosis

occur rarely among children under the age of 10 years;[32] however, burn encephalopathy, as characterized by lethargy, withdrawal, or coma, is a condition observed in children as well as adults.[35,36] EEGs in such cases typically reveal diffuse, nonspecific slow waves.[35,37] Causative factors probably are the same as those for delirium.[38] Although Andreasen et al.[39] report long-term neurological impairment following burn delirium in adults, other studies (and our own experience) do not find residual neurological effects following delirium or encephalopathy.[29–32,35,36] These symptoms, though apparently short-lived, are upsetting to a patient's family and treatment team when they do occur. Proper treatment must first address organic causes of delirium and/or encephalopathy. Vital signs must be stabilized and blood chemistries and glucose normalized. Also, oxygenation should be checked and sepsis investigated and treated. Pain must be addressed. Then psychotropic medications may be administered.

The use of antipsychotic phenothiazines in an acute burn unit is a common approach to address delirium and/or combative, uncooperative behavior such as pulling off dressings, attempting to get out of bed, or striking out at care takers.[40–43]

Pharmacologic control is preferable to physical restraints which tend to exacerbate a patient's distress and worsen the symptoms.[1] Haloperidol (Haldol) is the phenothiazine of choice, as it does not have significant cholinergic side-effects. The initial does is 1 or 2 mg of haloperidol, but doses as high as 5 or 10 mg may be administered. Since phenothiazines do not cause respiratory depression, they may be repeated hourly until symptoms begin to come under control. Usually, phenothiazines are administered in two or three doses per day.

Chlorpromazine (Thorazine) and thioridazine (Mellaril) may be used in place of haloperidol in the dosage range of 25–100 mg per dose. Chlorpromazine and thioridazine have strong sedative effects and interfere with learning, but are less likely than haloperidol to produce associated dystonia, pseudo-Parkinsonism, and akathisia. If more than 2 mg of haloperidol per day are used, attention must be given to simultaneous administration of 1 or 2 mg/day of benztropine (Cogentin) or 2–5 mg/day of trihexyphenidyl (Artane) in divided doses. Benztropine or trihexyphenidyl are used to avoid dystonia, pseudo-Parkinsonism, and akathisia.[41] Occasionally, dystonia takes the form of an oculogyric crisis, which resembles an acute neurological catastrophe[44] and can be a true medical emergency if respiration is impaired. These reactions are usually alleviated by 50 mg intravenous diphenhydramine (Benadryl).

There are two severe side-effects for which the patients on phenothiazine must be monitored: neuroleptic malignant syndrome[45] and tardive dyskinesia.[41] Neuroleptic malignant syndrome is a potentially life-threatening crisis characterized by fever, muscle rigidity, mental status changes, and autonomic dysfunction. Neuroleptics should be discontinued, and symptoms must be treated aggressively with supportive therapy, as well as benzodiazepines, dantrolene, bromocriptine, and anticholinergics. The long-term side-effect of greatest concern for patients who receive phenothiazine is tardive dyskinesia. This reaction can be permanent and is characterized by abnormal, involuntary, irregular choreiform, and athetoid movements. Usually, a patient is unaware of the writhing and twisting movements that most often involve the tongue, but can also involve the limbs and the trunk as well. The reaction typically occurs only in individuals who have received phenothiazines for extended periods of time, i.e. longer than 6 months. The risk of occurrence is 2–4% per year over the first 7 years in which phenothiazines are taken. Although it is a very unusual complication in individuals who receive phenothiazines for short periods of time, it has been reported.

Due to the problems associated with phenothiazines, benzodiazepines have been used to a greater extent in recent years for the combative, delirious patient.[41,46,47] The two most commonly used benzodiazepines are diazepam (Valium) and lorazepam (Ativan). Lorazepam (0.03 mg/kg) orally or intervenously, can usually be given every 4–8 hours; for a very combative patient it can be given hourly. A third benzodiazepine which is frequently used is midazolam (Versed) at 0.05 mg/kg intravenously, typically used in conjunction with morphine for procedures such as tubbing and staple removal. When using the benzodiazepine class of medications, a clinician must balance the desired effects of relaxation with oversedation. Visual and auditory hallucinations may occur if the dose of benzodiazepine is too high. In those cases, it should be reduced or replaced by another type of medication. In cases of excessive anxiety in the presence of adequate pain control, lorazepam can be added to a patient's treatment. Nighttime doses usually enhance sleep. Diazepam in doses of 2–10 mg per dose, depending on the size of an individual, may be used in place of lorazepam if simultaneous muscle relaxation is desired.[48] Diazepam has an extremely long half-life, 40 hours, and therefore should be used sparingly (see Chapter 58). To avoid excessive sedation by benzodiazepines, a patient should not be awakened for the next dose.

Acute stress and post-traumatic stress disorder symptoms

A significant number of burn survivors will experience post-traumatic stress disorder symptoms, including intrusive memories of the injury, during their acute recovery.[49,50] If anxiety is associated with other symptoms of post-traumatic stress, such as hypervigilance or poor sleep, an antidepressant tricyclic such as imipramine should be considered.[32,51] The usual starting dose of imipramine is 25 mg/day unless the patient weighs less than 25 kg. The beginning dose is 12.5 mg for those under 25 kg. The dose can be increased rapidly over the next few days to a dose of 1 mg/kg. Further increases should be monitored by blood levels and EKG changes. A dose can be divided and given twice a day, but such division is usually unnecessary. The preferable time of administration is in the evening to aid with sleep. Major side-effects of the tricyclics such as imipramine are anticholinergic effects (dry mouth and dry nasal passages, constipation, urinary hesitance, and occasional esophageal reflux).[41] Autonomic complications such as orthostatic hypotension, palpitations, and hypertension have been reported in adolescents with this medication.[40] Cardiac arrhythmias, associated with a prolonged PR interval, can be life-threatening.[52–54] Sudden death has been reported for teenagers and children receiving desipramine and other tricyclics.[55] Amitriptyline or doxepin may be used in place of imipramine. The dosages are similar; however, both these medications cause more sedation than imipramine.[41]

Sleep disturbances

Patients with significant sleep problems are common in an acute burn unit.[56,57] When sleep disturbance with nightmares is associated with post-traumatic anxiety, as described above, antidepressant medications are the drugs of choice. Imipramine[58] and doxepin are both sedating antidepressants that are effective treatments for sleep problems in burn patients. Trazodone and nefazodone are alternative medications for insomnia and do not appear to alter sleep architecture as much as other antidepressants. Sleep problems may be associated with stimulation from the caretaking staff who awaken a patient while checking vital signs and well-being throughout the night. Sometimes lights and televisions are left on throughout the day and night in a patient's room. These environmental factors can be destructive to a patient's sleep–wake cycle. As soon as physiologic conditions allow, a patient should be given as much undisturbed sleep time at night as possible, so as to allow natural sleep cycles to reestablish, and to maintain a normal circadian rhythm. Pain and itch are other problems that can interfere with sleep and should be addressed with appropriate analgesic or antipruritic medications. If a patient continues to have significant sleep problems, sleep can be induced with diphenhydramine. Diphenhydramine doses of 1.5 mg/kg are often used throughout the day for itching and may be used alone for sleep at night or as an adjunct to other sleep medications. Usually, doses of 25 or 50 mg in the evening are adequate.

Often, post-traumatic symptoms other than sleep disturbances are not evident. In such cases, chloral hydrate may also be used in doses of 1.5 mg/kg, up to a maximum of 1 g per single dose.[47] Doses of 250 mg are usually adequate for a child; however, we prefer to use benzodiazepine, imipramine, and/or diphenhydramine for sedation and sleep with pediatric patients because deaths have been reported in children taking chloral hydrate for sedation.[47] Also, in our experience, chloral hydrate does not alleviate nightmares as does imipramine.

Depression

For depression, tricyclics have been the medications of first choice and are given as described above by following symptoms and monitoring blood levels. Recently, fluoxetine (Prozac), 20–40 mg and other selective serotonin re-uptake inhibitors (SSRIs), are being used for impulsive, angry patients with depressive symptoms.[52,54] The SSRIs have the added advantage of being a safer drugs for outpatient treatment since an overdose is unlikely to cause significant cardiac problems as have been attributed to the tricyclics.[52] Side-effects of SSRIs include gastrointestinal upset, increased agitation, headaches, and sweating. They have, however, fewer instances of anticholinergic side-effects such as constipation. Patients should be monitored for hypomania or mania induced by antidepressant medications. When this occurs, the antidepressant dose should be lowered and lithium therapy or other mood stabilizer medication should be considered.

Pain

Symptoms of depression and agitation are often related to excessive pain and subside with adequate pain management (see Chapter 58). A patient's experience of pain is related to the extent and depth of injury and influenced by individual responses to analgesia, pain threshold, emotional state, cognitive functioning, cultural beliefs, interpersonal interactions, and expectations.[38,59–64] Chemical analgesics and anesthetics are as important in managing pain with burns as they are with other medical/surgical conditions. Care must be taken to consider the appropriate doses of medication and the most efficacious schedule of administration. Modifications should be continued until good control is achieved.[65,66] Around-the-clock or continuous administration of analgesics achieves better pain control than PRN administration.[67,68] This avoids the period of less than therapeutic levels of the drug with increased discomfort prior to the request for medication and ameliorates a patient's anxiety about whether the medication will be allowed. Postoperatively, patient-controlled analgesia (PCA) pumps are very effective in achieving around-the-clock pain control with minimal undesired side-effects for adults and for children.[69,70]

In-hospital Recuperation

After the initial postburn period, a patient progresses through a series of operative procedures interspersed with days of physical therapy in order to maintain physical activity and range of motion. Immediate operative sites (those grafted and those which donate) are painful. In addition, exercises are painful. A patient's world is one of pain or concern about possible pain in the near future. It must be remembered that many of the treatments and experience of hospitalization may be as traumatic psychologically as the original burn injury, especially for young children.[71] The patient's expectations for treatment are also very important. Those patients who have low expectation for further improvement and attach higher importance to outcome are at greater risk for psychological distress during recovery.[72] The major goal of therapy from the psychiatrist's point of view is to control the pain and maximize a patient's participation in the exercises and other aspects of care.

In addition to the pharmacological treatment described above, designing a psychological milieu that supports comfort and security is a primary task.[32] A specific daily treatment schedule is crucial to achieving these goals. The schedule provides specific times for pain medication to insure coverage at times of expected pain (e.g. tubbing and physical therapy), but avoids sedation during family, social, and educational activities. Time should be provided in the schedule for fun and diversionary activities. A pediatric patient must have time scheduled for school and play. Patients must be allowed to have expected 'safe' periods without procedures. Whenever possible, the patient, even a young child, should be included in planning the schedule. The schedule should be posted and followed as closely as possible. In order to motivate a patient to participate at a maximum level in rehabilitation, a reward system can be incorporated with rewards consisting of special treats as designated by the patient, such as extra videos or going out of the hospital.

As a latency age child, adolescent, or adult recovers, they often want to talk about the accident. A patient begins a long process of 'understanding' what has happened. Part of this process is learning to look at a 'new' self, literally and metaphorically. As part of the treatment plan, a regularly scheduled meeting with a psychotherapist is established. This special time for 'talking' therapy may vary in content from play therapy with a child or light banter with an adult to serious confrontation with the most difficult emotionally charged issues. The reliability of this safe time in which a patient can complain about everybody and everything, express anger, express fear and sadness, can be very therapeutic. It is important for a patient to have someone other than family who is accepting, safe, and neutral with whom to talk. Communication with the therapist and others may be difficult if the patient is suffering with symptoms of post-traumatic stress disorder or alexithymia, a condition characterized by problems in describing feeling and thoughts.[73,74]

A patient's experience in adapting to burn injury can be thought of as a grieving process. A patient has experienced a loss of self. Using a familiar paradigm, we can describe a patient as moving through several stages of adjustment to loss: shock, denial, anger, depression, and finally acceptance.[75] This formulation is useful in working with patients about their injury. In our experience, shock and denial predominate during the initial hospitalization; anger and depression often last for years as a patient continues treatment, faces reconstructive surgeries, and confronts a series of social experiences.

Psychiatric problems beyond acute hospitalization

The novice usually expresses a belief that all burned persons need to see a psychiatrist due to the nature of the injury. A number of approaches have been used to determine the incidence of psychiatric difficulties among survivors of major burns. These studies report with surprising consistency that large numbers of survivors do not suffer long-term major psychiatric disorders or psychosocial impairment.[76,77] Longitudinal studies have found about one-third of burn survivors develop post-traumatic stress disorder within 2 years of their injury.[78,79] It might be expected that the appearance of the burn scar might influence long-term adjustment, and Fukunishi[80] did find cosmetic disfigurement predictive for post-traumatic stress disorder symptoms of avoidance and emotional numbing in women with burn injuries. In contrast, Taal and Farber[81] found that neither the severity nor the visibility of burn scars influence long-term adjustment, but rather social introversion, which predicted the development of pathological shame.

Our own work has focused on children and adolescents who are at least 1 year postburn and are either outpatients or have returned for further reconstructive surgery. One method we have used has been to survey patients with questionnaires pointed at specific psychiatric symptom complexes. For instance, Koon et al.[82] surveyed adolescents with the Piers–Harris Children's Self-concept Scale and found that male pediatric burn survivors had significantly higher scores than the normative population. Females described themselves as less popular, although otherwise equal to the norm. Self-esteem did not appear to be related to other burn-related variables (i.e. age at burn or size of burn). With a similar goal of looking for specific symptoms, we hypothesized significant depression and utilized several standardized instruments, including the Suicide Probability Scale (SPS),[83] to assess depressive symptoms. This study revealed no increase above norm in depression or suicidality, but did reveal significant anger among adolescent burn survivors.

We use a variety of instruments to detect general psychiatric needs among the children that we follow. The Achenbach series of standardized behavioral checklists are useful screening tools.[84–86] They offer validity, reliability, and convenience of administration in a setting such as ours where we must assess many clinical variables in a brief period of time. The Child Behavior Checklist (CBCL)[84] is a 113-item rating of each child's current behavior problems and competencies as perceived by a parent. Complementary to the CBCL are the Teacher Report Form (TRF)[85] and the Youth Self Report (YSR),[86] which provide assessments of the same behaviors by different observers. Our data from these instruments indicate that about 20–25% of the children and adolescents who survive major thermal injury may develop a variety of significant behavioral problems as indicated, but good adjustment is achieved by the majority of individuals.[87,88] Blakeney[89] and Zeitlin[90] reported similar findings of only modest psychological sequela to pediatric burns in his long-term follow-up study.

Parents usually report more problems than do the children themselves or the teachers.[87,91] In one study, 60 children with burns (35 boys, 25 girls) were surveyed with the Achenbach instruments at least 1 year after burn injury. The parental perception on the CBCL revealed a statistically significant ($p < 0.05$) increase in problems and decrease in competency for most age groups and both sexes when compared with the normal reference population. In contrast, the TRF and the YSR revealed very few differences from the reference population. Burn size did not account for any of the differences. Item analysis of individual questions revealed excessive endorsement by parents of specific items on all scales compared to their respective reference populations.[92] These results could be explained by increased problems of the children following severe burns that would not be easily observed by persons who do not live with the patient, e.g. nocturnal enuresis or nightmares. Or, perhaps, the parents reporting increased behavioral problems are overly sensitive to any indication of difficulty for their children.

Our investigations have also considered outcomes for the parents of youth burn survivors. The Parental Stress Index (PSI)[93] revealed that parents who reported their children as troubled were themselves more stressed than the normal reference population, not only by their children's behaviors but in areas unrelated to their children.[94] In addition, on a measure of mood state, the Eight-state Questionnaire (8SQ),[95] mothers who reported troubled children more often felt depressed and guilty than did mothers of well-adjusted children.[94] In a separate study of mothers of children with burns, 52% met criteria for a diagnosis of post-traumatic stress disorder, larger burns were strongly correlated with symptoms in the mother.[96] Fukunishi[97] found higher rates of depressive and post-traumatic stress symptoms in the mothers of children with burns than in their offspring. These studies emphasize the need for psychological attention to parents of burned children, as well as to the children themselves.

Using a standardized psychiatric interview for children, Stoddard *et al.* reported a very high incidence of psychiatric disorders among 30 pediatric burn survivors.[98,99] In order to make a fair comparison with other populations, these authors compared the burn survivors with a group of survivors of flood trauma and a community sample. Burned children had significantly more phobic disorders, overanxious disorders, enuresis, encopresis, major depression, post-traumatic stress disorder (PTSD), and substance/ethanol abuse than the comparison groups.[99] Sleep disorders and psychotic disorders were also slightly more common among the burned children. Even though most burn survivors eventually make good adjustments, they can be expected, at some time during the adjustment process, to suffer psychiatric sequelae which might be attenuated by psychiatric treatment.

Phobias and Other Anxiety Disorders

Many patients continue beyond acute hospitalization to have periods during which they appear extremely anxious and express fear. These periods often recur in association with return to a hospital for reconstructive surgeries. Some are so anxious that they are constantly soliciting their families or others for comfort. Generalized anxiety disorder or overanxious disorder of childhood is characterized in the *Diagnostic and Statistical Manual of Mental Disorders* (DSM-IV) by the following criteria:

- excessive worry occurring more days than not for at least 6 months about a number of events;
- difficulty in controlling the anxiety;
- the anxiety causes clinically significant distress or impairment in social, occupation, or other important areas of functioning;
- anxiety and worry associated with three or more (only one for children) of the following symptoms (with some symptoms present for more days than not for the past 6 months): restlessness, feeling on edge, easily fatigued, difficulty concentrating or mind going blank, irritability, muscle tension, sleep disturbances.

In a burned patient, difficulty controlling anxiety which is so distressful that it interferes with important functioning, restlessness, and difficulty in concentrating are diagnostic of anxiety disorders since some other symptoms can be related to burn injuries specifically, e.g. being easily fatigued.

Not infrequently, anxiety spills over to other situations and/or becomes focused on specific objects; thus, phobias develop that are characterized by excessive persistent fear in response to specific stumuli. Although adults may express anxiety through 'panic' symptoms such as sweating, palpitations, trembling, or nausea, children may express anxiety by crying, tantrums, freezing, or clinging. A differential diagnosis of these anxiety disorders distinct from post-traumatic stress disorder is difficult and requires a careful interview. Burned patients suffering from post-traumatic stress often see the fire or aspects of their accidents whenever they close their eyes; they dream about their traumas. An overanxious patient is afraid of what might happen; the post-traumatic stress disorder patient fears what has happened. Most burn patients, certainly those who qualify for the diagnosis of generalized or overanxious disorder, benefit from lorazepam therapy in addition to supportive psychotherapy.

Acute Stress Disorder and Post-traumatic Stress Disorder

Acute stress disorder and PTSD are the most common psychiatric disorders seen in survivors of major burns.[100] The two disorders are very similar, differing only in how long the symptoms persist. Acute stress disorder symptoms appear immediately following the trauma, last for at least 2 days and resolve within 4 weeks after the trauma. If symptoms persist or appear more than 4 weeks after the trauma, then the appropriate diagnosis is post-traumatic stress disorder. These disorders are characterized in the *Diagnostic and Statistical Manual of Mental Disorders* (DSM-IV) by the following criteria:

- The person has experienced, witnessed, or was confronted with an event which involved actual or threatened death or serious injury to self or others, and the person's response involved intense fear, helplessness, or horror.
- The traumatic event is persistently re-experienced. Recurrent and intrusive thoughts of the event occur. Burned patients often complain of seeing the fire whenever they

close their eyes or when they try to go to sleep. Young children may relive the event over and over again in repetitive play. Nightmares about the event are common; in young children, frightening dreams occur without recognizable content. Feeling as if the event were recurring (e.g. flashback) is reported often. Intense reactivity, psychological and/or physiologic, occurs at exposure to internal or external cues that trigger associations with the traumatic incident, e.g. seeing a fire on television.

- There is continued avoidance of stimuli associated with the trauma or numbing of general responsiveness. Persons suffering from PTSD develop flat affect, memory problems, and withdrawal from others. Children's behavior may be regressed; children may lose recently acquired developmental skills such as toilet training or language skills.

- Persistent symptoms of increased arousal, which were not present before the trauma, may develop. These symptoms include sleep disturbance, irritability/anger, difficulty concentrating, hypervigilance, exaggerated startle response, and panic attacks. Patients have periods of feeling afraid and not knowing why.

Nightmares and altered sleep patterns are usually the symptoms first noted. Although one study found no correlation between psychiatric diagnosis emerging during acute hospitalization and later development of post-traumatic disorder,[101] the presence of avoidant post-traumatic disorder symptoms during the acute phase of recovery is reported to predict chronic post-traumatic disorder in burn patients.[78,102,103] Many of the other symptoms are described when a more complete history is taken. Patients should be given ample opportunity to explore their feelings and fears about the traumatic event. This process may persist for months. In addition, tricyclic medications are helpful in reducing the nightmares and improving the sleep pattern. Our preference among these medications has been imipramine. The initial dose is usually 25 mg at bed time. This may be increased in 25 mg increments until a dose of 1 mg/kg is reached. If the symptoms are still uncontrolled, the dose may be increased stepwise to 3 mg/kg, but only with frequent checking of the plasma level with each increment of dosage increase. Fluoxetine and the other SSRIs are alternative medications for treatment, especially if the patient has a cardiac condition that would contraindicate tricyclic antidepressants. Typically, the SSRIs are given in the morning rather than the evening as they may interfere with sleep onset. Usually a patient's sleep pattern improves quickly. Imipramine therapy must often be continued up to a year longer. When it is to be discontinued, the medication should be reduced over time, for suddenly stopping the medicine will cause a recurrence of sleep disturbance.

Major Depression and Dysthymia

Although depression is a reaction most observers would expect of burned patients, it is a rare long-term sequela of burn injury. According to Stoddard,[97] fewer than 50% of the children he surveyed had ever suffered major depression; dysthymia, another depressive disorder, occurred in only 10%. Outcome studies of adult burn survivors show a similar prevalence of major depression.[29,39,104–107]

To diagnose major depression, a patient must have five or more

of the following DSM-IV symptoms *for a period of at least 2 weeks, and they must represent a change from previous functioning*:

- depressed mood most of the day (may be an irritable mood in children and adolescents);
- markedly diminished interest or pleasure in most activities;
- significant change in appetite, resulting in either weight loss or gain (for children, failure to make expected weight gains);
- insomnia or hypersomnia;
- feelings of worthlessness or excessive/inappropriate guilt nearly every day;
- fatigue or loss of energy nearly every day;
- diminished concentration or enhanced indecisiveness nearly every day;
- psychomotor agitation or retardation observable by others; and
- recurrent thoughts of death, suicidal ideation, suicide attempt or plan.

This is an extremely difficult diagnosis to make during the acute burn period since many of the criteria are linked to physical symptoms. Even beyond the acute phase, the diagnosis is often complicated by grief following the loss of a loved one during a fire, and by sadness at one's altered body. The critical symptoms in a burned patient are depressed mood and anhedonia. Many times a patient's expressed interest in play or plans for the future rule out the diagnosis.

Major depression, with or without grief reaction, should be treated by a team approach. A patient should be involved in scheduled daily activities. Psychotherapy should begin to identify and address appropriate issues. Medication with tricyclics, as described for post-traumatic stress, is often helpful. After checking serum levels, the dose should be increased until it reaches therapeutic levels. This process involves frequent checking of serum levels as the dose is raised. A steady state is usually not reached until a given dose is maintained for 3–5 days. Again, the sleep pattern improves first. Therapy must often be continued for 6 months or longer. When discontinuing therapy, the medication should be slowly reduced rather than stopped suddenly so as to prevent dysphoria and sleep problems.

A smaller percentage of burned patients will develop a milder but more protracted type of depression called dysthymia. This condition must be present for *at least 2 years in adults*, or *1 year in children and adolescents* in order to be diagnosed. It is characterized by the following:

- depressed or irritable mood;
- appetite changes, sleep difficulties, fatigue, low self-esteem;
- poor concentration or difficulty making decisions; and
- feelings of hopelessness.

The same combination of medication and psychotherapy is recommended for dysthymic patients as for major depression.

Summary

Psychiatric symptoms occur commonly as part of the complex systemic response to burn injuries. Psychological and pharmacologic treatment are important in the successful recovery of a burned person, and perhaps mitigate against long-term psychiatric seque-lae of post-injury. It is important to note that psychological adaptation is a lengthy process occurring over months or years. During the postburn years, it is imperative that the burn team assess the mental and affective states of patients while assessing their physical recovery. Although most burned patients eventually make satisfactory adjustments, many continue for a long time to struggle with self-image, anger, and sadness. These disturbances often seem to be expressed through symptoms that are not easily observed by other than intimate friends and family of a patient.[108] Sleep disturbance, fear or withdrawal from previous activities are not behavioral disturbances which necessarily insure that a patient will attract psychiatric attention and treatment. They are, however, unhappy responses which can be ameliorated by treatment. It then becomes a responsibility of the expert in burn care and recovery to be aware of frequently occurring disturbed responses, to ask the right questions in order to assess a patient's status, and to assist a patient in receiving psychological and psychiatric assistance.

References

1. Mendelsohn IE. Liaison psychiatry and the burn center. *Psychosomatics* 1983; **24(3)**: 235–43.
2. Ochitill H. Psychiatric consultation to the burn unit: the psychiatrist's perspective. *Psychosomatics* 1984; **25(9)**: 689, 697–701.
3. Andreasen NJC, Nayes P, Hartford C. Factors influencing adjustment of burn patients during hospitalization. *Psychosom Med* 1972; **34(6)**: 517–25.
4. Noyes R, Frye S, Slymen D, Canter A. Stressful life events and burn injuries. *J Trauma* 1979; **19(3)**: 141–4.
5. Darko D, Wachtel T, Ward H, Frank H. Analysis of 585 burn patients hospitalized over a six-year period. Part III: Psychosocial data. *Burns* 1986; **12**: 395–401.
6. Vogtsberger K, Taylor E. Psychosocial factors in burn injury. *Texas Med* 1984; **80**: 43–6.
7. Barillo DJ, Goode R. Substance abuse in victims of fire. *J Burn Care Rehabil* 1996; **17**: 71–6.
8. Powers PS, Stevens B, Arias F, Cruse CW, Krizek T, Daniels S. Alcohol disorders among patients with burns: crisis and opportunity. *J Burn Care Rehabil* 1994; **15**: 386–91.
9. Grobmyer SR, Maniscalco SP, Purdue GF, Hunt JL. Alcohol, drug introxication, or both at the time of burn injury as a predictor of complications and mortality in hospitalized patients with burns. *J Burn Care Rehabil* 1996; **17**: 532–9.
10. Ho WS, To EWH, Chan ESY, King WWK. Burn injuries during paint thinner sniffing. *Burns* 1998; **24**: 757–59.
11. Sheridan RL. Burns with inhalation injury and petrol aspiration in adolescents seeking euphoria through hydrocarbon inhalation. *Burns* 1996; **22(7)**: 566–67.
12. Oh SJ, Lee SE, Burm JS *et al*. Explosive burns during abusive inhalation of butane gas. *Burns* 1999; **25**: 341–44.
13. Nielson JA, Kolman PBR, Wachtel TL. Suicide and parasuicide by burning. *J Burn Care Rehabil* 1984; **5(4)**: 335–8.
14. Davidson T, Brown L. Self-inflicted burns: a five-year retrospective study. *Burns* 1985; **11**: 157–60.
15. Stoddard FJ, Cahners SS. Suicide attempted by self-immolation during adolescence; II Psychiatric treatment and outcome. *J Adol Psychiatry* 1985; **12**: 266–80.
16. Krummen DM, James K, Klein RL. Suicide by burning: a retrospective review of the Akron Regional Burn Center. *Burns* 1998; **24**: 147–49.
17. Garcia-Sanchez V, Palao R, Legarre F. Self-inflicted burns. *Burns* 1994; **20(6)**: 537–8.
18. Erzurum VZ, Varcellotti J. Self-inflicted burn injuries. *J Burn Care Rehabil* 1999; **20**: 22–4.
19. Tuohig GM, Saffle JR, Sullivan JJ, Morris S, Lehto S. Self-inflicted patient burns: suicide versus mutilation. *J Burn Care Rehabil* 1995; **16**: 429–36.
20. Raskind SM. Suicide by burning: emotional needs of the suicidal adolescent on the burn unit. *Issues Compr Pediatr Nurs* 1986; **9**: 369–82.
21. Powers PS, Cruse CW, Boyd F. Psychiatric status, prevention, and outcome in patients with burns: a prospective study. *J Burn Care Rehabil* 2000; **21**: 85–8.
22. Van Der Does AJW, Hinderink EMC, Vloemans AFPM, Spinhoven P. Burn injuries, psychiatric disorders and length of hospitalization. *J Psychosomatic Res* 1997; **43(4)**: 431–35.
23. Fauerbach JA, Lawrence J, Haythornthwaite J, McGuire M, Munster A. Preinjury psychiatric illness and post injury adjustment in adult burn survivors. *The Acad Psychosomatic Med* 1996; **37(6)**.
24. Fauerbach JA, Lawrence J, Stevens S, Munster A. Work status and attrition from longitudinal studies are influenced by psychiatric disorder. *J Burn Care Rehabil* 1998; **19**: 247–52.
25. Fauerbach JA, Lawrence J, Haythornthwaite J, *et al*. Preburn psychiatric history affects post trauma morbidity. *Psychosomatics* 1997; **38**: 374–385.
26. Tasal LA, Faber AW. Dissociation as a predictor of psychopathology following burns injury. *Burns* 1997; **23(5)**: 400–03.
27. Tedstone JE, Tarrier N, Faragher EB. An investigation of the factors associated with an increased risk of psychological morbidity in burn injured patients. *Burns* 1998; **24**: 407–15.
28. Tedstone JE, Tarrier N. An investigation of the prevalence of psychological morbidity in burn-injured patients. *Burns* 1997; **23(7/8)**: 550–54.
29. Steiner H, Clark W. Psychiatric complications of burned adults: a classification. *J Trauma* 1977; **17**: 134–43.
30. Perry S, Blank K. Relationships of psychological processes during delirium to outcome. *Am J Psychiatry* 1984; **141**: 843–7.
31. Patterson D, Everett J, Bombardier C, Questad K, Lee V, Marvin J. Psychological effects of severe burn injuries. *Psychol Bull* 1993; **113(2)**: 362–78.
32. Blakeney P, Meyer W III. Psychological aspects of burn care. *Trauma Q* 1994; **II(2)**: 166–79.
33. Morton R, Gleason O, Yates W. Psychiatric effects of anabolic steroids after burn injuries. *Psychosomatics* 2000; **41**: 1 January-February.
34. Thomas C, Ganceres N, Behrends L, *et al*. Hallucinations and Burned Children. *Proc Am Burn Assoc* 1999.
35. Haynes B, Bright R. Burn coma: a syndrome associated with severe burn wound infection. *J Trauma* 1967; **7**: 46F75.
36. Antoon A, Volpe J, Crawford J. Burn encephalopathy in children. *Pediatrics* 1972; **50**: 609–16.
37. Hughes J, Cayaffa J, Boswick J. Seizures following burns to the skin: m. Electroencephalographic recordings. *Dis Nerv Syst* 1975; **36**: 443–7.
38. Stoddard E. Psychiatric management of the burned patient. In: Martyn JAJ, ed. *Acute Care of the Burn Patient*. Orlando, FL: Grune and Stratton, 1990: 256–72.
39. Andreasen NJC, Norris A, Hartford C. Incidence of long-term psychiatric complications in severely burned adults. *Ann Surg* 1971; **174(5)**: 785–93.
40. Teicher MH, Glod CA. Neuroleptic drags: indications and guidelines for their rational use in children and adolescents. *J Child Adole Psychopharmacol* 1990; **1**: 33–56.
41. Schatzberg AF, Cole JO. *Manual of Clinical Psychopharmacology*, 2nd edn. Washington, DC: American Psychiatric Press, 1991.
42. Kiely WE. Psychiatric syndromes in critically ill patients. *JAMA* 1976; **23S**: 2759–61.
43. Moore DP. Rapid treatment of delirium in critically ill patients. *Am J Psychiatry* 1977; **134**: 1431–2.
44. Huang V, Figge H, Demling R. Haloperidol in burn patients. *J Burn Care Rehabil* 1987; **8**: 269–73.
45. Still J, Friedman B, Law E, Deppe S, Epperly N, Orlet H. Neuroleptic malignant syndrome in a burn patient. *Burns* 1998; **24**: 573–5.
46. Coffey BJ. Anxiolytics for children and adolescents. Traditional and new drugs. *J Child Adol Psychopharmacol* 1990; **1**: 57–83.
47. USP DI Volume I: *Drug Information for the Health Care Professional*. Rockville, MD: United States Pharm Convention, Inc., 1994.
48. Martyn JAJ, Greenblatt DJ, Quinby WC. Diazepam kinetics in patients with severe burns. *Anesth Analg* 1983; **62**: 293–7.
49. Ehde DM, Patterson DR, Wiechman SA, Wilson LG. Post-traumatic stress symptoms and distress following acute burn injury. *Burns* 1999; **25**: 587–592.
50. Yu BH, Dimsdale JE. Posttraumatic stress disorder in patients with burn injuries. *J Burn Care Rehabil* 1999; **20**: 426–33.
51. Robert R, Blakeney P, Villarreal C, Rosenbert L, Meyer W III. Imipramine treatment in pediatric burn patients with symptoms of acute stress disorder: a pilot study. *J Acad Child Adol Psychiatry* 1999; **38(7)**: 873–82.
52. Glassman AH. The newer antidepressant drugs and their cardiovascular effects. *Psychopharmacol Bull* 1984; **20**: 272–9.
53. Glassman AH, Bigger JT Jr. Cardiovascular effects of therapeutic doses of tricyclic antidepressants. *Arch Gen Psychiatry* 1981; **38**: 815–20.
54. Ryan ND. Heterocyclic antidepressants in children and adolescents. *J Child Adol Psychopharmacol* 1990; **1**: 21–31.
55. Popper CW, Elliott GR. Sudden death and tricyclic antidepressants: clinical considerations for children. *J Child Adol Psychopharmacol* 1990; **1**: 125–32.
56. Lawrence JW, Fauerbach J, Eudell E, Ware L, Munster A. The 1998 clinical research award sleep disturbance after burn injury: a frequent yet understudied complication. *J Burn Care Rehabil* 1998; **19**: 480–86.

57. Rose M, Sanford A, Thomas C, Opp MR. Factors altering the sleep of burned children. *Sleep.*

58. Robert R, Meyer W III, Villarreal C, Blakeney PE, Desai M, Herndon D. *J Burn Care Rehabil* 1999; **20**: 250–8.

59. Szyfelbein S, Osgood P, Carr D. The assessment of pain and plasma B-endorphin immunoactivity in burned children. *Pain* 1985; **22**: 173–82.

60. Beales J. Factors influencing the expectation of pain among patients in a children's burns unit. *Burns* 1983; **9(3)**: 187–92.

61. Charlton J, Gragliardi G, Klein R, Heimbach D. Factors affecting pain in burned patients – a preliminary report. *Postgrad Med J* 1983; **59**: 604–7.

62. Difede J, Jaffe AB, Musngi G, Perry S, Yurt R. Determinants of pain expression in hospitalized burn patients. *Pain* 1997; **72**: 245–51.

63. Taal LA, Faber AW. Burn injuries, pain and distress: exploring the role of stress symptomatology. *Burns* 1997; **23(4)**: 288–90.

64. Taal LA, Faber AW. Post-traumatic stress, pain and anxiety in adult burn victims. *Burns* 1998; **23(7/8)**: 545–49.

65. Perq S. Undermedication for pain on a burn unit. *Gen Hosp Psychiatry* 1984; **6**: 308–16.

66. Watkins P, Cook E, May R, Ehleben C. Psychological stages in adaptation following burn injury: a method for facilitating psychological recovery of burn victims. *J Burn Care Rehabil* 1988; **9(4)**: 376–84.

67. Yaster M, Deshpande J, Maxwell L. The pharmacologic management of pain in children. *Therapy* 1989; **15(10)**: 14–26.

68. Colditz R. Management of pain in the newborn infant. *J Pediatr Child Health* 1991; **27**: 11–15.

69. Webb C, Stergios D, Rodgers B. Patient controlled antagesia as postoperative pain treatment for children. *J Pediatr Nurs* 1989; **4(3)**: 162–71.

70. Gaukroger P, Chapman M, Davey R. Pain control in pediatric burn the use of patient-controlled analgesia. *Burns* 1991; **17(5)**: 396–9.

71. Wintgens A, Boileau B, Robaey P. Posttraumatic stress symptoms and medical procedures in children. *Can J Psychiatry* 1997; **42**: 611–16.

72. Blalock SJ, Bunker BJ, DeVellis RF. Psychological distress among survivors of burn injury: the role of outcome expectations and perceptions of importance. *J Burn Care Rehabil* 1994; **15**: 421–7.

73. Fukunishi I, Yasunori C. Posttraumatic stress disorder and alexithymia in burn patients. *Psychol Rep* 1994; **75**: 1371–76.

74. Fukunishi I, Sasaki K, Chishima Y, Anze M, Saijo M. Emotional disturbances in trauma patients during the rehabilitation phase. *Gen Hosp Psychiatry* 1996; **18**: 121–27.

75. Knudson-Cooper M. Emotional care of the hospitalized burned child. *J Burn Care Rehabil* 1982; **3**: 109–16.

76. Shakespeare V. Effect of small burn injury on physical, social and psychological health at 3–4 months after discharge. *Burns* 1998; **24**: 739–44.

77. Kimmo Tanttula, Jyrki V, Sirpa AS. Health status after recovery from burn injury. *Burns* 1998; **24**: 293–98.

78. Bryant RA. Predictors of post-traumatic stress disorder following burns injury. *Burns* 1996; **22(2)**: 89–92.

79. Taal LA, Faber AW. Posttraumatic stress and maladjustment among adult burn survivors 1–2 years postburn. *Burns* 1998; **24**: 285–92.

80. Fukunishi I. Relationship of Cosmetic disfigurement to the severity of posttraumatic stress disorder in burn injury or digital amputation. *Psychotherapy Psychosom* 1999; **68**: 82–86.

81. Taal L, Faber AW. Posttraumatic stress and maladjustment among adult burn survivors 1 to 2 years postburn. Part II: the interview data. *Burns* 1998; **24**: 399–405.

82. Koon K, Blakeney P, Broemeling L, Moore P, Robson M, Herndon D. Self-esteem in pediatric burn patients. *Proc Am Burn Assoc* 1992; **24**: 112.

83. Cull JG, Gill WS. *Suicide Probability Scale Manual*. Los Angeles: Western Psychological Services, 1982.

84. Achenbach TM. *Manual for Child Behavior Checklist 4/18 and 1991 Profile*. Burlington, VT: University of Vermont Department of Psychiatry, 1991.

85. Achenbach TM. *Manual for the Teachers Report Forms and 1991 Profile*. Burlington, VT: University of Vermont Department of Psychiatry, 1991.

86. Achenbach TM. *Manual for the Youth Self-Report and 1991 Profile*. Burlington, VT: University of Vermont Department of Psychiatry, 1991.

87. Blakeney P, Meyer W, Moore P, et al. Social competence and behavioral problems of pediatric survivors of burns. *J Burn Care Rehabil* 1993; **14**: 65–72.

88. LeDoux J, Blakeney P, Meyer W, Herndon D. Relationships between parental emotional states, family environment and the behavioral adjustment of pediatric burn survivors. *Proc Am Burn Assoc* 1994; **26**: 134.

89. Blakeney P, Meyer III W, Robert R, Desai M, Wolf S, Herndon D. Long-term psychosocial adaptation of children who survive burns involving 80% or greater total body surface area. *J Trauma Infect Crit Care* 1998; **44(4)**: 625–34.

90. Zeitlin REK. Long-term psychosocial sequelae of pediatric burns. *Burns* 1997; **23(6)**: 467–72.

91. Blakeney P, Meyer W, Moore P, et al. Psychosocial sequelae of pediatric burns involving 80% or greater total body surface area. *J Burn Care Rehabil* 1993; **14**: 684–9.

92. Meyer W, Blakeney P, Moore P, et al. Inconsistencies in psychosocial assessment of children post major burn. *J Burn Care Rehabil* 1995 (in press).

93. Abidin RR. *Parental Stress Index Manual*. Charlottesville, VA: Pediatric Pathology Press, 1983.

94. Meyer W, Blakeney P, Moore P, Murphy L, Robson M, Herndon D. Parental well-being and behavioral adjustment of pediatric burn survivors. *J Burn Care Rehabil* 1994; **15**: 62–8.

95. Curran JP, Cattell RB. *Manual for the Eight-State Questionnaire (85Q)*. Champaign, IL: Institute for Personality and Ability Testing, 1976.

96. Rizzone LP, Stoddard FJ, Murphy JM, Kruger LJ. Posttraumatic stress disorder in mothers of children and adolescent with burns. *J Burn Care Rehabil* 1994; **15**: 158–63.

97. Fukunishi I. Post-traumatic stress symptoms and depression in mothers of children with severe burn injuries. *Psychol Rep* 1983; 331–35.

98. Stoddard FJ, Nomzan DK, Murphy M. A diagnosis outcome study of children and adolescents with severe burns. *J Trauma* 1989; **29**: 471–7.

99. Stoddard FJ, Nomzan DK, Murphy M, Beardslee WR. Psychiatric outcome of burned children and adolescents. *J Am Acad Child Adol Psychiatry* 1989; **28**: 589–95.

100. Baur KM, Hardy PE, Van Dorsten B. Posttraumatic stress disorder in burn populations: a critical review of the literature. *J Burn Care Rehabil* 1998; **19**: 230–40.

101. Powers PS, Cruse CW, Daniels S, Stevens B. Posttraumatic stress disorder in patients with burns. *J Burn Care Rehabil* 1994; **15**: 147–53.

102. Lawrence JW, Fauerbach J, Munster A. Early avoidance of traumatic stimuli predicts chronicity of intrusive thoughts following burn injury. *Behav Res Ther* 1996; **34(8)**: 643–46.

103. Difede J, Barocas D. Acute intrusive and avoidant PTSD symptoms as predictors of chronic PTSD following burn injury. *J Traumatic Stress* 1999; **12(2)**: 363–69.

104. Ward H, Moss R, Darko D, et al. Prevalence of post-burn depression following burn injury. *J Burn Care Rehabil* 1987; **8(4)**: 294–8.

105. Malt U. Long-term psychosocial follow-up studies of burned adults: review of the literature. *Burns* 1980; **6**: 190–7.

106. Malt U. A long-term psychosocial follow-up study of burned adults. *Acta Psychia Scand Suppl* 1989; **80(355)**: 94–102.

107. Faber A, Klasen H, Sauer E, Vuister E. Psychological and social problems in burn patients after discharge: a follow-up study. *Scand J Plast Reconstr Surg* 1987; **21(3)**: 307–9.

108. Meyer W, LeDoux J, Blakeney P, Herndon D. Diminished adaptive behaviors among pediatric burn survivors. *Proc Am Burn Assoc* 1994; **26**: 133.

Chapter 60

Abuse, neglect, and fire setting: when burn injury involves reporting to a safety officer

Rhonda Robert, Patricia Blakeney, David N Herndon

Introduction

As a subject of scientific investigation, violence, including that occurring within the family, has received much attention from professionals in sociology, mental health, medicine, and law.[1] Yet most health professionals, themselves devoted to healing and comforting others, are reluctant to believe that human beings will cause serious injury to others, especially to those who are significant members of their own family circle and most especially to those who are helpless such as young children or elderly parents. Caregiving professionals value the role of supportive other, and assessing for abuse and neglect can run counter to career training, values, and interests. The degree of uncertainty in identifying abuse or neglect is uncomfortable, and the family members typically do not validate suspicion. However, the evidence is overwhelming that people do behave brutally, and they do cause injury even to close family members. Sometimes the maltreatment involves burning. The problem of deliberate injury to children by burning has been identified and discussed in the professional literature for many years.[2]

Similar aggressive acts toward adults began to be recognized as a concern more recently; abuse of adults by burning has rarely been documented in empirical studies.[2–7] Three articles have been found reporting abuse to adults by burning.[2,5,6] It seems highly probable that burning as a form of violence against adults occurs with much greater frequency than reflected in the literature and has often been unrecognized. Unless adult patients are asked about abuse, they are unlikely to volunteer the information.[5] As burn care professionals become increasingly sensitive to the problem of abuse to adults the reported incidence will probably increase dramatically, replicating the pattern observed with child abuse, i.e. the more we ask, the more we will discover.[7]

The authors share the guilt of failing to be attuned to abuse in adults in the same way we alert to that possibility with children. Therefore, our clinical experience with known adult abuse by burning is limited to a few flagrant cases. Our experience with child abuse is extensive. Since the literature and our own experience are heavily weighted with information about child abuse, this chapter also represents that bias. The reader may, at times, be led to believe that the pediatric population is the only target for maltreatment. That is not an intention but rather a reflection of our current knowledge, and we caution the reader, as we remind ourselves, to avoid that misconception.

In this chapter, we have integrated our experience with available information to identify risk factors in the total population and to suggest therapeutic approaches to treating, in addition to the burn wounds, the complex social, interpersonal, and familial issues that both produce injury and complicate the recovery and rehabilitation of the patient.

We also have included at the end of this chapter a brief section on firesetting, another event that perplexes hospital staff for many of the same reasons that suspicious injuries cause concern. Discovering that a patient was injured while engaged in fire-setting activities, or by a fire set by a friend so engaged presents us with the same dilemma of whether to report the event to an outside agency. Although the family of the fire-setter may not be as defensive as in the case of abuse or neglect, they usually are not comfortable with reports to any official agency, and the hospital staff must decide whether to report and how to deal with the family's discomfort. Yet, because burn care professionals are likely to be the only entrée to help for the victims and the perpetrators and because we know what the 'worst case' outcomes can be, we bear the responsibility of finding ways to prevent further harm while maintaining a trusting relationship with the patient and with the patient's family.

Prevalence of abuse/neglect

During our pediatric hospital's staff orientation, participants are asked to estimate the percentage of children abused and neglected in the United States annually, as well as to estimate the percentage of children abused and neglected by burning. These health care professionals routinely underestimate the prevalence. No single participant has ever estimated higher than the official rate.

Approximately one and a half million people in the United States are believed abused and neglected.[8] Of children in the US suspected to have been abused, 80% of the injuries involved the skin.[9] Reports of child abuse by burning indicate that abuse or neglect is suspected in 30% of admissions to pediatric burn units, and, at minimum, one-third of the suspected cases are confirmed by investigating officials to have been caused by abuse or neglectful supervision.[8–20] Adult abuse by burning is reported less frequently. In one sample of adult burns, 4% of injuries were attributed to abuse or neglect.[6] Without intervention, abuse persists. Thirty percent of the children suffering recurrent abuse and neglect are eventually mortally injured.[13] Thus, many children are injured repeatedly in escalating severity, perhaps over years, until they die from abuse related injuries.

Dynamics of abuse

It is helpful when dealing with persons suspected of abuse to understand that abuse usually occurs as a multigenerational characteristic that is symptomatic of relationships impoverished of nurturance. Central to understanding abuse is understanding that abusers typically are individuals who were themselves denied adequate parenting and who experienced severe emotional deprivation. The infantile needs of the abuser were unmet; the adult abuser has not learned that it is possible to assert oneself appropriately and to meet one's own needs autonomously. Rather, the abuser looks to external sources to meet those needs to be cared for and comforted.

In some situations there are two 'abusers', i.e. the actual perpetrator and the overtly passive observer who does not stop the abuse. Both persons are elements of a psychosocial system that supports abuse, and usually both are from similar backgrounds with similar needs.[21]

Although violence may seem anything but passive, it often grows from a nonthinking, passive life position. Violent behaviors can be thought of as expressions of desperation from immature individuals who feel lost and helpless, incompetent to care for themselves, and who are in a constant quest for some external source of comfort. Their own experiences of parental neglect or abuse have taught them to mistrust others so that, as adults, they are typically socially isolated. This further decreases opportunities for comfort or for developing self-efficacy. Feeling helpless and inadequate, and predicting rejection in every interpersonal contact, such people also experience more difficulty in seeking and securing employment, thus frequently incurring a further stress of financial instability.

In an environment devoid of emotional support, abusers passively wait for comfort from a spouse, a lover, or a child. When those 'others' fail to gratify the abusers' needs or when a change in the situation imposes additional stress, these needful persons react in a child-like, nonthinking way to resolve frustration. Physical aggression and violence are often the end results of intense frustration.[22] A child, an elderly person, or a physically dependent adult is commonly an immediate precipitator of stress as well as an easily available target for physical aggression.[3,22,23]

This perceived helplessness and desperate needfulness also explain some of the other behaviors commonly attributed to abusers. They often fail to seek appropriate and timely medical treatment for an injured child, not only because they fear punishment but because of their learned helplessness and passivity. They discount the seriousness of the injury, as well as their ability to take care of the injury. 'I didn't think it was that bad' is an explanation often given for delay in seeking treatment. By diminishing the significance, they relieve themselves of responsibility to act. When the abuser does take the child for help, it is frequently first to a relative or neighbor rather than to a physician because the abuser does not believe in their own ability to decide whether to seek medical treatment. Abusers are observed to interact inappropriately with their children because they are preoccupied with having their own needs met. A child who is hurt and demanding is unlikely to reward the abuser with feelings of comfort that the abuser seeks, and so the abuser withdraws from the child. If the child is quiet and compliant, the abuser may be observed to ignore the child and sit passively, watching television for long periods until some external force acts as a stimulus to motivate the adult into action.

Justice and Justice,[24] in their work with families who abuse children, identified several erroneous belief systems that are commonly held by abusers; these are listed in **Table 60.1**. Since, as most authorities believe, violence is a multigeneration intrafamily pattern, then it is likely that the belief systems attributed to child abusers can be extrapolated to abusers of adults as well. The issues of dependency, lack of trust, felt inadequacy, frustration, and emotional pain recur in situations describing abuse spanning age groups.[3,24,25]

Table 60.1 Erroneous beliefs of abusers

Erroneous belief systems commonly contributing to the family system in which abuse occurs (Justice & Justice, 1990)[29]

- If my child cries, misbehaves or does not do what I want, he or she does not love me and I am a bad parent.
- My child should know what I want and want to do it.
- My child should take care of me like I took care of my parents.
- My spouse/lover should know what I want and meet all of my needs.
- If I have to ask, it does not count.
- You cannot trust anyone.

Assessment begins at admission

As with all patients and families, the therapeutic relationship with patients and families in which abuse or neglect is suspected is initiated at admission and developed through the process of assessment and treatment. Abusive and neglectful caregivers are aware that something is wrong in their lives, although they may be at an impasse in changing their behavior or limited in degree of personal awareness. The need for medical attention and the visible nature of the burn injury have the potential to heighten the caregiver's sense of vulnerability. This crisis can be utilized to bring positive changes for the family. Risk assessment should be discussed with the family members, including the suspected perpetrator. Once the concerns are presented, the individuals have the opportunity to engage in services from which the family could potentially benefit. The family should be apprised of any report to a protective agency and the events to expect thereafter. Remembering that an important factor in the typical abuser's character is reluctance to trust, it is essential that the hospital staff be truthful and nonavoidant. Frequent follow-up sessions with the family throughout the course of hospitalization and outpatient treatment are essential to maximizing family change (**Figure 60.1**). To facilitate a positive rela-

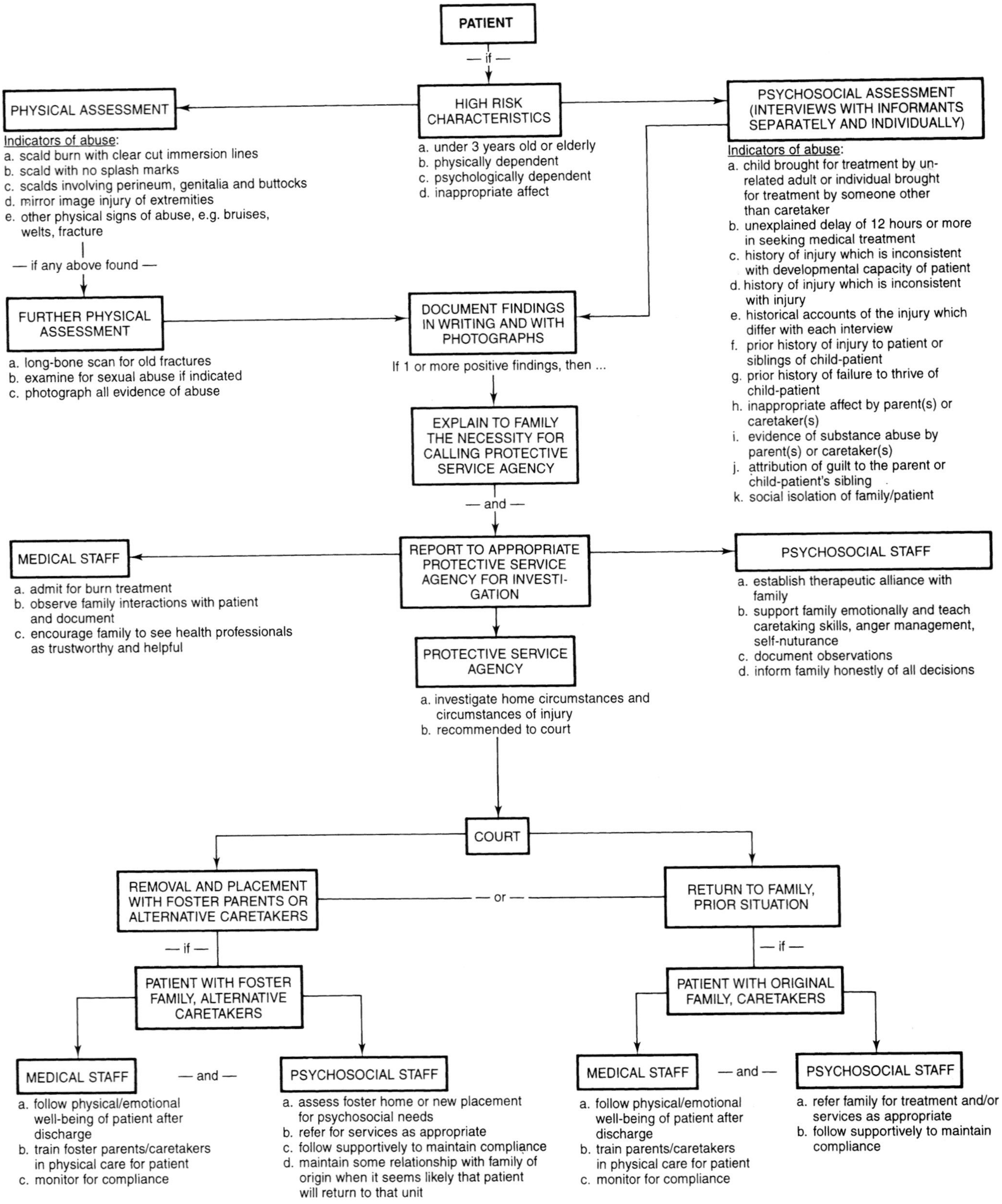

PATIENT

— if —

HIGH RISK CHARACTERISTICS

a. under 3 years old or elderly
b. physically dependent
c. psychologically dependent
d. inappropriate affect

PHYSICAL ASSESSMENT

Indicators of abuse:
a. scald burn with clear cut immersion lines
b. scald with no splash marks
c. scalds involving perineum, genitalia and buttocks
d. mirror image injury of extremities
e. other physical signs of abuse, e.g. bruises, welts, fracture

— if any above found —

FURTHER PHYSICAL ASSESSMENT

a. long-bone scan for old fractures
b. examine for sexual abuse if indicated
c. photograph all evidence of abuse

PSYCHOSOCIAL ASSESSMENT (INTERVIEWS WITH INFORMANTS SEPARATELY AND INDIVIDUALLY)

Indicators of abuse:
a. child brought for treatment by un-related adult or individual brought for treatment by someone other than caretaker
b. unexplained delay of 12 hours or more in seeking medical treatment
c. history of injury which is inconsistent with developmental capacity of patient
d. history of injury which is inconsistent with injury
e. historical accounts of the injury which differ with each interview
f. prior history of injury to patient or siblings of child-patient
g. prior history of failure to thrive of child-patient
h. inappropriate affect by parent(s) or caretaker(s)
i. evidence of substance abuse by parent(s) or caretaker(s)
j. attribution of guilt to the parent or child-patient's sibling
k. social isolation of family/patient

DOCUMENT FINDINGS IN WRITING AND WITH PHOTOGRAPHS

If 1 or more positive findings, then ...

EXPLAIN TO FAMILY THE NECESSITY FOR CALLING PROTECTIVE SERVICE AGENCY

— and —

REPORT TO APPROPRIATE PROTECTIVE SERVICE AGENCY FOR INVESTI-GATION

MEDICAL STAFF

a. admit for burn treatment
b. observe family interactions with patient and document
c. encourage family to see health professionals as trustworthy and helpful

PSYCHOSOCIAL STAFF

a. establish therapeutic alliance with family
b. support family emotionally and teach caretaking skills, anger management, self-nurturance
c. document observations
d. inform family honestly of all decisions

PROTECTIVE SERVICE AGENCY

a. investigate home circumstances and circumstances of injury
b. recommended to court

COURT

REMOVAL AND PLACEMENT WITH FOSTER PARENTS OR ALTERNATIVE CARETAKERS

— or —

RETURN TO FAMILY, PRIOR SITUATION

— if —

PATIENT WITH FOSTER FAMILY, ALTERNATIVE CARETAKERS

— if —

PATIENT WITH ORIGINAL FAMILY, CARETAKERS

MEDICAL STAFF

— and —

a. follow physical/emotional well-being of patient after discharge
b. train foster parents/caretakers in physical care for patient
c. monitor for compliance

PSYCHOSOCIAL STAFF

a. assess foster home or new placement for psychosocial needs
b. refer for services as appropriate
c. follow supportively to maintain compliance
d. maintain some relationship with family of origin when it seems likely that patient will return to that unit

MEDICAL STAFF

— and —

a. follow physical/emotional well-being of patient after discharge
b. train parents/caretakers in physical care for patient
c. monitor for compliance

PSYCHOSOCIAL STAFF

a. refer family for treatment and/or services as appropriate
b. follow supportively to maintain compliance

Fig. 60.1 Flow of activities toward treating victims of abuse.

tionship, the helping professional must be sensitive to the fear, pain, and sadness that are often the sources of the perpetrators' abusive behavior.[13]

Child abuse indicators

Most abusive burn injuries to children occur to the very young, aged 3 years and under, and are scald or contact burns[13–15,17] Most abused children live in poverty-level households headed by a young, single parent who has two or more children.[13,14,17,26] Abused burned children are reported to require longer hospitalization and to have higher rates of morbidity and mortality from their burns than nonabused children.[27–29]

Table 60.2 Exposure time to receive a severe burn in hot water			
Degrees in Celsius	Degrees in Fahrenheit	Time to Second Degree Burn	Time to Third Degree Burn
45	113.0	120 minutes	180.0 minutes
47	116.6	20 minutes	45.0 minutes
48	118.4	15 minutes	20.0 minutes
49*	120.0*	8 minutes	10.0 minutes
51	124.0	2 minutes	4.2 minutes
55	131.0	17 seconds	30 seconds
60	140.0	3 seconds	5 seconds

*Voluntary standard published by Consumer Product Safety Commission, American Journal of Public Health, and the plumbing industry.
Downward adjustments to time needed for young children.

Suspicion of child abuse may be prompted by observations of parental behavior. Parents who are not abusive typically report the details of the child's injury spontaneously and express concern about the treatment and prognosis. They exhibit a sense of guilt, ask questions about discharge data and follow-up care, visit the child frequently, and bring gifts. In contrast, abusive parents usually do not volunteer information, but are evasive or contradictory; they seem critical of the child and angry with the patient for being hurt. They do not seem to feel guilty or show remorse. They show no concern about the injury, treatment or prognosis. They seldom visit or play with the child, do not ask about discharge date or follow-up care, and appear to be preoccupied with themselves and unconcerned about the child.[22]

Prospective studies of abuse do not exist, and the ability to predict future injury is limited. However, factors associated with abuse and neglect have been reviewed retrospectively in a number of studies.[11,13,15,26,30,31] A comprehensive list of indicators of child abuse/neglect gleaned from these studies and our own experience is presented in **Table 60.3**. Utilizing these indicators provides an informed framework from which to begin assessing risk for abuse and neglect.[32] Any one of these indicators should elicit suspicion. The presence of two or more indicators has been found to identify 60% of abusive situations.[19]

When evaluating risk factors, consideration should be given to the cultural standards of the family's home community. Folk-healing practices should be queried, as well as use of traditional healers.[11,33] We have seen in the past year two newborns who were burned in hospitals in a country where improperly trained hospital personnel were tending to the infants.

Adult abuse and indicators

Abuse by burning of adults is, as noted earlier, much more rarely reported, probably because the index of suspicion for abuse of an adult is low and therefore injuries are more rarely questioned. Adult victims are also noted to be reluctant to report the circumstances of their injuries because of their fear of retaliation or because of shame and embarrassment.[23] Spousal[34] and elder abuse[4] are subpopulations within the adult population who are at risk for abuse by burning. Two studies describe burn injuries of adults due to violent assault.[5,6] Associated risk factors in these reports were substance abuse and domestic violence. Although Purdue and Hunt[6] report that there was no identifiable burn pattern, Krob et al.[5] described a pattern of scald injury to the anterior trunk and upper extremity. Males and females seem equally at risk for burning by assault.

Bowden et al.[2] describe a population of older adults made vulnerable by physical or mental impairment who were burned by abuse or neglect. All but three of their 26 subjects were burned while living in health care facilities or institutions. Although this single article identifies abuse of the elderly by burning as a problem, it is likely that such abuse occurs with greater frequency than presently documented, and that it occurs within family settings as well as the institutional settings which dominate this Michigan sample.

Elder abuse has been identified as a public concern in the United States only in the last 15 years. Relatively little, however, has been written about the subject in spite of the estimated 2.5 million person who suffer annually.[35] When such abuse does occur within the family, it is often perpetrated by an adult, child or spouse of the victim. The abusers are often intoxicated and were themselves abused as children.[3] Some abusers of the elderly are individuals with no prior history of pathology, but who have become exhausted by the demands of their lives, e.g. caring for an aged parent as well as a spouse and children of their own.[7,23] Passive neglect may also result in injury to an elderly or vulnerable person, particularly if that person is disoriented or is reluctant to ask for attention and physical care.[35] Risk factors of abuse or neglect for adults are similar to those for children and are listed in **Table 60.4**.[2,3,7,23,35]

Reporting and documenting suspected abuse or neglect

State legislatures in the United States first enacted reporting laws in 1963, and by 1967 every State had laws mandating professionals who work with children to report suspected abuse or neglect to designated authorities. A federal law, the Child Abuse Prevention and Treatment Act, was passed in 1974. The laws require professionals to report suspected abuse or neglect of a child when there is evidence that 'would lead a competent professional to believe abuse or neglect is reasonably likely'.[36] In the case of abuse and neglect, privileged communication typically only exists for attorney and client. If local laws are not known, staff at the governing protective agency, sourcebooks,[37] or the hospital attorneys will be able to provide necessary legal references.

There are no federal programs to specifically address reporting of suspected abuse in adults. Each State has its own set of definitions, reporting laws, and penalties.[23] Professionals who suspect abuse or malignant neglect of an adult should be guided by the same principles as in reporting suspicious injury to a child, comforted by the knowledge that it is the role of the health care profes-

Table 60.3 Risk factors for abuse/neglect by burning

I. Forced – Immersion Demarcation
- Symmetrical, mirror image burn of extremities
- Glove-like (burned in web spaces)
- Circumferential
- Minimal splash marks
- Uniform depth
- Full-thickness
- Clear line of demarcation, crisp margin
- Doughnut-shaped scars on buttocks/perineum (spared area forcibly compressed against container, decreasing contact with hot liquid, if container is not on a heated element)
- Flexion burns, 'zebra' demarcation to popliteal fossa, anterior hip area, or lower abdominal wall
- Injuries of restraint (e.g., bruises mimicking fingers and hands on upper extremities)[16]

II. Injury Demarcation, Other
- Incongruent with history of event
- Pattern of household appliance – note whether even pattern versus brushed, imperfect mark
- Scald
- Location of injury: palms, soles, buttocks, perineum, genitalia, posterior upper body
- Cigarette burn, if more than one on normally clothed body parts and if impetigo ruled out

III. History of Injury
- Evasive, implausible explanation
- Incompatible with child's developmental age
- Changes in story (across time, between reporters)
- Unexplained burn; discovered to be burned – rule out dermatologic epidermolysis bullosa (EB), dermatitis, dermatitis herpetiformis, chemical burn due to analgesic cream, phytophotodermatitis,[17] and birth marks, including Mongolian spots[18]
- Under-supervised – inadequate monitoring, impaired person supervising, inordinately young baby-sitter (< 12 years of age)
- Burn is older than history given
- Water outlet temperature greater than 120° F
- Mechanism of burn is incompatible with injury (e.g., exposure time, history of event, and degree burn are inconsistent (refer to www.antiscald.com/table; reproduced in Table 60.2).
- Patient's peri-event behavior displeasing to caregiver (e.g., inconsolable, failed to meet caregiver's expectations)
- Toileting events related to history of injury[19]
- Burn attributed to:
  - child or patient, as per caregiver
  - caregiver who is not present at the health care facility
  - caregiver, as per patient
- Delay in seeking medical treatment – note estimated time of delay

IV. Developmental Associations
- Pre-verbal, non-verbal person
- Vulnerable person (e.g., special need, failure to thrive, elderly)
- Caregiver expectations are inconsistent with patient's development; caregiver overestimates child's developmental skills and safety knowledge; caregiver unaware of patient's developmental capacity
- Patient has symptoms of mental disorder (e.g., ruminating, aggressive)
- Patient displays disturbing behaviors related to attachment (e.g., excessive crying, clinging, apathy/ lethargy, excessively withdrawn, listless, unemotional, submissive, polite, fearful, vacant stare)
- Hyper-sexualized language or behavior, as compared to same age peers

V. Caregiver-patient Relations
- History of interrupted caregiver-child bonding
- Adolescent caregiver(s) (e.g., child-child versus adult-child interactions)
- Strained interactions; inappropriate expectations of the patient by the caregiver
- Role reversal (rely on patient for support)
- Inappropriate or lack of caregiver concern
  - detached
  - lack of sympathy
  - lack of physical contact (e.g., fails to hold or pick up child)
  - inebriated during visits
  - infrequent visits

VI. Other Physical Signs of Abuse or Neglect
- Unrelated injuries:
  - fractures, dislocations; rupture to spleen, liver, or pancreas; point tenderness; impaired range of motion or function
  - signs of poisoning
  - ocular insult (edema, scleral hemorrhage, hyphema, bruise, blue sclera)
  - swelling, bogginess, depressions, cephalhematomas palpable on head or increased intracranial pressure at fontanel
  - blood, infection, or foreign body in ear
  - edema, bleeding, septal deviation of nose; foreign bodies in nose; cerebrospinal fluid rhinorrhea from nose
- Other injuries involving the skin: hematomas, soft tissue swelling, lacerations, fingernail markings, scars, bruises (check behind ear), welts, rope burns, strangulation marks, bites, alopecia – note color, size, shape, and location of each (scalp most visible while shampooing)
- Abdominal tenderness, guarding, rebound tenderness, or bruises
- Cardiac instability, tachycardia, murmurs, flow murmurs secondary to anemia, or palpable rib fractures
- Dehydration or malnutrition – note weight, height, and head circumference
- Previous burns
- Unkempt, e.g., severe diaper rash, dirt under nails or in axillae, odoriferous, dirt on plantar surfaces of feet in cold weather
- Inadequate or no immunization record
- Inadequate dental care (e.g., caries); trauma to lips, tongue, gums, frenula, palate, pharynx, or teeth
- Inadequate medical care
- Inappropriate dress
- Assess prior to invasive medical procedures
- Genital, urethral, vaginal, or anal bruising, bleeding
- Swollen, red vulva or perineum
- Foreign body in genital area
- Positive cultures for sexually transmitted diseases – if herpes develops, note whether lesions are on unburned body surface area, on genitals or Type II
- Pregnant minor
- Recurrent urinary tract infections, streptococcus pharyngitis, abdominal pain

VII. Family
- Caregiver abused or emotionally deprived during childhood
- Limited disciplinary practices (e.g., only physical punishment)
- Lack of external supports; isolation
- Mental illness; substance abuse; criminal history
- Lack of financial self-sufficiency
- Poor employment history
- Dependent caregiver; unable to cope with daily responsibilities; unorganized
- Violent couples; impulsive; easily frustrated
- Previous Department of Protective and Regulatory Services involvement[20]
- Prior accidents to dependents
- Acute family stressors
- No primary caregiver

Table 60.4 Indicators of abuse/neglect of adults
1. Physical dependence.
2. Psychological dependence.
3. Accessibility as a target for abuse as in institutional living or living with a 'caretaker'.
4. Caretaker(s) with a history of substance abuse, and/or other psychopathology.
5. Social isolation.
6. An injury that is not consistent with the story described.
7. Conflicting reports of the injury.
8. Scalds with clear-cut immersion lines and no splash marks.
9. Scalds that involve the anterior or posterior half of an extremity and/or the buttocks and genitals, or a flexion pattern.
10. Other physical signs of abuse/neglect.
11. History of related incidents.

sional to report suspicious injury in the interest of helping the patient stay safe and healthy. When abuse or neglect is suspected, a report must be made to the proper governing protective agency. In the United States, the protective agencies operate under the purview of the State Department of Health and Human Welfare. Most States' referrals are made to a statewide intake office. The numbers are located in all phone books. A National Child Abuse Hotline is available (800)-4-A-CHILD (800–422–4453). Telecommunications Device for the Deaf number is (800)-2-A-CHILD. At least two web sites have the 1–(800) numbers for statewide reporting: acf.dhhs.gov/programs/cb/rpt_abu and childhelpusa.org/report.

Health care professionals are often reluctant to report suspicious injuries because they feel as if they are condemning a person with uncertain evidence and because they have been trained to maintain patients' confidentiality. However, the medical professional is the sole point of possible intervention for most victims. The purpose of reporting a suspicious injury is to prevent further harm. Making a report is an official trigger requesting investigation and not a condemnation. It is not the health professional's job to prove culpability.

The ultimate decision about whether abuse has actually occurred is left to the investigating officials; however, the professionals reporting the incident must document the observed data to provide the investigating officials and/or the courts the information necessary to intervene appropriately. Professionals should document, for example, observations that render the caretaker's professed ignorance of the cause of injury questionable or that an explanation of cause is implausible given the nature of the injury. Observations of inappropriate behaviour or lack of interest in the child's treatment must be documented. Although any single observation may seem unimportant, the pattern of behaviors described by multiple observations may be very significant in obtaining protection for the victim and help for the perpetrator.[36] In addition to the documentation of first hand observations, the following tasks should be delegated:

- Examine the patient for other signs of abuse or neglect including a long bone radiological scan.
- Photograph any possible evidence.
- If the patient has been referred from another hospital,

access information from the staff at that hospital to determine whether they identified suspicious aspects of the injury and whether the injury was reported to an investigating agency. If so, ascertain the number assigned to the patient's case by the investigating agency. This number is needed for subsequent calls related to the patient.
- Interview the patient.
- Interview the family members or caretakers individually and together for thorough histories of the event, sensitive to the differences in the story or changes across time.
- Obtain a thorough family history, the patient's medical history and the developmental capacity of the patient.
- Gather other available collateral information, e.g. medical records from other places of treatment.[20]

Understanding that abuse does occur and is an expression of rage stemming from pain and sadness can enable the health care professional to begin the process of assessment as a critical observer and empathetic interviewer. The interviewer must not respond personally to apparent hostility from the informant(s) but recognize hostility as a defense against fear. Each informant should be interviewed separately, not only to check for conflicting stories, but also because there are likely to be tensions between the informants that inhibit the interviewer's ability to establish a relationship with each individual. The informants should also be interviewed together to provide the opportunity to observe tensions, conflicts, and alliances within the family group.

Interviewing the pediatric patient with suspicious injury

Interviews with the child-patient are especially important in cases of suspicious injury. Even children as young as 29 months often relate information with remarkable accuracy.[38] An interview with the child alone should be conducted by a professional who has established rapport with the child. The professional can first ask the child to recall specific past experiences which are thought to have no relationship to the current suspected abuse, such as a birthday party or Christmas celebration. The descriptions of these events provide some indication of the child's ability to recall and to describe memories either verbally or in drawings. Questions about the specific events leading to injury should initially be very general; e.g. 'how did you get hurt?' and the child should be encouraged to tell the story freely. Specific questions for clarification should be asked only after the child has told the story. If the child seems unwilling to talk about what happened, the interviewer can suggest the child raise a hand or wiggle a finger to signal that they know something but do not yet want to talk about it. Interviews with a young child are best conducted in several short sessions, giving the child an opportunity to feel safe in the hospital and with the interviewer.[39]

Interviews with the elderly or handicapped adult patient

When interviewing children or other vulnerable patients, special care must be taken to help them feel safe and comfortable with the interviewer and the hospital setting. The vulnerable adult may be frightened of retribution by the caretaker(s) or afraid of being placed in an institutional setting. The abused adult also may be embarrassed and ashamed of their victimization. If the perpetrator is an adult child, the victim may attempt to protect the perpetrator from detection and punishment. The interviewer must assess the circumstances of the injury and establish a relationship in which the patient can trust the hospital staff to act in the best interest of all concerned, i.e. the patient and the perpetrator(s).

Maintaining professional relationships with patient and family

Working therapeutically with a family suspected of abusing or mistreating the patient requires skill and diplomacy, not only because of a strong tendency on the part of health care professionals to be angry with anyone who would allow or inflict such maltreatment, but also because suspected perpetrators often appear hostile toward the professional staff. Yet establishing a therapeutic alliance with these families is extremely important, for, no matter how serious the injury, the patient will probably return to that same family, if not at the time of discharge from the hospital, then at a future time.

One careful study[40] to identify factors that determined which children would be removed from parental custody found that the nature of the abuse and the social worker's perception of the severity of maltreatment, as well as child, family, and environmental factors were poor predictors of those decisions. Referrals to protective agencies from police and the courts were more likely to result in foster home placement of the children than referrals from medical or school officials. The single most important determinant was the identity and/or location of the investigating agency. Although not mentioned in that study, our experience indicates that the availability of foster homes is a prime determinant. Agencies in large urban areas are much more likely to recommend foster home placement than agencies in rural areas even though burn injuries by abuse can always be considered as potentially lethal, regardless of where they occur. Even if the child is removed from parental custody, placement will often be made with another family member, such as a grandparent or aunt.

Such placement might seem illogical since the families of abusive patients are also probably abusive and since all family members are likely to share similar values and sympathies.[22] Nonetheless, a key provision of the United States federal law regarding child abuse requires that 'reasonable efforts' be made to prevent removal of neglected and abused children from their homes, and to reunify families when children are removed.[36] The intent of the law is to ensure that families are provided necessary services to enable them to become healthy and nurturing environments. However, 'reasonable efforts' is not defined. Thus, in conjunction with the large caseloads of most caseworkers in protective service agencies and the limited number of available foster homes, abiding by the law frequently results in children continuing to live with the same adults who hurt them. Adults who have been abused within the family often prefer returning to that family setting, especially if they believe the alternative to be institutions.[23] This means that, in order to protect the patient from future harm and to achieve good recovery and rehabilitation, the professionals who interact with the family suspected of violent abuse must establish therapeutic rapport.

Therapeutic interventions with abusive families

Ironically, the professionals of the burn team who identify and report suspected abuse also have an exceptional opportunity to intervene in the dynamic process that has led to the violence. During the days or weeks of the patient's hospitalization, the family is placed in a situation of coerced interaction with the burn team. At this time, the family is also in a state of crisis, i.e. their customary defenses have failed to protect them from external scrutiny. In a state of crisis, when their usual belief systems and defensive behaviors are failing, people are more likely to be amenable to new learning and change than during times of equilibrium.[41] Thus, if members of the burn team can interact with the abusive family in ways that invalidate, or at least cast serious doubt upon, the family beliefs, there is a good possibility that the family system will begin to change. As change is initiated, continued positive support for change can lead to further change.

In order to take advantage of this therapeutic opportunity, the members of the team must relate to abusers with honesty and compassion. This does not mean that the team should approve of the behaviors of the perpetrator(s) nor advocate for the perpetrator(s) to be given another opportunity to harm a victim. However, the team can work with perpetrators in a manner that encourages them to trust professional help. The team's behavior can demonstrate that not all people are self-serving and that it is possible to relate to others in ways that are more likely to lead to gratification of their needs for nurturance and comfort. To work effectively with these families, it is essential to control the expression of anger on the part of the health care team. The clinician who rages against abusers only reinforces the abusers' view of the world as a hostile, uncaring place against which one must battle for survival. To mitigate one's natural anger toward abusers, it is helpful to remember the sad histories of abusers as victims and to respond to them as the suffering, hurt children they once were. Beneath the hostile suspicious facade of the adult abuser is a frightened and lonely child who feels hopelessly unworthy of kindness. The clinician who is consistently honest, firm, and compassionate can develop a therapeutic alliance with a perpetrator even while explaining that a report is being made to the appropriate investigating agencies. It can be explained that this report is not only mandated by law, but also is a way to obtain helpful services for the family. The clinician then must assist the family during the process of investigation. It is important that the clinician continue to honestly inform the family of decisions that are made as a result of the investigation.

Even while explaining that parental rights are terminated or that criminal charges are being filed, a skillful clinician can maintain a therapeutic relationship with the perpetrator(s). By helping the perpetrator(s) perceive the situation as one in which there is hope and opportunity to receive help, the clinician can continue a therapeutic relationship that greatly enhances the likelihood that the abusive family will accept further assistance to continue the process of change.

The burn team can work with the community agencies to obtain help for abusive families. Many communities have programs that provide foster grandparents or parent aides, i.e. lay therapists who teach parenting skills and nurture the parent(s).[22,24] There also may be local self-help groups or telephone crisis intervention services for abusive families; concrete services such as financial assistance or transportation are available for most families in need in the

United States. If the burn team has succeeded in developing and maintaining the trust of the abusive family, they are in an advantageous position to encourage families whose prior experiences with social service agencies may have left them hostile and suspicious. Even when parental rights are terminated or the patient is removed from the home, the burn team's continued therapeutic support of the abuser(s) is advisable since the victim will likely return to that family eventually. In any event, perpetrators of violence against others are a risk to society, and health professionals have an obligation to use their knowledge and skills to diminish that risk.

Firesetting occurrence

Firesetting destroys and compromises human lives and is associated with other unsavory criminal acts. Some of the people setting fires are also the ones incurring burn injuries while offending. Though some firesetters are arsonists and need to be incarcerated, the majority of firesetters have a problem amenable to treatment. The burn-injured firesetter, however, is at risk for not having the firesetting behavior addressed. A typical belief is that having been burned, the firesetter will have learned a lesson and will cease the dangerous behavior – a belief that is not always justified. If the patient is a child, staff and family may want to shrug the event off as typical 'child's play', and that may be the case in the very young child. However, firesetting should be taken very seriously. Ignoring the behavior can have very serious consequences.[42] Again, if presented with sensitivity to the concerns of the family, education about possible consequences of continued dangerous behavior and about possible avenues for help will usually convince the family to permit a report to be made.

Given the severe devastation caused by firesetting, thought should be given to the role of hospital staff when treating patients suspected of having been involved either as an active or passive participant in firesetting. Though safety officer involvement in firesetting occurrence has great potential, the degree to which fire officials are involved is variable. Some States have no laws addressing the reporting of burn injuries to fire service officials, while others clearly regulate burn injury reporting. Such laws clarify a limitation to patient confidentiality. Massachusetts law mandates the reporting of all burn injuries ≥5% total body surface area. State police manage the Massachusetts Burn injury Reporting System (M-BIRS), which delineates procedures, forms, and education on both tollfree telephone and facsimile reporting. Excerpted below is the Massachusetts General Law Chapter 112, Section 12A, Amended by the Act of 1986:

> Every physician . . . examining or treating a person with a burn injury affecting five percent or more of the surface area of his body, or, whenever any such case is treated in a hospital, sanitarium or other institution, the manager, superintendent or other person in charge thereof, shall report such cases . . . at once to the commissioner of public safety and to the police in the community where the burn occurred.

Advocating for such legislation in all 50 States would be a meaningful mission, as has been accomplished with child abuse and neglect laws. A more immediate change may be accomplished through hospital policy. Patient confidentiality is the primary concern when establishing policies for reporting fire occurrence. Prior to creating related hospital policy, discussing questions such as those below with the hospital attorney will facilitate clarification of state laws relevant to fire-setting, privileged communication, and the reporting of firesetting occurrence.[43]

- In what cases is firesetting a criminal activity in your State?
- Does privileged communication apply to events involving this type of criminal activity?
- If future harm to self or others is likely, is confidentiality limited? Though predicting exactly which person will set another fire is not possible, 81% children who set a fire and do not engage in treatment will set another fire within 1 year.[42] The high likelihood of future firesetting behavior, combined with the potential for lethal injury, influences clinical practice.
- Is breaking confidentiality for the purpose of referring to a firesetter program justified? Juvenile firesetter treatment programs are typically affiliated with local fire departments. Referrals for the programs originate with the fire safety officer. In order to accomplish a clinically relevant treatment referral, the local fire department would need to be contacted. Some program's low recidivism rates have significantly increased the safety of entire communities.[44]

Preventing all burn injury perpetrated by a human offense is the ultimate goal. Involving the safety officer, whether consequent to abuse, neglect, or firesetting, is tertiary prevention in which hospital professionals can make a significant difference. Safety officer intervention due to a single injury could potentially prevent several other injuries, by means of external monitoring, intra-individual change, and/or familial change.[45]

References

1. Hansen JC, Barnhill LR. *Clinical Approaches to Family Violence.* Rockville, Maryland: Aspen, 1982; 157.
2. Bowden M, Grant S, Vogel B, Prasad J. The elderly, disabled and handicapped adult burned through abuse and neglect. *Burns* 1988; **14**(6): 447–50.
3. Rathbone-McCuan E. Elderly victims of family violence and neglect. *Social Casework: The Journal of Contemporary Social Work* 1980; 296–304.
4. Rathbone-McCuan E, Goodstein R. Elder abuse: clinical considerations. *Psychiatric Annals* 1985; **15**(5): 331–9.
5. Krob M, Johnson A, Jordan M. Burned and battered adults. *J Burn Care Rehabil* 1986; **7**(6): 529–31.
6. Purdue G, Hunt J. Adult assault as a mechanism of burn injury. *Arch Surg* 1990; **125**: 268–9.
7. Pedrick-Cornell C, Gelles RJ. Elder abuse: the status of current knowledge. *Family Relations* 1982; **31**: 457–65.
8. Kessler D. Physical, sexual, & emotional abuse of children. *Clin Symp* 1991; **43**(1): 1–32.
9. Johnson CF, Showers J. Injury variables in child abuse. *Child Abuse Neglect* 1985; **9**: 207–15.
10. Meagher DP. Burns. In: Raffensperger JG, ed. *Swenson's Pediatric Surgery* 5th edn. Norwalk, CT: Appleton & Lange, 1990; 317–37.
11. Giardino A, Christian C, Giardino E. *A Practical Guide to the Evaluation of Child Physical Abuse and Neglect.* Thousand Oaks, CA: Sage, 1997; 74–96.
12. Herndon D, Rutan R, Rutan T. Management of the pediatric patient with burns. *J Burn Care Rehabil* 1993; **14**(1): 3–8.
13. Weimer C, Goldfarb I, Slater H. Multidisciplinary approach to working with burn victims of child abuse. *J Burn Care Rehabil* 1988; **9**(1): 79–82.
14. Showers J, Garrison K. Burn abuse. A four-year study. *J Trauma* 1988; **28**(11): 1581–3.
15. Hight D, Bakalar H, Lloyd J. Inflicted burns in children. *J Am Med Assoc* 1979; **242**(6): 517–20.
16. Hobbs C. When are burns not accidental? *Arch Dis Childhood* 1986; **61**: 357–61.
17. Kumar P. Child abuse by thermal injury-a retrospective survey. *Burns* 1984; **10**: 344–8.
18. Rossignal A, Locke J, Burke J. Paediatric burn injuries in New England, USA. *Burns* 1990; **16**(1): 41–8.

19. Hammond J, Perez-Stable A, Ward C. Predictive value of historical and physical characteristics for the diagnosis of child abuse. *Southern Med J* 1991; **84(2)**: 166–8.

20. Rosenberg N, Marino D. Frequency of suspected abuse/neglect in burn patients. *Pediatr Emerg Care* 1989; **5(4)**: 219–21.

21. Kempe CH. Paediatric implications of the battered baby syndrome. *Arch Dis Childhood* 1971; **46**: 28–37.

22. Justice B, Justice R. *The Abusing Family*. New York: Human Services Press, 1976.

23. Fulmer T. Elder mistreatment: Progress in community detection and intervention. *Family Community Health* 1991; **14(2)**: 26–34.

24. Justice R, Justice B. Crisis intervention with abusing families: Short-term cognitive coercive group therapy using goal attainment scaling. In: Roberts AR, ed. *Crisis Intervention Handbook*. Belmont, CA: Wadsworth, 1990; 153–72.

25. Goldberg H. The dynamics of rage between the sexes in a bonded relationship. In: Hansen JC, Barnhill LR, eds. *Clinical Approaches to Family Violence*. Rockville, MD: Aspen, 1982; 61–7.

26. Bakalar H, Moore J, Lloyd J. Psychosocial dynamics of pediatric burn abuse. *Health Social Work* 1981; 27–31.

27. Watkins A, Gagan R, Cupoli J. Child abuse by burning. *J Florida Med Assoc* 1985; **72(7)**: 497–502.

28. Campbell J, LaClave L. Clinical depression in pediatric burn patients. *Burns* 1987; **13(3)**: 213–7.

29. Purdue G, Hunt J, Prescott P. Child abuse by burning – An index of suspicion. *J Trauma* 1988; **28(2)**: 221–4.

30. Rivara F. Developmental and behavioral issues in childhood injury prevention. *Dev Behav Pediatr* 1995; **16(5)**: 362–70.

31. Ayoub C, Pfeiffer D. Burns as a manifestation of child abuse and neglect. *Am J Dis Children* 1979; **133**: 910–4.

32. Doctor M. Abuse through burns. In: Carrougher G, ed. *Burn Care and Therapy*. St Louis, MO: Mosby, 1998; 359–80.

33. Forjuoh S. Pattern of intentional burns to children in Ghana. *Child Abuse Neglect* 1995; **19(7)**: 837–41.

34. Hendriks JH, Black D, Kaplan T. *When Father Kills Mother: Guiding Children Through Trauma & Grief*. New York: Routledge, 1993.

35. Sukosky DG. Elder abuse: A preliminary profile of abusers and the abused. *Family Violence and Sexual Assault Bulletin* 1992; **8(4)**: 23–6.

36. Myers JEB. *Legal Issues in Child Abuse and Neglect*. Newbury Park, CA: Sage, 1992; 102.

37. Hays JR, Costello R, eds. *Texas Law and the Practice of Psychology*. Austin, TX: Texas Psychological Association, 1994.

38. Fivush R. Developmental perspectives on autobiographical recall. In: Goodman GS, Bottoms BL, eds. *Child Victims, Child Witness: Understanding and Improving Testimony*. New York: Guilford Press, 1993; 1–24.

39. Yuille JC, Hunter R, Joffe R, Zaparniuk J. Interviewing children in sexual abuse cases. In: Goodman GS, Bottoms BL, eds. *Child Victims, Child Witness: Understanding and Improving Testimony*. New York: Guilford Press, 1993; 95–115.

40. Runyan DK. The emotional impact of societal intervention into child abuse. In: Goodman GS, Bottoms BL, eds. *Child Victims, Child Witness: Understanding and Improving Testimony*. New York: Guilford Press, 1993; 263–77.

41. Roberts AR. An overview of crisis theory and crisis intervention. In: Roberts AR, ed. *Crisis Intervention Handbook*. Belmont, CA: Wadsworth, 1990; 3–16.

42. Kolko D. *Juvenile Firesetter Intervention Clinical Training*. Pittsburg, PA: University of Pittsburgh School of Medicine, Department of Psychiatry, 2000.

43. Keith-Spiegel P, Koocher G. *Ethics in Psychology: Professional Standards and Cases*. New York: Random House, 1985.

44. Wilcox D, Pinsonneault I. *What is Juvenile Firesetting? The Scope and Complexity of the Problem*. Boston, MA: Harvard Medical School, Department of Psychiatry, 2000.

45. Yamamoto L, Wiebe R, Matthews WJ, Sia C. The Hawaii EMS-C project data: I. Reducing pediatric emergency morbidity and mortality; II. Statewide pediatric emergency registry to monitor morbidity and mortality. *Pediat Emerg Care*, 1992; **8(2)**: 70–8.

Chapter 61

Psychosocial recovery and reintegration of patients with burn injuries

Patricia E Blakeney, James A Fauerbach
Walter J Meyer III, Christopher R Thomas

Introduction

Burn treatment extends beyond patient survival to include recovery of optimal function for the whole person. The increased likelihood of physical survival[1,2] heightens concern for potential psychological morbidity for the burn survivor.[3–7] Even in emergency circumstances, burn care providers enact treatment plans based on an assumption of future life for the patient. Decisions about treatment are influenced by concerns for preserving function, optimizing cosmetic appearance, and restoring the psychological well-being. Psychological and social issues are integral parts of burn treatment from the time of injury through recovery and rehabilitation.

Burn survivors experience a series of traumatic assaults to the body and mind and the fabric of their social network which present extraordinary challenges to psychological resilience.[3,6,8,9] Contrary to what might be expected, empirical data regarding the long-term sequelae of burn injury indicate that many burn survivors do achieve a satisfying quality of life and that most are judged to be well-adjusted individuals. However, 30% of any given sample of adult burn survivors consistently demonstrate moderate to severe psychological and/or social difficulties.[10–13] Similarly, most pediatric burn survivors, even those with the most extensive and disfiguring injuries, adjust well.[14–18] The incidence of psychopathology among children may be somewhat higher than for adults.[9,19–27]

Empirical studies, as well as clinical observations and patient self-reports, suggest that burn care of the whole person can facilitate positive psychological adaptation to the challenges of traumatic injury, painful treatment, and permanent disfigurement.[9,18]

Yet, a significant minority of burn survivors report a diminished quality of life, including dissatisfaction with appearance and social or occupational difficulties.[28–30] Burn injury often leads to at least temporary reduction in social involvement[31] and vocational activity, with 50–60% of individuals requiring a change in employment status.[28] Decreased sexual satisfaction, particularly for women, may also occur and appears to relate to physical changes and body image more than burn size or location.[32]

Postburn adjustment is affected by quality of adjustment prior to injury, notably pre-burn psychiatric disorder.[33,34] Recently it has been demonstrated that even subclinical levels of post-traumic distress[35] and body image dissatisfaction[36] during the acute hospitalization can independently reduce health-related quality of life for prolonged periods. Importantly, baseline indices of psychosocial strength (absence of preburn psychopathology) and support (marital status and living arrangement) predicts psychological adjustment after a severe burn injury while burn severity (TBSA, burn location, trips to OR) does not.[22,23,37] For children and adolescents, several studies have found that postburn adjustment is determined primarily by the quality of parental and family support. Family cohesion, organization, and emphasis on spiritual/moral concerns have all been found to relate to positive adjustment of pediatric burn survivors.[22,23,38] For adolescent survivors, families of well-adjusted individuals valued and encouraged autonomy within the context of family cohesion.[22]

Psychological treatment concurrent with physical treatment

Burn injury treatment and rehabilitation requires interdisciplinary participation, with a complete spectrum of specialists involved to a greater or lesser extent at each phase of treatment. Specialists focus on specific systems or functional domains of each patient at each stage of treatment but the overall approach of the team is integrated and organized both vertically and horizontally throughout the entire process. The *horizontal organization* flows longitudinally, such that variables assessed in earlier phases impact in measurable ways the variables assessed in later phases. We categorize those factors which influence burn injury and recovery in terms of six horizontal (i.e. longitudinal) time phases (pre-injury, admission, critical care, in-hospital recuperation, reintegration, and rehabilitation). Burn care and rehabilitation also has a *vertical organization* in which each phase is further categorized by the domains of function directly related to health-related quality of life (physiological/anatomical, cognitive, psychological, social). The assessment and intervention provided in these domains involve the entire patient from the cellular level upwards in complexity of organization to the organ system level, then to the cognitive and psychological level, and finally to the social system level. The individual's functional ability within each domain is bi-directionally related to the other domains. The assessment and treatment by the various specialties is therefore interdisciplinary. Each specialist interacts with the patient, with significant others in the patient's social system, and with the other members of the burn care and rehabilitation team. Thus, the burn care and rehabilitation team comprises a true system that operates over six time phases (i.e. horizontal organization) and across four functional domains (i.e. vertical organization).

Clinicians with expertise in human behavior should be involved in the treatment program for all burned patients throughout the process.[5,9,39–43] In this chapter, these experts are called psychotherapists. Every person, however, who interacts with a patient impacts the psychosocial world of the patient. Any caregiver, including the patient's family, may be the instrument of psychotherapeutic intervention.[9] The role of the psychotherapist is to consult with caregivers about psychological and social issues and to suggest therapeutic interventions that any or all can act upon.[41–43] Furthermore, the psychotherapist on a burn team provides direct treatment to patients as appropriate to their changing concerns. As the needs of the patient evolve, the intensity of direct psychotherapeutic intervention varies according to those changing needs.

The family of a patient will always greatly influence a patient's recovery and must be considered as part of a patient's treatment plan. For the psychotherapist on the burn team, the family unit is often the 'patient'.[9,43–46] Each individual within a family, including the burn survivor, is an essential element of this unit which must adapt to change. The psychosocial issues and therapeutic tasks for the patient and family are much the same across the spectrum of ages from young children through the elderly, regardless of size and severity of injury.[9,10,43,44,47–50]

Assisting with Death

Treatment plans and programs must be based on an assumption of life beyond the hospital; however, death also occurs on the burn unit, and psychosocial treatment planning includes plans for assisting patients in living to the cessation of life.[9] As part of such a plan, the patient's family must be aided in preparing for and enduring bereavement.[51] In this event, supporting and enhancing whatever coping strengths the family manifests is the primary task for psychotherapy. Most families initially deny the possibility of death, appearing not to hear an unwanted prognosis. Staff can allow the family to maintain hope while subtly preparing them with honest statements which pose death as an outcome that is possible to accept.[9] Comforting the bereft and helping them to care for themselves, physically and spiritually, are essential elements of a plan that facilitates the family's ability to participate in the process. Keeping the family informed about changes in the patient's condition and actively supporting, sometimes instructing, them in continuing their relationships with the dying patient help the patient and family through this difficult event. At the time of death, the staff can psychologically support the family by assisting them through the necessary paperwork (e.g. signing consents for release of the body or for autopsy) and in allowing them quiet, private time with the deceased loved one before the body is removed. Bereft family members often want to hold on to something belonging to or representing the deceased. The staff should offer to assist in finding or creating such a tangible object for distraught family members who may not think to make the request. At the Shriners Hospital in Galveston, families typically say they do want a 'memory' item. When no such item is readily available, a hand or foot print on paper or a plaster cast model of the patient's hand or foot seems to bring solace to those feeling such loss.

A death occurring in the context of family acceptance is more easily accepted by staff. Nevertheless, death of a patient is always sad and may elicit a wide range of strong emotions among the members of the burn team. Structuring a time for de-briefing and validating the feelings of the staff can be extremely helpful in maintaining the morale of the team as a whole.

The 'enabling–disabling process' and the 'new paradigm' of rehabilitation research

The key terms in rehabilitation science are: injury, impairment, functional limitation, disabling condition, and disability. Uniform definitions of these terms are provided in an Institute of Medicine (IOM) report.[52] *Injury* (i.e., pathology) is any interference of normal bodily processes or structures. *Impairment* is a loss or abnormality of mental, emotional, physiological or anatomical structure or function. A *functional limitation* is a restriction in the ability to perform an action or activity in the manner or within the range considered 'normal' and which is attributable to impairment. *Disability* is a limitation in performing socially defined roles expected of individuals within the social and physical environments. Impairments and functional limitations represent potentially disabling conditions, while disability itself is a function of the interaction between the person's limits and the environment.[52] The IOM model describes the pathway along which a person with potentially disabling conditions may decline (i.e. experience less access and/or less integration) from injury to impairment, and from impairment to functional limitation. Factors that moderate the relations among these include:

biology (e.g. genetic, congenital, pathology), environment (e.g. physical, social, psychological), and lifestyle (e.g. behavior).

Enablement (i.e. the absence of disability) is represented by full social–environmental integration including access to social opportunities (i.e. roles) and physical space (i.e. absence of physical barriers). The goals of rehabilitation science are to remove barriers to social and physical integration by restoring function to the individual and/or enhancing access to the environment.

A new paradigm for rehabilitation-related research is based on the IOM model and recommendations (1997), and has been incorporated into the long-range plan of the National Institute on Disability and Rehabilitation Research (NIDRR).[53] NIDRR, the principal source of USA federal funds for burn rehabilitation research, espouses a 'new paradigm' for conceptualizing and conducting rehabilitation research that places environmental factors on an equal footing with person factors. The complex interaction of impairments and functional limitations with environmental structure is understood to determine the degree of disability that results from any given potentially disabling condition. Environmental structure is broadly understood as composed of physical space (e.g. architecture, transportation systems), intrapersonal structure (e.g. personality), interpersonal structure (e.g. social support), and socio-economic structure (e.g. insurance coverage, work, and training opportunities). It is important to note that one's abilities may interact with aspects of the physical and social environments to enable full function in certain environments or at certain times, but allow for only partial integration into other environments and/or at other times. NIDRR has identified five substantive research areas related to the goals of their long-range plan.[53] The outcome areas targeted in the NIDRR initiatives for rehabilitation research are:

- employment;
- community integration;
- technology for access and function;
- health and function; and
- associated disabilities.

The goals of rehabilitation science are to develop basic and applied programs of research that preserve or restore function either directly or via technological accommodation, and to enhance access to the physical and social environment by removing barriers to full integration in the community and the workplace.

The longitudinal pattern of psychological recovery

Psychological healing occurs across time commensurate with physical healing in a pattern which is relatively predictable and consistent.[8,9,43–47,54,55] Awareness of this pattern allows caregivers to anticipate the emergence of psychosocial issues and to prepare a patient for coping with those issues. Predicting problematic issues for patients enables them to view their concerns in a context of normal reactions rather than as symptoms of psychological impairment.[5,9] For convenience in describing this pattern, we have arbitrarily designated a pre-injury phase and five phases of recovery: admission, critical care, in-hospital recuperation, reintegration, and rehabilitation.

Pre-injury Adjustment
Psychosocial assessment is usually begun immediately upon arrival. However, preburn physical and psychological health,

coping skills, and family/social support are closely related to the behavior, distress and recovery of a patient.[9,22,33–38,56–58] Size or severity of burn, age at injury, and gender of the survivor are important variables in psychotherapy, but have little documented influence on the eventual outcome for a survivor.[13,22,56,59,60] Prior stressful events and coping strategies, risk factors, as well as psychosocial and economic strengths are included in a good history of a patient's premorbid lifestyle. A patient's history, a patient's position in the family, and the family's strenghts and weaknesses are often helpful pieces of information in guiding plans for treatment.

Because a patient will be dependent to some extent on family or other caretakers during recovery, it is essential to identify risk factors in the family system.[9] Historical risk factors which may predispose individuals to burn injury and which portend poor prognoses are physical illness, substance abuse, psychiatric illness, behavioral problems, poverty, inadequate social support, and heightened family disruption.[3,61–66] These factors are often causally related to the burn injury and to post-injury recovery. For example, a lifetime prevalence of psychiatric disorder is much more common among patients with burn injuries relative to published national data from a representative community sample.[67] This is particularly troublesome in that this history of psychiatric disorder is significantly related to postburn psychiatric complications and to poorer postburn health-related quality of life.[67] In addition to these risk factors, every family has its unique difficulties. The trauma of serious injury exacerbates preexisting problems.

Early identification of psychosocial strengths and vulnerabilities, including those which contributed to the circumstances of the burn injury, allow the team to develop treatment and discharge plans which will optimize the patient's recovery. The importance of assessing the circumstances of injury is emphasized in instances of abuse or malignant neglect. In addition, during early assessment interviews with a family, the staff initiates a therapeutic alliance with those who are most likely to be involved in assisting a patient's recovery.

Admission Crisis
At the time of admission, patients with burn injuries universally suffer pain and anxiety. Most are experiencing terror, confusion, and psychological shock. Events causing a serious burn injury are frightening, and the patient often believes that death is imminent. The hospital environment can also be confusing and frightening. While the physiologic emergency is being treated aggressively, the psychological crisis must also be addressed. On admission, the primary psychological tasks are to establish therapeutic rapport, diminish anxiety, and assess the psychosocial strengths and needs of the patient. The first two tasks are addressed immediately by orienting a patient, by assisting the patient to focus on immediate priorities, and by assuring the patient that the burn team is composed of knowledeable experts who will provide excellent care. The patient's heightened anxiety can be expected to interfere with their comprehension, so it is usually necessary to repeat statements of reassurance. To prevent a patient from becoming emotionally overwhelmed, it may be necessary to – at least temporarily – not talk about trauma-related content perhaps by asking objective, easily answered questions not directly related to the event or injury (e.g. hometown, favorite sports, etc).[68]

Psychotherapeutic rapport is developed as a patient associates the voice or touch of a therapist with increased comfort.

Techniques of hypnotherapy or relaxation with focused imagery can be very helpful in quickly assisting a patient to feel more comfortable. Patients during this crisis can be expected to be cognitively and emotionally regressed, and it may be important to respond to them at that regressed level. Touching patients in a soothing rhythm is often the most effective way to maintain a regressed patient's focus and communicate reassurance.

Members of the patient's family are also traumatized and may experience difficulty in eating and sleeping for the first several days. They, too, experience difficulty in concentrating and may require frequent repetition of information. They may feel a loss of control, a generalized sense of incompetence and helplessness in providing comfort for the patient. The psychotherapeutic tasks to be accomplished immediately with a family are similar to those for a patient (i.e. to establish a therapeutic relationship and to diminish anxiety). Both tasks can often be initiated by assisting them in orienting to the hospital and by providing relevant information about the normal responses to trauma. Explaining, for example, that people in this situation often have difficulty for a few days in eating, sleeping, and concentrating, communicates empathy and validates that their distress is acceptable and temporary.[4,9] The family members are important components of the therapeutic efforts for the patient, and it is important to say this explicitly. This helps to return to them a sense of purpose and control. Even on the day of admission, the staff begin shaping the family behaviors and support network by outlining some immediate concerns. Learning about the injury and its treatment helps to restore a family's sense of competence and provides opportunities for them to experience the reality of their roles in helping the patient.

The manner in which an individual and family will ultimately adjust to long-term sequelae of a burn injury (e.g. deformity, disfigurement) is often determined in the early stages. 'The loss of reinforcement resulting from the limitations imposed by the new disability on a wide range of life's activities, the aversive sequelae of disability such as pain and fatigue, the individual's cognitions regarding the negative aspects of disability, and the negative attitudes of others toward the disabled can combine to result in emotional catastrophe' (J Michael, 1970, paraphrased in Brockway and Fordyce, p. 158).[69] It is therefore of the utmost importance that respect for individuality and autonomy be demonstrated from the first interactions of the treatment team.

Critical Care Phase

From hospital admission until the majority of open wounds are covered, the emphasis in treatment of a burned patient is necessarily on intensive medical and surgical care to resolve physiologic crises. This period is psychologically critical as well. A patient experiences great anxiety during much of this time. Fear of death blends into fear of pain and fear of treatment procedures.[44] A multitude of organic factors stemming from both the injury and its treatment, as well as premorbid conditions, can all contribute to psychological symptoms of disorientation, confusion, sleep disturbance, transient psychosis and delirium which are commonly observed among adolescent and adult patients.[44,70,71] Psychological interventions as well as pharmacological interventions can diminish anxiety and confusion. Repeated statements of orientation to time, place, and person are mandatory. Objects that are familiar and comforting to a patient can be placed in the patient's view or so that the patient can touch them. The patient's environment

should be as soothing as possible. A schedule which approximates a regular wake/sleep cycle helps a patient begin to feel normal.[9,71] Visits from family and friends can provide familiarity and reassurance to a patient.

Staff who interact with patients during this phase must be willing to listen to patients' anxieties and reassure them that the nightmares and vivid memories are normal aspects of recovery.[4] Staff can help patients focus on the present time in which they are safe in the hospital and are healing. When a patient is withdrawn or in a coma, staff must remember that the patient may be hearing, although not responding, and must take care to talk to the patient. They must also be discreet in what is said within a patient's hearing range. Patients are often listening to determine what will happen to them; and, in their altered mental states, they may attribute unexpected meanings to what they hear. Although the staff should persist in attempting to orient a patient, they should not argue about the patient's description of reality. Arguments with a patient who is having vivid illusions, delusions, or hallucinations are usually counterproductive. Psychological interventions are aimed at diminishing anxiety and increasing comfort rather than correcting a patient's perceptions of reality.[9]

Often, the content of the patient's delirium can be used to facilitate reassurance and relaxation. For example, a man in this phase who believed he was on a boat was combative and remained agitated in spite of psychopharmacological attempts to calm him. The psychologist assisted during procedures by talking to the patient about being on the boat in the same manner used to induce hypnotic trance. As the patient engaged in the description of the boat, the psychologist described calming elements of their imaginary surroundings such as the rhythm of the waves, the cool breeze, the warm sun. For these temporary periods the patient could become calm and could follow the psychologist's instructions to allow procedures. Although the patient was, for several days, disoriented and intermittently agitated, the staff were able to provide the care he needed during this critical phase.

During the critical-care phase, family members usually become at ease with the routines of the hospital. They may, however, continue to experience some symptoms of acute traumatic stress, such as intrusive thoughts, difficulties with sleep, or avoidance behaviors.[72,73] They remain anxious about their relative's condition and eager for information about the patient's present and future status.[73,74] In addition, as they accept what has happened, family members begin to think of other concerns which elicit anxiety. They may find themselves thrust by the burn injury into new roles with new responsibilities. Often, especially if the hospital is at some distance from their home, they are without their customary support systems.

It is helpful to provide a family with information about what they may expect to observe with their burned relative in the immediate future and to guide the family as they respond to the patient. Families need instruction about how they can be helpful.[73,74] They may be reluctant to touch the burned person for fear of causing pain and are usually relieved when encouraged to do so. They may feel uncomfortable in talking aloud to a nonresponsive patient; the staff can suggest that their voices and words are extremely important to the patient even though the patient does not respond. The staff must find ways to allow family members to nurture their relative and provide instructions so that the family can begin to become comfortable in caring for the patient's needs. Staff members of critical-care units are very busy and may, at moments, want to send the family away so that tasks can be completed more efficiently. However, these first instructions to the family are of critical importance to the future of the patient who needs the expressions of care by loved ones. Taking the time to 'treat' the family is a very important part of treating the patient. In addition, this 'treatment' facilitates the family's resumption of feelings of competence and control, desensitizes them to the sights and odors of the burned person, and encourages the family to join with the burn team in the healing and rehabilitation of the patient.

The burn team must also emotionally support the family's defenses. Often, family members appear to deny or to cling to delusions about the critical nature of the patient's status or the extent of the patient's injuries. It is important to give a family honest information while allowing them to protect themselves from overwhelming despair.[57] A family must find reason to hope, and the staff can assist them by suggesting realistic and optimistic outcomes. For example, we display in our offices many photographs of burn survivors engaged in a variety of activities such as swimming, going to a prom, wedding pictures, pictures of survivors with their children. The snapshots convey a hopeful message even if nothing is said explicitly about them. Family members of acute patients usually can be observed looking at the photos, and at that point it is easy to discuss which of those survivors had injuries comparable to their relative. The message to be conveyed is that there is hope for a good outcome and that successful recovery requires arduous and painful work over a period of time.

Psychotherapeutic work with the family must also identify and plan for management of those family issues which may impede a patient's recovery and rehabilitation. Some of the common issues are financial support, family alliances, historical family events, and beliefs which influence current perceptions and behaviors. Management plans must support, to the extent possible, the physical and emotional well-being of all the members of the family during a period of time in which the burned patient's needs place unusual and urgent demands on the family system.[74–77]

Psychological factors play a significant role in pain management (see the chapter on managing discomfort, this volume). The scheduling of pain assessments and the choice of assessment tools utilized have psychological relevance. Regular, routine assessments of pain imply to a patient and a patient's family that the medical staff consider discomfort a valid issue that will be treated. This not only validates a patient's concerns, but sets an expectancy of relief when pain is a problem. The use of standardized scales provides the message that to experience a range of pain and comfort responses is normal and allows the patient to participate to some degree in mastering discomfort. When the staff assess comfort as routinely as vital signs and indicate that they believe the patients, patients are less likely to feel that they must complain loudly in order to convince the staff that their need for pain relief is legitimate. They also are less likely to feel hopeless and helpless and become depressed.

A supportive milieu that diminishes anxiety also enhances a patient's ability to gain increased comfort with both background and procedural pain. The presence of a supportive person is effective in decreasing pain.[78] Encouraging patient participation in self-care has been demonstrated to be effective in assisting a patient to become more comfortable.[4,79] In particular, patients who are hypervigilant and reluctant to trust seem to gain mastery over pain when they remove their own dressings or debride their own wounds. Behavioral interventions that enhance a patient's mastery or control, in general, seem to decrease pain and anxiety. For example, adults and children who are developmentally capable of understanding the relationship of treatment to healing better tolerate procedures when told the reason for each procedure.[80] The choice of words used in explanations of procedures can ameliorate anxiety and reduce the expectancy of pain; for example, one can say 'some people feel a poke; others feel a prick or a tingle – you tell me what you feel' rather than saying 'This is going to hurt now.'[9] Touch can be used as a distraction and to induce relaxation; continuous, rhythmic repetitive stroking of a noninjured and nonthreatening body part accompanied by comforting sounds assists relaxation of adults as well as children, including infants.[9,81] Music therapy can be an excellent adjunct to analgesia. Verbal praise and other tangible reinforcers facilitate learning to cope with painful stimuli by relaxing.[82]

Modeling for and instructing a family in soothing their patient is important. While outside the hospital, family members may know well how to calm their relative, they may need instruction and/or encouragement from the staff to be comforting within the hospital. Once involved, family members can be valuable assets in providing the 'placebo' that relieves a patient's distress.

Other, nonpharmacologic, interventions also can facilitate comfort. Distraction, deep breathing, progressive relaxation, and biofeedback have all been reported to be effective in decreasing pain and distress associated with burn treatment.[82–84] Hypnosis induces a relaxed and focused state of awareness which can be extremely helpful in facilitating comfort for adults and pediatric patients.[85–88] The use of hypnosis as an adjunctive analgesic appears to decrease a patient's use of medication.[88,89] Hypnosis may offer other benefits to a burned patient as well. Some studies suggest that hypnotic suggestions given early postburn modify the physiologic response to the injury and hasten healing.[90–93] Hypnosis also can be used to increase appetite, to decrease regressive behavior, and to enhance a patient's sense of well-being, self-confidence, and body image.[86–88] An inflexible protocol for hypnosis, however, will be no more effective than an inflexible regimen of medications. With each patient, hypnotic inductions and suggestions must be modified to facilitate a patient's use of imagery. Some patients will respond well to suggestions of imagining a 'favorite place'; others can more easily imagine switches to 'turn off sensation in selected body parts. Children aged 3 and over respond well to story telling with suggestions for comfort and mastery interwoven into the story.[94,95]

Providing good pain control enhances the burn care staff's effectiveness in promoting psychological recovery of a patient by allowing the staff to interact in more pleasant ways with happier patients. Comfortable patients who perceive themselves to have some power are less prone to regressive behavior. They are perceived by the staff as more likable which, in turn, reinforces the positive self-regard of the patients.

Manifestations of psychosocial distress

Many burn survivors, as well as their family, friends, and associates have difficulty in coming to terms with the manner in which the injury occurred and with the immediate and delayed consequences of the injury. There are several manifestations of psychosocial distress that are commonly observed in the burn unit in response to these sources of stress. Among the most common are: generalized distress (nonspecific anxious, depressed or irritable mood); acute traumatic distress (re-experiencing trauma, avoidance and hyperarousal related to the trauma); body image dissatisfaction (distress over the reactions of self and others related to changes in appearance and function); hopelessness depression (hopelessness, anhedonia, withdrawal/lowered motivation related to perceived difficulty in achieving future goals); and phobic avoidance (behavioral avoidance often related to aversive stimuli feared or experienced during or following rehabilitation tasks).

Acute and Post-trauma Distress

As described in the chapter on psychiatric disorders in this book, acute stress disorder (ASD) and post-traumatic stress disorder (PTSD) following exposure to trauma are common, with a lifetime prevalence in the US of 7.8%.[96] Certain classes of trauma are particularly likely to yield PTSD, including: combat,[97] natural disasters,[98] motor vehicle accidents,[99] crime or injury,[100] and severe burn injury.[67,101] ASD and PTSD are characterized by three symptom clusters:

- re-experiencing trauma – intrusive distressing thoughts of the traumatic event or vivid flashbacks of the event;
- avoidance – suppression of trauma-related stimuli; and
- hyper-arousal – persistent symptoms such as inability to sleep, chronic anxiety and irritability.

Between 25 and 38% of burn survivors meet criteria for PTSD in the first postburn year, and almost 50% of survivors meet criteria for at least one of the PTSD symptom clusters.[67,102–104] Post-trauma distress has been found to be associated with greater lengths of acute hospitalization,[67] enhanced sense of distress and impaired adjustment to injury.[35,105] It might be assumed that PTSD is related to adjustment because of greater initial injury; however, PTSD among burn survivors has not been found to be related to the severity of the injury.[106–108] On the other hand, high levels of acute post-trauma stress symptomatology have been shown to be positively related to perception of more intense pain among hospitalized burn patients.[101,109]

PTSD can impair long-term adjustment following severe burn injury.[67] Certain aspects of pretrauma adjustment (e.g. history of mood disorder) can clearly influence the risk of developing PTSD following trauma exposure.[67,110–112] Individuals with high levels of trait neuroticism appear to be at greater risk of PTSD symptomatology following burn injury while high levels of extraversion appear protective against PTSD.[102] Similarly, neuroticism was inversely related and extraversion was directly related to global satisfaction with life and functional recovery in male burn survivors.[113]

Body Image Dissatisfaction

The scarring, disfigurement, deformity, and loss of function that often result from a severe burn injury are likely to lead to significant perceptual and subjective body image changes.[114] Deformities or disfigurement of the face and other exposed areas may be obvious sources of distress. Disfigurement of areas such as the genitalia may be less apparent, but still highly relevant to body image satisfaction or self-esteem. In any case, changes in appearance or function may result in altered body image perception, a decrease in body image satisfaction and behavioral avoidance. The association of larger TBSA and facial involvement with body image dissatisfaction of adult survivors may represent the influence of physical injury on psychological disturbance (i.e. physical condition affecting psychological disturbance).[36,115] Perhaps those individuals who appraise their injuries as worse because of location (i.e. more physically unattractive because of facial burns) or severity (i.e. larger TBSA) are at greater risk of developing body image dissatisfaction. Conversely, it has been suggested that cognitive and affective factors may interact with the objective aspects of the burn to worsen the appraisal of physical impairment and disability following a burn injury (i.e. psychological disturbance affecting physical condition).

Etiology of Distress

The arousal associated with negative events culminates in the state of preparedness for action (i.e. fight or flight response). However, relatively little has been specified regarding the process by which people return to baseline arousal following termination of aversive stimuli. Patterson et al.[6] found that the presence of distress symptoms such as anxiety and depression are common in the acute postburn period. This period may be seen as the mobilization phase of responding to negative events, (i.e. exposure to a burn event, pain, medical and surgical procedures, disfigurement and delirium).[116] As Patterson et al. have noted, however, symptoms of distress 'tend to dissipate by the time of hospital discharge' (p. 374).[6] This may be a result of the minimization phase of responding that Taylor posits in recommending that research focus on understanding the exceptions to the mobilization-minimization hypothesis when 'rather than being minimized on the long term, a negative event may be seen as pivotal or symbolic in a person's life' (p. 80).[116]

Hopelessness Depression Model

The theoretical model of anxiety and depression we work from is grounded in experimental studies using an animal model. These studies show that when an aversive electrical stimulus was unavoidable and uncontrollable, the subject gave up and stopped responding; in many cases this response could not be unlearned, and the animal became chronically depressed. The theory of 'hopelessness depression' proposes that this experience of 'giving up' or 'hopelessness' is the proximal, sufficient cause of a subtype of depressive disorder they term Hopelessness Depression (HD).[117,118]

Hopelessness is made more likely when one believes that, as a consequence of the negative life event (e.g. hand burn), further highly aversive consequences are very probable, and/or that positive consequences are very improbable, and that the causes of those consequences are seen as uncontrollable (i.e. stable/permanent, and global/pervasive). An example of such *generalized hopelessness* can be seen in burned infants and toddlers, who have little control over what is done to them, no understanding of long-term benefits of painful procedures, and no concept that these painful circumstances may be temporary. They typically withdraw, exhibit blunted affective responses, and are described as 'depressed'.[119] It is easy to imagine that they feel hopeless, caught in a painful situation and unable to escape.

Circumscribed hopelessness (versus *generalized hopelessness*) should result when only one or a few negative events are seen as uncontrollable. Circumscribed hopelessness leads to less severe symptoms of depression than does generalized hopelessness.

Circumscribed HD is '. . . characterized primarily by a motivational deficit in the relevant domain' (Abrarnson *et al.*, p. 120).[118] Thus, for example, if as a result of a significant burn, one expects negative outcomes (e.g. poor hand functioning), and one holds the belief that little can be done to alter that outcome, then *circumscribed HD* should result and lead to a lower motivation to comply with rehabilitation plans. In the context of burn injury rehabilitation, we would expect to see sporadic performance or a decreasing trend towards accomplishing rehabilitation goals. This could be the result of a loss of hope that therapy will either lead to a desired goal (e.g. acceptable function or appearance) or prevent an undesirable outcome (social stigmatization). Similar beliefs about the hopelessness of regaining acceptable function and/or appearance in order to achieve pre-injury wage-earning capacity or social status may lead to depression and avoidance of co-workers or significant others.

The models of HD and of PTSD[120] present cogent arguments regarding the analogy between those symptoms elicited from experimental animals and those in evidence in patients with either PTSD or HD and suggested a common etiological pathway. The common element in each of the laboratory paradigms for investigating experimental neurosis is that 'environmental events of vital importance to the organism become unpredictable, uncontrollable, or both' (Mineka and Kihlstrom, p. 257).[121] The conclusions of the reviewers are that extensive experience with uncontrollable and unpredictable aversive stimuli lead to: persistent arousal and generalized fear, increased fear of specific stimuli, enduring opioid mediated analgesia and opioid system sensitization, an enhanced learning of passive avoidance, and a deficit in learning of active avoidance. Furthermore, they conclude that 'aversive stimuli lead to heightened stress to which, in the absence of an effective escape or avoidance response (i.e. uncontrollable) and in the absence of information regarding the occurrence of the stressor (i.e. unpredictable), the organism responds with . . . what appears as a passive coping style, or resignation' (Foa *et al.*, p. 230).[120]

The behavioral manifestations of lab animals subjected to uncontrollable and unpredictable aversive events thus closely parallel those of humans suffering from states of heightened anxiety and depression.[122,123] Perhaps those individuals who manifest adjustment difficulties following trauma and disfigurement can be distinguished from those who do not on the basis of having experienced more uncontrollable and unpredictable aversion during the event, or in the treatment and recovery phases. The perception of uncontrolled and unpredictable aversiveness may interact with premorbid patient characteristics, and post event injury, illness, treatment, and social characteristics to differentially predict adjustment. For example, if therapy or debridement is done in a fashion that the patient perceives no control over when that painful stimulation begins or ends, this may 'lock' the patient into the arousal pattern across all response systems characterizing the mobilization phase. Likewise, if medication is the principal means of relief from pain, and that medication is prescribed 'as needed' (rather than on a scheduled dosing) resulting in a widely varying schedule of relief, the absence of predictable relief may 'lock' the patient into the mobilization phase.

Specific Etiology of Distress Attributable to Coping Method

In a recent study, adult patient-participants who coped in the first few days following trauma by *both* suppressing and processing experienced severe, prolonged, posttrauma distress.[124] The frequent use of *both* suppression (mental distancing) *and* processing (focusing/expressing emotions) resulted in significantly more intrusive thoughts over the course of 24 hours and in significantly more intrusive thoughts, avoidance behaviors, and hyperarousal symptoms at the 2-month follow-up. Conversely, the use of *either* suppression (mental distancing) *or* processing (focusing on and expressing emotions) alone at baseline resulted in reduced intrusive thoughts over 24 hours as well as fewer intrusive, avoidance and hyperarousal symptoms at the 2-month follow-up.

Using *both* suppression and processing also contributed to significantly more body image distress than using *either* one or *neither* of the coping methods.[125] These 'maladaptive copers' had higher body image dissatisfaction related to nonfacial aspects of their appearance and perceived the social impact of their body image changes to be significantly worse 2 months following discharge. Of note, the 'maladaptive copers' were also significantly younger and had significantly larger burns than the other participants.

The effect of adaptive coping methods (i.e. acceptance, planning, active coping) on body image dissatisfaction was mediated by dispositional optimism. Interestingly, individuals with low optimism did better with infrequent use of the adaptive coping methods, while those high in optimism experienced less distress when using moderate levels of adaptive coping. Those who used high levels of adaptive coping experienced more distress regardless of their dispositional optimism.

The relationship of pre-injury psychopathology, personality structure, and coping behavior to the etiology of PTSD and body image dissatisfaction may be related to other findings in the literature. Perhaps vulnerable individuals with a dysfunctional Behavioral Activation System substrate, associated with both depression and the absence of the protective affect of high extraversion, fail to generate the energy, activity, incentive motivation and sensitivity to reward signals that are necessary in coping with the challenges that come with a severe burn injury.[126,127] Similarly, it may be that a dysfunctional Behavioral Inhibition System substrate promotes attention to threat-relevant stimuli leading to hyperarousal and intrusiveness, and encourages behavioral inhibition leading to avoidance of trauma-related stimuli.

In-Hospital Recuperation Phase

Paradoxically, as burned patients become physically stronger, open wounds almost healed and grafting near completion, their continued treatment presents additional, and perhaps more difficult, challenges to the burn team. Treatment at this stage cannot simply be imposed upon a relatively helpless patient; now the team must succeed in motivating the patient to participate in treatments and to assume responsibility for recovery. The patient who desires optimal recovery must comply with the medical team's orders and instructions, many of which require significant physical discomfort.

In this phase, patients are just beginning to comprehend the extent of their injury and to realize that their body, changed forever, is no longer congruent with their premorbid self-image. Their anxieties now are increasingly about the future and less about the past and present. Pain continues to be a concern; new experiences of pain must be addressed as patients become increasingly active in rehabilitative exercises. Patients are confronted with the new physical limitations imposed by their injuries; they experience their bodies now as incompetent and disfigured. Patients involved in this struggle shift rapidly in affective behaviors reflecting rapid shifts in cognition. Much of the time, patients experience themselves as the 'preburn self' (i.e. the 'real self'). When the body will not move as it did in the past or when the scarred skin is viewed, a patient remembers and grieves.[128] Patients slowly become aware of their changed appearance as they observe the responses of others and how these responses invalidate their former body image. Their concepts about their social roles may no longer fit with society's beliefs. Their pre-morbid identities no longer exist intact and new identities must incorporate remnants of the old, as well as the changed, physical body, thus further stripping them of their identities. In this confusing state, the patient may be expected to act out anger and fear.

In addition to physical limitations, the role of 'hospital patient' imposes a loss of control and autonomy on the survivor. After a period of realistic dependence on others, a patient may be frightened and ambivalent about resuming self-care.[57] The demanding schedule necessary for treatment during this period heightens a patient's feelings of inadequacy. A patient becomes easily fatigued yet must continue in a schedule of tasks determined primarily by the burn team, thus providing additional evidence of the patient's loss of autonomy and ability.

Emotional lability and cognitive and behavioral regression are typically observed in patients of all ages during this trying time.[9,129] Perhaps the most difficult behavior for patient, family, and staff is the patient's expression of anger. Patients, of course, have many reasons to be angry, and they need to express that anger in order to define and direct it adaptively;[44] however, there are significant limitations upon the availability of situations in which they can express anger. Patients have almost no privacy, nor can they relieve tension through physical activities such as running. Typically, family members and patient care staff, having devoted much time and energy to the patient, are prone to perceive the patient's angry behavior as a personal and unjust attack by an ungrateful patient. Certainly, the patient will direct rageful temper tantrums toward those who are the safest targets, usually a spouse or parent first and then a nurse or therapist. Angry attacks are best understood as necessary ventilation by the patient rather than sincere evaluations of the family or staff.

Expressions of rage are not only upsetting to family and staff; they also frighten patients who themselves perceive this loss of control as evidence of potential destruction of self or others on whom they are dependent. Following an outburst, a patient typically feels guilty and fears withdrawal of love and support by those who were earlier subjugated to the angry behavior. These fears are added to the patient's fears of being rejected because of the changed appearance. Turning anger now toward self, the patient may feel overwhelmed, hopeless, depressed, and even suicidal. If the hospitalization continues over several weeks, patients experience repetitive frustrations, and tend to feel hopeless and depressed more often.[9,44]

Much of the psychotherapeutic work during this phase is accomplished with the patient and the family together. The family during this time must learn how to assist a patient in adjusting to the new situation, and the family system itself must accommodate to the changed situation. Research has shown the high importance of strengthening the family unit, facilitating family closeness and supporting their attempts to organize their lives to incorporate the additional duties involved in providing continued care for their patient.[22,23,37,38] They must plan and implement adjustments in the family and home environment that will be necessary for the continuation of the patient's recovery and rehabilitation after discharge. Maintaining the integrity of the family unit while making needed adjustments is of high priority and is a challenge. Parents must learn to advocate for their injured child but to avoid overprotection by themselves or others. They must encourage the child to perform independently to the limits of physical and age-appropriate ability. Parents and spouses even of adult patients often struggle against desires to protect and infantilize their recovering loved one. Staff can model for the family behaviors that demonstrate respect and courtesy for each family member including the patient.

A psychotherapeutic challenge of this phase is to accept and validate the patient's emotional demonstrations as normal behaviors in the recovery process while also setting limits on the ways in which the emotional upheaval will be expressed. Early in this phase, as the patient begins to ask about the future, the psychotherapist can describe the predictable pattern of emotional vicissitudes indicating that, should such occur, they are normal; they can be endured and managed. The staff must demonstrate positive regard and acceptance of the patient while also helping the patient to exercise control over destructive behaviors. At times, they must impose external limits to protect the patient.

Another psychotherapeutic task with both patient and family is to titrate their denial with graded presentations of reality.[57] The staff can anticipate and assist a patient in asking questions about future disfigurement and functional abilities, including sexual activity. Without evading questions, a psychotherapist gives honest but hopeful appraisals that emphasize ability and minimize deformity and disability. For example, as a patient voices an unrealistic belief that time and/or plastic surgery will return the former appearance, one can state that burned skin will never look like unburned skin and that there will always be some scarring, but that the appearance will change with time. Allowing patients to hope, even for unrealistic outcomes, protects them from despair and enables them to continue to believe that there are reasons to endure the pain of rehabilitation.[42–44] Patients and families should be given the information that rehabilitation may require several years to achieve optimal satisfaction, but that the painful efforts usually obtain good results.[9]

The therapeutic message to be delivered is that survivors can find ways of achieving whatever goals they set for themselves; the process is lengthy and difficult, and survivors will often feel overwhelmed and hopeless. Expressing sadness and anger is to be expected and accepted; however, such feelings can never be allowed to stop a patient from participating in the necessary regimen to achieve full recovery. Being burned does not relieve a survivor of the responsibility of competence.

Many survivors have endured the process and discovered that they can enjoy their lives even though their early expectations were not, and could not have been, realized.[6] Introducing such a recovered survivor to the recuperative burned patient can be a very helpful intervention at this point.[44] The more experienced survivor can be heard as a trustworthy authority in a way the unburned professional cannot. Visual images of burn survivors telling their stores and presenting themselves in daily life activities on film or video can aid in accomplishing this purpose.[130–134] Groups of patients and/or families of burned patients at varying stages of recovery and rehabilitation have been helpful in providing information, emotional validation, and support as well as reinforcing the concept that it is possible to survive burns and live acceptably happy lives.[9,74,135]

Reintegration Phase

Although plans for a patient's discharge to outpatient status are developed from the time of admission, very specific plans must be made in the final days of hospitalization. A major objective at this time is to facilitate a patient's reentry and reintegration into life at home. Returning home signifies social interactions with the larger community of extended family, friends, and strangers. Patients as well as family must prepare for those encounters. Goodstein[57] appropriately labels this the 'social emergency' phase of treatment.

Families and patients alike are often ambivalent about leaving the safe environment of the hospital. Patients, including very young children, fear social rejection or ridicule because of their changed abilities or appearance.[136–138] Family members will probably feel, and may express, a desire to protect their patient from rejection or ridicule. Family members may also express concerns about their ability to continue the time-consuming physical care of the patient while resuming their usual responsibilities. Patients may doubt their abilities to resume former activities. As discharge approaches, anxieties intensify, and patients can be expected to evidence some regressive behaviors that, in turn, can reinforce the family's doubts.

Psychotherapeutic activities of this phase involve education of patient and family about the difficulties that can be anticipated at discharge. The therapist may assist in problem-solving to develop a repertoire of alternative behaviors to address those problems. Rather than accepting their assurance that problems will not arise, the psychotherapist can characterize such concerns as normal and 'usual', and proceed with a verbal rehearsal of problem solving … 'just in case' without condescending or judging. Issues such as recurrence of symptoms of post-traumatic stress, including sleep disturbance and irritability, or fear of resuming sexual activities, should be discussed during the days prior to discharge. This preparatory rehearsal enhances the probability that the patient/family will be less reluctant to ask for help if problems do occur; if problems do not occur, the staff has the opportunity to congratulate the patient/family on their strengths or skills in coping.[9]

Toward the end of inpatient treatment, patients are expected to resume increased autonomy; caretakers are supported in withdrawing assistance to the degree possible. It is helpful at this point to develop with patients/families a daily schedule to guide them in accomplishing necessary tasks. The burn team relinquishes performance of daily care so that the patient/family can assume care to the extent that they will be required to conduct it at home. The patient and family can benefit from the opportunity to rehearse out-patient care while still able to consult with the burn team for direction and support. Rehearsals are opportunities for all involved to experience difficulties in a safe environment and to plan corrective actions.

Important among these rehearsals are those of interpersonal interactions outside the hospital. Burn survivors have reported their most difficult experience at discharge involved observing the reactions of others.[128,138] Patients benefit from the opportunity to experience such reactions before discharge from the hospital. They may leave the hospital for brief outings and return to the hospital for reassurance, encouragement, and praise.[139,140] Patient/family

groups can be extremely helpful in the process of anticipating difficulties at discharge and rehearsing solutions while also providing emotional support.

In addition to preparing a patient and family for discharge, the burn team may also prepare the 'community' to which a patient will return. The 'community' may include extended family, neighbors, church groups, social clubs, a patient's workplace or, in the case of a school-age pediatric patient, the school. Instructing those unfamiliar with burns in what to say or do to ease a survivor's reentry may facilitate reintegration.[138–143]

A few well organized reentry programs for pediatric burned patients have been described in the literature.[138,141–143] Although there is no evidence that adult burn survivors are in less need of assistance with reintegrating into their social worlds, published information about organized reentry programs for adults is scarce.[139,144,145] Reentry programs for adults and children involve the same fundamental elements and address the same issues.[138] They educate the community in a developmentally sensitive fashion. They address both the intellectual and emotional aspects of burn injury, provide generic information about burn injuries and burn treatment, and emphasize a survivor's abilities as well as clarify the ways in which a survivor may need assistance. Homemade videotapes can be sent to target groups ahead of a patient, thus allowing a community the opportunity to see and hear the burn survivor, to anticipate difficulties, and to plan coping responses.[138,145] Educational information presented in pamphlets or letters can be directed to those who will play key roles in facilitating a patient's transition from hospital to home community.[146,147] If possible, one or more members of a burn team may visit the home community and speak to targeted groups, answering questions which people may be reluctant to ask of the patient or family. Although there are no empirical data to demonstrate that reentry programs do, in fact, facilitate reintegration, anecdotal reports and clinical experience suggest that survivors have benefited from such efforts.[138,148]

Rehabilitation Phase, Post-discharge

Discharge from inpatient treatment does not signify that a patient is well. A burn survivor's wounds are covered with sensitive and fragile skin which is vulnerable to breakdown and requires special care. Dressing changes, exercises, and application of special splints and pressure garments continue. Patients must confront anew their losses and may experience a delayed grief reaction. Upon leaving the protective hospital environment, symptoms of post-traumatic stress that had remitted in the hospital may recur. A survivor must continue in the arduous process of tedious, uncomfortable physical treatments while struggling to comprehend and incorporate the multitude of changes into an image of 'self' which the survivor can accept and value.

After survival is assured, quality of life is arguably the most important outcome to individuals who are seriously ill or injured. Health-related quality of life has been defined as a multifactorial construct that involves an individual's degree of satisfaction and level of functioning in several core domains of function including: physical-behavioral (e.g. ability to perform self-care behaviors) and psychological (i.e. subjective sense of contentment and the absence of emotional distress) well-being, social and role functioning (e.g. ability to fulfill family, work, and community responsibilities), and personal perception of health (i.e. satisfaction with one's health status).[149] Severe burn injuries can lead to negative psychological complications as well as both acute and chronic physical impairments. Although most attempts to assess outcomes following burns have focused on either physical or psychological status, recent research has begun to focus on the overall quality of life.[18] As discussed below, post-trauma distress and body image dissatisfaction are two secondary complications that can undermine recovery and rehabilitation.

Body image dissatisfaction at the time of discharge is associated with prolonged periods of poorer mental health-related quality of life among adult patients following disfiguring injuries.[102] Mental domain adjustment is affected by body image dissatisfaction above and beyond the impact of baseline quality of life, injury severity and negative affect (i.e. depression, trauma-specific distress). Perhaps those patients who make a positive postburn adjustment (i.e. no body image dissatisfaction) are protected by a relatively high preburn level of functioning. An alternative explanation is that the differences in reported adjustment may represent divergent attentional biases. For example, depressed individuals have been shown to be accurate in their appraisals, while nondepressed subjects overestimate both control and performance.[150,151] After controlling for the effect of distress, preburn physical health status and greater injury severity, body image dissatisfaction does not independently predict self-reported physical functioning. Thus, it may be that individuals who develop body image dissatisfaction appraise their physical impairment as a function of early distress.

Alternatively, perhaps there are readily available schemas in operation at the time of discharge, when wounds have just healed, that are involved with assimilating the changes in appearance and function related to injury. Two months later, after the wound has healed and only the residual disfiguring scars and reduced function remain, there may be no previously developed cognitive schema capable of assimilating the relatively chronic changes in body image. These scarring processes leave previously even-toned and smooth skin with altered pigmentation and contours that are both raised and irregular. Such disfigurement schema have important implications for integrating changes into the perceptual, subjective, and behavioral aspects of body image. The absence of such schema leave one deficient in cognitive, behavioral, and social skills necessary for adapting to new disfigurement. The impact of body image dissatisfaction on psychosocial quality of life independent of distress, injury, and pre-injury adjustment variables suggests the importance of early identification of populations at risk and the development of early intervention programs. Unfortunately, no controlled studies have been completed involving individuals with disfiguring injuries such as burns. The importance of developing such interventions for individuals who already have body image dissatisfaction as well as preventative interventions for groups at risk (e.g. patients with a larger TBSA or facial burns) cannot be over-emphasized.

Interestingly, three studies of self-regard by adolescent and adult burn survivors indicate that the survivors developed positive feelings of global self-worth even while rating themselves low on the characteristic of physical appearance.[152–154] They also ranked physical appearance as a less important domain in their value structures than job competence, romantic appeal, scholastic competence, and a number of other domains. Apparently, burn survivors develop the ability to focus on positive characteristics over which they have some control and deemphasize those factors over which they have little or no control. As one young survivor said

when explaining why she wanted no further reconstructive surgeries, 'I'll just have to get by with my GREAT personality!'

Post-trauma distress during the reintegration phase is also related to significant extended problems with adjustment during subsequent phases of recovery.[35,104] These problems are greater for those with post-trauma distress relative both to survivors without significant post-trauma distress, and, to published, normative data. Moreover, the effect of post-trauma distress on physical and psychological health-related quality of life is felt even after controlling for pre-injury level of adjustment. Post-trauma distress at the time of discharge is associated with poor psychosocial adjustment even when controlling for the influence of baseline state negative affectivity (i.e. depression, body image dissatisfaction), generalized optimistic–pessimistic expectancies and injury severity (face burn, TBSA, TBSA full-thickness) as well as pre-injury adjustment. On the other hand, the influence of post-trauma distress on physical adjustment appears to be moderated by generalized optimistic–pessimistic expectancies as well as by aspects of the burn injury itself.[104] This is consistent with the literature, indicating that negative affectivity or neuroticism (which covaries with state distress and generalized optimism–pessimism expectancies) may exacerbate symptom reporting and disability in physical illness.[155,156]

The long-term impact on the families of burn survivors has not been well studied, but clinical experience and scanty empirical data indicate the sequelae to be significant. Family members may continue to experience symptoms of post-traumatic stress after a patient has returned home.[72,73] Parents of survivors of massive injuries appeared extraordinarily stressed even several years after their children's recoveries.[18] A series of studies at the Shriner's Hospital for Children in Galveston found that parents of recovering pediatric burned patients reported significant depressive symptoms at 2 years post-injury and that they attributed their distress to their burned children.[157–159] Although parental distress appears to improve with time for most, parents of the most troubled burned children continued across time to be troubled themselves.[159] Parents also express concern for their unburned children whom some felt had been slighted of attention and time while the burned sibling presented an extensive drain on the family system. Even free medical and surgical care did not eliminate the burden of direct and indirect costs of burn injury and many families experience financial difficulties attendant to the injury and treatment of the burned child.[158] The National Institute on Disability and Rehabilitation Research has established a program of research geared towards improving our understanding of, and ability to intervene with determinants of physical/anatomical, cognitive, psychological, and social outcome following severe burn injury.

Approaches to intervention and assessment

We have described our general approach to the assessment and care of burn survivors throughout this chapter. A more concise description of some of these guidelines is given next with the purpose of presenting a coherent approach that is applicable to many of the problems encountered following severe burn injury.

The Behavioral Learning Model
Our approach to comprehensive medical rehabilitation is best expressed in Brockway and Fordyce.[69] The behavioral approach to rehabilitation is:

- based on learning principles;
- adjustment and maladjustment are quantitatively, not qualitatively, different;
- maladjusted behavior itself is the target of intervention; and
- assessment and treatment are integrally related.

Rehabilitation goals are specified in terms of target behaviors occurring in a specified setting at a specific rate. Challenges to the patient and professional are made more difficult since 'many behavior changes that are required owing to the disability are low-frequency, low-strength, low-value behaviors, having minimal inherent attractiveness to the patient or to the family' (p. 154).[69] The same is equally if not more valid for the behaviors required in burn injury rehabilitation, recovery from psychological traumatization, and adjustment to disfigurement or deformity.

Recovery from severe burn injury is complex as reflected in our model of burn care and rehabilitation as well as the IOM and NIDRR models of rehabilitation research described earlier in this chapter. Furthermore, 'adjustment to disability is a function of the behavioral repertoire acquired prior to the onset of the disability, the behavioral repertoire remaining to the patient after the onset of the disability, the meaning or value of the disability and losses to the patient, and the response of the environment to the patient with respect to the disability' (p. 157).[69] Hence, 'the greater the similarity between the patient's past behavior, and the patient's capabilities after disability, the less likely it is that the ensuing behavior changes will be perceived as low frequency, low strength, and low value' (p. 159). Similarly, 'the better the patient's coping skills are prior to the onset of the disability, the better equipped the patient will be to make the needed changes in behavior' (p. 159).[69]

Several principles of behavior change are useful in assessing patient and system strengths and in designing interventions. These are reviewed here:

- *Operant Conditioning* – A behavior increases based on the individual's experiences of the consequences (i.e. reinforcements) that follow it. Behavior increases when a desired state is achieved or an undesired state is avoided or withdrawn.
- *Reinforcement* – onset of positive consequence following given response (positive reinforcement) or cessation of negative state following a given response (negative reinforcement).
- *Punishment* – onset of an aversive consequence following a given response. 'The result of punishment is generally either a decrease in strength of the response it follows, or an increase in behaviors designed to escape or avoid the punishment' (p. 158).[69]
- *The Law of Effect* – 'high-frequency behavior can be used to strengthen low-frequency behavior'.
- *Discriminative Stimuli* – By repeatedly observing safety signals, signals that a desired state is attainable, or, signals of danger that an undesired state is possible. The individual gets to know when the 'coast is clear' and when 'danger is near'.
- *Shaping* – Challenging and complex new behaviors are best learned by successively setting and achieving smaller goals that move one closer and closer to the larger goal.

Intervention – The Behavioral Learning Model

The principles of behavioral change just described can form the basis of treatment planning regardless of whether the identified problem is related to physical rehabilitation, adjustment to disfigurement or recovery from psychological traumatization. A few simple steps have been identified which help in setting up a behavioral program (adapted from Rohe, 1998).[160]

1. define the target behavior;
2. define units of that behavior that can be readily measured;
3. record the rate of occurrence of the behavior over time (i.e. baseline rate);
4. identify potentially effective and controllable reinforcers;
5. establish a schedule of reinforcement (continuous, intermittent, variable ratio);
6. implement and evaluate the program; and
7. modify based on outcome (i.e., movement toward goals).

Goal-setting
Positive feelings are generated by achieving the goals one has established, and increase one's likelihood of repeating the effort. Treatment based on a work to quota versus work to tolerance basis establishes clear expectations, rewards adequate performance and consistently builds on prior achievements.[161]

Contingency
Reinforce desired behaviors (e.g. pressure garment use, walking on treadmill, reassuring self-statements when looking in a mirror at one's scars) by allowing access to usual behaviors (e.g. TV, rest, friends).

Session structure
Since success breeds success begin and end sessions with manageable tasks that generate positive feelings of achievement and mastery. In addition, it can be helpful to 'Always Leave 'em Laughing'. Relaxation, humor and ending on a good note in general are methods of following the desired response with a rewarding experience.

Hopelessness Depression Model
By making a few modifications, the behavioral treatment approach just described can incorporate aspects of cognition that are known determinants of anxiety, depression and adherence.

- *Appraisal of Control:* When stressors are controllable they are more tolerable. Include patient in goal-setting, planning, and evaluating rehabilitation.
- *Appraisal of Predictability:* Being able to reliably tell when a stressful task will start and end vastly improves comfort and tolerance of it. Combining patient control over start and end of a given task with clearly quantified goals for a given session enables predictability and controllability to aid patient adjustment.
- *Appraisal of Ability to do the Necessary Tasks:* Self-efficacy or confidence in one's ability is improved by setting meaningful, measurable and achievable goals for each session and attributing their achievement to the patient's effort.
- *Appraisal of Utility of Necessary Tasks:* Outcome efficacy or confidence in treatment improves adherence and effort. It

is enhanced by clearly describing the task, specifying the goal and delineating how the task leads to the goal. This is one reason why exposure to survivors with similar experiences aids the recovery of newly burned patients.

Methods for emphasizing the cognitive appraisal aspects of the behavioral program:

1. *Define the target behavior:* work with the patient to select a target behavior that is important.
2. *Define units of that behavior that can be readily observed and reliably measured:* shape complex behavior with smaller sequential steps. Approach long term goals (e.g. fitness defined as walking unassisted for 15 minutes on a treadmill set at 5 mph) with meaningful yet attainable intermediate goals (walking on a treadmill for 5 minutes at 2.5 mph and using handrails only for balance).
3. *Record the rate of occurrence of the behavior over time (i.e. baseline rate):* establish a baseline and set goals on less than the baseline (roughly 80%)[161] to establish early success and sense of mastery in the present and hope for continued success.
4. *Identify potentially effective and controllable reinforcers:* when reinforcing this success with praise, make your praise contingent on adequate performance, attribute that performance to the patient's own internal and specific experience (i.e. effort not motivation).
5. *Establish a schedule of reinforcement (continuous, intermittent, variable ratio):* predictability and controllability of stressors AND reinforcers are equally important. When providing the reinforcement, clearly repeat the contingency that was met BY THE PATIENT to earn the reinforcement.
6. *Implement and evaluate the program:* solicit feedback from patient as well as looking at progress toward established goals. Is the patient perceiving their effort and involvement as instrumental in their progress? Is the patient growing in self-confidence regarding the ability to do the target behavior? Is the patient growing in confidence that by getting better at performing the target behavior (e.g. prolonged wearing of pressure garments) they are also moving towards their own larger goals (e.g. flatter scars)?
8. *Modify based on outcome* (i.e. movement toward goals).

The above principles are incorporated into most psychotherapy programs that aim for cognitive and behavioral changes. Specific psychologically based treatment programs with empirically demonstrated efficacy for adults have been described to treat PTSD,[162] acute stress disorder,[163] and social skills training for coping with disfigurement.[164] A modified version of Partridge's curriculum is being used currently for small groups of adolescent burn survivors who have been identified as 'troubled' with a prime source of their difficulties being diminished social competence.[16,165] The Phoenix Society, an organization founded by burn survivors for burn survivors, has established a wide ranging support network for burn survivors and their significant others. A visit to their website[166] can be inspiring and informative, providing support, guidance, and information. In addition, a number of cognitive-behavioral treatments have been developed and demonstrated to be efficacious for

treating or preventing body image dissatisfaction in other populations;[167] and two recent volumes contribute to understanding how disfigurement impacts the individual and the group.[114,168]

Burn survivors and families may need psychotherapeutic attention for months or years as they adapt to new roles. Regular monitoring of psychosocial problems is important, especially for pediatric patients who continue to experience new problems related to burn scars as they mature.[9,13] The psychotherapist must help the patient to define a new self-image, incorporating and going beyond body image. In the early months, a patient may often be encouraged to overcompensate and enjoy the positive identification of 'hero'. The survivor is commended for rehabilitation gains and social accomplishments. Each victory is celebrated. As a patient's physical and psychological adaptation stabilize, the psychotherapist must assist the patient in resisting the temptation to remain satisfied with the identity of 'heroic survivor'. This role invites a survivor to achieve expectations which are unrealistic and to deny unhappiness or anger or pain. The task of the psychotherapist is to make explicit the expectation that each burn survivor is a human individual who can be strong and competent, optimistic and autonomous, and also can have moments of sadness, despair, or rage. Guiding the patient to accept vulnerabilities and flaws without detracting from the overall positive evaluation of 'self', the psychotherapist insist that the person who has been the 'heroic burn survivor' can become a competent, interesting individual who also once survived a serious burn injury.

Summary

Most burn survivors do eventually adapt well and resume lives of productive activity with satisfactory self-esteem and social interactions. Empirical data indicate that while the first year or so postburn is fraught with discomfort and distress, much of the difficulty is transient. The process of psychological adaptation continues for several months or even several years. The symptoms of disturbance that linger among burn survivors are likely to be such that only intimate friends and family members will observe them (e.g. nightmares, flashbacks, body image dissatisfaction, social anxiety), so it is valuable for persons with expertise in burn adaptation to periodically assess the survivor (especially pediatric survivors who change constantly) to ask about such common symptoms and to provide an opportunity for intervention.

That most burn survivors do amazingly well should never be interpreted as indicative of ease in adaptation. We would never want to diminish the pain and suffering they endure from physical and psychological wounds. As the psychotherapists to a large number of burn survivors, we know very well the struggles of survivors. They have moments of true despair and hopelessness, moments of rage, and moments of joy. Probably at some level, burn survivors always feel some sadness about their scars; eventually they attend to other things most of the time and do not obsess over their scars. Fortunate psychotherapists can know them through all the extremes – looking for glimmers of hope, validating their anger, celebrating their victories and gaining deep respect for the resilience of human beings.

References

1. Wolf S, Rose JK, Desai M, Mileski J, Barrow R, Herndon D. Mortality determinants in massive pediatric burns: an analysis of 103 children with ≥80% TBSA burns (≥70% full-thickness). *Ann Surg* 1997; 225(5): 554–69.

2. Ryan CM, Schoenfeld DA, Thorpe WP, Sheridan RL, Cassem EH, Tompkins RG. Objective estimates of the probability of death from burn injuries. *N Engl J Med* 1998; **338**: 362–6.

3. Andreasen NJC, Noyes P, Hartford C. Factors influencing adjustment of burned patients during hospitalization. *Psychosom Med* 1972; **34(6)**: 517–25.

4. Chang F, Herzog B. Burn morbidity: a follow-up study of physical and psychological disability. *Ann Surg* 1976; **183(1)**: 34–7.

5. Vanderplate C. An adaptive coping model of intervention with the severely burn-injured. *Intl J Psychiatr Med* 1984; **14(4)**: 331–41.

6. Patterson D, Everett J, Bombardier C, Questad K, Lee V, Marvin J. Psychological effects of severe burn injuries. *Psychol Bull* 1993; **113(2)**: 362–78.

7. Ward H, Moss R, Darko D, *et al.* Prevalence of post-burn depression following burn injury. *J Burn Care Rehabil* 1987; **8(4)**: 294–8.

8. Mendelsohn I. Liaison psychiatry and the burn center. *Psychosom* 1983; **24(3)**: 235–43.

9. Blakeney P, Meyer WJ. Psychological aspects of burn care. *Trauma Q* 1994; **11(2)**: 166–79.

10. Malt U. Long-term psychosocial follow-up of burned adults: review of the literature. *Burns* 1980; **6**: 190–7.

11. Andreasen NJC, Norris A, Hartford C. Incidence of long-term psychiatric complications in severely burned adults. *Ann Surg* 1971; **174(5)**: 785–93.

12. Malt U. A long-term psychosocial follow-up study of burned adults. *Acta Psychiatr Scand Suppl* 1989; **80(355)**: 94–102.

13. Faber A, Klasen H, Sauer E, Vuister F. Psychological and social problems in burn patients after discharge: a follow-up study. *Scand J Plast Reconstr Surg* 1987; **21(3)**: 307–9.

14. Blakeney P, Meyer W, Moore P, Broemeling L, Robson M, Herndon D. Psychosocial sequelae of pediatric burns involving 80% or greater TBSA. *J Burn Care Rehabil* 1993; **14**: 684–9.

15. Moore P, Moore M, Blakeney P, Meyer W, Murphy L, Herndon D. Competence and physical impairment of pediatric survivors of burns of more than 80% total body surface area. *J Burn Care Rehabil* 1996; **17**: 547–51.

16. Blakeney P, Meyer W, Robert R, Desai M, Wolf S, Herndon D. Long-Term Psychosocial adaptation of children who survive burns involving 80% or greater total body surface area. *J Trauma Inj Infect Crit Care* 1998; **44(4)**: 625–34.

17. Meyers-Paal R, Blakeney P, Murphy L, *et al.* 'Physical and psychological rehabilitation outcomes for pediatric patients who suffer >80% total body surface area burn and ≥ 70% 3rd degree burns.' *J Burn Care Rehabil* 2000; **21(1, Pt. 1)**, 43–9.

18. Sheridan RL, Hinson MI, Liang MH, *et al.* Long-term outcome of children surviving massive burns. *JAMA* 2000; **283(1)**: 69–73.

19. Stoddard F, Norman D, Murphy M. A diagnosis outcome study of children and adolescents with severe burns. *J Trauma* 1989; **29**: 471–7.

20. Stoddard F, Norman D, Murphy M, Beardslee W. Psychiatric outcome of burned children and adolescents. *J Am Acad Child Adol Psychiatry* 1989; **28**: 589–95.

21. Tarnowski K, Rasnake L, Linscheid T, Mulick J. Behavioral adjustment of pediatric burn victims. *J Pedia Psychol* 1989; **14**: 607–15.

22. Blakeney P, Herndon D, Desai M, Beard S, Wales-Sears P. Long-term psychological adjustment following burn injury. *J Burn Care Rehabil* 1988; **9(6)**: 661–5.

23. Blakeney P, Portman S, Rutan R. Familial values as factors influencing long-term psychosocial adjustment of children after severe burn injury. *J Burn Care Rehabil* 1990; **11(6)**: 472–5.

24. Moore P, Blakeney P, Broemeling L, Portman S, Herndon D, Robson M. Psychological adjustment after childhood burn injuries as predicted by personality traits. *J Burn Care Rehabil* 1993; **14**: 80–2.

25. Love B, Byrne C, Roberts J, Browne G, Brown B. Adult psychological adjustment following childhood injury: the effect of disfigurement. *J Burn Care Rehabil* 1987; **8**: 280–5.

26. DeWet B, Cywes S, Davies MRQ, Van der Riet L. Some aspects of post-treatment adustment in severely burned children. *Burns* 1979; **5**: 979–80.

27. Byrne C, Love B, Browne G, Brown B, Roberts J, Steiner D. The social competence of children following burn injury: a study of resilience. *J Burn Care Rehabil* 1986; **7**: 247–52.

28. Browne G, Byrne C, Brown B, *et al.* Psychosocial adjustment of burn survivors. *Burns* 1985; **12**: 28–35.

29. Blumenfeld M, Reddish P. Identification of psychologic impairment in patients with mild-moderate thermal injury: small burn, big problem. *Gen Hosp Psychiatry* 1987; **9**: 142–6.

30. Korloff B. Social and economic consequences of deep burns. In: Wallace AB, Wilkinson AW, eds. *Research in Burns: Transactions of the 2nd International Congress on Research in Burns*. Edinburgh: Livingstone, 1996.

31. Bernstein NR. Objective bodily damage: disfigurement and dignity. In: Cash TF, Pruzinsky T, eds. *Body Images; Development, Deviance, and Change*. New York: Guilford, 1990.

32. Tudahl LA, Blades BC, Munster AM: Sexual satisfaction in burn patients. *J Burn Care Rehabil* 1987; **8**: 292–3.

33. Fauerbach JA, Lawrence JW, Haythornthwaite J, McGuire M, Munster A. Preinjury psychiatric illness and postinjury adjustment in adult burn survivors. *Psychosom* 1996; **37(6)**: 547–55.

34. Sheffield CGI, Irons GB, Mucha PJ, Malec JF, Ilstrup DM, Stonnington HH: Physical and Psychological outcome after burns. *J Burn Care Rehabil* 1988; **9**: 172–7.

35. Fauerbach J, Lawrence J, Munster A, Palombo D, Richter D. Prolonged adjustment difficulties among those with acute post trauma distress following burn injury. *Behav Med* 1999; **22**: 359–78.

36. Fauerbach J, Heinberg L, Lawrence J, Munster A, Palombo D, Richter D. The effect of early body image dissatisfaction on subsequent psychological and physical adjustment following disfiguring injury. *Psychosom Med* 2000; **62**: 576–82.

37. Patterson D, Ptacek J, Cromes F, Fauerbach JA, Engrav L. Describing and predicting adjustment in burn survivors. *J Burn Care Rehabil* 2000; **21**.

38. LeDoux J, Meyer W, Blakeney P, Herndon D. Relationship between parental emotional states, family environment and the behavioral adjustment of pediatric burn survivors. *Burns* 1998; **24**: 425–32.

39. Kjaer G. Psychiatric aspects of thermal burns. *Northwest Med* 1969; **68**: 537–41.

40. Morris J, McFadd A. The mental health team on a burn unit. A multidisciplinary approach. *J Trauma* 1978; **18(9)**: 658–63.

41. Ochitill H. Psychiatric consultation to the burn unit. The psychiatrist's perspective. *Psychosom* 1984; **25(9)**: 689, 697–701.

42. Tucker P. The burn victim – a review of psychosocial issues. *Aust N Z J Psychiatry* 1986; **20**: 413–20.

43. Knudson-Cooper M. Emotional care of the hospitalized burned child. *J Burn Care Rehabil* 1982; **3**: 109–16.

44. Watkins P, Cook E, Mary R, Ehleben C. Psychological stages in adaptation following burn injury: a method for facilitating psychological recovery of burn victims. *J Burn Care Rehabil* 1988; **9(4)**: 376–84.

45. Tucker P. Psychosocial problems among adult burn victims. *Burns* 1987; **13(1)**: 7–14.

46. Shenkman B, Stechmiller J. Patient and family perception of projected functioning after discharge from a burn unit. *Heart Lung* 1987; **16(5)**: 490–6.

47. Luther S, Price J. Burns and their psychological effects on children. *J School Health* 1981; **51**: 419–22.

48. Wallace L. Abandoned to a 'social death?' *Nurs Times* 1988; **84(10)**: 34–7.

49. Davidson T, Bowden M, Feller I. Social support and post-burn adjustment. *Arch Phys Med Rehabil* 1981; **62**: 274–7.

50. Andreasen NJC, Norris A. Long-term adjustment and adaptation mechanisms in severely burned adults. *J Nerv Ment Dis* 1972; **154(5)**: 352–62.

51. Stoddard F. Psychiatric management of the burned patient. In: Martyn JAJ, ed. *Acute Care of the Burn Patient*. Orlando, FL: Grune and Stratton, 1990; 256–72.

52. Institute of Medicine. *Enabling America: Assessing the Role of Rehabilitation Science and Engineering*. Washington, DC: National Academy Press, 1997.

53. National Institute on Disability and Rehabilitation Research. Long Range Plan and the New Paradigm. NIDRR, 1999.

54. Blakeney P, Moore P, Meyer W, Murphy L, Herndon D. Early identification of long-term problems in the behavioral adjustment of pediatric burn survivors and their parents. *Proc Am Burn Assoc* 1995; **27**.

55. Meyer W, Murphy L, Robert R, Blakeney P. Changes in adaptive behavior among pediatric burn survivors over time. *Proc Am Burn Assoc* 1998; **19(1, part 2)** (Abstract #84).

56. Bowden L, Feller I, Tholen D, Davidson T, James M. Self-esteem of severely burned patients. *Arch Phys Med Rehabil* 1980; **61**: 449–52.

57. Goodstein R. Burns: an overview of clinical consequences affecting patient, staff, and family. *Compr Psychiatry* 1985; **26(1)**: 43–57.

58. Roberts J, Browne G, Streiner D, Byrne C, Brown B, Love B. Analyses of coping responses and adjustment: stability of conclusions. *Nurs Res* 1987; **36(2)**: 94–7.

59. Byrne C, Love B, Browne G, Brown B, Roberts J, Streiner D. The social competence of children following burn injury: a study of resilience. *J Burn Care Rehabil* 1986; **7**: 247–52.

60. Blakeney P, Meyer W, Moore P, *et al.* Social competence and behavioral problems of pediatric survivors of burns. *J Burn Care Rehabil* 1993; **14**: 65–72.

61. Darko D, Wachtel T, Ward H, Frank H. Analysis of 585 burn patients hospitalized over a 6-year period. Part III: Psychosocial data. *Burns* 1986; **12**: 395–401.

62. Davidson T, Brown L. Self-inflicted burns: a 5-year retrospective study. *Burns* 1985; **11**: 157–60.

63. Knudson-Cooper M, Leuchtag A. The stress of a family move as a precipating factor in children's burn accidents. *J Hum Stress* 1982; June: 32–8.

64. Noyes R, Frye S, Slyment D, Canter A. Stressful life events and burn injuries. *J Trauma* 1979; **19(3)**: 141–4.

65. Vogtsberger K, Taylor E. Psychosocial factors in burn injury. *Tex Med* 1984; **80**: 43–6.

66. Wilson G, Buckland R, Sully L. Childhood illness as an etiological factor in burns. *Burns* 1988; **14(3)**: 237–8.

67. Fauerbach JA, Lawrence J, Richter D, McGuire M, Schmidt C, Munster A. Preburn psychiatric history affects posttrauma morbidity. *Psychoso* 1997; **38(4)**: 374–85.

68. Blank K, Perry S. Relationship of psychological process during delirium to outcome. *Am J Psychiatry* 1984; **141**: 843–7.

69. Brockway JA, Fordyce WE. Psychological Assessment and Management. In: Kottke FJ, Lehmann JF, eds. *Krusen's Handbook of Physical Medicine and Rehabilitation*, 4th edn. Philadelphia: WB Saunders; 1990; 153–70.

70. Haynes B, Bright R. Burn coma: a syndrome associated with severe burn wound infection. *J Trauma* 1967; **7**: 464–75.

71. Steiner H, Clark W. Psychiatric complications of burned adults: a classification. *J Trauma* 1977; **17**: 134–43.

72. Cella D, Perry S, Kulchycky, Goodwin C. Stress and coping in relatives of burn patients: a longitudinal study. *Hosp Comm Psychiatry* 1988; **39(2)**: 159–66.

73. Cella D, Perry S, Poaz M, Amand R, Goodwin C. Depression and stress responses in parents of burned children. *J Pedia Psychol* 1988; **13(1)**: 87–99.

74. Rivlin E, Forshaw A, Polowyj G, Woodruff B. A multidisciplinary group approach to counseling the parents of burned children. *Burns* 1986; **12(7)**: 479–83.

75. Terry D. The needs of parents of hospitalized children. *Children's Health Care* 1987; **16(1)**: 18–20.

76. Kasper J, Nyamathi A. Parents of children in the pediatric intensive care unit: what are their needs? *Heart Lung* 1988; **17**: 574–81.

77. Reddish P, Blumenfield M. A typology of spousal response to the crisis of severe burn. *J Burn Care Rehabil* 1986; **7(4)**: 328–30.

78. Kelley M, Jarvie G, Middlebrook J, Mceer M, Drabman R. Decreasing burned children's pain behavior: impacting the trauma of hydrotherapy. *J App Behav Anal* 1984; **17(2)**: 147–58.

79. Kavanagh C. Psychological intervention with the severely burned child: report of an experimental comparison of two approaches and their effects on psychological sequelae. *J Am Acad Child Psychiatry* 1983; **22(2)**: 145–56.

80. Beales J. Factors influencing the expectation of pain among patients in a children's burns unit. *Burns* 1983; **9(3)**: 187–92.

81. Baker C, Wong D. Q.U.E.S.T.: a process of pain assessment in children. *Orthop Nurs* 1987; **6(1)**: 11–21.

82. Elliot C, Olson R. The management of children's distress in response to painful medical treatment for burn injuries. *Behav Res Ther* 1983; **21(6)**: 675–83.

83. Perry S. Undermedication for pain on a burn unit. *Gen Hosp Psychiatry* 1984; **6**: 308–16.

84. Knudson-Cooper M. Relaxation and biofeedback training in the treatment of severely burned children. *J Burn Care Rehabil* 1981; 103–10.

85. Zeltzer L, LeBaron I. Hypnosis and nonhypnotic techniques for reduction of pain and anxiety during painful procedures in children and adolescents with cancer. *Behav Pediatr* 1982; **101(6)**: 1032–5.

86. Crasilneck H, Stirman J, Wilson B, McVranie E, Fogelman M. Use of hypnosis in the management of patients with burns. *JAMA* 1955; **158**: 103–6.

87. Schafer D. Hypnosis on a burn unit. *Int J Clin Exp Hypn* 1975; **23(1)**: 1–14.

88. Wakeman R, Kapan J. An experimental study of hypnosis in painful burns. *Am J Clin Hypn* 1978; **21(1)**: 3–12.

89. Van der Does AJW, Van Dyck R, Spijker R. Hypnosis and pain in patients with severe burns: a pilot study. *Burns* 1988; **14(5)**: 399–404.

90. Ewin D. Emergency room hypnosis for the burned patient. *Am J Clin Hypn* 1986; **29(1)**: 8–12.

91. Hammond D, Keye W, Grant C. Hypnotic analgesia with burns: a initial study. *Am J Clin Hypn* 1983; **26(1)**: 56–9.

92. Margolis C, Domarque B, Ehliben C, Shrier L. Hypnosis is the early treatment of burns: a pilot study. *Am J Clin Hypn* 1983; **26(1)**: 9–15.

93. May S, DeClement F. Effects of early hypnosis on the cardiovascular and renal physiology of burn patients. *Burns* 1983; **9(4)**: 257–66.

94. Olness K. Imagery (self-hypnosis) as adjunct therapy on childhood cancer. *Am J Pediatr Hematol Oncol* 1981; **3(3)**: 313–20.

95. Kuttner L. Favorite stories: a hypnotic pain-reduction technique for children in acute pain. *Am J Clin Hypn* 1985; **28**: 289–95.

96. Kessler RC, Sonnega A, Bromet E, Nelson CB. Postraumatic stress disorder in the National Comorbidity Sample. *Arch Gen Psychiatry* 1995; **52**: 1048–60.

97. Kulka RA, Schlenger WE, Fairbank JA, Hough RL, Jordan BK, Marmar CR, Weiss DS. *Trauma and the Vietnam War Generation*. New York: Brunner/Mazel, 1990.

98. Green BL, Lindy JC, Grace MC, Leonard A. Chronic posttraumatic stress disorder and diagnostic comorbidity in a disaster sample. *J Nerv Ment Dis* 1992; **180**: 760–6.

99. Blanchard EB, Hickling AE, Taylor WR. Psychiatric comorbidity associated with motor vehicle accidents. *J Nerv Ment Dis* 1995; **183**: 495–9.

100. Resnick HS, Kilpatrick DG, Dansky BS, Saunders BE, Best CL. Prevalence of civilian trauma and postraumatic stress disorder in a representative national sample of women. *J Cons Clin Psychol* 1993; **61**: 984–91.

101. Taal LA, Faber AW. Post traumatic stress, pain and anxiety in adult burn victims 1998; *Burns* 23: 545–9.

102. Fauerbach JA, Lawrence J, Schmidt C, Munster A, Costa P. Personality predictors of injury-related PTSD. *J Nerve Ment Dis* 2000; **188**: 510–7.

103. Powers PS, Cruse CW, Daniels S, Stevens B. Posttraumatic stress disorder in patients with burns. *J Burn Care Rehabil* 1994; **15(2)**: 147–53.

104. Saxe G, Stoddard F, Sheridan R. PTSD in children with burns: a longitudinal study. *J Burn Care Rehabil* 1998; **19(1, part 2)**: S206.

105. Munster AM, Fauerbach JA, Lawrence JW. Development and utilization of a psychometric instrument for measuring quality of life in burn patients, 1976–1996. *Acta Chirurgiae Plastic* 1996; **4**: 128–31.

106. Bryant RA. Predictors of post-traumatic stress disorder following burn injury. *Burns* 1996; **22**: 89–92.

107. Perry S, DiFede J, Musngi G, Frances A, Jacobsberg L. Predictors of posttraumatic stress disorder after burn injury. *Am J Psychiatry* 1992; **149(7)**: 931–5.

108. Roca RP, Spence RJ, Munster AM. Posttraumatic adaptation and distress among adult burn survivors. *Am J Psychiatry* 1992; **149**: 1234–8.

109. Williams D, Kiecolt-Glaser J. Self-blame, compliance and distress among burn patients. *J Person Soc Psychol* 1987; **53**: 187–93.

110. Schnurr PP, Friedman MJ, Rosenberg SD. Premilitary MMPI scores as predictors of combat-related PTSD symptoms. *Am J Psychiatry* 1993; **150(3)**: 479–83.

111. Smith EM, North CS, McCool RE, Shea JM. Acute postdisaster psychiatric disorders: identification of persons at risk. *Am J Psychiatry* 1990; **147(2)**: 202–6.

112. Breslau N, Davis GC, Andreski P, Peterson EL. Traumatic events and posttraumatic stress disorder in an urban population of young adults. *Arch Gen Psychiatry* 1991; **48(3)**: 216–22.

113. Gilboa D, Bisk L, Montag I, Tsur H. Personality traits and psychosocial adjustment of patients with burns. *J Burn Care Rehabil* 1999; **20**: 340–6.

114. Heinberg LJ. Theories of body image: perceptual, developmental, and sociocultural factors, In: Thompson JK, ed. *Body Image, Eating Disorders, and Obesity: An Integrative Guide to Assessment and Treatment*. Washington, DC.: American Psychological Association. 1996.

115. Cohen S, Rodriguez MS. Pathways linking affective disturbances and physical disorders. *Health Psychol* 1995; **15**: 374–80.

116. Taylor S. Asymmetrical effects of positive and negative events: The mobilization-minimization hypothesis. *Psycho Bull* 1991; **110(1)**: 67–85.

117. Abramson LY, Metalsky GI, Alloy LB. Hopelessness depression: A theory-based subtype of depression. *Psycho Rev* 1989; **96**: 358–72.

118. Abramson LY, Alloy LB, Metalsky GI. Hopelessness depression. In: Buchanan GM, Seligman MEP, eds. Explanatory Style. Hillsdale, NJ: Lawrence Erlbaum Associates, 1995; 113–34.

119. Meyer WJ III, Robert R, Murphy L, Blakeney P. Evaluating the psychosocial adjustment of 2- and 3-year-old pediatric burn survivors. *J Burn Care Rehabil* 2000; **21(2)**: 179–84.

120. Foa E, Zinbarg R, Rothbaum B. Uncontrollability and unpredictability in post-traumatic stress disorder: An animal model. *Psychol Bull* 1992; **112(2)**: 218–38.

121. Mineka S, Kihlstrom J. Unpredictable and uncontrollable events: A new perspective on experimental neurosis. *J Ab Psychol* 1978; **2**: 256–71.

122. Maier SF, Seligman MP. Learned helplessness: theory and practice. *J Exper Psychol Gen* 1976; **195**: 30–46.

123. Abramson LY, Garber J, Seligman MP. Learned helplessness in humans: an attributional analysis. In: Garber J, Seligman MP, eds. *Human Helplessness: Theory and Applications.* 1980; New York: Academic Press.

124. Fauerbach JA, Heinberg L, Lawrence JW, Bryant AG, Richter L, Spence R. Coping with body image changes following disfiguring injury. Submitted a.

125. Fauerbach J, Richter L, Lawrence JW, Bryant AG, Richter D. Mental control processes in coping with trauma. Submitted b.

126. Fowles DC. A motivational theory of psychopathology. *Nebr Symp Motiv* 1994; **41**: 181–238.

127. Gray JA. The neuropsychology of anxiety: reprise. *Nebr Symp Motiv* 1996; **43**: 61–134.

128. Knudson-Cooper M. Adjustment to visible stigma: the case of the severely burned. *Soc Sci Med* 1981; **15**: 31–44.

129. Stoddard F. Body image development in the burned child. *J Am Acad Child Psychiatry* 1982; **21(5)**: 502–7.

130. Blakeney P, Washam K, Cahners S, Driscoll E. *Brandon.* Tampa, FL: Shriners Hospitals for Children, videotape, 1993.

131. Blakeney P, Washam K, Cahners S, Driscoll E. *Megan.* Tampa, FL: Shriners Hospitals for Children, videotape, 1993.

132. Doctor ME, Burne B, Jarecke D. *Through the Eyes of a Child: Burn Recovery.* Denver, CO: Children's Hospital, videotape, 1993.

133. Blakeney P, Washam K, Hendricks L, Cahners S, Driscoll E. *Sarah*. Tampa, FL: Shriners Hospitals for Children, videotape, 1994.

134. Blakeney P, Washam K, Hendricks L, Cahners S, Driscoll E. *Dennis and Alex*. Tampa, FL: Shriners Hospitals for Children, videotape, 1994.

135. Cahners S. Group meetings benefit families of burned children. *Scand J Plast Reconstr Surg* 1979; **13**: 169–71.

136. Langlois JH, Downs AC. Peer relations as a function of physical attractiveness: the eye of the beholder or behavioral reality? *Child Dev* 1979; **50**: 409–18.

137. Barden RC. The effects of crania-facial deformity, chronic illness, and physical handicaps on patient and familial adjustment: research and clinical perspectives. In: Lahey BB, Kazdin AE, eds. *Advances in Clinical Child Psychology*, Vol 13. New York: Plenum, 1990; 343–75.

138. Blakeney P. School reintegration. In: Tarnowski KJ ed. *Behavioral Aspects of Pediatric Burns*. New York, Plenum, 1994; 217–41.

139. Dobner D, Mitani M. Community reentry program. *J Burn Care Rehabil* 1988; **9(4)**: 420–1.

140. Stein J. Comments from Maricopa Medical Center, Phoenix. *J Burn Care Rehabil* 1988; **9(4)**: 418–9.

141. Cahners S. A strong hospital – school liaison: a necessity for good rehabilitation planning for disfigured children. *Scand J Plast Recorstr Surg* 1979; **13**: 167–8.

142. Doctor ME. Returning to school after a severe burn. In: Boswick JA Jr, ed. *The Art and Science of Burn Care*. Rockville, MD: Aspen Press, 1987; 323–8.

143. Walls Rosenstein DL. A school reentry program for burned children. Part I: Development and implementation of a school reentry program. *J Burn Care Rehabil* 1987; **8**: 319–22.

144. Blumenfield M, Schoeps M. Reintegrating the healed burned adult into society: psychological problems and solutions. *Clin Plast Surg* 1992; **19(3)**: 599–605.

145. Angermeier J. A desensitization process to facilitate first visits between burn scarred parents and young children. *J Burn Care Rehabil* 1991; **12(4)**: 344–5.

146. Shriners Burns Hospital. *Back to School Guidelines*. Cincinnati, OH: Shriners Hospitals for Children, 1993a.

147. Shriners Burns Hospital. *Back to School Guidelines for Parents*. Cincinnati, OH: Shriners Hospitals for Children, 1993b.

148. Blakeney P, Moore P, Meyer W, *et al.* Efficacy of school of reentry programs. *J Burn Care Rehabil* 1995; **16**: 469–72.

149. Ware JE, Snow KK, Kosinski M, Gandek B. *SF-36 Health Survey: Manual and Interpretation Guide*. Boston, MA: Nimrod Press, 1993.

150. Alloy LB, Abramson LY. Judgement of contingency in depressed and nondepressed students: Sadder by wiser? *J Exper Psychol: Gen* 1979; **108**: 441–85.

151. Alloy LB, Abramson LY. Learned helplessness, depression, and the illusion of control. *J Person Soc Psychol* 1982; **42**: 1114–26.

152. LeDoux JM, Meyer W, Blakeney P, Herndon D. Positive self-regard as a coping mechanism for pediatric burn survivors. *J Burn Care Rehabil* 1996; **17**: 472–6.

153. Clyne W, Turner S. Perceived changes and adaptations in self-concept following burn injury. *Proc Am Burn Assoc Sci Meeting*, #23. 1995.

154. Robert R, Bishop S, Murphy L, *et al.* The Evolution of Self-Perception in Children and Adolescents Post-Burn Injury. 8th Congress of the European Burns Association, Marathon-Attica, Greece, 1999.

155. Costa PTJ: Hypochondriasis, neuroticism, and aging. When are somatic complaints unfounded? *Am Psychol* 1985; **40**: 19–28.

156. Watson D, Pennebaker JW: Health complaints, stress and distress: Exploring the role of negative affectivity. *Psychol Rev* 1989; **96**: 234–54.

157. Blakeney P, Moore P, Broemeling L, Hunt R, Herndon D, Robson M. Parental stress as a cause and effect of pediatric burn injury. *J Burn Care Rehabil* 1993; **14(1)**: 73–9.

158. Blakeney P, Meyer W, Moore P, *et al.* Psychosocial sequelae of pediatric burns involving 80% or greater total body surface area. *J Burn Care Rehabil* 1993; **14**: 684–9.

159. Meyer W, Blakeney P, Moore P, Murphy L, Robson M, Herndon D. Parental well-being and behavioral adjustment of pediatric burn survivors. *J Burn Care Rehabil* 1994; **15**: 62–8.

160. Rohe DE. Psychological aspects of rehabilitation. In: DeLisa JA, Gans BM, eds. *Rehabilitation Medicine: Principles and Practice*, 3rd edn. Philadelphia: Lipincott-Ravens, 1998; 189–212.

161. Ehde DH, Patterson DR, Fordyce WE. The quota system in burn rehabilitation. *J Burn Care Rehabil* 1998; **19**: 436–40.

162. Foa EB, Keane TM, Friedman MJ. *Effective Treatments for PTSD*. New York: The Guilford Press, 2000.

163. Bryant RA, Harvey AG. *Acute Stress Disorder: A Handbook of Theory, Assessment and Treatment*. Washington, DC: *Proc of Am Psychol Assoc*; 2000.

164. Partridge J. *Changing Faces: The Challenge of Facial Disfigurement*. London, Penguin, 1998.

165. Meyer W, Blakeney P, Ledoux J, Herndon D. Diminished adaptive behaviors among pediatric survivors of burns. *J Burn Care Rehabil* 1995; **16**: 511–8.

166. The Phoenix Society's website: *www.phoenix-society.org*

167. Stormer S, Thompson JK: Explanations of body image disturbance: A test of maturational status, negative verbal commentary, social comparison, and sociocultural hypotheses. *Int J Eating Dis* 1996; **19**: 193–202.

168. Heatherton TF, Kleck RE, Hebl MR, Hull JG. *The Social Psychology of Stigma*. New York: Guilford Press, 2000.

Index

Entries are arranged in letter-by-letter alphabetical order. Page numbers in *italics* refer to tables and figures, those in **bold** indicate main discussion.

Intravenous access *see* Venous cannulation; Venous catheters
Intravenous fluids *see under* Fluid resuscitation
Iodine, as cause of burn injury, 22
Iron
nutritional needs, 277
reduced serum levels, 332
Irrigation, 43
following radiation exposure, 485
following vesicant exposure, 488
Ischemia-reperfusion phenomenon, 227–228, 383, 385, 503–504
gut, 447
Itching, 47–48
caused by vesicant agents, 488
measurement scale, 752
treatments, 48, 758–759

Janzekovic, Z, 6–7
Joint contractures, 614
surgical treatment, 700–705
evaluation, presurgical, 701
interpositional flap technique, 702–703, *704*
muscle or skin-muscle flap technique, 703–705
release techniques, 701
skin grafting, 702
wound coverage techniques, 701
z-plasty, 701
Joint dislocation, 602–605
positioning, 604
susceptible areas, 602–604
Joule's law, 456

Kallikrein-kinin system, 264
see also Kinins, as mediators of burn injury
Kaplan-Meier curves, *407*
Keloid *vs* hypertrophic scarring, 550, 553–554
Keratinocytes, 213
cultured, 530, 752
viral transfection of, 215
in wound healing, 524
Keraunoparalysis, following lightning injury, 459
Kerlix elastic gauze bandages, 45
Ketamine
anesthesia, 191–192, 197
in pain management, 757–758
Ketanserin, 89
Ketoconazole, 376
Kinins, as mediators of burn injury, 48, 82, 89, **264**
'Kissing lesions', 462
Klebsiella-Enterobacter (K-E) group, 130
in cholelithiasis, 147
susceptibility to antimicrobials, 141, *142, 143*, 161, 162
Klebsiella pneumoniae, 141, *143*, 145
Kling elastic gauze bandages, 45
Knee
positioning, 572, 604, 697, 699–700
stabilization, 577, *578*
skeletal traction technique, 700
susceptibility to dislocation, 603–604
three-point extension splint, 699–700
very large burns, 177

Labia majora burns, 179, 712, *713*
reconstruction of deformity, 715–717
Lactic acid dehydrogenase, 289
Lactic acid, as marker for tissue perfusion/oxygen delivery, 188
Laminar method *see* Tangential excision
Landis-Starling's equation, 79, 80, 264

Laryngeal mask airway (LMA), 192
Laser Doppler flowmetry, in estimation of burn depth, 103–104
Lavage *see* Irrigation
'Leaky capillary', 80, 90, 265, 443
Leishmania, treatment, 163–164
Leukocytes, 334–335, 352–353
in hypophosphatemia, 313
Leukocytosis, 334
Leukopenia, 334
Leukotrienes, 227, 228, 261, 519
types, 384
Lidocaine, 754–755
Lidocaine/prilocaine cream, 83, 754–755
Lightning injuries, 21
complications, 459
incidence, 21, 459
mortality rates, 21, 459
prognosis, 459
treatment, 459
Light reflectance, in estimation of burn depth, 104
Limb tourniquets, 116, 173
Lip deformities, correction of, 675
Lipid metabolism, role of liver, 291–292
Lipolysis, in hypermetabolism, 365
Lipopolysaccharide (LPS)-stimulated cytokine production, 351
Lipoxygenase pathway, 384, 388
Listeria monocytogenes, 128
Liver
autopsy findings, 508–512
biliary formation, 289–291
blood flow, 288
coagulation and clotting factors, 292–293
enzyme markers of liver damage, 289, 297
impairment, and drug clearance, 190
metabolic functions, 291–292
morphological changes, 288–289
vitamin metabolism, 292
see also Acute phase response, hepatic
Liver cell apoptosis, 289, *290*
Liver function tests, 288
Liver weight, 288–289
Lodoxamide tromethanine, 83
Lorazepam, 756–757
Lund, CC, 2–3
Lung pathology *see* Acute lung damage (ALD); Acute respiratory distress syndrome (ARDS); Alveolar damage; Inhalation injury; Pulmonary edema
Luteinizing hormone, 364
Lymphatic system
autopsy findings, *511*, 512
chronic impairment, 737
Lymph flow
animal models, 81, 227, 264–265
lung, 225, 227
Lymphocytes, 526
count and analysis, in radiation injuries, 485
see also B-cell; T-cell
Lysyl oxidase, 527, 532

MAC *see* Membrane attack complex (MAC)
McGill Pain Questionnaire, 749, 750
Macrophage colony-stimulating factor (M-CSF), 336, 337, 338
Macrophage inflammatory protein (MIP), 260
Macrophages/monocytes
in acute phase response, 335–338
in wound healing, 526
Macrostomia, 673, *674*
Mafenide acetate (Sulfamylon), 113, 152
history, 5

Magnesium
deficiency, 302
in hypophophatemia, 311
homeostatic control, 301
metabolic functions, 300
monitoring, 96
replacement therapy, in children, 432
Magnetic resonance imaging (MRI)
in burn depth estimation, 104
in cold injury, 472
in electrical injury, 458
hepatic, 288
Major histocompatability complex (MHC), 335
Malnutrition, in elderly, 439–440
Mandibular growth reduction, 666–671
Mandibular wires, 684
Mason, AD, 9
Massage, scar, 587–588
Massive burns
management
fascial excision, 178
recombinant human growth hormone (rHGH), 178
surgical wound closure, 177–178
temperature maintenance, 177
mortality and survival, 740
outcomes in children, 611–612, 734–735
Membrane attack complex (MAC), 261
Meperidine, 755
Metabolic acidosis, 349
Metabolic alkalosis, 310
Metabolic requirements, 272
Metacarpopharyngeal (MCP) joint *see* Finger, joint positioning; joint deformities
Metaproterenol, 244–245
Methadone, 755
Methane inhalation, 235
Methicillin-resistant *S. aureus* (MRSA), 124, 160
Methicillin-resistant *S. epidermidis* (MRSE), 124, 160
Metoprolol, 375–376
MHC *see* Major histocompatability complex (MHC)
Microcirculation
in cold injury, 471
Landis-Starling's equation, 79, 80, 264
normal function, 79
pulmonary, in inhalation injury, 225–226
Micrococcus spp., 123–123
Microstomia, 673, *674*
prevention, 564
Microthrombi formation, 332, 342
Microvascular permeability *see* Vascular permeability
Midazolam, 44, 756
Mifepristone, 376
Military personnel, 19
cold injury, 470
as high risk population, 19
role in disaster management, 59
Mineral metabolism
effect of burn injury, 301–302
normal, 300–301
Mineral supplementation
guidelines, *292*
for children, *434*
Mivacurium, 191
MODS *see* Multiple organ dysfunction syndrome (MODS)
Moisturizing creams, 48
Monitors, anesthetic management, 192–194
Monoclonal antibody trials, 262, 388, 389
Monocytopoiesis, 337–338, 352
norepinephrine influence, 353